Rook's
Textbook of
Dermatology

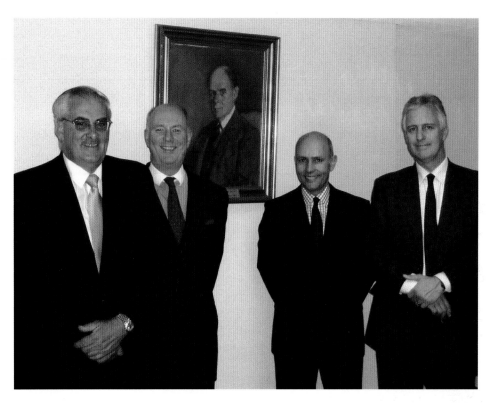

The Editors. From l to r, Tony Burns, Stephen Breathnach, Christopher Griffiths and Neil Cox standing in front of a portrait of Arthur Rook, the father of the *Textbook of Dermatology*.

Rook's
Textbook of
Dermatology

EDITED BY

Tony Burns
MB, BS, FRCP, FRCP(Edin)
Emeritus Consultant Dermatologist, Leicester Royal Infirmary, Leicester

Stephen Breathnach
MA, MB, BChir, MD, PhD, FRCP
Consultant Dermatologist and Senior Lecturer, St John's Institute of Dermatology, St Thomas' Hospital, London,
and Consultant Dermatologist, Epsom & St Helier University Hospitals NHS Trust, Epsom, Surrey

Neil Cox
BSc, MB, ChB, FRCP(Lond & Edin)
Consultant Dermatologist, Department of Dermatology, Cumberland Infirmary, Carlisle

Christopher Griffiths
BSc, MD, FRCP, FRCPath
Professor of Dermatology and Consultant Dermatologist, The Dermatology Centre, University of Manchester,
Hope Hospital, Salford, Manchester

IN FOUR VOLUMES
VOLUME 4

SEVENTH EDITION

Blackwell
Science

First published 1968   Fourth edition 1986
Reprinted 1969   Reprinted 1988, 1990
Second edition 1972   Fifth edition 1992
Reprinted 1975   Reprinted 1993, 1994
Third edition 1979   Sixth edition 1998
Reprinted 1982, 1984   Seventh edition 2004

Library of Congress Cataloging-in-Publication Data
Rook's textbook of dermatology.—7th ed. / edited by Tony Burns . . . [et al.].
    p. ; cm.
   title: Textbook of dermatology.
  Rev. ed. of: Rook/Wilkinson/Ebling textbook of dermatology. 6th ed. / edited by
R.H. Champion . . . [et al.] . c1998.
   Includes bibliographical references and index.
   ISBN 0-632-06429-3
   1. Skin—Diseases.   2. Dermatology.
   [DNLM: 1. Skin Diseases. WR 140 R77711 2004]   I. Title: Textbook of dermatology.
II. Rook, Arthur.   III. Burns, Tony, FRCP.   IV. Rook/Wilkinson/Ebling textbook of
dermatology.
RL71.R744   2004
616.5—dc22   2004010343

ISBN 0-632-06429-3
ISBN 1-4051-2974-3 (IE)

A catalogue record for this title is available from the British Library

Set in 9.5/12pt Palatino by Graphicraft Limited, Hong Kong
Printed and bound in Italy by G. Canale & C. SpA, Turin

Commissioning Editor: Stuart Taylor
Managing Editor: Rupal Malde
Editorial Assistant: Katrina Chandler
Production Editor: Nick Morgan
Production Controller: Chris Downs

For further information on Blackwell Publishing, visit our website:
http://www.blackwellpublishing.com

The publisher's policy is to use permanent paper from mills that operate a sustainable
forestry policy, and which has been manufactured from pulp processed using acid-free
and elementary chlorine-free practices. Furthermore, the publisher ensures that the text
paper and cover board used have met acceptable environmental accreditation standards.

Contents

Contributors

ADRIAANS, Beverley M.
MD, FRCP
Consultant Dermatologist, Department of Dermatology,
Gloucestershire Royal Hospital, Great Western Road, Gloucester
GL1 3NN
Co-author of
Chapter 27: Bacterial Infections

ANSTEY, Alexander V.
MB, BS, FRCP
Consultant Dermatologist, Royal Gwent Hospital, Cardiff Road,
Newport NP20 2UB, and Honorary Senior Lecturer, Academic
Department of Dermatology, University of Wales College of
Medicine, Heath Park, Cardiff CF14 4XN
Co-author of
Chapter 39: Disorders of Skin Colour

ARCHER, Clive B.
BSc, MB, BS, MD, PhD(Lond), FRCP(Lond & Edin)
Consultant Dermatologist and Clinical Senior Lecturer, Bristol
Dermatology Centre, Bristol Royal Infirmary, Marlborough Street,
Bristol BS2 8HW
Author of
Chapter 4: Functions of the Skin
Co-author of
Chapter 60: The Skin and the Nervous System

ATHERTON, David J.
MA, MB, BChir, FRCP
Consultant in Paediatric Dermatology, Department of Dermatology,
Great Ormond Street Hospital for Children, Great Ormond Street,
London WC1N 3JH
Co-author of
Chapter 14: The Neonate
Chapter 15: Naevi and other Developmental Defects

BARAN, Robert
MD
Head of Nail Disease Centre, Le Grand Palais, 42 rue des Serbes,
06400 Cannes, France
Co-author of
Chapter 62: Disorders of Nails

BARHAM, Kelly L.
MD
Resident Physician, Department of Dermatology, Wake Forest
University School of Medicine, Medical Center Boulevard,
Winston-Salem, NC 27157-1071, USA
Co-author of
Chapter 49: Vasculitis and Neutrophilic Vascular Reactions

BARKER, Jonathan N.W.N.
BSc, MD, FRCP, FRCPath
Professor of Clinical Dermatology, St John's Institute of
Dermatology, St Thomas' Hospital, Lambeth Palace Road,
London SE1 7EH
Co-author of
Chapter 35: Psoriasis

BARLOW, Richard J.
MD, FRCP
Consultant Dermatologist and Senior Lecturer, Dermatological
Surgery and Laser Unit, St John's Institute of Dermatology, St
Thomas' Hospital, Lambeth Palace Road, London SE1 7EH
Co-author of
Chapter 77: Physical and Laser Therapies

BECK, Michael H.
MB, ChB, FRCP
Consultant Dermatologist and Director of Contact Dermatitis
Investigation Unit, Dermatology Centre, University of
Manchester, Hope Hospital, Stott Lane, Salford, Manchester M6
8HD
Co-author of
Chapter 19: Contact Dermatitis: Irritant
Chapter 20: Contact Dermatitis: Allergic

BERTH-JONES, John
FRCP
Consultant Dermatologist, University Hospitals Coventry and
Warwickshire NHS Trust, Department of Dermatology,
Walsgrave Hospital, Clifford Bridge Road, Coventry CV2 2DX,
and Coventry and George Eliot Hospital NHS Trust, Nuneaton
Author of
Chapter 44: Rosacea, Perioral Dermatitis and Similar Dermatoses,
Flushing and Flushing Syndromes
Chapter 75: Topical Therapy
Co-author of
Chapter 17: Eczema, Lichenification, Prurigo and Erythroderma

BLACK, Martin M.
MD, FRCP, FRCPath
Consultant Dermatologist, St John's Institute of Dermatology, St
Thomas' Hospital, Lambeth Palace Road, London SE1 7EH
Co-author of
Chapter 42: Lichen Planus and Lichenoid Disorders
Chapter 55: Subcutaneous Fat

BLEEHEN, Stanley S.
MA, MB, BChir, FRCP
Emeritus Professor of Dermatology, University of Sheffield,
Sheffield, and Honorary Consultant Dermatologist, St John's

Institute of Dermatology, St Thomas' Hospital, Lambeth Palace Road, London SE1 7EH
Co-author of
   Chapter 39: Disorders of Skin Colour

BREATHNACH, Stephen M.
MA, MB, BChir, MD, PhD, FRCP
Consultant Dermatologist and Senior Lecturer, St John's Institute of Dermatology, St Thomas' Hospital, Lambeth Palace Road, London SE1 7EH, and Consultant Dermatologist, Epsom and St Helier University NHS Trust, Dorking Road, Epsom, Surrey KT18 7EG
Editor
Author of
   Chapter 73: Drug Reactions
   Chapter 74: Erythema Multiforme, Stevens–Johnson Syndrome and Toxic Epidermal Necrolysis
Co-author of
   Chapter 11: Wound Healing
   Chapter 42: Lichen Planus and Lichenoid Disorders
   Chapter 57: Metabolic and Nutritional Disorders
   Chapter 72: Systemic Therapy

BUNKER, Christopher B.
MA, MD, FRCP
Consultant Dermatologist, Chelsea & Westminster Hospital, Fulham Road, London SW10 9NH, and the Royal Marsden Hospital, Fulham Road, London SW3 6JJ, London, and Honorary Senior Lecturer, Imperial College School of Medicine, London
Co-author of
   Chapter 26: AIDS and the Skin
   Chapter 68: The Genital, Perianal and Umbilical Regions

BURD, D. Andrew R.
MD, FRCSEd, FHKAM
Chief of Division of Plastic and Reconstructive Surgery, Department of Surgery, Chinese University of Hong Kong, Prince of Wales Hospital, Shatin, Hong Kong
Co-author of
   Chapter 22: Mechanical and Thermal Injury

BURGE, Susan M.
BSc, DM, FRCP
Consultant Dermatologist, Department of Dermatology, Churchill Hospital, Old Road, Headington, Oxford OX3 7LJ
Co-author of
   Chapter 40: Genetic Blistering Diseases
   Chapter 41: Immunobullous Diseases

BURNAND, Kevin G.
MB, BS, FRCS, MS
Professor of Vascular Surgery, Head of Academic Department of Surgery, UMDS, St Thomas' Campus, Lambeth Palace Road, London SE1 7EH
Co-author of
   Chapter 50: Diseases of the Veins and Arteries: Leg Ulcers

BURNS, David Anthony
MB, BS, FRCP, FRCP(Edin)
Emeritus Consultant Dermatologist, Leicester Royal Infirmary, Leicester LE1 5WW
Editor
Author of
   Chapter 2: Comparative Dermatology
   Chapter 33: Diseases Caused by Arthropods and Other Noxious Animals
   Chapter 67: The Breast
Co-author of
   Chapter 1: Introduction and Historical Bibliography
   Chapter 57: Metabolic and Nutritional Disorders

BURROWS, Nigel P.
MD, FRCP
Consultant Dermatologist and Associate Lecturer, Department of Dermatology, Addenbrooke's Hospital, Hills Road, Cambridge CB2 2QQ
Co-author of
   Chapter 46: Disorders of Connective Tissue

CALONJE, Eduardo
MD, DipRCPath
Director of Diagnostic Dermatopathology, and Consultant and Honorary Senior Lecturer in Dermatology, St John's Institute of Dermatology, St Thomas' Hospital, Lambeth Palace Road, London SE1 7EH
Co-author of
   Chapter 7: Histopathology of the Skin: General Principles
   Chapter 37: Tumours of the Skin Appendages
   Chapter 53: Soft-Tissue Tumours and Tumour-like Conditions

CAMP, Richard D.R.
PhD, FRCP
Professor of Dermatology, Department of Infection, Immunity and Inflammation, Maurice Shock Medical Sciences Building, University of Leicester, University Road, Leicester LE1 9HN
Co-author of
   Chapter 35: Psoriasis

CANT, Andrew J.
BSc, MRCP, MD, FRCP, FRCPCH
Consultant in Paediatric Immunology and Infectious Diseases, and Honorary Clinical Senior Lecturer in Child Health, Newcastle General Hospital, Westgate Road, Newcastle upon Tyne NE4 6BE
Co-author of
   Chapter 14: The Neonate

CERIO, Rino
BSc, MB, BS, FRCP, FRCP(Edin), FRCPath
Consultant Dermatologist and Reader in Dermatopathology, Department of Dermatology and Institute of Pathology (QMUL), Bart's and Royal London Medical Schools, Whitechapel Road, London E1 1BB
Co-author of
   Chapter 7: Histopathology of the Skin: General Principles

CHALMERS, Robert J.G.
MB, FRCP
Consultant Dermatologist, University of Manchester, Dermatology Centre, Hope Hospital, Stott Lane, Salford, Manchester, M6 8HD
Co-author
   Chapter 72: Systemic Therapy

CHU, Anthony C.
FRCP
Senior Lecturer/Honorary Consultant Dermatologist, Imperial College, Hammersmith Campus, Hammersmith Hospital, Du Cane Road, London W12 0HS
Author of
   Chapter 52: Histiocytoses

CHURCH, Martin K.

MPharm, PhD, DSc

Professor of Immunopharmacology, Allergy and Inflammation
  Research, Southampton General Hospital, Tremona Road,
  Southampton SO16 6YD

Co-author

  Chapter 9: Inflammation

COTTERILL, John A.

BSc, MD, FRCP

Formerly Consultant Dermatologist, Department of Dermatology,
  Leeds General Infirmary, Leeds

Co-author

  Chapter 61: Psychocutaneous Disorders
  Chapter 71: General Aspects of Treatment

COULSON, Ian H.

BSc, MB, BS, FRCP

Consultant Dermatologist, Dermatology Unit, Burnley General
  Hospital, Casterton Avenue, Burnley, Lancashire BB10 2PQ

Author of

  Chapter 45: Disorders of Sweat Glands

Co-author

  Chapter 5: Diagnosis of Skin Disease

COX, Neil H.

BSc, MB, ChB, FRCP(Lond & Edin)

Consultant Dermatologist, Department of Dermatology,
  Cumberland Infirmary, Carlisle CA2 7HY

Editor

Co-author of

  Chapter 1: Introduction and Historical Bibliography
  Chapter 5: Diagnosis of Skin Disease
  Chapter 48: Purpura and Microvascular Occlusion
  Chapter 49: Vasculitis and Neutrophilic Vascular Reactions
  Chapter 59: Systemic Disease and the Skin

CUNLIFFE, William J.

MD, FRCP

Professor of Dermatology, Department of Dermatology, Leeds
  General Infirmary, Great George Street, Leeds LS1 3EX

Co-author

  Chapter 43: Disorders of the Sebaceous Glands
  Chapter 55: Subcutaneous Fat

DART, John K.G.

MA, DM, FRCS, FRCOphth

Consultant Ophthalmologist, Corneal External Disease and Cataract
  Services, Moorfields Eye Hospital, City Road, London EC1V 2PD

Co-author

  Chapter 64: The Skin and the Eyes

DAWBER, Rodney P.R.

MA, FRCP

Consultant Dermatologist, Department of Dermatology, Churchill
  Hospital, Old Road, Headington, Oxford OX2 7LJ

Co-author

  Chapter 62: Disorders of Nails

de BERKER, David A.R.

BA, MRCP

Consultant Dermatologist and Clinical Senior Lecturer, Bristol
  Dermatology Centre, Bristol Royal Infirmary, Marlborough Street,
  Bristol BS2 8HW

Co-author

  Chapter 62: Disorders of Nails
  Chapter 63: Disorders of Hair

DOWD, Pauline M.

BSc, MD, FRCP

Professor of Dermatology, Department of Dermatology, The
  Middlesex Hospital, Tottenham Street, London W1T 4NJ

Author of

  Chapter 23: Reactions to Cold

EADY, Robin A.J.

DSc, FRCP, FMedSci

Emeritus Professor of Experimental Dermatopathology, Division of
  Skin Sciences, Guy's, King's and St Thomas' School of Medicine,
  King's College London, and Honorary Consultant Dermatologist,
  St John's Institute of Dermatology, St Thomas' Hospital, Lambeth
  Palace Road, London SE1 7EH

Co-author of

  Chapter 3: Anatomy and Organization of Human Skin
  Chapter 13: Prenatal Diagnosis of Genetic Skin Disease
  Chapter 40: Genetic Blistering Diseases

EEDY, David J.

MD, FRCP

Consultant Dermatologist, Department of Dermatology, Craigavon
  Area Hospital Group Trust, 68 Lurgan Road, Portadown, Co.
  Armagh, Northern Ireland BT63 5QQ

Co-author of

  Chapter 60: The Skin and the Nervous System

ENGLISH, John S.C.

MB, BS, FRCP

Consultant Dermatologist, Department of Dermatology, Queen's
  Medical Centre, University Hospital, Clifton Boulevard,
  Nottingham NG7 2UH

Co-author of

  Chapter 21: Occupational Dermatoses

FERGUSON, James

MD, FRCP

Consultant Dermatologist, Photobiology Unit, Department
  of Dermatology, Ninewells Hospital and Medical School,
  Dundee DD1 9SY

Co-author of

  Chapter 24: Cutaneous Photobiology

FINE, Jo-David

MD, MPH, FACP

Professor of Medicine, University of Kentucky College of Medicine,
  and Dermatology Associates of Kentucky, PSC, 250 Fountain
  Court, Lexington, KY 40509, USA

Co-author of

  Chapter 40: Genetic Blistering Diseases

FINLAY, Andrew Y.

FRCP(Lond & Glasg)

Professor of Dermatology and Honorary Consultant Dermatologist,
  Department of Dermatology, University of Wales College of
  Medicine, Heath Park, Cardiff CF14 4XN

Co-author of

  Chapter 71: General Aspects of Treatment

FRIEDMANN, Peter S.
MD, FRCP, FMedSci
Professor of Dermatology, Dermatopharmacology Unit,
Southampton General Hospital, Tremona Road, Southampton
SO16 6YD
Co-author of
Chapter 18: Atopic Dermatitis

GAWKRODGER, David J.
MD, FRCP, FRCPE
Consultant Dermatologist and Honorary Senior Clinical Lecturer,
Department of Dermatology, Royal Hallamshire Hospital,
Glossop Road, Sheffield S10 2JF
Author of
Chapter 58: Sarcoidosis
Chapter 69: Racial Influences on Skin Disease

GENNERY, Andrew R.
MD, MRCP, MRCPCH, DCH, DipMedSci
Watson Clinical Senior Lecturer/Honorary Consultant in Paediatric
Immunology and Bone Marrow Transplantation, Newcastle
General Hospital, Westgate Road, Newcastle upon Tyne NE4 6BE
Co-author of
Chapter 14: The Neonate

GOODFIELD, Mark J.D.
MD, FRCP
Consultant Dermatologist, Department of Dermatology, Leeds
General Infirmary, Great George Street, Leeds LS1 3EX
Co-author of
Chapter 56: The 'Connective Tissue Diseases'

GOTCH, Frances
PhD, FRCPath
Professor of Immunology, Head of Department, Department of
Immunology, Imperial College School of Medicine, Chelsea &
Westminster Campus, Fulham Road, London SW10 9NH
Co-author of
Chapter 26: AIDS and the Skin

GRAHAM, Robert M.
MB, FRCP
Consultant Dermatologist, Department of Dermatology, James
Paget Healthcare NHS Trust, Lowestoft Road, Gorleston, Great
Yarmouth, Norfolk NR31 6LA
Co-author of
Chapter 59: Systemic Disease and the Skin

GRAHAM-BROWN, Robin A.C.
BSc, MB, BS, FRCP
Consultant and Honorary Senior Lecturer in Dermatology,
Department of Dermatology, Leicester Royal Infirmary, Leicester
LE1 5WW
Author of
Chapter 70: The Ages of Man and their Dermatoses

GRATTAN, Beth
MD
Resident Physician, Department of Dermatology, Medical
University of South Carolina, Charleston, SC 29425, Carolina,
USA
Co-author of
Chapter 49: Vasculitis and Neutrophilic Vascular Reactions

GRATTAN, Clive E.H.
MA, MD, FRCP
Consultant Dermatologist, Department of Dermatology, Norfolk
and Norwich University Hospital, Colney, Norfolk NR4 7UZ
Co-author of
Chapter 47: Urticaria and Mastocytosis

GREAVES, Malcolm W.
MD, PhD, FRCP
Professor of Dermatology, Department of Dermatology, Singapore
General Hospital, Outram Road, Singapore 169608
Author of
Chapter 16: Pruritus

GRIFFITHS, Christopher E.M.
BSc, MD, FRCP, FRCPath
Professor of Dermatology and Consultant Dermatologist, The
Dermatology Centre, University of Manchester, Irving Building,
Hope Hospital, Salford, Manchester M6 8HD
Editor
Co-author of
Chapter 9: Inflammation
Chapter 35: Psoriasis
Chapter 72: Systemic Therapy

HARPER, John I.
MD, FRCP, FRCPCH
Professor of Paediatric Dermatology, Great Ormond Street Hospital
for Children, Great Ormond Street, London WC1N 3JH
Co-author of
Chapter 12: Genetics and Genodermatoses

HAWK, John L.M.
BSc, MD, FRACP, FRCP
Consultant Dermatologist and Head, Department of Environmental
Dermatology, St John's Institute of Dermatology, St Thomas'
Hospital, Lambeth Palace Road, London SE1 7EH
Co-author of
Chapter 24: Cutaneous Photobiology

HAY, Roderick J.
DM, FRCP, FRCPath
Dean, Faculty of Medicine and Health Sciences, Queen's University
Belfast, Whitla Medical Building, 97 Lisburn Road, Belfast BT9
7BL
Co-author of
Chapter 27: Bacterial Infections
Chapter 31: Mycology
Chapter 32: Parasitic Worms and Protozoa
Chapter 72: Systemic Therapy

HOLDEN, Colin A.
BSc, MD, FRCP
Consultant Dermatologist, Epsom and St Helier University
Hospitals NHS Trust, St Helier Hospital, Wrythe Lane,
Carshalton, Surrey SM5 1AA
Co-author of
Chapter 17: Eczema, Lichenification, Prurigo and Erythroderma
Chapter 18: Atopic Dermatitis

JONES, Stephen K.
BMedSci, BM, BS, MD, FRCP(Lond & Edin)
Consultant Dermatologist, Department of Dermatology,
Clatterbridge Hospital, Bebington, Wirral CH63 4JY

Co-author of
 Chapter 56: The 'Connective Tissue Diseases'

JORIZZO, Joseph L.
MD
Professor and Former (Founding) Chair, Department of
 Dermatology, Wake Forest University School of Medicine,
 Medical Centre Boulevard, Winston-Salem, NC 27157-1071, USA
Co-author of
 Chapter 49: Vasculitis and Neutrophilic Vascular Reactions

JUDGE, Mary R.
MD, FRCP, DCH
Consultant Dermatologist, Department of Dermatology, Royal
 Bolton Hospital, Minerva Road, Farnworth, Bolton BL4 0JR, and
 Consultant Paediatric Dermatologist, Dermatology Centre, Hope
 Hospital, Stott Lane, Salford, Manchester M6 8HD
Co-author of
 Chapter 34: Disorders of Keratinization

KELLY, Charles G.
MSc, FRCP, FRCR
Consultant Clinical Oncologist, Northern Centre for Cancer
 Treatment, Newcastle General Hospital, Westgate Road,
 Newcastle upon Tyne NE4 6BE
Co-author of
 Chapter 76: Radiotherapy and Reactions to Ionizing Radiation

KENNEDY, Cameron T.C.
MA, MB, BChir, FRCP
Consultant Dermatologist and Clinical Senior Lecturer, Bristol
 Dermatology Centre, Bristol Royal Infirmary, Marlborough Street,
 Bristol BS2 8HW
Author of
 Chapter 65: The External Ear
Co-author of
 Chapter 22: Mechanical and Thermal Injury

KERDEL-VEGAS, Francisco
CBE, MD, MSc, DSc, FACP
Former Professor of Dermatology, Universidad Central de
 Venezuela, Caracas, and Fellow of the National Academy of
 Medicine and the Academy of Sciences of Venezuela, Central
 University of Venezuela, Apartado 60391, Caracas 1060-A,
 Venezuela
Co-author of
 Chapter 30: The Treponematoses

KINGHORN, George R.
MB, ChB, MD, FRCP
Clinical Director, Department of Genitourinary Medicine, Royal
 Hallamshire Hospital, Glossop Road, Sheffield S10 2JF
Co-author of
 Chapter 30: The Treponematoses

KOBZA BLACK, Anne
MD, FRCP
Consultant Dermatologist, St John's Institute of Dermatology, St
 Thomas' Hospital, Lambeth Palace Road, London SE1 7EH
Co-author of
 Chapter 47: Urticaria and Mastocytosis

LAWRENCE, Clifford M.
MD, FRCP

Consultant Dermatologist, Department of Dermatology, Royal
 Victoria Infirmary, Queen Victoria Road, Newcastle upon Tyne
 NE1 4LP
Co-author of
 Chapter 77: Physical and Laser Therapies
 Chapter 78: Dermatological Surgery

LEONARD, Jonathan N.
BSc, MD, FRCP
Consultant Dermatologist, Department of Dermatology, St Mary's
 Hospital, Praed Street, London W2 1NY
Co-author of
 Chapter 64: The Skin and the Eyes

LOCKWOOD, Diana N.J.
MD, FRCP
Consultant Physician and Leprologist, The Hospital for Tropical
 Diseases, Capper Street, London WC1E 6AU
Author of
 Chapter 29: Leprosy

LOVELL, Christopher R.
MD, FRCP
Department of Dermatology, Royal United Hospital, Coombe Park,
 Bath BA1 3NG
Co-author of
 Chapter 46: Disorders of Connective Tissue

LUGER, Thomas A.
MD
Professor and Chairman, Department of Dermatology, University of
 Münster, Von-Esmarch-Strasse 58, D-48149 Münster, Germany
Co-author of
 Chapter 9: Inflammation

MacKIE, Rona M.
CBE, FRSE, MD, DSc, FRCP, FRCPath
Senior Research Fellow, Public Health and Health Policy, University
 of Glasgow, 1 Lilybank Gardens, Glasgow G12 8RZ
Author of
 Chapter 38: Disorders of the Cutaneous Melanocyte
Co-author of
 Chapter 36: Non-Melanoma Skin Cancer and Other Epidermal
 Skin Tumours
 Chapter 37: Tumours of the Skin Appendages
 Chapter 53: Soft-Tissue Tumours and Tumour-like Conditions
 Chapter 54: Cutaneous Lymphomas and Lymphocytic Infiltrates

McGRATH, John A.
MD, FRCP
Professor of Molecular Dermatology, St John's Institute of
 Dermatology, St Thomas' Hospital, Lambeth Palace Road,
 London SE1 7EH
Co-author of
 Chapter 3: Anatomy and Organization of Human Skin
 Chapter 11: Wound Healing
 Chapter 13: Prenatal Diagnosis of Genetic Skin Disease

McLEAN, W.H. Irwin
PhD, DSc
Wellcome Trust Senior Research Fellow and Professor of Human
 Genetics, Human Genetics Unit, Division of Pathology and
 Neuroscience, Ninewells Hospital and Medical School, University
 of Dundee, Dundee DD1 9SY

Co-author of
Chapter 34: Disorders of Keratinization

MESSENGER, Andrew G.
MD, FRCP
Consultant Dermatologist, Department of Dermatology, Royal
Hallamshire Hospital, Glossop Road, Sheffield S10 2JF
Co-author of
Chapter 63: Disorders of Hair

MILLARD, Leslie G.
MD, FRCP(Lond & Edin)
Consultant in Dermatology and Cutaneous Surgery, Department of
Dermatology and Dermatological Surgery, Queen's Medical
Centre, University Hospital NHS Trust, Clifton Boulevard,
Nottingham NG7 2UH
Co-author of
Chapter 61: Psychocutaneous Disorders

MOORE, Mary K.
MA, PhD
Lecturer, Mycology Department, St John's Institute of Dermatology,
St Thomas' Hospital, Lambeth Palace Road, London SE1 7EH
Co-author of
Chapter 31: Mycology

MORTIMER, Peter S.
MD, FRCP
Professor of Dermatological Medicine, Dermatology Unit, St
George's Hospital Medical School, Cranmer Terrace, London
SW17 0RE
Author of
Chapter 51: Disorders of Lymphatic Vessels
Co-author of
Chapter 50: Diseases of the Veins and Arteries: Leg Ulcers

MORTON, Robert S. [Deceased]
MBE, MD, FRCP(Edin), DHMSA
Formerly Honorary Lecturer in History of Medicine, University of
Sheffield
Co-author of
Chapter 30: The Treponematoses

MOSS, Celia
DM, FRCP, MRCPCH
Consultant Dermatologist, Department of Dermatology,
Birmingham Children's Hospital, Steelhouse Lane, Birmingham
B4 6NL
Co-author of
Chapter 15: Naevi and other Developmental Defects

MUNRO, Colin S.
MD, FRCP(Glasg)
Consultant Dermatologist and Professor, Department of
Dermatology, South Glasgow University Hospitals NHS Trust,
Govan Road, Glasgow G51 4TF
Co-author of
Chapter 34: Disorders of Keratinization

NEILL, Sallie M.
FRCP
Consultant Dermatologist, St John's Dermatology Unit, Guy's and St
Thomas' NHS Trust, Lambeth Palace Road, London, SE1 7EH,
Chelsea and Westminster NHS Trust, Fulham Road, London

SW10 9NH and Ashford & St Peter's NHS Trust, Guildford Road,
Chertsey, Surrey KT16 0PZ
Co-author of
Chapter 68: The Genital, Perianal and Umbilical Regions

PIETTE, Warren W.
MD
Professor and Vice-Chair, Department of Dermatology, University
of Iowa Roy J. and Lucille A. Carver College of Medicine,
University of Iowa Hospitals and Clinics, 200 Hawkins Drive,
Iowa City, IA 52242-1090, USA
Co-author of
Chapter 48: Purpura and Microvascular Occlusion

POPE, F. Michael
MD, FRCP(Lond, Edin & Glasg)
Consultant Dermatologist, West Middlesex University Hospital,
Twickenham Road, Isleworth, Middlesex TW7 6AF, and the
Chelsea & Westminster Hospital, Fulham Road, London SW10
9NH, Professor of Medical Genetics and Honorary Consultant
Clinical Geneticist, Institute of Medical Genetics, University of
Wales College of Medicine and University Hospital of Wales,
Heath Park, Cardiff CF14 4XN
Co-author of
Chapter 3: Anatomy and Organization of Human Skin

QUINN, Anthony G.
BMSc, MB, ChB, PhD, FRCP
Director/Senior Principal Scientist, Experimental Medicine,
AstraZeneca R&D Charnwood, Bakewell Road, Loughborough,
Leicestershire LE11 5RH
Co-author of
Chapter 36: Non-Melanoma Skin Cancer and Other Epidermal
Skin Tumours

REES, Jonathan L.
BMedSci, MB, BS, FRCP, FMedSci
Grant Chair of Dermatology, Department of Dermatology, The
University of Edinburgh, Lauriston Building, Lauriston Place,
Edinburgh EH3 9HA
Author of
Chapter 8: Molecular Biology

ROOK, Graham A.W.
BA, MB, BChir, MD
Professor of Medical Microbiology, Department of Medical
Microbiology, Windeyer Institute of Medical Sciences, Royal Free
and University College Medical School, 46 Cleveland Street,
London W1T 4JF
Co-author of
Chapter 28: Mycobacterial Infections

SARKANY, Robert P.E.
BSc, MRCP, MD
Consultant Dermatologist, Department of Dermatology, St George's
Hospital, Blackshaw Road, London SW17 0QT
Co-author of
Chapter 57: Metabolic and Nutritional Disorders

SCHWARZ, Thomas
MD
Professor of Dermatology, Department of Dermatology, University
of Münster, Von-Esmarch-Strasse 58, D-48149 Münster, Germany
Co-author of
Chapter 10: Clinical Immunology, Allergy and Photoimmunology

SCULLY, Crispian
CBE, MD, PhD, MDS, MRCS, FDSRCS, FDSRCPS, FFDRCSI, FDSRCSE, FRCPath, FMedSci
President of the European Association of Oral Medicine, and Dean and Director of Studies and Research, Eastman Dental Institute for Oral Health Care Sciences, and International Centres for Excellence in Dentistry, University College London, 256 Gray's Inn Road, London WC1X 8LD
Author of
  Chapter 66: The Oral Cavity and Lips

SEYMOUR, Carol A.
MA(Oxon), MA(Cantab), PhD, FRCPath, FRCP
Emeritus Professor of Clinical Biochemistry and Metabolic Medicine, St George's Hospital Medical School, Blackshaw Road, London SW17 0QT
Co-author of
  Chapter 57: Metabolic and Nutritional Disorders

SIMPSON, Nicholas B.
MD, FRCP(Lond & Glasg)
Consultant Dermatologist, Department of Dermatology, Royal Victoria Infirmary, Queen Victoria Road, Newcastle upon Tyne NE1 4LP
Co-author of
  Chapter 43: Disorders of the Sebaceous Glands

SINCLAIR, Rodney D.
MB, BS, FACD
Senior Lecturer and Consultant Dermatologist, Skin and Cancer Foundation and St Vincent's Hospital Melbourne, Department of Dermatology, 41 Victoria Parade, Fitzroy, Victoria 3065, Australia
Co-author of
  Chapter 63: Disorders of Hair

SPICKETT, Gavin P.
MA, DPhil, FRCPath, FRCP(Lond)
Consultant Clinical Immunologist, Regional Department of Immunology, Royal Victoria Infirmary, Queen Victoria Road, Newcastle upon Tyne NE1 4LP
Co-author of
  Chapter 10: Clinical Immunology, Allergy and Photoimmunology

SPITTLE, Margaret F.
MSc, FRCP, FRCR, AKC
Consultant Clinical Oncologist, Meyerstein Institute of Oncology, The Middlesex Hospital, Mortimer Street, London W1N 8AA
Co-author of
  Chapter 76: Radiotherapy and Reactions to Ionizing Radiation

STEINHOFF, Martin
MD, PhD
Associate Professor, Department of Dermatology and Boltzmann Institute for Immunobiology of the Skin, University of Münster, Von-Esmarch-Strasse 58, D-48149 Münster, Germany
Co-author of
  Chapter 9: Inflammation

STERLING, Jane C.
MB, BChir, MA, FRCP, PhD
Honorary Consultant Dermatologist, Department of Dermatology, Addenbrooke's Hospital, Hills Road, Cambridge CB2 2QQ
Author of
  Chapter 25: Virus Infections

TELFER, Nicholas R.
FRCP
Consultant Dermatological Surgeon, Dermatology Centre, University of Manchester, Irving Building, Hope Hospital, Stott Lane, Salford, Manchester M6 8HD
Co-author of
  Chapter 78: Dermatological Surgery

TREMBATH, Richard C.
BSc, MB, BS, FRCP, FMedSci
Professor of Medical Genetics, Division of Medical Genetics, Adrian Building, University of Leicester, Leicester LE1 7RH
Co-author of
  Chapter 12: Genetics and Genodermatoses

VEALE, Douglas J.
MD, FRCPI, FRCP(Lond)
Consultant Dermatologist, Department of Rheumatology, St Vincent's University Hospital, Elm Park, Dublin 4, Republic of Ireland
Co-author of
  Chapter 56: The 'Connective Tissue Diseases'

VEGA-LÓPEZ, Francisco
MD, MSc, PhD
Consultant Dermatologist and Honorary Senior Lecturer, University College London Hospitals NHS Trust, London School of Hygiene and Tropical Medicine, Keppel Street, London WC1E 7HT, and Former Chair and Professor of Dermatology, National University (UNAM) and National Medical Centre (IMSS), Mexico City, Mexico
Co-author of
  Chapter 32: Parasitic Worms and Protozoa

VENNING, Vanessa A.
MA, DM(Oxon), FRCP
Consultant Dermatologist, Department of Dermatology, Churchill Hospital, Old Road, Headington, Oxford OX3 7LJ
Co-author of
  Chapter 41: Immunobullous Diseases

WALKER, Neil P.J.
BSc, MB, FRCP
Honorary Consultant Dermatologist, Department of Dermatology, Churchill Hospital, Old Road, Headington, Oxford OX3 7LJ
Co-author of
  Chapter 77: Physical and Laser Therapies
  Chapter 78: Dermatological Surgery

WEISMANN, Kaare
MD, PhD
Consultant Dermatologist and Professor of Dermatology, Clinic of Dermatology, Hørsholm Hospital, DK-2970 Hørsholm, Denmark
Co-author of
  Chapter 57: Metabolic and Nutritional Disorders

WHITTAKER, Sean J.
MD, FRCP
Head of Service for St John's Institute of Dermatology, Guy's and St Thomas' Hospitals NHS Trust, Lambeth Palace Road, London SE1 7EH, and Head of Skin Cancer Unit, Division of Skin Sciences, King's College London, London, UK
Co-author of
  Chapter 54: Cutaneous Lymphomas and Lymphocytic Infiltrates

WILKINSON, S. Mark
MD, FRCP

Consultant Dermatologist, Department of Dermatology, Leeds General Infirmary, Great George Street, Leeds LS1 3EX

Co-author of
Chapter 19: Contact Dermatitis: Irritant
Chapter 20: Contact Dermatitis: Allergic

WILLIAMS, Hywel C.
BSc, MB, BS, FRCP, MSc, PhD

Professor of Dermato-epidemiology, Department of Dermatology, Queen's Medical Centre, Clifton Boulevard, Nottingham NG7 2UH

Author of
Chapter 6: Epidemiology of Skin Disease

WOJNAROWSKA, Fenella
MSc, DM(Oxon), FRCP(UK)

Professor of Dermatology, Department of Dermatology, Churchill Hospital, Old Road, Headington, Oxford OX3 7LJ

Co-author of
Chapter 41: Immunobullous Diseases

YATES, Victoria M.
MB, ChB, FRCP

Consultant Dermatologist, Department of Dermatology, Royal Bolton Hospital, Minerva Road, Farnworth, Bolton BL4 0JR, and University Department of Dermatology, Hope Hospital, Stott Lane, Salford, Manchester M6 8HD

Co-author of
Chapter 28: Mycobacterial Infections

YOUNG, Antony R.
PhD

Deputy Head, St John's Institute of Dermatology, Guy's, King's and St Thomas' School of Medicine, King's College London, University of London, St Thomas' Hospital, Lambeth Palace Road, London SE1 7EH

Co-author of
Chapter 24: Cutaneous Photobiology

Preface to the Seventh Edition

Over thirty years have passed since the first edition of *Textbook of Dermatology* was published under the leadership of Arthur Rook, Darrell Wilkinson and John Ebling.

Arthur Rook, a wise clinician with an encyclopaedic knowledge of medical literature, and a man of great linguistic talent and enormous energy, died in 1991 (see Preface to the fifth edition).

John Ebling, who continued as an editor to the fifth edition, died in 1992. He occupied a unique position in British dermatology, as a full-time Professor of Zoology, a distinguished research worker and a man of enormous erudition and editorial skills. His breadth of knowledge covered the whole of biology and we owe him a great debt for his tremendous and untiring work over 25 years on this textbook.

The fifth edition, published in 1992, was edited by Champion, Burton and Ebling, with invaluable advice from Darrell Wilkinson. Bob Champion and John Burton continued to lead the editorial team into the sixth edition, published in 1998, and we are indebted to them for their expertise and dedicated hard work for many years.

For this seventh edition, Tony Burns and Stephen Breathnach have been joined by two new editors, Neil Cox and Christopher Griffiths. As always, we would all like to express our gratitude to the three original editors who laid the foundations and provided a framework upon which this book has developed through subsequent editions.

Our aim is to continue to provide a comprehensive reference guide to all recognized dermatological diseases, and to encourage understanding and development of scientific aspects of dermatology, although the book is not intended to provide details of research in the basic sciences.

For this edition, every chapter has been updated, and several have been completely rewritten. There are several new contributors, and a new chapter on AIDS and the skin is a reflection of the impact this disease has had in recent years. We would like to acknowledge our indebtedness to contributors to earlier editions, who have generously allowed some of their original material to be retained for the present edition.

We are also very grateful to all those colleagues who have donated colour photographs, and the origin of these is given in the legend to each figure. Where no acknowledgement is given the figures have been provided by the authors of that chapter.

Our wives and families deserve our thanks for their forbearance and support over many years.

We should also like to thank the staff of Blackwell Publishing for their efforts throughout the production of this edition, in particular Rupal Malde, Nick Morgan, Katrina Chandler and Stuart Taylor. We are once again extremely grateful to Caroline Sheard for her excellent index. Her index for the sixth edition deservedly won the Wheatley Prize (1998). Our heartfelt thanks also go to the team of copy editors and proof readers who, in deciphering and analysing reams of verbiage, are the ultimate refiners of these four volumes.

D.A. Burns
S.M. Breathnach
N.H. Cox
C.E.M. Griffiths

Preface to the First Edition

No comprehensive reference book on dermatology has been published in the English language for ten years and none in England for over a quarter of a century. The recent literature of dermatology is rich in shorter texts and in specialist monographs but the English-speaking dermatologist has long felt the need for a substantial text for regular reference and as a guide to the immense monographic and periodical literature. The editors have therefore planned the present volume primarily for the dermatologist in practice or in training, but have also considered the requirements of the specialist in other fields of medicine and of the many research workers interested in the skin in relation to toxicology or cosmetic science.

An attempt has been made throughout the book to integrate our growing knowledge of the biology of skin and of fundamental pathological processes with practical clinical problems. Often the gap is still very wide but the trends of basic research at least indicate how it may eventually be bridged. In a clinical textbook the space devoted to the basic sciences must necessarily be restricted but a special effort has been made to ensure that the short accounts which open many chapters are easily understood by the physician whose interests and experience are exclusively clinical.

For the benefit of the student we have encouraged our contributors to make each chapter readable as an independent entity, and have accepted that this must involve the repetition of some material.

The classification employed is conventional and pragmatic. Until our knowledge of the mechanisms of disease is more profound no truly scientific classification is possible. In so many clinical syndromes multiple aetiological factors are implicated. To emphasize one at the expense of others is often misleading. Most diseases are to some extent influenced by genetic factors and a large proportion of common skin reactions are modified by the emotional state of the patient. Our knowledge is in no way advanced by classifying hundreds of diseases as genodermatoses and dozens as psychosomatic.

The true prevalence of a disease may throw light on its aetiology but reported incidence figures are often unreliable and incorrectly interpreted. The scientific approach to the evaluation of racial and environmental factors has therefore been considered in some detail.

The effectiveness of any physician in practice must ultimately depend on his ability to make an accurate clinical diagnosis. Clinical descriptions are detailed and differential diagnosis is fully discussed. Histopathology is here considered mainly as an aid to diagnosis but references to fuller accounts are provided.

The approach to treatment is critical but practical. Many empirical measures are of proven value and should not be abandoned merely because their efficacy cannot yet be scientifically explained. However, many familiar remedies old and new have been omitted either because properly controlled clinical trials have shown them to be of no value or because they have been supplanted by more effective and safer preparations.

There are over nine hundred photographs but no attempt has been made to provide an illustration of every disease. To have done so would have increased the bulk and price of the book without increasing proportionately its practical value. The conditions selected for illustrations are those in which a photograph significantly enhances the verbal description. There are a few conditions we wished to illustrate, but of which we could not obtain unpublished photographs of satisfactory quality.

The lists of references have been selected to provide a guide to the literature. Important articles now of largely historical interest have usually been omitted, except where a knowledge of the history of a disease simplifies the understanding of present concepts and terminology. Books and articles provided with a substantial bibliography are marked with an asterisk.

Many of the chapters have been read and criticized by several members of the team and by other colleagues. Professor Wilson Jones, Dr R.S. Wells and Dr W.E. Parish have given valuable assistance with histopathological, genetic and immunological problems respectively. Many advisers, whose services are acknowledged in the following pages, have helped us with individual chapters. Any errors which have not been eliminated are, however, the responsibility of the editors and authors.

The editors hope that this book will prove of value to all those who are interested in the skin either as physicians or as research workers. They will welcome readers' criticisms and suggestions which may help them to make the second edition the book they hope to produce.

Chapter 61

Psychocutaneous Disorders

L.G. Millard & J.A. Cotterill

Introduction

An essential component of dermatological illness is the relationship that somatic dermatology has with the psychological status of the patient at the time. The influence that these psychological, psychosocial and sometimes psychiatric factors have can be conveniently assessed as:

1 Multifactorial dermatological disorders that can be substantially influenced by psychological factors (e.g. psoriasis)

2 Dermatological disorders as a result of psychiatric illness (e.g. factitious dermatoses, body dysmorphic disorder)

3 Psychiatric illness developing as a result of skin disease (e.g. reactive depression, adjustment disorder)

4 Comorbidity with other psychiatric disorder (e.g. alcoholism).

In large centres, this work can be refined and developed in specific clinics for psychosomatic dermatology [1]. Ideally, liaison psychiatry should be available together with help from clinical psychologists and social workers [2]. Research and dissemination of further knowledge in psychosomatic dermatology is supported in Europe by the European Society for Dermatology and Psychiatry (ESDaP) and in North America by the Association for Psychodermatological Medicine of North America (APMNA).

The dermatological consultation is substantially different from the psychiatric one. However, for those who feel intimidated, the consultation process and descriptive psychopathology of psychological medicine is well described for non-psychiatrists [3,4].

REFERENCES

1 Schneider G, Geiler U. Psychosomatic dermatology: state of the art. *Z Psychosom Med Psychother* 2001; **47** (4): 307–31.
2 Fritzche K, Ott J, Augusti M. Psychosomatic liaison service. *Dermatology* 2002; **203**: 27–31.
3 Neighbour R. *The Inner Consultation.* Lancaster: MTP Press, 1989.
4 Sims A. *Symptoms in the Mind: An Introduction to Descriptive Psychopathology,* 2nd edn. London: Saunders, 1995.

Emotional factors in diseases of the skin [1–4]

The narrative of clinical anecdote and experience held for a long time that emotional stress could be counted as an integral cause of skin disease or at least an exacerbating factor leading to increased disease morbidity [1].

It has been estimated that the effective management of at least one-third of patients attending skin departments depends upon the recognition and treatment of emotional factors [5]. While in disease such as dermatitis artefacta this influence is primary and pathogenic, the relationships between the mind and the skin are usually more complex than this. This intricate interaction may reveal that chronic insult hand dermatitis is the result of the hand-washing rituals of those with obsessive compulsive disorders [6], or that the intractability of atopic dermatitis is a response to an impaired parent–child relationship [7]. The narrative has been supported by an increasing evidence base showing, for example, that stressed patients with psoriasis have more prolonged disease and that simple counselling support can be an effective way of reducing disease severity [3].

The burgeoning science of psychoneuroimmunology has contributed enormously to an understanding of altered immune mechanisms in depression and anxiety. This knowledge might help to explain why pemphigus might be triggered by stress [8] or viral skin infections prolonged [9]. The concepts of the relationship between mind and body and mind and skin may have seemed rather nebulous in the past but measurement and analysis of these interconnections is established. Although the intricacies of the neuro-immuno-cutaneous–endocrine (NICE) network [10] remains rudimentary and science lags behind practice, practical applications in dermatology are effective using hypnosis or biofeedback [11]. Similarly, work on the relationship between mental activity and peripheral blood flow [12] may shed light on the exacerbation of some inflammatory dermatoses by stress, and perhaps on the effect of stress on itching. The influence of psyche upon the skin implies that there are chemical mediators that translate an emotion to a cutaneous lesion. These mediators are neurotransmitters and hormones that can be produced directly in skin by nerve fibres or by other cells such as keratinocytes, Langerhans' cells and perhaps Merkel cells [13]. Neuropeptides, substance P (SP), substance Y, vasoactive intestinal peptide (VIP), calcitonin gene-related peptide (CGRP), and melanocyte stimulating hormone (MSH) all bind to cell surface receptors.

Nevertheless, many of the conditions mentioned in this chapter form obvious groups, shading from one into another. One such spectrum ranges from natural anxiety over disfiguring skin lesions, through disproportionate worry over minor blemishes, to disturbances of body image that lead patients to become obsessed with their skin in the absence of any abnormality, and, finally, to psychotic delusions about their skin (e.g. of parasitosis), which may occasionally be caused by organic brain pathology [14]. These are dealt with in more detail on p. 61.8.

In any patient-centred medical specialty, physical symptoms often present as a manifestation of emotional distress. Somatization is defined as physical symptoms suggesting physical disorder for which there are no demonstrable organic findings and for which there are positive evidence that symptoms are linked to psychological factors or conflicts (Diagnostic and Statistical Manual of Mental Disorders, fourth edition; DSM-IV). In primary care practice, an emotionally distressed patient is more likely to present with physical symptoms than to complain about psychological or social problems [15]. Many studies confirm that this type of patient, with unrecognized psychiatric morbidity, is often passed on to medical and surgical clinics [16]. Surgeons see patients with somatic abdominal pain, physicians those with chest pain and breathlessness, and neurologists those with somatic or 'functional' headache. Dermatologists see a spectrum of those who, for example, may have symptoms as varied as psychogenic itch to those with intractable burning genitalia. Indeed, dermatology in-patients are known to have a higher prevalence of psychiatric disorders than general medical in-patients and dermatology outpatients a higher prevalence than the general population [17].

Somatizing patients may recognize psychological symptoms as part of their illness, but these are overshadowed by intense physical complaints that allow those reluctant to accept the stigma of mental illness still to occupy the 'sick role' [18]. Depression and anxiety are the most common underlying psychological disorders but their mood disturbance and characteristic patterns of thinking are not volunteered. Some somatic symptoms are amplifications of normal physiological sensations (e.g. itching), which tend to worsen under stress [19]; others relate to the physiological accompaniments of anxiety, such as excessive sweating. This type of behaviour merges imperceptibly with hypochondriasis. In some patients, this amplification of physical symptoms with symptom hyperbole is an enduring personality trait [20].

Those areas of overlap between psychiatry and dermatology are important, and a competent dermatologist should be able to pick up any emotional and psychological clues and cues that may be advanced by the patient during consultation. All patients are individual but individual patient personality styles present with recognizable distinctive verbal and body language [21].

REFERENCES

1 Koblenzer CS. Psychosomatic concepts in dermatology. *Arch Dermatol* 1983; **119**: 501–12.
2 Koo JYM. *Psychodermatology: Current Concepts Series.* Kalamazoo: Upjohn, 1989: 1–45.

3 Picardi A, Abeni D. Stressful life events and skin disease. *Psychother Psychosom* 2001; **70**: 118–36.
4 Panconesi E, Hautmann G. Psychophysiology of stress in dermatology: the psychologic pattern of psychosomatics. In: *Dermatol Clin* 1996; **3**: 399–421.
5 Sneddon J, Sneddon I. Acne excoriée: a protective device. *Clin Exp Dermatol* 1983; **8**: 65–8.
6 Rasmussen SA. Obsessive compulsive disorder in dermatologic practice. *J Am Acad Dermatol* 1985; **13**: 965–7.
7 Koblenzer CS, Koblenzer PJ. Chronic intractable atopic eczema: its occurrence as a physical sign of impaired parent–child relationships and psychologic developmental arrest—improvement through parent insight and education. *Arch Dermatol* 1988; **124**: 1673–7.
8 Brenner S, Bar-Nathan EA. Pemphigus vulgaris triggered by emotional stress. *J Am Acad Dermatol* 1984; **11**: 524–5.
9 Kalivas L, Penick E, Kalivas J. Personality factors as predictors of therapeutic response to cryosurgery in patients with warts. *J Am Acad Dermatol* 1989; **20**: 429–32.
10 O'Sullivan RL, Lipper G, Lerner EA. The neuro-immuno-cutaneous–endocrine network: relationship of mind and skin. *Arch Dermatol* 1998; **134**: 1431–5.
11 Bilkis MR, Mark KA. Mind–body medicine. *Arch Dermatol* 1998; **134**: 1437–41.
12 Wilkin JK, Trotter K. Cognitive activity and cutaneous blood flow. *Arch Dermatol* 1987; **123**: 1503–6.
13 Misery L. Are biochemical mediators the missing link between pschosomatics and dermatology? *Dermatol Psychosom* 2001; **2**: 178–83.
14 Shelley WB, Shelley ED. Delusions of parasitosis associated with coronary bypass surgery. *Br J Dermatol* 1988; **118**: 309–10.
15 Craig T, Boardman AP. Somatization in primary care settings. In: Bass CM, ed. *Somatization: Physical Symptoms and Psychological Illness*. Oxford: Blackwell Scientific Publications, 1990: 10–39.
16 Bass CM. Assessment and management of patients with functional somatic symptoms. In: Bass CM, ed. *Somatization: Physical Symptoms and Psychological Illness*. Oxford: Blackwell Scientific Publications, 1990: 40–72.
17 Woodruff PW, Higgins EM, du Vivier AW, Wessely S. Psychiatric illness in patients referred to a dermatology–psychiatry clinic. *Gen Hosp Psychiatry* 1997; **19**: 29–35.
18 Goldberg DP, Bridges K. Somatic presentation of psychiatric illness in a primary case setting. *J Psychosom Res* 1988; **32**: 137–44.
19 Fjellner B, Arnetz BB. Psychological predictors of pruritus during mental stress. *Acta Derm Venereol (Stockh)* 1985; **65**: 504–8.
20 Barsky AJ. Patients who amplify bodily symptoms. *Ann Intern Med* 1979; **91**: 63–70.
21 Putnam SM, Lipkin M, Lazare A, Kaplan C. Personality styles. In: Lipkin M, Putnam SM, Lazare A, eds. *The Medical Interview*. New York: Springer Verlag, 1995: 251–74.

Psychological importance of the skin [1–3]

Some cutaneous stimulation is a basic need. Newborn mammals require the stimulus of licking and stroking, and caressing favours emotional development. Massaged babies gain weight as much as 50% faster than unmassaged babies. The functions of swaddling clothes provide an environment of warmth, touch and decreased stress as demonstrated by reduced heart rate, better feeding and longer sleep patterns. Children who live in emotionally destructive homes may show growth arrest as a response to the withdrawal of love and touch. As an organ of touch, temperature and pain sensation, and as an erogenous zone, the skin has great psychological importance at all ages. Many of the alternative medical therapies such as aromatherapy and kinesthesiology show clinical effects related to the the measureable effects of touch. Furthermore, patients who are regularly touched by their carers

show quicker improvement than those who do not [3] and this effect is measureable at all ages and intelligences [4]. It is an organ of emotional expression and a site for the discharge of anxiety. Its texture and colour have meaning socially and politically, and its disorders carry with them a disproportionately heavy psychological punishment [5].

REFERENCES

1 Messeri P, Montagna W. Ethologic implications of the skin and its disturbances. In: Panconesi E, ed. *Clinics in Dermatology*. Vol. 2. *Psychosomatic Dermatology*. 1984: 27–36.
2 Montagu A. The skin, touch and human development. In: Panconesi E, ed. *Clinics in Dermatology*. Vol. 2. *Psychosomatic Dermatology*. 1984: 17–26.
3 Autton N. *Touch: An Exploration*. London: Dalton, Longman & Todd, 1989: 40–63.
4 Keiko T, Adachi Y, Yokota Y *et al.* Effects of body touching therapy on the elderly. *J Int Soc Life Science* 2000; **18**: 246–50.
5 Seville RH. Stress and psoriasis: the importance of insight and empathy in prognosis. *J Am Acad Dermatol* 1989; **20**: 97–100.

Body image [1,2]

Body image can be conceptualized by individuals in many different ways. There are a multiplicity of definitions, but the simplest is that of Critchley [3] who defined body image as 'the physical properties of a person carried into the imagery of himself'. It is important to remember that body image is completely abstract in conceptualization, depending on many factors, including memory, intellect, perception and early life experiences.

Body image may be conceptualized as the internal subjective representation of physical appearance and bodily experience [2]. This develops early, by the age of 3–4 years, with the drawing of the first recognizable figures by children [4]. Body image represents a view of ourselves not only physical but also has always had vital psychological and sociological importance [5]. There is a very significant cutaneous component, the most important areas of which include the face, scalp, hair, breasts in females and genital areas. A child's first recognizable body drawings are 'tadpole' figures, which emphasize the head with spindly legs and an absent body [4]. The nose, which is the central part of the face, is also focal to body-image conceptualization and it is not surprising therefore that skin disease manifesting itself even as a tiny spot on the nose, may produce disparate cosmetic distress, while a much larger lesion on an adjacent cheek may be completely ignored. As the face is both visible and in a very important body-image area, skin disease in this area can produce major distress and lowering of self-esteem. It has been shown that individuals with severe acne, particularly female, have a significant depression of their body image and self-esteem, which was reversible with successful treatment [6]. In addition, individuals with acne are less successful at gaining employment [7]. It may be that potential employers perceive individuals with acne as unattractive, but also the interviewees themselves may reflect their lower self-esteem and confidence at interviews. Eczema and psoriasis are both likely to produce the same sort of effects, particularly at times of life when the individual would normally be beginning to socialize [8]. Adolescence can be particularly difficult for the teenager with acne, facial psoriasis or eczema. This self-recognition also appears early in child drawings of their disfigurement. The stigmatization induced by a port-wine stain may also deter individuals, particularly males, from making any sort of contact with the opposite sex [9]. The older that patients were before treatment, the higher negative scores for most psychosocial parameters such as self-esteem, supporting the argument for early treatment on psychological grounds [10].

It is important to recognize that individuals with skin problems in important body-image areas may be manifestly depressed. These individuals can be helped both by effective treatment and also by an empathetic medical practitioner. In some instances, a clinical psychologist may help a person to come to terms with his or her problems while, in a minority, depression is severe enough to merit treatment with antidepressants and the help of a psychiatrist. A liaison clinic is particularly helpful in managing this type of patient, where at times there may be a definite risk of suicide or parasuicide [11].

REFERENCES

1 Morris D. *Bodywatching*. London: Jonathan Cape, 1986.
2 Cash T, Pruzinsky T. *Body Images: Development, Deviance and Change*. New York: Guildford, 1990.
3 Critchley M. Corporeal awareness: body image; body scheme. In: *The Divine Banquet of the Brain and Other Essays*. New York: Raven Press, 1980: 92–105.
4 Cox M. *Drawings of People by the Under-5s*. London: Falmer Press, 1997: 3–36.
5 Miller J. Self-recognition, self-regard, self-representation. In: *On Reflection*. London: National Gallery, 1998: 134–82.
6 Kellett SC, Gawkrodger DJ. The psychological and emotional impact of acne and the effect of treatment with isotretinoin. *Br J Dermatol* 1999; **140**: 273–82.
7 Cunliffe WJ. Acne and unemployment. *Br J Dermatol* 1986; **115**: 386.
8 Ginsburg IH, Link BG. Feelings of stigmatization in patients with psoriasis. *J Am Acad Dermatol* 1989; **20**: 53–63.
9 Lanigan S, Cotterill JA. Psychological disabilities amongst patients with port-wine stains. *Br J Dermatol* 1989; **121**: 209–15.
10 Troilius A, Wrangsjo B, Ljunngren B. Patients with port-wine stains and their psychosocial reactions after photothermolytic treatment. *Dermatol Surg* 2000; **26**: 190–6.
11 Schneider G, Geiler U. Psychosomatic dermatology: state of the art. *Z Psychosom Med Psychother* 2001; **47** (4): 307–31.

Psychoneuroimmunology [1–3]

The immune system and its relationship to cutaneous reponses is now established as part of the NICE system [1,2]. None of these processes can be be regarded as autonomous because immunoregulatory processes are part of an integrated system of defence [1]. Psychoneuroimmunology is the study of this integrated system and of behavioural–neuroendocrine–immune system interactions in particular.

The brain and immune system are linked by the autonomic nervous system and the neuroendocrine outflow via the hypothalamus and the pituitary gland. Communication between the immune system and the brain is bidirectional and probably largely mediated by neuropeptides [2]. More than 50 neuropeptides have now been identified, the smallest ones containing only two amino acids while the larger peptides contain 40 or more amino acids. Neuropeptides act not only as neurotransmitters, but also as neuromodulators.

Lymphoid tissue is innervated by noradrenergic postganglionic sympathetic nerve fibres, and peptidergic nerve fibres have also been identified in lymph nodes, thymus, spleen and bone marrow [3]. These nerve fibres form close neuroeffective junctions with lymphocytes and macrophages, which also possess receptors for neuropeptides [1].

Neuropeptides in the skin [2] are found not only in cutaneous nerves but also in most skin cells including keratinocytes, fibroblasts and Langerhans' cells. The role of vasoactive petides such as calcitonin gene-related peptide (CGRP), nocioceptive neurotransmitter SP, VIP, neuropeptide Y, and the newer pituitary adenylcyclate-activating peptide are increasingly evident in cutaneous inflammatory disease [3]; SP receptors found on mast cells, neutrophils and macrophages suggest a link between neurogenic stimuli and infiltration of the skin by inflammatory cells. CGRP has crucial immunomodulating effects on disease expression, perhaps by inhibition of antigen presentation by Langerhans' cells.

Moreover, lymphocytes have receptors for corticotrophin-releasing hormone (CRH), adrenocorticotrophic hormone (ACTH) and endogenous opioids, and both endorphins and enkephalins are known to directly influence antigen-specific and non-specific *in vivo* and *in vitro* responses [1].

Mind–body efferent immune interactions

Dermatologists have long recognized the relationship between stress and exacerbations of skin disease. With further knowledge of the psychoneuroimmunology of depression [4] and the further reviews of these effects in psychosomatic medicine [5], the efferent pathway from stress to disease is becoming clearer. Exposure to either naturally occurring or experimentally induced stress affect both humoral and cell-mediated immune responses. Bereavement is often associated with depression and many changes in immune function have been shown in depressed patients. Depression is associated with an increased number of circulating neutrophils, a decreased number of natural killer (NK) cells, T and B lymphocytes, and helper and suppressor cytotoxic T cells [6]. There are also alterations in B-cell function, manifest by increased antibody titres to herpes simplex and cytomegalovirus [1]. Changes in both humoral and cell-mediated immunity have been found following marital separation and divorce [7] and alterations in immune function may occur during examinations [2]. Slowing of human wound healing has also been shown to be associated with stress, possibly mediated by depression of local production of the cytokine interleukin 1B [8].

Raychaudhuri and Farber [9] have proposed a psychoneuroimmunological basis for psoriasis. Thus, psoriatic skin has been shown to have a significant increase in SP-containing nerves. Psoriatic lesions are rich in neuropeptides such as SP and VIP. Proliferation of keratinocytes, a central feature of psoriasis, could be triggered by release of both SP and VIP, while SP could also induce localized lymphocytic proliferation. Moreover, the initiation and maintenance of the lymphocytic infiltrate characteristic of psoriasis could be in part related to SP, CGRP and VIP; indeed, SP can induce the expression of E-selectin on endothelium. For patients with atopic eczema, both SP and VIP have been demonstrated in lesional skin [10]. Moreover, NPY, a very potent vasoconstrictor, has been detected in the Langerhans' cells of patients with atopic eczema, but not in normal control subjects.

Body–mind afferent immune reactions

The bidirectional communication between the central nervous system (CNS) and the immune system provides the basis not only for behaviourally induced alterations in immune function, but also for immunologically based changes in behaviour [1]. Those patients who present with diseases causing intense afferent stimuli such as scratching, rubbing or traction are probably in a NICE loop where the inflammatory reaction stimulates an immune response which in turn releases cytokines to activate CNS neurotransmitters. Endorphins, for example, modify not only the perception of pain, but also other sensory perceptions [11] such as beauty. The compulsive and irresistible nature of scratching, excoriating and picking may relate to the pleasureable release of endorphins. These pathways may explain how emotional stress influences a wide range of disorders.

REFERENCES

1 Alder R, Felten DL, eds. *Psychoneuroimmunology*, 3rd edn. San Diego: Academic Press, 2001.
2 Panconesi E, Hautmann G. Pathophysiology of stress in dermatology: the psychobiologic pattern of psychosomatics. *Dermatol Clin* 1996; **14**: 399–421.
3 O'Sullivan RL, Lipper G, Lerner EA. The neuro-immuno-cutaneous–endocrine network: relationship of mind and skin. *Arch Dermatol* 1998; **134**: 1431–5.
4 Irwin M. Psychoneuroimmunology of depression: clinical implications. *Brain Behav Immun* 2002; 16: 1–16.
5 Kiecolt-Glaser J, McGuire L, Robles T. Psychoneuroimmunology and psychosomatic medicine. *Psychosom Med* 2002; **64**: 15–28.
6 Sternberg EM. Neural-immune interactions in health and disease. *J Clin Invest* 1997; **100**: 2641–7.
7 Glaser R, Rice J, Sheridan J *et al.* Stress-related immune suppression: health implications. *Brain Behav Immun* 1987; **1**: 7–20.
8 Kiecolt-Glaser JK, Marucha PT, Malarkey WB *et al.* Slowing of wound healing by psychological stress. *Lancet* 1995; **346**: 1194–6.
9 Raychaudhuri SP, Farber EM. Neuroimmunologic aspects of psoriasis. *Cutis* 2000; **66**: 357–62.
10 Panconesi E, Hautmann G. Stress and emotions in skin disease. In: Koo J, Lee CS, eds. *Psychocutaneous Medicine*. New York: Dekker, 2003: 51–7.
11 Stefano GB, Salzet B, Fricchione GL. Enkelytin and opioid peptide association in invertebrates and vertebrates immune activation and pain. *Immunol Today* 1998; **19**: 265–8.

Emotional reactions to skin disease [1,2]

Skin disease causes physical problems and distress. The anthropological importance of the skin as an organ of communication both tactile and visual by touch and expression is well recorded [1]. With either real or imagined disfigurement comes shame and reclusiveness. These emotions are part of the arcane folk beliefs that most cutaneous disease is the result of infection with significant imputations of uncleanliness and self-neglect, even in Western cultures. The religious significance of leprosy in many cultures continues to exert an influence where the psychosocial stigma of depigmented skin in vitiligo may operate even in non-endemic populations. A poor self-image and low self-esteem is easily demonstrated by appropriate questionnaires [3]. Patients with psoriasis are aware that other people stare at them, particularly in socially revealing situations such as swimming, and experience much social distress [1,2]. Patients with vitiligo adjust better to their disorder than do those with psoriasis, but also tend to have low self-esteem [4]. There may be a hidden and unbroached difficulty with sexual expression and confidence [5], as skin disease frequently has a negative impact on sexual relationships [6], independent of extent but significantly related to site. The impaired self-image and psychological distress of patients with acne improve with successful treatment of the skin lesions [7].

One of the consistent correlates of the social isolation and low self-esteem is heavy alcohol consumption, which in male psoriatics correlates with both the physical severity of their skin disease and its duration [8]. Ten per cent of patients with psoriasis reported a death wish and 6% reported active suicidal ideation in one study [9]. Acne scarring can lead to profound depression and suicide [10].

Genital skin disease, particularly herpes and chronic candidosis, produces initial shock and emotional numbing at diagnosis followed by a frantic search for a cause, and later by a sense of loneliness and isolation. Some 10–15% of patients with genital herpes never adjust satisfactorily and continue to experience difficulties in all areas of their lives, which become increasingly reclusive and monastic [11].

The concept of stigma [12] is important in this context. It can be defined as a biological or social mark that sets a person apart from others, is discrediting and disrupts interactions with others [13]. In a study of adults with psoriasis, those who were older at the onset of the disease seemed less likely to anticipate rejection, and to be less sensitive to the opinions of others and to feelings of guilt, shame and secrecy [13]. Further, the perceptions of stigmatization were found to be related to psychological distress and degree of disability but not to clinical severity of involvement or anatomical area [14,15].

Atopic dermatitis in children is associated with high levels of psychological morbidity [13]. The disturbance was best predicted by the distribution of the eczema rather than its extent, with facial involvement in children showing particularly high levels of psychological distress. The additional effect of brief, simple, psychotherapy was sufficient to help those patients with high anxiety levels achieve normal remission [16].

With the approach of puberty, a disfiguring skin disease becomes an increasing anxiety to many children and may handicap them in developing easy relationships with the opposite sex [17]. Some children become increasingly introspective and solitary, while others become aggressive and uncooperative. The consultation process in these circumstances is most demanding. The best results are achieved by defusing the anger, which is usually the result of frustration and disappointment, by adopting a planned therapeutic and supportive role. This may be difficult but an organized programme with cooperation from parents, teachers and physicians can maintain optimism through established coping strategies [18]. With sensible and affectionate parents and intelligent teachers, children with disfiguring skin lesions will often adjust extremely well, form satisfactory sexual relationships and establish themselves in successful careers.

REFERENCES

1 Ginsburg IH. The psychosocial impact of skin disease: an overview. *Dermatol Clin* 1996; **14**: 473–84.
2 Papadopoulos L, Bor R. *Psychological Approaches to Dermatology*. Leicester: BPS Books, 1999: 47–63.
3 Cash TF. *The Body Image Automatic Thoughts Questionairre (BIATQ)*. Norfolk: Old Dominion University, 1990.
4 Porter JR, Beuf AH, Lerner A et al. Psychosocial effect of vitiligo. *J Am Acad Dermatol* 1986; **15**: 220–4.
5 Updike J. Personal history at war with my skin. *New Yorker* 1955; 2 September: 39–55.
6 Coen-Buckwater K. The influence of skin disorders on sexual expression. *Sex Disabil* 1982; **5**: 98–106.
7 Rubinov PR, Peck GL, Squillace KM et al. Reduced anxiety and depression in cystic acne patients after successful treatment with oral isotretinoin. *J Am Acad Dermatol* 1987; **17**: 25–32.
8 Melotti E, Herpeisen SM, Polenghi MM. Alcohol consumption in psoriasis. *Ann Ital Dermatol Clin Sper* 1987; **41**: 343–8.
9 Gupta MA, Schork NJ, Gupta AK et al. Suicidal ideation in psoriasis. *Int J Dermatol* 1993; **32**: 188–90.
10 Cotterill JA, Cunliffe WJ. Suicide in dermatological patients. *Br J Dermatol* 1997; **137**: 246–50.
11 Luby EB, Klinge V. Genital herpes: a pervasive psychosocial disorder. *Arch Dermatol* 1985; **121**: 494–7.
12 Goffman E. *Stigma: Notes on the Management of Spoiled Identity*. London: Penguin, 1999.
13 Jowett S, Ryan T. Skin disease and handicap: an analysis of the impact of skin conditions. *Soc Sci Med* 1985; **20**: 425–9.
14 Richards H, Fortune DG, Griffiths CEM. The contribution of perceptions of stigmatization to disability in patients with psoriasis. *J Psychosom Res* 2001; **50**: 11–5.
15 Ginsburg IH, Link BG. Feelings of stigmatization in patients with psoriasis. *J Am Acad Dermatol* 1989; **20**: 53–63.
16 Linnet J, Jemmec GB. Anxiety level and severity of skin condition and outcome of psychotherapy. *Int J Dermatol* 2001; **40**: 632–6.
17 Jacobs B, Green J, David TJ. A self-concept of children with atopic dermatitis. *Br J Dermatol* 1995; **133**: 1004.
18 Papadopoulos L, Bor R. *Psychological Approaches to Dermatology*. Leicester: BPS Books, 1999: 23–30.

Disability and quality of life [1,2]

This aspect of dermatology is covered in more detail in Chapter 71.

Quality of life is defined as an individual's perception of their position in life in the context of the culture and value system in which they live and in relation to their goals, expectations, standards and concerns. It is a broad-ranging concept affected in a complex way by the person's physical heath, psychological state, level of independence, social relationships and relationship to salient features of their environment.

Established dermatological medicine describes skin disorders in relatively enclosed diagnostic terms, which takes little account of the effect of a particular skin disease on the individual patient. The patient with disease needs to be understood not only in terms of mechanistic outcomes of the kind usually assessed in clinical practice but also those composed of the psychosocial (hermaneutic) constructs that are assessed from the patient's self-reports. It is important to try to determine these disparate degrees of disability that a particular skin disease confers because their recognition leads to greater patient compliance and a more positive response [1–3].

The concept of skin failure is just as valid as that of renal, heart or respiratory failure [2]. The effect on quality of life induced by psoriasis, eczema and acne have been assessed using disability indices that are readily accessible [4]. These scales can also be used to quantify reduction in disability before and after treatment. The newer indices of disability have successfully combined the physical and psychological measures to produce a more holistic assessment of disease as exemplified by the Salford Psoriasis Index [3,5]. For instance, the presence of relatively trivial amounts of psoriasis on an individual's face may induce disparate depression. There are other instruments available for atopic eczema [6], acne in adolescence [7] and hair loss [8], which continue this development.

Quality of life assessments are not related to health but to disease and are usually specific to a particular diagnosis. This is very different from the non-medical connotation of the meaning of the phrase, which is accepted to relate to a well state of contentedness of 'having a good time'. It has been proposed that in future the quality of life of ill people may need to take account of this difference because the patient's pathology involving release of cytokines and other mediators may affect their psychological state and thus response to questionnaires [9].

REFERENCES

1 Bowling A. *Measuring Disease: A Review of Disease-Specific Quality of Life Scales*. Buckingham: Open University Press, 2001.
2 Ryan TJ. Disability in dermatology. *Br J Hosp Med* 1991; **46**: 33–6.
3 Kirby B, Fortune DG, Bhushan M, Chalmers RJG, Griffiths CEM. The Salford Psoriasis Index: an holistic measure of psoriasis. *Br J Dermatol* 2000; **142**: 728–32.
4 Papadopoulos L, Bor R. *Psychological Approaches to Dermatology*. Leicester: BPS Books, 1999: 141–52.
5 Kirby B, Richards HL, Woo P *et al*. Physical and psychologic measures are necessary to assess overall psoriasis severity. *J Am Acad Dermatol* 2001; **45**: 72–6.
6 Buske-Kirchbaum A, Gieben A, Hellhammer D. Psychobiological aspects of atopic dermatitis: an overview. *Psychother Psychosom* 2001; **70**: 6–16.
7 Smith JA. The impact of skin disease on the quality of life in adolescents. *Adolesc Med* 2001; **12**: 343–53.
8 Williamson D, Gonzalez M, Finlay AY. The effect of hair loss on quality of life. *J Eur Acad Dermatol Venereol* 2000; **15**: 137–9.
9 Koller M, Lorenz W. Quality of life: a deconstruction for clinicians. *J R Soc Med* 2002; **95**: 451–88.

Classification [1,2]

There are two main internationally recognized classifications of psychiatric disorders. The first is produced by the American Psychiatric Association with disorders defined by diagnostic criteria describing their essential features. The DSM is modified regularly, the current revision dating from 2000 [1]. The current international classification and nomenclature system for medical and psychiatric disorder is published by the World Health Organization [2] and in many respects is similar to DSM. These classifications are part of the essential practice of psychiatry where the language and symptoms of disease and thus its subsequent treatment is to identify, for example, organic syndromes, schizophrenia, bipolar disorders, somatic and personality disorders. This may not be user friendly enough for clinical dermatologists in everyday practice. However, whatever the presenting features to dermatologists, it is signally important to remember that the symptoms are not a diagnosis and therefore should not be assumed to be amenable to the same treatment. For example, dermatitis artefacta may be a symptom of depression, personality disorder or an abnormal psychosocial situation; each requires different treatment. Various other classifications have their merits [3–5] but as our knowledge increases, overlap and clarification make changes inevitable. This classification is therefore pragmatic with an emphasis on usefulness for dermatologists.

Conditions that are primarily psychiatric but which commonly present to dermatologists

Delusional beliefs of skin
(i) Parasitosis (Ekbom's disease)
(ii) Smell
(iii) Impregnation and contamination
(iv) Folie à deux
Disorders of body image
(i) Body dysmorphic disorder (BDD) (syn. dysmorphophobia, dermatological non-disease)
(ii) Atypical pain disorders such as glossodynia and essential vulvodynia
(iii) Dermatological hypochondriasis
(iv) Cyberchondria
(v) Anorexia nervosa
(vi) Bigorexia
(vii) Tanorexia
Phobic states
(i) Venereophobia and acquired immune deficiency syndrome (AIDS) phobia
(ii) Mole phobia
(iii) Wart phobia
(iv) Erythrophobia
(v) Age phobia and botoxophilia
(vi) Ateroidphobia
Obsessive compulsive hand washing

Group and mass population reactions

Sick building syndrome
Epidemic hysteria

Dermatoses primarily factitious in origin

Dermatitis artefacta
Artefact by proxy
Witchcraft syndrome
Dermatological pathomimicry
Dermatitis simulata
Malingering
Compensation neurosis
Munchausen's syndrome
Munchausen's syndrome by proxy
Deliberate self-cutting
Self-mutilation
Religious stigmata and psychogenic purpura

Dermatoses aggravated by harmful habits and compulsions

Lichen simplex
Neurotic excoriations
Prurigo nodularis
Acne excoriée

Hair plucking
Trichotillomania
Trichophagia
Nail destruction
Onychotillomania
Lip-licking cheilitis
Knuckle biting
Disorders of neglect of self-care (syn. Diogenes syndrome)

Dermatoses caused by accentuated physiological responses

Hyperhidrosis
Blushing

Dermatoses in which emotional precipitating or perpetuating factors may be important

Vesicular eczema of the palms and soles
Atopic dermatitis in the adult
Seborrhoeic dermatitis
Psoriasis
Some cases of localized or generalized pruritus
Alopecia areata
Aphthosis
Rosacea
Chronic urticaria

This last group produces most debate and significant continuing research. Different views are held by dermatologists but while the early work relating skin disease to stress [6] was greeted with scepticism, the evolving body of evidence (see above) is a significant development to support the link.

REFERENCES

1 American Psychiatric Association. *Diagnostic and Statistical Manual of Mental Disorders*, 4th edn. Washington DC: American Psychiatric Association, 2000.
2 World Health Organization. *The ICD-10 Classification of Mental and Behavioural Disorders: Clinical Descriptions and Diagnostic Guidelines.* Geneva: World Health Organization, 1992.
3 Whitlock FA. *Psychophysiological Aspects of Skin Disease.* London: Saunders, 1976.
4 Koblenzer CS. Psychosomatic concepts in dermatology. *Arch Dermatol* 1983; **119**: 501–12.
5 Medansky RS, Handler RM. Dermatopsychosomatics: classification, physiology and therapeutic approaches. *J Am Acad Dermatol* 1981; **5**: 125–36.
6 Seville RH. Stress and psoriasis: the importance of insight and empathy in prognosis. *J Am Acad Dermatol* 1989; **20**: 97–100.

Dermatological delusional symptoms

[1,2]

A delusion is a disorder of the content of thinking. Delusions are beliefs that are false or not true to fact, cannot be corrected by an appeal to reason of the individual and are out of harmony with his or her educational and cultural background. Furthermore, the delusion can be further subclassified into [1,2]: (a) primary, where the delusion is the only psychological symptom; rather than (b) secondary functional, in which there is an underlying psychiatric condition such as depression; or (c) secondary organic, where there is physical illness such as dementia [3].

The dermatologist is most likely to see patients with delusions of parasitosis, which in itself is rare, rather than other cutaneous delusions. These are delusions of smell [2], of impregnation or of ocular or oral infestation, all of which are exceedingly uncommon. Equally so are patients who have a belief that they are ageing rapidly, the so-called Dorian Gray syndrome.

Delusions of parasitosis [4–6]

Definition. The patient with delusions of parasitosis (DP) has an unshakeable conviction that his or her skin is infested by parasites (this must be differentiated from parasitophobia—the *fear* of becoming infested).

Aetiology. Most patients with DP have a primary disorder defined as a monosymptomatic hypochondriacal psychosis being characterized by a single delusional system, relatively distinct from the remainder of the personality. The term monosymptomatic hypochondriacal psychosis may be applied to patients with a single, fixed, hypochondriacal delusion that is apparently not secondary to another psychiatric disorder [7]. Occasionally, there are associated visual hallucinations.

Secondary DP has been recorded as a feature of depression, bipolar disorder, paranoid states and schizophreniform illnesses [4–7]. It is therefore essential to define the full psychiatric spectrum in each patient. Those seen by psychiatrists are more likely to be labelled schizophrenic or depressed, or both. Such patients are often intelligent, and the professions are well represented, including doctors and even psychiatrists, but they are often rather solitary people and sometimes thought to be eccentric individuals. Lyell [4] has commented that it is hard to know where eccentricity ends and psychiatric illness begins. Moreover, some patients have a rather obsessional premorbid personality. Table 61.1 summarizes the secondary organic causes of DP [5]. Delusions of perception may follow disease in the non-dominant hemisphere, and so DP is sometimes seen in patients after a cerebrovascular accident involving that side of the brain. Similarly, DP may be part of the picture of dementia and should be considered when examining the elderly patient [8]. DP has also been described in pellagra, vitamin B_{12} deficiency, following coronary bypass surgery, as a side effect of phenelzine and in severe renal disease. DP in a young adult suggest illicit exposure to recreational drugs, in particular amphetamine or cocaine [9].

It is particularly important to exclude the possibility of

Table 61.1 Organic medical disorders associated with delusional parasitosis.

Neurological
Cerebrovascular disease
Dementia
Parkinson's disease
CNS tumours

Cardiovascular disorders
Arrhythmias
Heart failure
Coronary artery bypass

Endocrine disease
Diabetes mellitus
Hyperthyroidism
Hypoparathyroidism
Acromegaly

Nutritional disorders
Pellagra
Vitamin B$_{12}$ deficiency
Anorexia nervosa

Infectious diseases
Syphilis
AIDS
Tuberculosis (pulmonary)
Leprosy

Malignancy
Breast cancer
Lung cancer
Lymphoma
Chronic lymphatic leukaemia

Substance abuse
Amphetamines
Cocaine

Medicines
Corticosteroids
Phenelzine pargyline

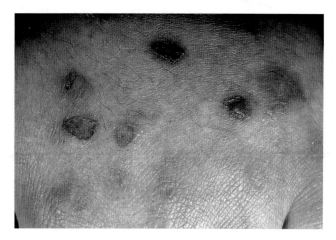

Fig. 61.1 Neurotic exoriations.

a real infestation. In 6% of one series, patients developed DP following real infestation [4] and 12% had a delusion shared with another member of the family (folie à deux; see below).

Incidence. Patients with DP are rare but the true prevalence is unknown. The condition affects both sexes equally below the age of 50 years, but after that age three times as many women are affected as men [3,10]. Although patients with DP are relatively easily recognized, it is possible to spend a lifetime as a dermatologist and never see such a patient. The young patient with DP should be regarded with the utmost concern for they may be drug abusers or the symptom may be the early signs of a major psychotic illness [9].

Clinical features. The presenting features of DP may be extremely variable. It can be as dramatic as an appeal from the primary care practitioner to see urgently a patient with an established delusion of infestation because they are disrupting everyone's life with constant demands, to an apparently benign, ill-defined, persistent itching with no immediate obvious delusional thoughts.

In the most established case, the patient may have consulted a series of specialist services to eradicate the imagined infestation. The family doctor is consulted repeatedly for even 'stronger' medicines to treat the 'bugs', the public health authorities called on many occasions to disinfest the home and the veterinary services recruited to scrutinize and treat pets. Eminent university personnel may have been consulted, both medical in infectious disease departments or scientific in zoology specialties. Specimens are sent to international institutions such as the British Museum for the ultimate examination. By the time the patient reaches the clinic there is always an inevitable degree of frustration, anger and impatience which makes the first consultation both difficult and vital.

The presenting symptoms may often be surprisingly ill-defined. Some speak of a sensation in their skin as though an insect or worm is crawling around, followed by a prolonged and elaborate description of the pathway the organism is taking. This agent may not be confined to the skin but also involve the genital, oral [11] or ocular [12] areas. They may describe and draw the insect or worm concerned but not uncommonly describe the infestation as invisible or dissolved in orificial secretions.

No obvious skin disease may be present, but excoriations are common and can be both extensive and very destructive (Fig. 61.1). These follow attempts by the patient to extract the 'parasites' and are therefore not artefactual lesions but produced in an apparently legitimate attempt at cure. Usually, the patient will bring samples to the clinic. Commonly, they proffer a small container, such as a matchbox or pill container, enclosing their 'insects' (Fig. 61.2). Some samples may be described as 'seeds', a guarded interpretation particularly in the patient who is

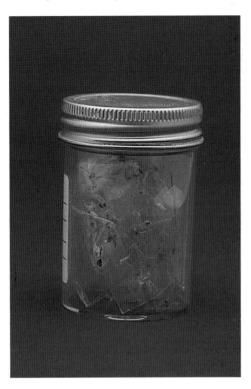

Fig. 61.2 Container of imaginary insects—from a patient with delusional parasitosis.

now cautious after seeing many doctors. Other samples that have been brought are collections of sweat, sellotape strippings of skin, folded elastoplast impregnated with debris and liquid samples collected from orifices. On microscopy these offerings are usually found to be fragments of skin and hair, samples of fabric and coagulated elements of serum, dust and detritus. The samples may include actual organisms such as ants, flies and sundry isolated fleas. The purification rituals that rapidly become established compel the patients to cleanse the skin and their environment with ever-increasing zeal. Their skin may smell of organic solvents such as benzyl benzoate or horticultural insecticide spray, the hands of bleach and disinfectant. A secondary general or localized chemically induced dermatitis is a feature. This irritant dermatitis is a further reinforcement of the delusional belief.

In 12% of cases, delusions are shared [2,7,13,14]: so-called folie à deux. This is defined in DSM-IV as a delusion developing in an individual in the context of a close relationship with another person, who has an established delusion. Once again this phenomenon is reported more often in women [14] and therefore the relationship between subjects is more often between sisters (34%), wife and husband (20%) and mother and child (20%). This contrasts with that reported between brothers (9%) and fathers and sons (2%). Rarely, the disorder can involve whole families [14].

Diagnosis. Although it is unlikely, the first task is to be certain there is no infestation; primarily scabies, rarely onchocerciasis. In most cases, the history, clinic behaviour, physical examination and presentation of specimens makes the diagnosis of DP obvious. It is also important to rule out underlying secondary organic disease, although this is rare. However, presentations in patients with secondary delusions as part of a depression or dementia may present in a more subtle fashion. The nature of depression may make the patient less communicative and more guilt-ridden. There may be a need to enquire actively about beliefs of infestation in a patient who complains of itching alone. Clinically, there may be a distinction between a true delusion and an overvalued idea [15]. The latter is an acceptable comprehensible idea carried on beyond the bounds of reason. It becomes so dominant that all other ideas are secondary. The patient's life becomes to revolve around this one idea. For example, a depressed bereaved widow who suddenly becomes a social isolate may come to believe that her itching is caused by insects. The nature of depression with feelings of unworthiness and guilt is part of this psychopathology.

Management. Musalek *et al.* [3] have emphasized the importance of establishing a psychiatric diagnosis before instituting treatment. Some patients with DP are depressed, and have been treated with conventional tricyclic antidepressants or serotonin reuptake inhibitors (SSRIs), often with pimozide. It should be remembered that suicide is an ever-attendant risk in these patients [1,4]. The management of patients with DP is always difficult. The basis of the consultation is to change the agenda from one of dermatological infestation as seen by the patient to one of psychiatric intervention. It is therefore essential to maintain a cohesive doctor–patient relationship. The full consultation process should be pursued, with adequate time given for the history, and proper care taken in the physical examination. All samples should be examined at the time and under the microscope. If you are perfunctory about this the patient will be less likely to continue with the same cooperation. Neither should you collude with the patient; it is better to say, 'I can't see any of the parasites today' than to tell the patient that you will treat 'them just in case' to get them out of the room. Neither is it helpful to say directly on the first visit that he or she has a mental problem. Sometimes, patients can be persuaded to accept the medication if told that it has helped previous patients with similar problems. Initially, it is often best to admit the patient to hospital. This reduces pressure at home on other family members and ensures compliance with medication. A psychiatric colleague can more easily be asked to see the patient in the dermatology ward. The further management is ideally a joint consultation with liaison psychiatry but the inevitable difficulty is to convince the patient that this is a psychiatric problem [16].

The response to pimozide is often good in these patients and the initial dose (2 mg) is increased weekly by 2-mg increments as necessary to a maximum of 12 mg/day [16,17]. On higher doses, patients may develop extrapyramidal symptoms which require addition of benzatropine 1–2 mg up to four times daily. With higher doses of pimozide there is a definite risk of ventricular arrhythmias and other electrocardiogram (ECG) abnormalities such as prolongation of the Q–T interval and T-wave changes. An ECG should be performed before pimozide therapy, and the drug should not be given to patients with a prolonged Q–T interval or to patients with a history of cardiac arrhythmia. Patients taking long-term pimozide should have a regular ECG at least once a year and if the Q–T interval is prolonged, treatment should be reviewed or withdrawn [10]. Moreover, concurrent treatment with other antipsychotics, tricyclic antidepressants and other drugs that prolong the Q–T interval, such as the antihistamines terfenadine and astemizole, antimalarials or drugs such as diuretics that alter the electrolyte status, should be avoided [17]. Hypokalaemia may predispose to the cardiotoxic effects of pimozide and care should be taken in patients with hepatic or renal dysfunction [16]. For most patients, pimozide is slightly stimulant so is best given in the morning. However, some find it hypnotic and this minority should take the drug in the evening.

Alternative effective therapy with a better side effect profile includes sulpiride 200–400 mg/day [18]. While this too may produce extrapyramidal side effects, there is no risk of arrhythmias. More recently, the antipsychotic risperidone has proved of use at a dosage of 4–8 mg/day [18,19]. When compliance is a problem, depot neuroleptics may be used [18].

Patients frequently defect from follow-up clinics with the risk of relapse and therefore strenuous efforts should be made to maintain contact either via the general practitioner or community psychiatric services.

REFERENCES

1 Sims A. *Symptoms in the Mind*. London: Saunders, 1995: 101–11.
2 Munro A. Paranoia or delusional disorder. In: Bhugra D, Munro A, eds. *Troublesome Disguises: Underdiagnosed Psychiatric Syndromes*. Oxford: Blackwell Scientific Publications, 1997: 24–51.
3 Musalek M, Bach M, Passweg V, Jaeger S. The position of delusional parasitosis in psychiatric nosology and classification. *Psychopathology* 1990; **23**: 115–24.
4 Lyell A. Delusions of parasitosis. *Br J Dermatol* 1983; **108**: 485–99.
5 Driscoll MS, Rothe MJ, Grant-Kels JM, Hale MS. Delusional parasitosis: a dermatologic, psychiatric, and pharmacologic approach. *J Am Acad Dermatol* 1993; **29**: 1023–33.
6 Trabert W. 100 years of delusional parasitosis: meta analysis of 1223 case reports. *Psychopathology* 1995; **28**: 238–46.
7 Munro A. Delusional parasitosis: a form of monosymptomatic hypochondriacal psychosis. *Semin Dermatol* 1983; **2**: 197–202.
8 Rasanen P, Erkonen K, Isaksson U *et al*. Delusional parasitosis in the elderly. *Int Psychogeriatr* 1997; **9**: 459–64.
9 Mitchell J, Vierkant AD. Delusions and hallucinations of cocaine abusers and paranoid schizophrenics: a comparative study. *J Psychol* 1991; **125**: 301–10.
10 Reilly TM, Batchelor DH. The presentation and treatment of delusional parasitosis: a dermatological perspective. *Clin Pschipharmacol* 1986; **1**: 340–53.
11 Maeda K, Yamamoto Y, Yasuda M, Ishii K. Delusions of oral parasitosis. *Prog Neuropsychol Psychiatry* 1998; **22**: 243–8.
12 Sherman MD, Holland GN, Holsclaw DS *et al*. Delusions of ocular parasitosis. *Am J Ophthalmol* 1998; **125**: 852–6.
13 Hughes TA, Sims A. Folie à deux. In: Bhugra D, Munro A, eds. *Troublesome Disguises: Underdiagnosed Psychiatric Syndromes*. Oxford: Blackwell Scientific Publications, 1997: 168–94.
14 Wykoff RE. Delusions of parasitosis. *Rev Infect Dis* 1987; **9**: 433–7.
15 Hopkinson G. The psychiatric syndrome of infestation. *Psychiatrica Clinica* 1973; **6**: 330–45.
16 Committee on Safety of Medicines. *Current Problems*. London: Medical Control Agency, 1990: 29.
17 Committee of Safety of Medicines. *Current Problems in Pharmacovigilance: Cardiac Arrhythmias with Pimozide (Orap)*. London: Medical Control Agency, 1995; **21**: 2.
18 Koo J, Lee CS. Delusions of parasitosis: a dermatologists' guide to treatment. *Am J Clin Dermatol* 2001; **2**: 285–90.
19 Elmer KB, George RM, Peterson K. Use of risperidone for the treatment of monosymptomatic hypochondriacal psychosis. *J Am Acad Dermatol* 2000; **43**: 683–6.

Delusions of smell [1,2]

In these cases, there is no actual olfactory hallucination but the patient 'knows' that they are emitting a foul odour. This is because they believe that other people avoid them and talk about them with evident disgust [1]. They believe that the origin of the smell is usually flatus and may see a gastroenterologist, or possibly foul sweat usually produced in excess from body folds and orifices. A subgroup complain of unbearable halitosis and seek dental advice. This delusion is commonly related to a chronic avoidant paranoid personality trait [2].

Two organic syndromes should be noted. First, delusions of smell have been associated with cerebral tumours and, secondly, the fish odour syndrome [3] where patients have suffered social exclusion because of the pungent smell. Occasionally, people who sweat excessively are made to feel unwanted, particularly if they are in an enclosed work environment. This form of social phobia may precipitate a more paranoid response.

REFERENCES

1 Videbech T. Chronic olfactory paranoid syndromes. *Acta Psychiatr Scand* 1966; **42**: 183–212.
2 Pryse-Phillips W. An olfactory reference syndrome. *Acta Psychiatr Scand* 1971; **47**: 485–509.
3 Ayesh R, Mitchell SC, Zhang A. The fish odour syndrome: biochemical, familial and clinical aspects. *BMJ* 1993; **307**: 655–7.

Body dysmorphic disorder [1–4]

SYN. DERMATOLOGICAL NON-DISEASE;
DYSMORPHOPHOBIA

The terms 'dysmorphophobia' and more recently 'dermatological non-disease' have been in use for over a century to describe patients who are rich in symptoms (especially in areas important in the body image) but poor in signs of organic skin disease [1]. All dermatology clinics contain these distressed patients whose chronic attendance is a reflection of their impaired family, social and occupational functioning. This somatoform disorder is defined in DSM-IV as body dysmorphic disorder (BDD), a preoccupation with an imagined defect in appearance; if a slight defect is present the person's concern is markedly excessive. Although BDD is classified as a somatoform disorder, there is a delusional variant which is recognized as a psychotic disorder.

Prevalence. This condition was originally thought to be uncommon, but screening research over the last decade has revealed a prevalence of 12% [2]. A point prevalence study of a community sample of women in the USA showed a frequency of 0.75% [5], while a study of German students revealed a prevalence of 5.3% [6]. Patients who present for plastic surgery show rates of up to 15% [7]. Subclinical BDD (patients who keep their beliefs covert) are found in approximately one-fifth of patients presenting to aesthetic medicine; there is an equal gender frequency [8].

Aetiology. The aetiology is unknown. Some patients may be examples of monosymptomatic hypochondriacal psychosis [9] in that they have an isolated delusion. Affected individuals are often solitary, unmarried or divorced. As a whole, they socialize poorly and do not like contact with other people [2,10]. Their symptoms may appear after severe emotional, especially marital, problems and perineal symptoms in men may follow imagined or real sexual exposure. The disorder most often comorbid with BDD is major depression; rates of 60% and a lifetime rate of up to 80% have been reported [2,11]. The depressive symptoms may be subclinical but is revealed on direct questioning. An obsessional premorbid personality is not unusual [10] and comorbidity with obsessional compulsive disorder may be found in 30% [10,12]. Dysmorphophobic symptoms in a teenager or adult may be the presentation of schizophrenia, while in an elderly patient dementia should be considered. Comorbid psychiatric conditions have also included social phobia, trichotillomania, substance abuse and avoidant personality disorder [12,13]. In a study of patients with anorexia nervosa, 39% were diagnosed with comorbid BDD unrelated to weight concerns. These individuals had higher levels of delusionality and lower levels of social functioning than those with eating disorders alone [14]. There is usually no evidence of any underlying organic disease.

Clinical features. Most patients are in their third decade although reported ages are from 5 to 80 years. In one study, the average age of onset was 15 years and the average duration of symptoms was 18 years [12]. Opinions differ whether BDD is more common in men or women

[2,10], although referral sources may affect the statistics. Many patients are unmarried and unemployed [15]. Dermatological non-disease presents with symptoms particularly in the face and head including the mouth and scalp. Facial symptoms include complaints of excessive redness, blushing, a burning feeling, scarring, large pores, excessive facial hair and facial greasiness. Patients with orodynia or glossodynia fit into this group with their defect in pain perception involving the mouth. Scalp symptoms include a feeling of intense burning, unremitting by day or night, and excessive hair loss. Those patients with facial and scalp problems are more often female, but those with perineal symptoms are more likely to be male. Perineal symptoms in males include complaints of an excessively red scrotum, discomfort in the genital area, often spreading on to the anterior thighs and making the wearing of clothes uncomfortable, described rather cumbersomely as the dysthaesic peno-scrotal syndrome [16]. The female equivalent, vulvodynia (the burning vulva syndrome) consists of several different clinical entities, including vulval dermatosis, cyclic vulvitis, vulval papillomatosis, the vulva vestibular syndrome and essential vulvodynia [17]. In essential vulvodynia, the discomfort may be so severe that the patient will neither sit down nor go to bed, and this drives every other member of the family to distraction. Women with essential vulvodynia are more distressed than patients with an identified physical cause of vulval pain [18] (see also Chapter 68).

A consultation with a patient with dermatological non-disease always takes much longer than one with a patient with organic disease. The same ground has to be gone over repeatedly and the patient never appreciates normal non-verbal communication emanating from the doctor. The content of the consultation is dominated by complaints of ugliness, unattractiveness and irreconcilable deformity. Any body part may be involved, although a minority may worry about more than one area. Their thoughts are dominated by the abnormality for up to 8 h daily, the distress is intense, self-esteem poor and insight minimal. They admit to compulsive behaviours with excessive grooming, clothes changes and mirror gazing [2]. Patients are driven by the desire to know what they look like, a desire that is made worse if they resist the urge. BDD patients invariably feel worse after mirror watching but cannot resist looking in other reflective surfaces such as shop windows, cutlery and shiny compact discs. The function of mirror watching may be to practise showing the best face to the public [19]. Other activities and behaviour may be stimulated by these beliefs with diet regimes, the purchase of enormous quantities of beauty products and the seeking of unending aesthetic treatments. Muscle dysmorphia describes the men who use illicit anabolic steroids and obsessive weight training to develop their bodies, so-called 'bigorexia'.

Patients with dermatological non-disease are 'doctor shoppers' and will have often seen many doctors over the years about their many problems. An individual patient is likely to return to the clinic within a few minutes of being seen and may repeatedly telephone the doctor asking questions that have already been answered many times in the immediate past. Uncommonly, the delusional type of BDD gives rise to familial BDD where the parent imposes a delusional idea upon the child who in turn develops BDD [20] or, even more rarely, the patient believes that their child has a bodily defect, BDD by proxy [21].

There is a definite risk of suicide in patients with dermatological non-disease [1,2,22,23] and in a large series of 30 patients with BDD, 29% had made a suicide attempt [24].

Dermatological and plastic-surgical treatment. Most patients with dysmorphophobia perceive the solution to their problems in dermatological or plastic-surgical terms and so come to haunt dermatologists and plastic surgeons rather than psychiatrists. It is interesting that a significant proportion of patients presenting with dysmorphophobia have previously received plastic surgery, most commonly to change the shape of their nose. However, occasionally plastic surgery in carefully selected cases may be helpful, but there is always a risk that the patients themselves may then move to a preoccupation with another part of the body. In a series of 30 patients, it was found that 30% of patients had received previous cosmetic surgery, with a mean of 2.0 ± 1.3 procedures and as many as six procedures had occurred in individual patients [24]. Furthermore, 81% of patients with BDD were either dissatisfied or very dissatisfied with their consultation and results of surgery [12]; therefore, if plastic surgery is planned in this group of patients it is very important to have careful preoperative psychiatric assessment. Those contemplating surgery should remember that some patients with BDD are angry and go to litigation relatively easily. A perfect cosmetic result may be perceived by a depressed dysmorphophobic patient as worse than the situation before surgery. Photography before and after surgery is important to refute such claims objectively.

Diagnosis [2,3]. It may be surprising that BDD is often diagnosed late because patients are reluctant to disclose their distress, shame and embarrassment. The clinical clue may be a persistent return to the clinic for a harmless small lesion. BDD should be asked about and stringent questionnaires are available to expose BDD-related thoughts and behaviours [2,3].

Management. The management of patients with dermatological delusional disease is always difficult. There are two treatments that are shown to be successful; first, pharmacotherapy with SSRIs and latterly with cognitive-behavioural therapy.

Treatment with SSRIs. Early studies showed that nearly 50% of patients may respond completely or partially to fluoxetine or clomipramine, whereas there was only a 5% response to all other medications [24]. Systematic review of trials [25] confirmed that over 60% of patients have significant improvement in symptoms. It is important that the medication be continued long term as discontinuation precipitates relapse in 80%. All SSRIs are equally effective and the choice depends on tolerability. In many patients there is a significant improvement in the social prognosis evidenced by an ability to return to school or work. This is accompanied by a reduction in ritualistic behaviour, such as mirror checking and skin picking. Phillips *et al.* [24] observed that only a small proportion of patients responding to SSRIs experience any change in insight.

It is important to note that the effective dosage of SSRIs is usually higher than the dosage conventionally used to treat depression (e.g. the dosage of fluoxetine and fluvoxamine are 50 and 260 mg/day, respectively). In short, the dosage of SSRI needs to be high and the duration of treatment is long term, with response taking on average 2–4 months. The duration of treatment is usually at least 1 year.

There are several pharmacological options for patients who fail to respond to this type of regimen, and the addition of low-dose clomipramine, buspirone 30–60 mg/day or other antipsychotics have been used by psychiatrists. Venlafaxine 37.5 mg/day can be substituted for the SSRI. The help of liaison psychiatry services can be very helpful at this stage.

Patients with somatic pain (e.g. vulvodynia and scrotodynia) may benefit from tricyclic antidepressants such as amitriptyline 50–150 mg/day or alternatively gabapentin 900–1500 mg/day.

Cognitive–behavioural therapy [2,26]. Simple behavioural treatment, such as encouraging patients to avoid ritualistic behaviour and mirror checking, and urging them to give up unnecessary cosmetic camouflage, while gradually exposing them to the most feared social situations, can be helpful, especially if combined with a cognitive approach involving self-esteem building and modification of distorted thinking, coupled with coping strategies. All these techniques are more likely to be effective when combined with SSRI treatment, and initially some patients may be too ill to benefit from a cognitive–behavioural approach. This needs the help of a skilled clinical psychologist but has the advantage that it is often more acceptable to the patient. Up to 77% response can be measured in stress and symptom reduction [26].

Supportive psychotherapy can be helpful in those patients with overvalued ideas who are not truly deluded, but it is very time-consuming and emotionally demanding. As a generalization, patients with BDD are poor communicators and difficulty with interpersonal relationships may be one of the central crucial and earliest features of this disorder. The physician therefore undertaking supportive psychotherapy has to be patient and very tolerant. Dysmorphophobic patients are poor attenders at clinics, but the consultation may, in some cases, be the only opportunity that they have to talk to another human being, a reflection of the isolated life these patients often lead.

REFERENCES

1 Cotterill JA. Dermatological non-disease: a common and potentially fatal disturbance of cutaneous body image. *Br J Dermatol* 1981; **104**: 611–8.
2 Phillips KA, ed. *Somatoform and Factitious Disorders: Review of Psychiatry*, Vol. 20. 2001; 67–88.
3 Phillips KA. *The Broken Mirror.* New York: Oxford University Press, 1996.
4 Cotterill JA. Dermatologic non-disease. *Dermatol Clin* 1996; **14**: 439–45.
5 Otto MW, Wilhelm S, Cohen LS. Prevalence of body dysmorphic disorder in a community sample of women. *Am J Psychiatry* 2001; **158**: 2061–3.
6 Bohne A, Wilhelm S, Keuthen N. Prevalence of body dysmorphic disorder in German students. *Psychiatry Res* 2002; **109**: 101–4.
7 Ishigooka J, Iwao M, Suzuki M *et al.* Demographic features of patients seeking cosmetic surgery. *Psychiatr Clin Neurosci* 1998; **52**: 283–7.
8 Altamura C, Paluello MM, Mundo E. Clinical and subclinical body dysmorphic disorder. *Eur Arch Psychiatry* 2001; **251**: 105–8.
9 Munro A. Delusional parasitosis: a form of monosymptomatic hypochondriacal psychosis. *Semin Dermatol* 1983; **2**: 197–202.
10 Zimmerman M, Mattia JI. Body dysmorphic disorder in psychiatric outpatients: recognition, prevalence, comorbidity demographic and clinical correlates. *Compr Psychiatry* 1998; **39**: 265–70.
11 Hardy GE, Cotterill JA. A study of depression and obsessionality in dysmorphophobic and psoriatic patients. *Br J Psychol* 1982; **140**: 19–20.
12 Veale D, Boocock A, Gournay K *et al.* Body dysmorphic disorder: a survey of 50 cases. *Br J Psychiatry* 1996; **169**: 169–201.
13 Phillips KA, McElroy SL. Personality disorders and traits in patients with body dysmorphic disorder. *Compr Psychiatry* 2000; **41**: 229–36.
14 Grant JE, Kim SW, Eckert ED. Body dysmorphic disorder in patients with anorexia nervosa: prevalence, clinical features and delusions of body image. *Int J Eat Disord* 2002; **32**: 291–300.
15 Phillips KA, Diaz SF. Gender differences in body dysmorphic disorder. *J Nerv Ment Dis* 1997; **185**: 570–7.
16 Markos AR. The male genital skin burning syndrome (dysthaesic peno/scrotodynia). *Int J STD AIDS* 2002; **13**: 271–4.
17 Stewart DE, Reicher AE, Gerulath AH, Boydell KM. Vulvodynia and psychological distress. *Obstet Gynecol* 1994; **84**: 587–90.
18 McKay M. Vulvodynia: a multifactorial clinical problem. *Arch Dermatol* 1989; **125**: 256–62.
19 Veale D, Riley S. The psychopathology of mirror gazing in body dysmorphic disorder. *Behav Res Ther* 2001; **39**: 1381–93.
20 Seaton ED, Baxter KF, Cunliffe WJ. Familial dysmorphophobia. *Br J Dermatol* 2001; **144**: 439–40.
21 Atiullah M, Phillips KA. Fatal body dysmorphic disorder by proxy. *J Clin Psychol* 2001; **62**: 204–5.
22 Cotterill JA. Body dysmorphic disorder. *Dermatol Clin* 1996; **14**: 457–63.
23 Hull SM, Cunliffe WJ, Hughes BR. Treatment of the depressed and dysmorphophobic acne patient. *Clin Exp Dermatol* 1991; **16**: 210–1.
24 Phillips KA, McElroy SL, Keck PE *et al.* Body dysmorphic disorder: 30 cases of imagined ugliness. *Am J Psychiatr* 1993; **150**: 302–8.
25 Phillips KA. Pharmacologic treatment of body dysmorphic disorder: a review of empirical data and a treatment algorism. *Psychiatr Clin North Am* 2000; 7: 59–82.
26 Cororve MB, Gleaves DH. Body dysmorphic disorder: a review of conceptualizations, assessment, and treatment strategies. *Clin Psychol Rev* 2001; **21**: 949–70.

Habituation to dressings

Liddell and Cotterill [1] described a group of patients who became habituated to occlusive bandages, which had been initially applied many years before as treatment for either gravitational ulcers or eczema of the legs. Although the skin in all patients had returned to complete normality, it was impossible to persuade the patients to abandon their occlusive therapy. The patients tended to be elderly, single, lonely and inadequate, and most were male.

It was thought that the behaviour in this group may be regarded as 'attention seeking' in that they derive some sympathy from others because of their problem. Avoidance of work may have been successfully accomplished by some of these patients.

Some patients seem to enjoy the social contact that regular attendance at the clinic brings and are reluctant to be discharged. Thus, it appears that occlusive dressings may support not only the legs, but in a minority of patients, the psyche too.

REFERENCE

1 Liddell K, Cotterill JA. Habituation to occlusive dressings. *Lancet* 1973; **i**: 1485–6.

Cutaneous phobias

A phobic disorder is said to exist when anxiety, often amounting to panic, is evoked only or predominantly in well-defined situations. Patients who are subject to obsessional and ruminative thoughts about contamination and infestation may formalize these specifically into phobias about warts, infestation, dirt or bodily secretions. Patients are afraid to touch anything in the consulting room; indeed, in the hospital occasionally. Such patients will wear gloves when shopping or filling their car with petrol, and even the sight of a wart on another person can induce acute panic. Wart-phobic patients will bring other family members to dermatologists, and attempts will be made to make the dermatologist collude with the phobia and treat a wide variety of minute skin lesions in both the patient and his or her immediate relatives. A sterile pack may be produced so that there is no question of the patient's bare feet coming in contact with anything in the consulting room. Tights and socks are abandoned on the consulting room floor because they are regarded as contaminated by the patient. While relatively few patients with obsessive–compulsive disorder present directly to psychiatrists, it has been claimed that up to 14% of anxious, itchy, dermatological patients have this psychiatric disorder [1]. The typical patient realizes that these persistent ideas are inappropriate, but they continue to engender much distress and anxiety. Attempts are made to ameliorate the anxiety resulting from the obsession by compulsive acts and rituals, which vary from rubbing, lip licking or touching the skin, to more complex rituals involving washing, cleaning, hair pulling, skin excoriation and other cutaneous damaging behaviour.

Patients' phobias about dirt and bacteria may present as hand eczema induced by repeated hand washing. This psychiatric diagnosis should be considered in all patients with refractory hand eczema. The obsessional ideas become heightened during periods of emotional stress.

Mole phobia has also become more common since the recent publicity campaigns about the early diagnosis of malignant melanoma. Affected individuals consult dermatologists repeatedly, along with their unwilling family members. This is often a response to an actual tragic death from malignant melanoma in family, friends or neighbours. Despite reassurances they present repeatedly at clinics [2] and often demand that all the moles are removed and if refused will find a private surgeon to do this [3]. Regularly timed appointments with responsibility given to the physician can be a simple way to defuse panic attacks.

Patients with an overvalued idea about the possibility of venereal disease, including AIDS and herpes simplex, may be anxious or depressed, and a rather obsessional personality trait is not unusual in this group of patients [4].

Although blushing itself is normal under certain circumstances, blushing that is grossly excessive in both frequency and extent is particularly seen in women and may be the cause of considerable embarrassment. The fear of easy and excessive blushing gives rise to erythrophobia [5], which has two components: first, the fear of blushing and, secondly, excessive reactive flushing. Patients with erythrophobia show abnormal autonomic regulation under mental stress [5]. It has also been shown that task training can reduce the phobic behaviour independent of facial coloration [6]. These patients frequently suffer emotional difficulties and inhibitions and can sometimes be helped by a sympathetic clinical psychologist. Flushing may be a manifestation of hyperthyroidism and the distinctive flushing of the carcinoid syndrome must also be excluded (see Chapter 44).

A patient presenting with 'multiple allergies' may have a fear of allergic reactions [7]. All minor skin complaints are misinterpreted by the phobic patient as allergies and the consequent avoidant behaviour may become socially destructive.

An unreasonable fear of topical steroids amounting to an overvalued negative idea prompts patients and parents to refuse treatment. This was based first on real fears of skin thinning but, secondly, in one-quarter of those questioned, on a belief that non-specifically there will be long-term bad effects [8]. Treatment compliance is greatly improved by close surveillance and reassurance.

REFERENCES

1 Hatch ML, Paradis C, Friedman S *et al.* Obsessive–compulsive disorder in patients with chronic pruritic conditions: case studies and discussion. *J Am Acad Dermatol* 1992; **26**: 549–51.
2 Allan SJ, Doherty VR. Naevophobia. *Clin Exp Dermatol* 1995; **20**: 499–501.
3 Williams HC. Malignant melanoma screening: excision of 57 moles. *Br J Dermatol* 1998; **138**: 262–3.
4 Oates JK, Gomaz J. Venereophobia. *Br J Hosp Med* 1984; **31**: 435–6.
5 Laederach HK, Mussgay L, Buechel B. Patients with erythrophobia show abnormal autonomic regulation. *Psychosom Med* 2002; **64**: 358–65.
6 Mulkens S, Boegels SM, deJong PJ *et al.* Fear of blushing. *J Anxiety Disord* 2001; **15**: 413–32.
7 Simmich T, Traencker I, Gieler U. Phobic neuroses presenting as 'intolerance reaction of the skin'. *Hautarzt* 2001; **52**: 712–6.
8 Charman CR *et al.* Topical corticosteroid phobia in patients with atopic eczema. *Br J Dermatol* 2000; **142**: 931–6.

Anorexia nervosa and bulimia [1–3]

Anorexia nervosa can be looked upon as a phobia about body weight. In the definition of anorexia nervosa in the International Statistical Classification of Diseases 10 (ICD-10), body image distortion is one of the essential features. There is a dread of fatness as an intrusive overvalued idea. There are associations with other psychodermatoses, BDD and self-injurious behaviours. Hair pulling, self-cutting, excoriations and bruising occurred in 44% of 134 female patients [4].

The nutritional consequences of anorexia nervosa are frequent and many dermatological sequelae have been described. The most frequent skin manifestation is xerosis (58%), with a particular form of branny scaling developing on the extensor surfaces of the limbs and flexures. Hair effluvium occurred in 50%, with nail deformities in 45% and cheilitis in 40%. Diffuse hypertrichosis, carotenoderma, poor wound healing and striae distensae were more common in the restrictive type of anorexia as opposed to the bulimic type where hair and nail changes and generalized pruritus were more prominent [3]. Severe perniosis is also seen in individuals with anorexia nervosa [5]. Drenching night sweats during weight recovery, possibly brought about by secondary changes in thermoregulation, which occur with rapid refeeding, have also recently been described in patients with eating disorders [6] as has acne [2].

A minority may develop melasma and seborrhoeic dermatitis. Brittle nails, dry skin and calluses on the fingers are produced by repetitive self-induced vomiting. In the mouth, there may be dental enamel erosion and gingivitis and some patients develop a Sjögren-like syndrome. Other cutaneous features may result from the use of laxatives, such as phenolphthalein, producing a fixed drug reaction, and thiazide diuretics, producing photosensitivity, while the use of the emetic ipecacuanha can be associated with a dermatomyositis-like syndrome [7]. Compulsive hand washing and trichotillomania may result from accompanying psychiatric illness.

The alert dermatologist should suspect anorexia nervosa when presented with these suggestive signs, particularly hair loss and xerosis in an underweight girl. A simple screening questionnaire (SCOFF) [8] is helpful for detecting eating disoders. The patient should be referred to the psychiatrist for specialized care.

REFERENCES

1 Gupta MA, Gupta AK. Dermatologic signs in anorexia nervosa and bulimia nervosa. *Arch Dermatol* 1987; **123**: 1386–90.
2 Marshman GM, Hanna MJ, Ben-Tovin DI, Walker MK. Cutaneous abnormalities in anorexia nervosa. *Australas J Dermatol* 1990; **31**: 9–12.
3 Strumia R, Varotti E, Manzano E *et al.* Skin signs in anorexia nervosa. *Dermatology* 2001; **203**: 314–7.
4 Claes L, Vandereycken W, Vertommen H. Self-injurious behaviours in eating disordered patients. *Eat Behav* 2001; **2**: 263–72.
5 Luck P, Wakerling A. Increased cutaneous vasoreactivity to cold in anorexia nervosa. *Clin Sci (Lond)* 1981; **61**: 559–67.
6 Tyler I, Wiseman MC, Crawford RI, Birmingham CL. Cutaneous manifestations of eating disorders. *J Cutan Med Surg* 2002; **6**: 345–53.
7 Gupta MA, Gupta AK. Psychodermatology: an update. *J Am Acad Dermatol* 1996; **34**: 1030–46.
8 Luck AJ, Morgan JF, Reid F *et al.* The SCOFF questionnaire and clinical interview for eating disorders in general practice. *BMJ* 2002; **325**: 755–6.

Group and mass population reactions [1]

Epidemic hysteria syndrome and occupational mass psychogenic illness

The modern nomenclature for hysteria is conversion or dissociation disorder. The implications of this classification are that the symptoms are psychogenic, that the causation is unconscious, and that symptoms may carry some advantage, either primary such as debilitating symptoms or secondary by being exempted from community responsibility or gaining public attention. Conversion implies the behaviour of physical illness without evidence of organic pathology, the patient being unaware of the psychopathology. The prime examples of this group response are epidemics occurring in the closed communities of workplace and school.

In 1978 there were two separate outbreaks of skin disorders among factory workers in a small town in northern England. In each outbreak, a central female figure with non-industrial dermatological problems fuelled an epidemic of what was thought to be dermatitis among several employees in a ceramics factory and a second epidemic in a textile factory. In the first outbreak 10 employees were affected and 17 in the second. No significant dermatological pathology of industrial origin was found [2]. A similar outbreak occurred in a warehouse, triggered by two severe cases of non-occupational eczema, combined with the idea that incoming aircraft parts to the warehouse from foreign countries might be 'dirty' in some way. This caused a heightened perception of the risk of skin disease, with increased frequency of hand washing. Overfrequent hand washing in a few employees resulted in precisely what the warehouse staff had been trying to avoid [3]. An outbreak in the pottery industry that began as isolated gum arabic sensitivity developed into a more widespread epidemic described as 'epidemic hysteria dermatologica' in eight female workers [4]. There was also a female preponderance in the outbreak at a textile factory where the skin problems were common dermatoses unrelated to work [5]. Most of these mass reactions involve female workers and to try to explain this it has been postulated that in stressful situations in boring, low-paid, repetitive jobs women are more likely to externalize their discontent as a conversion symptom than a direct complaint that may jeopardize their job [1].

Surveys of occupational mass psychogenic illness (OMPI) episodes stress that many outbreaks occur in dehumanizing jobs with poor management communication. Secondary compensation neurosis may follow to prolong the epidemic from those who feel particularly injured. It is clearly important, if possible, to visit a factory very early and examine all the complainants in an outbreak of alleged 'epidemic' industrial dermatitis.

In the other common closed community, schools, epidemic complaints of itch dry skin and transient rash were predominant [6–8]. These outbreaks involved 50–100 children aged 7–12 years. The symptoms lasted 2 weeks and no cause was found. Girls outnumbered boys by 3 to 1. It has been suggested that the precipitating factors may be illness in a favourite teacher or student, rigid teaching regimens and parental pressure for academic success.

REFERENCES

1 Bartholomew RE. *Little Green Men, Meowing Nuns and Head-Hunting Panics: A Study in Mass Psychogenic Illnesses*. North Carolina: MacFarland, 2001: 25–78.
2 McGuire A. Psychic possession among industrial workers. *Lancet* 1978; i: 376–8.
3 Ashworth J, Rycroft RJ, Waddy RS, Irvine D. Irritant contact dermatitis in warehouse employees. *Occup Med* 1993; **43**: 32–4.
4 Ilchyshyn A, Smith AG. Gum arabic sensitivity and epidemic hysteria dermatologica. *Contact Dermatitis* 1985; **13**: 282–3.
5 Cunliffe WJ. Psychic possession amongst textile workers. *Lancet* 1978; ii: 44.
6 Levine RJ. An outbreak of psychogenic illness at a rural elementary school. *Lancet* 1974; i: 1500–3.
7 Polk LD. Mass hysteria in an elementary school. *Clin Paediatr* 1974; **13**: 1013–4.
8 Robinson P, Haddy L, Jones P. Outbreak of itching and rash. *Arch Intern Med* 1984; **144**: 159–62.

Sick building syndrome [1,2]

The concept of building-related illness (BRI) [1] has grown from the rather vague and controversial grouping of symptoms that appear to be caused by a range of supposed allergic, toxic, irritative and possibly infectious causes, to a subject where objective evidence is beginning to define the multifactorial aetiology of this contemporary phenomenon. Both sick building syndrome (SBS) and BRI refer to illnesses related particularly to non-industrial premises such as large blocks of apartments or offices where people spend considerable periods of time in close association. These syndromes consist of a series of heterogeneous complaints such as irritable dry skin, dryness and cracking of mucous membranes of mouth, nose and eyes, recurrent sore throat, headache, fatigue and loss of concentration. In over half of patients the symptoms are dermatological but the lack of demonstrable biological correlates together with vague aetiological attributes makes precise definition of the problem difficult [2]. Patch testing is negative.

Much of the debate has centred on dampness, smell and ventilation in buildings. In a large review [2], symptoms were significantly associated with signs of dampness, condensation, water leakage, high humidity and mouldy odour. Furthermore, the symptomatology could be related more to mechanical ventilation systems and internal air conditioning than in buildings where there was efficient natural ventilation [3,4]. In addition, changing from artificial ventilation to a natural one reduced skin symptoms by one-third [5].

Workers may feel ill when exposed to odours from xenobiotic sources (cacosmia) [6]. The presence of a strange smell at work may precipitate symptoms in a significant number of previously healthy individuals. Subsequent exposure sets up a classical conditionary loop with somatic amplification of symptoms. Patients develop headache, itchy eyes, transient rash and congested nose or throat followed by sweating, faintness and tachycardia. In most cases, the odour is chemically harmless. A significant psychological component has been postulated, as was the case when 24 workers reported sensitivity to electricity in the workplace, causing itchy whealing of face and limbs [7]. The patients reported increased symptoms not only when they were exposed to an experimental electromagnetic field but also when they believed they were exposed, even though the field was turned off.

Not surprisingly therefore, work stress, manifested by role conflict, work overload, managerial difficulties and workplace building renovations have all been significantly associated with perceptions of poor workplace air quality and increased dermatological symptoms of SBS [8].

Symptoms were more common in those lower down the office hierarchy than in managers, and women had more symptoms than men, irrespective of their status [2].

REFERENCES

1 Menzies D, Bourbeau J. Building related illnesses. *N Engl J Med* 1997; **337**: 1524–31.
2 Worgocki PM, Sindell J, Bischoff W *et al*. Sick building syndrome: a review of 105 papers. *Indoor Air* 2002; **12**: 113–28.
3 Seppanen O, Fisk WJ. Association of ventilation system type with SBS symptoms in the office worker. *Indoor Air* 2002; **12**: 98–112.
4 Engvall K, Norrby C, Norbaek D. Sick building syndrome in relation to building dampness. *Int Arch Occup Environ Health* 2001; **74**: 270–8.
5 Bourbeau J, Brisson C, Allaire S. Prevalence of sick building syndrome before and after improved office ventilation. *Occup Environ Med* 1996; **53**: 204–10.
6 Magnavita M. Cacosmia in healthy workers. *B J Med Psychol* 2001; **74**: 121–7.
7 Lonne RS, Andersson B, Melin I *et al*. Provocation with stress and electricity of patients with 'sensitivity to electricity'. *J Occup Environ Med* 2000; **42**: 512–6.
8 Mendelson MB, Catano VM, Kelloway K. The role of stress and social support in sick building syndrome. *Work Stress* 2000; **14**: 137–55.

Self-inflicted and simulated skin disease

It is important to differentiate the dermatological diseases provoked by voluntary, admitted, self-traumatizing behaviour from those induced by covert deception to give the appearance of disease. The former group may range from a normal stress-related activity such as nail biting to a more disease-classifiable problem (e.g. trichotillomania or compulsive hair plucking). At no time is there an intention to falsify the origin of the skin-related damage or to actively obscure the part the patient plays in its production. This does not mean that the shame and self-reproach associated with these activities are not occasionally responsible for a reluctance to primarily volunteer the patient's part. However, this behaviour is significantly different from that of a true factitious disorder, which exhibits the essential elements of the intentional production or feigning of physical or psychological signs or symptoms and the continued denial of the disease origin to the physician. The motivation for this behaviour is assumed to be the sick role and an essential difference from malingering is that there is no external incentive for the behaviour such as economic, legal or employment advantage.

There are normal behaviour habits associated with the skin that appear repetitively at times of stress and anxiety. Picking, plucking, sucking, rubbing, biting and pulling behaviour on skin, nails and hair are stress-relieving activities, which may be reinforced by the release of endorphin-like substances as a neuroendocrine response.

Each of these behaviours is physically brief or spasmodic and, on most occasions, a conscious activity that does not intrude on normal skin function. However, when these habits become entrenched as a repetitive almost compulsive daily routine, or progress beyond the stage where they are an incidental stress-relieving activity, then they are recognizable as a number of dermatological disorders. Nail biting (onychophagia) has been recorded from the age of 15 months [1] but is more common after the age of 3 years and is present in over one-third of children between the ages of 7 and 10 years [2]. Up to half of adolescents continue to bite their nails, and 13.7% of older students and young adults [3,4] show continued body-focused repetitive behaviours (BFRBs), of which nail biting was the most frequent. In addition, those patients who continue with BFRBs also exhibit frequent somatizing activity in other illness. Obsessive onychophagia is well recorded [5]. Studies of college students [5,6] showed 1.5% of males and 3.4% of females continued hair pulling, but only 0.5% satisfied the DSM-IV-R criteria for trichotillomania.

Scratching and rubbing behaviour may progress to lichen simplex or nodular prurigo. Destructive picking activity may develop into neurotic excoriations or acne excoriée. Nose picking (rhinotillexomania) greater than

20 times per day may persist in 8% of adolescents [7] and while this may be a culture-bound syndrome, it is associated with multiple BFRBs in approximately 15% of individuals, usually men. In extreme cases, trigeminal trophic syndrome may follow herpes zoster in the nasal area. Persistent pluckers most commonly abuse their hair and can present with trichotillomania. Perioral dermatitis can be a consequence of chronic lip-licking behaviour and chronic cheilitis the result of lip biting (see Chapter 66). Chronic nail disease such as paronychia follows from nail biting and onychophagia (see Chapter 62).

REFERENCES

1 Illingworth RS. *Body Manipulations in the Normal Child*, 5th edn. Edinburgh: Churchill Livingstone, 1972: 318.
2 Leung AK, Robson WL. Nailbiting. *Clin Paediatr* 1990; **29**: 690–2.
3 Teng EJ, Woods DW, Twohig MP, Marcks BA. Body-focussed repetitive behaviour problems. *Behav Modif* 2002; **26**: 340–60.
4 Wilhelm S, Keuthen NJ, Jenike MA. Skin picking in German students. *Behav Modif* 2002; **26**: 320–39.
5 Leonard HL, Lenane MC, Swedo SE *et al.* Treatment of severe onychophagia. *Arch Gen Psychiatry* 1991; **48**: 821–7.
6 Christenson GA, Pyle RL, Mitchell JE. Estimated lifetime prevalence of trichotillomania in college students. *J Clin Psychiatry* 1991; **52**: 415–7.
7 Andrade C, Srihari BS. Rhinotillixomania in adolescence. *J Clin Psychiatry* 2001; **62**: 426–31.

Lichen simplex and neurodermatitis
(see Chapter 17)

Lichenification describes the characteristic pattern of response of the predisposed skin to repeated rubbing. In some instances, a minor initiating event, such as trauma, infection or insect bite, precipitates episodic insistent scratching and rubbing. Irresistable itching is the major complaint, scratching the chronic accompaniment. This behaviour takes the form of rubbing with either the hands, back of nails or knuckles and in extreme cases sometimes with the use of a convenient instrument such as a hairbrush, a pen or some other domestic implement. The actions may be subconscious and proceed without continuous conscious control. However, in some cases patients subject themselves to frenetic prolonged spasms of uncontrollable self-damage, which proceeds with increasing rapidity until the pruritus is replaced by soreness and pain. The change from itch to pain is quite sudden and this abrupt cessation has been described as orgasm cutanée. Lichen simplex and neurodermatitis are much less common in the elderly.

Regular rubbing and pressure on the skin produces the characteristic thickened, coarsely grained nodules on the skin with hyperpigmentation. The classic sites of involvement are within easy reach, particularly on the nape and sides of the neck, elbows, thighs, knees and ankles. It is unknown why these areas remain so discrete. These areas may be in varying stages of evolution, from early small violaceous papules with surface excoriations to chronic

areas that present as hyperkeratotic plaques with pigment changes, described as 'dermatological worry beads'. Localized patches of lichen simplex presenting as pruritus ani and vulvae are described in Chapters 17 and 68. These lesions are more often found in females and occur predominantly after puberty. They are found, very rarely, as isolated phenomena in children, even in atopics. They are more often seen in Afro-Caribbean patients.

Most authors have commented on the relationship of emotional tension to bouts of scratching [1]. Patients are usually described as stable but anxious individuals, whose reactions to stress are relieved by ritualized behaviour such as rubbing [2]. Aggression and hostility related to anxiety [3] caused by emotional disturbance may lead to itching. This maladaptive response has been treated successfully with behaviour therapy [3] to break the itch–scratch cycle.

Treatment with antihistamines is helpful, but antidepressants, particularly tricyclic compounds such as doxepin in dosage as low as 25–50 mg/day, have been shown to be more effective [4]. Non-psychotropic medication is also sometimes effective using thalidomide 50–100 mg/day for up to 2 months at a time.

REFERENCES

1 Allerhand ME, Gough HG, Grais ML. Personality factors in neurodermatitis. *Psychosom Med* 1950; **12**: 386–9.
2 Freid RG. Evaluation and treatment of psychogenic pruritus and self-excoriation. *J Am Acad Dermatol* 1994; **30**: 993–9.
3 Fried RG. Non-pharmacologic treatment in psychodermatology. *Dermatol Clin* 2002; **20**: 177–85.
4 Melin L, Noren P. Behavioural treatment of scratching in patients with atopic dermatitis. *Br J Dermatol* 1986; **115**: 467–74.

Psychogenic excoriations
SYN. NEUROTIC EXCORIATIONS; COMPULSIVE SKIN PICKING; DERMATILLOMANIA; ACNE EXCORIÉE [1,2]

The most common of the self-inflicted dermatoses are neurotic excoriations and acne excoriée. The differences between the two are more a matter of distribution than degree of severity of the lesions. The lesions differ from other artefactual disorders as those who suffer readily admit to an urge to pick and gouge at their skin. Both of these clinical syndromes are characterized by the preponderance of females, the destructive scarring nature of the lesions and the relationship to psychological stress. Some patients show features of both conditions and one condition may merge into the other.

Destructive excoriations are seen most frequently in middle-aged women, the average age of onset being between 30 and 50 years of age [1,4], but significantly the average duration of disease before presentation can be up to 10 years. This group make up the most severe cases, where the problem tends to be persistent and unremitting.

The picking and excoriation proceeds in bouts that exceed the bounds of simple habit. These patients are described as rather rigid and obsessional individuals with repressed emotions [3,5]. They have difficulty in verbalizing their problems and are aggressive but also insecure [4]. Depression was a very common feature in one series [2]. These patients describe picking, scratching, gouging and using implements on their skin, producing bleeding and pain during periods of low mood and self-esteem. There is a compulsive quality about the need to continue until pain is produced. The duration of these bouts may last for some hours and can be ritualized to a set time and place. Psychosocial stresses have been reported to precede exacerbations of excoriations in 30–90% of patients [1,4]. Immediately following such behaviour, patients are characteristically unhappy and guilty about the disfigurement.

Patients with psychogenic excoriations frequently have co-morbid disorders in the compulsivity–impulsivity spectrum, including BDD, substance abuse, eating disorders and trichotillomania [2]. The Skin Picking Impact Scale (SPIS) is a self-report instrument developed to assess the psychosocial consequences of repetitive skin picking. SPIS scores were significantly higher for those with self-injurious behaviour than those with reactive scratching from itchy dermatoses and correlated with anxiety and depression inventories [6].

Clinical features. Lesions can be seen in all stages of development. Clinically, the lesions are polymorphic, the newer lesions are angular crusted excoriated erosions with a serosanguinous crust, found predominantly on the sides of the neck, chin, upper chest shoulders and upper arms. The healing lesions are erythematous and depigmented, eventually with chronicity becoming white and atrophic centrally and commonly hyperpigmented at the periphery. They may be quite deep, extending into dermis, and are distributed symmetrically within reach of the hands. Older lesions show pink or red scars, some of which may be hypertrophic. Chronic lesions may also show atrophic scars, which merge and are eventually seen as linear coalescent areas. Lesions appear at all stages of development and may number from a few to several hundred (Fig. 61.1).

Differential diagnosis. It is important to exclude excoriations caused by generalized pruritus, bullous disorders such as pemphigus, and linear excoriated lesions, which may be the presenting signs of lichen planus or lupus erythematosus.

Treatment. Simple, empathic, supportive psychotherapy can produce significant improvement, whereas insight-orientated analysis may exacerbate symptoms [7]. Cognitive–behavioural therapy has improved some patients, although the management of underlying personality difficulties may require the specific skills of a psychotherapist [8,9]. Habit reversal programmes may also help [2]. The compulsive nature of this disorder responds well to antidepressants and in particular to SSRIs, such as fluoxetine, fluvoxamine and citalopram [2,6]. Clomipramine [10] and doxepin [11] have been reported to work well. While the condition eventually resolves, the most difficult cases are middle-aged women with established patterns of excoriation, which may have been present continuing for decades. It may be necessary to continue antidepressants in these patients for some years.

REFERENCES

1 Gupta M, Gupta A, Haberman H. Neurotic excoriations: a review and some new perspectives. *Compr Psychiatry* 1986; **27**: 381–6.
2 Arnold LM, Auchenbach MB, McElroy SL. Psychogenic excoriation: clinical features, proposed diagnostic criteria, epidemiology and approaches to treatment. *CNS Drugs* 2001; **5**: 351–9.
3 Nielsen H, Fruensgaard K, Hjorshoj A. Controlled neuropsychological investigations of patients with neurotic excoriations. *Psychother Psychosom* 1980; **34**: 52–61.
4 Fruensgaard K. Neurotic excoriations. *Int J Dermatol* 1987; **17**: 761–7.
5 Musaph H. Psychodermatology. In: Hill O, ed. *Modern Trends in Psychosomatic Medicine*. London: Butterworths, 1974: 216–9.
6 Keuthen NJ, Deckersbach T, Wilhelm S et al. The Skin Picking Impact Scale (SPIS). *Psychosomatics* 2001; **42**: 397–403.
7 Seitz PFD. Psychocutaneous aspects of persistent pruritus and excessive excoriation. *Arch Dermatol Syphiligr* 1951; **64**: 136–41.
8 Fried RG. Non-pharmacologic treatment in psychodermatology. *Dermatol Clin* 2002; **20**: 177–85.
9 Welkowitz LA, Held JL, Held AL. Management of neurotic scratching with behavioural therapy. *J Am Acad Dermatol* 1989; **21**: 802–4.
10 DeVeaugh-Geiss J, Landau P, Katz R. Preliminary results from a multicenter trial of clomipramine in obsessive compulsive disorder. *Pharmacol Bull* 1989; **25**: 36–40.
11 Harris BA, Sheretz EF, Flowers FP. Improvement of chronic neurotic excoriations with oral doxepin therapy. *Int J Dermatol* 1983; **26**: 541–3.

Acne excoriée (see Chapter 43) [1,2]

There is not one patient with acne who can resist squeezing and pinching of lesions. Brocq [3] in 1891 described acne excoriée particularly in adolescent girls under emotional stress who picked and squeezed acne spots. The condition should be considered to be a variant of psychogenic (neurotic) excoriation [2] with the lesions largely confined to the face. Acne excoriée is more common in women [1–4] and seen in an older age group than acne vulgaris, with a mean age of approximately 30 years [1,2,4]. Psychological studies have shown no diagnosable DSM-IV-R disorder [4,5], although associated phobic states [1] and depressive and delusional disorders [6,7] have been described.

The clinical lesions resemble those of excoriations. They are found predominantly around the hairline, forehead, pre-auricular cheek and chin areas. Extension to the neck and occipital hairline is common and with even more extensive lesions producing an overlap clinically with psychogenic pruritus. Chronic lesions characteristically show white atrophic scarring with peripheral hyperpigmentation.

A strong association with atopy has been suggested with resemblances to prurigo mitis.

Although patients with acne excoriée sometimes respond to simple topical acne therapy, most require systemic antibiotics and isotretinoin. The tetracyclines, in particular doxycycline, are better than the other antibiotics [1] and topically the patients prefer antibiotic roll-on preparations to the benzoyl peroxide creams, which are too irritant. While this may arrest the development of new lesions and scarring, the physical course of the disease is poor without psychological support [1]. These patients tend to be psychologically dependent, and the benefits of simple supportive consultation and psychotherapy should not be underestimated [8]. Compulsive behaviour that leads to further scarring may respond to cognitive and habit-reversal therapy [9].

REFERENCES

1 Sneddon J, Sneddon I. Acne excoriée: a protective device. *Clin Exp Dermatol* 1983; **8**: 65–8.
2 Wrong NM. Excoriated acne of young females. *Arch Dermatol Syphiligr* 1954; **70**: 574–82.
3 Brocq L, Jacquet L. Notes pour servir á l'histoire des neurodermites. *Arch Dermatol Syphiligr* 1891; **97**: 193–5.
4 Zadro-Jaeger S, Musalek M. Acne excoriée psychiatric studies. *Abstracts of the Third International Congress on Dermatology and Psychiatry.* Florence: Tipographia, 1991.
5 Bach M, Bach D. Psychiatric and psychometric issues in acne excoriée. *Psychother Psychosom* 1993; **60**: 207–8.
6 Koo JM, Smith LL. Psychologic aspects of acne. *Pediatr Dermatol* 1991; **8**: 185–9.
7 Ginsburg IH. The psychosocial impact of skin disease. *Dermatol Clin* 1996; **14**: 473–84.
8 Freid RG. Evaluation and treatment of psychogenic pruritus and self-excoriation. *J Am Acad Dermatol* 1994; **30**: 993–9.
9 Kent A, Drummond LM. Acne excoriée: a case report using habit reversal. *Clin Exp Dermatol* 1989; **14**: 163–4.

Psychogenic pruritus [1,2]

This subgroup of the psychopruritic disorders represents those with intractable or persistent itch for which no pruritic physical illness or dermatological illness can be found [1]. Musaph [2] pointed out that one mechanism for relieving everyday irritations is to scratch a little. The motorist stopped at a red traffic light almost invariably scratches some accessible site such as the neck and most of us develop a small itch from time to time during the day that is relieved by slight scratching. He called this the 'traffic-light phenomenon' and its function is a common way of relieving minor frustrations. Individuals who develop localized or generalized neurodermatitis may begin in this way, but their itch–scratch cycle gets out of hand. In some individuals, intense scratching can induce an ultimate feeling of pleasure and this may be related to the release of opioids centrally.

Enkephalins and endorphins are important as neurotransmitters in the CNS in mediating the sensation of itch because it has been recognized for many years that, although morphine may alleviate pain, it may aggravate itch. As itch and pain are thought to share common neurological pathways, the central elicitation of itch by morphine may result from binding to opioid receptors and this binding may mimic normal physiological binding of endorphins and enkephalins at these receptor sites [3]. Moreover, naloxone, an opioid antagonist, has been found to reduce or abolish histamine-provoked itch. It has been shown that naloxone can relieve itching experienced by patients with intrahepatic cholestasis and may also be effective in patients with generalized pruritus caused by chronic liver disease. This drug, however, did not produce a uniform reduction in itching in all patients. Patients with generalized pruritus who had responded well to placebo reported greater itching after naloxone, probably because of the abolition of the placebo response. Conversely, the placebo non-responders reported less itch after naloxone than the placebo responders, suggesting that naloxone may be competing with an endorphin system, thus modulating the individual's perception of itch [3,4].

There are more intricate relationships between allergic disease and neural mechanisms, which identify further mechanisms that produce central itch [5] including those selectively responsive to histamine [6].

The psychopruritic disorders have some common features that help to differentiate them from physical diseases. Pruritic episodes may be bizarre in onset and presentation with abrupt and sudden termination. This itching may occur commonly during relaxation or sometimes after nighttime waking [7]. Furthermore, localized itching may lead to generalized body itch within a short time. The episodes are chronic and relapsing and last variable lengths of time from hours to days.

Patients with psychogenic itch tend to be introverted and there may be a history of recent major psychological stress [8]. A psychiatric and psychodynamic investigation of patients with prurigo nodularis demonstrated an extraordinary propensity for these patients to suffer from psychological trauma, and a distinct correlation was claimed between the outbreak of the disease and the preceding loss of a human relationship detrimental to self-esteem [9]. A significant proportion of patients with generalized pruritus may be suffering from depression. Using the Beck depression inventory, significantly more patients with generalized pruritus (32.4%) had depressive symptomatology than controls [10].

Treatment with antihistamines is disappointing, although those that have phenothiazine activity, such as hydroxyzine 50–75 mg/day, may produce more relief. Doxepin used in dosage up to 125 mg/day is more effective, probably because of the combined effect of both antipruritic and antidepressant actions. SSRIs can also afford relief: typical dosage is paroxetine 20–40 mg/day, fluvoximine 100–200 mg/day or citalopram 20–40 mg/day [11].

Behaviour-orientated therapy may give some benefit but relies upon a receptive patient, and success will be limited and disappointing in those with significant mood shift or personality disorder [12].

REFERENCES

1 Musaph H. Psychogenic pruritus. *Dermatologica* 1967; **135**: 126–30.
2 Musaph H. Psychogenic pruritus. *Semin Dermatol* 1983; **2**: 217–22.
3 Bernstein JE, Swift R. Relief of intractible pruritus with naloxone. *Arch Dermatol* 1979; **115**: 1366–7.
4 Summerfield JA. Naloxone modulates the perception of itching. *Br J Clin Pharmacol* 1980; **10**: 180–3.
5 Undem BJ, Krajekar Hunter DD *et al*. Neural integration and allergic diseases. *J Allergy Clin Immunol* 2000; **106**: 213–20.
6 Andrew D, Craig AD. Spinothalamic lamina 1 neurones selectively sensitive to histamine: a central neural pathway for itch. *Nat Neurosci* 2000; **4**: 72–7.
7 Gupta MA, Gupta K, Kirkby S *et al*. Pruritus associated with night time waking. *J Am Acad Dermatol* 1989; **21**: 479–84.
8 Radmanesh M, Shafei S. Underlying psychopathologies of psychogenic pruritic disorders. *Dermatol Psychosom* 2001; **2**: 130–3.
9 Valtola J. A psychiatric and psychodynamic investigation of LCO (prurigo nodularis Hyde) patients. *Acta Derm Venereol Suppl (Stockh)* 1991; **156**: 49–52.
10 Sheehan-Dare RA, Henderson MJ, Cotterill JA. Anxiety and depression in patients with chronic urticaria and generalized pruritus. *Br J Dermatol* 1990; **123**: 769–74.
11 Gupta MA, Gupta AK. The use of antidepressant drugs in dermatology. *J Eur Acad Dermatol* 2001; **15**: 512–8.
12 Freid RG. Non-pharmacologic treatments in psychodermatology. *Dermatol Clin* 2002; **20**: 177–85.

Trichotillomania [1–3]

Definition. Trichotillomania is defined as the irresistable urge to pull out hair, accompanied by a sense of relief after the hair has been plucked. The term was firstly used by Hallopeau in 1889 and literally means a morbid craving to pull out hair. Originally, DSM-IV [4] listed trichotillomania under impulse–control disorders in company with compulsive gambling and kleptomania, but the broad spectrum of psychopathologies [1] prompted modifications to the definition. The revised DSM-IV-R [5] diagnostic criteria for trichotillomania are:
1 Recurrent pulling out of one's own hair resulting in hair loss
2 An increasing sense of tension immediately before pulling out the hair or when attempting to resist the behaviour
3 Pleasure, gratification or relief when pulling out the hair
4 The disturbance is not better accounted for by another mental disorder
5 The disturbance provokes clinically marked distress and/or impairment in occupational, social or other areas of functioning.
The ICD-10 definition [6] is consistent with this but does not mention distress or loss of functioning.

Aetiology and pathogenesis [1,2]. The epidemiology of this complaint is not absolutely clear, probably for the reason that this physical sign and response is a product of various psychopathologies. Studies of frequency show a wide variation. In an unselected population the incidence has been reported as below 1 in 1000 to as high as 1 in 200 by the age of 18 years [6]. However, there appear to be two distinct populations: those who present in childhood [2,7] and who probably represent the bulk of cases [6,8]; and fewer but more chronic cases who present as adults, who have continued hair-pulling activity from adolescence or developed the disorder in early adult life [2]. There is an estimated lifetime prevalence of 0.6% in college students [9], with equal sex incidence. If the criteria are based on ICD-10 then the prevalence increased to 3.4% in females and 1.5% in men. The number of affected children may be seven times that of adults [10] and preschool children are more likely to be boys (62%) although after this older boys and adolescents are 30% of the group [7]. This early-onset group, usually between the ages of 2 and 10 years, show benign self-limiting behaviour and most are probably suffering from a habit disorder, perhaps as an extension of hair twirling activity and childhood stress [11]. The association with nail biting and thumb sucking, skin picking, nose picking, lip biting and cheek chewing is well documented [12,13]. In children, there is an association with anxiety and dysthymia [12], learning disability and iron deficiency [8]. Emotional problems in the pre-adolescent group tend to be less severe, more a reflection of a stressful life event rather than serious psychopathology [13].

The adolescent age group, more likely to be girls, have more psychopathology related to parent relationships, school difficulties commonly bullying, body image changes and infrequently sexual abuse. It is more likely that there is an accompanying anxiety disorder although depression in children may be missed because the features are of somatic complaints and irritability [14].

The adult age groups are associated with greater psychopathology and show distinct female preponderance [1,2,7,], usually 4 : 1, but 15 : 1 being most evident in the oldest group [15]. This remains true for different racial groups [16–18]. The adult patients show more diverse psychopathology with depression, anxiety disorder, obsessive–compulsive disorder (OCD) and panic attacks prominent. Depression was present in 14% and anxiety in 15% [19]. Substance abuse (6%) and eating disorders may also be evident [2,3]. There is a significant debate about the relationship of trichotillomania to OCD [1]. While it has been proposed that adult chronic trichotillomania is a variant of OCD, with positive correlation in family studies [20], this definition is too narrow for many patients [2] and has not been supported by psychometric testing [21]. OCD compulsions are performed to avoid increased anxiety, are not pleasureable and are performed in full awareness. Patients with OCD have an explanation for their responses, whereas those with trichotillomania rarely justify their actions. In addition, the activity relieves stress for those with trichotillomania, although a small subset may have the typical disabling compulsive conscious behaviours [22]. A family history is present in 5–8%, which may represent either a genetic predisposition or, more likely, a continuing family psychosocial response [20].

Clinical features [1]. The hair pulling activity is usually not as a response to any skin symptoms but is either a conscious deliberate act or, more often, a subconscious act, in some children being part of a hypnogogic (dream-like) state. Most adult patients describe an increased sense of tension before hair pulling or a sense of relief after the act. Some patients may have incomplete awareness until the pattern has been established [23].

Hair pulling and plucking is most common from the scalp but only occasionally as a response to scalp symptoms. Most pull hair from the vertex, but temporal, occipital and frontal hair loss in children may be more obvious on the side of manual dominance. The hair loss may be minimal, commonly a solitary patch, but visible hair thinning may progress to virtual total depilation, significantly so in adult women. Typically, the hairs are short, irregular, broken and distorted. The hair feels like stubble because of the fractured hair shafts, in contrast to alopecia areata which is much smoother. The patterns of plucking activity are centrifugal from a single starting point or linear, in wave-like activity. In extreme cases, the centrifugal pattern removes all hair except the most difficult to access, namely the occiput. This shows as a 'tonsure pattern' [24] or 'Friar Tuck' [25] distribution. The eyelashes, eyebrows, facial and pubic hair may also be primarily affected. Children will pluck the eyebrows and eyelashes but adults almost exclusively pluck hair on the torso. Two-thirds of adults pulled hair from two or more sites and one-third from three areas [2,3]. Body and pubic hair plucking is more common in males and may become a ritualized activity, either alone or as a conjugal activity.

Younger patients will tend to pick and pluck the hair at times of leisure, when alone or when tired and in the evening. Adults have a more conscious structured activity, initially seeking thicker or distorted hair and then progressing to larger areas, taking longer and longer over the activity. This may become more like a compulsion with elaboration of the rituals using instruments. The more frequent the plucking episodes, the greater the body image dissatisfaction and the more likely the patient will have depression and anxiety.

Patients present in the clinic with bald patches but associated features are the use of wigs, false eyelashes and semi-permanent use of hats and scarves. Occasionally, the psychosocial effects of hair loss (e.g. reluctance to swim, date and do sports) may precipitate referral to clinical psychologists or psychiatrists. Chronic folliculitis of the neck, chin, chest, pubic areas or thighs as a result of plucking activity may also be the presenting complaint.

One of the secretive activities in many patients with trichotillomania is some degree of hair licking, chewing and eating (trichophagia). Children may pluck the hair, stroke or suck the hair root before chewing and swallowing the remainder. Occasionally, hair may be seen stuck between the teeth. Patients may swallow longer strands of hair and a small percentage develop gastrointestinal bezoars. There should be a high index of suspicion in children with trichotillomania who present with abdominal pain, weight loss, nausea, vomiting, anorexia and foul breath [7,8]. Gastric trichobezoars may cause intestinal bleeding, pancreatitis or obstructive jaundice [1,17]. If the hair bolus extends down the small intestine (Rapunzel syndrome), life-threatening intestinal obstruction necessitates a laparotomy [26]. It has been reported in over 10% of adults, who usually report no abdominal symptoms, and patients with learning disability [27].

Investigations. Scalp biopsy has been shown to be most useful [7,10]. The most important findings include multiple catagen hairs, pigment casts and traumatized hair bulbs.

Gastrointestinal bezoars have been investigated by conventional radiography, sonography, and computed tomography (CT) scanning. CT scan diagnosed all cases in both stomach and small intestine, while ultrasound was almost as accurate [28]. Conventional X-ray of bezoar was least helpful.

Differential diagnosis. See Chapter 63.

Treatment. Clinical assessment scales are helpful in the fuller evaluation of treatments but remain largely research tools [29]. For many adolescents and children, identification of stressful episodes with accompanying support and parent education is usually all that is necessary. It is essential to present the harmful habit in an atmosphere of non-blame or fault but to change the agenda to a positive one to negotiate change. Habit reversal [29] is effective as is behaviour therapy. This was effective in children [1,22,30] and reduced symptoms by 90% in 19 adults [29]. It is time consuming and needs expert clinical psychology support to maintain progress.

One study showed that tricyclic antidepressants were effective agents and further that clomipramine was more effective than desipramine [16], although relapse may be common unless treatment is continued for at least 1 year. SSRIs have been of benefit in open studies. In two further studies [31,32], fluoxetine in dosage of up to 80 mg/day decreased severity by 60%. In a double-blind study, citalopram reduced severity by 30% by week 12 [33]. Low-dose pimozide has been shown to augment this response [34] as has risperidone because relapse is common after 1 year if SSRIs are used as monotherapy [35].

REFERENCES

1 Hautmann G, Hercogova J, Lotti T. Trichtillomania. *J Am Acad Dermatol* 2002; **46**: 807–21.
2 Christenson GA, Mackenzie TB, Mitchell JE. Characteristics of 60 adult chronic hair pullers. *Am J Psychiatry* 1991; **148**: 365–70.
3 Swedo SE, Rapoport JL. Trichotillomania. *J Clin Psychol Psychiatry* 1991; **32**: 401–9.
4 American Psychiatric Association. *Diagnostic and Statistical Manual of Mental Disorders (DSM-IV)*, 4th edn. Washington DC: American Psychiatric Association, 1994.
5 American Psychiatric Association. *Diagnostic and Statistical Manual of Mental Disorders (DSM-IV)*, 4th edn revised. Washington DC: American Psychiatric Association, 2000.
6 Greenberg HR, Sarner CA. Trichotillomania. *Arch Gen Psychiatry* 1965; **12**: 482–9.
7 Muller SA. Trichotillomania: a histopathologic study in 66 patients. *J Am Acad Dermatol* 1990; **23**: 56–62.
8 Oranje AP, Peereboom-Wynia JD, DeRaeymacker DM. Trichotillomania in childhood. *J Am Acad Dermatol* 1986; **15**: 614–9.
9 Christenson GA, Pyle RL, Mitchell JE. Estimated lifetime prevalence of trichotillomania in college students. *J Clin Psychiatry* 1991; **52**: 415–7.
10 Mehregan AH. Trichotillomania: a clinicopathologic study. *Arch Dermatol* 1970; **102**: 129–33.
11 Deaver C, Miltenberger RG, Stricker JM. Functional analysis and treatment of hair twirling in children. *J Appl Behav Anal* 2001; **34**: 535–8.
12 Reeve EA, Bernstein GA, Christenson GA. Clinical characteristics and psychiatric comorbidity in children with trichotillomania. *J Am Acad Child Adolesc Psychiatry* 1992; **31**: 132–8.
13 Krishnan RRK, Davidson JRT, Guajardo C. Trichotillomania: a review. *Compr Psychiatry* 1985; **26**: 123–8.
14 Birmaher B, Ryan ND. Williamson DE *et al.* Childhood and adolescent depression: a 10 year review. *J Am Acad Child Adolesc Psychiatry* 1996; **35**: 1427–39.
15 Swedo S, Leonard HL, Rapoport JL. A double blind comparison of clomipramine and desipramine in the treatment of trichotillomania. *N Engl J Med* 1989; **321**: 497–501.
16 Bhatia MS, Singhal PK, Rastogi V, Dhar NK. Clinical profile of trichotillomania. *J Ind Med Assoc* 1991; **89**: 137–9.
17 Chang CH, Lee MB, Chiang YC, Lu YC. Trichotillomania: a clinical study of 36 patients. *J Formos Med Assoc* 1991; **90**: 176–80.
18 Hussein SH. Trichotillomania. *Psychopathology* 1992; **25**: 289–93.
19 Simeon D, Cohen LJ, Stein DJ. Co-morbid self-injurious behavior in 71 female hair pullers. *J Nerv Ment Dis* 1997; **185**: 117–9.
20 Lenane MC, Swedo SE, Rapoport JL *et al.* Rates of obsessive compulsive disorder in first-degree relatives of patients with trichotillomania. *J Clin Psychiatry* 1992; **33**: 925–33.
21 Stanley MA, Prather RC, Wagner AL *et al.* Can the Yale–Brown Obsessive Compulsive Scale be used to assess trichotillomania? *Behav Res Ther* 1993; **31**: 171–7.
22 Baer L. Behaviour therapy for OCD and trichotillomania. In: Chase TN, ed. *Advances in Neurology*, New York: Raven Press, 1992: 333–40.
23 Demaret A. Onychophagia, trichotillomania and grooming. *Ann Med Psychol (Paris)* 1973; **1**: 235–42.
24 Sanderson KV, Hall-Smith P. Tonsure trichotillomania. *Br J Dermatol* 1970; **82**: 343–50.
25 Dimino-Emme L, Camisa C. Trichotillomania associated with the 'Friar Tuck' sign and nail biting. *Cutis* 1991; **47**: 107–10.
26 Delsmann BM, Nikolaidis N, Schomacher PH. Trichobezoar as a rare cause of ileus. *Dtsche Med Wochenschr* 1993; **118**: 1361–4.
27 Wadlington WB, Rose M, Holcomb GW. Complications of trichobezoars: a 30-year experience. *South Med J* 1992; **85**: 1020–2.
28 Ripolles T, Garcia-Aguayo J, Martinez MJ, Gil P. Gastrointestinal bezoars: sonographic and CT characteristics. *Am J Roentgenol* 2001; **177**: 65–9.
29 Azrin NH. Treatment of hair-pulling: a comparative study of habit reversal and negative practice training. *J Behav Ther Exp Psychiatry* 1980; **11**: 80–5.
30 Vitulano LA, King RA, Scahill L, Cohen DJ. Behavioural treatment of children and adolescents with trichotillomania. *J Am Acad Child Adolesc Psychiatry* 1992; **31**: 139–46.
31 Koran LM, Ringold A, Hewlett W. Fluoxetine for trichotillomania. *Psychopharmacol Bull* 1992; **28**: 145–9.
32 Winchel RM, Jones JS, Stanley B *et al.* Clinical characteristics of trichotillomania and its response to fluoxetine. *J Clin Psychiatry* 1992; **53**: 304–8.
33 Stein DJ, Bouwer C, Maud CM. Use of citalopram in treatment of trichotillomania. *Eur Arch Psychiatry Clin Neurosci* 1997; **247**: 234–6.
34 Stein DJ, Hollander E. Low-dose pimozide augmentation of SSR blockers in trichotillomania. *J Clin Psychiatry* 1992; **53**: 123–6.
35 Gupta MA, Gupta AK. Use of psychotropic drugs in dermatology. *Dermatol Clin* 2000; **18**: 711–25.

Onychotillomania and onychophagia
(see Chapter 62) [1,2]

The compulsive habits of nail picking and nail biting have been shown to be common in children and adolescents [2,3]. The aetiologies suggested include stress, imitation of family members and a transference from the thumb sucking habit. Nail biting is usually confined to the fingernails, but nail picking, especially in adults, may involve all digits. Damage to cuticles and nails causes paronychia, nail dystrophy and longitudinal melanonychia [4]. In chronic cases, there is an association with trichotillomania [1]. Compulsive biting, tearing or picking with instruments such as scissors, knives or razorblades may lead to permanent destruction [5].

Onychotillomania is often denied by the patient but some admit to the habit. Of these, the most common problem is a compulsive action, not always at times of stress. Self-induced anonychia of the toenails was produced by one man who plucked out the nails with pliers rather than suffer recurrent paronychia of previously crushed toes [6]. DP may provoke self-destruction of the nails [7] as can a folie à deux in the confused elderly [8]. Successful response to treatment has been shown with clomipramine [9] and pimozide [8].

REFERENCES

1 Demaret A. Onychophagia, trichotillomania and grooming. *Ann Med Psychol (Paris)* 1973; **1**: 235–42.
2 Leung AK, Robson WL. Nailbiting. *Clin Paediatr* 1990; **29**: 690–2.
3 Odenrick B, Fattstrom V. Nailbiting: frequency and association with root resorption during orthodontic treatment. *Br J Orthod* 1985; **12**: 78–81.
4 Baran R. Nail biting and picking as a cause of longitudinal melanonychia. *Dermatologica* 1990; **181**: 126–8.
5 Sait MA, Reddy BSN, Garg BR. Onychotillomania. *Dermatologica* 1985; **171**: 200–2.
6 Hurley PT, Balu V. Self-inflicted anonychia. *Arch Dermatol* 1982; **118**: 956–7.
7 Alkiewicz J. Uber Onychotillomanie. *Dermatol Wochenschr* 1934; **98**: 519–21.
8 Hamman K. Onychotillomania treated with pimozide. *Acta Derm Venereol (Stockh)* 1982; **62**: 346–8.
9 Leonard HL, Lenane MC, Swedo SE *et al.* A double blind comparison of clomipramine and desipramine in severe onychophagia. *Arch Gen Psychiatry* 1991; **48**: 821–7.

Psychogenic purpuras [1,2]

This group of disorders is incompletely understood. The common features are the presence of purpura, bruising or frank bleeding in patients who show severe emotional disturbance. The patients are predominantly female. For clarification it is helpful to consider the following separate categories, although some overlap is apparent:

1 Autoerythrocyte sensitization syndrome (Gardner–Diamond syndrome) [3]
2 Psychogenic purpura without autoerythrocyte sensitization but with other abnormalities [4,5]
3 Psychogenic purpura with no measurable abnormality [6,7]
4 Purpura factitia [8–10]
5 Religious stigmata [2].

Autoerythrocyte sensitization syndrome [3]
SYN. GARDNER–DIAMOND SYNDROME

In this rare but well-recognized condition (see Chapter 48), exquisitely tender bruises arise after minimal trauma with or without a history of emotional disorders. In the original cases, it was noted there was a preceding history of an injury involving extensive bruising or major surgery. These bizarre tender lesions are most commonly located on the arms and legs [11,12]. Bruising is heralded by a burning or stinging sensation followed after a few hours by oedema and erythema. The bruising appears a day or so later [12]. Abdominal pain, bleeding from internal organs and neurological symptoms may occur [1]. Psychiatric symptoms were present in 21 of 30 cases reported [13]. Severe emotional disturbances are a constant feature and the relationship to religious stigmatization has been discussed [1,2,14]. The possible relationship of stress to altered fibrinolysis is conjectural but measureable effects have been found [2].

Typical bruising can be reproduced by the intradermal injection of the patient's own erythrocytes and in some cases red-cell phosphotidyl-L-serine [15]. Gomi and Miura [16] described a case with associated thrombocytosis where busulfan therapy produced a reduction in attacks. Increased fibrinolytic activity has also been noted at the onset of fresh lesions in some patients [5,17]. One case seemed to have been made worse by a copper-containing intrauterine contraceptive [18]. Psychiatric treatment using psychotherapy [1,11] or psychotropics [15] has been reported.

Psychogenic purpura without autoerythrocyte sensitization but with other abnormalities [4,5]

A very similar clinical syndrome has been reported but with a negative reaction to intradermal red cells. Rowell [5] described two women with painful bleeding and bruises in association with increased fibrinolytic activity and mental stress. A further condition in this group consists of autosensitivity to DNA [4] described as painful itchy eccymoses, which recurred over a number of years.

Psychogenic purpura with no measurable abnormality [6,7]

Sorensen *et al.* [7] considered that patients with psychogenic purpura with no abnormal tests shared the same emotional background and other clinical features and should be regarded as part of the same syndrome. The lesions may be less tender and dramatic [6].

Purpura factitia [8–10]

Bleeding, bruising and purpura have all been reported as artefactual disease. Agle [8] described malingerers who misuse anticoagulants, while aspirin has also been taken to similar effect. Mechanical purpuras are ingenious and well reported [9,10].

REFERENCES

1 Ratnoff OD. The psychogenic purpuras: a review of autoerythrocyte sensitization, autosensitization to DNA, 'hysterical' and factitious bleeding, and the religious stigmata. *Semin Hematol* 1980; **17**: 192–213.
2 Panconesi E, Hautman G. Stress, stigmatization and psychosomatic purpuras. *Int J Angiol* 1995; **14**: 130–7.
3 Gardner FH, Diamond LK. Autoerythrocyte sensitization: a form of purpura producing painful bruising following autosensitization to red blood cells in certain women. *Blood* 1955; **10**: 675–90.
4 Uthman IW, Moukarbel GV, Salman SM *et al.* Autoerythrocyte sensitization (Gardner–Diamond) syndrome. *Eur J Haematol* 2000; **65**: 144–7.
5 Rowell NR. A painful bleeding syndrome with increased fibrinolytic activity. *Br J Dermatol* 1974; **91**: 591–3.
6 Ogston D, Ogston WD, Bennett NB. Psychogenic purpura. *BMJ* 1971; i: 30.
7 Sorenson RU, Newman AJ, Gordon EM. Psychogenic purpura in adolescent patients. *Clin Paediatr* 1985; **21**: 700–4.
8 Agle D, Ratnoff OD, Spring GK. The anticoagulant malingerer. *Ann Intern Med* 1970; **73**: 67–72.
9 Sneddon IB. Simulated disease: problems in diagnosis and management. *J R Coll Phys Lond* 1983; **17**: 199–205.
10 Yates VM. Factitious purpura. *Clin Exp Dermatol* 1992; **17**: 238–9.
11 Berman DA, Roenigk HH, Green D. Autoerythrocyte sensitization syndrome (psychogenic purpura). *J Am Acad Dermatol* 1992; **27**: 829–32.
12 Verstraete M. Psychogenic haemorrhages. *Verh K Acad Geneeskd Belg* 1991; **53**: 5–28.
13 Hersle K, Mobacken H. Autoerythrocyte sensitization syndrome (psychogenic purpura): report of two cases and review of the literature. *Br J Dermatol* 1969; **81**: 574–87.
14 Whitlock FA. Self-inflicted and related dermatoses. In: Whitlock FA, ed. *Psychophysiological Aspects of Skin Disease.* London: Saunders, 1976: 98–107.
15 Strunecka A, Krpejsova L, Palecek J *et al.* Transbilayer redistribution of phosphatidylserine in erythrocytes of a patient with autoerythrocyte sensitization syndrome (psychogenic purpura). *Folia Haematol* 1990; **117**: 829–41.
16 Gomi H, Miura T. Autoerythrocyte sensitization syndrome with thrombocytosis. *Dermatology* 1994; **188**: 160–2.
17 Lotti T, Benci M, Sarti MG *et al.* Psychogenic purpura with abnormally increased tPA dependent cutaneous fibrinolytic activity. *Int J Dermatol* 1993; **32**: 521–3.
18 Grossman RA. Autoerythrocyte sensitization worsened by a copper containing IUD. *Obstet Gynecol* 1987; **70**: 526–8.

Factitious skin disease

The dermatologist, in common with most clinicians, is trained to believe what the patient says. Most physicians will maintain an endearing and undiscerning naivety even in the face of strong evidence of simulated or fraudulent illness. Clinical deception refers to a spectrum of illness that lies in a continuum which stretches from the unconscious processes (e.g. conversion and somatization) through the conscious and sporadic (e.g. dermatitis artefacta) to the falsification for deliberate gain (e.g. so-called malingering). The dilemma for the clinician is to determine the degree of voluntariness present in the patient for the consciousness of the action may not equate with the consciousness of the motive.

At a simple and elementary level, patients commonly exaggerate or minimize symptoms, may misattribute causation or have mistaken beliefs. This pattern is common and does not really constitute a fabrication although as a persistent behaviour it can alienate the clinician's objectivity. These distortions are singularly different from the factitious falsification of information (lying), the manufacture of skin lesions, the occult use of others (proxy disease) and disease produced for material profit or retribution.

The definition of factitious behaviour is not completely clear because the level of intention may vary, but for the dermatologist the definition by DSM-IV-TR criteria maintains the difference from malingering [1]. The DSM-IV-TR criteria for factitious disorder include:
1 Intentional feigning of physical or psychological signs or symptoms
2 The motivation is to assume the sick role
3 External incentives for the behaviour (such as economic gain, avoiding legal responsibility or improving physical well-being, as in malingering) are absent.
Dermatologists will encounter the subtype 300.19 presenting with predominantly physical signs and symptoms.

There are a series of recognized skin diseases characterized by the essential features that first are caused by the fully aware patient and, secondly, involve the desire to hide the cause from their doctors. This definition includes dermatitis artefacta, dermatological pathomimicry, dermatitis simulata and dermatitis passivata. These syndromes are additionally distinguishable from others where there is a secondary gain, such as Munchausen's syndrome, Munchausen's by proxy and malingering.

Dermatitis artefacta

Definition. Dermatitis artefacta is an artefactual skin disease caused entirely by the actions of the fully aware (not consciously impaired) patient on the skin, hair, nails or mucosae. These patients hide the responsibility for their actions from their doctors [2].

Epidemiology and aetiology. All studies have shown the preponderance of females, the ratio of female to male varying from 20 : 1 to 4 : 1 [2–6]. Lesions have been found in children from the age of 8 years [6], prepubertal children having an equal sex ratio rising to 3 : 1 female predominance by the early teens. In half of subjects the

lesions are on the face, particularly in children [3,6]. While these series confirm that the majority of cases commence in adolescence and in adults under 30 years of age, there is an important subgroup whose age of onset is significantly older. This subgroup is distinguished by being more likely to be male (male to female ratio 1 : 2) to produce more subtle skin lesions [3,4] and to have a past history of somatizing illness [7–9]. These complaints may take the form of pseudoseizures, abdominal pain, syncope, chronic fatigue and backache. Previous work has suggested that dermatitis artefacta is more common in health care workers and their families [5,10,11] because this environment provides not only a ready 'model to copy' but also a social structure where illness is always understood and allowed for. However, this bias may now be less obvious [3] in a well-informed society whose medical symptoms, pathology and disease are more available via the media and the Internet.

Much has been written about the motivation to assume the sick role and the psychopathology underlying the production of artefact [7,12–14]. The idea that the patient *wants* the sickness role is the essential pathology because the primary gain of *being* a patient is usually to be expected of all illness. The main additional gains can be summarized as:
1 Strong masochistic needs (e.g. self-hate and guilt)
2 A sickness that allows inappropriate regression and avoidance of adult (especially sexual) responsibilities (e.g. marital trauma)
3 An illness that symbolizes anger at or conflict with authority figures (e.g. school phobia)
4 Psychiatric or medical care that fulfills massive dependency needs (e.g. inadequate coping strategies)
5 An illness that symbolizes attempts at mastery of past trauma (repetitive compulsion) (e.g. childhood abuse).

In many cases, the psychosocial stress of a major life event may be apparent. Children and adolescents commonly show anxiety and immaturity of coping styles in response to a dysfunctional parent–child relationship, bullying, physical body changes, or sexual and substance abuse. Adults may be neurotic and react to adverse situations in an immature impulsive manner [2,13]. However, there may also be significant depression [2,3]. The more chronic patients tend to have a demonstrable personality disorder, more particularly borderline or hysterical in females and paranoid in males [3,7,11,13]. There is a significant literature on the relationship between factitious disorder and illness falsification in both children and adults and previous factitious disorder by proxy victimization (Munchausen's by proxy; see below).

Clinical features. The nature of the clinical symptomatology in dermatitis artefacta is the 'hollow history' [15]. The patient describes the sudden appearance of complete lesions with little or no prodrome. There is no complete description of the genesis of individual skin lesions. The signs invariably appear overnight, in a lunch break, on the way home from school or work. Lesions appear at the same identical stage in development in crops or groups, either symmetrically or scattered apparently at random. There is a significant lack of a history of a progression of lesions from an initial lesion to its fully developed state. By contrast, there is a prolonged and elaborate description of complications and failure to heal. Characteristically, established lesions may undergo sudden deterioration at the same time as new areas appear. It has been suggested that the patients show a 'belle indifference' to their predicament as part of a dissociative state and, in the presence of visible disease, manifest a nonchalance and innocence transmitted through an enigmatic 'Mona Lisa' smile. It is probably true to say that the patients are more often passive than aggressive, even though they have a widespread disfigurement. However, this is not always the case and considerable anger may be shown by the patient, but more particularly by parents, carers, husbands or partners, who rail at the incompetence of a succession of doctors. This may extend further to recruiting other doctors, university academics, nurses and social workers to support their case [3]. More than one person may be involved, as in the 'folie à deux' of two patients with factitious ulcers [16].

Clinical signs [5,11,15]. The most common site of involvement is the face, particularly cheeks. The dorsa of the hands rather than the palms are the next most common site then the forearms, most frequently the non-dominant limb. There is a particular covert pattern on covered skin where clothes hide significant mutilation of the breasts, abdominal areas and sometimes the genitalia. Involvement of the back, axillae and external ear is uncommon.

Cutaneous lesions are produced by every known means of damaging the skin. Crude destructive processes are the result of thermal, chemical or instrumental injury. Less commonly, dermal lesions from blunt trauma or injections are found. Oedema of limbs from constricting bands and hysterical dependent posture has been described (Secretan's syndrome) [17]. It is characteristic that one digit, usually a toe, will be constricted at a time while all others are healthy. A series of single ischaemic toes while all others are healthy should raise suspicion of artefact.

Excoriations may be made with nail files, sanding boards, wood or wire brushes to produce raw, crusty, linear or arciform lesions with characteristic angulated edges (Fig. 61.3). Punched out necrotic areas, sometimes with blisters developing into indurated necrotic scars are typical of thermal burns from cigarettes, soldering irons or ovens. These are usually uniform in size and scattered haphazardly. Urticarial lesions are initially produced by chemical damage and progress subsequently to crusting and scarring.

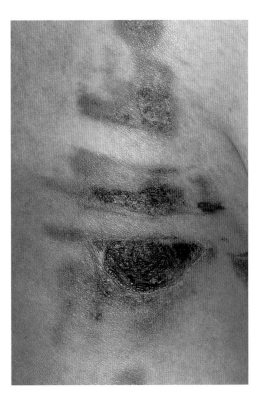

Fig. 61.3 Dermatitis artefacta: note the straight edges and sharp angulation of some of the lesions.

Characteristically, these areas may show the 'drip-sign', where corrosive liquids have been allowed to run over the skin (Fig. 61.4). Bleaches, soaps and household cleaners are most commonly employed by women; industrial acids and automotive fluids by men. These chemicals may produce a persistent detectable smell on the skin. Purpura and bruising are seen after suction, friction or blunt trauma. Children produce purpura on the chin by sucking on cups and on limbs by direct mouth suction or with the use of a toy or tool. Shearing stress also produces purpura, tending to present as linear lesions on the limbs.

Subtle artefact [3] is seen as fixed urticaria, vasculitis (Fig. 61.5), dermal nodules, panniculitis-type lesions and boggy fluctuant swellings. Considerable atrophy and pigment change occur with resolution. Careful examination may reveal the presence of a needle track where milk, air, faeces, urine, cooking oil, silicone, grease or engine oil has been injected [18,19].

In other specialties such as ophthalmology, oral medicine and otolaryngology artefact presents as non-healing infected wounds and excoriations [20–22].

The last common group is that presenting as non-healing surgical wounds. Commonly, this may follow a small operation after minor skin trauma, instrumentation such as an arthroscopy or breast biopsy. Unfortunately, further 'wound repairs' exacerbate and ligitimize the continuing wound. It is not unusual to see patients who

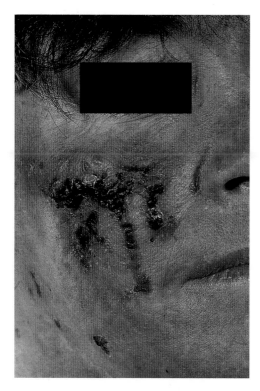

Fig. 61.4 Dermatitis artefacta showing the drip sign.

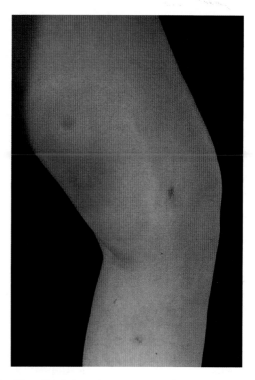

Fig. 61.5 Vasculitic lesions showing acute inflammatory lesions and old monomorphic atrophic scars.

have had up to eight operative revisions before a further referral is made to a dermatologist.

There may be unexpected complications to the artefactual damage leading to severe infection such as cerebral abscess [23] which may be life threatening [24].

Differential diagnosis. The distribution and physical characteristics of the crude dermatitis artefacta are diagnostic. However, blistering crusty lesions may simulate ecthyma, herpes simplex and bullous disorders. More subtle facial blisters may simulate porphyria cutanea tarda. The collagen–vascular diseases including vasculitis and pyoderma gangrenosum must be excluded in non-healing wounds as must atypical mycobacterial infections and imported tropical infections. The curious linear dermatoses such as Nékam's syndrome, cutaneous lymphomas and linear drug eruptions [25] must be excluded. The diverse hereditary sensory neuropathies can show chronic non-healing ulcers and be mistaken for artefact as can the cutaneous changes of reflex sympathetic dystrophy [26]. The purpuras and tissue purpuric reactions such as cutaneous amyloid can be perplexing and should be excluded [27].

REFERENCES

1 American Psychiatric Association. *Diagnostic and Statistical Manual of Mental Disorders (DSM-IV)*, 4th edn. Text revision. Washington DC: American Psychiatric Association, 2000: 517.

2 Koblenzer C. Dermatitis artefacta: clinical features and approaches to treatment. *Am J Clin Dermatol* 2000; **1**: 47–55.

3 Millard L. Dermatitis artefacta in the 1990s. *Br J Dermatol* 1996; **135** (Suppl. 47): 27.

4 Lyell A. Dermatitis artefacta in relation to the syndrome of contrived disease. *Clin Exp Dermatol* 1976; **1**: 109–26.

5 Cotterill J. Self-stigmatization: artefact dermatitis. *Br J Hosp Med* 1992; **47**: 115–9.

6 Rogers M, Fairley M, Santhaman R. Artefactual skin disease in children and adolescents. *Australas J Dermatol* 2001; **42**: 264–70.

7 Phillips KA, ed. *Somatoform and Factitious Disorders: Review of Psychiatry*, Vol. 20. 2001: 129–67.

8 Millard LG. Factitious dermatological disorders in the somatizing patient. *Abstracts of the Fifth International Meeting of the European Society for Dermatology and Psychiatry*. Bordeaux: European Society for Dermatology and Psychiatry, 1993.

9 Sneddon IB. Simulated disease: problems in diagnosis and management. *J R Coll Phys Lond* 1983; **17**: 199–205.

10 Fras I. Factitial disease: an update. *Psychosomatics* 1978; **19**: 119–22.

11 Sneddon I, Sneddon J. Self-inflicted injury: a follow-up study of 43 patients. *BMJ* 1975; **3**: 527–30.

12 Cunnien AJ. Psychiatric and medical syndromes associated with deception. In: Rogers R, ed. *Clinical Assessment of Malingering and Deception*. New York: Guildford Press, 1997: 23–46.

13 Fabisch W. Psychiatric aspects of dermatitis artefacta. *Br J Dermatol* 1980; **102**: 29–34.

14 Overholser JC. Differential diagnosis of malingering and factitious disorders with physical symptoms. *Behav Sci Law* 1990; **8**: 55–65.

15 Lyell A. Cutaneous artefactual disease. *J Am Acad Dermatol* 1979; **1**: 391–407.

16 Hubler WR, Hubler WRSr. Folie à deux factitious ulcers. *Arch Dermatol* 1980; **116**: 1303–4.

17 Smith RJ. Factitious lymphoedema of the hand. *J Bone Joint Surg* 1975; **57**: 89–94.

18 Aduan RP, Fauci AS, Dale DC *et al*. Factitious fever and self-induced infection. *Ann Intern Med* 1979; **90**: 230–42.

19 Behar TA, Anderson EE, Barwick WJ *et al*. Sclerosing lipogranulomatosis: a literature review of subcutaneous injection of oils. *Plast Reconst Surg* 1993; **91**: 352–61.

20 Ugurlu S, Bartley GB, Otley SCC. Factitious disease of periocular and facial skin. *Am J Ophthalmol* 1999; **127**: 196–201.

21 Ebeling O, Ott S, Michel O. Self-induced illness ENT medical practice. *HNO* 1996; **44**: 526–31.

22 Svirsky JA, Sawyer DR. Dermatitis artefacta of the paraoral region. *Oral Surg* 1987; **64**: 259–63.

23 Reed DH, Martin I. Dermatitis artefacta complicated by cerebral abscess. *Postgrad Med J* 1988; **64**: 976–8.

24 Murray SJ, Ross JB, Murray AH. Life-threatening dermatitis artefacta. *Cutis* 1987; **39**: 387–8.

25 Miori L, Vignini M, Rabbiosi G. Flagellate dermatitis after bleomycin. *Am J Dermatopathol* 1990; **12**: 598–602.

26 Buijs EJ, Klijn FA, Lindeman E. Reflex sympathetic dystrophy versus a factitious disorder. *Ned Tijdschr Geneeskd* 2000; **144**: 1614–20.

27 Mahood JM. Familial amyloid neuropathy. *Postgrad Med J* 1980; **56**: 658–9.

Factitious cheilitis (Fig. 61.6)

SYN. LE TIC DES LEVRES

Artefactual lesions of the lips are uncommon. Studies are small but it appears equally in males and females [1,2]. Such lesions manifest particularly as persistent inflammation with crusting and variable haemorrhage. This is caused by picking, biting, rubbing and licking [3]. Occasionally, young adolescents will develop a disuse crusting of the lips because they become dysmorphic about cleaning and washing their mouths [4].

Differential diagnosis includes contact dermatitis, actinic damage, chronic lip-licking habit and causes of granulomatous cheilitis.

REFERENCES

1 Crotty CP, Dicken CH. Factitious lip crusting. *Arch Dermatol* 1981; **117**: 338–40.

2 Thomas JR, Greene SL, Dicken CH. Factitious cheilitis. *J Am Acad Dermatol* 1983; **3**: 368–72.

3 Kuffer R. Cheilitis and lip lesions artificially induced. *Ann Dermatol Vénéréol* 1990; **117**: 477–86.

4 Calobrisi S, Baselga E, Miller ES. Factitious cheilitis in an adolescent. *Pediatr Dermatol* 1999; **31**: 128–33.

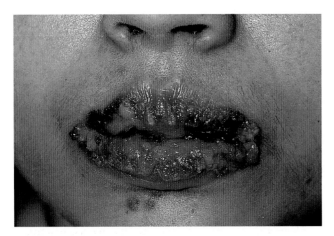

Fig. 61.6 Factitial cheilitis—a type of dermatitis artefacta of the lips.

Nail artefact

Chronic paronychia caused by the insertion of nails, pins or splinters has been recorded in soldiers avoiding duty and also in children [1]. The characteristic lesions show purpura and haemorrhage around the nail fold but also subungual haemorrhage and pustules. Similarly, Lyell [2] described a patient who induced haemorrhagic nail loss using a nail file. A significant sign is repeated traumatic nail loss occurring singly or multiply on one hand only. The differential diagnosis is described in Chapter 62.

REFERENCES

1 Sneddon IB. Simulated disease: problems in diagnosis and management. *J R Coll Phys Lond* 1983; **17**: 199–205.

2 Lyell A. Dermatitis artefacta and self-inflicted disease. *Scott Med J* 1972; **17**: 187–95.

Hair artefact

A bizarre pattern of hair loss may occur after cutting or shaving. It differs from the plucked appearance of trichotillomania and usually appears acutely, either as rough cropped areas of hair loss or unnatural patterned alopecia of scalp or eyebrows (Fig. 61.7).

Differential diagnosis. See Chapter 63.

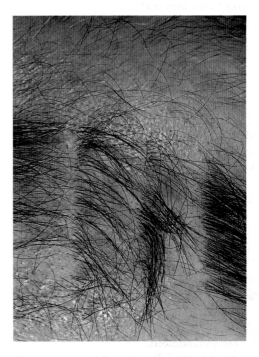

Fig. 61.7 Bizarre pattern of alopecia on the scalp with regimented rows of surviving hairs.

Artefact by proxy [1,2]

SYN. WITCHCRAFT SYNDROME

Artefact dermatitis can be provoked on an unknowing and unsuspecting victim by proxy. As an act of revenge, the daughter of a hairdresser applied benzyl ether of nicotinic acid to the customer's skin. This induced hyperaemia with some oedema within 10 min but not on the perpetrator because absorption of the agent is very low on the palm of the hand, so she could easily apply it to the customer's skin without harm to herself.

REFERENCES

1 Bandmann Wahl B. Contact urticaria artefacta (witchcraft syndrome). *Contact Dermatitis* 1982; **8**: 145–6.
2 Simani VK. Witchcraft syndrome. *Int J Dermatol* 1998; **37**: 229–31.

Dermatitis artefacta with artefact of patch tests [1]

Bullous dermatitis artefacta in a female veterinary assistant healed with occlusive dressings. New bullae on the other arm prompted the parents to demand 'allergy' tests. Ten patch tests to yellow petrolatum were applied to the back, which provoked a non-inflammatory bulla on one of the sites 2 days later. Two other cases are cited.

REFERENCE

1 Maurice PDL, Rivers JK, Jones C, Cronin E. Dermatitis artefacta with artefact of patch tests. *Clin Exp Dermatol* 1987; **12**: 204–6.

Investigations

The diagnosis of dermatitis artefacta is based upon major suspicions. In the absence of admission of deceit by the patient, suspicions are aroused by the presence of physiologically impossible symptoms, incompatable lesions, contradictory objective evidence and non-response to reasonable treatment. Other clinical diagnostic clues may be seen such as the sparing of decorative marks and areas of skin on the back [1]. While the diagnosis is based clinically upon a high index of suspicion, litmus paper has been reported as a valuable aid to diagnosis, because it detects strong alkali or acid, particularly in new lesions [2]. Ordinary histopathology will confirm the nature of skin damage in crude artefact, while deeper lesions of vasculitis and panniculitis may show injection tracks and foreign material [3–5]. It has also been shown that serial biopsy may be diagnostically helpful in sophisticated artefact [6].

There are psychometric tests that can be used for the assessment of factitial disorders, but these are essentially research tools [7].

REFERENCES

1 Joe EK, Li VW, Magro CM *et al.* Diagnostic clues to dermatitis artefacta. *Cutis* 1999; **63**: 209–14.
2 Sneddon IB. Simulated disease: problems in diagnosis and management. *J R Coll Phys Lond* 1983; **17**: 199–205.
3 Ackerman BA, Mosher DT, Schwamm HA. Factitial Weber–Christian syndrome. *JAMA* 1966; **198**: 155–60.
4 Winkelmann RK, Barker SM. Factitial traumatic panniculitis. *J Am Acad Dermatol* 1985; **13**: 988–94.
5 Raquena L, Sanchez YE. Panniculitis. *J Am Acad Dermatol* 2001; **45**: 325–61.
6 Weedon D. *Skin Pathology*. Edinburgh: Churchill Livingstone, 1998: 501–2.
7 Greene RL. Assessment of malingering and defensiveness. In: Rogers R, ed. *Clinical Assessment of Malingering and Deception*. New York: Guildford Press, 1997: 169–207.

Co-morbidity

There are common overlap syndromes and related disorders that should be investigated. Twenty per cent of patients have a somatization disorder [1] and hypochondriasis. These are co-morbid with anxiety, depression and substance abuse [2]. Borderline personality disorder is a factor for chronicity in both sexes [3].

REFERENCES

1 Fink P. Physical complaints and symptoms of somatizing patients. *J Psychosom Res* 1992; **36**: 125–36.
2 Barsky AJ. Overview: hypochondriasis, bodily complaints, and somatic styles. *Am J Psychiatry* 1992; **140**: 101–8.
3 Kapfhammer HP, Dobmeir P. Artefactual disorders between deception and self-mutilation. *Nervenartzt* 1998; **69**: 401–9.

Treatment. There are three therapeutic aims. The first is to treat the cutaneous damage. There is always significant skin damage, which will be both inflamed and infected. Topical and systemic antibiotics and anti-inflammatories establish the doctor–patient relationship and underlines to the patient that the physician is helpful, non-aggressive and sympathetic.

Secondly, there is a need to identify the nature and extent of the psychological problem. The dilemma has always been whether or not patients should be confronted [1]. In most cases, the urge to confrontation is stimulated by the aggression the physician feels because the doctor–patient relationship has apparently been betrayed. The doctor must avoid personalizing the episode and needs to consider the approach that is likely to change the patient's behaviour. Confrontation is a highly charged strategy and should only be done if the deliberate act is certain (e.g. if the self-damage has been witnessed) and there is sufficient support and advice available at the consultation. This will need the assistance of psychiatric advice and finally to effect a transference to psychiatric care if necessary. This catharsis can be achieved in a manner that allows the patient to express a positive decision to change without dwelling on the deception and precipitating an aggressive defensive response [2,3].

Not surprisingly, other workers disagree with this approach, citing the high failure rate and the risk that the patient will strive even harder to legitimize the illness and himself by seeing other doctors [4].

For many years, a non-confrontational and non-punitive approach has been favoured. This passive acceptance of 'a cry for help' has the merit of a non-aggressive interview in the short term but may paradoxically give the patient consent to continue in the abnormal sickness role, albeit as a psychiatric patient [5]. This approach has been unsuccessful; although for a dermatologist it is the most comfortable because there are no rows. Unfortunately, many patients usually default the clinic or are referred elsewhere.

Efficient occlusive bandaging will allow most lesions to heal, except for those of the most devious and determined. The psychological problems should be approached in a non-confrontational manner [6–11], allowing the patient to express their difficulties in a passive confidential environment. Children usually respond well to this approach, particularly if a cause of psychosocial pressure is identifiable. However, chronic persistent self-damage is predictive of long-term emotional illness and referral to a child psychiatrist is imperative [6].

For adults, a non-confrontational approach that also displays surprising robustness is the 'narrow escape', 'quasi-confession', 'recovery' or 'face-saving' strategy. This is the suggestion that the patient finds a solution to their illness by offering a rationale for recovery. This may take the form of a self-explanation, however fantastic, as a mechanism to escape without public retribution. The patient may claim that alternative medicine such as hypnosis, homoeopathy or fringe methods such as kinaesthetic manipulation has 'cured' them [12]. One additional technique is the double bind strategy where the physician explains that the treatment carries an expectation for recovery. If this does not occur then they will be forced to conclude that the problem is psychological or factitious [12].

The management and prognosis in adults is that of the primary psychological disorder [6]. Acute stress reaction can be addressed in a series of short consultations at the time when the dressings are changed. Patients with depression responded well in two series to tricyclics or SSRI antidepressants [7,8], even when no precipitating event was identifiable. Tacit acceptance that the cause of the rash has been identified, without further challenge, helps to make the transfer to formal psychiatric care easier if needed [10]. Between one-third and half of patients continue to develop chronic lesions [6,11]. Such cases usually have a personality disorder, commonly hysterical, paranoid or borderline [10,11] and need psychiatric assessment [13]. Unfortunately, this is frequently unacceptable to the patient.

REFERENCES

1 Phillips KA, ed. *Somatoform and Factitious Disorders. Review of Psychiatry*, Vol. 20. 2001: 152–4.
2 Bass C, May S. Chronic multiple functional somatic symptoms. In: Mayou R, Sharp M, eds. *The ABC of Psychological Medicine*. London: BMJ, 2002: 325–7.
3 Rogers R. Psychiatric and medical syndromes associated with deception. In: Rogers R, ed. *Clinical Assessment of Malingering and Deception*. New York: Guildford Press, 1997: 390–7.
4 van der Feltz-Cornelis CM. Confronting patients about a factitious disorder. *Ned Tidjschr Geneeskd* 2000; **144**: 545–8.
5 Feldman MD, Ford CV. Factitious disorders. In: Sadock BJ, Sadock VA, eds. *Comprehensive Psychiatry*, 7th edn. Baltimore: American Psychiatric Press, 1996: 175–94.
6 Lyell A. Dermatitis artefacta in relation to the syndrome of contrived disease. *Clin Exp Dermatol* 1976; **1**: 109–26.
7 Sneddon I, Sneddon J. Self-inflicted injury: a follow-up study of 43 patients. *BMJ* 1975; **3**: 527–30.
8 Consoli S. Dermatitis artefacta: a general review. *Eur J Dermatol* 1995; **5**: 5–11.
9 Fabisch W. Psychiatric aspects of dermatitis artefacta. *Br J Dermatol* 1980; **102**: 29–34.
10 Koblenzer C. Psychologic aspects of skin disease. In: Fitzpatrick TB, Eisen AZ, Wolff K, *et al*. eds. *Dermatology in General Medicine*. New York: McGraw-Hill, 1993: 14–26.
11 Millard L. Dermatitis artefacta in the 1990s. *Br J Dermatol* 1996; **135** (Suppl. 47): 27.
12 Eisendrath SJ. Factitious physical disorders without confrontation. *Psychosomatics* 1989; **30**: 383–7.
13 van Moffaert MM. Integration of medical and psychiatric management in self-mutilation. *Gen Hosp Psychiatry* 1991; **13**: 59–67.

Dermatological pathomimicry [1]

Some patients intentionally aggravate an existing dermatosis as an expression of their distress at the unresolved discomfort they feel towards their skin disease, or equally as a mechanism to recruit an existing sick role into another psychosocial situation. To this extent it is distinguishable from dermatitis artefacta because the disease appears as an exacerbation of established skin disease with none of the bizarre physical signs typical of mechanical, chemical or thermal interference. This is also to be differentiated from self-inflicted delayed healing of surgical and traumatic wounds that is achieved by external damage. However, a group of 13 patients who had deliberately caused recurrence of their existing skin disease by reintroducing the precipitating factor and invoking the original pathogenic mechanism have also been described [1,2]. The most common provocative agents were atopic allergens, contact allergens, drug sensitivities and irritants applied to chronic leg disorders. Other reports have described irritant contact dermatitis [3] and artificial oedema of an arm or leg [4]. Most patients were young women who had lost support from within their family group. More direct confrontational discussion without recrimination proved helpful and follow-up showed only minor recurrence in two patients 5 years later [2]. Since the original description there have been numerous reports of contrived exacerbations of common dermatoses. These include atopic eczema by deliberate exposure to individual known personal aeroallergens such as pet danders or food allergens such as milk. In one case this was done by proxy by a mother. A patient with psoriasis covertly retook atenolol, which previously had caused problems (Dr L. Stankler, personal communication).

REFERENCES

1 Millard LG. Dermatological pathomimicry: a form of patient maladjustment. *Lancet* 1984; **2**: 969–71.
2 Millard LG. Dermatological pathomimicry: a follow-up study. *Proceedings of the First International Symposium on Dermatology and Psychiatry*. Vienna: European Society for Dermatology and Psychiatry, 1987.
3 Condé-Salazar L, Gomez J, Meza B. Artefactual irritant dermatitis. *Contact Dermatitis* 1993; **28**: 246.
4 Stoberi C, Musalek M, Partsch H. Artificial oedema of the extremity. *Hautartz* 1994; **45**: 149–53.

Dermatitis simulata

Apparent skin disease can be represented by patients who are ingenious enough to use external disguise to simulate disease. Make-up has been used to paint on a rash [1], sugar to simulate chronic cheilitis, drugs to induce skin discoloration [2] and topical printing dyes to produce discolored sweat [3]. Red make-up has been used to simulate a port-wine stain on the face. These deceptions were clever enough to confuse doctors for months. Most of these patients were young and immature, but a somatizing illness was recorded in one older patient and previous treated depression in another.

REFERENCES

1 King MC, Chalmers RJG. Another aspect of contrived disease: 'dermatitis simulata'. *Cutis* 1984; **34**: 463–4.
2 Sneddon IB. Simulated disease: problems in diagnosis and management. *J R Coll Phys Lond* 1983; **17**: 199–205.
3 McSween R, Millard L. A green man: a case of artefact. *Arch Dermatol* 2000; **136**: 115–8.

Dermatitis passivata

The cessation of normal skin cleansing will produce an accumulation of keratinous crusts. This is commonly seen in geriatric or demented patients who suffer from self-neglect and has been called the Diogenes syndrome [1]. Lesions are usually found on the upper central chest, over the back both upper and sacral and accumulated as coagulated debris in the groin creases. However, a group of patients were described [2] who showed lesions on the scalp, face or arms. Notably, they were young adults who were invariably accompanied by parents or family. Significant psychopathology such as schizoid thought disorder or hysterical limb palsy was present. Specialist psychological therapy was usually necessary either as day care or community psychiatric support [3].

REFERENCES

1 Clark ANG, Mankikar GD, Gray I. Diogenes syndrome: a study of neglect in old age. *Lancet* 1975; **i**: 366–8.
2 Millard LG. Dermatitis passivata: the young Diogenes syndrome. *Cutis* 1997; **47**: 124–7.
3 Reyes-Ortiz CA. Diogenes syndrome: the self-neglect elderly. *Compr Ther* 2001; **27**: 117–21.

Munchausen's syndrome [1,2]

Asher [1] used this term to describe the notorious hospital hopper who presents with a dramatic and untruthful story of illness. This is a severe and chronic subtype of factitious disease [2]. The essential elements are the chronicity of the illness, and the frequency and similarity of the repetitive pattern of the complaint in different hospitals (peregrination). The simulated illnesses may be esoteric and rare. While dermatological complaints are uncommon in Munchausen's syndrome, patients with simulated porphyria and connective tissue disease, for example, may present to the dermatologist. The last element in the syndrome is pseudologica fantastica. This describes the telling of lies about past social history and connections, exploits, wealth and invention of an alias [3]. The patients are usually male, and travel widely from hospital to hospital complaining of abdominal pain, haemorrhage or some neurological incapacity. Skin lesions such as non-healing wounds, widespread blistering and multiple excoriations may be part of the syndrome of simulated disease [4]. The secondary gain is prolonged medical attention, although serious consequences such as septicaemia and paraplegia have occurred [5] from induced cutaneous ulceration. The Internet provides access to those interested in health and medicine and is a rich resource for the expansive personality of the Munchausen patient. Because the Internet offers 'virtual support groups', these individuals may offer 'virtual' factitious disorders. Four cases have been reported, showing the facility with which they can attract attention, mobilize sympathy and control others [6].

REFERENCES

1 Asher R. Munchausen's syndrome. *Lancet* 1951; **1**: 339–41.
2 Menninger K. Polysurgery and polysurgical addiction. *Psychoanal Q* 1934; **4**: 173–99.
3 Newmark N, Adityanjee KJ. Pseudologica fantastica and factitious disorder: review of the literature. *Compr Psychiatry* 1999; **40**: 89–95.
4 Eisendrath SJ. When Munchausen becomes malingering. *Bull Am Acad Psychiatry* 1996; **24**: 471–81.
5 Burket JM, Burket BA. Factitial dermatitis resulting in paraplegia. *J Am Acad Dermatol* 1987; **17**: 306–7.
6 Feldman MD. Munchausen by Internet: detecting factitious illness and crisis on the Internet. *South Med J* 2000; **93**: 669–72.

Munchausen's syndrome by proxy [1,2]

In 1977, Meadow [1] had the clinical acuity and personal courage to described the syndrome of Munchausen's by proxy where the illness is fabricated by the parent, usually the mother, or someone *in loco parentis*. Since then it is clear that not only do some parents harm their children but other carers may be involved and these may include health professionals. Doctors and others may not only fail to understand the origins of a child's symptoms but also institute further harm by inappropriate investigations, treatment and surgery [3]. The guidelines to identifying cases [2] mirror many of those discussed for dermatitis artefacta. The victims have a persistent or recurrent illness that cannot be readily explained. The diagnosis remains descriptive and not stringent. Symptoms do not respond and laboratory tests are incongruous. The reported symptoms are inconsistent with presenting health and the symptoms fail to appear in the absence of a certain parent (usually the mother). The perpretrator is reluctant to leave the child even for a few minutes, but remains oddly impassive even in an emergency. Characteristically, like patients with dermatitis artefacta, these carers attempt to make close relationships with medical staff with a blurring of the doctor–parent barrier. There may be fabrication of family details and a disturbed marital and social structure. Rarely, the parent exhibits the syndrome herself and produces proxy lesions on the child (Polle's syndrome) [4].

The victims are usually infants or toddlers with a mean age at diagnosis of 40 months [6]. The mean delay between presentation and diagnosis is 15 months. The signs and symptoms of illness were mostly produced in hospital. The most common presentation in one series was bleeding (44%), CNS depression (19%), apnoea (15%), diarrhoea (11%), vomiting (10%), fever (10%) and rash (9%) [6]. Skin lesions are usually crude forms of dermatitis artefacta [6,7] produced by scratching or caustic painting on skin. On one occasion the rash was the result of drug poisoning. A large review of countries outside English-speaking industrialized populations produced similar results in rather older children [8]. The long-term consequences of childhood victimization might contribute to the development of factitious disease in adult life. Elements of the child victim's experience, including feelings of powerlessness, lack of control and disappointment in the physician, are the suggested dynamics for the development of independent illness falsification [9].

Munchausen's by proxy may also rarely be seen in the elderly, mentally handicapped or other dependent persons [10], perpetrated by relatives, nurses and care home personnel.

REFERENCES

1 Meadow SR. Munchausen syndrome by proxy. *Arch Dis Child* 1982; **57**: 92–8.
2 Parnell TF. Guidelines for identifying cases. In: Parnell TF, Day DO, eds. *Munchausen by Proxy Syndrome*. California: Sage, 1998: 47–67.
3 McLure RJ, Davis PM, Meadow SR. Epidemiology of Munchausen syndrome by proxy. *Arch Dis Child* 1996; **75**: 57–61.
4 Verity CM, Winkworth C, Bruman D. Polle syndrome: children of Munchausen. *BMJ* 1979; **2**: 422–3.
5 Siebel MA. The physicians role in confirming the diagnosis. In: Parnell TF, Day DO, eds. *Munchausen by Proxy Syndrome*. California: Sage, 1998: 68–95.
6 Rosenberg D. Web of deceit Munchausen by proxy: a literature review. *Child Abuse Negl* 1987; **11**: 547–63.
7 Meadow SR. Who's to blame—mothers, Munchausen or medicine? *J R Coll Phys Lond* 1994; **28**: 332–7.
8 Feldman MD, Brown RMA. Munchausen by proxy in an international context. *Child Abuse Negl* 2002; **26**: 509–24.
9 Libow JA. Beyond collusion: active illness falsification. *Child Abuse Negl* 2002; **26**: 525–36.
10 Sigal MD, Altmark D, Carmel I. Munchausen syndrome by adult proxy. *J Nerv Ment Dis* 1986; **186**: 696–8.

Malingering [1]

Asher [1] defined malingering as the imitation, production or encouragement of illness for a deliberate end. The American Psychiatric Association DSM-IV definition is 'the intentional production of false or grossly exaggerated physical or psychological symptoms, motivated by external incentives'. However, the taxonomy of the malingering is difficult because of the moralistic overtones of criminality and false compensation litigation [2,3].

Malingering may be co-morbid with conversion disorders, personality disorders and other factitial behaviour. However, usually it differs from most factitial disease in being short term and opportunistic, whereas other illness falsification is chronic and persistent. Fear, desire and escape are the three main motives to produce false or grossly exaggerated physical or psychological symptoms. Soldiers feigning disease and disability hope to avoid duty, suspend transfer or be discharged from the service. Workers can prolong sick leave, delay corporate change of job or seek to obtain early retirement with an apparently extended illness. Some patients may seek compensation for some contrived illness (e.g. alleged burns) or aggravate and continue an existing disease (e.g. industrial dermatitis) out of a sense of grievance or retribution. Prolonged legal cases of supposed medical negligence are common in those with manufactured illness whose dissatisfaction with their doctors or the care they have received may lead to a financial settlement as a reward [4].

Cutaneous lesions are usually crude forms of artefact dermatitis [5]. Chronic non-healing postoperative scars are manipulated with instruments, or even faecal injection to maintain sepsis [6]. Hand dermatitis, both irritant and allergic contact dermatitis, may be perpetuated to seek higher compensation awards [7].

Treatment depends on the underlying psychiatric illness if significant psychopathology can be found, but the opportunist response in patients with an underlying personality disorder is poor [8].

REFERENCES

1 Asher R. *Talking Sense*. Bath: Pitman, 1973: 145–7.
2 Hutchinson GL. *Disorders of Simulation*. Madison: Psychosocial Press, 2001: 53–63.

3 Cunnien AJ. Psychiatric and medical syndromes associated with deception. In: Rogers R, ed. *Clinical Assessment of Malingering and Deception.* New York: Guildford Press, 1997: 33–46.

4 Eisendrath SJ. When Munchausen becomes malingering: factitious disorders that penetrate the legal system. *Bull Am Acad Psych Law* 1996; **24**: 471–81.

5 Lyell A. Cutaneous artefactual disease. *J Am Acad Dermatol* 1979; **1**: 391–407.

6 Reich P, Gottfreid LA. Factitious disorders in a teaching hospital. *Ann Intern Med* 1983; **99**: 240–7.

7 Condé-Salazar L, Gomez J, Meza B. Artefactual irritant dermatitis. *Contact Dermatitis* 1993; **28**: 246–7.

8 Hutchinson GL. *Disorders of Simulation.* Madison: Psychosocial Press, 2001: 195–221.

Self-mutilation

There is a transition between some forms of self-decorative behaviour such as piercings and the development of pathological self-mutilation (SM). This will depend upon the psychological state of the individual, the acceptable fashion norms and the peer group pressures to conform [1]. In a study of adolescents, of 14% engaged in SM two-thirds were girls. Self-cutting was most common followed by self-hitting, pinching, scratching and biting. These students with SM showed significantly more anxiety and depressive symptoms than non-mutilators.

Dermatologists are seldom asked to manage patients who admit to SM but it may be seen as an incidental clinical finding. A group of female patients perform delicate self-cutting, which leaves fine linear non-sutured scars on the wrist and forearm [2]. The cutting is a form of emotional release, both immediately physical often accompanied by euphoria and in the longer term as a control of anxiety [3]. The most common mutilators are young women who are wrist slashers [3]. They are described further as usually attractive, unmarried, easily addicted and unable to relate to others. The patient slashes her wrist at the slightest provocation but does not commit suicide. They tend to be depressed and obsessional, attached and dominated by their mothers, often in the absence of a father. Other impulse control disorders may be evident such as anorexia and bulimia [4]. It is suggested that this form of self-harm is a substitute for masturbation, a form of self-purifying catharsis which modulates stress and anger in patients who remain infantile in outlook [5]. Child abuse and family psychiatric history were frequent in some studies where genital mutilation predominated [6,7]. The more severe forms of SM leading to autocastration or enucleation of an eye are usually reported in association with schizophrenia [8,9].

REFERENCES

1 Ross S, Heath N. A study of self-mutilation in a community of adolescents. *J Youth Adolesc* 2002; 31: 67–77.

2 Doctors S. The symptom of delicate cutting in adolescent females. *Adolesc Psychiatry* 1981; **20**: 443–60.

3 Wewetzer G, Friese H, Warnke A. Open self-injury behaviour in children and adolescence. *Z Kinder Jugendpsychiatr Psychother* 1997; **25**: 95–105.

4 Ghaziuddin M, Tsai L, Naylor M, Ghaziuddin N. Mood disorder in a group of self-cutting adolescents. *Acta Paedopsychiatr* 1992; **55**: 103–5.

5 Lane RC. Anorexia, masochism, self-mutilation and autoeroticism. *Psychoanal Rev* 2002; **89**: 101–23.

6 Alao AO, Yolles JC. Female genital self-mutilation. *Psychosomatic Serv* 1999; **50**: 971–5.

7 Catalano G, Carroll KM. Repetitive male genital self-mutiltion. *J Sex Marital Ther* 2002; **28**: 27–37.

8 Gardner AR, Gardner AJ. Self-mutilation, obsessionality and narcissism. *Br J Psychiatry* 1975; **127**: 127–32.

9 Simpson MA. Self-mutilation. *Br J Hosp Med* 1976; **16**: 430–8.

Cutaneous disease and alcohol misuse [1,2]

Alcoholism and alcohol abuse rank among the three most common psychiatric disorders in the community. There are significant medical and economic consequences because of differing effects of alcohol on metabolism, health, treatment, behaviour and motivation [3]. Alcohol abuse can be missed as a diagnosis by experienced physicians even though the problem is common. Mechanisms for screening and brief interventions are well established and show robust stringency. The two-question screen consisting first of enquiry about past alcohol problems and, secondly, the period since the last drink shows 90% accuracy [4].

The psychosocial effects of chronic and disfiguring skin disease commonly produce feelings of stigma and rejection. Recreational substances, such as alcohol, are commonly used by affected patients [5]. A study of a large urban population suggested that male as well as female psoriatics showed an excess rate of alcoholism [6]. However, further studies suggested that while alcohol abuse was not a factor in the onset of psoriasis, it became significant in women after the disease was present and was significantly associated with the area of skin surface involvement [7] and severity, particularly in men [8]. Furthermore, a prospective study [9] showed that a daily intake of alcohol of more than 80 g was more frequently associated with less treatment-induced in-patient improvement in the percentage of the total body surface area affected by psoriasis. In two wide reviews [2,10], it appears that the changed character and distribution of psoriasis make it more difficult to treat. In studies of patients with psoriasis, alcohol abuse was not marked by elevated liver function tests. Alcohol abstinence helped to induce remission, and relapse was induced by reconsumption.

Discoid eczema appears to be more frequent in alcohol abusers and is a more reliable indicator of alcohol dependence, with significantly abnormal biochemistry and immunology related to alcohol excess. Atopic eczema appears to be unaffected by alcohol to the same degree. Seborrhoeic dermatitis is twice as common with alcohol abuse [11] and this may be related to immunosuppression and the effect on cutaneous microflora. The effects of alcohol on immune function and skin vasculature are thought to precipitate exacerbations of rosacea and post-adolescent acne.

Infestations of the skin and superficial skin infections were found more often in alcoholic vagrants than in non-alcoholics and those with other psychiatric disorders. This also suggests that more specific alcohol-related immune factors were active [12].

REFERENCES

1 Smith KE, Fenske NA. Cutaneous manifestations of alcohol abuse. *J Am Acad Dermatol* 2000; **43**: 1–16.
2 Higgins E, du Vivier A. Alcohol intake and other skin disorders. *Clin Dermatol* 1999; **17**: 437–41.
3 Volpicelli JR. Alcohol abuse and alcoholism: an overview. *J Clin Psychiatry* 2001; **62** (Suppl. 20): 4–10.
4 Fleming MF, Graham AW. Screening and brief interventions for alcohol use disorders in managed care settings. *Recent Dev Alcohol* 2001; **15**: 393–416.
5 Ginsburg IH, Link BG. Feelings of stigmatization in patients with psoriasis. *J Am Acad Dermatol* 1989; **20**: 53–60.
6 Lidegaard B. Disease associated with psoriasis in a population of middle aged urban native Swedes. *Dermatologica* 1986; **172**: 298–304.
7 Poikolinen K, Reunala T, Karvonen J. Smoking, alcohol and life events related to psoriasis among women. *Br J Dermatol* 1994; **130**: 473–7.
8 Monk BE, Neill SM. Alcohol consumption and psoriasis. *Dermatologica* 1986; **173**: 57–60.
9 Gupta MA, Schnork NJ, Gupta AK, Ellis CN. Alcohol intake and treatment responsiveness in psoriasis. *J Am Acad Dermatol* 1993; **28**: 730–5.
10 Higgins EM, du Vivier AW. Cutaneous disease and alcohol misuse. *Br Med Bull* 1994; **50**: 85–98.
11 Rosset M, Oki G. Skin disease in alcoholics. *Q J Stud Alcohol* 1971; **32**: 1017–24.
12 Arfi C, Dela L, Benassia E. Dermatologic consultation in a precarious situation. *Ann Dermatol Vénéréol* 1999; **126**: 682–6.

AIDS, HIV infection and psychological illness (see Chapter 26)

Human immunodeficiency virus (HIV) and AIDS cause cognitive, motor, behavioural and psychiatric symptoms in children and adults [1]. The impact is variable and the progression of disease unpredictable. Poor compliance with retroviral therapy is related to psychiatric morbidity [2] and suicidal ideation, which may be found in 60% of some groups of HIV patients. Most CNS involvement complicating HIV infection occurs in the late phase of the disease. Such patients have been usefully classified first into those with headache or meningitic symptoms; secondly, those with focal CNS symptoms or signs; and, lastly, those with non-focal cerebral and/or motor dysfunction [3]. This latter group present with mental illness where alertness is characteristically impaired because of metabolic or toxic encephalopathy. It refers to a distinct subcortical dementia characterized by retarded and imprecise cognition and motor control. New-onset delusions and hallucinations may be either a result of the metabolic encephalopathy of AIDS or an opportunist cerebral infection, rather than a psychological reaction to having HIV and/or AIDS *per se* [4]. Psychosis develops in patients with late HIV infection and immunosuppression, and has been shown to have a higher incidence in those with CD4 counts of less than 100/µL [5]. A con-

trolled study [6] showed that the neuropsychological deficit as measured by a broad range of cognitive functions was 44% in seropositive patients and up to 87% in those with AIDS.

Progression to AIDS is affected by many factors but significantly so by the effects of stress, lack of social support and depressive symptoms. The presence of all three made the progression to AIDS at least twice as likely [7]. Highly active antiretroviral therapy (HAART) has had a significant impact on patient survival but brings with it the psychosocial aspects of living with a chronic disease. While HAART therapy has a beneficial effect on the psychiatric manifestations of AIDS and HIV, depression responds to SSRI antidepressants used in tandem [1].

REFERENCES

1 Rausch DM, Storer ES. Neuroscience research in AIDS. *Rev Prog Neuropsychopharmacol Psychiatry* 2001; **25**: 231–57.
2 Gil F, Passik S. Psychological adjustment and suicidal ideation in patients with AIDS. *AIDS Care* 1998; **12**: 927–30.
3 Price RW. Neurological complications of HIV infection. *Lancet* 1996; **348**: 445–52.
4 Alcian A, Fusi A, Ferri A *et al.* New onset delusions and hallucinations in patients with HIV. *J Psychiatry Neurol* 2001; **26**: 229–34.
5 Price R. Management of AIDS dementia complex and HIV-1 infection of the nervous system. *AIDS* 1995; **9** (Suppl. A): S221–36.
6 Grant I, Atkinson JH. The evolution of neurobehavioural complications of HIV infection. *Psychol Med* 1990; **20**: 747–54.
7 Lesserman J, Jackson ED, Pettito JM *et al.* Progression to AIDS: effects of stress, depressive symptoms and social support. *Psychosom Med* 1999; **61**: 397–406.

Suicide in dermatological patients

Suicide refers to a range of self-destructive behaviours ranging from non-lethal acts which have been called suicidal gestures, attempted suicide, parasuicide and, more recently, self-injury. A lethal action in which a patient dies is defined as a completed suicide. The rates of completed suicide in the UK are 8–10 in 100 000 people. It is therefore one of the 10 most common causes of death in the UK [1]. Psychiatric disorders are the main risk factors but numerous studies have also identified physical illness as an important contributory factor [1,2]. Chronic illness is a risk factor in suicidal ideation and completed suicide and, not surprisingly, disfiguring chronic dermatoses have been shown to put patients at risk.

In a study of 217 patients with psoriasis, 10% of patients reported a death wish and 6% reported active suicidal ideation at the time of the study [3]. In another group, 2.5% of outpatients and 7.2% of in-patients with psoriasis expressed suicidal ideas. The severity of the psoriasis was reflected in the frequency of suicidal ideation and also measurable clinical depression [4]. Facial acne was also associated with significant risk (5.6%) of suicidal ideation, which is also higher than the levels reported in general medical patients [1]. Suicide ideation was found in seven of 11 patients with Darier's disease related to the disfigurement, the intractability, social exclusion and smell of the dermatosis [5].

Some dermatological patients become so disturbed that they do commit suicide successfully [6–8]. A group of 16 patients has been described [6]—seven males and nine females—who successfully committed suicide after presenting with dermatological problems to two dermatologists working in the same skin department. The majority of these patients had either body-image disorders (dysmorphophobia; BDD) or acne. It is important to recognize that patients with dermatological non-disease, and particularly females with facial complaints, may be extremely depressed and at risk of suicide [9]. Even more strikingly, BDD in children and adolescents carries a much larger risk; 67% experienced suicidal ideation and 21% had attempted suicide [10]. Acne scarring can have just as profound an effect, or even a more profound effect, on body image, self-esteem and confidence as inflammatory acne. The positive therapeutic role of isotretinoin was emphasized [1,11].

There is a definite risk of suicide in patients with active HIV disease [12], and rates of suicide for people with AIDS were 66 times higher than in the general population in New York City. Men with AIDS aged 20–59 years were 36 times more likely to commit suicide than their counterparts without such a diagnosis. Half of the people in this particular sample had expressed suicidal intents and one-quarter killed themselves by jumping from the windows of medical units in general hospitals. Assisted suicide has occurred in up to 23% of patients with AIDS [13].

REFERENCES

1 Diekstra RFW. The epidemiology of suicide and parasuicide. *Acta Psychiatr Scand* 1993; **371**: 9–20.
2 Carson AJ, Best S, Warlow C. Suicidal ideation among outpatients at general clinics. *BMJ* 2000; **320**: 1311–3.
3 Gupta MA, Schork NJ, Gupta AK *et al.* Suicidal ideation in psoriasis. *Int J Dermatol* 1993; **33**: 188–90.
4 Gupta MA, Gupta AK. Depression and suicidal ideation in dermatology patients with acne, alopecia areata, atopic dermatitis and psoriasis. *Br J Dermatol* 1998; **139**: 846–50.
5 Denicoff KD, Lehman ZA, Rubinow DR *et al.* Suicidal ideation in Darier's disease. *J Am Acad Dermatol* 1990; **22**: 196–8.
6 Cotterill JA, Cunliffe WJ. Suicide in dermatological patients. *Br J Dermatol* 1997; **137**: 246–50.
7 Ive FA, Magnus A, Warin RP, Wilson Jones E. 'Actinic reticuloid': a chronic dermatosis associated with severe photosensitivity and the histological resemblance to lymphoma. *Br J Dermatol* 1969; **81**: 469–85.
8 King MB. *AIDS, HIV and Mental Health*. Cambridge: Cambridge University Press, 1993: 32–6.
9 Cotterill JA. Skin and the psyche. *Proc R Coll Phys Edin* 1995; **25**: 29–33.
10 Albertini RS, Phillips KA. Thirty three cases of BDD in children and adolescents. *J Am Acad Child Adolesc Psychiatry* 1999; **38**: 453–9.
11 Kellett SC, Gawkrodger DJ. The psychological and emotional impact of acne and the effect of treatment with isotretinoin. *Br J Dermatol* 1999; **140**: 273–82.
12 Marzuk PM, Tieney H, Tardiff K *et al.* Increased risk of suicide in persons with AIDS. *JAMA* 1988; **259**: 1333–7.
13 Van den Boom FMLG, Mead C, Gremmen T, Roozenburg H. AIDS, euthanasia and grief [Abstract]. Paper presented at the VIIth International Conference on AIDS, Florence, 1991; **vi**: MD 55.

Treatment of psychocutaneous disorders [1]

General management

'Disease' is a perception of ill health rather than a physical entity. The same degree of physical damage will be translated into different 'diseases' by different patients. In many patients, psoriasis does not itch; in a few it is very itchy. The condition is the same; the perception and interpretation differ so that it is necessary first to understand the language in which the disease is expressed. Once translated, the key is provided for an understanding of a patient's particular concern, and for a valid channel of therapeutic communication.

When a rapid cure is possible, there is no great problem in management. However, where a disease is of unknown origin and unpredictable duration, it is likely to assume undue proportions in the patient's thoughts. In diseases of the skin, as in other spheres of life, the unknown is feared. The spots of acne are magnified in any mirror. The patient and the dermatologist see two different images. It is the patient rather than the spots that must be treated.

Psychiatry is not an exact science. Some anxiety or depression will be felt by many of the patients seen by a dermatologist. This may be unrelated to their skin disease but often plays some part in it or occasionally is the reason for its presentation. When the anxiety is reasonable and openly expressed—fear of cancer, ignorance of prognosis, anxiety about scarring and so on—it is sufficient to reassure the patient with a clear explanation, in easily understood terms. When anxiety is obviously present but at first denied, its nature must be elicited by careful questioning. Those whose conflicts are fully repressed, but whose skin lesions, often factitious in type, leave no doubt about the cause, present the most difficult problems.

All patients with skin disease respond to a receptive and sympathetic approach. Visible illness has a particularly disturbing emotional effect; itching intensifies this. The physician must have patience, sympathy and insight into human behaviour, and must inspire the patient to talk freely. Advice should be given sparingly and without expecting it always to be taken. The dermatologist must know when a psychological situation is out of control and must recognize organic mental disease and endogenous depression as such, and seek psychiatric help.

The therapeutic effect of the physician's personality is often underrated. The stronger this is, the less necessary are drugs. Even the act of touching a patient with skin disease relieves the anxiety of those who have marked feelings of guilt and ostracism. When it is necessary to draw out the patient's emotional difficulties, the 'listening ear' is as important as the 'seeing eye'. Tones of voice, hesitancy, a temporary stammer or an unguarded or ambiguous remark may provide the key to an important emotional difficulty. Initial explanations given by a patient are often 'cover stories' and are not intended to be believed.

The first aim in management must be to determine whether any significant emotional situation is present, the second is whether the reaction is one of anxiety, depression or hysteria, and, thirdly, how environmental stresses can be reduced or the patient's frustration, guilt or aggression can be eased or rechannelled. Hidden fears can often be remedied once they are expressed; anxiety about a child, spouse or parent may lie behind apparent rudeness. Fatigue alone may provide a 'stressful situation' and the adjustment of household burdens, insistence on holidays or proper periods of rest, and the provision of 'emotional bunkers' when the situation cannot be avoided, are matters of common sense and experience of what is feasible. Feelings of guilt, 'dirtiness' and inadequacy, frequently components of a depressive state, are more difficult to dispel and may require expert help. Obsessional behaviour and phobias are also usually beyond the reach of superficial psychotherapy.

The English language is perhaps deficient in words that are not themselves emotive but can be used to describe emotional disturbances. To ask if a patient has 'any worries' is to invite a denial, which is often misleading. It may be more fruitful to ask about tiredness or depression. The manner of the reply matters more than the phrasing.

When a fuller assessment of the social and domestic situation is required, the services of a trained medical social worker are called for to extract information about family relationships and stresses and to indicate where these can be helped or eased.

The help of relatives must also often be enlisted, although their concern is not always disinterested if they are themselves part of the emotional situation. The parents of children with hair pulling or adolescents with artefacts must be approached tactfully. It is not they who have raised the cry for help, but they are often the cause of it. They may feel their honour impugned and their pride at stake. Employers, schoolteachers and rehabilitation officers can give further information or material help in particular situations. To some patients, a priest's aid is invaluable.

Three further general points have to be made. The patient may present with a dermatosis that represents only one facet of a complex psychocutaneous situation. It serves its function in expressing an emotional disturbance. If 'cured' too quickly, without attention being paid to the underlying emotional problem, the patient may develop other less accessible ills. Secondly, psychiatrists themselves are of different persuasions. Their views on aetiology and their approach to treatment differ considerably. It is well for the dermatologist to be aware of this lest the patient loses confidence by being given different explanations and advice. Finally, there is a small but important group of patients who do not want to get better [2]. They are skilled at deceiving their doctors, their spouses and their friends. They suffer from 'too good' husbands and 'too kind' doctors. Many have an histrionic personality. Once recognized, certain principles of management should be followed, even then the prognosis is not good. The patient has too much to lose by recovering.

REFERENCES

1 Sarti MG, Cossidente A. Therapy in psychosomatic dermatology. *Clin Dermatol* 1984; **2**: 255–73.
2 Sneddon J. Patients who do not want to get better. *Semin Dermatol* 1983; **2**: 183–7.

Psychotropic drugs

The use of psychotropic drugs in dermatology has become much more refined as the diagnostic criteria for the psychodermatoses has clarified. In addition, the awareness and detection of psychological accompaniments to organic skin disease, particularly depression, has presented a greater need for the dermatologist to become familiar with the use of psychotropic drugs.

The most useful are the antidepressants, both SSRIs and tricyclics. These vary in their specific activity, which can be an advantage as a sedative action may be beneficial in some circumstances, or an anticompulsion effect may be helpful. The indications for antidepressants and suggested regimens are provided in Table 61.2.

There are excellent descriptions of the use of antidepressants in dermatology [1–4]. In general, the patient should be started on a low dosage, which has the benefit of helping compliance, and then to increase the dosage over the next month to the therapeutic range. SSRIs are usually well tolerated. The effects should be evident in 4–6 weeks. If the response is slow or side effects are too intolerable, then another SSRI or tricyclic should be substituted. This should be achieved by gradually tailing the dosage of the original and building the dosage of the new drug [5–7]. SSRIs should be continued for at least 6–12 months. They should be gradually withdrawn over 2–3 months to prevent the serotonin withdrawal syndrome [6]. Sudden withdrawal can precipitate dizziness, anxiety, agitation, insomnia, flu-like symptoms, abdominal cramps and mood swings.

There has been a healthy reaction in recent years against the overuse of benzodiazepine drugs in the management of patients with psychoneurotic disorders. However, short-term therapy with anxiolytics or sedatives may be as helpful to anxious, itching patients as analgesics are to those in pain. Sedative SSRIs and tricyclics are very effective for anxiety and if additional sedation is needed hydroxyzine can be added. Sleep deprivation is common, and the restoration of a normal pattern is an adequate reason for giving hypnotics.

Table 61.2 Antidepressant drugs: usage and dosage.

Drug class	Activity	Dose (min–max)	Particular side effect
Sertraline SSRI	Depression, obsession, compulsion, BDD, panic, anxiety	50–200 mg mane	Caution hepatic/renal disease
Fluvoxamine SSRI	Depression, BDD	100–300 mg mane	Weight loss, rash, drowsiness
Citalopram SSRI	Depression	10–40 mg mane	Dry mouth
Venlafaxine SSRI, norepinephrine (noradrenaline) RI	Depression, pain syndromes	12.5–100 mg mane	Hypertension
Amitriptyline tricyclic	Depression, anxiety, pruritus, dynias	10–100 mg hs	Dry mouth, visual blurring, sedation
Clomipramine tricyclic	Depression, phobias, compulsive behaviour	25–150 mg/day	As above
Doxepin tricyclic	Depression, pruritus, anxiety	25–100 mg hs	Sedative

hs, at bedtime; mane, in the morning.
BDD, body dysmorphic disorder; RI, reuptake inhibitors; SSRIs, serotonin reuptake inhibitors.

Most dermatologists will not need to prescribe antipsychotic drugs. The primary indications for antipsychotic drugs are schizophrenia, acute mania and other psychotic states including paranoid disorders. In dermatological use, the indications for use are cutaneous delusions, dysaesthesias, pain syndromes and the compulsive self-picking disorders [2]. Drugs include pimozide, sulpiride, olanzapine and risperidone. The major disadvantages are extrapyramidal symptoms, although at low dosage there are minimal side effects.

REFERENCES

1 Gupta MA, Gupta AK. The use of antidepressant drugs in dermatology. *J Eur Acad Dermatol* 2001; **15**: 512–8.
2 Koblenzer CS. The use of psychotropic drugs in dermatology. *Dermatol Psychosom* 2001; **2**: 167–76.
3 Gupta MA, Gupta AK, Haberman HF. Psychotrophic drugs in dermatology. *J Am Acad Dermatol* 1986; **14**: 633–45.
4 Koo J, Gamba C. Psychopharmacology for dermatologic patients. *Dermatol Clin* 1996; **14**: 509–25.
5 Edwards G, Anderson I. Systematic review and guide to selection of SSRIs. *Drugs* 1999; **57**: 507–33.
6 Taylor D, McConnell H, McConnell D, Kerwin R. *The Maudsley 2001 Prescribing Guidelines*, 6th edn. London: Martin Dunitz, 2001.
7 Kent JM. New antidepressants. *Lancet* 2000; **355**: 911–8.

Hypnosis [1]

Hypnosis has always had its adherents and detractors but until recently there has been little attempt at scientific evaluation. Thus, there have been claims that hypnosis could induce inflammatory change and blisters in skin [2], and more than 30 years ago it was shown that immediate type 1 reactions, and even a Mantoux reaction, could be modified by hypnotic suggestion. The diminution in the Mantoux response was shown to be caused by a reduction in oedema rather than in the cellular response [3]. Hypnotic suggestion has been used to treat various types of ichthyosis [4–7]. It was claimed that the depth of the trance-like state could be important in determining the response to therapy, at least as far as patients with ichthyosis are concerned, and that the best results were obtained in deep-trance rather than light-trance subjects [5].

There are also many case reports detailing the response of warts to hypnosis [8–11], the most striking case being that where only half of each subject's body was treated. Disappearance of the warts on the treated side was observed while other warts on the control side remained unchanged [12].

Adults with extensive atopic dermatitis, resistant to conventional treatment, were treated with hypnotherapy with statistically significant benefit, measured both subjectively and objectively [13]. More encouragingly, the benefit was maintained at follow-up for up to 2 years. Moreover, 20 children with severe resistant atopic dermatitis were also treated by hypnosis and all but one showed immediate improvement, which was maintained subsequently. In 12 of the 20 children whose families replied to a questionnaire up to 18 months after treatment, 10 of them maintained improvement in mood. Long-term studies showed that a smaller proportion of patients with atopic dermatitis could be maintained without second-line therapy with regular hypnosis [14].

It may be that improvement with hypnosis can be achieved more by anxiety reduction and stress management than direct suggestion. Psychodermatoses such as acne excoriée, neurodermatitis and trichotillomania may all respond to hypnosis [15]. Relaxation techniques, which approximate to light hypnotic states, led to some improvement in patients with chronic urticaria, although the number of their weals did not lessen [16].

REFERENCES

1 Cotterill JA. Hypnosis in dermatology. In: Champion RH, ed. *Recent Advances in Dermatology*, Vol. 7. Edinburgh: Churchill Livingstone, 1986: 256–7.
2 Wittkower E, Russell B. *Emotional Factors in Skin Disease*. London: Cassell, 1953: 13.
3 Black S. Inhibition of the immediate type hypersensitivity by direct suggestion under hypnosis. *BMJ* 1963; **1**: 925–8.
4 Bethune HD, Kidd CD. Psychophysiological mechanisms in skin disease. *Lancet* 1961; **2**: 1419–22.

5 Kidd CD. Congenital ichthyosiform erythroderma treated by hypnosis. *Br J Dermatol* 1996; **78**: 101–5.

6 Mason AA. Ichthyosis and hypnosis. *BMJ* 1955; **2**: 57–8.

7 Winck CAS. Congenital ichthyosiform erythroderma treated by hypnosis: a report of two cases. *BMJ* 1961; **2**: 741–3.

8 French AP. Treatment of warts by hypnosis. *Am J Obstet Gynecol* 1973; **116**: 887–8.

9 Sinclair-Gieben AHC, Chalmers D. The treatment of warts by hypnosis. *Lancet* 1959; **2**: 480–2.

10 Surman OS, Gottlieb SK, Hackett TP, Silverberg BL. Hypnosis in the treatment of warts. *Arch Gen Psychiatry* 1973; **28**: 439–41.

11 Tasini MF, Hackett TP. Hypnosis and the treatment of warts in immuno-deficient children. *Am J Clin Hypn* 1977; **17**: 152–4.

12 Ullman M, Budek S. On the psyche of warts: hypnotic suggestion and warts. *Psychosom Med* 1960; **22**: 68–76.

13 Stewart AC, Thomas SE. Hypnotherapy as a treatment for atopic dermatitis in adults and children. *Br J Dermatol* 1995; **113**: 778–83.

14 Shenefelt PD. Hypnosis in dermatology. *Arch Dermatol* 2000; **136**: 393–9.

15 Shenefelt PD. Complementary psychotherapy in dermatology, hypnosis and biofeedback. *Clin Dermatol* 2001; **20**: 595–60.

16 Hertzer CL, Lookingbill DP. Effects of relaxation therapy and hypnotizability in chronic urticaria. *Arch Dermatol* 1987; **123**: 913–6.

Miscellaneous therapies

Biofeedback techniques

In recent years interest has grown in biofeedback techniques, during which patients are given visual or auditory information about the level of a particular autonomic function and then learn, through mechanisms that are not yet clear, to exercise some voluntary control over it. Biofeedback has been used for dyshidrotic eczema [1] and for hyperhidrosis [2].

Behaviour therapy

Behaviour therapy has sometimes been useful for patients who scratch repeatedly. In one study [3], parents were trained to withdraw their attentions when their child scratched; in another [4] a patient was required to monitor his own scratching and, to gain his therapist's attention, intervals without scratching were required. These therapeutic methods require regular reinforcement until autonomy has been obtained. These interactions assume that there will eventually be recognition of the patient's problem and the acceptance that there is a somatic component to the illness. The therapy can be used to reinforce positive adaptive illness responses, to extinguish maladaptive habits like excoriations, or to foster self-control over intrusive ruminative thinking (e.g. BDD) [5]. Habit reversal therapy helped a group of patients with atopic eczema [6,7].

Group therapy

Group therapy has been tried in psoriasis [8] and eczema [9]. Small groups of psoriatics met to discuss their problems with a trained fellow patient and a physician; illness behaviour, anxiety and feelings of depression all decreased. Help along similar lines can come from self-help groups

[10]. A 6-week cognitive–behavioural therapy programme as an adjunct to pharmaceutical treatments produced significant improvement in severity of psoriasis as compared to pharmaceutical treatment alone [11].

REFERENCES

1 Miller RM, Coger RW. Skin conductance conditioning with dyshidrotic eczema patients. *Br J Dermatol* 1979; **101**: 435–40.

2 Shenefelt PD. Complementary psychotherapy in dermatology, hypnosis and biofeedback. *Clin Dermatol* 2001; **20**: 595–60.

3 Allen K, Harris FR. Elimination of a child's excessive scratching by training the mother in reinforcement procedures. *Behav Res Ther* 1966; **4**: 79–84.

4 Cataldo MF, Varni JW, Russo DC et al. Behaviour therapy techniques in treatment of exfoliative dermatitis. *Arch Dermatol* 1980; **116**: 919–22.

5 Panconesi E, Gallassi F, Saltini C. Biofeedback, cognitive–behavioural methods, hypnosis alternative therapy. *Clin Dermatol* 1998; **16**: 709–26.

6 Bridgett C, Noren P, Staughton R. *Atopic Skin Disease: a Manual for Practitioners.* Petersfield: Wrightson Biomedical, 1996.

7 Noren P, Melin L. The effect of combined topical steroids and habit-reversal treatment in patients with atopic dermatitis. *Br J Dermatol* 1989; **121**: 359–66.

8 Schulte MB, Cormane RH, van Dijk E et al. Group therapy of psoriasis. *J Am Acad Dermatol* 1985; **12**: 61–6.

9 Cole CC, Roth HL, Sachs LB. Group psychotherapy as an aid in the medical treatment of eczema. *J Am Acad Dermatol* 1988; **18**: 286–9.

10 Logan RA. Self-help groups for patients with chronic skin diseases. *Br J Dermatol* 1988; **118**: 505–8.

11 Fortune DG, Richards HL, Kirby B et al. A cognitive–behavioural symptom management programme as an adjunct in psoriasis therapy. *Br J Dermatol* 2002; **146**: 458–65.

Psychiatric problems caused by dermatological treatment

It is well known that systemic glucocorticoid therapy can induce either depression or hypomania in 5% of cases. Steroid-induced psychosis is more likely with larger dosage, in females and those with systemic lupus erythematosus (SLE) or a history of affective disorder [1,2]. It is less well known that antimalarials such as chloroquine and mefloquine [3] can induce psychosis, as can dapsone [4]. Aciclovir-induced psychosis has also been described in patients with impaired renal function [5]. There is also a report of a man who applied 70% diethyltoluamide, the most common insect repellant, immediately before a sauna, and developed an acute manic psychosis after 2 weeks [6].

REFERENCES

1 Lewis DA, Smith RE. Steroid-induced psychotic syndromes: review of literature. *J Affect Disord* 1983; **5**: 319–32.

2 Wada K, Yamada N, Scott T et al. Corticosteroid-induced psychotic and mood disorders. *Psychosomatics* 2001; **42**: 461–6.

3 Evans RL, Khalid S, Kinney JL. Antimalarial psychosis revisited. *Arch Dermatol* 1984; **120**: 765–7.

4 Daneshmend TK. The neurotoxicity of dapsone: adverse drug reactions. *Acute Poisoning Rev* 1984; **3**: 53–8.

5 Thomson CR, Goodship THJ, Rodger RSC. Psychiatric side-effects of acyclovir in patients with chronic renal failure. *Lancet* 1985; **ii**: 385–6.

6 Snyder JW, Poe RO, Stubbins JF et al. Acute manic psychosis following the dermal application of N,N-diethyl-m-toluamide (DEET) in an adult. *Clin Toxicol* 1986; **24**: 429–39.

Skin disease in patients with learning disability

Mental deficiency is not a disease in its own right but a condition resulting from a variety of causes, some inborn and others acquired. As a rough guide, some 3% of the population have learning difficulties, with an IQ of below 70, but the terms 'idiot', 'imbecile' and 'moron' are now obsolete in the professional sense. The class of subjects with higher grade learning disabilities shades into that of the less intelligent members of the ordinary population [1].

The number of syndromes in which cutaneous lesions and mental deficiency may be associated is large, and many of them have been delineated only during the last few years. Although many of these genetic or developmental conditions are rare, when put together they constitute a formidable part of present day paediatrics [2]. In addition, there are a number of other skin abnormalities that seem to affect those with learning disabilities in particular.

However, the available statistics must be interpreted with caution as they relate to patients in special institutions to which admission is largely determined by social factors. The proportion of patients with disabilities of the lowest grade, and of those of any grade with associated severe physical difficulties, is likely to be higher in such institutions than in the population of those with learning difficulties as a whole. In addition, institutional life itself may influence the prevalence of skin disease by allowing the rapid spread of infections, and other conditions may be favoured by unsuspected nutritional deficiencies.

The skin abnormalities of people with learning disabilities fall into three broad groups as outlined below.

Cutaneous lesions specifically associated with syndromes of genetic or developmental origin

Many of the numerous associations of this type are dealt with in detail elsewhere. Sometimes, the nature of the defect is understood at a biochemical level (Table 61.3) and sometimes chromosomal abnormalities have been demonstrated (Table 61.4) but, in most cases, the mechanism of both the cutaneous changes and mental impairment remains obscure (Table 61.5). The severity of the

Table 61.3 Some metabolic disorders that may be associated with mental defect and skin changes.

Anginosuccinic amino aciduria	Trichorrhexis nodosa
Cretinism	Coarse, dry skin and hair
Gangliosidosis (type 1) [3]	Extensive mongolian spots
Hartnup's disease	Photosensitivity
Homocystinuria	Fine hair, livedo reticularis
Hunter's syndrome [4]	Ivory white papules
Lesch–Nyhan syndrome	Self-mutilation
Lipoid proteinosis	Skin nodules and plaques
Phenylketonuria	Eczema, long eyelashes
Menkes' syndrome	Hair defects

mental defect and of the cutaneous involvement may run more or less in parallel as in epiloia, but in most of these conditions there is no such relationship and the prevalence and severity of the mental impairment are highly variable.

Non-specific cutaneous lesions showing an increased prevalence in patients with learning disability

Moniliform hamartoma (see Chapter 15). Beaded strands of papules, mainly on the forehead and temples, develop at puberty in some patients, more often in black people than in white people.

Atypical keratosis pilaris. A symmetrical eruption of erythematous follicular papules extending from the base of the neck to the lumbar region is seen in young adults in institutions for those with learning difficulties [13]. This might represent *Pityrosporum* folliculitis.

Abnormal hair patterns [14]. The frequency of abnormal patterns of hair growth has been emphasized and is confirmed by our experience. Fusion of the eyebrows and a low frontal hairline are often seen; the latter is characteristic of those with true microcephaly but occurs in those with other learning difficulties. Hypertrichosis of the trunk or limbs is not unusual. The significance of the abnormal patterns is unknown and further surveys are required.

Atopic dermatitis. Only one patient with atopic dermatitis was found among over 200 children with learning

Table 61.4 Some conditions in which chromosomal abnormalities may be associated with mental defect and skin changes.

Down's syndrome	Ichthyosis
Familial X/Y translocation [5]	Facial hypertrichosis
Partial trisomy 2P	Scalp defect, haemangiomas
Patau's syndrome (trisomy 13)	Depigmented spots, café-au-lait patches
Ring chromosome 14 [6]	Nail hypoplasia, lymphoedema
Trisomy 18	Pre-auricular skin tags, scalp defects, flame naevi
Wolf–Hirschhorn syndrome (4P deletion)	Acne
XYY syndrome (see Chapter 12)	

Albinism	Monilethrix
Alopecia/retardation syndromes [7]	Moynahan's syndrome
Anhidrotic ectodermal dysplasia	Naevus sebaceous syndrome
Apert's syndrome	Netherton's disease
Ataxia–telangiectasia	Neurofibromatosis
Basal cell naevus syndrome	Onchotrichodysplasia with neutropenia [8]
Cockayne's syndrome	Papillon–Léage syndrome
Coffin–Siris syndrome [9]	Poikiloderma congenitale
De Sanctis–Cacchione syndrome	Richner–Hanhart syndrome [10]
Dystrophia myotonica	Rubinstein–Taybi syndrome [11]
Fanconi's anaemia	Russell–Silver dwarfism
Focal dermal hypoplasia	Sjögren–Larsson syndrome [12]
Hallermann–Streiff syndrome	Spina bifida
IBIDS syndrome [1]	Sturge–Weber syndrome
Incontinentia pigmenti	Treacher Collins' syndrome
Leprechaunism	Werner's syndrome
Marfan's syndrome	Wyburn–Mason syndrome

Table 61.5 Some other conditions in which mental defect may be associated with skin abnormalities.

IBIDS syndrome, ichthyosis, brittle hair, impaired intelligence, decreased fertility and short stature.

difficulties examined (A.J. Rook, unpublished data, 1953). Others have noticed a low prevalence of eczema [14], but atopic dermatitis is frequent in patients with Down's syndrome and phenylketonuria.

Traumatic keratoses and hypertrichosis [15]. Those with severe disabilities develop the habit of biting or chewing the forearm, hand, fingers or lips when excited or angry. Repeated biting at the same site induces thickening, hyperpigmentation and hypertrichosis. More rarely, there may be atrophic scarring, particularly on the hands. Keratoses in unusual sites may result from the repeated adoption of the same posture.

Prader–Willi syndrome is a genetic disorder that affects multiple systems and results in a cluster of behaviours including hyperphagia, emotional lability and compulsive destructive skin picking [16].

Traumatic alopecia. This is the result of a hair pulling tic. The patch selected for plucking is usually in the frontoparietal region, but may be anywhere on the scalp and even in the pubic region (A.J. Rook, unpublished data, 1953). Multiple self-mutilations including traumatic alopecia are seen in children with familial sensory neuropathy.

Crusted scabies. The crusted form of scabies [17] (see Chapter 33) is particularly frequent in those with severe learning disabilities.

Bacterial infections. Pyogenic infections accounted for 34% of patients referred from an institution for a dermatologist's opinion. The high incidence suggests low resistance to pyogenic organisms but the part played by the unhygienic habits of the patients is difficult to evaluate. Folliculitis of the thighs occurred in children and adolescents of both sexes, predominantly in males. Chronic sup-

purative hidradenitis was seen exclusively in adolescent boys. Erythrasma has a high prevalence [18].

Mycoses. Trichophyton infections are often common and refractory in those with learning difficulties. It is possible that enzyme induction by other drugs administered reduces the efficacy of griseofulvin.

Intertrigo and perleche. Genitocrural intertrigo is common in incontinent patients, especially those who are bedridden. Perleche, frequently complicated by fissuring and secondary infection, is seen in a large proportion of patients who dribble constantly.

Primary irritant dermatitis. The failure to take reasonable care in the use of disinfectants and cleansing agents is responsible for a relatively high incidence of primary irritant dermatitis in those patients who are encouraged to carry out simple domestic duties. Allergic contact dermatitis is said to be uncommon [14], perhaps because exposure to potential sensitizing agents is limited.

Drug reactions. The higher incidence of epilepsy in those with learning difficulties accounts for the relative frequency of reactions to drugs.

Non-specific cutaneous lesions, the prevalence and cause of which are not proved to differ significantly from those of the general population

There is no reliable evidence that the other common dermatoses are either more or less frequent in those with learning difficulties than in normal individuals [17]. Doubt has been cast upon the widely accepted association between epilepsy and acne [19].

REFERENCES

1 Jorizzo JL, Atherton DJ, Crounse RG *et al.* Ichthyosis, brittle hair, impaired intelligence, decreased fertility and short stature (IBIDS syndrome). *Br J Dermatol* 1982; **106**: 705–10.

2 Ousted C. Mucocutaneous syndromes. In: Salmon MA, ed. *Developmental Defects and Syndromes.* Aylesbury: HM & M, 1978.

3 Weissbluth M, Esterly NB, Caro WA. Report of an infant with GMI gangliosidosis type 1 and extensive and unusual mongolian spots. *Br J Dermatol* 1981; **104**: 195–200.

4 Prystowsky SD, Maumenee IH, Freeman RG *et al.* A cutaneous marker in the Hunter syndrome: a report of four cases. *Arch Dermatol* 1977; **113**: 602–5.

5 Metaxotou C, Ikkos D, Panagiotopoulou P *et al.* A familial X/Y translocation in a boy with ichthyosis, hypogonadism and mental retardation. *Clin Genet* 1983; **24**: 380–3.

6 Schmidt R, Eviator L, Nitowsky HM *et al.* Ring chromosome 14: a distinct clinical entity. *J Med Genet* 1981; **18**: 304–20.

7 Baraitser M, Carter CO, Brett EM. Case reports of a new alopecia/mental retardation syndrome. *J Med Genet* 1983; **20**: 64–75.

8 Hernandez A, Olivares F, Cantu JM. Autosomal recessive onychotrichodysplasia, chronic neutropenia and mild mental retardation: delineation of the syndrome. *Clin Genet* 1979; **15**: 147–52.

9 Carey JC, Hall BD. The Coffin–Siris syndrome. *Am J Dis Child* 1978; **132**: 667–71.

10 Bohnert A, Anton-Lamprecht I. Richner–Hanhart's syndrome: ultrastructural abnormalities of epidermal keratinization indicating a causal relationship to high intracellular tyrosine levels. *J Invest Dermatol* 1982; **79**: 68–74.

11 Selmanowitz VJ, Stiller MJ. Rubinstein–Taybi syndrome: cutaneous manifestations and colossal keloids. *Arch Dermatol* 1981; **117**: 504–6.

12 Jagell S, Linden S. Ichthyosis in the Sjögren–Larsson syndrome. *Clin Genet* 1982; **21**: 243–52.

13 Coombs FP, Butterworth T. Atypical keratosis pilaris. *Arch Dermatol* 1950; **62**: 305–13.

14 Butterworth T, Wilson M Jr. Incidence of disease of the skin in feebleminded persons. *Arch Dermatol Syphilol* 1938; **38**: 203–9.

15 Ressmann A, Butterworth T. Localized acquired hypertrichosis. *Arch Dermatol Syphilol* 1952; **65**: 458–63.

16 Medved M, Percy M. Prader–Willi syndrome: a literature review. *J Dev Disabil* 2001; **8**: 41–55.

17 Kidd CB, Meenan JC. The neurodermatoses and intelligence. *Br J Dermatol* 1961; **73**: 134–6.

18 Savin JA, Somerville DA, Noble WC. The bacterial flora of trichomycosis axillaris. *J Med Microbiol* 1970; **3**: 352–6.

19 Greenwood R, Fenwick PBC, Cunliffe WJ. Acne and anticonvulsants. *BMJ* 1983; **287**: 1669–70.

Chapter 62

Disorders of Nails

D.A.R. de Berker, R. Baran & R.P.R. Dawber

Introduction

The epithelial part of the nail apparatus develops *in utero* from the primitive epidermis. In generalized integumentary diseases, such as psoriasis, the nail apparatus, hair follicle and epidermis may all be structurally and functionally affected, presumably because of their common tissue of origin.

The main function of the nail apparatus is to produce a strong, relatively inflexible, keratinous nail plate over the dorsal surface of the end of each digit. The nail plate acts as a protective covering for the fingertip. By exerting counter-pressure over the volar skin and pulp, the flat nail plate allows precision and delicacy when picking up small objects and in many other subtle finger functions [1–3]. Fingernails typically cover approximately one-fifth of the dorsal surface, whereas on the great toe the nail may cover up to 50% of the dorsum of the digit.

REFERENCES

1 Baran R, Dawber RPR, de Berker DAR, Haneke E, Tosti A, eds. *Baran and Dawber's Diseases of the Nails and Their Management*, 3rd edn. Oxford: Blackwell Science, 2001.
2 Scher RK, Daniel CR, eds. *Nails: Therapy, Diagnosis, Surgery*, 2nd edn. Philadelphia: Saunders, 1997.
3 Baran R, Dawber RPR, Haneke E, Tosti A, Bristow I. *A Text Atlas of Nail Disorders. Techniques in Investigation and Diagnosis*, 3rd edn. London: Martin Dunitz, 2003.

Anatomy and biology of the nail unit

Structure

Gross anatomy [1–5]

The component parts of the nail apparatus are shown diagrammatically in Fig. 62.1. The rectangular nail plate is the largest structure, resting on and firmly attached to the nail bed; it is less adherent proximally, apart from the posterolateral corners. Approximately one-quarter of the nail is covered by the proximal nail fold, and a narrow margin of the sides of the nail plate is often occluded by the lateral nail folds. Underlying the proximal part of the nail is the white lunula (half-moon lunule); this area represents the most distal region of the matrix [6]. It is most prominent on the thumb and great toe and may be partly or completely concealed by the proximal nail fold in other digits. The reason for the white colour is not known [7–9]. The natural shape of the free margin of the nail is the same as the contour of the distal border of the lunula. The nail plate distal to the lunula usually appears pink, due to its translucency, which allows the redness of the vascular nail bed to be seen through it. The proximal nail fold has two epithelial surfaces, dorsal and ventral; at the junction of the two, the cuticle projects distally onto the nail surface. The lateral nail folds are in continuity with the skin on the sides of the digit laterally, and medially they are joined by the nail bed. Some authorities term the lateral

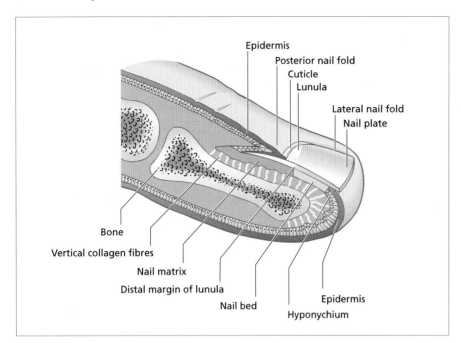

Fig. 62.1 Longitudinal section of a digit showing the dorsal nail apparatus.

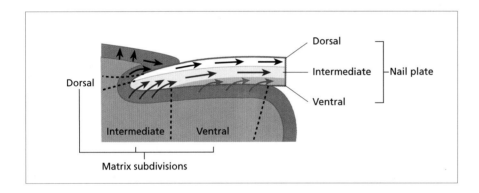

Fig. 62.2 Direction of differentiation and cell movement within the nail apparatus.

nail fold and adjacent tissue lateral to the nail fold the nail wall.

The definition of nail matrix is controversial [10]. There is common acceptance that there is a localized region beneath proximal nail which produces the major part of the normal nail plate. For those who consider this the sole source of nail it is termed simply the matrix, or germinal matrix. However, there is some evidence that other epithelial parts of the nail unit also contribute to the nail plate, and these are then also attributed matrix status. According to the histological criteria of Lewis and Montgomery [4] (Fig. 62.2), matrix can be subdivided into dorsal (ventral aspect of the proximal nail fold), intermediate (germinal matrix or matrix) and ventral (nail bed) sections. The nail bed is also termed the sterile matrix and its role in the production of nail is unclear. Although it appears that the nail plate may thicken by up to 30% as it passes from the distal margin of the lunula to the end of the nail bed [2], this is not associated with an increase in cell numbers and may represent compaction of the nail

from distal tip trauma rather than nail bed or nail plate production [11]. The situation may change in disease, where the nail bed changes its histological appearance to gain a granular layer [12] and may contribute a false nail of cornified epithelium to the undersurface of the nail [5].

At the point of separation of the nail plate from the nail bed, the proximal part of the hyponychium may be modified as the *solehorn* [13]. This is a central thickened structure with a dermal core. It is usually found on the toes of elderly people, where there are often associated vascular abnormalities. Beyond the solehorn region, the hyponychium terminates at the distal nail groove; the tip of the digit beyond this ridge assumes the structure of the epidermis elsewhere.

When the attached nail plate is viewed from above, two distinct areas may be visible: the proximal lunula and the larger pink zone. On close examination, two further distal zones can often be identified: the distal yellowish-white margin and immediately proximal to this the onychodermal band [14]. Terry describes this as a barely perceptible, narrow, transverse band 0.5–1.5 mm wide and more prominent in acrocyanosis. The exact anatomical basis for the onychodermal band is not known, but it appears to have a blood supply different from the main body of the nail bed; if the tip of the finger is pressed firmly, the band and an area just proximal to it blanch, and if the pressure is repeated several times the band reddens. Many changes in colour have been described in the onychodermal band in health and disease [13]. Histologically, it is defined as the most distal attachment of cornified epithelium to the undersurface of the nail. As such, it is structurally significant for the adherence of nail plate to the nail bed. Once breached, as in conditions such as psoriasis, separation of the nail bed from the nail plate can be progressive.

Microscopic anatomy [15]

Nail folds

The proximal nail folds are similar in structure to the adjacent skin but are normally devoid of dermatoglyphic markings and pilosebaceous glands. There is a normal granular layer. From the distal area of the proximal nail folds the cuticle adheres to the upper surface of the nail plate; it is composed of modified stratum corneum and serves to protect the structures at the base of the nail, particularly the germinal matrix, from environmental insults such as irritants, allergens and bacterial and fungal pathogens.

Nail matrix (intermediate matrix)

Nail matrix produces the nail plate in the absence of disease (Fig. 62.2). The basal compartment of the matrix is broader than the same region in normal epithelium or in other parts of the nail unit, such as the nail bed [10]. There is no granular layer, and cells differentiate with the expression of trichocyte 'hard' keratin as they become incorporated into the nail plate, alongside normal epithelial keratins [16,17]. During this process, they may retain their nuclei until more distal in the nail plate. These retained nuclei are called *pertinax bodies*. Apart from this, the detailed cytological changes seen in the matrix epithelium under the electron microscope are essentially the same as in the epidermis [18,19].

The nail matrix contains melanocytes in the lowest three cell layers and these donate pigment to the keratinocytes. The presence of 6.5 melanocytes per millimetre of matrix basement membrane can be used as a guide to a normal matrix melanocyte population [20]. The appearance of melanocytes separate from the basement membrane distinguishes them from those found in the nail folds, which are primarily basal [21]. Matrix melanocytes are further distinguished from those elsewhere by their failure to produce melanin in normal circumstances in white people.

This can change, with melanotic streaks presenting in local inflammatory, naevoid or neoplastic disease. In non-white people, brown streaks are common and are almost universal in Afro-Caribbeans by the age of 60 years.

Langerhans' cells are detectable in the matrix by CD1a staining, and the matrix appears to contain basement membrane components indistinguishable from normal skin [22].

Nail bed

Nail bed consists of epidermis with underlying connective tissue closely apposed to the periosteum of the distal phalanx. There is no subcutaneous fat in the nail bed, although scattered dermal fat cells may be visible microscopically.

The nail bed epidermis is usually no more than two or three cells thick, although there may be tongues of epithelium that extend obliquely down. The transitional zone from living keratinocyte to dead ventral nail plate cell is abrupt, occurring in the space of one horizontal cell layer; in this regard it closely resembles the Henle layer of the internal root sheath of the epidermis [23]. Nail bed cells do not have any independent movement, and it is yet to be clearly demonstrated whether they are incorporated into an overlying nail plate as it grows distally [24]. The process of nail bed keratinization has been likened to that seen in rat-tail epidermis, possibly being affected by pressure changes. The loss of the overlying nail results in the development of a granular layer, which is otherwise present only in disease states [12,25,26].

The nail bed dermal collagen is mainly orientated vertically, being directly attached to the phalangeal periosteum and the epidermal basal lamina. Within the connective tissue network lie blood vessels, lymphatics, a fine network of elastic fibres and scattered fat cells; at the distal margin, eccrine sweat glands have been seen [1].

Nail plate

The nail plate comprises three horizontal layers: a thin dorsal lamina, the thicker intermediate lamina and a ventral layer from the nail bed [4]. This is not always apparent with normal light microscopy using routine stains, where the nail demonstrates a transition between flattened cells dorsally and thicker cells on the ventral aspect. Electron microscopy shows squamous cells with tortuous interlocking plasma membranes [18,19]. At high magnification, the contents of each cell show a uniform fine granularity similar to the hair cuticle [23].

The nail plate contains significant amounts of phospholipid, mainly in the dorsal and intermediate layers, which contribute to its flexibility. The detectable free fats and long-chain fatty acids may be of extrinsic origin. For further details of these and other histochemical changes in the components of the nail apparatus, the reader is referred to more detailed texts [8,27].

The nail plate is rich in calcium, found as the phosphate in hydroxyapatite crystals; it is bound to phospholipids intracellularly [28]. The relevance of other metals (copper, manganese, zinc, iron and others), which are present in smaller amounts, is not known [25]. Calcium is present in a concentration of 0.1% by weight, 10 times greater than its concentration in hair. It is possible that calcium is not an intrinsic part of the nail but is incorporated from extrinsic sources. Calcium does not significantly contribute to the hardness of the nail [6].

Nail keratin

Nail keratin analysis shows essentially the same fractions as in hair:

1 fibrillar, low-sulphur protein;
2 globular, high-sulphur matrix protein;
3 high glycine–tyrosine-rich matrix protein.

Amino acid analysis shows higher cysteine, glutamic acid and serine and less tyrosine in nail compared with hair and wool [17,29].

An alternative classification of keratins defines them as 'soft' epithelial keratins or 'hard' trichocyte keratins. The latter are characteristic of hair and nail differentiation, where their high sulphur content is probably responsible for their rugged physical qualities. This is matched by the resistance of trichocyte keratins to dissolution in strong solvent.

Trichocyte and epithelial keratins are intermediate filaments representing the major cytoskeletal protein of epithelial cells. They share the normal classification into type I or type II based on gene hybridization, which reflects segregation on two-dimensional electrophoresis into acidic and basic proteins. Each acidic keratin is expressed in a tissue with a corresponding basic keratin to form specific heterodimers, which are assembled into higher-order protofibrils and protofilaments.

Keratin distribution in the nail and associated epithelium has been studied in adult [16,30], infant [17] and embryonic [31,32] digits. Immunohistochemistry of the epithelial structures of normal nail demonstrates that the suprabasal keratin pair K1/K10 is found on both aspects of the proximal nail fold and to a lesser degree in the matrix. However, it is absent from the nail bed. This is reversed when there is nail bed disease, such as onychomycosis or psoriasis, where a granular layer develops and K1/K10 becomes expressed at corresponding sites [23]. The nail bed contains keratin synthesized in normal basal layer epithelium, K5/K14, which is also found in nail matrix. An antibody marking the epitope characteristically associated with keratin expressed in the basal layer is found throughout the thickness of the nail bed, but only basally in the matrix [26].

Recent examination of the nail bed using monospecific monoclonal antibodies to the keratin pair K6/K16 demonstrates these proteins in the nail bed but not the germinal matrix [16]. This is paradoxical given our understanding that K6/K16 is characteristic of psoriasis and wound healing, where proliferation is a prominent feature. It has been shown that the nail bed has very low rates of proliferation [10,33], and it may be that K6/K16 more precisely illustrates a loss of differentiation, often associated with proliferation in skin but representing the resting state of nail bed epithelium.

The location of K6/K16 is reflected in the localization of the features of pachyonychia congenita. In this group of autosomal dominant disorders, there is thickening of the nail plate attributed to disease of the nail bed. In some forms of pachyonychia congenita, there is a missense mutation of the initiation peptide of K16 [34].

Trichocyte keratins can also be detected immunohistochemically within the epithelial structures of the nail unit. A monospecific antibody to Ha-1 has been created and characterized on nail, hair and skin. In the nail, it demonstrates a well-demarcated suprabasal region corresponding to the matrix [16]. Proximally, it does not extend onto the ventral aspect of the proximal nail fold, sometimes described as the dorsal matrix. Distally, the keratin expression is limited to a margin taken as corresponding to the lunula. Ha-1 is only one of at least 10 trichocyte keratins, but quantitatively it probably represents a large fraction of nail keratin. According to its distribution it appears to define a matrix consistent with the classic description of the germinal matrix.

Improved understanding of the distribution of keratins in the nail bed and matrix has accompanied further understanding of the molecular basis of pachyonychia congenita, where the various nail manifestations correlate with mutations within the keratin genes and corresponding phenotypes [35].

REFERENCES

1 Gonzalez-Serva A. The normal nail: structure and function. In: Scher RK, Daniel CR, eds. *Nails: Therapy, Diagnosis, Surgery*. Philadelphia: Saunders, 1990: 11–30.
2 Johnson M, Comaish JS, Shuster S. Nail is produced by the normal nail bed: a controversy resolved. *Br J Dermatol* 1991; **125**: 27–9.
3 Lewin K. The normal fingernail. *Br J Dermatol* 1965; **77**: 421–4.
4 Lewis BL, Montgomery H. The senile nail. *J Invest Dermatol* 1955; **24**: 11–8.
5 Samman PD. Anatomy and physiology. In: Samman PD, Fenton D, eds. *The Nails in Disease*. London: Heinemann, 1986: 1–20.
6 Cohen PR. The lunula. *J Am Acad Dermatol* 1996; **34**: 943–53.
7 Achten G. L'ongle normal et pathologique. *Dermatologica* 1963; **126**: 229–34.
8 Dawber RPR, de Berker D, Baran R. Science of the nail apparatus. In: Baran R, Dawber RPR, eds. *Diseases of the Nails and Their Management*, 2nd edn. Oxford: Blackwell Science, 1994: 1–34.
9 Burrows MT. The significance of the lunula of the nail. *Johns Hopkins Hosp Rep* 1919; **18**: 357–61.
10 de Berker D, Angus B. Markers of epidermal proliferation are limited to nail matrix in normal nail. *Br J Dermatol* 1996; **135**: 555–9.
11 de Berker DAR, MaWhinney B, Sviland L. Quantification of regional matrix nail production. *Br J Dermatol* 1996; **134**: 1083–6.

12 Fanti PA, Tosti A, Cameli N, Varotti C. Nail matrix hypergranulosis. *Am J Dermatopathol* 1994; **16**: 607–10.
13 Pinkus F. In: Jadassohn J, ed. *Handbuch der Haut und Geschlechtskrankheiten*. Berlin: Springer, 1927: 267–89.
14 Terry RB. The onychodermal band in health and disease. *Lancet* 1955; i: 179–81.
15 Lewis BL. Microscopic studies of foetal and mature nail and surrounding soft tissue. *Arch Dermatol* 1954; **70**: 732–6.
16 de Berker D, Wojnarowska F, Sviland L *et al*. Keratin expression in the normal nail unit: markers of regional differentiation. *Br J Dermatol* 2000; **142**: 89–96.
17 Westgate GE, Tidman N, de Berker D *et al*. Characterization of LHTric-1, a new monospecific monoclonal antibody to the trichocyte keratin Ha1. *Br J Dermatol* 1997; **137**: 24–30.
18 Hashimoto K. Ultrastructure of the human toenail. 1. Proximal nail matrix. *J Invest Dermatol* 1971; **56**: 235–46.
19 Hashimoto K. Ultrastructure of the human toenail. *Ultrastruct Res* 1971; **36**: 391–410.
20 Tosti A, Cameli N, Piraccini BM *et al*. Characterisation of nail matrix melanocytes with anti-PEP1, anti-PEP8, TMH-1 and HMB-45 antibodies. *J Am Acad Dermatol* 1994; **31**: 193–6.
21 de Berker D, Graham A, Dawber RPR, Thody A. Melanocytes are absent from the normal nail bed: the basis of a clinical dictum. *Br J Dermatol* 1996; **134**: 564.
22 Sinclair RD, Wojnarowska F, Leigh IM, Dawber RPR. The basement membrane zone of the nail. *Br J Dermatol* 1994; **131**: 499–505.
23 Achten G. L'ongle normal. *J Med Esth Chir Dermatol* 1988; **XV**: 193–200.
24 Zaias N. The movement of the nail bed. *J Invest Dermatol* 1967; **48**: 402–3.
25 Zaias N. *The Nail in Health and Disease*. New York: Spectrum Press, 1990: 6–7.
26 de Berker D, Sviland L, Angus BA. Suprabasal keratin expression in the nail bed: a marker of dystrophic nail bed differentiation. *Br J Dermatol* 1995; **133** (Suppl. 45): 16.
27 Sayag J, Jancovici E. Physiologie de l'ongle. In: Meynadier J, ed. *Précis de Physiologie Cutané*. Paris: Editions de le Porte Verte, 1980: 121–3.
28 Cane AK, Spearman RIC. A histochemical study of keratinisation in the domestic fowl. *J Zool* 1967; **153**: 337–44.
29 Baden HP, Goldsmith LA, Flemming BC. A comparative study of the physicochemical properties of human keratinised tissue. *Biochim Biophys Acta* 1973; **322**: 269–78.
30 Haneke E. The human nail matrix: flow cytometric and immuno-histochemical studies. In: *Clinical Dermatology in the Year 2000*. London: Book of Abstracts, 1990.
31 Heid WH, Moll I, Franke WW. Patterns of expression of trichocytic and epithelial cytokeratins in mammalian tissues. II. Concomitant and mutually exclusive synthesis of trichocytic and epithelial cytokeratins in diverse human and bovine tissues. *Differentiation* 1988; **37**: 215–30.
32 Moll I, Heid HW, Franke WW, Moll R. Patterns of expression of trichocytic and epithelial cytokeratins in mammalian tissues. *Differentiation* 1988; **39**: 167–84.
33 Zaias N, Alvarez J. The formation of the primate nail plate. An autoradiographic study in the squirrel monkey. *J Invest Dermatol* 1968; **51**: 120–36.
34 McLean WHI, Rugg EL, Lunny DP *et al*. Keratin 16 and keratin 17 mutations cause pachyonychia congenita. *Nat Genet* 1995; **9**: 273–8.
35 Irvine AD, McLean WH. Human keratin diseases: the increasing spectrum of disease and subtlety of the phenotype–genotype correlation. *Br J Dermatol* 1999; **140**: 815–28.

Development and comparative anatomy [1–3]

The nail apparatus develops and matures from the primitive epidermis between the ninth and 20th weeks of intrauterine growth. At 20 weeks, the matrix cells show postnatal-type cell division, differentiation and keratinization, and the nail plate begins to form and move distally [4,5]; the nail bed loses its granular layer at this stage [6]. By 36 weeks, the complete nail plate reaches the tip of the digit and is surrounded by prominent lateral nail folds and a well-formed cuticle.

The structure of claws and hooves and their evolutionary relationship to humans has been well reviewed [2,3,7]. In higher primates, nails have evolved with the acquisition of manual dexterity; other mammals do not possess such flattened claws from which nails have evolved. Claws and talons are harder than human nails, probably because of their high content of calcium phosphate as crystalline hydroxyapatite within keratinized cells compared with human nails [8]. The hard 'soft plate' under hooves is produced from an area equivalent to the subungual part of the claw. In some animals, cloven hooves have only developed on the 'digits' that touch the ground; in horses, the single large hoof is produced from the third digit. The keratin biochemistry of the human nail has many similarities to that of the anteater or pangolin [6,9].

REFERENCES

1 Breathnach AS. *An Atlas of the Ultrastructure of Human Skin*. London: Churchill Livingstone, 1971.
2 Moore K. *The Developing Human*, 4th edn. Philadelphia: Saunders, 1988.
3 Spearman RIC. The physiology of the nail. In: Jarrett A, ed. *The Physiology and Pathophysiology of the Skin*, Vol. 5. New York: Academic Press, 1978: 1827–41.
4 Zaias N. Embryology of the human nail. *Arch Dermatol* 1963; **87**: 37–42.
5 Zaias N. *The Nail in Health and Disease*. New York: Spectrum Press, 1990.
6 Baden HP, Kubilus J. A comparative study of the immunologic properties of hoof and nail fibrous proteins. *J Invest Dermatol* 1984; **83**: 327–31.
7 Hamrick MW. Development and evolution of the mammalian limb: adaptive diversification of nails, hooves, and claws. *Evol Dev* 2001; **3**: 355–63.
8 Chapman RE. Hair, wool, quill, nail, claw, hoof, horn. In: Bereiter Hahn J, Matoltsy AG, Richards KS, eds. *Biology of the Integument*, Vol. 2. Berlin: Springer, 1986.
9 Spearman RIC. On the nature of the horny scales of the pangolin. *J Linn Soc Zool* 1967; **46**: 267–9.

Blood supply [1]

There is a rich arterial blood supply to the nail bed and matrix derived from paired digital arteries, a large palmar and small dorsal digital artery on either side. The palmar arteries are supplied from the large superficial and deep palmar arcades [2]. The main supply passes into the pulp space of the distal phalanx before reaching the dorsum of the digit (Fig. 62.3). Distally, the arteries are extremely tortuous and coiled, which allows them to be distorted without kinking to occlude supply. An accessory supply arises further back on the digit and does not enter the pulp space [3]. There are two main arterial arches (proximal and distal) supplying the nail bed and matrix, formed from anastomoses of the branches of the digital arteries. In the event of damage to the main supply in the pulp space, such as may occur with infection or scleroderma, there may be sufficient blood from the accessory vessels to permit normal growth of the nail.

There is a capillary loop system to the whole of the nail fold but the loops to the roof and matrix are flatter than those below the exposed nail [4]. The loops run longitudinally in the axis of splinter haemorrhages. Those in the nail bed are longest [5]. There are many arteriovenous

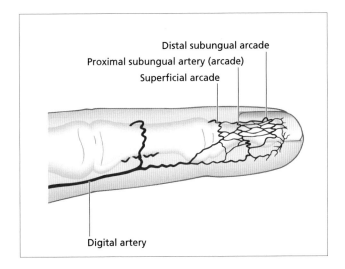

Fig. 62.3 Arterial supply of the distal finger.

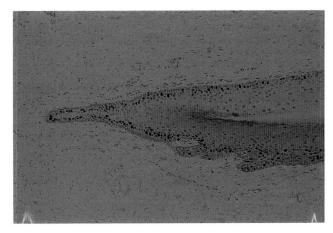

Fig. 62.4 Proliferating epithelial cells of the matrix and ventral aspect of the proximal nail fold, staining with the antibody MIB-1.

anastomoses beneath the nail—glomus bodies—which are concerned with heat regulation. Glomus bodies are important in maintaining acral circulation under cold conditions: arterioles constrict with cold but glomus bodies dilate [6]. These occupy the subdermal tissues and increase in number in a gradient towards the distal nail bed [7].

REFERENCES

1 Dawber RPR, de Berker DAR, Baran R. Science of the nail apparatus. In: Baran R, Dawber RPR, de Berker DAR, Haneke E, Tosti A, eds. *Diseases of the Nails and Their Management*, 3rd edn. Oxford: Blackwell Science, 2001: 1–47.
2 Smith DO, Oura C, Kimura C, Toshimuri K. Arterial anatomy and tortuosity in the distal finger. *J Hand Surg* 1991; **16A**: 297–302.
3 Flint MH. Some observations on the vascular supply of the nail bed and terminal segments of the finger. *Br J Plast Surg* 1955; **8**: 186–94.
4 Samman PD. The human toenail. Its genesis and blood supply. *Br J Dermatol* 1959; **71**: 296–301.
5 Hasegawa K, Pereira BP, Pho RW. The microvasculature of the nail bed, nail matrix, and nail fold of a normal human fingertip. *J Hand Surg* 2001; **26A**: 283–90.
6 Ryan TJ. The arteriovenous anastomoses. In: Jarrett A, ed. *The Physiology and Pathophysiology of the Skin*, Vol. 2. London: Academic Press, 1973: 612–4.
7 Wolfram-Gabel R, Sick H. Vascular networks of the periphery of the fingernail. *J Hand Surg* 1995; **20B**: 488–92.

Nail growth and morphology

Clinicians used to observing the slow rate of growth of diseased or damaged nails are apt to view the nail apparatus as inert, although it is biochemically and kinetically active throughout life. In this respect, it differs from the hair follicle, which undergoes periods of quiescence as part of the follicular cycle.

Cell kinetics

The kinetic activity of the matrix has been examined using many techniques. These include immunohistochemistry, autoradiography and direct measurement of matrix product (i.e. nail plate) by ultrasound [1], micrometer or histology.

There is a broad basal compartment of proliferating cells in the matrix, which can be detected immunohistochemically with antibodies to proliferating cell nuclear antigen and Ki-67 (Fig. 62.4); both antigens are associated with proliferating cells [2]. The matrix is also the site of maximal inclusion of tritiated thymidine if injected into the peritoneum of squirrel monkeys and followed subsequently by autoradiography [3]. Although there was some inclusion of thymidine into the nail bed, Zaias and Alvarez interpreted the findings as indicating that the nail bed had no role in creation of the nail plate. Norton [4] drew a similar conclusion from work with live human subjects where labelled thymidine and glycine were injected locally to act as markers of proliferating and metabolically active keratinocytes, and both primarily labelled the matrix.

However, the earlier work of Lewis [5] suggested on histological grounds that the nail plate is a trilaminar structure originating from three separate matrix zones: the dorsal matrix (ventral aspect of proximal nail fold), intermediate matrix (germinal matrix) and ventral matrix (nail bed). In support of this, Johnson *et al.* [6,7] demonstrated that 21% of the nail thickness is gained as it passes over the nail bed, implying that the nail bed is generating this fraction of the nail plate. De Berker *et al.* [2] noted that the increase in nail thickness did not coincide with corresponding increases of nail plate cells. This challenges the interpretation that nail thickens over the nail bed through the contribution from underlying structures. An alternative explanation may be appropriate, such as compaction arising through repetitive distal trauma. Others have also debated this issue [8], and although the nail bed may have a significant contribution to make in disease [9], the evidence for its contribution at other times is conflicting.

Table 62.1 Physiological and environmental factors affecting the rate of nail growth.

Faster	Slower
Daytime	Night
Pregnancy [25]	First day of life [14]
Right-hand nails	Left-hand nails [28,29]
Youth, increasing age	Old age [18,23,30]
Fingers	Toes [31]
Summer [18]	Winter or cold environment [32,33]
Middle, ring and index fingers	Thumb and little finger [28,31,34,35]
Male gender	Female gender [27,35]
Minor trauma/nail biting [26,27]	

Table 62.2 Pathological factors affecting the rate of nail growth.

Faster	Slower
Psoriasis [36]	Finger immobilization [41]
Normal nails [23]	
Pitting	
Onycholysis [37]	
Pityriasis rubra pilaris [21,38]	Fever [42]
	Beau's lines [43]
Etretinate, rarely [39]	Methotrexate [24], azathioprine [24], etretinate [39]
Idiopathic onycholysis of women [37]	Denervation [44]
Bullous ichthyosiform erythroderma [13]	Poor nutrition
	Kwashiorkor [45]
Hyperthyroidism [28]	Hypothyroidism [28]
Levodopa [40]	Yellow nail syndrome [13]
Arteriovenous shunts [28]	Relapsing polychondritis [46]

Nail morphology

Why the nail grows flat, rather than as a heaped-up keratinous mass, has generated much thought and discussion [10–14]. Several factors probably combine to produce a relatively flat nail plate: the orientation of the matrix rete pegs and papillae; the direction of cell differentiation [15]; and moulding of the direction of nail growth between the proximal nail fold and distal phalanx [16]. Containment laterally within the lateral nail folds assists this orientation, and the adherent nature of the nail bed is likely to be important. In diseases such as psoriasis, the nail bed can lose its adherent properties, exhibiting onycholysis. In addition, there may be subungual hyperkeratosis. These combined factors make psoriasis the most common pathology in which up-growing nails are seen. Onychogryphosis is characterized by upward growth of thickened nail. In this condition, the nail matrix may become bucket-shaped and the effect of the overlying proximal nail fold is lost.

Linear nail growth [17–19]

Over the last century, many studies have been carried out on the linear growth of the nail plate in health and disease; these have been reviewed [20,21] and are listed in Tables 62.1 and 62.2 [22]. Most of these studies have been performed by observing the distal movement of a reference mark etched on the nail plate over a fixed period of time; this may well correlate with matrix germinative cell kinetics but there is no direct proof that it does. However, studies on nail growth in psoriasis, and its inhibition by cytostatic drugs [23,24], suggest that cell kinetics and linear growth rate do have a direct correlation.

Fingernails grow approximately 1 cm every 3 months and toenails at one-third of this rate.

REFERENCES

1 Finlay AY, Moseley H, Duggan TC. Ultrasound transmission time: an *in vivo* guide to nail thickness. *Br J Dermatol* 1987; **117**: 765–70.
2 de Berker D, MaWhinney B, Sviland L. Quantification of regional matrix nail production. *Br J Dermatol* 1996; **134**: 1083–6.
3 Zaias N, Alvarez J. The formation of the primate nail plate. An autoradiographic study in squirrel monkeys. *J Invest Dermatol* 1968; **51**: 120–36.
4 Norton LA. Incorporation of thymidine ^{3}H and glycine-2 ^{3}H in the nail matrix and bed of humans. *J Invest Dermatol* 1971; **56**: 61–8.
5 Lewis BL. Microscopic studies of foetal and mature nail and surrounding soft tissue. *Arch Dermatol* 1954; **70**: 732–7.
6 Johnson M, Comaish JS, Shuster S. Nail is produced by the normal bed: a controversy resolved. *Br J Dermatol* 1991; **125**: 27–9.
7 Johnson M, Shuster S. Continuous formation of nail along the bed. *Br J Dermatol* 1993; **128**: 277–80.
8 Pinkus F. In: Jasassohn J, eds. *Handbuch der Haut und Geschlechtskrankheiten.* Berlin: Springer, 1927: 267–89.
9 Samman PD. The ventral nail. *Arch Dermatol* 1961; **84**: 192–5.
10 Baran R. Nail growth direction revisited. Why do nails grow out instead of up? *J Am Acad Dermatol* 1981; **4**: 78–84.
11 Kligman AM. Nail growth direction revisited. Why do nails grow out instead of up? Response. *J Am Acad Dermatol* 1981; **4**: 78–84.
12 Kligman AM. Why do nails grow out instead of up? *Arch Dermatol* 1961; **84**: 181–3.
13 Samman PD. *The Nails in Disease*, 3rd edn. London: Heinemann, 1978: 14.

14 Schmiegelow P, Lindner J, Puschmann M. Autoradiographische Quantifizierung dosisabhängiger 35S CystinbZW. *Aktuelle Dermatol* 1983; **2**: 62.

15 Hashimoto K. Ultrastructure of the human toenail. *Arch Dermatol Forsch* 1971; **240**: 1–22.

16 Kelikian H. *Congenital Deformities of the Hand and the Forearm*. Philadelphia: Saunders, 1974: 210–2.

17 Baran R, Dawber RPR, eds. *Guide Médico-Chirurgical des Onychopathies*. Paris: Arnette, 1990: 12.

18 Bean WB. Nail growth: 30 years of observations. *Arch Intern Med* 1974; **134**: 497–502.

19 Dawber R, Baran R. Nail growth. *Cutis* 1987; **39**: 99–102.

20 Dawber RPR, de Berker D, Baran R. Science of the nail apparatus. In: Baran R, Dawber RPR, eds. *Diseases of the Nails and Their Management*, 2nd edn. Oxford: Blackwell Science, 1994: 1–34.

21 Runne U, Orfanos CE. The human nail. *Curr Probl Dermatol* 1981; **9**: 102–49.

22 de Doncker P, Pierard GE. Acquired nail beading in patients receiving itraconazole: an indicator of faster nail growth? A study using optical profilometry. *Clin Exp Dermatol* 1994; **19**: 404–6.

23 Dawber RPR. Fingernail growth in normal and psoriatic subjects. *Br J Dermatol* 1970; **82**: 454–7.

24 Dawber RPR. The effect of methotrexate, corticosteroids and azathioprine on fingernail growth in psoriasis. *Br J Dermatol* 1970; **83**: 680–8.

25 Hewitt D, Hillman RW. Relation between rate of nail growth in pregnant women and estimated previous general growth rate. *Am J Clin Nutr* 1966; **19**: 436–9.

26 Gilchrist ML, Buxton LHD. The relation of fingernail growth to nutritional status. *J Anat* 1939; **73**: 575–81.

27 Hamilton JB, Tereda H, Mestler GE. Studies of growth throughout the lifespan in Japanese. *Gerontology* 1955; **10**: 401–10.

28 Orentreich N, Markofsky J, Vogelman JH. The effect of ageing on the rate of linear nail growth. *J Invest Dermatol* 1979; **73**: 126–30.

29 Pfister R. Das normale Onychodiagramm. *Z Haut Geschlechtskr* 1955; **18**: 132–7.

30 Lavelle CE. Nail growth. *Curr Probl Dermatol* 1981; **9**: 102–4.

31 Pfister R, Henera J. Wachstum und Gestaltung der Zehennagel bei Gesunden. *Arch Klin Exp Dermatol* 1965; **223**: 263–74.

32 Donovan KM. Antarctic environment and nail growth. *Br J Dermatol* 1977; **96**: 507–10.

33 Roberts DF, Sandford MR. A possible climatic effect on nail growth. *Appl Physiol* 1958; **13**: 135–7.

34 Knobloch VH. Das normale Wachstum der Fingernagel. *Dtsch Med Wochenschr* 1953; **78**: 743–5.

35 Le Gros-Clark WE, Buxton LHD. Studies in nail growth. *Br J Dermatol* 1938; **50**: 221–9.

36 Landherr G, Braun-Falco O, Hofmann C *et al*. Fingernagel Wachstum bei Psoriatitern unter PUVA-Therapie. *Hautarzt* 1982; **33**: 210–3.

37 Dawber RPR, Samman PD, Bottoms E. Fingernail growth in idiopathic and psoriatic onycholysis. *Br J Dermatol* 1971; **85**: 558–67.

38 Dawber RPR. The ultrastructure and growth of human nails. *Arch Dermatol Res* 1980; **269**: 197–204.

39 Baran R. Action thérapeutique et complications du rétinoïd aromatique sur l'appareil unguéal. *Ann Dermatol Vénéréol* 1982; **109**: 367–70.

40 Miller E. Levodopa and nail growth. *N Engl J Med* 1973; **288**: 916–9.

41 Dawber RPR. Effects of immobilisation on fingernail growth. *Clin Exp Dermatol* 1981; **6**: 1–4.

42 Sibinger MS. Observations on growth of fingernails in health and disease. *Pediatrics* 1959; **24**: 225–33.

43 Weismann K. Beau and his description of transverse depressions on nails. *Br J Dermatol* 1977; **97**: 571–2.

44 Head H, Sherrin J. The consequence of injury to peripheral nerves in man. *Brain* 1905; **28**: 116–8.

45 Babcock MJ. Methods of measuring fingernail growth in nutritional studies. *J Nutr* 1955; **55**: 323–38.

46 Estes SA. Relapsing polychondritis. *Cutis* 1983; **32**: 471–6.

Nails in childhood and old age

Childhood [1]

In early childhood, the nail plate is relatively thin and may show temporary koilonychia. This is particularly promin-

ent on the great toes. Under the age of 5 years, nails are also prone to terminal onychoschizia (lamellar splitting). This can be most prominent on the sucked thumb, but is also seen on the toes. Sucking may also lead to paronychia, which can be a troublesome condition in childhood, with pain and nail dystrophy. Ingrowing can also cause pain and may present in different forms. At birth, there is often a degree of distal ingrowing, particularly in the great toe, as the nail has not surmounted the tip of the digit in its development [2]. In a more gross form, this may present as congenital hypertrophic lip of the hallux, where soft-tissue overgrowth may resemble fibrous tumours of the digit before spontaneously disappearing [3]. Painful distal embedding can lead to infection, but as long as the toenail is properly orientated with respect to the underlying phalanx, the condition usually subsides. In one series of seven children, two needed surgery due to painful persistence of the problem [4]. The changes associated with congenital malalignment of the great toe may also subside within 5–10 years in about 50% of children. In this condition, there is deviation of the tip of the great toe nail laterally, rotating on the distal phalanx. The nail is yellow, triangular, thickened and has transverse ridges [5].

Fungal infection is relatively uncommon in children, with a prevalence of 0.44% in one study [6].

Beau's lines can be seen in up to 92% of normal infants between 8 and 9 weeks of age [7]. One child demonstrated a transverse depression through the whole nail thickness on all 20 digits [8]. Normal surface markings of the nail can differ in children from those seen in adults. A herringbone pattern is common and gradually diminishes with time [9], which may reflect a gradual change in the pattern of matrix maturation.

Old age

Many of the changes seen in old age may occur in younger age groups in association with impaired arterial blood supply. Elastic tissue changes diffusely affecting the nail bed epidermis are often seen histologically [10]; these changes may be due to the effects of UV radiation, although it has been stated that the nail plate is an efficient filter of UVB radiation [11]. The whole subungual area in old age may show thickening of blood vessel walls with vascular elastic tissue fragmentation. Pertinax bodies are often seen in the nail plate. Nail growth is inversely proportional to age [12]; related to this slower growth, corneocytes are larger in old age [13].

The nail plate becomes paler, dull and opaque with advancing years, and white nails similar to those seen in cirrhosis, uraemia and hypoalbuminaemia may be seen in normal subjects. Longitudinal ridging is present to some degree in most people after 50 years of age and this may give a 'sausage links' or beaded appearance.

For details of the common traumatic abnormalities and

changes due to inadequate pedicure or neglect, detailed texts should be consulted [1,12].

REFERENCES

1 Baran R, Barth J, Dawber RPR, eds. *Nail Disorders*. London: Dunitz, 1991: 78–101.
2 Tosti A, Peluso AM, Piraccini BM. Nail diseases in children. *Adv Dermatol* 1997; **13**: 353–73.
3 Hammerton MD, Shrank AB. Congenital hypertrophy of the lateral nail folds of the hallux. *Pediatr Dermatol* 1988; **5**: 243–5.
4 Piraccini BM, Parente GL, Varotti E, Tosti A. Congenital hypertrophy of the lateral nail folds of the hallux: clinical features and follow-up of seven cases. *Pediatr Dermatol* 2000; **17**: 348–51.
5 Baran R. Congenital malalignment of the toe nail. *Arch Dermatol* 1980; **116**: 1346.
6 Gupta AK, Sibbald RG, Lynde CW *et al*. Onychomycosis in children: prevalence and treatment strategies. *J Am Acad Dermatol* 1997; **36**: 395–402.
7 Turano AF. Beau's lines in infancy. *Pediatrics* 1968; **41**: 996–4.
8 Wolf D. Beau's lines in childhood. *Cutis* 1982; **29**: 191–4.
9 Parry EJ, Morley WN, Dawber RPR. Herringbone nails: an uncommon variant of nail growth in childhood. *Br J Dermatol* 1995; **132**: 1021–2.
10 Baran R. Nail care in the 'golden years' of life. *Curr Med Res Opin* 1982; **7**: 96–101.
11 Parker SG, Diffey BL. The transmission of optical radiation through human nails. *Br J Dermatol* 1983; **108**: 11–4.
12 Brauer E, Baran R. Cosmetics: the care and adornment of the nail. In: Baran R, Dawber RPR, de Berker DAR, Haneke E, Tosti A, eds. *Diseases of the Nails and Their Management*, 3rd edn. Oxford: Blackwell Science, 2001: 366–8.
13 Germann H, Barran W, Plewig G. Morphology of corneocytes from human nail plates. *J Invest Dermatol* 1980; **74**: 115–8.

Nail signs and systemic disease

It is important for clinicians to understand and accurately describe nail findings if they are to communicate accurately with their colleagues and avoid the vagueness that often surrounds nail pathology. Signs fall into categories of shape, surface and colour.

Abnormalities of shape

Clubbing

In clubbing there is increased transverse and longitudinal nail curvature with hypertrophy of the soft-tissue components of the digit pulp. Hyperplasia of the fibrovascular tissue at the base of the nail allows the nail to be 'rocked' and in causes associated with cardiopulmonary disease there may be local cyanosis.

There are three forms of geometric assessment that can be performed. *Lovibond's angle* is found at the junction between the nail plate and the proximal nail fold, and is normally less than 160°. This is altered to over 180° in clubbing (Fig. 62.5). *Curth's angle* at the distal interphalangeal joint is normally about 180°. This is diminished to less than 160° in clubbing (Fig. 62.6). *Schamroth's window* is seen when the dorsal aspects of two fingers from opposite hands are apposed, revealing a window of light, bordered laterally by the Lovibond angles. As this angle is obliterated in clubbing, the window closes [1]. Assessment of

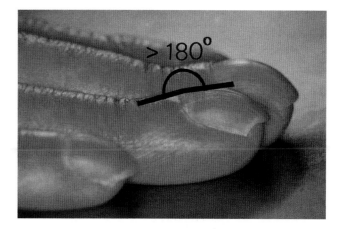

Fig. 62.5 Clubbing: Lovibond's profile sign. The angle is normally less than 160° but exceeds 180° in clubbing.

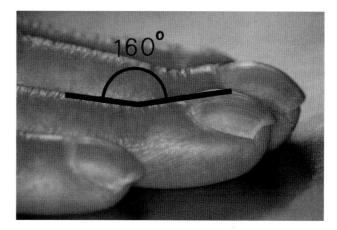

Fig. 62.6 Clubbing: Curth's modified profile sign.

clubbing at the bedside shows poor agreement between examiners [2] in milder cases and there are problems in firm morphometric analysis that do not lend themselves to routine clinical solutions [3].

Clubbing appears to be related more to increased blood flow through the vasodilated plexus of nail unit vasculature than to vessel hyperplasia. Altered vagal tone and microvascular infarcts have been implicated [4,5].

Pathological associations of clubbing include inflammatory bowel disease, carcinoma of the bronchus and cirrhosis. In forms associated with bronchiectasis or neoplasm, prominent inflammatory joint signs may also be seen, resulting in hypertrophic pulmonary osteoarthropathy. It has also been reported as a common finding in hemiplegic limbs [6] and can be a presenting feature of a subungual tumour when in a single digit [7]. In some cases of bronchiectasis, a variant of clubbing, *shell nail syndrome*, can be seen. This is distinguished from clubbing by the presence of atrophy of underlying bone and nail bed [8] and may have more in common with yellow nail syndrome than with clubbing.

REFERENCES

1 Lampe RM, Kagan A. Detection of clubbing: Schamroth's sign. *Clin Pediatr* 1983; **22**: 125.
2 Myers KA, Farquhar DR. The rational clinical examination. Does this patient have clubbing? *JAMA* 2001; **286**: 341–7.
3 Goyal S, Griffiths AD, Omarouayache S, Mohammedi R. An improved method of studying fingernail morphometry: application to the early detection of fingernail clubbing. *J Am Acad Dermatol* 1998; **39**: 640–2.
4 Currie AE, Gallagher PJ. The pathology of clubbing: vascular changes in the nail bed. *Br J Dis Chest* 1988; **82**: 382–5.
5 Silveri F, Carlino G, Cervini C. The endothelium/platelet unit in hypertrophic osteoarthropathy. *Clin Exp Rheumatol* 1992; **10** (Suppl. 7): 61–6.
6 Siragusa M, Schepis C, Cosentino FI *et al.* Nail pathology in patients with hemiplegia. *Br J Dermatol* 2001; **144**: 557–60.
7 Baran R, Perrin C. Subungual perineurioma: a peculiar location. *Br J Dermatol* 2002; **146**: 125–8.
8 Cornelius CE, Shelley WB. Shell nail syndrome associated with bronchiectasis. *Arch Dermatol* 1967; **96**: 694–5.

Koilonychia

In koilonychia (Greek: *koilos*, hollow; *onyx*, nail), there is reverse curvature in the transverse and longitudinal axes giving a concave dorsal aspect to the nail [1]. Fingers and toes may be affected, with signs most prominent in the thumb or great toe. The nail may be thickened, thinned, softened or unchanged in quality. Koilonychia is common in infancy as a benign feature of the great toenail, although in some infants its persistence may be associated with a deficiency of cysteine-rich keratin [2] in trichothiodystrophy. The most common systemic association is with iron deficiency [3] and haemochromatosis, although the majority of adults with koilonychia demonstrate a familial pattern which may be autosomal dominant [4]. In dermatoses such as psoriasis and dermatophyte infection, nail bed hyperkeratosis may push the nail up distally to produce a spoon-shaped nail. In mechanics, softening of the nail with oil may be a factor [5], and in hairdressers, permanent wave solutions may be causal [6].

REFERENCES

1 Stone OJ. Spoon nails and clubbing: significance and mechanisms. *Cutis* 1975; **16**: 235–41.
2 Jalili MA, Al-Kassab S. Koilonychia and cystine content of nails. *Lancet* 1959; **ii**: 108–10.
3 Hogan GR, Jones B. The relationship of koilonychia and iron deficiency in infants. *J Pediatr* 1970; **77**: 1054.
4 Bergeron JR, Stone OJ. Koilonychia. A report of familial spoon nails. *Arch Dermatol* 1967; **95**: 351.
5 Dawber RPR. Occupational koilonychia. *Br J Dermatol* 1974; **91** (Suppl. 10): 11.
6 Alanko K, Kanerva L, Estlander T *et al.* Hairdresser's koilonychia. *Am J Contact Dermatitis* 1997; **8**: 177–8.

Pincer nail

SYN. INVOLUTED OR TRUMPET NAIL

Pincer nail describes a dystrophy where nail growth is pitched towards the midline, combined with increased transverse curvature. Although the changes in matrix geometry may only be slight, their effect is amplified by longitudinal growth of the nail such that the free edge may take on the shape of the apex of a cone in extreme cases. Pain may arise due to embedding of the pincer nail in the lateral nail folds and nail bed, which becomes most pronounced distally. Thumbs and great toes are the most commonly affected digits, with a gradient of involvement to more lateral digits. It occurs in several patterns [1–3]. It is seen as an isolated familial abnormality that usually becomes manifest in adulthood. It is also seen in association with psoriasis. Isolated digits may be affected as a result of trauma, degenerative joint changes or a subungual tumour that is displacing the nail upwards in the midline. Rarely, single associations with unusual presentations are reported [4–6].

Assessment should include imaging. Treatment is usually by surgery to relieve the pain. In toes it is usually best to perform a lateral ablation of the most embedded margin. This will sometimes lead to a shift of the nail such that the other side no longer embeds. If both sides require ablation, the dimensions of the toenail may mean that it is better to ablate the entire matrix rather than to leave a central zone of nail. The alternative of corrective surgery in toes has only a modest chance of success and ablation may ultimately be required as a definitive procedure. When treating the thumbs or fingers, the chance of success with corrective surgery is higher and the cosmetic and functional handicap of ablation may not be acceptable. Again, a lateral ablation may be adequate, but more complex procedures entail altering the alignment of the matrix [2,7,8] and addressing any midline hypertrophy of the distal phalanx. Some surgeons advocate a combination of reconstruction and ablation [9]. Nail braces rarely produce long-term benefit.

REFERENCES

1 Baran R, Haneke E, Richert B. Pincer nails: definition and surgical treatment. *Dermatol Surg* 2001; **27**: 261–6.
2 Haneke E. Ingrown and pincer nails: evaluation and treatment. *Dermatol Ther* 2002; **15**: 148–58.
3 Mimouni D, Ben-Amitai D. Hereditary pincer nail. *Cutis* 2002; **69**: 51–3.
4 Hwang SM, Lee SH, Ahn SK. Pincer nail deformity and pseudo-Kaposi's sarcoma: complications of an artificial arteriovenous fistula for haemodialysis. *Br J Dermatol* 1999; **141**: 1129–32.
5 Vanderhooft SL, Vanderhooft JE. Pincer nail deformity after Kawasaki's disease. *J Am Acad Dermatol* 1999; **41**: 341–2.
6 Jemec GB, Thomsen K. Pincer nails and alopecia as markers of gastrointestinal malignancy. *J Dermatol* 1997; **24**: 479–81.
7 Plusje LG. Pincer nails: a new surgical treatment. *Dermatol Surg* 2001; **27**: 41–3.
8 Brown RE, Zook EG, Williams J. Correction of pincer-nail deformity using dermal grafting. *Plast Reconstr Surg* 2000; **105**: 1658–61.
9 Aksakal AB, Akar A, Erbil H, Onder M. A new surgical therapeutic approach to pincer nail deformity. *Dermatol Surg* 2001; **27**: 55–7.

Macronychia and micronychia

Macronychia and micronychia are conditions where a nail is considered too large or too small in comparison with

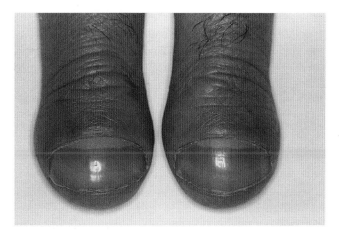

Fig. 62.7 Racket nail associated with clubbing.

other nails on nearby digits. The nail disorder is usually associated with an abnormal digit, arising from underlying bony abnormalities such as local gigantism causing macronychia or megadactyly [1]. This is also the basis of racket thumb (Fig. 62.7), the most common form of benign, dominantly inherited macronychia. Plexiform neurofibromas may cause nail changes, and duplication of the terminal phalanges may cause bifid or small nails [2].

REFERENCES

1 Barsky AJ. Macrodactyly. *J Bone Joint Surg* 1967; **49**: 1255–6.
2 Millman AJ, Strier RP. Congenital onychodysplasia of the index fingers. *J Am Acad Dermatol* 1982; **7**: 57–65.

Anonychia

Anonychia is absence of all or part of one or several nails [1]. The term implies a permanent state, which can be congenital and associated with underlying bony changes [2]. If there is residual nail matrix, there may be some vestigial nail or hyperkeratosis. Temporary anonychia may arise from onychomadesis (nail loss) associated with transient local or systemic upset. If local, the appearance of the nail unit may reflect the precipitating cause.

REFERENCES

1 Solammadivi SV. Simple anonychia. *South Med J* 1981; **74**: 1555.
2 Baran R, Juhlin L. Bone dependent nail formation. *Br J Dermatol* 1986; **114**: 371–5.

Abnormalities of nail attachment

Nail shedding

Nails can be lost through different mechanisms.
1 Complete loss of the nail plate due to proximal nail separation extending distally [1] is called onychomadesis and

is a progression of profound Beau's lines. This may reflect local or systemic disease and in the latter may result in temporary loss of all nails.
2 Local dermatoses such as the bullous disorders and paronychia may cause nail loss. Generalized dermatoses may be manifest, for example toxic epidermal necrolysis (TEN) and severe/rapid onset of pustular psoriasis. Scarring of the nail unit is seen in lichen planus and following TEN, which may both provoke nail loss.
3 Trauma is a common cause of recurrent loss and may reflect the nature of the activity, such as football, or some underlying abnormality of footwear [2] or pedal mechanics. It is often associated with subungual haemorrhage [3]. In the long term, athletes often develop thickened dystrophic nails matching a history of recurrent shedding.
4 Temporary loss has also been described due to retinoids [4], and large doses of cloxacillin and cephaloridine during the treatment of two anephric patients [5].
5 Onychoptosis defluvium or alopecia unguium describes atraumatic, familial, non-inflammatory nail loss [6]. It may be periodic and associated with dental amelogenesis imperfecta.
6 Nail shedding can be part of an inherited structural defect, most obviously in epidermolysis bullosa [7], although at times the diagnosis may be occult [8].

REFERENCES

1 Runne U, Orfanos CE. The human nail. *Curr Probl Dermatol* 1981; **9**: 102–49.
2 Almeyda J. Platform nails. *BMJ* 1973; **i**: 176.
3 Baran R, Barth J, Dawber RPR. *Nail Disorders*. London: Dunitz, 1991: 84–8.
4 Baran R. Retinoids and the nails. *J Dermatol Treat* 1990; **1**: 151–4.
5 Eastwood JB, Curtin JR, Smith EKM *et al.* Shedding of the nails apparently induced by large amounts of cephaloridine and cloxacillin in 2 anephric patients. *Br J Dermatol* 1969; **81**: 750–2.
6 Oliver WJ. Recurrent onychoptosis occurring as a family disorder. *Br J Dermatol* 1927; **26**: 59–68.
7 Bruckner-Tuderman L, Schnyder UW, Baran R. Nail changes in epidermolysis bullosa: clinical and pathogenetic considerations. *Br J Dermatol* 1995; **132**: 339–44.
8 Dharma B, Moss C, McGrath JA, Mellerio JE, Ilchyshyn A. Dominant dystrophic epidermolysis bullosa presenting as familial nail dystrophy. *Clin Exp Dermatol* 2001; **26**: 93–6.

Onycholysis

Onycholysis is the distal and/or lateral separation of the nail from the nail bed [1,2]. Psoriatic onycholysis can be considered the reference point for other forms of onycholysis where it is typically distal, with variable lateral involvement. Areas of separation appear white or yellow due to air beneath the nail and sequestered debris, shed squames and glycoprotein exudate. Isolated islands of onycholysis present as 'oily spots' or 'salmon patches' in the nail bed. At the border of onycholysis, the nail bed is usually reddish-brown, reflecting the underlying psoriatic inflammatory changes. All the common causes are associated with diminished adherence of nail to nail bed

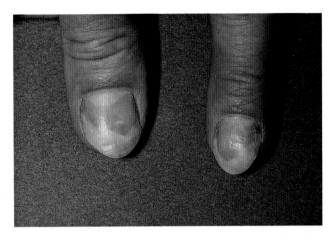

Fig. 62.8 Onycholysis: idiopathic type.

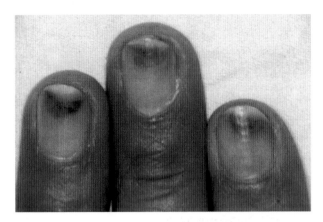

Fig. 62.9 Photo-onycholysis with a uniform pattern of discoloured onycholysis in the midline.

as a primary (idiopathic) or secondary event and include trauma, fungal infection, eczema and photo-onycholysis [3].

Idiopathic onycholysis

This is a painless separation of the nail from its bed, which occurs without apparent cause. Overzealous manicure, frequent wetting and cosmetic 'solvents' may be the cause but may not be admitted by the patient. There may, however, be a minor traumatic element, as the condition occurs rather more often in persons who keep their nails abnormally long. Maceration with water may also be a factor [3]. It must be distinguished from other causes of onycholysis (see below). The affected nails grow very quickly [4].

The condition usually starts at the tip of one or more nails and extends to involve the distal third of the nail bed (Fig. 62.8). Persistent manicure is attempted to remove the debris which accumulates within the onycholytic space, and this can result in a crescentic margin of onycholysis matching the onychocorneal band and appearing similar in all involved digits. Pain occurs only if there is further extension as a result of trauma or if active infection supervenes. More often there is microbial colonization of a mixed nature, including *Candida albicans* and several bacteria, of which *Pseudomonas pyocyanea* is the most common. If the condition persists for several months, the nail bed becomes dark and irregularly thickened.

The condition is mostly seen in women and many cases return to normal after a few months. The longer it lasts, the less likely is the nail to become reattached, due to keratinization of the exposed nail bed.

Treatment [5]. The patient should be advised to cut away as much as possible of the loosened nail and to apply a topical steroid preparation containing antibiotics and nystatin (e.g. Tri-Adcortyl cream) to the nail bed two or three

times a day, or to use miconazole/hydrocortisone cream twice a day [1]. Reattachment is slow, and the loosened nail should be recut several times if necessary. The object of treatment is to prevent infection becoming established beneath the loosened nail, because this leads to thickening of the nail bed and prevents reattachment. Some authorities still recommend 4% thymol in chloroform (not available in the USA) as a means of preventing infection and further maceration of the nail bed [6]; however, 2% thymol is often as strong as the patient can tolerate and is usually effective. Where antimicrobial therapy is needed for *Pseudomonas*, gentamicin eye drops can be useful. Drying under the onycholytic nails with a hair dryer has been advocated in order to desiccate the environment in which *Pseudomonas* would otherwise grow.

Secondary onycholysis

There are many other causes of onycholysis, which is one of the commonest nail signs [5,7–9]. Psoriasis, fungal infections and dermatitis are common causes; congenital ectodermal defect is a rare one. Onycholysis occurs in general medical conditions, including impaired peripheral circulation, hypothyroidism [10], hyperthyroidism [11], hyperhidrosis, yellow nail syndrome and shell nail syndrome. Minor trauma is a common cause, and many occupational cases are due to trauma [6,12]. Immersion of the hands in soap and water may be considered traumatic, as also may the use of certain nail cosmetics. It has also been described after the application of 5% 5-fluorouracil to the fingertips [13]. There is a condition of hereditary partial onycholysis associated with hard nails [14]. Photo-onycholysis (Fig. 62.9) may occur during treatment with psoralens, demethylchlortetracycline and doxycycline [15,16], and rarely other antibiotics. This is sometimes associated with cutaneous photosensitivity (see Chapter 24). Drugs such as retinoids [17] and cancer chemotherapy [18] can also be implicated.

REFERENCES

1 Ray L. Onycholysis: a classification and study. *Arch Dermatol* 1963; **88**: 181–5.
2 Taft EH. Onycholysis: a clinical review. *Australas J Dermatol* 1968; **2**: 345–51.
3 Baran R, Juhlin L. Drug-induced photo-onycholysis. Three subtypes identified in a study of 15 cases. *J Am Acad Dermatol* 1987; **17**: 1012–6.
4 Dawber RPR, Samman PD, Bottoms E. Fingernail growth in idiopathic and psoriatic onycholysis. *Br J Dermatol* 1971; **85**: 558–60.
5 Wilson JW. Paronychia and onycholysis: aetiology and therapy. *Arch Dermatol* 1965; **92**: 726–30.
6 Forck G, Kastner N. Onycholysis. *Hautarzt* 1967; **18**: 85–8.
7 Baran R, Barth J, Dawber RPR. *Nail Disorders.* London: Dunitz, 1991: 69–73.
8 Baran R, Dawber RPR. Physical signs. In: Baran R, Dawber RPR, eds. *Diseases of the Nails and Their Management.* Oxford: Blackwell Science, 1994: 58.
9 Kechijian P. Onycholysis of the fingernails: evaluation and management. *J Am Acad Dermatol* 1985; **12**: 552–60.
10 Fox EC. Diseases of the nails: report of cases of onycholysis. *Arch Dermatol Syphilol* 1940; **44**: 426–8.
11 Luria MN, Asper SP. Onycholysis in hyperthyroidism. *Ann Intern Med* 1958; **42**: 102–8.
12 Heinmann H, Silverberg MG. Onycholysis in fur workers. *Arch Dermatol Syphilol* 1941; **44**: 426–8.
13 Shelley WB. Onycholysis due to 5-fluorouracil. *Acta Derm Venereol (Stockh)* 1972; **52**: 320–2.
14 Schultz HD. Hereditary partial onycholysis and hard nails. *Dermatol Wochenschr* 1966; **152**: 766–8.
15 Franks SB, Coton HJ, Mirkin W. Photo-onycholysis due to tetracycline. *Arch Dermatol* 1971; **103**: 520.
16 Baran R, Juhlin L. Photoonycholysis. *Photodermatol Photoimmunol Photomed* 2002; **18**: 202–7.
17 Onder M, Oztas MO, Oztas P. Isotretinoin-induced nail fragility and onycholysis. *J Dermatol Treat* 2001; **12**: 115–6.
18 Chen GY, Chen YH, Hsu MM, Tsao CJ, Chen WC. Onychomadesis and onycholysis associated with capecitabine. *Br J Dermatol* 2001; **145**: 521–2.

Pterygium [1]

The term 'pterygium' describes the winged appearance achieved when a central fibrotic band divides a nail proximally in two. However, the fibrotic tissue may not always grossly alter the nail and can extend from the lateral nail fold as well as the more typical proximal nail fold. A large pterygium may destroy the whole nail.

An inflammatory destructive process precedes pterygium formation. There is fusion between the nail fold and underlying nail bed. The fibrotic band then obstructs normal nail growth. Superficial abnormal vessels may be seen and there are no skin markings. It most typically develops in trauma or lichen planus and its variants, including idiopathic atrophy of the nail [2] and graft-versus-host disease [3]. It can also occur in leprosy, where it may represent scarring secondary to neuropathic damage and secondary purulent infection [4].

REFERENCES

1 Richert BJ, Patki A, Baran RL. Pterygium of the nail. *Cutis* 2000; **66**: 343–6.
2 Samman PD. Idiopathic atrophy of the nails. *Br J Dermatol* 1969; **81**: 746–9.
3 Little BJ, Cowan MA. Lichen planus-like eruption and nail changes in a patient with graft-versus-host disease. *Br J Dermatol* 1990; **122**: 841–3.
4 Patki AH, Mehta JM. Pterygium unguis in a patient with recurrent type 2 lepra reaction. *Cutis* 1989; **44**: 311–2.

Ventral pterygium [1]

Ventral pterygium or pterygium inversum unguis [2] occurs on the distal undersurface of the nail, with forward extension of the nail bed epithelium dislocating the hyponychium and obscuring the distal groove. Causes include trauma, systemic sclerosis [2,3], Raynaud's phenomenon, lupus erythematosus, familial [4] and infective [5]. The overlying nail may be normal, but adjacent soft tissues can be painful.

REFERENCES

1 Drake L. Pterygium inversum unguis. *Arch Dermatol* 1976; **112**: 255–6.
2 Caputo R, Cappio F, Rigoni C *et al.* Pterygium inversum unguis. Report of 19 cases and review of the literature. *Arch Dermatol* 1993; **129**: 1307–9.
3 Patterson JW. Pterygium inversum unguis-like changes in scleroderma. *Arch Dermatol* 1977; **113**: 1429–30.
4 Amblard P, Reymond JL. Familial subungual pterygium. *Ann Dermatol Vénéréol* 1980; **107**: 949–50.
5 Patki AH. Pterygium inversum unguis in a patient with leprosy. *Arch Dermatol* 1990; **126**: 1110.

Subungual hyperkeratosis

Subungual hyperkeratosis entails hyperkeratosis of the nail bed and hyponychium and may occur in a range of conditions, including those where the primary diagnosis is not clear. Nail plate changes are variable, but thickening is common. Dry, white or yellow hyperkeratosis may crumble away from the overhanging nail. Hyperkeratosis may extend onto the digit pulp. Features of onychomycosis and wart virus infection (mainly toes) or psoriasis, pityriasis rubra pilaris and eczema (mainly fingers) may be found elsewhere to determine the aetiology.

The nail bed is an epithelium of low proliferative turnover. Any disease process that affects it is likely to result in an excess of squamous debris. The overlying nail prevents simple loss. The initial outcome is compaction of debris into layers of subungual hyperkeratosis. The only route of loss is by emerging distally with the growing nail.

Focal subungual keratoses are seen with Darier's disease, and keratotic debris beneath the nail in Norwegian (crusted) scabies may contain mites and eggs.

Nail thickening

Isolated thickening of the nail is associated with yellow discoloration as the nail bed vasculature is obscured. Common causes include psoriasis, eczema, trauma and onychomycosis, some of which may be associated with subungual hyperkeratosis. The shape of the nail may alter depending on the underlying cause, such as in yellow nail syndrome, where there is increased curvature in the longitudinal and transverse axes.

In the elderly and yellow nail syndrome, retarded longitudinal growth of the toenail is compensated for by increased thickness [1]. Yellow nail may also develop where the nail bed produces abnormal nail [2]. Onychogryphosis describes thickened nails, usually the great toenail, which commonly grow upwards in a spiral. It is attributed to chronic distorting trauma and can be treated surgically or by conservative methods. These include trimming with an electric drill, chemical destruction with 40% urea paste, phenolization of the matrix to achieve total ablation (phenol time reduced to 2 min) or carbon dioxide laser.

REFERENCES

1 Higashi N, Matsumura T. The aetiology of onychogryphosis of the great toe nail and of ingrowing nail. *Hifu* 1988; **30**: 620–3.
2 Schönfeld PH. The pachyonychia congenita syndrome. *Acta Derm Venereol (Stockh)* 1980; **60**: 45–9.

Changes in nail surface

Longitudinal grooves

Longitudinal grooves may run all or part of the length of the nail in the longitudinal axis, and need to be distinguished from ridges which are proud of the nail surface [1]. Grooves may be full or partial thickness.

The median canaliform dystrophy of Heller [2] is the most distinctive form [3]. The nail is split, usually in the midline, with a fir-tree-like appearance of ridges angled backwards. The thumbs are most commonly affected and the involvement may be symmetrical. The cuticle may be normal, as distinct from the cuticle in habit tic deformity (washboard nails). After a period of months or years the nails often return to normal, but relapse may occur [4] and a ridge may replace the original defect. Some patients give a definite history of trauma [1], or the disorder can be attributed to oral retinoids [5]. Familial cases have been recorded. Sutton [6] described involvement of a toenail in which a flabby filament of fleshy tissue was present in the canal. Treatment is unnecessary, although the patient should be advised to apply an emollient cream to the nail fold.

Physiological furrows and ridges are accentuated in lichen planus, rheumatoid arthritis, peripheral vascular disease, old age and Darier's disease. *Onychorrhexis* may occur where there are superficial grooves in the nail that lead to a distal split.

Tumours (warts, myxoid cysts) pressing on the matrix, or a proximal nail fold pterygium, may produce a longitudinal groove.

REFERENCES

1 Ronchese F. Peculiar nail anomalies. *Arch Dermatol* 1951; **63**: 565–9.
2 Heller J. Dystrophia unguium mediana canaliformis. *Dermatol Z* 1928; **51**: 416–7.

3 Zelger J, Wohlfarth P, Putz R. Dystrophia unguium mediana canaliformis Heller. *Hautarzt* 1974; **25**: 629.
4 Sweet RD. Dystrophia unguium mediana canaliformis. *Arch Dermatol Syphilol* 1951; **64**: 61–2.
5 Bottomley W, Cunliffe W. Median canaliform dystrophy associated with isotretinoin therapy. *Br J Dermatol* 1992; **127**: 447.
6 Sutton RJ Jr. Solenonychia: canaliform dystrophy of the nails. *South Med J* 1965; **58**: 1143–6.

Transverse grooves and Beau's lines [1]

Transverse grooves may be full or partial thickness through the nail. When they are endogenous they have an arcuate margin matching the lunula. If exogenous, such as those due to manicure, the margin may match the proximal nail fold and the grooves may be multiple as in washboard nails associated with a habit tic [2,3]. When multiple, it may be difficult to distinguish a habit tic from psoriasis. Transverse grooves may occur on isolated diseased digits (trauma, inflammation or neurological events) or may be generalized, reflecting a systemic event such as coronary thrombosis, measles, mumps or pneumonia. If endogenous, they are usually referred to as *Beau's lines* [4,5]. They arise through temporary interference with nail formation and become visible on the nail surface (Fig. 62.10) some weeks after the precipitant. The distance of the groove from the nail fold is related to the time since the onset of growth disturbance. The depth and width of the groove may be related to the severity and duration of disturbance, respectively. In many cases, grooves are seen on all 20 nails but are most prominent on the thumb and great toenail, and are deeper in the midline of the nail. Full-thickness grooves can be associated with distal extension

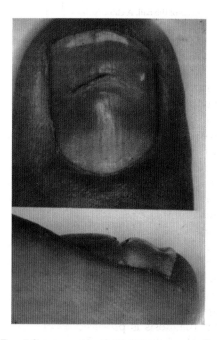

Fig. 62.10 Beau's lines present as transverse grooves in the nail matching the proximal margin of the nail matrix and lunula.

of the plane of separation of the nail plate. This can lead to nail loss, termed *onychomadesis*.

REFERENCES

1 Runne V, Orfanos CE. The human nail. *Curr Probl Dermatol* 1981; **9**: 102–49.
2 de Berker DAR. What is a Beau's line? *Int J Dermatol* 1994; **33**: 545–6.
3 Macaulay WL. Transverse ridging of the thumbnails. *Arch Dermatol* 1966; **93**: 421–3.
4 Beau JHS. Note sur certain caractères de séméiologie rétrospective présentés par les ongles. *Arch Gén Méd* 1846; **11**: 447–9.
5 Weismann K. Lines of Beau: possible markers of zinc deficiency. *Acta Derm Venereol (Stockh)* 1977; **57**: 88–90.

Pitting

Pitting presents as punctate erosions in the nail surface. Individual pits may be shallow or deep, with a regular or irregular outline. The individual pits of psoriasis are said to be less regular in form and in overall pattern than those of alopecia areata, but this is not always the case. When numerous, they appear randomly distributed upon the nail surface or have a geometric pattern. The latter may cause rippling or create a grid of pits. Extensive pitting combined with other surface irregularities results in the appearance of *trachyonychia*. An isolated large pit may produce a localized full-thickness defect in the nail plate termed *elkonyxis*, which is found in Reiter's disease, psoriasis and following trauma.

Histologically, pits represent foci of parakeratosis, reflecting isolated nail malformation [1].

REFERENCE

1 Zaias N. Psoriasis of the nail. A clinicopathologic study. *Arch Dermatol* 1969; **99**: 567–79.

Trachyonychia

Trachyonychia presents as a rough surface affecting all of the nail plate and up to 20 nails (20-nail dystrophy) [1]. The original French term was 'sand-blasted nails', which evokes the main clinical feature of a grey roughened surface (Fig. 62.11). It is mainly associated with alopecia areata [2], psoriasis and lichen planus, although the most common presentation is as an isolated nail abnormality. In the isolated form, histology shows spongiosis and a lymphocytic infiltrate [3] of the nail matrix. It may present as a self-limiting condition in childhood or as a more chronic problem in adulthood. There is some response to potent topical, locally injected and systemic steroids, but this may be temporary. Topical 5-fluorouracil has also been used to good effect [4], although it is important to be wary of associated onycholysis where the diagnosis is psoriasis, as onycholysis can be exacerbated by 5-fluorouracil. Childhood forms normally resolve spontaneously.

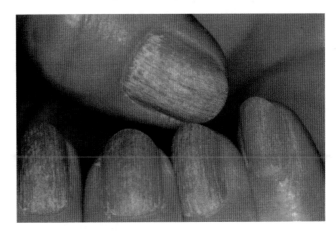

Fig. 62.11 Trachyonychia: roughened surface of up to 20 nails.

REFERENCES

1 Samman PD. Trachyonychia (rough nails). *Br J Dermatol* 1979; **101**: 701–5.
2 Baran R. Twenty nail dystrophy of alopecia areata (letter). *Arch Dermatol* 1981; **117**: 1.
3 Tosti A, Fanti PA, Morelli R *et al*. Spongiotic trachyonychia. *Arch Dermatol* 1991; **127**: 584–5.
4 Schissel DJ, Elston DM. Topical 5-fluorouracil treatment for psoriatic trachyonychia. *Cutis* 1998; **62**: 27–8.

Onychoschizia

Onychoschizia is also known as lamellar dystrophy and is characterized by transverse splitting into layers at or near the free edge (Fig. 62.12) in fingers and toes, especially in infants [1]. This can result in discoloration because of sequestration of debris between the layers.

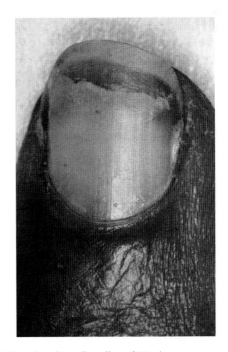

Fig. 62.12 Onychoschizia (lamellar splitting).

Variants include splitting at the lateral margins alone and multiple crenellated splits at the free edge. It is seldom associated with any systemic disorder, although it has been reported with polycythaemia [2], human immunodeficiency virus (HIV) infection [3] and glucagonoma [4].

Scanning electron microscopy illustrates the tendency of the lamellar structure of nail to separate after repeated immersion in water [5], although case–control studies show that occupation is not a major determinant of the condition [6]. However, efforts at retaining hydration (gloves, emollient and base coat with nail varnish) may help reverse clinical changes. Biotin has been used as systemic therapy, but the evidence for its efficacy is weak [7].

REFERENCES

1 Scher RK. Brittle nails. *Int J Dermatol* 1989; **28**: 515–6.
2 Graham-Brown RAC, Holmes R. Lamellar nail dystrophy with polycythaemia. *Clin Exp Dermatol* 1980; **5**: 209–12.
3 Cribier B, Mena ML, Rey D *et al*. Nail changes in patients infected with human immunodeficiency virus. A prospective controlled study. *Arch Dermatol* 1998; **134**: 1216–20.
4 Chao SC, Lee JY. Brittle nails and dyspareunia as first clues to recurrences of malignant glucagonoma. *Br J Dermatol* 2002; **146**: 1071–4.
5 Wallis MS, Bowen WR, Guin JR. Pathogenesis of onychoschizia (lamellar dystrophy). *J Am Acad Dermatol* 1991; **24**: 44–8.
6 Lubach D, Beckers P. Wet working conditions increase brittleness of nails but do not cause it. *Dermatology* 1992; **185**: 120–2.
7 Colombo VE, Gerber F, Bronhofer M *et al*. Treatment of brittle fingernails and onychoschizia with biotin: scanning electron microscopy. *J Am Acad Dermatol* 1990; **23**: 1127–32.

Brittle nails

Brittle nails [1–3] are often associated with onychoschizia and frequent immersion of the hands in water, especially if alkaline. Treatment is the same as for onychoschizia. Other common causes are iron deficiency anaemia and impaired peripheral circulation. A rare cause is disturbance of arginine metabolism, when it is also associated with diffuse alopecia [4].

REFERENCES

1 Baran R, Barth J, Dawber RPR. *Nail Disorders*. London: Dunitz, 1991: 137–44.
2 Kechijian P. Brittle fingernails. *Dermatol Clin* 1985; **3**: 421–9.
3 Scher RK. Brittle nails. *Int J Dermatol* 1989; **28**: 515–6.
4 Shelley WB, Rawnsley HM. Aminogenic alopecia: loss of hair associated with arginosuccinic aciduria. *Lancet* 1965; **ii**: 1327–8.

Beading and ridging

Beading and ridging have been described as occurring more often than normal in patients with rheumatoid arthritis [1]. More recently, increased beading has been examined using optical profilometry in patients taking itraconazole for onychomycosis [2]. Itraconazole is known to increase the rate of nail growth, and it was proposed that beading may be a feature of this increase. As beading

is more commonly a feature of old age, when nail growth rate slows down, one would not expect beading to correspond directly to faster linear nail growth. Both beading and ridging are common signs in normal ageing patients and at present their significance remains unclear.

REFERENCES

1 Hamilton EDB. Nail studies in rheumatoid arthritis. *Ann Rheum Dis* 1960; **19**: 167–73.
2 de Doncker P, Pierard GE. Acquired nail beading in patients receiving itraconazole: an indicator of faster nail growth? A study using optical profilometry. *Clin Exp Dermatol* 1994; **19**: 404–6.

Changes in colour [1–7]

Alteration in nail colour may occur because of changes affecting the dorsal nail surface, the substance of the nail plate, the undersurface of the nail or the nail bed.

Exogenous pigment

Exogenous pigment on the upper surface is easy to demonstrate by scraping the nail. If the proximal margin of the pigment is an arc matching the proximal nail fold, this is a further clue confirming an exogenous source. Often, the cuticle is less absorbent than nail and there will be a narrow proximal margin of unstained nail. This margin will broaden as the period since exposure lengthens. Hence the 'quitters' nail, which demonstrates the cessation of smoking and nicotine-free fingers for 2 months.

Exogenous pigment on the undersurface of the nail is less easy to demonstrate and may mean that part or all of the nail needs to be avulsed in order to scrape the undersurface and examine it separate from the nail bed. The green pigment of *Pseudomonas* infection [6] in association with onycholysis is a typical situation where partial avulsion is the best way to demonstrate the site of pigmentation, although it may not always be the best treatment.

Nail plate changes

The substance of the nail plate can be changed by the addition of pigment or the alteration of the normal cellular and intercellular organization such that there is loss of normal lucency. Pigment is typically added in the form of melanin produced by matrix melanocytes during nail formation. This produces a brown longitudinal streak the entire length of the nail. In white people this is abnormal and requires thorough assessment and, in some instances, biopsy. In darker-skinned people it is a common variant. The incorporation of heavy metals and some drugs into the nail via the matrix can also produce altered nail plate colour, such as the grey colour associated with silver. The disruption of normal nail plate formation by disease, chemotherapy, poisons or trauma can result in waves of parakeratotic nail cells or small splits between cells within the nail. Both make the nail less lucent and produce the white marks of true *leukonychia*. Transmission electron microscopy suggests that there is a change in collagen fibre organization, which might provide an intracellular basis for altered diffractive properties. This disruption can be achieved at nail formation or subsequently in the case of fungal nail infection, where discoloration may start distolaterally rather than via the matrix.

Nail bed changes

In addition to generalized vascular changes in the nail bed, there can be localized changes, as seen with nail bed tumours. In the instance of a glomus tumour, this may be the sole method of localization and arises because of the differential blood supply in the tumour and surrounding nail bed. Subungual hyperkeratosis or the incorporation of drugs (antimalarials, phenothiazines) may also change the apparent colour of the nail. Splinter haemorrhages, representing ruptured nail bed vessels, deposit haemoglobin on the undersurface of the nail, which grows out. Cyanosis makes the nail bed blue and carbon monoxide poisoning makes it bright red.

REFERENCES

1 Baran R. Longitudinal melanotic streaks as a clue to Laugier–Hunziker syndrome. *Arch Dermatol* 1979; **115**: 1448–9.
2 Daniel CR. Nail pigmentation abnormalities. *Dermatol Clin* 1985; **3**: 431–43.
3 Daniel CR, Zaias N. Pigmentary abnormalities of the nails with emphasis on systemic diseases. *Dermatol Clin* 1988; **6**: 305–13.
4 Higashi N. Melanonychia due to tinea unguium. *Hifu* 1990; **32**: 379–80.
5 Lovemann AB, Fliegelman MT. Discoloration of the nails. *Arch Dermatol* 1955; **72**: 153–6.
6 Shellow WVR, Koplon BS. Green striped nails: chromonychia due to *Pseudomonas aeruginosa. Arch Dermatol* 1963; **97**: 149–53.
7 Zaias N. Onychomycosis. *Arch Dermatol* 1972; **105**: 263–74.

True leukonychia

White discoloration of the nail attributable to matrix dysfunction occurs in a variety of patterns [1,2]. There is the rare, inherited form called total leukonychia, in which all nails are milky porcelain white [3]. In subtotal leukonychia, the proximal two-thirds are white, becoming pink distally. This is attributed to a delay in keratin maturation, and the nail may still appear white at the distal overhang (Fig. 62.13).

Transverse leukonychia (Mees' line) reflects a systemic disorder, such as chemotherapy or poisoning [4], or systemic infection [5] affecting matrix function. The 1–2-mm-wide transverse band is in the arcuate form of the lunula and is analogous to a Beau's line, with which it is occasionally found. Punctate leukonychia comprises white spots of 1–3 mm diameter attributed to minor matrix trauma (e.g. manicure) and is also seen in alopecia areata.

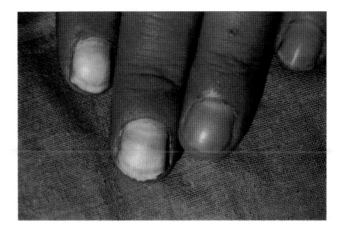

Fig. 62.13 True leukonychia with white nail in the distal free edge.

The pattern and number of spots may change as the nail grows. With longitudinal leukonychia, there is a parakeratotic focus in the matrix, sometimes attributable to Darier's disease or a small tumour.

REFERENCES

1 Albright SD, Wheeler CE. Leukonychia: total and partial leukonychia in a single family with review of the literature. *Arch Dermatol* 1964; **90**: 392–9.
2 Grossman M, Scher RK. Leukonychia: review and classification. *Int J Dermatol* 1990; **29**: 535–41.
3 Baran R, Dawber RPR. Physical signs. In: Baran R, Dawber RPR, eds. *Diseases of the Nails and Their Management*, 2nd edn. Oxford: Blackwell Science, 1994: 72.
4 Marino MT. Mees' lines. *Arch Dermatol* 1990; **126**: 827–8.
5 Mautner GH, Lu I, Ort RJ, Grossman ME. Transverse leukonychia with systemic infection. *Cutis* 2000; **65**: 318–20.

Apparent leukonychia

In apparent leukonychia, changes in the nail bed are responsible for the white appearance [1,2]. Nail bed pallor may be a non-specific sign of anaemia, oedema or vascular impairment. It may occur in particular patterns which have become associated with certain conditions.

Terry's nail

This is white proximally and normal distally and is attributed to cirrhosis, congestive cardiac failure and adult-onset diabetes mellitus [3]. Nail bed biopsy reveals only mild changes of increased vascularity. This is similar to *half-and-half nails*, where there is a proximal white zone and distal (20–60%) brownish sharp demarcation, the histology of which suggests an increase of vessel wall thickness and melanin deposition. It is seen in 9–50% of patients with chronic renal failure and after chemotherapy. It is unclear whether the variant *Neapolitan nails*, where there are bands of white, brown and red, is a version of half-and-half or Terry's nails, or a feature of old age.

Muehrcke's paired white bands

These bands are parallel to the lunula in the nail bed, with pink between two white lines. They are commonly associated with hypoalbuminaemia, the correction of which by albumin infusion can reverse the sign. They have also recently been reported following placement of a left ventricular assist device in a patient with congestive heart failure [4].

REFERENCES

1 Albright SD, Wheeler CE. Leukonychia: total and partial leukonychia in a single family with review of the literature. *Arch Dermatol* 1964; **90**: 392–9.
2 Grossman M, Scher RK. Leukonychia: review and classification. *Int J Dermatol* 1990; **29**: 535–41.
3 Holzberg M, Walker HK. Terry's nails: revised definition and new correlations. *Lancet* 1984; i: 896–9.
4 Alam M, Scher RK, Bickers DR. Muehrcke's lines in a heart transplant recipient. *J Am Acad Dermatol* 2001; **44**: 316–7.

Colour changes due to drugs [1]

There are a number of colour changes due to drugs. Yellowing of the nail is a rare occurrence in prolonged tetracycline therapy, which can also produce a pattern of dark distal photo-onycholysis associated with photosensitivity [2]. The whole nail is affected and returns to normal when the drug is discontinued. A similar effect, but of a bluish colour, is seen with mepacrine [3], the nails fluorescing yellow–green or white when viewed under Wood's light. Normal nails show slight fluorescence of violet–blue colour.

Chloroquine may produce blue-black pigmentation of the nail bed [4]. Other antimalarials may produce longitudinal or vertical bands of pigmentation on the nail bed or in the nail [5,6]. A fixed drug eruption of the nail bed can be dark blue [7]. Argyria may discolour the nails slate blue [8], and inorganic arsenic may produce longitudinal bands of pigment or transverse white stripes (*Mees' stripes*) across the nail.

Hyperpigmentation due to increased melanin in the nail and nail bed has been noted in children after 6 weeks of treatment with doxorubicin (adriamycin) [9,10]. Other similar cytotoxic drugs may cause a variety of patterns of increased pigmentation [1]. However, in acquired immune deficiency syndrome (AIDS), longitudinal melanonychia may be seen in untreated cases [11,12] as well as in those receiving zidovudine [9,13].

REFERENCES

1 Baran R, Dawber RPR, Richert B. Physical signs. In: Baran R, Dawber RPR, de Berker DAR, Haneke E, Tosti A, eds. *Diseases of the Nails and Their Management*, 3rd edn. Oxford: Blackwell Science, 2001: 86–103.
2 Orentreich N, Harber LC, Tromovitch TH. Photosensitivity and photo-onycholysis due to demethylchlortetracycline. *Arch Dermatol* 1961; **83**: 730–7.
3 Mallon E, Dawber RPR. Longitudinal melanonychia induced by minocycline. *Br J Dermatol* 1994; **130**: 794–5.
4 Tuffanelli D, Abraham RK, Dubois E. Pigmentation from antimalarial drugs. *Arch Dermatol* 1963; **88**: 419–26.
5 Colomb D. Antimalarial nail pigmentation. *Bull Soc Fr Dermatol Syphiligr* 1975; **82**: 319–22.
6 Maguire A. Antimalarial nail pigmentation. *Lancet* 1963; i: 667–71.
7 Wise F, Sulzberger MB. Drug eruptions. *Arch Dermatol Syphilol* 1933; **27**: 549–67.
8 Ramelli G. Argyria. *Cutis* 1972; **10**: 155–9.
9 Goark SP, Hood AF, Nelson K. Nail pigmentation associated with zidovudine. *J Am Acad Dermatol* 1984; **5**: 1032–3.
10 Pratt CB, Shanks EC. Hyperpigmentation of the nails due to doxorubicin. *JAMA* 1974; **228**: 460.
11 Fisher BK, Warner LC. Cutaneous manifestations of AIDS. *Int J Dermatol* 1987; **16**: 615–30.
12 Panwalker A. Nail pigmentation in AIDS. *Ann Intern Med* 1987; **107**: 943–4.
13 Gallais V, Lacour JPh, Perrin C *et al.* Acral hyperpigmented macules and longitudinal melanonychia in AIDS patients. *Br J Dermatol* 1992; **126**: 387–91.

Yellow nail syndrome

The nails in yellow nail syndrome are yellow due to thickening, sometimes with a tinge of green possibly due to secondary infection. The lunula is obscured and there is increased transverse and longitudinal curvature and loss of cuticle (Fig. 62.14). Occasionally, there is chronic paronychia with onycholysis and transverse ridging [1]. The condition usually presents in adults, but may occur as early as the age of 8 years [2]. Some of the clinical features may overlap with lichen planus [3,4], although the latter does not have the other systemic features normally seen in this syndrome. The features are usually accompanied by lymphoedema [5] at one or more sites and respiratory or nasal sinus disease. The nails grow at a greatly reduced rate: 0.1–0.25 mm/week for fingernails compared with the lowest normal rate of 0.5 mm/week. All 20 nails may be involved, although often a few are spared. Histologically, in the nail bed and matrix, dense fibrous tissue is found replacing subungual stroma, with numerous ectatic endothelium-lined vessels [6]. A foreign-body reaction has been noted [7]. It has been suggested that obstruction of lymphatics by this dense stroma leads to the abnormal lymphatic function found in the affected digits in some [8] but not all [9] cases.

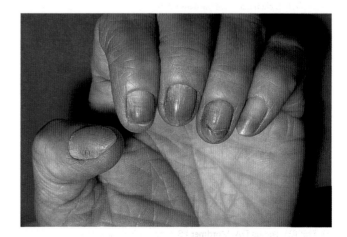

Fig. 62.14 Yellow nail syndrome.

The oedema most frequently affects the legs, and may not be seen for some months after the nail change has been noted. Less often it affects the face or hands and occasionally it is universal. Recurrent pleural effusions have been noted in a few cases [10,11]. Chronic bronchitis and bronchiectasis may also occur [12]. The oedema has been shown to be due to abnormalities of the lymphatics, either atresia or, in some cases, varicosity [11]. As other cases seem to have normal lymphatics, it is possible that a functional rather than an anatomical defect may be present [13], or perhaps only the smallest lymph vessels are defective. Although the nail changes may draw attention to the underlying lymphatic abnormality, they are found only in a minority of patients with congenital abnormality of the lymphatics. The condition may be associated with an increased incidence of malignant neoplasms [11,14,15]. Other associations include D-penicillamine therapy [5] and nephrotic syndrome [16]. In hypothyroidism and AIDS [17] there may be yellow nails, but it is debatable whether these represent yellow nail syndrome or simply the discoloration of nail associated with retarded growth [18].

Although the nail changes, once established, are usually permanent, complete reversion to normal may occur at times. Attempted treatments include oral [19] and topical [20] vitamin E, oral zinc [21] and treatment of chronic infection at other sites [22]. There is debate as to whether itraconazole is of value as treatment. The drug has been demonstrated to increase the rate of longitudinal growth, but an open trial in eight patients demonstrated that half gained no benefit with respect to nail changes [23]. It is reported that results are better when itraconazole or fluconazole are combined with oral vitamin E [24].

REFERENCES

1 Samman PD, White WF. The 'yellow nail' syndrome. *Br J Dermatol* 1964; **76**: 153–7.
2 Magid M, Esterly NB, Prendiville J, Fujisaki C. The yellow nail syndrome in an 8 year old girl. *Pediatr Dermatol* 1987; **4**: 90–3.
3 Tosti A, Piraccini BM, Cameli N. Nail changes in lichen planus may resemble those of yellow nail syndrome. *Br J Dermatol* 2000; **142**: 848–9.
4 Baran R. Lichen planus of the nails mimicking the yellow nail syndrome. *Br J Dermatol* 2000; **143**: 1117–8.
5 Ilchyshin A, Vickers CFH. Yellow nail syndrome associated with penicillamine therapy. *Acta Derm Venereol (Stockh)* 1983; **63**: 554–5.
6 De Coste SD, Imber MJ, Baden HP. Yellow nail syndrome. *J Am Acad Dermatol* 1990; **22**: 608–11.
7 Mallon E, Dawber RPR. Nail unit histopathology in the yellow nail syndrome. *Br J Dermatol* 1995; **133** (Suppl. 45): 55.
8 Fenton DA, Bull R, Gane J et al. Abnormal lymphatic function assessed by quantitative lymphoscintigraphy in the yellow nail syndrome. *Br J Dermatol* 1990; **123** (Suppl. 37): 32.
9 Ellis JP, Marks R, Pery BJ. Lymphatic function: the disappearance rate of 131albumin from the dermis. *Br J Dermatol* 1970; **82**: 593–9.
10 Emerson PA. Yellow nails, lymphoedema and pleural effusions. *Thorax* 1966; **21**: 247–53.
11 Miller E, Rosenow EC, Olsen AM. Pulmonary manifestations of the yellow nail syndrome. *Chest* 1972; **61**: 452–8.
12 Dilley JJ, Kierland RR, Randall RV, Schick RM. Primary lymphoedema associated with yellow nails and pleural effusions. *JAMA* 1968; **203**: 670–3.
13 Bull RH, Fenton DA, Mortimer PS. Lymphatic function in the yellow nail syndrome. *Br J Dermatol* 1996; **134**: 307–12.
14 Burrows NP, Russell Jones R. Yellow nail syndrome in association with carcinoma of the gall bladder. *Clin Exp Dermatol* 1991; **16**: 471–3.
15 Stosiek N, Peters KP, Hiller D et al. Yellow nail syndrome in a patient with mycosis fungoides. *J Am Acad Dermatol* 1993; **28**: 792–4.
16 Cockram CS, Richards P. Yellow nails and nephrotic syndrome. *Br J Dermatol* 1979; **101**: 707–9.
17 Chernosky ME, Finley VK. Yellow nail syndrome in patients with AIDS. *J Am Acad Dermatol* 1985; **13**: 731–6.
18 Scher RK. Acquired immunodeficiency syndrome and yellow nails. *J Am Acad Dermatol* 1988; **18**: 758–9.
19 Ayres S, Mihan R. Yellow nail syndrome. Response to vitamin E. *Arch Dermatol* 1973; **108**: 267–8.
20 Williams HC, Buffham R, du Vivier A. Successful use of topical vitamin E solution in the treatment of nail changes in yellow nail syndrome. *Arch Dermatol* 1991; **127**: 1023–8.
21 Arroyo JF, Cohen ML. Yellow nail syndrome cured by zinc supplementation. *Clin Exp Dermatol* 1993; **18**: 62–4.
22 Pang SM. Yellow nail syndrome resolution following treatment of pulmonary tuberculosis. *Int J Dermatol* 1993; **32**: 605–6.
23 Tosti A, Piraccini BM, Iorizzo M. Systemic itraconazole in the yellow nail syndrome. *Br J Dermatol* 2002; **146**: 1064–7.
24 Baran R. The new oral antifungal drugs in the treatment of the yellow nail syndrome. *Br J Dermatol* 2002; **147**: 189–91.

Red lunulae

Erythema of all or part of the lunula may affect all digits, but most prominently the thumb. Erythema is less intense in the distal lunula, where it can merge with the nail bed or be demarcated by a pale line, and can be obliterated by pressure on the nail plate. The appearance can fade over a few days. A single report of histological features failed to reveal vascular or epidermal changes [1]. Dotted red lunulae have been reported in psoriasis and alopecia areata, but otherwise the list of associations is so broad that it is unconvincing [2].

The exception to this is a red lunula seen in a single digit. In this setting, it often indicates a local disturbance of vascular flow, which is most likely to be a benign tumour. Glomus tumours and subungual myxoid cysts are the most common [3] and the colour may vary between blue and red.

REFERENCES

1 Cohen PR. Red lunulae: case report and review of the literature. *J Am Acad Dermatol* 1992; **26**: 292–4.
2 Wilkerson MG, Wilkin JK. Red lunulae revisited: a clinical and histopathologic examination. *J Am Acad Dermatol* 1989; **20**: 453–7.
3 de Berker D, Goettmann S, Baran R. Subungual myxoid cysts: clinical manifestations and response to therapy. *J Am Acad Dermatol* 2002; **46**: 394–8.

Longitudinal erythronychia (Fig. 62.15)

A longitudinal red streak in the nail can have several causes. All will have a corresponding band of thinned nail plate as part of the defect. The effect of this is a strip where the nail bed is less compressed by the overlying nail so that blood pools and is more apparent. Equally, the colour is more easily seen because the nail is thinner in this line. Splinter haemorrhages may lie longitudinally within the erythronychia.

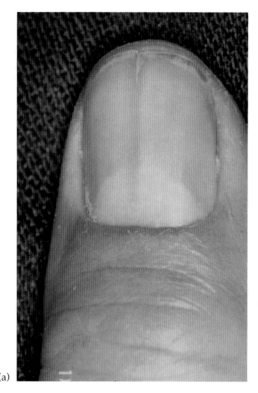
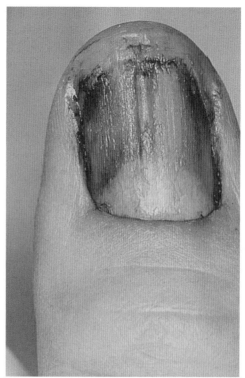

(a)

(b)

Fig. 62.15 (a) Longitudinal erythronychia. (b) The longitudinal ridge in the nail bed corresponds to the groove on the undersurface of the nail plate.

A strip of thinned nail arises because of focal reduction of matrix function. This can be due to direct matrix disease, such as an epidermal pathology, or as a result of pressure on the matrix with secondary loss of function. This second category contains the full range of dermal tumours as well as tumours of bone and cartilage that arise from the distal phalanx.

Matrix epidermal disease covers a spectrum of pathologies. One group of pathologies has histological features of acantholytic dyskeratosis and/or multinucleate giant cells [1]. The original model for this clinical presentation and histology is Darier's disease, where the thin longitudinal red streak may terminate at the free edge with a split and small subungual keratosis [2]. Acantholytic dyskeratotic naevus and warty subungual dyskeratoma [3] may both represent localized forms of Darier's disease. Acrokeratosis verruciformis of Hopf has a greater focus on nail fold disease, but also demonstrates longitudinal erythronychia and both clinical and pathological overlap with Darier's disease.

Baran has coined the term 'onychopapilloma' to describe the isolated benign warty distal nail bed lesions found in association with longitudinal erythronychia where the diagnosis lies outside those described above [4]. The papilloma is a secondary element, given that it is found distally in the nail bed while the cause lies proximally within the matrix. However, there is a category of this disease where the matrix disease remains unclear and the distal papilloma represents the identifiable entity. At other times, despite a similar clinical presentation with erythronychia and splinter haemorrhages, the matrix pathology may reveal a specific alternative diagnosis such as Bowen's disease [4] or basal cell carcinoma [5]. This means that an isolated longitudinal erythronychia needs careful assessment, and biopsy may be warranted if there is evolution.

Not all causes of longitudinal erythronychia conform to these rules. This is particularly the case where there are multiple red streaks associated with a dermatosis and additional nail changes. It can be a feature of lichenoid diseases of the nail unit, discoid lupus erythematosus, psoriasis, Langerhans' cell histiocytosis and a number of other diseases where there is patchy nail atrophy.

REFERENCES

1 Baran R, Perrin C. Localized multinucleate distal subungual keratosis. *Br J Dermatol* 1995; **133**: 77–82.
2 Zaias N, Ackerman AB. The nail in Darier–White disease. *Arch Dermatol* 1973; **107**: 193–9.
3 Baran R, Perrin C. Focal subungual warty dyskeratoma. *Dermatology* 1997; **195**: 278–80.
4 Baran R, Perrin C. Longitudinal erythronychia with distal subungual keratosis: onychopapilloma of the nail bed and Bowen's disease. *Br J Dermatol* 2000; **143**: 132–5.
5 Gee BC, Millard PR, Dawber RP. Onychopapilloma is not a distinct clinicopathological entity. *Br J Dermatol* 2002; **146**: 156–7.

Splinter haemorrhages

Splinter haemorrhages represent longitudinal haemorrhages in the nail bed conforming to the pattern of subungual vessels [1–4]. They are most frequently seen in the distal nail bed and on the fingers of the dominant hand, reflecting trauma as the cause. In dermatological practice, they are often found in association with psoriasis, dermatitis and fungal infection of the nails. As they occur under so many conditions, their importance as a sign of disease is often exaggerated. Focal pathology may also represent a cause, as in longitudinal erythronychia and onychomatricoma (see pp. 62.19 and 62.35).

Large numbers of proximal haemorrhages with no obvious traumatic origin may indicate a systemic cause [5], such as bacterial endocarditis or antiphospholipid syndrome [6]. Unilateral splinter haemorrhages may arise after arterial catheterization on the involved side. Examination under oil with a dermatoscope may reveal greater detail.

REFERENCES

1 Heath D, Williams DR. Nail haemorrhages. *Br Heart J* 1978; **40**: 1300–5.
2 Kilpatrick ZM, Greenberg PA, Sanford JP. Splinter haemorrhages, their clinical significance. *Arch Intern Med* 1965; **115**: 730–5.
3 Monk BE. The prevalence of splinter haemorrhages. *Br J Dermatol* 1980; **103**: 183–5.
4 Young JB, Will EJ, Mulley GP. Splinter haemorrhages: facts and fiction. *J R Coll Phys Lond* 1988; **22**: 240–3.
5 Gross NJ, Tall R. Clinical significance of splinter haemorrhages. *BMJ* 1963; ii: 1496–8.
6 Ames DE, Asherson RA, Aynes B et al. Bilateral adrenal infarction, hypoadrenalism and splinter haemorrhages in the primary antiphospholipid syndrome. *Br J Rheumatol* 1994; **31**: 117–20.

Developmental abnormalities of the nails [1,2]

Anonychia

Absence of the nails from birth is a rare congenital anomaly. It may occur as an isolated sign or be accompanied by other defects of the digits and other structures. Littman and Levin [3] described a girl with seven nails missing, and reported that her brother was similarly affected; it was suggested that this was a recessive trait. The mode of inheritance of most of these disorders has not yet been established with certainty. The condition described as anonychia with ectrodactylia [4] has been investigated more fully, however, and has been shown to be inherited as a dominant trait without sex linkage. In this condition, there is usually complete absence of the nails on the index and middle fingers, and when there is any nail on the thumb it is often present on the proximal lateral corners of the nail fold. On the ring fingers, the radial half of the nail is often absent, and the nail bed is also missing. In a minority of affected individuals there are striking and bizarre defects of the digits, sometimes restricted to one hand or foot. The defects usually take the form of absence of one or more digits. Two sisters in a sibship of five, whose parents were first cousins, are recorded as having rudimentary nails associated with congenital deafness. The parents showed neither abnormality [5]. Bart *et al.* [6] described a family with congenital absence of areas of skin, blistering of skin and mucous membranes, and absence or deformity of the nails, inherited as an autosomal dominant trait. It is now classified as a subtype of dominantly inherited dystrophic epidermolysis bullosa, with the responsible gene mapped to chromosome 3p [7]. Verbov [8] described a case with bizarre flexural pigmentation and anonychia, thought to be an autosomal dominant condition.

REFERENCES

1 Juhlin L, Baran R. Hereditary and congenital nail disorders. In: Baran R, Dawber RPR, eds. *Diseases of the Nails and Their Management*, 2nd edn. Oxford: Blackwell Science, 1994: 297–9.
2 Telfer NR, Barth JH, Dawber RPR. Congenital and hereditary nail dystrophies: an embryological approach to classification. *Clin Exp Dermatol* 1988; **13**: 160–3.
3 Littman A, Levin S. Autosomal recessive anonychia. *J Invest Dermatol* 1964; **42**: 177–80.
4 Lees DH. Anonychia and ectrodactylia. *Ann Hum Genet* 1957; **22**: 69–71.
5 Feinmesser M, Zelig S. Anonychia and congenital deafness. *Arch Otolaryngol* 1962; **74**: 507–10.
6 Bart BJ, Gorlin RJ, Anderson E et al. Congenital localised absence of skin: associated abnormalities resembling epidermolysis bullosa. *Arch Dermatol* 1966; **93**: 296–304.
7 Zelickson B, Matsumura K, Kist D et al. Bart's syndrome. *Arch Dermatol* 1995; **131**: 663–8.
8 Verbov J. Anonychia with bizarre flexural pigmentation: an autosomal dominant dermatosis. *Br J Dermatol* 1975; **92**: 469–74.

Nail–patella syndrome

This uncommon condition is of special interest because it involves abnormalities of ectodermal and mesodermal structure. It is inherited as an autosomal dominant trait. The disorder is caused by mutations in the LIM-homeodomain transcription factor β1 protein (LMX1B). This protein plays an important role in dorsoventral limb patterning during embryogenesis [1]. Gradients of expression of the protein determine the dominance of dorsal or ventral axon growth with concomitant trophic effects on mesoderm and ectoderm [2]. The gene maps to chromosome 9q34.1, with affected families showing a wide range of deletions and mutations [3]. In a typical case, the nails are grossly defective, being only one-third or half the normal size and never reaching the free edge of the finger [4]. In other cases, the thumbnails alone may be defective or only the ulnar half of each may be missing [5]. In every case, the thumbnails are most affected [6] and the remaining nails, if involved, are progressively less damaged from index to little finger. The lunulae may be triangular, with a distal peak (Fig. 62.16) in the midline [7]. Even when the

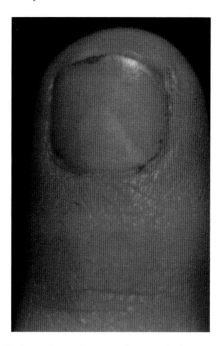

Fig. 62.16 Nail–patella syndrome with triangular lunula.

nail is completely missing, the nail bed is present. In addition to the nail changes, the patellae are smaller than normal and may be rudimentary, so that the knees are unstable. There are also bony spines arising from the posterior aspect of the iliac bones, visible on X-ray examination.

Other recorded features include hyperextension of the joints, skin laxity, hyperhidrosis [8] and renal abnormalities [9,10], and open angle glaucoma. LMX1B is known to influence transcription of genes affecting collagen IV in the glomerular basement membrane [11].

In 1965 there were 255 patients with this syndrome known to be living in the UK, and the prevalence is estimated at 1 per 22 million. The mutation rate is estimated at 1 per 1.9 million alleles per generation [12].

The condition must be distinguished from congenital ectodermal defects and pachyonychia congenita.

REFERENCES

1 Bongers EM, Gubler MC, Knoers NV. Nail–patella syndrome. Overview on clinical and molecular findings. *Pediatr Nephrol* 2002; **17**: 703–12.
2 Chen H, Lun Y, Ovchinnikov D *et al.* Limb and kidney defects in Lmx1b mutant mice suggest an involvement of LMX1B in human nail patella syndrome. *Nat Genet* 1998; **19**: 51–5.
3 Dreyer SD, Zhou G, Baldini A *et al.* Mutations in LMX1B cause abnormal skeletal patterning and renal dysplasia in nail patella syndrome. *Nat Genet* 1998; **19**: 47–50.
4 Renwick JH, Izatt MM. Some genetic parameters of the nail–patella locus. *Ann Hum Genet* 1965; **28**: 369–78.
5 Levan NE. Congenital defect of thumbnails. *Arch Dermatol Syphilol* 1961; **83**: 938–40.
6 Guidera KJ, Satterwhite Y, Ogden JA *et al.* Nail patella syndrome: a review of 44 orthopaedic patients. *J Paediatr Orthop* 1991; **11**: 737–42.
7 Daniel CR, Osment LS, Noojin RO. Triangular lunulae: a clue to nail patella syndrome. *Arch Dermatol* 1980; **116**: 448–9.
8 Pechman KJ, Bergfield WF. Hyperhidrosis in nail–patella syndrome. *J Am Acad Dermatol* 1980; **3**: 627–30.
9 Ben Bassat M. The glomerulo-basement membrane in nail–patella syndrome. *Arch Pathol* 1971; **92**: 350–5.
10 Goodman RM. Hereditary congenital deafness with onychodystrophy. *Arch Otolaryngol* 1959; **90**: 474–7.
11 Morello R, Zhou G, Dreyer SD *et al.* Regulation of glomerular basement membrane collagen expression by LMX1B contributes to renal disease in nail patella syndrome. *Nat Genet* 2001; **27**: 205–8.
12 Renwick JH, Lawler SD. Genetic linkage between the ABO and nail–patella loci. *Ann Hum Genet* 1955; **19**: 312–31.

Congenital onychodysplasia of the index fingers [1,2]

SYN. ISO KIKUCHI SYNDROME

In this condition, the nail of the index finger is absent, small or represented by two nails of unequal size. There may be a family history suggestive of autosomal dominant inheritance, although there is frequently no clear genetic pattern, and involvement of other digits has been reported [1,3,4]. Underlying changes in the distal phalanx can usually be demonstrated by lateral radiography, where bifurcation of the distal phalanx is the norm [4]. Syndactyly is an associated hand anomaly in some cases [2].

Variants include a similar form of onychodysplasia affecting other digits, including toes [5].

REFERENCES

1 Baran R. Syndrome d'Iso Kikuchi (COIF syndrome): 2 cas avec revue de la litérature. *Acta Derm Venereol (Stockh)* 1980; **107**: 431–5.
2 Miura T, Nakamura R. Congenital onychodysplasia of the index fingers. *J Hand Surg* 1990; **15A**: 793–7.
3 Kikuchi I, Horikawa S, Amano F. Congenital onychodysplasia of the index fingers. *Arch Dermatol* 1974; **110**: 743–6.
4 Kikuchi I. Congenital onychodysplasia of the index fingers: a case involving the thumb nails. *Semin Dermatol* 1991; **10**: 7–11.
5 Youn SH, Kwon OS, Park KC, Youn JI, Chung JH. Congenital onychodysplasia of the index fingers: Iso-Kikuchi syndrome. A case involving the second toenail. *Clin Exp Dermatol* 1996; **21**: 457–8.

Pachyonychia congenita (Fig. 62.17)

Pachyonychia congenita (PC) is a rare genodermatosis in which hypertrophy of the nails occurs, in some cases associated with nail bed and hyponychial hyperkeratosis [1,2]. Although Feinstein provides an excellent overview of the features, the disease divides best into two variants when the phenotype is interpreted in the light of the genotype. Autosomal dominant inheritance is the rule, although Haber and Rose [3] described cases transmitted in an autosomal recessive form.

The two variants of PC arise through mutations affecting the genes encoding keratins 6a and 16 in PC-1 [4,5] and 6b and 17 in PC-2 [6,7].

PC-1 (Jadassohn–Lewandosky type). The nails are normal at birth but within months they become discoloured and progressively thicken, more so on the hands than feet.

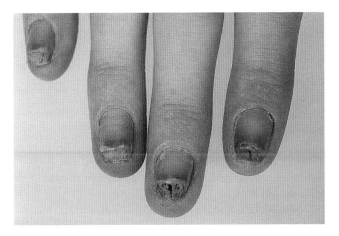

Fig. 62.17 Pachyonychia congenita.

Typical associated findings include palmar and plantar hyperkeratosis and warty skin lesions at various sites: knees, elbows, buttocks, legs, ankles and popliteal region. Acral bullae may be crippling and hyperhidrosis may be severe. Mouth and corneal dyskeratosis are less common findings.

PC-2 (Jackson–Lawler type). In this type, with less severe nail thickening and keratoses than type 1, many associations have been described: teeth may be present at birth; multiple epidermal cysts; sebocystomatosis; dry, lustreless and kinky scalp hair; eyebrows that stand straight out; and hamartomas.

The thickened nails can be treated surgically in some instances [8,9]. This is most likely to be warranted in PC-1. The localization of the four implicated keratins to the nail bed underlines that this is the main site of pathology [10]. Affected nails viewed end-on can appear almost normal, but with a dense wedge of subungual keratin, representing the focus of nail bed disease.

A range of associated features have been reported, including amyloidosis in one pedigree [11] and a case where PC coincided with tuberous sclerosis [12].

REFERENCES

1 Feinstein A, Friedman J, Schwach-Millet M. Pachyonychia congenita. *J Am Acad Dermatol* 1988; **19**: 705–11.
2 Samman PD. Developmental abnormalities. In: Samman PD, Fenton DA, eds. *The Nails in Disease*. London: Heinemann, 1986: 168–93.
3 Haber RM, Rose TH. Autosomal recessive pachyonychia congenita. *J Am Acad Dermatol* 1986; **122**: 919–23.
4 Bowden PE, Haley JL, Kansky A *et al.* Mutation of a type II keratin gene (K6a) in pachyonychia congenita. *Nat Genet* 1995; **10**: 363–78.
5 McLean WHI, Rugg EL, Lunny DP *et al.* Keratin 16 and keratin 17 mutations cause pachyonychia congenita. *Nat Genet* 1995; **9**: 273–8.
6 Smith FJD, Jonkman MF, van Goor H *et al.* A mutation in human keratin K6b produces a phenocopy of the K17 disorder pachyonychia congenita type 2. *Hum Mol Genet* 1998; **7**: 1143–8.
7 Covello SP, Smith FJD, Sillevis Smitt JH *et al.* Keratin 17 mutations cause either steatocystoma multiplex or pachyonychia congenita type 2. *Br J Dermatol* 1998; **138**: 475–80.
8 Cosman B, Symonds FC, Crikelair GF. Plastic surgery in pachyonychia congenita and other dyskeratoses. *Plast Reconstr Surg* 1964; **33**: 226–41.
9 Thomsen RJ, Zuehlke RL, Beckman BL. Pachyonychia congenita. Surgical management of the nail changes. *J Dermatol Surg Oncol* 1982; **8**: 24–8.
10 de Berker D, Wojnarowska F, Sviland L *et al.* Keratin expression in the normal nail unit: markers of regional differentiation. *Br J Dermatol* 2000; **142**: 89–96.
11 Tidman MJ, Wells RS, MacDonald DM. Pachyonychia congenita with cutaneous amyloidosis and hyperpigmentation: a distinct variant. *J Am Acad Dermatol* 1987; **16**: 935–40.
12 Sharma VK, Sharma R, Kaus S. Pachyonychia congenita with tuberous sclerosis. *Int J Dermatol* 1989; **28**: 332–3.

Infections of the nail and nail folds

Fungal nail infections

See Chapter 31.

Paronychia

Bacterial paronychia

Acute paronychia is a common complaint and is usually due to staphylococcal infection. It may result from local injuries, splits, splinters or nail biting, or there may be no preceding injury. It also occurs frequently as a complication of chronic paronychia, when other organisms may be involved, including streptococci, *Pseudomonas pyocyanea*, coliform organisms and *Proteus vulgaris*.

The condition presents as a painful swelling of the nail fold. If superficial it may point close to the nail and can easily be drained by incision with a size 11 scalpel, without anaesthesia [1]. Deeper lesions are best treated by antibiotics initially, but if they do not improve within 2 days, incision under local anaesthesia is required, particularly in childhood. A broad-spectrum antibiotic is preferred because it is unlikely that the organisms can be identified in advance. Some authorities recommend removing the proximal one-third of the nail plate without initial incisional drainage. This gives more rapid relief and more sustained drainage. There may be a place for treatment with topical steroid at the same time as antibiotic therapy [2].

REFERENCES

1 Keyser JJ, Littler JW, Eaton RG. Surgical treatment of infections and lesions of the perionychium. *Hand Clin* 1990; **6**: 137–53.
2 Wollina U. Acute paronychia: comparative treatment with topical antibiotic alone or in combination with corticosteroid. *J Eur Acad Dermatol Venereol* 2001; **15**: 82–4.

Chronic paronychia

This is one of the most common specific nail complaints met within dermatological practice. It ranks in importance

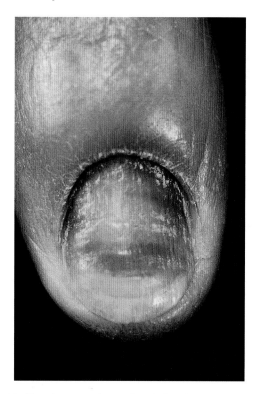

Fig. 62.18 Chronic paronychia with nail plate discoloration due to *Pseudomonas pyocyanea*.

with fungal infection and psoriasis as a cause of nail disease, but presents more commonly and is often misdiagnosed and mistreated. It is an inflammatory dermatosis of the nail folds, with secondary effects on the nail matrix, nail growth and soft-tissue attachments. It may be associated with infection on the background of the dermatosis. The dermatosis may be directly due to an irritant associated with wet work or caustic materials. Alternatively, it may be on the background of atopy or psoriasis, where minor provocation can result in active disease.

Wet cold hands are predisposed to chronic paronychia [1,2]. Wet foods are a combined source of factors, where the food may be an irritant [3]. It is predominantly a disease of domestic workers, bar staff, canteen workers and fishmongers [4]. The majority of cases are in patients between 30 and 60 years of age [1], although chronic paronychia is also seen in children, especially as a result of finger- or thumb-sucking [5].

Any finger may be involved, most often the index and middle fingers of the right hand and the middle finger of the left [4]. These fingers may be more subject to minor trauma than the remainder. The condition begins as a slight swelling at the base of one or more nails (Fig. 62.18), which is tender but much less so than in acute paronychia. The cuticle is soon lost and pus may form below the nail fold. Inflammation adjacent to the matrix disturbs nail growth, resulting in irregular transverse ridges and other surface irregularities, which may be combined with dis-

coloration (Fig. 62.18). There is some evidence that the darkening is due to the pigment from *Pseudomonas* infection of the nail [6]. In long-standing cases, the size of the nail may be reduced, and this reduction is exaggerated by bolstering of the fold all around the nail. Most of the nail deformity is due to the inflammation interfering with the formation of the nail, but a true *Candida* infection of the nail plate is occasionally seen.

There is a complex relationship with *Candida*, usually *Candida albicans* [7], which may be identified by swabs or scraping. Stone and Mullins [8] showed that chronic paronychia can be produced by non-viable *C. albicans* introduced into a relatively sterile nail fold. Much of the chronic inflammation seen in this disorder probably arises from an irritant reaction to material sequestered beneath the proximal nail fold. The loss of the cuticle means that detergent and other solvents may gain access to this tight space and act like a prolonged irritant patch test. This chronic non-infective inflammatory component is why topical steroids are useful in addition to antimicrobials as part of the treatment [9]. Acute exacerbations occur from time to time and are due to secondary bacterial infection. Various organisms may be found, including *Staphylococcus aureus* or *albus*, *Proteus vulgaris*, *Escherichia coli* and *Pseudomonas pyocyanea*. Barlow *et al.* [9] consider that *S. aureus* plays a more active part in initiating the process by penetrating the keratin at the base of the nail and opening up the nail fold. The role of *S. aureus* as a superantigen may also be relevant. Ingested allergens may also play a part [10].

Pemphigus [11] and squamous cell carcinoma [12] can present as chronic paronychia. The latter usually involves a single digit, and underlines the need for biopsy in isolated periungual conditions where the diagnosis is unclear. Cancer chemotherapy, antiretroviral medication and retinoids can provoke acute paronychia with features of pyogenic granuloma which may become chronic.

Treatment. Treatment is a combination of avoidance of precipitants, hand care and medication. Perhaps the most important part of the treatment, but the one most difficult to achieve, is to keep the hands dry. For all wet work the patients should be advised to wear cotton gloves under rubber gloves and avoid manicure of the proximal nail folds. Covering the affected fingers with porous surgical tape may afford some protection, but normal occlusion aggravates the problem. General hand care with emollient and protection during rough work is useful. If this stage of the therapy is not adequately pursued, the condition is likely to fail to settle whatever medical treatment is provided.

Topical therapy requires a combination of steroid [13] and antimicrobial. A potent steroid may be used for short periods when there is adequate antimicrobial cover. Injected triamcinolone (2.5 mg/mL) is useful in some instances. Topical imidazoles are usually sufficient to treat *Candida* and may provide a modest therapy against some bacteria. More potent topical antibacterials may be needed. Barlow *et al.* [9] suggest using gentamicin ointment during the day and nystatin ointment at night. When features are marked, oral antibiotics appropriate for *S. aureus* should be used. Because of the 'mixed' aetiology of the inflammation, many clinicians use antiseptic or antibiotic/anticandida/steroid creams in the chronic phase.

Incision is not indicated unless the condition enters an acute tender purulent phase, where removal of the proximal third of the nail may help. Attempting to clean out the nail fold with a sharpened orange stick is not recommended. If there is obvious candidal infection elsewhere, or *Candida* onychomycosis, this must also be treated. Surgical removal of the proximal nail fold and adjacent part of the lateral nail folds may cure recalcitrant cases [14].

REFERENCES

1 Esteves J. Chronic paronychia. *Dermatologica* 1959; **119**: 229–31.
2 Hellier FF. Chronic paronychia: aetiology and treatment. *BMJ* 1955; **ii**: 1358–60.
3 Tosti A, Buerra L, Mozelli R et al. Role of food in the pathogenesis of chronic paronychia. *J Am Acad Dermatol* 1992; **27**: 706–10.
4 Frain-Bell W. Chronic paronychia. Short review of 590 cases. *Trans St John's Hosp Dermatol Soc* 1957; **38**: 29–35.
5 Stone OJ, Mullins JF. Chronic paronychia in childhood. *Clin Pediatr* 1968; **7**: 104–7.
6 Samman PD. Management of disorders of the nails. *Clin Exp Dermatol* 1982; **7**: 189–94.
7 Marten RH. Chronic paronychia: a mycological and bacteriological study. *Br J Dermatol* 1959; **71**: 422–6.
8 Stone OJ, Mullins JF. Role of *Candida albicans* in chronic disease. *Arch Dermatol* 1965; **91**: 70–2.
9 Barlow AJE, Chattaway FW, Holgate ML et al. Chronic paronychia. *Br J Dermatol* 1970; **82**: 448–53.
10 Zaias N. *The Nail in Health and Disease*. Stanford, NJ: Appleton & Lange, 1990.
11 Engineer L, Norton LA, Ahmed AR. Nail involvement in pemphigus vulgaris. *J Am Acad Dermatol* 2000; **43**: 529–35.
12 Betti R, Vergani R, Inselvini E, Tolomio E, Crosti C. Guess what! Subungual squamous cell carcinoma mimicking chronic paronychia. *Eur J Dermatol* 2000; **10**: 149–50.
13 Tosti A, Piraccini BM, Ghetti E, Colombo MD. Topical steroids versus systemic antifungals in the treatment of chronic paronychia: an open, randomized double-blind and double dummy study. *J Am Acad Dermatol* 2002; **47**: 73–6.
14 Baran R, Bureau H. Surgical treatment of recalcitrant chronic paronychias of the fingers. *J Dermatol Surg Oncol* 1981; **7**: 106–9.

Pseudomonas infection

This is almost always a complication of onycholysis or chronic paronychia and is usually restricted to one or two nails (see Fig. 62.18). The nail plate has a characteristic bluish-black or green colour [1–3] and smells infected. This colour is due to accumulation of debris beneath the nail and the pigment pyocyanin adhering to the undersurface of the nail plate. Pigment may remain after the organism has been removed. In some cases, the nail plate appears to be invaded by the bacillus [2]. Subjects with nail extensions and nail wraps are susceptible to *Pseudomonas* colonization beneath the extensions. This has been documented as a risk factor for passing infection to patients in the medical setting [4]. Treatment [5] is as described for onycholysis or paronychia, whichever appears to be the prominent predisposing state. In addition, it is possible to treat with gentamicin or sulfacetamide (sulphacetamide) eye drops to eradicate the colonization where onycholysis is resistant to therapy.

REFERENCES

1 Bauer MF, Cohen BA. The role of *Pseudomonas aeruginosa* infections about the nails. *Arch Dermatol* 1957; **75**: 394–6.
2 Chernosky ME, Dukes CD. Green nails: importance of *Pseudomonas aeruginosa* in onychia. *Arch Dermatol* 1963; **88**: 548–53.
3 Goldman L, Fox H. Greenish pigmentation of nail plates from *Bacillus pyocyaneus*. *Arch Dermatol* 1944; **49**: 136–7.
4 Foca M, Jakob K, Whittier S et al. Endemic *Pseudomonas aeruginosa* infection in a neonatal intensive care unit. *N Engl J Med* 2000; **343**: 695–700.
5 Samman PD. Topical sulphacetamide for onycholysis. *Clin Exp Dermatol* 1982; **7**: 189–90.

Herpetic paronychia [1,2]

SYN. HERPETIC WHITLOW

This uncommon condition is due to primary inoculation of the herpes simplex virus and presents as single or grouped blisters close to the nail; it may give a honeycomb appearance. Clear at first, the blisters soon become purulent and may break and be replaced by crusts. It is usually very painful and takes about 3 weeks to resolve, with pain settling in half that time. Lymphangitis sometimes occurs and may precede vesiculation. Diagnosis may be established by recovering the virus from a recent blister and by cytological examination of the blister floor. Contact cases may occur.

Treatment probably does little to shorten the course of the disorder, but cleaning with 1/6000 potassium permanganate followed by application of a bland cream is recommended. Relapse may occur as with other primary herpetic infections. The value of thymidine analogues, such as 5% topical idoxuridine and oral or topical aciclovir, remains unproven at this site; if the lesion is seen within 2 days of onset, topical aciclovir may inhibit progression.

Numbness of the finger has been reported following infection [1] and persistent lymphoedema may occur. Persistent cases may have an atypical presentation in patients with HIV infection [3].

REFERENCES

1 Chang T, Gorbach SL. Primary and recurrent herpetic whitlow. *Int J Dermatol* 1977; **16**: 752–4.
2 Stern H, Elek SD, Millar DM et al. Herpetic whitlow: cross-infection in hospitals. *Lancet* 1958; **ii**: 871–4.
3 Robayna MG, Herranz P, Rubio FA et al. Destructive herpetic whitlow in AIDS: report of three cases. *Br J Dermatol* 1997; **137**: 812–5.

HIV infection

The most common nail changes in individuals with HIV infection are clubbing, transverse lines, onychoschizia, leukonychia and longitudinal melanonychia [1]. In addition, there is a lower threshold for infection with dermatophytes, yeasts and herpesvirus [1]. The patterns of infection may alter, such that proximal subungual white fungal infection is said to be a pointer to immunodeficiency and particularly HIV [2]. The nail folds may be red in the absence of infection [3] or be provoked into an appearance of pyogenic granuloma by retroviral therapy [4]. The nail can also manifest various patterns of melanonychia, which is usually ascribed to zidovudine therapy [5] but has also been attributed to hydroxycarbamide (hydroxyurea) [6].

REFERENCES

1 Cribier B, Mena ML, Rey D *et al*. Nail changes in patients infected with human immunodeficiency virus. A prospective controlled study. *Arch Dermatol* 1998; **134**: 1216–20.
2 Gupta AK, Taborda P, Taborda V *et al*. Epidemiology and prevalence of onychomycosis in HIV-positive individuals. *Int J Dermatol* 2000; **39**: 746–53.
3 Itin PH, Gilli L, Nüesch R *et al*. Erythema of the proximal nail fold in HIV-infected patients. *J Am Acad Dermatol* 1996; **35**: 631–3.
4 Tosti A, Piraccini BM, D'Antuono A, Marzaduri S, Bettoli V. Paronychia associated with antiretroviral therapy. *Br J Dermatol* 1999; **140**: 1165–8.
5 Bendick C, Heinrich R, Steigleder GK. Azidothymidine induced pigmentation of skin and nails. *Arch Dermatol* 1989; **125**: 1285–6.
6 Laughon SK, Shinn LL, Nunley JR. Melanonychia and mucocutaneous hyperpigmentation due to hydroxyurea use in an HIV-infected patient. *Int J Dermatol* 2000; **39**: 928–31.

Dermatoses affecting the nails

Psoriasis

Psoriasis is probably the most common disorder affecting fingernails, with consequent dystrophy. Between 1.5 and 3% of the population have psoriasis, and up to 50% of psoriatics have nail involvement [1]. Over a lifetime, this may cumulatively increase to 80–90% [2]. In children, nail involvement ranges from 7% [3] to 39% [4], and pitting has been observed in the first week of life in the offspring of a mother severely affected with psoriasis [5]. Psoriatic nail changes are prominent in the childhood nail disease of parakeratosis pustulosa. Approximately one-third of these children will develop the manifest diagnosis of psoriasis in time, a smaller fraction will have variants of eczema and half of the total will get better [6]. De Jong *et al*. [7] reported that 93% of those with nail psoriasis considered it a significant cosmetic handicap, 58% found that it interfered with their job and 52% described pain as a symptom.

Clinical features. In order of reducing frequency, nail signs of psoriasis include pits, onycholysis, subungual hyperkeratosis, nail plate discoloration, uneven nail surface,

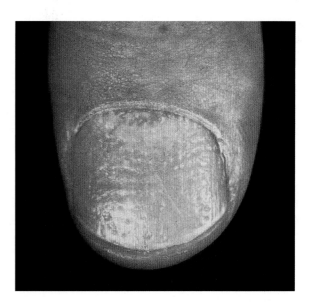

Fig. 62.19 Psoriasis: diffuse pitting.

splinter haemorrhages, acute and chronic paronychia, and transverse midline depressions in the thumbnails.

Pits. Pits more commonly affect fingers than toes (Fig. 62.19). They represent punctate surface depressions arising from proximal matrix disease (Table 62.3). Zaias [1,8] has demonstrated small columns of pathological parakeratotic nail falling off the upper surface of the nail plate to produce a pit. Some authorities advocate nail plate histology as a means of diagnosing nail psoriasis [9]. This can be useful for exclusion of fungal infection, although the specificity of nail plate changes in psoriasis is yet to be established. The origin of pits means that they can be influenced by disease in the proximal nail fold and it is thought that injection of triamcinolone into the nail fold alone can suppress this clinical feature. The pattern of pitting may be disorganized or occur in transverse/ longitudinal rows as seen in alopecia areata [2]. Pits may be shallow or large [8], to the point of leaving a punched-out hole in the nail plate (elkonyxis).

Onycholysis. Focal nail bed parakeratosis produces an 'oily spot' or 'salmon patch'. Extension of this area to the free edge gives onycholysis, which typically has a reddish-brown margin. Alternatively, onycholysis may commence at the distal edge (Fig. 62.20), representing disruption of the onychocorneal band [10]. Once this band of firm attachment has been breached, the condition is often progressive. Minor manicure, wet work and leverage from long nails exacerbates the condition.

Discoloration. Discoloration in psoriasis is multifactorial. The major factors are nail thickening and subungual hyperkeratosis. Both of these contribute to a yellow

Table 62.3 Relationship between clinical features and site of disease activity in psoriasis of the nail. (From Zaias [1].)

Clinical feature	Area of disease	Duration of disease
Changes in nail plate	*Matrix*	
Pits	Proximal matrix	Episodic: short
Transverse furrows	Proximal matrix; distal extension depends on depth of furrow	1–2 weeks
Crumbling nail plate	Entire matrix	Prolonged
Leukonychia with rough surface	Proximal matrix; leukonychia may involve distal matrix	Variable
Changes in nail bed and hyponychium	*Nail bed*	
Splinter haemorrhages	Nail bed dermal ridge haemorrhage	Short
Oily spot/onycholysis	Nail bed psoriasis	Prolonged
False nail following onychomadesis	Nail bed psoriasis	Prolonged
Subungual hyperkeratosis	Nail bed psoriasis	Prolonged
Yellow/green discoloration of nail bed	Secondary infection by yeasts or *Pseudomonas*	Prolonged

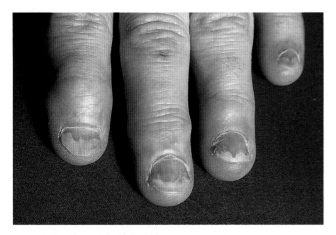

Fig. 62.20 Psoriasis: onycholysis.

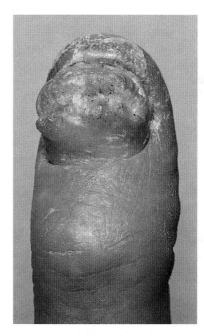

Fig. 62.21 Psoriasis: subungual hyperkeratosis.

appearance particularly common in the toes. It is possible that at this site repeated trauma elicits the isomorphic reaction, with local exacerbation of psoriasis. The coincidence of onychomycosis and psoriasis is also seen in the toenails [11] and can add to the pathological appearance. *Candida* spp. and *Pseudomonas* infection can result in green discoloration. While non-dermatophytes and bacteria are common, dermatophytes are rare [1].

Subungual hyperkeratosis. Subungual hyperkeratosis represents nail bed disease (Fig. 62.21). Substantial nail plate thickening may result from subungual hyperkeratosis, which is most marked distally and extends proximally. The fingertip may become very tender where there is gross subungual hyperkeratosis, as the nail plate attachment is greatly reduced and the nail can easily be caught and tug on the matrix attachment. Subungual hyperkeratosis is a prominent feature when pityriasis rubra pilaris affects the nail and is often seen with splinter haemorrhages [12,13].

Nail plate abnormalities. Splits, atrophy and fragility may be seen. The nail may also thicken, independent of subungual hyperkeratosis. Transverse midline depressions resembling the nail changes seen in 'washboard nails' [14] are also seen. Normally, they are attributed to the habit tic of disrupting the cuticle (Fig. 62.22) and although this may play a part in psoriasis, it appears that there is a lower threshold for the development of this midline feature in the presence of psoriasis.

Splinter haemorrhages. Splinter haemorrhages are seen in the nail bed of 42% of fingernails and 6% of toenails [15]. This may be due to the increased capillary prominence and fragility in nail bed dermis in psoriasis and the

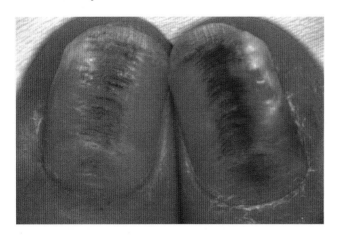

Fig. 62.22 Multiple transverse grooves of the thumbnails.

presence of dystrophy. Where transverse overcurvature occurs for reasons other than psoriasis, splinter haemorrhages are also common, suggesting that mechanical factors may contribute to splinter haemorrhage formation.

Subacute and chronic paronychia. Periungual involvement may be dramatic and inflammatory, giving rise to gross disruption of nail matrix. Loss of the nail may follow, with scaling of the nail bed or a deep transverse furrow.

Chronic psoriatic paronychia causes loss of the cuticle. The nail plate can become thin [16], although this may be offset by matrix disease, which can result in thickened nail. The nail fold may be scaly, in the form of psoriasis seen elsewhere.

Acropustulosis. This form of psoriasis involves destructive pustulation of the nail unit. It may present as part of pustular psoriasis, palmoplantar pustulosis [17], acrodermatitis continua of Hallopeau [18] or parakeratosis pustulosa (typically in young girls) on isolated digits. The nail plate may be lifted off by sterile pustules in the nail bed and matrix. There is associated erythema and discomfort of the end of the digit. There may be long-term nail loss, except in parakeratosis pustulosa, which usually resolves spontaneously. Parakeratosis pustulosa may affect only part of one digit. There is pitting and ridging combined with fine scaling erythema of the periunguium and only very rarely pustules. It is usually interpreted as a form of psoriasis [6], although it shares histological features with eczema [19], and some consider it a variant of eczema [20].

Acrodermatitis continua of Hallopeau can be very aggressive and result in resorptive osteolysis [21] or loss of toes and distal parts of fingers [22]. In a study of 20 patients with the condition, seven were male and 13 female, with a mean age of 46 years, and all had involvement of only one digit, with no features of psoriasis elsewhere [23].

Differential diagnosis. When the diagnosis of psoriatic nail dystrophy is in doubt, the main differential diagnoses are onychomycosis and lichen planus. In onychomycosis, the features usually present in the toes, whereas the fingernails are more commonly affected in psoriasis. Equally, there are often changes on the nail surface alone in psoriasis, whereas in onychomycosis features are usually within or beneath the nail plate. If there is fingernail involvement in onychomycosis, it is usually of only one or a minority of digits, in contrast with psoriasis where there are usually several digits affected.

Some forms of fingernail lichen planus and psoriasis are very difficult to distinguish. Both may result in roughened nails (trachyonychia) with subungual hyperkeratosis. If pits are prominent the diagnosis of psoriasis can be made, but if they are subtle and difficult to distinguish from other surface changes, they may be part of lichen planus. The nails in Reiter's disease and pityriasis rubra pilaris can also be difficult to distinguish from psoriasis [24,25], where distal subungual hyperkeratosis and splinter haemorrhages are common [8]. Aggressive forms of atypical nail psoriasis presenting in later life may represent acrokeratosis paraneoplastica. The patient is usually male, with subungual hyperkeratosis and scaling of the periunguium, ears and nose associated with malignancies of the upper gastrointestinal or respiratory tract [26–28].

Arthritis of the distal interphalangeal joint suggests a psoriatic cause of any associated dystrophy [29], with the exception of changes due to a myxoid pseudocyst associated with adjacent osteoarthritis. Baker *et al.* [30] found that there was no strict relationship between which joints are arthritic and which nails are dystrophic, although Jones *et al.* [31] noted that in a group of 100 psoriatics with arthritis, where there was nail involvement there was a significantly greater chance of joint disease in the adjacent distal interphalangeal joint. There was also a significant correlation between PASI (Psoriasis Area and Severity Index) score and scoring of nail disease, and nail disease increased with the duration of psoriasis. A variant of nail psoriasis presents with pain and soft-tissue swelling of the distal digit associated with psoriatic nail changes, and underlying bone erosion and periosteal reaction. This can be in the absence of joint involvement and has been termed 'psoriatic onycho-pachydermo-periostitis' [32].

Histopathology. Histopathology varies according to the clinical focus of the disease [1,33]. The matrix and nail bed develop a granular layer. Conversely, the hyponychium, where a granular layer is normally present, no longer has one [1]. Where there is subungual hyperkeratosis, there are mounds of parakeratotic keratinocytes beneath the nail plate. Neutrophils may be found throughout these mounds and Munro microabscesses may form. Similar features are seen in acrodermatitis continua of Hallopeau [23]. Amorphous material interpreted as glycoprotein may accumulate within the keratotic mass [1]. Acanthosis and elongation of the rete ridges is present, with increased dilatation and tortuosity of the capillaries of the dermal papillae. Where the nail is lost, the nail bed may form a false nail of compacted hyperkeratosis [34]. The matrix can become quiescent, which can be demonstrated immunohistochemically by the absence of synthesis of the hard keratin Ha-1, which is normally a major constituent of nail [35].

The nail plate may show faults, clinically manifest as transverse splits and pits, which are lined with parakeratotic cells. These probably originate from the most proximal part of the matrix, or the ventral aspect of the proximal nail fold [1].

Treatment [36]. General hand care is important to avoid provocation of the isomorphic (Koebner) response, whereby minor trauma may elicit psoriasis. These measures include avoiding manicure, keeping the nails short, wearing gloves for wet work and heavy or greasy manual work, avoiding direct exposure to solvents and encouraging emollient usage. Concealment with nail lacquer is a reasonable approach to milder forms of psoriasis, and surface irregularities can be smoothed by the use of nail gel. This is a polymer, applied by a beautician and hardened by exposure to a table-top UVA source. The gel can then be shaped and buffed. Gel or other forms of sculptured or adherent artificial nails have the potential for aggravating onycholysis and are not usually recommended if this is a prominent feature.

Active treatments are mainly directed at the more dystrophic forms of nail involvement and may sometimes help with onycholysis. Often the focus of therapy is the proximal nail fold, where active psoriasis is disturbing the underlying matrix and lack of cuticle is promoting chronic paronychia. Medical treatments include the following.

Local steroids. Clobetasol propionate ointment may be used without occlusion, rubbed into the nail fold. Duration of treatment is limited by local atrophy. It is useful for psoriatic paronychia where there are secondary nail plate changes. Onycholysis may benefit if the nail is clipped back to the point of nail plate attachment and the nail bed treated topically. *Candida* is a frequent colonizer of this space and warrants treatment at the same time. Triamcinolone acetonide may be used by injection into the nail fold or nail bed with regional or digital ring block. Using 0.1-mL injections of 10 mg/mL triamcinolone acetonide at matrix and nail bed sites, on no more than two or three occasions, de Berker and Lawrence [37] report a good response in subungual hyperkeratosis, nail plate thickening and ridging. However, onycholysis and pitting improved in only 50% of nails. Alternative regimens employ more dilute triamcinolone (2.5–5 mg/mL) and are routinely used more than two or three times per digit, infiltrating

the proximal nail fold alone and making a ring block optional. Triamcinolone has also been used with the Port-O-Jet or Dermojet, with improvement of pitting as well as other features [38]. There is a single anecdotal report that use of these devices has been associated with implantation epidermoid cysts, and many reports that local infection is more likely with this form of steroid delivery than with injection [39].

Topical vitamin D analogues. Calcipotriol can be useful where there is subungual hyperkeratosis and nail thickening [40]. It has also been used in combination with topical steroid on an alternating basis (a.m./p.m.) [41] and it is now possible to use it as a combined steroid and calcipotriol ointment. Calcipotriol has the advantage of avoiding the risk of atrophy with long-term use, but it is not as beneficial in treating the nail fold inflammation and consequent changes in proximal matrix function, which manifest as ridging and pitting.

Maintenance treatment with calcipotriol may also be one of the most effective topical therapies for pustular nail psoriasis [42].

Photochemotherapy. Subjects may improve as part of their general psoralen and UVA (PUVA) therapy or may have local PUVA to the nail unit. This can be done with topical or systemic psoralen. Specific high-dose handsets of UVA lamps have been advocated. As part of whole-body PUVA, 18 of 26 patients showed a greater than 50% improvement in nail changes, although pitting was unresponsive [43]. With local therapy, four of five patients improved: onycholysis was more responsive than pitting, but one patient with severe pitting showed improvement [44].

Retinoids. The nail plate is made thin by acitretin and etretinate. This reduces subungual hyperkeratosis. Pitting or onycholysis may be exacerbated [45,46]. Pustulation may be improved. Topical tazarotene 0.1% can be helpful for the treatment of onycholysis and pitting when applied under occlusion [47].

Others. Systemic methotrexate and ciclosporin (cyclosporin) may both help the nail unit but would not usually be advocated as therapy for this area of disease alone. Acrodermatitis continua of Hallopeau and psoriatic onychopachydermo-periostitis [48] are exceptions, and may respond to methotrexate.

Topical ciclosporin has been reported as useful in a single case report [49]. 5-Fluorouracil 1% has been used topically in 20% urea [50] and also in propylene glycol [51]. Pitting and subungual hyperkeratosis were thought to respond well to the former. Both are contraindicated in onycholysis.

Superficial radiotherapy [52] and electron-beam therapy [53] have been shown to be only of temporary benefit and are not usually recommended.

Treatment of coincident fungal infection may provide clinical benefit, although it is seldom a dermatophyte and positive cultures may only represent colonization.

REFERENCES

1 Zaias N. Psoriasis of the nail. A clinical–pathologic study. *Arch Dermatol* 1969; **99**: 567–79.
2 Samman PD. *The Nails in Disease*, 3rd edn. London: Heinemann, 1978.
3 Puissant A. Psoriasis in children under the age of 10: a study of 100 observations. *Gaz Sanita* 1970; **19**: 191.
4 Nanda A, Kaur S, Kaur I et al. Childhood psoriasis: an epidemiologic survey of 112 patients. *Pediatr Dermatol* 1990; **7**: 19–21.
5 Stankler L. Foetal psoriasis. *Br J Dermatol* 1988; **119**: 684.
6 Tosti A, Peluso AM, Zucchelli V. Clinical features and long-term follow-up of 20 cases of parakeratosis pustulosa. *Pediatr Dermatol* 1998; **15**: 259–63.
7 de Jong EM, Seegers BA, Gulinck MK, Boezeman JB, van de Kerkhof PC. Psoriasis of the nails associated with disability in a large number of patients: results of a recent interview with 1,728 patients. *Dermatology* 1996; **193**: 300–3.
8 Zaias N. Psoriasis of the nail unit. *Dermatol Clin* 1984; **2**: 493–505.
9 Grammer-West NY, Corvette DM, Giandoni MB, Fitzpatrick JE. Clinical pearl: nail plate biopsy for the diagnosis of psoriatic nails. *J Am Acad Dermatol* 1998; **38**: 260–2.
10 Sonnex TS, Griffiths WAD, Nicol WJ. The nature and significance of the transverse white band of human nails. *Semin Dermatol* 1991; **10**: 12–6.
11 Szepes E. Mycotic nail fold infection of psoriatic nails. *Mykosen* 1986; **29**: 82–4.
12 Griffiths WAD. Pityriasis rubra pilaris: an historical approach. 2. Clinical features. *Clin Exp Dermatol* 1976; **1**: 37–50.
13 Cohen PR, Prystowsky JH. PRP: a view of diagnosis and treatment. *J Am Acad Dermatol* 1989; **20**: 801–7.
14 Macaulay WL. Transverse ridging of the thumbnails. *Arch Dermatol* 1966; **93**: 421–3.
15 Calvert HT, Smith MA, Wells RS. Psoriasis and the nails. *Br J Dermatol* 1963; **75**: 415–8.
16 Ganor S. Chronic paronychia and psoriasis. *Br J Dermatol* 1975; **92**: 685–8.
17 Burden AD, Kemmett D. The spectrum of nail involvement in palmoplantar pustulosis. *Br J Dermatol* 1996; **134**: 1079–82.
18 Baran R. Hallopeau's acrodermatitis. *Arch Dermatol* 1979; **115**: 815–8.
19 Dulanto P, Armijo-Morens M, Camacho-Martinez F. Histological finding in parakeratosis pustulosa. *Acta Derm Venereol (Stockh)* 1974; **54**: 365–7.
20 Hjorth N, Thomsen K. Parakeratosis pustulosa. *Br J Dermatol* 1967; **79**: 527–32.
21 Miller JL, Soltani K, Toutellotte CD. Psoriatic acro-osteolysis without arthritis. *J Bone Joint Surg* 1971; **53A**: 371–4.
22 Mahowald ML, Parrish RM. Severe osteolytic arthritis mutilans pustular psoriasis. *Arch Dermatol* 1982; **118**: 434–7.
23 Pirracini BM, Fanti PA, Morelli R, Tosti A. Hallopeau's acrodermatitis continua of the nail apparatus: a clinical and pathological study of 20 patients. *Acta Derm Venereol (Stockh)* 1994; **74**: 65–7.
24 Lovy M, Bluhm G, Morales A. The occurrence of nail pitting in Reiter's syndrome. *J Am Acad Dermatol* 1980; **2**: 66–8.
25 Sonnex TS, Dawber RPR, Zachary CB et al. The nails in adult type I pityriasis rubra pilaris. A comparison with Sézary syndrome and psoriasis. *J Am Acad Dermatol* 1986; **15**: 956–60.
26 Bazex A, Griffiths A. Acrokeratosis paraneoplastica. A new cutaneous marker of malignancy. *Br J Dermatol* 1980; **103**: 301–6.
27 Richard M, Giroux JM. Acrokeratosis paraneoplastica (Bazex syndrome). *J Am Acad Dermatol* 1987; **16**: 178–83.
28 Handfield-Jones S, Matthews CNA, Ellis JP et al. Acrokeratosis paraneoplastica of Bazex. *J R Soc Med* 1992; **85**: 548–50.
29 Wright V, Roberts MC, Hill AGS. Dermatological manifestations in psoriatic arthritis. A follow up study. *Acta Derm Venereol (Stockh)* 1979; **59**: 235–40.
30 Baker H, Golding DN, Thompson M. The nails in psoriatic arthritis. *Br J Dermatol* 1964; **76**: 549–54.
31 Jones SM, Armas JB, Cohen MG et al. Psoriatic arthritis: outcome of disease subsets and relationship of joint disease to nail and skin disease. *Br J Rheumatol* 1994; **33**: 834–9.
32 Boisseau-Garsaud AM, Beylot-Barry M, Doutre MS et al. Psoriatic onycho-pachydermo-periostitis. *Arch Dermatol* 1996; **132**: 176–80.
33 Lewin K, Dewit S, Ferrington RA. Pathology of the fingernail in psoriasis. *Br J Dermatol* 1972; **86**: 555–63.
34 Samman PD. The ventral nail. *Arch Dermatol* 1961; **84**: 192–5.
35 de Berker D, Westgate G, Leigh I. Patterns of hard keratin (Ha-1) expression in nail matrix correspond to nail plate morphology (abstract). *Br J Dermatol* 1996; **134**: 584–5.
36 de Berker D. Management of nail psoriasis. *Clin Exp Dermatol* 2000; **25**: 357–62.
37 de Berker DA, Lawrence CM. A simplified protocol of steroid injection for psoriatic nail dystrophy. *Br J Dermatol* 1998; **138**: 90–5.
38 Peachey RDG, Pye RJ, Harman RR. The treatment of psoriatic nail dystrophy with intradermal steroid injections. *Br J Dermatol* 1976; **95**: 75–8.
39 Gottlieb NL, Riskin WG. Complications of local corticosteroid injections. *JAMA* 1980; **243**: 1547–8.
40 Tosti A, Piraccini BM, Cameli N et al. Calcipotriol ointment in nail psoriasis: a controlled double-blind comparison with betamethasone dipropionate and salicylic acid. *Br J Dermatol* 1998; **139**: 655–9.
41 Rigopoulos D, Ioannides D, Prastitis N, Katsambas A. Nail psoriasis: a combined treatment using calcipotriol cream and clobetasol propionate cream. *Acta Derm Venereol (Stockh)* 2002; **82**: 140.
42 Piraccini BM, Tosti A, Iorizzo M, Misciali C. Pustular psoriasis of the nails: treatment and long-term follow-up of 46 patients. *Br J Dermatol* 2001; **144**: 1000–5.
43 Marx JL, Scher RK. The response of psoriatic nails to photochemotherapy. *Arch Dermatol* 1980; **116**: 1023–4.
44 Handfield-Jones SE, Boyle J, Harman RRM. Local PUVA treatment for nail psoriasis. *Br J Dermatol* 1987; **116**: 280–1.
45 Baran R. Retinoids and the nails. *J Dermatol Treat* 1990; **1**: 151–4.
46 Ellis IN, Voohees JJ. Etretinate therapy. *J Am Acad Dermatol* 1987; **16**: 291–9.
47 Scher RK, Stiller M, Zhu YI. Tazarotene 0.1% gel in the treatment of fingernail psoriasis: a double blind, randomized, vehicle-controlled study. *Cutis* 2001; **68**: 355–8.
48 Bauza A, Redondo P, Aquerreta D. Psoriatic onycho-pachydermo periostitis: treatment with methotrexate. *Br J Dermatol* 2000; **143**: 901–2.
49 Tosti A, Guerra L, Bardazzi F, Lanzarini M. Topical cyclosporin in nail psoriasis. *Dermatologica* 1990; **180**: 110.
50 Fritz K. Psoriasis of the nail. Successful topical treatment with 5-fluorouracil. *Z Hautkr* 1988; **64**: 1083–8.
51 Friedriekson T. Topically applied fluorouracil in the treatment of psoriatic nails. *Arch Dermatol* 1974; **110**: 735–6.
52 Yu RCH, King CM. A double blind study of superficial radiotherapy in psoriatic nail dystrophy. *Acta Derm Venereol (Stockh)* 1992; **72**: 134–6.
53 Kwang TY, Nee TS, Seng KTH. A therapeutic study of nail psoriasis using electron beams. *Acta Derm Venereol (Stockh)* 1995; **75**: 90.

Darier's disease [1–5]

Nail involvement is common in Darier's disease; 96% of patients are reported to have acral changes, of which nail changes are the most common [2]. These include red and/or white longitudinal streaks in the nail, often terminating in a V-shaped nick (Fig. 62.23). The streak may represent a zone of fragile or thinned nail, which makes it prone to fragmentation at the tip with the consequent nick. In severe cases, the nails are almost lost by extension of the fragmentation process to involve the entire matrix. Subungual hyperkeratotic papules can be found in the hyponychium. Histologically, matrix and nail bed changes resemble the acantholysis seen in involved skin, with the addition of multinucleate giant cells and epithelial hyperplasia in the nail bed [5]. These histological features make it possible to diagnose Darier's disease when it is confined to the nail [1]. Excess ridging and a rough nail surface may also be found, as may total leukonychia. Occasionally, marked thickening of the nail plate occurs. It is probable

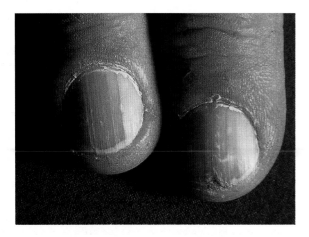

Fig. 62.23 Darier's disease: white and red longitudinal lines and distal notching.

that the nail is sometimes affected in the absence of disease elsewhere [1].

Hailey–Hailey disease has some histological similarities and may also present with longitudinal white streaks [2]. However, the disease does not have the same destructive effect and is not associated with hyperkeratoses or symptoms of the nail apparatus.

A case of squamous cell carcinoma developing in a nail bed with chronic changes of Darier's disease has been reported [6]. Pain or conspicuous uncharacteristic features in a nail apparatus affected by Darier's disease may therefore be indications for biopsy.

REFERENCES

1 Bingham EA, Burrows D. Darier's disease. *Br J Dermatol* 1984; **111** (Suppl. 26): 88–9.
2 Burge SM, Wilkinson JD. Darier–White disease: a review of the clinical features in 163 patients. *J Am Acad Dermatol* 1992; **27**: 40–50.
3 Ronchese F. The nail in Darier's disease. *Arch Dermatol* 1965; **91**: 617–8.
4 Schubert H. Darier's disease. *Z Haut Geschlechskr* 1966; **41**: 239–44.
5 Zaias N, Ackerman AB. The nail in Darier–White disease. *Arch Dermatol* 1973; **107**: 193–9.
6 Downs AM, Ward KA, Peachey RD. Subungual squamous cell carcinoma in Darier's disease. *Clin Exp Dermatol* 1997; **22**: 277–9.

Eczema

Nail changes in eczema may be seen in the context of eczema elsewhere or as an isolated finding. Endogenous and exogenous factors may contribute. The nail changes may reflect this division, in that they may be in response to a systemic atopic disposition, with pitting in the absence of inflammation, or may demonstrate the effects of local eczema in the nail unit influencing nail formation.

The common allergens such as nickel, fragrance and medicaments rarely have particular bearing on nail abnormalities. However, rubber, chrome and irritant dermatitis are significant factors in hand dermatitis. These materials, and hand dermatitis in general, are associated with particular occupations. Selective exposure to such allergens or strong irritants is as important as chronic low-grade irritation from milder agents, such as water, seen in catering workers.

Cyanoacrylates used in prosthetic nails can provoke local and distant allergic reactions. Formaldehyde, occasionally used as a nail hardener, can provoke painful onycholysis if the patient becomes sensitized, or sometimes when acting solely as an irritant. Some allergens may cause nail dystrophy without associated inflammation.

A combination of atopy and an exogenous irritant or allergic contact reaction is common.

Clinical features. Nail matrix disturbance is reflected in thickening, pits, nail loss, transverse ridges and furrows in a pattern similar to psoriatic nail disease (Table 62.4).

Nail bed disease can produce subungual hyperkeratosis, splinter haemorrhages, onycholysis and pain. Allergens and irritants can be sequestered beneath the free edge of the nail to achieve high concentrations and prolonged exposure.

Nail changes may betray eczema elsewhere and the nails may be buffed smooth and shiny, indicating their use as a tool for rubbing.

Associated hand dermatitis may show vesicles, scaling, erythema, cracks and swollen fingers, although the

Table 62.4 Differential diagnosis between four common nail disorders: fungal infections, psoriasis, chronic paronychia and dermatitis.

	Fungal infections	Psoriasis	Chronic paronychia	Dermatitis
Colour	Often yellow or brown; part or whole of nail	May be normal or yellow or brown	Edge of nail often discoloured brown or black	May be normal
Onycholysis	Frequent	Frequent	Usually absent	Confined to tip or absent
Pitting	Infrequent	Often present and fine	Uncommon	Coarse pits frequent
Filaments or spores in potash preparations	Filaments, usually abundant	Absent	May be spores in edge of nail; filaments and spores in scrapings from nail fold	Absent
Cross-ridging	Absent	Uncommon	Frequent	Frequent
Other	Associated fungal infections elsewhere	Associated psoriasis elsewhere or family history of psoriasis	Predominantly women; wet work and cold hands cause predisposition	Recent history of dermatitis on hands

presence of vesicles will not always distinguish the condition from psoriasis, which should be sought at other sites. The distribution on the hand or foot may give some clues as to possible local causes, such as gloves, shoes, prosthetic nails or nail varnish. Hands and feet should always be examined together, as the presence of disease in both diminishes the likelihood of a contact dermatitis.

Defining the presence of atopy or patch testing can be useful even in the absence of active eczema as subungual hyperkeratosis and discomfort may be disproportionate to the cutaneous features [1].

Treatment. General hand care is important, with the avoidance of soap, irritants, wet work and any identified cause. Protective gloves should be used, with copious emollient application. Barrier creams are not usually adequate protection once features have developed. Potent topical steroids may be needed, sometimes with additional topical or systemic antimicrobial therapy. These should be rubbed in around the nail folds. In the young, steroids may precipitate premature closure of the phalangeal epiphyses if too potent or used for too long [2]. Osteomyelitis has also been reported in children using potent topical steroids in this area.

Hand or foot PUVA can help.

REFERENCES

1 Marren P, de Berker DAR, Powell S. Occupational contact dermatitis due to Quaternium 15 presenting as nail dystrophy. *Contact Dermatitis* 1991; **25**: 253–5.
2 Boiko S, Kaufman RA, Lucky AW. Osteomyelitis of the distal phalanges in three children with severe atopic dermatitis. *Arch Dermatol* 1988; **124**: 418–23.

Lichen planus

Nails are involved in about 10% of cases of disseminated lichen planus [1]. In a study of 24 adults with nail lichen planus, nail changes were the sole manifestation of the disease in 75% [2,3], and the figure may be higher in children [4,5], in whom lichen planus of all types is rare. This suggests only a modest degree of overlap between the disease process in the nail unit and at other sites. Although the skin lesions may itch intensely, nail disease may be relatively asymptomatic except when nails are shed.

Clinical features. The disease can involve the proximal nail folds with bluish-red discoloration. Nail plate changes include thinning, onychorrhexis, brittleness, crumbling or fragmentation, and accentuation of surface longitudinal ridging. All these features are secondary to disease affecting the matrix, which can also produce transient or permanent longitudinal melanonychia [6] or leukonychia as a post-inflammatory phenomenon (Fig. 62.24). When inflammation is intense and widespread within the nail apparatus, nails may be shed. Single longitudinal depres-

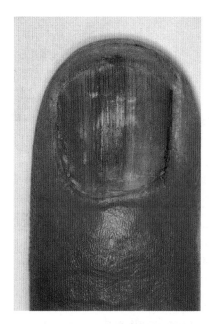

Fig. 62.24 Lichen planus with longitudinal melanonychia.

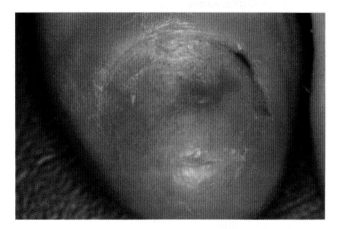

Fig. 62.25 Anonychia following lichen planus.

sions in the nail, with a distal notch or entire split, may arise from a pterygium. This is a fibrotic band of tissue fusing the proximal nail fold with the nail bed and matrix, following destructive local inflammation. Surviving proximal matrix is unable to push growing nail through the scar tissue, with a consequent split. Thickening, with features resembling yellow nail syndrome, is a less common pattern of presentation [7]. Where this occurs there is usually little difficulty in making the distinction in the fingernails as the prominent surface changes and/or atrophy of lichen planus are seen. However, these changes are less obvious in the toes, where yellow discoloration due to thickening can be marked [8].

Nail bed disease can produce subungual hyperkeratosis and onycholysis. Bullous lichen planus may affect the soles of the feet and in particular the toenails. Permanent anonychia may follow [9] (Fig. 62.25).

Twenty-nail dystrophy, with stippling of the nail plate (see Fig. 62.11) in up to 20 nails, is seen in a range of autoimmune diseases [10], alopecia areata [3], primary biliary cirrhosis and possibly in pemphigus [11]. In itself, it does not indicate the diagnosis of lichen planus, but is one of the recognized forms of the disease. It is one of the more common childhood patterns of presentation in which the nails feel rough and lose their lustre [12]. It has a reasonably good prognosis, in contrast with idiopathic atrophy of the nails, which may also occur in children. In this form, the surface change is less marked and the change in overall nail morphology greater, with thinning and shrivelling of the nail plate. Although nail biopsy is seldom undertaken in children, it may be warranted where the diagnosis of lichen planus needs to be explored. If destructive lichen planus is not treated in childhood, there will be lifelong loss of nails.

In the related disorder, lichen nitidus, numerous pits giving a fine rippling effect have been reported [13]. Longitudinal ridging, beads and thickening may occur and nails become brittle.

In keratosis lichenoides chronica, although the skin condition may resemble hyperkeratotic lichen planus, the nail changes may mimic psoriasis; 30% have nail involvement, with hyperkeratotic hypertrophy of periungual tissues.

Lichen planus nail changes are seen in graft-versus-host disease [14] and in the disseminated lichenoid papular dermatosis of AIDS. There can be an overlap between lichen planus and discoid lupus erythematosus, both in the skin and nails. Coexistence of skin and nail lichen sclerosus has been reported [15]. Lichen striatus may extend down a limb to the nails [16].

The differential diagnosis for the range of appearances of lichen planus in the nail unit includes Stevens–Johnson syndrome, infection, peripheral vascular disease, trauma and radiodermatitis.

Histology. In 20-nail dystrophy, there is a granular layer in the nail bed and matrix, with marked spongiosis [3]. The hypergranulosis is believed to reflect the disordered keratinization that causes both subungual hyperkeratosis and the poor nail plate formation. In other forms of nail lichen planus, in addition to hypergranulosis, there is occasionally saw-toothing of the rete pattern, and colloid bodies are rarely seen [2,17,18].

In 20-nail dystrophy it may be useful to perform a screen for organ-specific antibodies because of the association with alopecia areata and the related autoimmune diathesis [3].

Treatment. Potent topical steroids may help when rubbed into the nail folds in the active stage. Triamcinolone acetonide may be instilled into the proximal nail fold under local anaesthetic. In children, potent steroid therapy puts them at risk of premature closure of the phalangeal epi-physes. Oral steroids at up to 60 mg/day have been used to arrest severe scarring nail lichen planus [2]. Triamcinolone acetonide can be given intramuscularly at a dose of 0.5–1 mg/kg per month for 3–6 months [12]. Failure to deliver effective treatment in progressive disease may result in permanent nail loss or dystrophy. Ciclosporin can also be of benefit and azathioprine has been used to good effect in erosive disease [19]. Ulcerative lichen planus of the nail unit may benefit from grafting the nail bed.

REFERENCES

1 Samman PD. The nails in lichen planus. *Br J Dermatol* 1961; **73**: 288–92.
2 Tosti A, Peluso AM, Fanti PA *et al.* Nail lichen planus. Clinical and pathological study of 24 patients. *J Am Acad Dermatol* 1993; **28**: 724–30.
3 Tosti A, Fanti PA, Morelli R *et al.* Trachyonychia associated with alopecia areata. A clinical and pathological study. *J Am Acad Dermatol* 1991; **25**: 266–70.
4 de Berker D, Dawber RPR. Childhood lichen planus. *Clin Exp Dermatol* 1991; **16**: 233.
5 Milligan A, Graham-Brown RAC. Lichen planus in childhood: a review of six cases. *Clin Exp Dermatol* 1990; **15**: 340–2.
6 Baran R, Jancovici E, Sayag J, Dawber RPR. Longitudinal melanonychia in lichen planus. *Br J Dermatol* 1985; **113**: 369–74.
7 Baran R. Lichen planus of the nails mimicking the yellow nail syndrome. *Br J Dermatol* 2000; **143**: 1117–8.
8 Tosti A, Piraccini BM, Cameli N. Nail changes in lichen planus may resemble those of yellow nail syndrome. *Br J Dermatol* 2000; **142**: 848–9.
9 Cornelius CE, Shelley WB. Permanent anonychia due to lichen planus. *Arch Dermatol* 1967; **96**: 434–5.
10 Samman PD. Idiopathic atrophy of the nails. *Br J Dermatol* 1985; **81**: 746–9.
11 de Berker D, Dalziel K, Dawber RPR, Wojnarowska F. Pemphigus associated with nail dystrophy. *Br J Dermatol* 1993; **129**: 461–4.
12 Tosti A, Piraccini BM, Cambiaghi S, Jorizzo M. Nail lichen planus in children: clinical features, response to treatment, and long-term follow-up. *Arch Dermatol* 2001; **137**: 1027–32.
13 Munro CS, Cox NH, Marks JM *et al.* Lichen nitidus presenting as palmoplantar hyperkeratosis and nail dystrophy. *Clin Exp Dermatol* 1993; **18**: 381–3.
14 Saurat JH, Gluckman E. Lichen planus-like eruption following bone marow transplantation: a manifestation of the graft-versus-host disease. *Clin Exp Dermatol* 1977; **2**: 335–44.
15 Ramrakha-Jones VS, Paul M, McHenry P, Burden AD. Nail dystrophy due to lichen sclerosus? *Clin Exp Dermatol* 2001; **26**: 507–9.
16 Tosti A, Peluso AM, Misciali C, Cameli N. Nail lichen striatus: clinical features and long-term follow-up of five patients. *J Am Acad Dermatol* 1997; **36**: 908–13.
17 Barth JH, Millard PR, Dawber RPR. Idiopathic atrophy of the nails. A clinicopathological study. *Am J Dermatopathol* 1988; **10**: 514–7.
18 Zaias N. The nail in lichen planus. *Arch Dermatol* 1970; **101**: 264–71.
19 Lear JT, English JS. Erosive and generalized lichen planus responsive to azathioprine. *Clin Exp Dermatol* 1996; **21**: 56–7.

Tumours under or adjacent to the nail

Tumours of the nail apparatus and adjacent structures are relatively common. Neoplasms of the nail area can be divided into benign, benign but aggressive lesions (e.g. keratoacanthoma, recurring digital fibrous tumours of childhood and some warts) and malignant tumours.

Clinical diagnosis is often difficult because of traumatic factors, infection, pigmentation, and because the translucent nail plate masks physical signs in the nail bed. Also, common tumours, easily recognized at other sites, may behave differently in the nail apparatus. An X-ray

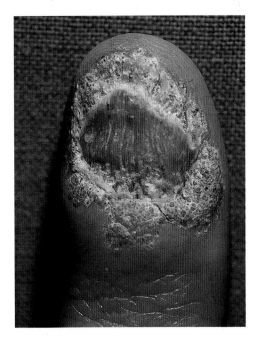

Fig. 62.26 The entire periunguium is affected by wart, with secondary nail changes.

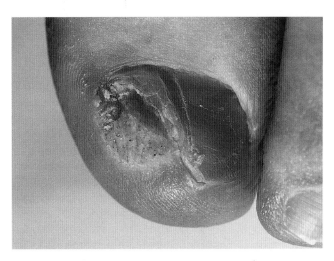

Fig. 62.27 Nail bed warts can cause onycholysis and nail plate disruption.

investigation should be carried out on all swellings in or around the nail apparatus, particularly those affecting a single digit, to exclude osteoma. Where changes are primarily in soft tissues, magnetic resonance imaging (MRI) may be preferable [1].

Benign tumours

Viral warts

This is the most common tumour involving the nail, usually found in one of the nail folds but also seen in the digit pulp and less commonly on the nail bed. In the lateral nail folds, there may be no nail plate changes, although proximal nail fold warts can result in longitudinal ridging and nail plate distortion (Fig. 62.26) and nail bed warts may cause onycholysis (Fig. 62.27). Erosion of underlying bone has also been reported.

The causal human papillomavirus is usually type 1, 2 or 4. Nail biting and certain occupations, such as butcher, may predispose to warts and complicate therapy. Warts are more common and difficult to eradicate in the immunosuppressed, particularly in organ-transplant recipients.

The most significant lesion from which warts need to be distinguished is squamous cell (epidermoid) carcinoma. However, this malignancy often destroys part of the matrix and nail bed and is usually painful; both features are uncommon in benign viral warts, unless aggressive cryosurgery has been used or there has been bacterial infection. Other disorders, such as syringometaplasia,

amyloid, subungual corn and verrucous epidermal naevus [2], may mimic viral warts.

Although most warts remit spontaneously, a wide range of therapies are available [3], including topical salicylic acid (paste, on plaster or in collodion), salicylic acid combined with abrasion [4], cryosurgery [4–7], bleomycin [8,9], cantharidin [10], imiquimod [11], curettage and carbon dioxide laser therapy [12,13], pulsed dye laser [14] and interferon [15]. Immunotherapy can be successful using sensitization to diphencyprone [16], or relying on naturally acquired immune sensitivity to pathogens such as mumps or *Candida* [17].

REFERENCES

1 Drapé JL, Idy-Peretti I, Goettmann S *et al*. Standard and high resolution MRI in glomus tumours of toes and fingertips. *J Am Acad Dermatol* 1996; **35**: 550–5.
2 Solomon LM, Fretzin DF, Dewald RL. The epidermal naevus syndrome. *Arch Dermatol* 1968; **97**: 273–85.
3 Gibbs S, Harvey I, Sterling J, Stark R. Local treatments for cutaneous warts: systematic review. *BMJ* 2002; **325**: 461.
4 Bunney MH, Nolan MW, Williams DA. An assessment of methods of treating viral warts by comparative trials based on a standard design. *Br J Dermatol* 1976; **94**: 667–79.
5 Colver GB, Dawber RPR. Cryosurgery: the principles and simple practice. *Clin Exp Dermatol* 1989; **14**: 1–6.
6 Dawber RPR, Colver GB, Jackson A. *Cutaneous Cryosurgery*, 2nd edn. London: Dunitz, 1997: 38–48.
7 Kuflik E. Cryosurgical treatment of periungual warts. *J Dermatol Surg Oncol* 1984; **10**: 673–6.
8 Munn SE, Higgins E, Marshall M, Clement M. A new method of intralesional bleomycin therapy in the treatment of recalcitrant warts. *Br J Dermatol* 1996; **135**: 969–72.
9 Shelley WB, Shelley ED. Intralesional bleomycin sulphate therapy for warts: a novel bifurcated needle puncture technique. *Arch Dermatol* 1991; **127**: 234–6.
10 Tkach JR. Finding and inventing alternative therapies. How I do it. *Dermatol Clin* 1989; **7**: 1–18.
11 Grussendorf-Conen EI, Jacobs S, Rubben A, Dethlefsen U. Topical 5% imiquimod long-term treatment of cutaneous warts resistant to standard therapy modalities. *Dermatology* 2002; **205**: 139–45.

12 Logan RO, Zachary CB. Outcome of carbon dioxide laser therapy for persistent cutaneous warts. *Br J Dermatol* 1989; **121**: 99–105.

13 Street ML, Roenigk RK. Recalcitrant periungual verrucae: the role of carbon dioxide laser vaporisation. *J Am Acad Dermatol* 1990; **23**: 115–20.

14 Kenton-Smith J, Tan ST. Pulsed dye laser therapy for viral warts. *Br J Plast Surg* 1999; **52**: 554–8.

15 Stadler R, Mayer-da-Silva A, Bratzke B *et al.* Interferons in dermatology. *J Am Acad Dermatol* 1989; **20**: 650–6.

16 Buckley DA, Keane FM, Munn SE *et al.* Recalcitrant viral warts treated by diphencyprone immunotherapy. *Br J Dermatol* 1999; **141**: 292–6.

17 Johnson SM, Roberson PK, Horn TD. Intralesional injection of mumps or *Candida* skin test antigens: a novel immunotherapy for warts. *Arch Dermatol* 2001; **137**: 451–5.

Fibrous tumours

There are several types of fibrous tumours of the nail apparatus, which can be differentiated on clinical and histological grounds [1,2]. Koenen tumours are associated with tuberous sclerosis and present at puberty as periungual fibromas. They are often multiple, large or small, elongated or nodular, and may produce a longitudinal groove in the nail plate due to matrix compression. Histologically, they show loose collagen with numerous small vessels distally, but with dense collagen and few vessels proximally.

Acquired periungual fibrokeratoma [3] is probably the same as acquired digital fibrokeratoma and garlic clove fibroma (Fig. 62.28). They are all benign asymptomatic fibromas with a hyperkeratotic tip and narrow base arising in the periunguium, especially at the proximal aspect of the matrix. They grow out along the nail resulting in a longitudinal groove. There are three histological variants:
1 thick, dense, closely packed collagen bundles;
2 similar to type 1, but with increased fibroblasts in the cutis;
3 oedematous and loose dermis.

Fibrous dermatofibroma is a true fibroma presenting as a smooth-edged tumour, commonly in the periungual tissues rather than within the nail unit. There is no collar of elevated skin as is often seen in acquired fibrokeratomas

and it lacks the hyperkeratotic tip. It is hypocellular but with prominent collagen bundles, and rarely has a histiocytic dermal component. Occasionally, fibromas can be confused with other lesions, such as Bowen's disease, exostosis, keloid, dermatofibrosarcoma, eccrine poroma, neurofibroma and verruca. Multiple soft fibromas presenting on the dorsal aspect of digits in childhood may be infantile digital fibromatosis. These are benign and resolve with age [4,5]. Periungual fibromas may act as a diagnostic clue for tuberous sclerosis, although they normally occur in association with at least one other feature such as hypomelanotic macules that allows corroboration [6]. They are rarely seen before the age of 5 years, but are present in 23% of subjects with tuberous sclerosis at 14 years, rising to 88% over 30 [6]. Presentation with a single periungual fibroma should lead to a full history and examination to establish whether it is a feature of undiagnosed tuberous sclerosis. However, if nothing else is found, it is unlikely that the tumour has broader significance [7].

Treatment is by excision. In acquired periungual fibrokeratoma arising in the proximal matrix, great care is needed to remove the origin of the tumour without damaging the matrix: there is a fine balance between allowing recurrence and producing long-term nail dystrophy. Koenen tumours are particularly prone to relapse, probably because of their dermal origin.

REFERENCES

1 Baran R, Perrin C, Baudet J, Requena L. Clinical and histological patterns of dermatofibromas (true fibromas) of the nail apparatus. *Clin Exp Dermatol* 1994; **19**: 31–5.

2 Kint A, Baran R. Histopathologic study of Koenen tumours. *J Am Acad Dermatol* 1988; **18**: 369–72.

3 Bart RS, Andrade R, Kopf AW, Leider M. Acquired digital fibrokeratomas. *Arch Dermatol* 1968; **97**: 120–9.

4 Cohen MM, Hayden PW. A newly recognised hamartomatous syndrome. *Birth Defects* 1979; **15**: 291–6.

5 Reye RDK. Recurring fibrous digital tumours of childhood. *Arch Pathol* 1965; **80**: 228–31.

6 Webb DW, Clarke A, Fryer A, Osborne JP. The cutaneous features of tuberous sclerosis: a population study. *Br J Dermatol* 1996; **135**: 1–5.

7 Zeller J, Friedmann D, Clerici T, Revuz J. The significance of a single periungual fibroma: report of seven cases. *Arch Dermatol* 1995; **131**: 1465–6.

Onychomatricoma

Onychomatricoma may be considered a form of fibroma of the proximal nail fold [1,2], closely associated with the matrix. Its location means that the main features are those of altered nail, which becomes thickened with increased longitudinal ridging (Fig. 62.29). There may be increased transverse and longitudinal curvature in larger tumours. Splinter haemorrhages within the zone of altered nail are common. When the onychomatricoma is small it may occupy only a narrow band of altered nail which is thickened and grey or yellow. As it enlarges, the band broadens

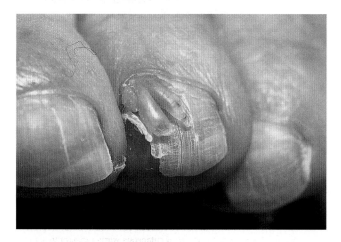
Fig. 62.28 Garlic clove fibroma.

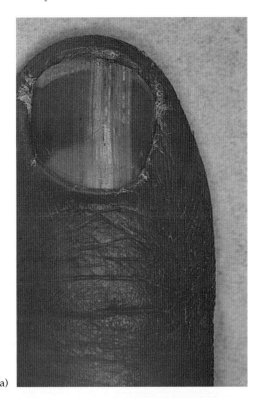

(a)

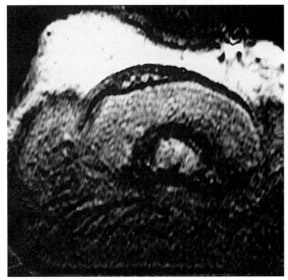

(b)

Fig. 62.29 (a) Subtle longitudinal thickening and opacity of the nail plate due to an onychomatricoma. (b) Onychomatricoma on MRI.

and thickens. When avulsed, the proximal aspect of the nail reveals multiple honeycomb channels corresponding to the digitations of the matrix, which has changed shape in response to the dermal matrix tumour. The tumour has normal immunohistochemical markers for a benign fibroma [2,3]. The matrix epithelium is normal in cytology and differentiation with respect to keratins [3]. Electron microscopy demonstrates decreased amounts of tonofilaments and desmosomes in basal epithelial cells [4]. It is the

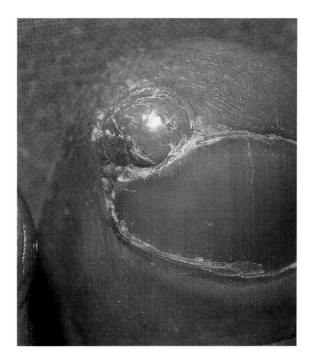

Fig. 62.30 Subungual exostosis.

marked change in shape that leads to the altered nail and characteristic clinical presentation.

Less classic presentations of the tumour may have nail features of melanonychia and onychomycosis [5].

Treatment is by excision. The margins need to include a proximal element of the proximal nail fold and extend down to bone and into proximal nail bed to obtain the whole tumour. This typically sacrifices a significant fraction of the matrix and may mean that total matrix excision is the best option.

REFERENCES

1 Perrin C, Goettmann S, Baran R. Onychomatricoma: clinical and histopathologic findings in 12 cases. *J Am Acad Dermatol* 1998; **39**: 560–4.
2 Fraga GR, Patterson JW, McHargue CA. Onychomatricoma: report of a case and its comparison with fibrokeratoma of the nailbed. *Am J Dermatopathol* 2001; **23**: 36–40.
3 Perrin C, Baran R, Pisani A, Ortonne JP, Michiels JF. The onychomatricoma: additional histologic criteria and immunohistochemical study. *Am J Dermatopathol* 2002; **24**: 199–203.
4 Kint A, Baran R, Geerts ML. The onychomatricoma: an electron microscopic study. *J Cutan Pathol* 1997; **24**: 183–8.
5 Fayol J, Baran R, Perrin C, Labrousse F. Onychomatricoma with misleading features. *Acta Derm Venereol (Stockh)* 2000; **80**: 370–2.

Subungual exostosis

A subungual exostosis is a benign bony outgrowth of the terminal phalanx. It is usually found on the great toe [1] or rarely a finger [2] in subjects between the ages of 10 and 35 years (Fig. 62.30). It is not clear whether trauma is causal or contributory. Where there are hereditary multiple exostoses, the problem is inherited in a dominant pattern and attributable to mutations of the *EXT1* and *EXT2* genes on chromosomes 8q and 11p, respectively. These genes encode the proteins exostosin 1 and 2, which are part of a family of glycosyltransferases required for the synthesis of heparan sulphate chains. Heparan sulphate is integral to the expression of proteoglycans on the cell surface and in the extracellular matrix [3]. Mutations of *EXT1* and *EXT2* are also found in specimens of solitary exostoses [3]. This corresponds to the absence of heparan sulphate in the chondrocyte zones of exostosis growth plates [4], consistent with the proposal that such changes in chondrocyte biology are associated with abnormal cell signalling.

Pain as a presenting feature is common. It is usually associated with trauma, but is also caused by ingrowing of the nail plate as it is displaced by the tumour [5]. The nail plate is elevated laterally but rarely damaged by the tumour. Radiography reveals an outgrowth of trabeculated bone [6], which may seem modest in comparison with the clinical complaint because of the large radiolucent cartilaginous cap. The X-ray examination should include a lateral view, as typically a view from above will miss the pathology.

Distinction from a subungual osteochondroma may be possible histologically because fibrous cartilage caps the bony outgrowth in exostosis and hyaline cartilage in osteochondroma [7]. Whereas this rule is often stated, it is not clear whether an absolute distinction can be made between the two lesions.

Where multiple exostoses exist, autosomal dominant multiple exostosis syndrome must be considered. The tumours in this condition are 'near the knee and far from the elbow' and can be destructive to nail [8]. The importance of making the diagnosis lies in the remote possibility of transformation of individual tumours to chondrosarcoma—an estimated figure for malignant change is 0.5% [9]. Older patients may have a different variety of exostosis, which represents hyperostosis of the distal tuft. This can cause elevation of the nail and pincer deformity, whereby the distal and lateral borders of the nail curve downward and inward to act as a pincer upon the nail bed.

Treatment. Treatment of subungual exostosis is by partial nail avulsion or fish-mouth elevation of nail bed and plate and removal of the tumour using bone nibblers or a chisel [7]. A margin of normal bone should be removed at the base to prevent recurrence. There is a 10% relapse rate following surgery, and children are more prone to relapse than adults [5]. Permanent matrix damage may follow surgery if tumours undermine the matrix.

REFERENCES

1 Landon GC, Johnson KA, Dahlin DC. Subungual exostoses. *J Bone Joint Surg* 1979; **61A**: 256–9.
2 Carroll RE, Chance JT, Inan Y. Subungual exostoses of the hand. *J Hand Surg* 1992; **17B**: 569–74.
3 Hall CR, Cole WG, Haynes R, Hecht JT. Reevaluation of a genetic model for the development of exostosis in hereditary multiple exostosis. *Am J Med Genet* 2002; **112**: 1–5.
4 Hecht JT, Hall CR, Snuggs M *et al*. Heparan sulfate abnormalities in exostosis growth plates. *Bone* 2002; **31**: 199–204.
5 de Berker DA, Langtry J. Treatment of subungual exostoses by elective day case surgery. *Br J Dermatol* 1999; **140**: 915–8.
6 Evison G, Price CHG. Subungual exostoses. *Br J Radiol* 1966; **39**: 451–5.
7 Dumontier CA, Abimelec P. Nail unit enchondromas and osteochondromas: a surgical approach. *Dermatol Surg* 2001; **27**: 274–9.
8 Baran R, Bureau H. Multiple exostoses syndrome presenting with anonychia on a single finger. *J Am Acad Dermatol* 1991; **25**: 333–5.
9 Voutsinas S, Wynne-Davies R. The infrequency of malignant disease in diaphyseal aclasis and neurofibromatosis. *J Med Genet* 1983; **20**: 345–9.

Other bone tumours

Enchondroma

An enchondroma is a cartilage tumour, which may present as a painful solitary tumour of the distal phalanx with clubbing, paronychia, nail thickening, discoloration, ridging and elevation of the nail, and pathological fractures [1]. In Ollier's disease, multiple digits are usually affected. In Maffuci's syndrome there are multiple subcutaneous angiomas and hard cartilaginous nodules of the epiphyseal line, which may distort the entire hand or foot [2].

X-ray shows lucent expansion of distal phalanges alone, with spotty calcification in simple enchondromas. In Maffuci's syndrome there is widespread lucency in many phalanges of all the digits. Treatment is by enucleation of the tumour and autologous cancellous bone grafting. All these tumours can be associated with chondrosarcoma, angiosarcoma being an additional risk in Maffuci's syndrome [3].

Osteoid osteoma [4–6]

Osteoid osteomas of the distal phalanx present with enlargement of the entire digit tip in a young adult, with thickening of nail, clubbing, increased local sweating and violaceous skin changes. A tender tumour may be palpated within the diffuse swelling, and the tumour may cause a nagging pain, characteristically relieved by non-steroidal anti-inflammatory drugs.

X-ray reveals a small area of rarefaction surrounded by sclerosis, although symptoms may precede this appearance and an isotope bone scan or MRI may show the focus earlier. Arteriography and thermography demonstrate the hypervascularity. Surgical treatment of this benign condition is by en bloc resection through a fish-mouth incision.

Implantation epidermoid cyst

Implantation epidermoid cyst may produce gradual enlargement of the tip of the digit, with the appearance of clubbing, or pincer nail. Pain may arise due to disturbance of the underlying bone where there is erosion, with distortion of cortical bone seen on X-ray, or a cyst may be demarcated on MRI. There is sometimes a history of previous trauma or surgery. Surgery is generally curative [7,8].

Metastases

Metastatic tumours present as inflamed swellings at the tip of a digit, with relatively few symptoms. X-ray reveals an osteolytic lesion, and systemic examination and investigation may reveal the primary focus; 50% will be from carcinoma of the lung [9,10].

REFERENCES

1 Yaffee HW. Peculiar nail dystrophy caused by an enchondroma. *Arch Dermatol* 1965; **91**: 361.
2 Monses B, Murphy WA. Distal phalangeal erosive lesions. *Arthritis Rheum* 1984; **27**: 449–55.
3 Lewis RJ, Ketcham AS. Maffuci's syndrome: functional and neoplastic significance. *J Bone Joint Surg* 1973; **55A**: 1465–79.
4 Bowen CVA, Dzus AK, Hardy DA. Osteoid osteomata of the distal phalanx. *J Hand Surg* 1987; **12B**: 387–90.
5 Brown RE, Russel JB, Zook EG. Osteoid osteoma of the distal phalanx of the finger: a diagnostic challenge. *Plast Reconstr Surg* 1991; **90**: 1016–21.
6 Jaffé HL. Osteoid osteoma. A benign osteoblastic tumour composed of osteoid and atypical bone. *Arch Surg* 1935; **31**: 709–28.
7 Baran R, Broutard JC. Epidermoid cyst of the thumb presenting as a pincer nail. *J Am Acad Dermatol* 1989; **19**: 143–4.
8 Schajowicz F, Alello CA, Slullitel I. Cystic and pseudo-cystic lesions of the terminal phalanx with special reference to epidermoid cyst. *Clin Orthop Rel Res* 1970; **68**: 84–92.
9 Baran R, Tosti A. Metastatic carcinoma to the terminal phalanx of the big toe: report of two cases and review of the literature. *J Am Acad Dermatol* 1994; **31**: 259–63.
10 Cohen PR. Metastatic tumors to the nail unit: subungual metastases. *Dermatol Surg* 2001; **27**: 280–93.

Vascular tumours

Glomus tumour

Glomus tumours are the most characteristic of vascular nail bed tumours. There is pain, which may be spontaneous or evoked by mild trauma or temperature change. Nail plate changes depend on the location of the tumour. Matrix tumours cause splitting and distortion of the nail plate. Nail bed lesions are most likely to appear as bluish or red foci, 1–5 mm in diameter, beneath the nail [1]. On X-ray, 36% show a depression in the underlying phalanx [1]; MRI can reveal the exact site of the tumour [2]. It is of particular value when there is pain after excision in order to help determine whether the pain is a complication of surgery or due to recurrent tumour [3]. High-resolution ultrasound has also been used with some success [4].

Histology is the definitive investigation and reveals vascular channels lined with endothelium and cuboidal glomus cells. These have dark nuclei and pale cytoplasm. Myelinated and non-myelinated nerves are found, which

may account for the associated symptoms; neuromas must be considered in the differential diagnosis [5].

Treatment. Excision is the treatment of choice. Some surgeons advocate approaching the pathology by a fish-mouth incision, expecially when the tumour is in the nail bed [6]. However, this assumes a clear knowledge as to the location and nature of the tumour before surgery. Often it is necessary to remove the nail for preliminary assessment and this also facilitates matrix repair [5,7]. Where there is persistent pain after treatment, it may be due to the earlier surgery or further tumour. MRI can help in assessing this [2]. Residual scarring of the nail may remain, depending on the nature of the surgery and the extent of preoperative damage.

REFERENCES

1 Van Geertruyden J, Lorea P, Goldschmidt D *et al.* Glomus tumours of the hand. A retrospective study of 51 cases. *J Hand Surg* 1996; **21B**: 257–60.
2 Drapé JL, Idy-Peretti I, Goettmann S *et al.* Standard and high resolution MRI in glomus tumours of toes and fingertips. *J Am Acad Dermatol* 1996; **35**: 550–5.
3 Theumann NH, Goettmann S, Le Viet D *et al.* Recurrent glomus tumors of fingertips: MR imaging evaluation. *Radiology* 2002; **223**: 143–51.
4 Fornage BD, Schernberg FL, Rifkin MD, Touche DH. Sonographic diagnosis of glomus tumour of the finger. *J Ultrasound Med* 1984; **3**: 523–4.
5 Shelley ED, Shelley WB. Exploratory nail plate removal as a diagnostic aid in painful subungual tumours: glomus tumour, neurofibroma and squamous cell carcinomas. *Cutis* 1986; **38**: 310–2.
6 Wegener EE. Glomus tumors of the nail unit: a plastic surgeon's approach. *Dermatol Surg* 2001; **27**: 240–1.
7 Takata H, Ikuta Y, Ishida O, Kimori K. Treatment of subungual glomus tumour. *Hand Surg* 2001; **6**: 25–7.

Pyogenic granuloma and periungual vascular lesions

Pyogenic granulomas are benign eruptive haemangiomas. They may involve the nail fold, with a prominent collar of epithelium, or be subungual and penetrate the nail plate (Fig. 62.31). In this location, they almost invariably arise from the matrix and produce a localized deformity of the nail plate, visible as the nail grows distally. Mild penetrating injury, friction [1] and immobilization of the limb in a cast [2] are physical causes. Medication can also be relevant. Retinoids [3], ciclosporin [4], cancer chemotherapy and antiretroviral treatment for HIV infection are all potential initiating factors. With these medications, the presentation is often of excessive granulation tissue on more than one digit as part of an ingrowing nail, rather than the classic isolated lesion puncturing the matrix and emerging from beneath the proximal nail fold. There may be features that blur the distinction between focal lesions and areas of hyperaemia with inflammation [5] and onycholysis [5–7]. Pain can be a significant feature [7] and docetaxel, used in breast and prostate cancer, has been implicated in such cases. Where antiretroviral medication is implicated, it is usually in association with nucleoside reverse transcriptase inhibitors [8,9].

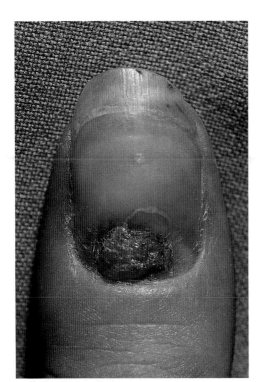

Fig. 62.31 Pyogenic granuloma penetrating the nail plate.

A pyogenic granuloma bleeds easily and must be distinguished from an amelanotic malignant melanoma, histiocytoid haemangioma [10], granulation tissue reaction to ingrowing nail and cavernous angioma. Where the clinical evolution is slow, the differential diagnosis includes squamous cell carcinoma and a range of benign tumours [11]. The possibility of malignancy and other progressive tumours makes histological examination important. Bacteriology is also required and may help with the diagnosis of coccal nail fold angiomatosis, which may resemble a pyogenic granuloma arising from the matrix. This can relapse locally and on other digits [12].

Treatment. Once histology is available, if the lesion persists, destructive therapy such as carbon dioxide laser or suppressive therapy such as a potent topical steroid can be used. The latter is preferable and adequate for matrix lesions where infection has been adequately treated. Potassium permanganate soaks, or local or systemic antibiotics, may be needed if there is secondary infection with excessive oozing.

REFERENCES

1 Richert B. Frictional pyogenic granuloma of the nail bed. *Dermatology* 2001; **202**: 80–1.
2 Tosti A, Piraccini BM, Camacho-Martinez F. Onychomadesis and pyogenic granuloma following cast immobilization. *Arch Dermatol* 2001; **137**: 231–2.
3 Baran R. Retinoids and the nails. *J Dermatol Treat* 1990; **1**: 151–4.

4 Higgins EM, Hughes JR, Snowden S, Pembroke AC. Cyclosporin-induced periungual granulation tissue. *Br J Dermatol* 1995; **132**: 829–30.
5 Nicolopoulos J, Howard A. Docetaxel-induced nail dystrophy. *Australas J Dermatol* 2002; **43**: 293–6.
6 Wasner G, Hilpert F, Schattschneider J et al. Docetaxel-induced nail changes: a neurogenic mechanism. A case report. *J Neurooncol* 2002; **58**: 167–74.
7 Stemmler HJ, Gutschow K, Sommer H et al. Weekly docetaxel (Taxotere) in patients with metastatic breast cancer. *Ann Oncol* 2001; **12**: 1393–8.
8 Ward HA, Russo GG, Shrum J. Cutaneous manifestations of antiretroviral therapy. *J Am Acad Dermatol* 2002; **46**: 284–93.
9 Heim M, Schapiro J, Wershavski M, Martinowitz U. Drug-induced and traumatic nail problems in the haemophilias. *Haemophilia* 2000; **6**: 191–4.
10 Tosti A, Peluso AM, Fanti PA et al. Histiocytoid haemangioma with prominent fingernail involvement. *Dermatology* 1994; **189**: 87–9.
11 Hassanein A, Telang G, Benedetto E, Spielvogel R. Subungual myxoid pleomorphic fibroma. *Am J Dermatopathol* 1998; **20**: 502–5.
12 Davies MG. Coccal nail fold angiomatosis. *Br J Dermatol* 1995; **132**: 162–3.

Arteriovenous abnormalities

Periungual and subungual arteriovenous tumours (cirsoid aneurysms) are firm, bluish, non-pulsatile nodules in a nail fold or penetrating the nail [1]. Treatment by excision reveals histology of thick-walled vascular channels with fibrous tissue boundaries and no internal elastic lamina. In the presence of a digital arteriovenous malformation, the digit and nail bed are purple, with gradual shrinkage and overcurvature of the nail plate [2]. Growth may be rapid in young people, in whom the digit may become bulbous and painful. X-ray may reveal aneurysmal destruction of the terminal phalanx, and more precise detail may be gained by MRI.

REFERENCES

1 Burge SM, Baran R, Dawber RPR, Verret JL. Periungual and subungual arteriovenous tumours. *Br J Dermatol* 1986; **115**: 361–6.
2 Enjolras O, Riché MC. *Hémangiomes et Malformations Vasculaires Superficielles.* New York: Medsi/McGraw-Hill, 1990.

Myxoid cyst
SYN. MYXOID OR MUCOID PSEUDOCYST

This benign cystic swelling has many names and is often termed a pseudocyst because a cellular cyst wall can seldom be demonstrated. It is usually located between the crease of the distal interphalangeal joint on the dorsal surface and the proximal nail fold. Less commonly it is found between the proximal nail fold and the nail plate, beneath the nail matrix or in the digit pulp. Pressure on the matrix results in a longitudinal groove or gutter in the nail plate (Fig. 62.32), which may have transverse ridges within it, reflecting episodes of decreased matrix pressure when the cyst is decompressed through discharge of its contents. When the tumour occupies the space between the nail and proximal nail fold, it may protrude from beneath the nail fold with what appears to be a keratotic tip, mimicking a fibrokeratoma. When located beneath the matrix, the nail becomes misshapen, with increased transverse curvature, and the lunula appears red [1].

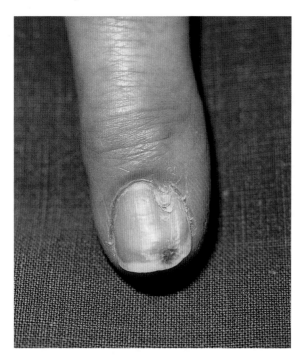

Fig. 62.32 Nail plate groove due to proximal myxoid cyst.

Myxoid cysts are more common in the fingers than the toes. They contain a clear gelatinous fluid that may discharge spontaneously or on minor trauma. This fluid may be the product of mucoid degeneration of connective tissue or be derived directly from the adjacent distal interphalangeal joint with which a communication is usually demonstrable by injection of methylene blue into the joint [2,3]. The condition of the joint is a major factor in the origin of the tumour, with osteoarthritic osteophytes damaging the joint capsule and provoking the flaw through which synovial fluid escapes. Infection of the ruptured pseudocyst may cause septic arthritis or local paronychia, although this is uncommon.

High-resolution ultrasound or MRI provides non-invasive visualization to confirm the diagnosis or to localize the pedicle in recurrent cases. However, it may be more practical to attempt transillumination with a pen torch. This will distinguish it from a giant cell tendon sheath tumour, which is usually found overlying the dorsal distal interphalangeal crease in women with osteoarthritis [4,5]. Giant cell tendon sheath tumours are often rubbery and fail to transilluminate. Alternatively, a myxoid cyst will easily puncture using a size 11 scalpel, with sterile technique, revealing the diagnostic gelatinous contents.

Histology usually reveals a pseudocyst cavity within a fibrous capsule containing a myxomatous stroma with scattered fibroblasts. Areas of myxomatous change may merge to form a multilobular pseudocyst. Some workers report a mesothelial lining to the pseudocyst, consistent with continuity with the synovial joint space. This is not always confirmed and may mean that there are different histological forms of myxoid pseudocysts.

Treatment. There are many conservative approaches to cure [6,7], none of which is definitive. These include incision and drainage (pricking with a sterile blade or needle) and which may be repeated by the patient [8], injected sclerosant [9] or steroid [10,11], cryosurgery [12,13], laser [14] and infrared photocoagulation [15].

Surgical therapy may entail removal of osteophytes involving the distal interphalangeal joint [16–19], excising the distal margin of the proximal nail fold if the tumour is located there [20], or tracing the communication between the joint and cyst with methylene blue and tying it off [3,21].

There is a high relapse rate after single treatments with less invasive therapies. More detailed surgical therapies are more effective [19,21].

REFERENCES

1 de Berker D, Goettman S, Baran R. Subungual myxoid cysts: clinical manifestations and response to therapy. *J Am Acad Dermatol* 2002; **46**: 394–8.
2 Kleinert HE, Kutz JE, Fishman JH *et al*. Etiology and treatment of the so-called mucous cyst of the finger. *J Bone Joint Surg* 1972; **54A**: 1455–8.
3 Newmeyer WL, Kilgore ES, Graham WP. Mucous cyst: the dorsal distal interphalangeal joint ganglion. *Plast Reconstr Surg* 1974; **53**: 313–5.
4 Averill RM, Smith RJ, Campbell CJ. Giant cell tumours of the bones of the hand. *J Hand Surg* 1980; **5**: 39–50.
5 Wright CJE. Benign giant-cell synovioma. An investigation of 85 cases. *Br J Surg* 1951; **38**: 257–71.
6 Baran R, Haneke E. Tumours of the nail apparatus and adjacent tissues. In: Baran R, Dawber RPR, eds. *Diseases of the Nails and Their Management*, 2nd edn. Oxford: Blackwell Science, 1994: 474–6.
7 de Berker DAR. Treatment of myxoid cysts. *J Dermatol Treat* 1995; **6**: 55–7.
8 Epstein E. A simple technique for managing digital mucous cysts. *Arch Dermatol* 1979; **115**: 1315–6.
9 Audebert C. Treatment of mucoid cysts of fingers and toes by injection of sclerosant. *Dermatol Clin* 1989; **7**: 179–81.
10 Epstein E. Steroid injection of myxoid finger cysts. *JAMA* 1965; **194**: 98–9.
11 Johnson WC, Graham JH, Helwig EB. Cutaneous myxoid cyst. A clinicopathological and histochemical study. *JAMA* 1965; **191**: 15–20.
12 Dawber RPR, Colver G, Jackson A. *Cutaneous Cryosurgery. Principles and Clinical Practice*. London: Dunitz, 1992: 71–2.
13 Dawber RPR. Myxoid cysts of the finger: treatment by liquid nitrogen spray cryosurgery. *Clin Exp Dermatol* 1983; **8**: 153–7.
14 Huerter CJ, Wheeland RG, Bailin PL, Ratz JL. Treatment of digital myxoid cysts with carbon dioxide laser vaporization. *J Dermatol Surg Oncol* 1987; **13**: 723–7.
15 Kemmett D, Colver GB. Myxoid cysts treated by infra-red photocoagulation. *Clin Exp Dermatol* 1994; **19**: 118–20.
16 Brown RE, Zook EG, Russell RC *et al*. Fingernail deformities secondary to ganglions of the distal interphalangeal joint (mucous cysts). *Plast Reconstr Surg* 1991; **87**: 718–25.
17 Gingrass MK, Brown RE, Zook EG. Treatment of fingernail deformities secondary to ganglions of the distal interphalangeal joint. *J Hand Surg* 1995; **20A**: 502–5.
18 Kasdan ML, Stallings SP, Leis V, Wolens D. Outcome of surgically treated mucous cysts of the hand. *J Hand Surg* 1994; **19A**: 504–7.
19 Mani-Sundaram D. Surgical correction of mucous cysts of the nail unit. *Dermatol Surg* 2001; **27**: 267–8.
20 Salasche SJ. Myxoid cysts of the proximal nail fold, a surgical approach. *J Dermatol Surg Oncol* 1984; **10**: 35–9.
21 de Berker D, Lawrence C. Ganglion of the distal interphalangeal joint (myxoid cyst): therapy by identification and repair of the leak of joint fluid. *Arch Dermatol* 2001; **137**: 607–10.

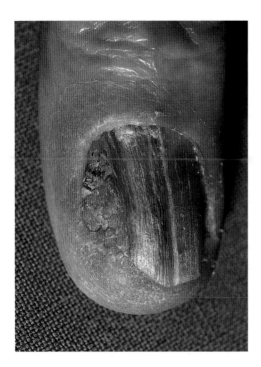

Fig. 62.33 Bowen's disease with melanonychia.

Squamous cell carcinoma

SYN. EPIDERMOID CARCINOMA

Squamous cell carcinoma of the nail unit includes *in situ* (Bowen's disease) and invasive forms (Fig. 62.33). A single biopsy may fail to make a distinction between them. A tumour that appears *in situ* at one site may be invasive elsewhere [1]. Periungual features include hyperkeratotic warty changes, erosions and fissuring, macerated cuticle, periungual swelling, erythema and occasional secondary infection. Subungual changes include onycholysis with a friable or warty nail bed, longitudinal melanonychia, nail dystrophy, ingrowing or loss. Some cases may be as subtle as a single red longitudinal streak [2] (see p. 62.19). Nodular change with ulceration and bleeding is a late development. The condition may affect many digits [3]. Common misdiagnoses include onychomycosis, periungual warts, recurrent paronychia, pyogenic granuloma and subungual exostosis. As some of these conditions do not warrant biopsy and clinicians seldom think of squamous cell carcinoma at this site, the diagnosis is frequently delayed. Mean periods of 52 months [4], 9 years [5] and 5 years [6] have been reported. This slow progression may mean that the diagnosis is never made on older people, with the consequent impression that the disease is less common than is the case [7].

Predisposing factors include radiation exposure [3,8], human papillomaviruses 16, 18 and 34 [4,5,8–10], and possibly ectodermal dysplasias and chronic trauma. Features of chronic radiation damage to the periunguium may precede the onset of malignancy [11]. History and examination should include a note of genital wart infection or cervical dysplasia in the patient or partner [8]. Appropriate investigation includes X-ray and biopsy of a large and representative area. Failed diagnosis can be attributed to poor diagnostic biopsy technique. Prognosis is good and there are only five cases of metastatic disease in the literature [9], two of which were in patients with ectodermal dysplasia [12,13].

Treatment. Mohs' micrographic surgery is the treatment of choice for ill-defined lesions, as long as there is no evidence of bone involvement [1,6,14]. The technique allows the digit to be preserved in most instances. Horizontal sections in the context of the complex three-dimensional anatomy and histology of the nail unit require careful and experienced interpretation [15]. Alternative treatments include local excision, digit amputation and radiotherapy [16].

REFERENCES

1 Mikhail G. Subungual epidermoid carcinoma. *J Am Acad Dermatol* 1984; **11**: 291–8.
2 Baran R, Perrin C. Longitudinal erythronychia with distal subungual keratosis: onychopapilloma of the nail bed and Bowen's disease. *Br J Dermatol* 2000; **143**: 132–5.
3 Baran RL, Gormley DE. Polydactylous Bowen's disease of the nail. *J Am Acad Dermatol* 1987; **17**: 201–4.
4 Sau P, McMarlin S, Sperling LC, Katz R. Bowen's disease of the nail bed and periungual area. *Arch Dermatol* 1994; **130**: 204–9.
5 Moy RL, Eliezri YD, Nuovo GJ *et al.* Human papillomavirus type 16 DNA in periungual squamous cell carcinomas. *JAMA* 1989; **261**: 2669–73.
6 Godlminz D, Bennett RG. Mohs micrographic surgery of the nail unit. *J Dermatol Surg Oncol* 1992; **18**: 721–6.
7 Virgili A, Rosaria Zampino M, Bacilieri S, Bettoli V, Chiarelli M. Squamous cell carcinoma of the nail bed: a rare disease or only misdiagnosed? *Acta Derm Venereol (Stockh)* 2001; **81**: 306–7.
8 Guitart J, Bergfeld WF, Tuthull RJ *et al.* Squamous cell carcinoma of the nail bed: a clinicopathological study of twelve cases. *Br J Dermatol* 1990; **123**: 215–22.
9 Ashinoff R, Jumli J, Jacobson M *et al.* Detection of HPV DNA in squamous cell carcinoma of the nail bed and finger determined by polymerase chain reaction. *Arch Dermatol* 1991; **127**: 1813–8.
10 McHugh RW, Hazen P, Eliezri YD, Nuovo GJ. Metastatic periungual squamous cell carcinoma: detection of human papillomavirus type 35 RNA in the digital tumour and axillary lymph node metastases. *J Am Acad Dermatol* 1996; **34**: 1080–2.
11 Richert B, de la Brassine M. Subungual chronic radiodermatitis. *Dermatology* 1993; **186**: 290–3.
12 Campbell J, Keokarn T. Squamous cell carcinoma of the nail bed in epidermal dysplasia. *J Bone Joint Dis* 1966; **48**: 92–9.
13 Mauro JA, Maslyn R, Stein AA. Squamous cell carcinoma of the nail bed in hereditary ectodermal dysplasia. *N Y State J Med* 1972; **72**: 1065–6.
14 de Berker DAR, Dahl MGC, Malcolm AJ, Lawrence CM. Micrographic surgery for subungual squamous cell carcinoma. *Br J Plast Surg* 1996; **49**: 414–9.
15 Zaiac MN, Weiss E. Mohs micrographic surgery of the nail unit and squamous cell carcinoma. *Dermatol Surg* 2001; **27**: 246–51.
16 Attiyeh FF, Shah J, Booker RJ *et al.* Subungual squamous cell carcinoma. *JAMA* 1979; **241**: 262–3.

Epithelioma cuniculatum [1,2]

Epithelioma cuniculatum is a slow-growing, locally destructive, low-grade tumour, histologically related to squamous cell carcinoma [1,2]. It is typically found on the sole of the foot, but may involve the periunguium, mucosal surfaces and other locations [3]. It is warty, with discharge of foul-smelling yellow material from nail bed sinuses. The overlying nail is disrupted by onycholysis or destruction at the matrix, and there may be paronychia. The underlying bone is usually affected and X-ray reveals destruction of the terminal phalanx in most cases. Biopsy confirms the diagnosis. A system of epithelium-lined channels within the tumour form fistulae extruding keratinous debris. Mitoses and dyskeratotic cells are rare and the benign appearance may lead to the misdiagnosis of pseudoepitheliomatous hyperplasia. Mohs' micrographic surgery is a useful treatment.

REFERENCES

1 McKee P, Wilkinson JD, Black MM *et al*. Carcinoma (epithelioma) cuniculatum: a clinicopathological study of nineteen cases and review of the literature. *Histopathology* 1986; **5**: 425–36.
2 Tosti A, Morelli R, Fanti PA *et al*. Carcinoma cuniculatum of the nail apparatus: report of 3 cases. *Dermatology* 1993; **186**: 217–21.
3 Schwartz RA. Verrucous carcinoma of the skin and mucosa. *J Am Acad Dermatol* 1995; **32**: 1–21.

Keratoacanthoma

Subungual or periungual keratoacanthomas are typically painful, rapidly enlarging lesions that are usually solitary [1,2]. They are often referred to by the acronym SUKA. Keratoacanthoma is a misleading term as there is no indication that the tumour follows the same pattern of involution seen in keratoacanthomas elsewhere; also, there is no apparent relationship with sun exposure. Although trauma and wire wool have been implicated [3], in most cases there is no obvious precipitating factor. Erosion of bone is seen on X-ray, which is an essential preliminary investigation [4–7]. This feature is likely to represent a pressure effect of rapid subungual expansion, rather than bone invasion. The diagnosis is made partly on the history but largely from the histology, which closely resembles that of a keratoacanthoma seen elsewhere but showing little or no squamous dysplasia [4]. Subungual wart, squamous cell carcinoma and subungual exostosis are among the differential diagnoses. Clinically, subungual keratotic incontinentia pigmenti tumours fall between the appearance of fibroma and keratoacanthoma [8,9]. They resemble the latter in often being painful and causing underlying bone changes. They are commonly multiple and seen with the other features of incontinentia pigmenti, which is usually lethal in males. These tumours can be treated with oral retinoids [10], but may eventually require surgery.

Treatment. Treatment of subungual keratoacanthoma can be by Mohs' micrographic surgery or curettage. More aggressive treatments, including amputation of the digit, have been employed in the past, but are not warranted. Given the concern that the tumour may represent a form of squamous cell carcinoma, micrographic surgery may be the treatment of choice.

REFERENCES

1 Baran R, Mikhail G, Costini B, Tosti A, Goettmann-Bonvallot S. Distal digital keratoacanthoma: two cases with a review of the literature. *Dermatol Surg* 2001; **27**: 575–9.
2 Baran R, Goettmann S. Distal digital keratoacanthoma: a report of 12 cases and a review of the literature. *Br J Dermatol* 1998; **139**: 512–5.
3 Fisher AA. Subungual keratoacanthoma: possible relationship of exposure to steel wool. *Cutis* 1990; **46**: 26–8.
4 Cramer SF. Subungual keratoacanthoma. A benign bone eroding neoplasm of the distal phalanx. *Am J Clin Pathol* 1981; **75**: 425–9.
5 Keeney GL, Banks PM, Linscheid RL. Subungual keratoacanthoma. Report of a case and review of the literature. *Arch Dermatol* 1990; **124**: 1074–6.
6 Oliwiecki S, Peachey RDG, Bradfield JWB *et al*. Subungual keratoacanthoma: a report of four cases and review of the literature. *Clin Exp Dermatol* 1994; **19**: 230–5.
7 Patel MR, Desai SS. Subungual keratoacanthoma in the hand. *J Hand Surg* 1989; **14A**: 139–42.
8 Adeniran A, Townsend PLG, Peachey RDG. Incontinentia pigmenti (Bloch–Sulzberger syndrome) manifesting as painful periungual and subungual tumours. *J Hand Surg* 1993; **18B**: 667–9.
9 Bessems PJM, Jagtman BA, Van de Staak W. Progressive, persistent, hyperkeratotic lesions in incontinentia pigmenti. *Arch Dermatol* 1988; **124**: 29–30.
10 Malvehy J, Palou J, Mascaro JM. Painful subungual tumour in incontinentia pigmenti. Response to treatment with etretinate. *Br J Dermatol* 1998; **138**: 554–5.

Melanocytic lesions

Benign melanocytic lesions usually present as longitudinal melanonychia (LM). This is also a common appearance of early malignant melanoma of the nail matrix [1]. An understanding of the causes of benign nail pigmentation is important in order to judge when biopsy is indicated to exclude melanoma.

Benign causes of LM

Laugier–Hunziker syndrome

Laugier–Hunziker syndrome gradually evolves with pale-brown LM on one or more digits [2,3]. There may be periungual involvement resembling Hutchinson's sign and the oral and genital mucosae may be affected with pigmented macules. The macules are amenable to laser treatment [4].

Subungual naevi

Subungual naevi may present in adulthood or early in life with LM or with naevoid melanosis of the nail plate [5] (Fig. 62.34). This has been described in European [6,7] and Japanese [8] adults and children.

Drug therapy

Drug therapy with minocycline, zidovudine [9] and antimalarials may produce brown streaks in the nail (see

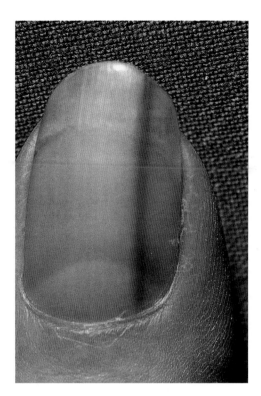

Fig. 62.34 Benign longitudinal melanonychia due to a subungual naevus.

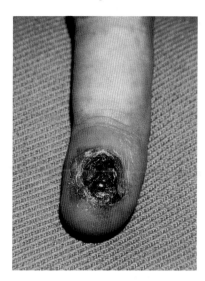

Fig. 62.35 Malignant melanoma arising in the nail matrix and invading the nail bed.

p. 62.18), as may dermatoses such as lichen planus [10] and onychomycosis [11], trauma [12] and non-melanocytic tumours such as squamous cell carcinoma *in situ* [13] (see Fig. 62.33). Subungual blood pigment may resemble melanin, but associated features in the history and appearance usually make it possible to distinguish the two.

Benign racial pigmentation

The most common cause of LM is racial variation; 77% of Afro-Caribbeans over 20 years of age have LM and this prevalence rises to almost 100% by the age of 50 years [14]. It is present in 10–20% of Japanese [15] and is more common in Mediterranean races than in northern Europeans. However, in this context, the percentage of malignant melanomas presenting in the nail unit is higher in Afro-Caribbeans (15–20%) [14] than in any other group (3% in white populations [16]). This contrasts with the low incidence of malignant melanoma at other skin sites in Afro-Caribbeans.

Malignant melanoma [17–20]

There are many features of LM that should suggest the possibility of malignant melanoma. These include the presence of brown-black periungual pigmentation (Hutchinson's sign) [21], especially when the pigmentation develops in a single digit in adult life and is evolving

to become darker and broader and has blurred edges. Hutchinson's sign needs careful assessment and does not necessarily carry a bad prognosis [2,22]. Dermatoscopic examination through the nail may help with diagnosis [23,24]. The suspicion of melanoma is raised further if the individual has any other risk factors for melanoma, if the involved digit is a thumb, great toe or index finger, and if the nail has become dystrophic.

Despite the importance of LM as a warning sign, 25% of subungual melanomas present as amelanotic tumours. This exceeds the percentage of melanomas presenting as an amelanotic tumour elsewhere. It is difficult to determine whether these tumours were always amelanotic [25] or whether loss of pigment is due to development of the disease process (Fig. 62.35). This form of melanoma usually has associated nail plate damage and easily bleeds. With this appearance, the differential diagnosis includes pyogenic granuloma, chronic paronychia and vascular tumour.

The assessment of pigmented streaks in children is complex. The earlier dictum that they were all benign and could be left has some ramifications. Indeed they are almost all benign [7], although very rare cases of melanoma are reported [26]. This alone may make diagnostic biopsy warranted in some or all. In addition, it is documented that pigmented streaks arising in childhood can evolve into melanoma, even after an initial biopsy with benign histology (S. Goettmann-Bonvallot, personal communication). The implication of this is that repeated biopsies may be needed as a pigmented streak evolves, and lifelong monitoring is required for children with such signs. Faced with this, complete excision of the matrix origin can sometimes be the best option, even when there is permanent loss of all or part of the nail.

The significance of preceding trauma is unclear [25]. Such a history is present in a large number of cases. It is thought that primary malignant melanoma of the nail unit arises only from within the matrix and not from the nail bed. This is consistent with the absence of antigenically identifiable melanocytes in the nail bed [27,28] and can provide some reassurance when assessing pigmented lesions not arising from the matrix. However, such lesions may arise from the nail folds, or be secondary malignant melanomas.

Biopsy of LM

Given the gravity of the potential cause of melanonychia, there should be a low threshold for biopsy. The type of biopsy can be determined by a range of factors [12].
1 Periungual pigmentation present. This indicates high risk of malignancy. If there are no other factors to account for this pigmentation, the whole area of affected nail unit should be removed en bloc down to bone with a 1-mm margin of normal tissue. Cosmetic considerations are secondary.
2 Lateral third of nail plate involved. This indicates lateral longitudinal biopsy. The cosmetic outcome is reasonable and the assurance provided by complete removal of the affected area is usually worthwhile.
3 Mid portion of the nail plate involved. The cosmetic outcome of complete excision at this site is potentially bad. This is particularly so if the origin of melanocytes is proximal in the matrix. This may be determined by sampling the free edge of the nail plate and performing a Masson–Fontana stain. Pigment in the lower part of the nail reflects a distal matrix origin, compared with ventral nail pigment reflecting an origin in the proximal matrix. The latter carries a high risk of scarring following excision.

For lesions less than 3 mm wide. The potential for postoperative dystrophy in midline lesions warrants preliminary investigation of thin (< 3 mm) pigmented streaks with a matrix punch biopsy unless the clinical evidence of malignancy is overwhelming. This technique involves:
1 reflection of proximal nail fold to visualize the origin of the pigment;
2 a 3-mm punch biopsy through the nail down to bone at the pigment origin, but leaving the biopsy *in situ*;
3 proximal hemi-avulsion, which will leave the 3-mm biopsy of nail remaining;
4 examination of fully exposed matrix;
5 careful removal of 3-mm biopsy of matrix and nail with iris scissors;
6 after gentle undermining, partial approximation and suture of the wound with 7/0 monofilament may be attempted for proximal matrix wounds.
Removal of the nail plate before biopsy can mean one loses the site of pigment origin once the clue of melanony-chia has gone. Removal of the 3-mm biopsy without hemi-avulsion of the surrounding nail is difficult and may result in damage to the specimen, which compromises histological interpretation. For these reasons, the method outlined above is preferred.

For lesions 3–6 mm wide. If the pigment arises from distal matrix, a transverse matrix biopsy can be performed. Proximal matrix pigment requires an en bloc removal and repair using a Schernberg and Amiel flap.

For lesions greater than 6 mm wide. Matrix punch or transverse biopsy is usually adequate as the preliminary investigation.

Treatment and prognosis

Nail unit melanoma has a record of delayed treatment and poor prognosis [29]. It affects light and dark skinned people, those of African origin representing 12% of patients in one North American series [30]. The most common pattern is of acral lentiginous melanoma [17], although one series reported the superficial spreading type as being marginally more common [31]. In the acral lentiginous form, there is lentiginous spread of pleomorphic, often dendritic, atypical melanocytes in the basal and suprabasal layers of the epidermis. Epidermal melanoma cells may be incorporated into the nail plate and seen on stained clippings of nail taken from the free edge. Dermal melanoma cells are pleomorphic, with spindle, epithelioid, polygonal, dendritic and bizarre shapes.

Hutchinson's sign is represented histologically by atypical melanocytes mainly in the basal layer, with a few higher in the epidermis. *In situ* subungual melanoma has junctional nests of melanoma cells. Nodular patterns of melanoma are rare.

Amputation of the digit is the routine treatment, although local excision is occasionally practised for small shallow lesions. Mohs' micrographic surgery is used in some centres, but is still at a relatively early stage of evaluation [32]. In one series of 14 patients, three had recurrence at the margins of treatment. Adjuvant isolated limb perfusion has failed to show benefit in stage 1 subungual melanoma [33], although use of a more aggressive regimen has possibly been associated with improved survival [34].

Recent British surveys suggest that the poor prognosis of subungual melanoma is related to the depth of invasion at diagnosis (4.7 mm). This reflects late diagnosis (3 months to 12 years) [31,35,36]. The mean 5-year survival was 41% compared with 61% for a control group of primary cutaneous malignant melanomas in the same study [35]. Other series have produced similar results, although recent Japanese evidence supports the idea that diagnosing subungual melanoma early, with a lower Breslow thickness, improves prognosis, with an 87% 5-year survival rate [34].

REFERENCES

1 Saida T, Oshima Y. Clinical and histopathologic characteristics of early lesions of subungual malignant melanoma. *Cancer* 1989; **63**: 556–60.
2 Baran R, Bariere H. Longitudinal melanonychia with spreading pigmentation in Laugier–Hunziker syndrome: a report of 2 cases. *Br J Dermatol* 1986; **115**: 707–10.
3 Veraldi S, Cavicchini S, Benelli C, Gasparini G. Laugier–Hunziker syndrome: a clinical, histopathologic and ultrastructural study of four cases and review of the literature. *J Am Acad Dermatol* 1991; **25**: 632–6.
4 Papadavid E, Walker NP. Q-switched Alexandrite laser in the treatment of pigmented macules in Laugier–Hunziker syndrome. *J Eur Acad Dermatol Venereol* 2001; **15**: 468–9.
5 Tosti A, Baran R, Piraccini BM *et al*. Nail matrix naevi: a clinical and histopathologic study of twenty-two patients. *J Am Acad Dermatol* 1996; **34**: 765–71.
6 Léauté-Labrèze C, Bioulac-Sage P, Taïeb A. Longitudinal melanonychia in children. *Arch Dermatol* 1996; **132**: 167–9.
7 Goettmann-Bonvallot S, Andre J, Belaich S. Longitudinal melanonychia in children: a clinical and histopathologic study of 40 cases. *J Am Acad Dermatol* 1999; **41**: 17–22.
8 Kikuchi I, Inoue S, Sakaguchi E *et al*. Nevoid nail area melanosis in childhood (cases which showed spontaneous regression). *Dermatology* 1993; **186**: 88–93.
9 Gallais V, Lacour JPH, Perrin C *et al*. Acral hyperpigmented macules and longitudinal melanonychia in AIDS patients. *Br J Dermatol* 1992; **126**: 387–91.
10 Juhlin L, Baran R. Longitudinal melanonychia after healing of lichen planus. *Acta Derm Venereol (Stockh)* 1989; **69**: 338–9.
11 Matsumoto T, Matsuda T, Padhye AA *et al*. Fungal melanonychia: ungual phaeohyphomycosis caused by *Wangiella dermatitidis*. *Clin Exp Dermatol* 1992; **17**: 83–6.
12 Haneke E, Baran R. Longitudinal melanonychia. *Dermatol Surg* 2001; **27**: 580–4.
13 Baran R, Simon C. Longitudinal melanonychia: a symptom of Bowen's disease. *J Am Acad Dermatol* 1988; **6**: 1359–6.
14 Monash S. Normal pigmentation in the nails of the negro. *Arch Dermatol* 1932; **25**: 876–81.
15 Kopf AW, Waldo E. Melanonychia striata. *Australas J Dermatol* 1980; **21**: 59–70.
16 Collins RJ. Melanomas in the Chinese among south western Indians. *Cancer* 1984; **55**: 2899–902.
17 Blessing K, Kernohan NM, Park KGM. Subungual malignant melanoma: clinicopathological features of 100 cases. *Histopathology* 1991; **19**: 425–9.
18 Baran R, Haneke E. Tumours of the nail apparatus and adjacent tissues. In: Baran R, Dawber RPR, eds. *Diseases of the Nails and Their Management*, 2nd edn. Oxford: Blackwell Science, 1994: 483–97.
19 Daly JM, Berlin R, Urmacher C. Subungual melanoma. *Ann Surg* 1987; **161**: 545–52.
20 Feibleman CE, Stoll H, Maize JC. Melanomas of the palm, sole and nailbed: a clinicopathologic study. *Cancer* 1980; **46**: 2492–504.
21 Kopf AW. Hutchinson's sign of subungual malignant melanoma. *Am J Dermatopathol* 1981; **3**: 201–2.
22 Baran R, Kechijian P. Hutchinson's sign: a reappraisal. *J Am Acad Dermatol* 1996; **34**: 87–90.
23 Ronger S, Touzet S, Ligeron C *et al*. Dermoscopic examination of nail pigmentation. *Arch Dermatol* 2002; **138**: 1327–33.
24 Kawabata Y, Ohara K, Hino H, Tamaki K. Two kinds of Hutchinson's sign, benign and malignant. *J Am Acad Dermatol* 2001; **44**: 305–7.
25 Miura S, Jimbow K. Clinical characteristics of subungual melanomas in Japan. *J Dermatol* 1985; **12**: 393–402.
26 Kiryu H. Malignant melanoma in situ arising in the nail unit of a child. *J Dermatol* 1998; **25**: 41–4.
27 de Berker D, Dawber RPR, Thody A, Graham A. Melanocytes are absent from normal nail bed: the basis of a clinical dictum. *Br J Dermatol* 1996; **134**: 564.
28 Perrin C, Michiels JF, Pisani A, Ortonne JP. Anatomic distribution of melanocytes in normal nail unit: an immunohistochemical investigation. *Am J Dermatopathol* 1997; **19**: 462–7.
29 Thai KE, Young R, Sinclair RD. Nail apparatus melanoma. *Australas J Dermatol* 2001; **42**: 71–83.
30 O'Leary JA, Berend KR, Johnson JL, Levin LS, Seigler HF. Subungual melanoma. A review of 93 cases with identification of prognostic variables. *Clin Orthop* 2000; **78**: 206–12.
31 Rigby HS, Briggs JC. Subungual melanoma: a clinicopathological study of 24 cases. *Br J Plast Surg* 1992; **45**: 275–8.
32 Brodland DG. The treatment of nail apparatus melanoma with Mohs micrographic surgery. *Dermatol Surg* 2001; **27**: 269–73.
33 Vrouenraets BC, Kroon BBR, Klaase JM *et al*. Regional isolated perfusion with melphalan for patients with subungual melanoma. *Eur J Surg Oncol* 1993; **19**: 37–42.
34 Kato T, Suetake T, Sugiyama Y *et al*. Epidemiology and prognosis of subungual melanoma in 34 Japanese patients. *Br J Dermatol* 1996; **134**: 383–7.
35 McLaren KM, Hunter JAA, Smyth JF *et al*. The Scottish Melanoma Group: a progress report. *J Pathol* 1989; **158**: 335A.
36 Banfield CC, Redburn JC, Dawber RP. The incidence and prognosis of nail apparatus melanoma. A retrospective study of 105 patients in four English regions. *Br J Dermatol* 1998; **139**: 276–9.

Nail surgery [1,2]

Nail surgery is delicate and requires attention to detail. It is important that anyone performing a nail biopsy appreciates the principles outlined in the preliminary section of this chapter on anatomy and physiology and that they obtain tuition in detailed technique. Once in this position, the outcome of nail unit surgery is usually excellent and provides useful and definitive diagnostic material [3].

For many procedures, the routine skin surgery pack needs to be supplemented by specialized instruments. These include a Freer septum elevator for finger work and a larger elevator for the great toenail. English nail splitters are essential for performing partial avulsion. They have a flat undersurface, which can be introduced beneath the nail to act as an anvil and a sharp upper part that cuts down upon the nail to meet the other half of the instrument. For bone surgery, such as removal of exostoses, bone rongeurs and McKindoes are needed.

Indications

A nail biopsy may perform several functions. It can provide useful positive diagnostic information or help exclude a malignant condition, such as squamous cell carcinoma of the nail bed. Painful conditions may be relieved by the drainage of pus with proximal hemi-avulsion, or ablation of an ingrowing toenail. Focal pathology, such as a glomus tumour or the origin of melanonychia, can be completely excised and provide the diagnosis. If a positive diagnostic and therapeutic attitude is taken to the nail disorder, a good outcome can be expected.

Diagnostic nail biopsy may be undertaken as part of the investigation of nail dystrophy of unknown cause in the presence of more than one negative mycology sample.

Biopsy of the nail plate alone, or with associated nail bed and occasionally matrix biopsy, may be needed to confirm fungal infection in atypical cases, although biopsies are more commonly directed at distinguishing between

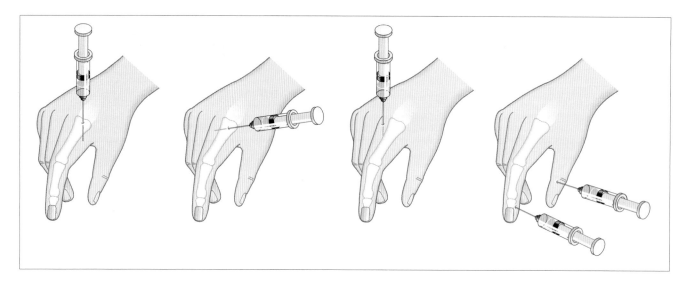

Fig. 62.36 Digital sites of injection for a ring block.

dermatoses affecting the nail, such as lichen planus, psoriasis or infiltrative disease. In instances of nail dystrophy of a single digit, it is appropriate to biopsy to exclude a neoplasm once necessary imaging has been performed.

Caution is needed in patients with relevant medical and circulatory problems. The latter are subject to poor reperfusion following the tourniquet and it may be necessary to abbreviate the procedure to ensure no inadvertent damage is done. The wound must be seen to bleed and the digit colour return before the dressing is applied in these cases, and this can take several minutes. This contrasts with the usual pace at which dressings are applied to prevent bleeding in a healthy digit. Diabetics may have ischaemia combined with immune impairment and frequently need attention to toenail problems. Paradoxically, they are cited as a group in whom cold steel surgery for nail problems is preferable to other techniques such as phenolic ablation or cryosurgery. This is because the course of healing in these wounds is predictable and often shorter than wounds produced by other therapies.

Preoperatively

It is essential to prepare the patient for the procedure by a discussion on a day separate from surgery. In this discussion, the patient must appreciate the potential benefits and problems of the biopsy. It is useful to make it clear that it will be painful and that they will have a degree of disability postoperatively for which they must make provision at home and at work. The best surgical technique can be utterly confounded by a patient who goes back to a dirty workplace the next day. Much of the information concerning scarring, the need for elevation, dressings and analgesia needs to be repeated on the day of the proced-

ure. The patient should have a means of transport home that does not involve them driving or standing for prolonged periods.

The affected digit should be soaked in warm antiseptic and scrubbed in a manner similar to that used by the surgeon prior to gloving. This will diminish the bacterial load beneath the free edge of the nail, which is a source of potential pathogens. Soaking for 10 min softens the nail and facilitates removal of parts of the nail plate, so avoiding complete avulsion. During this period, the local anaesthetic can take effect.

Anaesthetic (Fig. 62.36)

Lidocaine (lignocaine) 2% or equivalent can be used [4]. Bupivacaine can be used to provide prolonged analgesia. The use of epinephrine (adrenaline) in anaesthetic remains controversial. There are several publications illustrating how anaesthetic containing 1 in 200 000 epinephrine has been used safely [5]. The ischaemia and prolongation of anaesthesia is a potential advantage. If subjects with peripheral ischaemic or vasospastic disease are avoided, anaesthetic with 1 in 200 000 epinephrine appears safe. An alternative is to use ropivacaine. This local anaesthetic has physiological and pharmacological properties somewhere between bupivacaine and lidocaine. It has a moderately quick onset of action and can produce anaesthesia for over 12 h, combined with a modest short-term vasoconstrictive effect [6]. We use ropivacaine 7.5 mg/mL in the same way as lidocaine, with very good results. A 30-gauge needle causes less discomfort during injection than larger needles, and minimizes the risk of damage to digital nerves when inserting a ring block. Risk of nerve trauma may be reduced further by the use of nerve-block needles, which have less traumatic tips.

The most common form of anaesthesia is a ring block (digital nerve block), which is delivered by injection of

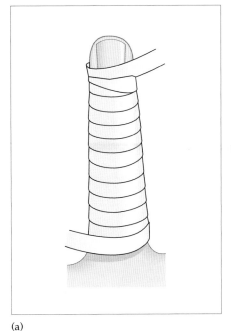

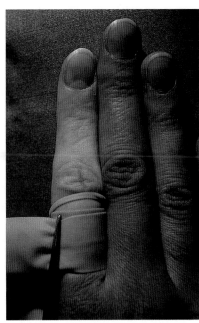

Fig. 62.37 (a) A Penrose drain is applied from the tip and wound down the digit achieving exsanguination. (b) The drain is then unwound from the top, with the base maintained secure with artery forceps.

(a)

(b)

anaesthetic into the dorsolateral aspect of the digit at the base, with about 1–2 mL on each side of the phalanx. Greater than 5 mL may impair circulation, but this can be assessed visually during the procedure and is very variable according to the bulk of individual digits. Anaesthesia may take 10–20 min to become total. In the great toe, additional anaesthetic should be placed ventrally. After 10 min, efficacy of the block can be assessed at the digit tip with the same needle; if the anaesthesia is incomplete, it can be supplemented by a small local injection at the site of surgery. However, this can increase tissue turgor and render fine manipulation difficult.

Other ring block techniques can be employed, including a method that aims to infiltrate the anaesthetic via the flexor tendon as a transthecal block [7,8]. An alternative is the distal 'wing' block given 2–3 mm proximal to the junction of the proximal and lateral nail folds. The injection is first directed distally into the lateral nail fold. After partial withdrawal, it is redirected over the proximal nail fold. Sufficient is used to produce blanching in both nail folds. The procedure is repeated on the other side to achieve complete block. The digit is more sensitive distally than proximally and it is often more comfortable to provide the traditional proximal digital nerve block.

For invasive procedures on many digits concurrently, more proximal or regional blocks can be employed [9]. In children it can be worthwhile to use a topical anaesthetic as a preliminary measure before ring block. Evidence of its efficacy in adults is mixed [10,11].

Tourniquet

It is important that the area of applied pressure beneath the tourniquet is as broad as possible to avoid pressure damage to underlying structures. In particular, neuritis may be a long-term complication of a narrow, tight, prolonged tourniquet. This effect can be exacerbated by topping up anaesthetic near the tourniquet after it is in place. Ischaemia can be tolerated in a normal digit for 20 min and possibly longer, with no complications as long as there is no local trauma from the tourniquet.

The standard tourniquet for local anaesthetic is the Penrose drain (Fig. 62.37), which may be wound around the digit from the tip proximally. This exsanguinates the digit and provides a tourniquet effect that can be maintained with a pair of artery forceps. A sterile glove is an alternative. It is worn by the patient and the tip of the glove digit at the site of surgery is snipped off. It is then rolled back to the base of the digit, exsanguinating it, providing a tourniquet, and avoiding contamination from adjacent digits peroperatively. With general anaesthetic, an exsanguinating cuff can be used on the forearm or calf.

Specimen

The specimen must be delivered to the pathologist undistorted and with the maximum of clinical and operative information. It is useful to allow the specimen to adhere lightly to a piece of paper before immersion in fixative, or to enclose it in a small plastic mesh cassette. This should be matched with a detailed drawing on the histopathology request form. It is helpful to work regularly with the same pathologist for nail specimens, as processing requires specialized understanding of specimen preparation and histological interpretation.

Postoperatively

Dressings should be ready before removal of the tourniquet. They must be firm and moderately bulky. An acceptable dressing includes an antimicrobial ointment under a greasy tulle, padding and a small bandage. Calcium alginate dressings can also be useful if there is an area that needs to heal by secondary intention. Dressings should be held in place with oblique or longitudinal sticky tape to avoid a tourniquet effect if the digit swells. A sling or plastic overshoe should be provided.

The frequency of change of dressings is determined by the nature of the procedure and the patient. An antiseptic soak is normally needed to remove the dressing and clean the wound. Infection should be treated vigorously with systemic antibiotics combined with daily antiseptic soaks.

It is good practice to provide a moderately strong analgesic and to recommend taking it regularly in the first 48 h. It may prove unnecessary, but the distress of unrelieved pain in the few who suffer warrants caution. Some patients need night-time sedation.

In most cases, it is wise to arrange review within 2 days of surgery to change the dressing, assess the wound and answer any questions which have arisen.

Complications

Pain can sometimes be disproportionate to the wound [12]. When it is severe, the patient is at risk of reflex sympathetic dystrophy [13]. They should receive regular potent analgesics, including non-steroidal anti-inflammatory agents, amitriptyline and sometimes an anxiolytic such as diazepam.

Bleeding is very common and should be accommodated by firm, bulky dressings. Once blood has clotted in these dressings they can be rock-like and represent an infection risk—good reasons for an early dressing change.

Infection is a potential problem and can be devastating to the matrix. Prophylactic antibiotics are a reasonable precaution when the surgical site is likely to be heavily colonized due to skin changes or a dystrophic nail. Children or patients with poor hygiene may also warrant antibiotics.

Longer term, complications are mainly related to scarring dystrophy and loss of function. The former is always a potential risk of any surgery involving the matrix and should be discussed preoperatively as part of the risk assessment with the patient. Loss of function can be modest, with a tendency for the nail to catch, or more significant if associated with pain or marked paraesthesia. Mild paraesthesia is quite common in the short term and is sometimes seen with cold sensitivity. Complications involving the tendons of the distal interphalangeal joint are very rare and usually related to more proximal surgery.

REFERENCES

1 Haneke E, Baran R. Nail surgery and traumatic abnormalities. In: Baran R, Dawber RPR, eds. *Diseases of the Nails and Their Management*, 2nd edn. Oxford: Blackwell Science, 1994: 345–415.
2 Salasche SJ, Peters VJ. Tips on nail surgery. *Cutis* 1985; **35**: 428–38.
3 de Berker D, Dahl MGC, Comaish JS, Lawrence CM. The value of nail unit surgery in dermatology. *Acta Derm Venereol (Stockh)* 1996; **76**: 484–7.
4 Abadir A. Use of local anaesthetics in dermatology. *J Dermatol Surg* 1975; **1**: 68–72.
5 Wilhelmi BJ, Blackwell SJ, Miller J, Mancoll JS, Phillips LG. Epinephrine in digital blocks: revisited. *Ann Plast Surg* 1998; **41**: 410–4.
6 Moffitt DL, de Berker DA, Kennedy CT, Shutt LE. Assessment of ropivacaine as a local anesthetic for skin infiltration in skin surgery. *Dermatol Surg* 2001; **27**: 437–40.
7 Chiu DTW. Transthecal digital block: flexor tendon sheath used for anaesthetic infusion. *J Hand Surg* 1990; **15A**: 471–3.
8 Brutus JP, Baeten Y, Chahidi N *et al.* Single injection digital block: comparison between three techniques. *Chir Main* 2002; **21**: 182–7.
9 Cohen SJ, Roegnik RK. Nerve blocks for cutaneous surgery on the foot. *J Dermatol Surg Oncol* 1991; **17**: 527–34.
10 Serour F, Ben-Yehuda Y, Boaz M. EMLA cream prior to digital nerve block for ingrown nail surgery does not reduce pain at injection of anesthetic solution. *Acta Anaesthesiol Scand* 2002; **46**: 203–6.
11 Browne J, Fung M, Donnelly M, Cooney C. The use of EMLA reduces the pain associated with digital ring block for ingrowing toenail correction. *Eur J Anaesthesiol* 2000; **17**: 182–4.
12 Moossavi M, Scher RK. Complications of nail surgery: a review of the literature. *Dermatol Surg* 2002; **27**: 225–8.
13 Ingram GJ, Scher RK, Lally EV. Reflex sympathetic dystrophy following nail biopsy. *J Am Acad Dermatol* 1987; **16**: 253–6.

Patterns of nail biopsy

Nail avulsion [1,2]

Nail avulsion can be performed in order to examine underlying tissues or to provide temporary relief in cases of soft-tissue trauma. In isolation, it is not a treatment for ingrowing toenails. The procedure requires a distal or ring block, and an elevator in addition to the routine instrument pack. For a partial avulsion, nail splitters are also needed.

To minimize the trauma of the procedure, soft-tissue nail attachments should be loosened at all sites prior to removal. This minimizes tearing damage to the nail folds. The cuticle may need disrupting with fine scissors or a blade, but all other detachments can be performed with a septum elevator. Once this is done, the nail is gripped with a pair of rugged artery forceps and removed by a mixed twisting and lifting action (Fig. 62.38).

With a lateral partial avulsion, the nail splitter is used to define the medial margin and only the attachments of the piece of nail to be removed need to be interrupted.

Proximal hemi-avulsion of the nail plate entails the following technique.
1 The origin of the nail and its proximal lateral aspects are undermined with a septum elevator.
2 In nails with a shallow lateral nail fold, a nail splitter may be inserted and the nail transversely bisected.
3 In nails with a deep lateral nail fold, a deep transverse score is placed with a scalpel across the nail halfway down.

4 The septum elevator is then fully inserted through the transverse score to loosen and elevate the proximal nail.

REFERENCES

1 Albom MJ. Avulsion of a nail plate. *J Dermatol Surg Oncol* 1977; **3**: 34–5.
2 Baran R. More on avulsion of nail plate. *J Dermatol Surg Oncol* 1981; **7**: 854.

Nail bed biopsy [1–4]

Biopsy of the nail bed is usually performed to investigate a focal abnormality of nail bed or changes in the nail plate arising distally. Occasionally, it may be appropriate to biopsy through the nail plate where the histological relationship between nail bed and plate is under investigation. More commonly, the nail bed is visualized first, following complete or partial avulsion. A thin ellipse is taken down to bone in the long axis of the digit (Fig. 62.39). An alternative is to employ a double punch technique, where a 6-mm hole can be made in the nail plate with a biopsy punch over the area of nail bed to be examined. The nail bed may then be sampled using a smaller punch.

If there has been nail avulsion, it is possible to close the wound, which may require gentle undermining. In small biopsies this may be unnecessary, and the wound will heal well by secondary intention. When the nail is left *in situ* or if the double punch technique is used, closure is not possible. After a double punch, as long as there is complete haemostasis, the original disc of nail plate can be returned after soaking in antiseptic; it may reattach or at least provide a natural dressing during the early healing phase.

No scarring is anticipated from this biopsy if it is small and does not extend into the nail matrix.

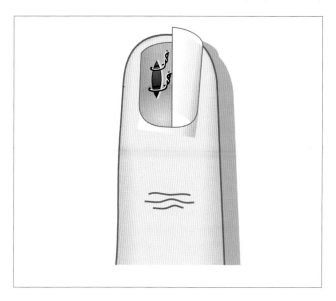

Fig. 62.39 After partial nail avulsion, the nail bed can be seen and biopsied along the longitudinal access.

REFERENCES

1 Baran R, Sayag J. Nail biopsy. Why, when, where, how? *J Dermatol Surg Oncol* 1976; **2**: 322–4.
2 Haneke E, Baran R. Nail surgery and traumatic abnormalities. In: Baran R, Dawber RPR, eds. *Diseases of the Nails and Their Management*, 2nd edn. Oxford: Blackwell Science, 1994: 345–415.
3 Hanno R, Mathes BM, Krull EA. Longitudinal nail biopsy in evaluation of acquired nail dystrophies. *J Am Acad Dermatol* 1986; **14**: 803–9.
4 Rich P. Nail biopsy: indications and methods. *J Dermatol Surg Oncol* 1992; **18**: 673–82.

Matrix biopsy

Lateral longitudinal nail biopsy [1,2]

Lateral longitudinal nail biopsy is the definitive method for sampling all the tissues of the nail unit. It is most commonly required when there is dystrophy affecting the whole nail or for the excision of a melanonychia. If focal

Fig. 62.38 The three stages of standard nail avulsion.

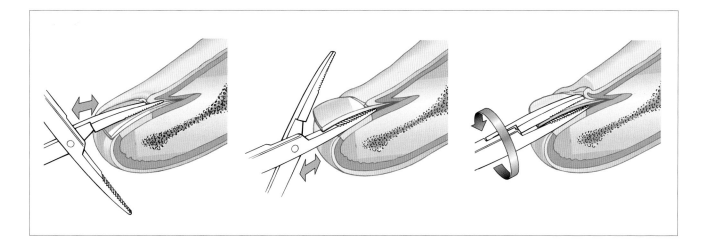

matrix pathology occurs laterally, longitudinal biopsy may be warranted to preserve the shape of the nail, which can otherwise be altered by local matrix surgery. Early literature suggested that longitudinal biopsies of less than 3 mm in width could be taken from the midline of the nail without scarring [3] but it is now accepted that this may produce long-term nail dystrophy.

The first incision starts in the lateral nail sulcus, between the nail and nail fold. The distal limit is just beneath the distal groove, in the tip of the digit. Proximally, the incision extends almost to the first of the transverse skin markings of the distal interphalangeal joint. The medial margin of the ellipse is formed by an incision through the nail plate, which has been softened by an antiseptic soak. Both incisions are down to bone and separated by 3 mm at the widest point. The specimen is released from its deep attachment from the distal point proximally. The nail can be lifted at the free edge with forceps, allowing the bottom of the specimen to be released with curved iris scissors. Particular care is needed at the proximal end to ensure that the matrix is fully sampled without damage.

A 3/0 or 4/0 monofilament suture is used for closure. One suture closes the wound through the proximal nail fold. One or two further sutures are needed through the nail plate and lateral nail fold. The suture is designed to elevate the lateral nail fold and enhance the embedding of the new nail edge in the nail fold (Fig. 62.40).

The nail will be permanently narrowed following this procedure and the contour of the lateral and proximal nail fold intersection is altered to provide a more acute angle. In spite of the specialized suture to elevate the lateral nail fold, the nail is seldom fully embedded in a new lateral sulcus. Where biopsies of greater than 3 mm width are taken, the nail may develop malalignment, with distal deviation towards the side of the biopsy [4].

REFERENCES

1 Rich P. Nail biopsy: indications and methods. *J Dermatol Surg Oncol* 1992; **18**: 673–82.
2 Salasche SJ, Peters VJ. Tips on nail surgery. *Cutis* 1985; **35**: 428–38.
3 Zaias N. The longitudinal nail biopsy. *J Invest Dermatol* 1967; **49**: 406–8.
4 de Berker D, Baran R. Acquired malalignment of the nail following broad lateral longitudinal nail biopsy. *Acta Derm Venereol (Stockh)* 1998; **78**: 468–70.

Transverse matrix biopsy (Fig. 62.41)

A transverse matrix biopsy may be performed to investigate focal abnormality of a nail dystrophy arising from the matrix.

The proximal nail fold is reflected following an oblique incision at the junction with the lateral nail folds and gentle separation of the proximal nail fold from the dorsal aspect of the nail plate. The matrix is then visualized by performing a proximal hemi-avulsion. A thin ellipse is

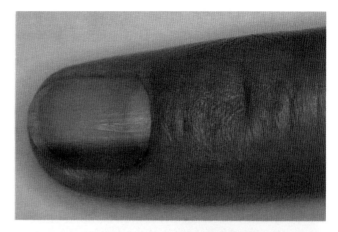
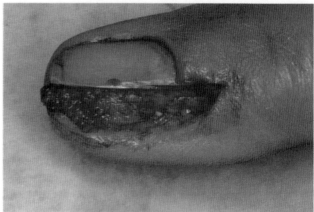
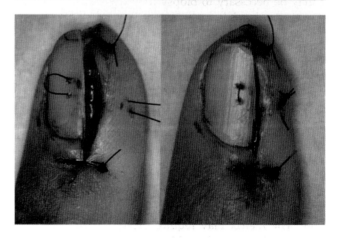

Fig. 62.40 A large, lateral, longitudinal nail biopsy is closed with sutures designed to reconstruct the lateral nail fold.

taken from the distal matrix with the distal margin of the excision matching the shape of the lunula.

The wound may be gently undermined, taking care with the extremely fragile matrix epithelium and undermining most on the distal nail bed margin. Loose sutures with resorbable 6/0 monofilament can be used.

Once healed, a blemish may remain in the margin of the lunula. The nail plate will show changes in thickness proportional to the extent of the biopsy.

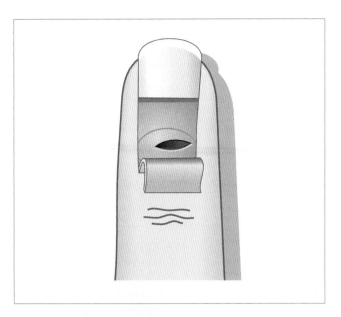

Fig. 62.41 Crescentic or narrow elliptical transverse matrix biopsy, which can be performed after removal of the proximal half of the nail plate alone.

Nail fold biopsy [1–4]

Proximal nail fold biopsy

It may be necessary to biopsy the proximal nail fold to investigate a local dermatosis, connective tissue disease or focal tumour. The biopsy can be taken in different axes, but preservation of the symmetry and curvature of the proximal nail fold is a priority. If sutures are to be used, a distal wing block should be avoided, as the tissues will become turgid and difficult to manipulate.

Transverse nail fold biopsy

A transverse ellipse (for connective tissue disease), a 2-mm punch (far from the free edge) or a shave biopsy are simple nail fold procedures. The transverse ellipse and punch biopsies are down to the dorsal aspect of the nail plate. The matrix may require protection from cutting trauma and this can be achieved by inserting a septum elevator between the nail fold and the nail.

The transverse biopsy requires 4/0 monofilament suture. Wounds from other biopsy methods can be left to heal by secondary intention. Postoperatively, a thin line may remain in the nail fold after the transverse biopsy; otherwise, these techniques leave little or no scarring. There is no nail plate change.

Crescentic nail fold biopsy (Fig. 62.42)

A larger nail fold biopsy can be taken as a distal crescentic wedge. A crescentic incision is performed just proximal to

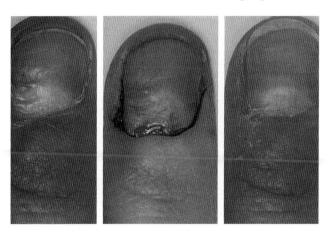

Fig. 62.42 Crescentic shave of the distal proximal nail fold and cuticle as treatment for chronic paronychia. Also provides histological specimen where biopsy relevant.

the cuticle with the blade bevelled to direct trauma away from the proximal matrix if the nail is penetrated. Additional matrix protection may be provided by inserting a septum elevator beneath the proximal nail fold. The distal fraction of the proximal nail fold (including the cuticle) can be removed, although the width of the specimen should not exceed 4–5 mm in the midline. The contour is aimed at recreating a new edge to the entire nail fold. The wound heals by secondary intention and a new cuticle usually reforms, depending upon the original problem. The amount of exposed nail is permanently enlarged, but the nail surface is unchanged unless ridging or grooves produced by the original pathology are reversed.

This technique can be used for the excision of chronic paronychia resistant to routine therapy. It has also been recommended for the excision of digital mucous cysts occupying the most distal margin of the nail fold. At this site, it is argued that the lesions are solely degenerative and do not communicate with the joint space [3,4].

Focal nail fold biopsy

Focal pathology in the nail fold can be excised by a V-shaped incision into the nail fold. The excision is through the entire thickness of the nail fold, but should not penetrate underlying nail. Relaxing incisions are made at one or both of the lateral margins of the proximal nail fold (Fig. 62.43). The primary defect is closed with 4/0 monofilament and the relaxing incisions heal by secondary intention. Wounds in the midline of the nail fold can leave some scarring, but the nail plate is usually unaffected.

REFERENCES

1 Baran R. Removal of the proximal nail fold. Why, when, how? *J Dermatol Surg Oncol* 1986; **12**: 234–6.

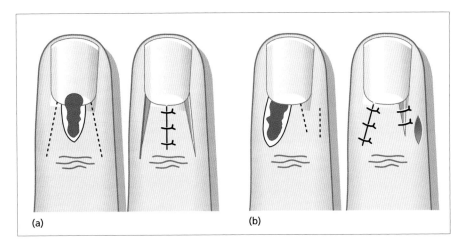

(a)   (b)

Fig. 62.43 Method for removing a small lesion from the proximal nail fold.

2 Haneke E, Baran R. Nail surgery and traumatic abnormalities. In: Baran R, Dawber RPR, eds. *Diseases of the Nails and Their Management*, 2nd edn. Oxford: Blackwell Science, 1994: 345–415.
3 Salasche SJ. Myxoid cysts of the proximal nail fold: a surgical approach. *J Dermatol Surg Oncol* 1984; **10**: 35–9.
4 Schnitzler L, Baran R, Civatte J et al. Biopsy of the proximal nail fold in collagen diseases. *J Dermatol Surg Oncol* 1976; **2**: 313–5.

Nail plate biopsy [1,2]

It is sometimes useful to biopsy the nail plate, with or without a small piece of the hyponychium. This may help differentiate between onychomycosis and psoriasis. If hyponychium is included, a small bleb of anaesthetic will be needed or a distal wing block can be performed. A chunk of distal nail plate of at least 3 mm width is then removed with large nail clippers. Subungual debris should also be obtained and a scalpel may be needed if hyponychium is attached. Hyponychial wounds heal by secondary intention after cautery haemostasis and leave no scarring.

REFERENCES

1 Suarez SM, Silvers DN, Scher RK. Histologic evaluation of nail clippings for diagnosing onychomycosis. *Arch Dermatol* 1991; **127**: 1517–9.
2 Grammer-West NY, Corvette DM, Giandoni MB, Fitzpatrick JE. Clinical pearl: nail plate biopsy for the diagnosis of psoriatic nails. *J Am Acad Dermatol* 1998; **38**: 260–2.

Lateral matrix phenolization [1,2]

Ingrowing nails, particularly toenails, are treated in many different ways [1–5]. However, phenolization is quick, relatively painless and has a high success rate [6]. Any area of matrix may be phenolized, including total ablation. The procedure yields no specimen other than the nail plate.

After anaesthetic, antiseptic soak and tourniquet, the margin of lateral ingrowing nail is avulsed using nail splitters to separate it from the rest of the nail plate. The nail folds are then protected with a layer of yellow soft paraffin and 85% aqueous phenol is applied on the end of an orange stick to the exposed matrix. This is done for 3 min (one stick per min), before douching with 70% alcohol to neutralize the chemical cautery. Although 3 min is common practice [1], in a series of 537 ingrowing nails, phenol was applied for 5–6 min and a 99% 1-year cure rate was achieved, with a mean healing period of 20 days [2].

As a result of this chemical burn, there is some ooze from the wound, which can occasionally last several weeks, but it is seldom infected and often pain-free. If the ooze is prominent, the toe should receive daily potassium permanganate or povidone–iodine soaks, after culture for specific microbes. The nail is permanently narrowed.

There is occasionally a small element of lateral nail regrowth, although further surgery is only indicated if there is repeated symptomatic ingrowing. Complete nail ablation can be achieved using the same technique applied to the entire matrix.

REFERENCES

1 Dagnall JC. The history, development and current status of nail matrix phenolisation. *Chiropodist* 1981; **36**: 315–24.
2 Kimata Y, Uetake M, Tsukada S, Harii K. Follow up study of patients treated for ingrown nails with the nail matrix phenol method. *Plast Reconstr Surg* 1995; **95**: 719–24.
3 Bose B. A technique for excision of nail fold for ingrowing toenail. *Surg Gynecol Obstet* 1971; **132**: 511–2.
4 Haneke E. Ingrown and pincer nails: evaluation and treatment. *Dermatol Ther* 2002; **15**: 148–58.
5 Johnson DB, Ceilley RI. A revised technique for the ablation of the matrix of a nail. *J Dermatol Surg Oncol* 1979; **5**: 642.
6 Rounding C, Hulm S. Surgical treatments for ingrowing toenails. *Cochrane Database Systematic Review* 2000; (2): CD001541.

Other surgical modalities

Mohs' micrographic surgery

This technique applied to the nail unit exploits the principle of maximum conservation of healthy tissue while ensuring tissue clearance of tumour. It is particularly useful in squamous cell carcinoma of the nail unit (see p. 62.41), where it should be offered as an alternative to digit amputation when there is no evidence of invasion of bone by tumour [1,2]. At this site, the conservation of normal tissue is of considerable functional significance. The place of Mohs' surgery in treatment of pigmented lesions of the nail apparatus remains to be fully explored. There is limited evidence of its use in nail melanoma [3].

Cryosurgery

Cryosurgery is widely used for the treatment of periungual warts. There is a small risk of damage to the tendons in the finger with aggressive freezing techniques. It is also used for myxoid cysts [4,5]. The cysts should be evacuated of their mucoid contents before a double 20-s freeze–thaw cycle. EMLA (eutectic mixture of local anaesthetics) or injected local anaesthetic may sometimes be needed. This regimen produces cure in approximately 25% of cases [5], although more aggressive freezing can produce better results [4].

Infrared photocoagulation

This has been used as a treatment for myxoid cysts of the proximal nail fold [6]. The contents are evacuated through a puncture wound before treatment.

Carbon dioxide laser

There is a range of indications for carbon dioxide laser [7–9], and its virtue may be in provision of a bloodless wound which allows a good view of the surgical procedure. This can only normally be provided in cold-steel surgery by an effective tourniquet.

The bulk of laser work on the nail unit is for subungual and periungual warts. This uses the defocused mode with a 1–2 mm spot at 5–10 W output and can be intermittent, in 0.05-s bursts, or continuous. Haemostasis may not be complete, and both anaesthetic and tourniquet are usually used with the laser.

It is also useful as a focused destructive instrument in the treatment of myxoid cysts [10] and ablation of abnormal nail in irreversible nail disorders. This includes partial destruction of the matrix of nails in ingrowing nails [11] and in pachyonychia congenita to reduce nail thickness.

REFERENCES

1 de Berker DAR, Dahl MGC, Malcolm AJ, Lawrence CM. Micrographic surgery for subungual squamous cell carcinoma. *Br J Plast Surg* 1996; **49**: 414–9.
2 Zaiac MN, Weiss E. Mohs micrographic surgery of the nail unit and squamous cell carcinoma. *Dermatol Surg* 2001; **27**: 246–51.
3 Brodland DG. The treatment of nail apparatus melanoma with Mohs micrographic surgery. *Dermatol Surg* 2001; **27**: 269–73.
4 Dawber RPR, Sonnex T, Leonard J, Ralfs I. Myxoid cysts of the finger: treatment by liquid nitrogen spray cryosurgery. *Clin Exp Dermatol* 1983; **8**: 153.
5 de Berker DAR, Lawrence CM. Cryosurgery for myxoid cysts. *Br J Dermatol* 1997; **137** (Suppl. 50): 27.
6 Kemmett D, Colver GB. Myxoid cysts treated by infra-red coagulation. *Clin Exp Dermatol* 1994; **19**: 118–20.
7 Apfelberg D, Maser M, Lash H, White D. Efficacy of the carbon dioxide laser in hand surgery. *Ann Plast Surg* 1984; **13**: 320–6.
8 Street M, Roegnik R. Recalcitrant periungual verrucae: the role of carbon dioxide laser vaporization. *J Am Acad Dermatol* 1990; **12**: 115–20.
9 Bennett G. Laser use in foot surgery. *Foot Ankle* 1989; **10**: 110–4.
10 Karrer S, Hohenleutner U, Szeimies RM, Landthaler M. Treatment of digital mucous cysts with a carbon dioxide laser. *Acta Derm Venereol (Stockh)* 1999; **79**: 224–5.
11 Lin YC, Su HY. A surgical approach to ingrown nail: partial matricectomy using CO_2 laser. *Dermatol Surg* 2002; **28**: 578–80.

Traumatic nail disorders

Nails may show signs of acute trauma, scars following acute trauma or chronic repetitive trauma.

Acute trauma

Acute trauma is classified with respect to severity, ranging from a small haematoma to digit amputation (Table 62.5).

Table 62.5 Classification of acute trauma. (From Van Beek *et al.* [1].)

Type	Effect	Therapy
I	Small haematoma associated with a small break in the nail bed	Fenestration of nail over the haematoma
II	Large haematoma with significant nail bed injury	Remove nail in order to identify site and nature of subungual damage
III	Large haematoma, nail plate displaced	X-ray may reveal fracture of terminal phalanx, usually in association with nail bed laceration which requires resorbable 6/0 suture
IV	Severe crush injury	Avulsion needed to reveal matrix, with multiple lacerations requiring careful reconstruction
V	Amputation of tip of digit, may include parts of matrix	If tip can be retrieved, it should be used as a graft. Otherwise nail bed from other sites may provide autologous grafts

Nail bed laceration

The nail bed may be lacerated by different forms of trauma, including incisions, crush and avulsion injuries. In simple injuries there is displacement of the nail plate, which may be found proximally avulsed but retaining distal attachment to the nail bed. In this form of trauma, and in many others, the nail plate can be used as a useful splint [1]. Initially, the nail bed damage should be assessed by avulsion, and then the nail can be replaced after any necessary nail bed repair has been performed; a small window for drainage of blood and exudate is made in the nail [2]. More complicated injuries may require flap or graft reconstructions and, in some instances, vascularized composite nail grafts are used with microvascular anastomoses. When the wounds arise from crush injury, fracture is relatively common. If the distal tuft has been fractured to leave fragments of bone dispersed in the soft tissues, it may prevent long-term morbidity if these are removed [3].

REFERENCES

1 Van Beek AL, Kassan MA, Adson MH *et al.* Management of acute fingernail injuries. *Hand Clin* 1990; **6**: 23–38.
2 Zook EG. Discussion of 'Management of acute nail bed avulsions'. *Hand Clin* 1990; **6**: 57–8.
3 Zook EG. Understanding the perionychium. *J Hand Ther* 2000; **13**: 269–75.

Delayed trauma

The most common kind of chronic deformity following an acute injury is a split nail or reduction in the length of the nail bed with consequent overcurvature of the tip of the nail.

Cure of a split-nail deformity is difficult, with only a modest chance of success [1]. Sometimes, there is an associated pterygium. Treatment entails excision of the nail bed and matrix scar and, in the case of a pterygium, a split-skin graft may be placed on the ventral aspect of the proximal nail fold to help prevent recurrence of the pterygium. It is important to keep the wounded aspects of nail bed or matrix separate from the overlying nail fold after surgery, and this is often best done by returning the nail plate after soaking it in antiseptic during the procedure.

If treatment is required for a shortened distal phalanx with nail bed changes, there are two choices [2]: the entire nail can be phenolized, or a V–Y advancement flap can be performed based on two neurovascular pedicles.

REFERENCES

1 Hoffman S. Correction of a split nail deformity. *Arch Dermatol* 1973; **108**: 568–9.
2 Haneke E, Baran R. Nail surgery and traumatic abnormalities. In: Baran R, Dawber RPR, eds. *Diseases of the Nails and Their Management*, 2nd edn. Oxford: Blackwell Science, 1994: 378–9.

Haematoma [1,2]

Subungual bleeding is a common sign. It may present as a feature of acute trauma, with pain due to the recent event in combination with pain arising from the pressure exerted by the subungual accumulation of blood. A haematoma arising within the matrix will be incorporated into the nail plate [3]. The only treatment that can be offered is to relieve the pressure, and if seen soon after the injury this can be done by puncturing the nail, for instance with a hot pointed implement, cautery or a small drill. This procedure will relieve pain and may save the nail. The possibility of an underlying fracture must be considered for larger haematomas [1]. As a general rule, if more than 25% of the visible nail is affected, the nail plate should be removed. However, there is evidence to challenge this rule. A comparison between two groups of children having exploration and repair or trephination alone showed fewer complications in the latter group and considerably less investment in medical time [4]. With less extreme trauma, a haematoma may not develop immediately and may be painless. This is most common in the toes and may give rise to clinical uncertainty as to whether it represents early subungual melanoma. A history of traumatic sporting hobbies is useful, and signs of symmetrical nail trauma and inappropriate footwear all point towards trauma as the cause of the appearance. In this situation, making a small punch in the surface of the nail may reveal old blood as the source of pigment. Malignancies can bleed and so confirmation of blood does not refute the possibility of a tumour; however, as an isolated finding in the absence of other clues, this test should be sufficient to obviate the need for surgical exploration. An alternative is to score a transverse groove in the nail at the proximal margin of the pigment and observe over a few weeks as the discoloration grows out. If pigment continues to spread proximal to the groove, surgical exploration is needed.

REFERENCES

1 Farrington H. Subungual haematoma: an evaluation of treatment. *BMJ* 1964; **i**: 742–4.
2 Mortimer PS, Dawber RPR. Trauma of the nail unit including sports injuries. *Dermatol Clin* 1985; **3**: 415–20.
3 Stone OJ, Mullins JF. The distal course of nail haemorrhage. *Arch Dermatol* 1963; **88**: 186–7.
4 Roser SE, Gellman H. Comparison of nail bed repair versus nail trephination for subungual hematomas in children. *J Hand Surg* 1999; **24A**: 1166–70.

Chronic repetitive trauma

Chronic repetitive trauma may take several forms. Some have been considered in other sections detailing transverse ridges produced by a habit tic (see Fig. 62.22, p. 62.28), the canaliform dystrophy of Heller (Fig. 62.44; see p. 62.55) and chronic paronychia (see Fig. 62.18, p. 62.24).

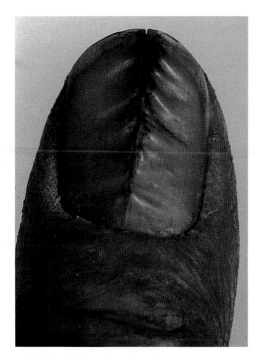

Fig. 62.44 Median canaliform dystrophy of Heller.

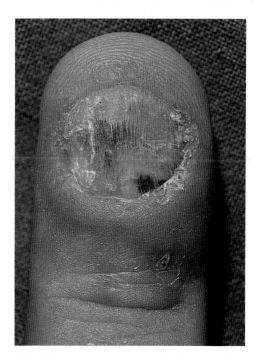

Fig. 62.45 Nail biting can be extensive, with damage to the nail folds and nail plate causing subungual haemorrhage.

Nail biting

The nail plate, periunguium and nail bed are all subject to nail biting and picking. Although fingers are most commonly involved, rarely toenails are also bitten [1]. This produces distinctive features, which are found in 60% of children, 45% of adolescents and 10% of adults [2]. The majority of moderate nail biters have no associated psychiatric disorder [3,4]. Focal abnormalities, such as viral warts, are often a complication, whether as a cause or as a result of the Koebner effect after biting. Severe damage may be associated with self-mutilating disorders such as Lesch–Nyhan syndrome.

The nails are typically short, with up to 50% of the nail bed exposed. The free edge may be even or ragged. Surface change may include splitting of the nail into layers or a sand-papered effect, and the nail may acquire a brown longitudinal streak [5]. The most aggressive nail biting (onychotillomania/onychophagia) can produce subungual haemorrhage, strips of nail loss, with residual spurs or loss of the entire nail (Fig. 62.45). Onychotillomania may be allied to parasitophobia when the patient picks off pieces claiming that they contain parasites [6]. A rough and irregular nail and nail fold may result. Many fingernails are involved. Oral pimozide may be beneficial [7].

Direct damage and secondary infection may make nail loss permanent or result in pterygium formation. The nail folds are sometimes bitten in addition to, or as a substitute for, the nail. This can lead to bleeding and chronic paronychia with acute infective exacerbations. This in turn may lead to nail plate damage or ridging and nail fold scarring.

In cases associated with infection, osteomyelitis of the terminal phalanx can develop [8,9]. Subjects will sometimes deny nail biting and attribute the appearance to a disease that stops nail growth. Transverse grooves scored proximally in the nail plate will confirm that the nail is growing by moving distally with time. In aggressive nail biting, the groove may be eroded from the surface.

Trauma is sometimes inflicted by other nails, with pushing back of the proximal nail fold as part of a habit tic (see p. 62.28). This results in serial transverse ridges and depressions running up the midline of the nail, associated with loss of the cuticle. In more conscious forms of self-damage, sharp instruments are used to produce dermatitis artefacta of the nail unit, and the nail fold is commonly preserved [10].

Treatment. Treatment is often unsuccessful and cure relies largely on the motivation of the patient. Local antiseptics and antimicrobial ointments may help settle the infection secondary to nail unit damage. Those with the most bitter taste are often prescribed in the belief that this will discourage biting. This is seldom the case. Antidepressants [11] and behavioural therapy [12] have been used with some success in limited studies.

REFERENCES

1 Hurley PT, Balu V. Self-inflicted anonychia. *Arch Dermatol* 1982; **118**: 956–7.
2 Malone AJ, Massler M. Index of nail biting in children. *J Abnorm Social Psychol* 1952; **47**: 193–202.

3 Ballinger BR. The presence of nail-biting in normal and abnormal populations. *Br J Psychol* 1970; **117**: 445–6.
4 Colver GB. Onychotillomania. *Br J Dermatol* 1987; **117**: 397–9.
5 Baran R. Nail biting and picking as a possible cause of longitudinal melanonychia. *Dermatologica* 1990; **181**: 126–8.
6 Combes FC, Scott MJ. Onychotillomania. *Arch Dermatol Syphilol* 1951; **63**: 778–80.
7 Hamann K. Onychotillomania treated with pimozide (Orap). *Acta Derm Venereol (Stockh)* 1982; **62**: 364–7.
8 Tosti A, Peluso AM, Bardazzi F *et al*. Phalangeal osteomyelitis due to nail biting. *Acta Derm Venereol (Stockh)* 1994; **74**: 206–7.
9 Waldmann BA. Osteomyelitis caused by nail biting. *Pediatr Dermatol* 1991; **7**: 189–90.
10 Norton L. Self-induced trauma to the nails. *Cutis* 1987; **40**: 223–7.
11 Leonard HL, Lenane MC, Swedo SC *et al*. A double blind comparison of clomipramine and desipramine treatment of severe onychophagia (nail biting). *Arch Gen Psychiatry* 1991; **48**: 821–7.
12 Silber KP, Haynes CE. Treating nailbiting: a comparative analysis of mild aversion and competing response therapies. *Behav Res Ther* 1992; **30**: 15–22.

Hang nails

These are due to hard pieces of epidermis breaking away from the lateral nail folds. Although often due to nail biting, they may result from many other minor injuries. The splits may be painful when they penetrate to the underlying dermis. They should be removed with sharp pointed scissors.

Nutcracker nails

Under this heading, Cohen [1] described splitting and onycholysis caused by the habit of separating the two halves of cracked walnuts over a period of 10 years.

REFERENCE

1 Cohen BH. Nutcracker nails. *Cutis* 1975; **16**: 141.

Damage from nail manicure instruments

Metal instruments, such as a nail file or scissors, wooden or plastic orange sticks, or nail whitener pencils may create acute or chronic injuries in the nail area. Onycholysis may result from using the sharp point for cleaning under the nail plate. Nails, however, are best cleaned with a nail brush and soap, because overzealous manicure, pushing back the cuticles, may result in white streaks across several nails. Cleaning around the nail with contaminated instruments may lead to acute or chronic paronychia. According to Brauer and Baran [1], it is not advisable to cut or clip the nail plate, as this produces a shearing action that weakens the natural layered structure and promotes fracturing and splitting. An emery board is preferred for shaping the fingernail by filing from the sides of the nail towards the centre.

REFERENCE

1 Brauer E, Baran R. Cosmetics: the care and adornment of the nail. In: Baran R, Dawber RPR, eds. *Diseases of the Nails and Their Management*, 2nd edn. Oxford: Blackwell Science, 1994: 285–95.

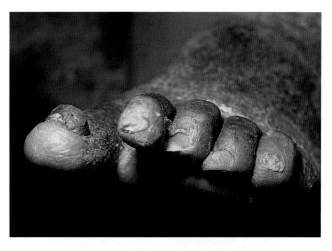

Fig. 62.46 Early onychogryphosis of the left great toenail.

Trauma from footwear

Onychogryphosis and nail hypertrophy [1–5]

Onychogryphosis is an acquired dystrophy usually affecting the great toenail, which is thickened, yellow and twisted. It is most commonly seen in the elderly [1,2,4], although trauma and biomechanical foot problems may precipitate similar changes in middle age or earlier.

At one time, onychogryphosis was known as ostlers' nail, owing to the fact that some cases could be traced to injury caused by a horse trampling on the foot of the ostler. Competitive sport is a more contemporary cause. The injury once sustained is aggravated by footwear and, as the nail becomes longer and thicker, the damage from the footwear becomes progressively more important. Nail hypertrophy implies thickening and increase in length, whereas onychogryphosis implies curvature also.

Some cases of nail hypertrophy are intrinsic, and this applies especially to toenails other than the nail of the great toe. The nail becomes thick and circular in cross-section instead of flat, and thus comes to resemble a claw. There are two possible explanations for this formation.
1 There is insufficient matrix under cover of the posterior fold to exert a flattening effect. The altered relationship between matrix and proximal nail fold in post-mortem specimens supports this.
2 The nail bed is contributing a greater quantity of keratin to the nail than usual. It is usually possible to exclude this on clinical grounds as there is often an element of onycholysis that separates the dystrophic nail from the nail bed. Hypertrophy of fingernails is usually traumatic in origin and is often the result of a single injury.

In onychogryphosis, one or more nails become greatly thickened (Fig. 62.46) and, with neglect, increase in length, becoming curved like a ram's horn. The nails of the great toes are most often involved, but no toenail is exempt. It is possible that the nail plate distortion produced by chronic untreated onychomycosis may be partly responsible for

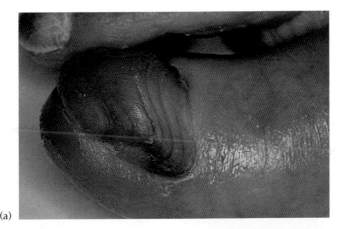

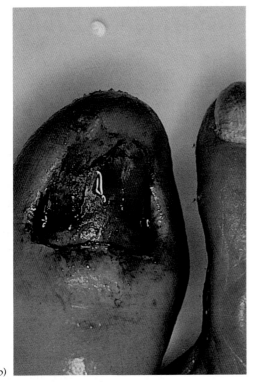

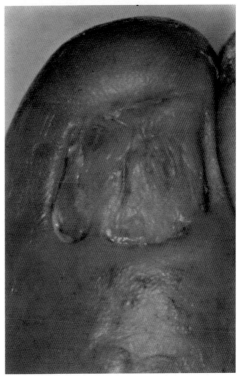

Fig. 62.47 (a–c) Onychogryphosis is often best treated with ablation of the nail matrix.

onychogryphosis at a later stage. In extreme cases, the free edge may press on or even re-enter the soft tissues of the foot.

Treatment of onychogryphosis and nail hypertrophy is either radical or palliative. Radical treatment consists of surgical removal of the nail and matrix and is recommended in those with good circulation (Fig. 62.47). Palliative treatment requires regular paring and trimming of the affected nails, usually by a chiropodist using nail clippers and a file or mechanical burr. The thickened nails are extremely hard and trimming is difficult. Not infrequently, the nail is invaded by granulation tissue from the

nail bed, and incision of this during trimming will result in pain and haemorrhage.

Other causes of thickened nails are psoriasis, pityriasis rubra pilaris, Darier's disease, fungal infections, pachyonychia congenita, congenital ectodermal defects and congenital malalignment of the great toenails [6].

REFERENCES

1 Cohen PR, Scher RK. Geriatric nail disorders: diagnosis and management. *J Am Acad Dermatol* 1992; **26**: 521–31.
2 Dawber RPR, Bristow I, Mooney J. *The Foot: Problems in Podiatry and Dermatology*. London: Dunitz, 1996.
3 Douglas MA, Krull EA. Diseases of the nails. In: Conn WB, ed. *Current Therapy*. Philadelphia: Saunders, 1981: 712.
4 Gilchrist AK. Common foot problems in the elderly. *Geriatrics* 1979; **34**: 67–70.
5 Lubach D. Erbliche onychogryphosis. *Hautarzt* 1982; **33**: 331–3.
6 Baran R, Bureau H. Congenital malalignment of the great toenail as a cause of ingrowing toenail in infancy. *Clin Exp Dermatol* 1983; **6**: 619–23.

Ingrowing toenail [1–3]

SYN. ONYCHOCRYPTOSIS

The soft tissue at the side of the nail (lateral nail fold) is penetrated by the edge of the nail plate, resulting in pain, sepsis and, later, the formation of granulation tissue [4]. Penetration is often caused by spicules of nail at the edge of the nail plate, which have been separated from the main portion of the nail. The great toes are those most often affected. The main cause for the deformity is compression of the toe from the side due to ill-fitting footwear, and the main contributory cause is cutting the toenails in a half-circle instead of straight across. Anatomical features, such as an abnormally long great toe and prominent lateral nail folds, are important in some cases. In recent years, the condition may have been caused in a minority of cases by the successful therapy of fungal infections of the nails with griseofulvin: a nail that has been infected for a long time is reduced in size, and the nail bed shrinks around it; when the infection is even partly overcome the nail plate is increased in size, the nail bed is no longer large enough to accommodate the whole of the new nail, and the lateral nail fold may be penetrated on each side.

In infancy, ingrowing toenail most commonly occurs before shoes are worn, associated with crawling, 'pedalling' or wearing undersized 'jumpsuits' [5]; acute paronychia may be associated [6]. Rarely, it is congenital [7] and even familial [2]. In children, ingrowing is commonly distal rather than lateral. Management is conservative in most instances, with topical steroid and antiseptic preparations. Surgery is occasionally required [8].

The first symptoms are pain and redness, shortly followed by swelling and pus formation. Granulation tissue then forms and adds to the swelling and discharge. More severe infection may follow. There is seldom any difficulty with diagnosis. Excess nail fold granulation tissue can also be a feature of amelanotic melanoma and reactions to medications such as retinoids, ciclosporin, antiretroviral drugs and chemotherapy [9–15].

Treatment. Treatment may be difficult and prolonged. The first essential is to insist on the patient wearing shoes sufficiently wide and pliable to remove lateral pressure [16]. Any abnormality of foot/toe function should be corrected. The patient must also be instructed to cut the nail straight across instead of in a semicircle. The nail must be allowed to grow until its edges are clear of the end of the toe before it is cut; this prevents the further formation of marginal spicules. In the early stages, the infection may be overcome by the application of antiseptics and by inserting a pledget of cotton-wool under the edge of the nail. Taping the toe or applying plastic gutters between nail edge and nail fold are alternatives [17]. Twice-daily warm-water baths followed by careful drying and powdering are helpful. If the infection is more severe and there is local cellulitis, an appropriate systemic antibiotic should be administered. When granulation tissue forms this should be destroyed by cauterization with a silver nitrate stick. It is important that an amelanotic melanoma is not missed [18], and if there are atypical features a biopsy should be performed.

If conservative measures fail, operative intervention will be necessary. Removing the nail alone is likely to result in recurrence of ingrowing when the nail returns [19] and so should be combined with a curative procedure such as phenolization of the relevant part of the matrix [4,20]. Although surgical excision of matrix can provide an excellent result, it is more dependent than phenolization on the skill of the practitioner. In large studies, phenol treatment results in a greater cure rate and less morbidity [19]. Where there is diabetes or impaired peripheral circulation, surgery may require avoidance of prolonged or tight tourniquet application, and close follow-up. Phenolization can be undertaken safely in diabetics [21]. Carbon dioxide laser has been used, although it lacks the analgesic properties intrinsic to phenol [22].

REFERENCES

1 Baran R, Bureau H. Congenital malalignment of the great toenail as a cause of ingrowing toenail in infancy. *Clin Exp Dermatol* 1983; **6**: 619–23.
2 Cambiaghi S, Pistritto G, Gelmeti C. Congenital hypertrophy of the lateral nail folds of the hallux in twins. *Br J Dermatol* 1997; **136**: 635–6.
3 Samman PD. Nail deformities due to trauma. In: Samman PD, Fenton DA, eds. *The Nails in Disease*. London: Heinemann, 1986: 148–9.
4 Baran R, Haneke E, Richert B. Pincer nails: definition and surgical treatment. *Dermatol Surg* 2001; **27**: 261–6.
5 Verbov J. Ingrowing toenails in infancy. *BMJ* 1978; **ii**: 1087.
6 Walker S. Paronychia of the great toe of infants. *Clin Pediatr* 1979; **18**: 247–8.
7 Katz A. Congenital ingrown toenails. *J Am Acad Dermatol* 1996; **34**: 519–20.
8 Piraccini BM, Parente GL, Varotti E, Tosti A. Congenital hypertrophy of the lateral nail folds of the hallux: clinical features and follow-up of seven cases. *Pediatr Dermatol* 2000; **17**: 348–51.
9 Baran R. Retinoids and the nails. *J Dermatol Treat* 1990; **1**: 151–4.
10 Higgins EM, Hughes JR, Snowden S, Pembroke AC. Cyclosporin-induced periungual granulation tissue. *Br J Dermatol* 1995; **132**: 829–30.
11 Nicolopoulos J, Howard A. Docetaxel-induced nail dystrophy. *Australas J Dermatol* 2002; **43**: 293–6.
12 Wasner G, Hilpert F, Schattschneider J *et al.* Docetaxel-induced nail changes: a neurogenic mechanism. A case report. *J Neurooncol* 2002; **58**: 167–74.
13 Stemmler HJ, Gutschow K, Sommer H *et al.* Weekly docetaxel (Taxotere) in patients with metastatic breast cancer. *Ann Oncol* 2001; **12**: 1393–8.
14 Ward HA, Russo GG, Shrum J. Cutaneous manifestations of antiretroviral therapy. *J Am Acad Dermatol* 2002; **46**: 284–93.
15 Heim M, Schapiro J, Wershavski M, Martinowitz U. Drug-induced and traumatic nail problems in the haemophilias. *Haemophilia* 2000; **6**: 191–4.
16 Wernick J, Gibbs RC. Pedal biomechanics and toenail disease. In: Scher RK, Daniel CR, eds. *Nails: Therapy, Diagnosis, Surgery*. Philadelphia: Saunders, 1990: 244–9.
17 Schulte KW, Neumann NJ, Ruzicka T. Surgical pearl: nail splinting by flexible tube—a new noninvasive treatment for ingrown toenails. *J Am Acad Dermatol* 1998; **39**: 629–30.
18 Lemont H, Brady J. Amelanotic melanoma masquerading as an ingrown toenail. *J Am Podiatr Med Assoc* 2002; **92**: 306–7.
19 Rounding C, Hulm S. Surgical treatments for ingrowing toenails. *Cochrane Database Systematic Review* 2000; (2): CD001541.
20 de Berker DA. Phenolic ablation of the nail matrix. *Australas J Dermatol* 2001; **42**: 59–61.
21 Giacalone VF. Phenol matricectomy in patients with diabetes. *J Foot Ankle Surg* 1997; **36**: 264–7.
22 Lin YC, Su HY. A surgical approach to ingrown nail: partial matricectomy using CO$_2$ laser. *Dermatol Surg* 2002; **28**: 578–80.

The nail and cosmetics

Dermatologists need to know the therapeutic options open to a patient when drugs or surgery may not provide the ideal aesthetic or functional solution to a medical problem. Professional cosmetic advice may be the most appropriate step in some cases, such as individuals with permanent unsightly dystrophy. However, the dermatologist may gain most experience of nail cosmetic products through their adverse effects, as they occasionally cause injury to the nail and surrounding tissues and may cause reactions at distant sites. In this section, the basic ingredients of nail preparations are considered together with the pathological changes sometimes induced by them [1,2]. In assessing eczematous and other periungual reactions, it is important also to realize that nail tissues, particularly the subungual and paronychial areas, may be 'reservoirs' for small amounts of cosmetic preparations applied by hand to other parts of the skin, leading to 'ectopic dermatitis'; these may also, rarely, be responsible for dystrophy of the nail apparatus.

Nail coatings represent an attractive nail enhancement. They may harden upon evaporation (nail polish) or polymerize (sculptured nails, gels, preformed artificial nails).

Coatings that harden upon evaporation

Nail polish

The term 'nail lacquer' is sometimes used to include enamels, top coats and base coats, either as separate entities or combined in one product. Although chemically similar, they contain different ratios of the same constituents to lend different characteristics. The base coat is used to improve the adhesion or bonding of enamel to the nail. A top coat improves the depth and lustre of the enamel and increases its resistance to chipping and abrasion. Nail polishes consist of solids and solvent ingredients, the former representing about 30%, the latter 70% of the product. The ingredients can be divided into six principal groups.
1 Cellulose film formers (e.g. nitrocellulose): provide gloss, body and gel structure.
2 Resins (e.g. toluene sulphonamide formaldehyde resin): improve the gloss and adhesion of the film.
3 Plasticizers (e.g. dibutylphthalate): give the film pliability, minimize shrinkage, and soften and plasticize the cellulose.
4 Thixotropic suspending agents (e.g. bentonite) for non-settling and flow: keep pigments in suspension on shaking.
5 Solvents and diluents (e.g. toluene): keep nitrocellulose, resin and plasticizer in the liquid state and control the application and drying time.
6 Colour substances: these are either inorganic (iron oxides) or a variety of certified organic colours (D and C yellow A1 lakes).

Recently, there has been a move away from toluene and formaldehyde resin, and most recently avoidance of dibutylphthalate due to potential health risk.

'Pearls' or 'frosts' are produced by bismuth oxychloride and titanium dioxide coated with mica and guanine (obtained from fish scales). 'Clears' contain a small tint.

The base coat is formulated in a manner similar to standard lacquer, but it has a lower non-volatile content (less nitrocellulose) and lower viscosity, because a thinner film is desirable; it may also contain hydrolysed gelatine. In the top coat the nitrocellulose content is increased and the resin is reduced. A slight increase in plasticizer content improves elasticity of the film. There is no pigment. The top coat often has an added sunscreen.

Reactions such as an allergic contact dermatitis to nail polish frequently appear on any part of the body accessible to the nails, with paradoxically no signs in or around the nail apparatus [3]. The commonest areas involved are the eyelids, the lower half of the face, the sides of the neck and the upper chest. Generalized dermatitis may rarely occur. Sometimes the use of nail polish on stockings to stop 'runs' or on nickel-plated costume jewellery to prevent nickel dermatitis may induce nail-polish dermatitis on the legs or at the site of metal contact. Nail-polish dermatitis may occur in the user's partner or other close contacts. Although any ingredient may account for distant allergic contact dermatitis, toluene sulphonamide formaldehyde resin is the most common culprit. After the nail polish is removed, the dermatitis usually clears rapidly unless secondary infection or lichenification has occurred. Metal pellets present in some bottles to maintain a liquid state may cause nickel reactions and onycholysis.

Nail plate staining from the use of polish is most commonly yellow/orange in colour. It typically starts near the cuticle, extends to the nail tip and becomes progressively darker from base to tip. With time, the dyes penetrate the nail too deeply to be removed. Injury to the nail plate from nail lacquers is rare. However, 'granulation' of nail keratin, a superficial friability, can be observed in some instances where individuals leave nail lacquer on for many weeks or where there is poor formulation of the product. For patch testing, several nail lacquers should be used and tested 'as is'; they should be allowed to dry for 15 min because the solvents and diluents may cause false-positive reactions. The following substances should be included in the test battery.

Toluene sulphonamide formaldehyde resin (10% in petrolatum)

Nickel (5% in petrolatum); dimethylglyoxime spot test for nickel

Glyceryl phthalate resin (polymer resin) (10% in petrolatum)

Pearly material: guanine powder (pure)

Formaldehyde (1% aqueous)

Colophony (20% in petrolatum); drometrizole (Tinuvin P) (1–5% in petrolatum).

The resin contains no free formaldehyde. Formaldehyde is merely the chemical moiety on which the resin is formed. Usually, formaldehyde-sensitive individuals do not cross-react with this resin. However, it has been suggested that there is always a small amount of free formaldehyde present in many preparations. Various cosmetic companies now make varnishes that are formulated without the sensitizing resin and are toluene-free.

Nail polish removers. These are composed of various solvents such as acetone. Occasionally, nail polish removers cause trouble by excessive drying of the nail plate and may be responsible for some inflammation of nail folds.

Coatings that polymerize [4,5]

Sculptured nails

The basic kit of sculptured nails is sold as a set containing a template, a liquid monomer and a powdered polymer. Self-curing acrylic resins are created by polymerization of methyl methacrylate monomer and polymethyl methacrylate powder with an organic peroxide and an accelerator. They harden at room temperature. The compound has to be moulded on the natural nail. The acrylic compound is applied to the nail, which has been roughened on the surface. When hardened, the compound produces a prosthetic nail that is enlarged and elongated by repeated applications. The prosthesis can be filed and manicured to shape; as the plate grows out, further applications of acrylic can be made to maintain a regular contour.

Technicians who sculpt nails should be instructed to wash their hands before touching the face or eye area. Usually, the area involved is the chin, which technicians tend to rest in their hands. Additionally, they should be warned to avoid contact with the dust of freshly applied product and to avoid using the wet product.

Allergic reactions. Allergic reactions due to sculptured nails may occur 2–4 months, and even as long as 16 months, after the first application. The first indication is an itch in the nail bed. Paronychia, which is usually present in allergic reactions, is associated with excruciating pain in the nail area, and sometimes with paraesthesia. The nail bed is dry and thickened, and there is usually onycholysis. The natural nail plate becomes thinner, split and sometimes discoloured. It takes several months for the nails to return to normal. Permanent nail loss is exceptional, as is intractable prolonged paraesthesia [6].

Patch tests most commonly show reactions to the acrylic liquid monomer and not to the polymer; this is similar to denture allergy (see Chapter 20).

Improper application and maintenance. With continued wear, the edges of the sculptured nails become loose. These must be clipped and then rebuilt to prevent the development of an environment prone to bacterial and, beneath the nail plate, candidal infection. In fact, this is a result of improper application and maintenance. Failure to file the prosthetic nail every 2 weeks will result in the creation of a lever arm that predisposes to traumatic onycholysis or damage to the natural nail. Onycholysis is very common with nail extensions that are too long.

Irritant reactions. Irritant reactions to monomers are possible. These manifest as a thickening of the nail bed's keratin layer, which can sometimes cause the entire nail bed to thicken with or without onycholysis. Nonetheless, the overwhelming majority of cases result from physical trauma or abuse.

Damage to the natural nail is not unusual after 2–4 months of wear of a sculptured nail. If it becomes yellow or crumbly, this means that the product was applied and maintained incorrectly. The patient should find a better-qualified nail technician. The problem may well not be the acrylic nail materials but rather the thinning of the nail due to excessive filing with heavy abrasives.

Primer (methacrylic acid) is a strong irritant, which may produce third-degree burns. It is hazardous if the cuticles are flooded or spills are not washed out immediately. Primer can permeate the plate and soak into the nail bed if the nails are too thin. Soap or baking soda, used with water, are excellent neutralizers. If primer gets into the eye, it should be flushed with water for at least 15 min, and a Poisons Information Centre should be contacted.

Premixed acrylic gels

Gel system products are premixed and either acrylic-based (14% of the market) or cyanoacrylate-based (1% or less of the market). Their virtual lack of odour makes gels popular in full-service beauty salons. UV light-cured gels are the best known of the different gel technologies. These gels contain urethanes and (meth)acrylate compounds, a photoinitiator and cellulose, which necessitates antiyellowing agents and a UV light unit. The gel remains in a semi-liquid form until cured in a photobonding box. The proportion of resins to monomers determines the gel consistency. When the gel is exposed to light of an appropriate wavelength, polymerization occurs, resulting in hardening of the gel. UV gels never involve catalysts and often do not employ primers.

Gel enhancement products shrink by up to 20%, which may result in lifting and tip cracking. As an effect of excessive shrinkage, clients may comment that the enhancement feels tight on the nail bed. Other symptoms include throbbing or warmth below the nail plate. This may lead to tender, sore fingertips. Photobonded acrylate has been observed to cause nail reactions, sometimes with nail loss and paraesthesia. Hemmer *et al.* [7] have patch tested 'hypoallergenic' commercial products in patients wearing photobonded acrylic nails who had perionychial and subungual eczema. Triethyleneglycol dimethacrylate, hydroxyfunctional methacrylates, and (meth)-acrylated urethanes proved to be relevant allergens in photobonded nail preparations. Meth-acrylated epoxy resin sensitization was not observed. The omission of irritant methacrylic acid in UV-curable gels does not reduce the high sensitizing potential of new acrylates. Contrary to the manufacturers' declarations, all 'hypoallergenic' products continue to include acrylate functional monomers and therefore continue to cause allergic sensitization. Gels and acrylics, being chemically distinct entities, will not necessarily cross-react.

Unreacted UV gel in the dusts and filings may produce distant allergic reactions. Although sensitization to butylhydroxytoluene is possible, gels usually contain acrylated oligomers and monomers. Acrylates are far more likely to cause sensitization than methacrylates or stabilizers.

Finally, thick ornately painted gel false nails that may be difficult to remove present a real challenge to pulse oximetry. It appears to be the polish more than the sculpted nail that interferes with the readings [8,9].

Preformed plastic nails

Preformed plastic nails are packaged in several shapes and sizes to conform to the normal nail plate configuration. Such nails are trimmed to fit the fingertip and are fixed with cyanoacrylate adhesive supplied with the kit. The usefulness of these prosthetic nails is limited by the need for some normal nail to be present for attachment. Normal physical and chemical insults to the nails cause the preformed plastic nails to loosen. If the preformed nails remain in place for more than 3 or 4 days, they may cause onycholysis and nail-surface damage. Eczematous, painful paronychia due to cyanoacrylate nail preparations may be observed after about 3 months. Dystrophy and discoloration of the nails may become apparent and last for several months. In some cases, distant contact dermatitis of the face and eyelids occurs. On patch testing, the patients react far more often to the adhesive than to the prosthetic nails. Suggested test substances are *p*-tertiary-butylphenol resin (1% in petrolatum), tricresyl ethyl phthalate (5% in petrolatum), cyanoacrylates and other glues (5% in methylethylketone).

Nail-mending kits

These include paper strips of a basic film-forming product to create a 'splint' for the partially fractured nail plate. The split is first bonded with cyanoacrylate glue, then the nail is painted with fibred clear nail polish. A piece of wrap fabric is cut and shaped to fit over the nail surface. This is then embedded in polish of high solid content, and several coats are applied.

Nail wrapping

In nail wrapping, the free edge of the nail should be long enough to be splinted with paper, silk, linen, plastic film or fibreglass and fixed with cyanoacrylate glue. After drying, the edge is shaped, and the nail is coated with enamel.

Removal of nail coatings that polymerize. The most commonly used solvent for removal of nail products is acetone. Warming the solvent with great care can cut product removal time in half. However, most gels are difficult to remove because they are highly cross-linked and resistant to many solvents. Therefore, if gel enhancements have to be removed, slowly file (not drill) the enhancement with a medium-grit file, leaving a very thin layer of product. Soak in warm product remover and, once softened, scrape the remaining product away with a wooden pusher stick.

Cuticle removers

These are lotions or gels containing approximately 0.4% sodium or potassium hydroxide. The lotion is left in place for 1–3 min and then washed off. Creams containing 1–5% lactic acid (pH 3–3.7) are also used.

Nail hardeners

Nail keratin can be hardened by tissue fixatives such as formaldehyde. These are not commercially available in the USA because of their toxic effects. Nail changes caused by such nail hardeners may include pain, subungual haemorrhage and bluish discoloration of the nail. The nail returns to normal when the offending agent is discontinued. Formaldehyde nail hardeners have been reported as causing onycholysis and allergic contact dermatitis; they may also act as irritants. Patch testing should be with formaldehyde (1% aqueous). Because of its irritant qualities, reactions should be interpreted with caution.

Silicone rubber nail prosthesis [10]

In a wide variety of cases, ranging from deformed nail to complete loss of the terminal phalanx, a silicone rubber, thimble-shaped finger-cover may be indicated. This prosthesis is easily fitted on the finger stump, encasing the entire distal phalanx; it must be fine and flexible to maintain pulp sensitivity and must have the same marking and colouring as the finger. The fixation is excellent and the nail form takes nail varnish well.

Nail cream

This is an ordinary water-in-oil moisturizing cream, with low water (30%) and high lipid content. It is applied, after cleaning the hands, to prevent or diminish brittleness.

Nail buffing

Weekly buffing may be indicated for removing small particles of nail debris, thus enhancing the lustre and smoothness of the nail plate. Buffing creams, which contain waxes and finely ground pumice, and buffing powders are abrasive and should not be overused on thin nails.

Nail whitener

This is a pencil-like device with a white clay (kaolin) core used to deposit colour on the undersurface of the free edge of the nail.

Infection risks

Secondary infection with *Candida* or bacteria is a hazard for anyone with an irritant or allergic contact dermatitis of the periunguium. Where this is associated with artificial nails, the prosthetic nails may be longer than usual and so reduce the ability to keep the area clean. Prosthetic nails are sometimes worn because there are underlying problems with the natural nails, such as cracks or onycholysis. These features may also lower the threshold to certain types of infection.

Medical staff with artificial nails may put patients at risk through carriage of pathogens [11] and it is a common operating theatre rule that artificial nails should not be worn [12]. Nail varnish is also thought to be associated with bacterial carriage when it becomes chipped, although the evidence for this is less strong [13]. Infection through nail salons and the manicuring process is a further factor that adds to the risks for those with artificial nails [14].

Conclusion

Nail beauty therapy may certainly produce an attractive enhancement and disguise unsightly nail conditions but it may also represent a potential hazard due to instrument damage, and is not recommended for psoriatic nails as it may provoke the Koebner phenomenon.

REFERENCES

1 Baran R. Nail beauty therapy: an attractive enhancement or a potential hazard? *J Cosmet Dermatol* 2002; **1**: 24–9.
2 Baran R. Allergy and irritation to nail cosmetics. *Am J Clin Dermatol* 2002; **3**: 547–55.
3 Liden C, Berg M, Färv G, Wrangsjö K. Nail varnish allergy with far-reaching consequences. *Br J Dermatol* 1993; **68**: 57–62.
4 Schoon D, Baran R. Cosmetics for nails. In: Barel AO, Paye M, Maibach HI, eds. *Handbook of Cosmetic Science and Technology*. New York: Marcel Dekker, 2001: 685–7.
5 Baran R, Schoon DD. Cosmetology of normal nails. In: Baran R, Maibach H, eds. *Textbook of Cosmetic Dermatology*, 2nd edn. London: Martin Dunitz, 1998: 233–44.
6 Baran RL, Schibli H. Permanent paresthesia to sculptured nails. A distressing problem. *Dermatol Clin* 1990; **8**: 139–41.
7 Hemmer W, Focke M, Wantke F *et al.* Allergic contact dermatitis to artificial fingernails prepared from UV light-cured acrylates. *J Am Acad Dermatol* 1996; **35**: 377–80.
8 Cote CJ, Goldstein EA, Fuchsman WH, Hoaglin DC. The effect of nail polish on pulse oximetry. *Anesth Analg* 1988; **67**: 683–6.
9 Peters SM. The effect of acrylic nails on the measurement of oxygen saturation as determined by pulse oximetry. *AANA J* 1997; **65**: 361–3.
10 Pillet J, Didierjean-Pillet A. Ungual prosthesis. *J Dermatol Treat* 2001; **12**: 41–6.
11 Hedderwick SA, McNeil SA, Lyons MJ, Kauffman CA. Pathogenic organisms associated with artificial fingernails worn by healthcare workers. *Infect Control Hosp Epidemiol* 2000; **21**: 505–9.
12 Toles A. Artificial nails: are they putting patients at risk? A review of the research. *J Pediatr Oncol Nurs* 2002; **19**: 164–71.
13 Arrowsmith VA, Maunder JA, Sargent RJ, Taylor R. Removal of nail polish and finger rings to prevent surgical infection. *Cochrane Database Systematic Review* 2001: CD003325.
14 Winthrop KL, Abrams M, Yakrus M *et al.* An outbreak of mycobacterial furunculosis associated with footbaths at a nail salon. *N Engl J Med* 2002; **346**: 1366–71.

Chapter 63

Disorders of Hair

D.A.R. de Berker, A.G. Messenger & R.D. Sinclair

Anatomy and physiology

[A.G. Messenger, pp. 63.1–63.18]

Introduction

Hair has no vital function in humans, yet its psychological functions are extremely important, as any clinical dermatologist or cosmetician can readily attest from routine daily practice. If the inevitability of scalp baldness makes it reluctantly tolerable to genetically disposed men, in women, loss of hair from the scalp is distressing as is the growth of body or facial hair in excess of the culturally accepted norm.

The evolutionary history of hair is no less enigmatic. Mammals probably evolved from Therapsid reptiles during the Late Triassic period over 200 million years ago (MyA). The earliest direct evidence of hair in mammals comes from fossilized casts and impressions in coprolites and pellets from the Late Paleocene beds of Inner Mongolia [1]. Hairs from at least four extinct mammalian taxa were identified, notably the multituberculate *Lambdopsalis bulla*, all showing striking preservation of the cuticular scale pattern. The three extant mammalian groups—monotremes, marsupials and placental mammals—all possess hair, indicating its presence prior to their divergence which probably took place 115–130 MyA [2]. The multituberculate lineage extends back into the Triassic, suggesting that hair is a very ancient and possibly defining feature of mammals. Whatever its origin, it is clear that the warm-blooded mammals owe much of their evolutionary success to the properties of the hairy pelage as a heat insulator. Paradoxically, Man's movement from the ancestral forest home to populate the globe is linked with a reversion to relative nudity and an ability to keep cool. Moreover, hair serves other purposes: in particular, it is concerned with sexual and social communication by constructing adornments such as the mane of the lion or the beard of the human male, or assisting in the dispersal of scents secreted by complexes of sebaceous or apocrine glands.

For these evolutionary reasons, hair follicles are not all under identical control mechanisms. To match the animal coat to seasonal changes in ambient temperature or environmental background requires moulting and replacement of the hairs. The process appears to involve an inherent follicular rhythm, modified by circulating hormones such as melatonin, prolactin, androgens or thyroxine, whose secretion is geared to environmental cues through the pineal gland, hypothalamus and pituitary.

The control of sexual hair growth must be clearly differentiated from that of the moult cycle. The development of pubic, axillary and other body hair is delayed until puberty because it is dependent upon androgens in both sexes; that 'male' hormones are, in contrast, also a prerequisite for the manifestation of androgenetic alopecia still defies adequate explanation.

In all mammals, including humans but with the possible exception of the merino sheep and the poodle dog, hair follicles show intermittent activity. Thus, each hair grows to a maximum length, is retained for a time without further growth, and is eventually shed and replaced.

Types of hair

Different types of hair may be produced by different kinds of follicle, and the type of hair produced in any particular follicle can change with age or under the influence of hormones. Animals characteristically have both an overcoat of stiff guard hairs and an undercoat of fine hairs [3], but many kinds of follicle and fibre have been described. Many species also have large vibrissae or sinus hairs, which are sensory and are produced from special follicles containing erectile tissue, but there are no strictly comparable follicles in humans. In humans, a prenatal coat of fine soft unmedullated and usually unpigmented hair, known as *lanugo*, is normally shed *in utero* in the eighth to ninth month of gestation. Postnatal hair may be divided at the extreme into two kinds: vellus, which is soft, unmedullated, occasionally pigmented and seldom more than 2 cm long; and terminal hair, which is longer, coarser and often medullated and pigmented. However, there is a range of intermediate kinds. Before puberty, terminal hair is normally limited to the scalp, eyebrows and eyelashes. After puberty, secondary sexual 'terminal' hair is developed from vellus hair in response to androgens.

Development and distribution of hair follicles

Human hair follicles appear first in the regions of the eyebrows, upper lip and chin at about 9 weeks of embryonic development, and in other regions in the fourth month [4]. Hair over most of the scalp passes through a complete cycle and is shed *in utero*, and follicles in these regions have re-entered anagen by the time of birth. In the occipital scalp, telogen is delayed until after birth and this may give rise to a patch of hair loss in this region in the neonatal period. A fuller account of embryonic development is given in Chapter 3.

In humans, the full complement of hair follicles is probably established by the time of birth. Follicle density is highest in the fetus, when it may be similar across the skin surface. With growth there is a progressive reduction in follicle density, which continues until adult life, as skin surface area increases (Table 63.1). This occurs to a greater degree over the trunk and limbs than over the head so that the reduction in follicle density is less marked on the head than elsewhere [5]. The highest hair follicle densities, in the region of 800/cm² are found on the forehead and cheeks, with rather lower values for visible vellus hairs on

Table 63.1 Hair follicle density in human fetal and adult skin. In adults, hair follicle density is highest on the head and much lower on the trunk and limbs. At 24 weeks' gestational age hair follicle density is similar in forehead and thigh skin. There is a pronounced reduction in thigh hair follicle density by adult life but only a small fall on the forehead. (Adapted from Szabo [5].)

| | Fetal skin | | | | Adult | |
| | 24 weeks | | Full term | | | |
	Mean	±	Mean	±	Mean	±
Cheek					830	40
Forehead	1060		1060	110	765	20
Scalp					350	50
Forearm					95	15
Thigh	1010	250	480	40	55	5
Lower leg					45	10
Abdomen					70	15
Chest					75	25

the forehead in young adults of both sexes, and on the cheeks in women (400–450/cm²) [6]. Lower hair densities of 50–100/cm² are found on the chest and back in both sexes [6,7], and follicle densities of approximately 50/cm² on the thigh and leg [5]. Published values for the average scalp hair density in white people vary between 250 and 320 hairs/cm² [8–11]. Scalp hair density shows a normal distribution in the population, with a wide range [11]. There is also racial variation in scalp hair density: average hair density in Africans (187/cm²) [12] and African Americans (171/cm²) [13] is lower than in white people, and it is lower still in Koreans (128/cm²) [14].

REFERENCES

1 Meng J, Wyss AR. Multituberculate and other mammal hair recovered from Palaeocene excreta. *Nature* 1997; **385**: 712–4.
2 Janke A, Xu X, Arnason U. The complete mitochondrial genome of the wallaroo (*Macropus robustus*) and the phylogenetic relationship among Monotremata, Marsupialia, and Eutheria. *Proc Nat Acad Sci USA* 1997; **94**: 1276–81.
3 Dry FW. The coat of the mouse (*Mus musculus*). *J Genet* 1925; **16**: 287–340.
4 Pinkus H. Embryology of hair. In: Ellis RA, ed. *The Biology of Hair Growth*. New York: Academic Press, 1958: 1–32.
5 Szabo G. The regional anatomy of the human integument with special reference to the distribution of hair follicles, sweat glands and melanocytes. *Philos Trans R Soc Lond B Biol Sci* 1967; **252**: 447–85.
6 Blume U, Ferracin J, Verschoore M *et al.* Physiology of the vellus hair follicle: hair growth and sebum excretion. *Br J Dermatol* 1991; **124**: 21–8.
7 Blume U, Verschoore M, Poncet M *et al.* The vellus hair follicle in acne: hair growth and sebum excretion. *Br J Dermatol* 1993; **129**: 23–7.
8 Barman JM, Astore I, Pecoraro V. The normal trichogram of the adult. *J Invest Dermatol* 1965; **44**: 233–6.
9 Rushton DH, Ramsay ID, James KC *et al.* Biochemical and trichological characterization of diffuse alopecia in women. *Br J Dermatol* 1990; **123**: 187–97.
10 Whiting DA. Diagnostic and predictive value of horizontal sections of scalp biopsy specimens in male pattern androgenetic alopecia. *J Am Acad Dermatol* 1993; **28**: 755–63.
11 Birch MP, Messenger JF, Messenger AG. Hair density, hair diameter and the prevalence of female pattern hair loss. *Br J Dermatol* 2001; **144**: 297–304.

12 Loussouarn G. African hair growth parameters. *Br J Dermatol* 2001; **145**: 294–7.
13 Sperling LC. Hair density in African Americans. *Arch Dermatol* 1999; **135**: 656–8.
14 Lee HJ, Ha SJ, Lee JH *et al*. Hair counts from scalp biopsy specimens in Asians. *J Am Acad Dermatol* 2002; **46**: 218–21.

Anatomy of the hair follicle (Fig. 63.1)

Hair is the keratinized product of the hair follicle, a tube-like structure continuous with the epidermis at its upper end. The follicles are sloped in the dermis, and longer follicles extend into the subcutaneous layer. An oblique muscle, the arrector pili, runs from the mid-region of the follicle wall to a point in the papillary dermis close to the dermal–epidermal junction. Above the muscle, one or more sebaceous glands, and in some regions of the body an apocrine gland also, open into the follicle. The hair fibre is made up of three cell layers: an outer cuticle, the cortex (which forms the bulk of the fibre in most hair types) and a variable central medulla, all of which derive from highly proliferative cells in the hair bulb at the base of the follicle. Cells in the hair bulb also give rise to the inner root sheath which surrounds the hair fibre and which disintegrates before the hair emerges from the skin. The inner root sheath is itself enclosed by the outer root sheath, which forms a continuous structure extending from the hair bulb to the epidermis, although the functions and microscopic structure of the outer root sheath vary along the length of the follicle. The hair follicle also has a specialized dermal component, which includes the dermal or connective tissue sheath surrounding the follicle, and the dermal papilla which invaginates the hair bulb.

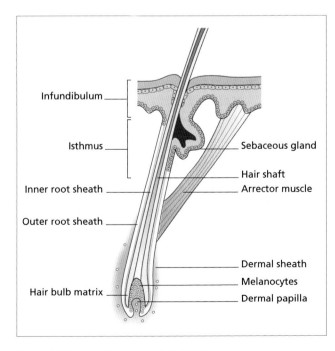

Fig. 63.1 Diagram of an anagen hair follicle.

Infundibulum

Isthmus

Inner root sheath

Outer root sheath

Hair bulb matrix

Sebaceous gland

Hair shaft

Arrector muscle

Dermal sheath

Melanocytes

Dermal papilla

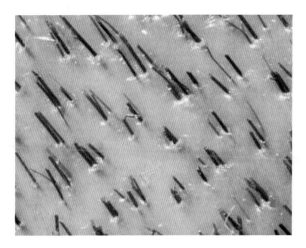

Fig. 63.2 Grouping of hairs in follicular units on human scalp. In some groups, multiple hairs emerge from a single follicular opening.

The hair follicle is conventionally divided into two regions: the upper part consisting of the infundibulum and isthmus and the lower part comprising the hair bulb and suprabulbar region. The upper follicle is a relatively constant structure, whereas the lower follicle undergoes repeated episodes of regression and regeneration during the hair cycle. On the scalp, and some other regions of the skin, hair follicles are arranged in groups of three or more follicles known as follicular units (Fig. 63.2). Several follicles within a follicular unit may coalesce so that hairs emerge through a common infundibulum.

The infundibulum

The infundibulum extends from the skin surface, where it merges with the epidermis, to the opening of the sebaceous duct at the junction with the isthmus. Infundibular epithelium differentiates in a similar manner to epidermis, producing a granular layer and stratum corneum which desquamates into the follicular lumen.

The isthmus

The isthmus extends from the opening of the sebaceous gland duct to the insertion of the arrector pili muscle. It consists of a multilayered outer root sheath that is continuous with the infundibulum but differs in its structure. The innermost cells lack a granular layer and undergo a pattern of differentiation known as trichilemmal keratinization. The keratinized inner root sheath, which lies within the outer root sheath, disintegrates at or about the level of the sebaceous duct. The arrector muscle loops around the follicle in the manner of a sling [1]. Each follicular unit is supplied by a single arrector muscle, which splits to encircle each follicle within the follicular unit [2].

Hair follicle stem cells are thought to reside in the lower part of the isthmus close to the insertion of the arrector

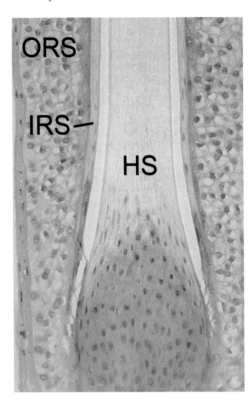

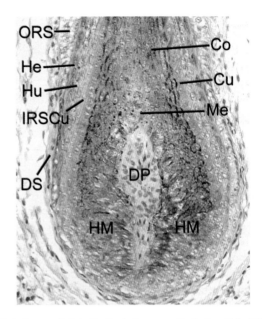

Fig. 63.4 Anagen hair bulb. Co, hair cortex; Cu, hair cuticle; DP, dermal papilla; DS, dermal sheath; He, Henle's layer; HM, hair matrix; Hu, Huxley's layer; IRSCu, inner root sheath cuticle; ORS, outer root sheath.

Fig. 63.3 Longitudinal section through suprabulbar region of an anagen follicle showing the keratogenous region of the hair shaft (HS). The inner root sheath (IRS) is keratinized at this level. ORS, outer root sheath.

muscle [3]. During embryogenesis, and in adult follicles in other species, this region shows a distinctive bulge, although a clearly defined bulge is often not seen in human adult hair follicles. Hair follicle stem cells show distinctive biochemical properties, they are slow cycling and proliferate only during the onset of anagen. Daughter cells, known as transient amplifying cells, input into the outer root sheath of the lower part of the hair follicle whence they migrate in a downward direction. On entering the hair bulb matrix, they proliferate and undergo terminal differentiation to form the hair shaft and inner root sheath [4]. The progeny of hair follicle stem cells may also migrate distally to form the sebaceous gland and, under certain circumstances such as wound healing, the epidermis.

The suprabulbar region (Fig. 63.3)

The suprabulbar region of the follicle, below the isthmus and above the hair bulb, is comprised of three layers from outermost to innermost: outer root sheath, inner root sheath and hair shaft. The outer root sheath is a multilayered epithelium enclosing the inner root sheath which, at this level, is a fully keratinized structure. Cells of the hair shaft, at the centre of the follicle, undergo terminal differ-

entiation within the keratogenous zone in the middle part of the suprabulbar region. Keratinization of the inner root sheath precedes that of the hair shaft, suggesting that the inner root sheath has a role in 'moulding' the shape of the hair fibre.

The hair bulb (Fig. 63.4)

In large terminal follicles, the deepest part of the follicle, the hair bulb, is situated in the subcutaneous fat. The hair bulb is invaginated at its base by the dermal papilla, which is connected to the perifollicular dermal sheath by a narrow stalk. The hair shaft and the inner root sheath are derived from epithelial cells surrounding the dermal papilla, a region known as the hair bulb matrix or germinative epithelium. These cells have a high mitotic rate, with a rate of cell turnover similar to that in the bone marrow. Daughter cells migrate in an upward direction and differentiate in a highly ordered fashion to form the concentric layers of the inner root sheath and the hair shaft. The inner root sheath derives from cells in the lower, more lateral part of the matrix, whereas the hair shaft is formed from the upper, centrally situated cells. In pigmented hair follicles, highly melanized melanocytes are situated amongst cells destined to form the hair cortex. Occasional Langerhans' cells may also be found in the matrix region. The outer root sheath surrounds the inner root sheath. At the level of the hair bulb it consists of a single layer of cells, which can be followed almost to the lower tip of the hair follicle.

The dermal papilla

In anagen follicles, the dermal papilla is a flask-shaped structure that invaginates the base of the hair follicle. It is made up of specialized fibroblast-like cells embedded in an extracellular matrix rich in basement-membrane proteins and proteoglycans, and in large follicles the dermal papilla often contains a loop of capillary blood vessels. It is connected to the dermal sheath surrounding the follicle by a narrow stalk. Both the dermal papilla and the dermal sheath are derived from a condensation of mesenchymal cells, which appear at an early stage in follicular embryogenesis. Tissue recombinant studies have shown that the dermal papilla plays an essential part in the induction and maintenance of follicular epithelial differentiation [5–8]. It is responsible for determining the follicle type, so that cultured dermal papilla cells derived from the rat vibrissae follicle induce the formation of a vibrissa-like follicle when implanted into ear skin [9]. The volume of the dermal papilla may also be responsible for controlling the size of the hair follicle, and that of the hair fibre [10,11]. This is of particular relevance to androgen-dependent changes in human hair growth, as the dermal papilla is probably the primary target of androgen action in the hair follicle.

The dermal sheath

The lower part of the hair follicle is enveloped by a collagenous layer known as the dermal or connective tissue sheath. Like dermal papilla cells, fibroblasts of the dermal sheath are highly specialized. In experimental circumstances, these cells can reconstitute the dermal papilla and induce the formation of new hair follicles in adult human skin [12]. As we move distally along the hair follicle, above the level of the arrector insertion, the dermal sheath becomes less distinct, both structurally and functionally, as it merges with the interfollicular dermis.

The inner root sheath

The inner root sheath consists of three layers (from outermost to innermost): Henle's layer, Huxley's layer and the inner root sheath cuticle. Inner root sheath cells accumulate filaments approximately 7 nm thick and, in contrast with the hair cortex, amorphous trichohyalin granules appear in the cytoplasm. As the cells move up the follicle towards the surface, the filaments become more abundant and the number and size of the granules increase. Each of the three layers of the inner root sheath undergoes abrupt keratinization. This occurs at different levels in each layer, although the patterns of change are identical. In the hardened cytoplasm, however, only filaments can be seen. The changes occur first in the outermost Henle's layer, then in the innermost cuticle and lastly in Huxley's layer, which is situated between them. Cells of the inner root sheath cuticle become flattened and overlap, with their free edges pointing downwards to interdigitate with the upwards-pointing cells of hair shaft cuticle, thus anchoring the hair shaft within the hair follicle. The inner root sheath hardens before the presumptive hair within it, and it is consequently thought to control the definitive shape of the hair shaft.

The outer root sheath

The outer root sheath forms the most peripheral layer of hair follicle epithelium, enclosing the inner root sheath. At the lower tip of the hair bulb it consists of a single layer of cuboidal cells, becoming multilayered in the region of the upper hair bulb. The cytoplasm of outer root sheath cells is rich in glycogen, giving a clear appearance with routine histological stains. In some follicles, particularly large beard follicles, there is a distinct single cell layer interposed between the outer and inner root sheaths, known as the companion layer [13]. Companion layer cells are flattened along the axis of the follicle and are relatively devoid of glycogen. They show numerous intercellular connections to the inner root sheath and are thought to migrate distally along with the inner root sheath to be lost in the isthmus region. The direction of movement of outer root sheath cells is unclear but they may migrate downwards towards the hair bulb, the companion layer forming the plane of slippage between the inner and outer root sheaths. The outer root sheath of the suprabulbar region merges imperceptibly with the isthmus where the innermost cells undergo tricholemmal keratinization.

The cuticle

The hair cuticle is formed initially as a single cell layer, but the cells become progressively imbricated (tile-like) as they move peripherally. The cells become flattened, first in a direction at right angles to the plane of the follicle, and then becoming progressively angulated so that the outer edges of the cells point in an upward direction. The flattened cells overlap, their free edges directed towards the tip (Fig. 63.5) and interlocking with the cuticle of the surrounding inner root sheath. In the fully formed hair shaft, the cuticle consists of 5–10 overlapping cell layers, each 350–450 nm thick (Fig. 63.6). The mature cells are thin scales consisting of compact cuticular keratin, associated with ultra-high sulphur proteins, which show three distinct layers by transmission electron microscopy: the outer A-layer, which is particularly rich in cystine; the exocuticle (also cystine-rich); and the inner endocuticle, which is virtually devoid of sulphur. The endocuticle has an irregular substructure of membrane-like elements which are probably the remnants of cytoplasmic structures [14].

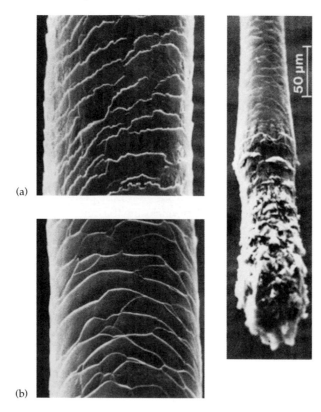

(a)

(b)

Fig. 63.5 (a) Surface view of weathered cuticular scales in the distal portion of the hair shaft. (b) Surface view of undamaged cuticular scales in proximal part of hair shaft. (Courtesy of Dr D. Jackson, University of Sheffield, Sheffield, UK.)

The outer surface of the cuticle is thought to be coated with long-chain (straight and branched) fatty acids linked to an underlying lipid–protein matrix [15]. This layer is 2–7 nm thick and is known as the fibre cuticle surface membrane or epicuticle. The cuticle has important protective properties. It acts as a barrier to physical and chemical insults, and also maintains the integrity of the hair shaft. Wear and tear (e.g. from cosmetic procedures) leads to gradual degradation of the cuticle ('weathering'), with breaking and lifting of the free margins of cuticular cells. Eventually this process may lead to exposure of the cortex and fracture of the hair shaft.

The cortex

Cells destined to form the cortex gradually become more fusiform in shape as they migrate upwards from the hair bulb. They develop a dense filamentous cytoskeleton in the upper hair bulb to become fully hyalinized in the suprabulbar region (the keratogenous zone) (Fig. 63.7). The hard α-keratin intermediate filaments (α-KIF) are the major structural component of the mammalian hair cortex. The molecule in α-KIF is an obligate heteropolymer containing a type I and a type II polypeptide chain [16,17], in which right-handed α-helices coil round one another in a left-handed manner to form a rod-like dimeric structure (a 'coiled coil') (Fig. 63.8). The 8-nm keratin filaments (microfibrils) are formed from multiple α-KIF molecules, on average 16 molecules or 32 chains in cross-section [18]. Keratin filaments are cross-linked to keratin-associated proteins, which form a matrix between the filaments. More than 60 hair keratin-associated proteins have been found in various species. They are classified into three major families: high sulphur, ultra-high sulphur and high glycine–tyrosine proteins [19]. In some species, notably the sheep, the cortex can be divided into two regions: the orthocortex and paracortex, which differ in the arrangement of KIFs and the proportion of keratin-associated

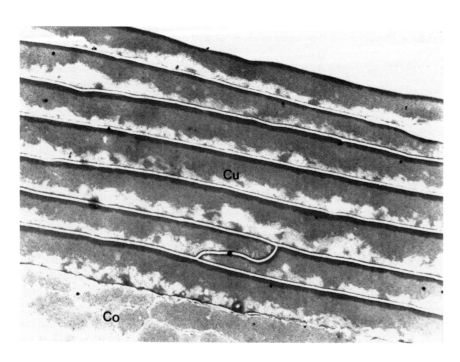

Cu

Co

Fig. 63.6 Cross-section through hair shaft showing cuticle layers (Cu) surrounding the central cortex (Co). (Transmission electron micrograph, silver methenamine stain.)

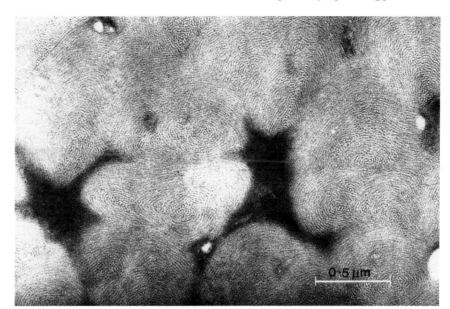

0·5 μm

Fig. 63.7 Cross-section of transformed cortical cells of human hair. The relatively translucent filaments, set in a more dense sulphur-rich matrix, appear as concentric lamellae (macrofibrils), giving a characteristic fingerprint pattern.

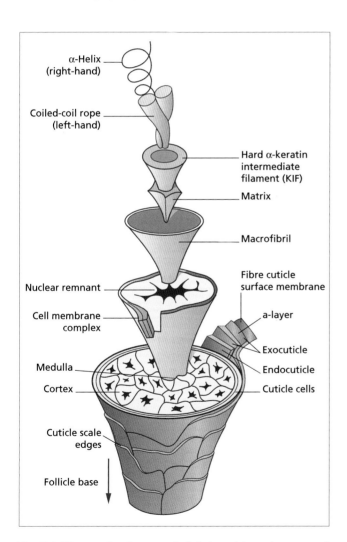

Fig. 63.8 Diagram showing an exploded view of the major structural components comprising a human hair fibre. Pigment granules that are normally dispersed throughout the cortex are not included. (Courtesy of Dr L. Jones [14].)

proteins. In humans, the hair cortex appears to contain mixtures of KIF arrangements within each cell.

The medulla

The medulla is a variable structure in human hairs, where it may be continuous, discontinuous or absent. Large diameter hairs are more likely to contain a medulla, although the relationship between hair diameter and medullation is not clear-cut. The medulla develops quite abruptly around the upper pole of the dermal papilla, without any obvious precursor cell population. Medullary cells contain distinctive eosinophilic granules that eventually form internal coatings within the membranes of mature cells. As these cells develop, arginine residues are converted to citrulline, and isopeptide bonds are formed to yield a highly insoluble protein complex [20]. Mature medulla cells have a spongy structure, with amorphous material bounding air spaces of varying sizes.

Hair follicle innervation

A plexus of longitudinally aligned sensory nerve fibres surrounds the isthmus region. Small nerve fibres may also be arranged in a circular fashion outside the longitudinal fibres. Several different types of nerve endings are found around human hair follicles, including free nerve endings, pilo-Ruffini nerve endings and Merkel nerve endings [21,22]. In other species, lamellated nerve endings are found in richly innervated sinus hair follicles (e.g. vibrissae follicles), which have specialized sensory function [22]. Merkel cells, with or without associated nerve endings, may be found within the bulge region epithelium and the surrounding connective tissue sheath, and it has been postulated that their secretions are involved in regulating the hair cycle [23].

REFERENCES

1 Narisawa Y, Kohda H. Arrector pili muscles surround human facial vellus hair follicles. *Br J Dermatol* 1993; **129**: 138–9.
2 Poblet E, Ortega F, Jimenez F. The arrector pili muscle and the follicular unit of the scalp: a microscopic anatomy study. *Dermatol Surg* 2002; **28**: 800–3.
3 Cotsarelis G, Sun TT, Lavker RM. Label-retaining cells reside in the bulge area of pilosebaceous unit: implications for follicular stem cells, hair cycle, and skin carcinogenesis. *Cell* 1990; **61**: 1329–37.
4 Oshima H, Rochat A, Kedzia C *et al.* Morphogenesis and renewal of hair follicles from adult multipotent stem cells. *Cell* 2001; **104**: 233–45.
5 Oliver RF. Whisker growth after removal of the dermal papilla and lengths of follicle in the hooded rat. *J Embryol Exp Morphol* 1966; **16**: 231–44.
6 Oliver RF. The experimental induction of whisker growth in the hooded rat by implantation of dermal papillae. *J Embryol Exp Morphol* 1967; **18**: 43–51.
7 Oliver RF. The induction of hair follicle formation in the adult hooded rat by vibrissa dermal papillae. *J Embryol Exp Morphol* 1970; **23**: 219–36.
8 Jahoda CA, Horne KA, Oliver RF. Induction of hair growth by implantation of cultured dermal papilla cells. *Nature* 1984; **311**: 560–2.
9 Jahoda CA, Reynolds AJ, Oliver RF. Induction of hair growth in ear wounds by cultured dermal papilla cells. *J Invest Dermatol* 1993; **101**: 584–90.
10 Van Scott EJ, Ekel TM. Geometric relationships between the matrix of the hair bulb and its dermal papilla in normal and alopecic scalp. *J Invest Dermatol* 1958; **31**: 281–7.
11 Ibrahim L, Wright EA. A quantitative study of hair growth using mouse and rat vibrissal follicles. I. Dermal papilla volume determines hair volume. *J Embryol Exp Morphol* 1982; **72**: 209–24.
12 Reynolds AJ, Lawrence C, Cserhalmi-Friedman PB *et al.* Trans-gender induction of hair follicles. *Nature* 1999; **402**: 33–4.
13 Rothnagel JA, Roop DR. Hair follicle companion layer: reacquainting an old friend. *J Invest Dermatol* 1995; **104**: 42S–3S.
14 Jones LN. Hair structure anatomy and comparative anatomy. *Clin Dermatol* 2001; **19**: 95–103.
15 Negri AP, Cornell HJ, Rivett DE. A model for the surface of keratin fibres. *Text Res J* 1993; **63**.
16 Langbein L, Rogers MA, Winter H *et al.* The catalog of human hair keratins. I. Expression of the nine type I members in the hair follicle. *J Biol Chem* 1999; **274**: 19874–84.
17 Langbein L, Rogers MA, Winter H *et al.* The catalog of human hair keratins. II. Expression of the six type II members in the hair follicle and the combined catalog of human type I and II keratins. *J Biol Chem* 2001; **276**: 35123–32.
18 Jones LN, Simon M, Watts NR *et al.* Intermediate filament structure: hard α-keratin. *Biophys Chem* 1997; **68**: 83–93.
19 Rogers GE, Powell BC. Organization and expression of hair follicle genes. *J Invest Dermatol* 1993; **101**: 50S–5S.
20 Harding HW, Rogers GE. Epsilon-(gamma-glutamyl)lysine cross-linkage in citrulline-containing protein fractions from hair. *Biochemistry (Mosc)* 1971; **10**: 624–30.
21 Hashimoto K, Ito M, Suzuki Y. Innervation and vasculature of the hair follicle. In: Orfanos CE, Happle R, eds. *Hair and Hair Diseases*. Berlin: Springer-Verlag, 1990: 117–47.
22 Halata Z. Specific nerve endings in vellus hair, guard hair and sinus hair. In: Orfanos CE, Happle R, eds. *Hair and Hair Diseases*. Berlin: Springer-Verlag, 1990: 149–64.
23 Narisawa Y, Hashimoto K, Nakamura Y *et al.* A high concentration of Merkel cells in the bulge prior to the attachment of the arrector pili muscle and the formation of the perifollicular nerve plexus in human fetal skin. *Arch Dermatol Res* 1993; **285**: 261.

The hair cycle (Fig. 63.9)

Hair follicles undergo a repetitive sequence of growth and rest known as the hair cycle. The timing of the phases of the hair cycle and its overall duration varies between

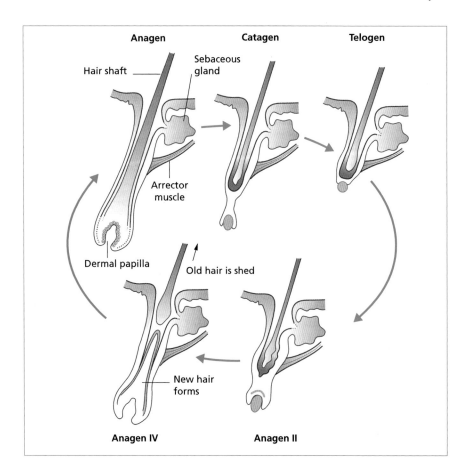

Fig. 63.9 The hair cycle. (From *Disorders of Hair Growth*, McGraw-Hill.)

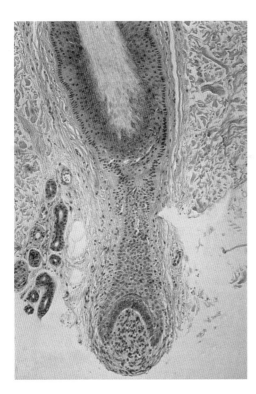

Fig. 63.10 Scalp hair follicle in Anagen 2 stage of development. The club hair from the previous cycle is still present within the follicle. (Courtesy of Dr A.J.G. McDonagh, Royal Hallamshire Hospital, Sheffield, UK.)

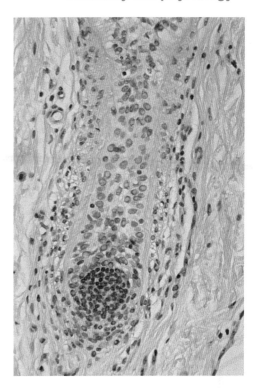

Fig. 63.11 Human hair follicle in mid-catagen. There is a prominent glassy membrane surrounding the regressing epithelial column. The dermal papilla has rounded and condensed. (Courtesy of McGraw-Hill.)

species, between follicles in different regions of the skin in the same species and, in some animals, between different follicle types, such as guard hairs and underhairs, in the same region of the skin.

The period of active hair growth is known as *anagen* and the duration of this phase is responsible for determining the final length of the hair. In most hair follicles in most animals, anagen is relatively brief, lasting a few weeks at most. In some hair follicles, such as those on human scalp, the horse's tail and wool follicles in the merino sheep, anagen may continue for several years, so that very long hairs are produced. Under normal circumstances, 80–90% of hair follicles on the human scalp are in anagen at any one time.

The entry of a resting hair follicle into anagen is heralded by the onset of mitotic activity in epithelial cells overlying the dermal papilla at the base of the follicle (the secondary epithelial germ). In most follicle types (vibrissa follicles are an exception), the lower part of the follicle elongates downwards along a preformed dermal tract (the stele). The developing hair bulb partly envelops the dermal papilla, and epithelial cells start to differentiate to form the inner root sheath and the hair shaft (Fig. 63.10). The dermal papilla expands from a tightly packed ball of cells into a flask-shaped structure where the cells become

separated by an extracellular matrix rich in proteoglycans and basement-membrane proteins. A network of capillary blood vessels develops around the lengthening follicle, extending into the dermal papilla in larger follicles. In the fully developed anagen follicle, epithelial cells in the hair bulb undergo vigorous proliferative activity. Their progeny move distally and differentiate in an ordered fashion to form the layers of the inner root sheath and the hair shaft. At the end of anagen, epithelial cell division declines and ceases, and the follicle enters an involutionary phase known as *catagen*. During catagen, the proximal end of the hair shaft keratinizes to form a club-shaped structure and the lower part of the follicle involutes by apoptosis (Fig. 63.11). The basement membrane surrounding the follicle becomes thickened and corrugated to form the 'glassy membrane'. The base of the follicle, together with its dermal papilla, moves upwards, eventually to lie just below the level of the arrector insertion. The period between the completion of follicular regression and the onset of the next anagen phase is termed *telogen*. The club hair lies within an epithelial sac to which it is attached by tricholemmal keratin. The club hair is eventually shed through an active process termed *exogen*. In many species, follicles re-enter anagen prior to shedding of the club hair so that the old hair is not shed until the follicle is well into its next growth phase. This may also be

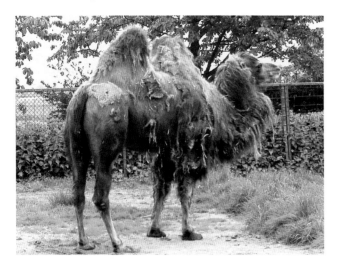

Fig. 63.12 Bactrian camel in spring moult.

seen in human follicles although it is unusual for a club hair to be retained much beyond the mid-stage of anagen development. In human scalp, hair follicles may remain in a state of latency for a prolonged period after the club hair is shed [1].

Control of the hair cycle

It is thought that hair cycling is controlled primarily within individual hair follicles but that this intrinsic rhythmic behaviour may be modulated by both local and systemic factors. In most newborn mammals, including humans, hair cycles are coordinated in a wave-like fashion (moult waves) across regions of the skin in the neonatal period. Moult waves are regulated within the skin and are accompanied by changes in other skin structures, such as epidermal and dermal thickness. Hence, skin flaps raised on the flanks of rats, rotated through 90–180° and then replaced, continue to moult in their original direction for a prolonged period [2,3]. Homografts between isogenic animals of different ages also retain the moult pattern of the donor, whereas autografts retain that of the recipient [4]. Hair cycles in homografts eventually come into phase with the surrounding skin as do those in rats of different ages joined parabiotically, suggesting that the factors regulating synchrony are able to diffuse into the grafted skin. In many mammals, living in their natural environment in temperate and higher latitudes, moult waves continue into adult life and occur on a seasonal basis. This allows adaptation of the thickness of the coat, and sometimes its colour, to different climatic conditions in summer and winter (Fig. 63.12). In humans, and some other mammals such as the guinea pig, synchronous hair cycling is lost rapidly with increasing age so that, beyond the neonatal period, hair follicles cycle independently of their neighbours. In these circumstances, hair cycling

must be regulated by mechanisms intrinsic to the hair follicle.

Seasonal hair growth

Seasonal moulting is regulated by the endocrine system under the influence of environmental signals. The most important of these is change in day length (the photoperiod) [5,6]. Temperature may act as a modifying factor in some species. Changing levels of melatonin production by the pineal gland have a key role in orchestrating endocrine control of seasonal hair growth [7–9]; pinealectomy prevents seasonal moulting, whereas administration of melatonin advances onset of the growth of the winter coat and prevents growth of the summer coat. Prolactin production by the pituitary correlates inversely with melatonin levels, being raised during the summer and falling during the winter. Pinealectomy abolishes the fall in prolactin level in animals kept in short day length conditions and prevents the development of the winter coat [10]. The same response is seen in animals treated with prolactin. Prolactin receptors have been identified in the hair follicle, suggesting that prolactin can affect hair growth directly [11]. Pineal and pituitary hormones may also act indirectly by modulating the activity of peripheral endocrine glands. In rats, estradiol, testosterone and adrenal steroids delay the onset of anagen, whereas gonadectomy and adrenalectomy have the opposite effect [12]. Conversely, thyroid hormones accelerate the onset of follicular activity, whereas thyroidectomy or treatment with propylthiouracil delays it. Seasonal moults are also delayed by testosterone and accelerated by thyroxine in other species [13]. Hormones also act on the anagen phase of hair growth [12]. Estradiol and thyroxine both reduce the duration of anagen in rats, but estradiol decreases the rate of hair growth, whereas thyroxine has the opposite effect, suggesting these hormones have different points of action. In the mouse, oestrogen receptors are expressed in the dermal papilla and the inhibitory effect of exogenous oestrogen on hair growth is prevented by topical treatment with an oestrogen receptor antagonist [14].

Vestiges of seasonal variation in hair growth are present in humans [15], although the magnitude is seldom sufficient to be noticeable. The best example of a systemic influence on the human hair growth cycle is pregnancy (Fig. 63.13) [16]. During pregnancy, there is an increase in the proportion of follicles in anagen, although it is not clear whether this is caused by prolongation of anagen or more rapid shedding of telogen hairs, as there is also a reduction in hair density during the second and third trimesters [17]. Following childbirth, large numbers of follicles enter telogen, leading to increased shedding from about 3 months postpartum (postpartum telogen effluvium). Telogen shedding may also be caused by a number of drugs and by febrile and other catabolic illnesses [18].

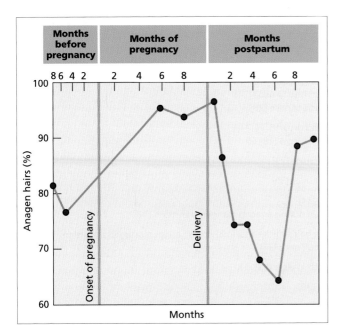

Fig. 63.13 Percentage of anagen hairs in a 25-year-old woman before, during and after pregnancy. (From Lynfield [16].)

Intrinsic control of the hair growth cycle

Although local and systemic factors modulate the hair cycle in some species, in humans and some other mammals hair cycling is asynchronous. Hair follicles in different regions of the skin may also cycle differently. In humans, for example, the duration of anagen on the scalp may last several years, whereas on the eyebrows anagen is very brief. Even in animals showing seasonal hair growth, hair cycles in different follicle types in the same skin region are not necessarily in phase. When scalp hair follicles are transplanted into other regions of the skin they retain the cyclical behaviour of the donor site, indicating that cycle control is determined within the follicle or its immediate tissue environment. Interactions between two key cell populations in the hair follicle, epithelial stem cells in the outer root sheath and mesenchymal cells in the dermal papilla and dermal sheath, are thought to underlie intrinsic control of hair cycling, and a large number of molecules have been implicated in this process. However, the location and the nature of the 'switch' that initiates and terminates anagen growth are unknown.

It has been known for many years that plucking of resting hairs from telogen follicles advances the onset of anagen. This led to the idea that the hair cycle is controlled by a locally active inhibitor which accumulates during anagen causing entry into catagen when present in sufficient concentration (the chalone hypothesis) [19]. The putative inhibitor would disperse during telogen, and plucking resting hairs could accelerate this process. The chalone hypothesis has been disputed because the plucking of resting hairs from follicles that have already entered

anagen does not prolong the anagen in progress, although it does advance the onset of the next anagen cycle [12]. There is one report that murine skin contains a factor that inhibits hair growth *in vivo* and *in vitro* [20]. This inhibitory factor, which has not been characterized, appeared to be derived from the epidermis and was present in telogen skin but not in anagen skin.

Cotsarelis *et al.* [21] have suggested that anagen is initiated by signals from the dermal papilla which stimulate mitosis in stem cells in the bulge region of the outer root sheath (the bulge activation hypothesis). As transient amplifying cells, daughter cells have a limited mitotic potential. When this is exhausted, hair growth ceases and the follicle enters catagen, thus determining the duration of anagen and the onset of catagen.

Several other ideas to explain hair cycle periodicity have been proposed [22] but, for the present, these remain at a theoretical level.

Molecular control of hair cycling

A wide variety of molecules and genes have been implicated in controlling the hair cycle (Table 63.2). These include developmental genes, several families of growth factors and their receptors, nuclear receptors, neurotrophins, cytokines and intracellular signalling pathways. These molecules have generally been studied in isolation, although they undoubtedly operate in a complex milieu of interactions and cross-talk about which little is currently known. The expression level of many of these molecules fluctuates during the hair cycle, and it is difficult to know whether this is of functional significance or is secondary to the metabolic and structural cycle-related changes in the hair follicle. However, there are some examples where there is convincing evidence of a physiological role.

The origin of the signals that initiate anagen has not been identified, and it is not known whether these signals are negative, as proposed in the chalone hypothesis, or positive, or both. Locally synthesized parathyroid hormone-related peptide (PTHrp) is a possible inhibitor of anagen, as injection of a PTHrp antagonist into murine skin accelerates the onset of anagen and delays catagen. Several growth factors appear to be involved in promoting anagen, including insulin-like growth factor 1 (IGF-1), hepatocyte growth factor, keratinocyte growth factor and vascular endothelial growth factor. The *sonic hedgehog* gene and its receptor *patched* also promote anagen in adult follicles as well as being essential for follicular development. Anagen development is a time of extensive remodelling of the follicle and its tissue environment. Follicles grown *in vitro* synthesize a variety of metalloproteinases, suggesting that this process involves degradation of the surrounding extracellular matrix. Hair follicles also express tissue inhibitor of matrix metalloproteinase 3 (TIMP-3) in the outer root sheath during anagen, implying

Table 63.2 Molecular mediators of hair cycle control.

Growth factor	Location	Function
FGF5	ORS	Terminates anagen [23]
FGF7 (KGF)	DP	Induces hair growth in athymic nude mice [24] Hair shaft defect in KGF deficient mice [25]
EGF/TGF-α		Inhibits hair development and growth [26,27] Stimulates ORS proliferation *in vitro* [28]
EGF-R	Hair bulb and ORS	Wavy hair in EGF-R deficient mice [29]
TGF-α		Wavy hair in TGF-α deficient mice [30]
TGF-β1, 2, 3		Inhibits hair growth *in vitro* [31] TGF-β mRNA expressed in skin during anagen/catagen transition [32]
TGF-β receptors		TGF-β receptors expressed in hair follicle—maximal during anagen/catagen transition [33] Delayed catagen in TGF-β1 null mice [34]
IGF-1	DP, hair bulb	Maintains hair follicle growth *in vitro* [35]
IGF-1 receptors	DP, pre-cortex, ORS	Down-regulated in catagen [36]
IGF BP-3, -4, -5	DP and DS [37]	
HGF		Stimulates hair growth when injected into mouse skin [38] Expression in skin varies during hair cycle: high in anagen, low in telogen [39]
VEGF	DP, ORS	Probably regulates perifollicular angiogenesis. Increased follicle size in transgenic mice which overexpress VEGF in ORS. Systemic VEGF antibody retards hair growth in mice [40]
IL-1α, IL-1β		Inhibit hair growth *in vitro* [41]
TNF-α		Inhibits hair growth *in vitro* [41]. TNF-α receptor mRNA expression increased in late anagen [36]
Sonic hedgehog (SHH)		Overexpression in skin accelerates entry into anagen [42] SHH antibody inhibits pelage (but not vibrissae) follicle development in mice. Inhibits anagen in postnatal cycles [43]
Hairless		Required for normal catagen [44]
PTHrp	Follicle epithelium	Inhibits initiation and maintenance of anagen. PTHrp antagonist induces and prolongs anagen [45]
RXR		Required for normal catagen? [46]
Vitamin D receptor	DP, ORS	Variable expression during hair cycle [47] Alopecia in vitamin D receptor knockout mice [48] and in human vitamin D-resistant rickets [49]
Oestrogen receptor	DP	Oestrogen inhibits hair growth in mice [50]
Neurotrophins	Follicle epithelium	NGF, brain-derived neurotrophic factor, neurotrophin-3, neurotrophin-4, and p75 neurotrophin receptor, TrkB receptors promote progression of catagen [51,52]
Mast cells		Increased degranulation at end of anagen and fall in number during telogen. May be involved in control of catagen [53]

DP, dermal papilla; DS, dermal sheath; EGF, epidermal growth factor; FGF, fibroblast growth factor; HGF, hepatocyte growth factor; IGF, insulin-like growth factor; IGF BP, IGF binding proteins; IL-1, interleukin-1; KGF, keratinocyte growth factor; ORS, outer root sheath; PTHrp, parathyroid hormone-related peptide; RXR, retinoid X receptor; TGF, transforming growth factor; TNF, tumour necrosis factor; VEGF, vascular endothelial growth factor.

that remodelling involves a carefully controlled sequence of positive and negative influences.

The end of anagen and transition into catagen is a key period in the hair cycle, as its timing determines the final length of the hair. Catagen may be initiated as a passive process through exhaustion of the mitotic potential of transient amplifying cells in the hair bulb or the loss of action of growth promoting agents. Also, several growth factors and cytokines, including transforming growth factor-β (TGF-β), interleukin-1α (IL-1α) and tumour necrosis factor-α (TNF-α) have an inhibitory effect on hair growth and may be actively involved in triggering catagen. Transgenic mice with a null mutation in the gene for fibroblast growth factor 5 (*FGF5*) show a delay in the onset of catagen and grow abnormally long hair. The phenotype is identical to the naturally occurring *angora* mouse which has a mutation in the *FGF5* gene, suggesting that this growth factor has an active role in terminating anagen

[23]. *FGF5* is expressed in the outer root sheath towards the end of anagen, in keeping with this idea. However, although anagen is delayed in *FGF5*-deficient mice, it is not delayed indefinitely, indicating that other factors must also be involved.

Catagen proceeds in an orderly fashion as cells are deleted from the regressing epithelial column by apoptosis. The expression levels of several proto-oncogenes associated with apoptosis, including c-*myc*, c-*jun* and c-*myb*, change immediately prior to or coincident with the onset of catagen [32]. The apoptosis-inhibitory proto-oncogene *bcl*-2 is expressed in cycling follicular epithelium during anagen, disappears during catagen and is absent in telogen. *Bcl*-2 is expressed in the dermal papilla throughout the hair cycle, suggesting a possible protective role in this site [54].

For the follicle to maintain the ability to cycle, it must maintain its integrity during catagen regression. In the *hairless* mouse, the first coat develops normally but the pelage is then lost. Towards the end of the first anagen phase, cells in the hair bulb undergo extensive premature apoptosis, and formation of the epithelial column is disrupted during catagen. The dermal papilla loses contact with the base of the hair follicle epithelium and the follicle is unable to re-enter anagen. Follicular remnants subsequently undergo cystic degeneration [44]. A similar pattern of hair loss is seen in the human disorder, atrichia with papular lesions, in which there is a mutation in the human homologue of the mouse *hairless* gene [55]. The function of *hairless* in the hair follicle is not fully established but there is some evidence that it acts as a co-repressor of the thyroid receptor (TR). Atrichia with papules also occurs in some families with vitamin D-resistant rickets [48], which is caused by a mutation in the vitamin D receptor (VDR) gene. Like the TR, the VDR is a transcription factor and a member of the nuclear hormone receptor superfamily. Both TR and VDR bind to response elements in target genes as heterodimers with the retinoid X receptor (RXR), another nuclear hormone receptor. Transgenic mice with a null mutation in the RXR gene also show a *hairless* phenotype [46], suggesting there is a common pathway involving nuclear hormone receptors that regulates entry into catagen.

Although generally regarded as a state of quiescence, it is possible that active mechanisms are also needed to maintain a follicle in telogen. For example, expression of the oestrogen receptor in dermal papillae of murine hair follicles is increased during telogen, and oestrogens inhibit entry into anagen [56], although the physiological relevance of this observation is unknown. Release of the club hair from the follicle, a process that has been termed *exogen* [57], does not necessarily coincide with re-entry of the follicle into anagen, and this has led to the idea that shedding is controlled separately from the hair cycle. The club root lies embedded in tricholemmal keratin and its release presumably requires local proteolysis. The cells surrounding the club root are also rich in desmosomes. Transgenic mice with a null mutation in the gene for the desmosomal protein desmoglein 3 show defective anchorage of the club hair [58].

Role of the immune system in hair cycling

Cells in the lower part of the hair follicle, below the arrector insertion, show reduced or absent expression of class I major histocompatibility complex (MHC) molecules [59]. In rat skin the expression of class I MHC in follicular epithelium increases during catagen, and this is associated with a perifollicular accumulation of activated macrophages and loss of the proteoglycan-rich extracellular matrix [60]. These observations led to the suggestion that an immune process mediated by macrophages contributes to control of the hair cycle but other studies have failed to confirm these findings [61]. However, there is experimental support for the idea that the lower part of the hair follicle is an immunologically 'privileged' site not subject to classic immune surveillance [62,63]. This is relevant to disease states, such as alopecia areata, which may be explained by a breakdown of putative immune privilege.

Rate of hair growth

The rate of hair growth varies from species to species, and within one species from region to region, as well as with sex and age. For example, in the rat it can be more than 1 mm/24 h [64] and in the guinea pig up to 0.6 mm/24 h, whereas in humans it is much less. The rate has been determined by direct measurement of marked hairs *in situ* [65], by shaving and clipping at selected intervals [66,67] or by pulse labelling with ^{35}S-cysteine [68–70]. Most investigators now use macrophotographic methods (phototrichography), which may be analysed using computerized systems. Comparable measurements are obtained by all methods. The average rate of growth of human hair has been stated to be approximately 0.03 mm/24 h for the vellus on the male forehead [71], 0.21 mm/24 h on the female thigh and 0.38 mm/24 h on the chin of a young male. On the crown of the scalp it averaged approximately 0.5 mm/24 h, being slightly less on the margins. In another study in which graduated capillary tubes were fitted around the growing hairs, the average growth in males was as follows: vertex 0.44 mm/24 h; temple 0.39 mm/24 h; chest 0.44 mm/24 h; beard 0.27 mm/24 h [72]. The average rate on the vertex of women was 0.45 mm/24 h and there were no variations diurnally or during the menstrual cycle. Although scalp hair grows faster in women than in men [72,73], the rate before puberty is greater in boys than in girls [74]. The average rate over the whole body is greater in men than in women [67]. Irrespective of sex, growth appears to be highest in the two decades between 50 and 69 years of age [67]. From studies on the guinea pig, it seems clear that the growth rate depends upon the time for which the activity of the follicle has been in progress [75].

There is agreement that shaving has no effect on the rate of growth [72,76]. Various endocrine factors have been shown to influence the rate of hair growth in animals; for example, oestrogens reduce it [64,77] and thyroxine increases it [78].

REFERENCES

1 Courtois M, Loussouarn G, Hourseau C. Aging and hair cycles. *Br J Dermatol* 1995; **132**: 86–93.
2 Durward A, Rudall KM. Studies on hair growth in the rat. *J Anat* 1949; **83**: 325–35.
3 Ebling FJ, Johnson E. Hair growth and its relation to vascular supply in rotated skin grafts and transposed flaps in the albino rat. *J Embryol Exp Morphol* 1959; **7**: 417–30.
4 Ebling FJ, Johnson E. Systemic influence on activity of hair follicles in skin homografts. *J Embryol Exp Morphol* 1961; **9**: 285–93.
5 Bissonnette TH. Relation of hair cycles in ferrets to changes in the anterior hypophysis and to light cycles. *Anat Rec* 1935; **63**: 159–68.
6 Harvey NE, MacFarlane VW. The effects of day length on the coat-shedding cycles, body weight, and reproduction of the ferret. *Aust J Biol Sci* 1958; **11**: 187–99.
7 Allain D, Rougeot J. Induction of autumn moult in mink (*Mustela vison* Peale and Beauvois) with melatonin. *Reprod Nutr Dev* 1980; **20**: 197–201.
8 Rose J, Stormshak F, Oldfield J et al. Induction of winter fur growth in mink (*Mustela vison*) with melatonin. *J Anim Sci* 1984; **58**: 57–61.
9 Rose J, Oldfield J, Stormshak F. Apparent role of melatonin and prolactin in initiating winter fur growth in mink. *Gen Comp Endocrinol* 1987; **65**: 212–5.
10 Badura LL, Goldman BD. Prolactin-dependent seasonal changes in pelage: role of the pineal gland and dopamine. *J Exp Zool* 1992; **261**: 27–33.
11 Choy VJ, Nixon AJ, Pearson AJ. Localization of receptors for prolactin in ovine skin. *J Endocrinol* 1995; **144**: 143–51.
12 Ebling FJ. The hormonal control of hair growth. In: Orfanos CE, Happle R, eds. *Hair and Hair Diseases*. Berlin: Springer-Verlag, 1990: 267–99.
13 Maurel D, Coutant C, Boissin J. Thyroid and gonadal regulation of hair growth during the seasonal molt in the male European badger, *Meles meles* L. *Gen Comp Endocrinol* 1987; **65**: 317–27.
14 Oh H-S, Smart RC. An estrogen receptor pathway regulates the telogen–anagen hair follicle transition and influences epidermal cell proliferation. *Proc Natl Acad Sci USA* 1996; **93**: 12525–30.
15 Randall VA, Ebling FJ. Seasonal changes in human hair growth. *Br J Dermatol* 1991; **124**: 146–51.
16 Lynfield YL. Effect of pregnancy on the human hair cycle. *J Invest Dermatol* 1960; **35**: 323–7.
17 Pecoraro V, Barman JM, Astore I. The normal trichogram of pregnant women. *Adv Biol Skin* 1967; **9**: 203–10.
18 Kligman AM. Pathologic dynamics of human hair loss. *Arch Dermatol* 1961; **83**: 175–98.
19 Chase HB. Growth of hair. *Physiol Rev* 1954; **34**: 113–26.
20 Paus R, Stenn KS, Link RE. Telogen skin contains an inhibitor of hair growth. *Br J Dermatol* 1990; **122**: 777–84.
21 Cotsarelis G, Sun TT, Lavker RM. Label-retaining cells reside in the bulge area of pilosebaceous unit: implications for follicular stem cells, hair cycle, and skin carcinogenesis. *Cell* 1990; **61**: 1329–37.
22 Paus R, Muller-Rover S, McKay I. Control of the hair follicle growth cycle. In: Camacho FM, Randall VA, Price VH, eds. *Hair and its Disorders*. London: Martin Dunitz, 2000: 83–94.
23 Hebert JM, Rosenquist T, Gotz J et al. FGF5 as a regulator of the hair growth cycle: evidence from targeted and spontaneous mutations. *Cell* 1994; **78**: 1017–25.
24 Danilenko DM, Ring BD, Yanagihara D et al. Keratinocyte growth factor is an important endogenous mediator of hair follicle growth, development, and differentiation: normalization of the nu/nu follicular differentiation

defect and amelioration of chemotherapy-induced alopecia. *Am J Pathol* 1995; **147**: 145–54.
25 Guo L, Degenstein L, Fuchs E. Keratinocyte growth factor is required for hair development but not for wound healing. *Genes Dev* 1996; **10**: 165–75.
26 Moore GP, Panaretto BA, Robertson D. Epidermal growth factor delays the development of the epidermis and hair follicles of mice during growth of the first coat. *Anat Rec* 1983; **205**: 47–55.
27 Hollis DE, Chapman RE, Panaretto BA et al. Morphological changes in the skin and wool fibres of Merino sheep infused with mouse epidermal growth factor. *Aust J Biol Sci* 1983; **36**: 419–34.
28 Philpott MP, Kealey T. Effects of EGF on the morphology and patterns of DNA synthesis in isolated human hair follicles. *J Invest Dermatol* 1994; **102**: 186–91.
29 Luetteke NC, Phillips HK, Qiu TH et al. The mouse waved-2 phenotype results from a point mutation in the EGF receptor tyrosine kinase. *Genes Dev* 1994; **8**: 399–413.
30 Luetteke NC, Qiu TH, Peiffer RL et al. TGF-α deficiency results in hair follicle and eye abnormalities in targeted and waved-1 mice. *Cell* 1993; **73**: 263–78.
31 Philpott MP, Green MR, Kealey T. Human hair growth *in vitro*. *J Cell Sci* 1990; **97**: 463–71.
32 Seiberg M, Marthinuss J, Stenn KS. Changes in expression of apoptosis-associated genes in skin mark early catagen. *J Invest Dermatol* 1995; **104**: 78–82.
33 Paus R, Foitzik K, Welker P et al. Transforming growth factor-β receptor type I and type II expression during murine hair follicle development and cycling. *J Invest Dermatol* 1997; **109**: 518–26.
34 Foitzik K, Lindner G, Mueller-Roever S et al. Control of murine hair follicle regression (catagen) by TGF-β1 *in vivo*. *FASEB J* 2000; **14**: 752–60.
35 Philpott MP, Sanders DA, Kealey T. Effects of insulin and insulin-like growth factors on cultured human hair follicles: IGF-I at physiologic concentrations is an important regulator of hair follicle growth *in vitro*. *J Invest Dermatol* 1994; **102**: 857–61.
36 Little JC, Redwood KL, Granger SP et al. *In vivo* cytokine and receptor gene expression during the rat hair growth cycle: analysis by semi-quantitative RT-PCR. *Exp Dermatol* 1996; **5**: 202–12.
37 Batch JA, Mercuri FA, Werther GA. Identification and localization of insulin-like growth factor-binding protein (IGFBP) messenger RNAs in human hair follicle dermal papilla. *J Invest Dermatol* 1996; **106**: 471–5.
38 Jindo T, Tsuboi R, Takamori K et al. Local injection of hepatocyte growth factor/scatter factor (HGF/SF) alters cyclic growth of murine hair follicles. *J Invest Dermatol* 1998; **110**: 338–42.
39 Yamazaki M, Tsuboi R, Lee YR et al. Hair cycle-dependent expression of hepatocyte growth factor (HGF) activator, other proteinases, and proteinase inhibitors correlates with the expression of HGF in rat hair follicles. *J Investig Dermatol Symp Proc* 1999; **4**: 312–5.
40 Yano K, Brown LF, Detmar M. Control of hair growth and follicle size by VEGF-mediated angiogenesis. *J Clin Invest* 2001; **107**: 409–17.
41 Philpott MP, Sanders DA, Bowen J et al. Effects of interleukins, colony-stimulating factor and tumour necrosis factor on human hair follicle growth *in vitro*: a possible role for interleukin-1 and tumour necrosis factor-α in alopecia areata. *Br J Dermatol* 1996; **135**: 942–8.
42 Sato N, Leopold PL, Crystal RG. Induction of the hair growth phase in postnatal mice by localized transient expression of Sonic hedgehog. *J Clin Invest* 1999; **104**: 855–64.
43 Wang LC, Liu ZY, Gambardella L et al. Conditional disruption of hedgehog signaling pathway defines its critical role in hair development and regeneration. *J Invest Dermatol* 2000; **114**: 901–8.
44 Panteleyev AA, Botchkareva NV, Sundberg JP et al. The role of the hairless (HR) gene in the regulation of hair follicle catagen transformation. *Am J Pathol* 1999; **155**: 159–71.
45 Schilli MB, Ray S, Paus R et al. Control of hair growth with parathyroid hormone (7–34). *J Invest Dermatol* 1997; **108**: 928–32.
46 Li M, Chiba H, Warot X et al. RXR-α ablation in skin keratinocytes results in alopecia and epidermal alterations. *Development* 2001; **128**: 675–88.
47 Reichrath J, Schilli M, Kerber A et al. Hair follicle expression of 1,25-dihydroxyvitamin D3 receptors during the murine hair cycle. *Br J Dermatol* 1994; **131**: 477–82.
48 Miller J, Djabali K, Chen T et al. Atrichia caused by mutations in the vitamin D receptor gene is a phenocopy of generalized atrichia caused by mutations in the hairless gene. *J Invest Dermatol* 2001; **117**: 612–7.
49 Li YC, Pirro AE, Amling M et al. Targeted ablation of the vitamin D receptor: an animal model of vitamin D-dependent rickets type II with alopecia. *Proc Natl Acad Sci USA* 1997; **94**: 9831–5.

50 Oh HS, Smart RC. An estrogen receptor pathway regulates the telogen-anagen hair follicle transition and influences epidermal cell proliferation. *Proc Natl Acad Sci USA* 1996; **93**: 12525–30.
51 Botchkarev VA, Botchkareva NV, Welker P et al. A new role for neurotrophins: involvement of brain-derived neurotrophic factor and neurotrophin-4 in hair cycle control. *FASEB J* 1999; **13**: 395–410.
52 Botchkarev VA, Botchkareva NV, Albers KM et al. A role for p75 neurotrophin receptor in the control of apoptosis-driven hair follicle regression. *FASEB J* 2000; **14**: 1931–42.
53 Maurer M, Fischer E, Handjiski B et al. Activated skin mast cells are involved in murine hair follicle regression (catagen). *Lab Invest* 1997; **77**: 319–32.
54 Stenn KS, Lawrence L, Veis D et al. Expression of the *bcl*-2 proto-oncogene in the cycling adult mouse hair follicle. *J Invest Dermatol* 1994; **103**: 107–11.
55 Ahmad W, Panteleyev AA, Christiano AM. The molecular basis of congenital atrichia in humans and mice: mutations in the hairless gene. *J Invest Dermatol Symp Proc* 1999; **4**: 240–3.
56 Smart RC, Oh HS, Chanda S et al. Effects of 17β-estradiol and ICI 182 780 on hair growth in various strains of mice. *J Invest Dermatol Symp Proc* 1999; **4**: 285–9.
57 Stenn KS, Paus R. Controls of hair follicle cycling. *Physiol Rev* 2001; **81**: 449–94.
58 Koch PJ, Mahoney MG, Cotsarelis G et al. Desmoglein 3 anchors telogen hair in the follicle. *J Cell Sci* 1998; **111**: 2529–37.
59 Harrist TJ, Ruiter DJ, Mihm MC et al. Distribution of major histocompatibility antigens in normal skin. *Br J Dermatol* 1983; **109**: 623–33.
60 Westgate GE, Craggs RI, Gibson WT. Immune privilege in hair growth. *J Invest Dermatol* 1991; **97**: 417–20.
61 Paus R, van der Veen C, Eichmuller S et al. Generation and cyclic remodeling of the hair follicle immune system in mice. *J Invest Dermatol* 1998; **111**: 7–18.
62 Barker CF, Billingham RE. Analysis of local anatomic factors that influence the survival times of pure epidermal and full-thickness skin homografts in guinea pigs. *Ann Surg* 1972; **176**: 597–604.
63 Reynolds AJ, Lawrence C, Cserhalmi-Friedman PB et al. Trans-gender induction of hair follicles. *Nature* 1999; **402**: 33–4.
64 Hale PA, Ebling FJ. The effect of epilation and hormones on the activity of rat hair follicles. *J Exp Zool* 1975; **191**: 49–61.
65 Trotter M. The life cycles of hair in selected regions of the body. *Am J Phys Anthropol* 1924; **7**: 427–37.
66 Ebling FJ, Thomas AK, Cooke ID et al. Effect of cyproterone acetate on hair growth, sebaceous secretion and endocrine parameters in a hirsute subject. *Br J Dermatol* 1977; **97**: 371–81.
67 Pelfini C, Cerimele D, Pisanu G. Aging of the skin and hair growth in man. In: Montagna W, Dobson RL, eds. *Advances in Biology of the Skin*. Oxford: Pergamon, 1969: 153–60.
68 Hale PA, Ebling FJ. The effects of epilation and hormones on the activity of rat hair follicles. *J Exp Zool* 1975; **191**: 49–62.
69 Comaish S. Autoradiographic studies of hair growth in various dermatoses: investigation of a possible circadian rhythm in human hair growth. *Br J Dermatol* 1969; **81**: 283–8.
70 Munro DD. Hair growth measurement using intradermal sulfur 35 cystine. *Arch Dermatol* 1966; **93**: 119–22.
71 Blume U, Ferracin J, Verschoore M et al. Physiology of the vellus hair follicle: hair growth and sebum excretion. *Br J Dermatol* 1991; **124**: 21–8.
72 Saitoh M, Uzuka M, Sakamoto M et al. Rate of hair growth. In: Montagna W, Dobson RL, eds. *Advances in Biology of Skin*. Vol. 9, *Hair Growth*. Oxford: Pergamon, 1969: 183–201.
73 Myers RJ, Hamilton JB. Regeneration and rate of growth of hairs in man. *Ann NY Acad Sci* 1951; **53**: 562–8.
74 Pecoraro V, Astore I, Barman JM et al. The normal trichogram in the child before the age of puberty. *J Invest Dermatol* 1961; **42**: 427–30.
75 Jackson D, Ebling FJ. The guinea-pig hair follicle as an object for experimental observation. *J Soc Cosmet Chem* 1971; **22**: 701–9.
76 Lynfield YL, MacWilliam P. Shaving and hair growth. *J Invest Dermatol* 1970; **55**: 170–2.
77 Johnson E. Quantitative studies of hair growth in the albino rat. II. The effect of sex hormones. *J Endocrinol* 1958; **16**: 351–9.
78 Ebling FJ, Johnson E. The action of hormones on spontaneous hair growth cycles in the rat. *J Endocrinol* 1964; **29**: 193–201.

Hair pigment and melanogenesis in the follicle

See p. 63.108.

Androgens and hair growth

Androgens influence hair growth in several ways. First, they participate in the endocrine control of moulting in animals that show seasonal hair growth [1]. Secondly, in some mammals, androgens stimulate the growth of hair follicles in certain regions of the skin following sexual maturity. Thirdly, in humans and some other primates, androgens are necessary for the development of balding on the scalp.

Androgen-stimulated hair growth

The growth of obvious facial, trunk and extremity hair in the male, and of pubic and axillary hair in both sexes, is clearly dependent on androgens. The development of such hair at puberty is, in broad terms and at least initially, in parallel with the rise in levels of androgen from testicular, adrenocortical and ovarian sources, which occurs in both sexes and is somewhat steeper in males. That testosterone from the interstitial cells of the testis is responsible for growth of beard and body hair in male adolescence and that testicular activity is itself initiated by gonadotrophic hormones of the pituitary is unquestioned. However, the findings that growth-hormone-deficient boys and girls are less than normally responsive to androgens, and that growth hormone is necessary as a synergistic factor to allow testosterone to be fully effective with respect to hair growth [2], as well as protein anabolism and growth promotion, suggest that hypophysial hormones also have a more direct role. Direct evidence of the role of testicular androgen is that castration reduces growth of the human beard [3], whereas testosterone stimulates it in eunuchs and elderly men. The role of androgen is further demonstrated in the treatment of hirsute women with the antiandrogen cyproterone acetate [4], which reduces the definitive length, rate of growth, diameter and extent of medullation of the thigh hairs [5].

At puberty, terminal hair gradually replaces vellus, starting in the pubic regions. In both sexes the first pubic hair is sparse, long, downy, slightly pigmented and almost straight. It later becomes darker, coarser, more curled and extends in area to form an inverse triangle. A British study showed that boys had the first recognizable pubic hair at an average age of 13.4 years, and the full adult 'male' pattern at 15.2 years, approximately 3.5 years after the start of development of the genitalia [6]. The corresponding mean ages for girls were considerably earlier, namely 11.7 years and 13.5 years [7]. In approximately 80% of men and 10% of women the pubic hair continues spreading until the mid-twenties or later; there is no absolute distinction between male and female patterns, only one of degree.

Axillary hair first appears approximately 2 years after the start of pubic hair growth. The amount, as measured by the weight of the fully grown mass, continues to increase until the late twenties in males as well as in females, in whom, however, it is less at any age [3]. The mean amounts grown per day increase from late puberty until the mid-twenties and thereafter decrease steadily.

Facial hair in boys first appears at about the same time as the axillary hair, starting at the corners of the upper lip, and spreading medially to complete the moustache and then the cheeks and beard.

Terminal hair development is continued in regular sequence on the legs, thighs, forearms, abdomen, buttocks, back, arms and shoulders [8]. The extent of terminal hair tends to increase throughout the years of sexual maturity, but most patterns occur over a wide age range. The adult pattern is not achieved until the fourth decade, when the androgen levels are already somewhat lower than in early adult life. Moreover, aural hairs do not appear until late middle age, and a study of coarse sternal hair in men showed that the hairs continue to increase in length and number from puberty to the fifth or sixth decade.

There is considerable racial variability in androgen-dependent hair growth. The growth of facial and body hair is greater in European men than in Chinese men [3] and there is also variation within these broad racial categories—southern European men tend to be hairier than men from northern Europe [9].

Androgenetic alopecia

It has been known since ancient times that eunuchs do not go bald. Hippocrates noted that 'eunuchs are not subject to gout nor do they become bald' (Aphorisms VI, 28). The role of testosterone in male balding was first recognized by James Hamilton, a US anatomist [10]. He observed that men castrated before puberty retain a prepubertal hairline and do not go bald. Of 12 such men who were treated with testosterone, four developed typical male hair loss. Castration later in life halted the progression of hair loss but did not result in regrowth of hair.

The prevalence and severity of male balding increase with age. All races are affected but the prevalence is higher in white males, reaching at least 80% in men aged over 70 years, than in African American [11] and in Japanese men [12]. Chinese and Korean men are also less likely to show frontal recession [13,14]. Genetic factors undoubtedly predispose to the development of male balding, but little is known of the genes involved and the mode of inheritance is also uncertain.

The loss of hair in male balding is the result of a gradual reduction in the duration of anagen and a prolongation of the latent period of the hair cycle [15], and miniaturization of terminal hair follicles [16].

Androgen synthesis and metabolism

The initial stages in the synthesis of steroid hormones from cholesterol occur exclusively in the gonads and the adrenal glands. Circulating androgens are also derived from the peripheral conversion of weak precursor hormones into potent androgens, a process that takes place in many tissues including the skin and hair follicles. The majority of androgens in the circulation are bound to plasma proteins, principally sex hormone-binding globulin (SHBG), with approximately 20% bound to albumin. The remaining 1–2% circulates in a free unbound form and this comprises the biologically active pool. Androgen bound to albumin dissociates readily and can replenish the free pool. SHBG binds androgen with high affinity and its plasma concentration therefore has an important effect on the free and albumin-bound pools. High levels of SHBG reduce the biologically active androgen level and low levels of SHBG have the reverse effect. Free androgen is thought to enter cells by passive diffusion where it binds to a specific intracellular androgen receptor.

Testosterone is the major circulating androgen, but in most body sites the effect of testosterone on hair growth is mediated by its more potent metabolite 5α-dihydrotestosterone (DHT). The conversion of testosterone to DHT is catalysed by the enzyme 5α-reductase. There are two isoforms of 5α-reductase, which are encoded by different genes [17]. Although both enzymes catalyse the conversion of testosterone to DHT they differ in their pH optima, substrate affinities and tissue distributions. Type 1 5α-reductase is widely distributed in the skin, but expression of the type 2 isoform is restricted to androgen target tissues such as the prostate and the epididymis. Much of our knowledge of the biological role of DHT in hair growth comes from studies of men with 5α-reductase deficiency (type II pseudohermaphroditism, pseudovaginal perineoscrotal hypospadias) [18,19], which is caused by mutations in the 5α-reductase 2 gene [20]. In this autosomal recessive disorder, genetic males (46XY) are born with normally differentiated but usually undescended testes. The external genitalia are ambiguous with a small hypospadic phallus, a bifid scrotum and a blind vagina. Partial virilization of the genitalia occurs at puberty, the voice deepens and the musculature assumes a typical male distribution. Circulating testosterone levels are within or above the normal male range but DHT levels remain low, with testosterone : DHT ratios 3.5–5 times higher than normal. Subjects show a female pattern of androgen-dependent hair growth, with terminal hair largely restricted to the axillae and the lower pubic triangle, suggesting that hair growth in these sites responds to less potent androgens. In the large group of subjects studied in the Dominican Republic, beard growth was absent or sparse. More facial hair has been observed in affected men from other parts of the world, perhaps reflecting underlying racial differences in normal androgen-dependent hair growth, although this was reduced compared with normal males in the same communities [21,22]. None of the cases studied has shown temporal recession of the hairline or balding. A role for DHT in balding is supported by studies in macaques in which treatment with 5α-reductase inhibitors prevented the development of balding [23] or increased scalp hair growth in balding animals [24], and a large clinical trial of the 5α-reductase type 2 inhibitor finasteride in balding men. This latter study showed that the progression of balding was prevented in almost all men taking finasteride orally, and about two-thirds showed an increase in hair growth [25].

Hair follicles possess 5α-reductase activity, suggesting that DHT acts as a paracrine or intracrine hormone (it is synthesized within or close to the target cell). It is possible that circulating DHT also contributes to androgen effects on hair growth. Other steroid metabolizing enzymes, including 3β- and 17β-hydroxysteroid dehydrogenase which interconvert weak and potent androgens, and aromatase which converts androgens to oestrogens, are also expressed in the hair follicle [26,27], but their role in hair growth is not currently known.

The androgen receptor

The tissue effects of androgens are mediated through binding to the intracellular androgen receptor. The androgen receptor is a nuclear hormone receptor [28], and like other members of the nuclear hormone receptor superfamily it acts as a gene transcription factor following ligand binding. Mutations in the androgen receptor gene are responsible for the androgen insensitivity syndrome [29]. Individuals with the complete form of the syndrome, in which there is failure of functional androgen receptor expression, have intra-abdominal testes but female external genitalia, breast development and psychosocial development. After puberty, circulating testosterone is in the normal or elevated male range but pubic and axillary hair fail to develop, there is no beard growth and no balding.

Mechanism of androgen action on the hair follicle

Hamilton [10] reported that balding did not progress following castration in older men but neither did it promote regrowth of hair. Similarly, although beard growth was prevented by castration before puberty and stimulated by subsequent treatment with testosterone, there was only partial regression of the beard in postpubertal men castrated before the age of 20 years and no effect in older men [3]. Hamilton's observations were relatively crude by modern standards and it is now clear from clinical trials of 5α-reductase inhibitors that some reversal of male balding is possible. However, the response is far from complete, indicating that androgens induce changes in gene expression in hair follicles that are only partially reversible in the absence of androgen and probably not at all once these changes are fully expressed.

The specificity of the response of hair follicles to androgens is determined within the skin. Hair follicles in occipital skin, a site that shows little or no response to androgens, retain their site-specific behaviour when transplanted into balding areas on the frontal scalp [30]. Conversely, hair follicles from balding scalp continue to regress when transplanted into skin of the forearm [31]. The success of micrografting techniques, in which individual follicles are transplanted, shows that androgen responsiveness is determined at the level of the follicle or its immediate tissue environment. Three lines of evidence suggest that the dermal papilla is the primary target of androgen action in the hair follicle.

1 Androgen receptor expression in the lower part of the follicle is restricted to dermal papilla cells [32,33]

2 The size of the hair follicle is probably determined by the volume of the dermal papilla [34–36]

3 Dermal papillae express 5α-reductase type 2 whereas hair follicle epithelium expresses only 5α-reductase type 1 [37].

However, it is not yet known how androgen action on dermal papilla cells causes changes in hair follicle size and hair cycling. Hence androgens may act on hair growth by altering the number of cells in the dermal papilla and its extracellular matrix [36]. Cells cultured from dermal papillae of human beard hair follicles also release growth factors in response to androgens that stimulate proliferation of keratinocytes [33,38], and the pattern of androgen metabolism by cultured and intact dermal papilla cells is consistent with that expected from their site of origin [39,40]. However, the molecular mechanisms whereby androgens inhibit hair growth on the scalp but stimulate growth in most other body sites are not yet understood.

REFERENCES

1 Ebling FJG. The hormonal control of hair growth. In: Orfanos CE, Happle R, eds. *Hair and Hair Diseases*. Berlin: Springer-Verlag, 1990: 267–99.

2 Blok GJ, de Boer H, Gooren LJ *et al.* Growth hormone substitution in adult growth hormone-deficient men augments androgen effects on the skin. *Clin Endocrinol (Oxf)* 1997; **47**: 29–36.

3 Hamilton JB. Age, sex and genetic factors in the regulation of hair growth in men: a comparison of Caucasian and Japanese populations. In: Montagna W, Ellis RA, eds. *The Biology of Hair Growth*. New York: Academic Press, 1958: 399.

4 Hammerstein J, Meckies J, Leo-Rossberg I *et al.* Use of cyproterone acetate (CPA) in the treatment of acne, hirsutism and virilism. *J Steroid Biochem* 1975; **6**: 827–36.

5 Ebling FJ, Thomas AK, Cooke ID *et al.* Effect of cyproterone acetate on hair growth, sebaceous secretion and endocrine parameters in a hirsute subject. *Br J Dermatol* 1977; **97**: 371–81.

6 Marshall WA, Tanner JM. Variations in pattern of pubertal changes in boys. *Arch Dis Child* 1970; **45**: 13–23.

7 Marshall WA, Tanner JM. Variations in pattern of pubertal changes in girls. *Arch Dis Child* 1969; **44**: 291–303.

8 Reynolds EL. The appearance of adult patterns of body hair in man. *Ann NY Acad Sci* 1951; **53**: 576–84.

9 Danforth CH, Trotter M. The distribution of body hair in white subjects. *Am J Phys Anthropol* 1922; **5**: 259–65.

10 Hamilton JB. Male hormone is prerequisite and an incitant in common baldness. *Am J Anat* 1942; **71**: 451–80.

11 Setty LR. Hair patterns on the scalp of white and negro males. *Am J Phy Anthropol* 1970; **33**: 49–55.

12 Takashima I, Iju M, Sudo M. Alopecia androgenetica: its incidence in Japanese and associated conditions. In: Orfanos CE, Montagna W, Stuttgen G, eds. *Hair Research Status and Future Aspects.* New York: Springer-Verlag, 1981: 287–93.

13 Hamilton JB. Patterned loss of hair in man: types and incidence. *Ann NY Acad Sci* 1951; **53**: 708–28.

14 Paik JH, Yoon JB, Sim WY *et al.* The prevalence and types of androgenetic alopecia in Korean men and women. *Br J Dermatol* 2001; **145**: 95–9.

15 Courtois M, Loussouarn G, Hourseau C. Ageing and hair cycles. *Br J Dermatol* 1995; **132**: 86–93.

16 Whiting DA. Diagnostic and predictive value of horizontal sections of scalp biopsy specimens in male pattern androgenetic alopecia. *J Am Acad Dermatol* 1993; **28**: 755–63.

17 Jenkins EP, Andersson S, Imperato-McGinley J *et al.* Genetic and pharmacological evidence for more than one human steroid 5α-reductase. *J Clin Invest* 1992; **89**: 293–300.

18 Imperato-McGinley J, Guerrero L, Gautier T *et al.* Steroid 5α-reductase deficiency in man: an inherited form of male pseudohermaphroditism. *Science* 1974; **186**: 1213–5.

19 Peterson RE, Imperato-McGinley J, Gautier T *et al.* Male pseudohermaphroditism due to steroid 5α-reductase deficiency. *Am J Med* 1977; **62**: 170–91.

20 Cai LQ, Zhu YS, Katz MD *et al.* 5α-Reductase-2 gene mutations in the Dominican Republic. *J Clin Endocrinol Metab* 1996; **81**: 1730–5.

21 Akgun S, Ertel NH, Imperato-McGinley J *et al.* Familial male pseudohermaphroditism due to 5α-reductase deficiency in a Turkish village. *Am J Med* 1986; **81**: 267–74.

22 Imperato-McGinley J, Miller M, Wilson JD *et al.* A cluster of male pseudohermaphrodites with 5α-reductase deficiency in Papua New Guinea. *Clin Endocrinol (Oxf)* 1991; **34**: 293–8.

23 Rittmaster RS, Uno H, Povar ML *et al.* The effects of N,N-diethyl-4-methyl-3-oxo-4-aza-5α-androstane-17β carboxamide, a 5α-reductase inhibitor and anti-androgen, on the development of baldness in the stumptail macaque. *J Clin Endocrinol Metab* 1987; **65**: 188–93.

24 Diani AR, Mulholland MJ, Shull KL *et al.* Hair growth effects of oral administration of finasteride, a steroid 5α-reductase inhibitor, alone and in combination with topical minoxidil in the balding stumptail macaque. *J Clin Endocrinol Metab* 1992; **74**: 345–50.

25 Kaufman KD, Olsen EA, Whiting D *et al.* Finasteride in the treatment of men with androgenetic alopecia. *J Am Acad Dermatol* 1998; **39**: 578–89.

26 Schweikert HU, Wilson JD. Regulation of hair growth by steroid hormones. I. Testosterone metabolism in isolated hairs. *J Clin Endocrinol Metab* 1974; **38**: 811–9.

27 Schweikert HU, Milewich L, Wilson JD. Aromatization of androstenedione by isolated human hairs. *J Clin Endocrinol Metab* 1975; **40**: 413–7.

28 Williams GR, Franklyn JA. Physiology of the steroid-thyroid hormone nuclear receptor superfamily. *Bailliere's Clin Endocrin Metab* 1994; **8**: 241–66.

29 Patterson MN, McPhaul MJ, Hughes IA. Androgen insensitivity syndrome. *Bailliere's Clin Endocrin Metab* 1994; **8**: 379–404.

30 Orentreich N. Autografts in alopecias and other selected dermatological conditions. *Ann NY Acad Sci* 1959; **83**: 463–79.

31 Nordström REA. Synchronous balding of scalp and hair-bearing grafts of scalp transplanted to the skin of the arm in male pattern baldness. *Acta Derm Venereol* 1979; **59**: 266–8.

32 Choudhry R, Hodgins MB, Van der Kwast TH *et al.* Localization of androgen receptors in human skin by immunohistochemistry: implications for the hormonal regulation of hair growth, sebaceous glands and sweat glands. *J Endocrinol* 1992; **133**: 467–75.

33 Itami S, Kurata S, Sonoda T *et al.* Interaction between dermal papilla cells and follicular epithelial cells *in vitro*: effect of androgen. *Br J Dermatol* 1995; **132**: 527–32.

34 Van Scott EJ, Ekel TM. Geometric relationships between the matrix of the hair bulb and its dermal papilla in normal and alopecic scalp. *J Invest Dermatol* 1958; **31**: 281–7.

35 Ibrahim L, Wright EA. A quantitative study of hair growth using mouse and rat vibrissal follicles. I. Dermal papilla volume determines hair volume. *J Embryol Exp Morphol* 1982; **72**: 209–24.

36 Elliott K, Stephenson TJ, Messenger AG. Differences in hair follicle dermal papilla volume are due to extracellular matrix volume and cell number: implications for the control of hair follicle size and androgen responses. *J Invest Dermatol* 1999; **113**: 873–7.

37 Asada Y, Sonoda T, Ojiro M *et al.* 5α-Reductase type 2 is constitutively expressed in the dermal papilla and connective tissue sheath of the hair follicle *in vivo* but not during culture *in vitro*. *J Clin Endocrinol Metab* 2001; **86**: 2875–80.

38 Itami S, Kurata S, Takayasu S. Androgen induction of follicular epithelial cell growth is mediated via insulin-like growth factor 1 from dermal papilla cells. *Biochem Biophys Res Commun* 1995; **212**: 988–94.

39 Itami S, Kurata S, Sonoda T *et al.* Characterization of 5α-reductase in cultured human dermal papilla cells from beard and occipital scalp hair. *J Invest Dermatol* 1991; **96**: 57–60.

40 Thornton MJ, Laing I, Hamada K *et al.* Differences in testosterone metabolism by beard and scalp hair follicle dermal papilla cells. *Clin Endocrinol (Oxf)* 1993; **39**: 633–9.

Alopecia

Common baldness and androgenetic alopecia

SYN. MALE PATTERN HAIR LOSS; FEMALE PATTERN HAIR LOSS; PATTERNED OR PREMATURE BALDNESS
[R.D. Sinclair, pp. 63.18–63.36]

Nomenclature. Common baldness is the result of a progressive patterned hair loss that only occurs in genetically predisposed individuals. The lack of balding in eunuchs, pseudohermaphrodites and individuals with androgen insensitivity syndrome confirms that androgens are a prerequisite for common baldness. As the pattern of hair loss differs between men and women, the terms male pattern hair loss and female pattern hair loss are also commonly used [1]. Whether someone is considered bald, and in particular prematurely bald, is in part a subjective assessment. The process by which common baldness occurs is androgen-mediated conversion of susceptible terminal hairs into vellus hairs, and has been termed androgenetic alopecia (AGA).

Aetiology. Most vertebrates show regional specificity in the induction and arrangement of skin appendages. The determinants of this are only beginning to be understood [2–4].

Four separate but interrelated factors determine whether an individual will become bald: susceptibility to AGA, age of onset, rate of progression and pattern of hair loss.

Hamilton [5] defined the progressive pattern of male baldness and produced the first useful grading scale. This classification was modified by Norwood [6], who added grades IIIa, III vertex, IVa and Va (Fig. 63.14). Although the grades are imprecise measures of the continuum of hair patterns that are seen in adult males, they are useful as diagnostic aides and in the classification of extent of hair loss in clinical investigations.

It is important to keep in mind that there is no gold standard for the diagnosis of early baldness. While it is safe to assume agreement that men with Hamilton–Norwood stage I are not balding and men with Hamilton–Norwood stage III are going bald, the fate of men who develop stage II pattern of scalp hair has not been followed prospectively.

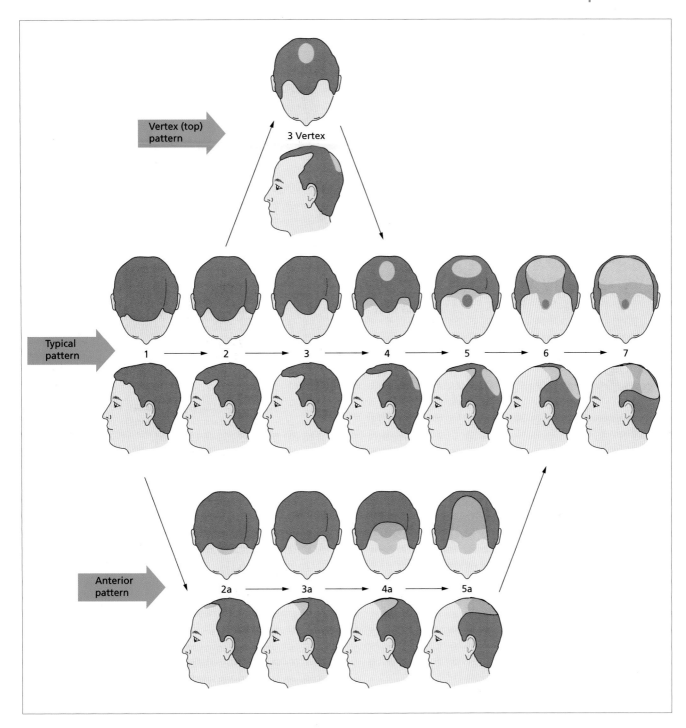

Fig. 63.14 Hamilton–Norwood scale for grading male patterned hair loss [2].

The lifetime risk of male pattern baldness (MPB) can be defined by studying hair patterns in men aged 80 years and above. In Norwood's cohort [6], 16% had a type I hair pattern and by definition are not bald. Fourteen per cent had a type 2 hair pattern, and although demonstrating at least some degree of AGA, would not be considered bald.

The remaining 70% had a type III (16%), IV (12%), V (12%), VI (13%) or VII (17%) pattern of hair loss and would be considered to demonstrate MPB.

At least 94% of adult men develop some degree of frontoparietal recession of the hairline after puberty [5]. As the histology of this hair loss shows increased vellus hairs, and as Hamilton observed that three males castrated at the age of 15 and 16 years failed to develop even minimal recession along the frontal hairline, it is likely that this hair loss occurs by androgen-mediated miniaturization of terminal follicles, and by definition is AGA [7]. However, 16% of 80-year-old men still have stage I hair density. Therefore, limited frontoparietal AGA does not always progress, and may be a benign manifestation of sexual maturity rather than a precursor of MPB.

The age of onset of MPB can also be determined by extrapolation of Norwood's data [6]. Sixty per cent of men aged 18–29 years, 36% aged 30–39 years, 33% aged 40–49 years, 28% aged 50–59 years, 19% aged 60–69 years, 17% aged 70–79 years and 16% of men aged 80 years or above were assessed as having no evidence of AGA. If early MPB is defined as stage II hair pattern, then 40% begin to develop MPB between the ages of 18 and 29, a further 24% first develop MPB in their thirties, 3% in their forties, 5% in their fifties, 9% in their sixties, 2% in their seventies and 1% at or beyond the age of 80 years. If this extrapolation of Norwood's data is valid, then a man with stage I hair at the age of 40 years has almost a 50% likelihood of still having stage I hair at the age of 80 years.

There is wide individual variation in the rate of progression of hair loss in MPB. A small number of men achieve type V or VI hair loss in their twenties, indicating a very rapid rate of progression. In contrast, approximately 25% of men with MPB show no visible hair loss on standardized clinical photographs over a 5-year period [8]. Norwood's data [6] also support the common observation that early-onset MPB progresses more rapidly. Men who develop MPB in their twenties tend to advance 1–2 stages per decade, whereas men with late-onset MPB may take two decades to progress a single stage. As stated above, not every man with AGA goes bald. Although 40% of men start losing their hair in their twenties, only 30% ever reach stage VI or VII. Hence, even for those with early-onset AGA complete baldness is not automatic.

Twin concordance studies in males indicate that susceptibility, age of onset, pattern and rate of progression of MPB are all under genetic influence [9,10]. The lower age-related prevalence of MPB and higher proportion of men with a Ludwig pattern hair loss among Koreans also confirms the profound influence of genes on susceptibility, age of onset and pattern of hair loss [11].

Patterned balding occurs in women, but the susceptibility, age of onset, rate of progression and pattern are different from men. Thirty-two per cent of women aged 80 years and above show no evidence of female pattern hair loss (FPHL). The age of onset of FPHL is later than that seen in men. Only 3% first develop clinically detectable FPHL by age 29 years, a further 13% first develop it by age 49 years, a further 8% by age 69 years and a further 6% after the age of 70 years. In addition, because many women wear their hair long, they are more aware of fluctuations in daily hair shedding. Women with AGA-related increased hair shedding often present prior to the development of reduction in hair volume over the crown (FPHL).

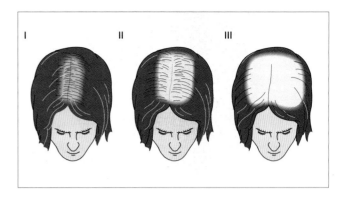

Fig. 63.15 Ludwig scale for grading female patterned hair loss [12].

Fewer than 1% of women progress to Hamilton–Norwood stage IV or above (equivalent to Ludwig stage III). Severe bitemporal recession (Hamilton–Norwood III) is uncommon and, as Ludwig pointed out, the most common pattern of hair loss seen in women is diffuse reduction of hair density over the crown with complete or near complete preservation of the frontal hairline [12]. Olsen observed the so-called Christmas-tree pattern, with widening of the central parting line most noticeably in the mid-frontal scalp. She also pointed out that the hair loss in women is often not confined to the crown but may extend ear to ear (Figs 63.15 & 63.16) [13].

The histology of the hair loss seen in women is indistinguishable from that seen in men. The process of FPHL involves androgen-mediated miniaturization of terminal hair follicles and therefore is AGA. The only caveat to this is that hair loss in an identical pattern has been observed in a female without androgens, indicating that other non-androgen-dependent mechanisms can produce hair loss that mimics AGA [14].

Minor bitemporal recession also occurs in more than 25% of women in their twenties and, as in men, is not necessarily a precursor of baldness, even though biopsy from these areas reveals AGA [15].

Inheritance. A familial tendency to MPB is well recognized, as is racial variation in the age-related prevalence of balding. A polygenic model of inheritance has been evoked in an attempt to explain the high prevalence of MPB in the population, the finding that baldness risk increases with the number of affected family members and, in particular, the high frequency of baldness in the fathers of balding men [16]. Of the 54 father–son relationships in the Victorian Family Heart Study, 81.5% of balding sons had fathers who had cosmetically significant balding.

Definition of MPB, particularly in its early stages, has confounded attempts to identify causative genes. By comparing DNA from young bald men with that of old non-bald men, Ellis *et al.* [17] identified an association of MPB with a polymorphism of the androgen receptor gene on the X chromosome. The androgen receptor gene *Stu1* restriction fragment length polymorphism (RFLP) was found in almost all (98.1%) young bald men, and most older bald men (92.3%), but only in 77% of non-bald men. This polymorphism appears to be necessary for the development of AGA, but its presence in non-bald men indicates that it is not sufficient for the development of AGA [17]. In addition, several shorter triplet repeat haplotypes were found in higher frequency in bald men than in normal controls. These RFLPs appear to be associated with a functional variant of the androgen receptor gene that is part of the polygenic inheritance of male common baldness. Of note is that the androgen receptor gene is located on the X chromosome, which is passed from the mother to a male child.

Current modelling suggests the involvement of at least four genes that combine to modify the age of onset, pattern of loss and rate of progression of MPB [16]. Other candidate gene and chromosomal regions have been examined. They include *SRDA1* and *SRDA5*, coding for the two variants of the 5α-reductase enzymes [18], the insulin gene [19], the aromatase gene, the gene for the Erα oestrogen receptor, the non-recombinant area of the Y chromosome and the type II IGF genes [16]. Thus far, no association has been found between any of the above-mentioned genetic areas and MPB.

Although a positive association between vertex balding and prostate cancer [20] has been identified, there is no clear association between MPB and dense hair patterns on the trunk [21], number of children [22] or coronary artery disease [23].

Regarding FPHL, Harrison examined DNA from 136 women with histologically proven AGA and compared them with 100 elderly female controls without hair loss, and suggested a possible role for both androgen receptor gene polymorphisms and polymorphisms in the aromatase gene in the development of FPHL [24].

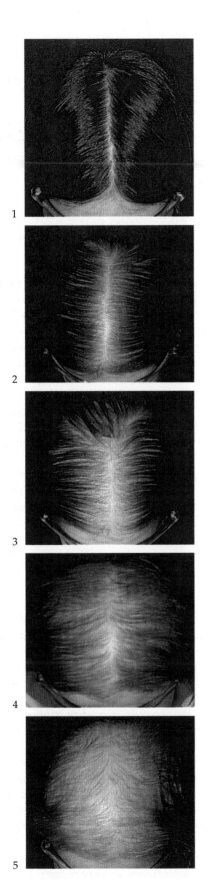

Fig. 63.16 Pattern of frontal hair loss in women with androgenetic alopecia. Stage 1 is normal.

REFERENCES

1 Sinclair RD. Male pattern androgenetic alopecia. *BMJ* 1998; **317**: 865–9.
2 Chodankar R, Chang CH, Yue Z *et al.* Shift of localized growth zones contributes to skin appendage morphogenesis: role of the Wnt/β-catenin pathway. *J Invest Dermatol* 2003; **120**: 20–6.
3 Chuong CM. Homeobox genes, fetal wound healing, and skin regional specificity. *J Invest Dermatol* 2003; **120**: 9–11.
4 Yu M, Wu P, Widelitz RB, Chuong CM. The morphogenesis of feathers. *Nature* 2002; **420**: 308–12.
5 Hamilton JB. Patterned hair loss in man: types and incidence. *Ann NY Acad Sci* 1951; **53**: 708–14.
6 Norwood O'TT. Male pattern baldness: classification and incidence. *South Med J* 1975; **68**: 1359–70.
7 Hamilton JB. Effect of castration in adolescent and young adult males upon further changes in the proportion of bald and hairy scalp. *J Clin Endocrinol Metab* 1960; **20**: 1309–18.
8 Kaufman K. Long term (5 year) multinational experience with finasteride in the treatment of men with androgenetic alopecia. *Eur J Dermatol* 2002: **12**; 38–49.

9 Stough DB, Rao N, Kaufman KD, Mitchell C. Finasteride improves male pattern hair loss in a randomized study in identical twins. *Eur J Dermatol* 2002; **12**: 32–7.

10 Nyholt DR, Gillespie NA, Heath AC, Martin NC. Genetic basis of male pattern baldness. *J Invest Dermatol* 2003; **121**: 1561–4.

11 Paik JH, Yoon JB, Sim WY, Kim BS, Kim BS. The prevalence and types of androgenetic alopecia in Korean men and women. *Br J Dermatol* 2001; **45**: 95–100.

12 Ludwig E. Classification of the types of androgenic alopecia (common baldness) arising in the female sex. *Br J Dermatol* 1977; **97**: 249–56.

13 Olsen E. Androgenetic alopecia. In: Olsen E, ed. *Disorders of Hair Growth*. New York: McGraw-Hill, 1994: 257–84.

14 Orme S, Cullen DR, Messenger AG. Diffuse female hair loss: are androgens necessary? *Br J Dermatol* 1999; **141**: 521–3.

15 Venning VA, Dawber R. Patterned androgenic alopecia. *J Am Acad Dermatol* 1988; **18**: 1073–8.

16 Ellis JA, Sinclair R, Harrap SB. Androgenetic alopecia: pathogenesis and potential for therapy. *Exp Rev Mol Med* 2002. http://www.expertreviews.org/

17 Ellis J, Stebbing M, Harrap S. Polymorphism of the androgen receptor gene is associated with male pattern baldness. *J Invest Dermatol* 2001; **116**: 452–5.

18 Ellis JA, Stebbing M, Harrap SB. Genetic analysis of male pattern baldness and the 5α-reductase genes. *J Invest Dermatol* 1998; **110**: 849–53.

19 Ellis J, Stebbing M, Harrap S. Insulin gene polymorphism and premature male pattern baldness in the general population. *Clin Sci* 1999; **96**: 659–62.

20 Giles GG, Saveri G, Sinclair RD *et al*. Androgenetic alopecia and prostate cancer: findings from an Australian case–control study. *Cancer Epidemiol Biomarkers Prev* 2002; **11**: 549–53.

21 Ellis JA, Stebbing M, Harrap SB. Male pattern baldness is not associated with established cardiovascular risk factors in the general population. *Clin Sci* 2001; **100**: 401–4.

22 Burton JL, Ben Halim MM, Meyrick G. Male pattern alopecia and masculinity. *Br J Dermatol* 1979; **100**: 507–12.

23 Damon A, Burr WA, Gerson DE. Baldness, fertility and number and sex ratio of children. *Hum Biol* 1965; **37**: 366–74.

24 Harrison S, Sinclair R, Ellis J, Harrap S. Female androgenetic alopecia and the androgen receptor gene. *Exp Dermatol* 2003; **12**: 222–3.

Hormonal influences

Systemic hormonal effects (see p. 63.15)

A number of studies have tried to identify increased circulating androgens in balding males, but no differences between patients and controls have been consistently found. Pitts [1] found elevated serum dihydroepiandrosterone sulphate (DHEA) but normal testosterone levels in 18 balding males compared with non-balding controls. A case–control study of 159 cases and 156 controls found a positive association between free testosterone and frontal and vertex baldness, compared with men who had only minimal hair loss [2]. The association with testosterone was also found in a cross-sectional study [3]. A positive association between IGF-1 and vertex balding has also been reported [4]. Sreekumar *et al*. [5] investigated a subset of patients with early-onset and advanced AGA and found no difference between patients and controls in the absolute levels of any androgens; however, the ratio of DHT : testosterone was elevated. All these studies suffer from a lack of reproducibility, and although differences in mean levels have been variously detected, the substantial overlap in the absolute levels of all androgens between cases and controls demonstrates that normal male levels of androgen are sufficient to make manifest the degree of baldness determined genetically for the individual.

The situation in women is more complex, as androgen-secreting tumours can trigger a sudden onset and rapidly progressive baldness [6]. Although hyperandrogenism was identified in 42 out of 109 women referred to an endocrinologist for hormonal evaluation of diffuse vertex alopecia, most of the abnormalities detected were inconsequential. For this survey, hyperandrogenism was defined as an increase in any plasma androgen. Of those 42 women, only 18 had polycystic ovary syndrome [7]. In contrast, no clinically significant hormone abnormality was found in 166 consecutive women with biopsy-proven AGA seen in a dermatology clinic [8].

Although the vast majority of women with FPHL have no discernible endocrine abnormality, in some women the hair loss may be accelerated by elevated circulating androgen levels [9–11]. Stated differently, androgens in the normal female range are sufficient to induce early baldness in women with a strong genetic predisposition. In women with a less strong genetic predisposition, balding will not occur until later in life unless androgen production is increased or drugs with androgen-like activity are taken. Some women with even grossly abnormal levels of androgen do not develop clinically significant baldness, although such patients are generally hirsute.

As there is no clear association between levels of circulating androgens and MPB, it is likely that the normal level of systemic androgen is adequate for the maximal production of dihydrotestosterone, and local factors determine individual susceptibility and severity of baldness. In females, local factors determine susceptibility, but severity is influenced by both local and systemic hormone factors.

Local hormonal effects

Beard dermal papilla cells are known to secrete growth-inducing autocrine growth factors in response to testosterone, leading to an increase in dermal papilla size and enlargement of the hair follicle and hair cortex. This response is not seen with occipital scalp hair follicles when subjected to the same testosterone challenge [12,13]. IGF-1 has been identified as a major component of secreted cytokines [14]. Similar investigations performed on dermal papilla cells from the balding scalp of the stump-tailed macaque showed that testosterone inhibited the growth and proliferation of keratinocytes [15]. TGF-β1 has been identified as a major component of the secreted cytokines in the vertex scalp and neutralizing anti-TGF-β1 antibody will reverse the androgen-induced inhibition of keratinocyte proliferation. It has been postulated that the androgen-induced anti-TGF-β1 derived from the dermal papilla cells mediates hair growth suppression in androgenetic alopecia [16]. Studies examining distribution and expression of androgen receptors have shown varying results. Two studies showed that androgen receptors are only found in the nuclei of dermal papilla cells [12,17].

However, another study found more extensive follicular distribution of receptors, including the hair bulb [18]. Comparing different anatomical sites, there appear to be higher numbers of androgen receptors in the pubic hair follicles and beard dermal papilla cells, with occipital scalp follicles expressing lower levels [19].

Hair loss on the scalp progresses in an orderly and reproducible pattern, and is a function of factors intrinsic to each hair follicle. *In vitro* experiments have shown that the hair follicles are able to self-regulate their response to androgens by regulating the expression of 5α-reductase and androgen receptors [20,21]. This self-regulation is postulated to produce the quantifiable difference in androgen receptor numbers [19,22] and 5α-reductase activity [20,23] that is observed between balding and non-balding areas of the scalp. This intrinsic regulation is best demonstrated in hair transplantation experiments; occipital hairs maintain their resistance to AGA when transplanted to the vertex, and scalp hairs from the vertex transplanted to the forearm miniaturize at the same pace as hairs neighbouring the donor site [24].

Hair cycle dynamics

In AGA, the duration of anagen decreases with each cycle, whereas the length of telogen remains constant or is prolonged. This results in a reduction of the anagen : telogen ratio. Balding patients often describe periods of excessive hair shedding, most noticeable while combing or washing. This is a result of the relative increase in numbers of follicles in telogen.

As the hair growth rate remains relatively constant, the duration of anagen growth determines hair length. Thus, with each successively foreshortened hair cycle, the length of each hair shaft is reduced. Ultimately, anagen duration becomes so short that the growing hair fails to achieve sufficient length to reach the surface of the skin, leaving an empty follicular pore. In addition, the latent phase is prolonged, reducing hair numbers, and further contributing to the balding process [25].

Hair follicle miniaturization

In addition to the changes in hair cycle dynamics, there is a stepwise miniaturization of entire follicles. It is not clear whether the same factors control the miniaturization and hair cycle changes. A significant proportion of men and women bald without ever being aware of increased hair shedding, but increased hair shedding can occur in the context of chronic telogen effluvium without associated follicular miniaturization.

As the dermal papilla is central to the maintenance and control of hair growth, it is likely to be the target of androgen-mediated events leading to follicle miniaturization and hair cycle changes [26–28]. The constant geometric relationship between the dermal papilla size and the size of the hair matrix [29] suggests that the size of the dermal papilla determines the size of the hair bulb and ultimately the hair shaft produced.

A greater than 10-fold reduction in overall cell numbers is likely to account for the decrease in hair follicle size [30]. The mechanism by which this decrease occurs is unexplained, and may be the result of either apoptotic cell death, cell displacement with loss of cellular adhesion leading to dermal papilla fibroblasts dropping off into the dermis, or migration of dermal papilla cells into the dermal sheath associated with the outer root sheath of the hair follicle [30].

In overall volumetric terms, change in the follicular extracellular matrix is unlikely to greatly affect follicle size. However, being a potential source of biologically active molecules, small changes in its volume may have significant effects on hair follicle function [31].

Smaller follicles result in finer hairs. The calibre of hair shafts reduces from 0.08 mm to less than 0.06 mm [32]. This is also followed by a reduction in pigment production. On the balding scalp, transitional indeterminate hairs represent the bridge between full-sized and miniaturized terminal hairs [33].

Follicular miniaturization has been traditionally thought to occur in a stepwise fashion. The cross-sectional area of individual hair shafts remains constant throughout fully developed anagen [31], indicating that the hair follicle, and its dermal papilla, remain the same size through each individual anagen stage of the cycle. Thus, miniaturization occurs between rather than within cycles.

In catagen, the entire bulb undergoes apoptosis and the base of the hair follicle retracts upwards to the level of the hair bulge. Entry into anagen occurs when the slow cycling stem cells in the bulge are activated, probably in response to signals from the dermal papilla. Daughter transient amplifying cells migrate downwards along the follicular stella, renew contact with the dermal papilla, and reform a new hair bulb and ultimately its differentiated cell product—the hair. This early part of the anagen cycle is the most likely point in time for miniaturization, and results in the stepwise reduction in follicle size between successive cycles [34].

Birch *et al.* [35] studied hair diameter in women in relation to hair density. The distribution of hair diameters showed wide variation between individual subjects, but narrow hair diameter was not associated with low hair density. They were not able to demonstrate a progressive reduction in the diameter of individual hairs with falling hair density, and concluded that miniaturization in FPHL occurs rapidly, possibly in the space of a single cycle.

Follicular miniaturization leaves behind stellae as dermal remnants of the full-sized follicle. These stellae, also known as fibrous tracts or streamers, extend from the subcutaneous tissue up the old follicular tract to the miniaturized hair and mark the formal position of the original terminal follicle. Arao–Perkins bodies may be seen with elastic stains within the follicular stellae. An Arao–Perkins body begins as a small cluster of elastic fibres in the neck of the dermal papilla. These clump in catagen and remain situated at the lowest point of origin of the follicular stellae. With the progressive shortening of anagen hair seen in AGA, multiple elastic clumps may be found in stellae, like the rungs of a ladder [36].

Follicular miniaturization is also a prominent feature of the histology of alopecia areata. It has been postulated that inflammation and fibrosis within the follicular stellae of AGA account for the difficulty of reversing the miniaturization in AGA.

REFERENCES

1 Pitts R. Serum elevation of dehydroepiandrosterone sulfate associated with male pattern baldness in young men. *J Am Acad Dermatol* 1987; **16**: 571–9.
2 Demark-Wahnefried W, Lesko SM, Conaway MR *et al.* Serum androgens: associations with prostate cancer risk and hair patterning. *J Androl* 1997; **18**: 495–500.
3 Platz EA, Pollak MN, Willett WC, Giovannucci E. Vertex balding, plasma insulin-like growth factor 1, and insulin-like growth factor binding protein 3. *J Am Acad Dermatol* 2000; **42**: 1003–7.
4 Signorello LB, Wuu J, Hsieh C *et al.* Hormones and hair patterning in men: a role for insulin-like growth factor 1? *J Am Acad Dermatol* 1999; **40**: 200–3.
5 Sreekumar GP, Pardinas J, Wong CQ *et al.* Serum androgens and genetic linkage analysis in early onset androgenetic alopecia. *J Invest Dermatol* 1999; **113**: 277–9.
6 Kim Y, Marjoniemi VM, Diamond T *et al.* Androgenetic alopecia in a postmenopausal woman as a result of ovarian hyperthecosis. *Australas J Dermatol* 2003; **44**: 62–6.
7 Futterweit W, Dunif A, Yeh HC *et al.* The prevalence of hyperandrogenism in 109 consecutive female patients with diffuse alopecia. *J Am Acad Dermatol* 1988; **19**: 831–7.
8 Mallari RS, Sinclair R. Diffuse hair loss in women: correlation of the clinical features and biopsy findings in 289 women seen at the Alfred Hospital and Skin and Cancer Foundation between 1997 and 1999. *Australas J Dermatol* 2000; **41**: A12.
9 De Villez RL, Dunn J. Female androgenic alopecia: the 3α, 17β-androstanediol glucuronide/sex hormone binding globulin ratio as a possible marker for female pattern baldness. *Arch Dermatol* 1986; **122**: 1011–4.
10 Miller J, Darley C, Karkavitas K *et al.* Low sex-hormone binding globulin levels in young women with diffuse hair loss. *Br J Dermatol* 1982; **106**: 331–5.
11 Moltz L. Hormonale Diagnostik der sogenannten androgenetischen Alopezie der Frau. *Geburts Frauenheil* 1988; **48**: 203–6.
12 Itami S, Kurata S, Sonoda T, Takayasu S. Interaction between dermal papilla cells and follicular epithelial cells *in vitro*: effect of androgen. *Br J Dermatol* 1995; **132**: 527–32.
13 Thornton MJ, Hamada K, Messenger AG *et al.* Androgen-dependent beard dermal papilla cells secrete autocrine growth factor(s) in response to testosterone unlike scalp cells. *J Invest Dermatol* 1998; **111**: 727–32.
14 Itami S, Kurata S, Takayasu S. Androgen induction of follicular epithelial cell growth is mediated via insulin-like growth factor 1 from dermal papilla cells. *Biochem Biophys Res Commun* 1995; **212**: 988–94.
15 Uno H, Adachi K, Montagna W. Morphological and biochemical studies of hair follicle in common baldness of stump-tailed macaque (*Macaca speciosa*). In: Montagna W, Dobson RL, eds. *Advances in Biology of Skin: Hair Growth*. Oxford: Pergamon, 1969: 221–45.
16 Inui S, Fukuzato Y, Nakajima T *et al.* Identification of androgen-inducible TGF-β1 derived from dermal papilla cells as a key mediator in androgenetic alopecia. *J Investig Dermatol Symp Proc* 2003; **8**: 69–71.
17 Choudhry R, Hodgins MB, van der Kwast TH, Brinkmann AO, Boersma WJ. Localization of androgen receptors in human skin by immunohistochemistry: implications for the hormonal regulation of hair growth, sebaceous glands and sweat glands. *J Endocrinol* 1992; **133**: 467–75.
18 Liang T, Hoyer S, Yu R *et al.* Immunocytochemical localization of androgen receptors in human skin using monoclonal antibodies against the androgen receptor. *J Invest Dermatol* 1993; **100**: 663–6.
19 Thornton MJ, Laing I, Hamada K *et al.* Differences in testosterone metabolism by beard and scalp hair follicle dermal papilla cells. *Clin Endocrinol* 1993; **39**: 633–9.
20 Itami S, Kurata S, Takayasu S. Differences in testosterone metabolism by beard and scalp hair follicle dermal papilla cells. *J Invest Dermatol* 1990; **94**: 150–2.
21 Boudou P, Reygagne P. Increased scalp and serum 5α-reductase reduced androgens in a man relevant to the acquired progressive kinky hair disorder and developing androgenetic alopecia. *Arch Dermatol* 1997; **133**: 1129–33.
22 Randall VA, Thornton MJ, Messenger AG. Cultured dermal papilla cells from androgen-dependent human hair follicles (e.g. beard) contain more androgen receptors than those from non-balding areas of scalp. *J Endocrinol* 1992; **133**: 141–7.
23 Sawaya ME, Price VE. Different levels of 5α-reductase type I and II, aromatase, and androgen receptors in hair follicles of men and women with androgenetic alopecia. *J Invest Dermatol* 1997; **109**: 296–300.
24 Orentreich N. Autografts in alopecias and other selected dermatological conditions. *Ann NY Acad Sci* 1959; **83**: 462.
25 Curtois M, Loussouarn G, Horseau C. Hair cycle and alopecia. *Skin Pharm* 1994; **7**: 84–9.
26 Obana NJ, Uno H. Dermal papilla cells in macaque alopecia trigger a testosterone-dependent inhibition of follicular cell proliferation. In: van Neste D, Randall VA, eds. *Hair Research in the Next Millennium*. Amsterdam: Elsevier, 1996: 307–10.
27 Oliver RF, Jahoda CAB. The dermal papilla and the maintenance of hair growth. In: Rogers GA, Reis Ward KA *et al.*, eds. *The Biology of Wool and Hair*. London: Chapman & Hall, 1989: 51–67.
28 Randall VA. The use of dermal papilla cells in studies of normal and abnormal hair follicle biology. *Dermatol Clin* 1996; **14**: 585–94.
29 van Scott EJ, Ekel TM. Geometric relationships between the matrix of the hair bulb and its dermal papilla in normal and alopecic scalp. *J Invest Dermatol* 1958; **31**: 281–7.
30 Jahoda CAB. Cellular and developmental aspects of androgenetic alopecia. *Exp Dermatol* 1998; **7**: 235–48.
31 Elliot K, Stephenson TJ, Messenger AG. Differences in hair follicle dermal papilla volume are due to extracellular matrix volume and cell number: implications for the control of hair follicle size and androgen responses. *J Invest Dermatol* 1999; **113**: 873–7.
32 Jackson D, Church RE, Ebling FJ. Hair diameter in female baldness. *Br J Dermatol* 1972; **84**: 361–7.
33 Sinclair RD. Male pattern androgenetic alopecia. *BMJ* 1998; **317**: 865–9.
34 Whiting D. Possible mechanisms of follicular miniaturization during androgenetic alopecia or pattern hair loss. *J Am Acad Dermatol* 2001; **45**: S81–6.
35 Birch MP, Messenger JF, Messenger AG. Hair density, hair diameter and prevalence of female pattern hair loss. *Br J Dermatol* 2001; **144**: 297–304.
36 Pinkus H. Differential patterns of elastic fibers in scarring and non-scarring alopecias. *J Cutan Pathol* 1978; **5**: 93–104.

Clinical features. The essential clinical feature of balding in both sexes is patterned hair loss over the crown. Pigmented terminal hairs are progressively replaced by finer hairs, which are short and virtually non-pigmented. This process may begin at any age after the onset of adrenarche and may precede pubarche.

Males. The clinical appearance of male androgenetic alopecia is instantly recognizable in most cases. The progression of the hair loss occurs in an orderly manner and has been well documented by Hamilton [1] and Norwood [2] (Fig. 63.14). The posterior and lateral scalp margins are spared, even in the most advanced cases, and even in old age. Twin concordance studies indicate that variations in the pattern are governed, at least in part, by genetic factors, as is the rate of progression [3].

The main significance of hair relates to socialization,

and hair is an essential part of an individual's self-image. Thus, the consequences of AGA are predominantly psychological. Bald men are likely to have fewer lifetime sexual partners than non-bald men, which may be a reflection of their physical attractiveness to the other sex [4]. Several studies have shown that the negative self-perception of balding patients appears to be consistent between Western [5,6] and Asian cultures [7]. The negative impact of AGA is often trivialized or ignored by the non-bald [8]. However, there is evidence that perception by others may compound the psychological problems suffered by balding men. A Korean study [7] of the perception of balding men by women and non-balding men found that their negative perception of men with AGA was similar to the psychosocial effects reported by the patients themselves. Of note was that a perception of bald men looking less attractive was found in more than 90% of subjects surveyed. Importantly, this view was more common in women than non-balding men. Such negative perceptions may further impair the social functioning of balding men.

However, it is important to note that most affected men cope well with AGA, and it does not have significant impact on their psychosocial function. Thus, those who do seek help are likely to be in greater emotional distress and to have been dissatisfied with any treatment they have received.

The most distressed balding men are those with more extensive hair loss, those who have very early onset, and those who regard their balding as progressive (often arising from observation of their father) and socially noticeable [5].

Females. The pattern of hair loss and the clinical presentation of AGA in women differ from men. Women may present with either an episodic or continuous increase in hair shedding without any noticeable reduction in hair volume, increased hair shedding with loss of hair volume over the crown or diffuse thinning over the crown with no history of hair shedding [9]. Women with FPHL commonly underestimate the severity of their loss [10]. Asking women with a loss of hair volume over the crown about the thickness of their ponytail often enables them to estimate and communicate the degree of hair loss. Diffuse thinning over the crown can be best detected when the hair is parted centrally. Widening of the central parting (part) often follows a Christmas tree pattern and can be used to grade the hair loss [11].

Ludwig [12] described the most common pattern of loss in women and his illustrations have been used as a grading scale. The earliest change (Ludwig grade I) is a rarefaction of the hair on the crown. This produces an oval area of alopecia encircled by a band of variable breadth with normal hair density. Frontally the fringe is narrow (1–3 cm) and at the sides the margin is 4–5 cm wide. Progression to Ludwig grade II results in further rarefaction of the crown, with preservation of the fringe. Grade III is near-complete baldness of the crown. As Ludwig only produced three illustrations (Fig. 63.15), other validated scales with more images should prove more useful for patient grading (Fig. 63.16) [13].

The relative incidence of Ludwig versus Hamilton pattern alopecia among balding women has been determined. Ludwig pattern I–III occurred in 87% of premenopausal women and Hamilton stage II–IV occurred in 13%. Among postmenopausal women, Ludwig I–III occurred in 63% and Hamilton II–V occurred in 37% [14].

In most women the hair loss is confined to the vertex scalp, but in a significant proportion hair loss also occurs diffusely over the parietal scalp. Generalized hair loss may preclude women from hair transplantation procedures because of a diminished donor population.

Most women who present with hair loss have no other evidence of virilization. However, if the hair loss is of sudden onset, rapidly progressive and advanced, a full medical history and examination, and endocrinological investigation are desirable to exclude virilization, which can rarely be caused by a virilizing tumour. Investigation is also indicated in women with AGA of gradual onset accompanied by menstrual disturbance, hirsutism or recrudescence of acne [15].

The principal differential diagnosis of early AGA is chronic telogen effluvium (CTE) [16]. Women with CTE present with chronic diffuse hair shedding without noticeable widening of the central parting. They may describe a loss in volume of the ponytail of up to one-third, and there is commonly mild bitemporal recession. Scalp biopsy of women who present in this fashion reveals AGA in approximately 60% of cases and CTE in 40% [13]. Scalp biopsy is not required in women who present with loss of hair volume either alone or associated with increased hair shedding.

REFERENCES

1 Hamilton JB. Patterned hair loss in man: types and incidence. *Ann NY Acad Sci* 1951; **53**: 708–14.
2 Norwood O'TT. Male pattern baldness: classification and incidence. *South Med J* 1975; **68**: 1359–70.
3 Nyhold DR, Gillespie NA, Heath AC, Martin NG. Genetic basis of male pattern baldness. *J Invest Dermatol* 2003; **121**: 1561–4.
4 Severi G, Sinclair R, Hopper JL *et al.* Androgenetic alopecia in men aged 40–69 years: prevalence and risk factors. *Br J Dermatol* 2003; **149**: 1207–12.
5 Cash TF. The psychology of hair loss and its implications for patient care. *Clin Dermatol* 2001; **19**: 161–6.
6 Budd D, Himmelberger D, Rhodes T *et al.* The effects of hair loss in European men: a survey in four countries. *Eur J Dermatol* 2000; **10**: 122–7.
7 Lee H-J, Ha S-J, Kim D, Kim H-O, Kim J-W. Perception of men with androgenetic alopecia by women and non-balding men in Korea: how the non-bald regard the bald. *Int J Dermatol* 2002; **41**: 867–9.
8 Passchier J. Quality of life issues in male pattern hair loss. *Dermatol* 1998; **197**: 217–8.
9 Sinclair RD, Dawber RPR. Androgenetic alopecia in men and women. *Clin Dermatol* 2001; **19**: 167–78.
10 Biondo S, Goble D, Sinclair R. Women who present with female pattern hair loss tend to underestimate the severity of their hair loss. *Br J Dermatol* 2004; **150**: 750–2.

11 Olsen EA. The midline part: an important physical clue to the diagnosis of androgenetic alopecia in women. *J Am Acad Dermatol* 1999; **40**: 106–9.

12 Ludwig E. Classification of the types of androgenic alopecia (common baldness) occurring in the female sex. *Br J Dermatol* 1977; **97**: 247–54.

13 Sinclair R, Jolley D, Mallari R, Magee J. The reliability of horizontally sectioned scalp biopsies in the diagnosis of chronic diffuse telogen hair loss in women. *J Am Acad Dermatol* (in press).

14 Venning V, Dawber R. Patterned androgenetic alopecia. *J Am Acad Dermatol* 1988; **18**: 1073–8.

15 Futterweit W, Dunif A, Yeh HC *et al.* The prevalence of hyperandrogenism in 109 consecutive female patients with diffuse alopecia. *J Am Acad Dermatol* 1988; **19**: 831–9.

16 Whiting DA. Chronic telogen effluvium. *Dermatol Clin* 1996; **14**: 723–32.

Pathology. The key elements of the histology of AGA are a marked reduction in terminal hairs, an increase in secondary vellus hair with associated angiofibrotic streamers, an increase in telogen and catagen hairs, and a mild or moderate perifollicular lymphohistiocytic infiltrate, with or without concentric layers of perifollicular collagen deposition (Fig. 63.17) [1].

A mild lymphohistiocytic inflammation is found in approximately one-third of cases of AGA and a similar number of controls, and is non-specific. In contrast, a moderate lymphohistiocytic inflammation is found in another one-third of cases of AGA, but in only 10% of controls [2]. Occasional eosinophils and mast cells can be seen. The cellular inflammatory changes also occur around lower follicles in some cases and occasionally involve follicular stellae. The diagnostic and prognostic significance of the degree of the inflammation is not known.

Many of these changes are best seen on horizontally sectioned scalp biopsies. Horizontal sections reveal numerous pseudovellus hair follicles in the papillary dermis, reflecting a miniaturization process. In the vast majority of cases there is no genuine reduction in the number of follicles, and follicular fibrosis is seen in less than 10% of cases. The presence of arrector pili muscles and angiofibrotic streamers distinguishes them from true vellus hairs. There is a change in the ratio of terminal : vellus hairs from greater than 8 : 1 to less than 4 : 1. Also, the anagen : telogen hair ratio reduces from 12 : 1 to 5 : 1 [3]. The increased proportion of catagen and telogen hairs reflects the shortened duration of anagen and the relative increase in telogen hairs.

As the balding scalp loses its protective covering of hair, solar degenerative changes may be seen. A reduction of blood supply has been observed [4], but whether it follows or precedes the hair loss is unknown.

The reduction in the size of the affected follicles, which is the essential histological feature of AGA, necessarily results in a reduction in the diameter of the hairs they produce. This reduction is said to be greater in women than in men [5,6]. Balding patients showed a wide spread of hair-shaft diameters, with peaks at 0.04 mm and 0.06 mm, whereas non-bald subjects showed a symmetrical distribution with a single peak at 0.08 mm. Increased hair

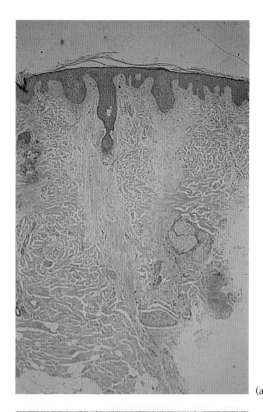

(a)

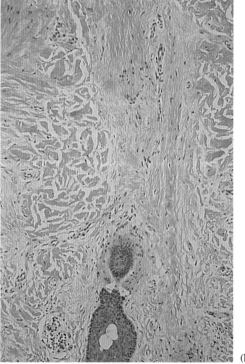

(b)

Fig. 63.17 Histology of androgenetic alopecia on vertically sectioned scalp biopsy. (a) The low-power photomicrograph shows a reduction in follicle number and size. (b) The high-power photomicrograph shows the follicular streamer and a light perifollicular inflammatory infiltrate.

diameter diversity has been used a diagnostic criterion for AGA [7].

REFERENCES

1 Kligman AM. The comparative histopathology of male pattern baldness and senescent baldness. *Clin Dermatol* 1988; **6**: 108–18.
2 Whiting D. Diagnostic and predictive value of horizontal sections of scalp biopsy specimens in male pattern androgenetic alopecia. *J Am Acad Dermatol* 1993; **28**: 755–63.
3 Whiting DA. Scalp biopsy as a diagnostic and prognostic tool in androgenetic alopecia. *Dermatol Ther* 1998; **8**: 24–33.
4 Klemp P, Peters K, Hansted B. Subcutaneous blood flow in early male pattern baldness. *J Invest Dermatol* 1989; **92**: 725–30.
5 Jackson D, Church RE, Ebling FJ. Hair diameter in female baldness. *Br J Dermatol* 1972; **87**: 361–7.
6 van Scott EJ, Ekel TM. Geometric relationships between the matrix of the hair bulb and its dermal papilla in normal and alopecic scalp. *J Invest Dermatol* 1958; **31**: 281–7.
7 de Lacharrière O, Deloche C, Misciali C *et al.* Hair diameter diversity: a clinical sign reflecting the follicle miniaturization. *Arch Dermatol* 2001; **137**: 641–6.

Pathogenesis. Any unifying hypothesis for AGA has to explain the following: the occurrence in humans and simian species; strong familial tendency; the involvement of both sexes; geographical patterning of hair loss on the scalp; the paradoxical effect of circulating and local androgens on scalp and body hairs; the phenomenon of donor dominance in hair transplantation; the alteration of hair cycle dynamics; follicular miniaturization; perifollicular inflammation; and the coexistence of greasy skin, acne and hirsutism in some women.

Treatment

Twenty-five years ago patterned baldness was thought to be irreversible, and although oral antiandrogens were advocated to arrest further hair loss for women, there were no medical treatments available for men. There are now a number of effective treatments to arrest the progression of the hair loss and stimulate regrowth in a significant proportion of individuals. Although the degree of regrowth achieved is often minor, a small proportion of men have a dramatic response to therapy.

As baldness is not life-threatening and the morbidity is variable, most people do not seek treatment. Some patients simply attend for a diagnosis, and when the currently available therapies are discussed, decline treatment. Without therapy baldness is progressive, although the rate of progression is extremely variable. Twenty-five per cent of men will have no visible progression after 5 years. Some will achieve Hamilton stage VII within 5 years, whereas others may take 50 years.

Before any patient embarks on therapy he or she should be counselled carefully and made aware of the need for maintenance therapy. It is preferable that advice is given by qualified medical practitioners who are fully aware of all the treatment options so that vulnerable individuals may be kept away from commercial centres where profit is the only motivation.

Surgery

All surgical procedures are attempts to spread parietal and occipital hairs thinly over the rest of the scalp. Hair can be redistributed using autografts or flaps. Either procedure can be performed alone or in combination with reduction of the bald area by excision and closure. Grafts may be as large as 4 mm in diameter, but better results are achieved with much smaller 'micrografts', which can be manipulated to produce a natural-looking frontal hairline. Reduction of the bald area by removal of an ellipse from the vault or repeated such operations may cover the top of the head by stretching the remaining parietal scalp. Expansion techniques have been used successfully to restore post-traumatic alopecia [1]. Hair transplantation techniques are constantly undergoing revision and improvement. They have been recently reviewed [2]. Artificial fibre implantation has been used for AGA but foreign body reactions and infections are potentially serious complications [3,4]. Use of artificial fibres has been banned in a number of countries.

Surgery is often performed long before the ultimate pattern of hair loss is clear. Without adjunctive medical therapy to prevent progression of the balding process, an unnatural appearance can evolve over time that may require further surgery to correct.

Camouflage and wigs

Camouflage is the simplest, easiest and cheapest way of dealing with mild AGA. Balding becomes most noticeable when the scalp can be seen through the hair. Camouflage treatments involve either adding small fibres held in place electrostatically or dyeing the scalp the same colour as the hair to create the illusion of thicker hair. Numerous brands are available, each in a range of colours. Although many of the newer agents are water-resistant, if the hair becomes wet in the rain the dye may still run.

Wigs are an alternative to scalp surgery. For many women, an alternative to a full wig is a smaller hair piece that can either be interwoven with existing hair or worn over the top of existing hair. Interwoven wigs tend to lift as the hair beneath grows, and they require periodic adjustment.

Wig hair is composed of either a synthetic acrylic fibre that withstands wear and tear very well, or natural fibre (usually Asian or European human hair). Natural fibre wigs look better, are easier to style and last longer, but are considerably more expensive. Wigs can be styled and washed, and modern wigs provide excellent coverage that looks natural. A drawback of wigs is that the head may be hot in the summer, and some patients find them difficult to wear for this reason.

Excellent advice on wigs is available from the alopecia patient support groups that exist in the UK, USA and Australia. In the UK, the National Health Service subsidizes wigs for 'medical hair loss'.

Medical management

Currently available medical management for women consists of oral antiandrogens and topical minoxidil. Antiandrogens may feminize males and therefore are not appropriate for use in balding men. They are potential teratogens, and women should be advised to take appropriate precautions to avoid pregnancy while taking these medications. Pharmacological therapy for men includes topical minoxidil and the 5α-reductase inhibitors finasteride and dutasteride. Finasteride and dutasteride are both teratogens with very long biological half-lives, and so should be avoided in women with child-bearing potential, as even if these agents were stopped as soon as a woman discovered she had become pregnant, activity may persist into the critical second trimester.

Medical treatment should be continued indefinitely, as the benefit is not maintained when therapy is stopped. Up to 1 year of treatment may be required before any clinical response is noticeable. The monitoring of this response can be problematic. Patients inspect their hair on a daily basis and subtle changes over time may not be readily observable. Doctors are essentially reliant upon the patient's subjective assessment of their hair density over time. Baseline photographs are helpful, but unlikely to detect changes of less than 20% in hair density. Periodic photography is useful for monitoring and maximizing patient compliance [5].

Management of male pattern baldness.
Many therapies given systemically for other reasons may produce general hypertrichosis and concurrent improvement in AGA (e.g. ciclosporin and psoralen with UVA therapy [PUVA]), but these cannot be used as treatment. Only minoxidil has been shown to enhance regrowth significantly when used topically. Minoxidil is a piperidinopyrimidine derivative and a potent vasodilator that is effective orally for severe hypertension. When applied topically as a 2% solution in an alcohol and water base containing 10% propylene glycol, minoxidil has shown conversion of vellus to terminal hair in up to 30% of individuals [6,7]. Terminal hair appeared to regrow at the margins, but complete covering of the bald areas was seen in less than 10% of responders. De Villez [8] suggested that bald men who responded best to minoxidil were those in whom the balding process was at an early stage, with a maximum diameter of the bald area of less than 10 cm and in whom the pretreatment hair density was in excess of 20 hairs/cm^2. There is a slight increase in benefit if the concentration is increased to 5%. The benefit is most pronounced in the first 6 months of therapy and thereafter is marginal.

Topical minoxidil appears to be a safe therapy with side effects only of local irritation and hypertrichosis of the temples, and there is a low incidence of contact dermatitis [9]. If treatment is stopped clinical regression occurs, after 3 months, to the state of baldness that would have existed if treatment had not been applied [10]. Patients should be warned that in order to maintain any beneficial effect, applications must continue twice daily for the rest of their lives [7]. Whether the benefits are maintained in the longer term is uncertain [11].

Finasteride is a synthetic aza-steroid that is a potent and highly selective antagonist of 5α-reductase type 2. Being a non-competitive antagonist, it binds irreversibly to the enzyme and inhibits the conversion of testosterone to DHT. Thus, although the pharmacokinetic half-life is about 8 h, the biological effect persists for much longer. The underlying principle for its use is the reduction of DHT production and thus limitation of the miniaturization of scalp hair follicles. A scalp biopsy study of patients with AGA found that after 12 months of finasteride treatment, terminal hair counts increase and vellus hair counts decrease, demonstrating the ability of finasteride to reverse the miniaturization process and to encourage the growth of terminal hairs [12].

An oral dosage of 1 mg/day reduces scalp DHT by 64% and serum DHT by 68% [13]. Finasteride is also approved for the treatment of benign prostatic hypertrophy in a dosage of 5 mg/day. Dose-ranging studies have found no significant difference in clinical benefit between 5 and 1 mg/day regimens [14], nor is there any significant further reduction of scalp or serum DHT levels.

At the end of 1 year, patients on finasteride have a 10% increase in the mean number of terminal hairs compared with baseline counts. After 5 years of continuous therapy, hair counts remained close to the 1-year level, whereas the counts in the placebo patients had dropped by 30%. Using global photography to assess scalp coverage, 48% of patients taking finasteride had increased hair density, compared with 7% of the placebo group at the end of 1 year. At 2 years [15], coverage continued to improve in the finasteride group, with 66% having increased density, whereas only 7% of the placebo subjects had increased coverage. By 5 years [16], 10% of treated patients had a lowered hair density, 42% had no change, and 22%, 21% and 5% were assessed as moderately, markedly and greatly improved, respectively. In contrast, 19%, 31% and 25% of patients in the placebo group were greatly, markedly or moderately worse. Nevertheless, 25% of the patients in the placebo group showed no deterioration over the 5-year period, reflecting the variable rate of progression of balding among males.

These data suggest that the maximal number of finasteride-responsive follicles are recruited by the end of 1 year, and further improvement in scalp coverage results from increase in hair length, diameter and pigmentation [16]. At the end of the first year, some finasteride patients were changed to placebo, resulting in a decrease in their hair counts after 12 months. Some in the placebo group were also crossed over, receiving finasteride for the second year; these subjects had an increase in their hair counts, although the average increase was less than that seen in the original group, indicating the potential for regrowth diminishes as the AGA progresses.

Studies using hair weight as the objective measure of outcome indicate that men on placebo had a reduction in hair weight of 9.2% of their hair at 48 weeks and 15.4% at 96 weeks, compared with the men on active treatment who had an increase of 25.6% at 48 weeks and 35.8% at 96 weeks. Factors that affect hair weight include the number of hairs, hair growth rate and hair thickness [17].

Work examining the effect of finasteride on frontal hair loss also confirmed efficacy here, albeit the magnitude of regrowth appears less [18].

Few adverse effects were reported in the phase III studies [15,16]. In the finasteride group, loss of libido was reported in 1.8% and erectile dysfunction in 1.3%. The placebo groups reported these same events, with frequencies of 1.3% and 0.7%, respectively. These events appeared to resolve on cessation of the drug and, in some cases, with continued treatment. It has been suggested that even these figures overstate the true incidence of sexual dysfunction [19].

Of note is that older men on finasteride experienced a 50% reduction in serum prostate-specific antigen (PSA) levels, which could result in an underestimation of prostatic cancer risk. It has been shown in the urology literature that PSA levels remain valid while patients are taking finasteride, but the value should be doubled to correct for the finasteride effect [20,21]. Men between 18 and 41 years of age have a negligible decrease in measured PSA [22].

Topical finasteride has been investigated as an alternative means of drug delivery. Although a 0.05% finasteride solution applied to the scalp was well absorbed and produced a 40% reduction in serum DHT, it had no effect on hair regrowth. One explanation is that inhibition of prostatic DHT production is an important factor in preventing hair loss with finasteride; a significant reduction in circulating DHT is required in addition to the local blockade of 5α-reductase at the hair follicle [23].

Finasteride is a teratogen. Male rats exposed to finasteride *in utero* develop hypospadias with cleft prepuce, decreased anogenital distance, reduced prostate weight and altered nipple formation [24]. As the drug is secreted in the semen and can be absorbed through the vagina during intercourse, it was originally advocated that men taking finasteride should avoid unprotected intercourse with pregnant women. In practice, the concentration of finasteride in the semen is well below the minimum effect dosage, and no recommendations regarding the use of condoms are made in the product information leaflet [25]. There are no reports of adverse pregnancy outcomes among women exposed to finasteride taken by their partners [26]. Finasteride has no effect on spermatogenesis or semen production [27].

With regard to long-term safety, finasteride has now been in widespread use for over 10 years. Many recipients are elderly men taking 5 mg/day. Very few side effects have been observed [28]. There is no effect of long-term use on bone mineral density [16,29]. Reversible painful gynaecomastia has been reported [30] and the incidence is thought to be approximately 0.001% [31]. The prostate cancer prevention trial has demonstrated that 5 mg daily of finasteride will reduce the incidence of prostate cancer by 25% among men aged 55 and over. More of the reduction occurred in low-grade prostate cancers (Gleason stage 2–6), whilst the incidence of high-grade cancers (Gleason stage 7–10) was increased [32].

Dutasteride is a combined type 1 and 2 5α-reductase inhibitor. There is a dose-dependent reduction in scalp DHT levels. At 0.5 mg/day a 53% reduction is scalp DHT is seen, and at 2.5 mg/day the reduction is 83%. The percentage reduction in scalp DHT seems to be the best indicator of clinical response. The drug is currently marketed at a 1 mg dosage for benign prostatic hypertrophy. Sexual side effects are more common with dutasteride than with finasteride, and are also dose related, but appear to be reversible on cessation.

Management of female pattern hair loss. Topical minoxidil has been demonstrated to either arrest hair loss or to induce mild to moderate hair regrowth in approximately 60% of women [33]. It may be used alone or in combination with oral antiandrogen therapy [34].

Oral antiandrogen therapy with cyproterone acetate, spironolactone and flutamide are of benefit in arresting AGA in women [35]. Most studies with these drugs have been performed in hirsutism and only a small number in AGA [36].

Spironolactone is a synthetic steroid, structurally related to aldosterone, which acts by competitively blocking cytoplasmic receptors for DHT. It also weakly inhibits androgen biosynthesis. Its primary use is as a diuretic and antihypertensive and many of its side effects and numerous drug interactions relate to this. Several studies have demonstrated the efficacy of spironolactone in the treatment of hirsutism [36], and some have found that it is also of benefit in AGA [37]. Dosage ranges from 100 to 300 mg/day, but most women require a minimum of 200 mg/day [38]. Side effects are dose related and include menstrual irregularities, postmenopausal bleeding, breast tenderness or enlargement, and fatigue [39]. Spironolactone has the potential to feminize a male fetus and women should not become pregnant while taking spironolactone. Concomitant use of oral contraceptives will reduce the hormonal side effects. The antialdosterone effect can result in an elevation of serum potassium and a slight reduction in blood pressure, although this is rarely significant in the absence of renal impairment. Rare cases of hepatocellular carcinoma and hepatitis have been reported, but with substantially higher doses [40,41].

Cyproterone acetate is an androgen receptor blocker and potent progestin [42]. It also has an antigonadotrophic effect. It has been in common usage for over 40 years. It has been shown to be of benefit in AGA [43] and is widely used to treat it in women. However, it appears more effective at arresting progression than stimulating hair regrowth [44]. Although low-dose therapy with 2 mg/day cyproterone acetate may be useful in hirsutism [45], higher doses, in the order of 100 mg/day for 10 days of each menstrual cycle, seem to be required in AGA [46]. For postmenopausal women, cyproterone acetate may be used continuously, with or without oestrogens. The average dosage required is 50 mg/day.

The side effects of cyproterone acetate are dose dependent and include lassitude, weight gain, breast tenderness, loss of libido, depression and nausea [47]. Shortness of breath is an uncommon side effect [48]. Feminization of a male fetus may occur and so patients should be advised to cease the medication before conception. The combination of cyproterone acetate and oral oestrogen therapy provides effective contraception and stabilizes menstrual irregularities.

Flutamide is a non-steroidal antiandrogen that acts by inhibiting androgen uptake and by inhibiting nuclear binding of androgen within the target tissue. One study suggested that flutamide is superior to cyproterone acetate and finasteride in the treatment of androgenetic alopecia [49]. However, rare but potentially fatal hepatotoxicity limits the use of flutamide for this condition [36].

In a double-blind placebo-controlled study involving almost 100 postmenopausal women, 1 mg finasteride was found to be no better than placebo [50]. Subsequently, a case report and a case series have shown idiosyncratic benefit [51,52].

REFERENCES

1 Masser MR. A twin tissue expander used in the elimination of alopecia. *Plast Reconstr Surg* 1988; **81**: 444–50.
2 Unger WP. Surgical approach to hair loss. In: Olsen EA, ed. *Disorders of Hair Growth. Diagnosis and Treatment*. New York: McGraw-Hill, 1994.
3 Auerback R. Dangers of synthetic fiber implantation for male pattern baldness. *Cutis* 1980; **26**: 416.
4 Lepaw M. Complications of implantation of synthetic fibres into scalps for 'hair' replacement: experience with 14 cases. *J Dermatol Surg Oncol* 1979; **5**: 201–4.
5 Trueb RM, Itin P, und Schweizerische Arbeitsgruppe fur Trichologie. Photographic documentation of the effectiveness of 1 mg oral finasteride in treatment of androgenic alopecia in the man in routine general practice in Switzerland. *Schweiz Rundsch Med Prax* 2001; **90**: 2087–93.
6 Reitschel RL, Duncan SH. Safety and efficacy of topical minoxidil in the management of androgenetic alopecia. *J Am Acad Dermatol* 1987; **16**: 677–85.
7 Olsen EA, Weiner MS, Amara LA *et al.* Five year follow-up of men with androgenetic alopecia treated with topical minoxidil. *J Am Acad Dermatol* 1990; **22**: 643–9.
8 De Villez RL. Topical minoxidil therapy in hereditary androgenetic alopecia. *Arch Dermatol* 1985; **121**: 197–202.
9 Tosti A, Bardazzi F, De Padova MP *et al.* Contact dermatitis to minoxidil. *Contact Dermatitis* 1985; **13**: 275–7.
10 Olsen EA, Delong ER, Weiner MS. Long-term follow-up of men with male pattern baldness treated with topical minoxidil. *J Am Acad Dermatol* 1987; **16**: 688–95.
11 Green J, Sinclair RD. Oral cyclosporin does not arrest progression of androgenetic alopecia. *Br J Dermatol* 2001; **145**: 842–4.
12 Whiting D, Waldstreicher J, Sanchez M, Kaufman K. Measuring reversal of hair miniaturization in androgenetic alopecia by follicular counts in horizontal sections of serial scalp biopsies: results of finasteride 1 mg treatment of men and postmenopausal women. *J Invest Dermatol Symp Proc* 1999; **4**: 282–4.
13 Drake L, Hordinsky M, Fieldler V *et al.* The effects of finasteride on scalp skin and serum androgen levels in men with androgenetic alopecia. *J Am Acad Dermatol* 1999; **41**: 550–4.
14 Roberts JN, Fieldler V, Imperato-McGinley J *et al.* Clinical dose ranging studies with finasteride, a type 2 5α-reductase inhibitor, in men with male pattern hair loss. *J Am Acad Dermatol* 1999; **41**: 555–63.
15 Kaufman KD, Olsen EA, Whiting D *et al.* Finasteride in the treatment of men with androgenetic alopecia. *J Am Acad Dermatol* 1998; **39**: 578–9.
16 Kaufman K. Long term (5 year) multinational experience with finasteride in the treatment of men with androgenetic alopecia. *Eur J Dermatol* 2002; **12**: 38–49.
17 Price VH, Menefee E, Sanchez M, Ruane P, Kaufman KD. Changes in hair weight and hair count in men with androgenetic alopecia after treatment with finasteride, 1 mg, daily. *J Am Acad Dermatol* 2002; **46**: 517–23.
18 Leyden J, Dunlap F, Miller B *et al.* Finasteride in the treatment of men with frontal male pattern hair loss. *J Am Acad Dermatol* 1999; **40**: 930–7.
19 Tosti A, Piraccini BM, Soli M. Evaluation of sexual function in subjects taking finasteride for the treatment of androgenetic alopecia. *J Eur Acad Dermatol Venereol* 2001; **15**: 418–21.
20 Matzkin H, Barak M, Braf Z. Effect of finasteride on free and total serum prostate-specific antigen in men with benign prostatic hyperplasia. *Br J Urol* 1996; **78**: 405–8.
21 Keetch DW, Andriole GL, Ratliff TL, Catalona WJ. Comparison of percent free prostate-specific antigen levels in men with benign prostatic hyperplasia treated with finasteride, terazosin, or watchful waiting. *Urology* 1997; **50**: 901–5.
22 Andriole GL, Guess HA, Epstein JI *et al.* Treatment with finasteride preserves usefulness of prostate-specific antigen in the detection of prostate cancer: results of a randomized, double-blind, placebo-controlled clinical trial. *Urology* 1998; **52**: 195–202.
23 Rushton DH, Norris MJ, Ramsay ID. Topical 0.05% finasteride significantly reduced serum DHT concentrations, but had no effect in preventing the expression of genetic hair loss in men. In: Van Neste D, Randall VA, eds. *Hair Research For The Next Millenium*. Amsterdam: Elsevier, 1996: 359–62.
24 Clark RL, Anderson CA, Prahalada S *et al.* Critical developmental periods for effects on male rat genitalia induced by finasteride, a 5α-reductase inhibitor. *Toxicol Appl Pharmacol* 1993; **119**: 34–40.
25 Physicians circular for Propecia. In: West Point: Merck, 1997.
26 Pole M, Koren G. Finasteride: does it affect spermatogenesis and pregnancy. *Can Fam Physician* 2001; **47**: 2469–70.
27 Overstreet JW, Fuh VL, Gould J *et al.* Chronic treatment with finasteride daily does not affect spermatogenesis or semen production in young men. *J Urol* 1999; **162**: 1295–300.
28 Marberger MJ. Long-term effects of finasteride in patients with benign prostatic hyperplasia: a double-blind placebo controlled, multicentre study. *Urology* 1998; **51**: 677–86.
29 Matsumoto AM, Tenover L, McClung M *et al.* The long-term effect of specific type II 5α-reductase inhibition with finasteride on bone mineral density in men: results of a 4-year placebo controlled trial. *J Urol* 2002; **167**: 2105–8.
30 Wade M, Sinclair R. Reversible painful gynaecomastia induced by low dose finasteride. *Australas J Dermatol* 2000; **41**:111–2.
31 Ferrando J, Grimalt R, Alsina M, Bulla F, Manasievska E. Unilateral gynecomastia induced by treatment with 1 mg of oral finasteride. *Arch Dermatol* 2002; **138**: 543–4.
32 Thompson IM, Goodman PJ, Tanger CM *et al.* The influence of finasteride on the development of prostate cancer. *N Engl J Med* 2003; **349**: 215–24.
33 DeVillez R, Jacobs J, Szpunar M *et al.* Androgenetic alopecia in the female: treatment with 2% minoxidil solution. *Arch Dermatol* 1994; **130**: 303–7.
34 Sinclair RD, Dawber RPR. Androgenetic alopecia in men and women. *Clin Dermatol* 2001; **19**: 167–78.

35 Olsen EA. Androgenetic alopecia. In: Olsen EA, ed. *Disorders of Hair Growth: Diagnosis and Treatment*. New York: McGraw-Hill, 1994.

36 Young R, Sinclair RD. Continuing medical education: hirsutes. II. *Australas J Dermatol* 1998; **39**: 151–7.

37 Burke BM, Cunliffe WJ. Oral spironolactone for female patients with acne, hirsutism or androgenetic alopecia. *Br J Dermatol* 1985; **112**: 124–5.

38 Adamopoulos DA, Karamertzanis M, Nickopoulou S, Gregoriou A. Beneficial effect of spironolactone on androgenetic alopecia. *Clin Endocrinol* 1997; **47**: 759–61.

39 Shaw JC. Spironolactone in dermatological therapy. *J Am Acad Dermatol* 1991; **24**: 236–43.

40 Barker DJP. The epidemiological evidence relating to spironolactone and malignant disease in man. *J Drug Develop* 1987; **1** (Suppl. 2): 22–5.

41 Thai KE, Sinclair RD. Spironolactone-induced hepatitis. *Australas J Dermatol* 2001; **42**: 180–2.

42 Neuman F. Pharmacological basis for clinical use of antiandrogens. *J Steroid Biochem* 1983; **19**: 391–402.

43 Pereboom-Wynia JD, van der Willigen AH, van Joost T, Stolz E. The effects of cyproterone acetate on hair roots and hair shaft diameter in androgenetic alopecia in females. *Acta Derm Venereol* 1989; **69**: 395–8.

44 Vexiau P, Chaspoux C, Boudou P *et al.* Effects of minoxidil 2% vs cyproterone acetate treatment of female androgenetic alopecia: a controlled 12 month randomized trial. *Br J Dermatol* 2002; **146**: 992–9.

45 Barth H, Cherry CA, Wojnarowska F. Cyproterone acetate for severe hirsutism: results of a double-blind dose-ranging study. *J Clin Endocrinol* 1991; **35**: 5–10.

46 Dawber RPR, Sonnex T, Ralfs I. Oral antiandrogen treatment of common baldness in women. *Br J Dermatol* 1982; **107** (Suppl. 22): 20.

47 Van Wayjen RG, Van den Ende A. Experience in the long-term treatment of patients with hirsutism and/or acne with cyproterone acetate-containing preparations: efficacy, metabolic and endocrine effects. *Exp Clin Endocrinol Diabetes* 1995; **103**: 241–51.

48 Mallari R, Sinclair RD. Shortness of breath: an uncommon side-effect of cyproterone acetate in the treatment of androgenetic alopecia. *Int J Dermatol* 2002; **41**: 946–7.

49 Carmina E, Lobo RA. Treatment of hyperandrogenetic alopecia in women. *Fertil Steril* 2003; **79**: 91–5.

50 Roberts J, Hordinsky M, Olsen E *et al.* The effects of finasteride on postmenopausal women with androgenetic alopecia. Hair Workshop, Brussels, May 2–5, 1998 (Abstr).

51 Thai KE, Sinclair RD. Finasteride for female androgenetic alopecia. *Br J Dermatol* 2002; **147**: 1–2.

52 Shum KW, Cullen DR, Messenger AG. Hair loss in women with hyperandrogenism: four cases responding to finasteride. *J Am Acad Dermatol* 2002; **47**: 733–9.

Disturbances of hair cycle

Telogen effluvium
SYN. TELOGEN DEFLUVIUM

Definition. The term telogen effluvium, first coined by Kligman in 1961 [1], refers to the loss of club (telogen) hair in disease states of the follicle. Kligman's hypothesis was that whatever the cause of the hair loss, the follicle tends to behave in a similar way; the premature termination of anagen. 'The follicle is precipitated into catagen and transforms into a resting stage that mimics telogen.' The observation of increased telogen hair shedding does not infer a cause. To establish a cause, one requires a history to identify known triggers, biochemical investigation to exclude endocrine, nutritional or autoimmune aetiologies and, in persistent cases, histology to identify the earliest stages of AGA. The duration of the hair shedding at presentation helps predict those patients in whom further investigation will have the greatest yield.

Follicular cycling within anatomical regions is synchronous in infancy, in that all neighbouring hairs grow together, involute together and are shed together, producing a moult wave. Whereas the moult wave persists indefinitely in many animals, in humans synchronous hair growth disappears in childhood. Rather than periodically shedding all 100 000 scalp hairs over the course of a few months, adult humans tend to lose a few hairs each day, and therefore are never normally bald [2].

Scalp trichography reveals 86% of plucked hairs are in anagen, 1% in catagen and 13% are in telogen, whereas data from analysis of horizontal scalp biopsies puts these figures at 93% of follicles in anagen and 7% in telogen [3]. Based on biopsy data, if the average number of scalp hairs is 100 000, then 7000 hairs should be in telogen at any one time. As the approximate duration of telogen is 100 days, 77 hairs should be shed each day, but most people are not aware of shedding anywhere near this amount. Although this number is likely to correspond to the absolute number of hairs that are shed each day, it still remains to be defined what amount is normally noticed and how introspection heightens one's powers of detection [4].

Pathogenesis. Headington [5] described five functional types of telogen effluvium based on different phases of the follicular cycle: immediate anagen release, delayed anagen release, short anagen syndrome, immediate telogen release and delayed telogen release.

Immediate anagen release is a short-onset effluvium where follicles are stimulated to leave anagen and enter telogen prematurely, resulting in increased hair shedding at the end of telogen approximately 2–3 months later. It is common after a physiological stress such as severe illness, and with drug-induced hair loss. Reversal is associated with resumption of the normal cycle. Delayed anagen release is the cause of postpartum hair loss. During pregnancy, hairs remain in prolonged anagen rather than cycling into telogen. If a large number of follicles are involved, postpartum telogen conversion will be accompanied by increased shedding some months later. Short anagen syndrome is caused by an idiopathic shortening of the duration of anagen and can cause a persistent telogen hair shedding in some individuals [5].

It is not known precisely how long a telogen hair remains in the follicle, but it is believed that club hairs are released 4–6 weeks after the onset of anagen. This may explain the different anagen : telogen rates seen on trichogram versus biopsy. Immediate telogen release results from a shortening of normal telogen, with release of club hairs as the follicles are stimulated to re-enter anagen. Drugs such as minoxidil can precipitate immediate telogen release. Delayed telogen release occurs after a prolonged telogen followed by transition to anagen. It occurs in animals with synchronous hair cycles during shedding

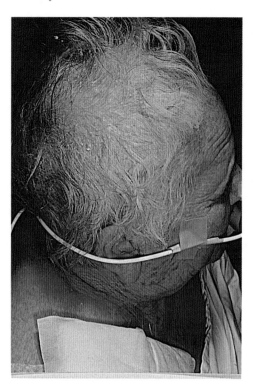

Fig. 63.18 Acute telogen effluvium.

of their winter coats. It may occur seasonally in some humans.

Acute telogen effluvium. Acute telogen effluvium is an acute-onset scalp hair loss that occurs 2–3 months after a triggering event such as a high fever, surgical trauma, sudden starvation or haemorrhage [2,4–6]. In approximately 33% of cases of acute telogen effluvium, no trigger can be identified. Acute telogen effluvium is commonly attributed to emotional stress, but the evidence for this is weak and there is no evidence that suggests the stresses of everyday life are sufficient to induce diffuse hair loss. The functional mechanism of shedding is immediate anagen release.

The patient may be particularly aware of increased loss on the brush or comb, or during shampooing. The daily loss ranges from under 100 to over 1000. If the lower rates of shedding are continued for only a short period there may be no obvious baldness, but if shedding occurs at higher rates, diffuse reduction in hair density is produced (Fig. 63.18). It may be severe but is never total. Unless the trigger is repeated, spontaneous complete regrowth occurs within 3–6 months. The proportion of follicles affected, and hence the severity of the subsequent alopecia, depends partly on the duration and severity of the precipitating cause and partly on unexplained individual variations in susceptibility.

Telogen gravidarum refers to the telogen hair loss seen 2–3 months after childbirth [7,8]. It is an example of delayed anagen release. It is universal to some degree, but is often subclinical. Most cases of telogen gravidarum resolve; however, a small proportion of women may experience persistent episodic shedding that may be diffuse or localized. It has been suggested that after pregnancy some hairs may not revert to an asynchronous growth pattern seen in normal adult hair follicles [5]. A similar state of affairs prevails when the contraceptive pill is discontinued after it has been taken continuously for some time [8,9].

Diagnosis. The diagnosis is usually simple. Abrupt-onset telogen effluvium is likely to be related to a specific event or trigger 6–16 weeks earlier. The hair pull test is positive, with normal club hairs. The hair loss is always diffuse and never total. Gradual onset or prolonged hair loss is more difficult to assess. Increased shedding of club hairs is a variable but often very obvious symptom of early AGA. Other differential diagnoses are discussed below under the heading of chronic diffuse telogen hair loss.

The hair pull test is notoriously difficult to interpret. In acute telogen effluvium, it is usually strongly positive for telogen hairs at the vertex and the scalp margins. However, a negative hair pull test does not exclude the diagnosis of telogen effluvium [10]. The trichogram from a hair pluck sample usually shows more than 25% of telogen hairs in acute telogen effluvium [2]. When an obvious explanation exists for a recent-onset telogen effluvium, expectant management and observation is appropriate. Shedding can be expected to cease within 3–6 months and thereafter recovery should be complete [2]. Histological examination shows no abnormality other than an increase in the proportion of follicles in telogen.

REFERENCES

1 Kligman AM. The human hair cycle. *J Invest Dermatol* 1959; **33**: 307–16.
2 Kligman AM. Pathologic dynamics of human hair loss. I. Telogen effluvium. *Arch Dermatol* 1961; **83**: 175–98.
3 Whiting DA. Chronic telogen effluvium. *Dermatol Clin* 1996; **14**: 723–31.
4 Harrison S, Sinclair RD. Telogen effluvium. *Clin Exp Dermatol* 2002; **27**: 389–95.
5 Headington JT. Telogen effluvium: new concepts and review. *Arch Dermatol* 1993; **129**: 556–8.
6 Dawber RPR, Simpson NB, Barth JH. Diffuse alopecia: endocrine, metabolic and chemical influences on the follicular cycle. In: Dawber RPR, ed. *Diseases of the Hair and Scalp*. Oxford: Blackwell Science, 1997: 123–50.
7 Schiff BL, Kern AB. Study of postpartum alopecia. *Arch Dermatol* 1963; **87**: 609–11.
8 Dawber RPR, Connor BL. Pregnancy, hair loss and the pill. *BMJ* 1971; **iv**: 234–5.
9 Griffiths WAD. Diffuse hair loss and oral contraceptives. *Br J Dermatol* 1973; **88**: 31–6.
10 Chong AH, Wade M, Sinclair RD. The hair pull test and hair pluck for analysis of hair abnormalities. *Mod Med Aust* 1999; **42**: 105–8.

Chronic diffuse telogen hair loss. A short-lived insult usually produces a sudden-onset diffuse shedding. If the insult is prolonged or repeated, shedding can develop insidiously. Chronic diffuse telogen hair loss refers to telogen hair shedding persisting for longer than 6 months. It can be a result of a primary chronic telogen effluvium or be secondary to a variety of causes. To be a true cause of chronic diffuse telogen hair loss, the relationship between the trigger and the hair loss must be reversible and reproducible. The requirements of proof include exclusion of other known causes of shedding, in particular AGA, reversal of the hair loss following correction of the causative factor, and relapse on rechallenge.

Accepted causes of chronic diffuse telogen hair loss are thyroid disorders (Fig. 63.19), profound iron deficiency anaemia, acrodermatitis enteropathica and malnutrition [1]. Both hyperthyroidism and hypothyroidism (including drug-induced hypothyroidism) cause a diffuse telogen hair loss in approximately 50% and 33% of patients, respectively [2,3]. The mechanism of telogen hair shedding in thyroid disorders still remains unclear [4]. Hair loss is reversible when the euthyroid state is restored, except in long-standing hypothyroidism where the hair follicles are said to have atrophied [3]. If replacement therapy fails to correct the hair loss, alternate causes should be sought [5].

Profound iron-deficiency anaemia can cause a diffuse telogen hair loss that is corrected by iron replacement. It is thought that hair follicles that have shed their hair at the end of telogen may temporarily fail to re-enter anagen —leading to a slow-onset diffuse hair loss [6]. The relationship between iron deficiency with no anaemia or only mild anaemia and chronic diffuse hair loss is, however, more complex and controversial [7–9]. Depending on how it is defined, low iron stores are a common finding in women of child-bearing age. AGA is also common in this age group and the shedding in the early stages of female AGA can be diffuse and episodic, and mimic a telogen effluvium. It is important not to focus on the treatment of a subclinical iron deficiency while neglecting the underlying AGA, especially when therapy for female AGA is more reliable in arresting hair loss than stimulating regrowth. It is not uncommon for women presenting with increased telogen hair shedding caused by AGA to co-incidentally have low iron stores. As the telogen hair loss in AGA can be episodic, it may even appear to abate with iron replacement. However, in patients with AGA the shedding tends to be chronic and relapsing, and recovery is generally incomplete. A punch biopsy can usually clarify the diagnosis.

Acrodermatitis enteropathica and acquired zinc deficiency (Fig. 63.20) brought about by long-standing parenteral nutrition can lead to a severe telogen effluvium [1,10]. However, low zinc levels found on routine blood biochemistry screening in patients being investigated for diffuse telogen hair loss are probably an incidental finding. Diffuse hair loss alone, with no other symptoms or signs, is never a result of dietary zinc deficiency [9]. Correction of a subclinical zinc deficiency often does not stop

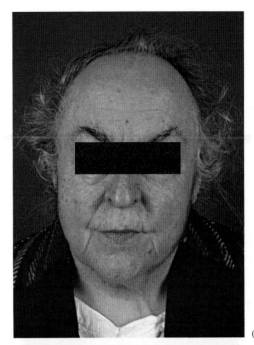

(a)

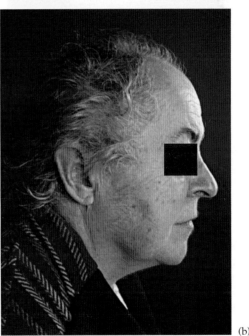

(b)

Fig. 63.19 Diffuse alopecia in association with hypothyroidism.

the increased hair shedding, and other forms of alopecia such as AGA or chronic telogen effluvium should be considered.

Crash dieting with severe protein-calorie restriction can precipitate hair loss [11,12]. Chronic starvation, especially marasmus, causes a diffuse telogen hair loss often accompanied by hair shaft abnormalities [13]. Hypoproteinaemia of metabolic as well as dietary origin can cause hair loss [1]. Pancreatic disease and other forms of

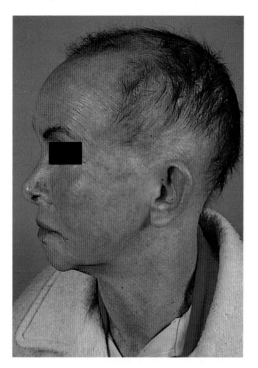

Fig. 63.20 Acquired zinc deficiency resulting from prolonged parenteral feeding and inadequate zinc supplementation.

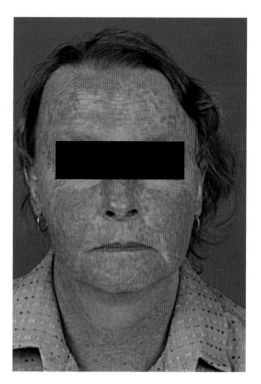

Fig. 63.21 Hair loss and photosensitivity caused by systemic lupus erythematosus.

malabsorption also cause a diffuse telogen hair loss [14], as do the essential fatty acid deficiencies seen in prolonged parenteral nutrition and hypervitaminosis A [15,16]. Metabolic disturbances such as liver disorders [1,17] and chronic renal failure can produce sparse scalp hair [18]. Hair loss in advanced malignant disease may be a result of hypoproteinaemia rather than the malignancy itself, but alopecia has occurred as an early sign of Hodgkin's disease [19]. Systemic lupus erythematosus (Fig. 63.21) and dermatomyositis can also cause telogen hair loss [20]. Diffuse hair loss may occur in secondary syphilis, but the characteristic moth-eaten appearance is not always present [21].

Drug-induced diffuse telogen hair loss usually starts 6–12 weeks after instigation of treatment and is progressive while the drug is continued [22,23]. It is most commonly a result of immediate anagen release [6]. The diagnosis of drug-induced telogen hair loss is made by demonstrating compatible chronology of drug exposure and the onset of the hair loss, and exclusion of the other causes of alopecia. Shedding can recur with drugs that are chemically unrelated, suggesting that true cross-reactivity is rare, and individual susceptibility exists to drug-induced telogen effluvium. CTE and AGA are important differential diagnoses. If a particular drug is suspected, testing involves stopping it for at least 3 months. Regrowth following discontinuation and recurrence on re-exposure to the drug supports the conclusion that the drug caused the alopecia. Many drugs have been said to cause a diffuse telogen hair loss but few have fulfilled the above criteria. A dose-related diffuse telogen hair loss is common with etretinate [24] and acitretin, but less common with isotretinoin. The retinoids appear to cause a telogen anchorage defect and reduce the duration of anagen. Occasionally, continued shedding is noted after retinoid-induced telogen effluvium, but such cases may be caused by coincidental AGA. Minoxidil has been reported to cause a short-lived telogen shedding by immediate telogen release [6,25].

REFERENCES

1 Dawber RPR, Simpson NB, Barth JH. Diffuse alopecia: endocrine, metabolic and chemical influences on the follicular cycle. In: Dawber RPR, ed. *Diseases of the Hair and Scalp.* Oxford: Blackwell Science, 1997: 123–50.
2 Rook A. Endocrine influences on hair growth. *BMJ* 1965; **1**: 609–14.
3 Church RE. Hypothyroid hair loss. *Br J Dermatol* 1956; **77**: 661–3.
4 Messenger AG. Thyroid hormone and hair growth. *Br J Dermatol* 2000; **142**: 631–5.
5 Sinclair R. Diffuse hair loss. *Int J Dermatol* 1999; **38** (Suppl. 1): 8–18.
6 Headington J. Telogen effluvium. New concepts and review. *Arch Dermatol* 1993; **129**: 356–63.
7 Rushton DH, Ramsey ID, James KC *et al.* Biochemical and trichological characterization of diffuse alopecia in women. *Br J Dermatol* 1990; **123**: 187–97.
8 Hard S. Non-anemic iron deficiency as an etiologic factor in diffuse hair loss of hair of the scalp in women. *Acta Derm Venereol (Stockh)* 1963; **43**: 562–9.
9 Sinclair R. There is no clear association between low serum ferritin and chronic diffuse telogen hair loss. *Br J Dermatol.* 2002; **147**: 982–4.
10 Weismann K. Zinc metabolism and the skin. In: Rook A, Savin J, eds. *Recent Advances in Dermatology*, 5th edn. Edinburgh: Churchill Livingstone, 1980: 109–29.

11 Goette DK, Odom RB. Alopecia in crash dieters. *JAMA* 1976; **235**: 2622–3.
12 Kaufman JP. Telogen effluvium secondary to starvation diet. *Arch Dermatol* 1976; **112**: 731–7.
13 Bradfield RB, Bailley MA. Hair root response to protein undernutrition. In: Montagna W, Dobson RC, eds. *Advances in Biology of the Skin,* Vol. IX. *Hair Growth.* Oxford: Pergamon, 1968: 109–11.
14 Wells G. Skin disorders in relation to malabsorption. *BMJ* 1962; **ii**: 937.
15 Skolnik P, Eaglstein WH, Ziboh VA. Human essential fatty acid deficiency. *Arch Dermatol* 1977; **113**: 939–41.
16 Stimson WH. Vitamin A intoxication in adults: report of a case with a summary of the literature. *N Engl J Med* 1961; **265**: 369–73.
17 Starzel TE, Putman CW, Groth CG, Corman JL, Taubman J. Alopecia ascites and incomplete regeneration after 85–95% liver resection. *Am J Surg* 1975; **129**: 587–8.
18 Scoggins RB, Harlan WR. Cutaneous manifestations of hyperlipidaemia and uraemia. *Postgrad Med J* 1967; **41**: 357–8.
19 Klein AW, Rudolf RI, Leydon JJ. Telogen effluvium as a sign of Hodgkin's disease. *Arch Dermatol* 1973; **108**: 702–3.
20 Dawber RPR, Simpson NB. Hair and scalp in systemic disease. In: Dawber RPR, ed. *Diseases of the Hair and Scalp.* Oxford: Blackwell Science, 1997: 483–527.
21 Kennedy C. Syphilis presenting as hair loss. *BMJ* 1976; **ii**: 854.
22 Brodin MB. Drug-related alopecia. *Dermatol Clin* 1987; **5**: 571–9.
23 Feidler VC, Gray AC. Diffuse alopecia: telogen hair loss. In: Olsen E, ed. *Disorders of Hair Growth, Diagnosis and Treatment,* 2nd edn. New York: McGraw-Hill, 2003: 3003–20.
24 Gupta AK, Goldfarb MT, Ellis CN, Vorhees JJ. Side-effect profile of acitretin therapy in psoriasis. *J Am Acad Dermatol* 1989; **20**: 1088–93.
25 Bardelli A, Rebora A. Telogen effluvium and minoxidil. *J Am Acad Dermatol* 1989; **21**: 572–3.

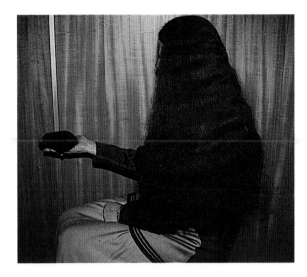

Fig. 63.22 Idiopathic chronic telogen effluvium.

Chronic telogen effluvium. CTE has become a term used to describe a pattern of presentation in middle-aged women that is distinct from androgenetic hair loss and is distinguished from chronic diffuse telogen effluvium and its organic causes [1,2]. It is described as an idiopathic self-limiting condition with increased telogen shedding of at least 6 months' duration, but with no widening of the central parting, and no miniaturization of hair follicles on scalp biopsy [1]. CTE contrasts with acute telogen effluvium by its prolonged fluctuating course and much less frequent occurrence. It is common in females between 30 and 50 years of age [2]. Hair shedding is much less obvious in males with short hair, and for unknown reasons few males with long hair present with increased hair shedding [3]. Although some cases of CTE follow an acute telogen effluvium with a known trigger, such as pregnancy or systemic illness, in most cases a trigger cannot be identified. Any of the functional types of telogen effluvium could account for CTE, but it is believed to be related to shortening of the anagen phase of the hair cycle [4].

The diagnosis of CTE is made by exclusion of other causes of diffuse telogen hair loss. A thorough history is required, including a detailed drug and dietary history. A full clinical examination should be performed, including scalp examination and hair pull testing. The routine work-up includes full blood count and thyroid function tests. Syphilis serology, antinuclear antibody titre, serum zinc levels and other investigations of nutritional status should be performed if clinically warranted.

Affected women commonly present with persistent severe shedding that runs a fluctuating course over several years [4] (Fig. 63.22). They often give a history of the ability to grow their hair very long in childhood, suggestive of a long anagen phase, and report a high hair density prior to the onset of hair loss [5,6]. They usually have a negative family history of AGA. Clinical examination reveals marked bitemporal recession, but no widening of the central hair parting, which if present would support the diagnosis of AGA. However, these criteria are not absolute, and AGA can mimic this presentation. A positive hair pull test is common over the vertex and occipital scalp, and patients may describe a reduction in the thickness of their ponytail volume, stating it has decreased by up to 50% [4]. A negative hair pull test does not exclude the diagnosis of CTE.

CTE has to be distinguished clinically from AGA as women with early AGA may present with periods of increased hair shedding without a discernible pattern to the loss. The mechanism of increased hair shedding in AGA is probably related to shortening of the anagen duration [7]. In an evaluation of 600 women presenting with chronic diffuse telogen hair shedding with little or no reduction of visible hair density, 60% were found on scalp biopsy to have hair miniaturization consistent with a diagnosis of AGA and 40% had CTE [8].

The natural history, prognosis and treatment of CTE and AGA differ [9]. The diagnosis of CTE can usually be suspected from the history and examination, but scalp biopsy is required to differentiate reliably between the two conditions [1]. The optimal scalp biopsy is a 4-mm punch biopsy taken from the vertex of the scalp for horizontal embedding. The vertex is the chosen site because AGA is a patterned disease that preferentially affects the vertex of the scalp, so diagnostic yields are greatest in this area. Histology of a scalp biopsy in CTE resembles normal scalp, but shows an anagen : telogen ratio of 8 : 1

compared with the ratio of 14 : 1 on normal scalp biopsies [1]. The total number of hairs in CTE is the same as that found in normal scalps and the terminal : vellus-like hair (miniaturized) ratio is similar in both, averaging eight terminal hairs per vellus-like hair [1]. These findings differ considerably from AGA. The mean terminal : vellus-like hair ratio in AGA is 1.9 : 1 [1].

Despite the assertion that CTE is a self-limiting process that does not evolve into AGA, its natural history remains poorly characterized, with only one published longitudinal study [9].

REFERENCES

1 Whiting DA. Chronic telogen effluvium. *Dermatol Clin* 1996; **14**: 723–73.
2 Whiting DA. Chronic telogen effluvium: increased scalp hair shedding in middle aged women. *J Am Acad Dermatol* 1996; **35**: 899–906.
3 Thai KE, Sinclair RD. Chronic telogen effluvium in a man. *J Am Acad Dermatol* 2002; **47**: 605–7.
4 Headington J. Telogen effluvium. New concepts and review. *Arch Dermatol* 1993; **129**: 356–63.
5 Sinclair, R. Diffuse hair loss. *Int J Dermatol* 1999; **38** (Suppl. 1): 8–18.
6 Rushton DH, Ramsey ID, James KC *et al.* Biochemical and trichological characterization of diffuse alopecia in women. *Br J Dermatol* 1990; **123**: 187–97.
7 Ludwig E. Classification of the types of androgenetic alopecia (common baldness) arising in the female sex. *Br J Dermatol* 1977; **97**: 247–54.
8 Sinclair R, Jolley D, Mallari R *et al.* Morphological approach to hair disorders. *J Invest Dermatol Symp Proc* 2003; **8**: 56.
9 Sinclair R. Chronic telogen effluvium: a study of 5 patients over 7 years. *J Am Acad Dermatol* (in press).

Alopecia in central nervous system disorders

Alopecia has been described in association with a number of diseases of the central nervous system, but in many instances the association was probably fortuitous. There are four forms of hair loss in which the association appears to be valid, although the mechanism is unknown.
1 Total and permanent alopecia has accompanied lesions of the mid-brain and brainstem [1]—a glioma in the region of the hypothalamus or post-encephalitic damage to the mid-brain.
2 Temporary diffuse alopecia may follow head injuries, particularly in children [2], and may be associated with reversible hirsutism.
3 Total loss of hair occurred at approximately annual intervals for 20 years in a patient with syringomyelia and syringobulbia [3].
4 Androgenetic baldness occurs early in myotonic dystrophy [4]. A genetic linkage rather than a direct effect of the neurological changes is probably concerned.

Piloerection [5]

Episodes of piloerection may occur in patients with lesions close to the hypothalamus or involving some portion of the limbic system, but the symptom has no precise localizing value.

REFERENCES

1 Hoff H, Riehl G. Alopecia in lesions of the midbrain and brain stem. *Arch Dermatol Syphilol* 1937; **176**: 196–9.
2 Tarnow G. Diffuse alopecia following a head injury. *Neurovis Relat* 1971; **X** (Suppl.): 549–51.
3 Mikula F, Stiedl L. Total alopecia in syringomyelia and syringobulbia. *Dermatol Wochenschr* 1961; **143**: 543–5.
4 Waring JJ, Walker CE. Studies in dystrophia myotonica. *Ann Intern Med* 1940; **65**: 763–99.
5 Brody LA. Piloerection associated with hypothalamic lesions. *Neurology* 1960; **10**: 993–4.

Alopecia areata
[A.G. Messenger, pp. 63.36–63.46]

Alopecia areata is a chronic inflammatory disease that involves the hair follicle and sometimes the nails. Current evidence indicates that hair follicle inflammation in alopecia areata is caused by a T-cell-mediated autoimmune mechanism occurring in genetically predisposed individuals. Environmental factors may be responsible for triggering the disease.

In the only formal population study of alopecia areata, from Olmsted County, Minnesota, USA, the incidence rate was 0.1–0.2% with a projected lifetime risk of 1.7% [1]. Several large case series of alopecia areata have been reported from Europe [2], North America [3,4] and Asia [5,6], but these have generally been drawn from hospital clinic attenders and no accurate indication of variation in disease rates between populations is available.

Aetiology

Genetic factors

The importance of genetic factors in alopecia areata is underlined by the high frequency of a positive family history in affected individuals [7]. In most reports, this ranges from 10 to 20% of cases, but mild cases are often overlooked or concealed and the true figure may be greater. The lifetime risk of alopecia areata in the children of a proband is approximately 6% [8]. Price and Colombe [9] found a family history of alopecia areata was more common in those with disease onset before the age of 30 years (37% compared with 7.1% in patients with onset after 30 years). There have been several case reports of alopecia areata in twins [10–12], but only a single study looking at concordance rates in monozygotic and dizygotic pairs [13]. In this investigation, there was a concordance rate of 55% for alopecia amongst monozygotic twins with no concordance among the dizygotic pairs. However, the numbers studied were insufficient to allow a precise estimate of the genetic contribution in alopecia areata. Except in occasional families, alopecia areata is not inherited in a simple Mendelian fashion and the genetic basis appears to be multifactorial.

Major histocompatibility complex genes. No consistent associations with MHC class I antigens have been reported, but several studies have shown an association between alopecia areata and the MHC class II antigens HLA-DR4, DR11 (DR5) and DQ3. Earlier studies using serological typing techniques suggested that DR4 and DR5 were associated with severe forms of alopecia areata [7]. This severity association was subsequently confirmed by molecular typing. Colombe *et al.* [14] found an increase in the broad antigen DQ3 in all patients in their study, suggesting this may act as a susceptibility factor. The DQB1*0301 allele (a subtype of DQ3 that is in linkage disequilibrium with DR5) was associated with severe alopecia but not with newly diagnosed patchy disease. There was also a strong association between alopecia totalis and universalis and the DR11 allele DRB1*1104 (relative risk 30.2), which was absent in milder disease. The association with DQB1*0301 had previously been reported by Morling *et al.* [15] and Welsh *et al.* [16]. The latter group also showed an increase in the frequency of DQ3, which was greater in alopecia totalis and universalis than in patchy alopecia. De Andrade *et al.* [17] confirmed the importance of DQB1*03 alleles, which were present in 85% of alopecia areata patients compared with 46% of controls. In the only family-based study of HLA association and linkage in alopecia areata, these authors reported an association between alleles of HLA-DQB1*0302, *0601, *0603 and HLA-DR4, DR6 using the transmission disequilibrium test [17]. Linkage analysis in 75 families supported linkage between alopecia areata and HLA class II loci, with maximal LOD scores of 2.42 for HLA-DQB at 5% recombination and 2.34 for HLA-DR at 0% recombination.

Cytokine genes. IL-1 is a primary cytokine involved in mediating inflammatory responses. The IL-1 gene cluster on chromosome 2 includes genes for the pro-inflammatory IL-1 proteins, their cell membrane receptors, the anti-inflammatory IL-1 receptor antagonist (*IL1RN*) and its homologue, *IL1F5* (*IL1L1*). Associations between the severity of alopecia areata and polymorphisms in *IL1RN* and *IL1F5* have been reported [18,19]. *IL1RN* variants are also associated with the severity of several other inflammatory autoimmune diseases, including ulcerative colitis, lichen sclerosus, psoriasis, myasthenia gravis, multiple sclerosis and rheumatoid disease. However, a later family-based study by Barahamani *et al.* [20] using 131 trios, failed to confirm the association of *IL1RN* genotypes with alopecia universalis.

Like IL-1, TNF-α has a potent inhibitory effect on hair growth *in vitro* [21]. TNF-α is encoded by a gene in the HLA class III region and a polymorphism of this gene has been shown to be strongly associated with certain autoimmune/inflammatory diseases including systemic lupus erythematosus (SLE), rheumatoid arthritis, dermatitis herpetiformis and coeliac disease. TNF-α polymor-

phisms were investigated in alopecia areata in a small study of 50 cases by Galbraith and Pandey [22], who demonstrated a significant difference in TNF-α genotypes between patients with patchy disease and those with alopecia totalis and universalis. However, there was no difference between disease and control groups overall.

Chromosome 21. The frequency of alopecia areata is increased in Down's syndrome, with up to 8.8% of patients affected [23,24], suggesting possible involvement of genes on chromosome 21. There is an even stronger association with the autosomal recessive disorder autoimmune polyglandular syndrome type 1 (APS-1, autoimmune polyendocrinopathy–candidiasis–ectodermal dystrophy), in which approximately 30% of patients have alopecia areata [25]. The defective gene in APS-1 maps to the Down's critical region on chromosome 21 [26,27]. A potentially functional exonic polymorphism in the APS-1 gene has been associated with alopecia universalis [28].

Atopy. Several studies have reported an association between alopecia areata and atopic disease [4,5,29,30], and have suggested that alopecia areata in atopic subjects tends to have an earlier age of onset and be more severe than in non-atopic subjects. However, none of these studies has used a control group to which the same criteria for defining atopy have been applied, and the association has been disputed in a study from India [31].

Autoimmunity

The idea that alopecia areata is an autoimmune disease was first suggested by Rothman following a paper presented by Van Scott [32]. Alopecia areata is associated with other autoimmune diseases, such as myxoedema and pernicious anaemia [4,33]. Intriguingly, the frequency of type 1 diabetes mellitus is increased in the relatives of patients with alopecia areata but not in the patients themselves [34], suggesting that the predisposition to alopecia areata protects against the development of diabetes. In most published series, patients with alopecia areata have had an increased frequency of circulating organ-specific and non-organ-specific autoantibodies compared with normal subjects, and a variety of non-specific abnormalities in peripheral T-cell numbers and function have also been reported (reviewed in [7]). Circulating autoantibodies to hair follicle tissue have been found in patients with alopecia areata [35]. These antibodies also occur in normal subjects but less frequently and at lower titre. They recognize various epithelial compartments within the hair follicle and appear to be targeted against intracellular antigens [36]. Antibody binding has not been demonstrated *in vivo* in humans, and their role in the pathogenesis is unclear. Passive immunization with alopecia areata serum failed to induce hair loss in human skin grafted on to nude mice

[37]. However, one study reported that serum from a horse with alopecia areata-like hair loss caused local inhibition of hair growth when injected into murine skin, whereas serum from a normal horse did not [38].

The most convincing evidence implicating circulating immune factors in the pathogenesis of alopecia areata comes from the transplantation experiments carried out by Gilhar *et al.* They first showed that hair growth recovered in alopecic skin transplanted on to athymic nude mice [39]. In their later experiments (in which SCID rather than athymic nude mice were used as graft recipients), alopecia was induced in grafted skin by the injection of autologous T lymphocytes incubated with hair follicle extracts and antigen-presenting cells [40]. T cells not incubated with hair follicle extracts failed to cause hair loss. Taken together with the immunopathological features of the disease, and with the T-cell depletion studies on the Dundee experimental bald rat (DEBR) model (see below) [41,42], the results of these experiments suggest that alopecia areata is a T-cell-mediated disease.

Environmental factors

The idea that alopecia areata is caused by infection, either directly or as a consequence of a remote 'focus of infection', has a long history and still cannot be ruled out. It was the predominant aetiological theory until well into the twentieth century, and sporadic reports connecting alopecia areata with infective agents continue to appear. Skinner *et al.* [43] reported finding mRNA for cytomegalovirus in alopecic lesions, but this was not confirmed in a subsequent study from Italy [44]. There are also reports of alopecia areata in husband and wife, although this may be coincidence [45,46]. The 'external' factor most frequently implicated in triggering alopecia areata is psychological stress [47–50]. The significance of such an association is difficult to establish because of the problems in performing a controlled investigation. The published evidence is also conflicting, with some studies failing to show any relationship between stressful events and onset of hair loss [51,52], to the extent that no firm conclusion can be reached.

Despite the anecdotal nature of much of the evidence it is possible that environmental factors are responsible for triggering alopecia areata in some patients. If so, it seems likely that a diversity of factors can operate in this way.

REFERENCES

1 Safavi KH, Muller SA, Suman VJ *et al.* Incidence of alopecia areata in Olmsted County, Minnesota, 1975 through 1989. *Mayo Clin Proc* 1995; **70**: 628–33.
2 Gip L, Lodin A, Molin L. Alopecia areata: a follow-up investigation of outpatient material. *Acta Derm Venereol* 1969; **49**: 180–8.
3 Walker SA, Rothman S. Alopecia areata: a statistical study and consideration of endocrine influences. *J Invest Dermatol* 1950; **14**: 403–13.
4 Muller SA, Winkelmann RK. Alopecia areata. *Arch Dermatol* 1963; **88**: 290–7.

5 Ikeda T. A new classification of alopecia areata. *Dermatologica* 1965; **131**: 421–45.
6 Ro BI. Alopecia areata in Korea (1982–1994). *J Dermatol* 1995; **22**: 858–64.
7 McDonagh AJG, Messenger AG. The pathogenesis of alopecia areata. *Dermatol Clin* 1996; **14**: 661–70.
8 van der Steen P, Traupe H, Happle R *et al.* The genetic risk for alopecia areata in first degree relatives of severely affected patients: an estimate. *Acta Derm Venereol* 1992; **72**: 373–5.
9 Price VH, Colombe BW. Heritable factors distinguish two types of alopecia areata. *Dermatol Clin* 1996; **14**: 679–89.
10 Omens DV, Omens HD. Alopecia areata in twins. *Arch Dermatol* 1946; **53**: 193.
11 Hendren OS. Identical alopecia areata in identical twins. *Arch Dermatol* 1949; **60**: 793–5.
12 Weidmann AI, Ziion LS, Mamelok AE. Alopecia areata occurring simultaneously in identical twins. *Arch Dermatol* 1956; **74**: 424–6.
13 Jackow C, Puffer N, Hordinsky M *et al.* Alopecia areata and cytomegalovirus infection in twins: genes versus environment? *J Am Acad Dermatol* 1998; **38**: 418–25.
14 Colombe BW, Price VH, Khoury EL *et al.* HLA class II antigen associations help to define two types of alopecia areata. *J Am Acad Dermatol* 1995; **33**: 757–64.
15 Morling N, Frentz G, Fugger L *et al.* DNA polymorphism of HLA class II genes in alopecia areata. *Dis Markers* 1991; **9**: 35–42.
16 Welsh EA, Clark HH, Epstein SZ *et al.* Human leukocyte antigen-DQB1*03 alleles are associated with alopecia areata. *J Invest Dermatol* 1994; **103**: 758–63.
17 de Andrade M, Jackow CM, Dahm N *et al.* Alopecia areata in families: association with the HLA locus. *J Investig Dermatol Symp Proc* 1999; **4**: 220–3.
18 Tarlow JK, Clay FE, Cork MJ *et al.* Severity of alopecia areata is associated with a polymorphism in the interleukin-1 receptor antagonist gene. *J Invest Dermatol* 1994; **103**: 387–90.
19 Tazi-Ahnini R, Cox A, McDonagh AJ *et al.* Genetic analysis of the interleukin-1 receptor antagonist and its homologue IL-1L1 in alopecia areata: strong severity association and possible gene interaction. *Eur J Immunogenet* 2002; **29**: 25–30.
20 Barahamani N, de Andrade M, Slusser J *et al.* Interleukin-1 receptor antagonist allele 2 and familial alopecia areata. *J Invest Dermatol* 2002; **118**: 335–7.
21 Philpott MP, Sanders DA, Bowen J *et al.* Effects of interleukins, colony-stimulating factor and tumour necrosis factor on human hair follicle growth *in vitro*: a possible role for interleukin-1 and tumour necrosis factor-α in alopecia areata. *Br J Dermatol* 1996; **135**: 942–8.
22 Galbraith GM, Pandey JP. Tumor necrosis factor α (TNF-α) gene polymorphism in alopecia areata. *Hum Genet* 1995; **96**: 433–6.
23 du Vivier A, Munro DD. Alopecia areata, autoimmunity and Down's syndrome. *BMJ* 1975; **i**: 191–2.
24 Carter DM, Jegasothy BV. Alopecia areata and Down syndrome. *Arch Dermatol* 1976; **112**: 1397–9.
25 Betterle C, Greggio NA, Volpato M. Autoimmune polyglandular syndrome type 1. *J Clin Endocrinol Metab* 1998; **83**: 1049–55.
26 The Finnish–German APECED Consortium. An autoimmune disease, APECED, caused by mutations in a novel gene featuring two PHD-type zinc-finger domains. The Finnish–German APECED Consortium. Autoimmune Polyendocrinopathy–Candidiasis–Ectodermal Dystrophy. *Nat Genet* 1997; **17**: 399–403.
27 Nagamine K, Peterson P, Scott HS *et al.* Positional cloning of the APECED gene. *Nat Genet* 1997; **17**: 393–8.
28 Tazi-Ahnini R, Cork MJ, Gawkrodger DJ *et al.* Role of the autoimmune regulator (AIRE) gene in alopecia areata: strong association of a potentially functional AIRE polymorphism with alopecia universalis. *Tissue Antigens* 2002; **60**: 489–95.
29 Penders AJM. Alopecia areata and atopy. *Dermatologica* 1968; **136**: 395–9.
30 Young E, Bruns HM, Berrens L. Alopecia areata and atopy. *Dermatologica* 1978; **156**: 306–8.
31 Sharma VK, Muralidhar S, Kumar B. Reappraisal of Ikeda's classification of alopecia areata: analysis of 356 cases from Chandigarh, India. *J Dermatol* 1998; **25**: 108–11.
32 Van Scott EJ. Morphologic changes in pilosebaceous units and anagen hairs in alopecia areata. *J Invest Dermatol* 1958; **31**: 35–43.
33 Cunliffe WJ, Hall R, Stevenson CJ *et al.* Alopecia areata, thyroid disease and autoimmunity. *Br J Dermatol* 1969; **81**: 877–81.
34 Wang SJ, Shohat T, Vadheim C *et al.* Increased risk for type I (insulin-dependent) diabetes in relatives of patients with alopecia areata (AA). *Am J Med Genet* 1994; **51**: 234–9.

35 Tobin DJ, Orentreich N, Fenton DA *et al*. Antibodies to hair follicles in alopecia areata. *J Invest Dermatol* 1994; **102**: 721–4.

36 Tobin DJ, Hann SK, Song MS *et al*. Hair follicle structures targeted by antibodies in patients with alopecia areata. *Arch Dermatol* 1997; **133**: 57–61.

37 Gilhar A, Pillar T, Assay B *et al*. Failure of passive transfer of serum from patients with alopecia areata and alopecia universalis to inhibit hair growth in transplants of human scalp skin grafted on to nude mice. *Br J Dermatol* 1992; **126**: 166–71.

38 Tobin DJ, Alhaidari Z, Olivry T. Equine alopecia areata autoantibodies target multiple hair follicle antigens and may alter hair growth: a preliminary study. *Exp Dermatol* 1998; **7**: 289–97.

39 Gilhar A, Krueger GG. Hair growth in scalp grafts from patients with alopecia areata and alopecia universalis grafted onto nude mice. *Arch Dermatol* 1987; **123**: 44–50.

40 Gilhar A, Ullmann Y, Berkutzki T *et al*. Autoimmune hair loss (alopecia areata) transferred by T lymphocytes to human scalp explants on SCID mice. *J Clin Invest* 1998; **101**: 62–7.

41 McElwee KJ, Spiers EM, Oliver RF. *In vivo* depletion of CD8+ T cells restores hair growth in the DEBR model for alopecia areata. *Br J Dermatol* 1996; **135**: 211–7.

42 McElwee KJ, Spiers EM, Oliver RF. Partial restoration of hair growth in the DEBR model for alopecia areata after *in vivo* depletion of CD4+ T cells. *Br J Dermatol* 1999; **140**: 432–7.

43 Skinner RB, Jr, Light WH, Bale GF *et al*. Alopecia areata and presence of cytomegalovirus DNA. *JAMA* 1995; **273**: 1419–20.

44 Tosti A, La Placa M, Placucci F *et al*. No correlation between cytomegalovirus and alopecia areata. *J Invest Dermatol* 1996; **107**: 443.

45 Swift S. Folie a deux? Simultaneous alopecia areata in a husband and wife. *Arch Dermatol* 1961; **84**: 94–6.

46 Zalka AD, Byarlay JA, Goldsmith LA. Alopecia à deux: simultaneous occurrence of alopecia in a husband and wife. *Arch Dermatol* 1994; **130**: 390–2.

47 Anderson I. Alopecia areata: a clinical study. *BMJ* 1950; **ii**: 1250–2.

48 Greenberg SI. Alopecia areata: a psychiatric survey. *Arch Dermatol* 1955; **72**: 454–7.

49 De Waard-van der Spek FB, Oranje AP, De Raeymaecker DM *et al*. Juvenile versus maturity-onset alopecia areata: a comparative retrospective clinical study. *Clin Exp Dermatol* 1989; **14**: 429–33.

50 Gupta MA, Gupta AK, Watteel GN. Stress and alopecia areata: a psychodermatologic study. *Acta Derm Venereol* 1997; **77**: 296–8.

51 MacAlpine I. Is alopecia areata psychosomatic? *Br J Dermatol* 1958; **70**: 117–31.

52 van der Steen P, Boezeman J, Duller P *et al*. Can alopecia areata be triggered by emotional stress? An uncontrolled evaluation of 178 patients with extensive hair loss. *Acta Derm Venereol* 1992; **72**: 279–80.

Pathogenesis

Pathology

Anagen follicles at the margins of expanding patches of alopecia areata characteristically show a perifollicular and intrafollicular inflammatory cell infiltrate, concentrated in and around the hair bulb (Fig. 63.23). The inflammatory infiltrate is composed mainly of activated T lymphocytes, with a preponderance of CD4 cells, and an admixture of macrophages and Langerhans' cells [1,2]. In contrast with the inflammatory scarring alopecias, little or none of the inflammatory infiltrate is seen around the isthmus of the hair follicle, the site for hair follicle stem cells [3]. This may explain why follicles are not destroyed in alopecia areata. Lymphocytic infiltration of the dermal papilla and bulbar epithelium may be accompanied by increased expression of HLA class I and II antigens and of intercellular adhesion molecule-1 (ICAM-1) [4–6], which are thought to be secondary to the local release of T-cell cytokines. Normal

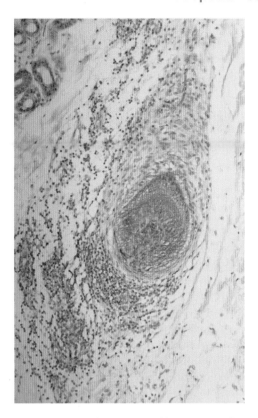

Fig. 63.23 Lymphocytic inflammatory infiltrate surrounding an anagen hair bulb in alopecia areata.

numbers of follicles are found in established bald patches and in alopecia universalis. Both anagen and telogen follicles are found in these sites, with a higher proportion in telogen than in normal scalp. Follicles are smaller than normal and anagen follicles do not develop beyond the Anagen 3–4 stage, when the hair shaft starts to be formed [7]. The inflammatory infiltrate tends to be less pronounced than in early lesions and is associated mainly with anagen follicles.

Pathodynamics

Eckert *et al*. [8] studied anagen : telogen ratios in hairs plucked from demarcated concentric zones around the periphery of expanding bald patches. They concluded that the initial event in alopecia areata is precipitation of anagen follicles into telogen. Less severely affected follicles may remain in anagen for a time but they produce a dystrophic hair and eventually also undergo telogen conversion. In keeping with these observations, biopsies from the margins of expanding lesions of alopecia areata show most follicles in catagen or telogen [9]. It is not clear whether follicles attain telogen via normal catagen. Exclamation mark hairs may have a well-formed club root identical to that of a normal telogen hair. However, the root is frequently narrowed and club hairs fall out more

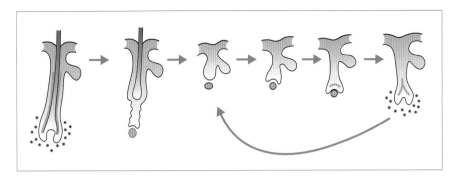

Fig. 63.24 Proposed pathodynamic changes in alopecia areata. An inflammatory attack on anagen follicles precipitates follicles into telogen. Follicles re-enter anagen but development is halted in Anagen 3–4 and follicles return to telogen prematurely.

readily than normal, suggesting that anchoring of the hair within the follicle is defective.

Van Scott [7] studied biopsies from patches of alopecia areata and found an average of 58% of follicles in anagen, suggesting that re-entry into anagen takes place. In early lesions there was a reduction in the size of the lower follicle, with preservation of the upper part of the follicle and the sebaceous gland. In long-standing disease, the entire follicle became smaller. The matrix of these miniaturized anagen follicles was mitotically active and produced a normal inner root sheath. However, the cortex was incompletely keratinized. Van Scott interpreted these changes as indicating arrest of follicle development in Anagen 4. A later study supported these findings and proposed that, while the disease is active, follicles are unable to develop beyond Anagen 3–4 and then return prematurely to telogen (Fig. 63.24) [9]. Follicles may pass through repeated truncated cycles until the disease activity subsides, and are then able to progress further into anagen.

Except in very long-standing alopecia, hair follicles are retained, even in clinically hairless scalp. When alopecia areata has persisted for many years, particularly in the universal form, there may be a decline in follicle density, possibly associated with fibrosis of the perifollicular connective tissues.

The hair follicle target

The inflammatory infiltrate in alopecia areata is concentrated in and around the bulbar region of anagen hair follicles. Cells of several different types and differentiation pathways are found in the hair bulb, but which of these is the primary focus of the pathology is unknown. Trichocytes in the hair bulb matrix undergoing early cortical differentiation may show vacuolar degeneration (Fig. 63.25) [10,11] and are also the predominant cell type showing aberrant class I and II MHC expression [4]. However, increased MHC expression is also seen in the dermal papilla, and pathological changes have been described in dermal papillae in clinically non-lesional sites [12]. Hence, it is possible that changes in the epithelial compartment of the hair follicle are secondary to dysfunction of the dermal papilla. The sparing of white hair sometimes seen in

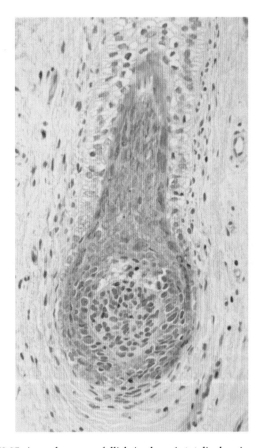

Fig. 63.25 An early anagen follicle in alopecia totalis showing vacuolation in the hair matrix epithelium around the upper pole of the dermal papilla.

alopecia areata has raised the possibility that alopecia areata is primarily a disease of hair bulb melanocytes. Alopecia areata may show other pigmentary features including reduced pigmentation in regrowing hairs and an association with vitiligo [13,14]. However, the melanocyte hypothesis does not explain why sparing of white hair is often a relative phenomenon and is sometimes absent.

Animal models

Alopecia areata occurs in mammals other than humans, including chimps, dogs, horses, rats and mice. Two rodent strains, in which alopecia areata is common, the Dundee experimental bald rat (DEBR) and the CH3/HeJ mouse, have been used as experimental models of the disease.

Dundee experimental bald rat

In this strain of the brown hooded rat, animals grow a normal first coat of hair but then become progressively hairless [15]. Skin histological examination confirms the persistence of hair follicles, mostly in a dystrophic anagen state. Perifollicular and intrafollicular lymphocytic infiltration is a prominent feature and vacuolar degeneration occurs in the cortex of some lesional anagen follicles. Increased expression of HLA class I and II molecules in the dermal papilla and precortical matrix is seen in a pattern similar to human alopecia areata [16]. Hair regrowth in DEBR alopecia can be stimulated by photochemotherapy (PUVA), topical minoxidil, systemic ciclosporin [17] and topical tacrolimus [18]. Partial regrowth can also be induced by depletion of circulating CD4 or CD8 cells using monoclonal antibodies, suggesting that T cells have an active role in the pathogenesis [19,20].

C3H/HeJ mouse

A diffuse non-scarring alopecia with clinical and pathological features similar to alopecia areata was reported by Sundberg *et al.* [21] in a large production colony of C3H/HeJ mice. On the dorsal skin, the alopecia developed in circular areas, with disease involvement restricted to anagen follicles. Pedigree analysis suggested the disease was inherited. Alopecia was more common in ageing animals, and the frequency was highest in mice selectively bred for inflammatory bowel disease. Subsequent studies have revealed considerable similarity in histopathology, immunological features and response to therapeutic agents between C3H/HeJ alopecia and human alopecia areata.

REFERENCES

1 Perret C, Wiesner-Menzel L, Happle R. Immunohistochemical analysis of T-cell subsets in the peribulbar and intrabulbar infiltrates of alopecia areata. *Acta Derm Venereol* 1984; **64**: 26–30.

2 Wiesner-Menzel L, Happle R. Intrabulbar and peribulbar accumulation of dendritic OKT 6-positive cells in alopecia areata. *Arch Dermatol Res* 1984; **276**: 333–4.

3 Cotsarelis G, Sun TT, Lavker RM. Label-retaining cells reside in the bulge area of pilosebaceous unit: implications for follicular stem cells, hair cycle, and skin carcinogenesis. *Cell* 1990; **61**: 1329–37.

4 Messenger AG, Bleehen SS. Expression of HLA-DR by anagen hair follicles in alopecia areata. *J Invest Dermatol* 1985; **85**: 569–72.

5 Brocker EB, Echternacht-Happle K, Hamm H *et al*. Abnormal expression of class I and class II major histocompatibility antigens in alopecia areata: modulation by topical immunotherapy. *J Invest Dermatol* 1987; **88**: 564–8.

6 McDonagh AJG, Snowden JA, Stierle C *et al*. HLA and ICAM-1 expression in alopecia areata *in vivo* and *in vitro*: the role of cytokines. *Br J Dermatol* 1993; **129**: 250–6.

7 Van Scott EJ. Morphologic changes in pilosebaceous units and anagen hairs in alopecia areata. *J Invest Dermatol* 1958; **31**: 35–43.

8 Eckert J, Church RE, Ebling FJ. The pathogenesis of alopecia areata. *Br J Dermatol* 1968; **80**: 203–10.

9 Messenger AG, Slater DN, Bleehen SS. Alopecia areata: alterations in the hair growth cycle and correlation with the follicular pathology. *Br J Dermatol* 1986; **114**: 337–47.

10 Thies W. Vergleichende histologische Untersuchungen bei Alopecia areata und narbig-atrophisierenden. *Arch Klin Exp Dermatol* 1966; **227**: 541–9.

11 Messenger AG, Bleehen SS. Alopecia areata: light and electron microscopic pathology of the regrowing white hair. *Br J Dermatol* 1984; **110**: 155–62.

12 MacDonald-Hull S, Nutbrown M, Pepall L *et al*. Immunohistologic and ultrastructural comparison of the dermal papilla and hair follicle bulb from 'active' and 'normal' areas of alopecia areata. *J Invest Dermatol* 1991; **96**: 673–81.

13 Anderson I. Alopecia areata: a clinical study. *BMJ* 1950; **ii**: 1250–2.

14 Muller SA, Winkelmann RK. Alopecia areata. *Arch Dermatol* 1963; **88**: 290–7.

15 Michie HJ, Jahoda CA, Oliver RF *et al*. The DEBR rat: an animal model of human alopecia areata. *Br J Dermatol* 1991; **125**: 94–100.

16 Zhang JG, Oliver RF. Immunohistological study of the development of the cellular infiltrate in the pelage follicles of the DEBR model for alopecia areata. *Br J Dermatol* 1994; **130**: 405–14.

17 Oliver RF, Lowe JG. Oral cyclosporin A restores hair growth in the DEBR rat model for alopecia areata. *Clin Exp Dermatol* 1995; **20**: 127–31.

18 McElwee KJ, Rushton DH, Trachy R *et al*. Topical FK506: a potent immunotherapy for alopecia areata? Studies using the Dundee experimental bald rat model. *Br J Dermatol* 1997; **137**: 491–7.

19 McElwee KJ, Spiers EM, Oliver RF. *In vivo* depletion of CD8+ T cells restores hair growth in the DEBR model for alopecia areata. *Br J Dermatol* 1996; **135**: 211–7.

20 McElwee KJ, Spiers EM, Oliver RF. Partial restoration of hair growth in the DEBR model for alopecia areata after *in vivo* depletion of CD4+ T cells. *Br J Dermatol* 1999; **140**: 432–7.

21 Sundberg JP, Boggess D, Montagutelli X *et al*. C3H/HeJ mouse model for alopecia areata. *J Invest Dermatol* 1995; **104**: 16S–7S.

Clinical features

The onset of alopecia areata may be at any age, peaking between the second and fourth decades. The sex incidence is probably equal. The characteristic initial lesion is a circumscribed, totally bald, smooth patch (Fig. 63.26). It is often noticed by chance by a parent, hairdresser or friend. The skin within the bald patch appears normal or slightly reddened. Short, easily extractable broken hairs, known as exclamation mark hairs, are often seen at the margins of the bald patches during active phases of the disease (Fig. 63.27). Subsequent progress is very varied; the initial patch may regrow within a few months, or further patches

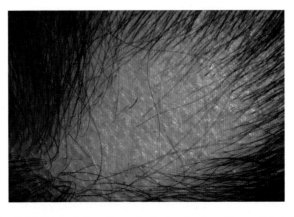

Fig. 63.26 Patch of alopecia areata. Broken 'exclamation mark hairs' are seen towards the margins of the patch.

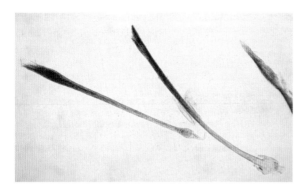

Fig. 63.27 Exclamation mark hairs.

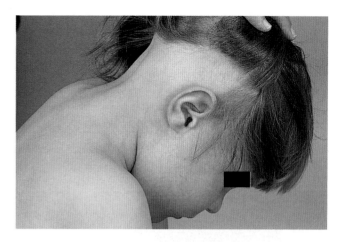

Fig. 63.29 The ophiasis pattern of alopecia areata.

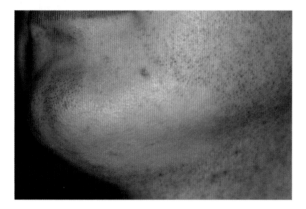

Fig. 63.28 Alopecia areata affecting the beard.

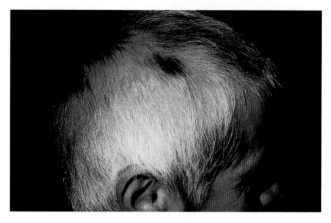

Fig. 63.30 Regrowth of hypopigmented hair in alopecia areata.

may appear after an interval of 3–6 weeks and then in a cyclical fashion. These intervals are of varying duration. A succession of discrete patches may rapidly become confluent by the diffuse loss of remaining hair. In some cases the initial hair loss is diffuse, and total denudation of the scalp has been reported within 48 h. However, diffuse hair loss may occur over part or the whole of the scalp without the development of bald areas. Regrowth is often at first fine and unpigmented, but usually the hairs gradually resume their normal calibre and colour. Regrowth in one region of the scalp may occur while the alopecia is extending in others.

The scalp is the first affected site in most cases, but any hair-bearing skin can be affected. In dark-haired men, patches in the beard are conspicuous and in such individuals are often the first to be noticed (Fig. 63.28). The eyebrows and eyelashes are lost in many cases of alopecia areata and may be the only sites affected. The term alopecia totalis is applied to total or almost total loss of scalp hair, and alopecia universalis is the loss of all body hair. The extension of alopecia along the scalp margin is known as ophiasis (Fig. 63.29).

An intriguing feature of alopecia areata is the sparing of white hairs. In patients with grey hair, which is an admixture of pigmented and non-pigmented hair, the disease process appears preferentially to affect pigmented hair, so that non-pigmented or white hair is spared. This may result in a dramatic change in hair colour if the alopecia progresses rapidly, and is probably the explanation for historical accounts of people 'going white overnight'. Sparing of white hair is a relative phenomenon and it is clear that the white hairs, although less susceptible to the disease, are not immune. During the regrowth phase hairs may be non- or hypopigmented (Fig. 63.30) but hair pigmentation usually recovers completely. In exceptional cases where regrowing hairs remain non-pigmented the possibility of concurrent vitiligo should be considered.

In 10–15% of cases referred for specialist opinion alopecia areata also involves the nails, usually in the context of severe hair loss. Classically, alopecia areata causes fine stippled pitting of the nails (Fig. 63.31), but some cases show less well-defined roughening of the nail plate (trachyonychia) or a non-specific atrophic dystrophy. For some patients, the latter problem is the most troublesome aspect of the disease.

Differential diagnosis

In children the main sources of difficulty are tinea capitis

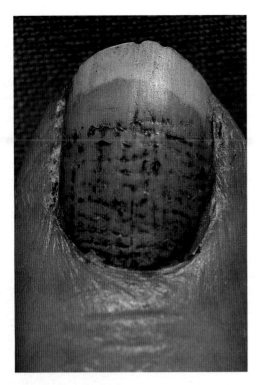

Fig. 63.31 An organized pattern of pitting present on all fingernails 8 months prior to onset of alopecia areata. Pits are highlighted with mascara.

and trichotillomania. Tinea capitis should always be considered in children presenting with patchy hair loss. There is usually evidence of scalp inflammation but this may be limited to mild scaling. The hair loss in trichotillomania may be asymmetrical or occur in artificial shapes. Broken hairs are usually present across the areas of hair loss, giving a bristly texture and, unlike exclamation mark hairs, are firmly anchored in the scalp. In most cases the true diagnosis will become evident with time; a biopsy is useful when doubt remains. Occasionally, the early stages of scarring alopecia can resemble alopecia areata. The diffuse form of alopecia areata is perhaps the most difficult to identify. A history of previous episodes of hair loss, nail dystrophy and the usually rapid progression may provide clues, but other causes of diffuse hair loss, such as SLE, may need to be excluded by appropriate serological tests and a scalp biopsy. Secondary syphilis sometimes presents with diffuse or patchy hair loss.

Prognosis

Alopecia areata does not destroy hair follicles, and the potential for regrowth of hair is retained for many years and is possibly lifelong. In some patients, patches of hair loss occur at infrequent intervals interspersed with long periods of normal hair growth. In others, alopecia areata is more persistent, so that new patches of hair loss con-

tinue to develop at the same time as regrowth occurs elsewhere. In a relatively small number of patients, hair loss progresses to involve all of the scalp (alopecia totalis) or the entire skin surface (alopecia universalis); in these cases, spontaneous recovery is the exception rather than the rule.

Data from secondary and tertiary referral centres indicate that 34–50% of patients will recover within 1 year, although almost all will experience more than one episode of the disease, and 14–25% progress to alopecia totalis or alopecia universalis, from which full recovery is unusual (less than 10%) [1,2]. One study from Japan reported that spontaneous remission within 1 year occurred in 80% of patients with a small number of circumscribed patches of hair loss [3]. The prognosis is less favourable when onset occurs during childhood [1,4–6] and in ophiasis [6]. The concurrence of atopic disease has been reported to be associated with a poor prognosis [3,6], but this was not found in a study from India [7].

REFERENCES

1 Walker SA, Rothman S. Alopecia areata: a statistical study and consideration of endocrine influences. *J Invest Dermatol* 1950; **14**: 403–13.
2 Gip L, Lodin A, Molin L. Alopecia areata: a follow-up investigation of outpatient material. *Acta Derm Venereol* 1969; **49**: 180–8.
3 Ikeda T. A new classification of alopecia areata. *Dermatologica* 1965; **131**: 421–45.
4 Anderson I. Alopecia areata: a clinical study. *BMJ* 1950; **ii**: 1250–2.
5 Muller SA, Winkelmann RK. Alopecia areata. *Arch Dermatol* 1963; **88**: 290–7.
6 De Waard-van der Spek FB, Oranje AP, De Raeymaecker DM *et al.* Juvenile versus maturity-onset alopecia areata: a comparative retrospective clinical study. *Clin Exp Dermatol* 1989; **14**: 429–33.
7 Sharma VK, Dawn G, Kumar B. Profile of alopecia areata in Northern India. *Int J Dermatol* 1996; **35**: 22–7.

Management

A number of treatments can induce hair growth in alopecia areata, but none has been shown to alter the course of the disease. The high rate of spontaneous remission makes it difficult to assess efficacy, particularly in mild forms of the disease. Some trials have been limited to patients with severe alopecia areata where spontaneous remission is unlikely. However, these patients tend to be resistant to all forms of treatment and the failure of a treatment in this setting does not exclude efficacy in mild alopecia areata. Few treatments have been subjected to randomized controlled trials and, except for contact immunotherapy, there are few published data on long-term outcomes. These difficulties mean that counselling of the patient and, where relevant, of their family, are of paramount importance. This should include discussion of the nature of the disease and its natural history, the treatments available and their chances of success. Some patients have great difficulty coping with alopecia areata and require considerable support. Sources of support may include the physician, other patients, formal patients' support groups and, in some circumstances, professional counselling services.

Treatment. Leaving alopecia areata untreated is a legitimate option for many patients. Spontaneous remission occurs in up to 80% of patients with limited patchy hair loss of short duration (less than 1 year) [1]. Such patients may be managed by reassurance alone, with advice that regrowth cannot be expected within 3 months of the development of any individual patch. The prognosis in long-standing extensive alopecia is less favourable. However, all treatments have a high failure rate in this group and some patients prefer not to be treated, other than wearing a wig if appropriate.

Corticosteroids. Intralesional depot corticosteroids have a small but useful role in the management of alopecia areata [2,3]. They can be used to accelerate regrowth in a circumscribed patch of alopecia areata that is cosmetically disfiguring or difficult to conceal, and can be useful for maintaining regrowth of the eyebrows in alopecia totalis; but great care must be exercised to avoid steroid side effects in the eye. Hydrocortisone acetate (25 mg/mL) and triamcinolone acetonide (5–10 mg/mL) are commonly used, either by needle injection or jet injection. Localized atrophy is a common complication, particularly if triamcinolone is used, but this is temporary and recovers within a few months.

Potent topical corticosteroids are widely used to treat alopecia areata but there is little evidence that they produce significant regrowth of hair. In some cases, a troublesome folliculitis may result.

Long-term daily treatment with oral corticosteroids will produce regrowth of hair in some patients. One small, partly controlled study reported that 30–47% of patients treated with a 6-week tapering course of oral prednisolone (starting at 40 mg/day) showed more than 25% hair regrowth [4]. Unfortunately, in most patients, continued treatment is needed to maintain hair growth and the response is usually insufficient to justify the risks [5]. There are several case series reporting response to high-dose pulsed corticosteroid treatment employing different oral and intravenous regimens [6–8]. However, these studies were uncontrolled and, although none reported significant side effects, the potential toxicity of systemic corticosteroids remains a serious concern.

Contact immunotherapy. Contact immunotherapy was introduced by Rosenberg in 1976 [9] and is the most effective and best-documented treatment for alopecia areata, but problems associated with its use mean that it is available in only a few centres. The patient is sensitized to a potent allergen and the same allergen is then applied to the scalp, usually at weekly intervals, in a concentration sufficient to induce a mild contact dermatitis. The contact

allergens that have been used in the treatment of alopecia areata include dinitrochlorobenzene (DNCB), squaric acid dibutylester (SADBE) and diphenylcyclopropenone (DPCP). Most centres now use DPCP [10]. A review of all the published studies of contact immunotherapy concluded that 50–60% of patients achieve a worthwhile response, but the range of response rates was very wide (9–87%) [11]. Patients with extensive hair loss are less likely to respond [12,13]. Other reported adverse prognostic features include the presence of nail changes, early onset and a positive family history [11]. In most studies treatment was discontinued after 6 months if no response was obtained. In one case series from Canada, clinically significant regrowth occurred in approximately 30% of patients after 6 months' treatment, but this increased to 78% after 32 months of treatment, suggesting that more prolonged treatment is worthwhile [14]. The response in patients with alopecia totalis and universalis was less favourable at 17% and this was not improved by treatment beyond 9 months. Relapses may occur following or during treatment. In the Canadian series, relapse following successful treatment occurred in 62% of patients. Two case report series of contact immunotherapy in children with alopecia areata reported response rates of 33% [15] and 32% [16]. A third study found a similar short-term response in children with severe alopecia areata, but less than 10% experienced sustained benefit [17].

Most patients will develop occipital and/or cervical lymphadenopathy during contact immunotherapy. This is usually temporary but may persist throughout the treatment period. Severe dermatitis is the most common adverse event, but the risk can be minimized by careful titration of the concentration. Uncommon adverse effects include urticaria [18], which may be severe [19], and vitiligo [20,21]. Cosmetically disabling pigmentary complications, both hyper- and hypopigmentation (including vitiligo), may occur if contact immunotherapy is used in patients with racially pigmented skin. Contact immunotherapy has been in use for 20 years and no long-term side effects have been reported.

The mode of action of contact immunotherapy is unknown. Happle [22] suggested that the contact allergen competes for CD4 cells, attracting them away from the perifollicular region ('antigenic competition'). Other suggested mechanisms include the non-specific stimulation of a local T-suppressor-cell response [23] and increased expression of TGF-β in the skin, which acts to suppress the immune response [24].

Photochemotherapy. There are several uncontrolled studies of photochemotherapy (PUVA) for alopecia areata, using all types of PUVA (oral or topical psoralen, local or whole body UVA irradiation) [25–28], claiming success rates of up to 60–65%. Two retrospective reviews have reported low response rates [29] or suggested that the response was no better than the natural course of the disease [30], although these observations were also uncontrolled. The relapse rate following treatment is high and continued treatment is usually needed to maintain hair growth, which may lead to an unacceptably high cumulative UVA dose.

Minoxidil. An early double-blind study reported a significantly greater frequency of hair regrowth in patchy alopecia areata in patients treated with topical 1% minoxidil compared with placebo [31]. Subsequent controlled trials in patients with extensive alopecia areata using 1% or 3% minoxidil failed to confirm these results [32–34]. Two of these studies reported a treatment response during an extended but uncontrolled part of the trial [33,34]. In one study comparing 5% and 1% minoxidil in extensive alopecia areata, regrowth of hair occurred more frequently in those receiving 5% minoxidil, but few subjects obtained a cosmetically worthwhile result [35]. Topical minoxidil is ineffective in alopecia totalis and universalis.

Dithranol. There are a small number of case report series of the use of dithranol (anthralin) or other irritants in the treatment of alopecia areata [36–38]. The lack of controls makes the response rates difficult to evaluate but only a small proportion of patients seem to achieve cosmetically worthwhile results. In one open study, 18% of patients with extensive alopecia areata achieved cosmetically worthwhile hair regrowth [36]. The published data indicate that dithranol needs to be applied sufficiently frequently and in a high enough concentration to produce a brisk irritant reaction in order to be effective.

Summary

Alopecia areata is difficult to treat and few treatments have been tested in randomized controlled trials. The tendency to spontaneous remission and the lack of adverse effects on general health are important considerations in management, and counselling, with no treatment, is the best option in many cases. Intralesional corticosteroids can be helpful in disease of limited extent, especially in cosmetically obvious sites. Topical corticosteroids, minoxidil lotion and dithranol are widely used but there is little convincing evidence of efficacy. Contact immunotherapy is the most effective treatment for extensive alopecia areata, although it is not widely available, and the response rate in alopecia totalis and universalis is low. The place of systemic corticosteroids is controversial. In view of the lack of evidence of sustained efficacy and the potential hazards, their routine use in alopecia areata cannot be recommended.

Alopecia areata may cause considerable psychological and social disability and, in some cases, particularly those seen in secondary care, it may be a chronic and persistent disease causing extensive or universal hair loss. If the prognosis is poor (e.g. in a prepubertal atopic child with total alopecia), a full explanation and help in adjusting to the problems of hair loss will be of far greater value than the raising of unwarranted hopes.

REFERENCES

1 Ikeda T. A new classification of alopecia areata. *Dermatologica* 1965; **131**: 421–45.
2 Abell E, Munro DD. Intralesional treatment of alopecia areata with triamcinolone acetonide by jet injector. *Br J Dermatol* 1973; **88**: 55–9.
3 Kubeyinje EP. Intralesional triamcinolone acetonide in alopecia areata amongst 62 Saudi Arabs. *East Afr Med J* 1994; **71**: 674–5.
4 Olsen EA, Carson SC, Turney EA. Systemic steroids with or without 2% topical minoxidil in the treatment of alopecia areata. *Arch Dermatol* 1992; **128**: 1467–73.
5 Winter RJ, Kern F, Blizzard RM. Prednisone therapy for alopecia areata: a follow-up report. *Arch Dermatol* 1976; **112**: 1549–52.
6 Sharma VK. Pulsed administration of corticosteroids in the treatment of alopecia areata. *Int J Dermatol* 1996; **35**: 133–6.
7 Kiesch N, Stene JJ, Goens J et al. Pulse steroid therapy for children's severe alopecia areata? *Dermatology* 1997; **194**: 395–7.
8 Friedli A, Labarthe MP, Engelhardt E et al. Pulse methylprednisolone therapy for severe alopecia areata: an open prospective study of 45 patients. *J Am Acad Dermatol* 1998; **39**: 597–602.
9 Rosenberg EW, Drake L. In discussion of Dunaway DA: Alopecia areata. *Arch Dermatol* 1976; **112**: 256.
10 Happle R, Hausen BM, Wiesner-Menzel L. Diphencyprone in the treatment of alopecia areata. *Acta Derm Venereol* 1983; **63**: 49–52.
11 Rokhsar CK, Shupack JL, Vafai JJ et al. Efficacy of topical sensitizers in the treatment of alopecia areata. *J Am Acad Dermatol* 1998; **39**: 751–61.
12 van der Steen PH, van Baar HM, Happle R et al. Prognostic factors in the treatment of alopecia areata with diphenylcyclopropenone. *J Am Acad Dermatol* 1991; **24**: 227–30.
13 Gordon PM, Aldrige RD, McVittie E et al. Topical diphencyprone for alopecia areata: evaluation of 48 cases after 30 months' follow-up. *Br J Dermatol* 1996; **134**: 869–71.
14 Wiseman M, Shapiro J, MacDonald N et al. Predictive model for immunotherapy of alopecia areata with diphencyprone. *Arch Dermatol* 2001; **137**: 1063–8.
15 Macdonald Hull SP, Pepall L, Cunliffe WJ. Alopecia areata in children: response to treatment with diphencyprone. *Br J Dermatol* 1991; **125**: 164–8.
16 Schuttelaar ML, Hamstra JJ, Plinck EP et al. Alopecia areata in children: treatment with diphencyprone. *Br J Dermatol* 1996; **135**: 581–5.
17 Tosti A, Guidetti MS, Bardazzi F et al. Long-term results of topical immunotherapy in children with alopecia totalis or alopecia universalis. *J Am Acad Dermatol* 1996; **35**: 199–201.
18 Tosti A, Guerra L, Bardazzi F. Contact urticaria during topical immunotherapy. *Contact Dermatitis* 1989; **21**: 196–7.
19 Alam M, Gross EA, Savin RC. Severe urticarial reaction to diphenylcyclopropenone therapy for alopecia areata. *J Am Acad Dermatol* 1999; **40**: 110–2.
20 Henderson C, Ilchyshyn A. Vitiligo complicating diphencyprone sensitization therapy for alopecia universalis [Letter]. *Br J Dermatol* 1995; **133**: 496–7.
21 Macdonald Hull SP, Norris JF, Cotterill JA. Vitiligo following sensitization with diphencyprone. *Br J Dermatol* 1989; **120**: 232.
22 Happle R. Antigenic competition as a therapeutic concept for alopecia areata. *Arch Dermatol Res* 1980; **267**: 109–14.
23 Bröcker EB, Echternacht-Happle K, Hamm H et al. Abnormal expression of class I and class II major histocompatibility antigens in alopecia areata. *J Invest Dermatol* 1987; **88**: 564–8.
24 Hoffmann R, Wenzel E, Huth A et al. Growth factor mRNA levels in alopecia areata before and after treatment with the contact allergen diphenylcyclopropenone. *Acta Derm Venereol* 1996; **76**: 17–20.
25 Claudy AL, Gagnaire D. PUVA treatment of alopecia areata. *Arch Dermatol* 1983; **119**: 975–8.
26 Lassus A, Eskelinen A, Johansson E. Treatment of alopecia areata with three different PUVA modalities. *Photodermatol* 1984; **1**: 141–4.
27 Mitchell AJ, Douglass MC. Topical photochemotherapy for alopecia areata. *J Am Acad Dermatol* 1985; **12**: 644–9.

28 van der Schaar WW, Sillevis SJ. An evaluation of PUVA-therapy for alopecia areata. *Dermatologica* 1984; **168**: 250–2.

29 Taylor CR, Hawk JL. PUVA treatment of alopecia areata partialis, totalis and universalis: audit of 10 years' experience at St John's Institute of Dermatology. *Br J Dermatol* 1995; **133**: 914–8.

30 Healy E, Rogers S. PUVA treatment for alopecia areata: does it work? A retrospective review of 102 cases. *Br J Dermatol* 1993; **129**: 42–4.

31 Fenton DA, Wilkinson JD. Topical minoxidil in the treatment of alopecia areata. *BMJ (Clin Res Ed)*. 1983; **287**: 1015–7.

32 Vestey JP, Savin JA. A trial of 1% minoxidil used topically for severe alopecia areata. *Acta Derm Venereol* 1986; **66**: 179–80.

33 Price VH. Double-blind, placebo-controlled evaluation of topical minoxidil in extensive alopecia areata. *J Am Acad Dermatol* 1987; **16**: 730–6.

34 Ranchoff RE, Bergfeld WF, Steck WD *et al*. Extensive alopecia areata: results of treatment with 3% topical minoxidil. *Cleve Clin J Med* 1989; **56**: 149–54.

35 Fiedler-Weiss VC. Topical minoxidil solution (1% and 5%) in the treatment of alopecia areata. *J Am Acad Dermatol* 1987; **16**: 745–8.

36 Fiedler-Weiss VC, Buys CM. Evaluation of anthralin in the treatment of alopecia areata. *Arch Dermatol* 1987; **123**: 1491–3.

37 Nelson DA, Spielvogel RL. Anthralin therapy for alopecia areata. *Int J Dermatol* 1985; **24**: 606–7.

38 Schmoeckel C, Weissmann I, Plewig G *et al*. Treatment of alopecia areata by anthralin-induced dermatitis. *Arch Dermatol* 1979; **115**: 1254–5.

Acquired cicatricial alopecia

[R.D. Sinclair, pp. 63.46–63.61]

Hair follicles are self-regenerating organs. A new and distinct hair bulb is produced for every anagen phase of the hair cycle. Stem cells located within the outer root sheath (ORS) at the level of insertion of the arrector pili muscle have the potential to induce not only hair bulb regeneration, but also sebaceous gland formation and re-epithelialization of the epidermis [1]. Selective damage to the ORS in the isthmus that destroys hair follicle stem cells will ultimately lead to loss of the entire pilosebaceous unit and replacement by a fibrous tract or stella. Other non-selective forms of hair follicle damage can produce a similar outcome.

Cicatricial alopecia is the generic term applied to permanent areas of hair loss that are associated with destruction of hair follicles. Following recovery from the initial injury or inflammatory insult, there is little if any potential for hair regrowth. Histologically, the follicles are replaced by fibrous stellae, but as there is no scar *per se* the alternative generic term *scarring alopecia* is not favoured [2]. Replacement of follicular structures by fibrous tissue is the common final pathway for a number of diverse conditions and it is commonly not possible to infer the cause of the hair loss.

Cicatricial alopecia is by no means rare. In Whiting's series of 5860 patients presenting with hair loss between 1989 and 1999, 427 (7.3%) had cicatricial alopecia [3]. One of the earliest descriptions of cicatricial alopecia was by Brocq in 1885 [4]. He described what later became known eponymously as pseudopelade of Brocq [5], which is now regarded as a syndrome in which destruction of follicles leading to permanent patchy baldness is not accompanied by any clinically evident inflammatory pathology. Quainquad [6] described folliculitis decalvans, a form of scarring alopecia in which pustular folliculitis of the advancing margin was a conspicuous feature.

Cicatricial alopecia may result from a disease that affects the follicles primarily or a disease process external to the follicle that damages them secondarily. Secondary causes include trauma, as in burns or radiodermatitis, infections such as favus, tuberculosis or syphilis, or benign or malignant tumours. Chemicals used to straighten or curl hair may also cause a secondary cicatricial alopecia in susceptible persons.

Once the preliminary diagnosis of cicatricial alopecia has been made, the scalp should be examined for other clues as to the cause of the hair loss such as folliculitis, follicular plugging or broken hairs. These signs may help to establish the cause of a cicatricial alopecia, but no single sign is pathognomonic for a particular disease, and clinicopathological correlation is usually needed to make a specific diagnosis. An occasional sterile pustule can even be seen in some cases of lichen planopilaris and chronic cutaneous lupus. Hairs, even if grossly normal in appearance, should be extracted from the edge of the bald area for microscopy and culture. Any pustule should be swabbed and the fluid cultured. If no firm diagnosis is achieved, general examination of the skin, nails and oral mucosa should be carried out. Up to 40% of patients with scalp lichen planus and 30% of patients with discoid lupus of the scalp will have cutaneous disease elsewhere either at presentation or during follow-up.

In most cases, a diagnostic biopsy is indicated. The site for biopsy must be carefully selected and an early lesion is preferable. Several punch biopsies are preferable to a single elliptical biopsy; in this way, the biopsies can be orientated along follicles, and different stages of the disease process can be investigated. Ideally, at least one 4-mm biopsy should be taken from a clinically active area, prepared for horizontal section and stained with haematoxylin and eosin. If vertical sections or immunofluorescence are desired, a second 4-mm biopsy specimen from an area of similar clinical activity should be obtained. Additional biopsies from the centre of a patch of alopecia to establish whether follicular loss has occurred or to assess potential regrowth are optional, as are further biopsies for special stains (e.g. elastin, mucin, periodic acid–Schiff [PAS]) [2].

Classification of the primary causes of cicatricial alopecia is difficult because of changing clinical and histological features as these conditions evolve. The most common identifiable causes among white people are lichen planopilaris (LPP), folliculitis decalvans and discoid lupus erythematosus. Among black people, especially in North America and Europe where hair-straightening procedures are common, the most common cause is central centrifugal alopecia (see p. 63.54). Tumours, in particular metastatic nodules from renal, breast and lung carcinomas, should not be forgotten as a rare but important cause of cicatricial alopecia.

Despite multiple investigations a specific diagnosis is not always possible and a generic diagnosis of cicatricial alopecia is the best that can be done. In such cases, a trial of oral steroids or antimalarials may be considered to assess the potential for regrowth. Surgical correction of small areas can be considered once the underlying disorder has burned out. This can be done either by follicle transplantation or excision of the area. Larger areas may require the prior use of tissue expanders [7].

Classification [2]. The causes of cicatricial alopecia are classified here into broad groups, and the individual causes then considered in greater detail. Many of the causes are discussed in other chapters where appropriate.

1 *Primary cicatricial alopecia*

Inflammatory	Lymphocytic	Chronic cutaneous lupus erythematosus
		Lichen planopilaris (LPP)
		Classic LPP
		Graham-Little syndrome
		Frontal fibrosing alopecia
		Pseudopelade of Brocq
		Central centrifugal cicatricial alopecia
		Alopecia mucinosa
		Keratosis pilaris spinulosa decalvans
		Morphoea/scleroderma
	Neutrophilic	Folliculitis decalvans (including tufted folliculitis)
		Dissecting cellulitis/folliculitis
	Mixed	Acne keloidalis
		Acne necrotica
		Erosive pustular dermatosis
	Non-specific or end-stage cicatricial alopecia	

2 *Secondary cicatricial alopecia*

Traumatic	Radiodermatitis
	Mechanical trauma
	Postoperative (flap necrosis)
	Burns
	Accidental alopecia
	Dermatitis artefacta
	Traction alopecia
	Hot comb alopecia
Sclerosing disorders	Morphoea
	Scleroderma
	Lichen sclerosus
	Sclerodermoid porphyria cutanea tarda
	Chronic graft-versus-host disease

Granulomatous	Sarcoidosis		
	Necrobiosis lipoidica		
	Infectious granulomas		
Infectious	Bacterial	Folliculitis	
		Carbuncle/furuncle	
	Fungal	Kerion	
		Favus	
		Tinea capitis (rarely scarring)	
	Viral	Shingles	
		Varicella	
		HIV	
	Protozoal	Leishmaniasis	
		Syphilis	
	Mycobacterial	Tuberculosis	
Neoplastic	Benign	Cylindroma	
		Other adnexal tumours	
	Malignant	Primary	Basal cell carcinoma
			Squamous cell carcinoma
			Cutaneous T-cell lymphoma
		Secondary	Renal, breast, lung, gastrointestinal
			Lymphoma, leukaemia

Developmental defects and hereditary disorders
Aplasia cutis
Facial hemiatrophy (Romberg's syndrome)
Epidermal naevi
Hair follicle hamartomas
Incontinentia pigmenti
Focal dermal hypoplasia of Goltz
Porokeratosis of Mibelli
Ichthyosis
Epidermolysis bullosa
Polyostotic fibrous dysplasia
Conradi–Hünermann syndrome (chondrodysplasia punctata)

REFERENCES

1 Dawber RPR. Cicatricial alopecia. In: Dawber RPR, ed. *Diseases of the Hair and Scalp*, 3rd edn. Oxford: Blackwell Science, 1997: 588–90.
2 Bergfeld WF, Elston DM. Cicatricial alopecia. In: Olsen E, ed. *Disorders of Hair Growth, Diagnosis and Treatment*, 2nd edn. New York: McGraw-Hill, 2003: 363–98.
3 Whiting DA. Cicatricial alopecia. *Clin Dermatol* 2001; **19**: 211–25.
4 Brocq L. Alopecia. *J Cutan Vener Dis* 1885; **3**: 49–56.
5 Brocq L, Lenglet E, Ayrignac J. Recherches sur l'alopecie atrophiante, varieté pseudopelade. *Ann Dermatol Syphiligr* 1905; **6**: 1, 97, 209–15.
6 Quainquad E. Folliculite epilante decalvante. *Ann Dermatol Syphiligr* 1889; **10**: 99–105.
7 Roenigk RK, Wheeland RG. Tissue expansion in cicatricial alopecia. *Arch Dermatol* 1987; **123**: 641–52.

Non-specific cicatricial alopecia

Aetiology. This is by far the most common diagnosis made among patients presenting with cicatricial alopecia. In Whiting's series of 358 patients who were biopsied because of cicatricial alopecia this was the diagnosis made in 32% of cases [1]. Although often called pseudopelade, this term is best avoided because of confusion with pseudopelade of Brocq, a specific and distinct clinical disease. This entity of non-specific cicatricial alopecia encompasses a range of idiopathic non-inflammatory irregular permanent alopecias that are often slowly progressive. Many primary cicatricial alopecias ultimately burn out and the final common pathway is an irregular area of cicatricial hair loss of the scalp with no distinguishing clinical or histological features. Various authorities have estimated that between 15% and 90% of cases of non-specific cicatricial alopecia result from LPP, but there is no way of confirming this. That a small minority of patients initially diagnosed as having non-specific cicatricial alopecia later develop associated cutaneous lichen planus confirms significant overlap between this condition and LPP.

Pathology. The histology is variable and non-specific. Scalp biopsies taken from hairy skin at the edge of a scarred patch may be either completely normal or show a non-specific lymphocytic infiltrate around follicular infundibulum and mid-follicle, with or without a light superficial perivascular infiltrate. Follicles may be depleted and replaced by fibrous tracts, and sebaceous glands and follicular units may be disrupted. In the centre of areas of alopecia, follicles are absent or dramatically diminished in number and the epidermis is atrophic. Concentric lamellar fibrosis and follicular atrophy is seen around residual follicles. The adjacent dermis is sclerotic. Follicle rupture can produce hair granulomas or pustules.

Clinical features. The initial patch often occurs over the crown, but may occur anywhere on the scalp. The lesions tend to be oval, and several foci may coalesce to form irregular bald areas. There is usually no erythema and the patches are smooth, shiny and slightly depressed. Within any patch, a small number of terminal hairs may persist. These are often irregularly twisted and sometimes easily extracted. Folliculitis is rarely seen. The hairs at the edge of the patch of alopecia are also often irregularly twisted and easily extracted, even when in anagen, which indicates active extension of the alopecia.

Prognosis. The prognosis is extremely variable and unpredictable. Some patches extend almost imperceptibly over many years, whereas others enlarge rapidly. Whether this condition ever truly burns out, or merely extends too slowly to be noticed is uncertain.

Treatment. Much has been tried empirically, but nothing has been shown to be effective.

Lichen planus (see Chapter 42)
SYN. LICHEN PLANOPILARIS; FRONTAL FIBROSING ALOPECIA

Aetiology. Lichen planus is an idiopathic inflammatory disease that may affect the skin, hair and nails. There are numerous cutaneous variants of lichen planus. On the scalp it tends to produce a cicatricial alopecia. Three variants of cicatricial alopecia resulting from lichen planus are recognized: LPP, Graham-Little syndrome and frontal fibrosing alopecia. In each of these conditions the scalp may be affected alone or in conjunction with lichen planus elsewhere.

Lichen planus occurs throughout the world, but there are marked regional variations in its incidence and in its clinical manifestations. In the USA, lichen planus accounts for at least 10% of cases of cicatricial alopecia and the mean age of onset is 44 years [1]. In Europe and Australia, where follicular degeneration syndrome is less common, the incidence is higher. Although drug-induced lichen planus is well recognized, drug-induced LPP is not recognized.

Pathology [2]. The initial abnormality is in the epidermis; fibrillar changes in the basal cells lead to the formation of colloid bodies and at an early stage these, and macrophages containing pigment, may be seen in the dermis. By immunofluorescence, fibrin and immunoglobulin M (IgM) may be detected in the upper dermis, and various components of complement in the basement-membrane zone. The damaged basal cells are continually replaced by the migration of cells from neighbouring normal epidermis. In the established lesion, the horny layer and granular layer are thickened and there is irregular acanthosis. Flattening of the rete pegs gives rise to a saw-tooth configuration. There is liquefaction degeneration of the basal cells. Close up against the epidermis is a dense infiltrate of lymphocytes and some histiocytes. In many sections, colloid bodies can be seen. If the process involves hair follicles, the infiltrate extends around them and the hairs are replaced by keratin plugs. The follicles may ultimately be totally destroyed (Figs 63.32 & 63.33).

AGA with associated fibrosis may be confused with patterned LPP, especially as mild to moderate lymphohistiocytic inflammation is commonly seen in AGA [3].

Clinical features [4]. Lichen planus occurs at any age, but in over 80% of cases the onset is between 30 and 70 years [5]. Significant involvement of the scalp is relatively infrequent—only 10 of 807 patients in one series [5]—but the incidence is probably rather higher than such figures suggest, because they tend to exclude those patients in whom alopecia, classified as pseudopelade, was the only

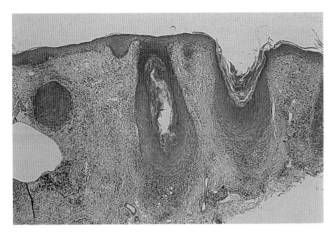

Fig. 63.32 Low-power photomicrograph showing lichen planopilaris. There is follicular plugging and a peri-appendageal inflammatory infiltrate.

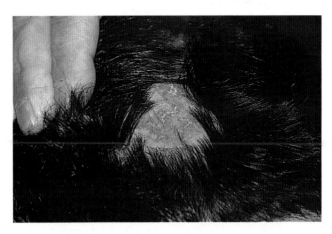

Fig. 63.34 Scarring alopecia caused by lichen planus showing active lesions.

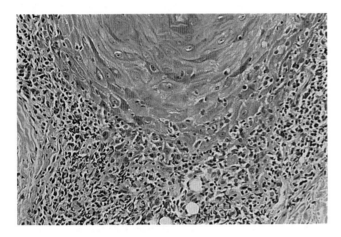

Fig. 63.33 Base of the hair follicle shows hydropic degeneration of the basal layer and a lichenoid mononuclear cell infiltrate.

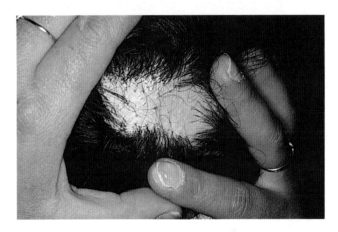

Fig. 63.35 More advanced lichen planus showing follicular plugs and scarring.

manifestation of the disease. Scalp involvement occurs in over 40% of patients with either of two unusual variants of lichen planus: the bullous or erosive form and LPP. Most patients seen with scalp lesions are middle-aged women, but a girl aged 13 years with scarring has been reported [6].

Recent scalp lesions may show violaceous papules, erythema and scaling (Fig. 63.34) [7]. These papules are replaced quickly by follicular plugs and scarring (Fig. 63.35). Eventually, the plugs are shed from the scarred area, which remains white, smooth and atrophic. Follicular orifices are absent within the area of alopecia. If the patch is extending, horny plugs may still be present in follicles around its margins, and the hair pull will be positive at the margins, with twisted anagen hairs being easily extracted by gentle traction.

Patients commonly present with pseudopelade-like patches of scarring that are non-specific. The diagnosis of lichen planus can be made only in the presence of unquestionable lesions elsewhere and lichen planus histology. These may take the form of bullous lichen planus with shedding of nails [8], of bullous lesions associated with typical lichen planus of the skin and mucous membranes [9], or of lichen planus of very limited extent involving, for example, the nails only [10].

One clinical variant of LPP is frontal fibrosing alopecia (Fig. 63.36) [11]. This condition superficially resembles AGA with frontal recession, but on close inspection there is loss of follicular orifices, and perifollicular erythema and hyperkeratosis at the marginal hairline. It typically occurs in postmenopausal women, although it can occur earlier. In contrast with AGA, the frontal hairline recedes in a straight line rather than bitemporally.

The natural history of frontal fibrosing alopecia is slow progression over many years. There is no effective treatment [11].

Prognosis. In some patients, the course of lichen planus of the scalp is slow and only a few inconspicuous patches are present after many years. However, particularly if the skin lesions are of bullous or planopilaris type, they may rapidly result in extensive and permanent baldness.

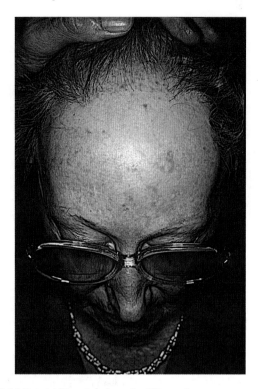

Fig. 63.36 Frontal fibrosing alopecia of Kossard.

Treatment. In some cases, a short course of systemic treatment with a corticosteroid may be desirable. In other cases, intralesional corticosteroids are helpful, but only at a stage when active inflammatory changes are still present. Potent topical steroids such as clobetasol propionate ointment twice daily usually relieve associated symptoms such as itch or pain, and may slightly inhibit the process [12]. Hydroxychloroquine and acitretin have been tried with variable success. Ciclosporin is very effective for cutaneous lichen planus, and has been reported as useful in Graham-Little syndrome [13], as has thalidomide [14,15].

REFERENCES

1 Whiting DA. Cicatricial alopecia. *Clin Dermatol* 2001; **19**: 211–25.
2 Headington JT. Cicatricial alopecia. *Dermatol Clin* 1996; **14**: 773–82.
3 Zinkernagel MS, Trueb RM. Fibrosing alopecia in a pattern distribution: patterned lichen planopilaris or androgenetic alopecia with a lichenoid tissue reaction pattern? *Arch Dermatol* 2000; **136**: 205–11.
4 Mehregan DA, Van Hale HM, Muller SA. Lichen planopilaris. *J Am Acad Dermatol* 1992; **27**: 935–7.
5 Altman J, Perry HO. The variations and course of lichen planus. *Arch Dermatol* 1961; **84**: 179–88.
6 Borda JM, Mazzini RHE, Ruiz DA. Liquen del cuero cabelludo. *Arch Argentin Dermatol* 1961; **11**: 257–61.
7 Sannicandro G. Etudes sur le lichen ruber planus typique et atypique ulcero-erosif, ulcerohemorragique, sclero-cicatriciel, alopecique et sur ses rapports avec les modifications de la protidopoiese. *Ann Dermatol Syphiligr* 1954; **81**: 380–6.
8 Cram DL, Kierland RR, Winkelmann RK. Ulcerative lichen planus of the feet. *Arch Dermatol* 1966; **93**: 692–5.
9 Ebner H. Lichen ruber planus mit Onychatrophie und narbiger Alopezie. *Dermatologica* 1973; **147**: 219–24.
10 Corsi H. Atrophy of hair follicle and nail matrix in lichen planus. *Br J Dermatol* 1937; **49**: 376–88.
11 Kossard S, Lee MS, Wilkinson B. Postmenopausal frontal fibrosing alopecia: a frontal variant of lichen planopilaris. *J Am Acad Dermatol.* 1997; **36**: 59–66.
12 Cheiregato C, Zini A, Barba A, Magnanini M, Rosina P. Lichen planopilaris: report of 30 cases and review of the literature. *Int J Dermatol* 2003; **42**: 342–5.
13 Bianchi L, Paro Vidolin P, Piemonte P, Carboni I, Chimenti S. Graham-Little–Piccardi–Lassueur syndrome: effective treatment with cyclosporin A. *Clin Exp Dermatol* 2001; **26**: 518–20.
14 George SJ, Hsu S. Lichen planopilaris treated with thalidomide. *J Am Acad Dermatol* 2001; **45**: 965–6.
15 Boyd AS, King LE. Thalidomide induced remission of lichen planopilaris. *J Am Acad Dermatol* 2002; **47**: 967–8.

Graham-Little syndrome [1,2]

In 1915, Graham-Little reported the case of a woman aged 55 years who had suffered for 10 years from slowly progressive cicatricial alopecia and for 5 months from groups of horny papules [3]. Since then many further cases have been reported. Whether this syndrome is or is not a form of lichen planus is still unresolved, although the immunofluorescence in typical cases strongly suggests lichen planus [4]. However, whatever its cause or causes, the syndrome is distinctive. It is known eponymously and variously as the Graham-Little, Lassueur–Graham-Little or Piccardi–Lassueur–Little syndrome.

Pathology. In the scalp, the mouths of affected follicles are filled by horny plugs. The underlying follicle is progressively destroyed and eventually an atrophic epidermis covers sclerotic dermis. In the axillae and pubic region, the follicles are likewise destroyed, although the skin does not appear clinically to be atrophic.

Clinical features. Most patients are women between the ages of 30 and 70 years. The essential features of the syndrome are progressive cicatricial alopecia of the scalp, loss of pubic and axillary hair without clinically evident scarring, and the rapid development of keratosis pilaris [5].

In most patients, the earliest change has been patchy cicatricial alopecia of the scalp. In general, the scalp alopecia precedes the widespread keratosis pilaris by months or years [6]. In some patients, the alopecia and the keratosis pilaris appear to have developed more or less simultaneously, or the keratosis pilaris has preceded the discovery of the alopecia [7].

The scalp changes are commonly described simply as patches of cicatricial alopecia. Some authors specifically mention associated follicular plugging of the scalp [7]; others refer to 'scaly red patches'.

The keratosis pilaris is referred to in early case reports as lichen spinulosus, which emphasizes that the horny papules are prolonged into conspicuous spines. In most cases they have developed aggressively over a period of weeks or months and have been grouped into plaques, often on the trunk, or the trunk and limbs, but occasionally involving the eyebrows and the sides of the face. Pruritus is an inconstant symptom; it was noted in several reported cases [8]. Thinning and ultimately total loss of pubic and axillary hair has been noted in many cases.

Treatment. None is universally effective. Ciclosporin was reported as useful in a single case [9].

REFERENCES

1 Arnozan X. Folliculite depilantes des partier glabres. *Bull Soc Fr Dermatol Syphiligr* 1982; **3**: 187–94.
2 Brocq L, Langlet E, Agrinac J. Recherches sur alopecie atrophisante, varieté pseudopelade. *Ann Dermatol Syphiligr* 1905; **6**: 1, 97, 209–13.
3 Graham-Little. Folliculitis decalvans et atrophicans. *Br J Dermatol* 1915; **27**: 183–90.
4 Horn RT, Goette DK, Odom RB *et al.* Immunofluorescent findings and clinical changes in two cases of follicular lichen planus. *J Am Acad Dermatol* 1982; **7**: 203–6.
5 Rongioletti F, Ghigliotti G, Gambina C *et al.* Agminate lichen follicularis with cysts and comedones. *Br J Dermatol* 1990; **122**: 844–9.
6 Pages F, Lapyre J, Misson R. Syndrome de Lassueur–Graham-Little. *Ann Dermatol* 1961; **88**: 272–80.
7 Reiss F, Reisch M, Buncke CM. Keratodermatitis folliculitis decalvans. *Arch Dermatol* 1958; **78**: 616–22.
8 Kubba R, Rook A. The Graham-Little syndrome. *Br J Dermatol* 1975; **93** (Suppl. 11): 53.
9 Bianchi L, Paro Vidolin P, Piemonte P, Carboni I, Chimenti S. Graham-Little–Piccardi–Lassueur syndrome: effective treatment with cyclosporin A. *Clin Exp Dermatol* 2001; **26**: 518–20.

Discoid lupus erythematosus [1]

Lupus erythematosus (LE) is an autoimmune connective tissue disease characterized by the presence of circulating non-organ-specific autoantibodies to cell nuclear antigens. Three different forms of LE are described: systemic (SLE), subacute and discoid (DLE) lupus. However, only DLE regularly produces cicatricial alopecia. Inflammation of the infundibular region of the hair follicle that contains the stem cells is thought to be the basis of the scarring alopecia that occurs in DLE, but this does not explain why the identical pattern of inflammation seen in SLE does not scar. The diffuse hair shedding that accompanies SLE is believed to be an acute telogen effluvium.

Pathology [2]. The histology of DLE, in common with SLE, shows hyperkeratosis with follicular plugging, a perivascular and periadnexal lymphoid infiltrate, which may be sparse, moderate or heavy, and the essential feature of focal basal layer vacuolar degeneration (Figs 63.37–63.39). This may be associated with colloid body formation, pigmentary incontinence, papillary dermal oedema, thickening of the basement-membrane zone and exocytosis of lymphocytes into the epidermis and follicular epithelium. Mucin can be seen in the dermis as a faint blue tinge between widely separated collagen bundles. Scarring only occurs in DLE and manifests as homogenized collagen fibres running parallel to the surface, a loss

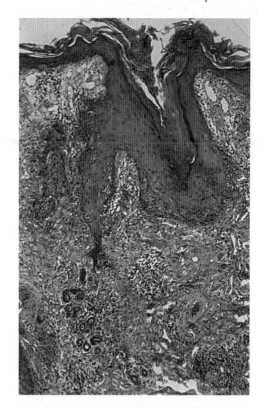

Fig. 63.37 Discoid lupus erythematosus. Low-power photomicrograph showing follicular plugging, superficial and deep perivascular and peri-appendageal lymphocytic infiltrate. (Courtesy of Dr G. Mason, Melbourne, Australia.)

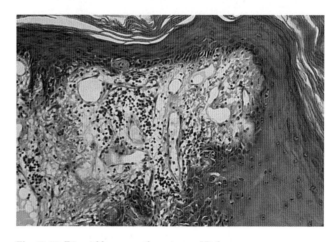

Fig. 63.38 Discoid lupus erythematosus. High-power photomicrograph showing the hydropic degeneration of the basal layer and the mononuclear cell infiltrate. (Courtesy of Dr G. Mason, Melbourne, Australia.)

of appendages and lone arrector pili muscles. Staining for elastin shows that elastic fibres are absent from the scar.

Hypergranulosis, saw-toothed rete ridges, perifollicular fibrosis and clefts are not seen in lupus, and this helps to distinguish it from lichen planus. However, frequently it is not possible to separate these two conditions on routine histological examination and in such cases

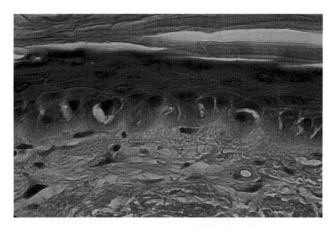

Fig. 63.39 Discoid lupus erythematosus. High-power photomicrograph showing the hydropic degeneration of the basal layer. (Courtesy of Dr G. Mason, Melbourne, Australia.)

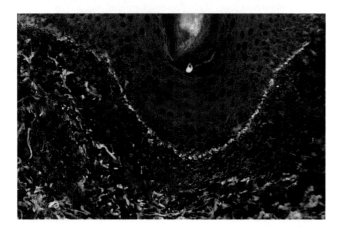

Fig. 63.40 Positive linear immunofluorescence to IgG: the lupus band test. (Courtesy of Dr G. Mason, Melbourne, Australia.)

immunofluorescence may be decisive. There is linear staining of deposits of complement (C3), IgM and IgG on the basement membrane in more than 80% of cases of LE, but not in lichen planus. Direct immunofluorescence is also positive in non-lesional skin in approximately 50–75% of cases of SLE, depending on whether sun-exposed or non-exposed skin is chosen. Only approximately 20% of cases of DLE will have positive immunofluorescence of uninvolved skin. A weak false-positive immunofluorescence to IgM can occur on the head and neck and is a source of confusion. Only positivity to IgG or very strong positivity to IgM (Fig. 63.40) should be used as supportive evidence of lupus on the scalp, as this only rarely occurs in the absence of lupus.

In old burnt-out lesions, the histology and immunofluorescence may be inconclusive and in such cases a non-specific diagnosis such as scarring alopecia is all that can be made.

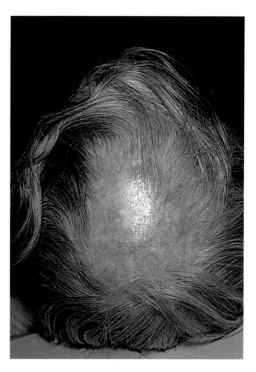

Fig. 63.41 Discoid lupus erythematosus producing cicatricial alopecia.

Clinical features [2]. DLE occurs most commonly in women (8 : 1 for SLE and 2 : 1 for DLE) and is about three times more common in African Americans than in white people. The incidence is approximately 1 in 2000. Familial cases occur in approximately 10%. The peak age of onset is around 40 years.

Scarring alopecia occurs in 20% of men and 50% of women affected with DLE, and the scalp is the only area affected in a significant number of patients. Patches on the scalp are often itchy. Areas of erythema and scaling with follicular plugging extend irregularly across the scalp and produce scarring (Fig. 63.41). Sometimes patches of scarring alopecia develop with little in the way of preceding inflammation and then resemble pseudopelade of Brocq. Ultimately, large areas of alopecia may form. Some cases burn out after 1–2 years, but others continue to progress for many years.

Pigmentary disturbance, particularly in dark-skinned people is common. Rarely, calcification occurs in the patches. Squamous cell carcinoma has been reported in chronic cicatricial LE of the scalp [3].

Antinuclear antibody (ANA) is positive in approximately 35% of patients with DLE. Anti-Ro antibodies are found in 10%. DLE may occur on its own or associated with SLE. If the initial DLE is confined to the head and neck, the risk is 1–2%, whereas if the lesions are generalized the risk is 22%. SLE first presents with DLE in 10% of cases and DLE can be found at some stage during the course of SLE in 33%.

Treatment [4]. Potent topical corticosteroids, intralesional triamcinolone and systemic prednisolone (1 mg/kg) may halt progression of active DLE. Antimalarials form the mainstay of treatment in chronic cases refractory to topical steroids. Hydroxychloroquine in a regimen of 200–400 mg/day produces a remission within 3 months in the majority and the dosage can then be tapered gradually. Scarring is permanent, but early treatment may produce a surprising amount of regrowth. Chloroquine, acitretin, dapsone, thalidomide or a combination of these medications may be useful in refractory cases. Cyclophosphamide, methotrexate and ciclosporin have also been used in severe, rapidly progressive cases where all other treatments have failed.

REFERENCES

1 Drake LA, Dinehart SM, Farmer ER *et al*. Guidelines of care for chronic cutaneous lupus erythematosus. *J Am Acad Dermatol* 1996; **34**: 830–6.
2 Whiting DA. Cicatricial alopecia. *Clin Dermatol* 2001; **19**: 211–25.
3 Onayemi O, Soyinka F. Squamous cell carcinoma of the scalp following a chemical burn and chronic discoid lupus erythematosus. *Br J Dermatol* 1996; **135**: 342–3.
4 Ter Pooten M, Theirs B. Discoid lupus erythematosus. In: Lebwohl M, Heymann WR, Berth Jones J, Coulson I, eds. *Treatment of Skin Disease*. London: Mosby, 2002: 166–8.

Pseudopelade of Brocq [1]

Pseudopelade of Brocq is an idiopathic, chronic, slowly progressive, patchy cicatricial alopecia that occurs without any evidence of inflammation. It is primarily an atrophy rather than an inflammatory folliculitis. The term pseudopelade was first used by Brocq to distinguish this condition from the 'pelade' of alopecia areata. The French term pelade had been in use at that time for more than 200 years and is derived from *pelage*—the fur, hair, wool, etc. of a mammal. In recent times, the term pseudopelade has been used to describe a generic scarring alopecia, the end result of any number of different pathological processes, and the interchangeable use by some of 'pseudopelade' and 'pseudopelade of Brocq' has led to confusion in the literature.

Pathology [2]. Early lesions may have a light lymphocytic infiltrate around the upper two-thirds of the hair follicle (including the hair bulge) that spares the epidermis and eccrine glands [3]. This infiltrate invades the walls of the follicles and sebaceous glands and eventually destroys the entire pilosebaceous unit. Single hairs may survive within a patch for many years.

Later patches are smooth, soft and slightly depressed and histological examination reveals only a thin atrophic epidermis overlying a sclerotic dermis containing fibrotic streams extending into the subcutis. There are no inflammatory changes at this stage. These fibrotic streams are follicular 'ghosts'. Arrector pili muscles may be seen

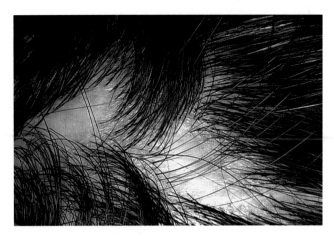

Fig. 63.42 Pseudopelade of Brocq.

inserting into these fibrous remnants of hair follicles. Elastic stains are important in differentiating pseudopelade of Brocq from lichen planus, DLE and other scarring alopecias. With an acid–alcohol orcein stain, elastic fibres are seen around the lower part of the follicle, whereas in all the other scarring alopecias the scar tissue consists of collagen devoid of elastin.

Clinical features [1]. Pseudopelade of Brocq may occur in both sexes at any age. Most commonly, women over 40 years are affected. Childhood cases are rare [4]. The aetiology and pathogenesis are unknown. The condition is almost always sporadic, but the occurrence in two brothers suggests a genetic factor may be important. There is no doubt that lichen planus can produce a very similar clinical picture and there are some authorities who maintain, on the basis of associated skin lesions and histopathological findings, that 90% of cases of 'pseudopelade' are caused by lichen planus [5].

The alopecia is asymptomatic and is often discovered by chance. It always remains confined to the scalp. The initial patch is often on the vertex but may occur anywhere (Fig. 63.42). On examination, the affected patches are smooth, soft and slightly depressed. At an early stage in the development of any individual patch there may be some erythema. The patches tend to be small and round or oval, but irregular bald patches may be formed by the confluence of many lesions. The hair in uninvolved scalp is normal, but if the process is active the hairs at the edges of each patch are very easily extracted.

The course is extremely variable. Most often there is slow development over many years of small round patches of alopecia that ultimately converge to produce larger irregular areas of hair loss. The hair in the uninvolved scalp is normal and the progression is sufficiently slow that even after 15–20 years patients may still be able to arrange their hair in such a way as to conceal the bald areas. The entire process can burn out spontaneously at

Table 63.3 Diagnostic criteria for pseudopelade of Brocq. (After Braun-Falco *et al.* [1].)

Clinical criteria
Irregularly defined and confluent patches of alopecia
Moderate atrophy (late stage)
Mild perifollicular erythema (early stage)
Female : male ratio = 3 : 1
Long course (more than 2 years)
Slow progression with spontaneous termination possible

Direct immunofluorescence
Negative (or only weak IgM on sun-exposed skin)

Histological criteria
Absence of marked inflammation
Absence of widespread scarring (best seen with elastin stain)
Absence of significant follicular plugging
Absence, or at least a decrease of sebaceous glands
Presence of normal epidermis (only occasional atrophy)
Fibrotic streams into the dermis

any stage, leaving behind only relatively small areas of alopecia.

The diagnostic criteria of Braun-Falco *et al.* [1] shown in Table 63.3, and based on the histological criteria of Pinkus [6], should be fulfilled before this specific diagnosis is made. Cases that do not fulfil these criteria should be diagnosed generically as scarring alopecia.

Treatment. The alopecia is irreversible and does not respond to topical or intralesional corticosteroids. No treatment is known to arrest progression. If the disfigurement is considerable and no active inflammatory changes are present, autografting from unaffected to scarred scalp may be considered [7], or surgical 'expansion' techniques in severe cases.

REFERENCES

1 Braun-Falco, Imei S, Schmoeckel C *et al.* Pseudopelade of Brocq. *Dermatologica* 1986; **172**: 18–26.
2 Degos R, Rabut R, Duperrat B *et al.* L'etat pseudopeladique. *Ann Dermatol Syphiligr* 1954; **81**: 5–12.
3 Pincelli C, Girolomoni G, Benassi L. Pseudopelade of Brocq: an immunologically mediated disease? *Dermatologica* 1987; **176**: 49–57.
4 Reinertson RP. Pseudopelade with nail dystrophy. *Arch Dermatol* 1958; **78**: 282–7.
5 Gay Prieto J. Pseudopelade of Brocq: its relationship to some forms of cicatricial alopecia and to lichen planus. *J Invest Dermatol* 1955; **24**: 323–34.
6 Headington JT. Cicatricial alopecia. *Dermatol Clin* 1996; **14**: 773–82.
7 Stough DB, Berger RA, Orentreich N. Surgical improvement of cicatricial alopecia of diverse etiology. *Arch Dermatol* 1968; **97**: 331–5.

Follicular degeneration syndrome [1]

This condition begins as a single focus of cicatricial alopecia over the vertex scalp in black women that gradually spreads outwards in a centrifugal pattern, but remains unifocal. It was originally called hot comb alopecia, but many patients have no preceding history of hot comb usage. A possible relationship to other hair-straightening procedures is postulated, but not conclusively proven. The name 'central centrifugal alopecia' has also been proposed, and this focuses attention on the clinical appearance of the hair loss rather than the histological identification of premature degeneration of the inner root sheath, which is variable and not entirely specific [2].

Pathology. A superficial perivascular and perifollicular lymphocytic infiltrate is seen in active areas. There is no associated interface change. Sebaceous glands are lost early, but eccrine glands are spared. Premature disintegration of the inner root sheath epithelium has been emphasized, but is not always found. Hair follicle destruction is severe and widespread and leaves prominent concentric lamellar fibrosis. Release of hair fragments into the dermis results in granulomatous inflammation.

Clinical features. Most patients are middle-aged black females who chemically straighten their hair. The alopecia is slowly progressive and the symmetrical forward progression follows a pattern similar to female pattern hair loss.

Treatment. Minimal hair grooming is recommended, but many patients find this difficult. No treatment has been found to help. Many patients resort to wearing a suitable hair piece.

REFERENCES

1 Sperling LC, Sau P. The follicular degeneration syndrome in black patients: hot comb alopecia revisited and revised. *Arch Dermatol* 1992; **128**: 68–74.
2 Whiting DA. Cicatricial alopecia. *Clin Dermatol* 2001; **19**: 211–25.

Folliculitis decalvans and tufted folliculitis [1]

Under the general term folliculitis decalvans we group the various syndromes in which clinically evident chronic folliculitis leads to progressive scarring. This is probably a heterogeneous group.

Aetiology. The cause of folliculitis decalvans is still uncertain. *Staphylococcus aureus* may be grown from the pustules. In the vast majority of people who develop a bacterial pustular folliculitis of the scalp it is transient, resolves with antibiotics and heals without scarring. In some, the folliculitis is more persistent, tends to recur in the same site after apparently successful treatment with antibiotics and produces a scarring alopecia. An abnormal host response to *Staph. aureus* is postulated, which may be the result of a defect in cell-mediated immunity.

Shitara *et al.* [2] reported severe folliculitis decalvans in two siblings who also had chronic candidiasis; defective cell-mediated immunity was demonstrated. Douwes *et al.* [3] reported simultaneous occurence in identical twins, with no identifiable immune abnormality.

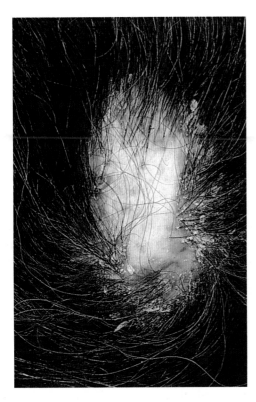

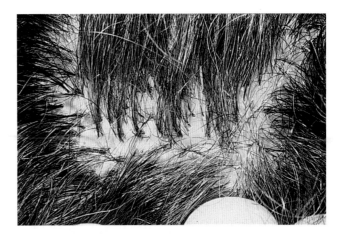

Fig. 63.44 Tufted folliculitis.

Fig. 63.43 Folliculitis decalvans showing active pustulation and scarring.

Pathology [1,4,5]. Histology reveals follicular abscesses, with a dense perifollicular polymorphonuclear infiltrate and scattered eosinophils and plasma cells. Foreign-body granulomas occur in response to follicular disruption, which is succeeded by scarring. Eventually all that remains of the follicle is extensive fibrosis.

Clinical features [1]. Men may be affected from adolescence onwards, whereas women tend not to develop this condition until their thirties. Following a pustular folliculitis of the scalp, usually one, but occasionally more, rounded patches of alopecia develop, each surrounded by crusting and a few follicular pustules. Successive crops of pustules appear and are followed by progressive destruction of the affected follicles (Fig. 63.43). In some cases the folliculitis spreads along the scalp margin in a coronal pattern, or along the edge of an AGA. The severity of the inflammatory changes fluctuates, but the course is prolonged.

Tufted folliculitis is a variant of folliculitis decalvans where circumscribed areas of scalp inflammation heal with scarring characterized by tufts of up to 15 hairs emerging from a single orifice (Fig. 63.44) [6–8]. The tufts consist of a central anagen hair surrounded by telogen hairs, each arising from independent follicles, converging towards a common dilated follicular infundibulum. Cases in which the tufts were comprised of only anagen hairs

have also been described. Based on an animal model, it is suggested that erythema and scaling are the initial events and the tufting is a consequence of the emergence of hairs from beneath the free edge of the scales.

A scalp biopsy is required to confirm the diagnosis and swabs should be taken of any pustules. Investigation for an underlying defect in cell-mediated immunity is generally unrewarding, and only indicated when there is additional evidence of impaired immunity. As fungal kerion may mimic folliculitis decalvans, hairs should be plucked for fungal culture and a PAS stain should be performed on the scalp biopsy.

Treatment [1]. Essentially, treatment consists of attempts to eradicate *Staph. aureus* from the scalp. Prolonged courses of flucloxacillin induce remission, but relapse occurs when the antibiotics are stopped. For localized areas, topical clindamycin is useful. Tetracyclines are also commonly effective. Isotretinoin has been used to alter the follicular environment to make it less suitable for *Staph. aureus* colonization, but it may increase cutaneous carriage of this organism and make the condition worse. The only treatment shown to induce prolonged remission is rifampicin in a dosage of 300 mg twice daily. This should be given in combination with other antibiotics to prevent the emergence of resistant organisms. Drugs commonly used in combination include clindamycin 300 mg twice daily, fucidic acid 150 mg three times daily, ciprofloxacin, doxycycline and clarithromycin.

Tufting may be reduced by measures directed at reducing the scale, such as the use of tar shampoos and topical keratolytics.

REFERENCES

1 Powell JJ, Dawber RPR, Gatter K. Folliculitis decalvans and tufted folliculitis: clinical, histological and therapeutic findings. *Br J Dermatol* 1999; **140**: 328–33.

2 Shitara A, Igareshi R, Morohashi M. Folliculitis decalvans and cellular immunity: two brothers with oral candidiasis. *Jpn J Dermatol* 1974; **28**: 133 [in Japanese].
3 Douwes KE, Landthaler M, Szeimies RM. Simultaneous occurrence of folliculitis decalvans capillitii in identical twins. *Br J Dermatol* 2000; **143**: 195–7.
4 Headington JT. Cicatricial alopecia. *Dermatol Clin* 1996; **14**: 773–82.
5 Whiting DA. Cicatricial alopecia. *Clin Dermatol* 2001; **19**: 211–25.
6 Dalziel K, Telfer N, Dawber RPR. Tufted folliculitis. *Am J Dermatopathol* 1990; **12**: 37–41.
7 Tong AKF, Baden H. Tufted folliculitis. *J Am Acad Dermatol* 1989; **21**: 1096–9.
8 Khalifen L, Todd DJ. Tufted folliculitis in Jordanian patients. *Int J Dermatol* 1996; **35**: 280–2.

Dissecting cellulitis of the scalp [1]
SYN. DISSECTING FOLLICULITIS;
PERIFOLLICULITIS CAPITIS ABSCEDENS ET
SUFFODIENS

This rare condition manifests with a perifolliculitis of the scalp, deep and superficial abscesses in the dermis, sinus tract formation and extensive scarring. It occurs predominantly in black males aged between 18 and 40 years. Familial cases are exceptional, as is childhood onset.

Aetiology. The aetiology of this inflammatory condition is unknown. Although staphylococci, streptococci and *Pseudomonas* may be cultured from various lesions, no specific causative organism has been isolated. Dissecting cellulitis associates with hidradenitis suppurativa and acne conglobata in the follicular occlusion triad [2]. Other reported associations include pilonidal sinus and spondyloarthropathy. The activity of the arthritis parallels the activity of the skin.

Clinical features. Painful, firm, skin-coloured nodules develop near the vertex of the scalp and later become softer and fluctuant (Fig. 63.45). Confluent nodules form tubular ridges with an irregular cerebriform pattern, on a red and oedematous background. Thin blood-stained pus exudes from crusted sinuses, and pressure on one region

of the scalp may cause discharge of pus from a neighbouring intercommunicating ridge. Cervical adenitis is present in some cases, but is more remarkable for its absence in many others. Progressive scarring and permanent alopecia occur. Characteristically, hair is lost from the summits of these inflammatory lesions and retained in the valleys. The condition is chronic, with frequent acute exacerbations. Fatal squamous cell carcinoma has developed within the areas of scarring after many years [3].

Pathology [4]. Histology shows a perifolliculitis with a heavy infiltrate of lymphocytes, histiocytes and polymorphonuclear cells. Abscess formation results, and leads to destruction of the pilosebaceous follicles initially, and eventually the other cutaneous appendages. Keratin fragments induce a granulomatous reaction, with foreign-body giant cells, lymphoid and plasma cells. Special stains for bacteria, fungi and mycobacteria are negative.

Investigations. Culture from affected areas often grows bacterial organisms. Fungal cultures and a scalp biopsy for routine histology and direct immunofluorescence will exclude other causes of scarring alopecia.

Treatment. Although systemic antibiotics and topical or intralesional corticosteroids are sometimes helpful, relapses are frequent and the course is usually protracted. Isotretinoin in full dosage (1 mg/kg), in combination with prednisolone (1 mg/kg) and erythromycin 500 mg four times daily, may induce a rapid remission and significant hair regrowth in areas not yet irreversibly damaged [5]. Because the inflammation is predominantly perifollicular, a surprising amount of regrowth may occur. The antibiotics can be stopped after 4 weeks and the prednisolone gradually tailed off and replaced by topical steroids. The isotretinoin should be continued for at least 6 months, and reintroduced if the condition relapses. In recalcitrant cases, widespread excision and grafting may be considered, or alternatively in an older patient, X-ray epilation has been used with success [6]. Improvement has also been noted following laser-assisted hair removal [7].

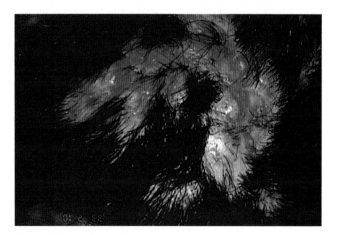

Fig. 63.45 Dissecting cellulitis of the scalp. (Courtesy of Dr D. Dyall-Smith and the *Australasian Journal of Dermatology* [5].)

REFERENCES

1 Wise F, Parkhurst HJ. A rare form of suppurating cicatrizing disease of the scalp (perifolliculitis capitis abscedens et suffodiens). *Arch Dermatol Syphilol* 1921; **4**: 750–8.
2 Chicarilli ZN. Follicular occlusion triad: hidradenitis suppurativa, acne conglobata, and dissecting cellulitis of the scalp. *Ann Plast Surg* 1987; **18**: 230–7.
3 Camisa C. Squamous cell carcinoma arising in acne conglobata. *Cutis* 1984; **33**: 185–7, 190.
4 Whiting DA. Cicatricial alopecia. *Clin Dermatol* 2001; **19**: 211–25.
5 Dyall-Smith D. Signs, syndromes and diagnoses in dermatology: dissecting cellulitis of the scalp. *Australas J Dermatol* 1993; **34**: 81–2.
6 Scheinfeld NS. A case of dissecting cellulitis and a review of the literature. *Dermatol Online J* 2003; **9**: 8.
7 Chui CT, Berger TG, Price VH, Zachary CB. Recalcitrant scarring follicular disorders treated by laser-assisted hair removal: a preliminary report. *Dermatol Surg* 1999; **25**: 34–7.

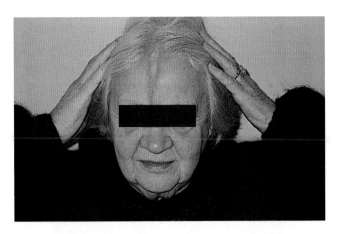

Fig. 63.46 Linear morphoea (en coup de sabre). After having this lesion since adolescence this lady recently developed biopsy-proven lichen sclerosus of the vulva.

Circumscribed scleroderma and linear morphoea

Circumscribed scleroderma is rare in the scalp, but may occur there as single or multiple lesions. The hair is shed at an early stage to leave a cicatricial alopecia. The diagnosis must be confirmed histologically. Linear circumscribed morphoea in the frontal region—'en coup de sabre' morphoea (Fig. 63.46)—is slightly more common (see Chapter 56). It has been suggested that lesions may follow the lines of Blaschko [1]. Histological examination of both conditions shows chronic inflammation of the upper and mid-follicle, and prominent fibrosis [2]. Linear morphoea has been associated with hereditary deficiency of complement C2 [3].

REFERENCES

1 McKennna DB, Benton EC. A tri-linear pattern of scleroderma 'en coup de sabre' following Blaschko's lines. *Clin Exp Dermatol* 1999; **24**: 467–8.
2 Whiting DA. Cicatricial alopecia. *Clin Dermatol* 2001; **19**: 211–25.
3 Hulsmans RFHJ, Asghar SS, Siddiqui AH, Cormane RH. Hereditary deficiency of C2 in association with linear scleroderma, 'en coup de sabre'. *Arch Dermatol* 1986; **122**: 76–80.

Cicatricial pemphigoid

SYN. BENIGN MUCOSAL PEMPHIGOID

Cicatricial pemphigoid affects predominantly the elderly, and women more than men [1,2]. It is associated with autoantibodies to the basement-membrane-zone adhesion complex (see Chapter 41).

Bullae are formed at the dermal–epidermal junction. Direct immunocytochemical studies show that linear deposits of IgG, IgA, C3 and C4 may be found in the basement-membrane zone, but circulating basement-membrane-zone antibodies (IgG or IgA) are not always demonstrable [3,4].

Although the disease affects predominantly the ocular and/or genital mucous membrane, the skin is involved in 40–50% of cases, and skin lesions may precede the mucosal lesions by months or years [5]. The skin lesions repeatedly recur and leave scars. The favoured sites are the face and upper trunk, the scalp being involved in approximately 10% of cases [6]. Skin lesions, predominantly on the head and neck, are the major feature of the Brunsting–Perry variant.

Management is often dictated by the need to control mucosal lesions. If recurrent bullae in a localized area of skin are troublesome, excision and grafting may be successful [6]. Whether to prescribe oral corticosteroids or immunosuppressive drugs for skin lesions alone is controversial, but topical clobetasol propionate cream may inhibit the process to some degree.

REFERENCES

1 Pearson RW. Advances in the diagnosis and treatment of blistering diseases: a selective review. In: Malkinson F, Pearson RW, eds. *Year Book of Dermatology*. Chicago: Year Book, 1977: 7.
2 Kurzhals G, Stolz W, Maciejewski W, Kurpati S. Localized cicatricial pemphigoid. *Arch Dermatol* 1995; **131**: 580–1.
3 Holubar K, Honigsmann H, Wolff K. Cicatricial pemphigoid. *Arch Dermatol* 1973; **108**: 50–6.
4 Whiting DA. Cicatricial alopecia. *Clin Dermatol* 2001; **19**: 211–25.
5 Leenutaphong V, von Kries R, Plewig G. Localized cicatricial pemphigoid (Brunsting–Perry) electron microscopic study. *J Am Acad Dermatol* 1989; **21**: 1089–93.
6 Slepyan AH, Burks JW, Fox J. Persistent denudation of the scalp in cicatricial pemphigoid: treatment by skin grafting. *Arch Dermatol* 1961; **84**: 444–51.

Erosive pustular dermatosis of the scalp

This clinical entity particularly affects the elderly [1,2]. Its cause is unknown but Grattan *et al.* [3], in their study of 12 cases, suggested that local trauma and sun damage are important. Surgery, cryosurgery, skin grafting and radiation therapy may all precipitate this condition [4].

Pathology. Histological examination shows areas of epidermal erosion, a chronic inflammatory cell infiltration in the dermis consisting predominantly of lymphocytes and plasma cells, and sometimes small foci of foreign body giant cells where hair follicles have been destroyed.

Clinical features. This condition almost always occurs in association with AGA. Initially, a small area of scalp becomes red, crusted and irritable; crusting and superficial pustulation overlie a moist eroded surface (Fig. 63.47). As the condition extends, areas of activity coexist with areas of scarring. Squamous carcinoma has developed in the scars [5].

Differential diagnosis. Pyogenic and yeast infection is excluded by bacteriological examination and the lack of response to antibacterial or antifungal agents. Biopsy may be necessary to exclude pustular psoriasis, cicatricial

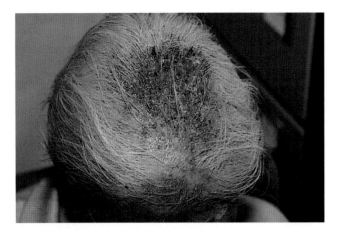

Fig. 63.47 Erosive pustular dermatosis of the scalp occurring on a sun-exposed bald scalp.

pemphigoid, 'irritated' solar keratosis or squamous cell carcinoma.

Treatment. The stronger topical corticosteroids (e.g. 0.05% clobetasol propionate) will suppress the inflammatory changes. Gradual reduction in the potency of topical steroid over a 6-month period may result in cure. Maintenance therapy with sun protection and intermittent moderate potency steroid can provide long-term relief. Ikeda *et al.* [6] suggested oral zinc sulphate and Boffa [7] suggested topical calcipotriol can be curative in some cases.

REFERENCES

1 Caputo R, Veraldi S. Erosive pustular dermatosis of the scalp. *J Am Acad Dermatol* 1993; **28**: 96–7.
2 Pye RJ, Peachey RDG, Burton JL. Erosive pustular dermatosis of the scalp. *Br J Dermatol* 1979; **100**: 559–63.
3 Grattan CEH, Peachey RD, Boon A. Evidence for a role of local trauma in the pathogenesis of erosive pustular dermatosis of the scalp. *Clin Exp Dermatol* 1988; **13**: 7–12.
4 Rongioletti F, Delmonte S, Rossi ME, Strani GF, Rebora A. Erosive pustular dermatosis of the scalp following cryotherapy and topical tretinoin for actinic keratoses. *Clin Exp Dermatol* 1999; **24**: 499–500.
5 Lovell CR, Harman RRM, Bradfield JWB. Cutaneous carcinoma arising in erosive pustular dermatosis of the scalp. *Br J Dermatol* 1980; **102**: 325–30.
6 Ikeda M, Arata J, Isaka H. Erosive dermatosis of the scalp successfully treated with oral zinc sulphate. *Br J Dermatol* 1983; **105**: 742–7.
7 Boffa MJ. Erosive pustular dermatosis of the scalp successfully treated with calcipotriol cream. *Br J Dermatol* 2003; **148**: 593–5.

Necrobiosis lipoidica, granuloma annulare and sarcoidosis

Necrobiosis lipoidica occurs in 0.2–0.3% of cases of diabetes mellitus, and approximately 70% of patients with necrobiosis have diabetes. The diabetic cases begin in childhood or early adult life, and the non-diabetic cases rather later and usually in women.

The oval atrophic plaques classically occur on the shins but may be seen on other parts of the body including the

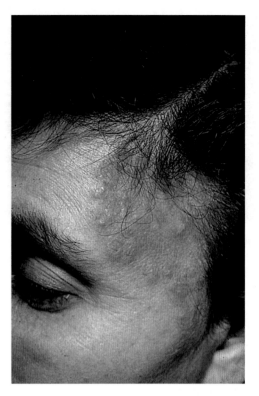

Fig. 63.48 Sarcoidosis of the scalp.

scalp. The patches are glazed and yellowish, often with conspicuous telangiectases. Scarring may be dense. The clinical features in the scalp vary from large plaques of cicatricial alopecia to multiple small areas of scarring [1].

An atrophic form affecting predominantly the forehead and the scalp has been described [2,3]. In general, the differential diagnosis is from sarcoidosis and granuloma annulare [4–6].

Cutaneous sarcoidosis may produce plaques or nodules on the scalp as well as both cicatricial and non-cicatricial alopecia (Fig. 63.48) [7]. Affected areas may itch. There is a marked preponderance of females amongst reported cases. The histology is distinctive, with non-caseating granulomatous inflammation [5].

REFERENCES

1 Gertmann H, Dickmans-Burmeister D. Ungewohnliche Hautveran-derungen bei einem 4 jahrigen Kinde mit Diabetes mellitus: 'Nekrobiosis diabetica acute parvimaculata'. *Hautarzt* 1969; **20**: 265–72.
2 Navaratnam A, Hodgson CA. Necrobiosis lipoidica presenting on the face and scalp. *Br J Dermatol* 1973; **89** (Suppl. 9): 100–1.
3 Wilson Jones E. Necrobiosis lipoidica presenting on the face and scalp. *Trans St John's Hosp Dermatol Soc* 1971; **57**: 202–9.
4 Maurice DDL, Goolamali SK. Sarcoidosis of the scalp presenting as scarring alopecia. *Br J Dermatol* 1988; **119**: 116–8.
5 Katta R, Nelson B, Chen D, Roenigk H. Sarcoidosis of the scalp: a case series and review of the literature. *J Am Acad Dermatol* 2000; **42**: 690–2.
6 Wong GA, Verbov JL. Subcutaneous granuloma annulare of the scalp in a diabetic child. *Pediatr Dermatol* 2002; **19**: 276–7.
7 Sinclair RD, Banfield C, Dawber RPR. *Handbook of Diseases of the Hair and Scalp*. Oxford: Blackwell Science, 1999.

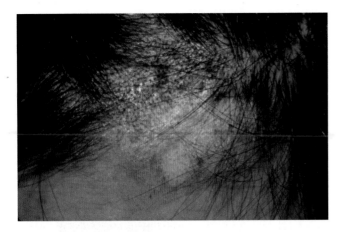

Fig. 63.49 Lichen sclerosus.

Lichen sclerosus et atrophicus

This disease affects females 10 times more often than males [1]. Lichen sclerosus of the scalp appears to be rare (Fig. 63.49). It may cause an extensive cicatricial alopecia that is relatively nondescript clinically, but which has all the characteristic features histologically. Associated lesions are usually found on the trunk and vulva [2,3].

REFERENCES

1 Wallace HI. Lichen sclerosis et atrophicus. *Trans St John's Hosp Dermatol Soc* 1972; **57**: 148–60.
2 Foulds IS. Lichen sclerosus et atrophicus of the scalp. *Br J Dermatol* 1980; **103**: 197–9.
3 Sinclair RD, Banfield C, Dawber RPR. *Handbook of Diseases of the Hair and Scalp*. Oxford: Blackwell Science, 1999.

Developmental defects and hereditary disorders

Scarring follicular keratosis

Numerous syndromes have been described and elaborately named, all of them characterized by keratosis pilaris associated with some degree of inflammatory change leading to destruction of the affected follicles [1].

Only detailed clinical and genetic studies can provide the essential facts to allow reliable differentiation of syndromes that some authorities regard as forms or degrees of a single state and others accept as distinct entities. For the time being, the reported cases can be conveniently classified in three groups; in addition, certain apparently well-defined entities can be recognized.

1 *Atrophoderma vermiculata* (acne vermiculata, folliculitis ulerythematosa reticulata). There is honeycomb atrophy of the cheeks. Scarring alopecia may occur, but rarely.
2 *Keratosis pilaris atrophicans faciei* (ulerythema oophryogenes). The process is more or less confined to the eyebrow region.

3 *Keratosis pilaris decalvans* (keratosis follicularis spinulosa decalvans, follicular ichthyosis). Keratosis pilaris of variable extent is associated with cicatricial alopecia [2].
All these conditions are assumed to be genetically determined, although many cases occur sporadically. Such genetic data as are available are considered under the individual forms.

The follicles are initially distended by horny plugs, the dermis is oedematous and there is some lymphocytic infiltration around follicles and vessels. Later, the follicles are destroyed. Small epithelial cysts may be numerous, particularly in keratosis pilaris atrophicans faciei.

Clinical features. Atrophoderma vermiculata usually begins in childhood. Follicular plugs, often in the preauricular regions, are gradually shed to leave reticulate atrophy. On the face, the extent of the process is variable. Exceptionally, cicatricial alopecia of the scalp may be associated [3].

Keratosis pilaris atrophicans faciei (ulerythema oophryogenes) is present from early infancy. Erythema and horny plugs begin in the outer halves of the eyebrows, which they eventually destroy, and then advance medially and to a variable extent on the cheeks. Involvement of the scalp has apparently not been reported in cases in which the eyebrows are predominantly involved. However, there are reports of cases to which this diagnosis has been applied, but which appear to be more rationally classified in one of the other categories, in which alopecia has occurred. Such cases emphasize the need for improved diagnostic criteria.

Keratosis pilaris decalvans is also such a variable syndrome that several genotypes must be considered. Keratosis pilaris begins in infancy or childhood, often on the face. Ultimately, it may be confined to the face or to face and limbs, or may be more or less universal. It is often succeeded by atrophy on the face, but rarely on the limbs or trunk. Cicatricial alopecia is noted from early childhood or later, and may be localized or extensive [4]. Familial cases without significant eyebrow involvement are reported [5].

Three members of one family developed keratosis pilaris of the face in early childhood [6] and then extensively on the back and limbs, and on the scalp, where horny papules replaced hairs. A similar syndrome was reported in a young man who had keratosis pilaris and severe cicatricial alopecia [7]. The occurrence of cases similar to those reported by MacLeod [6] in other siblings, born of normal parents, suggested recessive inheritance but the evidence was incomplete. The pattern of hair loss in the family reported by Ullmo [8] was in the distribution of the Marie–Unna type of congenital alopecia, apart from the presence of keratosis pilaris on the face.

What may be another distinct syndrome associates extremely severe keratosis pilaris—'closely woven bristles'

—with almost complete alopecia, reduced sweating and deafness [9].

Treatment. Only symptomatic measures are available. Retinoic acid deserves a trial. The status of oral retinoids remains controversial, although anecdotal response has been noted.

REFERENCES

1 Rand RE, Arndt KA. Follicular syndromes with inflammation and atrophy. In: Fitzpatrick TB, Eisen AZ, Wolff K *et al.*, eds. *Dermatology in General Medicine*, 3rd edn. New York: McGraw-Hill, 1987: 717–32.
2 Rand RE, Baden H. Keratosis follicularis spinulosa decalvans: report of two cases and review of the literature. *Arch Dermatol* 1983; **119**: 22–9.
3 Fisher AA. Keratosis pilaris rubra atrophicans faciei with diffuse alopecia of the scalp. *Arch Dermatol* 1957; **75**: 283–9.
4 Dawber RPR, Van Neste D. *Hair and Scalp Disorders*. London: Dunitz, 1995: 118–39.
5 Khumalo NP, Loo WJ, Hollowood K et·al. Keratosis pilaris atrophicans in mother and daughter. *J Eur Acad Dermatol Venereol* 2002; **16**: 397–400.
6 MacLeod JMH. Three cases of 'ichthyosis follicularis' associated with baldness. *Br J Dermatol* 1909; **21**: 165–71.
7 Kubba R, Mitchell JNS, Rook A. Keratosis pilaris with recurrent folliculitis decalvans. *Br J Dermatol* 1975; **93** (Suppl. 11): 55.
8 Ullmo A. Un nouveau type d'agenesie et de dystrophie pilaire familiale et hereditare. *Dermatologica* 1944; **90**: 74–8.
9 Morris J, Ackerman AB, Koblenzer PJ. Generalized spiny hyperkeratosis, universal alopecia and deafness. *Arch Dermatol* 1969; **100**: 692–7.

Porokeratosis of Mibelli

Porokeratosis of Mibelli commonly begins in childhood but may first appear at any age. It is most frequent on the limbs, particularly the hands and feet, the neck, the shoulders and the face, but may occur anywhere, including the scalp [1]. The initial lesion is a crateriform horny papule that gradually extends to form a circinate or irregular atrophic plaque with a raised horny margin, which may be surmounted by a furrow from which the lamina of horn projects. In the scalp there is loss of hair in the atrophic phase.

REFERENCE

1 Sehgal VM, Dube B. Porokeratosis (Mibelli) in a family. *Dermatologica* 1967; **134**: 269–72.

Incontinentia pigmenti

Cicatricial alopecia has been present in at least 25% of reported cases of incontinentia pigmenti; it appears in early infancy and ceases to extend after a variable period of up to 2 years, but the loss of hair is permanent. Other hair defects present in some cases have been hypoplasia of the eyebrows and eyelashes, and woolly hair naevus of the scalp [1].

REFERENCE

1 Wiklund DA, Weston WL. Incontinentia pigmenti. *Arch Dermatol* 1960; **115**: 701–5.

Generalized follicular hamartoma

Cicatricial alopecia beginning in childhood was a feature of a syndrome described by Mehregan and Hardin [1]. Their patient was a woman aged 23 years. From infancy, she had widespread horny plugs over the trunk and limbs and small pits on the palms and soles. She later developed cicatricial alopecia, in which, from the age of 8 years, appeared follicular tumours. The tumours of the scalp were proliferating tricholemmal cysts. The lesions of palms and soles showed funnel-shaped dilatation of sweat ducts, which were plugged with parakeratotic material containing acid mucopolysaccharide. Ridley and Smith [2] described this entity with alopecia and myasthenia gravis.

REFERENCES

1 Mehregan AH, Hardin I. Generalized follicular hamartoma. *Arch Dermatol* 1973; **107**: 435–40.
2 Ridley CM, Smith NP. Generalized hair follicle hamartoma associated with alopecia and myasthenia gravis. *Clin Exp Dermatol* 1981; **6**: 283–6.

Epidermolysis bullosa

The term epidermolysis bullosa is applied to a group of distinct, genetically determined disorders characterized by the formation of bullae of skin, and often also of mucous membranes, in response to trauma, or spontaneously (see Chapter 40). Only one of these diseases is accompanied by abnormalities of scalp or hair—recessive dystrophic epidermolysis bullosa. However, Gamborg Nielsen and Sjolund [1] described a new syndrome of localized epidermolysis bullosa simplex associated with hair, nail and teeth abnormalities. Alopecia may also occur in junctional epidermolysis bullosa.

Bullae form at the dermal–epidermal junction and fragments of dermis may adhere to the roof.

The inexorable blistering of skin and mucous membranes dominates the picture. The blisters are followed by atrophic scarring. This may give rise to more or less extensive cicatricial alopecia of the scalp [2,3]. Of 30 cases studied by Videl [4], three had cicatricial alopecia.

REFERENCES

1 Gamborg Nielsen P, Sjolund E. Epidermolysis bullosa simplex: localization associated with anodontia, hair and nail abnormalities. *Acta Derm Venereol (Stockh)* 1985; **65**: 526–31.
2 Wagner W. Alopezia und Nagelveranderungen bei Epidermolysis bullosa hereditaria. *Z Haut Geschlechtskr* 1956; **20**: 270–4.
3 Vuorinen E. Uber ein Zwillingspaar mit Epidermolysis bullosa dystrophica polydysplastica. *Dermatologica* 1970; **140** (Suppl.): 3–5.
4 Videl J. Epidermolysis ampollares. *Acta Derm Sifiliogr* 1974; **65**: 3–7.

Cleft lip-palate, ectodermal dysplasia and syndactyly

This rare or rarely recognized syndrome is probably

hereditary, and determined by an autosomal recessive gene.

The constant features of the syndrome are mental retardation, cleft palate, genital hypoplasia, cicatricial alopecia, defective teeth and syndactyly [1].

REFERENCE

1 Brown P, Armstrong HB. Ectodermal dysplasia, mental retardation, cleft lip/palate and other anomalies in three sibs. *Clin Genet* 1976; **9**: 35–40.

Polyostotic fibrous dysplasia

The progressive enlargement over a period of 10 years of a bald patch present since childhood was shown histologically to be caused by the replacement of the follicles by coils of fibrous tissue. The patient had polyostotic fibrous dysplasia [1].

REFERENCE

1 Shelley WB, Wood MG. Alopecia with fibrous dysplasia and osteomas of the skin. *Arch Dermatol* 1976; **112**: 715–9.

Infections
[A.G. Messenger]

Tinea capitis

See Chapter 31.

Infestations

See Chapter 33.

Syphilis

Hair loss occurs in approximately 10% of cases of secondary syphilis and may be the presenting feature [1,2]. The hair loss typically has a 'moth-eaten' appearance but may be diffuse in nature [3]. Other features of secondary syphilis are present in most cases, particularly lymph node enlargement and hepatomegaly, but hair loss has been reported as the only sign of the disease [4]. Histological features include an increase in catagen and telogen forms, and a peribulbar lymphocytic infiltrate, similar to the changes seen in alopecia areata [3]. Additional features in syphilis include lymphocytic infiltration of the isthmus region, parabulbar lymphoid aggregates and the presence of plasma cells within the infiltrate.

The serpiginous nodulo-squamous syphilide of tertiary syphilis may affect the scalp and the syphilitic gumma is a cause of scarring alopecia.

Human immunodeficiency virus (see Chapter 26)

A variety of alterations in hair growth have been described in patients with HIV infection. Telogen effluvium is a common cause of hair loss [5]. Causes include chronic HIV-1 infection itself, secondary infections, nutritional deficiencies and drugs. Hair loss has been reported with several antiretroviral drugs, particularly indinavir [6], which may cause loss of hair on the body as well as the scalp. There are also reports of alopecia areata occurring in patients with HIV infection [7–9].

There are several reports of hypertrichosis of the eyelashes (eyelash trichomegaly) in HIV infection [9–11]. The cause of this striking and unusual feature is not known. It is usually associated with advanced disease and has been noted to regress with antiretroviral treatment [11].

Straightening of the hair is a common feature of HIV infection in black patients [12].

Various forms of folliculitis are seen in HIV infection, including acneiform eruptions, staphylococcal folliculitis and eosinophilic pustular folliculitis.

Leprosy

Loss of eyebrow and body hair may occur in lepromatous leprosy but the scalp is rarely involved.

REFERENCES

1 Kennedy C. Syphilis presenting as hair loss. *BMJ* 1976; **2**: 854.
2 Hira SK, Patel JS, Bhat SG *et al.* Clinical manifestations of secondary syphilis. *Int J Dermatol* 1987; **26**: 103–7.
3 Lee JY, Hsu ML. Alopecia syphilitica, a simulator of alopecia areata: histopathology and differential diagnosis. *J Cutan Pathol* 1991; **18**: 87–92.
4 Cuozzo DW, Benson PM, Sperling LC *et al.* Essential syphilitic alopecia revisited. *J Am Acad Dermatol* 1995; **32**: 840–3.
5 Smith KJ, Skelton HG, DeRusso D *et al.* Clinical and histopathologic features of hair loss in patients with HIV-1 infection. *J Am Acad Dermatol* 1996; **34**: 63–8.
6 Calista D, Boschini A. Cutaneous side-effects induced by indinavir. *Eur J Dermatol* 2000; **10**: 292–6.
7 Ostlere LS, Langtry JA, Staughton RC *et al.* Alopecia universalis in a patient seropositive for the human immunodeficiency virus. *J Am Acad Dermatol* 1992; **27**: 630–1.
8 Stewart MI, Smoller BR. Alopecia universalis in an HIV-positive patient: possible insight into pathogenesis. *J Cutan Pathol* 1993; **20**: 180–3.
9 Grossman MC, Cohen PR, Grossman ME. Acquired eyelash trichomegaly and alopecia areata in a human immunodeficiency virus-infected patient. *Dermatology* 1996; **193**: 52–3.
10 Casanova JM, Puig T, Rubio M. Hypertrichosis of the eyelashes in acquired immunodeficiency syndrome. *Arch Dermatol* 1987; **123**: 1599–601.
11 Kaplan MH, Sadick NS, Talmor M. Acquired trichomegaly of the eyelashes: a cutaneous marker of acquired immunodeficiency syndrome. *J Am Acad Dermatol* 1991; **25**: 801–4.
12 Leonidas JR. Hair alteration in black patients with the acquired immunodeficiency syndrome. *Cutis* 1987; **39**: 537–8.

Artefactual alopecia
[D.A.R. de Berker, pp. 63.61–63.65]

Cosmetic alopecia

The dictates of religion, custom and fashion have imposed an immense variety of physical stresses on human hair. Two types of hair loss occur as a result of cosmetic

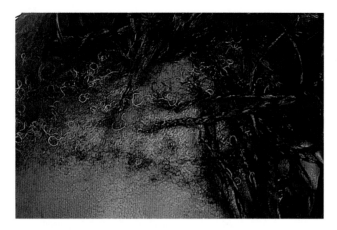

Fig. 63.50 Traction alopecia from braiding.

practices: those characterized by structural damage to the hair shaft leading to excessive weathering and breakage, and those where hair follicles are injured by prolonged traction from hair styling. A third type, centrifugal cicatricial alopecia or follicular degeneration syndrome, which occurs in women of African extraction, has been ascribed to cosmetic procedures, but this is controversial.

Traction alopecia

Traction alopecia is brought about by hair styles that impose sustained pulling on the hair roots. The clinical features in the many variants of this syndrome include folliculitis, reduction in hair density with vellus hairs and sometimes broken hairs in the affected areas, and eventually scarring alopecia. Keratin cylinders ('hair casts') may surround many hairs just above the scalp surface [1]. The pattern of the hair loss is often distinctive and reflects the distribution of the traction.

Traction alopecia is seen most commonly in Afro-Caribbean hair styles where the hair is tightly braided. The hair loss commonly begins in the temporal regions and in front of and above the ears, but may involve other parts of the scalp margin, or even linear areas in other parts of the scalp (Fig. 63.50). If continued long term, permanent scarring alopecia may occur [2]. The use of rollers may cause alopecia in the frontal and temporal regions, as may 'ponytail' styles. Frontal and parietal traction alopecia has been reported in young Sikh boys as a result of twisting their uncut hair tightly on top of the head [3], and tight braiding and wooden combs produce traction alopecia in the Sudan; frontal loss is reported in Libyan women as a result of traction from a tight scarf [4].

Treatment. The diagnosis of traction alopecia is usually not difficult, provided the possibility is considered. The cause is not always recognized by the patient and may be received with suspicion. The patient, or parents of affected children, need to be educated to adopt hair styles that do not pull the hair tight [2].

Follicular degeneration syndrome

See p. 63.54.

REFERENCES

1 Rollins TG. Traction folliculitis with hair casts and alopecia. *Am J Dis Child* 1961; **101**: 609–13.
2 Wilborn WS. Disorders of hair growth in African Americans. In: Olsen E, ed. *Disorders of Hair Growth*, 2nd edn. New York: McGraw-Hill, 2003: 497–518.
3 Singh G. Traction alopecia in Sikh boys. *Br J Dermatol* 1975; **92**: 232–8.
4 Malhotra YK, Kanwar AJ. Traumatic alopecia among Libyan women. *Arch Dermatol* 1980; **116**: 987–90.

Physical trauma

The diagnosis and treatment of the consequences of physical injuries of the scalp will seldom confront dermatologists, but they may be consulted as to the cause of an apparent physical injury (e.g. aplasia cutis may be falsely attributed to forceps injury at childbirth). The attachment of an electrode to the scalp for monitoring the fetal heartbeat during labour may occasionally cause some superficial damage, and this may be followed by a small scar. Aplasia cutis has sometimes been mistaken for such a lesion [1].

An unusual case of cicatricial alopecia in a boy aged 13 years was caused by injury to the scalp by an intravenous infusion given in infancy for gastroenteritis [2]. Exceptionally, self-inflicted injuries may involve the scalp and leave scars.

Halo scalp ring [3]

A type of alopecia, which may be temporary or permanent, is an area of scalp hair loss resulting from prolonged pressure on the vertex by the uterine cervix during or prior to delivery, resulting in a haemorrhagic form of caput succedaneum.

Scalp necrosis after surgical embolization

Adler *et al.* [4] described a case in which ischaemic necrosis of the occipital scalp occurred following embolization and surgery for a large convexity meningioma.

Women who had undergone prolonged pelvic operations in the Trendelenburg position developed, 12–26 days later, a vertical patch of alopecia, which was preceded by oedema, exudation and crusting. Pressure ischaemia during the operation was considered to be the cause of the alopecia [5]. In one large clinic, over a period of 3 years, 60 cases of occipital pressure alopecia were observed after open-heart surgery [6]. In 29 of these cases, the hair loss was permanent. Temporary alopecia followed prolonged pressure on the scalp by a foam rubber ring used to prevent such an occurrence [7].

REFERENCES

1 Brown ZA, Jung AL, Stenehuver MA. Aplasia cutis congenita and the fetal scalp electrode. *Am J Obstet Gynecol* 1977; **129**: 351–60.
2 Strong AMM. Extensive cicatricial alopecia following a scalp vein infusion. *Clin Exp Dermatol* 1979; **4**: 197–9.
3 Prendiville JS, Esterly NB. Halo scalp ring: a cause of scarring alopecia. *Arch Dermatol* 1987; **123**: 992–4.
4 Adler JR, Upton J, Wallman J *et al.* Management and prevention of necrosis of the scalp after embolization and surgery for meningioma. *Surg Neurol* 1988; **25**: 357–66.
5 Abel RR. Postoperative (pressure) alopecia. *Anesthesiology* 1964; **25**: 869–71.
6 Lawson NW, Mills NL, Ochsner NL. Occipital alopecia following cardiopulmonary bypass. *J Thorac Cardiovasc Surg* 1976; **71**: 342–5.
7 Patel KD, Henschel EO. Postoperative alopecia. *Anesth Analg* 1980; **59**: 311–4.

Chronic radiodermatitis [1,2]

Roentgen discovered X-rays in 1895. X-ray epilation of the face for hirsutism was frequently employed during the first two decades of the 20th century and, although Schultz [3] condemned this treatment, it continued to be so widely used that Cipollaro and Einhorn [4] entitled their paper: 'The use of X-rays for the treatment of hypertrichosis is dangerous'.

X-ray epilation for the treatment of scalp ringworm was introduced in Paris in 1904. The discovery of griseofulvin in 1958 gradually made X-ray epilation unnecessary, but it has been estimated that between 1904 and 1959 some 300 000 children throughout the world were treated with X-rays for ringworm of the scalp. Correct dosage did not cause toxicity; however, technical errors were frequent, from inadequate and poorly calibrated apparatus. The treatment produced complete epilation in approximately 3 weeks and regrowth after 2 months. The follow-up of 2043 patients treated in childhood showed a higher incidence of cancer in the patients than in a control group [1]. Radiodermatitis of the scalp may occur also as an unavoidable consequence of skin damage during the treatment of both internal malignant disease and malignant disease of the skin.

The use of X-rays for epilation depends on the high susceptibility of anagen hairs to radiation. Epilating and subepilating doses produced dystrophic changes in human hairs as early as the fourth day after exposure [5]. Chronic radiodermatitis may follow acute radiodermatitis, but may develop only slowly as degenerative changes induced by sun exposure and ageing become superimposed. In chronic radiodermatitis, the epidermis is generally atrophic, with loss of hair follicles and sebaceous glands, but there are also irregular areas of acanthosis. Degenerative changes and nuclear abnormalities are frequent in the epidermis. Dermal collagen stains irregularly. Superficial small vessels are telangiectatic, but deeper vessels are partially or completely occluded by fibrosis.

Clinical features. The development of a basal cell carcinoma in middle age or later in an area of the scalp should lead the dermatologist to enquire about X-ray epilation for ringworm in childhood [6]. In other cases, the patient complains of hair loss, which is apparently accentuated in certain areas, and these areas are found to show both AGA and reduction of follicle population as a result of the earlier radiation.

Chronic radiodermatitis produced by radiation therapy of a malignant tumour of the scalp presents a circumscribed area of cicatricial alopecia. Radiation necrosis may simulate a recurrence of carcinoma, but the edges of the necrotic ulcer are not raised. The diagnosis should be confirmed by a biopsy. Superficial X-ray of Grenz ray type does not penetrate deeply enough to damage scalp follicles. Malignant tumours arising in radiodermatitis should be excised [7].

REFERENCES

1 Albert RE, Omran AR. Follow-up study of patients treated with X-ray epilation for tinea capitis. I. Population characteristics, post-treatment illness and mortality experience. *Arch Environ Health* 1968; **17**: 899–905.
2 Getzrow PL. Chronic radiodermatitis and skin cancer. In: Andrade R, Gumport SL, Popkin GL *et al.*, eds. *Cancer of the Skin*. Philadelphia: Saunders, 1976: 458–67.
3 Schultz F, ed. *The X-ray Treatment of Skin Diseases*. London: Rebman, 1912: 135–51.
4 Cipollaro AC, Einhorn MB. The use of X-rays for the treatment of hypertrichosis is dangerous. *JAMA* 1947; **135**: 349–54.
5 Van Scott EJ, Reinertson RP. Detection of radiation effects on hair roots of the human scalp. *J Invest Dermatol* 1957; **29**: 205–16.
6 Ridley CM. Basal cell carcinoma following X-ray epilation of the scalp. *Br J Dermatol* 1962; **74**: 222–7.
7 Conway H, Hugo NE. Radiation dermatitis and malignancy. *Plast Reconstruct Surg* 1966; **38**: 255–9.

Trichotillomania (see also Chapter 61)

First described by Hallopeau in 1889 [1], trichotillomania is a psychiatric disorder with dermatological expression, in which there is a compulsive habit of pulling out the hair. It is probably a symptom of several different psychopathologies [2].

Pathology. The histological changes vary according to the severity and duration of the hair plucking. Numerous empty canals are the most consistent feature. Some follicles are severely damaged; there are clefts in the hair matrix, the follicular epithelium is separated from the connective tissue sheath, and there are intraepithelial and perifollicular haemorrhages and intrafollicular pigment casts (Fig. 63.51) [3]. Injured follicles may form only soft twisted hairs—a process that has been described as a separate entity under the name of trichomalacia [4]. Many follicles are in catagen, with very few or no follicles in

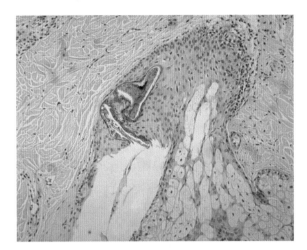

Fig. 63.51 Histology of trichotillomania showing fragmentation of the hair shaft.

Table 63.4 DSM-IV criteria for trichotillomania.

Recurrent pulling out of one's hair resulting in noticeable hair loss
An increasing sense of tension immediately before pulling out the hair or when attempting to resist the behaviour
Pleasure, gratification or relief when pulling out the hair
The disturbance is not better accounted for by another mental disorder and is not due to a general medical condition (e.g. a dermatological condition)
The disturbance causes clinically significant distress or impairment in social, occupational or other important areas of functioning

telogen. Some dilated follicular infundibula contain horny plugs [5].

Aetiology and psychopathology. Trichotillomania occurs in two main forms. In infants and young children it is usually a habit akin to thumb-sucking and nail biting. It seems slightly more common in boys and usually resolves spontaneously or with minimal treatment. Parents who have not noticed hair-pulling behaviour in their offspring may deny the diagnosis. In older children and adults trichotillomania is usually a chronic psychiatric problem, although periods of remission occur in some patients. This form occurs predominantly in females, with women outnumbering men by up to 7 : 1, although this figure may be skewed by a greater likelihood of women presenting for medical advice [2]. The American Psychiatric Association classifies trichotillomania as an impulse control disorder. Their diagnostic criteria are given in the fourth edition of the Diagnostic and Statistical Manual of Mental Disorders (DSM-IV), and are listed in Table 63.4, although not all patients with trichotillomania fit these criteria.

Trichotillomania shares some features of obsessive–compulsive disorder (OCD), but some authorities consider it may be the result of a number of psychopathologies including OCD, personality disorders, body dysmorpho-

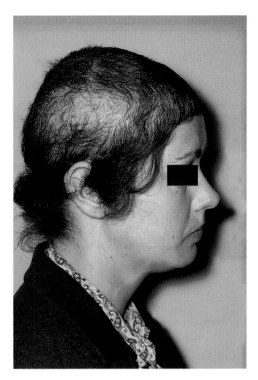

Fig. 63.52 Trichotillomania. Characteristic 'tonsure' pattern with scalp margin hair spared.

phobic disorders, mental retardation and psychosis. There is an extensive psychiatric literature on trichotillomania, but this may be biased because psychiatric help is likely to be sought only in those patients who accept that it is a self-inflicted problem. This is not true of all patients presenting to dermatologists.

Clinical features. In young children, the hair-pulling tic develops gradually and unconsciously. Hair is plucked most frequently from one frontoparietal region. This results in a patch of hair loss, often in a bizarre or angular pattern, in which the hairs are twisted and broken at various distances from the clinically normal scalp. Older patients present with an area of scalp on which the hair has been reduced to coarse stubble uniformly 2.5–3 mm long. The plucked area may be asymmetrical or cover the entire scalp apart from the margin (Fig. 63.52). It is unusual for hair to be lost completely within the affected area (in contrast with alopecia areata). The scalp skin appears normal. Over time the extent of hair loss can vary, and hair growth may recover temporarily.

Hair in sites other than the scalp can also be affected, such as eyelashes, eyebrows and beard. Exceptionally, the patient may pluck hair also, or only, from other regions of the body, such as the mons pubis and perianal region.

A hairball (trichobezoar) is a rare accompaniment of trichotillomania in those who also eat the plucked hair (trichophagia) [6,7].

Differential diagnosis. The minor form in young children can be confused with ringworm or with alopecia areata. In ringworm, the texture of the infected hairs is abnormal and the scalp surface may be scaly. Alopecia areata may be difficult to exclude with certainty at the first examination, but the course of the condition usually establishes the correct diagnosis. Unlike alopecia areata, it is unusual for hair to be lost completely in trichotillomania and, in contrast with exclamation mark hairs, the broken hairs of trichotillomania are firmly anchored in the scalp. Where doubt remains a skin biopsy will usually establish the correct diagnosis. However, there are reports of the co-existence of alopecia areata and trichotillomania [8]. In rare cases, genetic disorders characterized by increased hair fragility, such as monilethrix, may resemble trichotillomania and should be excluded by hair microscopy.

Treatment. The establishment of a relationship between the physician and the patient, or with the parents of an affected child, is an important step in management of trichotillomania. A confident diagnosis is essential, but this is not always easy and may require observation over time and sometimes a scalp biopsy. The habit tic in young children is often self-limiting, but input from a paediatric psychologist can be very helpful. Trichotillomania in adolescents and adults is a different proposition, and can be an intractable problem [9]. Patients with insight should be referred to a psychiatrist or clinical psychologist. A number of psychotherapeutic approaches have been used, particularly behaviour therapy aimed at habit reversal, but none is uniformly successful. Various drugs have been reported to be helpful, including clomipramine [10] and neuroleptic agents [11], but relapse rates are high. Promising results have also been claimed for the selective serotonin reuptake inhibitor fluoxetine [12], but this was not confirmed in controlled trials [13,14]. Behavioural therapy appears more effective than either clomipramine [15] or fluoxetine [16]. Some patients are helped by contact with fellow patients, and there are several patient support groups and Internet websites devoted to trichotillomania. Patients who fail to admit the self-inflicted nature of the hair loss present particular difficulties, as they are unlikely to accept psychiatric referral and, like dermatitis artefacta, a confrontational approach will probably be unsuccessful. Management should be aimed at helping the patient recognize the cause for themselves. This can be a long and slow process requiring skill and empathy on the part of the physician.

REFERENCES

1 Hallopeau H. Alopécie par grattage (trichomanie ou trichotillomanie). *Ann Dermatol Syphiligr (Paris).* 1889; **10**: 440–6.
2 Hautmann G, Hercogova J, Lotti T. Trichotillomania. *J Am Acad Dermatol* 2002; **46**: 807–21; quiz 22–6.
3 Mehregan AH. Trichotillomania: a clinicopathologic study. *Arch Dermatol* 1970; **102**: 129–33.
4 Lachapelle JM, Pierard GE. Traumatic alopecia in trichotillomania: a pathogenic interpretation of histologic lesions in the pilosebaceous unit. *J Cutan Pathol* 1977; **4**: 51–67.
5 Muller SA. Trichotillomania: a histopathologic study in 66 patients. *J Am Acad Dermatol* 1990; **23**: 56–62.
6 Lamerton AJ. Trichobezoar: two case reports—a new physical sign. *Am J Gastroenterol* 1984; **79**: 354–6.
7 Bouwer C, Stein DJ. Trichobezoars in trichotillomania: case report and literature overview. *Psychosom Med* 1998; **60**: 658–60.
8 Trueb RM, Cavegn B. Trichotillomania in connection with alopecia areata. *Cutis* 1996; **58**: 67–70.
9 Cohen LJ, Stein DJ, Simeon D *et al.* Clinical profile, comorbidity, and treatment history in 123 hair pullers: a survey study. *J Clin Psychiatry* 1995; **56**: 319–26.
10 Swedo SE, Leonard HL, Rapoport JL *et al.* A double-blind comparison of clomipramine and desipramine in the treatment of trichotillomania (hair pulling). *N Engl J Med* 1989; **321**: 497–501.
11 Stewart RS, Nejtek VA. An open-label, flexible-dose study of olanzapine in the treatment of trichotillomania. *J Clin Psychiatry* 2003; **64**: 49–52.
12 Koran LM, Ringold A, Hewlett W. Fluoxetine for trichotillomania: an open clinical trial. *Psychopharmacol Bull* 1992; **28**: 145–9.
13 Christenson GA, Mackenzie TB, Mitchell JE *et al.* A placebo-controlled, double-blind crossover study of fluoxetine in trichotillomania. *Am J Psychiatry* 1991; **148**: 1566–71.
14 Streichenwein SM, Thornby JI. A long-term, double-blind, placebo-controlled crossover trial of the efficacy of fluoxetine for trichotillomania. *Am J Psychiatry* 1995; **152**: 1192–6.
15 Ninan PT, Rothbaum BO, Marsteller FA *et al.* A placebo-controlled trial of cognitive–behavioral therapy and clomipramine in trichotillomania. *J Clin Psychiatry* 2000; **61**: 47–50.
16 van Minnen A, Hoogduin KA, Keijsers GP *et al.* Treatment of trichotillomania with behavioral therapy or fluoxetine: a randomized, waiting-list controlled study. *Arch Gen Psychiatry* 2003; **60**: 517–22.

Scaling disorders of the scalp
[A.G. Messenger, pp. 63.65–63.67]

Scaling of the scalp is a feature of a number of clinical disorders including dandruff (pityriasis capitis), seborrhoeic dermatitis, psoriasis and pityriasis amiantacea. These disorders show overlapping clinical and histological features and, when confined to the scalp, it can be difficult to distinguish between them. Scalp scaling is also seen in other inflammatory dermatoses such as atopic dermatitis, tinea capitis, discoid lupus erythematosus and cutaneous T-cell lymphoma.

Pityriasis capitis

Pityriasis capitis, or dandruff, and seborrhoeic dermatitis confined to the scalp are generally regarded as the same entity, with dandruff representing the mild non-inflammatory end of a spectrum of scalp scaling. Its peak incidence and severity are reached at the age of approximately 20 years, and it becomes less frequent after 50 years of age. At age 20 years, some 50% of white people are affected to some degree. Although previously thought to be uncommon in children, an epidemiological study from Australia found that approximately 40% of children under the age of 6 years showed at least mild pityriasis capitis, and 10% of neonates had seborrhoeic dermatitis of the scalp [1].

Aetiology [2]. It is reasonably well established that pityriasis capitis and seborrhoeic dermatitis are related, in some way, to the presence on the skin of lipophilic yeasts of the genus *Malassezia*, previously known as *Pityrosporum*. This idea, which evolved in the 19th century when these organisms were first identified [3–5], is based largely on the clinical observations of improvement with antifungal treatment. For a time during the 1960s and 1970s the microbial hypothesis was disputed [6], but it became re-established with the advent of azole antifungal agents [7–9]. Treatment of patients with seborrhoeic dermatitis with azole antifungal agents such as ketoconazole is associated with improvement of the rash, a reduction in colonization of the skin by *Malassezia*, and relapse as the skin is recolonized following treatment [10]. Scalp skin affected by dandruff or seborrhoeic dermatitis tends to be more heavily colonized by *Malassezia* species than normal scalp [11] although, in seborrhoeic dermatitis, the colonization rates are highly variable and there is no clear relationship between the number of organisms present on the skin and disease activity [12]. As *Malassezia* is present on normal skin there must be other factors involved that lead to scalp scaling. Possible explanations have included a direct inflammatory effect of toxins released by the organisms and an altered immune response to *Malassezia* [2].

Clinical features. Small, white or grey scales accumulate on the surface of the scalp in localized, more or less segmental patches or more diffusely. After removal with an effective shampoo, the scales form again within 4–7 days. The condition first becomes a cosmetic problem during the second and third decades, but there are long- and short-term variations in its severity, without obvious cause. There are also variations in the ease with which the scales become detached and drift unaesthetically among the hair shafts or fall on the collar and shoulders. Although pityriasis usually clears spontaneously during the fifth or sixth decade, it may persist in old age. Pityriasis merges, almost imperceptibly, into seborrhoeic dermatitis where signs of inflammation and itching are also present, and other skin sites may be involved. Pruritus is not a feature of simple pityriasis.

Diagnosis. Asymptomatic scalp scaling in children also occurs in pediculosis and in tinea capitis. The latter is typically associated with broken hair shafts and patchy hair loss, but these features may be absent in carriers of anthropophilic dermatophyte infections. Pediculosis should also be considered in adults with scalp scaling. Other than in the neonatal period, seborrhoeic dermatitis is uncommon in children, and psoriasis should be considered in the presence of significant scalp inflammation. Differentiation between seborrhoeic dermatitis and scalp psoriasis can be difficult at any age. Psoriasis is suggested by more demarcated plaques, extension of lesions beyond the hairline and the silvery character of the scaling. Occasionally, atopic dermatitis is confined to the scalp, when pruritus is usually a major feature. Profuse adherent silvery scale should suggest pityriasis amiantacea.

Treatment. Pityriasis in its milder forms is a physiological process. The object of treatment is to control it at the lowest possible cost and inconvenience to the patient, appreciating that any procedure found to be effective will need to be repeated at regular intervals.

Shampoos containing the anti-yeast agents ketoconazole or zinc pyrithione are effective in most cases of pityriasis capitis. One controlled trial reported an excellent response in 88% of subjects using ketoconazole [13]. Another study showed a 71% reduction in the dandruff score after 4 weeks of treatment with ketoconazole shampoo and a 67% reduction in subjects using a shampoo containing zinc pyrithione [14]. The scaling will return if treatment is discontinued, but the frequency of relapse can be reduced by prophylactic treatment (e.g. once weekly treatment with ketoconazole shampoo [13]). Shampoos containing selenium sulphide or tar have also been widely used to treat pityriasis capitis. Topical steroids may be used in patients with seborrhoeic dermatitis who do not respond to a shampoo. Salicylic acid-containing preparations (e.g. sulphur and salicylic acid cream) can be helpful for heavy scaling.

REFERENCES

1 Foley P, Zuo Y, Plunkett A *et al.* The frequency of common skin conditions in preschool-aged children in Australia: seborrheic dermatitis and pityriasis capitis (cradle cap). *Arch Dermatol* 2003; **139**: 318–22.

2 Hay RJ, Graham-Brown RA. Dandruff and seborrhoeic dermatitis: causes and management. *Clin Exp Dermatol* 1997; **22**: 3–6.

3 Malassez L. Notes sur le champignon de la pilade. *Arch Physiol Normal Pathol* 1874; **1**.

4 Unna PG. Seborrhoeic eczema. *J Cutan Dis* 1887; **5**.

5 Moore M, Kile RL, Engman MF. *Pityrosporum ovale* (bacillus of Unna, spore of Malassez): cultivation and possible role in seborrhoeic dermatitis. *Arch Dermatol Syphilogr* 1936; **33**.

6 Leyden JJ, McGinley KJ, Kligman AM. Role of microorganisms in dandruff. *Arch Dermatol* 1976; **112**: 333–8.

7 Aron-Brunetiere R, Dompmartin-Pernot D, Drouhet E. Treatment of pityriasis capitis (dandruff) with econazole nitrate. *Acta Derm Venereol* 1977; **57**: 77–80.

8 Ford GP, Farr PM, Ive FA *et al.* The response of seborrhoeic dermatitis to ketoconazole. *Br J Dermatol* 1984; **111**: 603–7.

9 Shuster S. The aetiology of dandruff and the mode of action of therapeutic agents. *Br J Dermatol* 1984; **111**: 235–42.

10 Cauwenbergh G. International experience with ketoconazole shampoo in the treatment of seborrhoeic dermatitis and dandruff. In: Shuster S, Blatchford N, eds. *Seborrhoeic Dermatitis and Dandruff: a Fungal Disease.* London: Royal Society of Medicine, 1988: 35–42.

11 McGinley KJ, Leyden JJ, Marples RR *et al.* Quantitative microbiology of the scalp in non-dandruff, dandruff, and seborrheic dermatitis. *J Invest Dermatol* 1975; **64**: 401–5.

12 Bergbrant IM, Faergemann J. Seborrhoeic dermatitis and *Pityrosporum ovale*: a cultural and immunological study. *Acta Derm Venereol* 1989; **69**: 332–5.

13 Peter RU, Richarz-Barthauer U. Successful treatment and prophylaxis of scalp seborrhoeic dermatitis and dandruff with 2% ketoconazole shampoo: results of a multicentre, double-blind, placebo-controlled trial. *Br J Dermatol* 1995; **132**: 441–5.

14 Pierard-Franchimont C, Goffin V, Decroix J *et al.* A multicenter randomized trial of ketoconazole 2% and zinc pyrithione 1% shampoos in severe dandruff and seborrheic dermatitis. *Skin Pharmacol Appl Skin Physiol* 2002; **15**: 434–41.

Pityriasis amiantacea

Pityriasis amiantacea is an inflammatory scaling reaction of the scalp, often without evident cause. One Scandinavian follow-up study reported that psoriasis occurred in 15% of patients with pityriasis amiantacea [1]. Another study failed to show an association with psoriasis but suggested that seborrhoeic dermatitis was more common [2]. In Knight's study of 71 patients, two had associated psoriasis and nine had eczema [3]; he pointed out that pityriasis amiantacea may occur at any age, but the average age was 25 years (range 5–40 years).

Pathology. Biopsies from 18 patients were examined by Knight [3]. The most consistent findings were spongiosis, parakeratosis, migration of lymphocytes into the epidermis and a variable degree of acanthosis. The essential features responsible for the asbestos-like scaling are diffuse hyperkeratosis and parakeratosis together with follicular keratosis, which surrounds each hair with a sheath of horn.

Clinical features. Masses of adherent silvery scales, overlapping like the tiles on a roof, adhere to the scalp and are attached in layers to the shafts of the hairs, which they surround (Fig. 63.53). The underlying scalp is usually reddened. The disease may be confined to discrete areas of the scalp, or may be very extensive, either involving a large area diffusely or affecting a number of small patches. The majority of patients notice some hair loss in areas of severe scaling. The hair regrows when the scaling is effectively treated, although scarring alopecia has been reported following pityriasis amiantacea [4].

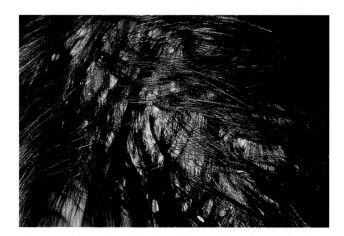

Fig. 63.53 Pityriasis amiantacea.

Diagnosis. The distinctive clinical appearance usually makes the diagnosis easy, but the identification of the underlying disease may not be straightforward; indeed, none may be established.

Treatment. Generous applications of an oil-based product are needed to remove the scales. Tar or salicylic acid ointments are commonly used. The preparation is left on the scalp for several hours and then washed out. The scales may be gently removed using a metal-toothed comb. Once the scaling is controlled an antidandruff or tar-based shampoo may help to maintain remission, but most patients will need to re-treat with an ointment from time to time. Potent topical corticosteroid lotions are beneficial in some cases, but are not effective in removing thick scales.

REFERENCES

1 Hansted B, Lindskov R. Pityriasis amiantacea and psoriasis: a follow-up study. *Dermatologica* 1983; **166**: 314–5.
2 Hersle K, Lindholm A, Mobacken H *et al.* Relationship of pityriasis amiantacea to psoriasis: a follow-up study. *Dermatologica* 1979; **159**: 245–50.
3 Knight AG. Pityriasis amiantacea: a clinical and histopathological investigation. *Clin Exp Dermatol* 1977; **2**: 137–43.
4 Langtry JA, Ive FA. Pityriasis amiantacea, an unrecognized cause of scarring alopecia, described in four patients. *Acta Derm Venereol* 1991; **71**: 352–3.

Folliculitis

See Chapter 27.

Keloidalis nuchae

See Chapter 27.

Pseudofolliculitis

See Chapter 27.

Thickened scalp disorders
[D.A.R. de Berker, pp. 63.67–63.69]

Cutis verticis gyrata

The term cutis verticis gyrata (CVG) describes a morphological syndrome in which there is hypertrophy and folding of the skin of the scalp to present a gyrate or cerebriform appearance. Polan and Butterworth [1] established the classification of CVG, dividing it into primary and secondary forms. The classification was later modified by Garden and Robinson [2] who subdivided the primary form into primary essential CVG, in which there are no associated features, and primary non-essential CVG, which is associated with a wide range of mental, cerebral and ophthalmological abnormalities.

Primary CVG. The aetiology of primary CVG is not known. Most cases appear to be sporadic although familial forms have been reported in the context of complex syndromes [3,4]. The skin changes typically develop after puberty and usually before 30 years of age. It is more common in men, with a male : female ratio of 5 : 1 or 6 : 1. There is a strong association with mental retardation. Akesson [5] found 47 cases (3.4%) of CVG in institutionalized mentally retarded subjects in Sweden, and CVG was observed in 22 out of 494 (4.5%) patients in an Italian psychiatric institution [6]. Cytogenetic analyses in the latter study showed chromosome fragile sites in nine subjects (chromosomes 9, 12 and X).

Secondary CVG. This has been described with a wide range of underlying causes. Congenital melanocytic naevi appear to be the most common but other naevoid abnormalities, such as naevus lipomatosus and connective tissue naevi, and acquired lesions such as neurofibroma, may also cause CVG [7–9]. CVG has been described in association with a variety of endocrine and genetic disorders, including acromegaly [10,11], myxoedema [12], insulin resistance [13] and Turner's syndrome [14,15]. The age of onset is more variable than in primary CVG and, in the naevoid forms, it may be present at birth.

Pachydermoperiostosis. This genetically determined syndrome also occurs mainly in men and has often been confused with CVG. It differs from it in several particulars. The scalp is folded but the skin of the face is affected, as is that of the hands and feet. The cutaneous changes, which are accompanied by thickening of the phalanges and of the long bones of the limbs, progress for 10–15 years, then become static.

Pathology. The essential abnormality appears to be overgrowth of the scalp in relation to the underlying skull. In primary CVG, the histology appears normal in most cases. The histopathology in the secondary form depends on the nature of the underlying pathology.

Clinical features. CVG typically affects the vertex and occipital scalp but it may involve the entire scalp. The folds are usually arranged in an antero-posterior direction but may be transverse over the occiput. Hair density may be reduced over the convexities of the folds.

Treatment. Investigations are aimed at identifying underlying causes. These may include neurological, endocrine, ophthalmological and cytogenetic studies. In early-onset CVG, a biopsy is advisable to identify those cases caused by a structural lesion, such as a melanocytic naevus. In the majority of cases treatment is symptomatic. Patients should be educated in scalp hygiene to avoid accumulation of skin debris and secretions in the furrows. Surgical correction can be helpful in selected cases, and may be indicated in cerebriform naevi.

REFERENCES

1 Polan S, Butterworth T. Cutis verticis gyrata: a review with report of seven new cases. *Am J Ment Defic* 1953; **57**: 613–31.
2 Garden JM, Robinson JK. Essential primary cutis verticis gyrata: treatment with the scalp reduction procedure. *Arch Dermatol* 1984; **120**: 1480–3.
3 Rosenthal JW, Kloepfer HW. An acromegaloid, cutis verticis gyrata, corneal leukoma syndrome. *Arch Ophthal* 1962; **68**: 722–6.
4 Megarbane A, Waked N, Chouery E *et al.* Microcephaly, cutis verticis gyrata of the scalp, retinitis pigmentosa, cataracts, sensorineural deafness, and mental retardation in two brothers. *Am J Med Genet* 2001; **98**: 244–9.
5 Akesson HO. Cutis verticis gyrata and mental deficiency in Sweden. I. Epidemiologic and clinical aspects. *Acta Med Scand* 1964; **175**: 115–27.
6 Schepis C, Palazzo R, Cannavo SP *et al.* Prevalence of primary cutis verticis gyrata in a psychiatric population: association with chromosomal fragile sites. *Acta Derm Venereol* 1990; **70**: 483–6.
7 Commens CA, Greaves MW. Cutis verticis gyrata due to an intradermal naevus with an underlying neurofibroma. *Clin Exp Dermatol* 1978; **3**: 319–22.
8 Orkin M, Frichot BC III, Zelickson AS. Cerebriform intradermal nevus: a cause of cutis verticis gyrata. *Arch Dermatol* 1974; **110**: 575–82.
9 Jeanfils S, Tennstedt D, Lachapelle JM. Cerebriform intradermal nevus: a clinical pattern resembling cutis verticis gyrata. *Dermatology* 1993; **186**: 294–7.
10 Zeisler EP, Wieder LJ. Cutis verticis gyrata and acromegaly. *Arch Dermatol Syphilogr* 1940; **42**: 1092–9.
11 O'Reilly FM, Sliney I, O'Loughlin S. Acromegaly and cutis verticis gyrata. *J R Soc Med* 1997; **90**: 79.
12 Corbalan-Velez R, Perez-Ferriols A, Aliaga-Bouiche A. Cutis verticis gyrata secondary to hypothyroid myxedema. *Int J Dermatol* 1999; **38**: 781–3.
13 Woollons A, Darley CR, Lee PJ *et al.* Cutis verticis gyrata of the scalp in a patient with autosomal dominant insulin resistance syndrome. *Clin Exp Dermatol* 2000; **25**: 125–8.
14 Parolin Marinoni L, Taniguchi K, Giraldi S *et al.* Cutis verticis gyrata in a child with Turner syndrome. *Pediatr Dermatol* 1999; **16**: 242–3.
15 Larralde M, Gardner SS, Torrado MV *et al.* Lymphoedema as a postulated cause of cutis verticis gyrata in Turner syndrome. *Pediatr Dermatol* 1998; **15**: 18–22.

Lumpy scalp syndrome [1]

The inheritance of this syndrome is determined by an autosomal dominant gene of variable expressivity. Raw areas are present in the scalp at birth. They heal to leave irregular nodules of connective tissue that, on histological examination, are not keloidal in structure. The pinnae are deformed; the tragus, antitragus and lobule are small or rudimentary. The nipples are rudimentary or absent, and only areolae are present.

REFERENCE

1 Finlay AY, Marks R. An hereditary syndrome of lumpy scalp, odd ears and rudimentary nipples. *Clin Exp Dermatol* 1989; **15**: 240.

Lipoedematous alopecia [1,2]

Lipoedematous alopecia is a rare condition of unknown aetiology. It is characterized by a thick boggy scalp with varying degrees of hair loss. This syndrome has been recognized mainly in black women. There is slowly progressive diffuse alopecia and obvious thickening of the scalp, with associated pruritus [3]. There are no associated medical or physiological conditions. The fundamental pathological finding consists of an approximate doubling in scalp thickness resulting from expansion of the subcutaneous fat layer in the absence of adipose tissue hypertrophy or hyperplasia. There is associated atrophy and fibrous replacement of many hair follicles. Light and electron microscopy suggests that the increase in scalp thickness is caused by localized oedema, with disruption and degeneration of adipose tissue. Mucin is not seen [4].

REFERENCES

1 Coskey RJ, Fosnaugh R, Fire G. Lipoedematous alopecia. *Arch Dermatol* 1961; **84**: 619–22.
2 Curtis JW, Heising RA. Lipoedematous alopecia associated with skin hyperelasticity. *Arch Dermatol* 1964; **89**: 819–20.
3 Tiscornia JE, Molezzi A, Hernandez MI, Kien MC, Chouela EM. Lipoedematous alopecia in a white woman. *Arch Dermatol* 2002; **138**: 1517–8.
4 Fair KP, Knoell KA, Patterson JW, Rudd RJ, Greer KE. Lipoedematous alopecia: a clinicopathologic, histologic and ultrastructural study. *J Cutan Pathol* 2000; **27**: 49–53.

Congenital alopecia and hypotrichosis
[R.D. Sinclair, pp. 63.69–63.72]

Total or partial absence of hair of developmental origin occurs in a bewildering variety of clinical forms, either as an apparently isolated defect or in association with a wide range of other anomalies. A logical classification must be based on detailed histological and genetic investigations and these, unfortunately, are seldom carried out. Provisionally, a purely clinical classification is useful to enable the clinician at least to understand the clearly defined types [1].

REFERENCE

1 Sinclair R, de Berker D. Hereditary and congenital alopecia and hypotrichosis. In: Dawber RPR, ed. *Diseases of the Hair and Scalp*, 3rd edn. Oxford: Blackwell Science, 1997: 252–397.

Total alopecia
SYN. ATRICHIA CONGENITA

As an isolated abnormality [1,2]

Aetiology. Total alopecia as an apparently isolated defect is usually determined by an autosomal recessive gene. Some pedigrees have been traced back to the early 19th century [1]. Dominant or irregular dominant inheritance has occurred in some families [3,4]. The two genotypes seem to be phenotypically indistinguishable, but detailed investigation would probably reveal differences. The term 'total' is relative, but if any hairs are present they are extremely few. Many isolated cases and families reported under the diagnosis of congenital alopecia are found on review of the original reports to be unquestionably examples of other syndromes; many were hidrotic ectodermal dysplasia.

Pathology. The hair follicles are absent in adult life, even when the fetal hair coat has been normal. Sebaceous glands are smaller than normal. When a few stray hairs have survived, the structure of the shaft appears to be normal.

Clinical features [4,5]. The scalp hair is often normal at birth but is shed between the first and sixth months, after which no further growth occurs. In some cases the scalp has been totally hairless at birth and has remained so [5]. Eyebrows, eyelashes and body hair may also be absent [6], but more often there are a few straggling pubic and axillary hairs and scanty eyebrows and eyelashes. Teeth and nails are normal, and general health, intelligence and life expectancy are unimpaired.

With associated defects

Total or almost total alopecia is unusual in hereditary syndromes.

Papular atrichia [7]. This rare autosomal recessive syndrome is associated with mutations in the zinc finger domain of the hairless gene [8]. Patients are born with hair that falls out and is not replaced. They are completely devoid of eyebrows, eyelashes, and axillary and pubic hair. Histological studies show the presence of the infundibular portion of the hair follicles, but the middle and lower portions of the follicle are replaced by small keratinizing epithelial cysts. No hair shafts are formed. At any age between 1 and 10 years, numerous small horny papules appear, first on the face, neck and scalp, and then gradually over the greater part of the limbs and trunk. Histologically, the papules are thick-walled keratin cysts [7]. Whitish hypopigmented streaks can be found on the scalp. Nails, teeth, sweating, growth and development are normal.

The underlying disorder in papular atrichia appears to be that towards the end of the first anagen phase the hair bulb, proximal inner root sheath and outer root sheath all undergo premature and massive apoptosis and disintegrate into separate cell clusters that lose contact with the dermal papilla. As a result the dermal papilla fibroblasts fail to migrate upward, and break up into clusters of shrunken cells stranded in the reticular dermis as dermal cyst precursors, and the follicle loses the ability to cycle [9].

The genetics are complex. Apart from cases of pseudodominant inheritance [10], there is phenotypic and genetic heterogeneity in inherited atrichias caused by mutations in the *hr* gene, suggesting different roles for the regions mutated in atrichia with papular lesions and in other forms of congenital atrichia during hair development [11]. Furthermore, mutations in a number of genes such as the vitamin D receptor [12], ornithine decarboxylase [13] and RXR-α genes result in a similar phenotype.

Progeria [14]. Scalp and body hair is totally deficient in this exceedingly rare syndrome, which is caused by mutation in the lamin A gene.

Hidrotic ectodermal dysplasia [15]. Total or almost total alopecia is associated with palmoplantar keratoderma and thickened discolored nails. Any hairs that are present are structurally normal but are often finer than the average. Mutations in the *GJB6* gene encoding the gap junction protein connexin 30 have been shown to cause this disorder.

Moynahan's syndrome [16]. This autosomal recessive syndrome, reported in male siblings, is associated with mental retardation, epilepsy and total baldness of the scalp; the hair may regrow in childhood between 2 and 4 years of age.

Baraitser's syndrome [17]. This autosomal recessive syndrome presents as almost total alopecia following the loss of some downy scalp hair present at birth.

Three cases are reported in an inbred family [9]; all had almost total alopecia of all sites, including eyebrows and lashes. There were occasional isolated hairs. Mental and physical retardation were associated.

REFERENCES

1 Calvo Melendro J. Atriquia congenita total y permanente. *Med Clin* 1955; **24**: 253–7.
2 Sinclair R, de Berker D. Hereditary and congenital alopecia and hypotrichosis. In: Dawber RPR, ed. *Diseases of the Hair and Scalp*, 3rd edn. Oxford: Blackwell Science, 1997: 252–397.
3 Birke G. Über Atrichia congenita und Erbgang. *Arch Dermatol Syphilol* 1954; **197**: 322–5.
4 Tillman WG. Alopecia congenita. *BMJ* 1952; **ii**: 428–9.
5 Linn HW. Congenital atrichia. *Australas J Dermatol* 1964; **7**; 223–5.
6 Friederich HC. Zur Kenntnis der Kongenitale Hypertrichosis. *Dermatol Wochenschr* 1950; **121**: 408–10.
7 Zlotogorski A, Panteleyev AA, Aita VM, Christiano AM. Clinical and molecular diagnostic criteria of congenital atrichia with papular lesions. *J Invest Dermatol* 2002; **118**: 887–90.
8 Ahmad W, Irvine AD, Lam H *et al.* A missense mutation in the zinc-finger domain of the human hairless gene underlies congenital atrichia in a family of Irish travellers. *Am J Hum Genet* 1998; **63**: 984–91.
9 Panteleyev AA, Botchkareva NV, Sundberg JP, Christiano AM, Paus R. The role of the hairless (*hr*) gene in the regulation of hair follicle catagen transformation. *Am J Pathol* 1999; **155**: 159–71.
10 Zlotogorski A, Martinez-Mir A, Green J *et al.* Evidence for pseudodominant inheritance of atrichia with papular lesions. *J Invest Dermatol* 2002; **118**: 881–4.
11 Klein I, Bergman R, Indelman M, Sprecher E. A novel missense mutation affecting the human hairless thyroid receptor interacting domain 2 causes congenital atrichia. *J Invest Dermatol* 2002; **119**: 920–2.
12 Miller J, Djabali K, Chen T *et al.* Atrichia caused by mutations in the vitamin D receptor gene is a phenocopy of generalized atrichia caused by mutations in the hairless gene. *J Invest Dermatol* 2001; **117**: 612–7.
13 Panteleyev AA, Christiano AM, O'Brien TG, Sundberg JP. Ornithine decarboxylase transgenic mice as a model for human atrichia with papular lesions. *Exp Dermatol* 2000; **9**: 146–51.
14 Eriksson M, Brown WT, Gordon LB *et al.* Recurrent *de novo* point mutations in lamin A cause Hutchinson–Gilford progeria syndrome. *Nature* 2003; **423**: 293–8.
15 Smith FJ, Morley SM, McLean WH. A novel connexin 30 mutation in Clouston syndrome. *J Invest Dermatol* 2002; **118**: 530–2.
16 Moynahan EJ. Familial congenital alopecia. *Proc R Soc Med* 1962; **55**: 411–2.
17 Baraitser M, Carter C, Brett EM. A new alopecia/mental retardation syndrome. *J Med Genet* 1983; **20**: 64–75.

Hypotrichosis [1,2]

Aetiology and pathology. Congenital hypotrichosis of sufficient degree to cause social embarrassment is not uncommon, and is probably determined by an autosomal dominant gene. There are a number of distinct syndromes, but the two most common are hypotrichosis simplex [3] and hereditary hypotrichosis simplex of the scalp [4]. Both conditions are autosomal dominant.

Hypotrichosis simplex maps to 18p11.32-p11.23 [5] and is characterized by reduced hair growth on the scalp and body, although eyelashes, eyebrows and male beards are normal. In contrast, hypotrichosis simplex of the scalp only [6] is associated with mutations in the *CDSN* gene located on 6p21.3. *CDSN* encodes a protein called corneodesmosin that is exclusively expressed in cornified squamous epithelia.

Hypotrichosis is also a relatively common feature of many hereditary syndromes, usually in association with other ectodermal defects. In the majority, the hair is not only sparse but is structurally abnormal. Where hypotrichosis is the most prominent manifestation and the structural defect is distinctive and well characterized, it has given its name to the syndrome, as in monilethrix and pili torti. In other syndromes, the scanty scalp hair is a minor and sometimes inconstant manifestation, and the shaft defect is usually less specific, although often gross. The follicles are sparse and are reduced in size, and the hair shafts are brittle and deficient in pigment. The nature of the disturbance in keratinization is not known.

Clinical features [7]. When hypotrichosis occurs as an isolated abnormality, the scalp hair at birth is normal in quantity and quality, but is shed during the first 6 months and never adequately replaced. It is sparse, fine, dry and brittle, and seldom exceeds 10 cm in length. The eyebrows, eyelashes and vellus may be absent, sparse or normal. In exceptional cases, improvement or recovery has taken place at puberty, but the condition is usually permanent.

In some families, the hair is normal until the age of 5 years or later, when growth becomes retarded and the scalp is progressively denuded so that baldness is almost total by the age of 25 years [4].

There are many hereditary syndromes of which hypotrichosis is a constant or frequent feature. In the majority, the hair is not only sparse but fine and brittle, and is often hypopigmented. The hair shafts are often defective, but may show no consistent well-characterized structural abnormality. As the hypotrichosis is not the most prominent feature of these syndromes, they are described more fully in other chapters.

There are also other syndromes, as yet incompletely investigated, in which hypotrichosis is associated with other defects.

Hypohidrotic ectodermal dysplasia [8]. Affected males show hypotrichosis, abnormal teeth and absent sweat glands. The hair is fine and silky but thin and short. Both X-linked and autosomal dominant forms exist, with the X-linked condition being caused by mutations in the ectodysplasin gene and the autosomal dominant form because of mutations in the downless gene that encodes a member of the TNF receptor superfamily, which is an ectodysplasin receptor. Mutations in either the ectodysplasin gene or its receptor disrupt ectodysplasin-mediated cell–cell signalling, which regulates the morphogenesis of ectodermal appendages.

Hypotrichosis resulting from short anagen [9]. This autosomal dominant condition is characterized by hair that is fine and short from birth. While the growth rate is normal, shortening of the duration of the anagen phase limits hair length to a few centimetres.

Hypotrichosis with keratosis pilaris [10]. The hair is apparently normal at birth, but after the birth coat has been shed, between the second and sixth months, it fails to grow satisfactorily and remains sparse, short, brittle and poorly pigmented. Eyebrows and eyelashes may be normal or sparse. Keratosis pilaris is present on the occipital region and neck, and sometimes on the trunk and limbs. Nails, teeth and general physical development are normal. The hairs show no beading or other distinctive abnormality.

Hypotrichosis with keratosis pilaris and lentiginosis [10]. Seven females in three generations in a family of three males and 13 females developed hypotrichosis at or just after puberty, which progressed until the menopause. Axillary and pubic hair was completely lost. There was keratosis pilaris of the scalp and axillae, brittleness and longitudinal striation of the nails, and centrofacial lentiginosis.

Eyelid cysts, hypodontia and hypotrichosis. See [11].

Hypomelia, hypotrichosis, facial haemangioma syndrome [12]. This 'pseudothalidomide' syndrome, which is probably determined by an autosomal recessive gene, associates gross reduction defects of the limbs, a mid-facial capillary naevus and sparse silver–blonde hair.

Hypotrichosis, Marie–Unna type [13–15]. In this rare but very distinctive syndrome the hair in affected individuals may be normal, sparse or absent at birth. If present, it remains fine and sparse until during the second or third year when it becomes coarse and twisted. The coarse wiry unruly hair may resemble a poor quality wig.

Unna described two patterns of alopecia. In the more severe form, the child's hair is always sparse and is progressively lost, so that alopecia is advanced by puberty. In the other, milder form, the hair is initially thick and the hair loss only commences in the second or third decade. At puberty, progressive loss begins over the parietal scalp bilaterally and progresses from anterior to posterior. Ultimately, the hair loss joins up centrally over the vertex to resemble Hamilton stage VIII androgenetic alopecia. There is usually also a subtle simultaneous loss from around the scalp margins.

The eyelashes, eyebrows and body hair are typically absent from birth, and after puberty any axillary or pubic hair that develops is also sparse. General physical and mental development is normal. Scanning electron microscopy shows that the hair shafts are coarse, irregularly twisted and fluted [13].

Although a distinct gene close to the hairless locus on chromosome 8p underlies hereditary Marie–Unna hypotrichosis, it has not yet been identified [16]. Other disorders clinically very similar to Marie–Unna hypotrichosis, but genetically distinct, are now recognized and indicate that more than one form of progressive patterned alopecia with wiry hair exists [17].

Hypotrichosis in disorders of amino acid metabolism. In many disorders with amino aciduria, the hair is hypopigmented and is often also fine, friable and sometimes sparse. Fine sparse hair has been reported in phenylketonuria, arginosuccinic aciduria and hyperlysinaemia.

A number of case reports associate hypotrichosis with a variety of ectodermal defects. Some such cases may represent partial forms of recognized syndromes but it is probable that many additional distinct syndromes remain to be identified and characterized.

Differential diagnosis. Microscopy of plucked hairs will exclude the more distinctive structural defects (pili torti, monilethrix and pili annulati). Other ectodermal defects should be carefully sought and relatives should be examined.

REFERENCES

1 Happle R. Genetic defects involving the hair. In: Orfanos CE, Happle R, eds. *Hair and Hair Diseases.* Berlin: Springer-Verlag, 1989: 325–62.
2 Sinclair R, de Berker D. Hereditary and congenital alopecia and hypotrichosis. In: Dawber RPR, ed. *Diseases of the Hair and Scalp,* 3rd edn. Oxford: Blackwell Science, 1997: 252–394.
3 Brain RT. Hereditary hypotrichosis. *Proc R Soc Med* 1938; **32:** 87.
4 Toribo J, Quinones PA. Hereditary hypotrichosis simplex of the scalp. *Br J Dermatol* 1974; **91:** 687–96.
5 Baumer A, Belli S, Trueb RM, Schinzel A. An autosomal dominant form of hereditary hypotrichosis simplex maps to 18p11.32-p11.23 in an Italian family. *Eur J Hum Genet* 2000; **8:** 443–8.

6 Levy-Nissenbaum E, Betz RC, Frydman M *et al.* Hypotrichosis simplex of the scalp is associated with nonsense mutations in *CDSN* encoding corneodesmosin. *Nat Genet* 2003; **34**: 151–3.
7 Sinclair RD. Congenital and hereditary alopecia and hypotrichosis. In: Sinclair RD, Banfield CC, Dawber RPR. *Diseases of the Hair and Scalp.* Oxford: Blackwell Science, 1999: 129–55.
8 Barsh G. Of ancient tales and hairless tails. *Nat Genet* 1999; **22**: 315–6.
9 Barraud-Klenovsek MM, Trueb RM. Congenital hypotrichosis due to short anagen. *Br J Dermatol* 2000; **143**: 612–7.
10 Greither A. Hypotrichosis with keratosis pilaris and lentiginosis. *Arch Klin Exp Dermatol* 1960; **210**: 123–7.
11 Burkett JM. Eyelid cysts, hypodontia and hypotrichosis. *J Am Acad Dermatol* 1984; **10**: 922–5.
12 Hall BD, Greenberg MH. Hypomelia, hypotrichosis, facial haemangioma syndrome. *Am J Dis Child* 1972; **123**: 602–6.
13 Peachey RDG, Wells RS. Hereditary hypotrichosis (Marie–Unna type). *Trans St John's Hosp Dermatol Soc* 1971; **57**: 157–66.
14 Solomon LM, Esterly M, Medenica M. Hereditary trichodysplasia: Marie–Unna syndrome. *J Invest Dermatol* 1971; **57**: 389–400.
15 Stevanovic DV. Hereditary hypertrichosis congenita: Marie–Unna syndrome. *Br J Dermatol* 1970; **83**: 331–3.
16 van Steensel M, Smith FJD, Steijlen PM *et al.* The gene for hypertrichosis of Marie–Unna maps between D8S258 and D8S298: exclusion of the *hr* gene by cDNA and genomic sequencing. *Am J Hum Genet* 1999; **65**: 413–9.
17 Green J, Fitzpatrick E, de Berker D, Forrest SM, Sinclair RD. Progressive patterned scalp hypotrichosis, with wiry hair, onycholysis, and intermittently associated cleft lip and palate: clinical and genetic distinction from Marie Unna. *J Invest Dermatol Symp Proc* 2003; **8**: 121–5.

Circumscribed alopecia of congenital origin [1,2]

The differential diagnosis of circumscribed alopecia of congenital origin presents little difficulty if a reliable history is available. Without it, alopecia areata and the acquired cicatricial alopecias must be considered.

The most common forms are naevoid. Epidermal naevi are usually devoid of hair and present as warty or smooth but slightly indurated plaques. A zone of non-cicatricial alopecia sometimes develops around melanocytic naevi.

Aplasia of all layers of the skin gives rise to a congenital defect, usually a circular or rectilinear area of scarring, somewhat depressed below the scalp surface and commonly on the vertex.

Irregular areas of cicatricial alopecia not preceded by clinically apparent inflammatory changes produce the syndrome known as pseudopelade. Pseudopelade may develop during early infancy in association with certain hereditary syndromes (e.g. incontinentia pigmenti and Conradi's syndrome).

Circumscribed non-cicatricial alopecia is uncommon. It is the result of hypoplasia or aplasia of a group of follicles. The scalp is clinically normal and histologically shows no change other than a reduced number of follicles. Any follicles present are usually small and of vellus rather than terminal type. The first hair coat is normal and the patches develop between the third and sixth months, although if they are small and not completely bald they may not be noticed by the parents until considerably later.

Several clinical forms occur [1,2]. In *vertical alopecia*, a small and often irregular patch of alopecia is present on the vertex at birth. It has been confused with aplasia cutis, but the skin is normal apart from the absence of appendages. In *sutural alopecia*, which is one component of the Hallermann–Streiff syndrome, multiple patches overlie the cranial sutures. *Triangular alopecia* [3–6] was first recognized by Sabouraud. In the usual form, a triangular area overlying the frontotemporal suture just inside the anterior hairline, and with its base directed forwards, is completely bald or covered by sparse vellus hairs. Rarely, similar triangular patches have occurred on the nape of the neck.

Single or multiple small patches of total alopecia or hypotrichosis may occasionally occur in other sites, but are often inconspicuous.

REFERENCES

1 Barth JH. Circumscribed alopecia of infancy. In: Dawber RPR, ed. *Diseases of the Hair and Scalp*, 3rd edn. Oxford: Blackwell Science, 1997.
2 Frieden IJ. Aplasia cutis congenita. *J Am Acad Dermatol* 1986; **14**: 646–60.
3 Canizares O. Alopecia triangularis congenita. *Arch Dermatol Syphilol* 1941; **44**: 1106–9.
4 Fuerman EJ. Congenital triangular alopecia. *Cutis* 1981; **28**: 196–7.
5 Kubba R, Rook A. Congenital triangular alopecia. *Br J Dermatol* 1976; **95**: 657–9.
6 Tosti A. Congenital triangular alopecia. *J Am Acad Dermatol* 1987; **16**: 991–3.

Abnormalities of hair shaft
[D.A.R. de Berker, pp. 63.72–63.120]

Structural defects of the hair shaft may be sufficient in degree to cause significant cosmetic disability, or they may render the hair abnormally susceptible to injury by minor degrees of trauma (excessive weathering). Hair microscopy can be a useful part of clinical assessment in some situations [1], including a range of hereditary or acquired metabolic disorders, where the hair shaft can sometimes provide clues to the diagnosis [2].

Price [3] classified anomalies of the shaft into those that are associated with increased fragility, and those that are not. This distinction is useful because only the former present clinically as patchy or diffuse alopecia. Price's classification will be followed throughout the present section. Whiting [4] and Rogers [5] have reviewed the structural abnormalities.

REFERENCES

1 de Berker D. Clinical relevance of hair microscopy in alopecia. *Clin Exp Dermatol* 2002; **27**: 366–72.
2 de Berker D, Sinclair R. Defects of the hair shaft. In: Dawber RPR, ed. *Diseases of the Hair and Scalp*, 3rd edn. Oxford: Blackwell Science, 1997: 396–489.
3 Price VH. Strukturanomalien des Haarschaftes. In: Orfanos CE, ed. *Haar und Haarkrankheiten*. Stuttgart: Fischer, 1979: 387–446.
4 Whiting DA. Structural abnormalities of the hair shaft. *J Am Acad Dermatol* 1987; **16**: 1–34.
5 Rogers M. Hair shaft abnormalities: Part II. *Australas J Dermatol* 1996; **37**: 1–11.

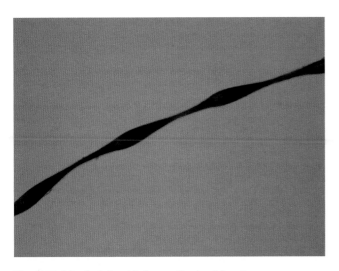

Fig. 63.54 Monilethrix with the swollen (node) and narrow (internode) fluctuations in hair bore.

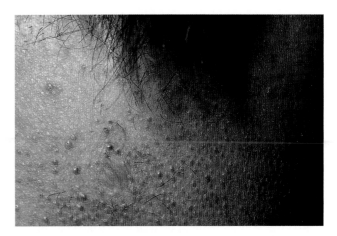

Fig. 63.55 Monilethrix. Nape of the neck showing follicular keratoses and short broken hairs.

Structural defects with increased fragility

Monilethrix (beading of hair)

Smith [1] initially called this condition 'a rare nodose condition of the hair'. Radcliffe Crocker subsequently suggested the term monilethrix. Nevertheless, some early reports, and even some more recent ones, confuse monilethrix with other shaft defects (e.g. trichorrhexis nodosa) when 'weathering' is severe.

Aetiology. Autosomal dominant transmission has been demonstrated in numerous large pedigrees [2–4]. The alleged occurrence of normal carriers of the dominant gene has not been proven, as a parent with only 5% of abnormal follicles is easily passed as normal [5]. Several pedigrees have suggested an autosomal recessive trait [6], but this is probably a result of the difficulty in making the diagnosis in a parent where the manifestations are subtle. Monilethrix can be a heterogeneous condition [7]. The abnormality is attributable to mutations in the genes coding for the human hair keratins hHb1 and hHb6. There is no clear correlation between the severity of the phenotype and the mutation responsible [8].

Pathology. The hair shaft is beaded and breaks easily (Fig. 63.54). Elliptical nodes 0.7–1 mm apart, are separated by narrower internodes with a form resembling the body and neck of a skittle. The widths of the nodes and the distances between them vary between the hairs of an individual and between members of the same family. The nodes and some of the internodes show a normal imbricated scale pattern, but most internodes show longitudinal ridging [9,10].

Histologically, the follicle shows wide and narrow zones corresponding to the nodes and internodes [11], but the general structure of the follicle is otherwise normal. Salamon and Schneyder [3] and Gummer *et al.* [12] noted that changes were visible in the zone of keratinization; the cell membranes of the deeper hair shaft cuticular cells are thrown into folds, particularly at the narrower internodes where breakage occurs.

Attempts have been made to investigate the mechanism of node formation and to relate it to the diurnal rate of hair growth. Klingmuller [13] claimed to have found a 48-h cycle in two patients. Baker [14] studied four cases in which he found that a complete nodal complex was formed in 24 h. Comaish [9] found no daily rhythm and no simple time cycle. Lubach and Traintos [15] showed no regular rhythm of node formation.

Intermittent administration of an antimitotic agent can give rise to zones of constriction alternating with zones of normal diameter [16].

Studies with the electron microscope [17] have shown that increased susceptibility of the hair shaft to the effects of trauma—premature weathering—is an important factor in the failure of the hair to attain a normal length.

Clinical features. Monilethrix shows considerable variation in age of onset, severity and course [18].

The hair may be obviously abnormal at birth but is most commonly normal, and is progressively replaced by abnormal hair during the first months of life; in other cases, normal hair is succeeded by horny follicular papules from the summit of which emerge fragile beaded hairs. The follicular keratoses and the abnormal hairs are most frequent on the nape and occiput but may involve the entire scalp. In a typical case, the short stubble of brittle hairs and rough horny plugs give a distinctive appearance (Fig. 63.55). In some cases, the eyebrows and eyelashes, pubic and axillary hair and general body hair may be affected.

In many patients, the condition persists with little change throughout life [4]. Spontaneous improvement or complete recovery has occurred [1] and has been reported during pregnancy [19]. Griseofulvin also has temporarily restored normal hair growth [20].

Associated defects. Some investigators thought the association with oligophrenia and with nail and tooth defects was significant [3]. It has been proposed that such associations may be a feature of the recessive phenotype, as oligophrenia and poor physical development were noted also in two siblings with monilethrix [21]. Association with juvenile cataract has been reported [22].

Reports of abnormalities of amino acid metabolism are conflicting. Argininosuccinic aciduria has been reported [23], but a technical error was subsequently detected [24]. No abnormality in the urinary amino acid pattern was found in the autosomal dominant type [19] or in an isolated case [25]. An apparent excess of aspartic acid and arginine in the urine of an affected mother and daughter was described by Marques Llagaria *et al.* [26].

Treatment. None is available, but Tamayo [27] has suggested that oral retinoids can induce some hair regrowth. This may result from a therapeutic effect on the keratosis pilaris, which lessens in combination with a reduction of shaft beading and modest increase in overall hair length [28]. Although improvement has been attributed to the hormone changes of menarche in one report [29], male and female cases may both improve at puberty. Iron supplementation has been reported to be of value in the presence of iron deficiency [30]. Reduction of hairdressing trauma may be followed by some improvement, by lessening the 'weathering' from chemical and physical insults.

REFERENCES

1 Smith WG. A rare nodose condition of the hair. *BMJ* 1879; **11**: 291–6.
2 Rodemund OE. Zur Monilethrix. *Z Haut Geschlectskr* 1969; **44**: 291–9.
3 Salamon T, Schneyder UW. Über die Monilethrix. *Arch Klin Exp Dermatol* 1962; **215**: 105–10.
4 Solomon IL, Green OC. Monilethrix. *N Engl J Med* 1963; **269**: 1279–85.
5 Deraemaeker R. Monilethrix: report of a family with special reference to some problems concerning inheritance. *Am J Hum Genet* 1957; **9**: 195–201.
6 Hanhert E. Erstmaliger Hinweis auf das Vorkommen einer Monohybrid-rezessivere Erbgangs bei Monilethrix (Moniletrichosis). *Arch Julius-Klaus Stift Verebungsforsch* 1955; **30**: 1.
7 Korge BP, Hamm H, Jury CS et al. Identification of novel mutations in basic hair keratins hHb1 and hHb6 in monilethrix: implications for protein structure and clinical phenotype. *J Invest Dermatol* 1999; **113**: 607–12.
8 Horev L, Glaser B, Metzker A et al. Monilethrix: mutational hotspot in the helix termination motif of the human hairbasic keratin 6. *Hum Hered* 2000; **50**: 325–30.
9 Comaish S. Autoradiographic studies of hair growth and rhythm in monilethrix. *Br J Dermatol* 1969; **81**: 443–9.
10 Dawber RPR. Weathering of hair in some genetic hair shaft abnormalities. In: Brown A, Crosin RG, eds. *Hair: Trace Elements and Human Illness*. New York: Praeger, 1980: 95–102.
11 de Berker D, Ferguson DJP, Dawber RPR. Monilethrix: a clinicopathological demonstration of the defect. *Br J Dermatol* 1993; **128**: 327–9.
12 Gummer CL, Dawber RPR, Swift JA. Monilethrix: an electron microscopic and electron histochemical study. *Br J Dermatol* 1981; **105**: 529–36.
13 Klingmuller G. Monilethrix mit 48 Studen-Rhythmus. *Hautarzt* 1954; **5**: 23–7.
14 Baker H. An investigation of monilethrix. *Br J Dermatol* 1962; **74**: 24–30.
15 Lubach D, Triantos N. Untersuchungen uber die Monilethrix. *Hautarzt* 1979; **30**: 253–9.
16 Van Scott EJ, Reinhertson RP, Steinmuller R. The growing hair roots of the human scalp and morphologic changes therein following aminopterin therapy. *J Invest Dermatol* 1957; **29**: 197–209.
17 Dawber RPR. Weathering of hair in monilethrix and pili torti. *Clin Exp Dermatol* 1977; **2**: 271–80.
18 Amichai B, Grunwald MH, Halevy S. Hair loss in a 6-month-old child. *Arch Dermatol* 1996; **132**: 577–8.
19 Summerly R, Donaldson EM. Monilethrix. *Br J Dermatol* 1962; **74**: 387–94.
20 Keipert JA. The effect of griseofulvin on hair growth in monilethrix. *Med J Aust* 1973; **ii**: 1236–8.
21 Sfaello H, Hariga J. Monilothrix associé à la debilité mental; étude d'une famille. *Arch Belges Derm Syph* 1967; **23**: 363.
22 Thiel E. Monilethrix und Fruhstar. *Hautarzt* 1959; **10**: 271–9.
23 Grosfeld JCM, Mighorst JA, Moolhuysen TMGF. Argininosuccinic aciduria in monilethrix. *Lancet* 1964; **ii**: 789–91.
24 Efron ML, Hoefnagel D. Argininosuccinic acid in monilethrix. *Lancet* 1966; **i**: 321.
25 Mader AK, Rose JH. Monilethrix und Argininbersteinsaure-Ausscheidung. *Dermatol Monatschr* 1969; **155**: 409–16.
26 Marques Llagaria E, Calap Calatynd J, Torres Peris V. Monilethrix: Estudio apropositio de dos casos familares. *Acta Derm Sifiligr* 1973; **64**: 203–12.
27 Tamayo L. Monilethrix: treated with the oral retinoid Ro-10-9359 (Tigason). *Clin Exp Dermatol* 1983; **8**: 393–6.
28 de Berker DAR, Dawber RPR. Monilethrix treated with oral retinoids. *Clin Exp Dermatol* 1990; **16**: 226–8.
29 Gebhardt M, Fischer T, Claussen U, Wollina U, Elsner P. Monilethrix: improvement by hormonal influences? *Pediatr Dermatol* 1999; **16**: 297–300.
30 Karaman GC, Sendur N, Basar H, Bozkurt Savk E. Localized monilethrix with improvement after treatment of iron deficiency anaemia. *J Eur Acad Dermatol Venereol* 2001; **15**: 362–4.

Pseudomonilethrix

It is not uncommon to see patients who complain that their hair is of poor quality or brittle. Microscopy of the hair to exclude the classical shaft defects is a routine procedure. Bentley-Phillips and Bayles [1] described a condition which they termed 'pseudomonilethrix' in South Africans of European or Indian descent. The status of the diagnosis is uncertain; some of the shaft deformities may be artefactual.

The patients present with alopecia starting in childhood. The family history suggests inheritance is determined by an autosomal dominant gene. The defect renders the hair so fragile that it readily breaks with the trauma of brushing, combing or other hairdressing procedures.

On microscopy, one, or occasionally two, of three abnormalities can be seen:

1 Pseudomonilethrix—irregular nodes, which on electron microscopy prove to be the protruding edges of depressions in the shaft
2 Irregular twists of 25–200° without flattening of the shaft
3 Breaks with brush-like ends in an apparently normal shaft.

There is no keratosis pilaris. Most authorities now believe that pseudomonilethrix microscopic changes are

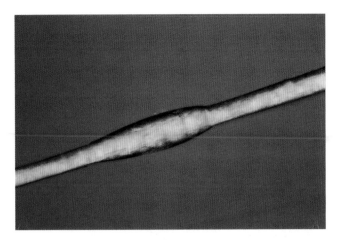

Fig. 63.56 Hair lacquer can cause fusiform bulges along the hair shaft.

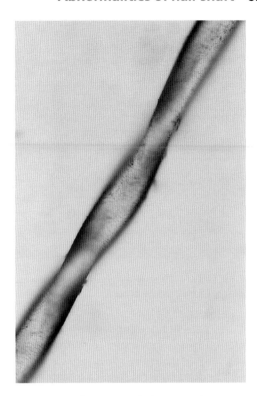

Fig. 63.57 Pili torti. Light micrograph showing 180° twists.

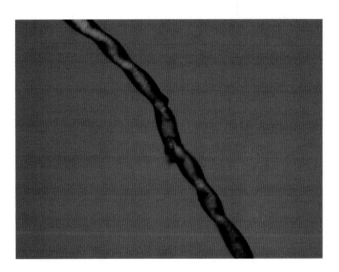

Fig. 63.58 Pili torti in a 6-month-old boy with Menkes' disease.

artefactual. They can be produced in normal hairs by trauma from tweezers or forceps, or compressing overlapping hairs between two glass slides; the indentation in one shaft caused by another overlying hair exactly mimics the appearance of pseudomonilethrix [2]. Hair lacquer and gel can also cause beading visible under the light microscope (Fig. 63.56) [3].

REFERENCES

1 Bentley-Phillips B, Bayles MAH. Pseudomonilethrix. *Br J Dermatol* 1975; **92**: 113–20.
2 Zitelli JA. Pseudomonilethrix: an artefact. *Arch Dermatol* 1986; **122**: 688–92.
3 Itin PH, Schiller P, Mathys D, Guggenheim R. Cosmetically induced hair beads. *J Am Acad Dermatol* 1997; **36**: 260–1.

Pili torti (twisting of hair)

The first definite description of pili torti was given by Schutz [1], although earlier authors had referred to the condition. Ormsby and Mitchell [2] twice presented the same patient to the Chicago Dermatological Society; on the first occasion the diagnosis was 'atrophia pilorum'; monilethrix. In discussion, attention was drawn to the fact that the hairs were twisted and not beaded. Galewsky [3] suggested the term 'pili torti', which was also adopted by Ronchese [4] in the USA.

In pili torti, the hairs are flattened and at irregular intervals completely rotated through 180° around their long axis (Fig. 63.57). True pili torti of Menkes' syndrome and the isolated expression of the abnormality in an otherwise unaffected person, demonstrate the same distinct twisting (Figs 63.58 & 63.59). Scanning electron microscopy has made it clear that twisted hairs occur in many distinct forms, and that the twisting may be associated with a number of other shaft defects. Occasional twists of varying angle should not be taken to be this distinctive genetically 'fixed' abnormality of pili torti—many dystrophies and distortions of the follicular zone of keratinization will vary the hair shaft 'bore', sometimes showing less than 180° irregular twists.

Syndromes in which twisted hair is a feature

Menkes' syndrome. Light-coloured twisted hair is a manifestation of a hereditary defect of intestinal copper transport; the inheritance is of sex-linked recessive type. Accumulation of copper in the neonatal period leads to brain damage, mental retardation and fitting. The latter

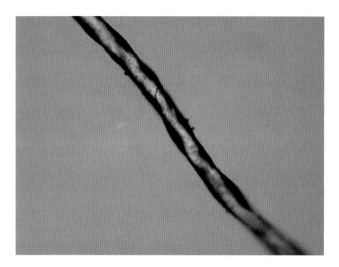

Fig. 63.59 Pili torti in a 27-year-old woman with no personal or family history of associated disorders.

may be the presenting complaint, with the diagnosis made later on hair microscopy. The twisting of the hair microscopically is generally exactly the same as in pili torti [5,6]. The disorder is caused by a mutation in the gene encoding Cu^{2+} transporting ATPase, α-polypeptide. The occipital horn syndrome is caused by mutation in the same gene.

Björnstad's syndrome (see below). Twisted hair with sensorineural deafness; probable autosomal dominant inheritance.

Crandall's syndrome. Twisted hair and deafness are associated with hypogonadism; probable sex-linked recessive inheritance. This may be a variant of Björnstad's syndrome.

Bazex syndrome. Twisted hair, with basal carcinomas of the face and follicular atrophoderma. Although this condition has come to be associated with the term pili torti, it illustrates how features of hair microscopy can be termed with low precision. The hair changes are probably more a form of irregular twisting than the tight distinctive changes seen with pili torti [7]. Vabres *et al.* [8] found evidence for X-linkage and regional assignment to Xq24–q27.

Hypohidrotic ectodermal dysplasia. Twisted hairs associated with characteristic facies and dental defects. The hairs are twisted irregularly and are not true pili torti.

Pseudomonilethrix. Twisted hair is associated, in the individual or the family, with apparently beaded hairs of autosomal dominant inheritance. However, the twists are irregular and the beads may be part of trauma sustained by the hair when plucked.

When patients with these syndromes are excluded, only

pili torti remains, but there is evidence that it does not constitute a homogeneous entity: the hairs show considerable variation from patient to patient in their ability to withstand breaking and pulling; the hairs in some patients weather badly, but in others they do not [9].

Pollitt *et al.* [10] reported siblings with mental retardation, pili torti and trichorrhexis nodosa; their hair keratin was deficient in cysteine. However, dystrophic pili torti may occur with a normal cysteine content [11]. Reduction in cysteine implies the diagnosis of trichothiodystrophy, where the hairs are flattened and single twists are common—again illustrating the care needed to make a precise morphological diagnosis of pili torti rather than referring to isolated or heterogeneous twists by this term.

Aetiology. In those cases in which classic pili torti of early onset appears to have occurred as an isolated defect, inheritance has usually been determined by an autosomal dominant gene [12]. There are many reports of apparently sporadic cases [13]. However, there are also cases in which the siblings of consanguineous parents have been affected and in which recessive inheritance must be suspected [14].

Local inflammatory processes that distort the follicles can result in distorted and twisted hairs, such as may be found around the edges of patches of cicatricial alopecia [15]. Acquired pili torti-type changes may be produced by retinoids [16], but the hair is more 'kinked' than twisted. Non-scarring acquired pili torti has also been recorded in anorexia nervosa [17].

Pathology. The earlier reports emphasized that the affected hairs were flattened and twisted through 180° around their long axis at irregular intervals along the shaft. The load-extension curve (breaking stress analysis) resembles that of the wool of merino sheep; the hairs breaking more easily than normal. Histologically, the only abnormality is some curvature of the hair follicles. With the scanning electron microscope, the cuticle of the hair shaft appears normal [18], although severe weathering changes are not uncommon.

Clinical features. The hair is usually normal at birth, but is gradually replaced by abnormal hair, which becomes clinically evident as early as the third month, or not until the second or third year. There is a wide variation from case to case in the fragility of the hair, and hence in the clinical picture. Affected hairs are brittle and may break off at a length of 5 cm or less, or grow longer in areas of the scalp less subject to trauma. There may therefore be only a short coarse stubble over the whole scalp or there may be circumscribed baldness, irregularly patchy or occipital. Affected hairs have a spangled appearance in reflected light. The cosmetic appearance of isolated pili torti can improve greatly with transition from childhood to early adulthood [19].

The diagnosis should be suspected if the hair is brittle and dry. The typical spangled appearance in reflected light is present only if the hair is at least moderately severely affected, yet is not so brittle that it breaks to leave only a sparse stubble. Microscopic examination of several hairs must be made to confirm the diagnosis.

Other ectodermal defects may be associated with pili torti. Keratosis pilaris is the most recently reported, but nail dystrophies, dental abnormalities, corneal opacities and mental retardation have all been described [20]. The syndrome described as corkscrew hair [21] is microscopically separate, with an intrinsic spiral both in the axis of the hair and around the axis.

REFERENCES

1 Schutz J. Pili moniliformis. *Arch Dermatol Syphilol* 1946; **53**: 69–73.
2 Ormsby OS, Mitchell JH. Atrophia pilorum. *Arch Dermatol Syphilol* 1925; **12**: 146–52.
3 Galewsky E. Pili torti. *Arch Dermatol Syphilol* 1932; **26**: 659–66.
4 Ronchese F. Twisted hairs (pili torti). *Arch Dermatol Syphilol* 1932; **26**: 98–104.
5 Dupre A, Enjolras O. Syndrome de Menkes avec pilotortoge alternante. *Ann Dermatol Vénéréol* 1980; **102**: 269–71.
6 Menkes JH, Alter M, Steigleder GK *et al.* A sex-linked recessive disorder with retardation of growth, peculiar hair and focal cerebral and cerebellar degeneration. *Paediatrics* 1962; **29**: 764–79.
7 Oley CA, Sharpe H, Chenevix-Trench G. Basal cell carcinomas, coarse sparse hair, and milia. *Am J Med Genet* 1992; **43**: 799–804.
8 Vabres P, Lacombe D, Rabinowitz LG *et al.* The gene for Bazex–Dupre–Christol syndrome maps to chromosome Xq. *J Invest Dermatol* 1995; **105**: 87–91.
9 Dawber RPR. Weathering of hair in monilethrix and pili torti. *Clin Exp Dermatol* 1977; **2**: 271–9.
10 Pollitt RJ, Jenner FA, Davis M. Sibs with mental and physical retardation, with abnormal amino-acid composition of the hair. *Arch Dis Child* 1968; **43**: 211–20.
11 Gedda L, Cavalieri R. Relievi genetici delle Distrofie congenita dei capelli. *Cronache Inst Dermopat Immacol* 1962; **17**: 3–8.
12 Rief PH, Patrizi A, Piraccini BM. Autosomal dominant pili torti. *Eur J Dermatol* 1996; **6**: 385–7.
13 Laub D, Horan RF, Yaffe H *et al.* A child with hair loss: pili torti, apparently unassociated with other abnormalities. *Arch Dermatol* 1987; **123**: 1071–7.
14 Pierini LE, Borda JMC. Pili torti. *Rev Argent Dermatosifil* 1947; **31**: 75–9.
15 Kurwa AR, Abdel-Aziz AHM. Pili torti: congenital and acquired. *Acta Derm Venereol (Stockh)* 1973; **10**: 34–8.
16 Hays SC, Camisa C. Acquired pili torti in two patients treated with synthetic retinoids. *Cutis* 1985; **35**: 466–70.
17 Lurie R, Danziger Y, Kaplan Y. Acquired pili torti in anorexia nervosa. *Cutis* 1996; **57**: 151–2.
18 Dawber RPR, Comaish S. Scanning electron microscopy of normal and abnormal hair shafts. *Arch Dermatol* 1970; **101**: 316–23.
19 Telfer NR, Cutler TP, Dawber RP. The natural history of 'dystrophic' pili torti. *Br J Dermatol* 1989; **120**: 323–5.
20 Friederich HC, Seitz R. Uber eine forme der ektodermalen Dysplasie unter dem Bilde der Pili torti mit Augenbeteilung und Storung der Schweissekretion. *Dermatol Wochenschr* 1955; **131**: 277–81.
21 Argenziano G, Monsurro MR, Pazienza R, Delfino M. A case of probable autosomal recessive ectodermal dysplasia with corkscrew hairs and mental retardation in a family with tuberous sclerosis. *J Am Acad Dermatol* 1998; **38**: 344–8.

Björnstad's syndrome [1,2]

SYN. CRANDALL'S SYNDROME

In this syndrome, pili torti is associated with sensorineural hearing loss. The loss of hair usually begins in infancy but in one case it was not noticed until the age of 8 years [3]. There is a correlation between the severity of the hair defect and the degree of hearing loss. On microscopy, the hair shafts show longitudinal ridging and irregular twisting. Pedigrees have suggested both dominant and recessive inheritance [4,5]. The disease gene maps to chromosome 2q34–q36 [5].

Two brothers were investigated after they had reached puberty and were found to have secondary hypogonadism [6] with deficiency of luteinizing and of growth hormones.

REFERENCES

1 Björnstad RT. Pili torti and sensory neural loss of hearing. *Proc Fennoscand Assoc Dermatol* Copenhagen, 1965: 3–6.
2 Petit A, Dontenwille MM, Blanchet-Bardon C, Civatte J. Pili torti with congenital deafness (Björnstad's syndrome): report of three cases in one family suggesting autosomal dominant transmission. *Clin Exp Dermatol* 1993; **18**: 94–6.
3 Voigtlander V. Pili torti with deafness (Björnstad syndrome). *Dermatologica* 1979; **159**: 50–7.
4 Richards KA, Mancini AJ. Three members of a family with pili torti and sensorineural hearing loss: the Björnstad syndrome. *J Am Acad Dermatol* 2002; **46**: 301–3.
5 Lubianca Neto JF, Lu L, Eavey RD *et al.* The Björnstad syndrome (sensorineural hearing loss and pili torti) disease gene maps to chromosome 2q34–36. *Am J Hum Genet* 1998; **62**: 1107–12.
6 Crandall BF, Samec L, Sparkes RS *et al.* A familial syndrome of deafness, alopecia and hypogonadism. *J Pediatr* 1973; **82**: 461–5.

Netherton's syndrome (bamboo hair) [1–4]

Netherton [5] observed bamboo-like nodes in the fragile hairs of a girl with 'erythematous scaly dermatitis'. It has gradually become apparent that ichthyosis linearis circumflexa (ILC) and 'bamboo hairs' (trichorrhexis invaginata) (Fig. 63.60) are two features of a single syndrome [6]. Most cases of Netherton's syndrome have had ILC but some have ichthyosis vulgaris [7] or both conditions, or ichthyosiform erythroderma. Features of ILC may be seen in variants of psoriasis. It is controversial as to whether it occurs as an isolated disease in the absence of Netherton's

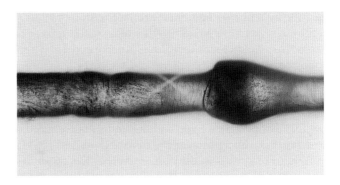

Fig. 63.60 Light microscopy revealing a trichorrhexis invaginata node likened to bamboo.

syndrome, or whether it is the fluctuating prevalence of the hair shaft changes that leads to difficulty in detecting both characteristics at the same time in some patients.

ILC is thus an almost constant feature of the syndrome, with hair shaft defects of various types and degrees of severity. Some authorities [8] question the variability of the syndrome.

The inheritance of Netherton's syndrome appears to be determined by an autosomal recessive gene of variable expressivity. Girls are affected more than boys. The underlying defect has been localized to a gene on chromosome 5q32, known as SPINK5, an acronym for serum protease inhibitor. The gene product is termed LEKTI (lympho-epithelial kazal-type-related inhibitor), as the gene is expressed in several lympho-epithelial tissues [9,10]. The protein has antitrypsin activities, but the mechanistic significance of this is not clear [11]. Examination of the SPINK5 gene in 13 families revealed 11 mutations, nine of which were associated with RNA instability. This is consistent with the low levels of SPINK5 gene product in those with the disease, where relevant RNA has decayed [12]. Immunohistochemical techniques are under development to allow tissue diagnosis of Netherton's syndrome on the basis of absence of LEKTI immunostaining. Identification of the gene has allowed prenatal diagnosis [13].

Pathology. As Netherton's syndrome results in fragile hair, samples should be cut at the scalp surface thus reducing the chances that the hair will break at the point of diagnostic interest, making diagnosis more difficult. Light microscopy is the best tool for detecting features of Netherton's syndrome in hair. However, an individual may have multiple hairs with characteristic changes in one sample and then no features in another sample taken some months later. Because of this it is important that samples of at least 100 hairs are carefully examined on several occasions before a definite negative is asserted. Alternatively, finding a single trichorrhexis invaginata node in a single hair is a conclusive positive (Figs 63.61 & 63.62).

To assess such large numbers of hairs it is necessary to use the light microscope, as electron microscopy will only allow assessment of small lengths of a small number of hairs. Detail of the surface features is enhanced using partially crossed polarizing filters, and the cortical anatomy of the hair is revealed if the hair is prepared on a slide in histological mounting medium. Scanning electron microscopy of the hair shafts shows focal defects that produce the development of torsion nodules, invaginated nodules (trichorrhexis invaginata) and trichorrhexis nodosa [14,15].

Where diagnosis is difficult, sampling the eyebrows may provide confirmation [16]. The proximal remnant of an invaginate node may resemble a golf tee and can allow diagnosis where classic nodes are absent [4].

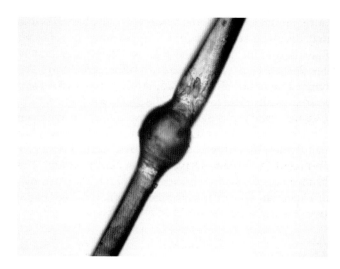

Fig. 63.61 Netherton's syndrome with an invaginate node showing partial twisting of the hair at the upper pole.

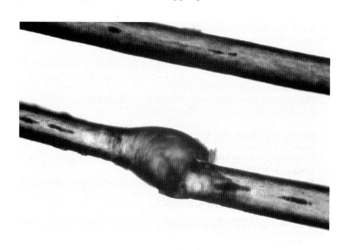

Fig. 63.62 Netherton's syndrome with the invaginate node acting as a point of weakness in the hair shaft.

Clinical features [17]. The patient may present primarily either with cutaneous changes or complaining of sparse and fragile hairs. Generalized scaling and erythema are present from birth or early infancy, but the degree, extent and persistence of the erythema are very variable. In some cases, the erythema may be slight and transient. In many it has the characteristics of atopic eczema accompanied by an elevated IgE. On the trunk and limbs, the fine dry scales are associated with a polycyclic and serpiginous eruption whose horny margin slowly changes its pattern.

The hair defects may be detected only if deliberately sought, but in most cases are readily apparent clinically [17]. The hair is short, dry, lustreless and brittle, and the eyebrows and lashes are sparse or absent. Jones *et al.* [18] described two cases in which neonatal hypernatraemia occurred. The severity of the phenotype does not show strict correlation with the mutation, and members of the same kindred may share a mutation but have different degrees of disease [19].

Treatment. There is no specific effective skin treatment. Copious emollient use is standard. In spite of features shared with atopic eczema, there is a disappointing response of the skin to topical steroid, and persistence with this therapy can lead to systemic side effects. Topical tacrolimus 0.1% ointment has been used. Although the therapeutic response was reasonable, monitoring of blood levels revealed them to be at or above levels considered safe in organ transplant patients [20]. This raises the question as to whether it would represent a useful systemic therapy. Nagata [21] described some response to photochemotherapy. Oral retinoids, even at low dosage [17], do not produce significant benefit and can result in deterioration. Hair management entails avoiding chemical and physical trauma.

REFERENCES

1 Altman J, Stroud J. Netherton's syndrome and ichthyosis linearis circumflexa. *Arch Dermatol* 1969; **100**: 550–5.
2 Ito M, Ito K, Hashimoto K. Pathogenesis of trichorrhexis invaginata (bamboo hair). *J Invest Dermatol* 1984; **83**: 1–7.
3 Salamon T, Lazovic O, Stenek S. Über das Netherton-Syndrome. *Hautarzt* 1972; **23**: 66–72.
4 de Berker D, Paige DG, Ferguson DJP, Dawber RPR. Golf-tee hairs in Netherton disease. *Pediatr Dermatol* 1995; **12**: 7–8.
5 Netherton GW. A unique case of trichorrhexis nodosa: 'bamboo hairs'. *Arch Dermatol* 1958; **78**: 482–90.
6 Mevorah B, Frenk E, Brooke EM. Ichthyosis linearis circumflexa Comel. *Dermatologica* 1974; **149**: 201–6.
7 Brodin MMB, Porter PS. Netherton's syndrome. *Cutis* 1980; **26**: 185–92.
8 Hurwitz S, Kirsch N, McGuire J. Re-evaluation of ichthyosis and hair shaft anomalies. *Arch Dermatol* 1971; **103**: 266–73.
9 Magert HJ, Kreutzmann P, Standker L *et al.* LEKTI: a multidomain serine proteinase inhibitor with pathophysiological relevance. *Int J Biochem Cell Biol* 2002; **34**: 573–6.
10 Chavanas S, Garner C, Bodemer C *et al.* Localization of the Netherton syndrome gene to chromosome 5q32, by linkage analysis and homozygosity mapping. *Am J Hum Genet* 2000; **66**: 914–21.
11 Walden M, Kreutzmann P, Drogemuller K *et al.* Biochemical features, molecular biology and clinical relevance of the human 15-domain serine proteinase inhibitor LEKTI. *Biol Chem* 2002; **383**: 1139–41.
12 Chavanas S, Bodemer C, Rochat A *et al.* Mutations in SPINK5, encoding a serine protease inhibitor, cause Netherton syndrome. *Nat Genet* 2000; **25**: 141–2.
13 Muller FB, Hausser I, Berg D *et al.* Genetic analysis of a severe case of Netherton syndrome and application for prenatal testing. *Br J Dermatol* 2002; **146**: 495–9.
14 Murphy GM, Griffiths WAD, Grice K. Netherton's syndrome. *J R Soc Med* 1989; **82**: 683–5.
15 Orfanos CE, Mahrle G, Salamon T. Netherton-Syndrome. *Hautarzt* 1971; **22**: 397–404.
16 Powell J. Increasing the likelihood of early diagnosis of Netherton syndrome by simple examination of eyebrow hairs. *Arch Dermatol* 2000; **136**: 423–4.
17 Judge MR, Morgan G, Harper JL. A clinical and immunological study of Netherton's syndrome. *Br J Dermatol* 1994; **131**: 615–9.
18 Jones SK, Thomason LM, Surbrugg SK *et al.* Neonatal hypernatraemia in two siblings with Netherton's syndrome. *Br J Dermatol* 1986; **114**: 741–4.
19 Bitoun E, Chavanas S, Irvine AD *et al.* Netherton syndrome: disease expression and spectrum of SPINK5 mutations in 21 families. *J Invest Dermatol* 2002; **118**: 352–61.
20 Allen A, Siegfried E, Silverman R *et al.* Significant absorption of topical

tacrolimus in three patients with Netherton syndrome. *Arch Dermatol* 2001; **137**: 747–50.
21 Nagata T. Netherton's syndrome which responded to photochemotherapy. *Dermatologica* 1980; **161**: 51–60.

Trichorrhexis nodosa

Trichorrhexis is best regarded as a distinctive response of the hair shaft to injury [1]. If the degree or frequency of the injury is sufficient, it can be induced in normal hair [2], and this is probably the most common scenario. The cuticular cells become disrupted, allowing the cortical cells to splay out to form nodes [3]. If, however, the hair is abnormally fragile, trichorrhexis may follow relatively trivial injury. The trauma of hairdressing procedures has often been incriminated [4]. Scratching may produce identical changes in pubic hairs [4]; and the severity of experimentally induced trichorrhexis nodosa is related to the degree of trauma in patients with or without preexisting trichorrhexis. The cumulative effect of shampooing, brushing, sea bathing and sunlight has led to seasonal summer recurrences [5].

Congenital and hereditary defects of the hair shaft resulting in fragility can predispose to trichorrhexis nodosa.

Trichorrhexis nodosa is a feature of the rare metabolic defect argininosuccinic aciduria, in which it is associated with mental retardation [6]; there is a deficiency of the enzyme argininosuccinase. Some 20 patients have been reported [7,8]. The hair tends to be dry, brittle and lustreless and may show trichorrhexis nodosa, but it does not occur in all patients with this metabolic disorder.

Trichorrhexis nodosa may occur in certain families as an apparently isolated defect of the hair; node formation and fracture are induced by minimal trauma and develop during the early months of life. Wolff *et al.* [9] described as 'trichorrhexis congenita' the presence from birth of trichorrhexis nodosa confined to the scalp, with normal teeth and nails.

In a case of generalized trichorrhexis nodosa in a male adult [10], electron histochemical study showed evidence of a disorder in the formation of α-keratin chains within the globular matrix of the hair cortex with respect to cysteine.

Pathology. In simple trichorrhexis nodosa, the shaft may appear normal with the light or electron microscope, except at the nodes; or the shaft, apart from the proximal 1 cm, may show signs of abnormal wear and tear [3]. At the nodes, the cuticle bulges and is split by longitudinal fissures (Fig. 63.63). If fracture occurs transversely through a node (trichoclasis), the end of the hair resembles a small paintbrush.

Clinical features. In trichorrhexis nodosa complicating a congenital defect of the hair shaft, the hair breaks so easily

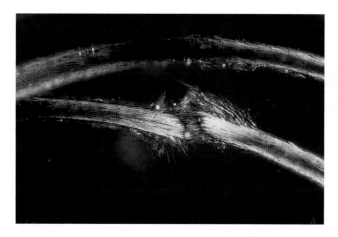

Fig. 63.63 Trichorrhexis nodosa. Polarized light examination demonstrates the splayed cortical fibres radiating from the transverse fracture in a trichorrhexis node.

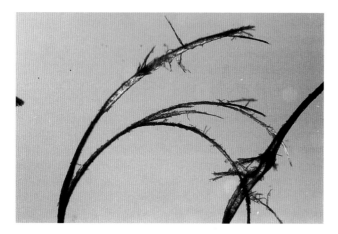

Fig. 63.64 Proximal trichorrhexis nodes and dramatic split ends (trichoptilosis) are visible in hair from an Afro-Caribbean woman.

that large or small portions of the scalp show only broken stumps and alopecia may be gross. However, the common situation is where trauma plays a major part and predisposition has a relatively minor role. In this setting there are three principal clinical presentations [11].

1 Distal trichorrhexis nodosa occurs in all races. Often it is discovered incidentally, and only a few whitish nodules are seen near the ends of scattered hairs. If many hairs are affected, the patient may complain that the hair is dry, dull or brittle. The longer the hair, the more likely it is to occur.

2 There is a generalized variant seen in Afro-Caribbean women called proximal trichorrhexis nodosa. The scalp hair is universally short and brittle and demonstrates severe weathering on light microscopic examination (Fig. 63.64). There may be an association with the follicular degeneration syndrome where there is a central scarring alopecia in the absence of an overt inflammatory process [12].

3 The third clinical form was well described by Sab-

ouraud [13] but it appears now to be rare. In a localized area of scalp, moustache or beard, some hairs are broken and others show from one to five or six nodules [14].

Diagnosis. The congenital forms must be differentiated from other shaft defects. The distal acquired form may simulate dandruff or even pediculosis. In all cases, diagnosis depends on careful microscopy. Excessive physical and chemical (cosmetic) trauma must be avoided, apart from shampooing.

REFERENCES

1 Whiting DA. Structural abnormalities of the hair shaft. *J Am Acad Dermatol* 1987; **16**: 1–24.
2 Dawber RPR, ed. *Diseases of the Hair and Scalp*, 3rd edn. Oxford: Blackwell Science, 1997: 401–13.
3 Dawber RPR, Comaish JS. Scanning electron microscopy of normal and abnormal hair shafts. *Arch Dermatol* 1970; **101**: 316–22.
4 Chernosky ME, Owens DW. Trichorrhexis nodosa. *Arch Dermatol* 1966; **94**: 577–81.
5 Papa CM, Mills OH, Hanshaw W. Seasonal trichorrhexis nodosa. *Arch Dermatol* 1972; **106**: 888–92.
6 Allan JD, Cusworth DC, Dent CE *et al*. A disease, probably hereditary, characterized by severe mental deficiency and a constant gross abnormality of amino acid metabolism. *Lancet* 1958; **i**: 182–7.
7 Brenton DP, Cusworth DC, Harley S *et al*. Argininosuccinic aciduria: clinical, metabolic and dietary study. *J Ment Defic Res* 1974; **18**: 1–13.
8 Shih VE. Early dietary management in an infant with arginino-succinase deficiency: preliminary report. *J Pediatr* 1972; **80**: 645–51.
9 Wolff HH, Vigl E, Braun-Falco O. Trichorrhexis congenita. *Hautarzt* 1975; **26**: 576–81.
10 Leonard JN, Gummer CL, Dawber RPR. Generalized trichorrhexis nodosa. *Br J Dermatol* 1980; **103**: 85–8.
11 Price V. Office diagnosis of structural hair anomalies. *Cutis* 1975; **15**: 213–39.
12 Sperling LC. Scarring alopecia and the dermatopathologist. *J Cutan Pathol* 2001; **28**: 333–42.
13 Sabouraud R. Trichoclasie, trichorrhexie et trichopilose. *Ann Dermatol Syphiligr* 1921; **2**: 445–50.
14 Camacho-Martinez FF. Localized trichorrhexis nodosa. *J Am Acad Dermatol* 1989; **20**: 696–8.

Trichothiodystrophy

The term trichothiodystrophy (TTD) was coined [1,2] to describe brittle hair with an abnormally low sulphur content [3]. The term covers a range of phenotypes, with low sulphur fragile hair representing the central defining criterion [4–10]. TTD can be classified according to the constellation of features that accompany the hair changes [4].

Using current criteria, approximately 50% of those with TTD are photosensitive. In this group, there is phenotypic and genetic crossover with xeroderma pigmentosum (XP). Of the different complementation groups within XP, most of the photosensitive TTDs share features with XP complementation group D, some with XP complementation group B and a small group represent an isolated photosensitive category, termed TTD-A. The common genetic defect in XPD and photosensitive TTD is within the ERCC2 (excision repair cross-complementation 2) gene on chromosome 19q as defined by *in vitro* complementation studies. Mutations of the ERCC3 gene on chromosome 2q

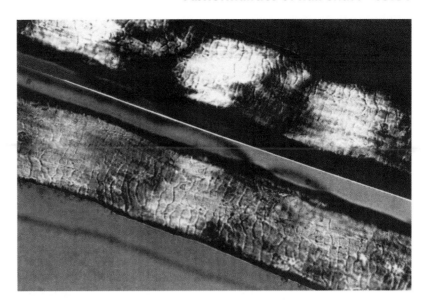

Fig. 63.65 Trichothiodystrophy. Alternating bright and dark zones in the polarizing microscope. (Courtesy of D. Van Neste, Brussels.)

have a corresponding role in XPB. These genes code for a transcription factor TFIIH, which has a dual function. First it acts as a helicase, which unravels the double helix of segments of photodamaged DNA as part of nucleotide excision and repair (NER). Secondly, it acts to enable transcription of segments of DNA to produce RNA and gene expression. A range of mutations in this gene can lead to changes in function of TFIIH. Where defects in NER occur, there is cumulative photodamage to the DNA, which is clinically expressed as photoageing and dysplasia. In XP, this ultimately predisposes to skin cancer, but not in TTD. Equally, the genetic basis for TTD can result in neuroectodermal changes that are not part of XP. A further mystery is that the genetic defect in Cockayne's syndrome arises within the same gene and affects the same transcription factor, but results in a different phenotype [5].

Currently, the genetic basis of the non-photosensitive forms of TTD has not been established.

Pathology. The hair is brittle and weathers badly [6]. With trauma it may fracture with a clean transverse break (trichoschisis) or may form nodes somewhat resembling trichorrhexis nodosa but without conspicuous release of individual spindle cells [1,2]. The hairs are flattened and can be twisted into various appearances—rather like a ribbon or shoe lace. Details of these changes are clarified by scanning electron microscopy. The shaft is irregular, with ridging and fluting, and the cuticular scales are patchily absent. Using crossed polarizing filters with a light microscope the hairs show alternating bright and dark zones (Fig. 63.65). This feature alone is not diagnostic of TTD and may occur in a range of genetic and acquired disorders where the longitudinal organization of cortical fibres within the hair is thrown into a sine wave pattern through loss of rigidity. As a sign, it may arise at different stages in infancy. In one instance it has been used prognostically

when identified in a fetal eyebrow biopsy obtained *in utero* [7]. Other cases illustrate that the sign may fail to develop until a few months of age [8].

Using transmission electron microscopy, Gummer and Dawber [9] showed a decrease in high-sulphur protein staining in the hair shaft and a reduction of this protein in the exocuticular part of the cuticle cells. Gillespie and Marshall [10] demonstrated a quantitative reduction in high sulphur proteins in the hair shaft. A large proportion of these are termed keratin-associated proteins (KAPs), of which there are at least 11 classes. KAPs 1–5 are highest in cysteine and are the likely targets of a condition where this amino acid is deficient.

Clinical features. There is a wide range of phenotypic characteristics, depending on the variant of TTD (Table 63.5). The hair is sparse, short and brittle, but the degree of alopecia varies considerably. There may be lamellar ichthyosis. The nails may be dystrophic. Mental and physical development may be normal but one or both may be slightly, moderately or severely retarded. The central feature of altered hair remains the basis of diagnosis, but the mechanism linking the associated features requires further elucidation.

REFERENCES

1 Price VH, Odom RB, Jones FT *et al.* Trichothiodystrophy: sulfur-deficient brittle hair. In: Brown AC, Crounse RG, eds. *Hair, Trace Elements and Human Illness.* New York: Praeger, 1980: 22–7.
2 Price VH, Odom RB, Ward WH *et al.* Trichothiodystrophy; sulfur deficient brittle hair as a marker for a neuroectodermal symptom complex. *Arch Dermatol* 1980; **166**: 1375–86.
3 Van Neste D, Degreef H, van Haute N *et al.* High sulfur protein deficient hair. *J Am Acad Dermatol* 1989; **20**: 195–202.
4 Itin PH, Sarasin A, Pittelkow MR. Trichothiodystrophy: update on the sulfur-deficient brittle hair syndromes. *J Am Acad Dermatol* 2001; **44**: 891–920.
5 Bergmann E, Egly JM. Trichothiodystrophy, a transcription syndrome. *Trends Genet* 2001; **17**: 279–86.

Table 63.5 Classification of trichothiodystrophy.

Type	Findings	Eponym/acronym
A	Hair +/– nails	
B	Hair +/– nails + mental retardation	Sabinas
C	Hair +/– nails + mental retardation, folliculitis, retarded bone age +/– caries	Pollitt
D	Brittle hair +/– nails, infertility, developmental delay, short stature	BIDS
E	Ichthyosis, BIDS. Hair +/– nails, mental retardation, short stature +/– decreased gonadal function +/– lenticular opacities/cataracts + failure to thrive/'progeria' + microcephaly +/– ataxia +/– calcifications of the basal ganglia + erythroderma and scale	Tay and IBIDS
F	Photosensitivity and IBIDS	PIBIDS
G	TTD with immune defects. Hair +/– mental retardation + chronic neutropenia or immunoglobulin deficiency	Itin
H	Trichothiodystrophy with severe intrauterine growth retardation and failure to thrive, developmental delay, recurrent infections, cataracts, hepatic angioendotheliomas	

6 Venning VA, Dawber RPR, Ferguson JDP *et al.* Weathering of hair in trichothiodystrophy. *Br J Dermatol* 1986; **114**: 591–9.
7 Quintero RA, Morales WJ, Gilbert-Barness E *et al.* In utero diagnosis of trichothiodystrophy by endoscopically guided fetal eyebrow biopsy. *Fetal Diagn Ther* 2000; **15**: 152–5.
8 Brusasco A, Restano L. The typical 'tiger tail' pattern of the hair shaft in trichothiodystrophy may not be evident at birth. *Arch Dermatol* 1997; **133**: 249.
9 Gummer CL, Dawber RPR. Trichothiodystrophy: an ultrastructural study of the hair follicle. *Br J Dermatol* 1985; **113**: 273–80.
10 Gillespie JM, Marshall RC. Comparison of the proteins of normal and trichothiodystrophic human hair. *J Invest Dermatol* 1983; **80**: 195–205.

Marinesco–Sjögren syndrome

This rare syndrome, of autosomal recessive inheritance, has as its principal features cerebellar ataxia, dysarthria, retarded physical and mental development, and congenital cataracts [1]. The teeth are abnormally formed and the lateral incisors may be absent. The nails are flat, thin and fragile.

The hair is sparse, fine, light in colour, short and brittle. On microscopy, transverse fractures (trichoschisis) can be seen at the sites of impending breaks. In polarized light the hair is irregularly birefringent. Scalp biopsy shows normal anagen follicles, but with incomplete keratinization of the internal root sheath [2]. The combination of neurological and physical retardation with fragile hair is reminiscent of non-photosensitive trichothiodystrophy, although there are no skin changes in Marinesco–Sjögren syndrome.

REFERENCES

1 Norwood WF. The Marinesco–Sjögren syndrome. *J Pediatr* 1964; **65**: 431–7.
2 Porter PS. The genetics of human hair growth. *Birth Defects* (Original Article Series) 1971; **7**: 69–81.

Structural defects without increased fragility

Pili annulati (ringed hair) [1,2]

Aetiology. This abnormality is characterized by hair showing alternate light and dark bands along its length, but which is otherwise normal. The inheritance of ringed hair has been shown in many extensive pedigrees to be determined by an autosomal dominant gene [3,4]. One pedigree was compatible with autosomal recessive inheritance [5]; sporadic cases have been described [6]. Blue naevus and ringed hair were associated in some members of a family, but the two conditions segregated [3].

Pathology and pathogenesis [7]. With the light microscope the abnormal dark bands alternating with normal light bands are reversed. The bright appearance of the abnormal bands in reflected light is caused by air spaces in the cortex (Fig. 63.66) [8]. Detection of the cortical defect is made easier if the hair is mounted in histological mounting medium because this enhances transmission of light through the hair.

The rate of growth has been measured in one case [3] and found to be 0.16 mm/day, which is less than half the average normal rate, but in our experience this is not a consistent finding. Breaking stress analysis showed no significant abnormality in ringed hair, but fractures were always in the normal bands. More recent studies have revealed protrusion of cortical fibres through the cuticle where there are cortical defects. Although this illustrates that the pathology can result in structural weakness, it only rarely leads to a clinical complaint of fragility [9].

Electron microscopic studies [10] showed that the clusters of air-filled cavities, randomly distributed throughout the cortex in the abnormal bands, lie partly within cortical cells and between macrofibrils, or in the case of larger cavities appear to replace cortical cells. Hairs from the family described by Dawber [3] showed an abnormal surface cuticle, which appeared 'cobble-stoned' on scanning electron microscopy. Electron histochemical methods confirmed this finding: cuticle cells are thrown into folds [11]. The pathogenesis of ringed hair remains uncertain. The abnormal alternating bands appear to be produced at random and not cyclically in relation to specific periods of growth [3].

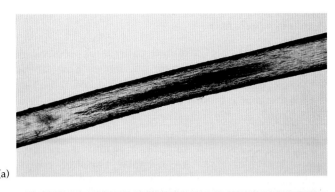

(a)

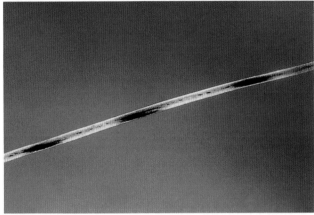

(b)

Fig. 63.66 (a) Pili annulati. Hair shaft by transmitted light showing an abnormal dark band (central part) caused by multiple cortical air spaces. This corresponds to a bright region as seen by reflected light. (b) The abnormality is intermittent, causing the beaded or ringed appearance.

Clinical features. Pili annulati is normally diagnosed as a coincidental finding or as part of pursuance of the unusual, but quite attractive, spangled appearance. The condition has been reported in association with alopecia areata on several occasions. It is uncertain whether this represents a genuine association or if medical scrutiny reveals the otherwise subtle diagnosis [12]. If many hairs are affected and fragility is great, then short hair may attract attention in early life and the 'banded' and sandy appearance of the shafts in reflected light can be readily detected. The axillary hair is occasionally affected [13].

The diagnosis is readily established on microscopy of affected hair. A defect in which partially twisted shafts have an elliptical cross-section has been named pseudo-pili annulati because such hair may give an impression of alternating light and dark bands [14].

Prognosis and treatment. The prognosis is good in the sense that severity of the defect does not increase with age.

REFERENCES

1 Karsch A. De Capillitiri humani coloiebus quardan. Cited by Landois, 1866.

2 Landois L. Das plötzliche Ergrauen der Haupthaare. *Arch Pathol Anat Physiol* 1866; **35**: 575–99.
3 Dawber R. Investigation of a family with pili annulati associated with blue naevus. *Trans St John's Hosp Dermatol Soc* 1972; **58**: 51–62.
4 Tomedei M, Ghetti P, Puiatti P *et al.* Pili annulati: family study. *G Ital Dermatol Venereol* 1987; **122**: 427–36.
5 Ebbing HC. Gibt es auch bei Ringelhaaren (pili annulati) einen einfach-rezessiven Erbgang? *Homo* 1957; **8**: 35–43.
6 Dini G, Casigliani R, Rindi L *et al.* Pili annulati. *Int J Dermatol* 1988; **27**: 256–61.
7 Amichai B, Grunwald MH, Halevy S. Hair abnormality present since birth. *Arch Dermatol* 1996; **132**: 577–8.
8 Cady LOP, Trotter M. Study of ringed hair. *Arch Dermatol Syphilol* 1922; **6**: 301–11.
9 Feldmann KA, Dawber RP, Pittelkow MR, Ferguson DJ. Newly described weathering pattern in pili annulati hair shafts: a scanning electron microscopic study. *J Am Acad Dermatol* 2001; **45**: 625–7.
10 Price VH, Thomas RS, Jones FT. Pili annulati. *Arch Dermatol* 1968; **98**: 640–8.
11 Gummer CL, Dawber RPR. Pili annulati: electron histochemical studies on affected hairs. *Br J Dermatol* 1981; **105**: 303–10.
12 Moffitt DL, Lear JT, de Berker DA, Peachey RD. Pili annulati coincident with alopecia areata. *Pediatr Dermatol* 1998; **15**: 271–3.
13 Montgomery RM, Binder AI. Ringed hair. *Arch Dermatol Syphilol* 1948; **58**: 177–91.
14 Price VH, Thomas RS, Jones FT. Pseudo-pili annulati: an unusual variant of normal hair. *Arch Dermatol* 1970; **102**: 354–8.

Woolly hair

History and nomenclature. Woolly hair is more or less tightly coiled hair occurring over the entire scalp or part of it. In those of African origin, woolly hair is the norm and is dominantly inherited. Tight coiling, knots and fractures are common [1]. The investigation by Hutchinson *et al.* [2] was important in delineating the clinical types.

The types may be classified as follows:
1 *Dominant woolly hair.* Some families have woolly hair inherited as an autosomal dominant trait.
2 *Recessive woolly hair.* Early genetic evidence is inconclusive but the condition has occurred in siblings whose parents were normal. Autosomal recessive inheritance is probable. Kindreds manifesting woolly hair as part of two different syndromes with heart disease have demonstrated an autosomal recessive inheritance [3].
3 *Acquired woolly hair.* This is usually circumscribed, occurs from adolescence onwards, and is also termed acquired progressive kinking of hair.
4 *Woolly hair naevus.* This is a circumscribed developmental defect, present at or near birth.
In a further uncommon variant, there are woolly hairs interspersed with otherwise normal hair [4].

Hair microscopy in all the woolly hair disorders reveals non-specific features that are consistent with a woolly, stiff hair phenotype. This usually arises in association with grooves, partial twists, irregularity of bore and sometimes features of trauma. When a hair shaft has an irregular shape and is stiffer, it is more prone to damage. The changes are often subtle, and are better appreciated on assessment of at least 20 and preferably 50 hairs or more. Isolated reports describing hair morphology often fall into the trap of describing individual hairs rather than the population of hairs as a whole. This mistake can be compounded by using scanning electron microscopy for the main assessment rather than as a supplementary tool. Although electron microscopy is excellent for revealing great detail in a small number of hairs, it is very poor at showing the characteristics of a population of hairs, which is the usual determinant of a phenotype.

Dominant woolly hair

In some pedigrees, the shaft diameter in affected individuals is reduced; the hair is fragile and may show trichorrhexis nodosa. Excessively curly hair is evident at birth or in early infancy; it has sometimes been described as negroid in appearance. Anderson [5] considered that the hair, although tightly coiled, was not negroid. The degree of variation in severity within a family is inconstant [1]. The hair shaft may be twisted [6]. In some cases the hair is brittle and breaks readily.

On the island of Naxos in Greece, a dominantly inherited condition has been identified, which now bears the name of the island. Naxos disease is characterized by woolly hair, palmoplantar keratoderma and a right ventricular cardiomyopathy that causes arrhythmia, heart failure and sudden death. The gene responsible for the disorder has been mapped to 17q21, which is the plakoglobin gene. Plakoglobin is an important constituent of desmosomes and adherens junction. Its loss in heart muscle leads to tissue replacement with fibrofatty material. The role in hair morphology is less clear [7]. A recent Dutch kindred were reported as having woolly hair as part of an ectodermal dysplasia, with dominant inheritance [8]. However, it should be noted that there are problems with terminology in hair science and genetics, and there is a type of hair change sometimes seen in ectodermal dysplasia that can be described as 'wiry' rather than 'woolly'.

In some cases of loose anagen syndrome, there may be associated woolly hair [9].

Recessive woolly hair

The hair is reported as brittle and on scanning electron microscopy shows signs of cuticular wear and tear [2]. In three cases [2], fine, tightly curled, poorly pigmented hair was present from birth; in two of them the hair never achieved a length of more than 2 or 3 cm. Eyebrows and body hair were sparse.

Two different variants of recessively inherited woolly hair have been defined in association with palmoplantar keratoderma and mutations causing defects in desmoplakin. One variant was associated with cardiomyopathy [10] and the other not [11].

Acquired woolly hair

There are a range of acquired patterns of woolly hair which have different and confusing names. They divide into those that develop as part of ageing and those that are attributable to trauma or drugs. The appearances may be indistinguishable when the drug is simply eliciting or catalysing an underlying process. Whisker hair describes the appearance seen in some cases, mainly males, from adolescence onwards. An irregular band of coarse, whisker-like hair extends around the edge of the scalp from above the ears towards the occipital region [12]. The hair shaft features are indistinguishable from acquired progressive kinking of hair [13], although the pattern and history may be different when drugs are implicated. Retinoids are most commonly cited [14,15]. In all these conditions the patient gradually becomes aware that the hair is changing in texture in one or more areas. On examination, the hair of the scalp is wiry, kinky, unruly, dry and lustreless. There are no sharply defined boundaries between normal and abnormal hair, although the appearance may be most marked in the frontal margins. In some of the cases described, the acquired kinking preceded hair loss, whether drug-induced or as part of the development of AGA [1].

Woolly hair naevus [16,17]

The hair in a circumscribed area of the scalp is woolly or curly and contrasts in colour and coarseness with the surrounding hair. The affected hair is usually finer at the outset, which also makes it more vulnerable to trauma. In time the contrasts may reverse, with hair in the naevoid patch becoming darker and coarser than the surrounding hair. The size of the affected area usually increases only proportionately with general growth. The abnormal hair is usually paler than that of the rest of the scalp [18]. In over half of the reported cases, a pigmented or epidermal naevus has been present, but not always at the same site. A woolly hair naevus has been reported in association with ocular defects [19], and with precocious puberty [20]. In the latter case the naevus was not limited to the scalp.

REFERENCES

1 Khumalo NP, Doe PT, Dawber RP, Ferguson DJ. What is normal black African hair? A light and scanning electron-microscopic study. *J Am Acad Dermatol* 2000; **43**: 814–20.
2 Hutchinson PE, Cairns RJ, Wells RS. Woolly hair. *Trans St John's Hosp Dermatol Soc* 1974; **60**: 160–76.
3 Carvajal-Huerta L. Epidermolytic palmoplantar keratoderma with woolly hair and dilated cardiomyopathy. *J Am Acad Dermatol* 1998; **39**: 418–21.
4 Ormerod AD, Main RA, Ryder ML, Gregory DW. A family with diffuse partial woolly hair. *Br J Dermatol* 1987; **116**: 401–5.
5 Anderson E. An American pedigree for woolly hair. *J Hered* 1936; **27**: 444–9.
6 Verbov J. Woolly hair: study of a family. *Dermatologica* 1978; **157**: 42–8.

7 McKoy G, Protonotarios N, Crosby A *et al.* Identification of a deletion in plakoglobin in arrhythmogenic right ventricular cardiomyopathy with palmoplantar keratoderma and woolly hair (Naxos disease). *Lancet* 2000; **355**: 2119–246.

8 van Steensel MA, Koedam MI, Swinkels OQ, Rietveld F, Steijlen PM. Woolly hair, premature loss of teeth, nail dystrophy, acral hyperkeratosis and facial abnormalities: possible new syndrome in a Dutch kindred. *Br J Dermatol* 2001; **145**: 157–61.

9 Chapalain V, Winter H, Langbein L *et al.* Is the loose anagen hair syndrome a keratin disorder? A clinical and molecular study. *Arch Dermatol* 2002; **138**: 501–6.

10 Norgett EE, Hatsell SJ, Carvajal-Huerta L *et al.* Recessive mutation in desmoplakin disrupts desmoplakin-intermediate filament interactions and causes dilated cardiomyopathy, woolly hair and keratoderma. *Hum Mol Genet* 2000; **9**: 2761–6.

11 Whittock NV, Wan H, Morley SM *et al.* Compound heterozygosity for nonsense and mis-sense mutations in desmoplakin underlies skin fragility/woolly hair syndrome. *J Invest Dermatol* 2002; **118**: 232–8.

12 Norwood OT. Whisker hair. *Arch Dermatol* 1979; **115**: 930–5.

13 Mortimer PS, Gummer CL, English J *et al.* Acquired progressive kinking of hair: report of six cases and review of the literature. *Arch Dermatol* 1985; **121**: 1031–7.

14 Bunker CB, Maurice PD, Dowd PM. Isotretinoin and curly hair. *Clin Exp Dermatol* 1990; **15**: 143–5.

15 Berth-Jones J, Shuttleworth D, Hutchinson PE. A study of etretinate alopecia. *Br J Dermatol* 1990; **122**: 751–5.

16 Reda AM, Rogers RS, Peters MS. Woolly hair naevus. *J Am Acad Dermatol* 1990; **22**: 377–81.

17 Lantis SD, Pepper MC. Woolly hair nevus: two case reports and a discussion of unruly hair forms. *Arch Dermatol* 1978; **114**: 233–8.

18 Amichai B, Grunwald MH, Halevy S. A child with a localized hair abnormality. *Arch Dermatol* 1996; **132**: 577–8.

19 Jacobson KV, Lewis M. Woolly hair naevus with ocular involvement. *Dermatologica* 1975; **151**: 249–56.

20 Tay YK, Weston WL, Ganong CA, Klingensmith GJ. Epidermal nevus syndrome: association with central precocious puberty and woolly hair nevus. *J Am Acad Dermatol* 1996; **35**: 839–42.

Uncombable hair syndrome

SYN. SPUN-GLASS HAIR; CHEVEUX INCOIFFABLES; PILI TRIANGULI ET CANALICULI

Aetiology [1]. This is a combination of a striking clinical presentation and distinctive hair shaft defect first described by Dupré *et al.* [2]. Since then, many more cases have been reported, some of them under the name of 'spun-glass hair'. Others have preferred the term pili trianguli et canaliculi, with emphasis on the triangular cross-section and longitudinal groove that is commonly found on microscopy. The mode of inheritance is probably autosomal dominant [3].

Pathology. Light microscopy reveals the features in a hair shaft that makes it rigid: the triangular cross-section (Fig. 63.67) and longitudinal grooving (Fig. 63.68). Twisting can also be present and contributes to stiffness to a minor degree. The first two features are best sought using partially crossed polarizing filters with air-mounted hair. If a histological mountant is used, the surface contours of the hair are not seen. On histological (horizontal sections) examination of the scalp hair, cross-sectional characteristics are more easily seen but preparation is time consuming. Scanning electron microscopy can be helpful on

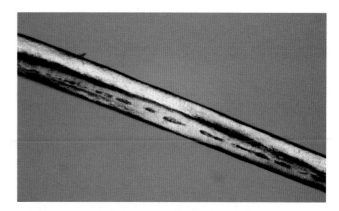

Fig. 63.67 Triangular cross-section of the hair contributes to stiffness.

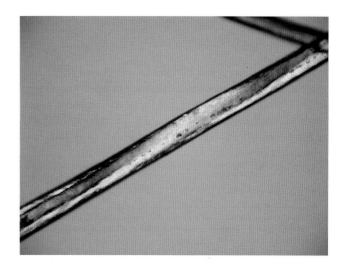

Fig. 63.68 Light microscopy reveals grooving when using partially crossed polarizing filters.

selected hairs (Fig. 63.69) [4–6]. The term 'pili trianguli et canaliculi' has been proposed for these defects. The pili canaliculi are present in all cases, pili trianguli in the majority and pili torti in a few [6]. Van Neste *et al.* [7] have suggested that the misshapen dermal papilla alters the shape of the internal root sheath, which hardens (before the hair within) in a triangular cross-sectional shape; the hair then hardens into a shape complementing the root sheath. The defect resembles the 'straight hair naevus' of which it may be a diffuse form.

Clinical features [4,5]. The abnormality may first become obvious from 3 months to 12 years of age. The hair is normal in quantity and sometimes also in length, but its wild disorderly appearance totally resists all efforts to control it with brush or comb. In some cases, these efforts lead to the hair breaking, but increased fragility is not a constant feature [8]. The hair is often a rather distinctive silvery blonde colour. The eyebrows and eyelashes are normal. The appearance becomes less marked with time [9].

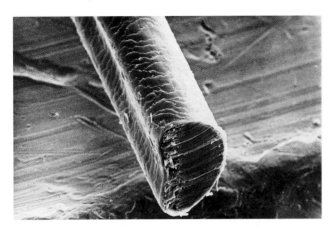

Fig. 63.69 Uncombable hair syndrome. Scanning electron micrograph showing essentially triangular cross-section and canalicular depression or gutter along one side.

The clinical appearance is usually distinctive. With light microscopy the diagnosis is dependent upon the experience of the microscopist as the three-dimensional aspect of the shaft changes can be difficult to establish. No treatment is known, although oral biotin therapy has been suggested [10].

REFERENCES

1 Mallon E, Dawber RPR, de Berker DAR, Ferguson DJP. Cheveux incoiffables: diagnostic, clinical and hair microscopic findings, and pathogenetic studies. *Br J Dermatol* 1994; **131**: 608–14.
2 Dupré A, Rochiccidi P, Bonafe J-L. 'Cheveux incoiffables': anomalie congenitale des cheveux. *Bull Soc Fr Dermatol Syphiligr* 1973; **80**: 111–7.
3 Herbert AA, Charrow J, Esterly NB *et al.* Uncombable hair (pili trianguli et canaliculi): evidence for dominant inheritance with complete penetrance. *Am J Med Genet* 1987; **28**: 185–91.
4 Dupré A, Bonafe J-L. Le syndrome des cheveux incoiffables: pili trianguli et canaliculi. *Ann Dermatol Vénéréol* 1978; **105**: 627–32.
5 Dupré A, Bonafe J-L. A new type of pilar dysplasia: the uncombable hair syndrome with pili trianguli et canaliculi. *Arch Dermatol Res* 1978; **261**: 217–23.
6 Ferrando J, Fontarnau R, Gratacos MR *et al.* Pili canaliculi ('cheveux incoiffables' ou 'cheveux en fibre de verre'): dix nouveaux cas avec étude au microscope électronique à balayage. *Ann Dermatol Vénéréol* 1989; **107**: 243–7.
7 Van Neste D, Armijo-Subieta F, Tennstedt D *et al.* The uncombable hair syndrome; four non-familial cases. *Arch Dermatol Res* 1981; **217**: 223–4.
8 Baden HP, Schoenfeld RJ, Stroud JD *et al.* Physicochemical properties of spunglass hair. *Acta Derm Venereol (Stockh)* 1981; **61**: 441–6.
9 Garty B, Metzker A, Mimouni M, Varsano I. Uncombable hair: a condition with autosomal dominant inheritance. *Arch Dis Child* 1982; **57**: 710–2.
10 Shelley WB, Shelley ED. Uncombable hair syndrome: observations on response to biotin. *J Am Acad Dermatol* 1985; **13**: 97–100.

Straight-hair naevus

In the straight-hair naevus, the hairs in a circumscribed area of a negroid scalp are straight, and are round in cross-section. The abnormal hair may be associated with an epidermal naevus [1,2]. With the scanning electron microscope, the cuticular scales may appear small and their pattern disorganized.

It has been suggested that this is a localized form of cheveux incoiffables.

REFERENCES

1 Downham TF, Chapel TA, Lupulescu AP. Straight hair naevus syndrome: a case report with scanning electron microscope findings of hair morphology. *Int J Dermatol* 1976; **15**: 498–501.
2 Gibbs RL, Berger RA. The straight hair naevus. *Int J Dermatol* 1970; **9**: 47–9.

Loose anagen hair syndrome [1]

This condition features anagen hairs that are loosely anchored and easily pulled from the scalp [2–4]. The majority of cases are fair-haired children, aged 2–9 years, mostly girls. There is usually a pattern of autosomal dominant inheritance. They typically have slightly unruly hair, which is of uneven length and patchy in quality. Variants of this include those with stiff, uncombable hair and those in whom shedding is the primary complaint. All three phenotypes may coexist within the same family [5]. The children may present with patchy alopecia, leading to a misdiagnosis of alopecia areata, but which, in fact, represents modest hair pulling. The child is well, and there are no other ectodermal abnormalities.

Hair is usually easily and painlessly plucked with the hair-pull test, although this is not a constant or specific finding [6]. Microscopy of plucked hair may show ruffling of the cuticle adjacent to the anagen bulb, giving the appearance of a 'floppy sock'. The hair shaft may have twists and grooves, and be angular in cross-section. The root sheath is absent or there may be a small everted remnant.

The hair becomes more normal with age, although the pull test may still yield abnormally large numbers of hairs into adulthood [7].

There have been isolated reports of loose anagen syndrome associated with hypohidrotic ectodermal dysplasia [8] and ocular coloboma [9].

Histological examination shows premature keratinization of the inner root sheath layers of Huxley and Henle. Trichograms show 98–100% anagen hairs. Keratin 6irs is an inner root sheath keratin proposed as a protein that might control manifestations of the disorder [10]. In one report, mutations in the gene coding for such a keratin supported this possibility [11].

Some authorities have had good results with 5% topical minoxidil [11], although it is not commonly employed and is not of clear value.

REFERENCES

1 Piraccini BM, Tosti A. Loose anagen hair syndrome and loose anagen hair. *Arch Dermatol* 2002; **38**: 521–2.
2 Price VH, Gummer CL. Loose anagen syndrome. *J Am Acad Dermatol* 1989; **20**: 249–58.

3 Hamm H, Traupe H. Loose anagen hair of children. *J Am Acad Dermatol* 1989; **20**: 242–8.

4 Baden HP, Kvedar C, Magro CM. Loose anagen hair syndrome as a cause of hereditary hair loss in children. *Arch Dermatol* 1992; **128**: 1349–50.

5 Chong AH, Sinclair R. Loose anagen syndrome: a prospective study of three families. *Australas J Dermatol* 2002; **43**: 120–4.

6 Chapman DM, Miller RA. An objective measurement of the anchoring strength of anagen hair in an adult with loose anagen hair syndrome. *J Cutan Pathol* 1996; **23**: 288–92.

7 Tosti A, Peluso AM, Misciali C *et al.* Loose anagen hair. *Arch Dermatol* 1997; **133**: 1089–93.

8 Azon-Masoliver A, Ferrando J. Loose anagen hair in hypohidrotic ectodermal dysplasia. *Pediatr Dermatol* 1996; **13**: 29–32.

9 Murphy MF, McGinnity FG, Allen GE. New familial association between ocular coloboma and loose anagen syndrome. *Clin Genet* 1995; **47**: 214–6.

10 Porter RM, Corden LD, Lunny DP *et al.* Keratin K6irs is specific to the inner root sheath of hair follicles in mice and humans. *Br J Dermatol* 2001; **145**: 558–68.

11 Chapalain V, Winter H, Langbein L *et al.* Is the loose anagen hair syndrome a keratin disorder? A clinical and molecular study. *Arch Dermatol* 2002; **138**: 501–6.

Other abnormalities of the shaft

Trichoclasis

Trichoclasis is the common 'greenstick' fracture of the hair shaft. Transverse fractures of the shaft occur, partly splinted by intact cuticle. Cuticle, cortex and sulphur content are normal. This sign may be seen in a variety of congenital and acquired 'fragile' hair states.

In the condition termed trichorrhexis blastysis [1], with unusual facies, failure to thrive, unexplained diarrhoea and abnormal hairs, the scanning electron micrographs showed features resembling trichoclasis.

REFERENCE

1 Stankler L, Lloyd D, Pollitt RJ *et al.* Unexplained diarrhoea and failure to thrive in two siblings with unusual hair. *Arch Dis Child* 1982; **57**: 212–4.

Trichoptilosis

History and nomenclature. The term trichoptilosis describes longitudinal splitting of the hair shaft from the tip. The patient often refers to the condition as 'split ends'.

Aetiology. Trichoptilosis is the most common macroscopic response of the hair shaft to the cumulative effects of chemical and physical trauma. It can readily be produced experimentally by vigorous brushing of normal hair, and it occurs in the nodes of pili torti. It is one component of the 'weathering' process particularly seen in long hair in normal individuals and in any congenital 'brittle hair' syndrome.

Pathology. The distal end of the hair shaft is split longitudinally into two or several divisions. Other microscopic evidence of hair damage may be present. The split surface often lacks cuticle, and the split commences from the dis-tal tip, thus distinguishing the problem from pili bifurcati or multigemini. The latter are abnormalities of hair genesis, rather than the results of hair damage.

Clinical features. Trichoptilosis is often an incidental finding in a person who complains that their hair is dry and brittle. Trichorrhexis nodosa and trichoclasis are often also present. Central trichoptilosis, a longitudinal split in the hair shaft without involvement of the tip, sometimes occurs [1]. Such a finding would be in the context of general hair damage and other more classic forms of trichoptilosis, which would distinguish it from pili bifurcati.

Treatment. Careful explanation is necessary to encourage the patient to avoid further hair trauma, because otherwise the condition will inevitably recur. Short hair and frequent trimming usually solve the problem.

REFERENCE

1 Burkhart CG, Huttner JJ, Bruner J. Central trichoptilosis. *J Am Acad Dermatol* 1981; **5**: 703–8.

Circle hairs [1,2]

Circle and spiral hairs occur in middle-aged men on the back, abdomen and thighs as small dark circles next to hair follicles. They are an unusual form of ingrown hair lying in a coiled track just below the stratum corneum, and can be easily extracted. Keratin follicular plugging is not associated (cf. scurvy, which may demonstrate keratosis pilaris with rolled and 'corkscrew' hairs).

REFERENCES

1 Levit F, Scott MJJR. Circle hairs. *J Am Acad Dermatol* 1983; **8**: 423–7.

2 Contreras-Ruiz J, Duran-McKinster C, Tamayo-Sanchez L, Orozco-Covarrubias L, Ruiz-Maldonado R. Circle hairs: a clinical curiosity. *J Eur Acad Dermatol Venereol* 2000; **14**: 495–7.

Trichomalacia

Miescher [1] described as trichomalacia a patchy alopecia in which some follicles are plugged and contain soft deformed swollen hairs. The changes have been attributed to the repeated trauma resulting from a hair-pulling tic [2,3], and subsequent histological studies in trichotillomania confirm this opinion.

Pathology. Above the bulb, the cells of the hair shaft appear to be disconnected and the hair is shapeless or partially disintegrated. High in the follicle, the shaft is thin and may be coiled. Whiting [4] described biopsy specimens as showing partially avulsed hair roots that are deformed and twisted. Clefting occurs between matrix cells and between hair bulb and outer connective tissue sheath. There is no inflammatory reaction; these changes are said to be pathognomonic of trichotillomania. One study of 26 patients with trichotillomania recorded trichomalacia in horizontal sections of 57% [5].

REFERENCES

1 Miescher G. Trichomalacie. *Arch Dermatol Syphilol* 1942; **183**: 117–29.
2 Haensch R, Blaich W. Trichomalacia und Trichotillomania. *Arch Klin Exp Dermatol* 1960; **210**: 447–52.
3 Miescher G, Schmuziger P. Trichomalacie und Trichotillomanie. *Dermatologica* 1957; **114**: 199–206.
4 Whiting DA. Structural abnormalities of the hair shaft. *J Am Acad Dermatol* 1987; **16**: 1–24.
5 Bergfeld W, Mulinari-Brenner F, McCarron K, Embi C. The combined utilization of clinical and histological findings in the diagnosis of trichotillomania. *J Cutan Pathol* 2002; **29**: 207–14.

Trichoschisis [1]

Trichoschisis is a clean transverse fracture across the hair shaft through cuticle and cortex; the fracture is associated with localized absence (loss) of cuticular cells. It is said to be a characteristic microscopic finding of trichothiodystrophy. It probably represents a clean fracture through hair with decreased high-sulphur matrix protein content and, in particular, a similar decrease in the exocuticle and A layer of cuticular cells. It may be prominent in the sulphur deficiency syndromes but it should not be considered as specific or pathognomonic.

REFERENCE

1 Brown AC, Belsher RB, Crounse RG *et al*. A congenital hair defect; trichoschisis and alternating birefringence and low-sulfur content. *J Invest Dermatol* 1970; **54**: 496–504.

Pohl–Pinkus constriction [1]

In some individuals, a zone of decreased shaft diameter coincides in time with a surgical operation, an illness or the administration of folic acid antagonists or other drugs that inhibit mitosis; it was first described by Pohl in 1894—he later changed his name to Pinkus. The proportion of affected hairs is variable and it seems probable that hairs in early anagen are most susceptible to a period of hypoproteinaemia or disturbed protein synthesis. This phenomenon was present in 21 of 100 hospitalized patients [2]; whether the illness or operation had been associated with pyrexia was not a relevant factor.

These constrictions in the hair shaft have been considered to be analogous to the transverse furrows in the nails (Beau's lines), which also coincide with episodes of ill health. Longer narrowings, resembling monilethrix, may occur with 'bolus' doses of cytotoxic drugs that do not lead to anagen effluvium.

REFERENCES

1 Pinkus H, ed. *Die Einwirking von Krankheiten auf das Kopfhaar des Menschen.* Berlin: Karger, 1971.
2 Sims RT. Reduction of hair shaft diameter associated with illness. *Br J Dermatol* 1967; **79**: 43–50.

Tapered hairs

Tapered hairs are those with a distal end that resembles the tip of a javelin. Most commonly, tapered hair is seen in any condition where there are many hairs regrowing after an effluvium, or where anagen is short. Regrowth after telogen effluvium, alopecia areata and trichotillomania may result in hairs with tapered ends. At body sites where the hairs are always short, such as the eyelashes, they are tapered. When scalp hair has a short anagen, such as in hypotrichosis simplex [1], the ends are also tapered. This is also the case in the newborn, as the duration of anagen has only been a few months from commencement *in utero*. As a feature on microscopy, tapered hairs are a useful sign that short hair is caused by the length of anagen rather than intrinsic hair shaft fragility.

REFERENCE

1 de Berker D. Congenital hypotrichosis. *Int J Dermatol* 1999; **38** (Suppl. 1): 25–33.

Bayonet hairs

Bayonet hairs are characterized by a 2–3 mm spindle-shaped hyperpigmented expansion of the hair cortex just proximal to a tapered tip, and may be associated with hyperkeratinization of the upper third of the follicle.

Trichonodosis

Michelson [1] first proposed the term noduli laqueati, and noted that naturally curly hair was most frequently affected. The term trichonodosis was popularized later by Kren [2], who found the condition in 35 out of 64 consecutively examined patients with skin disease.

Aetiology. The knotting of the hair shafts is induced by trauma. Short curly hair of relatively flat diameter is most readily affected [3]. Knots were seen most frequently in hair from people of African origin [4] and in short curly hair in white people; none was seen in long straight hair.

Some knotting is caused by braids and cosmetic manipulation. These knots are of a different form and scale to the inadvertent knotting brought about by hair type and random trauma. However, it is capable of inducing marked changes in the cuticle, which in turn results in a lower threshold for hair fracture.

Pathology. The only abnormalities are secondary to the knotting and are localized to that part of the shaft that forms the knot [3]. With the scanning electron microscope, the cuticle shows longitudinal fissuring and fractures, and cuticle scales are lost.

Clinical features [3]. Trichonodosis is usually an incidental finding, because it is inconspicuous and must be deliberately sought. One or few hairs are affected. The trauma of brushing or combing may cause the shaft to break at the site of the knot.

REFERENCES

1 Michelson P. Anomalien des Haarwachstums und der Haarfarbung. In: *Handbuch der speziellen Pathologie und Therapie* 1884; **14**: 89–93.
2 Kren O. Trichonodosis. *Wien Klin Wochenschr* 1907; **20**: 916–23.
3 Dawber RPR. Knotting of scalp hair. *Br J Dermatol* 1974; **91**: 169–74.
4 Khumalo NP, Doe PT, Dawber RP, Ferguson DJ. What is normal black African hair? A light and scanning electron-microscopic study. *J Am Acad Dermatol* 2000; **43**: 814–2.

Trichostasis spinulosa

This is probably a normal age-related phenomenon—easily overlooked—in which successive telogen hairs are retained in predominantly sebaceous follicles [1]. When it was specifically sought, 51 cases were seen in 1 month in Madras [2].

Aetiology. Ladany [3] thought trichostasis was no more than a variant of the comedo, and pointed out that 85% of comedones contain from one to 10 or more vellus hairs. Trichostasis is found most commonly in the middle-aged or elderly and is said by most authors to occur particularly on the nose and face [3]. Other sites were perhaps not always examined, for others have found it to be not uncommon on the trunk, limbs [4] and interscapular area [5].

Pathology. The affected follicles contain up to 50 vellus hairs embedded in a keratinous plug. A mild perifolliculitis is often present. The condition must be differentiated from the 'multiple hairs' of Flemming—Giovannini in which up to seven hairs grow from a composite papilla with a common outer root sheath [6]. Follicles may contain *Malassezia* yeasts and *Propionibacterium acnes* [5].

Clinical features [7]. Those reported to be affected have ranged in age from 17 to over 60 years. The lesions, which closely resemble comedones, may occur predominantly on the nose, forehead and cheeks, or the face may be spared and the nape, back, shoulders, upper arms and chest may be affected. The lesions vary greatly in number. On inspection with a hand lens, the 'comedones' seem to be unusually prominent and in some cases a tuft of hairs may be seen projecting through the horny plug.

Treatment. Keratolytic preparations have often been recommended but we have found them of little value. The most effective treatment is topical retinoic acid [8], which should be used as in the treatment of acne. Depilatory wax has also been successfully employed [7], and specialized cleaning pads have been advocated [9].

REFERENCES

1 Goldschmidt H, Hajyo-Tomoka MJ, Kligman AM. Trichostasis spinulosa: a common inapparent follicular disorder of the aged. In: Brown AC, ed. *First Human Hair Symposium*. New York: Medcom Press, 1974: 50–6.
2 Kailasam V, Kailasam A, Thambiah AS. Trichostasis spinulosa. *Int J Dermatol* 1979; **18**: 297–300.
3 Ladany E. Trichostasis spinulosa. *J Invest Dermatol* 1954; **23**: 33–4.
4 Young MC, Jorizzo JL, Sanchez RL *et al.* Trichostasis spinulosa. *Int J Dermatol* 1985; **24**: 575–80.
5 Chung TA, Lee JB, Jang HS, Kwon KS, Oh CK. A clinical, microbiological, and histopathologic study of trichostasis spinulosa. *J Dermatol* 1998; **25**: 697–702.
6 Pinkus H. Multiple hairs (Flemming–Giovannini). *J Invest Dermatol* 1951; **17**: 291–7.
7 Sarkany I, Gaylarde PM. Trichostasis spinulosa and its management. *Br J Dermatol* 1971; **84**: 311–16.
8 Mills OH, Kligman AM. Topically applied tretinoin in the treatment of trichostasis spinulosa. *Arch Dermatol* 1973; **108**: 378–81.
9 Elston DM, White LC. Treatment of trichostasis spinulosa with a hydroactive adhesive pad. *Cutis* 2000; **66**: 77–8.

Pili multigemini
SYN. PILI BIFURCATI

The term pili multigemini [1] describes an uncommon developmental defect of hair follicles as a result of which multiple matrices and papillae form hairs that emerge through a single pilosebaceous canal. The incidence of multigeminate hairs in the general population is unknown. Numerous follicles showing this defect have been seen in a patient with cleidocranial dysostosis [2].

Pathology. From two to eight matrices and papillae, each with its internal root sheath, form hairs that are often flattened, ovoid or triangular in configuration and may be grooved. In the follicular canal, contiguous hairs may adhere, bifurcate and then re-adhere.

Clinical features. Multigeminate follicles occur mainly on the face, especially along the lines of the jaw. Tufts of hair may be seen emerging from a few or many follicles. Their discovery is often a matter of chance, but the patient may complain of recurrent inflammatory nodules, leaving scars.

Treatment. If the hairs are plucked, they regrow [2]. A single report of ablation after three treatments with a ruby laser may indicate that this is a therapeutic option [3].

REFERENCES

1 Pinkus H. Multiple hairs (Flemming–Giovannini). *J Invest Dermatol* 1951; **17**: 291–7.

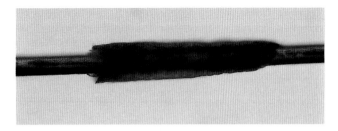

Fig. 63.70 Circumferential keratin cast resembling a cuff around the hair shaft.

2 Mehregan AH, Thompson WS. Pili multigemini: report of a case in association with cleidocranial dysotosis. *Br J Dermatol* 1979; **100**: 315–20.
3 Naysmith L, de Berker D, Munro CS. Multigeminate beard hairs and folliculitis. *Br J Dermatol* 2001; **144**: 427–8.

Hair casts

Hair casts (peripilar keratin casts) are firm yellowish white accretions ensheathing, but not attached to, scalp hairs. They freely move up and down the affected shafts [1]. Such casts are often found in scaly and seborrhoeic disorders of the scalp, and in children with hairstyles requiring traction [2].

Pathology. In cross-section, casts are composed of a central layer of retained internal root sheath and an outer thick keratinous layer. Scalp histology shows the follicular openings packed with parakeratotic squames, which break off at intervals to form hair casts.

Casts are found quite commonly in scaly, mainly parakeratotic conditions of the scalp such as psoriasis and pityriasis amiantacea [3]. Cases have been described in association with traction hairstyles [2,4,5] and hair sprays [6].

Clinical features. Hair casts (Fig. 63.70) may occur as an isolated abnormality unrelated to any overt scalp disease and may mimic pediculosis capitis [7]—hence the designation 'pseudonits' [8,9]. Girls and young women are most commonly affected; hundreds of casts may develop within a few days. No cause is known, but sex-linked inheritance has been suggested [1]. It is possible that this type may represent an unusual manifestation of psoriasis.

If patients with scaly parakeratotic diseases of the scalp complain of persistent dandruff that resists apparently adequate treatment, this is likely to be caused by multiple hair casts.

Diagnosis. In the absence of associated scalp disease, casts may be mistaken for pediculosis capitis, trichorrhexis nodosa or hair knots [10]. Of these nodal shaft abnormalities, only hair casts are freely movable along the hair.

Treatment. Any causative scalp disease must be treated.

Keratolytic preparations and shampoos that readily improve scalp scaling frequently fail to remove casts; prolonged brushing and combing is necessary to slide casts off the affected hairs [3,11].

REFERENCES

1 Kligman AM. Hair casts. *Arch Dermatol* 1957; **75**: 509–13.
2 Zhang W. Epidemiological and aetiological studies on hair casts. *Clin Exp Dermatol* 1995; **20**: 202–7.
3 Dawber RPR. The scalp and hair care in psoriasis. *J Psoriasis Assoc* 1979; **16**: 5–13.
4 Crovato F, Rebora A, Crosti C. Hair casts. *Dermatologica* 1980; **160**: 281–6.
5 Rollins TG. Traction folliculitis with hair casts and alopecia. *Am J Dis Child* 1961; **101**: 131–6.
6 Scott MJ. Peripilar keratin casts. *Arch Dermatol* 1959; **79**: 654–8.
7 Brunner MJ, Facq JM. A pseudoparasite of scalp hair. *Arch Dermatol* 1957; **75**: 583–7.
8 Kohn SR. Hair casts or pseudonits. *JAMA* 1977; **238**: 2058–9.
9 Keipert JA. Peripilar keratin casts (pseudonits) and psoriasis. *Med J Aust* 1974; **1**: 218–22.
10 Dawber RPR. Knotting of scalp hair. *Br J Dermatol* 1974; **91**: 169–74.
11 Bowyer A. Peripilar keratin casts. *Br J Dermatol* 1974; **90**: 231–6.

Weathering of the hair shaft [1,2]

All hair fibres undergo some degree of cuticular and secondary cortical breakdown from root to tip before being shed during the telogen or early anagen phase of the hair cycle. The term 'weathering' of hair has been limited by some authorities to structural changes in the hair shaft resulting from cosmetic procedures; indeed, both *in vivo* and *in vitro* studies carried out by cosmetic scientists have shown the type of damage that factors such as combing, brushing, bleaching and permanent waving can cause [3,4]. However, in considering the degeneration of hair fibres, cosmetic and other influences such as natural friction, wetting and UV radiation are so interwoven that it is more useful in practice to define weathering as the degeneration of hair from root to tip because of a variety of environmental and cosmetic factors. Scalp hair, having a long anagen phase and being subject to more frictional damage and cosmetic treatment, shows more deep cuticular and cortical degeneration than fibres from other sites.

Weathering of scalp hair has been studied in greater detail than hair from other sites. At the root end, surface cuticle cells are closely apposed to deeper layers. Within a few centimetres of the scalp, the free margin of these cells lifts up and breaks irregularly [5]. Increasing scale loss leads to surface areas denuded of cuticle. Many fibres show complete loss of overlapping scales well proximal to the tip (Fig. 63.71). This is particularly common on long hair shafts, which frequently have a frayed tip. Proximal to terminal fraying, longitudinal fissures may be present between exposed cortical cells. Hairs subjected to considerable friction damage may show transverse fissures and some nodes of the type seen in trichorrhexis nodosa [6,7]. Hair that has been bleached or permanently waved may show shaft distortion. The most severe changes are mostly

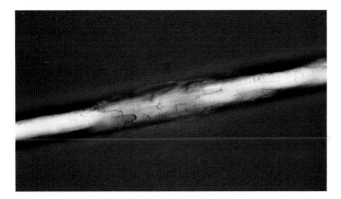

Fig. 63.71 Focal loss of cuticle in a weathered hair.

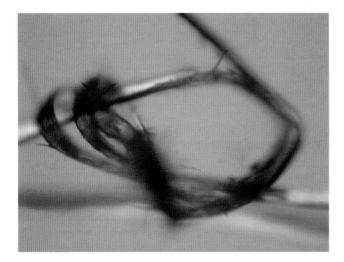

Fig. 63.72 Knotting of single and multiple hairs contributes to hair shaft trauma.

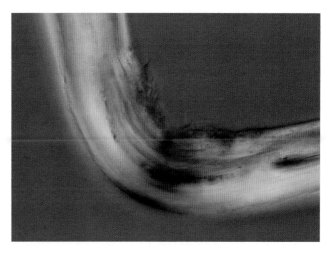

Fig. 63.73 Braiding damages hair shaft cuticle.

4 Robinson VNE. A study of damaged hair. *J Soc Cosmet Chem* 1976; **27**: 155–62.
5 Garcia ML, Epps JH, Yare RS. Normal cuticle wear patterns in human hair. *J Soc Cosmet Chem* 1978; **29**: 155–64.
6 Chernosky ME. Acquired trichorrhexis nodosa. In: Brown AC, ed. *The First Human Hair Symposium*. New York: Medcom Press, 1974.
7 Dawber RPR, Comaish S. Scanning electron microscopy of normal and abnormal hair shafts. *Arch Dermatol* 1970; **101**: 316–23.
8 Politt RJ, Jenner FA, Davies M. Sibs with mental and physical retardation and trichorrhexis nodosa with abnormal amino-acid composition of the hair. *Arch Dis Child* 1968; **42**: 211–20.
9 Lyon JB, Dawber RPR. A sporadic case of dystrophic pili torti. *Br J Dermatol* 1977; **96**: 197–9.
10 Camacho-Martinez F. Localized trichorrhexis nodosa. *J Am Acad Dermatol* 1989; **20**: 696–700.

Bubble hair

Brown [1] reported an unusual case of an acquired, localized, reversible hair shaft defect with intrinsic 'bubbles' within hairs, thought to be caused by repeated cosmetic trauma. Subsequent reports [2,3] have demonstrated that the bubbles are a sign of thermal injury, particularly of damp hair [3]. This may be because of poor thermostat control of a hair dryer, but most of us suffer bubble hairs by singeing over the cooker (Fig. 63.74).

REFERENCES

1 Brown VM, Crounse RG, Abele DC. An unusual new hair shaft abnormality, 'bubble hair'. *J Am Acad Dermatol* 1986; **15**: 1113–6.
2 Detwiles SP, Carson JL, Woosley JT *et al.* Bubble hair. *J Am Acad Dermatol* 1994; **30**: 54–60.
3 Gummer CL. Bubble hair: a cosmetic abnormality caused by brief, focal heating of damp hair fibres. *Br J Dermatol* 1994; **131**: 901–3.

Excessive growth of hair [1–3]

Growth of hair that in any given site is coarser, longer or more profuse than is normal for the age, sex and race of the individual is regarded as excessive. The terms hirsutism and hypertrichosis are often confused and applied

seen near the distal part of the hair shaft in normal scalp hair.

Hair knotting (Fig. 63.72) and braids (Fig. 63.73) are a significant source of hair shaft trauma, with loss of cuticle and damage to cortical fibres.

Trichorrhexis nodosa is the most severe form of weathering. Many of the changes seen in normal hair towards the tip are visible more proximally in congenitally weakened hair [8,9] and in trichorrhexis nodosa caused by overuse of cosmetic treatments [10].

In some hair structural abnormalities such as monilethrix and pili torti, specific weathering patterns may be seen.

REFERENCES

1 de Berker D, Sinclair R. Defects of the hair shaft. In: Dawber RPR, ed. *Diseases of the Hair and Scalp*, 3rd edn. Oxford: Blackwell Science, 1997: 427–9.
2 Dawber RPR. Weathering of hair in some genetic hair dystrophies. In: Brown AC, Crounse RG, eds. *Hair, Trace Elements and Human Illness*. New York: Praeger, 1980.
3 Brown AG, Swift JA. Hair breakage; the scanning electron microscope as a diagnostic tool. *J Soc Cosmet Chem* 1985; **26**: 289–98.

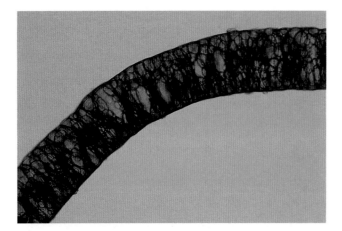

Fig. 63.74 Appearance of normal scalp hair after exposure to naked flame. Bubbles form within the cortex.

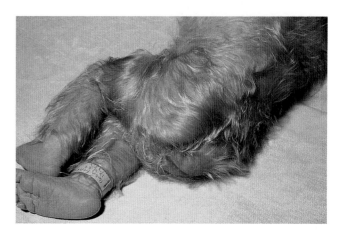

Fig. 63.75 Congenital hypertrichosis lanuginosa. (Courtesy of Dr Partridge, Leamington, UK.)

interchangeably and indiscriminately to excessive hair growth of any type in any distribution. On phylogenetic grounds, and on the basis of its specific androgenic induction, the growth in the female of coarse terminal hair in the adult male pattern should be differentiated clearly from the numerous other forms of excessive hair growth of widely varying aetiology. The term hirsutism will be restricted to androgen-dependent hair patterns of typically terminal hair and the term hypertrichosis will be applied to other patterns of excessive hair growth, typically vellus. In some areas it is difficult to make the distinction, such as in the excess facial hair in porphyria cutanea tarda. This is typically referred to as hypertrichosis, but the point can be argued.

There is much confusion in the literature concerning generalized congenital hypertrichosis because of a plethora of names such as apeman, bearman, dogman, manlion and wildman [4].

REFERENCES

1 Barth JH, Dawber RPR. Hypertrichosis. In: Dawber RPR, ed. *Diseases of the Hair and Scalp*, 3rd edn. Oxford: Blackwell Science, 1997: 490–3.
2 Rittmaster RS. Hirsutism. *Lancet* 1997; **349**: 191–5.
3 Dawber RP, Sinclair RD. Hirsuties. *Clin Dermatol* 2001; **19**: 189–99.
4 Bondeson J, Miles AEW. The hairy family of Burma. *J R Soc Med* 1996; **89**: 403–5.

Hypertrichosis

The terminology used in describing different patterns of hypertrichosis is inconsistent as reports have given synonymous terms to clinically different forms of the problem. Baumeister *et al.* [1] sought to unravel the matter. Hypertrichosis usually conforms to the classification of localized or generalized of congenital or acquired pattern, where congenital is loosely interpreted as that seen in early infancy.

REFERENCE

1 Baumeister FAM, Schwarz HP, Stengel-Rutkowski S. Childhood hypertrichosis: diagnosis and management. *Arch Dis Childhood* 1995; **72**: 457–9.

Congenital generalized hypertrichosis

Hypertrichosis lanuginosa

In congenital hypertrichosis, the fetal pelage is not replaced by vellus and terminal hair but persists, grows excessively and is constantly renewed throughout life. In the acquired form, the previously normal follicles of all types revert at any age to the production of hair with lanugo characteristics [1].

Aetiology. Traditionally, cases of congenital hypertrichosis have been classified into two groups—'dog faced' and 'simian'—but a survey [2] suggests that there may be only a single genotype, with considerable interfamily variation in the phenotype. With one exception [3], all published pedigrees suggest autosomal dominant inheritance.

Clinical features [2,4–7]. The child is usually noticed to be excessively hairy at birth (Fig. 63.75). The hair gradually lengthens until by early childhood the entire skin, apart from the palms and soles, is covered by silky hair, which may be 10 cm or more long. Long eyelashes and thick eyebrows are conspicuous features. Some affected individuals are normal at birth and sometimes for the first few years of life, before the universal replacement of other hair types by lanugo. Once established, the hypertrichosis is permanent, but some diminution of hairiness of trunk and limbs may be noted in later childhood. At puberty, axillary, pubic and beard hairs retain their downy character. Hypodontia or anodontia and deformities of the external ear are apparently associated in some families, but the physical and mental development of most patients has been normal. In a Mexican family, hypertrichosis was associated with an osteochondral dysplasia [8].

The status of the apparently recessive form is still more uncertain. Three children of a normal mother were densely hairy at birth and died within a week. Neonatal shaving was of cosmetic benefit in one rare case [6].

Treatment of children with long-pulsed ruby laser can result in a useful reduction of hair, although the benefits tend to wane over 6–12 months. Morley reported a 63% reduction in hair counts at 6 months [9].

Universal hypertrichosis

Not all people with congenital universal hypertrichosis will represent the same entity. If it is possible to make the distinction between lanugo and vellus hair, those with vellus hair may be classified as a form of universal hypertrichosis known as the Ambras syndrome, in which there are dysmorphic features. There is a debate concerning the distinction between Ambras syndrome and other forms of generalized hypertrichosis. Baumeister [10] argues that the uniformity of facial growth and the hypertrichosis of the external ear help set Ambras syndrome apart from other extreme forms of universal hypertrichosis where facial hair is not uniformly distributed and the ear hair growth is less marked. Although those outside the diagnosis of Ambras syndrome may have other associated features, such as gingival hyperplasia [11], there are some areas of overlap with respect to rearrangements on chromosome 8 [12,13].

There are also individuals who might be classified as demonstrating universal hypertrichosis, but with less extreme manifestations and without associated or dysmorphic features. The hair pattern is normal but in any site the hairs are larger and coarser than usual. The eyebrows may be double. Inheritance is determined by an autosomal dominant gene. The features begin to merge into what is considered the normal spectrum.

REFERENCES

1 Barth JH, Dawber RPR. Hypertrichosis. In: Dawber RPR, ed. *Diseases of the Hair and Scalp*, 3rd edn. Oxford: Blackwell Science, 1997: 490–3.
2 Felgenhauer WR. Hypertrichosis lanuginosa universalis. *J Génet Humaine* 1969; **17**: 10–3.
3 Jansen TAE, De Lange C. Familial hypertrichosis totalis. *Acta Paediatr Scand* 1945; **33**: 69–85.
4 Barth JH, Wilkinson JD, Dawber RPR. Prepubertal hypertrichosis. *Arch Dis Child* 1987; **63**: 666–70.
5 Beighton P. Congenital hypertrichosis lanuginosa. *Arch Dermatol* 1970; **101**: 669–72.
6 Partridge JW. Congenital hypertrichosis lanuginosa: neonatal shaving. *Arch Dis Child* 1987; **62**: 623–6.
7 Tourain A, ed. *L'Hérédité en Médecine*. Paris: Masson, 1995: 525–34.
8 Cantu JM, Sanchez-Corona J, Hernandez A. A distinct osteochondrodysplasia with hypertrichosis. *Hum Genet* 1982; **60**: 36–40.
9 Morley S, Gault DJ. Hair removal using the long-pulsed ruby laser in children. *J Clin Laser Med Surg* 2000; **18**: 277–80.
10 Baumeister FA. Differentiation of Ambras syndrome from hypertrichosis universalis. *Clin Genet* 2000; **57**: 157–8.
11 Lee IJ, Im SB, Kim D-K. Hypertrichosis universalis congenita: a separate entity or the same disease as gingival fibromatosis. *Pediatr Dermatol* 1993; **10**: 263–5.
12 Tadin M, Braverman E, Cianfarani S et al. Complex cytogenetic rearrangement of chromosome 8q in a case of Ambras syndrome. *Am J Med Genet* 2001; **102**: 100–4.
13 Baumeister FA. Diagnosis of Ambras syndrome: comments on complex cytogenetic rearrangement of chromosome 8q in a case of Ambras syndrome. *Am J Med Genet* 2002; **109**: 77–8.

Congenital generalized hypertrichosis associated with other syndromes

Hurler's syndrome and other mucopolysaccharidoses (see Chapter 12). Hypertrichosis is usually present from early infancy or early childhood on the face, trunk and limbs and may be a conspicuous feature. The eyebrows are often bushy and confluent. In abortive forms, the hair growth may first appear after puberty and be more limited in extent.

Congenital macrogingivae (see Chapter 66) [1]. Exuberant overgrowth of the gingivae as an isolated congenital defect is not uncommon. The association with profuse hypertrichosis of trunk, limbs and lower face has been reported on several occasions. Some patients have markedly acromegaloid features [2] or thyroid disease [3].

Cornelia de Lange syndrome (see Chapter 12). These mildly microcephalic, mentally defective children have a low hairline and profuse overgrowth of the eyebrows. The forehead is covered with long fine hair. Hypertrichosis is usually also conspicuous on the lower back, and may be generalized.

Winchester syndrome. This rare hereditary disorder is characterized by dwarfism, joint destruction and corneal opacities. The skin in many parts of the body becomes thickened, hyperpigmented and hypertrichotic [4,5].

Berardinelli's syndrome [6]. From early life, growth and maturation are accelerated and there is lipodystrophy with muscular hypertrophy. Enlargement of the liver and hyperlipidaemia are other constant features. The skin is coarse and often hypertrichotic.

Trisomy 18 (see Chapter 12). Generalized hypertrichosis of variable degree is present in these patients.

Hypertrichosis has been reported in the rare hereditary globoid leukodystrophy, Krabbe's disease. Most patients die in infancy [4].

Teratogenic syndromes

Fetal alcohol syndrome [7]. Mental and physical retardation affects the infants of many mothers with chronic alcoholism. The cutaneous changes include hypertrichosis and capillary haemangiomatosis.

REFERENCES

1 Byars LT, Jurkiewicz M. Congenital macrogingivae and hypertrichosis. *Plast Reconstr Surg* 1962; **27**: 608–12.
2 Vontobel F. Idiopathic gingival hyperplasia and hypertrichosis associated with acromegaloid features. *Helv Paediatr Acta* 1973; **28**: 401–11.
3 Gohlich-Ratmann G, Lackner A, Schaper J, Voit T, Gillessen-Kaesbach G. Syndrome of gingival hypertrophy, hirsutism, mental retardation and brachymetacarpia in two sisters: specific entity or variant of a described condition? *Am J Med Genet* 2000; **95**: 241–6.
4 Cohen AH, Hollister DW, Reed WB. The skin and the Winchester syndrome. *Arch Dermatol* 1975; **111**: 230–6.
5 Winchester P, Grossman H, Lim WN *et al*. A new acid mucopolysaccharidosis with skeletal deformities. *Am J Roentgenol* 1969; **106**: 121–8.
6 Beradinelli W. An undiagnosed endocrinopathy syndrome. *J Clin Endocrinol Metab* 1954; **14**: 193–204.
7 Hanson JW, Jones KL, Smith DW. Fetal alcohol syndrome. *JAMA* 1976; **235**: 1458–60.

Congenital localized hypertrichosis

Naevoid hypertrichosis

The growth of hair abnormal for the site and the age of the patient in its length, shaft diameter and colour may occur as a circumscribed developmental defect, either isolated or associated with other naevoid abnormalities [1], such as duplication of the thumb [2].

Melanocytic naevi (see Chapter 38) may be accompanied by a vigorous growth of coarse hair. The hair may be present from infancy or may develop at puberty. Less often, circumscribed hypertrichosis may occur as the only clinical abnormality. Histologically, the epidermis is acanthotic and the follicles are large, but there is no excess of melanocytes.

Hypertrichosis is a characteristic feature of Becker's naevus (see Chapter 15). The coarse hairs develop in the same body regions as the pigmentation, usually the thoracic or pelvic girdle, but pigmentation and hypertrichosis are not coextensive. It has been suggested that this naevus is a functional one, being androgen dependent; acne may also occur in the same site [3]. It has also rarely been reported in association with limb asymmetry and other ipsilateral anatomical abnormalities [4].

True linear hypertrichotic naevi are rare and hair growth may not be sustained [5].

A tuft of hair in the lumbosacral region, the so-called faun-tail naevus, is often associated with diastematomyelia (Fig. 63.76).

REFERENCES

1 Rupert LS, Bechtel M, Pellegrini A. Naevoid hypertrichosis. *Pediatr Dermatol* 1994; **11**: 49–50.
2 Taskapan O, Dogan B, Cekmen S, Baloglu H, Harmanyeri Y. Nevoid hypertrichosis associated with duplication of the right thumb. *J Am Acad Dermatol* 1998; **39**: 114–5.

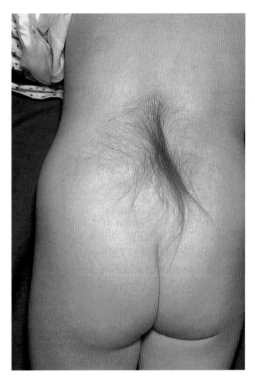

Fig. 63.76 Lumbosacral hypertrichosis ('faun tail'), here associated with diastematomyelia.

3 Downs AM, Mehta R, Lear JT, Peachey RD. Acne in a Becker's naevus: an androgen-mediated link? *Clin Exp Dermatol* 1998; **23**: 191–2.
4 Crone AM, James MP. Giant Becker's naevus with ipsilateral areolar hypoplasia and limb asymmetry. *Clin Exp Dermatol* 1997; **22**: 240–1.
5 Dudding TE, Rogers M, Roddick LG, Relic J, Edwards MJ. Nevoid hypertrichosis with multiple patches of hair that underwent almost complete spontaneous resolution. *Am J Med Genet* 1998; **79**: 195–6.

Acquired generalized hypertrichosis

Acquired hypertrichosis lanuginosa associated with malignancy

Aetiology. In its most dramatic severe form, this syndrome is rare. It usually accompanies a serious and often fatal illness. Fine downy hair grows over a large area of the body, replacing normal hair and primary and secondary vellus. Approximately 60 cases have been reported and all except two (in which there was no follow-up) were suffering from malignant disease of the gastrointestinal tract, bronchus, breast, gall bladder, uterus, bladder or other organs [1–5]. One patient with lymphatic leukaemia had acquired ichthyosis as well as hypertrichosis, and one had a lymphoma. The hypertrichosis may precede the diagnosis of a neoplasm by several years [6].

Pathology. In one case [7] the lanugo follicles lay almost parallel to the surface, and were apparently derived from mantle follicles.

Clinical features [8–10]. In the milder forms ('malignant down' [7]), hair is confined to the face, where it attracts attention by its appearance on the nose and eyelids and other sites that normally are clinically hairless. As the growth of hair continues, it may ultimately involve the entire body, apart from the palms and soles. Existing terminal hair of scalp, beard and pubes may not be replaced, and may contrast in colour and texture with the very fine white or blonde lanugo. Such hair may grow abundantly, even on the previously bald scalp. The hair may grow exceedingly rapidly, up to 2.5 cm/week, and may be more than 10 cm long.

REFERENCES

1 Hegedus SI, Schorr WF. Acquired hypertrichosis lanuginosa and malignancy. *Arch Dermatol* 1970; **106**: 84–8.
2 Hensley GT, Glynn KP. Hypertrichosis lanuginosa as a sign of internal malignancy. *Cancer* 1969; **24**: 1051–3.
3 Jemec GBE. Hypertrichosis lanuginosa acquisita: report of a case and review of the literature. *Arch Dermatol* 1986; **122**: 805–8.
4 Knowling MA, Meakin JW, Hradsky NS. Hypertrichosis associated with carcinoma of the lung. *Can Med Assoc J* 1982; **126**: 1308–10.
5 Ricken KH. Hypertrichosis lanuginosa bei chronische lymphatische Leukämie. *Z Hautkr* 1979; **54**: 819–24.
6 Farina MC, Tarin N, Grilli R *et al.* Acquired hypertrichosis lanuginosa: case report and review of the literature. *J Surg Oncol* 1998; **68**: 199–203.
7 Davis RA, Newman DM, Phillips MJ. Acquired hypertrichosis lanuginosa. *Can Med Assoc J* 1978; **118**: 1090–6.
8 Gonzales JJ, Ungaro PC, Hooper JW. Acquired hypertrichosis lanuginosa. *Arch Intern Med* 1980; **140**: 969–70.
9 Goodfellow A, Calvert H, Bohn G. Hypertrichosis lanuginosa acquisita. *Br J Dermatol* 1980; **103**: 431–3.
10 Sindhupak W, Vibhagool A. Acquired hypertrichosis lanuginosa. *Int J Dermatol* 1983; **21**: 599–603.

Non-malignant acquired generalized hypertrichosis

There is a range of non-malignant systemic diseases in which hypertrichosis may develop. Generally, the hair is coarser and less profuse than the lanugo hair associated with systemic malignancy. However, at any single point early in the process, the distinction may not always be obvious.

Endocrine disturbances

Hypothyroidism [1]. A profuse growth of hair on the back and the extensor aspects of the limbs develops in some children with hypothyroidism.

Hyperthyroidism. Coarse hair often grows over the plaques of pretibial myxoedema as it may over other forms of inflammation on the anterior shin.

Possible diencephalic or pituitary mechanisms. Severe generalized hypertrichosis has been reported in young children after encephalitis [2] and after mumps followed by the sudden onset of obesity [3]. A diencephalic disturbance is postulated. Generalized hypertrichosis occurred in a girl after traumatic shock [4] and remitted in 6 months. There are many reports of hypertrichosis after head injuries, especially in children. The hair growth is first noticed 4–12 weeks after the injury (which seems to be of no consistent type) and appears as fine silky hair on the forehead, cheeks, back, arms and legs, and may be asymmetrical. It is sometimes shed after a few months, but may persist.

Other conditions

Malnutrition [5]. Gross malnutrition, which may be primary or occur in coeliac disease or other malabsorption states or in severe infections, may cause profuse generalized hypertrichosis in children.

Anorexia nervosa [6]. An increased growth of fine downy hair on the face, trunk and arms, sometimes of severe degree, has been reported in 20–77% of adult cases [7,8], and is also seen in children [9]. The prevalence of hypertrichosis in bulimia is reported to be half of that in anorexia, and both are associated with approximately 60% prevalence of scalp alopecia [7].

Acrodynia [5]. Some increased growth of hair on the limbs is common. In severe cases, the hypertrichosis is very conspicuous on the face, trunk and limbs. One child was described as monkey-like.

Dermatomyositis [10]. Excessive hair growth has been noted mainly in children and principally on the forearms, legs and temples, but it may be more extensive.

Epidermolysis bullosa. Gross hypertrichosis of the face and limbs has occurred in association with epidermolysis bullosa of the dystrophic type, although this is rare (see Chapter 40).

Hypertrichosis is seen affecting the extensor surface of the arm (Fig. 63.77) in a sporadic or familial form in children, resolving in adolescence. Although associations with

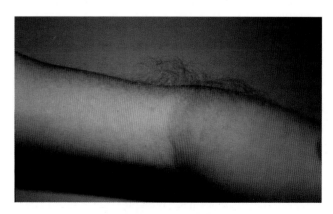

Fig. 63.77 Hypertrichosis of the elbows in a child.

other disorders have been sought, it appears as a largely isolated finding [11].

REFERENCES

1 Perloff WH. Hirsutism: a manifestation of juvenile hypothyroidism. *JAMA* 1955; **157**: 651–2.
2 Stegano G, Vignetti P. Considerazione su di ipertricosi con cerebropatia. *Arch Ital Pediatr Puericolt* 1955; **17**: 421–4.
3 Lesne E. Mumps hypertrichosis. *Bull Soc Pediatr* 1930; **28**: 94–6.
4 Robinson RCV. Temporary acquired hypertrichosis following traumatic shock. *Arch Dermatol* 1955; **71**: 401–2.
5 Holzel A. Hypertrichosis in childhood. *Acta Paediatr Scand* 1951; **40**: 59–69.
6 Ryle JA. Anorexia nervosa. *Lancet* 1936; **ii**: 140–4.
7 Glorio R, Allevato M, De Pablo A *et al.* Prevalence of cutaneous manifestations in 200 patients with eating disorders. *Int J Dermatol* 2000; **39**: 348–53.
8 Hediger C, Rost B, Itin P. Cutaneous manifestations in anorexia nervosa. *Schweiz Med Wochenschr* 2000; **130**: 565–75.
9 Schulze UM, Pettke-Rank CV, Kreienkamp M *et al.* Dermatologic findings in anorexia and bulimia nervosa of childhood and adolescence. *Pediatr Dermatol* 1999; **16**: 90–4.
10 Reich MG, Reinhart JB. Dermatomyositis associated with hypertrichosis. *Arch Dermatol Syphilol* 1948; **57**: 725–32.
11 Escalonilla P, Aguilar A, Gallego M *et al.* A new case of hairy elbows syndrome (hypertrichosis cubiti). *Pediatr Dermatol* 1996; **13**: 303–5.

Iatrogenic hypertrichosis

In iatrogenic hypertrichosis, there is a uniform increased growth of fine hair over extensive areas of the trunk, hands and face, unrelated to androgen-dependent hair growth.

The mode of action of the offending drugs on hair follicles is not known; the same mechanism is not involved in all cases. Cortisone, diphenylhydantoin and penicillamine are all known to affect connective tissue, but in different ways. Psoralens presumably induce hypertrichosis in predisposed subjects by accentuating the tendency of sunlight to induce this temporary change. The stimulation of hair growth on sun-exposed sites by benoxaprofen may have a similar mechanism. Existing vellus hairs increase in length and less so in diameter. The hairs are seldom more than 3 cm in length and are considerably finer than terminal hair.

Diphenylhydantoin induces hypertrichosis after 2–3 months. It affects the extensor aspects of the limbs, then the face and trunk, and clears within a year of cessation of therapy [1].

Diazoxide produces hypertrichosis in all of those treated but it seems to be a cosmetic problem in only half [2,3]; in adults, the anagen phase may last longer [4]. There are no associated changes in the sebaceous glands [2].

Minoxidil commonly induces hypertrichosis [5]. It is apparent after a few weeks' therapy [6].

Hypertrichosis of some degree develops in 60% of patients treated with ciclosporin [7–9]. Keratosis pilaris may precede the appearance of thick pigmented hair on the face, trunk and limbs. Changes in other parts of the pilosebaceous unit occur: keratosis pilaris (21%), sebaceous hyperplasia (10%) and acne (15%) [8].

Benoxaprofen induced a fine downy growth of hair on the face and exposed extremities after only a few weeks [10].

Streptomycin caused hypertrichosis in 22 of 27 children who had received 1 g/day for miliary tuberculous meningitis [11,12].

Prolonged administration of cortisone may induce hypertrichosis, most marked on the forehead, the temples and the sides of the cheeks, but also on the back and the extensor aspects of the limbs.

Penicillamine appears to cause lengthening and coarsening of hair on the trunk and limbs.

Psoralens, used in the treatment of vitiligo and psoriasis, may induce temporary hypertrichosis of light-exposed skin [13].

Latanoprost eye drops used for glaucoma may cause hypertrichosis of eyelashes and increased vellus hair on the eyelid skin [14]. This prostaglandin receptor agonist is the subject of current research in the sphere of hair regrowth products [15].

REFERENCES

1 Livingstone S, Peterson D, Bohs LL. Hypertrichosis occurring in association with dilantin therapy. *J Pediatr* 1955; **47**: 351–2.
2 Koblenzer PJ, Baker L. Hypertrichosis lanuginosa associated with diazoxide therapy in prepubertal children: a clinicopathological study. *Ann NY Acad Sci* 1968; **150**: 373–9.
3 Prigent F, Gantzer A, Romain O *et al.* Hypertrichose diffuse acquisé au cours d'un traitment par diazoxide chez un nouveau-né. *Ann Dermatol Vénéréol* 1988; **115**: 191–2.
4 Burton JL, Schutt WH, Caldwell IW. Hypertrichosis due to diazoxide. *Br J Dermatol* 1975; **93**: 707–9.
5 Burton JL, Marchall A. Hypertrichosis due to minoxidil. *Br J Dermatol* 1979; **101**: 593–5.
6 Lorette G, Nivet H. Hypertrichose diffuse au minoxidil chez un enfant de deux ans et demi. *Ann Dermatol Vénéréol* 1985; **112**: 527–8.
7 Bencini PL, Montagnino G, Sala F *et al.* Cutaneous lesions in 67 cyclosporin-treated renal transplant recipients. *Dermatologica* 1986; **172**: 24–31.
8 Bencini PL, Montagnino G, Crosti C *et al.* Acne in a kidney transplant patient treated with cyclosporin A. *Br J Dermatol* 1986; **114**: 396.
9 Griffiths CEM, Powles AV, Leonard JN *et al.* Clearance of psoriasis with low-dose cyclosporin. *BMJ* 1986; **293**: 731–3.
10 Fenton DA, English JS, Wilkinson JD. Reversal of male pattern baldness, hypertrichosis, and accelerated hair and nail growth in patients receiving benoxaprofen. *BMJ* 1982; **248**: 1228–9.
11 Fono R. Appearance of hypertrichosis during streptomycin treatment. *Ann Paediatr* 1950; **174**: 389–92.
12 Buffoni L. Streptomicini e ipertricosi. *Minerva Pediatr* 1951; **3**: 710–2.
13 Singh G, Lal S. Hypertrichosis and hyperpigmentation with systemic psoralen treatment. *Br J Dermatol* 1967; **79**: 501–2.
14 Demitsu T, Manabe M, Harima N *et al.* Hypertrichosis induced by latanoprost. *J Am Acad Dermatol* 2001; **44**: 721–3.
15 Uno H, Zimbric ML, Albert DM, Stjernschantz J. Effect of latanoprost on hair growth in the bald scalp of the stump-tailed macaque: a pilot study. *Acta Derm Venereol* 2002; **82**: 7–12.

Acquired localized hypertrichosis

Cutting or shaving the hair influences neither its rate of growth nor the calibre of the hair shaft. However, repeated or long-continued inflammatory changes involving the dermis, whether or not clinically evident scarring is produced, may result in the growth of long and coarse hair at

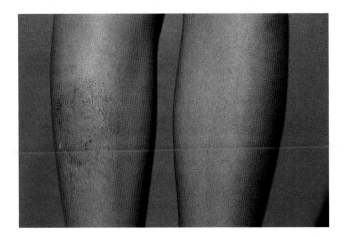

Fig. 63.78 Circumscribed hypertrichosis in an area of steroid-treated lichen simplex.

the site. The cause of the hair growth is usually obvious but may be overlooked when the trauma is occupational; for example, circumscribed patches of hypertrichosis on the left shoulder in people frequently carrying heavy sacks [1] or religious items during holy week in Spain [2]. A patch of hypertrichosis on one forearm has been reported in those with mental retardation who have acquired the habit of chewing the site [3]. Sometimes, hypertrichosis develops at the site of an accidental wound or a vaccination scar [4]. It has developed on the back of the hand and fingers 3 months after the excision of warts [5]. It has been reported also in an irregular pattern on the legs in chronic venous insufficiency [6], around the edges of a burn [7] and at the site of multiple clusters of excoriated insect bites [8]. Hypertrichosis of this type may occur near inflamed joints and has been reported particularly in association with gonococcal arthritis [9] and in the skin overlying chronic osteomyelitis of the tibia [10]. Very exceptionally, inflammatory dermatoses, especially in children, may induce a temporary overgrowth of hair; for example after eczema (Fig. 63.78) [11] and varicella [12]. A linear pattern of hypertrichosis on the leg has been described after recurrent thrombophlebitis that persisted for a year [13]. Hypertrichosis may occur in the indurated skin in melorheostotic scleroderma [14]. The damaged skin in epidermolysis bullosa may also become hypertrichotic [15]. Children have developed itching eczema and local hypertrichosis at the site of injection of diphtheria–tetanus vaccine adsorbed on aluminium chloride [16].

Hypertrichosis of one leg or forearm after a prolonged period of occlusion by plaster of Paris is a phenomenon well known to orthopaedic surgeons. It is seen in association with 55% of cases of reflex sympathetic dystrophy and may be accompanied by Beau's lines [17]. It occurs mainly in children. The hypertrichosis is likely to result from prolongation of anagen. It is not clear whether this is

caused by local vascular changes, as occurs with hypertrichosis associated with areas of skin inflammation.

Porphyria (see Chapter 57). Hypertrichosis of exposed skin is a common feature of the very rare erythropoietic porphyria; appearing first on the forehead, it later extends to the cheeks and chin and, to a lesser degree, to other exposed areas. It is also present in many cases of the much more common erythropoietic protoporphyria [18].

In porphyria cutanea tarda, hypertrichosis is an inconstant finding, but may accompany the pigmentation, plethora, blistering and scleroderma-like changes on exposed skin, and is marked in some children with the disease [19]. Darkening of scalp hair in a subject with white hair at the onset of porphyria cutanea tarda has been reported [20], and hypertrichosis has been reported as the presenting complaint in one subject in whom porphyria cutanea tarda was the underlying cause [21]. In black people, hypertrichosis and pigmentation may be present without blistering [22].

The most extreme degree of hypertrichosis is seen in children with hepatic porphyria induced by hexachlorobenzene or other chemicals. Hypertrichosis is frequent in porphyria variegata. The temples, forehead and cheeks are covered with downy hair. There is also increased pigmentation.

Some forms of localized hypertrichosis are caused by the local application or effect of drugs and are discussed in the section on iatrogenic causes of hypertrichosis (see p. 63.96).

REFERENCES

1 Csillag J. Über Beruishypertricose. *Arch Dermatol Syphilol* 1921; **134**: 147–8.
2 Camacho F. Acquired circumscribed hypertrichosis in the 'costaleros' who bear the 'pasos' during Holy Week in Seville, Spain. *Arch Dermatol* 1995; **131**: 361–3.
3 Ressmann AC, Butterworth T. Localized acquired hypertrichosis (as a result of biting in mentally deficient). *Arch Dermatol Syphilol* 1952; **65**: 458–60.
4 Linser A. Demonstrationen: patient mit einer Hypertrichosis irritative. *Klin Wochenschr* 1926; **115**: 149–50.
5 Friederich HC, Gloor M. Postoperativ 'irritative' Hypertrichose. *Z Haut Geschlechts* 1970; **45**: 10–1.
6 Schraibman IG. Localized hirsutism. *Postgrad Med J* 1967; **43**: 545–6.
7 Shafir R, Tsur H. Local hirsutism at the periphery of burned skin. *Br J Plast Surg* 1979; **32**: 93–5.
8 Tisocco LA, Del Campo DV, Bennin B *et al.* Acquired localized hypertrichosis. *Arch Dermatol* 1981; **117**: 129–31.
9 Heidemann H. Et tifaelde af hypertrichose opstaalt i tilknytning til en gonorrhoisk ledaffektasion. *Ugeskr Laeger* 1934; **96**: 553–5.
10 Schuller PA, Frost JA. Osteomilitis cronica de perone e hipertrichosis localizada. *Medicina* 1956; **24**: 360–1.
11 Edel K. Hypertrichosis als verwikkeling bij eczeem. *Ned Tijdschr Geneeskd* 1938; **82**: 2466–7.
12 Naveh Y, Friedman A. Transient circumscribed hypertrichosis following chicken pox. *Paediatrics* 1972; **50**: 487–8.
13 Soyuer U, Aktas E, Ozesmi M. Post-phlebitic localized hypertrichosis. *Arch Dermatol* 1988; **124**: 30–1.
14 Miyachi Y, Hori T, Yamada A *et al.* Linear melorheostotic scleroderma and hypertrichosis. *Arch Dermatol* 1979; **115**: 1233–4.
15 Cofano AR. Su un caso di epidermolisi bollosa distrofica con accentuada ipertricosi. *Ann Ital Dermatol* 1995; **10**: 195–6.

16 Pembroke AC, Marten RH. Unusual reactions following diphtheria and tetanus immunization. *Clin Exp Dermatol* 1979; **4**: 345–7.
17 Veldman PHJM, Reynen HM, Arntz IE, Goris RJA. Signs and symptoms of reflex sympathetic dystrophy: prospective study of 829 patients. *Lancet* 1993; **342**: 1012–6.
18 Dean G, ed. *The Porphyrias*. London: Pitman, 1963.
19 Pinol Aguade J, Lecha M, Almeida J *et al*. Porfiria cutanea tarda en miños. *Med Cutanea* 1973; **7**: 37–42.
20 Shaffrali FC, McDonagh AJ, Messenger AG. Hair darkening in porphyria cutanea tarda. *Br J Dermatol* 2002; **146**: 325–9.
21 Boffa MJ, Reed P, Weinkove C, Ead RD. Hypertrichosis as the presenting feature of porphyria cutanea tarda. *Clin Exp Dermatol* 1995; **20**: 62–4.
22 Zeligman J. Patterns of porphyria in the American Negro. *Arch Dermatol* 1963; **88**: 616–26.

Hirsutism

Perception of hirsutism is by definition subjective, and women present with a wide variation in severity [1]. Both the severity of the hirsutism and the degree of its acceptance are dependent on racial, cultural and social factors. Even the criteria for the definition of hirsutism used by physicians vary widely [2–6]. In order to resolve this issue, different groups have evolved different grading schemes for body hair growth. The scheme employed in the study by Ferriman and Gallwey [3], which has become the standard grading system, defined hirsutism purely on quantitative grounds. Hirsutism is graded as numerical scores beyond an upper limit of twice the standard deviation from the mean. Scoring can be on a global basis assessing 8–11 body sites, or it can be based on a single site. Others have examined women complaining of hirsutism and compared them with controls; they have demonstrated that there is a considerable overlap in the grades of hirsutism between the two groups [4,6]. Hair on the face, chest or upper back is a good discriminating factor between hirsute women and controls with similar hair growth scores. In clinical practice, it has often been suggested that 'real' hirsutism is simply that which the woman in question thinks is excessive.

Facial and body hair is less commonly seen on oriental people [7], black people and native Americans than on white people [8]. Even among white people there are differences; hair growth is heavier on those of Mediterranean than those of Nordic ancestry [9]. The pattern of hair growth in hirsutism within different racial groups is identical [3–6]. However, different criteria have made the determination of the comparative incidence and severity within these groups difficult to assess. Only one study of a random population stated how many women considered themselves to be hirsute. McKnight [5] examined 400 unselected students, 60% of whom were Welsh: 9% were considered by both the women and investigator to be hirsute and 4% were considered to be disfigured by their facial hair growth. This investigation also included studies of hair growth in women who were not complaining of hirsutism. It is important to the definition of hirsutism that a sizeable proportion of normal women have some terminal hairs on their face, breasts or lower abdomen.

Lorenzo [10] studied 90 hirsute women and found an increased incidence of hirsutism in their female relatives compared with control populations. McKnight [5] reported that 14% of hirsute Welsh women gave a positive family history. This tendency to familial clustering in hirsutism might be anticipated, as some of the underlying disorders that result in hyperandrogenism have a familial basis. For example, congenital adrenal hyperplasia is autosomal recessive and linked to MHC [11], and a very strong family relationship has been reported in the polycystic ovary syndrome (PCOS) [12].

In hirsutism, one role of society is to determine the threshold level for normality and this is now determined by the media. Women receive a barrage of advertisements for cosmetics that are based on the premise that only a woman with a hairless body can be normal, healthy and attractive. To some extent, men are falling victim to the same media aesthetic, with the advent of laser techniques capable of removing hair from large areas.

There have been few studies on the psychological status of hirsute women. Meyer and Zerssen [13] concluded on the basis of a small sample of patients studied within a psychoanalytic framework that many suffered reactive psychological problems. A small controlled study [14] revealed increased levels of anxiety. In contrast, Callan *et al.* [15] were unable to detect significant differences in comparison with normal.

Another approach to the psychological aspect of hirsutism has been to implicate 'stress' as an aetiological factor. Segre [16] states, in his monograph on the hirsute female, that: 'Lack of peace of mind appears at the core of the problem. We believe it to be both a cause and result of hirsutism.' This view has been endorsed [17]. The onset of hirsutism in four of 10 hirsute women was noted to coincide with a period of emotional stress [18]. Bush and Mahesh [19] reported stress-induced hirsutism in a young woman whose unstressed twin was not hirsute. Objective before and after data on this observation are difficult to identify.

REFERENCES

1 Hughes CL. Hirsutism. In: Olsen EA, ed. *Disorders of Hair Growth*. New York: McGraw-Hill, 2003: 431–52.
2 Editorial. Endocrine treatment in hirsutism. *BMJ* 1975; **ii**: 461–2.
3 Ferriman D, Gallwey JD. Clinical assessment of body hair growth in women. *J Clin Endocrinol* 1961; **21**: 1440–9.
4 Lunde O, Grottum P. Body hair growth in women; normal or hirsute. *Am J Phys Anthropol* 1984; **64**: 307–12.
5 McKnight E. The prevalence of 'hirsutism' in young women. *Lancet* 1964; **i**: 410–2.
6 Shah PN. Human body hair: a quantitative study. *Am J Obstet Gynecol* 1957; **73**: 1255–61.
7 Hamilton JE. Age, sex and genetic factors in the regulation of hair growth in men: a comparison of Caucasian and Japanese populations. In: Montagna W, Ellis RA, eds. *The Biology of Hair Growth*. New York: Academic Press, 1958: 399–417.
8 Danforth CH, Trotter M. The distribution of body hair in white subjects. *Am J Phys Anthropol* 1922; **5**: 259–65.
9 Greenblatt RB. Hirsutism: ancestral curse or endocrinopathy. In: Mahesh

VB, Greenblatt RB, eds. *Hirsutism and Virilism.* Boston: John Wright, 1983: 1–9.

10 Lorenzo EM. Familial study of hirsutism. *J Clin Endocrinol Metab* 1970; **31**: 556–60.

11 Gordon MT, Conway DI, Anderson DC et al. Genetics and biochemical variability of variants of 21 hydroxylase deficiency. *J Med Genet* 1985; **22**: 354–7.

12 Hague WM, Adams J, Reeders ST et al. Familial polycystic ovaries: a genetic disease? *Clin Endocrinol* 1988; **29**: 593–6.

13 Meyer AE, Zerssen DV. Frauen mit sogenanntem idiopathischem Hirsutismus. *J Psychosom Res* 1960; **4**: 206–10.

14 Rabinowitz S, Cohen R, Le Roith D. Anxiety and hirsutism. *Psychol Rep* 1983; **53**: 827–33.

15 Callan A, Dennerstein L, Burrows GD et al. The psychoendocrinology of hirsutism. In: Dennerstein L, Burrows GD, eds. *Obstetrics, Gynaecology and Psychiatry.* Melbourne: University of Melbourne, 1980: 43–51.

16 Segre EJ, ed. *Androgens, Virilization and the Hirsute Female.* Springfield: Thomas, 1967: 92–4.

17 Rook AJ. Aspects of cutaneous androgen-dependent syndromes. *Int J Dermatol* 1980; **19**: 357–60.

18 Merivale WH. The excretion of pregnanediol and 17-ketosteroids during the menstrual cycle in benign hirsutism. *J Clin Pathol* 1951; **4**: 78–83.

19 Bush IE, Mahesh VB. Adrenocortical hyperfunction with sudden onset of hirsutism. *J Endocrinol* 1959; **18**: 1–7.

Endocrine factors and hirsutism [1]

Hirsutism attracts a wide range of endocrine investigations, which differ according to the presentation and the specialty background of the clinician. However, the assumption that hirsutism is wholly related to androgens can be challenged on an individual and general level. The increasing awareness of insulin metabolism and hirsutism has highlighted this and, on an individual level, it is very clear that many women with unwanted hair have no endocrinological disturbance.

There have been several attempts to correlate hair growth in women with plasma androgen levels but these reports have yielded conflicting results. Reingold and Rosenfield [2] noted a considerable variability between hair growth scores and free testosterone, but no significant relationship. Ruutiainen et al. [3] have calculated a complex formula for multiple plasma androgen levels:

Testosterone/SHBG + androstenedione/100 + dehydroepiandrosterone sulphate/100.

This correlates with hair growth only in women with idiopathic hirsutism. In a further study, the same group [4] found a relationship between hair growth and salivary testosterone levels, but in this study no selection of patients was required. A different ratio has been determined for female baldness [5]:

3α-androstanediol glucuronide/SHBG.

Both equations demonstrate the significance of SHBG as a factor modifying the effects of circulating androgen.

The first sign of androgen production in women occurs 2–3 years before the menarche and is caused by adrenal secretion [6]. The major androgens secreted by the adrenal are androstenedione, dehydroepiandrosterone (DHA) and DHA sulphate (DHAS). Their control during postpubertal life is unknown, but it is thought that androstenedione and

DHA may be controlled by adrenocorticotrophic hormone (ACTH), as their serum levels mirror those of cortisol [7,8].

Ovarian androgen production begins under the influence of the pubertal secretion of luteinizing hormone (LH) and takes place in the theca cells. The predominant androgen secreted by the ovaries is androstenedione during the reproductive years, and testosterone after the menopause. Androgen secretion continues throughout the menstrual cycle but peaks at the middle of an ovulatory cycle [9]. Androstenedione secretion is greater from the ovary containing the dominant follicle [10].

In normal women, the majority of testosterone production (50–70%) is derived from peripheral conversion of androstenedione in skin and other extrasplanchnic sites [11–13]. The remaining proportion is secreted directly by the adrenals and ovaries. The relative proportion estimated from each gland varies between reported studies: 5–20% from the ovary and 0–30% from the adrenal [13,14]. DHA is the source of less than 10% of circulating androstenedione and 1% of circulating testosterone [15,16].

Androgen transport proteins

In non-pregnant women, the majority of circulating androgens are bound to a high-affinity β-globulin, SHBG. A further 20–25% is transported loosely bound to albumin, and approximately 1% circulates freely. The free steroid is believed to be active, and the binding protein is therefore of paramount importance. The affinity of the androgens for SHBG is proportional to their biological activity.

The function of SHBG is unknown. It is probable that its main role is to buffer acute changes in unbound androgen levels and to protect androgens from degradation. Burke and Anderson [17] suggested that it also acts as a biological amplifier. High oestrogen levels increase SHBG and therefore reduce available androgen; high androgen levels reduce SHBG and increase available free androgen.

REFERENCES

1 Rittmaster RS. Hirsutism. *Lancet* 1997; **349**: 191–5.

2 Reingold SB, Rosenfield RL. The relationship of mild hirsutism or acne in women to androgens. *Arch Dermatol* 1987; **123**: 209–14.

3 Ruutiainen K, Erkola R, Kaihola HL et al. The grade of hirsutism correlated to serum androgen levels and hormonal indices. *Acta Obstet Gynecol Scand* 1985; **64**: 629–34.

4 Ruutiainen K, Sannika E, Santii R et al. Salivary testosterone in hirsutism: correlations with serum testosterone and the degree of hair growth. *J Clin Endocrinol Metab* 1987; **64**: 1015–20.

5 De Villez RL, Dunn J. Female androgenic alopecia; the 3α, 17β-androstanediol glucuronide : sex hormone binding globulin ratio as a possible marker for female pattern baldness. *Arch Dermatol* 1986; **122**: 1011–7.

6 Reiter EO, Fuldauer VG, Root AW. Secretion of the adrenal androgen dehydroepiandrosterone sulphate, during normal infancy, childhood, and adolescence, in sick infants and children with endocrinological abnormalities. *J Pediatr* 1977; **90**: 766–70.

7 James VHT, Tunbridge D, Wilson GA et al. Central control of steroid hormone secretion. *J Steroid Biochem* 1978; **9**: 429–34.

8 Rosenfeld RS, Rosenburg BJ, Fukushima DK et al. 24-Hour secretory pattern of dehydroisoandrosterone and dehydroisoandrosterone sulphate. *J Clin Endocrinol Metab* 1975; **40**: 850–8.

9 Vermeuler A, Verdonck L. Plasma androgen levels during the menstrual cycle. *Am J Obstet Gynecol* 1976; **125**: 491–8.
10 Baird DT, Burger PE, Heaven-Jones GD *et al.* The site of secretion of androstenedione in non-pregnant women. *J Endocrinol* 1974; **63**: 201.
11 Horton R. Markers of peripheral androgen production. In: Serio M, Motta M, Martini L, eds. *Sexual Differentiation; Basic and Clinical Aspects.* New York: Raven Press, 1984: 261–85.
12 Horton R, Tait JF. Androstenedione production and interconversion rates measured in peripheral blood and studies on the possible site of its conversion to testosterone. *J Clin Invest* 1966; **45**: 301–6.
13 Kirschner MA, Bardin CW. Androgen production and metabolism in normal and virilized women. *Metabolism* 1972; **21**: 667–73.
14 Moltz L, Sorensen R, Schwartz U *et al.* Ovarian and adrenal vein steroids in healthy women with ovulatory cycles: selective catheterization findings. *J Steroid Biochem* 1984; **20**: 901–8.
15 Horton R, Tait JF. *In vivo* conversion of dehydroisoandrosterone to plasma androstenedione and testosterone in man. *J Clin Endocrinol Metab* 1967; **27**: 79–85.
16 Kirschner MA, Sinhamahapatra S, Zucker IR *et al.* The production, origin and role of dehydroepiandrosterone and 5-androstenediol as androgen prehormones in hirsute women. *J Clin Endocrinol Metab* 1973; **37**: 183–8.
17 Burke CW, Anderson DC. Sex-hormone binding globulin is an oestrogen amplifier. *Nature* 1972; **240**: 38.

Androgen pathophysiology in hirsutism [1,2]

The growth of normal secondary sexual hair is a response of the hair follicles to androgens. Abnormal degrees of hair growth are therefore often seen in endocrine disorders characterized by hyperandrogenism. However, not all women with greater amounts of secondary sexual hair will have abnormal androgens. Many will lie within the range of normal for their age and ethnic origin—albeit possibly at an extreme of the spectrum. For those objectively classified as hirsute, many will have underlying PCOS. Most of the others will have no detectable hormonal abnormality and are usually classified as having 'idiopathic' hirsutism. This subgroup is gradually becoming smaller as diagnostic techniques for PCOS become more refined.

Polycystic ovary syndrome [3–5].

The perception of PCOS has changed dramatically since it was first described by Stein and Leventhal in 1935 [6]. They defined a syndrome consisting of obesity, amenorrhoea, hirsutism and infertility associated with enlarged polycystic ovaries. This diagnosis is complicated by the fact that it is defined by the appearance of organs that are difficult to visualize. This has led to the use of multiple diagnostic formulations based on clinical and biochemical abnormalities. A more fundamental issue has been raised by modern imaging techniques, which have revealed the presence of polycystic ovaries in normal women [7] or mildly polycystic ovaries in hirsute women with normal menses [8]. The latter finding has led to the inclusion of women who were previously labelled as having idiopathic hirsutism under the diagnosis of PCOS. An estimated one-third of women in the UK have polycystic ovaries—defined as 10 or more follicles/ovary detected on ultrasound [9]. One-third of these women will suffer from PCOS, which is now formally defined in the UK as the presence of polycystic ovaries in the presence of one or more of hirsutism, male pattern baldness, acne, oligomenorrhoea or amenorrhoea, obesity, or raised serum concentrations of testosterone and/or luteinizing hormone [10]. The pattern of these features will depend upon the presenting complaint, be it dermatological, endocrinological or gynaecological. Using ultrasound visualization of polycystic ovaries as the diagnostic criterion in those presenting to a gynaecologist, Conway *et al.* [11] found the following clinical features in a series of 556 patients: hirsutism (61%), acne (24%), alopecia (8%), acanthosis nigricans (2%), obesity (35%), menorrhagia (1%), oligomenorrhoea (45%), amenorrhoea (26%) and infertility (over 29%). However, those patients who present to a dermatologist will almost invariably have acne and/or hirsutism.

Laboratory investigations in PCOS usually reveal an elevated level of LH, often with an increased LH : follicle-stimulating hormone (FSH) ratio, and testosterone, androstenedione and oestradiol levels are also often raised [12], although these tests are neither wholly sensitive nor specific. The demonstration by ultrasound examination of multiple peripheral ovarian cysts around a dense central core will depend on the expertise of the operator [13].

Ideas concerning the pathogenesis of PCOS have been as controversial as the diagnosis, and different authorities embrace beliefs that it is primarily caused by an ovarian abnormality, inappropriate gonodotrophin secretion, a disorder of the adrenal glands or increased peripheral aromatase activity resulting in hyperoestrogenaemia [14]. Whether the increased androgen is of adrenal or ovarian origin remains unclear [15]. However, in addition to the presence of elevated testosterone, commonly in the range of 2.6–4.8 nmol/L [4], 50% or more of patients will have hyperinsulinaemia of varying degrees [16]. This appears to be the case for both the classically obese and the non-obese PCOS patient [17]. Insulin acts to inhibit production of SHBG and stimulates ovarian testosterone production. Both effects amplify androgenic features in PCOS. Excess insulin production is related to the feedback loop of peripheral insulin resistance which increases in PCOS. This is characteristic of type 2 diabetes mellitus, which is a disease more common in PCOS. Consistent with this association, PCOS patients are also at higher risk of dyslipidaemias and coronary artery disease [18]. Altered glucose tolerance, hyperinsulinaemia and hirsutism are all exacerbated by obesity, and the relationship between diabetes and hyperandrogenism in women, or 'diabetes of bearded women', has been recognized for many years [19].

Such features are not invariably part of PCOS. Hyperinsulinaemia may be an autonomous process causing acanthosis nigricans (AN), which acts as a cutaneous marker for the insulin resistance (IR). The combination of AN and IR occurs in 5% of women with hyperandrogenism (HA) [20] and in 7% of women presenting with hirsutism [21]. Women with HAIR-AN have marked features of virilism: muscular physique, acne, alopecia and hidradenitis suppurativa [21]. The cause of hyperinsulinaemia is not always apparent, but its effects can be partly reversed by troglitazone [22], and its significance is illustrated by the evolution of HAIR-AN syndrome with an insulin-secreting tumour, cured by partial pancreatectomy [23].

Leptin is a protein secreted by adipocytes that increases energy expenditure and decreases appetite [24]. In genetically obese *ob/ob* mice, leptin is functionally deficient and the mice develop obesity, insulin resistance, diabetes and infertility. In recent years, there has been much interest in determining the role of this protein in PCOS. High serum levels appear primarily related to obesity rather than the diagnosis of PCOS alone [25] and there is evidence that its fluctuations are synchronized with those of luteinizing hormone [26]. However, although there is some correlation between polymorphisms of the leptin gene and insulin regulation, no mutation specific to PCOS has yet been identified [27]. Although family studies of PCOS suggest an autosomal dominant inheritance, no single gene has been defined. Linkage has been found to the follistatin gene on 5q (follistatin is a peptide with the ability to inhibit release of FSH). PCOS is also strongly associated with polymorphisms of the gene for cytochrome P-450, CYP, on chromosome 15q [28], and a susceptibility gene for PCOS located on chromosome 19p13.3, in the insulin receptor gene region, has been demonstrated [29].

SAHA syndrome. The term SAHA syndrome is used by some to describe the constellation of features that arise with cutaneous virilization [30]. The acronym stands for *sebor-rhoea, acne, hirsutism* and *androgenetic alopecia.* The term does not suggest any specific aetiology; all the causes of hirsutism need to be considered and investigated where clinically indicated. As with all women with hirsutism, androgen receptor sensitivity can be implicated where there are no apparent endocrine abnormalities. The four features exist together in only 20% of women embraced by this diagnosis, but the concept is favoured by some as a clinical label encompassing the range of problems associated with the diagnosis of hirsutism.

Ovarian tumours. Hirsutism is an almost universal feature in virilizing ovarian tumours; however, functioning tumours that cause virilization represent approximately 1% of ovarian tumours [31]. Amenorrhoea or oligomenorrhoea develop in all premenopausal patients, and alopecia, clitoromegaly, deepening of the voice and a male habitus develop in approximately half of the patients [32,33]. The majority of patients with virilizing ovarian tumours have raised plasma testosterone levels [31,33]. As a rule, these levels exceed double the upper limit of normal and combine with the more extreme and evolving

clinical picture to distinguish these women from those with PCOS.

Hirsutism in pregnancy. Hirsutism has only rarely been reported to develop during pregnancy; it may be caused by the development of PCOS or a virilizing tumour. PCOS has been reported to present with virilization during the first or third trimester and may regress postpartum [34]. Androgens freely cross the placenta and virilization of a female fetus may occur [35]. The range of tumours occurring during pregnancy has been reviewed by Novak *et al.* [36].

Congenital adrenal hyperplasia. Cholesterol is metabolized in the adrenal cortex, via a complex pathway, into aldosterone, cortisol, androgens and oestrogens. A defect in cortisol synthesis results in redistribution of the precursors to other pathways, which results in overproduction of the other hormones. In approximately 95% of cases, 21-hydroxylation is impaired [37] so that 17-hydroxyprogesterone (17-OHP) is not converted to 11-deoxycortisol. Because of defective cortisol synthesis, ACTH levels increase, resulting in overproduction and accumulation of cortisol precursors, particularly 17-OHP. This causes excessive production of androgens, resulting in virilization.

Congenital adrenal hyperplasia (CAH) is divided into four categories:
1 Salt-losing, which presents in infancy with dehydration
2 Simple virilizing, in which children present with precocious puberty and short stature
3 Non-classic, attenuated or acquired, and it is this variant that is likely to present to the dermatologist with degrees of hirsutism in otherwise well women
4 Cryptic.

The diagnosis of non-classic late-onset CAH (LO-CAH) cannot be made clinically, and dynamic endocrine investigations are required to differentiate between it, PCOS and idiopathic hirsutism. These women may have only mild degrees of hirsutism, normal physique, normal menses and no metabolic sequelae to the changes in cortisol pathways; however, approximately 80% will have polycystic ovaries [38].

21-Hydroxylase deficiency is the most common defect found with (more than 90%) LO-CAH. As many as 3–6% of women presenting with hirsutism may be affected with this form. It is an allelic variant of the classic childhood salt-wasting type. It is associated with a mutation of the gene controlling cytochrome P-450, CYP 21 on chromosome 6 [39]. Among a group of 56 women with LO-CAH, a range of mutations was found. Some put the woman at risk of progeny with classic salt-losing CAH if the father is heterozygous for the same mutation. This raises the significance of detailed analysis of this pathway in such women and the genotypic basis in the woman and male partner [40]. 3β- and 11β-hydroxylase deficiencies are less common forms of CAH and are consequently less frequently found in hirsute women [41]. This is not a diagnosis made in men, although we must presume that they are equally affected and that it is not of any metabolic significance. Where men are heterozygous for mutations relevant to the salt-losing variant, the genotype of the mother will be relevant.

Acquired adrenocortical disease. Adrenal carcinomas usually present with abdominal swelling or pain; however, 10% of both adenomas and carcinomas may present with isolated virilization [42]. The combination of virilization and Cushing's syndrome strongly suggests the presence of a carcinoma. The testosterone level is usually markedly raised in the latter.

Patients with Cushing's syndrome are said to have both hypertrichosis, a generalized diffuse growth of fine hair resulting from hypercortisolaemia, and androgen-induced coarse hair in the usual male pattern [43].

Gonadal dysgenesis. Moltz *et al.* [44] described six patients with 46XY gonadal dysgenesis. All had unambiguously female genitalia but male skeletal characteristics: wide-span broad shoulders and chest; two were hirsute, two had temporal recession and three had deep voices. Rosen *et al.* [45] reported a further 30 patients with gonadal dysgenesis, of whom three (with Y chromosome material) presented with slowly progressive hirsutism and secondary amenorrhoea.

Hyperprolactinaemia. The exact relationship between prolactin and hirsutism is not clear. The incidence of hirsutism in the amenorrhoea–galactorrhoea syndrome has been reported as 22–60% [46]. This may be caused by a direct effect of prolactin on adrenal androgen production or to PCOS, with which it is frequently associated; prolactin has also been reported to attenuate cutaneous 5α-reductase activity both *in vivo* and *in vitro* [47].

Idiopathic hirsutism (Fig. 63.79). Idiopathic hirsutism is the diagnostic label given to those hirsute women in whom no overt underlying endocrine disorder can be detected. There are a number of subtle dynamic alterations in the androgen metabolism of some hirsute women compared with non-hirsute women: daily testosterone production can be increased 3.5–5-fold; the majority of androgen is secreted as testosterone (hirsute 75%, versus normal less than 40%) rather than as androstenedione [48]; increased androgens in hirsute women are associated with lower levels of SHBG, which binds less testosterone and increases its free level [49]. More free testosterone is therefore available for peripheral metabolism and clearance; these two factors disguise the increased rates of testosterone production.

Normal values for total testosterone are found in 25–60% of hirsute women and in 80% of those with regular

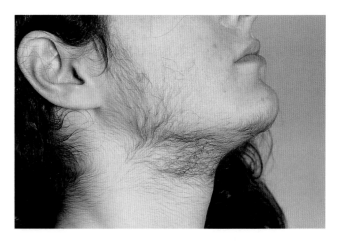

Fig. 63.79 Facial hirsutism: in this case not associated with any systemic disease or detectable biochemical endocrine abnormality.

menstrual cycles [50]. This may be a result of the effect of SHBG or to the wide fluctuations in plasma testosterone seen in hirsute women, or it may reflect the role of androgen receptor sensitivity. The finding of a small elevation of testosterone is not a holy grail, and the tendency to repeat the test many times in the setting of hirsutism is only warranted in progressive or extreme cases where a neoplasm is suspected. Although many women classified as having idiopathic hirsutism may have subtle PCOS, others may be completely normal.

REFERENCES

1 Oake RJ, Davies SJ, McLachlan MSF *et al.* Plasma testosterone in adrenal and ovarian vein blood of hirsute women. *Q J Med* 1974; **43**: 603–14.
2 Simpson NB, Barth JH. Hair patterns: hirsuties and androgenetic alopecia. In: Dawber RPR, ed. *Diseases of the Hair and Scalp*, 3rd edn. Oxford: Blackwell Science, 1997: 140–55.
3 Stahl NL, Teeslink CR, Greenblatt RB. Ovarian, adrenal, and peripheral testosterone levels in the polycystic ovary syndrome. *Am J Obstet Gynecol* 1973; **117**: 194–9.
4 Balen AH, Conway GS, Kaltsas G *et al.* Polycystic ovary syndrome: the spectrum of the disorder in 1741 patients. *Hum Reprod* 1995; **10**: 2107–11.
5 Anonymous. Tackling polycystic ovary syndrome. *Drug Ther Bull* 2001; **39**: 1–5.
6 Stein IF, Leventhal MC. Amenorrhoea associated with bilateral polycystic ovaries. *Am J Obstet Gynecol* 1935; **29**: 181–4.
7 Polson DW, Adams J, Wadsworth J *et al.* Polycystic ovaries: a common finding in normal women. *Lancet* 1988; **i**: 870–2.
8 Carmina E, Lobo RA. Polycystic ovaries in hirsute women with normal menses. *Am J Med* 2001; **111**: 602–6.
9 Balen A. Pathogenesis of polycystic ovary syndrome: the enigma unravels? *Lancet* 1999; **354**: 966–7.
10 Balen AH, Conway GS, Kaltsas G *et al.* Polycystic ovary syndrome: the spectrum of the disorder in 1741 patients. *Hum Reprod* 1995; **10**: 2107–11.
11 Conway GS, Honour JW, Jacobs HS. Heterogeneity of the polycystic ovary syndrome: clinical, endocrine and ultrasound features in 556 patients. *Clin Endocrinol* 1989; **30**: 459–64.
12 Coney P. Polycystic ovarian disease: current concepts of pathophysiology and therapy. *Fertil Steril* 1984; **42**: 667–72.
13 Adams J, Polson DW, Franks S. Prevalence of polycystic ovaries in women with anovulation and idiopathic hirsutism. *BMJ* 1986; **293**: 355–7.
14 McKenna TJ. Current concepts: pathogenesis and treatment of polycystic ovary syndrome. *N Engl J Med* 1988; **318**: 558–69.

15 Polson DW, Reed MJ, Franks S et al. Serum 11β-hydroxyandrostenedione as an indicator of the source of excess androgen production in women with polycystic ovaries. J Clin Endocrinol Metab 1988; **66**: 946–50.

16 Pugeat M, Ducluzeau PH, Mallion-Donadieu M. Association of insulin resistance with hyperandrogenaemia in women. Horm Res 2000; **54**: 322–6.

17 Marsden PJ, Murdoch AP, Taylor R. Tissue insulin sensitivity and body weight in polycystic ovary syndrome. Clin Endocrinol (Oxf) 2001; **55**: 191–9.

18 Conway GS, Jacobs HS. Clinical implications of hyperinsulinaemia in women. Clin Endocrinol 1993; **39**: 623–32.

19 Achard C, Thiers S. Insuffisance glycolytique associée au virilisme pilaire (diabète des femmes à barbe). Bull Acad Nat Méd 1921; **136**: 58–63.

20 Flier JS, Eastman RC, Minaker KL et al. Acanthosis nigricans in obese women with hyperandrogenism: characterization of an insulin-resistant state distinct from the type A and B syndromes. Diabetes 1985; **34**: 101–5.

21 Barth JH, Wojnarowska F, Dawber RPR. Acanthosis nigricans, insulin resistance and cutaneous virilism. Br J Dermatol 1988; **118**: 613–20.

22 Elkind-Hirsch KE, McWilliams RB. Pregnancy after treatment with the insulin-sensitizing agent troglitazone in an obese woman with the hyperandrogenic, insulin-resistant acanthosis nigricans syndrome. Fertil Steril 1999; **71**: 943–7.

23 Pfeifer SL, Wilson RM, Gawkrodger DJ. Clearance of acanthosis nigricans associated with the HAIR-AN syndrome after partial pancreatectomy: an 11-year follow-up. Postgrad Med J 1999; **75**: 421–2.

24 Jacobs HS, Conway GS. Leptin, polycystic ovaries and polycystic ovary syndrome. Hum Reprod Update 1999; **5**: 166–71.

25 Takeuchi T, Tsutsumi O. Basal leptin concentrations in women with normal and dysfunctional ovarian conditions. Int J Gynaecol Obstet 2000; **69**: 127–33.

26 Sir-Petermann T, Piwonka V, Perez F et al. Are circulating leptin and luteinizing hormone synchronized in patients with polycystic ovary syndrome? Hum Reprod 1999; **14**: 1435–9.

27 Oksanen L, Tiitinen A, Kaprio J et al. No evidence for mutations of the leptin or leptin receptor genes in women with polycystic ovary syndrome. Mol Hum Reprod 2000; **6**: 873–6.

28 Gharani N, Waterworth DM, Batty S et al. Association of the steroid synthesis gene CYP 11a with polycystic ovary syndrome and hyperandrogenism. Hum Mol Genet 1997; **6**: 397–402.

29 Tucci S, Futterweit W, Concepcion ES et al. Evidence for association of polycystic ovary syndrome in Caucasian women with a marker at the insulin receptor gene locus. J Clin Endocrinol Metab 2001; **86**: 446–9.

30 Orfanos, CE, Adler YD, Zouboulis CC. The SAHA syndrome. Horm Res 2000; **54**: 251–8.

31 Woodruff JD, Parmley TH. Virilizing ovarian tumors. In: Mahesh VB, Greenblatt RB, eds. Hirsutism and Virilism: Pathogenesis and Management. Boston: John Wright, 1983: 129–45.

32 Sandberg EC, Jackson JR. A clinical analysis of ovarian virilizing tumors. Am J Surg 1963; **105**: 784–95.

33 Moltz L, Pickartz H, Sorensen R et al. Ovarian and adrenal vein steroids in seven patients with androgen-secreting ovarian neoplasm: selective catheterization findings. Fertil Steril 1984; **42**: 585–96.

34 Shortle BE, Warren MP, Tsin D. Recurrent androgenicity in pregnancy: a case report and literature review. Obstet Gynecol 1987; **70**: 462–8.

35 Fayez JA, Bunch TR, Miller GL. Virilization in pregnancy associated with polycystic ovary disease. Obstet Gynecol 1974; **44**: 511–5.

36 Novak DJ, Lauchlan SC, McCawley JC et al. Virilization during pregnancy: case report and review of the literature. Am J Med 1970; **49**: 281–90.

37 Dewailly D, Vantyghem-Haudiquet MC, Saintard C et al. Clinical and biological phenotypes in late-onset 21-hydroxylase deficiency. J Clin Endocrinol Metab 1986; **63**: 418–23.

38 Hague WM, Adams J, Rodda C et al. Prevalence of ultrasonically detected polycystic ovaries in females with congenital adrenal hyperplasia. J Endocrinol 1986; **111** (Suppl.): 46–7.

39 Blanche H, Vexiau P, Clauin S et al. Exhaustive screening of the 21-hydroxylase gene in a population of hyperandrogenic women. Hum Genet 1997; **101**: 56–60.

40 Deneux C, Tardy V, Dib A et al. Phenotype–genotype correlation in 56 women with non-classical congenital adrenal hyperplasia due to 21-hydroxylase deficiency. J Clin Endocrinol Metab 2001; **86**: 207–13.

41 Pang S, Lerner AJ, Stoner E et al. Late-onset adrenal steroid 3β-hydroxysteroid dehydrogenase deficiency. I. A cause of hirsutism in pubertal and postpubertal women. J Clin Endocrinol Metab 1985; **60**: 428–33.

42 King DR, Lack EE. Adrenal cortical carcinoma: a clinical and pathologic study of 49 cases. Cancer 1979; **44**: 239–49.

43 Griffing GT, Melby JC. Cushing's syndrome. In: Mahesh VB, Greenblatt RB, eds. Hirsutism and Virilism. Boston: John Wright 1983: 63–78.

44 Moltz L, Schwartz U, Pickartz H et al. XY gonadal dysgenesis: aberrant testicular differentiation in the presence of H-Y antigen. Obstet Gynecol 1981; **58**: 17–23.

45 Rosen GF, Kaplan B, Lobo RA. Menstrual function and hirsutism in patients with gonadal dysgenesis. Obstet Gynecol 1988; **71**: 677–83.

46 Robyn C, Tukumbane M. Hyperprolactinemia and hirsuties. In: Mahesh VB, Greenblatt RB, eds. Hirsutism and Virilism. Boston: John Wright, 1983: 189–211.

47 Serafini P, Lobo RA. Prolactin modulates peripheral androgen metabolism. Fertil Steril 1986; **45**: 41–50.

48 Kirschner MA, Bardin CW. Androgen production and metabolism in normal and virilized women. Metabolism 1972; **21**: 667–77.

49 Hauner H, Ditschuneit SB, Pal SB et al. Fat distribution, endocrine and metabolic profile of obese women with and without hirsutism. Metabolism 1988; **37**: 281–6.

50 Cummings DC, Wall SR. Non-sex-hormone binding globulin-bound testosterone as a marker for hyperandrogenism. J Clin Endocrinol Metab 1985; **61**: 873–80.

Diagnostic approach to the hirsute woman

Most hirsute women have noted excess hair since puberty; some will give a shorter history but it will be in the order of years. It is important to obtain information from the history regarding patterns of hirsutism, alopecia, other features of cutaneous virilism and evidence for PCOS, in particular irregular menses or infertility. A family history of childhood dehydration or precocious puberty in a brother might be a feature of CAH. A drug history may point to an ingested source of androgens (e.g. glucocorticoid or anabolic steroids) and those used to enhance athletic performance. The progestogenic components of many contraceptive preparations are relatively androgenic and this is often cited as a cause of hirsutism, but it has not been a major factor in our experience.

The cutaneous examination should include the pattern and severity of hair growth and the associated presence of acne, androgenetic alopecia and acanthosis nigricans. Systemic virilization is very rare, and likely to indicate significant pathology such as a testosterone-secreting tumour. Features include a deepening voice, increased muscle bulk and loss of the smooth skin contours, hypertension, striae distensae and clitoromegaly. Clitoromegaly is probably the most important physical sign of systemic virilization. These changes are set apart from cutaneous virilism, and if evolving over a short period (e.g. 12–18 months) they warrant detailed investigation.

The extent to which it is necessary for hirsute women without suspicious signs or history to be investigated is debatable. The main reason cited for investigation of most hirsute women is the inability to differentiate between idiopathic hirsutism, PCOS and LO-CAH on clinical grounds. Not all dermatologists consider it necessary to pursue a diagnosis of PCOS and its ramifications in a woman with normal menses who is not attempting to conceive. Equally, the value of pursuing a diagnosis of LO-CAH is doubtful when there is no clinical metabolic problem, and the therapeutic tools available at present are too clumsy to warrant such diagnostic sensitivity [1,2]. However, it remains an overriding priority to exclude a virilizing tumour if this is suggested by the history and examination.

If it is necessary to undertake investigations, these should be directed by the presenting complaint and diagnostic objectives. In addition to clinical assessment, abnormal menses represent a trigger for investigation. The best screening test for an androgen-secreting tumour is plasma total testosterone. Mild elevations will usually occur in individuals with PCOS, and those in whom the level is more than twice the upper limit of normal require further investigation to exclude a neoplasm. However, if confirmation of a diagnosis of PCOS is required, estimation of plasma LH and FSH and pelvic ultrasound are indicated. In addition, the metabolic aspects of PCOS warrant a fasting glucose and lipid profile. Some authorities would suggest a full glucose tolerance test in those with established PCOS.

Prolactin levels, and assessment of adrenal and thyroid status would normally be undertaken if there were clinical clues suggesting abnormality of these systems. Pursuance of the diagnosis of LO-CAH is controversial. There is no record of women with this disorder being at risk of any significant salt-losing process. However, there may be reduced fertility [3] and if the woman is heterozygous for a mutation that predisposes to the salt-losing variant, her progeny may be at risk if their father is heterozygous for the same mutation [4]. This last point raises the question of whether the diagnosis should be sought more rigorously. Although it may not alter clinical management of the hirsutism, it may be of significance to the reproductive plans of the woman. At present, defining whether the woman is heterozygous for a mutation of the CYP 21 gene that can lead to the salt-losing variant of CAH in offspring is limited to gene analysis. The phenotype and endocrine investigations are not sufficiently sensitive to distinguish between heterozygosity for a range of CAH mutations of differing significance. The standard screening test for such mutations is estimation of the basal plasma 17-hydroxyprogesterone level.

REFERENCES

1 Barth JH. Investigations in the assessment and management of patients with hirsutism. *Curr Opin Obstet Gynecol* 1997; **9**: 187–92.
2 Marshburn PB, Carr BR. Hirsutism and virilization: a systematic approach to benign and potentially serious causes. *Postgrad Med* 1995; **97**: 99–106.
3 Premawardhana LD, Hughes IA, Read GF, Scanlon MF. Longer term outcome in females with congenital adrenal hyperplasia (CAH): the Cardiff experience. *Clin Endocrinol (Oxf)* 1997; **46**: 327–32.
4 Deneux C, Tardy V, Dib A *et al.* Phenotype–genotype correlation in 56 women with non-classical congenital adrenal hyperplasia due to 21-hydroxylase deficiency. *J Clin Endocrinol Metab* 2001; **86**: 207–13.

Treatment [1–4]

For most women, medical consultation concerning excess hair is on two levels. First it is necessary to determine whether the pattern is pathological and related to a definable aetiology. For some, weight loss will contribute to a reduction of insulin resistance, hyperinsulinaemia and hyperandrogenism. Often, medical intervention is not needed. However, the next level concerns whether there is a medical avenue for providing help, even with the acknowledgement that treatment is not for a disease, but in order to achieve a cosmetic norm.

Cosmetic measures

Where a woman has failed to make full use of physical methods of hair removal it is helpful if the dermatologist is familiar with what is available [4] or can direct her to a reliable beautician or other expert in cosmetic care for advice. The easiest measure is to bleach the hair with hydrogen peroxide. This produces a yellow hue because of the native colour of keratin. Hair plucking is widely performed, but the act of plucking not only removes the hair shaft but also stimulates the root into the anagen phase and there is only a brief delay while the shaft grows through the epidermis. Shaving avoids this problem by removing all the hairs but is followed by growth only of the hairs that were previously in anagen.

Depilatory creams contain thioglycolates that dissolve sulphur bonds within keratin molecules, making the hair gelatinous. They are irritant and require care in terms of strength of preparation and duration of exposure. It is often the case that the patient has used a depilatory cream once and given up because she became sore or it did not work. Results can be improved by employing the cream much in the same way that one might use dithranol when treating psoriasis, using small test areas to gain experience.

Waxing is performed by the application of a sheet of soft wax to the skin and, as soon as it has hardened with the hair shafts embedded, it is abruptly peeled off, removing all the shafts. This is a painful method and is often complicated by folliculitis. Certain natural sugars, long used in parts of the Middle East, are becoming popular in place of waxes as they appear to depilate as effectively, but with less trauma. Both methods require the hair to be long enough for the wax, resin or sugar to gain sufficient purchase on the hair shaft.

Electrolysis is a more permanent method of hair removal [4]. A fine electrical wire is introduced down the hair shaft to the papilla, which is destroyed by an electrical current. Laser thermolytic hair removal is now widely used. Although its long-term efficacy is not yet known [5], laser-assisted hair removal has been in use for sufficient time to allow a reasonable estimate of its efficacy and safety. Most practitioners will select patients for dark hair and light skin. This maximizes the absorption of laser energy by the hair and minimizes absorption by the skin. Nevertheless, it is still possible for soreness and crusting to occur following treatment. In darker skin this can be associated with post-inflammatory pigmentary changes. Treatments are usually administered as part of a course of at least three visits separated by several weeks. This reflects the biology of the follicle, which is most responsive to abalation when in anagen. The gap between treatments allows those hairs initially in telogen to move into anagen. Sommer *et al.* [6] compared the hair counts 36 weeks after four treatments to the face with a normal pulse ruby laser with the effects of a single pulse. Hair counts were reduced by 61% and 41%, respectively. As well as laser techniques, there are alternatives to the use of lasers. Broad-band intense pulsed light represents a cheaper technology with less restriction on the licensing of those who use it. There are no good comparative studies of laser and pulsed light, but results from open trials of the latter suggest it is useful [7]. In a study of pulsed light therapy of hirsutism, 76% hair clearance was reported following a mean of 3.7 treatments [8].

Drug therapy [9]

Because hirsutism is a condition mediated by androgens, attempts have been made to reduce the growth of hair with antiandrogens. The complete spectrum of therapeutic agents evaluated in the treatment of hirsutism is described in the following text. However, it is our practice to use cyproterone acetate in combination with ethinylestradiol as first-line therapy for women whose hirsutism is so severe as to warrant systemic therapy. Spironolactone is the next alternative [1]. The oral contraceptive can be useful to avoid conception during therapy with antiandrogens. At the same time, it will increase the amount of SHBG and reduce free androgen. A progestogen in the oral contraceptive, such as norethisterone, is best avoided in favour of one of the synthetic progestogens to avoid any potential intrinsic androgenic effect.

It is important that hirsute women are carefully assessed prior to initiating therapy for the following reasons. First, the effect on hair growth takes several months to become apparent and only partial improvement may be expected. Secondly, antiandrogens feminize a male fetus and it is essential that the women do not become pregnant during therapy. Thirdly, these drugs only have a suppressive, and not curative, effect that wears off a few months after cessation of therapy [10]. Consequently, it may be necessary to take therapy indefinitely if improvement occurs. Finally, the long-term safety of these drugs is unknown and tumours in laboratory animals have been reported with several of the following agents.

Cyproterone acetate [11,12]. Cyproterone acetate (CPA) is a synthetic progestogen that acts as both an antiandrogen and an inhibitor of gonadotrophin secretion. It reduces androgen production, increases the metabolic clearance of testosterone and binds to the androgen receptor; in addition, long-term therapy is associated with a reduction

in the activity of cutaneous 5α-reductase. Although CPA is a potent progestogen it does not reliably inhibit ovulation. It is usually administered with cyclical oestrogens in order to maintain regular menstruation and to prevent conception in view of the risk of feminizing a male fetus.

Several regimens have been advocated. Low-dose therapy (Dianette; Schering AG) is an oral contraceptive containing 35 µg ethinylestradiol and 2 mg CPA, taken daily for 21 in every 28 days. However, many of the dose-ranging and efficacy studies have been performed using the preparation that contained 50 µg ethinylestradiol; this may be relevant, as only the higher dose of oestrogen increases SHBG. Current dosage recommendations for CPA usually advise that 50 mg or 100 mg CPA should be administered for 10 days/cycle (e.g. day 1–10 or 5–15). However, there have now been many dose-ranging studies that suggest that there is no dose effect. Objective studies comparing Dianette with and without extra CPA found no difference in the reduction of overall hirsutism grades, although the rate of onset of benefit was faster with the additional cyproterone [13].

Side effects of CPA include weight gain, fatigue, loss of libido, breast tenderness, nausea, headaches and depression. All these side effects are more frequent with higher dosage. As with all medication for a cosmetic problem, safety can be a concern for those needing long-term treatment. Contraindications to its use are the same as for the contraceptive pill and include cigarette smoking, age, obesity and hypertension. Venous thromboembolism is the adverse effect of greatest medical significance. A case–controlled study indicated that risk of this was four times greater in women taking an oral contraceptive containing CPA as the progestogen in comparison with those containing levonorgestrel [14].

One retrospective study of 188 women taking CPA 50–100 mg/day, described side effects in 23%. Nine per cent of the total group stopped therapy on account of these effects, but it is difficult to discern whether the problems were a result of the CPA or ethinylestradiol that many also took. Most of the problems were related to mood, weight or menstrual disturbance. Within the group, 24 had been treated for 5 years or more, nine for 10 years or more and two for 15 years [15].

Spironolactone [16,17]. Spironolactone is a popular and relatively safe treatment for hirsutism. Formal proof of its efficacy is not to the highest standards, although a Cochrane review concluded that it was of some value [18]. The discovery of its benefit in hirsutism was serendipitous—a 19-year-old hirsute woman with PCOS was treated with spironolactone (200 mg/day) for concurrent hypertension and she noted after 3 months the need to shave less frequently.

Spironolactone has several antiandrogenic pharmacological properties. It reduces the bioavailability of testosterone by interfering with its production and increases its metabolic clearance. It binds to the androgen receptor and, like CPA, long-term therapy is associated with a reduction in cutaneous 5α-reductase activity [19]. Different regimens of spironolactone have been studied, varying between 50 and 200 mg taken either daily or cyclically (daily for 3 weeks in every 4). Within this dosage range, the one chosen will depend on the severity of the hirsutism. A 3 out of 4 week cycle will result in a withdrawal bleed in the fourth week which is similar to that seen with the oral contraceptive. However, spironolactone cannot be relied on as a contraceptive and care must be taken to avoid conception while on the drug.

Spritzer *et al.* [20] compared the relative benefits of a combination of CPA 50 mg/day and ethinylestradiol 35 μg/day with spironolactone 200 mg/day over 12 months. Both groups were stratified for those with PCOS and idiopathic hirsutism. In both groups, those with idiopathic hirsutism did equally well. However, those with PCOS did significantly better with the CPA/ethinylestradiol combination. Where spironolactone is used in combination with ethinylestradiol 35 μg and CPA 2 mg, there may be some modest advantage [21].

When compared with finasteride 5 mg, spironolactone 100 mg produced a significantly greater improvement during a 9-month trial [22]. Spironolactone may feminize a male fetus. Long-term high-dose spironolactone has been shown to produce tumours in rodents. Some clinicians feel that this finding makes long-term use inappropriate in healthy young patients with hirsutism.

5α-Reductase inhibitors. 5α-Reductase inhibitors are a potential systemic therapy for hirsutism. Finasteride inhibits the type 2 isoenzyme of 5α-reductase and has been assessed in small placebo-controlled trials, with some benefit after 6 months' therapy. In open trials, maximal benefit was seen in idiopathic hirsutism after 12 months [23]. Controlled comparative trials suggest that flutamide [24] and spironolactone [22] are more effective. Topical finasteride has been trialled with mixed results [25]. Other similar systemic and topical 5α-reductase inhibitors are likely to be available in the near future. This group of drugs feminizes a male fetus, which is a drawback in the therapy of women of child-bearing potential and has precluded a drug licence for the treatment of hirsutism.

Corticosteroids. Corticosteroids have a logical place in the treatment of LO-CAH. However, any benefits that they may have in this setting need to be balanced against their well-described side effects. Although their use is justified on the basis of physiological replacement, it is likely that pharmacological regimens will far exceed this, with consequent problems. Spritzer *et al.* [26] demonstrated the superiority of ethinylestradiol 35 μg with CPA 2 mg over hydrocortisone in treatment of hirsutism associated with LO-CAH [26].

Metformin. Metformin is a biguanide originally used in the treatment of type 2 diabetes mellitus. It has found a place in the treatment of hirsutism associated with hyperinsulinaemia and insulin resistance. In this setting, it can reduce levels of insulin, increase insulin sensitivity and, particularly when associated with a low-calorie diet, result in weight loss [27]. In many, this constellation of problems will be part of PCOS, and metformin has also been shown to assist in normalization of menstruation and improvement in lipid profiles [28]. These broader metabolic effects can make it a useful therapy where hirsutism is not the only problem, although its use in PCOS requires further assessment [29,30].

Eflornithine. Eflornithine was originally used orally in the treatment of hyperactivity in childhood. It is an inhibitor of ornithine decarboxylase and is able to delay the initiation of anagen [31]. Consequently, it can help to keep hair in telogen. Limited studies show some reduction in hirsutism when used as a cream on women's faces [32].

Medroxyprogesterone acetate. Medroxyprogesterone acetate (MPA) is a synthetic progestogen that was introduced as an anovulatory agent because of its ability to block gonadotrophin secretion. It lowers androgen levels by reducing the production of testosterone and increasing its metabolic clearance.

A comparison of topical (0.2% ointment) with systemic therapy, either by intramuscular injection of MPA (150 mg every 6 weeks) or subcutaneous injection (100 mg every 6 weeks), was said to give a beneficial response in most patients [33]. MPA given alone may result in menorrhagia.

Desogestrel. This is the progestogen used in the Marvelon® contraceptive pill (Organon Ltd), which contains 30 μg ethinylestradiol and 150 mg desogestrel. All the studies undertaken have reported subjective and/or objective reductions in hair growth of 20–25% after 6–9 months' therapy, with a high degree of patient satisfaction [34].

Ketoconazole. This is a potent inhibitor of adrenal and ovarian steroid synthesis. There have been only isolated reports of its use in hirsutism but these have demonstrated a marked reduction in hair growth after 6 months [35]. However, this treatment cannot be recommended in view of the risks of hepatic toxicity during long-term therapy.

Flutamide [36]. This acts as a pure antiandrogen and works by binding to androgen receptors. However, it has no antigonadotrophic effect, and the result of binding to central androgen receptors is that it prevents the negative feedback effect of testosterone, and consequently androgen levels rise. There has been a single study in hirsutism in which flutamide (250 mg twice daily) was administered with an oral contraceptive for 7 months; 12 out of 13 patients demonstrated a subjective reduction in hair growth and improvement in acne [37]. Flutamide is potentially hepatotoxic and requires close monitoring to avoid liver complications. This has limited its use.

Gonadotrophin-releasing hormone agonists. Gonadotrophin-releasing hormone (GnRH) agonists inhibit LH production and this results in profound suppression of ovarian androgen production. These agents are presently under investigation, but preliminary studies suggest that they effectively reduce hair growth and acne in women with PCOS [38] and may be superior to finasteride [39]. Drawbacks are cost and the need for monthly injections.

Cimetidine. Cimetidine is an H_2 receptor blocker, and weak antiandrogen as indicated by androgen receptor-binding studies. A study of patients with idiopathic hirsutism demonstrated a marked reduction in hair growth using hair weight, whereas no such effect was seen in controls given only a placebo [40].

Bromocriptine. This is a dopamine agonist, and long-term therapy with bromocriptine regulates menstrual cycle length, but 12 months' therapy produced no measurable effect on linear hair growth in women with polycystic ovaries [41].

REFERENCES

1 Young R, Sinclair R. Hirsutes. II. Treatment. *Australas J Dermatol* 1998; **39**: 151–7.
2 Bergfeld WF. Hirsutism in women: effective therapy that is safe for long-term use. *Postgrad Med* 2000; **107**: 93–104.
3 Lanigan SW. Management of unwanted hair in females. *Clin Exp Dermatol* 2001; **26**: 644–7.
4 Olsen EA. Methods of hair removal. *J Am Acad Dermatol* 1999; **40**: 154–5.
5 Grossman MC, Dierickx C, Farinelli W et al. Damage to hair follicles by normal mode ruby laser pulses. *J Am Acad Dermatol* 1996; **35**: 889–94.
6 Sommer S, Render C, Sheehan-Dare R. Facial hirsutism treated with the normal-mode ruby laser: results of a 12-month follow-up study. *J Am Acad Dermatol* 1999; **41**: 974–9.
7 Lask G, Eckhouse S, Slatkine M et al. The role of laser and intense light sources in photo-epilation: a comparative evaluation. *J Cutan Laser Ther* 1999; **1**: 3–13.
8 Sadick NS, Weiss RA, Shea CR et al. Long-term photoepilation using a broad-spectrum intense pulsed light source. *Arch Dermatol* 2000; **136**: 1336–40.
9 Rittmaster RS. Antiandrogen treatment of polycystic ovary syndrome. *Endocrinol Metab Clin North Am* 1999; **28**: 409–21.
10 Yücelten D, Erenus M, Gürbüz O, Durmusoglu F. Recurrence rate of hirsutism after three different antiandrogen therapies. *J Am Acad Dermatol* 1999; **41**: 64–8.
11 Jones DB, Ibraham I, Edwards CRW. Hair growth and androgen responses in hirsute women treated with continuous cyproterone acetate and cyclical ethinyl oestradiol. *Acta Endocrinol* 1987; **116**: 497–503.
12 Jones KR, Katz M, Keyzer C et al. Effect of cyproterone acetate on rate of hair growth in hirsute females. *Br J Dermatol* 1981; **105**: 685–91.
13 Barth JH, Cherry CA, Wojnarowska F et al. Cyproterone acetate for severe hirsutism: results of a double-blind dose-ranging study. *J Clin Endocrinol Metab* 1991; **35**: 5–10.
14 Vasilakis-Scaramozza C, Jick H. Risk of venous thromboembolism with cyproterone or levonorgestrel contraceptives. *Lancet* 2001; **358**: 1427–9.
15 Van Wayjen RG, van den Ende A. Experience in the long-term treatment of patients with hirsutism and/or acne with cyproterone acetate-containing preparations: efficacy, metabolic and endocrine effects. *Exp Clin Endocrinol* 1995; **103**: 241–51.
16 Barth JH, Cherry CA, Wojnarowska F et al. Spironolactone is an effective and well-tolerated systemic antiandrogen therapy for hirsute women. *J Clin Endocrinol Metab* 1989; **68**: 96–102.
17 Ober KP, Hennessy JF. Spironolactone therapy for hirsutism in a hyperandrogenic woman. *Ann Intern Med* 1987; **98**: 643–51.
18 Farquhar C, Lee O, Toomath R, Jepson R. *Cochrane Database Syst Rev* 2001; **4**: CD000194.
19 Serafini P, Catalino J, Lobo RA. The effect of spironolactone on genital skin 5α-reductase. *J Steroid Biochem* 1985; **23**: 191.
20 Spritzer PM, Lisboa KO, Mattiello S, Lhullier F. Spironolactone as a single agent for long-term therapy of hirsute patients. *Clin Endocrinol (Oxf)* 2000; **52**: 587–94.
21 Kelestimur F, Sahin Y. Comparison of Diane 35 and Diane 35 plus spironolactone in the treatment of hirsutism. *Fertil Steril* 1998; **69**: 66–9.
22 Erenus M, Yucelten D, Durmusoglu F, Gurbuz O. Comparison of finasteride versus spironolactone in the treatment of idiopathic hirsutism. *Fertil Steril* 1997; **68**: 1000–3.
23 Petrone A, Civitillo RM, Galante L et al. Usefulness of a 12-month treatment with finasteride in idiophathic and polycystic ovary syndrome-associated hirsutism. *Clin Exp Obstet Gynecol* 1999; **26**: 213–6.
24 Falsetti L, Gambera A, Legrenzi L, Iacobello C, Bugari G. Comparison of finasteride versus flutamide in the treatment of hirsutism. *Eur J Endocrinol* 1999; **141**: 361–7.
25 Lucas KJ. Finasteride cream in hirsutism. *Endocr Pract* 2001; **7**: 5–10.
26 Spritzer P, Billaud L, Thalabard JC et al. Cyproterone acetate versus hydrocortisone treatment in late-onset adrenal hyperplasia. *J Clin Endocrinol Metab* 1990; **70**: 642–6.
27 Pasquali R, Gambineri A, Biscotti D et al. Effect of long-term treatment with metformin added to hypocaloric diet on body composition, fat distribution, and androgen and insulin levels in abdominally obese women with and without the polycystic ovary syndrome. *J Clin Endocrinol Metab* 2000; **85**: 2767–74.
28 Ibanez L, Valls C, Potau N, Marcos MV, de Zegher F. Sensitization to insulin in adolescent girls to normalize hirsutism, hyperandrogenism, oligomenorrhea, dyslipidemia, and hyperinsulinism after precocious pubarche. *J Clin Endocrinol Metab* 2000; **85**: 3526–30.
29 Harborne L, Fleming R, Lyall H, Norman J, Sattar N. Descriptive review of the evidence for the use of metformin in polycystic ovary syndrome. *Lancet* 2003; **361**: 1894–901.
30 Lord JM, Flight IHK, Normal RJ. Metformin in polycystic ovary syndrome: systematic review and meta-analysis. *BMJ* 2003; **327**: 951–5.
31 Coyne PE Jr. The eflornithine story. *J Am Acad Dermatol* 2001; **45**: 784–6.
32 Balfour JA, McClellan K. Topical eflornithine. *Am J Clin Dermatol* 2001; **2**: 197–201.
33 Schmidt JB, Huber J, Spona J. Medroxyprogesterone acetate therapy in hirsutism. *Br J Dermatol* 1985; **113**: 161–6.
34 Ruutianen K. The effect of an oral contraceptive containing ethinylestradiol and desogestrel on hair growth and hormonal parameters of hirsute women. *Int J Gynaecol Obstet* 1986; **24**: 361–70.
35 Martikainen H, Heikkinen J, Ruokonen A et al. Hormonal and clinical effects of ketoconazole in hirsute women. *J Clin Endocrinol Metab* 1988; **66**: 987–94.
36 Erenus M, Gurbuz O, Durmusoglu E. Comparison of the efficacy of spironolactone versus flutamide in the treatment of hirsutism. *Fertil Steril* 1994; **61**: 613–6.
37 Cusan L, Dupont A, Tremblay R et al. Treatment of hirsutism with the pure antiandrogen flutamide. *Proc Int Soc Gynaecol Endocrinol* 1988: 74–95.
38 Rittmaster RS. Differential suppression of testosterone and estradiol in hirsute women with the superactive gonadotrophin-releasing hormone agonist leuprolide. *J Clin Endocrinol Metab* 1988; **67**: 651–6.
39 Bayhan G, Bahceci M, Demirkol T et al. A comparative study of a gonadotropin-releasing hormone agonist and finasteride on idiopathic hirsutism. *Clin Exp Obstet Gynecol* 2000; **27**: 203–6.
40 Grandesso R, Spandri P, Gangemi M et al. Hormonal changes and hair growth during treatment of hirsutism with cimetidine. *Clin Exp Obstet Gynaecol* 1984; **11**: 105–10.
41 Murdoch AP, McClean KG, Watson MJ et al. Treatment of hirsutism in polycystic ovary syndrome with bromocriptine. *Br J Obstet Gynaecol* 1987; **94**: 358–67.

Hair pigmentation [1–3]

In humans, hair pigmentation depends entirely on the presence of melanin from melanocytes. The perceived colour will depend also on physical phenomena. The range of colours produced by melanins is limited to shades of grey, yellow, brown, red and black, depending on the amount and ratio of eumelanin (black) and phaeomelanin (red).

It is important to remember that much of the research on melanogenesis and its cellular control is in relation to epidermis outside the follicle. Many aspects of hair bulb melanogenesis are likely to be the same. Hair melanin is formed by melanocytes situated in the hair bulb epithelium around the upper half of the dermal papilla amongst cells destined to form the hair cortex. Ultrastructurally, hair bulb melanocytes appear more melanogenic than epidermal melanocytes and their population density is much greater than in the epidermis (approximately one melanocyte to four basal keratinocytes in the upper hair bulb compared with a ratio of 1 : 25 in the basal layer of the epidermis [4]). Melanocytes are also present in the basal layer of the infundibulum and, in small numbers, in the outer root sheath of the lower part of the follicle. These latter cells are DOPA-negative and non-melanized and are thought to form a melanocyte reservoir in the skin. Under certain circumstances (e.g. during repigmentation of vitiligo), outer root sheath melanocytes proliferate and migrate to the epidermis [5]. In humans, hair bulb melanocytes donate pigment almost exclusively to cells undergoing early differentiation to form the hair cortex (Fig. 63.80). Therefore there is a close spatial and functional relationship between hair bulb melanocytes and the cells that act as pigment receptors (cortical keratinocytes).

Melanogenic activity in the hair follicle is closely linked to the hair cycle. In the telogen follicle, non-melanogenic melanocytes are found in the basal layer of the outer root sheath and in the secondary germ region [6]. These cells are assumed to be the precursors of active melanocytes during the next anagen phase and either migrate or are carried into the hair bulb in early anagen development. They congregate in the upper part of the anagen hair bulb amongst cells destined to form the hair cortex. Melanogenesis begins well after epithelial proliferation has started and coincides with the onset of morphological evidence of cortical differentiation. Tyrosinase activity becomes apparent in Anagen 3 and pigment transfer to cortical epithelium begins in the Anagen 4 stage of development [7–9]. In pigmented hair follicles, intense melanogenesis continues throughout the remainder of anagen (Anagen 5 and 6) and then ceases with the onset of catagen. The close anatomical and functional association of hair bulb melanocytes with cells to which pigment is donated, cells destined to form the hair cortex, suggests that interaction between these two cell types has a key role in regulating

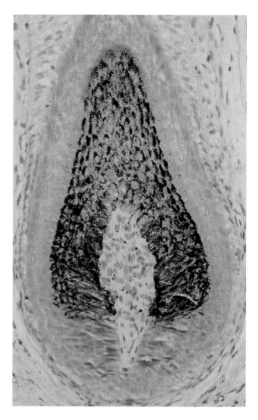

Fig. 63.80 Human anagen follicle showing pigment donation to the hair cortex. There is pigment incontinence in the dermal papilla (Masson–Fontana stain).

pigmentary activity. The fate of hair bulb melanocytes during catagen is uncertain. Non-melanizing melanocytes have been observed in the regressing epithelial column in human catagen follicles [10] but apoptotic deletion of follicular melanocytes has also been described during this stage of the hair cycle [11].

REFERENCES

1 Messenger AG. Control of hair growth and pigmentation. In: Olsen E, ed. *Disorders of Hair Growth*. New York: McGraw-Hill, 1994: 39–58.
2 Bolognia JL, Pawelek JM. Biology of hypopigmentation. *J Am Acad Dermatol* 1988; **19**: 217–25.
3 Castanet J, Ortonne J-P. Hair melanin and hair colour. In: Jollès P, Zahn H, eds. *Formation and Structure of Human Hair*. Basel: Birkhäuser Verlag, 1997: 209–25.
4 Cesarini JP. Hair melanin and hair color. In: Orfanos CE, Happle R, eds. *Hair and Hair Diseases*. Berlin: Springer-Verlag, 1990: 165–97.
5 Cui J, Shen LY, Wang GC. Role of hair follicles in the repigmentation of vitiligo. *J Invest Dermatol* 1991; **97**: 410–6.
6 Silver AF, Chase HB, Potten CS. Melanocyte precursor cells in the hair follicle germ during the dormant stage (telogen). *Experientia* 1969; **25**: 299–301.
7 Kukita A. Changes in tyrosinase activity during melanocyte proliferation in the hair growth cycle. *J Invest Dermatol* 1957; **28**: 273–4.
8 Fitzpatrick TB, Brunet P, Kukita A. The nature of hair pigment. In: Montagna W, Ellis RA, eds. *The Biology of Hair Growth*. New York: Academic Press, 1958: 255–303.
9 Slominski A, Paus R. Melanogenesis is coupled to murine anagen: toward new concepts for the role of melanocytes and the regulation of melanogenesis in hair growth. *J Invest Dermatol* 1993; **101**: 90S–7S.
10 Commo S, Bernard BA. Melanocyte subpopulation turnover during the

human hair cycle: an immunohistochemical study. *Pigment Cell Res* 2000; **13**: 253–9.

11 Tobin DJ, Hagen E, Botchkarev VA *et al.* Do hair bulb melanocytes undergo apoptosis during hair follicle regression (catagen)? *J Invest Dermatol* 1998; **111**: 941–7.

Melanogenesis [1–3]

Functional melanocytes respond to the peptide hormones α-melanocyte stimulating hormone (α-MSH) or ACTH through the MC1R receptor to stimulate melanin production. This receptor is a transmembrane G-protein. When bound to melanocortin peptides, intracellular cyclic adenosine monophosphate (AMP) rises, resulting in tyrosinase gene expression, melanocyte proliferation and increased dendricity. There may also be switching of melanin type. Loss of function mutations in the *MC1R* gene are associated with a switch from eumelanin (dark) to phaeomelanin (red) production [4,5]. The phaeomelanosome, containing the key enzyme of the tyrosinase pathway, produces light red-yellowish melanin, whereas the eumelanosome produces darker melanins via induction of additional TYRP1, TYRP2, SILV enzymes, and the P-protein. Intramelanosomal pH, governed by the P-protein, may act as a critical determinant of tyrosinase enzyme activity. There is significant genetic variation in the genes from which these proteins arise. Over 30 variant alleles have been identified in the *MC1R* gene alone. Functional correlation of *MC1R* alleles with skin and hair colour provides evidence that this receptor molecule is a principal component underlying normal human pigment variation.

In black hair follicles, deposition of melanin within melanosomes continues until the whole unit is uniformly dense. Lighter coloured hair shows less melanin deposition, and blonde hair follicles show melanosomes with a moth-eaten appearance. Red and blonde hair follicles have spherical melanosomes; those in brown and black hair are ellipsoidal.

Pigment is incorporated into hair cortex. No pigment is donated to presumptive cuticular and internal root sheath cells, although pigment granules have been detected in the cuticle of human nostril hair and in the coats of many animals [6]. Melanocytes are functional only during the anagen phase of the hair cycle. They were formerly thought to disappear during telogen but it is now known that they remain at the surface of the papilla in a shrunken adendritic form. Jimbow *et al.* [7] found melanocytes with mature melanosomes in resting (telogen) feather follicles. It is possible that the full complement of melanocytes present during successive anagen phases is the result not only of reactivation of 'dormant' cells, but also of new cells resulting from melanocyte replication [8].

Hair colour resulting from physical phenomena

The whiteness of hair seen when melanin is absent is an optical effect resulting from reflection and refraction of incident light from various interfaces at which zones of different refractive index meet. Thus, in general, non-pigmented hair with a broad medulla appears paler than non-medullated hair. Normal 'weathering' of hair along its length may lead to the terminal part appearing lighter than the rest as a result of a similar mechanism—the cortex and cuticle become disrupted and form numerous interfaces from internal reflection and refraction of light. This also applies in trichorrhexis nodosa (excessive 'weathering'), in which patients often note a lightening in colour of the brittle hair, and in the white bands of pili annulati. Because these optical lightening effects are caused by reflection and refraction of incident light, when such hairs are viewed by transmitted light microscopy they appear dark. Newly formed unpigmented hair with no medulla appears yellowish rather than white. This is probably the intrinsic colour of dense keratin as orientated in hair fibres. Findlay [9] showed that the perceived colour is affected by the physical characteristics of the hair shaft and may bear little relationship to the true chromaticity of the shaft.

Hair fibre tryptophan content increases with age and within age groups, and is higher in dark hair than fair hair. The exception is with white hair and the significance of these findings is uncertain [10].

Lanugo hair present *in utero* is unpigmented. Vellus hair is also typically unpigmented but, in men in particular, some vellus fibres may pigment slightly after puberty. Hair colour varies according to body site in most people. Eyelashes are usually the darkest. Scalp hair is generally lighter than genital hair, which often has a reddish tint even in subjects having essentially brown hair. Grobbelaar [11] showed that hair on the lower and lateral scrotal surfaces is lighter than on the pubes. Apart from individuals with red scalp hair, a red tint to axillary hair is most common in brown-haired individuals.

Hairs on exposed parts may be bleached by sunlight. Very dark hair first lightens to a brownish red colour but rarely becomes blonde even after strong sunlight exposure; brown hair, however, may be bleached white.

REFERENCES

1 Montagna W, Parakkal PK. *The Structure and Function of Skin*. New York: Academic Press, 1974: 232–9.

2 Orfanos C, Ruska H. Die Feinstruktur des menschlichen Haares. III. Das Haarpigment. *Arch Klin Exp Dermatol* 1968; **231**: 279–80.

3 Rees JL. The melanocortin 1 receptor (MC1R): more than just red hair. *Pigment Cell Res* 2000; **13**: 135–40.

4 Schaffer JV, Bolognia JL. The melanocortin-1 receptor: red hair and beyond. *Arch Dermatol* 2001; **137**: 1477–85.

5 Sturm RA, Teasdale RD, Box NF. Human pigmentation genes: identification, structure and consequences of polymorphic variation. *Gene* 2001; **277**: 49–62.

6 Swift JA. The histology of keratin fibres. In: Asquith RS, ed. *The Chemistry of Natural Protein Fibres*. London: Wiley, 1977.

7 Jimbow K, Roth S, Fitzpatrick TB. Ultrastructural investigation of autophagocytosis of melanosomes and programmed death of melanocytes in white Leghorn feathers. *Dev Biol* 1974; **36**: 8–14.

8 Jimbow K, Roth S, Fitzpatrick TB *et al.* Mitotic activity in non-neoplastic melanocytes *in vivo* as determined by histochemical, autoradiographic and electron microscopic studies. *J Cell Biol* 1975; **66**: 663–77.

9 Findlay G. An optical study of human hair colour in normal and abnormal conditions. *Br J Dermatol* 1982; **107**: 517–23.

10 Biasiolo M, Bertazzo A, Costa CV, Allegri G. Correlation between tryptophan and hair pigmentation in human hair. *Adv Exp Med Biol* 1999; **467**: 653–7.

11 Grobbelaar CS. The distribution of, and correlation between eye, hair and skin colour in male students at the University of Stellenbosch. *Ann Univ Stellenbosch* 1952; **28**: Sect a/1, 12.

Variation in hair colour

Genetic and racial aspects [1–3]

Ethnic differences in hair colour are very conspicuous, as are the differences in hair morphology, although colour and hair form are inherited separately [4]. Dark hair predominates in the world. Among white people there is wide variation in colour within geographical regions. Blonde hair is most frequent in northern Europe and black hair in southern and eastern Europe; foci of blondeness are to be found even in North Africa, the Middle East and in some Australoids. Congoid, Capoid, Mongoloid and Australoid hair is mainly black.

Red hair (rutilism)

This has attracted more attention than other colours because it is less common and because it is so distinctive. The pigment is phaeomelanin, not eumelanin. In Italy, and in the UK excluding East Anglia, the distribution of red hair is similar to that of blood group O [5]. The incidence of red hair varies from 0.3% in northern Germany to as high as 11% in parts of Scotland. Like hair of many other colours, red hair often darkens with age from red through brown to sandy or auburn in the adult. The skin of redheads is generally pale, burns easily in sunlight and pigments very little even after prolonged and frequent sun exposure. The loss of eumelanin production is caused by a range of mutations in the *MCR1* gene that alter the function of the receptor and consequently melanin synthesis.

Heterochromia

This implies the growth of hair of two distinct colours in the same individual. A colour difference between scalp and moustache is not uncommon. In fair-haired individuals, pubic and axillary hair, eyebrows and eyelashes are much darker than scalp hair. In humans, eyelashes are generally the most darkly pigmented hairs.

In general, scalp hair darkens with age. Rarely, a circumscribed patch of hair occurs of different colour. This generally has a genetic basis, although the type of inheritance is not known in humans. Patchy differences of hair colour are of six types.

1 Tufts of very dark hair growing from a melanocytic naevus

2 Hereditary, usually autosomal dominant heterochromia (e.g. tufts of red hair at the temples in a black-haired subject or a single black patch in a blonde)

3 Perhaps as a result of somatic mosaicism; partial asymmetry of hair and eye colour may occur sporadically

4 The white forelock of piebaldism

5 The 'flag' sign in kwashiorkor

6 Fair fine woolly hair growing from a scalp woolly hair naevus.

Greying of hair (canities)

Greying of hair is usually a manifestation of the ageing process and results from a progressive reduction in melanocyte function [6]. The larger medullary spaces of older people may contribute to the process.

There is a gradual dilution of pigment in greying hairs: the full range of colour from normal to white can be seen both along individual hairs and from hair to hair. Loss of hair-shaft colour is associated with decrease and eventual cessation of tyrosinase activity in the lower bulb [7]. In white hairs, melanocytes are infrequent or absent [8] or possibly dormant. It has been suggested that autoimmunity plays a part in the pathogenesis of greying; grey hair certainly has an association with the autoimmune disease pernicious anaemia (see below) [9,10].

The age of onset of canities is primarily dependent on the genotype of the individual although acquired factors may play a part. The visual impression of greyness is more obvious (seen earlier) in the fair-haired. In white races, white hair first appears at the age of 34.2 ± 9.6 years, and by the age of 50 years 50% of the population have at least 50% grey hairs [14]. The onset in black people is 43.9 ± 10.3 years, and in Japanese between 30 and 34 years in men and between 35 and 39 years in women. The beard and moustache areas commonly become grey before scalp or body hair. On the scalp, the temples usually show greying first, followed by a wave of greyness spreading to the crown and later to the occipital area.

Rapid onset, allegedly 'overnight', greying of the hair has excited the literary, medical and anthropological worlds for centuries [11,12]. Many reports have been over-dramatized but it certainly occurs. Historical examples often quoted include Sir Thomas More and Marie Antoinette whose hair became grey over the night preceding their executions. The probable mechanism for rapid greying is the selective shedding of pigmented hairs in diffuse alopecia areata, the non-pigmented hairs being retained (Figs 63.81 & 63.82).

Despite occasional reports to the contrary, in general, greying of hair is progressive and permanent, although melanogenesis during anagen may be intermittent for a time before finally stopping. Most of the reports of the

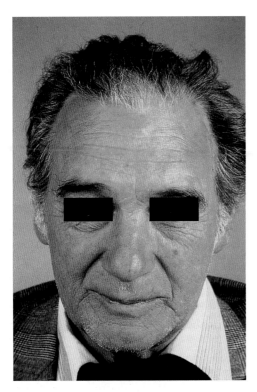

Fig. 63.81 Slight greying of hair. (Courtesy of Dr D. Fenton, St Thomas' Hospital, London, UK.)

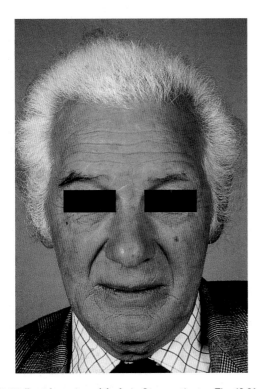

Fig. 63.82 Rapid greying of the hair. Same patient as Fig. 63.81 taken 1 week later. Caused by alopecia areata. (Courtesy of Dr D. Fenton, St Thomas' Hospital, London, UK.)

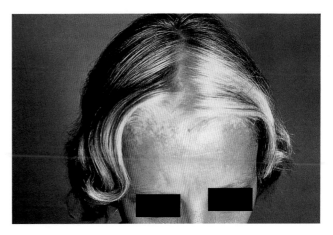

Fig. 63.83 Premature greying of hair, which commenced at 19 years of age in this individual.

return of normal hair colour from grey are examples of a pigmented regrowth following alopecia areata, which eventually repigments in many cases. The reported repigmentation of grey hair in association with Addisonian hypoadrenalism may result from a mechanism similar to that in alopecia areata or vitiligo, in view of the known association between these diseases [13–16]. Darkening of grey hair may occur following large doses of p-aminobenzoic acid [17].

Premature greying (Fig. 63.83)

Premature greying of hair has been defined as onset of greying before 20 years of age in white people and 30 years of age in black people. It probably has a genetic basis and occasionally occurs as an isolated autosomal dominant condition. The association between premature greying and certain organ-specific autoimmune diseases is well documented. The relationship is probably not one of common pathogenesis but on the basis of genetic linkage. It is often stated that premature greying may be an early sign of pernicious anaemia, hyperthyroidism and, less commonly, hypothyroidism, and all autoimmune diseases that have a genetic predisposition. In a controlled study of the integumentary associations of pernicious anaemia, 11% had premature greying [9]. In Book's syndrome, an autosomal dominant trait, premature greying is associated with premolar hypodontia and palmoplantar hyperhidrosis [18]. In the early stages, it may be partially reversible [19].

The premature ageing syndromes, progeria and Werner's syndrome (pangeria), may have very early greying as a prominent feature. It does not occur in metageria or total lipodystrophy [17]. In progeria it is associated with marked loss of scalp hair as early as 2 years of age.

In dystrophia myotonica the onset of grey hair may precede the myotonia and muscle wasting.

Premature canities is an inconstant feature of the Rothmund–Thomson syndrome; when present, it typically commences in adolescence.

One-third of patients with chromosome 5p syndrome (cri du chat syndrome) have prematurely grey hair [20].

Poliosis

Poliosis is defined as the presence of a localized patch of white hair resulting from the absence or deficiency of melanin in a group of neighbouring follicles. Essentially, the changes in melanogenesis are the same in the hair follicle as in the affected epidermis. Pigment absence can be congenital or acquired. In many cases of the former it is brought about by physically or functionally abnormal melanocytes from birth, or abnormal migration during embryogenesis. Such migratory defects may be restricted to the skin, but there can be associated abnormalities in other organs such as the ear or eye, where melanocytes or related neural crest cells have an important role.

Acquired forms of poliosis have more varied causes, although some of the most significant relate to autoimmunity where the melanocyte has attracted autoimmune attack.

Hereditary defects [21]

Piebaldism (white spotting or partial albinism) is an autosomal dominant abnormality with patches of skin totally devoid of pigment, which remain unchanged throughout life. The borders of unpigmented areas are hyperpigmented. Heterochromia iridis occurs in some. Most commonly, a frontal white patch occurs—the white forelock—which may be the only sign. Melanocytes are decreased in number, but are morphologically abnormal and contain normal non-melanized premelanosomes, and also premelanosomes and melanosomes of abnormal appearance [22]. Piebaldism can be caused by mutation in the *KIT* proto-oncogene [23] mapping to chromosome 4q12. In one kindred with a severe and progressive phenotype, the *KIT* mutation affected function of tyrosine kinase [24].

Similar pathological changes are seen in Tietz's syndrome of generalized 'white spot' loss of skin and hair pigment, complete deaf mutism and eyebrow hypoplasia [25]. This disease can be caused by a mutation in the microphthalmia-associated transcription factor gene, and mutations in other regions of this gene have been found to produce Waardenburg's syndrome (WS) type 2 [26].

WS [27] is a heterogeneous condition, usually divided into four types, with absence of melanocytes from cochlear, skin, eye, hair and other structures. Features are present at birth. Type 1 WS is characterized by dystopia canthorum with lateral displacement of the medial canthi, hypertrophy of the nasal root and hyperplasia of the inner third of the eyebrows with confluent brows [28,29]. Total

or partial iridial heterochromia may occur, as may perceptive deafness. The white forelock is present in 20% of cases. Premature greying may develop with or without the white forelock [30]; a minority have piebaldism and congenital nerve deafness but no other overt signs of WS, suggesting that this association may be genetically distinct. Type 1 WS is caused by loss of function mutations in the *PAX3* gene which plays a part in control of neural crest cells during embryogenesis. Type 3 WS (Klein–Waardenburg syndrome, with abnormalities of the arms) is an extreme presentation of type 1, and affected individuals are usually homozygotes. Type 4 WS (Shah–Waardenburg syndrome with Hirschsprung's disease) can be caused by mutations in the genes for endothelin-3 or one of its receptors, EDNRB. Type 2 WS is a heterogeneous group, approximately 15% of whom are heterozygous for mutations in the *MITF* (microphthalmia-associated transcription factor) gene. All these forms show marked variability even within families, and at present it is not possible to predict the severity, even when a mutation is detected.

In vitiligo, the white patches of skin frequently have white hairs within them. The histological changes are consistent with an 'autoimmune injury' to the melanocytes.

Alezzandrini's syndrome combines unilateral facial vitiligo, retinitis and poliosis of eyebrows and eyelashes [31]; perceptive deafness is rarely associated.

In alopecia areata, regrowing hair is frequently white. It may remain so, particularly in cases of late onset. Although absent hair pigment is only evident at the stage of resolution, melanocytes are lost from the hair bulb quite early and migrate to the dermal papilla.

Poliosis occurs in 60% of people with tuberous sclerosis. Depigmented hair may be the earliest sign of the disease [32].

The pathognomonic signs of Von Recklinghausen's neurofibromatosis relate to hyperpigmented areas—café-au-lait macules and axillary and perineal freckling. Scalp hypopigmented patches must not be mistaken for vitiliginous changes.

Acquired defects [33]

Permanent pigmentary loss may be induced by inflammatory processes that damage melanocytes (e.g. herpes zoster). X-irradiation often causes permanent hair loss but less intense treatment leads to hypopigmented and, rarely, hyperpigmented hair. Patchy white hair may develop on the beard area after dental treatment.

The Vogt–Koyanagi–Harada syndrome [34,35] consists of a post-febrile condition comprising bilateral uveitis, labrynthine deafness, tinnitus and vitiligo, poliosis and alopecia areata. It is likely to be an autoimmune disease, with the melanocyte, tyrosinase or tyrosinase-related protein as targets.

Albinism [36]

In autosomal recessive oculocutaneous albinism (complete, perfect or generalized albinism) changes in the hair bulb melanocytes are similar to those in the epidermis [25]. This applies to tyrosine-positive and -negative types. Melanocytes are structurally normal and active in producing melanosomes of grades I and II. However, they are enzymically inactive. The melanocyte system is never completely devoid of melanin. In white people, the hair is typically yellowish white, although it might be cream, yellow, yellowish red or vibrant red. This range of colour parallels that seen in normal blonde white people. In Negroid albinos, the hair colour is white or yellowish brown.

Chediak–Higashi syndrome

This syndrome is basically an autosomal recessive defect of the membrane-bound organelles of several cell types [37]. It combines oculocutaneous hypopigmentation with a defect of leukocytes, which is lethal in some forms, but other affected individuals live to adulthood. The defect lies in the lysosome trafficking regulator gene found on 1q [36]. The hair is silvery grey or light blonde and may be sparse.

Colour changes induced by drugs and other chemicals

Some topical agents temporarily change hair colour. Dithranol and chrysarobin stain light-coloured or grey hair mahogany brown. Resorcin, formerly used a great deal in a variety of skin diseases, colours black or white hair yellow or yellowish brown.

Some systemic drugs alter hair colour by interfering with the eumelanin or phaeomelanin pathway; in others, the mechanism is not known. Chloroquine interferes with phaeomelanin synthesis [38] and affects only blonde and red-haired individuals; the changes are completely reversible. Mephenesin, a glycerol ether used for diseases with muscle spasms, causes pigmentary loss in dark-haired people [39]. Triparanol, an anticholesterolaemic drug, and fluorobutyrophenone, an antipsychotic drug, both interfere with keratinization and cause hypopigmentation and sparse hair. Minoxidil and diazoxide [40,27], two potent antihypertensive agents, both cause hypertrichosis and darkening of hair. The colour produced by diazoxide is reddish, whereas minoxidil darkens hair mainly by converting vellus hair to terminal hair. Hydroquinone and phenylthiourea interfere with tyrosine activity, causing hypopigmentation of skin and hair [41].

Darkening of white hair occurred in a patient with Parkinson's disease following the addition of carbidopa and bromocriptine therapy [42].

Colour changes induced by nutritional deficiencies

Because specific dietary deficiencies are rare in humans, most clinical knowledge of their effects is derived from laboratory and animal studies. Copper deficiency in cattle causes achromotrichia because it is the prosthetic group of tyrosinase; loss of hair colour from this mechanism occurs in humans as Menkes' kinky hair syndrome. In protein malnutrition, exemplified by kwashiorkor, hair colour changes are a prominent feature; normal black hair becomes brown or reddish, and brown hair becomes blonde [43,44]. Intermittent protein malnutrition leads to the 'flag' sign of kwashiorkor (signe de la bandera). Alternating white (abnormal) and dark bands occur along individual hairs. Changes similar to those in kwashiorkor have been described in severe ulcerative colitis and after extensive bowel resection.

The lightening of hair colour from black to brown described in severe iron-deficiency anaemia may be an effect on keratinization rather than on melanocytic function [45].

Noppakun and Swasdikul [46] described a case of reversible white hair in vitamin B_{12} deficiency and commented on a variety of reversible and other hair colour changes in adult coeliac disease.

Hair colour in metabolic disorders

Phenylketonuria is an autosomal recessive disorder in which the tissues are unable to metabolize phenylalanine to tyrosine because of phenylalanine hydroxylase deficiency. Mental retardation, fits and decreased pigmentation of the skin, eyes and hair occur with eczema and dermographism. Black hair may become brown, and older institutionalized patients with phenylketonuria may have pale blonde or grey hair. Tyrosine treatment causes darkening towards normal colour within 1–2 months.

The paling of hair seen in homocystinuria is probably caused by keratinization changes resulting from the error in methionine metabolism.

Light, almost white hair and recurrent oedema are manifestations of the hair condition, 'oast house' disease. Methionine concentration in the blood is raised.

Darkening of grey hair has been reported in porphyria cutanea tarda [47].

Accidental hair discoloration

Hair avidly binds many inorganic elements and thus hair colour changes are occasionally seen after exposure to certain substances.

Exposure to high concentrates of copper in industry or from inadvertently high concentrations in tap water [48] or in swimming pools may cause green hair, particularly visible in blonde-haired subjects [49,50]. Cobalt workers may develop bright blue hair and a deep blue tint may be seen in indigo handlers [51]. A yellowish hair colour is not uncommon in white- or grey-haired heavy smokers resulting from the tar in cigarette smoke; yellow staining may also occur from picric acid and dithranol. Trinitrotoluene (TNT) workers sometimes develop yellow skin and reddish brown hair.

REFERENCES

1 Castanet J, Ortonne J-P. Hair melanin and hair colour. In: Jollès P, Zahn H, eds. *Formation and Structure of Human Hair.* Basel: Birkhäuser Verlag, 1997: 209–25.
2 Rees JL. The melanocortin 1 receptor (MC1R): more than just red hair. *Pigment Cell Res* 2000; **13**: 135–40.
3 Sturm RA, Teasdale RD, Box NF. Human pigmentation genes: identification, structure and consequences of polymorphic variation. *Gene* 2001; **277**: 49–62.
4 Trotter M, Duggins OH. Age changes in head hair from birth to maturity. *Am J Phys Anthropol* 1950; **8**: 467–77.
5 Harrison GA, Weiner JS, Tanner JM et al. *Human Biology: An Introduction to Human Evolution, Variation and Growth.* London: Oxford University Press, 1964.
6 Kligman AM. Pathologic dynamics of human hair loss. *Arch Dermatol* 1961; **83**: 175–82.
7 Kukita A, Fitzpatrick TB. The demonstration of tyrosinase in melanocytes of the human hair matrix by autoradiography. *Science* 1955; **121**: 893–904.
8 Hertzberg J, Gusck W. Das Ergrauen des Kapfhaares: eine histo-und fermentschemische sowie elektronen-mikroskopische Studie. *Arch Klin Exp Dermatol* 1970; **236**: 368–75.
9 Dawber RPR. Integumentary associations of pernicious anaemia. *Br J Dermatol* 1970; **82**: 221–6.
10 Klaus SN. Acquired pigment dilution of the skin and hair; a sign of pancreatic disease in the tropics. *Int J Dermatol* 1980; **19**: 508–11.
11 Keough EV, Walsh RJ. Rate of greying human hair. *Nature* 1965; **207**: 877–80.
12 Jelinek JE. Sudden whitening of hair. *Bull NY Acad Med* 1972; **48**: 1003–6.
13 Cunliffe WJ, Hall R, Newell DJ et al. Vitiligo, thyroid disease and autoimmunity. *Br J Dermatol* 1968; **80**: 135–42.
14 Dunlop D. Eighty-six cases of Addisons's disease. *BMJ* 1963; **ii**: 887–99.
15 Main RA, Robbie RB, Gray ES et al. Smooth muscle antibodies and alopecia areata. *Br J Dermatol* 1975; **92**: 289–95.
16 Sieve BF. Darkening of grey hair following para-aminobenzoic acid. *Science* 1941; **94**: 257–60.
17 Gilkes JJH, Sharvill DE, Wells RS. The premature ageing syndromes: report of eight cases and descriptions of a new entity named metageria. *Br J Dermatol* 1974; **91**: 243–52.
18 Book JA. Clinical and genetic studies of hypodontia. I. Premolar aplasia, hyperhidrosis and canities prematura: a new hereditary syndrome in man. *Am J Hum Genet* 1950; **2**: 240–1.
19 Tobin DJ, Cargnello JA. Partial reversal of canities in a 22-year-old normal Chinese male. *Arch Dermatol* 1993; **129**: 789–90.
20 Breg WR. Abnormalities of chromosomes 4 and 5. In: Gardner LI, ed. *Endocrine and Genetic Diseases of Childhood and Adolescence.* Philadelphia: Saunders, 1975.
21 Mosher DB, Fitzpatrick TB. Piebaldism. *Arch Dermatol* 1988; **124**: 245–50.
22 Grupper C, Prunieras M, Hincky M et al. Albinisme partiel familial (piebaldisme): étude ultrastructurale. *Ann Dermatol Syphilol* 1970; **97**: 267–86.
23 Giebel LB, Spritz RA. Mutation of the KIT (mast/stem cell growth factor receptor) proto-oncogene in human piebaldism. *Proc Natl Acad Sci USA* 1991; **88**: 8696–9.
24 Richards KA, Fukai K, Oiso N, Paller AS. A novel *KIT* mutation results in piebaldism with progressive depigmentation. *J Am Acad Dermatol* 2001; **44**: 288–92.
25 Witkop CJ Jr. Albinism. In: Harris H, Hirschom K, eds. *Advances in Human Genetics.* New York: Plenum Press, 1971.
26 Smith SD, Kelley PM, Kenyon JB, Hoover D. Tietz syndrome (hypopigmentation/deafness) caused by mutation of *MITF*. *J Med Genet* 2000; **37**: 446–8.

27 Read AP, Newton VE. Waardenburg syndrome. *J Med Genet* 1997; **34**: 656–65.
28 Burton JL, Marshall A. Hypertrichosis due to minoxidil. *Br J Dermatol* 1979; **101**: 593–6.
29 Waardenburg PJ. New syndrome combining developmental abnormalities of the eyelid, eyebrows, nose root, with pigmentary defects of the iris and head hair and with congenital deafness. *Am J Hum Genet* 1951; **3**: 195–202.
30 Rugel SJ, Keats EU. Waardenburg's syndrome in six generations of one family. *Am J Dis Child* 1965; **109**: 579–89.
31 Alezzandrini AA. Manifestations unilaterales de degenerescence tapetoretinienne de vitiligo, de poliose, de cheveux blancs et hypoacousie. *Ophthalmologica* 1964; **147**: 409–15.
32 McWilliam TS, Stephenson JBP. Depigmented hair; the earliest sign of tuberose sclerosis. *Arch Dis Child* 1978; **53**: 961–9.
33 Prunieras M. Melanocytes, melanogenesis and inflammation. *Int J Dermatol* 1986; **25**: 624–8.
34 Read RW, Rao NA, Cunningham ET. Vogt–Koyanagi–Harada disease. *Curr Opin Ophthalmol* 2000; **11**: 437–42.
35 Tsuruta D, Hamada T, Teramae H, Mito H, Ishii M. Inflammatory vitiligo in Vogt–Koyanagi–Harada disease. *J Am Acad Dermatol* 2001; **44**: 129–31.
36 Oetting WS, King RA. Molecular basis of albinism: mutations and polymorphisms of pigmentation genes associated with albinism. *Hum Mutat* 1999; **13**: 99–115.
37 White JG, Clawson CC. The Chediak–Higashi syndrome: the nature of the giant neutrophil granules and their interaction with cytoplasm and foreign particles. *Am J Pathol* 1980; **48**: 151–9.
38 Saunders TS, Fitzpatrick LE, Seji M et al. Decrease in human hair colour, and feather pigment of fowl following chloroquine diphosphate. *J Invest Dermatol* 1959; **33**: 87–98.
39 Spillane JD. Brunette to blond: depigmentation of hair during treatment with oral mephenesin. *BMJ* 1963; **i**: 997–8.
40 Ridgley GV, Kassassieh SD. Minoxidil. *Lahey Clin Found Bull* 1979; **28**: 80–6.
41 Dieke SH. Pigmentation and hair growth in black rats as modified by the chronic administration of thiourea, phenylthiourea and α-naphthylthiourea. *Endocrinology* 1947; **40**: 123–30.
42 Reynolds NJ, Crossley J, Ferguson I et al. Darkening of white hair in Parkinson's disease. *Clin Exp Dermatol* 1989; **14**: 317–20.
43 Bradfield RB. Hair tissue as a medium for the differential diagnosis of protein-calorie malnutrition: a commentary. *J Pediatr* 1974; **84**: 294–9.
44 Bradfield RB, Jellife DB. Hair colour changes in kwashiorkor. *Lancet* 1974; **i**: 461–3.
45 Sato S, Jitsukawa K, Sato H et al. Segmental heterochromia in black scalp hair associated with Fe-deficiency anaemia. *Arch Dermatol* 1989; **125**: 531–8.
46 Noppakun N, Swasdikul D. Hyperpigmentation of skin and nails with white hair due to vitamin B_{12} deficiency. *Arch Dermatol* 1986; **122**: 896–904.
47 Shaffrali FC, McDonagh AJ, Messenger AG. Hair darkening in porphyria cutanea tarda. *Br J Dermatol* 2002; **146**: 325–9.
48 Goldschmidt H. Green hair. *Arch Dermatol* 1979; **115**: 1288–90.
49 Blanc D, Zultak M, Rochefort A. Les cheveux vert: étude clinique, chimique et epidemiologique. *Ann Dermatol Vénéréol* 1988; **115**: 807–12.
50 Melnik BC, Plewig G, Daldrup T. Green hair: guidelines for diagnosis and therapy. *J Am Acad Dermatol* 1986; **15**: 1065–9.
51 Beigel H. Blue hair in indigo handlers. *Arch Pathol Anat Physiol* 1965; **83**: 324–8.

Hair cosmetics [1,2]

Women and men have always been concerned about their hair, and have sought to modify it by grooming, colouring, cutting and wigs. There are references in Egyptian papyruses to the importance of arranging the hair prior to seduction [3,4]. Now, hair care and hair cosmetics are big business and many of the advances have come from cosmetic science laboratories [5,6]. Some aspects of cosmetic management can lead to secondary hair problems, such as traction alopecia (see p. 63.62) or follicular degeneration syndrome (see p. 63.54).

REFERENCES

1 Draelos Z. The biology of hair care. *Dermatol Clin* 2000; **18**: 651–8.
2 Bolduc C, Shapiro J. Hair care products: waving, straightening, conditioning and coloring. *Clin Dermatol* 2001; **19**: 431–6.
3 Pomey-Rey D. Hair and psychology. In: Zviak C, ed. *The Science of Hair Care*. New York: Marcel Dekker, 1986.
4 Gummer C, Dawber RPR. Hair cosmetics. In: Dawber RPR, ed. *Diseases of the Hair and Scalp*, 3rd edn. Oxford: Blackwell Science, 1997: 732–59.
5 Zviak C, Dawber RPR. Hair structure, function and physicochemical properties. In: Zviak C, ed. *The Science of Hair Care*. New York: Marcel Dekker, 1986: 1–34.
6 Schoen LA, ed. *Skin and Hair Care*, 1st English edn. Harmondsworth: Penguin, 1978.

Shampoos [1–5]

In modern terms, a shampoo may be defined as a suitable detergent for washing hair that leaves the hair in good condition. Originally, shampoos were used solely for cleansing hair, but their range of function has extended in recent years to include conditioning, and the treatment of some hair and scalp diseases.

In principle, to wash hair a shampoo must remove grease, as it is the latter that attracts dirt and other particulate matter. The polar group of a detergent achieves this by displacing oil from the hair surface. The evaluation of shampoo detergency is difficult and complicated. The consumer tends to equate detergency with foaming; in Western society, few shampoos sell unless they possess good foaming power. In the evaluation of detergents as shampoos no single criterion can be used, although instrumental methods have been devised. Efficacy can be based only on the subjective impression of the consumer.

Shampoo formulations

These vary enormously but the basic ingredients can be resolved into a few groups: water, detergent and some fatty material. Soap shampoos are made from vegetable or animal fats and remove dirt and grease as efficiently as detergents; however, a scum forms with hard water and most shampoos contain detergents as the principal washing ingredient. Detergents are synthetic petroleum products and form no hard-water scum.

Shampoos contain:
1 Principal surfactants for detergency and foaming power
2 Secondary surfactants to improve and 'condition' hair
3 Functional additives to control pH and viscosity, or ingredients such as tar or antifungal agents
4 Preservatives
5 Aesthetic additives such as colourants and fragrance.
Whatever the claims of some manufacturers, most special additives end up down the sink [6]!

In general, cosmetic shampoos can be dry (powder types), liquid, solid cream, aerosol or oily. Antidandruff, 'medicated' and scalp treatment shampoos contain antiseptics and active agents such as coal- and wood-tar fractions or selenium sulphide. Clear liquid shampoos are the most popular, including 'cleansing' types, sold for treating greasy hair, and 'cosmetic' types having good conditioning action and popular among women with dry or 'normal' hair. For details of other specific formulas, the reader is recommended to read more specialized texts [3,4,7].

Shampoo safety

Shampoos obviously must be non-toxic, and at concentrations used by the consumer not irritate either skin or eyes. New shampoo formulations are tested exhaustively prior to marketing, particularly to assess their propensity to cause eye irritation, scarring and corneal opacities. Skin irritation is not usually encountered from shampoos that have low eye irritancy potential. Eye safety is assessed by the technique known as the Draize test; standard solutions of shampoo are instilled into the conjunctival sac of an albino rabbit. In general, the eye irritancy of detergents is greatest with cationics, followed by anionics, and least with non-anionics. There are exceptions to this, suggesting that shampoo irritancy may be caused by properties other than detergency including surface activity, pH, wetting power, foaming power (Ross–Miles test), and wetting and foaming power together. Most shampoos are, in fact, irritant but not dangerously so. Allergic contact dermatitis resulting from biocides does occur (see Chapters 20 and 21).

Conditioners

Dry hair lacks gloss and lustre and is difficult to style. This results from natural weathering and is worsened by chemical and physical processes applied to the hair. Conditioners have a range of characteristics that may contribute to shine, reduction of static electricity, protection from ultraviolet radiation and possibly increased hair strength [8]. Conditioners comprise fatty acids and alcohols: natural triglycerides (e.g. almond, avocado, corn and olive oil); waxes (e.g. beeswax, jojoba oil, mink oil, lanolin); phospholipids (e.g. egg yolk and soya bean); vitamins A, B and E, protein hydrolysates of silk, collagen, keratin (horn and hoof), gelatin and other proteins; and cationic polymers. Conditioners are available in a variety of forms and are widely used. They provide lubrication and gloss and render the hair easier to comb and style. The most commonly used are those combined with a shampoo as a 2-in-1 preparation. These cationic chemicals bind with the hair at the negatively charged surface and areas of weathering. In so doing they reduce static by electrically neutralizing the hair and provide a physical coating to the areas of damaged hair shaft with materials such as dimethicone. Other forms of conditioner may be applied as a separate procedure and can take the form of creams and emulsions applied for a few minutes after washing and then rinsed off. Deep conditioners are left on for up to 30 min, often with damp heat. Fluids, gels and aerosol foams aid styling. Hair oils are traditional conditioners. Men may use brilliantines, greases or oils to leave the hair glossy and sleek [3].

Where the hair is significantly dry or damaged, or the scalp is inflamed or eczematous, conditioner may be used as a shampoo substitute in the same manner that one might advocate an emollient as soap substitute on the skin of someone with eczema. The conditioner will mix with water to remove surface dirt and odour, but will not subject the hair and scalp to the powerful solvent effects of the shampoo.

REFERENCES

1 Corbett JP. The chemistry of hair-care products. *J Soc Dyers Colourists* 1976; **92**: 285–93.
2 Robbins CR, ed. *Chemical and Physical Behaviour of Human Hair*, 1st edn. New York: Van Nostrand Reinhold, 1979.
3 Zviak C, Bouillon C. Hair treatment and hair care products. In: Zviak C, ed. *The Science of Hair Care*. New York: Marcel Dekker, 1986: 210–24.
4 Zviak C, Vanderberghe G. Scalp and hair hygiene: shampoos. In: Zviak C, ed. *The Science of Hair Care*. New York: Marcel Dekker, 1986: 224–41.
5 Bouillon C. *Clin Dermatol* 1996; **14**: 113–21.
6 Spoor HJ. Shampoos. *Cutis* 1973; **12**: 671–6.
7 Gummer C, Dawber RPR. Hair cosmetics. In: Dawber RPR, ed. *Diseases of the Hair and Scalp*, 3rd edn. Oxford: Blackwell Science, 1997: 732–59.
8 Fox C. An introduction to the formulation of shampoos. *Cosmet Toilet* 1988; **103**: 25–38.

Cosmetic hair colouring [1–4]

Since the days of the pharaohs, women in particular have used hair dyes to hide grey hair. Use has increased enormously during the past 50 years and now men are using hair dyes. Or perhaps they always did!

The penetration of dyes into hair depends on molecular size and the aqueous swelling of the hair at the time of application of the dye; basicity of the dye is also important. The most successful dyes are relatively small molecules.

Excluding bleaches, hair-colouring materials can be divided into three groups: vegetable, metallic and synthetic organic dyes. Synthetic organic materials are thought to give more 'natural' colours than those obtained with vegetable and metallic hair colourants.

Vegetable dyes

Henna may be used to give reddish auburn shades. It is obtained from shrubs found in North Africa and the Middle East: *Lawsonia alba*, *L. spinosa* and *L. inermis*. The dye is produced from dried leaves, which are removed before the plant flowers. The active principle is an acidic naphthoquinone (lawsone). Traditionally, it is applied as a thick paste 'pack', which is left *in situ* for 5–60 min. The effects last for up to 10 weeks. This process is non-toxic but

messy, and fingernails may become stained. Henna rinses are mixtures of henna and powdered indigo leaves that produce blue-black shades. A wide range of products containing compound henna exist [5]. Ground flower heads of a Roman or German chamomile yield a yellow dye: 1,3,4,-trihydroxyflavone (apigenin). It stains only the cuticle and can be used to lighten or brighten hair. Other vegetable dyes include extracts from logwood and walnut shell and these can be used by patients who are *para*-phenylenediamine sensitive. These products are obtainable at herbalists and beauty shops.

Metallic dyes

Traditionally, hair dyes for men have been of this type, as the colour changes occur less rapidly and are not as immediately obvious as with the oxidative dyes. Inorganic salts are used, which are altered by the hair and coat the surface as either oxides from reduction of the metal salts by keratin, or sulphides from the action of the sulphur in keratin on the metal. They all give a rather dull (metallic) appearance and may cause brittle or damaged hair if used too often.

Lead acetate, with precipitated sulphur or sodium thiosulphate, gives brown to black shades; grey hair may be changed through yellow to brown or black. Silver nitrate used alone produces a greenish black colour; pyrogallol is used as developer. Colours from ash blonde to black are possible by mixing silver nitrate variously with copper, cobalt or nickel; brownish black skin staining is the great disadvantage. Bismuth salts give shades of brown. Newer metallic dyes, containing a metal plus an organic ligand, are used on textile fibres and in some hair-dye patents. Metallic dyes cannot be removed without hair damage and should be left to grow out.

Synthetic organic dyes

This group has now been in use for more than 60 years. They are the most important type because of the comprehensive range of 'natural' colours that can be obtained. Most penetrate the hair cuticle so are potentially permanent, but in recent years less permanent types have been introduced.

Synthetic organic colourants are of three types:
1 *Temporary*. These wash out with one shampoo and last no longer than 1 week. Many temporary rinses belong to this group, including fashionable unnatural colours used by avant-garde sects and groups. They are available in aerosol sprays by incorporation into transparent polymeric plastics such as PVP; the disadvantage of such vehicles is their tendency to flake off on to clothing.
2 *Semipermanent*. In the UK, these have the widest appeal. They are used frequently at home and also in salons to brighten or subdue a natural colour, modify a permanent

or bleached colour, or modify white or grey. They are of sufficiently small molecular size to penetrate the cortex. They are intrinsically coloured; no developing is required (see the oxidative permanent group). They are relatively easy to wash out with shampoos containing ammonia; other shampoos must be used 6–10 times to remove them. Some semipermanent dyes have an affinity for thioglycolate-waved hair. Many are now used in colour shampoos.

3 *Permanent* (developed or oxidation dyes). These do not rely on the natural colour of a single chemical dye-stuff, (see semipermanents), but require an oxidative developer —hydrogen peroxide—to produce the final colour:

Paraphenylenediamine (PPD) and/or
paratoluenediamine (PTD)
+
Hydrogen peroxide
↓
Applied to hair
↓
Quinone diamine (small molecule)
↓
Penetrate hair—to cortex
↓
Large molecules produced
(by diamine 'self' condensation and modifiers,
e.g. pyrogallol)

Other substances may be included in specific formulations to give greater intensity to the dye (e.g. resorcinol and polyhidric phenols).

Oxidative dyes are potentially hazardous. The need for hydrogen peroxide enables lighter shades to be obtained and is chiefly responsible for the structural damage to hair that may occur if care is not exercised. Additives such as pyrogallol and resorcinol are potential irritants. The greatest problem is the potential of PPD (less so with PTD) to cause allergic dermatitis. Up to 10% of users may develop type IV allergy [6,7]. All dyes in this group are therefore sold with instructions to carry out preliminary patch testing 24–48 h before the proposed dye is used. Thus, the dye system is applied to skin either behind one ear or on the forearm—any redness, swelling or blistering implies allergy and the dyeing should not therefore proceed. A negative patch test does not mean that subsequent allergy cannot develop; it simply shows the subject is not allergic at the time the test is carried out. If allergy is shown, it is not sufficient merely to stop all future use of oxidative dyes; unfortunately, cross-sensitization also occurs with other aromatic benzenes (e.g. sulphonamides and some local anaesthetics), which must also be avoided for life. Modern formulations seem to cause less problems with allergy [8]. Hair dyes of this group have been incriminated as possible carcinogens [9]. Chromosome breaks have occurred under experimental conditions [10] and an increased incidence of tumours has been found in regular users [11]. It has also been intimated that aplastic anaemia could be produced by hair dyes [12]. None of these reports is sufficiently conclusive to warrant the withdrawal of such dyes.

Permanent dyes last for several months; they must not be applied more frequently than every 2–3 weeks because hair damage will occur. Permanently dyed hair must therefore be allowed to grow out. However, if a light shade has been produced and the subject wishes a darker shade, then temporary rinses may safely be used as these only coat the hair surface and have no propensity to cause structural damage.

For less commonly used permanent dye formulations, such as 'highlights', the reader is referred to specialized texts [4].

Bleaches [13–15]

Women have bleached their hair since Roman times. Bleaching is used both to lighten hair and to prepare it to take up hair dyes. Bleaching is an oxidative alkaline treatment that oxidizes and bleaches melanin. The hair lightens to reddish or yellow tones, depending on the underlying hair colour, and ultimately to platinum. Bleaching is very damaging to the hair, rendering it dry, porous and more prone to tangle. Overuse may cause disruption and fracture of the hair. Thus, it is advisable to perform permanent waving before bleaching. Home bleaching is usually performed with 6% hydrogen peroxide (20 volumes) with ammonia to speed the reaction, which otherwise takes 12 h. Salons use more powerful bleaching creams, powders and pastes, which are much faster. They are often applied to individual strands of hair, others being left untreated to give highlights, which lessens the problem of the darkened roots. Bleaching is terminated by shampooing or an acid rinse. The human eye perceives a more aesthetically acceptable blonde ('platinum' blonde) when the bleached hair is treated with a blue or lilac colourant.

REFERENCES

1 Corbett JF, Menkart T. Hair colouring. *Cutis* 1973; **12**: 190–5.
2 Kalopesis G. Toxicology and hair dyes. In: Zviak C, ed. *The Science of Hair Care*. New York: Marcel Dekker, 1986; 287–305.
3 Zviak C. Hair coloring: non-oxidation coloring. In: Zviak C, ed. *The Science of Hair Care*. New York: Marcel Dekker, 1986; 235–62.
4 Zviak C. Oxidation coloring. In: Zviak C, ed. *The Science of Hair Care*. New York: Marcel Dekker, 1986; 263–86.
5 Natow AJ. Henna. *Cutis* 1986; **38**: 21–5.
6 Blohm SG, Rajka G. The allergenicity of paraphenylene diamine. *Acta Derm Venereol (Stockh)* 1970; **50**: 49–55.
7 Lubowe I. Allergic dermatitis and cosmetics. *Cutis* 1973; **11**: 431–5.
8 Calnan C. Adverse reactions to hair products. In: Zviak C, ed. *The Science of Hair Care*. New York: Marcel Dekker, 1986; 409–24.
9 Burnett CM. Evaluation of toxicity and carcinogenicity of hair dyes. *J Toxicol Environ Health* 1980; **6**: 247–51.
10 Kirkland DJ, Lawler SD, Venitt S. Chromosome damage and hair dyes. *Lancet* 1978; **ii**: 124–6.

11 Burnett CM, Menkart T. Hair dyes and breast cancer. *N Engl J Med* 1978; **299**: 1253–60.
12 Burnett CM, Corbett JF, Lanman BM. Hair dyes and aplastic anaemia. *Drug Chem Toxicol* 1978; **1**: 45–7.
13 Natow AJ. Hair bleach. *Cutis* 1986; **37**: 28–31.
14 Wolfram LJ, Hall K, Hui I. The mechanism of hair bleaching. *J Soc Cosmet Chem* 1970; **21**: 875–85.
15 Zviak C. Hair bleaching. In: Zviak C, ed. *The Science of Hair Care*. New York: Marcel Dekker, 1986: 213–34.

Permanent waving [1–3]

Permanent waving is often referred to as 'a perm'. It has been defined as the process of changing the shape of the hair so that the new shape persists through several shampoos. During the last 70 years, increasing knowledge of keratin chemistry has enabled semipermanent chemical methods to be developed. Whatever the process used, three stages are involved in hair waving:

1 Physical or chemical softening of the hair
2 Reshaping
3 Hardening of fibres to retain the reshaped position.

Softening

Water can extend the hydrogen bonds between adjacent polypeptides in the keratin molecule, allowing temporary reshaping to be carried out—exposure to high humidity or rewetting immediately reverses the process. To obtain a more durable effect from water, steam may be used which, in a limited way, disrupts disulphide bonds. Heat and steam alone are rarely acceptable to modern women because their effects are temporary and the treatment is uncomfortable. Heat can be more effectively employed in conjunction with ammonium hydroxide and potassium bisulphite or triethanolamine as agents to reduce disulphide bonds; great skill is involved in this process as failure to judge the time of application of chemicals and heat may cause severe damage.

Since 1945, cold wave processes using substituted thiosulphates (thioglycolates) have largely superseded hot waving. Thioglycolates are potent reducers of disulphide bonds in the keratin molecule:

$$-S=S- \rightarrow 2-SH.$$

A typical cold waving lotion contains thioglycolic acid plus ammonia or monoethanolamine.

Acid permanent waves have recently become popular for salon use. They contain glyceryl monothioglycolate and produce a softer curl, and can be used on damaged and bleached hair. Their disadvantage is the high frequency of sensitization in the hairdressers using the product and, occasionally, sensitization of the client [4].

Reshaping

The type of rollers or curlers used to reshape the softened hair depends on the training of the hairdresser and the fashion desired. The degree of curl or tightness of the permanent wave depends both on the diameter of the roller and the size of the strand wound round the roller. Increasing the time of the exposure to the perming solution up to 20 min increases the curl, but longer times do not give a further increase. The strength of the solution used depends on the hair type, texture and previous bleaching. Home permanent waves are weaker and cannot achieve the same degree of curl. 'Tepid' waving involves using a weaker thioglycolate solution plus warm air. Neutralization is carried out initially with the curlers in place and again after they have been carefully removed. The reshaping stage is thus a great test of hairdressing skill and experience.

Hardening (neutralizing or setting)

In general, this process involves a reversal of the softening (reduction) stages:

$$\text{oxidation}$$
$$2-SH \rightarrow -S=S-.$$

It is important to note that complete reversal to presoftened 'strength' cannot occur because many free SH groups may not be in a position for oxidation to be effective, for example:

$$2-SH \rightarrow -S-C-S- \quad (C = carbon)$$
$$2-SH \rightarrow -S-Ba-S- \quad (Ba = barium)$$

Atmospheric oxidation may efficiently neutralize the waving process. This method is slow and rollers must be left in position for several hours overnight. Chemical oxidation is now the rule. Hairdressers generally use hydrogen peroxide whereas most solutions for home use contain sodium perborate or percarbonate (UK) or sodium or potassium bromate (USA). This is why hair is lighter after permanent waving. Some neutralizers contain shellac, which may react with alcohol groups to cause hair discoloration.

Practical procedures

Hot waving

This is almost never used. The procedure is:
1 Shampooing
2 Hair divided and rollers or curlers applied under slight tension
3 Waving solution applied
4 Heating.

Heating varies according to the solution used or the type of wave required. Electric rollers or exothermic reactive chemicals may be used. The latter allow free head movement during the waving. The skill of this procedure lies in good hair sectioning, judging the right amount of solution, correct winding tension and appropriate steaming time.

Cold waving

This also involves initial shampooing, hair division into locks, moistening with waving lotion and application of croquignole curlers. Further solution may then be applied. The softening time is 10–20 min. Occasionally, mild heat is included, using exothermic chemicals or the natural heat from the head by enclosing the scalp in a plastic bag. These may add to the comfort of the process. Rinsing then takes place, followed by neutralization with the oxidizing solution for up to 10 min. After removing the curlers, further 'hardening' solution is usually applied. 'Loose' curl waves last for no more than a few weeks but 'tight' curl styles may persist for 4–12 months.

REFERENCES

1 Zviak C. Permanent waving and hair straightening. In: Zviak C, ed. *The Science of Hair Care*. New York: Marcel Dekker, 1986: 183–212.
2 Wickett RR. Permanent waving and straightening of hair. *Cutis* 1987; **39**: 496–500.
3 Bolduc C, Shapiro J. Hair care products: waving, straightening, conditioning and coloring. *Clin Dermatol* 2001; **19**: 431–6.
4 Morrison LH, Storrs FJ. Persistence of an allergen in hair after glyceryl monothioglycolate-containing permanent wave solutions. *J Am Acad Dermatol* 1988; **19**: 52–9.

Hair straightening (relaxing) [1,2]

In principle, the methods used to straighten hair are similar to those used in permanent waving. The practice is almost exclusively used to straighten negroid hair and is also called relaxing. One survey found that relaxing formulations were used in 45% of black American women [3]. These practices are associated with a range of problems and ultimately may contribute to scarring alopecia [4].

Pomades

These are mostly used by men with relatively short hair. They are greasy and act by 'plastering' hair into position.

Hot-comb methods

Shampooing is carried out and the hair is towelled dry; oil is then applied (e.g. petroleum jelly or liquid paraffin), which acts as a heat-transferring agent. Heat pressing with hot combing is then used (148–260°F), causing breakage and reforming of disulphide bonds, allowing the hair to be moulded straight. Structural damage (and breakage) of hair is common with this process and scarring alopecia may occur as a result of hot waxes entering the follicles. Sweating and rain reverse this procedure.

Cold methods

The chemical methods employed use alkaline reducing agents (caustics), thioglycolates, ammonium carbonate or sodium bisulphite. Caustic soda preparations are usually creams and require the application of protective scalp oil or wax. They are combed through the hair and left for 15–20 min; the hair is combed and straightened again, then rinsed and neutralized. These preparations are limited to salon use because of their potential to cause irritant dermatitis and damage to the hair. Thioglycolate creams are the most common agents used; the cream is applied liberally to the hair, which is then combed until it is straight. The cream is then washed off and a neutralizer (oxidizing agent) applied. Other straighteners ('relaxers') do not contain thioglycolates (e.g. sodium bisulphite and ammonium carbonate, acidic ethylene glycol or 1,3-propylene glycol). Bisulphite straighteners are suitable for home use in combination with alkaline stabilizers.

REFERENCES

1 Wickett RR. Permanent waving and straightening of hair. *Cutis* 1987; **39**: 496–500.
2 Zviak C. Permanent waving and hair straightening. In: Zviak C, ed. *The Science of Hair Care*. New York: Marcel Dekker, 1986: 183–212.
3 Grimes PE. Skin and hair cosmetic issues in women of colour. *Dermatol Clin* 2000; **18**: 659–65.
4 Wilborn WS. Disorders of hair growth in African Americans. In: Olsen E, ed. *Disorders of Hair Growth, Diagnosis and Treatment*. New York: McGraw Hill, 1994: 389–407.

Hair setting [1]

Setting lotions have changed considerably in recent years. The traditional semiliquid gels based on water-soluble gums (e.g. tragacanth, karaya and acasia) have been replaced by various synthetic polymers in a bewildering array of forms—aerosol foams and sprays, liquids and gels. Most are based on PVP in a gelled aqueous solution and give an attractive glossy non-greasy appearance [2]. Some preparations incorporate other ingredients to condition or to add antistatic action, lustre or sheen.

Setting lotion and spray formulations are considered safe, after early reports of foreign body granulomatous inflammation [3,4] had been questioned and not supported by further cases. Hair sprays were incriminated as a possible cause of peripilar casts [5] but this was not confirmed by later work [6].

REFERENCES

1 Zviak C. Hair setting. In: Zviak C, ed. *The Science of Hair Care*. New York: Marcel Dekker, 1986: 149–82.
2 Friefeld M, Lyons J, Martinelli AT. Polyvinylpyrrolidone in cosmetics. *Am Perfumery* 1962; **77**: 25.
3 Edelson BG. Thesaurosis following inhalation of hair spray [Letter]. *Lancet* 1959; **ii**: 465–6.

4 Bergmann M, Flance IJ, Blumenthal AT. Thesaurosis following inhalation of hair spray: a clinical and experimental study. *N Engl J Med* 1958; **258**: 471–6.
5 Scott MJ. Peripilar keratin casts. *Arch Dermatol* 1959; **79**: 654–9.
6 Dawber RPR. Hair cast. *Br J Dermatol* 1979; **100**: 417–20.

Methylolated compounds

Many cosmetic preparations, by their action on the keratin molecule, irreversibly weaken the hair. The cosmetic scientist has produced chemicals that attempt to combat this problem. The formulations contain methylolated compounds of varying strength depending on the type of hair under treatment and the solubility of the compound. Most preparations containing alkylated methylol compounds have greater stability and release very little formaldehyde [1].

REFERENCE

1 Zviak C, Bouillon C. Hair treatment and hair care products. In: Zviak C, ed. *The Science of Hair Care*. New York: Marcel Dekker, 1986: 87–148.

Complications

Hair loss is often attributed to cosmetics, with relatively little evidence in support [1]. Matting of scalp hair is most commonly a sudden, usually irreversible, tangling of scalp hair resulting from shampooing [2]. Excessive bleaching, permanent waving and straightening procedures may induce excessive weathering and fragility of hair.

Complications from the use of synthetic hair fibre implantation for male pattern balding can be severe [3].

REFERENCES

1 Gummer CL. Cosmetics and hair loss. *Clin Exp Dermatol* 2002; **27**: 418–21.
2 Wilson CL, Ferguson DJ, Dawber RPR. Matting of scalp hair during shampooing: a new look. *Clin Exp Dermatol* 1990; **15**: 139–41.
3 Lepaw MI. Complications of implantation of synthetic fibres into scalps for 'hair' replacement: experience with 14 cases. *J Dermatol Surg Oncol* 1979; **5**: 201–4.

Chapter 64

The Skin and the Eyes

J.N. Leonard & J.K.G. Dart

Introduction

This chapter is not intended to be a comprehensive account of all diseases that affect the skin and eyes, for which there are several reviews [1–6]. The main focus is on those conditions that commonly occur in clinical practice and present a problem with management. It is also intended to alert the dermatologist to conditions that might threaten visual acuity and require urgent referral to an ophthalmologist. Also, many systemic diseases affect both the skin and eyes, and ophthalmic assessment will be of help in making the correct diagnosis and in long-term management of the patient.

REFERENCES

1 Easty DI, Sparrow JM, eds. *Oxford Textbook of Ophthalmology*. Oxford: Oxford University Press, 1999.
2 Hoang-Xuan T, Baudouin C, Creuzot-Garcher C, eds. *Inflammatory Diseases of the Conjunctiva*. Stuttgart: Thieme, 2001.
3 Kanski JJ. *Clinical Ophthalmology. A Systematic Approach*, 4th edn. Oxford: Butterworth–Heinemann, 1999.
4 Pepose JS, Holland GN, Wilhelmus KR, eds. *Ocular Infection and Immunity*. St Louis: Mosby, 1996.
5 Theirs BH, Grant-Kels JM, Rothe MJ *et al.*, eds. *Dermatology Clinics—Oculocutaneous Diseases, I & II*, Vol. 10; Nos 3 & 4. Philadelphia: WB Saunders, 1992.
6 Mannis MJ, Macsai MS, Huntley AC, eds. *Eye and Skin Disease*. New York: Lippincott-Raven, 1996.

Anatomy and physiology of the eye [1,2]

The eye and skin share a common embryological origin. The structure of the lid, conjunctiva, the lacrimal gland and associated drainage apparatus are of surface ecto-dermal origin while the remainder of the eye arises from epithelium of the ectodermal neural plate. The only meso-dermal contribution to the eye is the myoblasts of the extra-ocular muscles. The anatomy of the eye is shown in Fig. 64.1. The eye appendages are as follows.

The eyebrows

This hair-bearing area rests on a very mobile fat and muscle pad overlying the superior orbital ridge. Its mobility is important as a means of facial expression. The eyebrows help protect the eye from bright light and sweat.

The eyelids

The eyelids have distinct anatomical layers, comprising the skin with subcutaneous tissue, the tarsal plate and conjunctiva, and striated muscles that effect lid movement (Fig. 64.2).

The skin is thin and modified in several ways to protect the eyeball. It contains sebaceous glands associated with

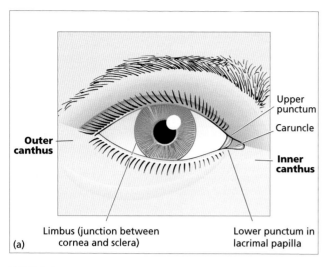

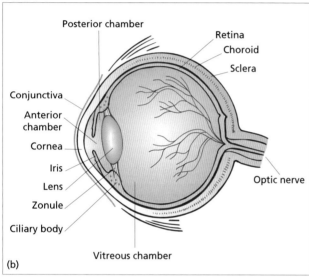

Fig. 64.1 Anatomy of normal eye. (a) The external appearance of the right eye. (b) Cross-section of the human eye.

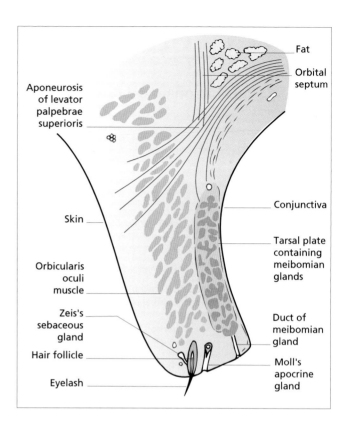

Fig. 64.2 Cross-section of upper eyelid.

the fine hairs of the eyelashes (cilia) and both apocrine and eccrine sweat glands. There are about 300 eyelashes arising in two rows along the eyelid margin, two thirds of which are in the upper lid. They have no associated erector muscles, but rudimentary sebaceous glands (of Zeis) are present. Some lashes, particularly those of the lower lid, are associated with ancillary apocrine sweat glands (of Moll). The ducts of these glands open both into the lash follicles and directly onto the anterior lid margin between the lashes. The eyelashes help to protect foreign bodies from impinging on the eyeball. Each lash follicle has a rich nerve plexus, which is easily excited and light touch initiates reflex closure.

The tarsal plate of each eyelid gives the palpebral aperture shape and stability. They comprise dense, fibrous tissue surrounding modified sebaceous glands (meibomian glands). These secrete the outer lipid layer of the precorneal tear film through openings along the mucocutaneous junction of the eyelid margin. This lipid helps stabilize the tear film and reduce evaporation. There are about 30 glands in the upper tarsal plate and 20 in the lower. Meibomian glands have up to 20 acini surrounding a central vertical duct and are visible through the conjunctiva.

The eyelids are lined by a mucous membrane called the palpebral conjunctiva. It is reflected over the anterior portion of the eyeball up to the edge of the cornea as the bulbar conjunctiva. The folds formed by the reflection of the conjunctiva from the lids onto the eyeball are called the superior and inferior palpebral fornices. The conjunctiva contains numerous goblet cells secreting mucin into the tear film. It also contains about 50 accessory lacrimal glands and its substantia propria contains neural tissue, mast cells, lymphocytes and lymphoid follicles, which are important in mediating local immunological reactions.

The striated muscle of the levator palpebrae superioris opens the eye, and the striated orbicularis oculi muscle closes it. Both are innervated by the facial nerve. Two divisions of the trigeminal nerve supply sensation to the eyelids; the upper lid and medial canthus are supplied by the ophthalmic division, and the remainder of the lower lid by the maxillary division.

The eyelid has a rich blood supply mainly through the medial and lateral palpebral arteries, which are branches of the ophthalmic artery. There is also a rich anastomosis

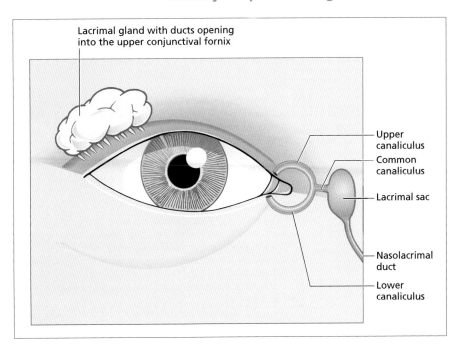

Lacrimal gland with ducts opening
into the upper conjunctival fornix

Upper
canaliculus
Common
canaliculus
Lacrimal sac
Nasolacrimal
duct
Lower
canaliculus

Fig. 64.3 The lacrimal apparatus of the
right eye.

between adjacent arteries arising from the internal and external carotid. The blood drains through a network of veins to the facial and orbital veins and the cavernous sinus. Lymphatics drain the conjunctiva and tarsal plate to the post-tarsal plexus and the skin and orbicularis to the pre-tarsal plexus. The medial canthus and lower lid subsequently drain to the submandibular nodes whilst the lateral canthus and upper lid drain to the parotid and preauricular nodes.

The lacrimal glands

The main lacrimal gland is a modified sweat gland located in the lacrimal fossa, a bony depression just under the upper and outer margin of the orbit. It produces an aqueous secretion, which discharges through a network of ductules onto the conjunctiva of the palpebral conjunctiva. In addition, there are a variable number of accessory lacrimal glands in the upper and lower conjunctival fornices. The lacrimal gland is innervated whereas the accessory glands are not.

The pre-corneal tear film

The eyelids make a vital contribution to the composition and stability of the precorneal tear film, which is about 40 μm thick. It is a three-layered structure consisting of a lower hydrophilic mucin layer secreted by goblet cells of the conjunctiva, a central aqueous layer secreted by the lacrimal gland, and a surface hydrophobic lipid layer secreted by the meibomian glands (as discussed above). Blinking consists of a lateral to medial movement of the eyelids, which enables resurfacing of the tear film of the

cornea and propels the tears to the punctum of the tear duct; from here, they are actively removed by the lacrimal pump mechanism through the lacrimal canaliculi into the common canaliculius and lacrimal sac, and then via the nasolacrimal duct into the nose (Fig. 64.3).

The tear film has a number of functions:

1 To supply oxygen and other nutrients to the cornea
2 To remove particulate matter from the surface of the eye
3 To prevent drying of the eye
4 To act as a lubricant and prevent adhesion of the palpebral to the bulbar conjunctiva
5 To protect the eye surface through its antibacterial role. It contains white blood cells, various proteins, lysozyme and immunoglobulins.

REFERENCES

1 Burns RP. Eyelids lacrimal apparatus and conjunctiva. *Arch Ophthalmol* 1968; **79**: 211–25.
2 Dickinson AJ. Anatomy physiology and malformation of the eyelids. In: Easty DL, Sparrow JM, eds. *Oxford Textbook of Ophthalmology*. Oxford: Oxford University Press, 1999: 355–60.

Glossary of ophthalmological terms

A glossary is provided in Table 64.1.

Disorders affecting the eyebrows and eyelashes

There is a wide variation in the colour distribution and density of the eyebrow hairs. The inheritance of the appearance of the eyebrows is polygenic. Some hereditary variations are of no known significance, but others are

Table 64.1 Glossary of ophthalmological terms.

Astichiasis	Absence of lashes
Anophthalmia	Absence of eye
Blepharitis	Inflammation of the eyelid margin
Blepharochalasis	Elastic tissue atrophy causing loose eyelid skin
Bruch's membrane	The retinal layer sandwiched between the retinal pigment epithelium and the vascular choroid
Coloboma	Congenital cleft created by failure of development of a portion of the eye or adnexal structures
Dermatochalasis	Laxness of the skin of the eyelids
Distichiasis	Accessory row of eyelashes
Ectropion	Eversion of the eyelid
Entropion	Inversion of the eyelid
Epicanthal fold	Accessory fold of skin at the inner canthal region of the eye
Epicanthus inversus	Lower lid fold larger than upper lid fold
Epiphora	Excess tearing
Episcleritis	Inflammation of the superficial scleral tissues
Hypertelorism	Increased distance between the two eyes measured radiologically
Hypopyon	The presence of pus in the anterior chamber
Keratopathy	Corneal abnormalities including: *exposure keratopathy*—from corneal exposure and drying of the cornea
Keratitis	Inflammation of the cornea—various types are recognized, including *filamentary keratitis*—the development of epithelialized mucous filaments on the corneal surface; *interstitial keratitis*—inflammation of the corneal stromal layer
Keratoconjunctivitis sicca	Corneal and conjunctival inflammation associated with impaired tear secretion and ocular dryness
Keratoconus	Conical distortion of the central cornea as a result of a degenerative process in the stroma
Lagophthalmos	Persistent exposure of the eyeball despite closure of the eyelid
Limbus	Boundary between the cornea and sclera
Madarosis	Loss of the eyelashes
Pannus	Vascularized corneal scar
Phlyctenule	Wedge-shaped, peripheral corneal or conjunctival, nodule
Preseptal cellulitis	Cellulitis of the eyelids that has not penetrated through the orbital septum to involve the orbit
Symblepharon	Adhesions between the bulbar and palpebral conjunctiva resulting in complete or partial obliteration of the eyelid fornices
Telecanthus	Increased distance between the inner canthi
Trichiasis	Lashes that turn inward toward the cornea usually as a result of entropion
Uveitis	Inflammation of the uveal tract. It is subdivided into anterior uveitis, which is the most common, intermediate uveitis, posterior uveitis and pan uveitis. *Anterior uveitis* is subdivided into iritis, in which the inflammation predominantly affects the iris, and iridocyclitis, in which both the iris and the anterior part of the ciliary body (pars plicata) are equally involved. *Intermediate uveitis* involves the posterior part of the ciliary body (pars plana) and the extreme periphery of the choroid and retina. *Posterior uveitis* is inflammation located behind the vitreous base. *Pan uveitis* is involvement of the entire uveal tract

associated with other development defects or are part of a recognized syndrome.

Disorders of the eyebrows [1]

Synophrys

This term is applied when the eyebrows are profuse with a tendency to meet in the centre of the face. Synophrys is a feature of some genodermatoses (Chapter 12). The eyebrows also tend to become more bushy in the ageing male for reasons that are unknown. Bushy eyebrows may also occur in other acquired forms of hypertrichosis, for example due to drugs such as diazoxide, and fusion of the eyebrows has been reported in kwashiorkor.

Hypoplasia of eyebrows

Some inherited diseases are characterized by hypoplasia

of the eyebrows (Chapter 12). Acquired conditions can cause sparsity of the eyebrows. They may be the only site affected in alopecia areata. Thinning of the eyebrows also occurs in hypothyroidism, erythroderma, follicular mucinosis and secondary syphilis. Lepromatous leprosy causes thinning of the outer third of the eyebrows in the early stages, often with depigmentation, and this progresses to total loss of the brows and lashes. Tuberculoid leprosy, by contrast, does not cause loss of the eyebrows. Plucking the eyebrows for cosmetic reasons is common, but true trichotillomania of the eyebrows is unusual.

Inflammatory disorders affecting the eyebrows

The eyebrows are often involved in seborrhoeic dermatitis and psoriasis. Post-inflammatory cicatricial alopecia from discoid lupus erythematosus, folliculitis decalvans, lupus vulgaris or tertiary syphilis may cause eyebrow loss. Scarring with loss of eyebrows may also follow chemical and thermal burns or radiation. Loss of eyebrows can be camouflaged by the use of eyebrow pencils, permanent tattooing or by a hair prosthesis glued in place daily.

Disorders of the eyelashes

Trichomegaly [2–4]

This may be due to a genetic trait. Increased growth of the eyelashes has also been described in human immunodeficiency virus (HIV) infection and related to various drugs including ciclosporin, zidovudine or interferon. Long lashes also occur in some patients with phenylketonuria.

Madarosis [1]

Madarosis is a decrease in the number or complete loss of lashes. A number of causes have been recognized and include alopecia areata, chronic anterior lid margin blepharitis, infiltrating tumours of the lid, burns, cryotherapy and radiotherapy, trichotillomania and discoid lupus erythematosus. Systemic diseases such as hypothyroidism and syphilis may also be responsible.

REFERENCES

1 Draelos ZK, Yeatts RP. Eyebrow loss, eyelash loss and dermatochalasis. *Dermatol Clin* 1992; **10**: 793–8.
2 Casanova JM, Puig T, Rubro M. Hypertrichosis of the eyelashes in acquired immunodeficiency syndrome. *Arch Dermatol* 1987; **123**: 1599–601.
3 Klutman NE, Hinthorn DR. Excessive growth of eyelashes in a patient with AIDS being treated with zidovudine. *N Engl J Med* 1991; **324**: 1896.
4 Foon KA, Dougher G. Increased growth of the lashes in a patient given leukocyte A interferon. *N Engl J Med* 1984; **311**: 1259.

Abnormality of the eyelids

These include dermatochalasis, blepharochalasis and lid laxity. Numerous developmental defects can affect the palpabral fissure or size and shape of the eyelids. A number of hereditary dermatoses affect the eyelids (Chapter 12).

Ptosis

Drooping of the eyelids on one or both sides is a common genetic defect. Mild ptosis commonly develops in the elderly due to the laxity of the connective tissue. There are many important acquired causes, such as third nerve palsy, Horner's syndrome and myasthenia gravis, which require neurological referral. Ptosis may be associated with other ocular abnormalities.

Skin diseases affecting the eyelids

A large number of dermatological conditions can affect the eyelids as part of a generalized process. Usually there is little diagnostic difficulty as the diagnosis is made by examination of the rest of the skin. Psoriasis and lichen planus can both involve the lids and cause considerable irritation. These are chronic diseases and management can become a problem with use of potent topical corticosteroids on the eyelids over a prolonged period of time. Use of the new topical immunosuppressants such as tacrolimus and pimecrolimus may offer some promise for the future in reducing topical corticosteroid exposure. Unilateral involvement of an eyelid raises the possibility of infective conditions, including tinea and mycobacterial infections.

Psoriasis [1]

Eyelid involvement can occur in about 10% of patients with psoriasis. Men are more susceptible to ocular disease. Involvement of the eyelid gives rise to blepharitis, madarosis and development of psoriatic plaques. Chronic non-specific conjunctivitis may occur over time and lead eventually to keratoconjunctivitis sicca with symblepharon formation and trichiasis. Conjunctivitis usually complicates eyelid margin involvement; white or yellow psoriatic plaques can spread from the lid on to the conjunctiva itself. Corneal changes are rare and are most commonly related to exposure and trichiasis. Anterior uveitis is rare but has been reported in patients with psoriatic arthritis and is similar to that seen in Reiter's syndrome. Ocular psoriasis is treated with use of lubricants and topical corticosteroids. Patients with chronic eyelid involvement should be referred for ophthalmological assessment.

Contact dermatitis [2–8]

Contact dermatitis is the responsible cause in approximately half of patients with an eyelid dermatitis. The remainder have manifestations of atopic or seborrhoeic dermatitis. The eyelid skin is very sensitive to primary irritants. These can cause a dermatitis in their own right or can aggravate an underlying constitutional tendency in patients with either atopic or seborrhoeic dermatitis.

Allergic contact dermatitis can present after many years of exposure to the culpable allergen. Clinically it is characterized by severe itching, erythema and swelling of the eyelid, progressing to formation of vesicles. A large variety of allergens have been reported as causing an allergic contact dermatitis of the lid and include preservatives (used in cosmetics, topical medications and contact lens cleaning solutions), fragrances and the resin used in nail polish. Patients with suspected contact dermatitis of the eyelids should be patch tested. Careful history taking is of paramount importance to make sure the relevant allergens are included in the test battery. The possibility of transferring antigen from the hands to the eyelids needs to be considered. Maibach described the upper eyelid dermatosis syndrome in which patients have discomfort of the eyelids with or without dermatitis; it is thought to be unrelated to use of cosmetics.

Periorbital oedema [9]

The subcutaneous tissue of the eyelids is lax and prone to oedema. There are many systemic and dermatological causes of eyelid oedema that need to be considered. Systemic causes include angio-oedema, glomerulonephritis, hypoalbuminaemia (especially nephrotic syndrome), cardiac failure, superior venocaval obstruction and thyroid disease. Some systemic infections such as infectious mononucleosis and scarlatina cause periorbital oedema. It may be the presenting feature of dermatomyositis and has been reported in systemic lupus erythematosus.

The most common dermatological causes of periorbital oedema are angio-oedema, lymphoedema, allergic contact dermatitis and blepharochalasis; they are usually distinguished by the history. Angio-oedema is transient and often part of a more generalized urticarial eruption. Lymphoedema is permanent and tends to be worse first thing in the morning and improves during the day; it may be associated with underlying sinus disease or a chronic inflammatory condition such as granulomatous rosacea. Allergic contact dermatitis presents acutely with swelling, redness and itching. Blepharochalasis is an uncommon condition which may be inherited (autosomal dominant) or sporadic; it presents in the second decade with recurrent episodes of painless lid oedema, resulting in the development of excess skin and thickened subcutaneous tissue which may require treatment by blepharoplasty. Senile orbital fat prolapse through a deficient orbital septum may mimic periorbital oedema but is differentiated by the fact that there is minimal fluctuation in the associated swelling.

Changes in pigmentation [10–14]

There are considerable racial and familial variations of the degree of pigmentation of the eyelids (Chapter 39). Marked periorbital melanosis is seen as a genetic trait. Pigmentation of the periorbital skin can also be post-traumatic, post-inflammatory or can accompany melanocyte-stimulating hormone-induced melanosis of any cause. Chemical pigmentation can occur from prolonged use of a mercurial or silver preparation producing a slate-blue or grey-brown discoloration. Mauve discoloration of the eyelids and periorbital area is an early part of chrysiasis from parenteral gold therapy. A grey discoloration can complicate long-term treatment with minocycline. Local increase in pigmentation may also be due to cosmetics containing phototoxic agents, usually psoralens. Increased pigmentation can also follow inflammatory dermatoses such as eczema and lichen planus. The eyelids may be involved in vitiligo. Hypopigmentation can complicate

the use of topical medications including thiotepa eye drops and mercurial ointments.

REFERENCES

1 Steiner G, Arffa RC. Psoriasis, ichthyosis and porphyria. *Int Ophthalmol Clin* 1997; **37**: 41–61.
2 Guin JD. Eyelid dermatitis: experience in 203 cases. *J Am Acad Dermatol* 2002; **47**: 755–65.
3 Nethercott JR, Nield G, Holmes DL. A review of 79 cases of eyelid dermatitis. *J Am Acad Dermatol* 1989; **21**: 223–30.
4 Valecchi R, Imberti G, Martinod D, Carnelli T. Eyelid dermatitis—an evaluation of 150 patients. *Contact Dermatitis* 1992; **27**: 143–7.
5 Shah M, Lewis FM, Gawkrodger DJ. Facial dermatitis and eyelid dermatitis—a comparison of patch tests results and final diagnosis. *Contact Dermatitis* 1992; **27**: 143–7.
6 Rapaport M. Contact dermatitis secondary to chlorhexidine in contact lens cleansing solution. *Am J Contact Dermat* 1991; **2**: 65–6.
7 Herbst RA, Maibach HI. Contact dermatitis caused by allergy to ophthalmic drugs and contact lens solutions. *Contact Dermatitis* 1991; **25**: 305–12.
8 Maibach HI, Engasser P, Ostler B. Upper eyelid dermatosis syndrome. *Dermatol Clin* 1992; **10**: 549–54.
9 Jarek MJ, Finger DR, Gillil UR, Giandoni MB. Periorbital oedema and Mees' lines in systemic lupus erythematosus. Non-specific but disease-related skin lesions. *J Clin Rheumatol* 1996; **2**: 156–9.
10 Hunzinger N. Apropos of familial hyperpigmentation of the eyelid. *J Genet Hum* 1962; **11**: 16–21.
11 Aguilera Diaz L. Hyperpigmentation of the eyelids. *Ann Dermatol Syphiligr (Paris)* 1972; **99**: 43–6.
12 Smith RW, Leppard B, Barnett NL et al. Chrysiasis revisited a clinical and pathological study. *Br J Dermatol* 1995; **133**: 671–8.
13 Cowan CI, Halder RM, Grimes PE. Ocular disturbances in vitiligo. *J Am Acad Dermatol* 1986; **15**: 17–24.
14 Harben DJ, Cooper PH, Rodman OG. Thiotepa induced leucoderma. *Arch Dermatol* 1979; **115**: 973–4.

Chronic blepharitis, rosacea and seborrhoeic dermatitis [1–4]

Description. Chronic blepharitis is a term that is used to describe a group of disorders in which the lid margin is always involved. These disorders often occur simultaneously. Not all of them result in inflammation of the lid margin. They are frequently associated with a conjunctivitis or keratoconjunctivitis. Chronic blepharitis may occur in the absence of any significant dermatological association and its classification is further complicated, both by the variable association of chronic blepharitis with rosacea and seborrhoeic dermatitis, and also by the term ocular rosacea, a condition which may occur in the absence of dermatological rosacea.

It is hardly surprising that this classification causes confusion amongst practitioners. This situation has arisen partly because there is no consensus about the terminology (although most modern authors use similar classifications based on McCulley's modification of Thygeson's classification) and, more probably, because the pathogenesis is very poorly understood with few unifying concepts.

Table 64.2 summarizes a current classification, associations and features. It includes ocular rosacea amongst the meibomian gland disorders with which it is always

Table 64.2 Classification of types of chronic blepharitis (lid margin disorders).

Anterior lid margin*		Posterior lid margin*		
Staphylococcal blepharitis	Seborrhoeic blepharitis	Meibomitis/ocular rosacea	Meibomian gland dysfunction	Meibomian seborrhoea
Associations with other types of blepharitis				
Secondary meibomitis	Any posterior lid margin condition	Staphylococcal & seborrhoeic blepharitis	Seborrhoeic blepharitis	Seborrhoeic blepharitis
Associated skin disease				
Atopic eczema Impetigo Rosacea (rare)	Seborrhoea Rosacea (rare)	Acne rosacea in up to 50% of cases	Acne rosacea in up to 50% of cases	
Associated eye disease				
Dry eye Atopic kerato-conjunctivitis		Scleritis and episcleritis in ocular rosacea		
Main features				
Symptoms Burning Itching Photophobia	Minimal	Foreign body sensation Burning Discomfort Photophobia with ocular rosacea	Variable: Foreign body sensation Burning Discomfort	Variable: Foreign body sensation Burning Discomfort
Lid signs Unilateral/patchy lid margin involvement (Fig. 64.4d) Brittle fibrinous scales bleed when detached, form collarettes at lash base (Fig. 64.4a) Dilated vessels, styes Poliosis and madarosis (Fig. 64.4b)	Bilateral greasy scales (not fibrinous)	Chalazia (Fig. 64.5b) Irregular lid margins Distorted meibomian orifices Inspissated secretions Expression difficult Surrounding inflammation For lid signs in ocular rosacea see Table 64.3		Plugged and elevated orifices without inflammation
Conjunctival & corneal signs Follicles, papillae and hyperaemia of lower tarsal conjunctiva and fornix (Fig. 64.4c) Coarse punctate keratitis in lower third of cornea. Marginal keratitis (Fig. 64.4e) and vascularization. Conjunctival scarring (Fig. 64.5a)		Early tear break up time Foam/debris in tears Punctate keratitis (dry eye) For conjunctival and corneal signs in ocular rosacea see Table 64.3		Minimal injection ± Foamy tear film

* The anterior lid margin is the portion anterior to the meibomian gland orifices and the posterior lid margin is behind this, including the meibomian glands. Anterior and posterior lid margin disorders are commonly mixed; frequent associations are shown in the table.

associated. Table 64.2 classifies the five types of blepharitis (including ocular rosacea) into those principally affecting the anterior lid margin structures (cutaneous margin with lash-bearing skin and associated glands) or the posterior lid margin (mucocutaneous junction, meibomian orifices). This classification simplifies the treatment because this differs between the anterior- and posterior-lid margin disorders but not between the individual conditions within the anterior- and posterior-lid margin groups. The commoner clinical signs of staphylococcal blepharitis are shown in Fig. 64.4. Ocular rosacea (Table 64.3, Fig. 64.5) is an important condition because of its severity and wide spectrum of clinical features.

In addition to these very common types of blepharitis, there are other chronic causes in which the pathogenesis is clear. These are all uncommon and are often misdiagnosed as one of the types of chronic blepharitis described in Table 64.2. They include fungal infection (e.g. *Candida*), parasitic infection (e.g. phthiriasis), protozoal infection (e.g. leishmaniasis), some neoplasms, and autoimmune conditions such as lupus erythematosus; some of these are illustrated in Fig. 64.6. They should be considered when therapy for conventional blepharitis fails.

Acute blepharitis is a clearly defined group of conditions, which may overlap with the chronic blepharitis causes summarized in Table 64.4.

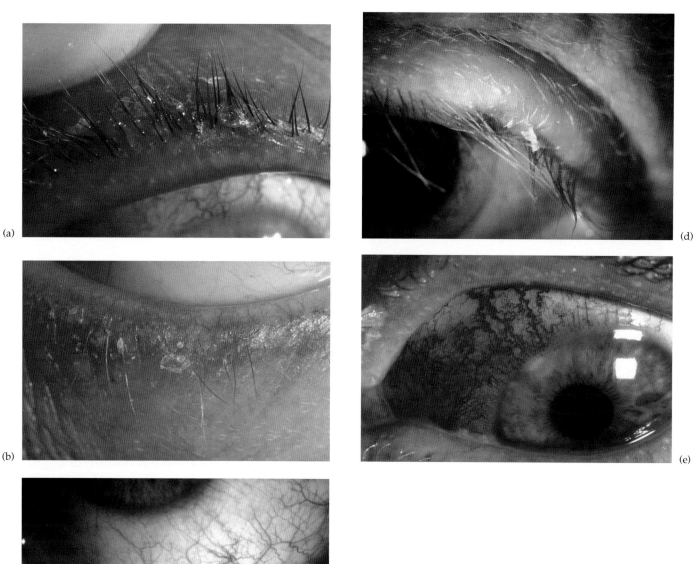

(a)

(b)

(c)

(d)

(e)

Fig. 64.4 Staphylococcal blepharitis. (a) Fibrinous 'collarettes' lifting away from the skin as the lashes grow. (b) Fibrinous scales on the anterior lid margin with the madarosis (loss of lashes) and poliosis (white lashes) that accompanies chronic blepharitis. (c) Follicular conjunctivitis with arrows showing the white/yellow follicles. (d) Localized ulcerative blepharitis. Sectoral disease like this is quite common in staphylococcal blepharitis which can also be largely unilateral. (e) Marginal ulceration, a common corneal complication of staphylococcal blepharitis.

Epidemiology

The epidemiology has been dogged by difficulties of disease definition and the different perspectives of dermatologists and ophthalmologists. Chronic blepharitis is one of the commonest disorders in both ophthalmic and general medical practice. In general medical practice it makes up about 70% of ophthalmic referrals, which themselves account for between 2% and 7% of all outpatient

consultations. Meibomian gland dysfunction is probably the commonest type of blepharitis and affects 20–40% of all patients consulting ophthalmologists for routine eye examinations. Between 3% and 58% of patients with rosacea have ocular involvement, this wide variation being the result of differences in disease definition. Approximately half the patients with rosacea have signs of ocular rosacea whereas one quarter of patients with ocular rosacea have no dermatological disease.

Table 64.3 Clinical signs of ocular rosacea.

Signs	Common	Uncommon	Rare
Lid	Meibomitis (Fig. 64.5a) Seborrhoeic blepharitis Lid margin telangiectasia Lid notching Retroplacement of the mucocutaneous junction Chalazia (Fig. 64.5b) Hordeoleum	Entropion	
Conjunctiva	Conjunctival hyperaemia Papillary conjunctivitis	Reticular and linear tarsal scarring and fornix shortening	
Cornea	Phlyctenular keratoconjunctivitis Marginal corneal infiltration and ulceration (Fig. 64.5d,e)	Pseudopterygium	Corneal perforation
Sclera and episclera		Episcleritis	Scleritis

Immunopathogenesis [5]

There is some evidence to support hypotheses of pathogenesis in staphylococcal blepharitis and in meibomian dysfunction, but the pathogenesis is even more poorly understood in the other types of chronic blepharitis.

Staphylococcal blepharitis

In staphylococcal blepharitis [6–13] there is an association with *Staphylococcus aureus* and *S. epidermidis* colonization of the lid margins, although colonization by *S. aureus* is often transient and the numbers of either organism are often no greater than in normal controls. Although folliculitis, styes and lid margin ulcers may be due to infection by *S. aureus*, the persistence of lid inflammation after treatment and the sterile marginal ulcers are not explained by infection alone. The importance of cell-mediated immunity in the pathogenesis of the disease was shown by experimental studies in rabbits; when these were immunized with either whole *S. aureus* or with cell wall ribitol–teichoic acid, both ulcerative keratitis, phlyctenules and marginal corneal ulcers developed after secondary challenge, providing evidence for the hypothesis that these changes were due to the development of hypersensitivity to both viable and killed organisms. These finding could not be reproduced for *S. epidermidis*. However the evidence for a similar pathogenesis in humans is lacking; the relationship between the clinical signs of staphylococcal blepharitis and hypersensitivity to subcutaneous injections of either whole *S. aureus* or of *S. aureus* cell wall protein A is poor. *Staphylococcus epidermidis* is more often isolated than *S. aureus* from the lids of patients with staphylococcal blepharitis, but the evidence of the role of a hypersensitivity response is assumed and not supported by any data. The pathogenesis of the, often severe, follicular and papillary conjunctivitis that accompanies this condition is assumed to be due to a combination of transient infection and hypersensitivity.

Meibomian gland disease (MGD) [14–16]

The meibomian lipids (meibum) are a complex mixture of cholesterol esters and esterified unsaturated fatty acids. These lipids are responsible for maintaining a stable tear film, reducing tear film evaporation and, therefore, drying of the ocular surface, preventing tear spill over the lid margins by lowering surface tension and reducing ocular surface contamination, by sebum, from the cutaneous surface of the lids which otherwise forms dry spots.

Three factors have been invoked as contributing to MGD: (i) keratinization of the meibomian ductules; (ii) the effect of bacterial lipases on the meibum at the lid margin; and (iii) primary abnormalities in the production of meibum by individuals with MGD.

Normal meibomian gland ducts open just anterior to the mucocutaneous junction. As the duct lining is partially keratinized, abnormalities of keratinization, analogous to those present in the sebaceous glands of patients with rosacea, may be important in the pathogenesis of MGD by altering gland function. Bacterial lipases are produced by all the bacteria that colonize the lid margin and have the potential to break down meibum into free fatty acids that will destabilize the tear film. These bacteria colonize the gland orifices and expression of lipid from deeper within the glands can stabilize the tear film. Meibomian lipids differ between individuals and, as analytical methods increase in sensitivity, the relative roles of primary abnormalities of meibum, and those secondary to the effects of bacterial lipases in the pathogenesis of MGD, are likely to become clearer.

Neither the pathogenesis of the conjunctival inflammation that is common in meibomitis (and which is a feature of ocular rosacea), nor that of the keratitis in ocular rosacea, has been explained.

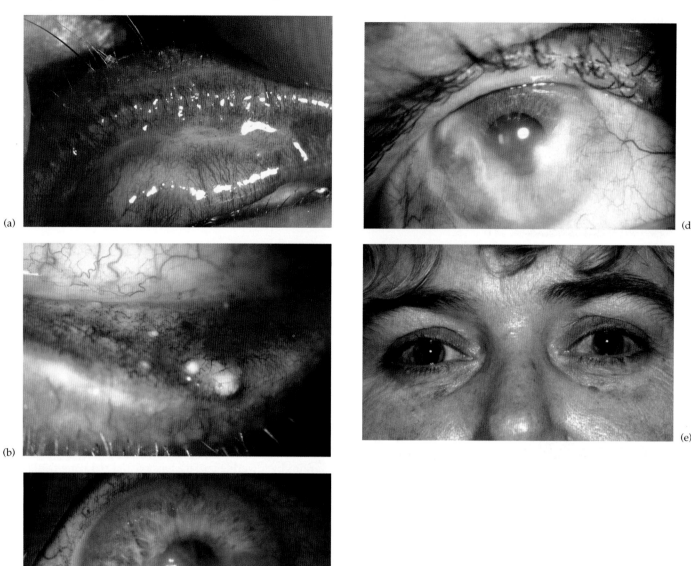

(a)

(b)

(c)

(d)

(e)

Fig. 64.5 Ocular rosacea. (a) Scales on the anterior lid margin, meibomitis with posterior migration of the orifices associated with loss of the normal posterior lid margin architecture and scarring in the superior tarsal marginal sulcus. Entropion and trichiasis may result from this degree of scarring. (b) Meibomian dysfunction with blocked glands and small chalazia. (c) Marginal ulceration complicated by frank bacterial superinfection with an hypopyon ulcer. (d,e) Rosacea keratitis showing the right cornea (d) of the patient whose eyes are shown in (e).

Treatment [17–23]

The treatment of blepharitis is that of the underlying cause, if a specific cause can be identified. Treatment for the principal causes of chronic blepharitis is outlined in Table 64.5. The blepharitis should initially be classified into either anterior or posterior lid disease or both (Table 64.2). It is important to decide whether blepharitis is the cause of the symptoms; seborrhoea rarely causes symp-

toms and should not be used as a scapegoat to explain away symptoms possibly due to other, or undiagnosable, conditions. Other conditions that give rise to similar symptoms and signs (Table 64.2) should be excluded or treated. Symptoms of dry eye and associated skin disorders should also be treated.

Diffuse folliculitis is generally caused by *S. aureus* and requires a course of an appropriate systemic antibiotic. Laboratory investigations are of limited value—bacteriology

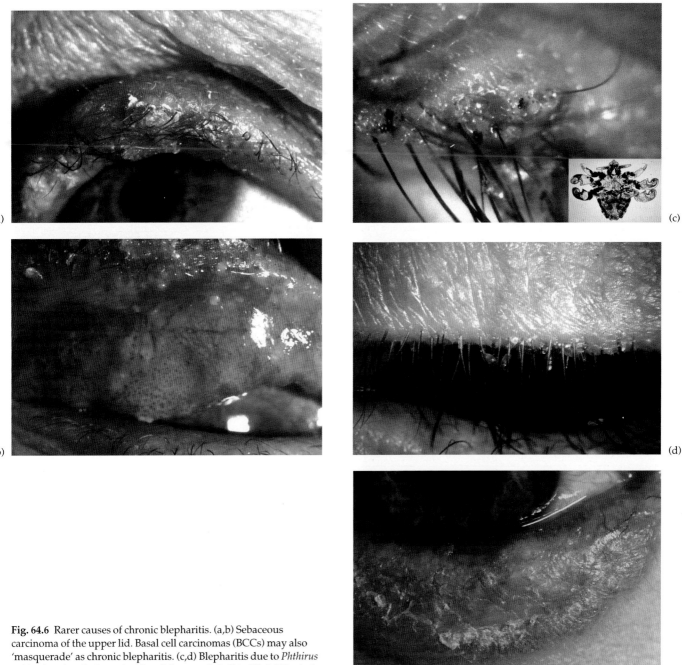

Fig. 64.6 Rarer causes of chronic blepharitis. (a,b) Sebaceous carcinoma of the upper lid. Basal cell carcinomas (BCCs) may also 'masquerade' as chronic blepharitis. (c,d) Blepharitis due to *Phthirus pubis*, showing the louse in (c) and the eggs ('nits') in (d). (e) Typical lid lesion of discoid lupus.

Table 64.4 Causes of acute blepharitis.

Acute anterior lid margin	Folliculitis (infected lash follicles)
	External hordeoleum (stye)
	Angular (at lateral canthus)
	Impetigo
	Pustular (herpes infections)
Acute posterior lid margin	Chalazion
	Internal hordeoleum
Generalized anterior and posterior	Necrotizing fasciitis

samples can be taken from lid margins using swabs dipped in trypsin digest broth, but are usually only performed for recurrent disease that has not responded to initial therapy.

Chalazion will resolve in time, approximately 60% of lesions will resolve in 6 months and the remainder will resolve spontaneously given longer. Resolution of chalazia can be hastened by incision and curettage; the lid is incised, usually from the conjunctival surface under local anaesthesia, and the necrotic granulomatous tissue in the

Table 64.5 Treatment of chronic blepharitis.

Aims of treatment	Therapeutic guidelines
For anterior lid margin disease (ALMD)	
Treat infection	Staphylococcal and mixed staphylococcal/seborrhoeic groups
	Topical antibiotics—chloramphenicol or fucidic acid—four times daily to lid margins
	Oral oxytetracycline or erythromycin 500 mg b.d. for 10 days
Clean lid margins	'Lid scrubs': 1–2 times daily with cotton wool bud dampened in boiled water or with proprietary lid cleaning pads, to remove debris
Lid hyperaemia and exudate	Topical chloramphenicol and hydrocortisone 0.5–1.0% to lid margins 2–4 times daily for 1 month
For posterior lid margin disease (PLMD)	
Mechanically unblock meibomian glands	Apply hot compresses for 3–5 min to liquefy meibomian secretions, followed by massage* of tarsal plate with cotton wool bud (or finger), to express lipid from glands, 1–2 times daily
Alter meibomian secretions	Oral oxytetracycline (doxycycline 100 mg o.d.) or erythromycin 250–500 mg b.d. for 12 weeks minimum
For the tear film	
Restore tear film	Artificial tears—drops 2–4 hrly, or Viscotears 3–4 times daily
For associated conjunctivitis (papillary or mixed follicular and papillary)	
Reduce inflammation	Fluoromethalone 0.1% four times daily for 1 week, progressively reducing to one time daily over a further 4 weeks
Treat associated skin disease	Seborrhoea—medicated soap and shampoo (ideally containing glycolic acid 10–15%)
	Rosacea—oral oxytetracycline (or doxycycline 100 mg) or erythromycin 250–500 mg b.d. for 12 weeks
For keratitis	
Coarse punctate keratitis and/or marginal keratoconjunctivitis	Fluoromethalone 0.1% four times daily for 1 week, progressively reducing to once daily over a further four weeks†
Corneal thinning and perforation	Exclude and treat any concomitant microbial keratitis and establish disease control by methods summarized above, apply tissue glue to perforations. Carry out tectonic keratoplasty, if necessary, once the inflammation is controlled.

* Lid scrubs, lid massage and low dose systemic antibiotics take about 4–6 weeks to start to work. DO NOT assume treatment has failed until at least 8 weeks on treatment has elapsed, and continue the regime for a minimum of 2–3 months if benefit is shown. Then advise a maintenance regime of lid scrubs (for ALMD), hot compresses and tarsal massage (for PLMD), ± artificial tears. In the case of relapse, repeat a 3-month course of oral antibiotic treatment.

† More prolonged courses of corticosteroid or more potent corticosteroids may be needed under specialist ophthalmological supervision.

centre of the lesion removed with a curette. This leaves a linear conjunctival and tarsal scar. It is only recommended for cosmetic reasons or to improve vision in large lesions affecting the upper lid which can cause temporary astigmatism.

Practice points for dermatologists are that the association between blepharitis and skin disease is variable, that treatment with tetracyclines may be beneficial for both the ocular and dermatological manifestations of these disorders, and that ocular rosacea and staphylococcal blepharitis may produce sight-threatening complications.

REFERENCES

1 McCulley JP, Dougherty JM, Deneau DG. Classification of chronic blepharitis. *Ophthalmology* 1982; **89**: 1173–80.
2 Browning DJ, Proia AD. Ocular rosacea. *Surv Ophthalmol* 1986; **31**: 145–58.
3 Akpek EK, Merchant A, Pinar V, Foster CS. Ocular rosacea. *Ophthalmology* 1997; **104**: 1863–7.
4 Erzurum SA, Feder RS, Greenwald MJ. Acne rosacea with keratitis in childhood. *Arch Ophthalmol* 1993; **111**: 228–30.
5 Huang-Xuan T, Rodriguez A, Zaltas MM, Rice B, Foster CS. Ocular rosacea. A histologic and immunopathologic study. *Ophthalmology* 1990; **97**: 1468–75.
6 Mondino BJ, Brawman-Mintsev O, Adamu S. Corneal antibody levels to ribitol teichoic acid in rabbits immunised with staphylococcal antigen using various routes. *Invest Ophthalmol Vis Sci* 1987; **28**: 1553–8.
7 Mondino BJ, Caster AI, Dethlefs B. A rabbit model of staphylococcal blepharitis. *Arch Ophthalmol* 1987; **105**: 409–12.
8 Mondino BJ, Dethlefs B. Occurrence of phylctenules after immunisation with ribitol teichoic acid of *S. aureus*. *Arch Ophthalmol* 1984; **102**: 461–3.
9 Mondino BJ, Kowalski R, Ratajczak HV *et al.* Rabbit model of phylctenulosis and catarrhal infiltrates. *Arch Ophthalmol* 1981; **99**: 891–5.
10 Shine WE, Silvany R, McCulley JP. Relation of cholesterol stimulated *Staphylococcus aureus* growth to chronic blepharitis. *Invest Ophthalmol Vis Sci* 1993; **34**: 2291–6.
11 Dougherty JM, McCulley JP. Comparative bacteriology of chronic blepharitis. *Br J Dermatol* 1984; **68**: 524–8.
12 Dougherty JM, McCulley JP. Bacterial lipases and chronic blepharitis. *Invest Ophthalmol Vis Sci* 1986; **27**: 484–91.
13 Thygeson P. Complications of staphylococcal blepharitis. *Am J Ophthalmol* 1969; **68**: 446–9.
14 McCulley JP, Scialis GF. Meibomian keratoconjunctivitis. *Am J Ophthalmol* 1977; **84**: 788–93.
15 Mathers WD. Ocular evaporation in meibomian gland dysfunction and dry eye. *Ophthalmology* 1993; **10**: 347–51.

16 Yokoi N, Mossa F, Tiffany JM, Bron AJ. Assessment of meibomian gland function in dry eye using meibometry. *Arch Ophthalmol* 1999; **117**: 723–9.

17 Huber-Spitzy V, Baumgartner I, Bohler-Sommeregger K, Grabner G. Blepharitis—a diagnostic and therapeutic challenge: a report on 407 consecutive cases. *Graefes Arch Clin Exp Ophthalmol* 1991; **229**: 224–7.

18 Thygeson S. Etiology and treatment of blepharitis: a study in military personnel. *Arch Ophthalmol* 1946; **36**: 445–77.

19 Brown SI, Shahinian L Jr. Diagnosis and treatment of ocular rosacea. *Ophthalmology* 1978; **85**: 779–86.

20 Bartholomew RS, Reid BJ, Cheeseborough MJ, McDonald M, Galloway NR. Oxytetracycline in the treatment of ocular rosacea: a double blind trial. *Br J Ophthalmol* 1982; **66**: 386–8.

21 Frucht-Pery J, Sagi E, Hemo I, Ever-Hadani P. Effficacy of doxycycline and tetracycline on ocular rosacea. *Am J Ophthalmol* 1993; **116**: 88–92.

22 Dougherty JM, McCulley JP, Silvany RE, Meyer DR. The role of tetracycline in chronic blepharitis. Inhibition of lipase production in staphylococci. *Invest Ophthalmol Vis Sci* 1991; **32**: 2970–5.

23 Lemp MA, Mahmood MA, Weiler HH. Association of ocular rosacea and keratoconjunctivitis sicca. *Arch Ophthalmol* 1984; **102**: 556–7.

Atopy and atopic eye disease

Description and epidemiology [1–5]

This group of disorders, usually known as the allergic eye diseases, is better termed the atopic eye diseases to distinguish them from disorders which result from other hypersensitivity mechanisms. The atopic eye diseases comprise a group of disorders which have in common a papillary conjunctivitis and evidence of a type 1 allergic mechanism; the immunopathogenesis has recently been shown to be more complex than this. Table 64.6 summarizes these disorders and Fig. 64.7 shows the commoner clinical signs.

Of these disorders only atopic keratoconjunctivitis (AKC) (Figs 64.7b,g), atopic blepharoconjunctivitis (ABC) and vernal keratoconjunctivitis (VKC) (Figs 64.7c,d) are of interest to the dermatologist because of their association with atopic dermatitis and will be described here. Of these AKC and VKC are sight-threatening disorders that are often difficult to treat; VKC occurs in children and 90% of cases resolve in adult life. All of these diseases are uncommon. Only a small proportion of patients with atopic dermatitis have ocular disease. The severity of symptoms is closely related to disease activity, and patients with minimal symptoms will respond to simple treatment with antihistamines and/or mast cell stabilizers that have an excellent safety profile. However, acute exacerbations of AKC and VKC must be recognized and treated promptly as these may develop within hours and can lead to blinding corneal complications within 1–2 days.

Symptoms are similar for all of these atopic eye diseases. Typically there is itching, watering and the production of a sticky white and stringy mucous discharge. During exacerbations the symptoms increase in severity very rapidly—the itching may be superseded by extreme discomfort with soreness and a foreign body sensation, and the vision deteriorates. The lids may be difficult to open in the morning because of a combination of discomfort and discharge.

Signs that can be seen without a slit-lamp examination are thickened lids; in AKC and ABC the lid margins are usually inflamed, crusted and excoriated with madarosis (Fig. 64.7g). Lid margin signs are uncommon in VKC. The bulbar conjunctiva is inflamed during exacerbations but otherwise grossly normal except for the limbal region which may be thickened and nodular (Fig. 64.7d) with the presence of pinpoint Trantas' dots at the apices of the nodules; these may be present in AKC and in the limbal type of VKC. The distinction between limbal and palpebral VKC is principally of interest to the ophthalmologist; in the UK the limbal form of the disease is generally easier to manage although this may not be the case in Africa. The lower tarsal conjunctiva is usually less abnormal than that of the upper lid, which can be seen to be thickened and velvety when the lid is everted. In VKC, and in some cases of AKC, 'giant' compound papillae are easily seen (Fig. 64.7c). In adults with long-standing disease there is sheet-like scarring of the upper tarsal conjunctiva and shortening of the lower conjunctival fornix. During exacerbations the tarsal conjunctiva becomes very inflamed and covered in adherent mucous. The corneal signs, with the exception of plaque (Fig. 64.7e) or ulceration due to superadded infection (Fig. 64.7f), are difficult to see without a slit lamp but fluorescein staining is diffuse during flare-ups of disease.

Diagnosis

The clinical features, together with a personal or family history of atopy, are usually sufficient for diagnosis. Laboratory investigations are only needed in patients who do not respond to therapy or who require topical (or systemic) immunosuppressive therapy for relief of symptoms, or when the diagnosis is uncertain. Serum IgE and skin prick tests have no value in the diagnosis of atopic conjunctivitis as the results do not indicate the antigens precipitating the eye disease. Ophthalmic investigations are the province of the ophthalmologist and are summarized in Table 64.6.

Immunopathogenesis [6–9]

Recent advances in the understanding of these diseases have come from investigations of the humoral mediators of inflammation in the tears, and analysis of the cellular components by immunostaining and *in situ* hybridization. These techniques have shown that seasonal allergic conjunctivitis (SAC) and perennial allergic conjunctivitis (PAC) are primarily typical type 1 hypersensitivity diseases, whereas the others show varying degrees of a coexisting type 4 hypersensitivity response. SAC and PAC show mast cells and eosinophils in the conjunctival mucosa and submucosa, with high levels of locally produced IgE to specific allergens being present in the tears.

Table 64.6 Clinical characteristics and distinguishing features and diagnosis of the atopic eye diseases.

Disease	Disease course	Conjunctival signs	Corneal signs	Disease associations	Diagnostic tests
Seasonal allergic conjunctivitis (SAC)	Onset 5–20 years Spontaneous remissions common Rare in old age Strikingly seasonal	Hyperaemia. Stringy white discharge. Oedema Micropapillae if severe	None	Personal or family history of atopy including atopic dermatitis	*Cytology:* usually normal. Serum & tear IgE often elevated but not diagnostic
Perennial allergic conjunctivitis (PAC)	As for SAC but symptoms all year round with seasonal exacerbations	Hyperaemia, stringy white discharge, micropapillae common	None	Personal or family history of atopy including atopic dermatitis	
Atopic keratoconjunctivitis (AKC)	Onset between 20–50 years. Chronic course over many years (Fig. 64.7g). Spontaneous resolution in old age Non-seasonal	Micropapillae with intense infiltrate (Fig. 64.7b). Reticular and sheet scarring. Shortened fornices in some cases Trantas' dots*	Punctate epithelial keratopathy, pannus, macroerosion† and plaque‡ Pseudogerontoxon§. Herpes keratitis and bacterial keratitis (Fig. 64.7f) common	*Systemic:* atopy and atopic dermatitis in all cases *Ocular:* staphylococcal lid disease, cataract, keratoconus, herpes simplex keratitis (often bilateral)	*Cytology:* shows eosinophils and mast cells. Serum IgE elevated. Skin prick tests positive to many allergens but not diagnostic *Upper tarsal conjunctival punch biopsy:* the gold standard for disease confirmation after a 2 week abstention from use of topical corticosteroids *Tear IgE:* useful unless the serum IgE is very high; an office test is now available (*Lacrytest* from Adiatec SA, France)
Atopic blepharoconjunctivitis (ABC)	As for AKC	Micropapillae with intense infiltrate, reticular scarring	None	Personal or family history of atopy	
Vernal keratoconjunctivitis (VKC)—*palpebral, limbal and mixed forms*	Onset between 5–15 years. Spontaneous resolution in 95% after 10 years Seasonal exacerbations usual	*Palpebral form:* giant upper tarsal papillae (Fig. 64.7c) often bilaterally asymetrical *Limbal form:* micropapillae on upper tarsus but gelatinous macropapillae at limbus (Fig. 64.7d). Trantas' dots in both *Mixed form:* combines features of both diseases	*Palpebral form:* punctate epithelial keratopathy affecting upper half of cornea. Adherent mucous appearing as superficial syncytial opacity progressing to macroerosion and vernal plaque (Fig. 64.7e) *Limbal form:* keratopathy extending in from limbus with associated epithelial dysplasia	*Ocular:* keratoconus and cataract *Systemic:* atopy in variable proportions from 0–100% depending on geographical location (atopy common in Northern Europe but rare in Middle East)	

* Trantas' dots: white pinhead sized dots consisting of eosinophils and necrotic epithelial cells.
† Macroerosion: large epithelial erosions usually in upper half of cornea.
‡ Plaque (vernal plaque): laminated structure of protein and polysaccharide adherent to the anterior stroma with destruction of Bowman's layer.
§ Pseudogerontoxon: arcus-like appearance in relation to limbal pannus; may disappear in remissions.

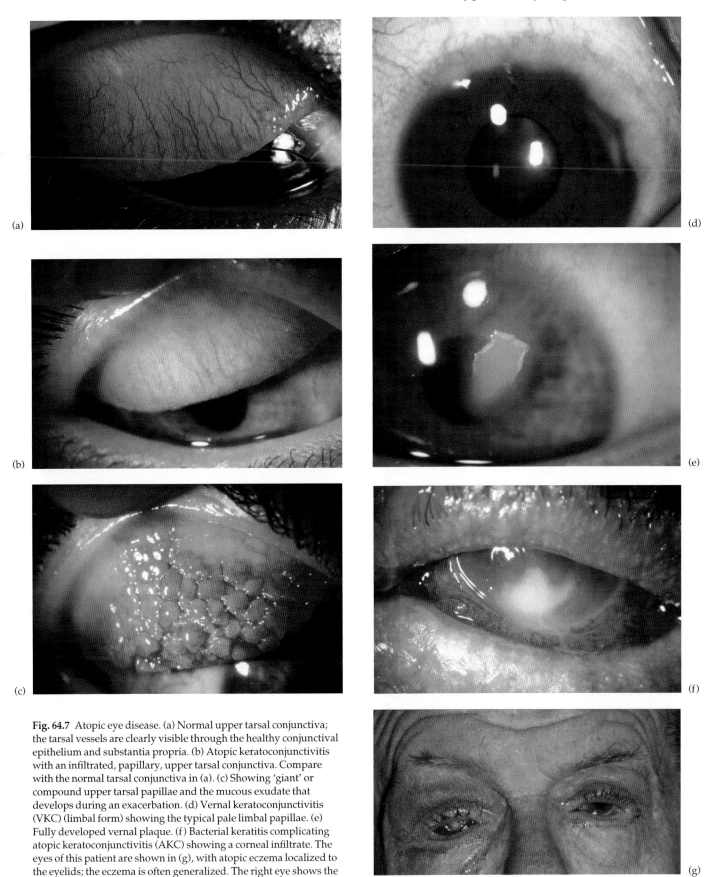

Fig. 64.7 Atopic eye disease. (a) Normal upper tarsal conjunctiva; the tarsal vessels are clearly visible through the healthy conjunctival epithelium and substantia propria. (b) Atopic keratoconjunctivitis with an infiltrated, papillary, upper tarsal conjunctiva. Compare with the normal tarsal conjunctiva in (a). (c) Showing 'giant' or compound upper tarsal papillae and the mucous exudate that develops during an exacerbation. (d) Vernal keratoconjunctivitis (VKC) (limbal form) showing the typical pale limbal papillae. (e) Fully developed vernal plaque. (f) Bacterial keratitis complicating atopic keratoconjunctivitis (AKC) showing a corneal infiltrate. The eyes of this patient are shown in (g), with atopic eczema localized to the eyelids; the eczema is often generalized. The right eye shows the infection in (f).

The diseases can be mimicked by topical instillation of antigen; this reaction is blocked by drugs that are active against mast cells. AKC and VKC show both the cellular components present in SAC and VKC but also connective tissue hyperplasia, CD4 T lymphocytes and plasma cells, together with different subsets of mast cells. The T cells are probably important inducers of the cellular inflammatory response in these diseases. Differences in AKC and VKC phenotypes may be explained by differences in the predominance of T-helper subsets; the Th1 subset, predominant in delayed type hypersensitivity responses and inactivated by ciclosporin, is more predominant in AKC than in VKC, in which the Th2 subset, with a B-cell-helper role, may be more important. Mast cells and eosinophils are found in larger numbers in VKC than in AKC and functional heterogeneity in their populations may also be determinants of disease phenotype.

These effector cell types are known to cause atopic eye diseases by the following mechanisms. Mast cells release preformed mediators by exocytosis when they degranulate in response to binding of IgE with allergen. The important mediators released are histamine, resulting in hyperaemia, oedema and mucous production, and prostaglandins. Histamine has been detected in the tears in these diseases. Eosinophils release cationic proteins including major basic protein, which is epitheliotoxic and has been identified in the tears in VKC. It is probably a major factor responsible for the development of corneal epithelial erosions and macroerosion. The presence of the latter, with the mucous and debris present in an acute exacerbation of keratopathy, accounts for the formation of plaque. B cells produce IgE locally in atopic conjunctivitis; locally produced IgE is an important factor in the pathogenesis of SAC, PAC and some cases of VKC, but less so in AKC and ABC.

Management [10,11]

The management of VKC and AKC requires specialized ophthalmological care, as these diseases are uncommon, and some of the management strategies are outside the remit of the general ophthalmologist. Topical cromones (sodium cromoglycate 2–4% or the more recently introduced nedocromil or lodoxamide) are the first-line treatment given 1–4 times daily depending on symptoms. The newer cromones have been more effective in trials of SAC. Addition of a potent topical antihistamine (levocabastine or emedastine) or a systemic antihistamine may help relieve itch. These treatments are very safe and do not require ophthalmological supervision but are only effective for very mild disease. Cromones are often not tolerated until the inflammation is brought under control with high dose topical corticosteroids such as dexamethasone 0.1% or prednisolone acetate 1%. These will precipitate glaucoma in 10% of patients as well as contributing to cataract;

as soon as the disease is brought under control, a 'safe' corticosteroid with a lower risk of precipitating glaucoma (about 1% risk) should be substituted (fluoromethalone, rimexolone or clobetasone). Cromones are used topically, whenever possible, as corticosteroid-sparing drugs.

Topical ciclosporin is not yet available commercially, although a preparation designed for use in dry eye is expected to be available soon (Restasis, Allergan, USA). It has shown promise in trials for AKC. Trials of ciclosporin 2% (available from some hospital pharmacies) have been very encouraging and a 0.02% veterinary ointment (Optimmune, Schering) has been successfully used by the authors. Adverse effects, apart from stinging, are infrequent and introduction of the drug as a corticosteroid sparing agent, for patients requiring high doses of topical corticosteroids, has allowed reduction or complete withdrawal of corticosteroids in many cases. Topical ciclosporin is most successfully tolerated if introduced during remissions.

Systemic immunosuppression is needed in severe exacerbations of disease; a 3–4 week course of systemic corticosteroids starting at a prednisolone dose of 60 mg daily, may be necessary to bring the disease under control while topical therapy is introduced. These also carry a risk of glaucoma. Patients with a previous history of labial or ocular herpes simplex (HSV), or serological evidence of previous exposure to HSV, should be aware that they may develop herpetic keratitis while on systemic or topical corticosteroids. Patients who have had previous episodes of ocular HSV should receive prophylaxis with oral aciclovir 400 mg b.d. (or valaciclovir 500 mg o.d.); topical prophylaxis is unnecessary and may complicate the clinical signs in patients with a complex keratoconjunctivitis. Patients with AKC are predisposed to bilateral herpes keratitis and prophylactic antivirals are advisable when they are using corticosteroids.

For a small number of patients, systemic ciclosporin (usually starting at 5 mg/kg) can be very helpful. Patients who need systemic ciclosporin for management of their atopic eczema will usually obtain substantial collateral ocular benefits.

Severe staphylococcal blepharitis often accompanies AKC and ABC and can be treated with a course of azithromycin followed by local therapy with an antibiotic ointment to which the skin flora is sensitive, usually chloramphenicol, together with a topical ophthalmic corticosteroid ointment such as hydrocortisone 0.5% or 1.0%. Combined preparations often contain aminoglycosides which frequently cause toxicity or allergy and should be avoided.

The management of the corneal complications that often accompany these conditions (vernal plaque, bacterial keratitis and herpes keratitis) are beyond the scope of this summary but present challenging management problems in the context of these conditions.

Practice points for dermatologists are that the dermatologist should be aware that any sudden deterioration in vision may herald one of the blinding complications of these diseases and should be treated as an emergency. Good control of the underlying condition aims to reduce the frequency with which the blinding corneal complications develop, whilst minimizing the potentially serious side effects of corticosteroid treatment.

The interaction of drugs used for the management of atopic eye disease and atopic dermatitis

Most cases of atopic eye disease are managed with topical ocular therapy which has no effect on the dermatological aspects of the disorder. However treatment with courses of systemic corticosteroid and/or ciclosporin, when needed either for the dermatological or ophthalmological aspects of atopy, are beneficial to the management of both. The risk of glaucoma from systemic corticosteroids, while occurring, is very low whereas topical application of corticosteroid around the eyelids probably constitutes a higher risk; patients who chronically use corticosteroid cream around the eyes should have glaucoma screening.

REFERENCES

1 Friedlander MH. Conjunctivitis of allergic origin: clinical presentation and differential diagnosis. *Surv Ophthalmol* 1993; **38**: 105–14.
2 Tuft SJ, Kemeney DM, Dart JKG, Buckley RJ. Clinical features of atopic keratoconjunctivitis. *Ophthalmology* 1991; **98**: 150–8.
3 Power WJ, Tughal-Tutkun I, Foster CS. Long-term follow up of patients with atopic keratoconjunctivitis. *Ophthalmology* 1998; **105**: 637–42.
4 Tuft SJ, Dart JKG. Limbal vernal keratoconjunctivitis. Clinical characteristics and IgE expression compared with palpebral vernal. *Eye* 1989; **3**: 420–7.
5 Dart JKG, Buckley RJ, Monnickendam M, Prasad J. Perennial allergic conjunctivitis. Definition, clinical characteristics and prevalence. *Trans Ophthalmol Soc UK* 1986; **105**: 513–20.
6 Abelson M, Schaefer K. Conjunctivitis of allergic origin: immunologic mechanisms and current approaches to therapy. *Surv Ophthalmol* 1993; **38**: 115–32.
7 Tuft SJ, Ramakrishnan M, Seal DV, Kemeny DM, Buckley RJ. Role of *Staphylococcus aureus* in chronic allergic conjunctivitis. *Ophthalmology* 1992; **99**: 180–4.
8 Montan PG, van Hage-Hamsten M. Eosinophil cationic protein in tears in allergic conjunctivitis. *Br J Ophthalmol* 1980: 556–60.
9 Whitcup SM, Chan CC, Luyo DA, Bo P, Li Q. Topical cyclosporine inhibits mast cell mediated conjunctivitis. *Invest Ophthalmol Vis Sci* 1996; **37**: 2686–93.
10 Hoang-Xuan T, Prisant O, Hannouche D, Robin H. Systemic cyclosporine A in severe atopic keratoconjunctivitis. *Ophthalmology* 1997; **104**: 1300–5.
11 Bleik JH, Tabbara KF. Topical cyclosporine in vernal keratoconjunctivitis. *Ophthalmology* 1991; **98**: 1679–84.

Cicatrizing conjunctivitis and the immunobullous disorders

Description and epidemiology [1–4]

Cicatrizing conjunctivitis, although uncommon, is one of the most difficult management problems in ophthalmology because of the widespread effects on the ocular surface leading to corneal blindness in many victims. The classification of the conjunctival disorders follows the

Table 64.7 Immunobullous diseases (those associated with conjunctivitis are shown in italics).

Intraepithelial	Subepithelial
• Pemphigus	• Pemphigoid
vulgaris	*Bullous*
vegetans	*Cicatricial* (Fig. 64.8a–f)
sebhorreic	• Pemphigoid gestationis
• Pemphigus foliaceous	• *Epidermolysis bullosa aquisita*
• Pemphigus erythematosis	• Bullous systemic lupus erythematosis
• Brazilian pemphigus	• *Linear IgA disease*
• *Paraneoplastic pemphigus*	• *Dermatitis herpetiformis*
	• *Lichen planus*

Graft-versus-host disease

Erythema multiforme
• Minor
• *Major (Stevens–Johnson syndrome)*

Toxic epidermal necrolysis (Lyell syndrome)

dermatological classification although not all the dermatological disorders are associated with conjunctivitis (Table 64.7).

The severity of the conjunctival involvement varies but is mild, without scarring, in pemphigus vulgaris, and with variable degrees of scarring and severity in the remainder.

Cicatricial pemphigoid (CP) [5–9]

CP is the commonest of these rare disorders. It is a systemic disease with involvement of the skin (25% of cases), oro-pharyngeal mucosa (85% of cases) and conjunctiva (65% of cases) and may be localized to one of these sites alone. About 70% of patients presenting to a dermatologist will have conjunctival involvement, in addition to skin disease, whereas disease confined to the conjunctiva alone is found in 50% of patients in ophthalmology clinics and is known as ocular cicatricial pemphigoid (OCP). Some authorities feel that the term mucous membrane pemphigoid should be adopted but this belies the scarring nature of the disease when it affects the eye and will not be used in this discussion.

Epidemiology of CP

Unambiguous data on the epidemiology of the disease is difficult to obtain because studies have been based on the site of involvement. However the incidence of dermatological disease is about 1/million/year. This is likely to be an underestimate of the disease as a whole because mucosal presentations are more common. In ophthalmology centres CP affects between 1 : 8000 and 1 : 46 000 patients. The male : female ratio is 1 : 3 and age range

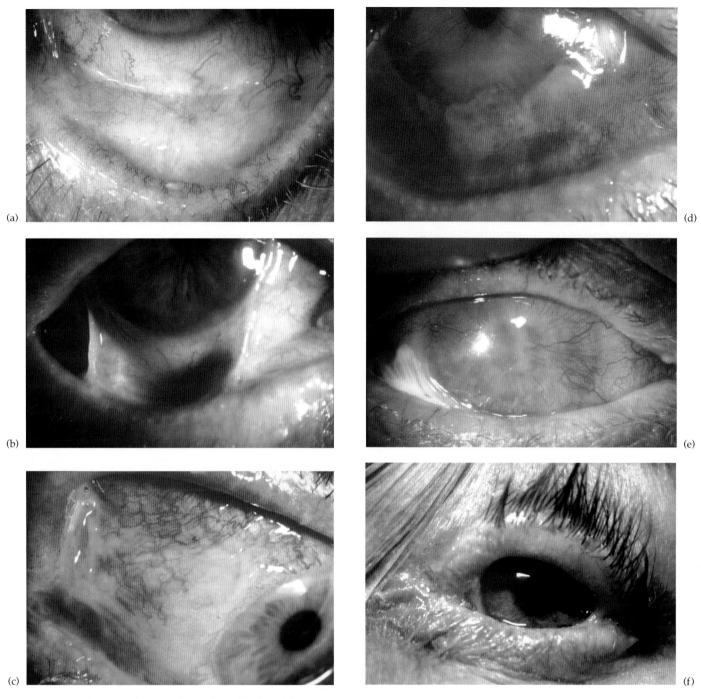

Fig. 64.8 Ocular signs of cicatricial pemphigoid (CP). (a) Inferior fornix shortening and subconjunctival scarring. (b) Conjunctival symblepharon tethering the globe to the lower lid. (c) Acute exacerbation of conjunctival CP showing conjunctival ulceration. This occurs in only 10% of patients presenting with CP affecting the eye. (d) Severe conjunctival inflammation and limbitis. This leads rapidly to the ocular surface failure and corneal blindness shown in (e) unless it is promptly controlled with adequate immunosuppressive therapy. (e) Ocular surface failure and keratinization (the white area) in advanced pemphigoid. This eye is blind. (f) Advanced ocular pemphigoid showing loss of the medial canthal structures (plica and caruncle) with a reduced interpalpebral aperture secondary to shortening of the fornices (as in (a)) and fusion of the tarsal and bulbar conjunctiva.

30–90 years with peak onset in the seventh decade, although patients may rarely present in childhood and in extreme old age. At presentation between 25 and 38% of patients with ocular disease have significant visual loss and about 30% become legally blind. Treatment has been shown to slow disease progression. A genetic predisposition has been found in an association with the *DQw7* gene and expression of the HLA-DR4 antigen.

Clinical features [10]

Most patients with OCP have progressive disease. However, early presenting disease is usually milder and progresses more slowly than late-presenting disease. Current aggressive treatment regimens, with systemic immunosuppression, have been shown to reduce the rate of progression by about 50%. Because patients can occasionally progress to blindness within months from the onset, both early diagnosis and effective treatment are critical in improving the prognosis.

In most patients the onset is insidious, with non-specific conjunctival symptoms including irritation, hyperaemia and discharge. Dry eye and mucous deficiency are late signs. Acute disease occurs in about 20% of new patients with severe inflammation and conjunctival ulceration; this presentation may follow lid surgery for entropion on undiagnosed cases.

Signs, in order of progression, often start at the medial canthus with loss of the plica and later of the caruncle (Fig. 64.8f), subepithelial reticular fibrosis of tarsal conjunctiva (Fig. 64.8a), conjunctival infiltrate due to increased cellularity and collagen formation (Figs 64.8c.d), hyperaemia, shortening of the fornices (Fig. 64.8a), symblepharon (Fig. 64.8b), blepharitis, trichiasis and entropion, punctate keratopathy, limbitis, conjunctival and corneal keratinization, and corneal surface failure (Fig. 64.8e). Late disease results in fusion of the lids and globe (Fig. 64.8f), and may obscure the cornea completely. Persistent epithelial defect, microbial keratitis and corneal perforation are common and, with the corneal surface failure, account for the management challenges posed by the disease. Cicatricial pemphigoid is associated with the autoimmune diseases rheumatoid arthritis, systemic lupus erythematosus and polyarteritis nodosa.

Diagnosis

Laboratory investigations [11–13] require specialized services and are only positive in 40–60% of cases so that for practical purposes a clinical diagnosis, based on a history of progression and the presence of the typical clinical signs, is adequate in most cases outside a clinical research setting. However, laboratory investigations for OCP may be useful. Indirect immunofluorescence for circulating antibodies to conjunctival basement membrane are present in 50% of cases of CP but the ability to perform this test requires a constant source of conjunctival substrate. The sensitivity of indirect immunofluorescence can be significantly increased using 1.0 mol/L sodium chloride split skin as the substrate.

Bulbar conjunctival biopsy is easy and safe providing the inferior fornix is avoided. Routine histopathology is of little value in the diagnosis because the conjunctiva is fragile and detection of basement membrane zone cleav-

Table 64.8 Causes of non-autoimmune cicatrizing conjunctivitis.

Infective conjunctivitis
Trachoma
Corynebacterium diphtheriae conjunctivitis
Streptococcal conjunctivitis
Adenoviral keratoconjunctivitis

Systemic diseases
Sarcoidosis
Progressive systemic sclerosis
Sjögren's syndrome
Atopic keratoconjunctivitis

Trauma
Iatrogenic conjunctivitis (pseudo-pemphigoid)
Chemical, thermal or mechanical trauma
Factitious (self-induced) conjunctival trauma

Others
Ocular rosacea
Staphylococcal blepharoconjunctivitis

age unreliable. Squamous metaplasia of the conjunctival epithelium and a reduction in goblet cells are non-specific findings as is an increased inflammatory cell infiltrate. In acute disease there is a neutrophil-rich infiltrate. Direct immunofluorescence for IgA, IgG, IgM, and complement is positive with linear staining at the conjunctival basement membrane in 50% of cases and is characteristic of OCP. However biopsies are often negative in acute disease and may revert to normal in time or after treatment.

Differential diagnosis

The conjunctival signs in CP and OCP may be identical to those produced by the other immunobullous disorders that are summarized in Table 64.7. However, in these conditions the skin disease precedes the ocular disease so that there is rarely any confusion. In erythema multiforme major, exacerbations of conjunctival inflammation can occur many years after the acute disease leading to a condition indistinguishable from OCP both in terms of the clinical signs and immunopathology. The principal problems in differential diagnosis relate to diseases other than the immunobullous disorders, that may also cause cicatrizing conjunctivitis (Table 64.8). Patients with conjunctival cicatrization secondary to infective causes are sometimes referred for investigation of what has been longstanding conjunctival scarring, following a long forgotten episode of infection, in whom the absence of a recent history of inflammation, or of progressive symptoms, usually indicates static disease. Patients with sarcoidosis or systemic sclerosis normally have a well-established diagnosis by the time conjunctival scarring develops. However, Sjögren's syndrome may mimic early OCP but can usually be differentiated by the presence of Sjögren's specific antibodies and/or a positive labial biopsy. AKC can occasionally be difficult to differentiate from slowly progressive OCP but the history and clinical signs of severe eczema, and a tarsal conjunctival biopsy (performed after withdrawal of topical corticosteroids for 2 weeks) that shows excessive numbers of mast cells and eosinophils, can confirm the diagnosis. Iatrogenic conjunctivitis is non-progressive, except in the case of drug-induced OCP, which is indistinguishable from classical OCP. Awareness that conjunctival scarring can occur in ocular rosacea and in staphylococcal bleph-aroconjunctivitis (see Fig. 64.5a) is usually enough to distinguish these conditions from OCP. Factitious conjunctival trauma is rare and usually more focal than classical OCP but can mimic OCP while the self-trauma is active.

Pathogenesis [14,15]

OCP is probably primarily an autoimmune disease directed at the conjunctival basement membrane; progression occurs as a result of inflammatory disease and cicatrization, secondary ocular surface disease, infection and treatment toxicity. Drug-induced pemphigoid (pseudopemphigoid), and Stevens–Johnson syndrome lead to an identical situation, suggesting that conjunctival damage may precipitate OCP. OCP may be the final common pathway for one type of conjunctival insult.

Inflammatory mechanisms in OCP are reasonably well understood and provide a rationale for immunosuppressive therapy. In chronic disease macrophages and T cells are present, of which the Th1 subset is active, as demonstrated by the presence of the cytokines, interleukin-2 and interferon-γ, as opposed to the Th2 subset that is involved in B-cell activation. This, coupled with the low numbers of B cells but increased number of plasma cells, suggests that B-cell activation must be occurring in the extraocular tissues with homing of mature plasma cells to the conjunctiva. Major histocompatibility complex (MHC) class II expression is increased, suggesting the potential for local antigen presentation to T-helper cells. There is a slight increase in activated T cells, which are involved in the recruitment of fibroblasts and macrophages. In acute disease, neutrophils and antigen-presenting (dendritic) cells are also present together with an increase in CD4 (helper) T cells, which probably reflects their role in recruiting other inflammatory cells.

Growth factors including fibroblast growth factor (FGF), platelet-derived growth factor (PDGF) and transforming growth factor-β (TGF-β) are all present in OCP. PGDF up-regulates the extracellular matrix component (ECM) thrombospondin, which is itself important in activating latent TGF-β. PDGF is a powerful chemoattractant for macrophages and fibroblasts and is probably pivotal to the scarring response. However only TGF-β is

capable of stimulating fibroblasts to produce collagen and ECM components. It also blocks matrix degradation by decreasing protease synthesis and increasing protease inhibition. In acute disease, TGF-β is significantly increased and is produced by macrophages and fibroblasts in OCP conjunctiva. Once macrophages and fibroblasts are present in large numbers and activated they may become self regulating; T-cell deficient models have shown that T cells are not necessary for wound healing to occur, and fibroblasts from OCP conjunctiva display abnormal activity in cell culture after several passages.

This inflammatory cell infiltrate is also associated with the presence of increased amounts of an abnormal type II 'curly' collagen.

Implications of immunopathological findings for therapy

Inflammation is important in acute disease; severe inflammation is associated clinically with rapid scarring and therefore demands effective immunosuppression to reduce scarring. Inflammation may also play a role in chronic disease although scarring often continues even in the presence of minimal inflammation, suggesting that growth factor production by macrophages and fibroblasts is relatively independent of the other inflammatory cells. Therefore modulation of growth factor activity, collagen metabolism or fibroblast activity may be necessary to halt the disease process. Of these, growth factor activity can potentially be specifically blocked or inhibited, thus holding promise for new treatments.

Other subepithelial immunobullous disorders and conjunctivitis [16]

Other immunobullous disorders are much less frequently associated with conjunctival cicatrization. As a result little is known about the pathogenesis of the conjunctival disease as opposed to the events in the skin. Bullous pemphigoid generally results in mild conjunctivitis although severe cicatrization has been reported. Epidermolysis bullosa aquisita, linear IgA disease, dermatitis herpetiformis and lichen planus may all be associated with progressive conjunctival scarring indistiguishable from that of CP.

Erythema multiforme major and toxic epidermal necrolysis [17–21]

The ocular complications of these two conditions are identical (Table 64.9); about 70–80% of patients admitted for treatment of these diseases will develop eye disease. It is the eye disease which leads to the most profound long-term morbidity in many such patients. In addition the eye disease, unlike the lesions affecting the remaining

Table 64.9 Ocular effects of Stevens–Johnson syndrome and toxic epidermal necrolysis.

Ocular effects	Resulting symptoms and signs
Loss of goblet cells	Disrupted tear film leading to poor vision and punctate keratopathy (Fig. 64.9b)
Loss of accessory lacrimal glands	
Scarring of meibomian gland orifices	
Metaplasia of meibomian gland epithelium with development of metaplastic lashes	Trichiasis secondary to metaplastic lashes (Fig. 64.9b)
Conjunctival scarring and obliteration of lacrimal gland ductules	Very dry eye with secondary conjunctival and corneal squamous metaplasia (Fig. 64.9b)
Keratinization due to squamous metaplasia	Exacerbates drying and discomfort
Conjunctival scarring with fornix shortening and symblepharon formation	May cause lagophthalmos
Retroplacement of meibomian gland orifices	Disrupts tear film
Entropion of upper and lower lids with trichiasis of both metaplastic and normal lashes	
Lid shortening	
Corneal epithelial failure secondary to limbal inflammation	Blindness

mucosal surfaces, may progress years after the acute episode has resolved.

Acute ocular complications usually occur concurrently with the skin disease but may sometimes precede it by several days. The conjunctivitis varies from a papillary reaction with watery discharge (Fig. 64.9a) to a membranous conjunctivitis with sloughing of the conjunctival epithelium. Corneal epithelial defects are common and may progress to corneal ulceration with or without bacterial superinfection. The morbidity of the disease may be due to the acute corneal complications but is more usually due to conjunctival scarring.

Chronic ocular complications are numerous. The severe conjunctival inflammation leads to loss of goblet cells and the accessory conjunctival lacrimal glands as well as disruption of the meibomian gland orifices leading to MGD. This results in a disrupted tear film and a secondary punctate keratinopathy. In mildly affected patients this causes chronic mild discomfort, photophobia and slightly reduced vision. In more severely affected patients the conjunctival inflammation leads to cicatrization of the lacrimal ductules resulting in a severely dry eye accompanied by squamous metaplasia and keratinization of both the conjunctival and corneal components of the ocular surface, resulting in more severe discomfort and loss of vision (Fig. 64.9b). In addition the meibomian gland ductal epithelium undergoes metaplasia resulting in the development of fine metaplastic lashes. The conjunctival shortening leads both to entropion, resulting in ocular surface abrasion by normal as well as by any metaplastic lashes, and may also cause lid shortening leading to reduced eye closure (lagophthalmos) which is easily overlooked. Lash abrasion and trichiasis lead to the development of corneal epithelial defects which, as

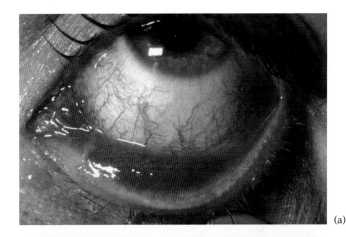

(a)

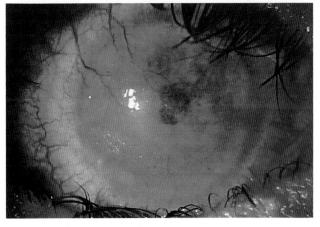

(b)

Fig. 64.9 Ocular disease in Stevens–Johnson syndrome. (a) Acute conjunctivitis in a patient with mild Stevens–Johnson syndrome. The conjunctiva is hyperaemic with a papillary reaction and mucopurulent discharge. (b) The late ocular complications of Stevens–Johnson syndrome showing entropion, a dry eye with ocular surface failure (in this case an opaque keratinized epithelium).

a result of the poor tear film, may persist. Persistent epithelial defect predisposes to corneal stromal melts and perforation, which are often precipitated by infection. The severe inflammation may also lead to ocular surface failure, not only as a result of squamous metaplasia, but also by loss of corneal epithelial progenitor cells (stem cells). This evolution of changes is not the direct consequence of the acute disease but is secondary to the effects on the tear film and lids, compounded in some cases by chronic or acute episodes of inflammation for which the pathogenesis is obscure. Late onset scleritis may also occur.

Graft-versus-host disease [22–28]

Ocular complications are common in patients with graft-versus-host disease (GVHD) and result from involvement of both the conjunctiva and the lacrimal gland. In acute GVHD, conjunctivitis ranges from hyperaemia through chemosis to a pseudomembranous conjunctivitis, with or without corneal epithelial sloughing. Severe conjunctival involvement is a marker for the severity of acute GVHD and was found to occur in 12% of patients in one study; this subset had 90% mortality [26]. In chronic GVHD the same study found conjunctival involvement in 11% of patients for whom it was also associated with disease severity. Some of these patients develop a severe scarring response like that of CP. Lacrimal gland involvement occurs in about 50% of patients with chronic GVHD who develop a Sjögren type picture of dry eyes.

The pathogenesis of the conjunctival disease has been examined in a few cases and appears to be similar to that in the skin.

Treatment of cicatrizing conjunctivitis and the ocular complications of the immunobullous disorders [29–35]

The same strategies can be used to treat the ocular aspects of all these disorders. The three principal treatment aims are: (i) management of the ocular surface disease; (ii) eliminating or minimizing treatment toxicity; and (iii) suppressing inflammation.

These three components of the treatment strategy are not required for all of these diseases. For example, in Stevens–Johnson syndrome most patients have relatively little inflammation once the surface disease has been treated, and any treatment toxicity eliminated, so that it is the minority of these patients, with recurrent inflammation or progressive cicatrization, who require suppression of inflammation. On the other hand most, but not all, OCP patients require use of all three components with 80% of patients requiring systemic immunosuppressive therapy to control inflammation that persists once the surface disease and toxicity has been controlled.

Successful management demands identification and treatment of all of the components of the disorder, including surface disease, treatment toxicity and inflammation related to activity of the underlying disease, as well as the early detection and treatment of secondary corneal infection.

Management of the ocular surface disease

The ocular surface disease is secondary to previous or current lid and conjunctival scarring and inflammation. The surface disease causes much of the damage to the cornea and is responsible for additional inflammation. Trichiasis and entropion, blepharitis, dry eye and filamentary keratitis, keratinization, persistent epithelial defect, microbial keratitis and corneal perforation may all result from a combination of a poor tear film, poor lid closure, and corneal damage secondary to trichiasis. These are treated as follows:

Trichiasis: epilate in the short term, use electrolysis or laser for odd lashes, cryotherapy for misdirected lashes and surgery for entropion (inferior retractor plication for lower lid and anterior lamellar reposition for upper lid).

Blepharitis: use oral tetracyclines and institute a lid hygiene regimen.

Dry eye and filaments: use non-preserved lubricants, topical acetylcysteine 5–10% as a mucolytic, and punctal occlusion to conserve tears (once any blepharitis has been controlled).

Keratinization: topical retinoic acid is effective in 30% but only available in specialized centres.

Persistent corneal epithelial defect: exclude infection, treat ingrowing lashes, use non-preserved lubricants, therapeutic lenses (silicone rubber or silicone hydrogel in dry eyes) and, if these measures are unsuccessful, close the eye with a botulinum toxin protective ptosis or with temporary tarsorraphy. Other more specialized treatments may be needed.

Corneal perforation: temporize with therapeutic contact lenses and/or corneal glue followed by keratoplasty only if absolutely necessary.

Eliminating or minimizing treatment toxicity

Treatment toxicity results principally from the preservative benzalkonium chloride, a component of most reusable bottles of eye drop preparations as well as of topical glaucoma medications and aminoglycoside eye drops.

Unnecessary topical treatment should therefore be avoided and unpreserved drops or saline used as far as possible. The effects of topical treatment toxicity are hard to distinguish from those of the ocular surface disease. After withdrawal of toxic topical therapy the mean recovery period is 2 weeks but may extend to 3 months.

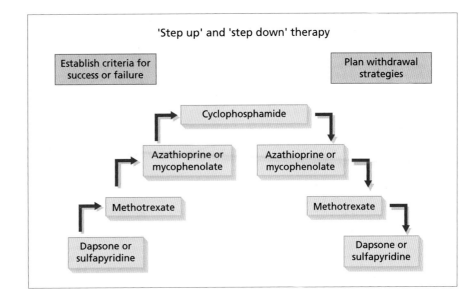

Fig. 64.10 Immunosuppressive therapy for progressive conjunctival cicatrization. 'Step up' and 'step down' therapy. For acute severe disease start at the top of the stepladder and 'step down' to the right (the withdrawal strategy). For less severe disease step up from the bottom left of the figure. The criterion for success is a reduction in inflammation when the surface disease, that may be contributing to it, has been controlled.

Suppressing inflammation—immunosuppressive therapy

Monitoring and side effects of the main immunosuppressive agents are discussed in Chapter 72 and are not repeated here.

In *mild disease* (*hyperaemia and oedema*), low-dose topical corticosteroid may be helpful for a few cases.

For *moderate disease* (*hyperaemia, intense infiltration*), sulphapyridine 500 mg daily for 2 weeks then 1 g daily (sulfasalazine 1–2 g daily is an alternative). Fifty-five per cent of patients respond in 1–2 months, but 15% develop an allergic reaction. If response is poor, dapsone 75 mg daily, increased each month by 25 mg daily to 125 mg, can be used; there is a 70% response in 1–2 months reducing to 50% after 1 year. Other agents that may be considered are azathioprine (1–2 mg/kg/day), methotrexate (7.5–25.0 mg once weekly) or mycophenolate mofetil (1–2 g daily) depending on the severity of the disease.

For *severe disease* (*hyperaemia, limbitis, conjunctival ulceration*), start prednisolone 1 mg/kg/day, reduce the dose after 2 weeks and tail off after 2–4 months. This is ineffective at low doses in the long term and a steroid-sparing immunosuppressive agent is generally added for long-term disease control. The most effective currently is cyclophosphamide 1 mg/kg/day. The dose is adjusted until the lymphocyte count is between 0.5 and 1.0×10^9; other haematological parameters should remain normal. Cyclophosphamide therapy is usually discontinued after 1 year and substituted by sulphonamides or immunosuppressive agents as described above.

Most of this therapy is empirical and a sulphonamide (dapsone or sulphapyridine) is often used together with an alkylating agent (cyclophosphamide) or an antimetabolite (azathioprine, methotrexate or mycophenolate) to control inflammation. This immunosuppressive strategy is summarized in Fig. 64.10, and can be modified as necessary for all these disorders; generally any systemic therapy will benefit the underlying disease.

REFERENCES

1 Bernauer W, Elder MJ, Dart JKG, eds. *Cicatrising Conjunctivitis. Developments in Ophthalmology*, Vol. 28. Basel: Karger, 1997.
2 Bernauer W, Elder MJ, Dart JK. Introduction to cicatrising conjunctivitis. *Dev Ophthalmol* 1997; **28**: 1–10.
3 Wright PW. Cicatrizing conjunctivitis. *Trans Ophthalmol Soc UK* 1986; **105**: 1–17.
4 Meyers SJ, Varley GA, Meisler DM, Camisa C, Wander AH. Conjunctival involvement in paraneoplastic pemphigus. *Am J Ophthalmol* 1992; **114**: 621–4.
5 Foster CS. Cicatricial pemphigoid. *Trans Am Ophthalmol Soc* 1986; **84**: 527–663.
6 Fiore PM, Jacobs IH, Goldberg DB. Drug induced ocular pemphigoid. A spectrum of disease. *Arch Ophthalmol* 1987; **105**: 1660–3.
7 Hoang-Xuan T, Robin H, Demers PE *et al.* Pure ocular cicatricial pemphigoid. A distinct immunopathologic subset of cicatricial pemphigoid. *Ophthalmology* 1999; **106**: 355–61.
8 Frith PA, Venning VA, Wojnarowska F, Millard PR, Bron AJ. Conjunctival involvement in cicatricial and bullous pemphigoid: a clinical and immuno-pathological study. *Br J Ophthalmol* 1989; **73**: 52–6.
9 Chan LS, Ahmed AR, Anhalt GJ *et al.* The first international consensus on mucous membrane pemphigoid. *Arch Dermatol* 2002; **138**: 370–9.
10 Elder MJ, Bernauer W, Leonard J, Dart JKG. Progression of disease in ocular cicatricial pemphigoid. *Br J Ophthalmol* 1996; **80**: 292–6.
11 Leonard JN, Hobday CM, Haffenden GP *et al.* Immunofluorescence studies in ocular cicatricial pemphigoid. *Br J Dermatol* 1988; **118**: 209–17.
12 Bernauer W, Elder M, Leonard JN, Wright P, Dart JK. The value of biopsies in the evaluation of chronic progressive conjunctivial cicatrisation. *Graefes Arch Clin Exp Ophthalmol* 1994; **232**: 533–7.
13 Sarret Y, Hall R, Cobo M *et al.* Salt split human skin substrate for the immunofluorescent screening of serum from patients with cicatricial pemphigoid and a new method of immunoprecipitation with IgA antibodies. *J Am Acad Dermatol* 1991; **24**: 952–8.
14 Elder MJ, Dart JK, Lightman S. Conjunctival fibrosis in ocular cicatricial pemphigoid—the role of cytokines. *Exp Eye Res* 1997; **65**(2): 165–76.
15 Bernauer W, Wright P, Dart JKG, Leonard JN, Lightman S. The conjunctiva in acute and chronic mucous membrane pemphigoid: an immunohisto-chemical analysis. *Ophthalmology* 1993; **100**: 339–46.
16 Leonard JN, Wright P, Williams DDM. The relationship between linear IgA disease and benign mucous membrane pemphigoid. *Br J Dermatol* 1984; **110**: 307–14.

17 Wright P, Collin JRO. The ocular complications of erythema multifirme (Stevens–Johnson syndrome) and their management. *Trans Ophthalmol Soc UK* 1983; **103**: 338–41.

18 Foster CS, Fong LP, Azar D, Kenyon KR. Episodic conjunctival inflammation after Stevens–Johnson syndrome. *Ophthalmology* 1988; **95**: 453–62.

19 Mondino BJ. Cicatricial pemphigoid and erythema multiforme. *Ophthalmology* 1990; **97**: 939–52.

20 Chan LS, Soong HK, Foster CS. Ocular cicatricial pemphigoid occurring as a sequela of Stevens–Johnson syndrome. *JAMA* 1991; **266**: 1543–6.

21 Power WJ, Ghorashi M, Merayo-Lloves J *et al*. Analysis of the acute ophthalmic manifestations of the erythema multiforme/Stevens–Johnson syndrome/toxic epidermal necrolysis disease spectrum. *Ophthalmology* 1995; **102**: 1669–76.

22 Franklin RM, Kenyon KR, Tutschka PJ *et al*. Ocular manifestations of graft-vs-host disease. *Ophthalmology* 1983; **90**: 4–13.

23 Hirst LW, Jabs DA, Tutschka PJ *et al*. The eye in bone marrow transplantation. I. Clinical study. *Arch Ophthalmol* 1983; **101**: 580–4.

24 Jabs DA, Hirst LW, Green WR *et al*. The eye in bone marrow transplantation. II. Histology. *Arch Ophthalmol* 1983; **101**: 585–90.

25 Jack MK, Jack GM, Sale GE *et al*. Ocular manifestations of graft-vs-host disease. *Arch Ophthalmol* 1983; **101**: 1080–4.

26 Jabs DA, Wingard JR, Green WR *et al*. The eye in bone marrow transplantation. III. Conjunctival graft-vs-host disease. *Arch Ophthalmol* 1989; **107**: 1342–8.

27 Bray LC, Carey PJ, Proctor SJ *et al*. Ocular complications of bone marrow transplantation. *Br J Ophthalmol* 1991; **75**: 611–4.

28 Lopez PF, Sternberg P, Dabbs CK *et al*. Bone marrow transplant retinopathy. *Am J Ophthalmol* 1991; **112**: 635–46.

29 Elder MJ, Bernauer W, Dart JK. General considerations in the management of chronic progressive conjunctival cicatrisation. *Dev Ophthalmol* 1997; **28**: 192–5.

30 Elder MJ, Bernauer W, Dart JK. The management of ocular surface disease. *Dev Ophthalmol* 1997; **28**: 219–27.

31 Elder MJ, Lightman SL, Dart JK. The role of cyclophosphamide and high dose steroid in ocular cicatricial pemphigoid. *Br J Ophthalmol* 1995; **79**: 264–6.

32 Elder MJ, Leonard J, Dart JKG. Sulphapyridine—a new agent for the treatment of ocular cicatricial pemphigoid. *Br J Ophthalmol* 1996; **80**(6): 549–52.

33 Foster CS, Neumann R, Tauber J. Long-term results of systemic chemotherapy for ocular cicatricial pemphigoid. *Doc Ophthalmol* 1992; **82**: 223–9.

34 Shimazaki J, Shimmura S, Fujishima H *et al*. Association of preoperative tear function with surgical outcome in severe Stevens–Johnson syndrome. *Ophthalmology* 2000; **107**: 1518–23.

35 Dart JKG. Corneal toxicity. The epithelium and stroma in iatrogenic and factitious disease. *Eye* 2003; **17**: 886–92.

Systemic diseases with skin and eye involvement

Some multisystem diseases affect both the skin and the eye [1–23]. It is not possible to catalogue every complication of all these diseases but the most frequent are summarized in Table 64.10.

REFERENCES

1 Callen JP, Mahl CF. Oculocutaneous manifestation observed in multisystem disorders. *Dermatol Clin* 1992; **10**: 709–16.

2 Krzystolik M, Power WJ, Foster CS. Diagnostic and therapeutic challenges of sarcoidosis. *Int Ophthalmol Clin* 1998; **38**: 61–76.

3 Smith JA, Foster CS. Sarcoidosis and its ocular manifestations. *Int Ophthalmol Clin* 1996; **36**: 109–25.

4 Newman LS, Rose CS, Maier LA. Sarcoidosis. *N Engl J Med* 1997; **336**: 1224–34.

5 Ghabral R, McCluskey FJ, Wakefield D. Spectrum of sarcoidosis involving the eye and brain. *Aust NZ J Ophthalmol* 1997; **25**: 221–4.

6 English JC, Patel PJ, Greer KE. Sarcoidosis. *J Am Acad Dermatol* 2001: 725–43.

7 Giuffrida TJ, Kerdel FA. Sarcoidosis. *Dermatol Clin* 2002; **20**: 435–47.

8 Burgess SM, Frith PA, Frith RP *et al*. Mucosal involvement in systemic and chronic lupus erythematosus. *Br J Dermatol* 1989; **121**: 727–41.

9 Foster CS. Systemic lupus erythematosus, discoid lupus erythematosus and progressive systemic sclerosis. *Int Ophthalmol Clinic* 1997; **37**: 93–110.

10 Quan DN, Foster CS. Systemic lupus erythematosus and the eye. *Int Ophthalmol Clin* 1998; **38**: 33–60.

11 Friedlander MH. Ocular manifestations of Sjögren syndrome: keratoconjunctivitis sicca. *Rheum Dis Clin North Am* 1992; **18**: 591–608.

12 Whallett AJ, Thurairajan G, Hamburger J *et al*. Behçet's syndrome: a multidisciplinary approach to clinical care. *QJM* 1999; **92**: 727–4.

13 Ando K, Fujino Y, Hijikata K *et al*. Epidemiological features and visual prognosis of Behçet's disease. *Jpn J Ophthalmol* 1999; **43**: 312–7.

14 Bernstein CN, Blanchard JF, Rawsthorne P, Yu N. The prevalence of extraintestinal diseases in inflammatory bowel disease: a population-based study. *Am J Gastroenterol* 2001; **96**: 1116–22.

15 Orchard TJ, Chua CN, Ahmed T *et al*. Uveitis and erythema nodosum in inflammatory bowel disease: clinical features and the role of *HLA* genes. *Gastroenterology* 2002; **123**: 714–8.

16 Blumenkranz MS, Penneys NS. Acquired immunodeficiency syndrome and the eye. *Dermatol Clin* 1992; **10**: 777–91.

17 Neves RA, Rodriguez A, Power WJ *et al*. Herpes zoster peripheral ulcerative keratitis in patients with the acquired immunodeficiency syndrome. *Cornea* 1996; **15**: 446–50.

18 Sarraf D, Ernest JT. AIDS and the eyes. *Lancet* 1996; **348**: 525–8.

19 Cunningham ET, Margolis TP. Ocular manifestations of HIV infection. *N Engl J Med* 1998; **339**: 236–44.

20 Mansour AM, Saad AJ, Haque AK *et al*. Ocular pathology in acquired immunodeficiency syndrome. *Ann Ophthalmol* 2002; **34**: 137–41.

21 Sober AJ, Grove AS Jr, Muhlbauer JE. Cicatricial ectropion and lacrimal obstruction with porphyria cutanea tarda. *Am J Ophthalmol* 1984; **91**: 396–400.

22 DeFrancisco M, Savino PJ, Schatz NJ. Optic atrophy in acute intermittent porphyria. *Am J Ophthalmol* 1976; **87**: 221–4.

23 Vassallo M, Shepherd RJ, Iqbal P, Feehally I. Age related variations in presentation and outcome in Wegener's granulomatous. *J R Coll Physicians Lond* 1977; **31**: 396–400.

Infections

A number of infections involve the eyelids, but the following are important to recognize because they are common or require urgent therapy or referral to an ophthalmologist [1].

Viral infections

Warts

These are common and are found on the eyelid margins often as a long thin projection. Lesions in this site are best treated with careful cryotherapy and accurate application of liquid nitrogen to the tip of the lesion using a cotton wool bud rather than cryospray.

Molluscum contagiosum [2]

This condition mainly affects children and young adults. It is also prevalent in patients with acquired immune deficiency syndrome (AIDS), who may develop multiple lesions around the eyelids. Lesions may grow in the lash line as well as on the lid skin and, occasionally, on the mucocutaneous junction. Lesions can be easily overlooked or mistaken for a sebaceous cyst; this condition must always be considered in the differential diagnosis of

Table 64.10 Systemic diseases with skin and eye involvement.

Systemic disease	Eye disease
Sarcoidosis *Epidemiology*: ocular involvement the presenting feature in 10%. 20–30% of patients have eye disease at some stage [1–7]	*Lids & orbital findings*: clusters of granulomatous eyelid swellings. Proptosis from orbital granulomas. Dry eye from lacrimal gland involvement *Heerfordt's syndrome*: (uveo-parotid fever) consists of uveitis and parotid gland enlargement, fever and facial nerve palsy. *Lofgren's syndrome*: acute iritis, bilateral hilar lymphadenopathy, erythema nodosum and arthralgia. *Mikulicz's syndrome*: bilateral swelling of lacrimal and salivary glands *Anterior segment findings*: *conjunctivitis*: occasionally a granulomatous conjunctivitis mimicking a follicular conjunctivitis. *Uveitis*: usually, but not always, bilateral granulomatous anterior uveitis in 80% of patients with eye manifestations with redness, pain, photophobia and blurred vision with floaters *Posterior segment findings*: rare
Systemic lupus erythematosus [8–10]	*Anterior segment findings*: dry eye, peripheral corneal ulcers. Scleritis is rare. Episcleritis occurs in 10% causing a red eye *Posterior segment findings*: retinal vasculitis common during exacerbations of systemic disease with flame shaped haemorrhages and cotton wool spots. May be associated with severe central nervous system vasculitis or lupus nephritis
Sjögren's syndrome [11]	*Lids & orbital findings*: lacrimal gland inflammation causing dry eye *Anterior segment findings*: symptoms: often severe with chronic discomfort, foreign body sensation, dryness and blurred vision. *Conjunctiva*: conjunctivitis and scarring in some cases. *Cornea*: punctate keratopathy, persistent corneal epithelial defects leading to corneal ulceration and perforation or corneal infection
Reiter's syndrome *Epidemiology*: ocular involvement in about 30% of patients [1]	*Anterior segment findings*: symptoms: red irritable eyes resolving spontaneously within 7–10 days *Conjunctiva*: bilateral mucopurulent conjunctivitis is the most frequent manifestation affecting approximately 30% of patients; this usually follows a urethritis by about 2 weeks and precedes the onset of arthritis. *Cornea*: keratitis may occur in isolation and is rare. *Uveitis*: anterior uveitis (iritis) occurs in about 20% of patients either with the first attack of Reiter's syndrome or during a recurrence
Behçet's syndrome *Epidemiology*: ocular involvement in 60% to 70% of patients [12, 13]	*Anterior segment findings*: external eye diseases: conjunctivitis, keratitis and episcleritis may occur but are not specific for the condition. *Uveitis*: is the commonest manifestation of the disease *Posterior segment findings*: visual impairment or blindness is a frequent complication of Behçet's syndrome as a result of the retinal ischaemia
Inflammatory bowel disease *Epidemiology*: ocular manifestations in about 5% of patients [14,15]	*Anterior segment findings*: external eye diseases: conjunctivitis, limbitis, peripheral corneal infiltrates and episcleritis may occur. *Uveitis*: acute iritis in about 5% of patients which may occur at the same time as exacerbation of colitis
Acquired immune deficiency syndrome (AIDS) *Epidemiology*: ocular complications occur in about 75% of patients [16,19]	*Common features*: (i) opportunistic infections with viruses mycobacteria and fungi; (ii) malignancies e.g. Kaposi's sarcoma; (iii) retinal microangiopathy; and (iv) neuro-ophthalmic lesions with intracranial infections and tumours. *Anterior segment findings*: external eye diseases: *Molluscum contagiosum* is a common ocular finding in patients with AIDS, they tend to be large and when located on the lid margin can give rise to follicular conjunctivitis. The lesions can be complicated by epithelial keratitis with associated pannus formation. Kaposi's sarcoma may involve the lids and conjunctiva. *Herpes simplex* keratitis tends to be severe with more frequent relapses. The peripheral cornea is more often involved in contrast to central disease in immunocompetent patients. *Herpes zoster ophthalmicus* is common and may be a presenting feature of HIV infection, especially if severe disease presents in young patients *Posterior segment findings*: retinal microangiopathy is common and characterized by retinal haemorrhages, microaneurysms and cotton wool spots. *Cytomegalovirus* retinitis and *Pneumocystis carinii* choroiditis are serious ophthalmic complications signifying severe systemic involvement
Porphyria [20, 21]	*Common feature*: ocular involvement results from either photosensitization and/or neurological dysfunction. Photosensitization can affect the eyelids, conjunctiva, cornea, sclera and possibly the retina. *Lids & orbital findings*: inflammation can lead to vesicle and bulla formation, secondary infection scarring with ectropion and hyperpigmentation *Neuro-ophthalmic complications*: include optic neuritis, optic atrophy, ptosis and cranial nerve palsies
Wegener's granulomatosis [22]	Episcleritis is very common in active stages. Also retinal vasculitis, optic neuritis, orbital pseudotumour
Polyarteritis nodosa	Episcleritis scleritis and keratitis

HIV, human immunodeficiency virus.

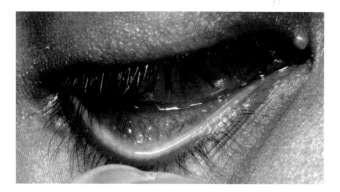

Fig. 64.11 Molluscum contagiosum. Molluscum contagiosum at medial aspect of the upper lid margin with an associated follicular conjunctivitis.

patients with unilateral or bilateral follicular conjunctivitis. There is associated conjunctival discharge and a variable, often severe, follicular conjunctival response (Fig. 64.11). A superficial epithelial keratitis may develop in long-standing cases, which can progress to pannus formation across the cornea. Treatment involves removal of the lesions by curettage; cryotherapy is also effective, but either of these will cause depigmentation in pigmented skins and are unnecessary for the management of a few localized lesions. In a co-operative adult this can be done under local anaesthetic, but for children a general anaesthetic is required.

Herpes simplex virus [3,4]

Primary HSV infection is asymptomatic in many patients; in others it causes blepharoconjunctivitis. However most of the ocular manifestations of HSV infection are due to reactivation of latent infection in the trigeminal ganglion. Both the primary infection, and reactivation of latent disease, may be particularly severe in patients with atopic dermatitis or with immunodeficiency. The blepharoconjunctivitis of HSV usually results in crops of small vesicles, which may be associated with mild oedema of the lids with or without a conjunctivitis. As with HSV elsewhere, the vesicles dry to a crust and heal within a few days. The conjunctivitis can be treated with aciclovir ointment five times daily for 5 days or with oral aciclovir 400 mg three times daily. Neither the blepharitis nor conjunctivitis present a serious problem for most patients. The serious and sight-threatening ocular complications of HSV infection of the eye are due to recurrent keratitis or keratouveitis. Herpetic keratitis may affect the epithelium alone (dendritic keratitis), the stroma (in stromal herpetic keratitis, geographical corneal ulceration and metaherpetic keratitis), or the endothelium (disciform keratitis or herpetic endotheliitis). Dendritic keratitis is in itself a benign disease unless treated with topical corticosteroids when the disease will rapidly spread, resulting in geo-

graphical keratitis, which may cause destructive corneal disease. Most cases of corneal disease represent reactivation of latent HSV and patients may develop any of the corneal manifestations. Stromal and endothelial disease can progress to blinding corneal vascularization, scarring and ulceration. Fortunately the disease is normally unilateral except in atopic individuals when it may often be bilateral. The management of the stromal and endothelial keratitis is beyond the scope of this review except to state that this involves the judicious use of topical corticosteroids with systemic or topical antivirals. Keratouveitis involves the endothelium and stroma and may also be associated with secondary glaucoma. Dendritic keratitis may occur during treatment with topical corticosteroids. Because of the difficulties of managing the ocular manifestations of this disease, patients with suspect HSV involvement of the eye should be referred for urgent ophthalmological assessment. Topical corticosteroids must not be used alone as these will mask the symptoms and signs, leading to spread of the ulcer and corneal perforation with catastrophic consequences for the patient's vision.

Herpes zoster [5]

Herpes zoster of the ophthalmic division (HZO) of the trigeminal nerve is an important condition to recognize. As with other sites, it often presents with a non-specific flu-like illness with fever and malaise and symptoms of unilateral neuralgia. This develops over the distribution of the affected nerve and varies in severity from a mild tingling in the skin to a deep severe pain. The characteristic lesions of herpes zoster may appear up to a week after the initial symptoms. Erythematous macules develop into clusters of papules and vesicles becoming pustular and haemorrhagic after 3–4 days. The lesions then scab and are dry by 7–14 days, separating to leave pitted scars. Involvement of the nasociliary nerve, which supplies the skin on the side of the nose (Hutchinson's sign), occurs in about 35% of patients and carries a high risk of ophthalmic complications. Ocular involvement may occur in the absence of nasociliary involvement but it is usually milder. Patients whose eyes cannot be examined due to persistent lid oedema, or those with ocular signs and symptoms, should be referred for urgent ophthalmological assessment. The disease can affect any part of the eye, including the orbit, extraocular muscles, optic nerve and cornea, and may give rise to long-term complications including severe relapsing keratitis, glaucoma and cataract.

Oral aciclovir is indicated when given within 3 days of the onset of the rash; using it later in the course of the disease is probably valueless. Topical aciclovir is also unhelpful. Topical corticosteroid therapy is needed to control the numerous corneal manifestations of the disease and may need to be continued for several years. Some of these complications may be delayed and occur months after the initial skin eruption.

Prolonged or severe post-herpetic neuralgia is a painful and unpleasant sequel to herpes zoster infection. It occurs in about half of elderly patients but is rare in children. There is some evidence that the use of amitriptyline in the early stages of infection is helpful in reducing the incidence and severity.

Bacterial infection

Staphylococcal infection

Impetigo

Impetigo is a common skin infection that mainly affects children. It can involve the eyelids, but usually as part of a general infection over the face. It presents as rapidly spreading erythematous macules, developing into flaccid vesicles that subsequently rupture to give rise to surface crusting. The lesions need to be swabbed for bacteriology and appropriate oral and topical antibiotics given.

Hordeolum

External hordeolum (stye) is caused by staphylococcal infection of an eyelash follicle and its associated glands. It presents with a tender, red, inflamed swelling on the lid margin, which subsequently points anteriorly and discharges close to the lash roots. No treatment is usually required beyond the application of local soothing compresses and removal of the affected lash. If there is a local cellulitis then systemic antibiotics should be given. An internal hordeolum is a staphylococcal abscess of the meibomian glands and needs incision and drainage.

Streptococcal infection

Erysipelas [6]

This represents subcutaneous spreading cellulitis, usually caused by β-haemolytic *Streptococcus*. It usually presents with a rigor followed by a red, raised, erythematous plaque with a well-demarcated edge that spreads rapidly over the skin. Erysipelas is a serious skin infection that needs to be treated urgently with appropriate systemic antibiotics.

Necrotizing fasciitis [7]

This is a very rare condition, most commonly caused by *Streptococcus*, which mainly affects elderly or debilitated patients. A spreading purple discoloration of the eyelid rapidly progresses to gangrene. Unlike erysipelas the periorbital tissue is not usually affected. Early recognition, immediate institution of intravenous antibiotics and referral to an ophthalmic plastic surgeon for debridement of the necrotic tissue are mandatory as the condition carries a high mortality.

Mycobacterial infection

Tuberculosis [8,9]

There are no specific ocular findings in tuberculosis, and diagnosis is often based on indirect evidence such as intractable uveitis that is unresponsive to corticosteroid therapy, with negative findings for other causes of uveitis, and in the presence of tuberculosis at a distant body site. Chronic iridocyclitis, which is usually granulomatous, is the commonest feature. Choroiditis and retinal vasculitis may occur.

Leprosy [8,9]

Ocular complications of leprosy are common, most frequently madarosis, conjunctivitis, episcleritis or scleritis. Keratitis results from a combination of corneal anaesthesia, lagophthalmus, trichiasis and secondary infection. Iritis and its complications are the most common causes of blindness and leprosy. Lepromatous disease is more commonly associated with uveitis than is tuberculoid leprosy.

Treponemal infection

Syphilis [10]

Ocular syphilis is very rare and there are no pathognomonic signs. Eye involvement mainly occurs during the secondary and tertiary stages, though primary chancre of the conjunctiva may occur. External features include madarosis, scleritis and interstitial keratitis. Uveitis and chorioretinitis are rare but serious complications of syphilis and lead to blindness. Neuro-ophthalmic features include Argyll Robertson pupils, optic nerve lesions, and palsies of the third and sixth cranial nerves. Gummatous involvement of the brain can cause visual field defects.

Lyme disease [11,12]

Ocular manifestations of Lyme disease involve all parts of the eye. As with syphilis, the ocular manifestations vary according to the stage of the disease. In stage 1, a localized conjunctivitis with photophobia occurs in 10% of patients. This is mild and brief and ophthalmologists are rarely consulted. In stage 2, various ophthalmic complications have been described including cranial nerve palsies; these may occur within 1 month of the rash appearing. It is in the late stage 3 that most of the severe ocular complications are seen, including episcleritis, symblepharon, interstitial keratitis, uveitis, chorioretinitis and retinal vasculitis.

Parasitic infection

Phthiriasis (lice) [13]

An infestation of the eyelashes by the pubic louse, *Phthirus pubis*. It mainly affects children and causes chronic itching, irritation and rubbing of the lids. As with louse infection elsewhere, the adult lice can be difficult to see, though nits and their shells are visible adhering to the eyelashes (see Fig. 64.6c,d). The skin nearest to the base of the lashes may show small bluish spots due to the louse bites (maculae caeruleae). A number of measures have been used to treat louse infestation of the eyelids, including mechanical removal with forceps, epilation of infested lashes, and application of fluorescein, yellow mercuric oxide ointment, physostigmine or aqueous malathion.

Filiriasis (onchocerciasis) [14]

Onchocerciasis or river blindness is caused by the filarial organism, *Onchocerca volvulus*. It is the second most common cause of preventable blindness in sub-Saharan Africa with an estimated prevalence of 500 000 cases with visual impairment and 270 000 with blindness. It appears that *Wolbachia endobacteria*, a bacterial symbiont, produces an endotoxin-like product which constitutes a major pro-inflammatory stimulus in the eye, causing corneal inflammation and sclerosing keratitis.

Protozoal infection

Ocular disease may complicate leishmaniasis. In *Leishmania donovani* infection, bilateral retinal haemorrhages may be a feature. In *L. tropica* and *L. braziliasis* infection, eyelid and corneal lesions occur, and subsequent destruction may lead to loss of the eye. In trypanosomiasis, unilateral oedema of the lids may occur.

REFERENCES

1 Holzberg M, Stulting RD, Drake LA. Ocular and periocular infections. *Dermatol Clin* 1992; **10**: 741–61.
2 Vannas S, Lapinleimu K. Molluscum contagiosum in the skin, caruncle and conjunctiva. *Acta Ophthalmol (Copenh)* 1967; **45**: 314–6.
3 Liesegang TJ, Melton J, Daly PJ. Epidemiology of herpes simplex: incidence in Rochester, Minnesota 1950 through 1982. *Arch Ophthalmol* 1987; **107**: 1160–5.
4 Herpetic Eye Disease Study Group. Oral acyclovir for herpes simplex virus eye disease. Effect on prevention of epithelial keratitis and stromal keratitis. *Arch Ophthalmol* 2000; **118**: 1030–6.
5 Marsh RJ. Ophthalmic zoster. *Lancet* 1991; **338**: 1527.
6 Jackson K, Baker SR. Periorbital cellulitis. *Head Neck Surg* 1987; **9**: 227–34.
7 Walters R. A fatal case of necrotizing fasciitis of the eyelid. *Br J Ophthalmol* 1988; **72**: 428–31.
8 John D, Daniel E. Infectious keratitis in leprosy. *Br J Ophthalmol* 1999; **83**: 173–6.
9 Dana MR, Hochman MA, Viana MA *et al.* Ocular manifestations of leprosy in the USA. *Arch Ophthalmol* 1994; **112**: 626–9.
10 Schlaegel TF Jr, Kao SF. A review (1970–1980) of 28 presumptive cases of syphilis uveitis. *Am J Ophthalmol* 1982; **93**: 412–4.

11 Zaidman GW. The ocular manifestation of Lyme disease. *Int Ophthalmol Clin* 1997; **37**: 13–28.
12 Lesser RI. Ocular manifestations of Lyme disease. *Am J Med* 1995; **98**: 605–25.
13 Burns DA. The treatment of pthirus pubis infestation of the eyelashes. *Br J Dermatol* 1987; **117**: 741–3.
14 Hoerauf A, Buttner DW, Adjei O, Pearlman E. Onchocerciasis. *BMJ* 2003; **326**: 207–10.

Inherited disorders

A large number of inherited disorders affect the skin and eyes. Major reference texts are cited [1–3]. The main ocular features are summarized in Table 64.11 [4–51].

REFERENCES

1 Harper J. *Inherited Skin Disorders—the Genodermatoses*. Oxford: Butterworth–Heinemann, 1996.
2 Wiedemann HR, Kunze J, eds. *Clinical Syndromes*. London: Mosby Wolfe, 1997.
3 Grant-Kels JM, Rothe MJ, Kels BD, eds. *Oculocutaneous Disease*, Vol. 10. Philadelphia, WB Saunders, Dermatologic Clinics, 1992.
4 Neldener KH, Hambridge KM, Walravens PA. Acrodermatitis enteropathica. *Int J Dermatol* 1978; **17**: 380–7.
5 Beighton P. Serious ophthalmological complications in the Ehlers–Danlos syndrome. *Br J Ophthalmol* 1970; **54**: 263–8.
6 Maumenee IH. The eye in the Marfan syndrome. *Trans Am Ophthalmol Soc* 1981; **79**: 684–733.
7 Neldner KH. Pseudoxanthoma elasticum. *Int J Dermatol* 1988; **27**: 98–100.
8 Pellegrino JE, Schnurr RE, Boghosian-Sell LE *et al.* Ablepharon macrostomia syndrome with associated cutis laxa: possible localisation to 18q. *Hum Genet* 1996; **97**: 532–6.
9 Leung RSC, Beer WE, Menta HK. Aplasia cutis congenita presenting as a familial triad of atrophic alopecia, ocular defects and a peculiar scarring tendency of the skin. *Br J Dermatol* 1988; **118**: 715–20.
10 Oley C, Baraitser M. Blepharophimosis, ptosis, epicanthus inversus syndrome. (BPES syndrome). Syndrome of the month. *J Med Genet* 1988; **25**: 47–51.
11 Nance MA, Berry SA. Cockayne syndrome. Review of 140 cases. *Am J Med Genet* 1992; **42**: 68–84.
12 Davidson HR, Connor JM. Dyskeratosis congenita. *J Med Genet* 1988; **25**: 843–6.
13 Pinheiro M, Freire-Maia N. Ectodermal dysplasias. In: Harper J, ed. *Inherited Skin Disorders—the Genodermatoses*. Oxford: Butterworth–Heinemann, 1996: 126–45.
14 Thomas JV, Yoshizumi MO, Beyer CK *et al.* Ocular manifestations of focal dermal hypoplasia syndrome. *Arch Ophthalmol* 1977; **95**: 1997–2001.
15 Gattuso J, Patton MA, Baraitser M. The clinical spectrum of the Fraser syndrome. *J Med Genet* 1987; **24**: 549–55.
16 Frydman M, Curran HA, Carmon G, Savir H. Autosomal recessive blepharophimosis ptosis V—esotrophic syndactyly and short stature. *Clin Genet* 1992; **41**: 57–61.
17 11th Annual David W. Smith Workshop on Malformations and Morphogenesis. Symposium on the Hallerman–Streiff syndrome. *Am J Med Genet* 1991; **41**: 487–523.
18 Happle R, Daniels D, Koopman RJJ. Midas syndrome (microphthalmia dermal aplasia and sclerocornea): an X-linked phenotype distinct from Golz syndrome. *Am J Med Genet* 1993; **47**: 710–3.
19 Su WPD, Chun IS, Hammond DL *et al.* Pachyonychia congenita. A clinical study of 12 cases and review of the literature. *Pediatr Dermatol* 1990; **7**: 33–8.
20 Jackson LG. Lange syndrome (editorial). *Am J Med Genet* 1992; **42**: 377–8.
21 Solomon IL, Green OC. Monilethrix. *N Engl J Med* 1963; **269**: 1279–85.
22 Galewsky E. Pili torti. *Arch Dermatol Syphilol* 1932; **26**: 659–66.
23 Bennett CP, Berry AC, Maxwell DJ, Seller MJ. Chondodysplasia punctata: another possible X-linked recessive case. *Am J Med Genet* 1992; **44**: 795–9.
24 Joy B, Black RK, Wells RS. Ocular manifestations of ichthyosis. *Br J Ophthalmol* 1968; **52**: 217–6.
25 Skinner BA, Greist MC, Norins AL. The keratitis ichthyosis and deafness (KID) syndrome. *Arch Dermatol* 1981; **117**: 285–9.

Table 64.11 Inherited disorders affecting the skin and eyes.

Group	Condition	Inheritance	Ocular features
Bullous disorders	Acrodermatitis enteropathica [4]	AR (MIM #201100)	Loss of eyebrows and eyelashes, conjunctivitis, blepharitis, photophobia
Connective tissue disorder	Ehlers–Danlos syndrome [5]	Mainly AD (see MIM 130000)	Lax eyelid skin with redundant folds, epicanthal folds, hypertelorism, strabismus, blue sclera, corneal abnormalities including keratoconus, angioid streaks, ectopic lens. Retinal detachments occasionally occur
	Marfan's syndrome [6]	AD (MIM #154700)	Subluxation of lens—60–80% of patients in early childhood. Amblyopia, myopia, cataract, corneal abnormalities, glaucoma. Retinal detachment is most serious complication
	Pseudoxanthoma elasticum [7]	Types I & II AR (MIM #264800, 264810) Types III & IV AD (MIM #177850, 177860)	Angioid streaks (breaks in Bruch's membrane) in majority. Haemorrhagic maculopathy after trauma may cause visual loss
Dysplasias, hyperplasia, atrophies and aplasias	Ablepharon macrostomia [8] syndrome	Unknown (MIM 200110)	Absent eyelids and ectropion
	Aplasia cutis congenita [9]	AD (MIM #107600) AR (MIM 207700)	Congenital absence of skin leading to eyelid colobomas, corneal opacities, scleral dermoids and lamellar cataracts
	Blepharophimosis ptosis epicanthus inversus syndrome [10]	AD (MIM #110100)	Blepharophimosis, ptosis, epicanthus inversus, telecanthus. Amblyopia in 50% of patients
	Cockayne's syndrome [11]	AR (MIM *216400)	Corneal opacities, cataracts in 30%, retinitis pigmentosa, optic atrophy, strabismus, photophobia
	Dyskeratosis congenita [12]	XR (MIM #305000)	Obliteration of the lacrimal puncta in 80% of cases, conjunctivitis, blepharitis, ectropion, loss of eyelashes and eyebrows
	Ectodermal dysplasias—a complex group of disorders with various inheritance patterns and a variety of ocular findings [13] Examples are given:		
	(i) Christ–Siemans–Touraine syndrome	XR	Photophobia dry eye
	(ii) Fischer–Jacobson–Clouston syndrome	AD	Usually normal
	(iii) Ellis–van Cleveld syndrome	AR (MIM #225500)	Coloboma of iris, microphthalmia occasional cataract
	Focal dermal hypoplasia (Golz's syndrome) [14]	XD (MIM *305600)	40% have ocular abnormalities, the commonest being colobomas of iris choroid retina or optic nerve
	Fraser's syndrome [15]	AR (MIM *219000)	Bilateral or unilateral absence of palpebral fissure with loss of eyebrows, anophthalmia, microphthalmia
	Frydman's syndrome [16]	AR	Synophrys, blepharophimosis, weakness of extra-ocular and frontal muscles
	Hallerman–Streiff syndrome [17]	Unknown (MIM *264090)	Loss of hair of eyebrows and eyelashes, microphthalmos, cataracts, amblyopia and nystagmus
	MIDAS syndrome [18]	XD	Microphthalmia, sclerocorneal
	Pachyonychia congenita [19]	AD (PC1 MIM #167200 PC2 MIM #167210)	Cataract and corneal dyskeratosis
Hair disorders	Brachmann–Lang syndrome [20]	AR	Synophrys thick, long eyelashes, narrow palpebral fissure, myopia, nystagmus and strabismus
	Monilethrix [21]	AD (MIM #158000)	Loss of eyebrows and lashes

(*continued overleaf*)

Table 64.11 (cont'd)

Group	Condition	Inheritance	Ocular features
	Pili torti [22]	AR (MIM 261900)	Loss of eyebrows and lashes
	Chondrodysplasia punctata [23]	AD (MIM 215105) XR (MIM #302950)	Cataracts Ocular albinism, cataracts, microphthalmia
Keratinization disorders	The ichthyoses [24] (i) Ichthyosis congenita gravis	AR (MIM *242500)	Severe ectropion
	(ii) Ichthyosiform erythroderma	AD (MIM 242100)	Early development of ectropion is characteristic
	(iii) Lamellar ichthyosis	AR (various types)	Cicatricial ectropion with exposure keratitis Direct conjunctival involvement may occur
	(iv) X-linked ichthyosis	XL (MIM *308100)	Deep corneal opacities
	KID syndrome [25]	XD (MIM #148210)	Keratitis
	Refsum's syndrome [26]	AR (MIM #266500)	Night blindness, posterior subcapsular cataracts develop in most cases
	Sjögren–Larson syndrome [27]	AR (MIM *270200)	Blepharitis, conjunctivitis, punctate corneal erosions and pigmentary degeneration of the retina
	Ulerythema ophryogenes [28]	AD	Erythema and perifollicular papules on eye to eyebrows spreading medially causing thinning of eyebrows
Metabolic disorders	Alkaptonuria [29]	AR (MIM #203500)	Scleral pigmentation is early sign, eyelid pigmentation
	Angiokeratoma corporis diffusum [30]	XL (MIM *301500)	Angiokeratomas of conjunctiva, corneal opacities, posterior capsular cataracts
	Homocystinuria [31]	AR (MIM *236200)	Myopia, cataracts, subluxation of lens, secondary glaucoma, retinal detachment
	Hurler's syndrome [32]	AR (MIM *252800)	Early clouding of cornea
Neurocutaneous syndromes	Richner–Hanhart syndrome [33]	AR (MIM 276600)	Corneal lesions vary from erosions to deep ulcers Nystagmus and lens opacities
	Neurofibromatosis type I [34]	AD (MIM *162200)	Neurofibromas of eyelid, corneal clouding, Lisch nodules of iris, optic nerve glioma, palsies from cranial nerve involvement
	Neurofibromatosis type II	AD (MIM #101000)	Cataract fundus lesions. Extraocular motility abnormalities
Photosensitive disorders	Tuberous sclerosis [35]	AD (MIM #191100)	Tumours of the lids or nodules on conjunctiva and retina
	Basal cell naevus syndrome [36]	AD (MIM #109400)	Basal cell carcinoma of eyelid and periorbital area, hypertelorism, strabismus, colobomas of the choroid, cataracts, glaucomas in 5–10%
	Bloom's syndrome [37]	AD (MIM #210900)	Telangiectasis on lower lids, blistering and scarring lower eyelids
	Rothmund–Thomson syndrome [38]	AR (MIM #268400)	Sparse eyebrows and eyelashes, degenerative changes in cornea, 50% of patients have bilateral cataracts which develop in childhood, strabismus
	Xeroderma pigmentosum [39]	AR (various types)	Angiomas, keratoses, papillomas, carcinomas develop on eyelids, sometimes extending on to conjunctiva and cornea, scarring and atrophy of lids with exposure keratitis leading to corneal ulceration symblepharon formation. Ocular melanoma
	Chediak–Higashi syndrome [40]	AR (MIM #214500)	Oculocutaneous albinism, corneal opacities

(continued)

Table 64.11 (*cont'd*)

Group	Condition	Inheritance	Ocular features
Pigmentation disorders	Cross syndrome [41]	AR (MIM *257800)	Microphthalmia, small opaque cornea, coarse nystagmus
	Epidermal naevus syndrome [42]	Sporadic	Ocular melanocytic naevi, coloboma of the lids, iris and choroid. Lipodermoid of conjunctiva or choroid
	Incontinentia pigmenti [43]	XD (MIM #308300)	35% of patients have eye abnormalities including strabismus, cataract and microphthalmia. Retinal detachment may occur
	Hypomelanosis of Ito [44]	Sporadic (MIM *300337)	Hypertelorism, strabismus, myopia
	Oculocutaneous albinism [45]	AR (various types; Chapter 39)	Total loss of pigment in eyes, nystagmus, absence of binocular vision
	Piebaldism [46]	AD (MIM #172800)	Absent pigmentation medially of eyebrows, eyelids and eyelashes, heterochromia of iris
	Waardenberg's syndrome [47]	AD (MIM #193150)	Telecanthus, synophrys, partial albinism, heterochromia of iris
Vascular and haematological syndromes	Congenital telangiectatic cutis marmorata [48]	Unknown (MIM 219250)	Clouding of cornea, glaucoma
	Fanconi pancytopenia syndrome [49]	AR (MIM #227650)	Microphthalmia strabismus, nystagmus and colobomas
	Lymphoedema–distichiasis syndrome [50]	AD (MIM #153400)	Double row of eyelashes on upper and lower eyelids
	Sturge–Weber syndrome [51]	Sporadic (MIM 185300)	50% of patients have angiotomatous changes of the ipsilateral choroid causing glaucoma

AD, autosomal dominant; AR, autosomal recessive; XD, X-linked dominant; XL, X-linked; XR, X-linked recessive.

26 Refsum S. Herdopathia atactica polyneuritiformis phytanic acid storage disease (Refsum's disease) with a particular reference to ophthalmological disturbances. *Metab Ophthalmol* 1977; **1**: 73–9.

27 Gilbert WR, Smith JL, Nyhan WY. The Sjögren–Larsson syndrome. *Arch Ophthalmol* 1968; **80**: 308–16.

28 Burnett JW, Schwartz MF, Berbian BJ. Ulerythema ophryogenes with multiple congenital abnormalities. *J Am Acad Dermatol* 1988; **18**: 437–40.

29 O'Brien WM, La Du BN, Bunim JJ. Biochemical pathologic and clinical aspects of alkaptonuria, ochronosis and ochronotic arthropathy. Review of world literature. *Am J Med* 1963; **34**: 813–38.

30 Wallace HJ. Anderson–Fabry disease. *Br J Dermatol* 1973; **88**: 1–23.

31 Carson NAJ, Cusworth DC, Dent CE et al. Homocystinuric. *Arch Dis Child* 1963; **38**: 425–36.

32 Burk RD, Valle D, Thomas GH et al. Early manifestations of multiple sulphatase deficiency. *J Pediatr* 1984; **104**: 574–8.

33 Goldsmith LA, Reed J. Tyrosine induced eye and skin lesions: a treatable genetic disease. *JAMA* 1976; **236**: 382–4.

34 Brownstein S, Little JM. Ocular neurofibromatosis. *Ophthalmology* 1983; **90**: 1595–9.

35 Greenwald MJ, Weiss A. Ocular manifestations of the neurocutaneous syndromes. *Pediatr Dermatol* 1984; **2**: 98–117.

36 Gorlin RJ. The naevoid basal cell carcinoma syndrome. *Medicine* 1987; **66**: 98–113.

37 Gretzula JC, Hevia O, Weber PJ. Bloom's syndrome. *J Am Acad Dermatol* 1987; **17**: 479–88.

38 Moss C. Rothmund–Thomson syndrome. A report of two patients and review of the literature. *Br J Dermatol* 1990; **122**: 821–3.

39 Kraemer KH, Lee MM, Scotto J. Xeroderma pigmentosum cutaneous ocular and neurologic abnormalities in 830 published cases. *Arch Dermatol* 1987; **123**: 241–50.

40 Blume RS, Wolff SM. The Chediak–Higashi syndrome. *Br J Dermatol* 1971; **85**: 336–47.

41 Cross HE, McKusick VA, Breen W. A new oculocerebral syndrome with hyperpigmentation. *J Pediatr* 1967; **70**: 396–406.

42 Rogers M, McCrossin I, Commons C. Epidermal naevi and the epidermal naevus syndrome. A review of 131 cases. *J Am Acad Dermatol* 1989; **20**: 476–88.

43 Berlin AL, Paller AS, Chan LS. Incontinentia pigmenti. A review and update on the molecular basis of pathophysiology. *J Am Acad Dermatol* 2002; **47**: 169–87.

44 Glover MT, Brett EM, Atherton DJ. Hypomelanosis of Ito: spectrum of the disease. *J Pediatr* 1989; **115**: 75–80.

45 Witkop CJ, Hill CW, Desnick S et al. Ophthalmologic biochemical platelet and ultrastructural defects in the various types of oculocutaneous albinism. *J Invest Dermatol* 1973; **60**: 443–56.

46 Winship I, Young K, Martell R et al. Piebaldism: an autonomous autosomal dominant entity. *Clin Genet* 1991: 330–7.

47 Goldberg MF. Waardenburg's syndrome with fundus and other anomalies. *Arch Ophthalmol* 1966; **76**: 797–810.

48 Pehr K, Moroz B. Cutis marmorata telangiectatica congenita. Long term follow up review of the literature and report of a case in conjunction with congenital hypothyroidism. *Pediatr Dermatol* 1993; **10**: 6–11.

49 Auerbach AD. Fanconi's anaemia. *Dermatol Clin* 1995; **13**: 41–9.

50 Kolin T, Johns KJ, Wadlington WB et al. Hereditary lymphoedema and distichiasis. *Arch Ophthalmol* 1991; **109**: 980–1.

51 Phelps CD. The pathogenesis of glaucoma in Sturge–Weber syndrome. *Ophthalmology* 1978; **85**: 276–8.

Ocular complications of dermatological therapy

A number of drugs used by dermatologists have significant side effects on the eye and require careful monitoring.

Corticosteroids [1–15]

The use of corticosteroids can cause significant side effects on the eye. Both systemic and topical corticosteroids are responsible, though the greatest risk is to those receiving prednisolone at a dose of 10–15 mg a day for over a year.

Continuous therapy is more likely to cause side effects than intermittent therapy.

Posterior subcapsular cataracts are induced by long-term systemic corticosteroids in as many as 30% of patients. They rarely occur at doses less than 10 mg/day and for less than 1 year. Children are particularly vulnerable. Reversibility of cataracts is not common and progression of cataracts may occur in spite of reduction or discontinuation of corticosteroid therapy.

Patients also risk developing open angle glaucoma, particularly if genetically predisposed. The precise mechanism is unknown, though it is thought to be due to decreased aqueous outflow. Particular risk factors include type 1 diabetes, high myopia, connective tissue disorders and a family history of glaucoma. Topical corticosteroids induce a rise in intraocular pressure more quickly than systemic corticosteroids. Medium or high potency dermatological corticosteroids applied for long periods to, or near, the eyelids may spread over the lid margin and are absorbed through the cornea, reaching sufficient concentrations to elevate ocular pressures. Patients on long-term topical or systemic corticosteroids need to have their eye pressures monitored regularly at 1–6 monthly intervals depending on their degree of risk.

Topical corticosteroids predispose patients to cataract, glaucoma and secondary surface infection. Injudicious use in HSV infection masks the clinical signs of dendritic ulcer and risks perforation. Wearing a soft contact lens is a contraindication to topical ocular corticosteroid usage. Other ocular complications from corticosteroids include angioneurotic oedema, papilloedema from raised intracranial pressure and toxic amblyopia. Systemic treatment with corticosteroids may cause serous chorioretinopathy or diffuse retinal pigment epitheliopathy.

Oral retinoids [16–22]

Both isotretinoin and acitretin can cause ocular side effects. The most common is dry eye with associated conjunctivitis and blepharoconjunctivitis giving rise to blurred vision. The blepharoconjunctivitis is frequently associated with staphylococcal infection. Exposure keratopathy and corneal ulceration rarely occur; asymptomatic corneal opacities may develop but resolve after 6–8 weeks. Patients should be warned that they may be unable to tolerate contact lenses whilst on retinoid therapy. Use of tear substitutes, humidification of the environment and lid hygiene measures help. Retinal abnormalities may also occur, with poor night vision and increased sensitivity to glare, and can be a significant problem in those who drive at night. The cause is unknown but may be due to competitive inhibition of ocular retinol dehydrogenase causing local vitamin A deficiency and reduction in rhodopsin formation. More serious side effects include papilloedema from raised

intracranial pressure, optic atrophy and cataract. Although these are rare, a history of visual disturbance should be asked for when patients come for follow-up. Severe headache early in the course of treatment is significant. The ocular manifestations are dose-dependent and usually reversible, provided they are recognized and the treatment regimen adjusted. However, there have been reports of the dry eye syndrome and night blindness persisting after retinoids have been discontinued.

Antimalarials [23–27]

The most serious potential side effect of antimalarial drugs is retinopathy. The mechanism is uncertain but seems to depend on the ability of the drug to bind the retinal pigment epithelium. Ocular side effects from antimalarials are much less common now that hydroxychloroquine rather than chloroquine is the drug of choice. However, both drugs should be used with caution in patients with hepatic or renal impairment. The Royal College of Ophthalmologists and American Academy of Ophthalmologists have issued clear guidelines on screening protocols for use of chloroquine and hydroxychloroquine. Baseline ophthalmic assessment of patients, for whom these drugs are proposed, is carried out by the dermatologist and requires questioning the patient about any known visual impairment (uncorrected by spectacles) and the recording of near visual acuity using a test type. If visual impairment is reported or detected then referral to an optometrist is advised; the optometrist will refer any patient with abnormal findings to an ophthalmologist. Patients should not be treated with more than the maximum daily dosage (hydroxychloroquine at a maximum dosage of 6.5 mg/kg or chloroquine phosphate not exceeding 4 mg/kg daily) and should have this visual screening repeated annually and recorded in their notes. Referral to an ophthalmologist is appropriate if visual impairment is detected at baseline, if changes are detected on the annual screening or if the patient develops visual symptoms. The ophthalmologist will then carry out a range of tests including visual acuity, colour vision, visual fields, Amsler fields, corneal and retinal examinations. If long-term treatment is required, for more than 5 years, the risks of ocular complications are increased; in this instance, individual arrangements for screening should be agreed with a local ophthalmologist. No screening is recommended for mepacrine as it is not associated with ophthalmological side effects.

Antibiotics for acne [28–32]

Oxytetracycline, minocycline and doxycycline can all cause raised intracranial pressure. The mechanism is unknown but is thought to be related to interference with energy-dependent absorption mechanism of cerebrospinal fluid, which is mediated by cyclic adenosine monophosphate (AMP) at the arachnoid granulations. Patients who complain of headache should be examined carefully with fundoscopy through dilated pupils to look for papilloedema, and should have formal testing of visual acuity and of visual fields. The condition is far from benign; permanent visual field loss can occur if the condition is not recognized early and the drug stopped. Sometimes treatment with acetazolamide is required to reduce the pressure. Erythromycin or trimethoprim may cause erythema multiforme and associated ocular changes. Pigmentation due to minocycline can occur in the skin (Chapter 39) and has also been reported in the sclera.

Psoralens [33–44]

Psoralens have been shown to bind to the lens proteins, and some animal studies have shown induction of anterior cortical opacities though others have not. 8-Methoxypsoralen can be detected in the human lens 12 h after oral ingestion. There has been a longstanding concern about the risk of cataract in patients having psoralen and long-wave UV radiation (PUVA) therapy. Although PUVA has been used in treatment of skin diseases for 30 years, and clinical studies have not yet shown any convincing evidence of an increase in cataract as compared with the general population, it is still recommended that ultraviolet light A (UVA)-filtered spectacles are used for 12 h after ingestion of psoralens in case significant long-term sequelae eventually develop. Care must be taken to ensue that the spectacles are suitable for ultraviolet protection.

Botulinum toxin [45]

With the increased use of botulinum toxin for the treatment of facial wrinkling and eyebrow position dermatologists need to be aware of the potential side effects. These include haematoma, ptosis, ectropion, diplopia and eyelid drooping, and are often related to poor injection technique.

REFERENCES

1 David D, Berkowitz J. Ocular effects of topical and systemic corticosteroids. *Lancet* 1969; **i**: 149–51.
2 Agaarwal RK, Potamitis T, Chong NHV. Extensive visual loss with topical facial steroids. *Eye* 1993; **7**: 664–6.
3 Black RL, Oglesby RB, von Sallman L *et al.* Posterior subcapsular cataracts induced by corticosteroids in patients with rheumatoid arthritis. *JAMA* 1960; **174**: 166–71.
4 Giles C, Mason G, Dugg I *et al.* The association of cataract formation and systemic corticosteroid therapy. *JAMA* 1962; **182**: 719–22.
5 Shiono H, Oonishi M, Yamaguchi M *et al.* Posterior subcapsular cataracts associated with long term oral corticosteroids therapy. *Clin Pediatr (Phila)* 1977; **16**: 726–8.
6 Branco N, Branco BC, Maibach HI. Cutaneous corticosteroids therapy and cataract in men. *J Toxicol Cutaneous Ocul Toxicol* 2002; **21**: 161–8.

7 First C, Smiley WK, Arsell BM. Steroid cataract. *Ann Rheum Dis* 1983; **25**: 364–8.
8 Armaly MF. Effect of corticosteroids on intraocular pressure and fluid dynamics. I. The effect of dexamethasone in the normal eye. *Arch Ophthalmol* 1963; **70**: 482–6.
9 Rentro L, Snow JS. Ocular effects of topical and systemic steroids. *Dermatol Clin* 1992; **10**: 505–12.
10 Kwok AKH, Lam DJC, Ng JSK *et al.* Ocular hypertensive response to topical steroids in children. *Ophthalmology* 1997; **104**: 2112–6.
11 Chua JK, Fan DS, Leung AT, Lam DS. Accelerated ocular hypertensive response after application of corticosteroid ointment to a child's eye. *Mayo Clin Proc* 2000; **75**: 539–48.
12 Cubey RB. Glaucoma following the application of corticosteroids. *Br J Dermatol* 1976; **95**: 207–9.
13 Zigerman C, Saunders D, Levit F. Glaucoma from topically applied steroids. *Arch Dermatol* 1976; **112**: 1362–6.
14 Brown SI, Blomfield S, Pearce DB, Tragakis M. Infections with the therapeutic soft lens. *Arch Ophthalmol* 1973; **91**: 275–7.
15 Sprawl CW, Lang GE, Lang GK. Retinal pigment epithelial changes associated with systemic corticosteroids treatment. Report of cases and review of the literature. *Ophthalmologica* 1998; **212**: 142–8.
16 Palestine AG. Transient acute myopia resulting from isotretinoin (acutane) therapy. *Ann Ophthalmol* 1984; **16**: 660–2.
17 Bigby M, Stein RSL. Adverse reactions to isotretinoin. A report from the adverse drug reaction reporting system. *J Am Acad Dermatol* 1988; **18**: 543–52.
18 Goulden V, Layton AM, Cunliffe WJ. Long term safety of isotretinoin as a treatment for acne vulgaris. *Br J Dermatol* 1994; **131**: 360–3.
19 Lerman S. Ocular side effects of accutane therapy. *Lens Eye Toxic Res* 1992; **9**: 429–38.
20 Leyden JJ. The role of isotretinoin in the treatment of acne: personal observation. *J Am Acad Dermatol* 1998; **39**: 545–9.
21 Weleber R, Denman S, Hanifin J, Cunningham WJ. Abnormal retinal function associated with isotretinoin therapy for acne. *Arch Opthalmol* 1986; **104**: 831–7.
22 Fraunfelder FT, Fraunfelder FW, Edwards R. Ocular side effects possibly associated with isotretinoin usage. *Am J Ophthalmol* 2001; **132**: 299–305.
23 Easterbrook M. Ocular side effects and safety of antimalarial agents. *Am J Med* 1988; **85**: 23–9.
24 Cox NH, Paterson WD. Ocular toxicity of antimalarials in dermatology: a survey of current practice. *Br J Dermatol* 1994; **131**: 878–82.
25 Browning DJ. Hydroxychloroquine and chloroquine retinopathy: screening for drug toxicity. *Am J Ophthalmol* 2002; **135**: 649–56.
26 Fielder A, Graham E, Jones S *et al.* Royal College of Ophthalmologists guidelines: ocular toxicity and hydroxychloroquine. *Eye* 1998; **12**: 907–9.
27 Marmor MF, Carr RE, Easterbrook M *et al.* Recommendations on screening for chloroquine and hydroxychloroquine retinopathy. A report by the American Academy of Ophthalmology. *Ophthalmology* 2002; **109**: 1377–82.
28 Digre KB. Not so benign intracranial hypertension. *BMJ* 2003; **326**: 613–4.
29 Elston J, Lochhead J. Doxycycline induced intracranial hypertension. *BMJ* 2003; **326**: 641–2.
30 Sabroe RA, Archer CB, Harlow D *et al.* Minocycline induced discolouration of the sclerae. *Br J Dermatol* 1996; **135**: 314–6.
31 Fraunfelder FT, Randall JA. Minocin induced scleral pigmentation. *Ophthalmology* 1997; **104**: 936–8.
32 Morrow GL, Abbott RL. Minocycline—induced scleral dental and dermol pigmentation. *Am J Ophthalmol* 1998; **125**: 396–7.
33 Boettner EA, Woffer JR. Transmission of the ocular media. *Invest Ophthalmol Vis Sci* 1962; **i**: 776–83.
34 Parrish JA, Chylack LT, Woehler ME *et al.* Dermatological and ocular examination in rabbits chronically photosensitised with methoxsalen. *J Invest Dermatol* 1979; **73**: 256–8.
35 Basis O, Hollstrom E, Lidor S *et al.* Absence of cataract 10 years after treatment with 8-methoxypsoralen. *Acta Derm Venereol Suppl (Stockh)* 1980; **60**: 79–80.
36 Hammershoy O, Jessen F. A retrospective study of cataract formation in 96 patients treated with PUVA. *Acta Derm Venereol Suppl (Stockh)* 1982; **62**: 444–6.
37 Stern RC, Parrish JA, Fitzpatrick TB. Ocular findings in patients treated with PUVA. *J Invest Dermatol* 1985; **85**: 269–73.
38 Lerman S, Megaw J, Gardner K *et al.* PUVA therapy and human cataractogenesis. *Invest Ophthalmol Vis Sci* 1982; **23**: 801–4.

39 Calzavara-Pinton PG, Carlino A, Manfredi E *et al.* Ocular side effects of PUVA treated patients refusing eye sun protection. *Acta Derm Venereol Suppl (Stockh)* 1994; **186**: 164–5.

40 Stern RS. Ocular lens findings in patients treated with PUVA. *J Invest Dermatol* 1994; **103**: 534–8.

41 See JA, Weller P. Ocular complications of PUVA therapy. *Australas J Dermatol* 1993; **34**: 1–4.

42 Prytowsky JH, Keen MS, Rabinowitz AU *et al.* Present status of eyelid phototherapy: clinical efficacy and transmittance of ultra violet and visible radiation through human eyelids. *J Am Acad Dermatol* 1992; **26**: 607–13.

43 Moseley H, Cox NH, MacKie RM. The suitability of sunglasses used by patients following ingestion of psoralens. *Br J Dermatol* 1988; **118**: 247–53.

44 Moseley H, Jones SK. Clear ultraviolet blocking lenses for use by PUVA patients. *Br J Dermatol* 1990; **123**: 775–81.

45 Huang W, Foster JA, Rogachefsky AJ. Pharmacology of botulinum toxin. *J Am Acad Dermatol* 2000; **43**: 249–59.

Tumours

Benign tumours of the eyelid

As would be expected of such complex tissue, the eyelid gives rise to a large number of skin tumours. Tumours can arise from the epidermis and dermis in addition to the adnexal structures, which include the meibomian and Zeis sebaceous glands, eccrine and Moll's apocrine sweat glands, and the specialized hair follicles of the eyelashes. They may also originate from lymphoid neural and vascular tissue found in the preseptal tissues of the eyelid. Although optimal treatment of the tumours begins with accurate diagnosis, many are rather non-specific in their appearance and are only diagnosed with certainty by histology.

Keratoses

Both seborrhoeic and actinic keratoses occur on the eyelid. They have similar clinical features to those elsewhere on the skin and are treated in the same way with local destructive measures, using carefully applied cryotherapy, curettage and cautery or laser ablation under local anaesthetic. Recurrent actinic keratosis should be biopsied and sent for histological examination to make sure it is not a deceptive manifestation of an early skin cancer.

Xanthelasma [1,2]

These present as yellowish cutaneous plaques, most commonly located on the medial part of the eyelids. They are usually bilateral and are much more common in elderly patients. About 60% of patients have an associated hypercholesterolaemia and lipid levels should be measured. Patients often request treatment for cosmetic reasons. Although 90% trichloroacetic acid applied with a cotton wool bud is used there is a significant risk of spillage into the eye. More effective treatment is by surgical excision or ablation with carbon dioxide laser. Necrobiotic xanthogranuloma may look similar to xanthelasma but they are thicker and more nodular. These lesions may involve

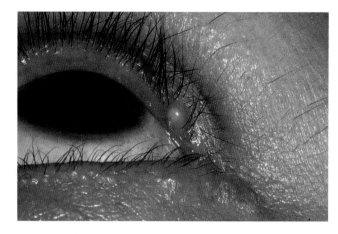

Fig. 64.12 Cyst of Moll. Small translucent cyst on anterior lid margin. (Courtesy of Mr N. Joshi, Chelsea & Westminster Hospital/ Medical Illustration UK, London, UK.)

the conjunctiva and sclera. On the rare occasions that they infiltrate the orbit they may cause proptosis.

Juvenile xanthogranuloma [3]

These lesions occasionally involve the eyelid, conjunctiva or uveal tract. They may be associated with glaucoma and threaten sight. Patients need screening by an ophthalmologist.

Adnexal tumours [4]

Syringomas, milia, trichoepitheliomas and tricholemmomas present as small papules around the eyelids. They can be very difficult to distinguish from each other. Syringomas are the most common, but histology from a biopsy is the only way to make a definite diagnosis. Treatment is by local destruction of the lesions. Eccrine hidrocystomas can present in an eruptive fashion on the face and eyelids; they may respond to topical atropine.

Benign cysts of the eyelid

Retention cysts may arise from either the glands of Moll or of Zeis. A cyst of Moll usually presents as a small translucent lesion on the anterior lid margin close to the lacrimal punctum (Fig. 64.12). Glands of Zeis are sebaceous glands and their retention cysts contain oily secretions and are more opaque than a cyst of Moll. An eccrine gland hidrocystoma is similar in appearance to a cyst of Moll but is not confined to the lid margin. These cysts are treated by excision.

Chalazion [5]

This lesion represents a chronic granulomatous inflammatory reaction around a blocked sebaceous gland.

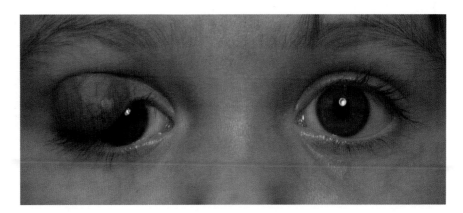

Fig. 64.13 Capillary haemangioma. Enlarging lesion on right upper lid starting to occlude vision. (Courtesy of Mr N. Joshi, Chelsea & Westminster Hospital/Medical Illustration UK, London, UK.)

Patients with seborrhoeic dermatitis and rosacea are at increased risk of chalazion formation. A chalazion presents as a firm lump in the eyelid, which is clearly visible when the lid is everted; an association with chronic posterior blepharitis is common. Large and troublesome lesions can be treated by everting the lid with a special clamp, incising the cyst and curetting the contents through the tarsal plate. Patients who develop recurrent chalazion associated with seborrhoeic dermatitis and rosacea benefit from long-term antibiotic treatment using tetracyclines. Hot saline compresses reduce the inflammation.

Pigmented naevi

The skin on the eyelid can develop pigmented naevi. Their appearance, classification and potential malignant change applies as elsewhere on the skin.

Naevus of Ota

This lesion affects the eyelids, conjunctiva and sclera. Occasionally the pigmentation is confined to the eye with no cutaneous involvement. Naevus of Ota carries an increased risk of ocular melanoma and glaucoma and patients need to be referred for ophthalmic examination and long-term review.

Melanoacanthoma [6]

These are small, shining, black papules situated along the line of the lashes and are a form of dermatosis papulosa nigricans.

Vascular naevi [7–10]

Strawberry naevus (capillary haemangioma) can affect the eyelids. It is more common on the upper lid and presents as a unilateral red raised lesion, which grows quickly during the first year of life (Fig. 64.13). Spontaneous involution occurs usually by age 9 years. Amblyopia is the main complication of larger periorbital lesions and results either from physical closure of the eye and occlusion of the pupil, giving rise to stimulus deprivation, or from refractive errors caused by changes in local pressure. Both systemic and intralesional corticosteroids can reduce the bulk of the haemangioma. Surgical resection or laser therapy is helpful in certain cases.

Port-wine stain

This is a rare congenital vascular lesion, which may affect the eyelids. It presents as a sharply demarcated red patch. Extensive lesions involving the periocular region have a high risk of central nervous involvement and of ipsilateral glaucoma (especially if the upper lid is involved), which may not develop until adult life.

Keratoacanthoma

Keratoacanthomas may develop on the eyelid. They present as a small papule, which grows rapidly developing a characteristic keratin-filled crater and may reach up to 3 cm in diameter (Fig. 64.14). The lesions then stop growing and remain static for 2 or 3 months before spontaneously involuting, which can lead to significant scarring of the eyelid. Because of this, the lesion should be excised at an early stage.

Malignant tumours of the eyelid [11,12]

Basal cell carcinomas (BCCs), squamous cell carcinomas (SCCs) and malignant melanomas all occur on the eyelid as on other areas of the skin. The same rules for management apply on the eyelid as at any site, but the eyelid poses specific problems in preserving good cosmesis and residual function. Clinical examination is an unreliable way of determining the extent of many of these lesions, particularly sclerosing BCC. Early referral to an oculoplastic surgeon is advisable with a view to Mohs micrographic surgery if appropriate.

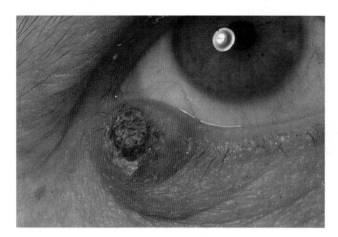

Fig. 64.14 Keratoacanthoma. Keratin-filled crater on lid margin. (Courtesy of Mr N. Joshi, Chelsea & Westminster Hospital/Medical Illustration UK, London, UK.)

Basal cell carcinomas [13–16]

These are the most common skin malignancy and in most series account for 90% of malignant tumours. They rarely metastasize but cause problems by local tissue destruction and invasion of periorbital tissue. Over 70% arise on the lower eyelid followed in order of frequency by the medial canthus, upper eyelid and lateral canthus. Tumours located near to the medial canthus can invade the orbit and sinuses. They are more difficult to excise than those elsewhere, because of the high risk of damaging the tear duct. The majority of BCCs are solid or cystic and fairly straightforward to recognize (Fig. 64.15). Sclerosing or morphoeic BCCs are less common and can be difficult to diagnose as they infiltrate beneath the epidermis forming a flat indurated plaque with indistinct margins, which may simulate a localized area of chronic dermatitis. The paucity of reticular dermis and subcutaneous fat to resist deep invasion presents a particular problem with the eye. Once the orbital septum is penetrated the BCC can rapidly invade, threatening the orbit. At the medial canthus the lacrimal sac and the rich anastomosis of blood vessels offers little barrier. Curettage and cautery is generally not advised for the treatment of eyelid lesions. The skin is thin and tears easily and the sensitivity of the curette is lost in the soft tissue. Successful initial treatment with surgery and accurate margin assessment to ensure complete excision is mandatory in management of these tumours. Mohs' micrographic surgery is usually the treatment of choice where margins are in doubt. Radiotherapy damages and scars the eyelid tissues and lacrimal system and should be reserved for situations when surgery is otherwise inappropriate. Cryotherapy is best avoided due to the risk of leaving residual tumour.

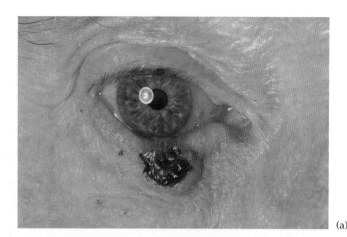

(a)

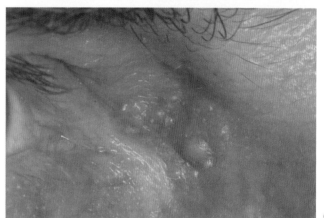

(b)

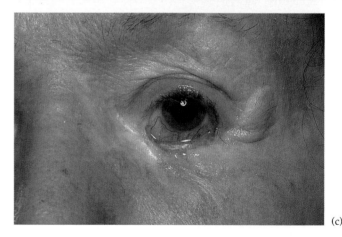

(c)

Fig. 64.15 Basal cell carcinoma (BCC). (a) Ulcerated BCC on lower lid. (b) Poorly defined BCC at medial canthus. (c) Morphoeic BCC along lower lid. (Courtesy of Mr N. Joshi, Chelsea & Westminster Hospital/Medical Illustration UK, London, UK.)

Squamous cell carcinomas [17]

This is much less common than BCCs, accounting for between 5 and 10% of eyelid malignancies. SCCs occur on a background of marked actinic damage. They mainly affect the lower eyelid and lid margin, and may arise *de*

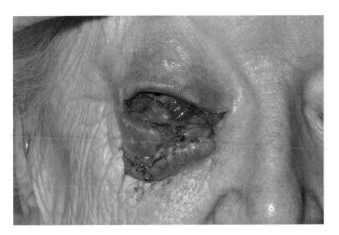

Fig. 64.16 Squamous cell carcinoma (SCC). Infiltrating ulcerated SCC on lower lid. (Courtesy of Mr N. Joshi, Chelsea & Westminster Hospital/Medical Illustration UK, London, UK.)

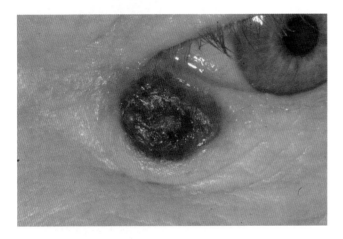

Fig. 64.17 Malignant melanoma. Irregularly pigmented lesion on lower lid. (Courtesy of Mr N. Joshi, Chelsea & Westminster Hospital/Medical Illustration UK, London, UK.)

novo or from pre-existing actinic keratoses. SCC of the eyelids may be nodular, plaque like or ulcerated (Fig. 64.16). Excision with adequate margins is the treatment of choice. Tumours greater than 2 cm in diameter and those with deep penetration have a higher risk of metastasis. Histological evidence of poor differentiation or of perineural invasion are also poor prognostic factors requiring more aggressive treatment. Mohs' surgery is indicated where the initial margins are not free of tumour and offers a good long-term prognosis. As with BCC, cryotherapy and radiotherapy are reserved for situations where surgery is inappropriate.

Malignant melanoma

This may occur on the eyelids or conjunctiva. As elsewhere, melanomas are characterized by a change in size, shape or colour of a pigmented lesion (Fig. 64.17). However, a sig-

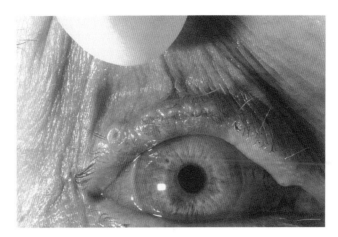

Fig. 64.18 Sebaceous gland carcinoma. Infiltrating lesion on upper lid. (Courtesy of Mr N. Joshi, Chelsea & Westminster Hospital/Medical Illustration UK, London, UK.)

nificant proportion of lid melanomas are amelanotic and this may give rise to difficulties with clinical diagnosis.

Sebaceous gland carcinoma and epithelioma [18,19]

These are very rare tumours, accounting for less than 1–5% of malignant tumours of the eyelid. Sebaceous gland carcinoma usually arises from the meibomian glands, occasionally from the glands of Zeis. In contrast to BCC or SCC, the majority of lesions affect the upper lid. Most lesions are nodular and look very much like a chalazion (see Figs 64.6a, 64.6b & 64.18), causing delay in diagnosis; a sebaceous tumour should always be suspected if a 'chalazion' lasts for more than 6 months, and a 'chalazion' that recurs should be viewed with great suspicion, excised and sent for histology. Because of late diagnosis, sebaceous gland carcinoma carries a significantly mortality. Wide local excision is the treatment of choice. The multicentric nature of the tumour may limit the use of Mohs' surgery.

Eccrine carcinoma [20]

These are rare cancers of the eye and may present as an indurated thicking of the lid or with a signet-ring appearance. They are commonest in middle-aged or elderly men and recur after excision.

Merkel cell carcinoma

A very rare tumour. It can also mimic a chalazion in its early stages, with delay in diagnosis. It is highly malignant and has often metastasized by the time of excision.

Kaposi's sarcoma

A vascular malignancy. It presents as a purple lesion on

the eyelid or conjunctiva and can be mistaken for a benign haemangioma. However, it grows rapidly and may ulcerate and bleed. When it presents on the eyelid it is associated with AIDS, of which it may be the sole manifestation at the time of presentation. These lesions are very radiosensitive, and this is the preferred mode of treatment once a biopsy has been taken to confirm the diagnosis.

REFERENCES

1 Watanabe A. Serum lipids lipoprotein lipids and coronary heart disease in patients with xanthelasma palpebrarum. *Atherosclerosis* 1981; **38**: 283–90.

2 Codere F, Lee RD, Anderson RL. Necrobiotic xanthogranuloma of the eyelid. *Arch Ophthalmol* 1983; **101**: 60–3.

3 Dapling RB, Nelson ME. Ocular lesions in patients with juvenile xanthogranuloma. *Br J Dermatol* 1994; **130**: 260–1.

4 Armstrong DK, Walsh MY, Corbet JR. Multiple facial eccrine hidrocystomas —effective topical treatment with atropine. *Br J Dermatol* 1998; **139**: 558–9.

5 Coskey RJ, Liroi J, Rossini T. Diagnosis and treatment of chalazia. *J Am Acad Dermatol* 1986; **15**: 345–7.

6 Spott D, Heaton CL, Word MG. Melanoacanthoma of the eyelid. *Arch Dermatol* 1972; **105**: 898–9.

7 Goldberg NS, Rosanova M. Periorbital haemangioma. *Dermatol Clin* 1992; **10**: 653–61.

8 Stigmar G, Crawford JS, Ward CM *et al.* Ophthalmological sequelae of infantile haemangiomas of the eyelids and orbit. *Am J Ophthalmol* 1978; **85**: 806–13.

9 Bruckner AL, Frieden IJ. Haemangiomas of infancy. *J Am Acad Dermatol* 2003; **48**: 477–93.

10 Boyd MJ, Collin JRO. Capillary haemangiomas: an approach to their management. *Br J Ophthalmol* 1991; **75**: 298–300.

11 Salasche SJ, Shore JW, Olbricht SM. Periocular tumours. *Dermatol Clin* 1992; **10**: 669–85.

12 Char DH. The management of lid and conjunctival malignancies. *Surv Ophthalmol* 1980; **24**: 679–80.

13 Tesluk GC. Eyelid lesions. Incidence and comparison of benign and malignant lesions. *Ann Ophthalmol* 1985; **17**: 704–7.

14 Anderson RL. A warning on cryosurgery for eyelid malignancies. *Arch Ophthalmol* 1978; **96**: 1289–90.

15 Mohs FE. Microscopically controlled excision of medial canthal carcinomas. *Ann Plast Surg* 1981; **7**: 308–11.

16 Mohs FE. Micrographic surgery for the microscopically controlled excision of eyelid cancers. *Arch Ophthalmol* 1986; **104**: 901–9.

17 Rosin P, Drubow LM, Rigel DJ. Squamous cell carcinoma healed by Mohs' surgery: an experience with 414 cases in a period of 15 years. *J Dermatol Surg Oncol* 1981; **7**: 800–1.

18 Rao NA, Hidyet A, McClean JW *et al.* Sebaceous carcinoma of the ocular adnexae. A clinicopathologic study of 104 cases with a 5-year follow up date. *Hum Pathol* 1982; **13**: 113–22.

19 Spencer JM, Nossa R, Tse DT, Sequerra M. Sebaceous carcinoma of the eyelid treated with Mohs' micrographic surgery. *J Am Acad Dermatol* 2001; **45**: 1004–9.

20 Ni C, Dryja TP, Albert DM. Sweat gland tumours of the eyelids. A clinicopathological analysis of 55 cases. *Int Ophthalmol Clin* 1982; **22**: 1–22.

Chapter 65

The External Ear

C.T.C. Kennedy

Anatomy and physiology [1–3]

The external ear consists of the auricle, the external auditory canal and the outer layer of the tympanic membrane.

The auricle, or pinna (Fig. 65.1), is a convoluted, elastic and cartilaginous plate covered by skin which is continuous medially with the lining of the external auditory canal. Except on the non-cartilaginous lobe and at the back of the ear, the skin is bound firmly to the cartilage. The auricle is attached to the head by fibrous ligaments and three vestigial auricularis muscles. The size and general detail of the auricle can vary greatly between individuals, and may be characteristically affected in a number of congenital syndromes. In humans, the auricle is largely functionless and motionless.

The epidermis of the ear has a complex dermal–epidermal junction, a conspicuous stratum granulosum and a thick, compact stratum corneum [4]. The dermis contains abundant elastic tissue. Sebaceous glands are numerous, particularly on the tragus and lobe, and fine vellus or terminal hairs occur over the entire surface, but are especially prominent on the helix and tragus. Coarser terminal hair is seen in some men as a Y-linked and androgen-dependent inherited trait (Fig. 65.2). Eccrine sweat glands are sparsely and irregularly distributed except in the external auditory canal, which has, instead, a large number of modified apocrine or ceruminous glands. The pinna has a variably thick fatty layer that extends between the perichondrium and the reticular dermis and that also forms the main fibrofatty core of the lobe of the ear.

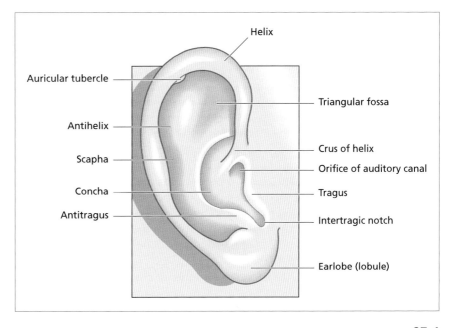

Fig. 65.1 Anatomical landmarks of the auricle.

Helix
Auricular tubercle
Antihelix
Scapha
Concha
Antitragus
Triangular fossa
Crus of helix
Orifice of auditory canal
Tragus
Intertragic notch
Earlobe (lobule)

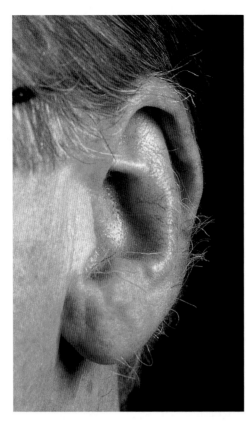

Fig. 65.2 Coarse terminal hair on the auricle: a trait associated with the Y chromosome.

The blood supply to the auricle is provided by anastomosing branches of the superficial temporal and posterior auricular arteries, which drain via posterior auricular and superficial temporal veins into the external jugular vein and via the superficial temporal, maxillary and facial veins into the internal jugular vein. Lymphatic drainage is to the superficial parotid, retro-auricular and superficial cervical lymph nodes. Embryonic fusion planes and minute deficiencies in the cartilaginous portion of the external auditory canal provide potential pathways for the spread of infection and tumours.

There is a complex nerve supply to the ear involving elements of the Vth, VIIth, IXth and Xth cranial nerves as well as cervical branches of the greater and lesser auricular nerves. The back of the ear is supplied by the greater auricular nerve (C2,3), the concha by the auricular branch of the vagus (Xth) and the anterior part of the pinna and the external auditory canal by the auriculotemporal branch of the Vth cranial nerve. Intercommunicating branches of the VIIth, IXth and Xth supply the deeper parts of the ear. With this complicated nerve supply, otalgia is more commonly due to referred pain than to disease in the ear itself [5]. Within the dermis, the nerve supply is abundant, especially around hair follicles where there are complicated basket-like networks of acetylcholinesterase and butyrylcholinesterase nerve fibres [4]. Free nerve endings are also present, but there are no organized nerve endings as occur on glabrous skin elsewhere [6].

The external auditory canal extends upwards and backwards in an S-shaped curve from the concha to the tympanic membrane. The angle of curvature varies between races and individuals, being more marked in white people than in black people or Polynesians. This has a bearing on trauma, infection and the retention of moisture. The length of the canal is 2.5 cm as measured from the concha to drum. The outer third of the canal is cartilaginous and is lined by a thicker layer of skin than the inner portion within the temporal bone. Anteroinferiorly there are two horizontal fissures in the cartilaginous canal, the fissures of Santorini. These can allow infection or tumour to pass beyond the external auditory canal, for example to the parotid gland. Subcutaneous tissue is scanty, and the epithelium is firmly bound to the perichondrium. Sebaceous glands are plentiful, and open into the follicles of extremely fine vellus hairs. Occasionally, larger terminal hairs (tragi) arise in the canal or around the meatus and these, if they become matted with wax or debris, may interfere with normal epidermal 'migration' and ventilation of the ear and hence may play a part in the development of 'hot-weather ear' (see p. 65.22).

Eccrine sweat glands are not present in the auditory canal but modified apocrine (ceruminous) glands are numerous. They increase in size and activity at puberty. There is great individual and racial variability, and although concentrated in the cartilaginous part of the canal, they may also occur, albeit sparsely, in the osseous portion.

The inner osseous part of the acoustic canal constitutes two-thirds of its total length. The skin is firmly bound to the periosteum, subcutaneous tissue being nearly absent and only 30–50 μm thick. The epidermis here is thin and easily traumatized, and rete ridges are absent [1]. The skin of the external auditory canal and tympanic membrane is unique in that there is no frictional loss of stratum corneum; cerumen (wax) and epithelial debris have therefore to be removed by a special 'migratory' property of the external ear canal epithelium [7]. A slight narrowing of the canal, the isthmus, occurs at or just medial to the junction of the two parts. When marked, it may impede the flow of cerumen to the exterior. Just medial to the isthmus, inferiorly and anteriorly, is the tympanic sulcus. Debris often collects here, especially in patients with chronic external otitis.

The surface pH of the auditory canal varies from 5.6–5.8 at the concha to 7.3–7.5 at 5–10 mm within the canal. With inflammation, the pH becomes slightly more acid [8].

Microbiology

The skin of the external auditory canal in most healthy

individuals supports the growth of multiple bacterial species, especially *Staphylococcus epidermidis*, *Corynebacterium* spp., *Bacillus* spp. and less often *Staphylococcus aureus*. *Pseudomonas aeruginosa*, often relevant to external otitis, and fungi are not normally found [3]. The normal flora can include organisms such as *Turicella otidis*, which can cause otitis media [9].

Cerumen (wax) [10]

Cerumen is the combined product of sebaceous and apocrine glands. It contains both squalene and insoluble fatty acids. Analysis by flash pyrolysis–gas chromatography/ mass spectrometry has shown numerous diterpenoids [11]. Its main function is to waterproof the external auditory canal. Extrusion is aided by mastication and by the peripheral movement and desquamation of the epithelial cells of the canal. It is impeded if the ear canal is too narrow or tortuous, or when inflammation interferes with the normal process of 'migration'.

There are genetically determined differences in cerumen composition and character: so-called 'dry' ear wax is light grey, dry and flaky; 'wet' ear wax is golden brown and sticky. The former is very common in Asians. Wax phenotype is determined by a single gene pair, the wet wax allele being dominant [10]. Cerumen darkens with exposure to air.

Although not bactericidal, cerumen does not encourage bacterial or fungal growth. Possible reasons include the presence of lysozyme, immunoglobulins and polyunsaturated fatty acids.

Two populations have been shown to have excessive production and/or impaction of cerumen: individuals with mental retardation and the elderly [10]. An increased secretion of cerumen occurs in patients treated with aromatic retinoids [12,13].

If wax becomes impacted or adherent, it can cause various symptoms such as hearing loss, tinnitus, vertigo, pain and itching, and can be a contributory factor to external otitis. It may be removed by irrigation techniques or suction under direct vision [14]. Although it is generally thought that cerumenolytics such as 10% aqueous sodium bicarbonate or 2.5% aqueous acetic acid are of little value, they may have a use in children [15]. Docusate sodium is more effective than some traditional agents [16]. Although not yet studied in controlled trials, the bile acids may be very effective for removing ear wax [11].

Contact dermatitis from medicaments or irritant cerumenolytics [17] is well recognized. Inflammation interferes with normal epidermal migration and tends therefore both to induce and to encourage the retention of scale. The pruritus associated with excess cerumen, and the low-grade inflammation that often accompanies this, frequently leads to a persistent form of low-grade neurodermatitis.

REFERENCES

1 Perry ET. *The Human Ear Canal*. Springfield, IL: Thomas, 1957.
2 Lucente FE. Anatomy, histology and physiology. In: Lucente FE, Lawson W, Novick NL, eds. *The External Ear*. Philadelphia: Saunders, 1995: 1–17.
3 Kelly KE, Mohs DC. The external auditory canal: anatomy and physiology. *Otolaryngol Clin North Am* 1996; **29**: 725–9.
4 Montagna W, Giacometti L. Histology and cytochemistry of human skin. XXXII. The external ear. *Arch Dermatol* 1969; **99**: 757–67.
5 Al-Sheikhli ARJ. Pain in the ear: with special reference to referred pain. *J Laryngol Otol* 1980; **94**: 1433–40.
6 Sinclair DC, Weddell G, Zander E. The relationship of cutaneous sensibility to neurohistology in the human pinna. *J Anat* 1952; **86**: 402–11.
7 Alberti PWRM. Epithelial migration on the tympanic membrane. *J Laryngol Otol* 1964; **78**: 808–30.
8 Fabricant ND. The pH factor in the treatment of otitis externa. *Arch Otolaryngol* 1957; **65**: 11–2.
9 Stroman DW, Roland PS, Dohar J, Burt W. Microbiology of normal external auditory canal. *Laryngoscope* 2001; **111**: 2054–9.
10 Roeser RJ, Ballachanda BB. Physiology, pathophysiology, and anthropology/ epidemiology of human earcanal secretions. *J Am Acad Audiol* 1997; **8**: 391–400.
11 Burkhart CN, Kruge MA, Burkhart CG, Black C. Cerumen composition by flash pyrolysis–gas chromatography/mass spectrometry. *Otol Neurotol* 2001; **22**: 715–22.
12 Burge SM, Wilkinson JD, Miller AJ *et al*. The efficacy of an aromatic retinoid, Tigason, in the treatment of Darier's disease. *Br J Dermatol* 1981; **104**: 675–9.
13 Kramer M. Excessive cerumen production due to the aromatic retinoid Tigason in a patient with Darier's disease. *Acta Derm Venereol (Stockh)* 1981; **62**: 267–8.
14 Grossan M. Cerumen removal: current challenges. *Ear Nose Throat J* 1998; **77**: 541–8.
15 Carr MM, Smith RL. Ceruminolytic efficacy in adults versus children. *J Otolaryngol* 2001; **30**: 154–6.
16 Singer AJ, Sauris E, Viccellio AW. Ceruminolytic effects of docusate sodium: a randomized controlled trial. *Ann Emerg Med* 2000; **36**: 228–32.
17 Holmes RC, Johns AN, Wilkinson JD *et al*. Medicament contact dermatitis in patients with chronic inflammatory ear disease. *J R Soc Med* 1982; **75**: 27–30.

Examination [1]

As well as examining the pinna, the dermatologist may need to examine the ear canal. Equipment available should include a headlight or equivalent, otoscope, several sizes of ear speculae, ear curettes, metal applicators, bayonet forceps, ear irrigation apparatus and cotton.

General inspection of the auricles should take account of their symmetry, size, shape and position, and completeness of development.

The ear canal is best inspected when the auricle is pulled gently upwards, outwards and backwards, and the largest possible speculum is used. It is essential to avoid traumatizing the thin skin of the canal, particularly beyond the isthmus. If inspection reveals accumulation of cerumenous debris, this can sometimes be removed carefully using a curette or wire loop along the posterior wall. If the material is against the drum, gentle suction may be feasible. Irrigation should only be used if the drum is known to be intact.

Samples may need to be taken for bacteriology, mycology and histology. If a biopsy is required from the canal, this should be devolved to a surgeon with the necessary expertise.

REFERENCE

1 Lucente FE. Techniques of examination. In: Lucente FE, Lawson W, Novick NL, eds. *The External Ear*. Philadelphia: Saunders, 1995: 18–24.

Developmental defects

The auricle begins to develop at the end of the fifth week of embryonic life in the first branchial groove, contributed to by the first (mandibular) and second (hyoid) arches [1]. Six hillocks appear on these arches and later fuse to form the complex shape of the fully developed auricle.

Developmental defects are considered in detail in Chapter 15. Only those defects of the ear sufficiently common to constitute a part of general dermatological practice are therefore considered here, together with some general principles relating to congenital ear abnormalities and their more important medical and otological associations [2–6]. Pinna abnormalities are associated sufficiently often with conductive hearing loss that screening tests should be carried out [7].

About 30% of infants with external ear anomalies have a renal anomaly identifiable by ultrasound examination, and this combination is a strong pointer towards a multiple congenital anomaly syndrome, in particular Townes–Brocks, CHARGE, branchio-oto-renal, Nager and diabetic embryopathy syndromes [8].

Many developmental defects are of unknown aetiology. Some, however, are associated with chromosomal abnormalities, for example those occurring in Down's syndrome, or are associated with syndromes that have well-recognized Mendelian inheritance patterns, for example the *e*ctrodactyly, *e*ctodermal dysplasia and *c*left lip–palate (EEC) syndrome. Environmental factors may be implicated as in fetal alcohol syndrome and fetal hydantoin syndrome, and maternal exposure to isotretinoin and thalidomide.

Congenital ear abnormalities exhibit great variability, even within syndromes or families, and any one aetiological factor may be associated with a variety of ear malformations. External ear malformations as part of a genetic syndrome account for less than 10% of all external ear abnormalities; isolated cases of ear malformation may either be non-genetic in origin or have a genetic basis but with poor gene penetrance [9].

Microtia (small ears)

Microtia designates a spectrum of underdevelopment of the pinna, from small ears to absence of an ear or ears. Small ears are often associated with hearing deficit and may be a feature of many syndromes. In addition to being small, the pinna may be rudimentary, resembling the hillocks from which it is embryologically derived. The more primitive the appearance, the greater the likelihood of hearing abnormalities, usually due to defects or atresia of the ossicles. There may also be a narrowing or atresia of the auditory canal [9–11] and various abnormalities of the middle ear [12] and inner ear [5]. A wide variety of non-aural abnormalities are associated with small ears, multiple malformations occurring in 56% in one large series [13]. Small ears are a feature of many syndromes, including Down's syndrome, Treacher Collins syndrome, Goldenhar's syndrome, Apert's syndrome, various first and second branchial arch and first branchial cleft syndromes, Mohr's orofaciodigital syndrome, Duane's retraction syndrome and thalidomide embryopathy [5,6,14].

Familial microtia inherited as an autosomal dominant trait has been described [15]. Microtia is one of the birth defects that occurs more on the right than the left side [16].

Macrotia (large ears)

Macrotia is a developmental variation in which the amount of tissue between the helix and antihelix is increased, causing the ears to wing out. The ear may also be diffusely enlarged, or elongated. Such changes are common in Turner's syndrome, and there may be associated sensorineural deafness. Larger ears are well described in fragile X syndrome [17] and Kabuki's syndrome, although in the latter they may also be smaller than normal [18]. Generally enlarged ears are sometimes seen in patients with the XXXXY chromosome defect. The cartilaginous parts of the ears are enlarged and soft in Laband's syndrome [19,20]. In this rare disorder the ears are large and floppy, in association with a bulbous soft nose, gingival fibromatosis and a variety of other findings including absence or dysplasia of nails and/or of terminal phalanges, hyperextensibility of joints, hepatosplenomegaly, and rarely hypertrichosis and mental retardation.

Low-set ears

Normally, the top of the helix is at the same level as the eyebrow, the earlobe is above the angle of the mandible and the external auditory meatus is at the level of the ala nasi. Low-set ears may in addition be posteriorly rotated, and are often small. The condition is usually bilateral. Although it may be isolated, it is often associated with major middle-ear or systemic malformations, appearing for example in Turner's, Noonan's, Patau's and Crouzon's syndromes.

Peri-auricular anomalies

Pre-auricular pits, sinuses (Fig. 65.3) and tags are relatively common, with an incidence of approximately 1% [9,21]. Lesions on or near the tragus are probably best

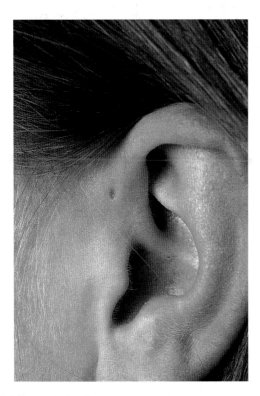

Fig. 65.3 Pre-auricular sinus.

termed 'accessory tragus' [22]. The term 'accessory auricle' is sometimes used for this, and for similar firm elevations of skin and cartilage just near the ascending crus of the helix. They may be single or multiple and may occur anywhere in a line from the tragus to the angle of the mouth. Accessory auricles, congenital fistulae and other external ear manifestations may occur alone or may be associated with more widespread first and second branchial arch abnormalities, for example Treacher Collins and Goldenhar's syndromes [3,4,8,21], or with developmental abnormalities of the genito-urinary tract [8,21], as well as with isolated hearing defects.

Variations in the shape of the pinna

Minor variations in size and shape are common and not usually associated with any other abnormality. These include *bat ear* or protruding ear, in which the antihelix lacks the usual bulge; *lop ear*, in which there is an unrolled helix, a poorly developed antihelix and scapha, and a large concha resulting in a somewhat floppy ear; and *prominent auricular (Darwin's) tubercle*. Variations in the contour of the helix and antihelix to produce a bulge of the anterosuperior part of the pinna account for so-called *Mozart's ear*, and in *Wildemuth's ear* the antihelix is prominent and the formation of the helix is poor. These minor ear anomalies can be a syndromic feature or can be associated with conductive and occasionally sensorineural hearing loss, but in most instances they are isolated. They may, however, be inherited, as in the Mozart family. A distinctive *railroad track abnormality* with marked prominence of the crus of the helix is said to occur in up to 30% of children with fetal alcohol syndrome [10,14] and a protruding auricle may, rarely, be a sign of neuromuscular disease [23]. Various abnormalities of the configuration of the pinna have been described in the distinctive *lumpy scalp syndrome* [24], in which other features include absent or rudimentary nipples and dermal nodules on the scalp [25]. The lobule can show isolated abnormalities, for example pits and clefts. Absence of the lobule is, however, usually associated with a syndrome of a more serious nature [6]. Diagonal linear creases in the lobule are seen in Beckwith–Wiedemann syndrome, and in adult life in association with some degenerative diseases (see p. 65.6), although they are a common finding in normal individuals.

Developmental anomalies of ear hair

Hypertrichosis of the pinnae was originally described as a Y chromosome-linked trait [26]. An autosomal dominant genetic basis for hairy ears has also been noted in South Indians [27] and Maltese [28]. Acquired hairy ears have been described in infants born of diabetic mothers [29,30] and in association with human immunodeficiency virus (HIV) infection [31].

Management [32]

The infant with obvious malformation of the pinna that might have auditory system or other associations should be assessed by a paediatrician. The history may reveal exposure to a teratogen (e.g. isotretinoin) or family history of a syndrome and examination may show evidence of other anomalies. Investigations may include radiological evaluation [33], an auditory brainstem evoked response hearing test and a renal ultrasound. It may be appropriate for an ear, nose and throat (ENT) specialist and plastic surgeon [34,35] to become involved with correction of complications and the physical deformity, respectively.

REFERENCES

1 Bowden REM. Development of the middle and external ear in man. *Proc R Soc Med* 1977; **70**: 807–15.
2 Anson BJ, Donaldson JA, eds. Clinical significance of developmental anatomy. In: *Surgical Anatomy of the Temporal Bone and Ear, Part II. The Ear: Developmental Anatomy*, 2nd edn. Philadelphia: Saunders, 1973: 17–50.
3 Bellucci RJ. Congenital aural malformations: diagnosis and treatment. Symposium on Congenital Disorders in Otolaryngology. *Otolaryngol Clin North Am* 1981; **14**: 95–124.
4 Melnick M. The etiology of external ear malformations and its relation to abnormalities of the middle ear, inner ear, and other organ systems. *Birth Defects* 1980; **16**: 303–31.
5 Bergstrom LB. Anomalies of the ear. In: English GM, ed. *Otolaryngology*, Vol. 1. Philadelphia: Lippincott, 1990: 1–35.

6 Sakashita T, Sando I, Kamerer DB. Congenital anomalies of the external and middle ears. In: Bluestone CD, Stool SE, Kenna MA, eds. *Pediatric Otolaryngology*, 3rd edn. Philadelphia: Saunders, 1996: 333–70.

7 Jaffe BF. Pinna anomalies associated with congenital conductive hearing loss. *Pediatrics* 1976; **57**: 332–41.

8 Wang RY, Earl DL, Ruder RO, Graham JM. Syndromic ear anomalies and renal ultrasounds. *Pediatrics* 2001; **108**: 32.

9 Melnick M, Myrianthopoulos NC. External ear malformations: epidemiology, genetics and natural history. *Birth Defects* 1979; **15**: 1–139.

10 Jahrsdoerfer RA. Congenital atresia of the ear. *Laryngoscope* 1978; **88** (Suppl. 13): 1–48.

11 Okajima H, Takeichi Y, Umeda K, Baba S. Clinical analysis of 592 patients with microtia. *Acta Otolaryngol (Stockh)* 1996; **525**: 18–24.

12 Kountakis SE, Helidonis E, Oarhsdoerfer RA. Microtia grade as an indicator of middle ear development in aural atresia. *Arch Otolaryngol Head Neck Surg* 1995; **121**: 885–6.

13 Jafek BW, Nager GT, Stife J *et al*. Congenital aural atresia: an analysis of 311 cases. *Trans Am Acad Ophthalmol Otolaryngol* 1975; **80**: 588–95.

14 Aase JM. Microtia: clinical observations. *Birth Defects* 1980; **16**: 289–97.

15 Balci S, Boduroglu K, Kaya S. Familial microtia in four generations with variable expressivity and incomplete penetrance in association with type I syndactyly. *Turkish J Pediatr* 2001; **43**: 362–5.

16 Paulozzi LJ, Lary JM. Laterality patterns in infants with external birth defects. *Teratology* 1999; **60**: 265–71.

17 Loesch DZ, Sampson ML. Effect of the fragile X anomaly on body proportions estimated by pedigree analysis. *Clin Genet* 1993; **44**: 82–8.

18 Fong C-T, Wang M, Young EC *et al*. Microtia associated with the Kabuki (Niikawa–Kuraki) syndrome. *Otolaryngol Head Neck Surg* 2001; **125**: 557–8.

19 Laband PF, Habib G, Humphreys GC. Hereditary gingival fibromatosis. Report of an affected family with associated splenomegaly and soft tissue abnormalities. *Oral Surg Oral Med Oral Pathol* 1964; **17**: 339–51.

20 Bazopoulou-Kyrkanidou E, Papagianoulis L, Papanicolaou S, Mavrou A. Laband syndrome: a case report. *J Otol Pathol Med* 1990; **19**: 385–7.

21 Melnick M. Hereditary hearing loss and ear dysplasia–renal adysplasia syndromes: syndrome delineation and possible pathogenesis. *Birth Defects* 1980; **16**: 59–72.

22 Jansen T, Romiti R, Altmeyer MD. Accessory tragus: report of two cases and review of the literature. *Pediatr Dermatol* 2000; **17**: 391–4.

23 Smith DW, Takashima H. Protruding auricle: a neuromuscular sign. *Lancet* 1978; **i**: 747–9.

24 Steinberg RD, Ethington J, Esterly NB. Lumpy scalp syndrome. *Int J Dermatol* 1990; **29**: 657–8.

25 Finlay AY, Marks R. An hereditary syndrome of lumpy scalp, odd ears and rudimentary nipples. *Br J Dermatol* 1978; **99**: 423–30.

26 Dronamrajn KR. Hypertrichosis of the pinnae of the human ear, Y-linked pedigrees. *J Genet* 1961; **51**: 230–43.

27 Kamalan A, Thambiah AS. Genetics of hairy ears in South Indians. *Clin Exp Dermatol* 1990; **15**: 192–4.

28 Ruggles Gates R, Vella F. Hairy pinnae in Malta. *Lancet* 1962; **ii**: 357.

29 Woods DL, Malan AF, Coetzee EJ. Intra-uterine growth in infants of diabetic mothers. *S Afr Med J* 1980; **58**: 441–3.

30 Rafaat M. Hypertrichosis pinnae in babies of diabetic mothers. *Pediatrics* 1981; **68**: 745–6.

31 Tosti A, Gaddoni G, Peluso AM *et al*. Acquired hairy pinnae in a patient infected with the human immunodeficiency virus. *J Am Acad Dermatol* 1993; **28**: 513.

32 Eavey RD. Ear malformations. What a pediatrician can do to assist with auricular reconstruction. *Pediatr Otolaryngol* 1996; **43**: 1233–43.

33 Calzolari F, Garani G, Sensi A, Martini A. Clinical and radiological evaluation in children with microtia. *Br J Audiol* 1999; **33**: 303–12.

34 Meyer R, de Goumoens R, Derder S. Combined aesthetic and functional treatment of microtia. *Aesthetic Plast Surg* 1997; **21**: 159–67.

35 Aguilar EF. Auricular reconstruction in congenital anomalies of the ear. *Facial Plast Surg Clin North Am* 2001; **9**: 159–69.

Ageing changes

Many changes seen on the skin of the pinna attributed to ageing are a result of its exposure to environmental factors, especially UV radiation, cold (perniosis) and infrared radiation. The elderly exposed pinna often shows varying degrees of dermal and epidermal atrophy, solar keratoses and lentigines, solar elastosis, telangiectasia and venous lakes. If the pinna is at least partially light protected, as in many women, the skin may still appear somewhat thinned due to intrinsic ageing changes.

Ear length

It is recognized in Chinese culture that length of the ear in men is a predictor for longevity [1]. Two studies would appear to confirm this: one from Kent, UK [2], and one from Japan [3]. The increase in length of the male ear from the age of 30 years onwards may have a 7-year periodicity [4].

Earlobe creases

First described in 1973 [5], and now known as Frank's sign, a diagonal crease in the earlobes of adults has been associated in many studies with an increased risk for atherosclerotic coronary artery disease. A meta-analysis in 1983 gave a relative risk of 2.06 for heart disease if there are bilateral creases [6] and there is approximately double the risk for death from heart disease [7,8]. The crease can be graded in terms of length and depth, and deeper longer creases have the strongest association. The ear crease appears to be separate from other risk factors for coronary artery disease, and is not simply a function of age [9]. A more recent case–control series suggests a relative risk of 1.37 for myocardial infarction [10] and a lower specificity for the sign than previously estimated [11].

Diagonal earlobe creases are seen in other contexts, for example Beckwith–Wiedemann syndrome [12] (Fig. 65.4),

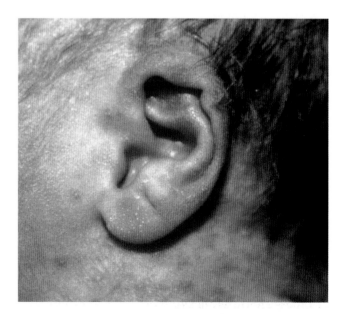

Fig. 65.4 Diagonal earlobe crease in an infant with Beckwith–Wiedemann syndrome.

and do not seem to be associated with coronary artery disease in Hawaiians [13], native Americans [14] or Chinese [15].

Earlobe creases have also been associated with primary open-angle glaucoma [16].

REFERENCES

1 Woo Pick-Ngor, Lip Peck-Lin. Why do old men have big ears? (letter) *BMJ* 1996; **312**: 586.
2 Heathcote JA. Why do old men have big ears? (letter) *BMJ* 1996; **311**: 1668.
3 Asai Y, Yoshimura M, Nago N, Yamada T. Correlation of ear length with age in Japan (letter). *BMJ* 1996; **312**: 582.
4 Verhulst J, Onghena P. Circaseptennial rhythm in ear growth. *BMJ* 1996; **313**: 1597–8.
5 Frank ST. Aural sign of coronary artery disease. *N Engl J Med* 1973; **289**: 327–8.
6 Elliott WJ. Earlobe crease and coronary artery disease: 1000 patients and review of the literature. *Am J Med* 1983; **75**: 1024–32.
7 Kirkham N, Murrells T, Melcher DH, Morrison EA. Diagonal earlobe creases and fatal cardiovascular disease: a necropsy study. *Br Heart J* 1989; **61**: 361–4.
8 Patel V, Champ C, Andrews PS *et al*. Diagonal earlobe creases and atheromatous disease: a post mortem study. *J R Coll Physicians Lond* 1992; **26**: 274–7.
9 Tranchesi B, Barbosa V, de Albuquerque CP *et al*. Diagonal earlobe creases as a marker of the presence and extent of coronary atherosclerosis. *Am J Cardiol* 1992; **70**: 1417–20.
10 Miric D, Fabijanic D, Giunio L *et al*. Dermatological indicators of coronary risk: a case–control study. *Int J Cardiol* 1998; **67**: 251–5.
11 Motamed M, Pelekoudas N. The predictive value of diagonal ear-lobe crease sign. *Int J Clin Pract* 1998; **52**: 305–6.
12 Weidemann HR. Earlobe creases, congenital and acquired (letter). *N Engl J Med* 1979; **301**: 111.
13 Rhoads GG, Klein K, Yano K, Preston H. The earlobe crease sign of obesity in middle-aged Japanese men. *Hawaii Med J* 1977; **36**: 74–7.
14 Fisher JR, Sievers ML. Earlobe crease in American Indians (letter). *Ann Intern Med* 1980; **93**: 512.
15 Cheng TO. Diagonal earlobe creases (letter). *J R Coll Physicians Lond* 1992; **26**: 460.
16 Hawksworth NR. Diagonal earlobe creases: an association with primary open angle glaucoma (letter). *J R Coll Physicians Lond* 1992; **26**: 459–60.

Traumatic conditions

Contusion and haematoma

Bruises of the ear are usually due to blunt trauma and are common in contact sports, such as boxing, wrestling and rugby. In children, physical abuse may need to be excluded [1,2]. A distinctive condition known as *tin ear syndrome* has been considered pathognomonic of child abuse: a triad of isolated ear bruising, haemorrhagic retinopathy and a small ipsilateral subdural haematoma [3].

Following trauma, blood and serum collects in the plane between perichondrium and cartilage, and will undergo fibrosis if not removed early. The patient should be carefully examined for concurrent auditory canal, middle ear, parotid and central nervous system trauma.

Repeated trauma may result in the distorted nodular deformity known as *cauliflower ear*, which is due to varying degrees of cartilage necrosis, fibrosis and dystrophic calcification.

Treatment. Subperichondrial haematomas must be treated promptly, with full aseptic technique to avoid secondary perichondritis. Small collections of fluid can sometimes be aspirated by syringe, but usually need to be drained through a small incision and a laterally placed pressure dressing applied to prevent reaccumulation [4,5]. Another useful technique is to use a through-and-through suture technique to maintain bolsters over the area where the haematoma has been evacuated [6]. Other approaches include a posterior incision and suction drainage [7], or fenestrations in the cartilage to promote adhesion of the opposing perichondrial layers [8]. Prophylactic antibiotics are sometimes given. Improvement of cauliflower ear usually requires multiple corrective procedures.

REFERENCES

1 Manning SC, Casselbrant M, Lammers D. Otolaryngologic manifestations of child abuse. *Int J Pediatr Otorhinolaryngol* 1990; **20**: 7–16.
2 Willner A, Ledereich PS, de Vries EJ. Auricular injury as a presentation of child abuse. *Arch Otolaryngol Head Neck Surg* 1992; **118**: 634–7.
3 Hanigan WC, Peterson RA, Njus G. Tin ear syndrome: rotational acceleration in pediatric head injuries. *Pediatrics* 1987; **80**: 618–22.
4 Germon WH. The care and management of acute haematoma of the external ear. *Laryngoscope* 1980; **90**: 881–5.
5 Lee D, Sperling N. Initial management of auricular trauma. *Am Fam Physician* 1996; **53**: 2339–44.
6 Schuller DE, Dankle SD, Strauss RH. A technique to treat wrestler's auricular hematoma without interrupting training or competition. *Arch Otolaryngol Head Neck Surg* 1989; **115**: 202–6.
7 Bull PD, Lancer JM. Treatment of auricular haematoma by suction drainage. *Clin Otolaryngol* 1984; **9**: 355–60.
8 Tenta LT, Keyes GR. Reconstructive surgery of the external ear. *Otolaryngol Clin North Am* 1981; **14**: 917–38.

Laceration and avulsion

Lacerations of the pinna vary from the trivial to amputation [1]. Because of the risk of cartilage infection, potentially dirty wounds should always be carefully cleaned and a course of prophylactic antibiotic given. It is probably best to avoid suturing the cartilage itself unless pieces overlap or are severely displaced [2]. Injuries that expose cartilage will need to be covered with a skin graft, for example taken from behind the ear or the upper eyelid. If the anterior perichondrium is destroyed, cartilage may need to be excised so that the graft can be placed on the posterior perichondrium. If the post-auricular area is not injured, a pedicled island flap of post-auricular skin may be pulled through the area of excised cartilage and sutured into place. If the helix or antihelix is exposed, it may be possible to cover it with an advancement or rotation flap from the posterior surface of the auricle. Large areas may need to be covered with a pedicled flap of temporoparietal fascia, which in turn is covered with a split-skin graft. The lobule of the ear can be repaired by direct closure, although a cosmetically superior result may be obtained by a broken line repair or Z-plasty [3]. Many techniques have been described for repair of major trauma, including even complete avulsion of the pinna [1,4,5], but these are likely to be beyond the scope of the dermatologist. Following total ear replantation there is lack of cutaneous sensation and this may explain the cold intolerance that can occur [6].

REFERENCES

1 Templer J, Renner GJ. Injuries of the external ear. *Otolaryngol Clin North Am* 1990; **23**: 1003–18.
2 Mladick RA. Salvage of the ear in acute trauma. *Clin Plast Surg* 1978; **5**: 427–35.
3 Walike J, Larrabee WF. Repair of the cleft earlobe. *Laryngoscope* 1985; **95**: 876–7.
4 Lawson W. Management of acute trauma. In: Lucente FE, Lawson W, Norvick NL, eds. *The External Ear*. Philadelphia: Saunders, 1996: 177–82.
5 Kind GM, Buncke GM. Total ear replantation. *Plast Reconstr Surg* 1997; **99**: 1858–67.
6 Finical SJ, Keller KM, Lovett JE. Postoperative ramifications of total ear replantation. *Ann Plast Surg* 1998; **41**: 667–70.

Dermatitis artefacta

The ear is occasionally the sole site for self-mutilation and there may be underlying psychodynamic reasons for this [1].

REFERENCE

1 Paar GH. Excerpt from the treatment of a patient with otitis externa artefacta. *Psychother Psychosom* 1994; **62**: 135–9.

Ear piercing

Earrings have been worn by men and women since antiquity, and tend to follow the dictates of fashion. Current trends include using rings or studs in almost all parts of the body, the use of up to 10 or more in a single ear, and the piercing of cartilage.

Complications are very common, with rates of about 30% whether the procedure is carried out by medical personnel, friend or relative, or in a store; they are also independent of technique, there being little difference in frequency of complications from piercing by needle, staple gun or sharpened stud [1]. Minor infection is the most common adverse effect, with contact dermatitis, keloid and traumatic tear occurring less often [2]; other consequences occur occasionally. Although case series indicate that so-called 'high' ear piercing, i.e. through cartilage, has a significant risk for perichondritis [3,4] and chondritis [5], such events were not found in a population study of 1000 nurses [2]. Embedding of the earring seems to be a common problem in children [6].

The ear is also pierced in acupuncture as used in traditional medicine, and complications have been reported [7,8].

Complications. Various infections and reactions may occur after ear piercing.

Localized bacterial infection, usually with Gram-positive cocci, is common; predisposing factors include skin disease, such as atopic or contact dermatitis. Life-threatening septicaemia has been described [9]. Infants with unsuspected immunodeficiency and individuals with valvular heart disease may be at particular risk. When cartilage is pierced the usual bacterial infection is with *Ps. aeruginosa*, which causes perichondritis [3] or chondritis [5], and for which the best treatment is ciprofloxacin [4]. Any purulent material should be cultured, since other pathogens have been described (e.g. *Lactobacillus* [10]). Primary tuberculosis has been described [11].

Viral hepatitis may also be a hazard [12,13].

Oedema and haematoma [1,14] usually respond to cold compresses, pressure and removal of the earring. Haematoma may require incision and drainage [15].

Trauma can occur from pressure on the lobe and post-auricular skin, or from inaccurate insertion of the post of the earring. Heavy earrings can tear the earlobe, sometimes making it bifid. Repair of the latter is probably best by excision of the cleft and simple closure with eversion of the edges [16], although a staggered repair such as a Z-plasty may be appropriate in some cases.

Sensitization to nickel from earrings remains a major problem, and ear piercing is one explanation for the higher incidence of nickel allergy in females [17]. Even stainless steel studs and clasps, which can produce irritant as well as allergic effects, may release sufficient nickel to elicit contact dermatitis [18]. Gold sensitization, although less common [19], can be a protracted cause of dermatitis even after the earrings are removed [20]. Contact dermatitis from other materials used in earrings, such as olive wood [21], copper [22], cobalt [23,24] and chromium [25], has been described, and may also occur from the use of topical antiseptics, antibiotics and dressings used to treat infection.

Granulomatous and lymphoid reactions. Reddish brown and purple papules and nodules at sites of ear piercing may denote a granulomatous response to gold [26,27] and a lymphocytoma cutis-like reaction has been described [28–30]. Sarcoidosis has presented after ear piercing [31].

Embedded earrings. The spring-loaded gun method of ear piercing can result in the earring backing becoming embedded in the back of the ear [32]. The 'vanishing earring' [33] can resemble a keloid [34]. The embedded metal can usually be pulled out, or if necessary an incision can be made to locate it.

Epidermoid cyst formation. Implantation epidermoid cysts due to ear piercing often present as tender, chronic,

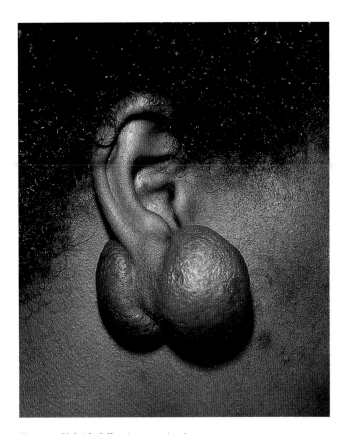

Fig. 65.5 Keloids following ear piercing.

inflammatory swellings, sometimes with drainage. There is usually an epithelial lined track as well as cysts, and all epithelial tissue must be removed, for example with a skin punch [35].

Keloids quite commonly follow ear piercing, especially in those ethnic groups with a predisposition (Fig. 65.5). The keloids seem to occur more on the back surface than the front of the earlobe [36]. As well as being unsightly, they can itch and be painful.

Treatment options include intralesional steroid, pressure [37], and excision with or without concurrent use of intralesional steroid [38] or radiotherapy (see Chapter 76) [39]. Prospective controlled trials are needed to assess these approaches.

A recent study has shown efficacy and acceptability of intralesional steroid followed by Zimmer splints which can be decorated to look like earrings [40].

Localized argyria. Bluish macules have been described on the posterior surface of the earlobe [41,42].

Frostbite has followed the use of ethyl chloride topical anaesthesia [43].

Measures to prevent complications [44]. Many of the complications of ear piercing are avoidable. The procedure is best not carried out on children under the age of 5 years or those with immunodeficiency, valvular heart disease or sarcoidosis, and there is clearly a risk if the individual has a tendency to keloid formation. For a dermatologist who wishes to pierce ears or instruct others, a simple method with a low likelihood of complications has been described [45]. The use of a surgical-grade, stainless steel, one-piece earring with an interlocking groove has been recommended. Gold-plated or gold-alloy earrings should be avoided for at least 6 weeks after the ear has been pierced. Sterile technique is important. Piercing of cartilage should be avoided. Only nickel-free earrings should be used. Large or heavy earrings should be removed prior to activities that may result in tearing the earlobes. A technique using a piece of intravenous catheter to avoid reactions in metal-sensitive individuals has been described [46].

REFERENCES

1 Biggar RJ, Haughie GE. Medical problems of ear piercing. *N Y State J Med* 1975; **75**: 1460–2.
2 Simplot TC, Hoffman HT. Comparison between cartilage and soft tissue ear piercing complications. *Am J Otol* 1998; **19**: 305–10.
3 Cumberworth VL, Hogarth TB. Hazards of ear-piercing procedures which traverse cartilage: a report of *Pseudomonas* perichondritis and review of other complications. *Br J Clin Pract* 1990; **44**: 512–3.
4 Hanif J, Frosh A, Marnane C *et al.* 'High' ear piercing and the rising incidence of perichondritis of the pinna. *BMJ* 2001; **322**: 906–7.
5 Turkeltaub SH, Habal MB. Acute *Pseudomonas* chondritis as a sequel to ear piercing. *Ann Plast Surg* 1990; **24**: 279–82.
6 Macgregor DM. The risks of ear piercing in children. *Scott Med J* 2001; **46**: 9–10.
7 Allison G, Kravitz E. Auricular chondritis secondary to acupuncture. *N Engl J Med* 1975; **293**: 780.
8 Davis O, Powell M. Auricular perichondritis secondary to acupuncture. *Arch Otolaryngol* 1985; **111**: 770–1.
9 Lovejoy FH Jr, Smith DH. Life-threatening staphylococcal disease following ear piercing. *Pediatrics* 1970; **46**: 301–3.
10 Razavi B, Schilling M. Chondritis attributable to *Lactobacillus* after ear piercing. *Diagn Microbiol Infect Dis* 2000; **37**: 75–6.
11 Morgan LG. Primary tuberculosis inoculation of an earlobe: report of an unusual case and review of the literature. *J Pediatr* 1952; **40**: 482–5.
12 Van Sciver AE. Hepatitis from ear piercing. *JAMA* 1969; **207**: 2285.
13 Johnson CJ, Anderson H, Spearman J. Viral hepatitis in young women after ear piercing. *MMWR* 1973; **22**: 390–5.
14 Jay AL. Ear piercing problems. *BMJ* 1977; **2**: 574–5.
15 Ellis DAF. Complication and correction of the pierced ear. *J Otolaryngol* 1976; **5**: 247–50.
16 Apesos J, Kane M. Treatment of traumatic earlobe clefts. *Aesthetic Plast Surg* 1993; **17**: 253–5.
17 Larsson-Stymne B, Widstrom L. Ear piercing: a cause of nickel allergy in school girls? *Contact Dermatitis* 1985; **13**: 289–93.
18 Fischer T, Fregert S, Gruvberger B. Nickel release from ear-piercing kits and earrings. *Contact Dermatitis* 1984; **10**: 39–41.
19 Nakada T, Iijima M, Nakayama H, Maibach HI. Role of ear piercing in metal allergic contact dermatitis. *Contact Dermatitis* 1997; **36**: 233–6.
20 Fisher AA. Allergic contact dermatitis due to gold earrings. *Cutis* 1990; **39**: 473–5.
21 Hausen BM, Rothenborg HW. Allergic contact dermatitis caused by olive wood jewelry. *Arch Dermatol* 1981; **17**: 732–4.
22 Karlberg AT, Boman A, Wahlberg JE. Copper: a rare sensitizer. *Contact Dermatitis* 1983; **9**: 134–9.
23 Menné T. Relationship between cobalt and nickel sensitization in females. *Contact Dermatitis* 1980; **3**: 337–40.
24 Lammintausta K, Pitkanen OP, Kalino K *et al.* Interrelationship of nickel and cobalt contact sensitization. *Contact Dermatitis* 1985; **13**: 148–52.
25 Burrows D. The dichromate problem. *Int J Dermatol* 1984; **23**: 215–20.

26 Fisher AA. Metallic gold: the cause of a persistent allergic 'dermal' contact dermatitis. *Cutis* 1974; **14**: 177–80.

27 Aoshima T, Oguchi M. Intracytoplasmic crystalline inclusions in dermal infiltrating cells of granulomatous contact dermatitis due to gold earrings. *Acta Derm Venereol (Stockh)* 1988; **68**: 261–4.

28 Iwatsuki K, Tagami H, Moriguichi T *et al.* Lymphadenoid structure induced by gold hypersensitivity. *Arch Dermatol* 1982; **118**: 608–11.

29 Iwatsuki K, Yamada M, Tagigawa M *et al.* Benign lymphoplasia of the earlobes induced by gold earrings: immunohistologic study on the cellular infiltrates. *J Am Acad Dermatol* 1987; **16**: 83–8.

30 Zilinsky I, Tsur H, Trau H, Orenstein A. Pseudolymphoma of the earlobes due to ear piercing. *J Dermatol Surg Oncol* 1989; **15**: 666–8.

31 Mann RJ, Peachey RDG. Sarcoidal tissue reaction: another complication of ear piercing. *Clin Exp Dermatol* 1983; **8**: 199–200.

32 Muntz HR, Cui DJ, Asher BA. Embedded earrings: a complication of the ear-piercing gun. *Int J Pediatr Otorhinolaryngol* 1990; **19**: 73–6.

33 de San Lazaro C, Jackson RH. Vanishing earrings. *Arch Dis Child* 1986; **61**: 606–7.

34 Saleeby ER, Rubin MG, Youshock E *et al.* Embedded foreign bodies presenting as earlobe keloids. *J Dermatol Surg Oncol* 1984; **10**: 902–4.

35 Ellis DAF. Complications and corrections of the pierced ear. *J Otolaryngol* 1976; **5**: 247–50.

36 Slobodkin D. Why more keloids on back than front of earlobe? *Lancet* 1990; **335**: 335–6.

37 Brent B. The role of pressure therapy in the management of earlobe keloids: a preliminary report of a controlled study. *Ann Plast Surg* 1978; **1**: 579–81.

38 Chowdri NA, Mattoo MMA, Darzi MA. Keloids and hypotrophic scars: results with intra-operative and serial post-operative corticosteroid injection therapy. *Aust N Z J Surg* 1999; **69**: 655–9.

39 Chaudry MR, Akhtar S, Duvalsaint F *et al.* Ear lobe keloids, surgical excision followed by radiation therapy: a 10-year experience. *Ear Nose Throat J* 1994; **73**: 779–81.

40 Russell R, Horlock N, Gault D. Zimmer splintage: a simple effective treatment for keloids following ear-piercing. *Br J Plast Surg* 2001; **54**: 509–10.

41 van den Nieuwenhuijsen IJ, Calame JJ, Brynzeel DP. Localised argyria caused by silver earrings. *Dermatologica* 1988; **177**: 189–91.

42 Shall L, Stevens A, Millard LG. An unusual case of acquired localised argyria. *Br J Dermatol* 1990; **123**: 403–7.

43 Noble DA. Another hazard of pierced ears. *BMJ* 1979; **1**: 125.

44 Hendricks WM. Complications of ear piercing: treatment and prevention. *Cutis* 1991; **48**: 386–94.

45 Landeck A, Newman N, Breadon J *et al.* A simple technique for ear piercing. *J Am Acad Dermatol* 1998; **39**: 795–6.

46 Cornetta AJ, Reiter D. Ear piercing for individuals with metal hypersensitivity. *Otolaryngol Head Neck Surg* 2001; **125**: 93–5.

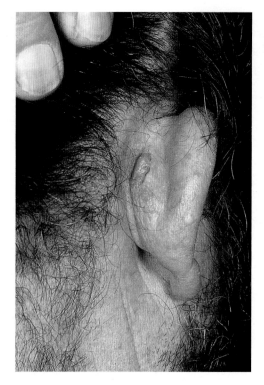

Fig. 65.6 Acanthoma fissuratum. Nodular thickening behind the pinna superficially resembling basal cell carcinoma.

Acanthoma fissuratum

This chronic response to friction and pressure from the spectacle frame can present with papules or nodules, sometimes with ulceration, in the supra-auricular or retro-auricular folds (Fig. 65.6); even when bilateral, basal cell carcinoma is a differential diagnosis. Acanthoma fissuratum is discussed in Chapter 22.

Cold injury

The ears are extremely susceptible to cold, and the pinna may be affected by chilblains in winter (Fig. 65.7). Extreme cold will cause frostbite (see Chapter 23). Similar changes have also been reported as a consequence of using excessive amounts of ethylchloride spray for ear piercing [1]. Frostbite may result in vesiculation, blisters and ischaemic necrosis of both skin and cartilage. Ears that have previously been damaged by cold may subsequently become calcified and even ossified [2,3].

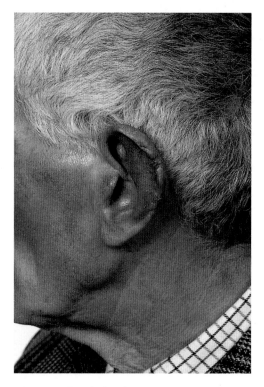

Fig. 65.7 Perniosis. Purple discoloration, soft-tissue loss and crusting due to acute-on-chronic cold injury.

Cold is also a provoking factor in many conditions that can affect the ear, for example chondrodermatitis nodularis helicis, chilblain lupus erythematosus and cryoglobulinaemia.

The ear subjected to frostbite should be thawed rapidly by the application of wet, sterile cotton pledgets warmed to 38–42°C for about 20 min [4] with adequate analgesic cover.

Emollients have traditionally been thought to protect against frostbite [5], at least in Finland. However, those who use them experience more frostbite, probably through conferring a false sense of safety, and only thermal protection from clothing can be expected to have protective value [6].

REFERENCES

1 Noble DA. Another hazard of pierced ears (use of ethylchloride spray anaesthetic with children) (letter). *BMJ* 1979; **1**: 125.
2 Di Bartolomeo JR. The petrified auricle: comments on ossification, calcification and exostoses of the external ear. *Laryngoscope* 1985; **95**: 566–75.
3 Yeatman JM, Varigos GA. Auricular ossification. *Australas J Dermatol* 1999; **39**: 268–70.
4 Sessions DG, Stallings JO, Mills WJ, Beal DD. Frostbite of the ear. *Laryngoscope* 1971; **81**: 1223–32.
5 Lehmuskallio E. Cold protecting ointments and frostbite. *Acta Derm Venereol (Stockh)* 1999; **79**: 67–70.
6 Lehmuskallio E. Emollients in the prevention of frostbite. *Int J Circumpolar Health* 2000; **59**: 122–30.

Solar damage

The external ear is often exposed to solar radiation and is therefore liable to acute and chronic sequelae. A significant hazard from severe sunburn is the development of perichondritis (see below). Many photosensitivity disorders will present on the ear, for example polymorphic light eruption, juvenile spring eruption, lupus erythematosus and porphyria (see Chapter 24).

The full gamut of chronic solar damage is frequently seen on the ears, including erythema, telangiectasia, atrophy, blotchy pigmentation, solar keratoses and cutaneous malignancies. As on the lower lip, venous lakes may be seen (Fig. 65.8). Solar elastosis is often evident, and distinctive elastotic nodules may be seen particularly on the anterior crus of the antihelix [1–3]. These lesions are usually bilateral and asymptomatic, and present as pale papules or nodules. Occasionally, they can occur on the helix and be painful, simulating chondrodermatitis nodularis. They differ from 'weathering' nodules (Fig. 65.9), which, like chondrodermatitis nodularis, occur on the helix of the ear [4].

For treatment of mild acute sunburn, cold compresses may be sufficient. More severe cases may benefit from a course of systemic corticosteroid, given for 5 days and then tapered. Preventive measures are discussed in Chapter 24.

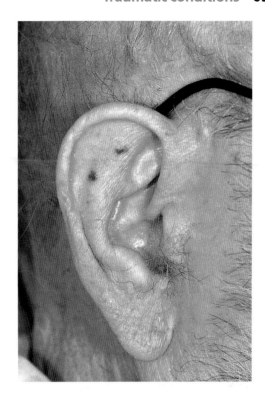

Fig. 65.8 Venous lakes on a sun-damaged pinna.

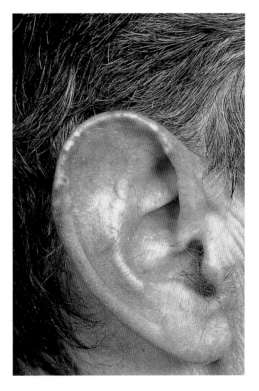

Fig. 65.9 Several firm, white, 'weathering' nodules on the helical rim.

REFERENCES

1 Carter VH, Constantine VS, Poole WL. Elastotic nodules of the antihelix. *Arch Dermatol* 1969; **100**: 282–5.
2 Kocsard E, Ofner F, Turner B. Elastotic nodules of the antihelix. *Arch Dermatol* 1970; **101**: 370.
3 Weedon D. Elastotic nodules of the ear. *J Cutan Pathol* 1980; **8**: 429–33.
4 Kavanagh GM, Bradfield JWB, Collins CMP, Kennedy CTC. Weathering nodules of the ear: a clinicopathological study. *Br J Dermatol* 1996; **135**: 550–4.

Altitude injury

A distinctive presentation of petechiae and haemorrhagic bullae in the skin of the external auditory canal and tympanic membrane has been described in air pilots descending from high altitudes or in pressure chambers while wearing well-sealed earplugs as noise protectors [1].

For treatment, a steroid–antibiotic ear drop has been advised, and if sizeable clots are present they can be gently dislodged by suction after the application of hydrogen peroxide. Preventive methods include the use of perforated earplugs on high-altitude descent.

REFERENCE

1 Senturia BH, Peugnet HB. Aero-otitis externa. *Laryngoscope* 1946; **56**: 225–36.

Radiation injury

Therapeutic use of radiation may result in characteristic acute and chronic changes (see Chapter 76). The cartilage can be susceptible to destruction if inappropriate techniques are used. Post-radiation changes on the external auditory canal include thickening of the canal epithelium, subepithelial fibrosis and resorption of underlying bone, as well as ulceration of the epithelium and the development of cholesteatoma [1].

REFERENCE

1 Adler M, Hawke M, Berger G et al. Radiation effects on the external auditory canal. *J Otolaryngol* 1985; **14**: 226–32.

Foreign bodies

A variety of vegetable, animal and mineral substances may be encountered lodged in the external ear and external auditory canal, and are frequently unsuspected. Presenting symptoms include pain, hearing loss, inflammation and discharge.

Vegetable matter, such as beans, peas and cotton, tends to absorb water and swell, impacting in the ear canal. Arthropods are the commonest animal material. While alive, their motion within the ear can produce distinctive symptoms, even vertigo. Flies can deposit eggs in the external auditory canal and the resulting myiasis has produced severe complications [1]; larvae in the triangular fossa of the pinna can also cause marked inflammation [2]. Mineral materials include beads, sand and pebbles, fragments of plaster and metallic substances. Even batteries have been found lodged in the ear and can produce serious consequences [3–5]. Impacted cerumen can behave like a foreign body in the ear canal. Loose hairs in the ear canal have been reported as a cause of noise [6].

Retrieval of foreign bodies should only be undertaken if appropriate instrumentation and expertise is available. For children, with whom the problem is more common, general anaesthesia is required. Small foreign bodies can usually be extracted with a curette or alligator forceps. Live insects should first be killed by drowning, for example in 2% lidocaine (lignocaine) [7], ether, chloroform or spirit. If some vegetable materials have absorbed water and become impacted, it may be necessary to divide the foreign body *in situ* and remove the fragments. It may be necessary to control bleeding from the skin of the canal, for example with epinephrine (adrenaline)-soaked gauze, and the canal should then be packed with an antibiotic-impregnated dressing. In cases of a battery lodged in the ear canal, it is essential that an ENT surgeon is involved in the management, because of the likelihood of serious destructive change to the middle ear and beyond.

REFERENCES

1 Mendivil JA, El Shammaa NA. Aural myiasis caused by *Cochliomyia hominivorax*: case report. *Milit Med* 1979; **144**: 261–2.
2 Kron MA. Human infestation with *Cochliomyia hominivorax*, the New World screwworm. *J Am Acad Dermatol* 1992; **27**: 264–5.
3 Rachlin LS. Assault with battery. *N Engl J Med* 1984; **311**: 921–2.
4 Kavanagh KT, Litovitz T. Miniature battery foreign bodies in auditory and nasal cavities. *JAMA* 1986; **255**: 1470–2.
5 Capo JM, Lucente FE. Alkaline battery foreign bodies of the ear and nose. *Arch Otolaryngol Head Neck Surg* 1986; **112**: 562–3.
6 Goldman G, Toher L. A hair in the ear as a cause of noise (letter). *N Engl J Med* 1982; **306**: 1553.
7 Schittek A. Insect in the external auditory canal: a new way out. *JAMA* 1980; **243**: 331.

Chondrodermatitis nodularis

This painful condition usually involves the superior portion of the helix, but may appear on the antihelix, concha, tragus and antitragus. It has formerly been known as painful nodule of the ear [1].

Aetiology. The principal factors in its pathogenesis are pressure and a compromised local blood supply. It is much more common in patients who habitually sleep on one side at night but can be triggered off by other factors, including cold, and by other types of pressure (e.g. from headgear, earphones). Alteration of connective tissue by chronic sun exposure may also be a factor [2]. The age of onset is over 40 years in most cases and the condition is commoner in males than females. We have encountered chondrodermatitis nodularis in juveniles, but only when there is an abnormality such as marked prominence of the antihelix or a history of injury (e.g. from contact sports). Chondrodermatitis nodularis has been reported in a series of patients with systemic sclerosis [3] and in childhood dermatomyositis [4].

Pathology [5,6]. A typical lesion of chondrodermatitis nodularis consists of a nodule of degenerate homogeneous collagen surrounded by vascular granulation tissue with an overlying acanthotic epidermis, and there may be a central ulcer through which the damaged collagen is extruded. In nearly all cases there is inflammation and fibrosis of the underlying perichondrium, and degenerative changes may be seen in the cartilage. Although many authors view the condition as an example of transepidermal elimination of altered connective tissue, it has been suggested that the infundibular portion of the hair follicle is primarily involved, with perforation of the follicular contents into the dermis [7,8].

Clinical features. The patient, usually a middle-aged to elderly man, seeks advice on account of pain. The more stoical may postpone consultation until the lesion interferes with sleep. The pain, which is sometimes severe, is initiated by pressure and occasionally by cold. It may be brief but can persist and throb for an hour or more. Occasionally, and particularly in women, there is little discomfort. The lesion is a globular or oval nodule, about 0.5–2 cm in diameter, raised above the often hyperaemic surrounding skin (Fig. 65.10). The surface is frequently scaly or crusted, concealing a small ulcer.

In men, nearly 90% of nodules are situated on the helix, usually at the upper pole and more frequently on the right, but may occur on the antihelix [9], tragus, concha and antitragus, in order of decreasing frequency [10]. Occasionally, there are multiple nodules or lesions, and they may occur bilaterally [11]. In women, the left and right ears are affected equally and the proportion of lesions on the antihelix and tragus is greater [12]. The nodules attain a maximum size in a few months and then remain unchanged indefinitely.

Diagnosis. Although the associated pain and tenderness are characteristic, the lesion is often misdiagnosed. Differential diagnosis includes basal and squamous cell carcinomas, solar keratosis, calcification of the pinna, elastotic nodules and 'weathering nodules' [13].

Treatment. For chondrodermatitis nodularis of the helix, excision with a narrow margin of normal skin has been recommended as standard treatment [14,15] and the approach can usefully be modified by the additional use of a curette, to define the extent of necrotic cartilage [16]. Cosmetic results are often poor and long-term recurrence rates rarely reported. Removal of cartilage only can pro-

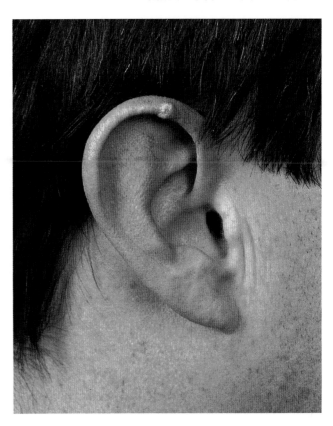

Fig. 65.10 Chondrodermatitis nodularis of the helix. A superficially ulcerated, exquisitely tender nodule.

vide excellent results and this technique can be applied to other sites such as the antihelix and tragus. The results are often cosmetically superior [17]; long-term cure rates in excess of 80% have been reported [18]. Other treatments include intralesional steroid therapy [19], liquid nitrogen cryotherapy and carbon dioxide laser [20,21]. In all patients, efforts must be made to reduce pressure or trauma to the helix. Where facilities exist for construction of individualized pressure-relieving devices, these can be useful [22].

REFERENCES

1 Forster OH. Painful nodular growth of the ear. *Arch Dermatol* 1925; **11**: 149–65.
2 Goette DK. Chondrodermatitis nodularis chronica helicis: a perforating necrobiotic granuloma. *J Am Acad Dermatol* 1980; **2**: 148–54.
3 Bottomley WW, Goodfield MDJ. Chondrodermatitis nodularis helicis occurring with systemic sclerosis: an under-reported association? *Clin Exp Dermatol* 1994; **19**: 219–20.
4 Sasaki T, Nishizawa H, Sugita Y. Chondrodermatitis nodularis helicis in childhood dermatomyositis. *Br J Dermatol* 1999; **141**: 363–5.
5 Shuman R, Helwig EB. Chondrodermatitis nodularis helicis chronica. *Am J Clin Pathol* 1954; **24**: 126–44.
6 Santa Cruz DJ. Chondrodermatitis nodularis helicis: a transepidermal perforating disorder. *J Cutan Pathol* 1980; **7**: 70–6.
7 Hurwitz RM. Painful papule of the ear: a follicular disorder. *J Dermatol Surg Oncol* 1987; **13**: 270–4.
8 Hurwitz RM. Pseudocarcinomatous or infundibular hyperplasia. *Am J Dermatopathol* 1989; **11**: 189–91.

9 Burns DA, Calnan CD. Chondrodermatitis nodularis antihelicis. *Clin Exp Dermatol* 1978; **3**: 207–8.

10 Barker LP, Young AW, Sachs W. Chondrodermatitis of the ears: a differential study of nodules of the helix and antihelix. *Arch Dermatol* 1960; **81**: 53–63.

11 Cannon CR. Bilateral chondrodermatitis helicis: case presentation and review of the literature. *Am J Otol* 1985; **6**: 164–6.

12 Yaffee HS. Perichondritis in nuns caused by a change of head-dress. *Arch Dermatol* 1963; **87**: 735.

13 Kavanagh GM, Bradfield JWB, Collins CMP, Kennedy CTC. Weathering nodules of the ear: a clinicopathological study. *Br J Dermatol* 1996; **135**: 550–4.

14 Zimmerman MC. Removal of chondrodermatitis nodularis helicis. In: Epstein E, Epstein E Jr, eds. *Skin Surgery*, 5th edn. Springfield, IL: Thomas, 1982: 1137–9.

15 Ceilly RI. Surgical treatment of chondrodermatitis nodularis chronica helicis. In: Roenigk RK, Roenigk HH Jr, eds. *Dermatologic Surgery: Principles and Practice*. New York: Marcel Dekker, 1988: 373–5.

16 Coldiron BM. The surgical management of chondrodermatitis nodularis helicis chronica. *J Dermatol Surg Oncol* 1991; **17**: 902–4.

17 Lawrence CM. The treatment of chondrodermatitis nodularis with cartilage removal alone. *Arch Dermatol* 1991; **127**: 530–5.

18 Hudson-Peacock MJ, Cox NH, Lawrence CM. The long-term results of cartilage removal alone for the treatment of chondrodermatitis nodularis. *Br J Dermatol* 1999; **141**: 703–5.

19 Wade TR. Chondrodermatitis nodularis helicis: a review with emphasis on steroid therapy. *Cutis* 1979; **24**: 406–9.

20 Karam F, Bauman T. Carbon dioxide laser treatment for chondrodermatitis nodularis chronica helicis. *Ear Nose Throat J* 1988; **67**: 757–63.

21 Taylor MB. Chondrodermatitis nodularis chronica helicis: successful treatment with the carbon dioxide laser. *J Dermatol Surg Oncol* 1991; **17**: 862–4.

22 Allen DL, Swinson PA, Arnstein PA. Auricular pressure relieving cushions for chondrodermatitis nodularis helicus. *J Maxillofac Prosthet Technol* 1998; **2**: 5–10.

Pseudocyst of the ear

SYN. ENDOCHONDRIAL PSEUDOCYST; IDIOPATHIC CYSTIC CHONDROMALACIA

A non-inflammatory, fluid-filled cavity within the cartilage of the ear.

Aetiology. Although the cause is unknown in most cases, trauma is likely to be important at least in some, as in fracture in the ear cartilage [1], habit-twisting of the ears [2] and rubbing due to atopic eczema [3]. Most speculations about the pathogenesis include an underlying malformation of the cartilage [4] and degeneration due to release of lysosomal enzymes from chondrocytes. A role for cytokines has also been suggested [5].

Pathology. There is a cavity within the cartilage, the walls of which show the presence of eosinophilic amorphous material [6,7]. There may be focal fibrosis, especially in older lesions.

Clinical features. Most cases are young men, although the condition is seen over a wide age range [8] including infants [9]. Occasional cases have been recorded in females [4]. All races are affected [10]. There may be a predilection for Chinese, although this could be reporting bias [11,12]. The condition is usually unilateral and presents as an asymptomatic swelling, which is non-tender and fluctuant. Occasionally, there are signs of inflammation and some tenderness. The commonest location is on

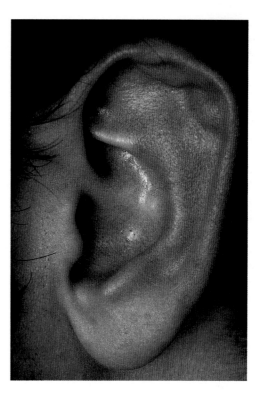

Fig. 65.11 Pseudocyst. Asymptomatic fluctuant swellings on the upper pinna.

the upper half of the ear (Fig. 65.11), on the scapha, less commonly over the helix and antihelix. Sometimes, coalescent swellings are seen. Aspiration usually yields serous fluid, which soon reaccumulates.

Diagnosis. The differential diagnosis includes traumatic perichondritis, relapsing polychondritis (see Chapter 46), haematoma, dermoid cyst and epidermoid cyst, and various benign and malignant tumours; any of these can if necessary be excluded by histological examination.

Treatment. Needle aspiration followed by the introduction of a few drops of 1% tincture of iodine [10] or corticosteroid [13] and then application of a contour pressure bandage is often successful. Thermoplastic material as used for mobilizing extremities can be used to provide the pressure [14].

For recurrences, excision of the anterior wall of the cyst, suturing the skin flap back and use of a pressure dressing can produce a cosmetically satisfactory result in most cases [12].

REFERENCES

1 Grabski WJ, Salasche SJ, McCollough ML, Angeloni VL. Pseudocyst of the auricle associated with trauma. *Arch Dermatol* 1989; **125**: 528–30.

2 Gonzales M, Raton JA, Manzano D *et al.* Pseudocyst of the ear. *Acta Derm Venereol (Stockh)* 1993; **73**: 212–3.

3 Devlin J, Harrison CJ, Whitby DJ, David TJ. Cartilaginous pseudocyst of the

external auricle in children with atopic eczema. *Br J Dermatol* 1990; **122**: 699–704.

4 Santos VB, Polisar IA, Ruffy ML. Bilateral pseudocysts of the auricle in a female. *Ann Otol Rhinol Laryngol* 1974; **83**: 9–11.

5 Yamamoto T, Yokoyama A, Umeda T. Cytokine profile of bilateral pseudocyst of the auricle. *Acta Derm Venereol (Stockh)* 1995; **76**: 92–3.

6 Glamb R, Kim R. Pseudocyst of the auricle. *J Am Acad Dermatol* 1984; **11**: 58–63.

7 Heffner DK, Hyams VJ. Cystic chondromalacia (endochondral pseudocyst) of the auricle. *Arch Pathol Lab Med* 1986; **110**: 740–3.

8 Lazar RH, Heffner DK, Hughes GB, Hyams VK. Pseudocyst of the auricle: a review of 21 cases. *Otolaryngol Head Neck Surg* 1986; **94**: 360–1.

9 Santos AD, Kelley PE. Bilateral pseudocyst of the auricle in an infant girl. *Pediatr Dermatol* 1995; **12**: 152–5.

10 Cohen PR, Grossman ME. Pseudocyst of the auricle: case report and world literature review. *Arch Otolaryngol Head Neck Surg* 1990; **116**: 1202–4.

11 Engel D. Pseudocyst of the auricle in Chinese. *Arch Otolaryngol* 1996; **83**: 29–34.

12 Choi S, Lam K, Chan K, Ghadially F. Enchondral pseudocyst of the auricle in Chinese. *Arch Otolaryngol Head Neck Surg* 1984; **110**: 792–6.

13 Myamoto H, Dida M, Onuma S, Uchiyama M. Steroid injection therapy for pseudocyst of the auricle. *Acta Derm Venereol (Stockh)* 1994; **74**: 140–2.

14 Schulte KW, Neumann NJ, Ruzicka T. Surgical pearl: the close-fitting ear cover cast. A noninvasive treatment for pseudocyst of the ear. *J Am Acad Dermatol* 2001; **44**: 285–6.

Dermatoses and the external ear

Atopic dermatitis

A crusted eczematous fissure at the junction of the earlobe and the face is a common finding in atopics, and can be regarded as a reliable feature of atopy [1–3]. In the series of Tada *et al.* [3], 45 of their 46 patients with severe atopic dermatitis had infra-auricular fissures. In addition to involvement of the infra-auricular crease, the tragal notch and sometimes the whole of the pinna may be commonly involved. Treatment of eczema and the secondary infection that often accompanies it is discussed in Chapter 18.

Seborrhoeic dermatitis

In its mildest form, seborrhoeic dermatitis simply causes a little scaling and inflammation at the entrance to the external auditory meatus, in the concha or in the auricular folds. When severe, the whole pinna may be affected and there may be infective eczematoid dermatitis both in and around the ear or post-auricularly. The relationship between seborrhoeic dermatitis and otitis externa is discussed in Chapter 17.

Asteatotic eczema

The exposed position of the ear renders it vunerable to the climatic changes that can induce asteatotic eczema (see Chapter 17). This common cause of a dry itchy ear is mainly seen in the elderly. Aggravating factors include overzealous cleansing, cold, windy weather, low humidity indoors and air-conditioned air during the summer. There may be little to see other than slight scaling. Similar changes can occur in the ear canal, where additional factors include drying vehicles used in ear drops, for example alcohol and acetone. Management will include avoidance of provocative factors, and use of emollients.

Contact dermatitis

The external ear is commonly affected by both irritant and allergic contact dermatitis [4]. Causes of contact allergy may be grouped as follows.

1 Products used for the hair and scalp: hairspray, shampoos, hair dyes, hair nets, bathing caps.
2 Items worn or placed in or on the ear: jewellery, especially nickel alloys (see p. 65.8).
3 Plastic, rubber or metal ear appliances, for example hearing aids, spectacles, headphones, telephone receivers, earplugs, hair nets.
4 Objects used to clean or scratch the ear, for example hairpins, matches.
5 Cosmetics and toiletries: make-up, perfumes, soaps and creams.
6 Topical medicaments.
7 Others (transferred to the ear by fingers): nail varnish, plant resins (e.g. poison ivy, oak or sumac).

The role of occult allergic contact dermatitis in patients with otitis externa is discussed on p. 65.24.

Psoriasis

Both guttate and plaque psoriasis involve the external ear. Sometimes this is by extension from the scalp, face or neck. Like seborrhoeic dermatitis, psoriasis often involves the concha and distal part of the external auditory canal, but usually its colour, the nature of the scaling and the presence of psoriasis elsewhere allow it to be differentiated. Sometimes both conditions appear to coexist.

Acne

Comedones frequently involve the concha, and are occasionally found on the helix, tragus or earlobe. Inflammatory cysts may be found on the lobe, at the entrance to the external auditory canal, or in both the pre- and post-auricular areas. Pressure from spectacle frames, telephone receivers or headsets can aggravate acne lesions.

Darier's disease

Occasionally, Darier's disease can present with involvement of the external ear as the principal affected site, with erythema, oedema and crusting mimicking an eczematous reaction [5].

Transepithelial elimination disorders

The ear may occasionally be the site for lesions of Kyrle's

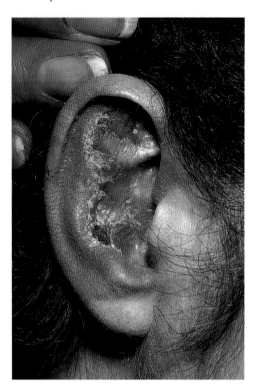

Fig. 65.12 Cutaneous lupus erythematosus. Acute erythema and erosions following sun exposure.

disease, elastosis perforans serpiginosa, perforating folliculitis and perforating papules of diabetic dialysis patients. These conditions are discussed in Chapter 46.

Lupus erythematosus (Fig. 65.12)

Although most parts of the pinna may be involved in lupus erythematosus, pits and scarring in the concha are distinctive features [6,7]. Atrophy often occurs, and even perforation of the pinna [8].

Mudi-chood

This distinctive dermatosis, which typically affects the nape of the neck and upper shoulders of girls and young women in the state of Kerala in South India, can occur on the ears. It is thought to be the result of the frictional and occlusive effects of moist oily hair in a hot and humid environment. Individual lesions are hyperpigmented papules with a thin surrounding rim of scale, occurring on the posterolateral aspects of the pinnae [9].

Lymphocytoma cutis

When the ear is involved, the lobe is characteristically affected, often with a large single nodule. Possible causative factors include *Borrelia burgdorferi* infection [10] and gold earrings [11,12].

Jessner's benign lymphocytic infiltration

This condition occasionally involves the ear and post-auricular region, and sunlight may precipitate or worsen the eruption.

Granuloma annulare

Typical papular and annular dermal lesions of granuloma annulare may involve the pinna, sometimes in the absence of lesions elsewhere [13].

Primary cutaneous amyloidosis

Asymptomatic papules on the helix and concha of the ear have been described as the sole manifestation of cutaneous amyloidosis [14]; such lesions can also occur with more generalized papular amyloid [15] and with macular amyloid of the back [16].

Angiolymphoid hyperplasia with eosinophilia
SYN. PSEUDOPYOGENIC GRANULOMA; NODULAR ANGIOBLASTIC HYPERPLASIA WITH EOSINOPHILIA

This is a reactive proliferative disorder of blood vessels with a variable component of inflammatory cells [17]. Opinions vary as to whether it is identical with Kimura's disease, a condition mainly found in Eastern orientals (see Chapter 53). Angiolymphoid hyperplasia with eosinophilia occurs in both a dermal [18] and a subcutaneous [19] form, and is most commonly found on the head and neck. The two forms are regarded as variants of the same condition [20–22].

Aetiological factors include trauma, pregnancy and immunization procedures [23].

Histology. There are circumscribed collections of vessels whose endothelial cells are epithelioid, i.e. have abundant eosinophilic cytoplasm and large nuclei. These cells sometimes proliferate into the lumen, and may occur in solid clumps. The associated inflammatory infiltrate consists of lymphocytes, sometimes lymphoid follicles, and there are varying numbers of eosinophils. At least in some cases there may be an underlying associated arteriovenous malformation [24]. In typical Kimura's disease there is more prominent lymphoid hyperplasia.

Clinical features. The dermal form commonly affects the pinna, external auditory meatus (Fig. 65.13) and post-auricular area. The lesions are red-brown papules or nodules. Occasionally, they itch and can be painful or pulsatile [23]. The condition mainly affects young to middle-aged adults, and in some series there is a female preponderance [25].

Kimura's disease has been reported as involving the

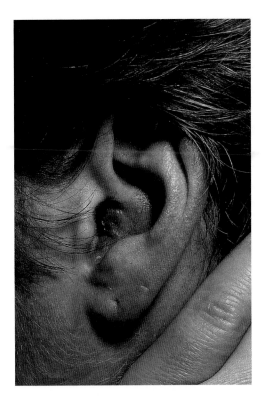

Fig. 65.13 Angiolymphoid hyperplasia with eosinophilia. Firm red-brown nodules at the entrance to the external auditory canal.

ears [26,27] but more commonly produces subcutaneous, lymph node and salivary gland-related masses in the head and neck.

Differential diagnosis includes pyogenic granuloma (rare at this site), bacillary angiomatosis and angiosarcoma.

Treatment. The treatment of choice is surgical excision, although there is often recurrence. Intralesional corticosteroids, pulsed dye laser [28], radiotherapy or oral immunosuppressive agents have been used in some cases with benefit.

Skin reactions to osseo-integrated implants

Restoration of the pinna following traumatic loss or congenital absence may be achieved using an osseo-integrated skin-penetrating titanium fixture. About 10% of such patients have skin reactions [29,30]. The reaction consists of erythema and crusting, sometimes with significant infection, which should be adequately treated.

Elephantiasis of the external ears

Chronically red swollen ears may occur for a number of reasons, including long-standing eczema, psoriasis [31] and chronic streptococcal infection. Long-standing head louse infection has also been reported as a cause [32].

Psychocutaneous disorders

Dermatitis artefacta and delusions of parasitosis (see Chapter 65) may occasionally result in self-induced lesions on the ears and even in the ear canals.

Granuloma faciale

The ear is an occasional site for this distinctive disorder [33].

Bullous diseases

Pemphigus, pemphigoid, dermatitis herpetiformis and epidermolysis bullosa aquisita may all involve the ear, and occasionally the auditory canal. Blistering of the pinna and stenosis of the canal can occur in dystrophic epidermolysis bullosa [34].

Verruciform xanthoma

This uncommon condition is typically found in the mouth but has been reported on the ear, where it can mimic squamous cell carcinoma [35].

Adult-onset xanthogranuloma

Symmetrical yellow-red nodular lesions with the same histology as juvenile xanthogranuloma have been described on the earlobes [36].

REFERENCES

1 Voss M, Voss E, Schubert H. Schuppung der Ohren: ein Leitsymtom der Ichthyosis gruppe? *Dermatol Monatsschr* 1982; **168**: 394–7.
2 Sampson HA. Atopic dermatitis. *Ann Allergy* 1992; **69**: 469–81.
3 Tada J, Toi Y, Akiyama H, Arata J. Infra-auricular fissures in atopic dermatitis. *Acta Derm Venereol (Stockh)* 1994; **74**: 129–31.
4 Jones EH. Allergy of the external ear and canal. *Otolaryngol Clin North Am* 1974; **7**: 735–48.
5 Thompson AC, Shall L, Moralee SJ. Darier's disease of the external ear. *J Laryngol Otol* 1992; **106**: 725–6.
6 Shuster S. A simple sign of discoid lupus erythematosus. *Br J Dermatol* 1981; **104**: 350–1.
7 Rebora A. Scarring of the concha as a sign of lupus erythematosus. *Br J Dermatol* 1982; **106**: 122.
8 Lucky PA. Lupus erythematosus with perforation of the pinna. *Cutis* 1983; **32**: 554–7.
9 Sugathan P. Mudi-chood on the pinnae. *Br J Dermatol* 1976; **95**: 197–8.
10 Albrecht A, Hofstadter S, Artsob H *et al.* Lymphadenosis benigna cutis resulting from *Borrelia* infection (*Borrelia* lymphocytoma). *J Am Acad Dermatol* 1991; **24**: 621–5.
11 Murata J, Toyoda H, Nogita T *et al.* A case of lymphadenosis benigna cutis of the earlobe: an immunohistochemical study. *J Dermatol* 1992; **19**: 186–9.
12 Kobayashi J, Nanko H, Nakamura J, Mizoguchi M. Lymphocytoma cutis induced by gold earrings. *J Am Acad Dermatol* 1992; **27**: 457–8.
13 Muhlbauer JE. Granuloma annulare. *J Am Acad Dermatol* 1980; **3**: 217–30.
14 Hicks BC, Weber PJ, Hashimoto K *et al.* Primary cutaneous amyloidosis of the auricular concha. *J Am Acad Dermatol* 1988; **18**: 19–25.
15 Bakos L, Weissbluth ML, Pires AKS, Muller LFB. Primary amyloidosis of the concha (letter). *J Am Acad Dermatol* 1989; **20**: 524–5.

16 Barnadas M, Perez M, Esquius J et al. Papules in the auricular concha: lichen amyloidosus in a case of biphasic amyloidosis. *Dermatologica* 1990; **181**: 149–51.

17 Rosai J. Angiolymphoid hyperplasia with eosinophilia of the skin. *Am J Dermatopathol* 1982; **4**: 175–84.

18 Wilson Jones E, Bleehen SS. Inflammatory angiomatous nodules with abnormal blood vessels occurring about the ears and scalp (pseudo and atypical pyogenic granuloma). *Br J Dermatol* 1969; **81**: 804–16.

19 Wells GC, Whimster IW. Subcutaneous lymphoid hyperplasia with eosinophilia. *Br J Dermatol* 1969; **81**: 1–15.

20 Kandil E. Dermal angiolymphoid hyperplasia with eosinophilia versus pseudopyogenic granuloma. *Br J Dermatol* 1970; **83**: 405–8.

21 Mehregan AH, Shapiro L. Angiolymphoid hyperplasia with eosinophilia. *Arch Dermatol* 1971; **103**: 50–7.

22 Reed RJ, Terezakis N. Subcutaneous angioblastic lymphoid hyperplasia with eosinophilia (Kimura's disease). *Cancer* 1972; **29**: 489–97.

23 Olsen TG, Helwig EB. Angiolymphoid hyperplasia with eosinophilia. A clinicopathologic study of 116 patients. *J Am Acad Dermatol* 1985; **12**: 781–96.

24 Onishi Y, Ohara K. Angiolymphoid hyperplasia with eosinophilia associated with arteriovenous malformation: a clinicopathological correlation with angiography and serial estimation of serum levels of renin, eosinophil cationic protein and interleukin 5. *Br J Dermatol* 1999; **140**: 1153–6.

25 Henry PG, Burnett JW. Angiolymphoid hyperplasia with eosinophilia. *Arch Dermatol* 1978; **114**: 1168–72.

26 Chan KM, Mok JSW, Ng SK, Abdullah V. Kimura's disease of the auricle. *Otolaryngol Head Neck Surg* 2001; **124**: 598–9.

27 Hiwatashi A, Hasuo K, Shiina T et al. Kimura's disease with bilateral auricular masses. *Am J Neuroradiol* 1999; **20**: 1976–8.

28 Lertzman BH, McMeekin T, Gaspari AA. Pulsed dye laser treatment of angiolymphoid hyperplasia with eosinophilia lesions. *Arch Dermatol* 1997; **133**: 920–1.

29 Jacobsson M, Tjellstrom A, Fine L, Andersson H. A retrospective study of osseointegrated skin-penetrating titanium fixtures used for retaining facial prostheses. *Int J Oral Maxillofac Implants* 1992; **7**: 523–8.

30 Gitto CA, Plata WG, Schaaf NG. Evaluation of the peri-implant epithelial tissue of percutaneous implant abutments supporting maxillofacial prostheses. *Int J Oral Maxillofac Implants* 1994; **9**: 197–206.

31 Grant JM. Elephantiasis nostras verrucosa of the ears. *Cutis* 1982; **29**: 441–4.

32 Mahzoon S, Azadeh B. Elephantiasis of external ears: a rare manifestation of pediculosis capitis. *Acta Derm Venereol (Stockh)* 1983; **63**: 363–5.

33 Foss MH. Granuloma faciale: report on a case. *Acta Derm Venereol (Stockh)* 1957; **37**: 473–82.

34 Kastanioudakis I, Bassioukas K, Ziavra N, Skevas A. External ear involvement in epidermolysis bullosa. *Otolaryngol Head Neck Surg* 2000; **122**: 618.

35 Jensen JL, Liao SY, Jeffes EW III. Verruciform xanthoma of the ear with coexisting epidermal dysplasia. *Am J Dermatopathol* 1992; **14**: 426–30.

36 Sueki H, Saito T, Iijima M, Fujisawa R. Adult onset xanthogranuloma appearing symmetrically on the ear lobes. *J Am Acad Dermatol* 1995; **32**: 372–4.

Systemic disease and the external ear

Many conditions described more fully elsewhere will occasionally present on the external ear with lesions of diagnostic value.

Granulomatous disorders

These include sarcoidosis [1,2], especially the lupus pernio variety. Metastatic Crohn's disease may rarely involve the ear [3]. Atypical facial necrobiosis may involve the ear, as well as the more typical location on the face and scalp. Wegener's granulomatosis can present with serous or suppurative otitis and conductive or sensorineural deafness [4,5]. A similar allergic granulomatosis affected both ears in a young black South African who died from glomerulonephritis [6]. Infective granulomatous diseases involve the ear, notably leprosy, in which the earlobe is a valuable site for taking smears [7]. Lupus vulgaris, other manifestations of tuberculosis, atypical mycobacterial infection (e.g. *Mycobacterium marinum* from swimming-pool injuries), deep fungal infections and even syphilis [8] can involve the ear.

Collagen vascular diseases

As well as discoid lupus, subacute cutaneous lupus erythematosus and systemic lupus erythematosus may also involve the ears. Scleroderma can produce pallor and telangiectasia of the auditory canal. Rheumatoid disease is characterized by nodules, which can occur on the ear, where they may ulcerate due to pressure from the pillow or spectacles. Redness, tenderness and swelling of the ear, but sparing the lobe, is characteristic of relapsing polychondritis (see Chapter 46).

Pyoderma gangrenosum

The ear is an occasional presenting site [9] for this primary ulcerative disorder, discussed in Chapter 49. Vasculitis and factitial disease may be mimicked.

Metabolic disorders

Xanthomas occasionally occur on the ears, presenting as yellow nodules. Gouty tophi frequently involve the pinna (Fig. 65.14), and may antedate the onset of joint disease or

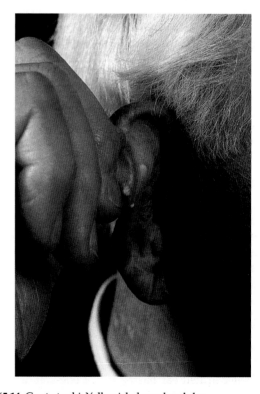

Fig. 65.14 Gouty tophi. Yellowish dermal nodules.

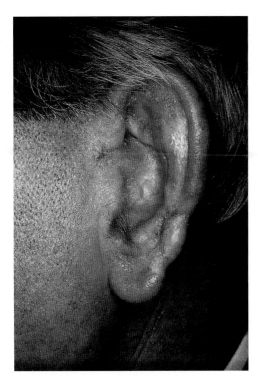

Fig. 65.15 Porphyria cutanea tarda. Firm, whitish, sclerodermoid changes at the site of repeated blistering.

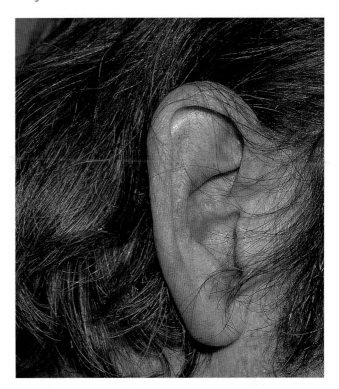

Fig. 65.16 Alkaptonuria. The auricular cartilage has a distinctive blue colour. (Courtesy of Dr P. Hollingworth, Southmead Hospital, Bristol, UK.)

appear decades after the initial attack. The helix and anti-helix are typical sites. Histology is distinctive. Porphyria cutanea tarda (Fig. 65.15) may present with vesicles and bullae, often on a background of scarring, hyperpigmentation, milia, sclerodermoid plaques and hypertrichosis. Pseudocysts of the auricle and perichondritis may be simulated [10].

Diseases of connective tissue

Cutis laxa may result in distinctive pendulous earlobes [11].

Alkaptonuria
SYN. OCHRONOSIS

This is typically associated with a bluish discoloration of the auricular cartilage due to oxidation of bound homogentisic acid (Fig. 65.16). The cerumen in such patients may be very dark, a finding that can precede other clinical manifestations.

Calcium deposition

Calcium deposition may occur in many circumstances (see Chapter 57) and occasionally the ear is involved. The so-called petrified ear has been described in association with diabetes mellitus [12]. Usually, calcium deposits in the ear occur for local reasons, for example degenerative changes in the cartilage. In infants, congenital nodular calcification of Winer should be considered [13].

Endocrine disorders

In Addison's disease, the pigmentary changes may involve the ear, and ossification of the auricular cartilage may occur [14]. In acromegaly, there is usually enlargement of the auricular cartilage and coarsening of the overlying skin.

Paraneoplastic syndromes

Bazex's syndrome (acrokeratosis paraneoplastica) (see Chapter 59) commonly affects the ears and is an important marker for internal malignancy [15].

Drug-related effects

Purpura of the ears has been described in a series of children receiving levamisole for nephritic syndrome [16]. Both vasculitis and thrombotic changes occurred, and there was an association with circulating autoantibodies.

Hypertrophy of the retro-auricular folds may be seen as a consequence of phenytoin therapy [17]. Hypertrichosis of the ear canal due to minoxidil therapy can be a predisposing factor for external otitis [18].

Lymphoma

Systemic lymphoma can occasionally present as an isolated lesion on the ear [19].

REFERENCES

1 Nova A. Sarcoidosis of the ear. *Ear Nose Throat J* 1981; **60**: 307–8.
2 Swansson-Beck H, Goos M, Christophers E. Ohrlappchengranuloma. *Hautarzt* 1982; **33**: 115–6.
3 McCallum DI, Gray WM. Metastatic Crohn's disease. *Br J Dermatol* 1976; **95**: 551–4.
4 McCaffrey TU, McDonald TJ, Facer GW *et al.* Otologic manifestation of Wegener's granulomatosis. *Otolaryngol Head Neck Surg* 1980; **88**: 586–93.
5 Kornblut AD, Wolffs M, Fauci AS. Ear disease in patients with Wegener's granulomatosis. *Laryngoscope* 1982; **92**: 713–7.
6 Bentley-Phillips B, Bayler MA. Destructive granuloma of the ear. *Int J Dermatol* 1980; **19**: 336–9.
7 Mansfield RE, Storkan MA, Cliff IS. Evaluation of the earlobe in leprosy. A clinical and histopathological study. *Arch Dermatol* 1969; **100**: 407–12.
8 Wilcox JR. An atypical case of secondary syphilis. *Br J Venere Dis* 1981; **57**: 30–2.
9 Lysy J, Zimmerman J, Ackerman Z, Reifen E. Atypical auricular pyoderma-gangrenosum simulating fungal infection. *J Clin Gastroenterol* 1989; **11**: 561–4.
10 Bukachevsky R, Kimmelman CP. Otolaryngologic manifestations of porphyria cutanea tarda. *Otolaryngol Head Neck Surg* 1989; **101**: 402–3.
11 Ghigliotti G, Parodi A, Borgiani L *et al.* Acquired cutis laxa confined to the face. *J Am Acad Dermatol* 1991; **24**: 504–5.
12 Strumia R, Lombardi AR, Altieri E. The petrified ear: a manifestation of dystrophic calcification. *Dermatology* 1997; **194**: 371–3.
13 Azon-Masoliver A, Ferrando J, Navarra E, Mascaro JE. Solitary congenital nodular calcification of Winer located on the ear: report of two cases. *Pediatr Dermatol* 1989; **6**: 191–3.
14 Chadwick JM, Downham TF. Auricular calcification. *Int J Dermatol* 1978; **17**: 799–801.
15 Bazex A, Griffiths A. Acrokeratosis paraneoplastica: a new cutaneous marker of malignancy. *Br J Dermatol* 1980; **102**: 301–6.
16 Rongioletti F, Ghio L, Ginevri F *et al.* Purpura of the ears: a distinctive vasculopathy with circulating autoantibodies complicating long-term treatment with levamisole in children. *Br J Dermatol* 1999; **140**: 948–51.
17 Trunnell TN, Waisman M. Hypertrophied retroauricular folds attributable to diphenylhydantoin therapy. *Cutis* 1982; **30**: 207–9.
18 Toriumi DM, Konior RJ, Berktold RE. Severe hypertrichosis of the external ear canal during minoxidil therapy. *Arch Otolaryngol Head Neck Surg* 1988; **114**: 918–9.
19 Darvay A, Russell-Jones R, Acland KM *et al.* Systemic B-cell lymphoma presenting as an isolated lesion on the ear. *Clin Exp Dermatol* 2001; **26**: 166–9.

Infection

The anatomy of the ear, with its many folds and the semi-occluded nature of the external auditory canal, make it particularly susceptible to intertriginous infection, especially with Gram-negative organisms. The close anatomical relationship between the middle and external ear means that infections can pass relatively easily from one to the other, and the eardrum should always be examined. The cartilaginous and bony structures close to the skin are particularly vulnerable to infection. Although chondritis and perichondritis may have other causes, they are included in this section.

Infections of the pinna

Staphylococcus aureus, alone or in association with group A β-haemolytic *Streptococcus*, may cause impetigo contagiosum of the ear. This is a relatively common site for infection in infants and young children. *Staphylococcus aureus* is also the most common causative organism of furuncles (boils) and carbuncles, which are more common in the external auditory canal than on the pinna. Cracks and fissures around the auricle are often the portal of entry for β-haemolytic streptococcal infection manifesting as erysipelas. This is more common in the elderly, the newborn and those suffering from malnutrition, disability, alcoholism, diabetes or immune deficiency states.

Erysipelas typically begins with high fever and constitutional upset, including malaise, vomiting and headache, and there is rapidly spreading erythema and oedema from the pinna on to the face. There is often lymphadenopathy. Recurrent attacks of cellulitis of the face may have the same predisposing factors as at other body sites. Recurrent attacks of cellulitis lead to fibrosis and lymphoedema. Treatment of erysipelas and cellulitis is discussed in Chapter 27.

Necrotizing fasciitis has rarely been described arising from an initial infection of the pinna [1].

The term *infective eczematoid dermatitis* is still used for an oozing, crusted, eczematous condition occurring on and often below the pinna in association with chronic discharge from the ear. Coagulase-positive staphylococci are the most frequently isolated bacteria. The ear canal is oedematous and erythematous, and purulent discharge may be seen coming from a perforated tympanic membrane. The condition should be differentiated from impetigo, secondarily infected contact dermatitis, seborrhoeic dermatitis and atopic dermatitis.

Treatment. Primary infection of the ear must be treated appropriately, usually with a systemic antibiotic; any associated chronic otitis media or mastoiditis is likely to be managed by an otologist. Involved skin can be cleansed with saline, 1 in 10 000 potassium permanganate or dilute aluminium acetate soaks and then treated with a topical steroid. Surgical intervention will be required for necrotizing fasciitis.

Perichondritis and chondritis

Inflammation of the cartilage itself (chondritis), or more commonly the vascularized lining (perichondritis), can be indistinguishable from infection of these structures, and infection is a common complication whatever the cause [2,3].

Aetiology. There are many causes, including physical trauma (Fig. 65.17), thermal and chemical burns, frostbite, pressure (e.g. from tight headphones and head-dresses [4]) and ear piercing (see p. 65.8) including acupuncture [5,6]. Perichondritis may occasionally follow superficial

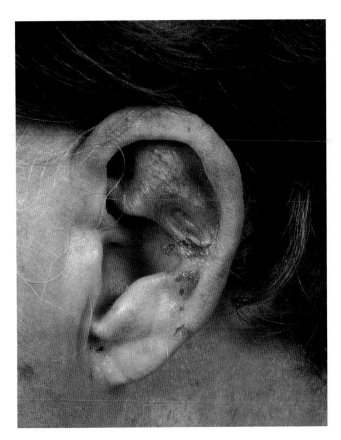

Fig. 65.17 Pressure ulcer exposing cartilage, a potential cause of chondritis.

infections of the ear such as furunculosis or otitis externa. The most common infecting organism is *Ps. aeruginosa*, although other Gram-negative organisms or staphylococci may at times be responsible.

Clinical features. Chondritis and perichondritis are typically painful. The pinna becomes hot, painful and swollen, with loss of normal contour due to oedema, and there may be accumulation of pus in the subperichondrial layer. Constitutional symptoms are common. The inflammation can spread back to the adjoining face. The destruction of cartilage results in deformity of the ear, which may be severe. Necrotizing fasciitis can follow perichondritis of the pinna [1], and if suspected must be treated by urgent débridement.

Diagnosis. Perichondritis may be difficult to distinguish from cellulitis, although perichondritis is usually more painful and does not involve the lobule of the ear, which lacks cartilage. Relapsing polychondritis (see Chapter 46) usually also involves cartilage at other body sites, and is often recurrent.

Treatment. Treatment should be instituted promptly. If an abscess has developed, early drainage is necessary.

Ciprofloxacin or other quinolones are probably the treatment of choice [7,8]. Necrotic cartilage may subsequently need to be excised, and fluid collections aspirated.

REFERENCES

1 Skorina J, Kaufman D. Necrotizing fasciitis originating from pinna perichondritis. *Otolaryngol Head Neck Surg* 1995; **113**: 467–73.
2 Martin R, Yonkers AJ, Yarington CT Jr. Perichondritis of the ear. *Laryngoscope* 1976; **86**: 664–73.
3 Bassiouny A. Perichondritis of the auricle. *Laryngoscope* 1981; **91**: 422–31.
4 Williams HC. Turban ear. *Arch Dermatol* 1994; **130**: 117–9.
5 Allison G, Kravitz E. Auricular chondritis secondary to acupuncture. *N Engl J Med* 1975; **293**: 780.
6 Davis O, Powell M. Auricular perichondritis secondary to acupuncture. *Arch Otolaryngol* 1985; **111**: 770–1.
7 Noel SB, Scattan P, Meadors MC *et al.* Treatment of *Pseudomonas aeruginosa* auricular perichondritis is with oral ciprofloxacin. *J Dermatol Surg Oncol* 1989; **15**: 633–7.
8 Thomas JN, Swanson N. Treatment of perichondritis with a quinolone derivative: norfloxacin. *J Dermatol Surg Oncol* 1988; **14**: 447–9.

Other bacterial infections of the pinna

Mycobacterial infection can rarely involve the external ear. Lupus vulgaris can produce extensive destruction [1] and mimic other conditions [2]. Secondary involvement from underlying lymph-node disease (scrofuloderma) can present with hearing loss, tinnitus and peri-auricular lymphadenopathy, with only minimal secretion in the ear canal [3].

Atypical mycobacteria that may involve the ear include *M. marinum* acquired from swimming-pool injuries.

In leprosy, the ear is almost always involved in the lepromatous type, and there may be evident infiltration of the skin. The earlobe is often used for taking smears [4].

Syphilis may occasionally involve the ear, usually in the secondary stage [5].

REFERENCES

1 Fasal P. But it was not leprosy. *Cutis* 1975; **15**: 499–509.
2 Okazaki M, Sakurai MD. Lupus vulgaris of the earlobe. *Ann Plast Surg* 1997; **39**: 643–6.
3 Hunsaker DH. Conchomeatoplasty for chronic otitis externa. *Arch Otolaryngol Head Neck Surg* 1988; **114**: 395–8.
4 Mansfield RE, Storkan MA, Cliff IS. Evaluation of the earlobe in leprosy. A clinical and histopathological study. *Arch Dermatol* 1969; **100**: 407–12.
5 Wilcox JR. An atypical case of secondary syphilis. *Br J Venereol Dis* 1981; **57**: 30–2.

Viral infections

Herpes simplex occasionally involves the ear. It is often transmitted during contact sports such as rugby and wrestling. Herpes zoster may present as an isolated herpetiform eruption of the external ear or may be associated with ipsilateral facial palsy and auditory symptoms (Ramsay–Hunt syndrome; geniculate herpes). The condition usually begins with pain and may initially be mistaken for erysipelas. Vesicles usually appear on about the fifth day and involve the pinna, the external auditory meatus and, rarely, the tympanic membrane. There is usually malaise, pyrexia and lymphadenopathy. Facial palsy, when it occurs, is usually transient, but more severe and persistent cases do occur. Taste and lacrimation may also be affected. Compression damage to the VIIIth cranial nerve may lead to tinnitus, vertigo, nystagmus, nausea and deafness. Management of herpes zoster is discussed in Chapter 25. Orf affecting the ear has been described, presenting as an inflammatory nodule on the tragus [1].

REFERENCE

1 Shinkwin CA, Holmes AH, Freeland AP. Orf of the pinna. *J Laryngol Otol* 1991; **105**: 947–9.

Superficial and deep mycoses

Dermatophyte fungi may rarely involve the ear, and when present can simulate granulomatous disease [1] and chondritis [2].

Pityriasis versicolor may involve the ears, but is usually easy to diagnose.

In cases of ulcerative granulomatous disease of the ear, deep fungal infections, for example sporotrichosis [3], should be considered. Biopsy, examination of smears, cultures and serological studies should enable accurate diagnosis. Deep fungal infection may prompt an enquiry for underlying immune deficiency.

Otomycosis is discussed under otitis externa.

REFERENCES

1 Verbov J. Granulomatous *Trichophyton rubrum* infection of the pinnae. *Br J Dermatol* 1973; **89**: 212–3.
2 Bishop M, Rist TE. Tinea of the ear mimicking chondritis. *Cutis* 1979; **23**: 638–9.
3 Cox RL, Reller LB. Auricular sporotrichosis in a brick mason. *Arch Dermatol* 1979; **115**: 1229–30.

Infections of the external auditory canal and meatus

External otitis
SYN. OTITIS EXTERNA

Otitis externa [1] is a loose term that embraces more than one disease process. Aetiologically, it is rarely unifactorial [2]; constitutional, traumatic, environmental and microbial factors usually coexist. The condition is characterized by inflammation of the canal epithelium and by varying degrees of pain, itch, deafness and discharge. The term 'external otitis' sometimes includes furunculosis of the ear canal, and is then subclassified as acute localized external otitis; furunculosis is described separately below.

Pathogenesis. Otitis externa can be divided, for convenience, into two main groups [3]: (i) a *reactive* group consisting of patients suffering from eczema, psoriasis or seborrhoeic dermatitis; and (ii) a predominantly *infective* group in which either bacteria or fungi are involved. However, the two components often coexist. The cause in many cases is not apparent [4] but the following predisposing factors appear to be important.

Genetic and constitutional. There are significant racial and individual differences in susceptibility to otitis externa. This may be due to anatomical differences in the curvature of the external auditory canal or narrowing of the isthmus—natives of New Guinea with wide straight canals only rarely suffer from external otitis [5]—or, possibly, to differences in the type, amount or composition of cerumen, whose waxy consistency and low pH are protective against bacteria. *Pseudomonas aeruginosa*, the commonest bacterial pathogen in external otitis, binds to cells by a lectin-mediated process, and binding occurs more in individuals expressing blood group A on their epithelial cells [6].

Abundant tragal hair or plugs of wax and debris increase the relative humidity and reduce ventilation of the external auditory canal so that the canal epithelium becomes macerated and more susceptible to infection. Hypertrichosis of the canal due to minoxidil has been associated with external otitis [7]. Dental abnormalities and poor mastication [8] may also retard expulsion of wax and epithelial squames.

The atopic and seborrhoeic states predispose to external otitis not only by interfering with the integrity of the auricular epithelium but also by encouraging scratching and secondary infection. Both too much and too little cerumen and alterations in skin pH have at times been held responsible [9].

Environmental. Heat, humidity and moisture are undoubtedly important in 'hot-weather ear' or 'swimmer's ear' [10]. This condition is common, especially among white people in tropical and subtropical regions. High temperature, high relative humidity and swimming [11] all encourage maceration and secondary bacterial or fungal infections of the canal epithelium. Freshwater swimming appears to be a particular risk factor [12]. Failure to dry the ears completely after swimming, shampooing or showering may also be a factor in some cases [4].

Traumatic. Trauma, in the opinion of many investigators [2,11,13,14], is one of the prime factors in both the initiation and the persistence of many cases. In one series of 113 patients, 58 admitted using wool-tipped matches, two admitted using bare matches and seven used hairgrips to relieve itching [2]. Patients suffering from eczema or those with neurodermatitis tend to scratch, rub or 'fiddle' with their ears; other patients appear obsessed about cleaning their ears and by doing so excessively they interfere with the normal homeostatic and self-cleaning properties [15]. Impacted cerumen may cause irritation, which is often increased by inexpert attempts to remove it; pressure from hearing aids and transistor ear pieces may also cause irritation and, especially with the 'internal' hearing aid, a combination of pressure and occlusion often leads to the development of external otitis.

Bacterial and mycotic infection. The epidermis of the external auditory canal is normally fairly resistant to infection. The bacterial flora, although varying with race, geography and season, tends to resemble that of the skin but with a higher likelihood of finding *Ps. aeruginosa* [16]. In hot humid environments, however, and particularly among swimmers, whose ears are habitually wet, the incidence of *Ps. aeruginosa* and other Gram-negative infections rises substantially [17,18] as does the frequency with which *Aspergillus* or *Candida* species are isolated [13]. An outbreak of *Pseudomonas* otitis has been reported in association with contaminated pool water [19] but a source has rarely been found in other series, and it is assumed that *Pseudomonas* infections are of endogenous origin.

In more temperate climates, *S. aureus* is often isolated. This may be associated with evidence of skin disease elsewhere or with staphylococcal carriage. Certainly, patients with recurrent staphylococcal otitis externa should have nasal and perianal swabs sent for bacterial culture; occasionally it may be necessary to swab and 'destaph' the whole family. In other cases, there may be an underlying tympanic perforation or coexistent otitis media. The eardrums should therefore always be examined, especially in patients with unilateral or recurrent disease. Occasionally, infection spreads out from the ear canal and causes impetigo or infective eczema of the auricle and surrounding skin.

In the tropics, mycotic infections of the external ear canal are relatively common [20,21]. *Aspergillus*, *Candida*, *Penicillium* and *Mucor* spp. are the organisms most often incriminated, most cases being due to either *Aspergillus niger* or *Candida albicans*. There is some debate, however, as to whether these fungi are pathogenic, opportunistic, saprophytic or simply commensal [21–24].

REFERENCES

1 Lucente FE. Diseases due to infection. In: Lucente FE, Lawson W, Novick NL, eds. *The External Ear*. Philadelphia: Saunders, 1996: 48–97.
2 McKelvie M, McKelvie P. Some aetiological factors in otitis externa. *Br J Dermatol* 1966; **78**: 227–31.
3 Mawson SR, Ludman H, eds. *Diseases of the Ear*, 4th edn. London: Arnold, 1979.
4 Russell JD, Donnelly M, McShane DP *et al*. What causes acute otitis externa? *J Laryngol Otol* 1993; **107**: 898–901.
5 Quayle AF. Otitis externa in New Guinea. *Med J Aust* 1944; **2**: 228–31.
6 Steuer MK, Hofstadter F, Probster L *et al*. Are ABH antigenic determinants

on human outer ear canal epithelium responsible for *Pseudomonas aeruginosa* infections? *Otorhinolaryngology* 1995; **57**: 148–52.
7 Toriumi DM, Konior RJ, Berktold RE. Severe hypertrichosis of the external ear canal during minoxidil therapy. *Arch Otolaryngol Head Neck Surg* 1988; **114**: 918–9.
8 Dunn B. Otitis externa and malposed third molars. *J Laryngol Otol* 1962; **76**: 981–4.
9 McLaurin JW, Raggio TP, Simmons M. Persistent external otitis. *Laryngoscope* 1965; **75**: 1699–707.
10 Calderon R, Mood EW. An epidemiological assessment of water quality and 'swimmers' ear'. *Arch Environ Health* 1982; **37**: 300–5.
11 Strauss NB, Dierker RL. Otitis externa associated with aquatic activities (swimmer's ear). *Clin Dermatol* 1987; **5**: 103–11.
12 Springer GL, Shapiro EA. Fresh water swimming as a risk factor for otitis externa: a case–control study. *Arch Environ Health* 1985; **40**: 202–6.
13 Wright DN, Alexander JM. Effect of water on the bacterial flora of swimmers' ears. *Arch Otolaryngol* 1974; **99**: 15–8.
14 Hirsch BE. Infections of the external ear. *Am J Otolaryngol* 1992; **13**: 145–55.
15 Alberti PWRM. Epithelial migration on the tympanic membrane. *J Laryngol* 1964; **78**: 808–30.
16 Brook I. Microbiological studies of bacterial flora of the external auditory canal in children. *Acta Otolaryngol (Stockh)* 1981; **91**: 285–7.
17 Hoadley AW, Knight DE. External otitis among swimmers and non-swimmers. *Arch Environ Health* 1975; **30**: 445–8.
18 Lambert IJ. A comparison of the treatment of otitis externa with 'Otosporin' and aluminium acetate: a report from a services practice in Cyprus. *J R Coll Gen Pract* 1981; **31**: 291–4.
19 Weingarten MA. Otitis externa due to *Pseudomonas* in swimming pool bathers. *J R Coll Gen Pract* 1977; **27**: 359–60.
20 Beaney GRE, Broughton A. Tropical otomycosis. *J Laryngol Otol* 1967; **81**: 987–97.
21 Youssef YA, Abdou MH. Studies on fungus infection of the external ear. I. Mycological and clinical observations. *J Laryngol Otol* 1967; **81**: 401–12.
22 Haley LD. Etiology of otomycosis II. Bacterial flora of the ear. *Arch Otolaryngol* 1950; **52**: 208–13.
23 Gregson AEW, La Touche CJ. Otomycosis: a neglected disease. *J Laryngol Otol* 1961; **75**: 45–69.
24 Smyth GDL. Fungal infection in otology. *Br J Dermatol* 1964; **76**: 425–8.

Histopathology [1–4]. In most cases of external otitis, there is acanthosis, elongation of the rete ridges and an increase in orthokeratosis and parakeratosis. Spongiosis occurs in eczematous and seborrhoeic forms. The nature of the dermal infiltrate varies with both cause and chronicity. The histopathology is seldom diagnostic except when fungal mycelia are seen.

Clinical features. The condition can be acute, subacute or chronic. In patients seen at hospital, it tends to be severe, chronic or chronic relapsing, but in the community it is less severe and recalcitrant [5,6].

Mild attacks may present with pain or itching without discharge and with a minimally congested or swollen meatus. The degree of irritation or discomfort is often out of all proportion to the appearance. This stage probably represents early damage to the meatal skin [7]. Most cases of this type will resolve with simple therapeutic measures, but a minority, perhaps due to trauma, secondary infection or failure to keep the ear dry and clean, progress to more severe disease.

Fully developed acute external otitis (diffuse otitis externa) is characterized by a sudden onset of ear pain, itching, a sense of fullness or stuffiness if there is significant oedema, and a variable degree of hearing loss. The otalgia is often exacerbated by jaw movements. With progression, there is usually drainage of malodorous pus, which tends to be bluish-green in colour if *Ps. aeruginosa* is the dominant infecting organism. Examination shows erythema and swelling, which may spread from the external auditory meatus to involve the concha or beyond. The external auditory canal shows erythema and oedema, and there is macerated debris and perhaps greenish pus present. In severe cases, inflammation can extend to involve the tympanic membrane. Hearing loss is due to oedema of the canal, and this may be sufficient to obscure vision of its full length. Traction on the pinna to examine the canal and pressure over the tragus characteristically elicit pain. There may be associated fever, malaise and regional lymphadenopathy.

It is important to gently remove debris in the process of a full examination, and to try to determine whether the disease is secondary to otitis media and whether or not the tympanic membrane is intact.

Bullous external otitis [8] is an uncommon variant in which there is a sudden onset of severe pain followed by discharge of blood from the ear canal. Bluish-red haemorrhagic bullae are visible on the osseous canal walls.

In granular external otitis the lining of the meatus and canal is replaced in part or whole by granulation tissue, which can project inwards as pedunculated masses. These are usually found near the tympanic membrane, arising from the osseous end of the canal. Granular external otitis is associated with a severe or neglected course [9,10].

The term 'chronic external otitis' is sometimes used for cases that have had persistent symptoms for more than 2 months [11]. Microbiological assessment has shown a significant organism in 82% in one series: *S. aureus* in one-third, *Pseudomonas* in one-third and various other Gram-negative and Gram-positive organisms in the remainder. In addition, 17 of the 99 patients had fungal disease alone [12]. There is often a dry canal due to lack of cerumen. It is likely that in most cases of chronic otitis externa, particularly when treatment has been used for the acute attack and symptoms have continued, concurrent dermatological disorders are present (Fig. 65.18). Patients in whom the disorder behaves in a recalcitrant manner may have an underlying systemic disease such as acquired immune deficiency syndrome (AIDS), malnutrition or uncontrolled diabetes mellitus; poor therapeutic response is also seen in patients treated with high-dose steroids or chemotherapeutic agents [13].

Seborrhoeic dermatitis, atopic dermatitis and psoriasis usually occur only at the meatus but may sometimes extend further into the canal. Seborrhoeic otitis externa is extremely common and has been regarded by some dermatologists as the basis for most cases of otitis externa. The symptoms and signs, however, are normally mild unless complicated by secondary factors and usually consist of no more than superficial scaling and a little discom-

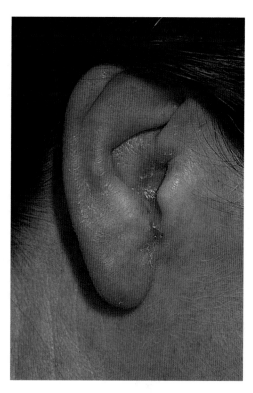

Fig. 65.18 Chronic otitis externa in an atopic patient with a history of recurrent streptococcal infection and resultant lymphoedema contributing to narrowing of the canal.

fort or itching. Signs of pityriasis capitis or seborrhoeic dermatitis elsewhere are usually present. The condition may deteriorate at times of stress or fatigue. Secondary bacterial infection is common. In this 'reactive' group the appearance is often that of a dermatitis spreading into the ear, in contrast with those cases with a primarily 'infective' aetiology where infection and/or inflammation often appears to be spreading out from the ear and where the entire length of the canal is often affected. The clinical appearance, however, is often non-diagnostic.

In infective eczema there is usually intense pruritus associated with exudate. The condition may complicate both otitis media and otitis externa and is usually associated with some degree of otorrhoea. In others it appears to develop from seborrhoeic dermatitis that has become secondarily infected. The condition may affect the meatus, concha, lobe and peri-auricular skin and often spreads widely. The post-auricular fold is commonly affected. The symptoms and signs are those of eczema with an accompanying or preceding aural discharge. In seborrhoeic individuals, other areas may be involved at the same time. Fissures and cellulitis are common complications.

Contact dermatitis is often occult [14] and easily overlooked. Sensitivity to topically applied medicaments is common in chronic otitis externa. Occlusion, the recurrent nature of the disease and frequent use of antibiotics on an already damaged skin probably account for the high incidence of contact dermatitis at this site. Other sensitivities include nickel from hair pins, metal implements, chromate and phosphorus sesquisulphide in matches, and nail varnish. It is characteristic that the degree of itching and burning is often markedly out of proportion to the amount of erythema and oedema present. Contact dermatitis may also rarely occur with ear moulds [15]. Clinically, it is often difficult to differentiate neurodermatitis from contact dermatitis.

Lichen simplex (neurodermatitis) may be localized to one area of the meatus or may occur more diffusely over the tragus, triangular fossa and adjoining skin. The condition is usually diagnosed by the history rather than the signs. Itching is intense, but often intermittent. The need to scratch or rub is compulsive, although often denied. Signs of inflammation are often minimal, but some degree of oedema and scaling is common. Complications from trauma, infection and sensitization are frequent. Intermittent itching of the external auditory canal (non-specific external otitis [2]) can also occur, irregularly and over a long period, without any obvious cause and with minimal signs of disease.

Whatever the primary aetiology, with the passage of time chronic external otitis becomes an increasingly complex diagnostic and therapeutic problem.

REFERENCES

1 Senturia BH. *Disease of the External Ear*. Springfield, IL: Thomas, 1957.
2 Jones EH. *External Otitis*. Springfield, IL: Thomas, 1965.
3 Perry ET. *The Human Ear Canal*. Springfield, IL: Thomas, 1957.
4 Peterkin GAG. Otitis externa. *J Laryngol Otol* 1974; **88**: 15–21.
5 Price J. Otitis externa in children. *J R Coll Gen Pract* 1976; **26**: 610–5.
6 Lambert IJ. A comparison of the treatment of otitis externa with 'Otosporin' and aluminium acetate: a report from a services practice in Cyprus. *J R Coll Gen Pract* 1981; **31**: 291–4.
7 Wright DN, Alexander JM. Effect of water on the bacterial flora of swimmers' ears. *Arch Otolaryngol* 1974; **99**: 15–8.
8 Senturia BH. External otitis, acute diffuse. *Ann Otol Rhinol Laryngol* 1973; **82** (Suppl. 8): 1–23.
9 Moffett AJ. Granulating myringitis: unusual affection of the eardrum. *J Laryngol Otol* 1943; **58**: 453–6.
10 Lucente FE. Diseases due to infection. In: Lucente FE, Lawson W, Novick NL, eds. *The External Ear*. Philadelphia: Saunders, 1996: 48–97.
11 Hirsch BE. Infections of the external ear. *Am J Otolaryngol* 1992; **13**: 145–55.
12 Hawke M, Wong J, Krajden S. Clinical and microbiological features of otitis externa. *J Otolaryngol* 1984; **13**: 289–95.
13 Selesnick SH. Otitis externa: management of the recalcitrant case. *Am J Otol* 1994; **15**: 408–12.
14 Holmes RC, Wilkinson JD, Johns AN *et al.* Medicament contact dermatitis in patients with chronic inflammatory ear disease. *J R Soc Med* 1982; **75**: 27–30.
15 Cockerill D. Allergies to ear moulds. A study of reactions encountered by hearing aid users to some ear mould materials. *Br J Audiol* 1987; **21**: 145.

Differential diagnosis. The part played by trauma, environment, infection, sensitization and altered physiology and anatomy must be assessed and evaluated as accurately as possible. Difficulties often arise in the interpretation of bacteriological and mycological findings. 'Hearing-aid dermatitis' is more often due to traumatic and physical factors than to allergic sensitivity. Sensitivity to topical antibiotics may be occult, especially when they are prescribed in combination with corticosteroids, and are one cause of chronicity. Contact hypersensitivity to aural treatments (see below) may produce eczema that extends onto facial skin anterior to, or below, the ear. The importance of perineal and nasal transfer of infection should not be underestimated, and mechanical interference with the external auditory canal in patients with otitis externa tends to be the rule rather than the exception.

External otitis is unlikely to be confused with any other condition except perhaps psoriasis and eczema, and these, of course, may coexist. Middle-ear disease, past and present, should always be excluded.

Swabs should be taken for bacteriological culture and epithelial debris examined and sent for mycological culture. Potassium hydroxide preparations showing evidence of epithelial invasion with hyphae are probably more important in this respect than a positive culture, which may simply indicate commensal or saprophytic infection.

In any long-standing or resistant case, patch testing with a special 'ear battery' [1] should be undertaken to rule out unsuspected contact dermatitis. If there is excess granulation, middle-ear disease should be ruled out, and if the patient is diabetic, debilitated, very young, elderly or immunosuppressed, malignant otitis externa must also be excluded.

Another condition that may need to be considered is *bullous myringitis*, an uncommon condition probably due to upper respiratory tract viral infection (e.g. influenza), which presents with single or multiple bullae on the tympanic membrane and adjacent canal wall. It can resemble bullous external otitis, which is usually due to *Pseudomonas*. Sudden severe pain is a feature, but this resolves rapidly after rupture of the bullae. Furuncles of the external auditory canal are described below. Other bacteria may be a rare cause, for example gonococcal otitis externa [2].

Complications. Recurrent otitis externa may also develop into hypertrophic otitis externa or localized elephantiasis nostra [3] of the ears as a result of the effects of chronic lymphatic obstruction. The resultant narrowing of the external acoustic canal coupled with the underlying lymphoedema makes recurrent and repeated infections even more likely.

Secondary trauma. Once an irritable focus occurs in the canal, energetic attempts to remove wax or debris or to satisfy the urge to rub or scratch the infected area often intensify the inflammation. Cotton buds, although frequently regarded as safe, are a common cause of tympanic perforation [4].

Secondary sensitization. This is usually a consequence of treatment or a reaction to objects placed in the ear to alleviate itching. Therapeutic agents may therefore enhance and perpetuate the condition for which they were prescribed. Penicillin, neomycin, framycetin (Soframycin) and chloramphenicol are all well-known topical sensitizers, but even gentamicin, Vioform (chinoform), polymyxin and bacitracin may sensitize at times [1]; allergy to topical corticosteroids used in the ear may also occur [5]. Allergy to topical medicaments is found in as many as 40% of patients with chronic or treatment-resistant otitis externa [1,6]. In only about 20% of cases is there improvement after discontinuing topical agents to which patients have been shown to be allergic [5].

Sensitivity to nail varnish may be misconstrued as lichen simplex and, in women who are nickel sensitive, otitis externa may be aggravated by using metal objects to alleviate itching or to clear the ear. Otoscopes themselves may release nickel. Another source of contact dermatitis is chromate [7] or phosphorus sesquisulphide in match heads, which some people use to scratch their ears.

Benign non-necrotizing otitis externa. This usually presents as chronic, non-painful otorrhoea with an ulcer present in the floor of the external canal. Surgery may be a better alternative than long-term medical management [8].

Allergic and 'ide' reactions [9,10]. A few well-documented cases have been reported in which recurrent pruritus, oedema and scaling of the ear canal have occurred in response to fungal infection at a distant body site, or associated with food or drug allergies. Some such cases also have an 'ide' reaction affecting the hands or other areas.

REFERENCES

1 Holmes RC, Wilkinson JD, Johns AN *et al.* Medicament contact dermatitis in patients with chronic inflammatory ear disease. *J R Soc Med* 1982; **75**: 27–30.
2 Pareek SS. Gonococcal otitis externa (letter). *N Engl J Med* 1979; **300**: 1490.
3 Grant JM. Elephantiasis nostra verrucosa of the ears. *Cutis* 1982; **29**: 441–4.
4 Robertson MS. A critical comment on the use of cotton buds. *N Z Med J* 1971; **86**: 102–3.
5 Devos SA, Mulder JJS, van der Valk PGM. The relevance of positive patch test reactions in chronic otitis externa. *Contact Dermatitis* 2000; **42**: 354–5.
6 Fraki JE, Kalimo K, Tuohimaa P *et al.* Contact allergy to various components of topical preparations for treatment of external otitis. *Acta Otolaryngol (Stockh)* 1985; **100**: 414–8.
7 McKelvie M, McKelvie P. Some aetiological factors in otitis externa. *Br J Dermatol* 1966; **78**: 227–31.
8 Wormald PJ. Surgical management of benign necrotizing otitis externa. *J Laryngol Otol* 1994; **108**: 101–5.
9 Brown WH. Some observations on neurodermatitis of the scalp, with particular reference to tinea amiantacea. *Br J Dermatol Syphil* 1948; **60**: 81–90.
10 Jones EH. *External Otitis.* Springfield, IL: Thomas, 1965.

Treatment [1]. The general principles of treatment of otitis externa are to relieve pain, reduce itching, prevent trauma and avoid known or potential sensitizers. Significant infective organisms should be identified and treated appropriately.

Many mild cases of otitis externa will respond to simple aural toilet, optimally with careful suction and under direct vision, followed by the use of an acidifying and drying agent. Moderately severe cases are likely to require antibiotic or antiseptic drops.

When there is coexistent eczema, combined steroid–antiseptic or steroid–antibiotic drops or wicks can be used. It should be noted, however, that many of the common infecting organisms are frequently antibiotic resistant; swabs for culture and sensitivity should therefore be taken before prescribing topical or systemic antibiotics. When *S. aureus* is the infecting organism, this is increasingly likely to be methicillin-resistant *S. aureus* (MRSA), especially when there has been recent hospital exposure [2]. In chronic cases, a great variety of treatments will already have been given and medicament contact dermatitis will therefore be more likely. Because this is often occult, patch testing should be done in all patients with chronic disease.

Pain is often severe, especially with acute staphylococcal infections, and strong analgesics may be required. Local heat also often helps. Bed rest and daily wicks or dressing may be needed in the more severe case.

If there is significant pyrexia (> 38.3°C), lymphadenopathy or failure to improve with topical therapy, an oral antibiotic should be used, for example a cephalosporin or fluoroquinolone. If pain is very severe, granulations are present in the canal or the patient is diabetic or immunocompromised, there should be suspicion for invasive (necrotizing) otitis (see p. 65.27).

Topical treatment. This is the essential part of therapy and the most difficult to carry out satisfactorily. Ear drops are of less value than regular cleaning of the ear, and this initially needs to be done daily by a doctor or an experienced nurse. Less severe cases may be treated once a week. Having cleaned the ear of debris and wax, preferably by suction under direct vision, a wick may be inserted or the patient instructed to apply ear drops regularly. When the cartilaginous portion of the canal alone is involved, the patient can be shown how to apply the prescribed medicament by holding a loose wool-tipped orange stick 2.5 cm from its end and inserting this until the fingers touch the tragus.

If wax is impacted, this can be softened with oil, glycerine or sodium bicarbonate eardrops and then removed either manually or by syringing, as long as the drum can be visualized and there is no perforation. Obstinate cases should be referred to an otologist. Some proprietary cerumenolytics are irritant and should be left in the ear for only 15–30 min before syringing.

In most chronic or complicated cases, treatment must be continued regularly for some weeks after apparent cure. Care must be taken to prevent cross-infection from other body sites, especially from the anterior vestibule of the nose or the perineum, and the ear should be kept as dry and as clean as possible.

A very large number of medicaments have been used in the treatment of otitis externa. Alcohol 70–85% (isopropyl alcohol), 1–2% acetic acid, aluminium subacetate solution and 2% salicylic acid in 60% spirit are all safe and effective, aluminium acetate solution being especially useful against the expected pathogens [3]. If acidic ear drops cause a burning sensation, ophthalmic hydrogen peroxide drops are a practical substitute. Wicks with 8–13% aluminium acetate, 0.25–0.5% silver nitrate, or glycerine and ichthyol are used to treat hypertrophic otitis externa. Although the use of corticosteroids with or without antimicrobials is a common practice, the evidence to support their use is controversial [4]. Neomycin, framycetin (Soframycin), gentamicin and polymyxin are probably acceptable as short-term treatments for acute otitis externa but the risk of sensitization and cross-sensitization increases with more protracted usage. The combination of neomycin and polymyxin will cover both *S. aureus* and *Ps. aeruginosa*. Topical ofloxacin is as effective and only has to be used twice daily [5]. For patients with chronic or chronic relapsing otitis externa, iodochlorhydroxyquinoline (Vioform, chinoform) can be used alone or in combination with corticosteroids.

The imidazoles have largely replaced nystatin and amphotericin as antifungal agents, as they are active against *Aspergillus* as well as *Candida*, although acetic acid, boric acid and 25% *m*-cresyl acetate may still at times be useful; 2% salicylic acid in spirit is useful for prophylaxis. Several ear-drops, for example the aminoglycosides, chlorhexidine, polymyxin and chloramphenicol, are potentially ototoxic [6,7] and should be avoided in the presence of tympanic perforation.

In all cases of external otitis, treatment should be prolonged beyond the time of apparent recovery and patients should be advised how best to avoid recurrence and about the dangers of indiscriminate or prolonged self-medication.

Surgical treatments. Occasionally, chronic otitis externa is due to narrowing of the external auditory meatus. Surgical enlargement of the meatus can then bring about resolution [8,9].

REFERENCES

1 Roland PS. External otitis: a challenge in management. *Curr Infect Dis Rep* 2000; **2**: 160–7.
2 Walshe P, Rowley H, Timon C. A worrying development in the microbiology of otitis externa. *Clin Otolaryngol* 2001; **26**: 218–20.
3 Thorpe MA, Kruger J, Oliver S et al. The antibacterial activity of acetic acid and Burow's solution as topical otological preparations. *J Laryngol Otol* 1998; **112**: 925–8.
4 Holten KB, Gick J. Management of the patient with otitis externa. *J Fam Pract* 2001; **50**: 353–60.
5 Ruben RJ. Efficacy of ofloxacin and other otic preparations for otitis externa. *Pediatr Infect Dis J* 2001; **20**: 108–10.
6 Brummett RE, Harris RF, Lindgren JA. Detection of ototoxicity from drugs applied topically to the middle ear space. *Laryngoscope* 1976; **86**: 1177–87.
7 Mittelman H. Ototoxicity of 'ototopical' antibiotics: past, present, and future. *Trans Am Acad Ophthalmol Otolaryngol* 1977; **76**: 1432–43.
8 Hunsaker DH. Conchomeatoplasty for chronic otitis externa. *Arch Otolaryngol Head Neck Surg* 1988; **114**: 395–8.
9 Roland PS. Chronic external otitis. *Ear Nose Throat J* 2001; **80** (6 Suppl.): 12–6.

Invasive external otitis [1,2]
SYN. MALIGNANT EXTERNAL OTITIS; NECROTIZING EXTERNAL OTITIS

This is an infection of the skin of the external ear canal that spreads to deeper structures and causes necrosis.

Aetiology. In most cases, the infecting organism is *Ps. aeruginosa*, although occasionally other organisms have been involved: *S. aureus* [3], *S. epidermidis* [4], *Klebsiella oxytoca* [5], *Aspergillus* [6–10], *Malassezia sympodialis* [11], *Scedosporium apiospermum* [12] and *Actinomycetes*. The condition characteristically occurs in elderly diabetics [13–16] but is also seen with some frequency in the immunocompromised, including patients with HIV infection [1,16,17]; it has also been reported in association with diabetes insipidus [18]. Cases have been reported in children [19–21] in whom chronic illness or immunosuppression are usually present. In diabetics, microangiopathy may be important in the pathogenesis [1]. It is possible that abnormalities of cellular immunity and polymorphonuclear function are important in some cases [22,23], but in many instances the pathogenesis is poorly understood.

Pathology. In most cases, there is evidence of osteomyelitis [5]. An early event is acellular necrosis of cartilage [24].

Clinical features. Quite often there is a preceding history of irrigation of the ear. The commonest presenting symptom is pain, which is usually very severe and persistent. It may spread from the region of the ear to the vertex, temporal or occipital areas, and there may be temporomandibular joint pain. Pain progresses more quickly in children than adults. The second most common symptom is discharge from the ear. In up to 50% there is some degree of hearing loss. Systemic symptoms, including fever, are uncommon [1]. There may be symptoms due to involvement of cranial nerves, particularly dysphagia.

On examination the external auditory canal is always abnormal, with varying degrees of oedema and erythema, and extensive granulation tissue formation is evident. This is particularly seen on the posterior and inferior aspect of the wall and at the junction between the bony and cartilaginous segments of the canal. There may be swelling of the soft tissues around the ear. The tympanic membrane is frequently necrotic in children but characteristically spared in adults [21]. Cranial neuropathies may be found in up to 40% of patients [1,17]. Facial palsy is the most common finding but involvement of cranial nerves

IV, VI, VIII, IX, X and XII may be variably present. When such nerve involvement is found, the disease is more extensive.

Investigations usually show elevation of the erythrocyte sedimentation rate, but the white-cell count is often normal.

Diagnosis. Invasive external otitis is usually diagnosed on clinical suspicion. It is essential to obtain material for culture to determine the infective cause, and samples should be taken from the ear canal, granulations, soft tissue and bone, depending on the case. Blood cultures may also be valuable.

Imaging techniques can be helpful, particularly in diagnosing bony involvement and following progress of the disease, and should enable granular external otitis to be distinguished from the much more serious invasive external otitis. Plain films, computed tomography (CT), bone scans and magnetic resonance imaging (MRI) have all been used. MRI with or without gadolinium enhancement is probably the best technique for imaging soft-tissue involvement, and for evaluation of the meninges and changes within the osseous medullary cavity, although CT is preferred for the initial diagnosis and recognition of cortical bone erosion [25,26].

Complications. Spread of the disease can produce parotitis, mastoiditis or osteomyelitis of the base of the skull and thence spread to the contralateral side. Meningitis can occur, and is an important cause of death. Cranial nerve paralysis may result in aspiration pneumonia. A rare complication is destructive osteomyelitis of the temporomandibular joint [27]. Overall, there is a mortality of 10–20%; in the presence of cranial neuropathies the mortality is 70% [1,17].

Treatment. Because of the range of possible infections, it is essential to base treatment on the result of culture. For *Pseudomonas*, the traditional approach has been to use an extended-spectrum antipseudomonal penicillin for 4–8 weeks and an aminoglycoside for 4–6 weeks [1]. Ciprofloxacin [28,29] can be successful if used early in the course of disease. When there is evidence of extensive bone destruction, removal of necrotic material is necessary. Some cases fail to respond to antibiotic therapy and, if the facility is available, hyperbaric oxygen can improve the outlook [30]. Ascorbic acid has also been recorded as an adjuvant therapy [22].

When the infective cause is bacteria other than *Pseudomonas* or is a fungus, advice on the choice of antimicrobial agent should be taken from a microbiologist.

REFERENCES

1 Doroghazi RM, Nadol JB Jr, Hyslop NE Jr *et al.* Invasive external otitis. Report of 21 cases and review of the literature. *Am J Med* 1981; **71**: 603–14.
2 Chandler JR. Malignant external otitis. *Laryngoscope* 1967; **78**: 1257–94.
3 Keay DG, Murray AM. Clinical records: malignant external otitis due to *Staphylococcus* infection. *J Laryngol Otol* 1988; **102**: 926–7.
4 Barrow HN, Levenson MJ. Necrotizing 'malignant' external otitis caused by *Staphylococcus epidermidis*. *Arch Otolaryngol Head Neck Surg* 1992; **118**: 94–6.
5 Bernheim J, Sade J. Histopathology of the soft parts in 50 patients with malignant external otitis. *J Laryngol Otol* 1989; **103**: 366–8.
6 Cunningham M, Yu VL, Turner J *et al.* Necrotizing otitis externa due to *Aspergillus* in an immunocompetent patient. *Arch Otolaryngol Head Neck Surg* 1988; **114**: 554–6.
7 Bickley LS, Betts RF, Parkins CW. Atypical invasive external otitis. *Arch Otolaryngol Head Neck Surg* 1988; **114**: 1024–8.
8 Phillips P, Bryce G, Sheperd J *et al.* Invasive external otitis caused by *Aspergillus*. *Rev Infect Dis* 1990; **12**: 277–81.
9 Gordon G, Giddings NA. Invasive otitis externa due to *Aspergillus* species: case report and review. *Clin Infect Dis* 1994; **19**: 866–70.
10 Anderson LL, Giandoni MB, Keller RA, Grabski WJ. Surgical wound healing complicated by *Aspergillus* infection in a non-immunocompromised host. *Dermatol Surg* 1995; **21**: 799–801.
11 Chai FC, Auret K, Christiansen K *et al.* Malignant otitis externa caused by *Malassezia sympodialis*. *Head Neck* 2000; **22**: 87–9.
12 Yao M, Messner AH. Fungal malignant otitis externa due to *Scedosporium apiospermum*. *Ann Otol Rhinol Laryngol* 2001; **110**: 377–80.
13 Meyerhoff WL, Gates GA, Montalbo PJ. *Pseudomonas* mastoiditis. *Laryngoscope* 1977; **87**: 483–92.
14 Johnson MP, Ramphal R. Malignant external otitis. Report on therapy with ceftazidime and review of therapy and prognosis. *Rev Infect Dis* 1990; **12**: 173–80.
15 Lang R, Goshen S, Kitzes-Cohen R *et al.* Successful treatment of malignant external otitis with oral ciprofloxacin: report of experience with 23 patients. *J Infect Dis* 1990; **161**: 537–40.
16 Kielhofner M, Atmar RL, Hamill RJ. Life-threatening *Pseudomonas aeruginosa* infections in patients with human immunodeficiency virus infection. *Clin Infect Dis* 1992; **14**: 403–11.
17 Rubin J, Yu VL. Malignant external otitis: insights into pathogenesis, clinical manifestations, diagnosis and therapy. *Am J Med* 1988; **85**: 391–8.
18 Giguere P, Rouillard G. Otite externe maligne bilatérale chez une fillete de 10 ans. *J Otolaryngol* 1976; **5**: 159–66.
19 Coser PL, Stamm AEC, Lobo RC *et al.* Malignant external otitis in infants. *Laryngoscope* 1980; **90**: 312–6.
20 Joachims HZ. Malignant external otitis in children. *Arch Otolaryngol* 1976; **102**: 236–7.
21 Rubin J, Yu VL, Stool SE. Malignant external otitis in children. *J Pediatr* 1988; **113**: 965–70.
22 Corberand J, Nguyen F, Fraysse B *et al.* Malignant external otitis and polymorphonuclear leukocyte migration impairment: improvement with ascorbic acid. *Arch Otolaryngol* 1982; **108**: 122–4.
23 Yust I, Radiano C, Tartakovsky B *et al.* Impairment of cellular immunity in patients with malignant external otitis. *Acta Otolaryngol* 1980; **90**: 398–403.
24 Ostfeld E, Segal M, Czernobilsky B. Malignant external otitis: early histopathologic changes and pathogenic mechanism. *Laryngoscope* 1981; **91**: 965–70.
25 Gherini SG, Brackmann DE, Bradley WG. Magnetic resonance imaging and computerized tomography in malignant otitis externa. *Laryngoscope* 1986; **96**: 542–8.
26 Grandis JR, Curtin HD, Yu VL. Necrotizing (malignant) external otitis: prospective comparison of CT and MR imaging in diagnosis and follow-up. *Radiology* 1995; **196**: 499–504.
27 Midwinter KI, Gill KS, Spencer JA, Fraser ID. Osteomyelitis of the temporomandibular joint in patients with malignant otitis externa. *J Laryngol Otol* 1999; **113**: 451–3.
28 Brody T, Pensak ML. The fluoroquinolones. *Am J Otol* 1991; **12**: 477–9.
29 Morrison GAJ, Bailey CM. Relapsing malignant otitis externa successfully treated with ciprofloxacin. *J Laryngol Otol* 1988; **102**: 872–6.
30 Davis JC, Gates GA, Lerner C *et al.* Adjuvant hyperbaric oxygen in malignant external otitis. *Arch Otolaryngol Head Neck Surg* 1992; **118**: 89–93.

Furunculosis

SYN. ACUTE LOCALIZED EXTERNAL OTITIS

A furuncle is a staphylococcal infection of a hair follicle [1]. A common site is between the junction of the tragus and the anterior crus of the helix. Furuncles also may occur in the skin of the external auditory canal at the junction with the concha. Coalescence of adjacent infected follicles results in a carbuncle.

The patient presents with pain, which can be aggravated by chewing if there is involvement of the anterior wall of the canal. There may be sufficient swelling to obstruct the entrance to the canal. There is often regional lymphadenopathy and sometimes fever.

Furunculosis can usually be distinguished from external otitis by the normal appearance of the canal epithelium and an absence of discharge; the two conditions can, however, coexist. If possible the tympanic membrane should be examined, in order to exclude otitis media and mastoiditis.

Localized lesions associated with mild swelling usually respond to an oral antistaphylococcal antibiotic [1]. If an abscess or carbuncle is present, incision and drainage is usually necessary. The latter can be achieved with a wick. Any draining material should be sent for culture and antibacterial sensitivities.

REFERENCE

1 Hirsch BE. Infection of the external ear. *Am J Otolaryngol* 1992; **13**: 145–55.

Otomycosis

Otomycosis is an inflammatory process due to a variety of yeast and fungal organisms as the primary aetiological agent. The same range of fungi may be found in patients with multifactorial or bacterial external otitis (see above).

Aetiology. The species of fungus and yeast involved vary somewhat depending on ambient climate. In most tropical regions of the world *Aspergillus* species account for the majority of isolates, whereas in temperate areas *Candida albicans* is the most frequent [1]. Others include phycomycetes, *Rhizopus*, *Actinomyces* and *Penicillium*. The fact that these organisms can be pathogenic as well as saprophytic has been confirmed in a number of studies [2–5].

The factors that convert organisms that are normally saprophytic into pathogens are similar to those that apply to bacterial external otitis. Heat and humidity are foremost, and account for the frequency of otomycosis in the tropics and in those using hearing aids or occlusive ear moulds. Diabetes mellitus, immunosuppression, systemic and topical antibiotics, and steroids are also important.

Clinical features. The principal symptom is usually itching, which can have a quality of being deep inside the ear. This is often accompanied by a sensation of fullness. Pain is uncommon, in contrast to bacterial external otitis. Discharge, if any, is usually slight. There may be hearing loss of a conductive type. Because of the irritation, patients are liable to traumatize the canal and may then initiate the symptoms and signs of bacterial external otitis. The most important complication is perforation of the eardrum [6].

On examination the dominant feature is the presence of wispy filamentous masses, which may be isolated or diffusely present in the canal. These masses are white, grey or stippled black if *Aspergillus* is present. Inflammation of the canal epithelium is usually mild. There may be some epithelial debris, which may be either moist or dry.

Diagnosis. The clinical appearance is usually distinctive. As always with external canal disorders it is important to check for other pathology. Material can be taken for mycological examination and culture.

Treatment [7]. Careful cleaning followed by drying is a prerequisite to successful management. The canal can then be wiped out, for example with *m*-cresyl acetate or 1% thymol in 70% alcohol, and the specific treatment applied on a wick. Treatment should be changed daily until a satisfactory result has been achieved. Many agents have been advocated for otomycosis, but there is little evidence to promote one above the others. They include aluminium acetate, acetic acid, *m*-cresyl acetate, thiomersal, gentian violet, clioquinol, nystatin, amphotericin and the imidazoles.

In rare situations, usually in immunosuppressed patients, there may be cellulitis of the surrounding soft tissues directly due to fungal infection. In such cases, itraconazole is likely to be the treatment of choice. Oral terbinafine has also been used when other treatments have failed [8].

REFERENCES

1 Lucente FE. Fungal infections of the external ear. *Otolaryngol Clin North Am* 1993; **26**: 995–1006.
2 Nielsen PG. Fungi isolated from chronic external ear disorders. *Mykosen* 1985; **28**: 234–7.
3 Sood VB, Sinha A, Mohaoatra LN. Otomycosis: a clinical entity—clinical and experimental study. *J Laryngol Otol* 1988; **81**: 999–1173.
4 Stern JC, Lucente FE. Otomycosis. *Ear Nose Throat J* 1988; **67**: 804–10.
5 Talwar P, Chakrabarti A, Kaur P et al. Fungal infection of ear with special reference to chronic suppurative otitis media. *Mycopathologia* 1988; **104**: 47–50.
6 Hurst WB. Outcome of 22 cases of perforated tympanic membrane caused by otomycosis. *J Laryngol Otol* 2001; **115**: 879–80.
7 Lucente FE. Diseases due to infection. In: Lucente FE, Lawson W, Novick NL, eds. *The External Ear*. Philadelphia: Saunders, 1995: 81–6.
8 Rotoli M, Sascaro G, Cavalier S. *Aspergillus versicolor* infection of the external auditory canal successfully treated with terbinafine. *Dermatology* 2001; **202**: 143.

AIDS and the external ear

The consequences of HIV infection will at times be seen on the pinna and in the external auditory canal [1]. The ear is a relatively common site for manifestation of Kaposi's sarcoma. Florid seborrhoeic dermatitis is often a presenting feature of AIDS. The occurrence of molluscum contagiosum lesions in an adult should prompt a suspicion of immunodeficiency; on the ear the lesions can resemble basal cell carcinoma. Bacillary angiomatosis may produce vascular papules and nodules on the ear. Herpes simplex and zoster can be more florid in patients with AIDS. Polyps in the external auditory canal due to *Pneumocystis carinii* have been described [2] and can invade the middle ear and middle cranial fossa [3]. Invasive external otitis (see p. 65.27) is a well-recognized consequence of HIV-related immunosuppression [4]. Excessive growth of ear hair has been noted [5].

REFERENCES

1 Lucente FE. Diseases due to infection. In: Lucente FE, Lawson W, Novick NL, eds. *The External Ear*. Philadelphia: Saunders, 1995: 95–6.
2 Gherman CR, Ward RR, Bassis ML. *Pneumocystis carinii* otitis media and mastoiditis as the initial manifestation of the acquired immunodeficiency syndrome. *Am J Med* 1988; **85**: 250–2.
3 Patel SK, Philpott JM, McPartlin DW. An unusual case of *Pneumocystis carinii* presenting as an aural mass. *J Laryngol Otol* 1999; **113**: 555–7.
4 Hern JD, Almeyda J, Thomas DM *et al*. Malignant otitis externa in HIV and AIDS. *J Laryngol Otol* 1996; **110**: 770–5.
5 Tosti A, Gaddoni G, Peluso AM *et al*. Acquired hairy pinnae in a patient infected with the human immunodeficiency virus. *J Am Acad Dermatol* 1993; **28**: 513.

Tumours of the pinna and external auditory canal [1]

Benign tumours

On the pinna, these will present as papules or nodules, sometimes with distinctive morphology. In the external auditory canal, benign tumours tend to present with hearing loss and may predispose to infection [2].

Benign tumours found on the pinna include melanocytic naevus, seborrhoeic keratosis (Fig. 65.19), squamous cell papilloma, pilomatrixoma [3,4], trichoepithelioma [5], trichofolliculoma [6,7], Winer's dilated pore [8], myoma, chondroma, osteoma, fibroma [9], neurofibroma [10], neurilemmoma [11], granular cell tumour, haemangioma (Fig. 65.20) and lymphangioma [12]. Benign glandular tumours may occur on the pinna, but are more common in the canal, especially sebaceous adenoma. Occasional unique lesions have been described [13].

Benign mass lesions in the canal include exostosis and osteoma, fibrous dysplasia both monostotic and polyostotic (Albright's syndrome), eosinophilic granuloma, cholesteatoma and keratosis obturans (see p. 65.36), benign ceruminous gland tumours (see p. 65.31) and temporomandibular joint herniation [14].

Papillomatosis of the external auditory canal presents with multiple rounded papules; it has been associated with human papillomavirus (HPV) 6 [15].

Extra-adrenal paraganglioma (glomus jugulare tumour) of the temporal bone can manifest in the external ear canal as a friable haemorrhagic neoplasm and can cause conductive hearing loss [1]. This tumour can be locally aggressive, and there are rare instances of metastasis.

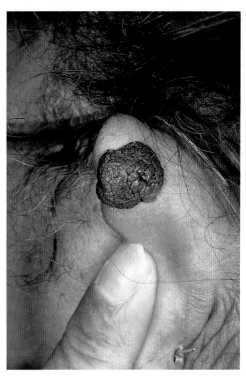

Fig. 65.19 Seborrhoeic keratosis (basal cell papilloma) of the pinna.

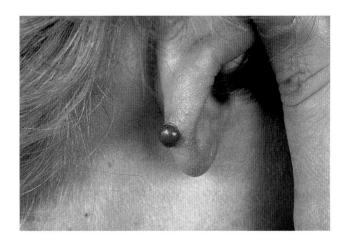

Fig. 65.20 Lobulated capillary haemangioma (pyogenic granuloma). A bright-red nodule with a surrounding collarette of keratin.

Various conditions can mimic benign tumours. On the pinna, these include cysts of various types, viral warts and molluscum contagiosum, chondrodermatitis, elastotic and weathering nodules, keloids, congenital malformations such as accessory tragi, nodular calcinosis [16], gouty tophi, deposits of amyloid, angiolymphoid hyperplasia with eosinophilia and 'pseudolymphoma', inflammatory polyps, hamartomas [17], choristomas [18] and congenital cysts of branchial arch origin in the external auditory canal. Cholesteatoma (see p. 65.36) may also occur in the external canal.

REFERENCES

1 Hyams VJ. Pathology of tumours of the external ear. In: Lucente FE, Lawson W, Novick NL, eds. *The External Ear.* Philadelphia: Saunders, 1995: 108–48.
2 Tran LP, Grundfast KM, Selesnick SH. Benign lesions of the external auditory canal. *Otolaryngol Clin North Am* 1996; **29**: 807–25.
3 Vinayak BC, Cox GJ, Ashton-Key M. Pilomatrixoma of the external auditory meatus. *J Laryngol Otol* 1993; **107**: 333–4.
4 Sevin K, Can Z, Yilmaz S, Saray A, Yormuk E. Pilomatrixoma of the earlobe. *Dermatol Surg* 1995; **21**: 245–6.
5 Ferlito A, Recher G, Polidero F *et al.* Solitary trichoepithelioma and epithelioma adenoides cysticum of Brooke involving the external auditory meatus. *J Laryngol Otol* 1981; **95**: 835–41.
6 O'Mahony JJ. Trichofolliculoma of the external auditory meatus. Report of a case and review of the literature. *J Laryngol Otol* 1981; **95**: 623–5.
7 Srivastava RN, Ajwani KD. Trichofolliculoma. *Ear Nose Throat J* 1979; **58**: 159–60.
8 Ayoub OM, Timms MS, Mene A. Winer's dilated pore: rare presentation in the external ear canal. *Auris Nasus Larynx* 2001; **28**: 349–52.
9 Varletzides E, Grigoriades S, Tsiliguri E. An unusual localization of fibroma on the lobe of the ear. *Panminerva Med* 1980; **22**: 37–9.
10 Trevisani TP, Pohl AL, Matloub HS. Neurofibroma of the ear: function and aesthetics. *Plast Reconstr Surg* 1982; **70**: 217–9.
11 Fodor RI, Pastore PN, Frable MA. Neurilemmoma of the auricle: a case report. *Laryngoscope* 1977; **87**: 1760–4.
12 Grabb WC, Dingman RO, Oneal RM *et al.* Facial hamartomas in children: neurofibroma, lymphangioma and hemangioma. *Plast Reconstr Surg* 1980; **66**: 509–27.
13 Donati P, Balus L. Folliculosebaceous cystic hamartoma: reported case with a neural component. *Am J Dermatopathol* 1993; **15**: 277–9.
14 Tran LP, Grundfast KM, Selesnick SH. Benign lesions of the external auditory canal. *Otolaryngol Clin North Am* 1996; **29**: 807–25.
15 Xia M-Y, Zhu W-Y, Lu J-Y *et al.* Ultrastructure and human papillomavirus DNA in papillomatosis of external auditory canal. *Int J Dermatol* 1996; **35**: 337–9.
16 Kacker SK, Dasgupta G. Hamartomas of the ear and nose. *J Laryngol Otol* 1973; **87**: 801–5.
17 Hansen KK, Segura AD, Esterly NB. Solitary congenital nodule on the ear of an infant. *Pediatr Dermatol* 1993; **10**: 88–90.
18 Braun GA, Lowry D, Meyers A. Bilateral choristomas of the external auditory canals. *Arch Otolaryngol* 1978; **104**: 467–8.

Exostosis and osteoma

Exostoses of the external auditory canal are usually bilateral, symmetrical, multiple, diffuse, broadly based growths of bone arising from the tympanic bone in the external auditory canal [1,2]. Frequent exposure to cold water is an aetiological factor in nearly all cases [3]. Exostoses are very common in surfers, especially those who have surfed for more than 10 years [4,5].

Osteomas can usually be differentiated by their solitary and unilateral distribution, although they may be similar to exostoses histologically [6]. They are often attached by a narrow pedicle to the tympanosquamous or tympanomastoid suture line [1].

Occasionally other fibro-osseous lesions are found which are neither exostosis nor osteoma [7,8].

Osteomas and exostoses are normally asymptomatic unless they enlarge sufficiently to block the external auditory canal [9]. Surgical removal may be indicated [10].

REFERENCES

1 Graham MD. Osteomas and exostoses of the external auditory canal. A clinical, histopathologic and scanning electron microscopic study. *Ann Otol Rhinol Laryngol* 1979; **88**: 566–72.
2 Sheehy JL. Diffuse exostoses and osteomata of the external auditory canal: a report of 100 operations. *Otolaryngol Head Neck Surg* 1982; **90**: 337–42.
3 di Bartolomeo JR. Exostoses of the external auditory canal. *Ann Otol Rhinol Laryngol* 1979; **88** (Suppl. 61): 2–20.
4 Chaplin JM, Stewart IA. The prevalence of exostoses in the external auditory meatus of surfers. *Clin Otolaryngol* 1998; **23**: 326–30.
5 Wong BJ, Cervantes W, Doyle KJ *et al.* Prevalence of external auditory canal exostoses in surfers. *Arch Otolaryngol Head Neck Surg* 1999; **125**: 969–72.
6 Fenton JE, Turner J, Fagan PA. A histopathologic review of temporal bone exostoses and osteomata. *Laryngoscope* 1996; **106**: 624–8.
7 Tran LP, Grundfast KM, Selesnick SH. Benign lesions of the external auditory canal. *Otolaryngol Clin North Am* 1996; **29**: 807–25.
8 Ramirez-Camacho R, Vicente J, Berrocal JRG *et al.* Fibro-osseous lesions of the external auditory canal. *Laryngoscope* 1999; **109**: 488–91.
9 Kemink JL, Graham MD. Osteomas and exostoses of the external auditory canal: medical and surgical management. *J Otolaryngol* 1982; **11**: 101–6.
10 Whitaker SR, Cordier A, Kosjakov S, Charbonneau R. Treatment of external auditory canal exostoses. *Laryngoscope* 1998; **108**: 195–9.

Glandular tumours

Tumours of the ceruminous glands are rare. It is often difficult to distinguish between adenoma and carcinoma on histological grounds [1–3] and the term 'ceruminoma' [4] is probably best avoided. The tumours comprise benign and pleomorphic adenomas, adenocarcinomas, adenoid cystic carcinomas and perhaps others including mucoepidermoid carcinomas. Tumours of the cerumen glands have been reported in association with other sweat gland tumours elsewhere [5].

Isolated cases of syringocystadenoma papilliferum, apocrine cystadenoma, benign eccrine cylindroma, hidradenoma papilliferum and carcinomas of eccrine and sebaceous origin have also been reported [6,7].

Extramammary Paget's disease of the external ear and/or canal resembles Bowen's disease or a dermatosis [8].

Benign tumours produce symptoms of obstruction and hearing loss. Pain is the usual presenting feature of the more malignant tumours. They are usually seen as polypoid masses in the canal. Other symptoms include bleeding, otorrhoea and, with spread of the neoplasm, nerve palsies.

Treatment is the province of the otorhinolaryngologist. Because of the potential for malignant behaviour, all ceruminous gland tumours should be fully excised with an adequate margin of normal tissue [9].

REFERENCES

1 Wetli CV, Pardo V, Millard M, Gerston K. Tumors of ceruminous glands. *Cancer* 1972; **29**: 1169–78.
2 Pulec JL. Glandular tumours of the external auditory canal. *Laryngoscope* 1977; **87**: 1601–12.
3 Lynde CW, McLean DI, Wood WS. Tumors of the ceruminous glands. *J Am Acad Dermatol* 1984; **11**: 841–7.
4 Neldner KH. Ceruminoma. *Arch Dermatol* 1968; **98**: 344–8.

5 Habib MA. Ceruminoma in association with other sweat gland tumours. *J Laryngol Otol* 1981; **95**: 415–20.
6 Dehner LP, Chen KTK. Primary tumours of the external and middle ear: benign and malignant glandular neoplasms. *Arch Otolaryngol* 1980; **106**: 13–9.
7 Nissim F, Czernobilsky B, Ostfeld E. Hidradenoma papilliferum of the external auditory canal. *J Laryngol Otol* 1981; **95**: 843–8.
8 Gonzalez-Castro J, Iranza P, Palou J, Mascaro JM. Extramammary Paget's disease of the external ear. *Br J Dermatol* 1998; **138**: 914–5.
9 Mansour P, George MK, Pahor AL. Ceruminous gland tumours: a reappraisal. *J Laryngol Otol* 1992; **106**: 727–32.

Premalignant epithelial neoplasms of the auricle

Because of its high level of exposure to UV radiation [1], especially in men, the auricle is a common site for premalignant and malignant lesions of epidermal origin. Other predisposing factors include prior ionizing radiation, a chronic dermatosis such as lupus vulgaris, and genetic factors such as xeroderma pigmentosum and Gorlin's syndrome.

The commonest premalignant lesion is the solar keratosis, which can occur on all sun-exposed aspects of the auricle, but is especially common on the upper surface of the helix [2,3]. The clinical presentations include an erythematous telangiectatic patch, a focal area of scaling or hyperkeratosis, or a cutaneous horn. Solar keratoses on the auricle are often multiple. Solar elastosis may be evident in the surrounding skin. On the auricle, progression to squamous carcinoma from solar keratosis may occur more readily than at other sites [4].

Other premalignant lesions include Bowen's disease, radiation and tar keratoses and, rarely, keratoacanthoma [5,6].

Treatment. Several forms of treatment can eradicate premalignant lesions from the auricle, but there are no adequate data to compare them. They include excision, curettage, electrosurgery, cryotherapy, 5-fluorouracil and photodynamic therapy. The choice will depend on a number of factors, including the need for a tissue diagnosis, size and location of the lesion, likely cosmetic outcome and the available facilities. Follow-up is important for detection of recurrences and the appearance of new lesions. Lesions closely resembling squamous carcinoma, such as keratoacanthoma, should probably be totally excised to ensure accurate diagnosis [6].

REFERENCES

1 Green A, Williams G. Ultraviolet radiation and skin cancer: epidemiological data from Australia. In: Young AR, Moan J, Bjorn LO, Nultsch W, eds. *Environmental UV Photobiology*. New York: Plenum Press, 1993: 233–54.
2 Byers R, Kesler K, Redman B *et al*. Squamous carcinoma of the external ear. *Am J Surg* 1983; **146**: 447–50.
3 Freedlander E, Chung FF. Squamous cell carcinoma of the pinna. *Br J Plast Surg* 1983; **36**: 171–5.
4 Blake GB, Wilson SP. Malignant tumours of the ear and their treatment: 1. Tumours of the auricle. *Br J Plast Surg* 1974; **27**: 67–76.
5 Patterson HC. Facial keratoacanthoma. *Otolaryngol Head Neck Surg* 1983; **91**: 263–70.
6 Moriyama M, Watanabe T, Sakamoto N *et al*. A case of giant keratoacanthoma of the auricle. *Auris Nasus Larynx* 2000; **27**: 185–8.

Squamous cell carcinoma of the auricle

Although the ratio of basal cell carcinoma (BCC) to squamous cell carcinoma (SCC) is about 4 : 1 on the head and neck generally, on the ear SCC is relatively more common (BCC : SCC, 1.3 : 1) [1].

In most instances, SCC evolves from a premalignant lesion, usually a solar keratosis, and occurs predominantly in elderly white men, although at a younger age in the immunosuppressed. The most common site is the helix [2]. Early SCC may be suspected when there is induration of the base of a scaly papule, nodule or cutaneous horn. With progression, SCC usually ulcerates and with invasion of cartilage can become grossly destructive (Fig. 65.21). Local spread along perichondrial, periosteal and neurovascular planes can make SCC of the auricle very difficult to control. With the exception of the lip, auricular SCC is more likely to metastasize than is SCC at any other sun-exposed site (11% compared with 2%) [3]. There is a small but significant mortality [2,4,5]. Adverse prognostic factors for both local recurrence and metastasis of SCC include size (> 2 cm), depth of invasion (> 4 mm, Clark levels 4 and 5), perineural involvement and poor differentiation of the tumour [6]. The pre-auricular site

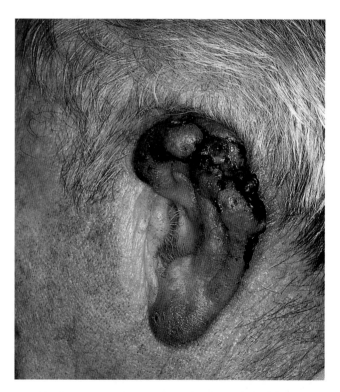

Fig. 65.21 Squamous carcinoma of the auricle. An advanced tumour with extensive destruction of the ear cartilage. (Courtesy of Mr D. Baldwin, Southmead Hospital, Bristol, UK.)

may also confer a poor prognosis [7]. It is not clear, however, to what extent these are independent variables; shallow lesions with large surface area (i.e. > 2 cm diameter) do not seem to have a poor prognosis. If SCC recurs after primary treatment, there is a much greater risk for further recurrence and metastasis [6].

Treatment. It is important to achieve control of the disease with the initial treatment for SCC. For small, minimally invasive lesions, simple excision, cryotherapy or curettage with cautery/electrodesiccation may be adequate. Excellent results have been reported from the combination of curettage and cryotherapy for carefully selected cases [8]. For larger lesions, and especially for those with adverse prognostic factors, the choice is likely to be between wide margin excision, Mohs micrographic surgery and radiation therapy.

The surgical procedure used will depend on the location and extent of the tumour. Smaller lesions can often be removed by wedge excision with primary repair by advancement flaps. Larger and ill-defined lesions are best closed by temporary grafts pending a histopathological assessment of the margins before definitive repair is carried out. Partial or total amputation may be needed for large tumours. If there is spread beyond the pinna, resection of the parotid, temporal bone, temporomandibular joint or mandibular ramus may be be required, with appropriate repair.

Several authors have recommended minimal resection margins, for example 1 cm [9], 6 mm with frozen section control [10], 8 mm for 1-cm-diameter tumours and 1.5 cm for 3-cm-diameter tumours [11], all with removal of the underlying cartilage. Overall, there is an incidence of 18.7% recurrence during follow-up for 5 years or more with non-Mohs modalities compared with 5.3% for Mohs micrographic surgery, suggesting that the latter is the treatment of choice [6,12].

SCCs in the tragal and pretragal location appear to have a greater tendency to spread along embryonic fusion planes and may only be curable by radical surgery, for example parotidectomy in association with removal of the tumour [7,13].

Various techniques are needed to reconstruct the ear after curative surgery [14–19].

Radiotherapy can be successful as a primary treatment for SCC of the auricle [20], with megavoltage electron-beam therapy having therapeutic and cosmetic advantages over conventional orthovoltage X-ray treatment [21]. There may, however, be a higher recurrence rate [22,23] compared with surgery, particularly for large tumours [2,24,25]. Radiation therapy can be complicated by damage to the cartilage and associated chronic infection; deformity of the pinna is another long-term consequence. Radiotherapy may improve the outlook for cases with extensive local spread requiring radical surgery.

The management of SCC with metastasis to regional lymph nodes and beyond is outside the scope of the dermatologist.

REFERENCES

1 Ahmad I, Das Gupta AR. Epidemiology of basal cell carcinoma and squamous cell carcinoma of the pinna. *J Laryngol Otol* 2001; **115**: 85–6.
2 Thomas SS, Matthews RN. Squamous cell carcinoma of the pinna: a 6-year study. *Br J Plastic Surg* 1994; **47**: 81–5.
3 Johnson TM, Rowe DE, Nelson BR, Swanson NA. Squamous carcinoma of the skin (excluding lip and oral mucosa). *J Am Acad Dermatol* 1992; **26**: 467–84.
4 Byers R, Kesler K, Redman B *et al*. Squamous carcinoma of the external ear. *Am J Surg* 1983; **146**: 447–50.
5 Freedlander E, Chung FF. Squamous cell carcinoma of the pinna. *Br J Plast Surg* 1983; **36**: 171–5.
6 Rowe DE, Carroll RJ, Day CL. Prognostic factors for local recurrence, metastasis and survival rates in squamous carcinoma of the skin, ear and lip. *J Am Acad Dermatol* 1992; **26**: 976–90.
7 Lee D, Nash M, Har-El G. Regional spread of auricular and periauricular cutaneous malignancies. *Laryngoscope* 1996; **106**: 998–1001.
8 Nordin P. Curettage–cryosurgery for non-melanoma skin cancer of the external ear: excellent 5-year results. *Br J Dermatol* 1999; **140**: 291–3.
9 Pless J. Carcinoma of the external ear. *Scand J Plast Reconstr Surg* 1976; **10**: 147–51.
10 Kitchens GG. Auricular wedge resection and reconstruction. *Ear Nose Throat J* 1989; **68**: 673–4, 677–9, 683.
11 Levine HL, Kinney SE, Bailin PL, Roberts JK. Cancer of the periauricular region. *Dermatol Clin* 1989; **7**: 781–95.
12 Mohs F, Larson P, Iriondo M. Micrographic surgery for the microscopically controlled excision of carcinoma of the external ear. *J Am Acad Dermatol* 1988; **19**: 729–37.
13 Niparko JK, Swanson NA, Baker SR *et al*. Local control of auricular, periauricular, and external canal malignancies with Mohs' surgery. *Laryngoscope* 1990; **100**: 1047–51.
14 Menick FJ. Reconstruction of the ear after tumor excision. *Clin Plast Surg* 1990; **17**: 405–15.
15 Johnson TM, Fader DJ. The staged retroauricular to auricular direct pedicle (interpolation) flap for helical ear reconstruction. *J Am Acad Dermatol* 1997; **37**: 975–8.
16 Yotsuyanagi T, Nihei Y, Sawada Y. Reconstruction of defects involving the upper one-third of the auricle. *Plast Reconstr Surg* 1998; **102**: 988–92.
17 Martinez JM, Alconchel MD, Olivares C, Cimorra GA. Reconstruction of the tragus after tumour excision. *Br J Plast Surg* 1997; **50**: 552–4.
18 van der Lei B, Spronk CA. Reconstruction of non-marginal ear defect by a postauricular wedge transposition flap. *Br J Plast Surg* 1998; **51**: 14–6.
19 Majumdar A, Townend J. Helix rim advancement for reconstruction of marginal defects of the pinna. *Br J Oral Maxillofac Surg* 2000; **38**: 3–7.
20 Avila J, Bosch A, Aristizabal S *et al*. Carcinoma of the pinna. *Cancer* 1977; **40**: 2891–5.
21 Hunter RD, Pereira DTM, Pointon RCS. Megavoltage electron beam therapy in the treatment of basal and squamous cell carcinomata of the pinna. *Clin Radiol* 1982; **33**: 341–5.
22 Blake GB, Wilson JSP. Malignant tumours of the ear and their treatment: 1. Tumours of the auricle. *Br J Plast Surg* 1974; **27**: 67–76.
23 Schewe EJ, Pappalardo C. Cancer of the external ear. *Am J Surg* 1962; **104**: 753–5.
24 Mazeron JJ, Ghalie R, Zeller J *et al*. Radiation therapy for carcinoma of the pinna using iridium 192 wires: a series of 70 patients. *Int J Radiat Oncol Biol Phys* 1986; **12**: 1757–63.
25 Silva JJ, Tsang RW, Panzarella T *et al*. Results of radiotherapy for epithelial skin cancer of the pinna: the Princess Margaret Hospital experience, 1982–1993. *Int J Radiat Oncol Biol Phys* 2000; **47**: 451–9.

Basal cell carcinoma of the auricle

BCC of the auricle is somewhat less common than SCC (Fig. 65.22). It is also mainly due to the effects of solar

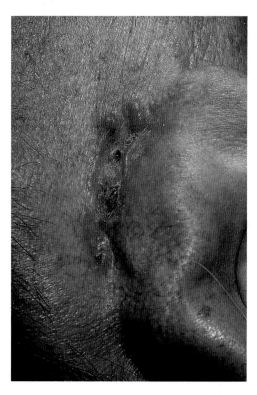

Fig. 65.22 Basal cell carcinoma. Translucent ulcerated nodules in the retro-auricular fold.

radiation, but is much less liable to metastasize [1,2]. Presentation is generally as for BCC elsewhere, although could be missed when resembling a cleft earlobe [3].

The approach to treatment is essentially similar to that outlined for SCC. Mohs micrographic surgery is the most likely modality to achieve cure with lesions that are extensive, deeply invasive or recurrent, or which have a morphoeic growth pattern.

REFERENCES

1 Blake GB, Wilson JSP. Malignant tumours of the ear and their treatment: 1. Tumours of the auricle. *Br J Plast Surg* 1974; **27**: 67–76.
2 Small CS, Hawkins FD. Basal cell carcinoma with metastases. *Arch Pathol* 1949; **47**: 196–204.
3 Altchek ED. Basal cell carcinoma presenting as a cleft earlobe. *Plast Reconstr Surg* 1998; **102**: 1758.

Squamous and basal cell carcinoma of the external auditory canal

Non-glandular carcinomas of the external auditory canal are uncommon. Most are squamous in type (Fig. 65.23). They affect a younger age group (50–65 years) and, in contrast to SCC of the auricle, there is much less of a male preponderance. A preceding history of chronic otitis is common [1,2]. Pseudo-epitheliomatous hyperplasia secondary to chronic infection or inflammation can sometimes be difficult to distinguish from SCC [3].

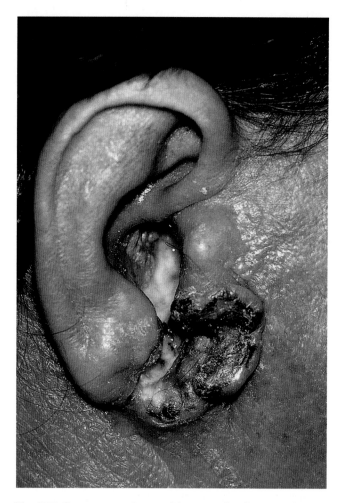

Fig. 65.23 Squamous carcinoma of the external auditory canal. Purulent discharge, inflammation and destruction of the meatus. (Courtesy of Mr D. Baldwin, Southmead Hospital, Bristol, UK.)

Most squamous carcinoma of the canal has an infiltrative growth pattern. It tends to grow along the canal, escaping anteriorly through Santorini's fissures in the cartilaginous segment and Huschke's foramen in the bony portion, into the temporomandibular joint and parotid. Spread also occurs posteriorly into the mastoid, and through the tympanic membrane into the middle ear and thence to the carotid canal, apex of the petrous temple bone, the internal auditory canal, base of the skull and the dura. Metastasis to lymph nodes and distantly is common.

Overall, there is a much poorer prognosis than for SCC of the pinna, with 5-year survival rates of about 40% [4]. Adverse factors are a large lesion, invasion of cartilage or bone, facial nerve palsy, spread to the middle ear and beyond, and lymph node metastasis. The extent of the disease can be determined accurately by CT [5]. Staging using clinical and imaging data is important for assessing prognosis and the likelihood of benefit from adjuvant radiotherapy [6,7].

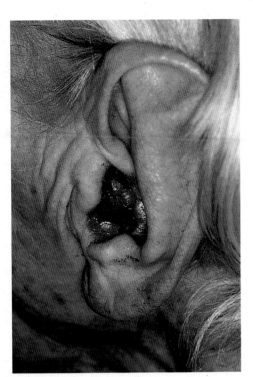

Fig. 65.24 Basal cell carcinoma of the external auditory canal. An erythematous tumour presenting as obstruction at the entrance of the canal. (Courtesy of Mr M. Birchill, Southmead Hospital, Bristol, UK.)

Verrucous carcinoma of the external auditory canal is an uncommon variant that can appear cytologically banal but nevertheless invade bone, by a pushing rather than an infiltrative growth pattern [8,9].

BCC of the external auditory canal can be locally destructive (Fig. 65.24), but does not metastasize and has a much better prognosis than SCC [10].

The most common symptoms of invasive SCC of the canal are purulent and bloody discharge from the ear, followed by pain, hearing loss and facial paralysis. Examination reveals a friable tumour, partially or completely obstructing the external auditory canal.

Treatment. Surgery has been regarded as the treatment of choice, the extent determined by an assessment of the limits of tumour growth. However, radiotherapy alone may be as effective if the disease is limited to the site of origin, i.e. there is no evidence of nerve or bone involvement [11]. Post-operative radiotherapy improves the outlook [6,7,12–15], but for lesions that have spread deeply or have metastasized cure is most unlikely.

REFERENCES

1 Lederman M. Malignant tumours of the ear. *J Laryngol Otolaryngol* 1965; **79**: 85–119.
2 Paaske PB, Witten J, Schwer S, Hansen HS. Results in treatment of carcinoma of the external auditory canal and middle ear. *Cancer* 1987; **59**: 156–60.

3 Gacek MR, Gacek RR, Gantz B *et al.* Pseudoepitheliomatous hyperplasia versus squamous cell carcinoma of the external auditory canal. *Laryngoscope* 1998; **108**: 620–3.
4 Chen KTK, Dehner LP. Primary tumors of the external and middle ear. I. Introduction and clinicopathologic study of squamous cell carcinoma. *Arch Otolaryngol* 1978; **104**: 244–52.
5 Arriaga M, Curtin H, Takashi H *et al.* Staging proposal for external auditory meatus carcinoma based on pre-operative clinical examination and computed tomography findings. *Ann Otol Rhinol Laryngol* 1990; **99**: 714–21.
6 Testa JRG, Fukuda Y, Kowalski LP. Prognostic factors in carcinoma of the external auditory canal. *Arch Otolaryngol Head Neck Surg* 1997; **123**: 720–4.
7 Moody SA, Hirsch BE, Myers EN. Squamous cell carcinoma of the external auditory canal: an evaluation of a staging system. *Am J Otol* 2000; **21**: 582–8.
8 Stafford DN, Frootko NJ. Verrucous carcinoma in the external auditory canal. *Am J Otol* 1986; **7**: 443–5.
9 Proops DW, Hawke WM, Van Nostrand AW *et al.* Verrucous carcinoma of the ear. Case report. *Ann Otol Rhinol Laryngol* 1984; **93**: 385–8.
10 Stell PM. Basal cell carcinoma of the external auditory meatus. *Clin Otolaryngol* 1984; **9**: 187–90.
11 Hashi N, Shirato H, Omatsu T *et al.* The role of radiotherapy in treating squamous cell carcinoma of the external auditory canal, especially in early stages of disease. *Radiother Oncol* 2000; **56**: 221–5.
12 Hahn SS, Kim JA, Goodchild N, Constable WD. Carcinoma of the middle ear and external auditory canal. *Int J Radiat Oncol Biol Phys* 1983; **9**: 1003–7.
13 Lewis JS. Cancer of the ear. *Cancer* 1987; **37**: 78–87.
14 Kinney SE. Squamous cell carcinoma of the external auditory canal. *Am J Otol* 1989; **10**: 111–6.
15 Shih L, Crabtree JA. Carcinoma of the external auditory canal: an update. *Laryngoscope* 1990; **100**: 1215–8.

Malignant melanoma

Malignant melanoma of the external ear is relatively uncommon, constituting about 1% of all cutaneous melanomas [1]. It accounted for 4.8% of all auricular malignancies in one series [2] and represented 7% of all melanomas in another series [3]. Melanomas at this site are about three times more common in males than females [3,4]. Melanoma is found in a similar frequency distribution on the ear as SCC and its precursors, i.e. about half occur on the helix and one-quarter on the antihelix [3], but they are rarely found in the external auditory canal [5,6]. Most melanomas on the ear are of superficial spreading or nodular type, the latter being relatively more common than at other head and neck sites [7,8]. The major determinant for prognosis is Breslow thickness [4].

Treatment is in principle no different from malignant melanoma elsewhere (see Chapter 38), and relatively conservative excision followed by reconstruction can be safe [9]. Sentinel lymph node mapping may be valuable for accurate staging, particularly for melanoma of the ear, since its lymphatic drainage is notoriously unpredictable [10].

REFERENCES

1 Hudson DA, Krige JEJ, Strover RM, King HS. Malignant melanoma of the external ear. *Br J Plast Surg* 1990; **43**: 608–11.
2 Blake GB, Wilson SP. Malignant tumours of the ear and their treatment: 1. Tumours of the auricle. *Br J Plast Surg* 1974; **27**: 67–76.
3 Pack GT, Conley J, Oropeza R. Melanoma of the external ear. *Arch Otolaryngol* 1970; **92**: 106–13.
4 Cox NH, Aitchison TC, Sirel JM, MacKie RM. Comparison between lentigo maligna melanoma and other histogenetic types of malignant melanoma of the head and neck. *Br J Cancer* 1996; **73**: 940–4.

5 Langman AW, Yarington T, Patterson SD. Malignant melanoma of the external auditory canal. *Otolaryngol Head Neck Surg* 1996; **114**: 645–8.

6 Milbrath MM, Campbell BH, Madiedo G, Janjan NA. Malignant melanoma of the external auditory canal. *Am J Clin Oncol* 1998; **21**: 28–30.

7 Davidson A, Hellquist HB, Villman K, Westman G. Malignant melanoma of the ear. *J Laryngol Otol* 1993; **107**: 798–802.

8 Cox NH, Jones SK, MacKie RM. Malignant melanoma of the head and neck in Scotland: an eight year analysis of trends in prevalance, distribution and prognosis. *Q J Med* 1987; **64**: 661–70.

9 Narayan D, Ariyan S. Surgical considerations in the management of malignant melanoma of the ear. *Plast Reconstr Surg* 2001; **107**: 20–4.

10 Wey PD, de la Cruz C, Goydos JS *et al*. Sentinel lymph node mapping in melanoma of the ear. *Ann Plast Surg* 1998; **40**: 506–9.

Other malignant tumours

Other malignant tumours involving the external ear or the external auditory canal are all rare. The pathology is reviewed in Friedman and Arnold's monograph [1]. The dermatologist may encounter sebaceous carcinoma [2], atypical fibroxanthoma, trichilemmal carcinoma [3], Merkel cell tumour [4], Kaposi's sarcoma [5,6] or rhabdomyosarcoma (mainly in children) [7–9]. Angiosarcoma of the pinna has the same gloomy outlook as it does on the scalp [10]. Other sarcomas have been recorded but are exceptionally rare. Lymphomas may occur on the external ear [11], particularly mycosis fungoides [12]. Perichondritis can be mimicked by non-Hodgkin's lymphoma [13,14], and both lymphoma [15,16] and myeloma [17] can present with an external auditory canal tumour. The ear may be involved by direct extension from tumours nearby, for example the parotid, and also by metastases from distant sites [18].

REFERENCES

1 Friedman I, Arnold W. *Pathology of the Ear*. Edinburgh: Churchill Livingstone, 1993.

2 Ray J, Schofield JB, Shotton JC, Al-Ayoubi A. Rapidly invading sebaceous carcinoma of the external auditory canal. *J Laryngol Otol* 1999; **113**: 578–80.

3 Billingsley EM, Davidowski TA, Maloney ME. Trichilemmal carcinoma. *J Am Acad Dermatol* 1997; **36**: 106–7.

4 Hanna GS, Ali MH, Akosa AB, Maher EJ. Merkel-cell carcinoma of the pinna. *J Laryngol Otol* 1988; **102**: 607–11.

5 Gnepp DR, Chandler W, Hyams VJ. Primary Kaposi's sarcoma of the head and neck. *Ann Med* 1984; **100**: 107–14.

6 Delbrouck C, Kampouridis S, Chantrain G. An unusual localisation of Kaposi's sarcoma: the external auditory canal. *Acta Otorhinolaryngol Belg* 1998; **52**: 29–36.

7 Jaffe N, Fuller RM, Farber S. Rhabdomyosarcoma in children: improved outlook with a multidisciplinary approach. *Am J Surg* 1973; **125**: 482–7.

8 Maurer HM. Rhabdomyosarcoma in childhood and adolescence. *Curr Probl Cancer* 1978; **2**: 3–36.

9 Feldman BA. Rhabdomyosarcoma of the head and neck. *Laryngoscope* 1982; **92**: 424–40.

10 Leighton SE, Levine TP. Angiosarcoma of the external ear: a case report. *Am J Otol* 1991; **12**: 54–6.

11 Darvay A, Russell-Jones R, Acland KM *et al*. Systemic B-cell lymphoma presenting as an isolated lesion on the ear. *Clin Exp Dermatol* 2001; **26**: 166–9.

12 Baumgartner BJ, Eusterman V, Myers J, Massengill P. Initial report of a cutaneous T-cell lymphoma appearing on the auricular helix. *Ear Nose Throat J* 2000; **79**: 391–4.

13 Levin RJ, Henick DH, Cohen AF. Human immunodeficiency virus-associated non-Hodgkin's lymphoma presenting as an auricular perichondritis. *Otolaryngol Head Neck Surg* 1995; **112**: 493–5.

14 Indudharan R, Arni T, Myint KK, Jackson N. Lymphoblastic lymphoma/leukaemia presenting as perichondritis of the pinna. *J Laryngol Otol* 1998; **112**: 592–4.

15 Kieserman SP, Finn DG. Non-Hodgkin's lymphoma of the external auditory canal in an HIV-positive patient. *J Laryngol Otol* 1995; **109**: 751–4.

16 Angeli SI, Brackmann DE, Xenellis JE *et al*. Primary lymphoma of the internal auditory canal. *Ann Otol Rhinol Laryngol* 1998; **107**: 17–21.

17 Quinodoz D, Dulguerov P, Kurt AM *et al*. Multiple myeloma presenting with external ear canal mass. *J Laryngol Otol* 1998; **112**: 469–71.

18 Golding-Wood DG, Quiney RE, Cheesman AD. Carcinoma of the ear: retrospective analysis of 61 patients. *J Laryngol Otol* 1989; **103**: 653–6.

Miscellaneous conditions

Cholesteatoma of the external auditory canal

Cholesteatoma of the middle ear space is accumulation of keratinous debris within a sac-like squamous epithelial lining. It can grow at the expense of normal structures and if it ruptures, the associated foreign body-type inflammatory reaction can produce serious damage.

A similar condition occurs rarely in the external auditory canal, although its status as a true cholesteatoma is disputed [1,2]. The accumulation of stratum corneum occurs within a cyst-like penetration of the bony portion of the canal wall by the epithelial lining. There is localized ulceration of the skin of the floor of the canal, with underlying osteitis and sometimes necrosis of bone. A necrotic sequestrum may become incorporated into the cholesteatoma. The cause is unknown, although trauma, for example from hard wax and manipulation of the canal, seems important in some cases [3].

Cholesteatoma usually occurs in patients over the age of 40 years. Symptoms are a dull pain in one ear and otorrhoea. Examination shows a white cystic mass protruding into the canal. The main differential diagnosis is from neoplasms and keratosis obturans [4,5]. External auditory canal cholesteatoma can occasionally behave aggressively, and may erode into the mastoid cavity, middle ear, temporomandibular joint and adjacent soft tissue. CT can be useful to assess the extent of the disease. Treatment is within the province of the otorhinolaryngologist.

Keratosis obturans

In this uncommon condition there is a localized accumulation of desquamated keratin in the ear canal. It may be due to a defect in the normal epithelial migration [6]. It is usually bilateral and typically occurs in younger patients than those presenting with external auditory canal cholesteatoma, which it can resemble. There is conductive hearing loss, sometimes with otalgia. Keratosis obturans can be associated with paranasal sinus disease and bronchitis; it has also been described in association with the yellow nail syndrome [7]. Treatment consists of careful removal of the accumulated keratin. Irrigation with water should be avoided [4,5].

REFERENCES

1 Friedman I, Arnold W. *Pathology of the Ear*. Edinburgh: Churchill Livingstone, 1993: 30–1.
2 Sismanis A, Williams GH, Abedi E. External auditory meatus cholesteatoma. In: Tos M, Thomas J, Peitersen E, eds. *Cholesteatoma and Mastoid Surgery*. Amsterdam: Kugler and Ghedini, 1984: 577–82.
3 Holt JJ. Ear canal cholesteatoma. *Laryngoscope* 1992; **102**: 608–13.
4 Corbridge RJ, Michaels L, Wright T. Epithelial migration in keratosis obturans. *Am J Otol* 1996; **17**: 411–4.
5 Armitage JM, Lane DJ, Stradling JR, Burton M. Ear involvement in the yellow nail syndrome. *Chest* 1990; **98**: 1534–5.
6 Piepergerdes JC, Kramer BM, Behnke EE. Keratosis obturans and external auditory canal cholesteatoma. *Laryngoscope* 1980; **90**: 383–90.
7 Shire JR, Donegan JO. Cholesteatoma of the external auditory canal and keratosis obturans. *Am J Otol* 1986; **7**: 361–4.

Referred pain

Due to the complicated nerve supply to the ear, referred pain is commoner than pain due to lesions in the ear itself [1]. Non-otological causes of such pain include the otomandibular syndrome [2] due to dysfunction of the temporomandibular joint, cervical arthritis with involvement of the cervical nerves, tonsillitis and carcinoma of the pharynx. Hair in the ear canal is an occasional cause [3]. Psychogenic otalgia has also been reported [4].

REFERENCES

1 Sheikhi AARJ. Pain in the ear: with special reference to referred pain. *J Laryngol Otol* 1980; **94**: 1433–40.
2 Arlen H. The otomandibular syndrome: diagnosis. *Ear Nose Throat J* 1978; **57**: 553–6.
3 Papay FA, Levine HL, Schiavone WA. Facial fuzz and funny feelings. *Cleve Clin J Med* 1989; **56**: 273–6.
4 Dight R. Psychogenic earache. An unusual cause of otalgia. *Med J Aust* 1980; i: 76–7.

Chapter 66

The Oral Cavity and Lips

Crispian Scully CBE

Introduction

Oral lesions are usually the result of local disease but may be the early signs of systemic disease, including dermatological disorders, and in some instances may cause the main symptoms. This chapter mainly discusses disorders of the dental, periodontal and mucosal tissues that may be related to skin disease and that may present at a dermatology clinic. It should be borne in mind that the professionals most competent in diagnosing and treating oral diseases are dentally qualified; few without this formal training and education are in a position to understand the full complexities of the region.

The chapter is an overview only and is divided into a brief discussion of the biology of the mouth, an overview of the more common signs and symptoms affecting specific oral tissues, discussion of the disorders of the oral mucosa of most relevance to dermatology and a tabulated review of oral manifestations of systemic diseases. Diseases affecting the jaws or temporomandibular joint are not discussed in any depth.

Only the more classic oral lesions are illustrated. About 20 of the colour illustrations are from the *Colour Atlas of Oral and Maxillofacial Disease*, 1996 (reproduced by kind permission of C. Scully, S. Flint, S.R. Porter and K. Moos, and publishers Martin Dunitz, London). More detail of histology is available elsewhere [1].

Biology of the mouth

Oral epithelium

The oral epithelium consists of a *functional compartment* —the progenitor cells (basal and parabasal cells)—which is the site of cell division; a *maturation compartment* (spinous and granular cells) where the cells become more terminally differentiated; and a superficial *cornified compartment* of squames and areas of keratinization, either orthokeratotic or parakeratotic. In the non-keratinized regions such as the buccal (cheek) and floor-of-mouth mucosae, overt keratinization and granular cells are absent and the surface cells are flattened, with elongated nuclei [2].

66.1

Lips

The lips extend from the lower end of the nose to the upper end of the chin. They mainly consist of bundles of striated muscle, particularly the *orbicularis oris* muscle, with skin on the external surface and mucous membrane on the inner surface, which has a profusion of minor salivary glands.

The vermilion zone, the transitional zone between the glabrous skin and the mucous membrane, is found only in humans. The vermilion zone contains no hair or sweat glands but does contain sebaceous glands (Fordyce spots, see below). The epithelium of the vermilion is distinctive, with a prominent stratum lucidum and a very thin stratum corneum. The dermal papillae are numerous at this site, with a rich capillary supply, which produces the reddish-pink colour of the lips in white people. Melanocytes are abundant in the basal layer of the vermilion of pigmented skin, but are infrequent in white skin.

The *oral commissures* are the angles where the upper and lower lip meet. The upper lip includes the *philtrum*, a midline depression, extending from the columella of the nose to the superior edge of the vermilion zone [3].

Oral mucosa

The mucosa is divided into masticatory, lining and specialized types. *Masticatory mucosa* (hard palate, gingiva) is adapted to the forces of pressure and friction and is keratinized, with numerous tall rete ridges and connective tissue papillae and little submucosa. *Lining mucosa* (buccal, labial and alveolar mucosa, floor of mouth, ventral surface of tongue, soft palate, lips) is non-keratinized, with broad rete ridges and connective tissue papillae and abundant elastic fibres in the lamina propria [4,5].

Specialized mucosa on the dorsum of the tongue, adapted for taste and mastication, is keratinized, with numerous rete ridges and connective tissue papillae, abundant elastic and collagen fibres in the lamina propria and no submucosa. The tongue is divided by a V-shaped groove, the *sulcus terminalis*, into an anterior two-thirds and a posterior third. Various papillae on the dorsum include the *filiform papillae*, which cover the entire anterior surface and form an abrasive surface to control the food bolus as it is pressed against the palate, and the *fungiform papillae*. The latter are mushroom-shaped, red structures covered by non-keratinized epithelium. They are scattered between the filiform papillae and have taste buds on their surface. Adjacent and anterior to the sulcus terminalis are eight to 12 large *circumvallate papillae*, each surrounded by a deep groove into which open the ducts of serous minor salivary glands. The lateral walls of these papillae contain taste buds.

The *foliate papillae* consist of four to 11 parallel ridges, alternating with deep grooves in the mucosa, on the lateral margins on the posterior part of the tongue. There are taste buds on their lateral walls. The *lingual tonsils* are round or oval prominences with intervening lingual crypts lined by non-keratinized epithelium. They are part of *Waldeyer's oropharyngeal ring* of lymphoid tissue. The lingual tonsil is a mass of lymphoid tissue in the posterior third of the tongue, between the epiglottis posteriorly and the circumvallate papillae anteriorly. It is usually divided in the midline by a ligament.

Teeth

The teeth develop from neuroectoderm [6]. Tooth development begins in the fetus, at about 28 days *in utero*. Indeed, all the deciduous and some of the permanent dentitions commence development in the fetus. At around the sixth week of intrauterine life the oral epithelium proliferates over the maxillary and mandibular ridge areas to form primary epithelial bands that project into the mesoderm, and produce a dental lamina in which discrete swellings appear—the enamel organs of developing teeth. Each enamel organ eventually produces tooth enamel, and the mesenchyme, which condenses beneath the enamel organ (actually neuroectoderm), forms a dental papilla that produces the dentine and pulp of the tooth. The enamel organ together with the dental papilla constitute the tooth germ, and this becomes surrounded by a mesenchymal dental follicle, from which the periodontium forms, ultimately to anchor the tooth in its bony socket. Mineralization of the primary dentition commences at about 14 weeks *in utero* and all primary teeth are mineralizing by birth. Permanent incisor and first molar teeth begin to mineralize at, or close to, the time of birth, mineralization of other permanent teeth starting later. Tooth eruption occurs after crown formation and mineralization is largely complete but before the roots are fully formed.

Teeth comprise a crown of insensitive enamel, surrounding sensitive dentine, and a root which has no enamel covering (Fig. 66.1). Teeth contain a vital pulp (nerve) and are supported by the periodontal ligament via which roots are attached into sockets in the alveolar process of the jaws (maxilla and mandible). The fibres of the periodontal ligament attach through cementum to the dentine surface. The alveolus is covered by the gingivae, or gum, which in health are pink, stippled and tightly bound down, and form a close-fitting cuff, with a small sulcus (gingival crevice), round the neck of each tooth.

The first or primary (deciduous or milk) dentition comprises two incisors, a canine and two molars in each of the four mouth quadrants (total 20 teeth). There are 10 deciduous (primary or milk) teeth in each jaw: all are fully

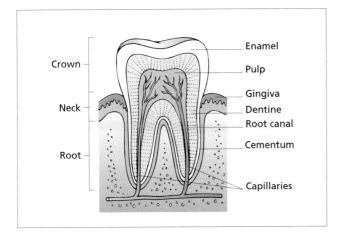

Fig. 66.1 Tooth structure.

Table 66.1 Tooth eruption timings (average timings; there is a wide range).

	Upper	Lower
Deciduous (primary) teeth		
A Central incisors	8–13 months	6–10 months
B Lateral incisors	8–13 months	10–16 months
C Canines (cuspids)	16–23 months	16–23 months
D First molars	13–19 months	13–19 months
E Second molars	25–33 months	23–31 months
Permanent teeth		
1 Central incisors	7–8 years	6–7 years
2 Lateral incisors	8–9 years	7–8 years
3 Canines (cuspids)	11–12 years	9–10 years
4 First premolars (bicuspids)	10–11 years	10–12 years
5 Second premolars (bicuspids)	10–12 years	11–12 years
6 First molars	6–7 years	6–7 years
7 Second molars	12–13 years	11–13 years
8 Third molars	17–21 years	17–21 years

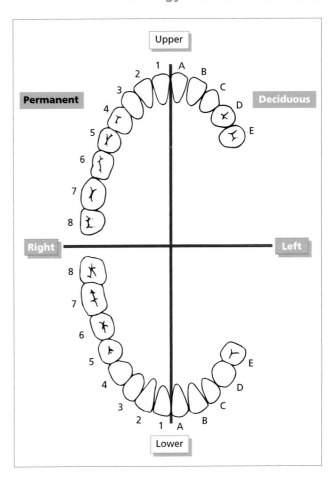

Fig. 66.2 Tooth notations.

erupted by the age of about 3 years (Fig. 66.2; Table 66.1). The secondary or permanent teeth begin to erupt at about the age of 6–7 years and the deciduous teeth begin to be slowly lost by normal root resorption.

The normal permanent (adult) dentition comprises two incisors, a canine, two premolars and three molars in each quadrant (total 32 teeth). The full permanent dentition consists of 16 teeth in each jaw: normally most have erupted by about 12–14 years of age. However, some milk teeth may still be present at the age of 12–13 years. The last molars (third molars or wisdom teeth), if present, often erupt later or may impact and never appear in the mouth.

Junction of the mucosa with the teeth

The dentogingival junction represents a unique anatomical feature concerned with the attachment of the gingival (gum) mucosa to the tooth. Non-keratinized gingival epithelium forms a cuff surrounding the tooth, and at its lowest point on the tooth is adherent to the enamel or cement. This 'junctional' epithelium is unique in being bounded both on its tooth and lamina propria aspects by basement membranes. Above this is a shallow sulcus or crevice (up to 2 mm deep), the gingival sulcus or crevice. Neutrophils continually migrate into the gingival crevice, and there is also a slow exudate of plasma (crevicular fluid).

Immunity in the oral cavity

Movement of the soft tissues during speech and swallowing, and salivation, ensures that much foreign material is swallowed. The need for this cleaning mechanism is clearly apparent in patients with facial paralysis, or in those with xerostomia, in whom there is accumulation of oral debris and subsequent infection.

Saliva also aggregates bacteria and deters their attachment to surfaces. Salivary lysozyme, thiocyanate, peroxides and various mucins and other components may be antimicrobial and saliva is inhibitory to various microbial agents including, for example, human immunodeficiency virus (HIV).

Salivary tissue derives its B cells from the gut-associated lymphoid tissue (GALT) system [7]. Salivary acinar cells produce secretory component (transport piece) needed for transport of IgA into the saliva and its stability in the presence of salivary or gastric proteolytic enzymes. Although the exact contribution to oral defence made by salivary IgA antibodies is difficult to assess, some patients who have IgA deficiency suffer from oral infections, and in animals it is possible to induce protective salivary IgA antibodies to caries-producing organisms such as *Streptococcus mutans*.

Neutrophils and other leukocytes are particularly essential for oral health as shown by the fact that patients with HIV infection, neutropenia, agranulocytopenia, leukaemia or chronic granulomatous disease are predisposed to severe gingivitis and rapid periodontal breakdown, as well as mouth ulceration and infections.

REFERENCES

1 Eveson JW, Scully C. *Colour Atlas of Oral Pathology*. London: Mosby, 1995.
2 Hume WJ, Potten CS. Advances in epithelial kinetics: an oral view. *J Oral Pathol* 1979; **8**: 3–22.
3 Zugerman C. The lips: anatomy and differential diagnosis. *Cutis* 1986; **38**: 116–20.
4 Meyer J, Squier CA, Gerson SJ. *The Structure and Function of Oral Mucosa*. Oxford: Pergamon Press, 1984.
5 Prime SS. Development, structure and function of oral mucosa. In: Scully C, ed. *The Mouth in Health and Disease*. Oxford: Heinemann Medical, 1989: 124–44.
6 Ten Cate AR. *Oral Histology*, 2nd edn. St Louis: Mosby, 1985.
7 Lamey PJ, Scully C. Salivary gland development, anatomy and physiology. In: Scully C, ed. *The Mouth in Health and Disease*. Oxford: Heinemann Medical, 1989: 283–8.

Examination of the mouth and perioral region

Examination includes inspection and palpation of the lymph nodes, temporomandibular joints, jaws, salivary glands and oral cavity.

Lymph nodes (Table 66.2)

Lymph from the superficial tissue of the head and neck generally drains first to groups of superficially placed lymph nodes, then to the deep cervical lymph nodes.
• Systematically, each region needs to be examined lightly with the pulps of the fingers, trying to roll the lymph nodes against harder underlying structures.
• Parotid, mastoid and occipital lymph nodes can be palpated simultaneously using both hands.
• Superficial cervical lymph nodes are examined with lighter palpation as they can only be compressed against the softer sternomastoid muscle.
• Submental lymph nodes are examined by tipping the patient's head forward and rolling the lymph nodes against the inner aspect of the mandible.

Table 66.2 Drainage areas of cervical lymph nodes.

Area	Draining lymph nodes
Scalp, temporal region	Superficial parotid
Scalp, posterior	Occipital
Scalp, parietal region	Mastoid
Ear, external	Superficial cervical over upper part of sternomastoid muscle
Ear, middle	Parotid
Over angle of mandible	Superficial cervical over upper part of sternomastoid muscle
Medial part of frontal region, medial eyelids, skin of nose	Submandibular
Lateral part of frontal region and lateral part of eyelids	Parotid
Cheek	Submandibular
Upper lip	Submandibular
Lower lip	Submental
Lower lip, lateral part	Submandibular
Mandibular gingivae	Submandibular
Maxillary teeth	Deep cervical
Maxillary gingivae	Deep cervical
Tongue tip	Submental; remainder drains to submandibular nodes
Tongue, anterior two-thirds	Submandibular; some midline cross-over of lymphatic drainage
Tongue, posterior third	Deep cervical
Tongue, ventrum	Deep cervical
Floor of mouth	Submandibular
Palate, hard	Deep cervical
Palate, soft	Retropharyngeal and deep cervical
Tonsil	Jugulodigastric

• Submandibular lymph nodes are examined in the same way with the patient's head tipped to the side being examined. Differentiation needs to be made between the submandibular salivary gland and submandibular lymph glands. Bimanual examination with one finger in the floor of the mouth may help.

• The deep cervical lymph nodes which project anterior or posterior to the sternomastoid muscle can be palpated. The jugulodigastric lymph node should be specifically examined, as this is the most common lymph node involved in tonsillar infections.

• The supraclavicular region should be examined at the same time as the rest of the neck; lymph nodes here may extend up into the posterior triangle of the neck on the scalene muscles, behind the sternomastoid.

• Parapharyngeal and tracheal lymph nodes can be compressed lightly against the trachea.

• Some information can be gained by the texture and nature of the lymphadenopathy.

• Tenderness and swelling should be documented. Lymph nodes that are tender may be inflammatory (lymphadenitis). Consistency should be noted. Nodes that are increasing in size and are hard or fixed to adjacent tissues may be malignant.

• Both anterior and posterior cervical nodes should be examined as well as other nodes, liver and spleen if systemic disease is a possibility.

Temporomandibular joints and muscles of mastication

Although disorders that affect the temporomandibular joint often appear to be unilateral, the joint should not be viewed in isolation but always considered together with its opposite joint, as part of the stomatognathic system. The area should be examined as follows.

Inspection

• Facial symmetry.
• Evidence of enlarged masseter muscles (masseteric hypertrophy) suggestive of clenching or bruxism.
• Mandibular opening and closing paths.
• Mandibular opening extent: (i) measure the interincisal distance at maximum mouth opening; (ii) measure the amount of lateral excursions achievable; (iii) listen for joint noises (a stethoscope placed over the joint can help).

Palpation

• Both condyles: via the external auditory meatus to detect tenderness posteriorly, and by using a single finger placed over the joints in front of the ears to detect pain, abnormal movements or clicking within the joint.
• Masticatory muscles on both sides.

Masseters: by intraoral/extraoral compression between finger and thumb. Palpate the masseter bimanually by placing a finger of one hand intraorally and the index and middle fingers of the other hand on the cheek over the masseter over the lower mandibular ramus.

Temporalis: by direct palpation of the temporal region. Palpate the temporal origin of the temporalis muscle by asking the patient to clench the teeth. Palpate the insertion of the temporalis tendon intraorally along the anterior border of the ascending mandibular ramus.

Lateral pterygoid (lower head): by placing a little finger up behind the maxillary tuberosity (the 'pterygoid sign'). Examine the lateral pterygoid muscle, which cannot readily be palpated, indirectly by asking the patient to open the jaw against resistance and to move the jaw to one side while a gentle resistance force is applied.

Medial pterygoid muscle intraorally lingually to the mandibular ramus.

Some palpate using a pressure algometer to standardize the force used, and undertake range-of-movement measurements.

• Examination of the dentition and occlusion: this may require monitoring of study models on a semi-adjustable or fully adjustable articulator. Note particularly missing premolars or molars, and attrition.

• Examination of the mucosa: note particularly occlusal lines and scalloping of the tongue margins, which may indicate bruxism and tongue pressure.

Jaws

There is wide normal individual variation in morphology of the face. Most individuals have facial asymmetry but of a degree that cannot be regarded as abnormal.

• Maxillary, mandibular or zygomatic deformities or lumps may be more reliably confirmed by inspection from above (maxillae/zygomas) or behind (mandible). The jaws should be palpated to detect swelling or tenderness.

• Maxillary air sinuses can be examined by palpation for tenderness over the maxillary antrum, which may indicate sinus infection. Transillumination or endoscopy can be helpful.

Salivary glands

Inspect and palpate the major salivary glands (parotid and submandibular) for:
• symmetry;
• evidence of enlarged glands;
• evidence of salivary flow from salivary ducts;
• appearance of saliva.

Parotid glands. Palpate by placing fingers over the preauricular glands, to detect pain or swelling. Early enlargement of the parotid gland is characterized by outward deflection of the lower part of the earlobe, which is best observed by looking at the patient from behind. This simple sign may allow distinction from simple obesity. Swelling of the parotid sometimes causes trismus. Swellings may affect the whole or part of a gland or tenderness may be elicited. The parotid duct (Stensen's duct) is most readily palpated with the jaws clenched firmly since it runs horizontally across the upper masseter where it can be gently rolled; the duct opens at a papilla on the buccal mucosa opposite the upper molars.

Submandibular glands. Bimanually palpate using fingers inside the mouth and extraorally. The submandibular gland is best palpated with a finger of one hand in the floor of the mouth lingual to the lower molar teeth, and a finger of the other hand placed over the submandibular triangle. The submandibular duct (Wharton's duct) runs anteromedially across the floor of the mouth to open at the side of the lingual fraenum.

Intraoral examination

The examination should be conducted in a systematic fashion to ensure that all areas are included. If the patient wears any removable prostheses or appliances, these should be removed in the first instance, although it may be necessary later to replace the appliance to assess fit, function and relationship to any lesion.

Complete visualization with a good source of light is essential. All mucosal surfaces should be examined, starting away from the location of any known lesions or the focus of complaint. The lips should be inspected first. The labial mucosa, buccal (cheek) mucosae, floor of mouth and ventrum of tongue, dorsal surface of the tongue, hard and soft palates, gingivae and teeth should then be examined in sequence and lesions noted on a diagram of the oral cavity (Fig. 66.3).

Lips. Features such as cyanosis are seen mainly in the lips in cardiac or respiratory disease; angular cheilitis (stomatitis) is seen mainly in oral candidiasis or in iron, vitamin or immune deficiencies. Examination is facilitated if the mouth is gently closed at this stage, so that the lips can then be everted to examine the mucosa.

Labial mucosa. Normally appears moist with a fairly prominent vascular arcade. In the lower lip, the many minor salivary glands which are often exuding mucus are easily visible. The lips therefore feel slightly nodular and the labial arteries are readily felt. Many adults have a few yellowish pinhead-sized papules in the vermilion border (particularly of the upper lip) and at the commissures; these are usually ectopic sebaceous glands (Fordyce spots), and may be numerous especially as age advances.

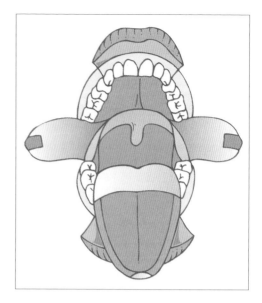

Fig. 66.3 Diagram of oral cavity.

Cheek (buccal) mucosa. This is readily inspected if the mouth is held half open. The vascular pattern and minor salivary glands so prominent in the labial mucosa are not obvious in the buccal mucosa but Fordyce spots may be conspicuous, particularly near the commissures and retromolar regions in adults. Place the surface of a dental mirror against the buccal mucosa. The mirror should lift off easily; if it adheres to the mucosa, then xerostomia is present.

Floor of mouth and ventrum of tongue. These are best examined by asking the patient to push the tongue first into the palate then into each cheek in turn. This raises for inspection the floor of the mouth, an area where tumours may start (the 'coffin' or 'graveyard' area of the mouth). Its posterior part is the most difficult area to examine well and one where lesions are most easily missed. Lingual veins are prominent and, in the elderly, may be conspicuous (lingual varices). Bony lumps on the alveolar ridge lingual to the premolars are most often tori (torus mandibularis). During this part of the examination the quantity and consistency of saliva should be assessed. Examine for the normal pooling of saliva in the floor of the mouth; normally there is a pool of saliva in the floor of the mouth.

Dorsum of tongue. This is best inspected by protrusion, when it can be held with gauze. The anterior two-thirds is embryologically and anatomically distinct from the posterior third, and separated by a dozen or so large circumvallate papillae. The anterior two-thirds is coated with many filiform but relatively few fungiform papillae. Behind the circumvallate papillae, the tongue contains several large lymphoid masses (lingual tonsil) and the foliate papillae lie on the lateral borders posteriorly. These are often mistaken for tumours. The tongue may be fissured (scrotal) but this is usually regarded as a developmental anomaly. A healthy child's tongue is rarely coated but a mild coating is not uncommon in healthy adults. The voluntary tongue movements and sense of taste should be formally tested. Abnormalities of tongue movement (neurological or muscular disease) may be obvious from dysarthria or involuntary movements and any fibrillation or wasting noted. Hypoglossal palsy may lead to deviation of the tongue towards the affected side on protrusion. Taste sensation can be tested by placing the tongue across the terminals of a pocket torch battery when a metallic taste may be obvious. Formal testing with salt, sweet, sour and bitter should be carried out by applying solutions of salt, sugar, dilute acetic acid and 5% citric acid to the tongue on a cotton swab or cotton bud.

Palate and fauces. These consist of an anterior hard and posterior soft palate, and the tonsillar area and oropharynx. The mucosa of the hard palate is firmly bound down as a mucoperiosteum (similar to the gingivae) and with no obvious vascular arcades. Rugae are present anteriorly on either side of the incisive papilla that overlies the incisive foramen. Bony lumps in the posterior centre of the vault of the hard palate are usually tori (torus palatinus). Patients may complain of lumps distal to the upper molars that they think are unerupted teeth but the pterygoid hamulus or tuberosity is usually responsible for this complaint. The soft palate and fauces may show a faint vascular arcade. Just posterior to the junction with the hard palate is a conglomeration of minor salivary glands. This region is often also yellowish. The palate should be inspected and movements examined when the patient says 'Aah'. Using a mirror, this also permits inspection of the posterior tongue, tonsils, oropharynx, and can even offer a glimpse of the larynx. Glossopharyngeal palsy may lead to uvula deviation to the contralateral side.

Gingivae. In health they are firm, pale pink, with a stippled surface, and have sharp gingival papillae reaching up between the adjacent teeth to the tooth contact point. Look for gingival redness, swelling or bleeding on gently probing the gingival margin. The 'keratinized' attached gingivae (pale pink) are normally clearly demarcated from the non-keratinized alveolar mucosa (vascular) that runs into the vestibule or sulcus. Bands of tissue which may contain muscle attachments run centrally from the labial mucosa onto the alveolar mucosa and from the buccal mucosa in the premolar region onto the alveolar mucosa (fraena).

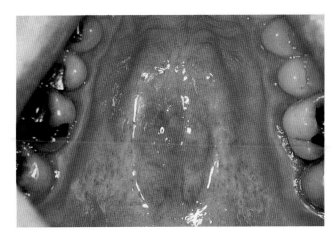

Fig. 66.4 Torus palatinus.

Teeth. The dentition should be checked to make sure that the expected complement of teeth is present for the patient's age. Extra teeth (supernumerary teeth) or deficiency of teeth (partial loss or hypodontia; oligodontia; complete loss or anodontia) can be features of many syndromes but teeth are far more frequently missing because they are unerupted, or lost as a result of caries or periodontal disease. The teeth should be fully examined for signs of disease, either malformations such as hypoplasia or abnormal colour, or acquired disorders such as dental caries, erosion or abrasion. The occlusion of the teeth should also be checked; it may show attrition or may be disturbed, as in some jaw fractures or dislocation of the mandibular condyles.

Anatomical variants

Patients sometimes become concerned after noticing various anatomical variants in the mouth. These include tori and exostoses [1,2], which are developmental bony lumps seen especially in Mongoloid and Negroid races. Most common is torus palatinus, a slow-growing, asymptomatic, benign bony lump in the midline of the palate (Fig. 66.4). Torus mandibularis are bilateral, asymptomatic, benign bony lumps lingual to the premolars.

The diagnosis is confirmed by radiography. Surgery is rarely indicated. These are excised or reduced only if causing severe difficulties with dentures.

REFERENCES

1 Eggen S, Natvig B. Relationship between torus mandibularis and number of present teeth. *Scand J Dent Res* 1986; **94**: 233–40.
2 Rezai RF. Torus palatinus, an exostosis of unknown aetiology: review of the literature. *Compend Contin Educ Dent* 1985; **6**: 149–52.

Disorders affecting the teeth

Disorders of tooth eruption

Teething

'Teething' in infancy is a poorly understood condition and the soreness and fever is often due to infection such as herpes simplex stomatitis. Nevertheless, there may be a very minor degree of pyrexia around the time of tooth eruption [1].

REFERENCE

1 Jaber L, Cohen IJ, Mor A. Fever associated with teething. *Arch Dis Child* 1992; **67**: 233–4.

Premature eruption of teeth [1–4]

Erupted teeth, particularly in the mandibular central incisor region, may be present at birth (natal teeth) or appear within the first few days or weeks of life (neonatal teeth). This rare event (about 0.1% of live births) occasionally has a familial basis or is associated with some other developmental anomaly. Such teeth occasionally cause ulceration of the infant's tongue or mother's nipple but usually they can be safely left *in situ*.

Retarded eruption of teeth

Congenital hypopituitarism, congenital hypothyroidism (cretinism), Down's syndrome, cleidocranial dysplasia, cytotoxic drugs and radiotherapy may cause retarded eruption of teeth, but most cases are of local aetiology (e.g. impactions).

Extra teeth

Extra (supernumerary) teeth are uncommon and usually of an unknown cause. They are generally found in the premaxilla. Supernumerary teeth are common in cleidocranial dysplasia.

Missing teeth

It is important to remember that teeth may be apparently missing simply because they are unerupted.

Dental aplasia
SYN. HYPODONTIA; ANODONTIA

Wisdom teeth (third molars), second premolars and upper lateral incisors are sometimes absent in otherwise normal individuals, probably because of some unidentified genetic trait. Up to 25% of white people lack a third molar. Absence of several teeth may indicate systemic disease such as cleidocranial dysplasia, incontinentia pigmenti or ectodermal dysplasia.

Hypodontia is often associated with microdontia and is often bilaterally symmetrical.

REFERENCES

1 Scully C. *ABC of Oral Health*. London: BMJ Books, 2000.
2 Laskaris G, Scully C, eds. *Periodontal Manifestations of Local and Systemic Diseases*. Berlin: Springer, 2003.
3 Scully C. *Handbook of Oral Disease: Diagnosis and Management*. London: Martin Dunitz, 1999.
4 Scully C, Flint S, Porter SR, Moos K. *Oral and Maxillofacial Diseases*. London: Martin Dunitz, 1996.

Loosening and early loss of teeth (Table 66.3)

Early loss of teeth is usually caused by trauma, dental caries or destructive periodontal disease, as discussed below [1,2]. Congenital disorders that may predispose to periodontal breakdown include Down's syndrome, Papillon–Lefèvre syndrome, neutropenia and other immune defects. Acquired disorders such as diabetes mellitus or immune defects also predispose to periodontal breakdown. Teeth are also lost early in other rare systemic disorders, for example eosinophilic granuloma or hypophosphatasia.

REFERENCES

1 Watanabe K. Prepubertal periodontitis: a review of diagnostic criteria, pathogenesis and differential diagnosis. *J Periodont Res* 1990; **25**: 31–48.
2 Hartsfield JK Jr. Premature exfoliation of teeth in childhood and adolescence. *Adv Pediatr* 1994; **41**: 453–70.

Table 66.3 Pathological causes of loosening and early loss of the teeth.

Local causes
Trauma
Periodontitis
Neoplasms

Systemic causes
Disorders with some immune deficit
  Down's syndrome
  Diabetes mellitus
  Leukopenia or leukocyte defects
  Human immunodeficiency virus disease
  Juvenile periodontitis
  Rapidly progressive periodontitis
  Papillon–Lefèvre syndrome
Hypophosphatasia
Ehlers–Danlos syndrome (type VIII)

Others
Acrodynia
Neoplasms
Eosinophilic granuloma

Table 66.4 Causes of discoloration of teeth.

Extrinsic
Poor oral hygiene
Smoking
Beverages/food
Drugs, e.g. iron, chlorhexidine, sweetened medication
Stains, e.g. from betel chewing

Intrinsic
Trauma
Caries
Restorative materials, e.g. amalgam
Pink spot (internal resorption)
Drugs: mainly tetracyclines
Fluorosis
Dentinogenesis imperfecta
Amelogenesis imperfecta
Porphyria
Kernicterus (severe neonatal jaundice)

Malformed and discoloured teeth (Table 66.4)

There is a wide range of normal variation in tooth morphology and colour, especially between races.

Most dental discoloration is caused by smoking, foods and beverages (such as tea), medicines such as iron or chlorhexidine, or poor oral hygiene. The regular use of sweetened medication at night (e.g. trimeprazine syrup in a child with eczema) can cause discoloration due to dental caries. Erosion of teeth may occur because of the repeated use of acidic drinks or sucking citrus fruits, or as a feature of gastric regurgitation in bulimia, anorexia nervosa or alcoholism.

Teeth may be malformed for genetic reasons. Peg-shaped teeth may be normal variants (Fig. 66.5) or may be found in some ectodermal dysplasias (see p. 66.11). Taurodontism (see below) can be found in a range of dermatological disorders [1]. Genetic defects that may cause tooth discoloration include dentinogenesis imperfecta

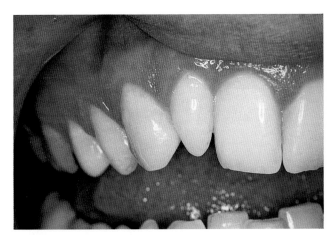

Fig. 66.5 A peg-shaped maxillary lateral incisor, a fairly common variant.

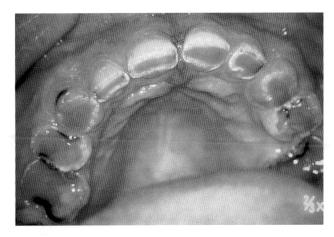

Fig. 66.6 Dentinogenesis imperfecta: staining and severe attrition.

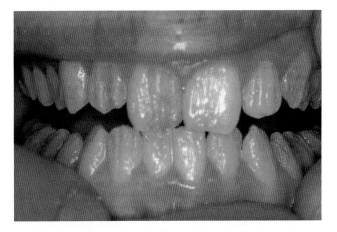

Fig. 66.7 Amelogenesis imperfecta: one variant showing longitudinal ridging of teeth.

(Fig. 66.6), which may be seen in some patients with osteogenesis imperfecta, and amelogenesis imperfecta (Fig. 66.7) [2,3].

Teeth may be damaged during their development. Local infection or trauma, or unknown factors, may cause malformation of a single tooth (or a few). The lower premolars are usually affected because there is caries and periapical infection related to their deciduous predecessors; such hypoplastic teeth are termed *Turner's teeth*. The upper permanent incisors may be malformed if there is trauma to the deciduous incisors. Radiotherapy or cytotoxic therapy may cause hypoplasia, as may congenital rubella or cytomegalovirus infection. However, classical *Hutchinsonian (screwdriver-shaped) incisors* and *Moon's (or mulberry) molars* of congenital syphilis are extremely rare.

Hypoplasia is relatively common in apparently healthy persons [4–7] and is also seen in early-onset malabsorption syndromes, many severe childhood illnesses (Fig. 66.8) and organ transplantation [8–10] and in some forms of epidermolysis bullosa (see below). Neonatal jaundice can produce greenish teeth.

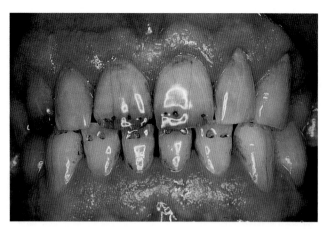

Fig. 66.8 Hypoplasia of teeth related to severe childhood respiratory infection.

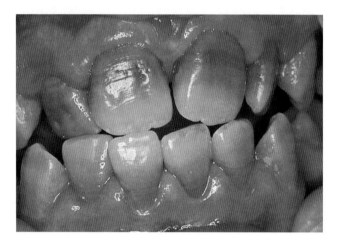

Fig. 66.9 Pronounced intrinsic tooth discoloration from use of tetracyclines in childhood.

Fluoride, at the concentrations present in water supplies in Western countries or given prophylactically, may occasionally produce inconsequential minute white flecks; however, concentrations over 2 ppm may produce significant fluorosis. Tetracyclines given to a pregnant or lactating mother may discolour the child's teeth and, if given to a child, particularly one under the age of 12 years, may cause significant brown intrinsic tooth staining (Fig. 66.9).

REFERENCES

1 Hill FJ, Winter GB. The teeth in dermatological diseases. In: Champion RH, ed. *Recent Advances in Dermatology*. London: Livingstone, 1986: 103–26.
2 Scully C, Welbury R, Flaitz C, Almeida OPD. *A Color Atlas of Orofacial Health and Disease in Children and Adolescents*. London: Martin Dunitz, 2001.
3 Seow WK. Enamel hypoplasia in the primary dentition: a review. *J Dent Child* 1991; **58**: 441–52.
4 Lukacs JR, Walimbe SR, Floyd B. Epidemiology of enamel hypoplasia in deciduous teeth: explaining variation in prevalence in western India. *Am J Hum Biol* 2001; **13**: 788–807.

5 Jalevik B. Enamel hypomineralization in permanent first molars. A clinical, histo-morphological and biochemical study. *Swed Dent J Suppl* 2001; **149**: 1–86.
6 Jalevik B, Klingberg G, Barregard L, Noren JG. The prevalence of demarcated opacities in permanent first molars in a group of Swedish children. *Acta Odontol Scand* 2001; **59**: 255–60.
7 Lukacs JR. Interproximal contact hypoplasia in primary teeth: a new enamel defect with anthropological and clinical relevance. *Am J Hum Biol* 1999; **11**: 718–34.
8 Hosey MT, Gordon G, Kelly DA, Shaw L. Oral findings in children with liver transplants. *Int J Paediatr Dent* 1995; **5**: 29–34.
9 Morisaki I, Abe K, Tong LS *et al*. Dental findings of children with biliary atresia. *J Dent Child* 1990; **57**: 220–3.
10 Wondimu B, Nemeth A, Modeer T. Oral health in liver transplant children administered cyclosporin A or tacrolimus. *Int J Paediatr Dent* 2001; **11**: 424–9.

Taurodontism

Taurodont teeth have an enlarged pulp chamber and a more inferiorly placed root furcation in premolars and molars. They are not readily detectable on clinical examination and are therefore most easily diagnosed on radiographs (Fig. 66.10). However, on clinical examination, lack of constriction of the tooth at the neck may be suggestive of taurodontism. Taurodontism is generally most obvious in molars of both deciduous and permanent dentitions, and may be found in single or several teeth, with or without evidence of other disorders.

Most studies have shown an overall prevalence of the order of 2% with no sex predilection, but oriental people and some other racial groups are especially affected [1–3]. XXY and other syndromes with additional X chromosomes may be affected [4–6] as may other chromosomal anomalies [7–9]. Dermatological conditions with which taurodontism may be associated are shown in Table 66.5 [10].

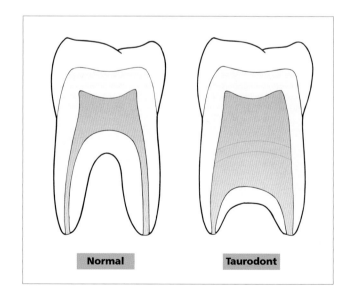

Fig. 66.10 Taurodontism.

Table 66.5 Dermatological disorders in which taurodontism may occasionally be found.

Some ectodermal dysplasias
Trichodento-osseous syndrome
Tricho-onychodental syndrome
Epidermolysis bullosa
Dental oculocutaneous syndrome
Otodental dysplasia
Orofacial digital syndrome type II
Dyskeratosis congenita

REFERENCES

1 Constant DA, Grine FE. A review of taurodontism with new data on indigenous southern African populations. *Arch Oral Biol* 2001; **46**: 1021–9.
2 Toure B, Kane AW, Sarr M, Wone MM, Fall F. Prevalence of taurodontism at the level of the molar in the black Senegalese population 15–19 years of age. *Odontostomatol Trop* 2000; **23**: 36–9.
3 Sarr M, Toure B, Kane AW, Fall F, Wone MM. Taurodontism and the pyramidal tooth at the level of the molar. Prevalence in the Senegalese population 15–19 years of age. *Odontostomatol Trop* 2000; **23**: 31–4.
4 Backman B, Wahlin YB. Variations in number and morphology of permanent teeth in 7-year-old Swedish children. *Int J Paediatr Dent* 2001; **11**: 11–7.
5 Varrela J, Alvesalo L. Taurodontism in 47,XXY males: an effect of the extra X chromosome on root development. *J Dent Res* 1988; **67**: 501–2.
6 Hata S, Maruyama Y, Fujita Y, Mayanagi H. The dentofacial manifestations of XXXXY syndrome: a case report. *Int J Paediatr Dent* 2001; **11**: 138–42.
7 Breen GH. Taurodontism, an unreported dental finding in Wolf–Hirschhorn (4p–) syndrome. *ASDC J Dent Child* 1998; **65**: 344–5, 356.
8 Tatakis DN, Milledge JT. Severe gingival recession in trisomy 18 primary dentition. A clinicopathologic case report of self-inflicted injury associated with mental retardation. *J Periodontol* 2000; **71**: 1181–6.
9 Rajic Z, Mestrovic SR. Taurodontism in Down's syndrome. *Coll Antropol* 1998; **22** (Suppl.): 63–7.
10 Ogden GR. Taurodontism in dermatologic disease. *Int J Dermatol* 1988; **27**: 360–4.

Ectodermal dysplasia

Ectodermal dysplasia is typically characterized by developmental abnormalities in at least two different ectodermally derived systems. Oral abnormalities are common, especially missing teeth and abnormally shaped teeth (Fig. 66.11). There are many variations, as discussed in the following sections and in Chapter 12.

X-linked hypohidrotic ectodermal dysplasia [1–3]

Hypodontia is common in X-linked hypohidrotic ectodermal dysplasia. Some anterior teeth are usually present but their crowns are typically conical or peg-shaped. The posterior teeth, when present, are smaller but otherwise normal. Overclosure of the jaws, together with maxillary hypoplasia and frontal bossing, give a characteristic facial appearance. There may be a degree of impaired salivary gland function.

Female carriers of this syndrome may have hypodontia and/or microdontia.

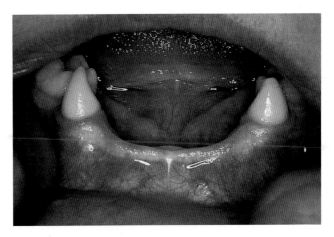

Fig. 66.11 Hypodontia and malformed teeth are common in ectodermal dysplasia.

Autosomal recessive ectodermal dysplasia [1,4]

Dental and oral anomalies in this condition are identical to those in the X-linked form of ectodermal dysplasia, although relatives may have a normal dentition.

Hypodontia, taurodontism and sparse hair [5]

There are a few reports of a variant of ectodermal dysplasia where there is taurodontism, and somewhat lesser hypodontia than in the more classic forms of ectodermal dysplasia.

Autosomal dominant hypodontia with nail dysgenesis [6]

Hypodontia, conical deciduous and permanent teeth, and dysplastic nails characterize this variant of ectodermal dysplasia.

Incontinentia pigmenti [7]
SYN. BLOCH–SULZBERGER SYNDROME

Hypodontia and retarded eruption affect both dentitions and the anterior teeth are small. The teeth tend also to be conical, often with accessory cusps.

Chondroectodermal dysplasia [8–10]
SYN. ELLIS–VAN CREVELD SYNDROME

Ellis–van Creveld syndrome, also called chondroectodermal dysplasia, is a rare autosomal recessive condition that manifests with chondrodysplasia of tubular bones resulting in disproportionate dwarfism, polydactyly and syndactyly of hands and feet, severe dystrophic nails, anomalous teeth, bilateral partial clefts of the alveolar bone and malocclusion. Half of the cases have cardiac malformations.

The most obvious oral anomalies are the multiple fraena extending from the lips and buccal mucosae to the alveolar ridges of both jaws. Natal teeth, mild hypodontia or hyperdontia, malformed or small teeth and accessory cusps are common.

Cranioectodermal dysplasia [11]

Deciduous teeth are small and may have dysplastic enamel, although the condition is so rare that the permanent teeth have not been clearly described. There may be hypodontia or taurodontism. Dolicocephaly, hair anomalies and shortened arms, fingers and toes are associated.

Nance–Horan syndrome [12]

X-linked congenital cataracts with supernumerary teeth constitute the Nance–Horan syndrome. The incisor teeth may also be morphologically abnormal and can resemble Hutchinson's incisors of congenital syphilis.

Trichodental syndrome [13,14]

The trichodental syndrome is a rare dominantly inherited condition in which there is fine short hair, thinning of the lateral ends of the eyebrows, hypodontia and/or conical teeth.

Trichodento-osseous syndrome [15–18]

Tight curly hair, sclerotic cortical bone and oral anomalies (especially thin enamel) are found in this autosomal dominant condition. The hypoplasia–hypomaturation type of amelogenesis imperfecta, enamel hypoplasia, unerupted teeth and taurodontism may be associated.

Trichonychodental syndrome [19]

This autosomal dominant trait of fine curly hair and thin dysplastic nails may be associated with taurodontism and enamel or dentinal developmental defects.

Curry–Hall syndrome [20]

Deciduous teeth are small and conical, and the incisors are often retained since their permanent successors may be congenitally absent. The remaining permanent teeth do erupt but are small. Other features include short limbs, polydactyly and nail dysplasia.

Otodental dysplasia [21–23]

Globe-shaped posterior teeth (globodontia) in both dentitions are the most common oral feature of this autosomal dominant condition, which is associated with sensorineu-ral hearing loss. The incisors are not affected and the patients are otherwise well.

Other oral anomalies may include taurodontism, microdontia and hypodontia.

Clouston syndrome [24] (see Chapter 12)

Palmoplantar hyperkeratosis, hair defects, nail dysplasia and oral white lesions characterize this autosomal dominant form of hidrotic ectodermal dysplasia. There may be diffuse white lesions in the buccal mucosa, palate, tongue and elsewhere but reports of malignancy are rare.

REFERENCES

1 Levin LS. Dental and oral abnormalities in selected ectodermal dysplasia syndromes. *Birth Defects* 1988; **24**: 205–27.
2 Sofaer JA. Hypodontia and sweat pore counts in detecting carriers of X-linked hypohidrotic ectodermal dysplasia. *Br Dent J* 1981; **151**: 327–30.
3 Glavina D, Majstorovic M, Lulic-Dukic O, Juric H. Hypohidrotic ectodermal dysplasia: dental features and carriers detection. *Coll Antropol* 2001; **25**: 303–10.
4 Bartlett RC, Eversole LR, Adkins RS. Autosomal recessive hypohidrotic ectodermal dysplasia: dental manifestations. *Oral Surg* 1972; **33**: 736–42.
5 Stenvik A, Zachrisson BU, Svatum B. Taurodontism and concomitant hypodontia in siblings. *Oral Surg* 1972; **33**: 841–5.
6 Hudson CD, Witkop CJ. Autosomal dominant hypodontia with nail dysgenesis. Report of twenty-nine cases in six families. *Oral Surg* 1975; **39**: 409–23.
7 Gorlin RJ, Anderson JA. The characteristic dentition of incontinentia pigmenti: a diagnostic aid. *J Pediatr* 1960; **57**: 78–85.
8 Sarnant H, Amir E, Legum CP. Development dental anomalies in chondroectodermal dysplasia (Ellis–Van-Creveld syndrome). *J Dent Child* 1980; **47**: 28–31.
9 Hattab FN, Yassin OM, Sasa IS. Oral manifestations of Ellis–van Creveld syndrome: report of two siblings with unusual dental anomalies. *J Clin Pediatr Dent* 1998; **22**: 159–65.
10 Hunter ML, Roberts GJ. Oral and dental anomalies in Ellis van Creveld syndrome (chondroectodermal dysplasia): report of a case. *Int J Paediatr Dent* 1998; **8**: 153–7.
11 Levin LS, Perrin JCS, Ose L et al. A heritable syndrome of craniosynostosis, short thin hair, dental abnormalities, and short limbs: cranioectodermal dysplasia. *J Pediatr* 1977; **90**: 55–61.
12 Bixler D, Higgins M, Hartsfield J. The Nance–Horan syndrome: a rare X-linked ocular–dental trait with expression in heterozygous females. *Clin Genet* 1984; **26**: 303–35.
13 Kersey PJW. Tricho-dental syndrome: a disorder with a short hair cycle. *Br J Dermatol* 1987; **116**: 259–63.
14 Salinas CF, Spector M. Tricho-dental syndrome. In: Brown AC, Crounse RG, eds. *Hair, Trace Elements and Human Illness*. New York: Praeger, 1980: 240–56.
15 Jorgenson RJ, Warson RW. Dental abnormalities in the trichodento-osseous (TDO) syndrome. *Oral Surg* 1973; **36**: 696–700.
16 Wright JT, Roberts MW, Wilson AR, Kudhail R. Tricho-dento-osseous syndrome. *Oral Surg* 1994; **77**: 487–93.
17 Spangler GS, Hall KI, Kula K, Hart TC, Wright JT. Enamel structure and composition in the tricho-dento-osseous syndrome. *Connect Tissue Res* 1998; **39**: 165–75; discussion 187–94.
18 Price JA, Wright JT, Walker SJ, Crawford PJ, Aldred MJ, Hart TC. Trichodento-osseous syndrome and amelogenesis imperfecta with taurodontism are genetically distinct conditions. *Clin Genet* 1999; **56**: 35–40.
19 Koshiba H, Kimura O, Nakata M. Clinical, genetic and histologic features of the trichonychodental (TOD) syndrome. *Oral Surg* 1978; **46**: 376–85.
20 Shapiro SD, Jorgenson RJ, Salinas CF. Brief clinical report: Curry–Hall syndrome. *Am J Med Genet* 1984; **17**: 579–83.
21 Levin LS, Jorgenson RJ, Cook RA. Otodental dysplasia: a 'new' ectodermal dysplasia. *Clin Genet* 1975; **8**: 136–44.
22 Witkop CJ, Gudlach KH, Street WJ et al. Globodontia in the otodental syndrome. *Oral Surg* 1976; **41**: 472–83.

Table 66.6 Oral features in rare ectodermal dysplasia variants [1–3].

Syndrome	Oral manifestations	Facial manifestations	Other features
GAPO (growth retardation, alopecia, pseudoanodontia, optic atrophy)	Failure of both dentitions to erupt	Frontal bossing Midface hypoplasia	*See left-hand column*
Johanson–Blizzard	Hypodontia in both dentitions Roots of deciduous teeth are short and deformed, crowns are conical	Microcephaly Hypoplastic alae nasi	Hearing loss Pancreatic dysfunction Learning disability
Waardenburg	–	Cleft lip/palate	Deafness Hair depigmentation
LEOPARD (*l*entigines, *e*lectrocardiographic anomalies, *o*cular hypertelorism, *p*ulmonary stenosis, *a*bnormal genitalia, *r*etarded growth, *d*eafness)	No mucosal lentigines	Triangular face with hypertelorism and ptosis, may be granular cell tumour	*See left-hand column*
Congenital erythrokeratoderma with sensorineural hearing loss	Hyperkeratosis Occasional carcinoma	–	*See left-hand column*

23 Sedano HO, Moreira LC, de Souza RA, Moleri AB. Otodental syndrome: a case report and genetic considerations. *Oral Surg Oral Med Oral Pathol Oral Radiol Endod* 2001; **92**: 312–7.

24 George DI, Escobar VH. Oral findings of Clouston's syndrome (hidrotic ectodermal dysplasia). *Oral Surg* 1984; **57**: 258–62.

Other rare ectodermal dysplasias [1]

Other rare ectodermal dysplasias and pachonychia congenita are discussed in Chapter 12. Others are summarized in Table 66.6.

REFERENCE

1 Gorlin RJ. Selected ectodermal dysplasias. *Birth Defects* 1988; **24**: 123–48.

Alstrom syndrome

Alstrom syndrome is a rare disorder characterized by early obesity, diabetes mellitus, loss of central vision, hearing loss and short stature. Light yellow-brown discolored enamel bands have been observed on the anterior teeth in some patients [1].

REFERENCE

1 Koray F, Dorter C, Benderli Y *et al*. Alstrom syndrome: a case report. *J Oral Sci* 2001; **43**: 221–4.

Disorders affecting the periodontium

Gingival disorders affecting the periodontium

Bleeding

Bleeding from the gingival margins is common, usually a consequence of inadequate oral hygiene leading to the accumulation of dental bacterial plaque and thus gingiv-

Table 66.7 Causes of gingival bleeding.

Local
Chronic gingivitis
Chronic periodontitis
Acute necrotizing gingivitis

Systemic
Any condition causing exacerbation of gingivitis (e.g. pregnancy)
Leukaemia
Human immunodeficiency virus infection
Other causes of purpura
Clotting defects
Drugs, e.g. anticoagulants
Scurvy

itis (Table 66.7). The tendency to gingivitis is slightly increased in patients taking oral contraceptives and in some pregnant women (especially during the second trimester).

Gingival haemorrhage may, however, also be an early feature in some vascular or platelet disorders and is commonly a problem, for example, in leukaemic patients.

Swelling

Localized gingival swellings (epulides) may be of local aetiology or can be manifestations of pregnancy, a neoplasm or systemic disease (Table 66.8).

Gingival swelling affecting many areas is most commonly seen in chronic gingivitis, may be produced by drugs such as phenytoin, ciclosporin (cyclosporin) and calcium channel blockers (Fig. 66.12), and is occasionally hereditary. Gingival swelling is seen with hypertrichosis in both drug-induced hyperplasias and hereditary gingival fibromatosis.

A degree of gingival swelling may also be seen in herpetic stomatitis, pregnancy, leukaemia, Crohn's disease,

Table 66.8 Causes of gingival swelling.

	Generalized swelling	Localized swelling
Local	Chronic gingivitis Hyperplastic gingivitis due to mouth breathing	Abscesses Cysts Pyogenic granuloma Neoplasms and warts (various)
Systemic	Hereditary gingival fibromatosis and associated syndromes Drugs (phenytoin, ciclosporin, nifedipine, diltiazem) Pregnancy Sarcoidosis Crohn's disease Leukaemia Wegener's granulomatosis Scurvy Amyloidosis Mucopolysaccharidoses Mucolipidosis Lipoid proteinosis Juvenile hyaline fibromatosis Hypoplasminogenaemia	Pregnancy Sarcoidosis Orofacial granulomatosis Crohn's disease Wegener's granulomatosis Amyloidosis Neoplasms (various)

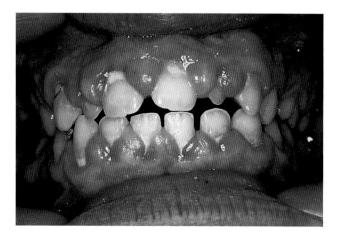

Fig. 66.12 Gingival hyperplasia in phenytoin therapy. Concomitant folate deficiency in this patient also caused mouth ulcers, seen in the maxillary buccal vestibule.

scurvy, Wegener's granulomatosis, sarcoidosis, amyloidosis, lipoid proteinosis, hypoplasminogenaemia, mucopolysaccharidoses and other disorders.

Redness

Chronic marginal gingivitis is the usual cause of gingival redness, and then is usually restricted to the gingival margins and interdental papillae.

More widespread erythema, particularly if associated with soreness, is usually caused by primary herpes simplex stomatitis, desquamative gingivitis (usually due to lichen planus or mucous membrane pemphigoid), rarely by pemphigus or other dermatoses, or occasionally by allergic responses.

Telangiectasia may be a manifestation of hereditary haemorrhagic telangiectasia, primary biliary cirrhosis or systemic sclerosis, or may follow radiotherapy. Haemangiomas are usually isolated but may occasionally extend deeply and rarely involve the ipsilateral meninges, producing a facial angioma and epilepsy, sometimes with learning disability (Sturge–Weber syndrome). Intraoral haemangiomas may be seen in Maffucci's syndrome.

Localized red areas may represent erythroplasia, carcinoma, candidiasis, lichen planus or lupus erythematosus. Kaposi's sarcoma may present as a red, purple, brown or bluish macule or nodule as may epithelioid angiomatosis. Hereditary mucoepithelial dysplasia is a rare cause of oral erythema. Irradiation-induced mucositis is a further cause of a red sore mouth.

White patches (Table 66.9)

Thrush (acute candidiasis) is a 'disease of the diseased' and produces oral white patches.

Leukoplakia is often associated with friction or smoking, occasionally with syphilis, candidiasis or chronic renal failure, but most cases are idiopathic. Lichen planus and lupus erythematosus may present as white lesions. Rarely, lichenoid lesions are associated with various drugs, liver disease or graft-versus-host disease (GVHD). Carcinoma may present as a white lesion.

Inherited causes of white patches, such as white sponge naevus and dyskeratosis congenita, are rare [1,2].

Pigmentation

Gingival pigmentation is usually seen in dark-skinned races (but may be seen even in white people) (Fig. 66.13).

Table 66.9 Main causes of oral white lesions.

Local
Frictional keratosis
Smoker's keratosis
Idiopathic keratosis
Carcinoma
Burns
Skin grafts

Systemic
Candidiasis
Lichen planus
Lupus erythematosus
Papillomas (some)
Hairy leukoplakia (mainly human immunodeficiency virus disease)
Syphilitic keratosis
Chronic renal failure
Inherited lesions (e.g. white-sponge naevus)

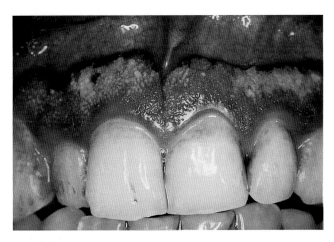

Fig. 66.13 Gingival hyperpigmentation of racial origin. The white lesion is due to accumulated oral debris—oral hygiene is very poor.

Other common causes include amalgam tattoo and melanotic macules.

Addison's disease, Kaposi's sarcoma and melanoma are the most important acquired causes of pigmented lesions but drugs such as hydroxychloroquine and minocycline may also cause hyperpigmentation.

Ulcers

Gingival ulcers are sometimes self-induced (artefactual) [1,2]. Herpesviruses can cause gingival ulceration, often with ulcers elsewhere in the mouth. Acute ulcerative (necrotizing) gingivitis causes ulceration of the interdental papillae and though usually a consequence of poor oral hygiene, it or a similar disorder is a rare complication of HIV infection, neutropenia or leukaemia, and in the malnourished or some immunosuppressed patients may spread to the cheek (*noma*, or *cancrum oris*). Other bacterial infections (e.g. syphilis, tuberculosis) and mycoses (deep mycoses) are uncommon causes of ulceration. Aphthae

Table 66.10 Main causes of mouth ulcers associated with systemic disease.

Microbial disease
Herpetic stomatitis
Chickenpox
Herpes zoster
Hand, foot and mouth disease
Herpangina
Infectious mononucleosis
Human immunodeficiency virus disease
Tuberculosis
Syphilis
Rarely fungal infections

Malignant neoplasms

Cutaneous disease
Erosive lichen planus and chronic ulcerative stomatitis
Pemphigus
Pemphigoid
Erythema multiforme
Dermatitis herpetiformis and linear IgA disease
Epidermolysis bullosa
Other dermatoses

Blood disorders
Anaemia
Leukaemia
Neutropenia
Other white cell dyscrasias

Gastrointestinal diseases
Coeliac disease
Crohn's disease
Ulcerative colitis

Rheumatic diseases
Lupus erythematosus
Behçet's syndrome
Sweet's syndrome
Reiter's disease

Drugs
Cytotoxic, NSAIDs, nicorandil, alendronate and other agents
Acrodynia

Radiotherapy

Disorders of uncertain pathogenesis
Angina bullosa haemorrhagica
Hypereosinophilic syndrome
Eosinophilic ulcer
Necrotizing sialometaplasia

(sometimes) and other causes of mouth ulcers (rarely) involve the gingiva (Table 66.10).

Blisters

Blisters may be seen as a result of burns or mucoceles, but the most important vesiculobullous disorders affecting the gingivae are pemphigoid (including cicatricial pemphigoid) and pemphigus and the typical presentation is of desquamative gingivitis. Vesicles may be seen in viral infections, especially in herpes simplex stomatitis, chickenpox, herpangina and hand, foot and mouth disease [3–6].

REFERENCES

1 Scully C, Porter SR. Disorders of the gums and periodontium. *Med Int* 1990; **76**: 3150–3.
2 Scully C, Porter SR. Oral medicine 1. Teeth and the periodontium. *Postgrad Dent* 1992; **2**: 93–100.
3 Scully C. *ABC of Oral Health*. London: BMJ Books, 2000.
4 Laskaris G, Scully C, eds. *Periodontal Manifestations of Local and Systemic Disease*. Berlin: Springer, 2003.
5 Scully C. *Handbook of Oral Disease: Diagnosis and Management*. London: Martin Dunitz, 1999.
6 Scully C, Flint S, Porter SR, Moos K. *Oral and Maxillofacial Diseases*. London: Martin Dunitz, 2004.

Genetic disorders affecting the periodontium

Hereditary gingival fibromatosis

Aetiology. An autosomal dominant condition due to chromosome 2 or 5 anomalies, resulting in transforming growth factor (TGF)-β1 autocrine stimulation of fibroblast proliferation with alteration in expression of matrix metalloproteinases (MMP)-1 and MMP-2 [1–14].

Pathology. The gingival connective tissue is mainly composed of thick interlacing collagen fibres forming a dense, almost avascular, mass in which many fibrocytes have dark shrunken nuclei. Mucoid material and some giant cells may be found.

Clinical features. There is generalized gingival enlargement, especially obvious over the anterior maxilla and during the transition from deciduous to permanent dentitions [1]. If the enlargement is gross, it may move or cover the teeth and even protrude from the mouth. The changes initially involve the gingival papillae and later the attached gingiva. The affected gingiva is usually of normal colour but firm in consistency, and the surface becomes coarsely stippled. Patients may also be hirsute, as may patients with drug-induced gingival hyperplasia. The prognosis is good, but gingival surgery is often indicated.

Although most patients have only gingival fibromatosis, there are occasional associations with supernumerary teeth [15] or with Zimmermann–Laband, Rutherford's, Cowden's and Cross's syndromes [16–18].

REFERENCES

1 Bozzo L, Almeida O, Scully C, Aldred M. Familial gingival fibromatosis: report of an extensive four generation pedigree. *Oral Surg* 1994; **78**: 452–4.
2 Bozzo L, Machado MA, de Almeida OP, Lopes MA, Coletta RD. Hereditary gingival fibromatosis: report of three cases. *J Clin Pediatr Dent* 2000; **25**: 41–6.
3 Hart TC, Pallos D, Bozzo L et al. Evidence of genetic heterogeneity for hereditary gingival fibromatosis. *J Dent Res* 2000; **79**: 1758–64.
4 de Andrade CR, Cotrin P, Graner E et al. Transforming growth factor-beta1 autocrine stimulation regulates fibroblast proliferation in hereditary gingival fibromatosis. *J Periodontol* 2001; **72**: 1726–33.

5 Xiao S, Bu L, Zhu L et al. A new locus for hereditary gingival fibromatosis (GINGF2) maps to 5q13–q22. *Genomics* 2001; **74**: 180–5.
6 Xiao S, Wang X, Qu B et al. Refinement of the locus for autosomal dominant hereditary gingival fibromatosis (GINGF) to a 3.8-cM region on 2p21. *Genomics* 2000; **68**: 247–52.
7 Hart TC, Pallos D, Bowden DW et al. Genetic linkage of hereditary gingival fibromatosis to chromosome 2p21. *Am J Hum Genet* 1998; **62**: 876–83.
8 Wright HJ, Chapple IL, Matthews JB. TGF-beta isoforms and TGF-beta receptors in drug-induced and hereditary gingival overgrowth. *J Oral Pathol Med* 2001; **30**: 281–9.
9 Coletta RD, Almeida OP, Ferreira LR, Reynolds MA, Sauk JJ. Increase in expression of Hsp47 and collagen in hereditary gingival fibromatosis is modulated by stress and terminal procollagen N-propeptides. *Connect Tissue Res* 1999; **40**: 237–49.
10 Coletta RD, Almeida OP, Reynolds MA, Sauk JJ. Alteration in expression of MMP-1 and MMP-2 but not TIMP-1 and TIMP-2 in hereditary gingival fibromatosis is mediated by TGF-beta 1 autocrine stimulation. *J Periodontal Res* 1999; **34**: 457–63.
11 Coletta RD, Almeida OP, Graner E, Page RC, Bozzo L. Differential proliferation of fibroblasts cultured from hereditary gingival fibromatosis and normal gingiva. *J Periodontal Res* 1998; **33**: 469–75.
12 Tipton DA, Dabbous MK. Autocrine transforming growth factor beta stimulation of extracellular matrix production by fibroblasts from fibrotic human gingiva. *J Periodontol* 1998; **69**: 609–19.
13 Gould AR, Escobar VH. Symmetrical gingival fibromatosis. *Oral Surg* 1981; **51**: 62–7.
14 Clark D. Gingival fibromatosis and related syndromes. *J Can Dent Assoc* 1987; **53**: 137–40.
15 Wynne SE, Aldred ME, Bartold M. Hereditary gingival fibromatosis associated with hearing loss and supernumerary teeth: a new syndrome. *J Periodontol* 1995; **66**: 75–9.
16 Bazoupoulou-Kyrkanidou E, Papagianoulis L, Papanicoliou S, Mavrou A. Laband syndrome: a case report. *J Oral Pathol Med* 1990; **19**: 385–7.
17 Bakaeen G, Scully C. Hereditary gingival fibromatosis and the Zimmermann–Laband syndrome. *J Oral Pathol Med* 1991; **20**: 456–9.
18 Chadwick B, Hunter B, Hunter L et al. Laband syndrome: report of two cases, review of the literature and identification of additional manifestations. *Oral Surg* 1994; **78**: 57–63.

Juvenile hyaline fibromatosis (see Chapter 46)
SYN. MURRAY–PURETIC–DRESCHER SYNDROME

Gingival enlargement may be seen in juvenile hyaline fibromatosis. It may precede tooth eruption or may present only in the first decade. It increases with age. Histology shows dilated capillaries in a hyaline PAS (periodic acid–Schiff)-positive matrix with pseudocartilaginous cells [1–5].

REFERENCES

1 Aldred MJ, Crawford PJM. Juvenile hyaline fibromatosis. *Oral Surg* 1987; **63**: 71–7.
2 Sciubba JJ, Nieblom T. Juvenile hyaline fibromatosis (Murray–Puretic–Drescher syndrome): oral and systemic findings in siblings. *Oral Surg* 1986; **62**: 397–409.
3 Bedford CD, Sills JA, Sommelet-Olive D et al. Juvenile hyaline fibromatosis: a report of two severe cases. *J Pediatr* 1991; **119**: 404–10.
4 Piattelli A, Scarano A, Di Bellucci A, Matarasso S. Juvenile hyaline fibromatosis of gingiva: a case report. *J Periodontol* 1996; **67**: 451–3.
5 Kawasaki G, Yanamoto S, Mizuno A, Fujita S. Juvenile hyaline fibromatosis complicated with oral squamous cell carcinoma: a case report. *Oral Surg Oral Med Oral Pathol Oral Radiol Endod* 2001; **91**: 200–4.

Hypoplasminogenaemia

Gingival swelling and ulceration may be seen in this disorder in which there can also be ligneous conjunctivitis [1].

REFERENCE

1 Scully C, Gokbuget AY, Allen C *et al.* Oral manifestations indicative of plasminogen deficiency (hypoplasminogenemia). *Oral Surg Oral Med Oral Pathol Oral Radiol Endod* 2001; **91**: 344–7.

Neutrophil defects (see p. 66.56)

A number of genetic disorders affecting neutrophil counts or function can lead to early-onset periodontitis, often with oral ulceration [1] (see p. 66.56).

REFERENCE

1 Defraia E, Marinelli A. Oral manifestations of congenital neutropenia or Kostmann syndrome. *J Clin Pediatr Dent* 2001; **26**: 99–102.

Leukocyte adhesion deficiency

Defects in cell-surface receptors on neutrophils and other leukocytes result in a range of disorders, especially recurrent cutaneous, respiratory and middle-ear infection, as well as periodontal destruction in both dentitions.

Local efforts to preserve the dentition, using débridement together with antimicrobials have been of little value [1–4].

REFERENCES

1 Meyle J. Leukocyte adhesion deficiency and prepubertal periodontitis. *Periodontology* 1994; **6**: 26–36.
2 Waldrop TC, Anderson DC, Hallmon WW *et al.* Periodontal manifestations of the heritable Mac-1, LFA-1 deficiency syndrome. *J Periodontol* 1987; **58**: 400–16.
3 Majorana A, Notarangelo LD, Savoldi E, Gastaldi G, Lozada-Nur F. Leukocyte adhesion deficiency in a child with severe oral involvement. *Oral Surg Oral Med Oral Pathol Oral Radiol Endod* 1999; **87**: 691–4.
4 Roberts MW, Atkinson JC. Oral manifestations associated with leukocyte adhesion deficiency: a five-year case study. *Pediatr Dent* 1990; **12**: 107–11.

Papillon–Lefèvre syndrome (see Chapter 34)

This is a rare, autosomal recessive condition of palmoplantar hyperkeratosis with periodontal breakdown (periodontosis or periodontoclasia) that manifests from childhood [1–3] and is related to a defect in cathepsin C [4] with defective polymorphonuclear leukocyte function [5].

The major oral feature of Papillon–Lefèvre syndrome is premature periodontal breakdown. The teeth develop and erupt normally in both the deciduous and permanent dentitions but the gingiva become red, swollen and bleed easily with the formation of periodontal pockets, loss of alveolar bone, loosening and loss of the teeth. The teeth are involved roughly in the order they erupt. The deciduous teeth are often lost by the age of 5 years and the permanent teeth are almost invariably lost by the age of 16 years. There are no obvious abnormalities in either the tooth cementum or dentine.

Hyperkeratosis of the palms and particularly the soles appears at about the age of 3–5 years, concurrent with periodontal breakdown of the deciduous dentition. Similar plaques may also be seen on the lips, cheeks and eyelids. The affected skin shows diffuse hyperkeratosis, hypergranulosis and acanthosis. There may also be calcification of the dura and some patients have recurrent pyogenic infections [6].

Similar syndromes include Haim–Munk syndrome [7], late-onset Papillon–Lefèvre syndrome [8], a condition including arachnodactyly and acro-osteolysis [9], and Unna–Thost syndrome (see below).

Diagnosis is on clinical and radiographic grounds. Intensive dental care is needed. Retinoids may be useful in suppressing oral and cutaneous lesions and minimizing the pyogenic infections [6,10,11] and it is possible to retain the dentition for some years [12].

REFERENCES

1 Efeoglu J, Porter SR, Mutlu S *et al.* Papillon–Lefèvre syndrome affecting two siblings. *Br J Pediatr Dent* 1990; **6**: 115–20.
2 Haneke E. The Papillon–Lefèvre syndrome: keratosis palmoplantaris with periodontopathy: report of a case and review of cases in the literature. *Hum Genet* 1979; **51**: 1–35.
3 Smith P, Rosenzweig KA. Seven cases of Papillon–Lefèvre syndrome. *Periodontics* 1967; **5**: 42–6.
4 Zhang Y, Lundgren T, Renvert S *et al.* Evidence of a founder effect for four cathepsin C gene mutations in Papillon–Lefevre syndrome patients. *J Med Genet* 2001; **38**: 96–101.
5 Van Dyke TE, Taubman MA, Ebersole JL *et al.* The Papillon–Lefèvre syndrome: neutrophil dysfunction with severe periodontal disease. *Clin Immunol Immunopathol* 1984; **31**: 419–29.
6 Bergman R, Friedman-Birnbaum R. Papillon–Lefèvre syndrome: a study of the long term clinical course of recurrent pyogenic infections and the effects of etretinate treatment. *Br J Dermatol* 1988; **119**: 731–6.
7 Hart TC, Hart PS, Michalec MD *et al.* Haim–Munk syndrome and Papillon–Lefèvre syndrome are allelic mutations in cathepsin C. *J Med Genet* 2000; **37**: 88–94.
8 Brown RS, Hays GL, Flaitz CM *et al.* A possible late-onset variation of Papillon–Lefèvre syndrome. *J Periodontol* 1993; **64**: 379–86.
9 Puliyel JM, Sridharanlyer KS. A syndrome of keratosis palmoplantaris congenita, pes planus, onychogryphosis, periodontosis, arachnodactyly and a peculiar acrosteolysis. *Br J Dermatol* 1986; **115**: 243–8.
10 El Darouti MA, Al Raubaie SM, Eiada MA. Papillon–Lefèvre syndrome: successful treatment with oral retinoids in three patients. *Int J Dermatol* 1988; **27**: 63–6.
11 Gelmetti C, Nazzaro V, Cerri D, Fracasso L. Long-term preservation of permanent teeth in a patient with Papillon–Lefèvre syndrome treated with etretinate. *Pediatr Dermatol* 1989; **6**: 222–5.
12 Wiebe CB, Hakkinen L, Putnins EE, Walsh P, Larjava HS. Successful periodontal maintenance of a case with Papillon–Lefevre syndrome: 12-year follow-up and review of the literature. *J Periodontol* 2001; **72**: 824–30.

Unna–Thost syndrome (hereditary palmoplantar keratoderma)

The Unna–Thost variety of hereditary palmoplantar keratoderma may be associated with oral keratosis and/or periodontitis [1–3].

REFERENCES

1 Ergorov HA. Unna–Thost syndrome in four generations. *Vestn Dermatol Venerol* 1978; **7**: 68–71.

2 Nikolov D, Lazarevska B, Arsovski T. Hereditary palmo-plantar kerato-derma Unna–Thost with periodontitis. *God Med Fak Skopje* 1976; **22**: 415–24.
3 Rode M. Soft and hard tissue changes in the oral cavity of patients with Unna–Thost syndrome. *Zobozdrav Vestn* 1986; **41**: 65–8.

Ehlers–Danlos syndrome [1–5]

Early-onset periodontitis is seen in Ehlers–Danlos syndrome, particularly type VIII (see Chapter 46).

REFERENCES

1 Stewart RE, Hollister DW, Rimoin DL *et al*. A new variant of Ehlers–Danlos syndrome: an autosomal dominant disorder of fragile skin, abnormal scarring and generalized periodontitis. *Birth Defects* 1977; **13**: 85–93.
2 Letourneau Y, Perusse R, Buithieu H. Oral manifestations of Ehlers–Danlos syndrome. *J Can Dent Assoc* 2001; **67**: 330–4.
3 Reichert S, Riemann D, Plaschka B, Machulla HK. Early-onset periodontitis in a patient with Ehlers–Danlos syndrome type III. *Quintessence Int* 1999; **30**: 785–90.
4 Fridrich KL, Fridrich HH, Kempf KK, Moline DO. Dental implications in Ehlers–Danlos syndrome. A case report. *Oral Surg Oral Med Oral Pathol* 1990; **69**: 431–5.
5 Leung AK, Barksy RL, Lewkonia RM. Oral manifestations of Ehlers–Danlos syndrome. *J Am Dent Assoc* 1989; **119**: 696.

Down's syndrome [1,2]

Early-onset periodontitis is common in Down's syndrome.

REFERENCES

1 Saxen L, Aula S. Periodontal bone loss in patients with Down's syndrome. *J Periodontol* 1982; **53**: 158–62.
2 Amano A, Kishima T, Akiyama S *et al*. Relationship of periodontopathic bacteria with early-onset periodontitis in Down's syndrome. *J Periodontol* 2001; **72**: 368–73.

Prader–Willi syndrome [1–3]

Early-onset periodontitis has been recorded in Prader–Willi syndrome, presumably as a consequence of the diabetes.

REFERENCES

1 Greenwood RE, Small ICB. Case report of the Prader–Willi syndrome. *J Clin Periodontol* 1990; **17**: 61–3.
2 Bazopoulou-Kyrkanidou E, Papagiannoulis L. Prader–Willi syndrome: report of a case with special emphasis on oral problems. *J Clin Pediatr Dent* 1992; **17**: 37–40.
3 Salako NO, Ghafouri HM. Oral findings in a child with Prader–Labhart–Willi syndrome. *Quintessence Int* 1995; **26**: 339–41.

Congenital epulis
SYN. GRANULAR CELL TUMOUR OR MYOBLASTOMA

Epulis is the term applied to a swelling on the gingiva. Congenital epulis is a rare, benign, pedunculated, firm pink swelling on the maxillary alveolus, seen in an infant [1,2]. It can be a prenatal ultrasonographic diagnosis [3,4]. There is an 8 : 1 female predominance.

It is probably a reactive mesenchymal lesion and is usually treated by excision. Histology shows large polygonal cells with a fine granular eosinophilic cytoplasm.

REFERENCES

1 Fuhr AH, Krogh PHJ. Congenital epulis of the newborn: centennial review of the literature and case report. *J Oral Surg* 1972; **30**: 30–5.
2 Webb JD, Wescott WB, Corell RW. Firm swelling on the anterior maxillary gingiva in an infant. *J Am Dent Assoc* 1984; **109**: 307–8.
3 Lopez de Lacalle JM, Aguirre I, Irizabal JC, Nogues A. Congenital epulis: prenatal diagnosis by ultrasound. *Pediatr Radiol* 2001; **31**: 453–4.
4 Meizner I, Shalev J, Mashiach R, Vardimon D, Ben-Rafael Z. Prenatal ultrasonographic diagnosis of congenital oral granular cell myoblastoma. *J Ultrasound Med* 2000; **19**: 337–9.

Epstein's pearls
SYN. GINGIVAL CYSTS OF THE NEWBORN

Epstein's pearls are superficial, white, keratin-containing cysts seen on the palatal or alveolar mucosa of about 80% of neonates. They are symptomless and inconsequential, usually being shed within a few weeks, sometimes found with cleft lip and palate [1–3].

REFERENCES

1 Gilhar A, Winsterstein G, Godfried E. Gingival cysts of the newborn. *Int Dent J* 1988; **27**: 261–2.
2 Hayes PA. Hamartomas, eruption cyst, natal tooth and Epstein pearls in a newborn. *ASDC J Dent Child* 2000; **67**: 365–8.
3 Richard BM, Qiu CX, Ferguson MW. Neonatal palatal cysts and their morphology in cleft lip and palate. *Br J Plast Surg* 2000; **53**: 555–8.

Acquired disorders affecting the periodontium

Chronic gingivitis

This is an extremely common condition. Over 90% of dentate adults exhibit some degree of gingivitis. The accumulation of dental bacterial plaque because of inadequate oral hygiene produces non-specific chronic inflammation. It is painless but may manifest with bleeding from the gingival crevice. The gingival margins are red and slightly swollen [1].

Dental advice on improved oral hygiene is needed. If untreated it may progress to periodontitis and tooth loss.

REFERENCE

1 Page RC. Gingivitis. *J Clin Periodontol* 1986; **13**: 345–59.

Chronic periodontitis

Chronic periodontitis (inflammation of the gingiva and periodontal membrane) may be a sequel of chronic gingivitis usually because of plaque accumulation and calculus (tartar) [1]. Smoking is a risk factor. The gingiva

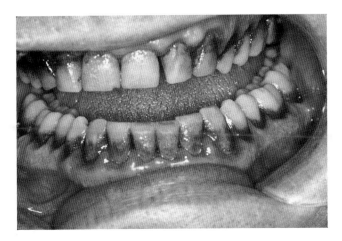

Fig. 66.14 Periodontitis.

detaches from the tooth neck, the periodontal membrane and alveolar bone are damaged, and an abnormal gap (pocket) develops between the tooth and gum. The tooth may slowly loosen and eventually be lost (Fig. 66.14).

Diagnosis. Chronic periodontitis is typically seen in adults. It is painless but may be associated with bleeding, halitosis and a foul taste. Debris and pus may be expressed from the pockets (pyorrhoea), and there may be increasing tooth mobility.

Management. Although periodontal disease has a bacterial component, systemic antibiotics have no place in routine treatment. Management comprises improvement in oral hygiene, although in this case plaque accumulates below the gumline, within periodontal pockets. Toothbrushing and mouthwashes have effect only above, or very slightly below, the gum level and are therefore ineffective in the treatment of periodontitis. Surgical removal of the pocket wall and removal of diseased tissue may be needed to facilitate future cleansing, or attempts to regenerate lost periodontal tissue (such as guided tissue regeneration) may be indicated. Periodontal attention is therefore required.

REFERENCE

1 Page RC. Gingivitis. *J Clin Periodontol* 1986; **13**: 345–59.

Early-onset periodontitis

Periodontal breakdown (periodontitis) is usually a consequence of inflammatory destruction as a result of poor oral hygiene and the subsequent accumulation of dental bacterial plaque [1] and is seen mainly in adults. The host response and periodontal microbiota can both be implicated in a heterogeneous group of causes of early-onset periodontitis [2–10]. If present in children or adolescents,

it can be a manifestation of severely neglected oral hygiene, such as seen in some patients with learning disability, or may be a feature of an immunocompromised host.

That host defences are extremely important in maintaining periodontal health is demonstrated well in the periodontal breakdown that may accompany leukaemias, leukocyte defects, diabetes and HIV infection. Periodontal breakdown is also a feature of Down's syndrome, Ehlers–Danlos syndrome type VIII and Papillon–Lefèvre syndrome.

Periodontal breakdown in a child or adolescent who is capable of maintaining good oral hygiene almost invariably suggests an immune or other systemic defect.

REFERENCES

1 Meyle J, Gonzales JR. Influences of systemic diseases on periodontitis in children and adolescents. *Periodontology* 2001; **26**: 92–112.
2 Mooney J, Hodge PJ, Kinane DF. Humoral immune response in early-onset periodontitis: influence of smoking. *J Periodontal Res* 2001; **36**: 227–32.
3 Seifert R, Wenzel-Seifert K. Defective Gi protein coupling in two formyl peptide receptor mutants associated with localized juvenile periodontitis. *J Biol Chem* 2001; **276**: 42043–9.
4 Shibata K, Warbington ML, Gordon BJ, Kurihara H, Van Dyke TE. Nitric oxide synthase activity in neutrophils from patients with localized aggressive periodontitis. *J Periodontol* 2001; **72**: 1052–8.
5 Haubek D, Ennibi OK, Poulsen K *et al.* Early-onset periodontitis in Morocco is associated with the highly leukotoxic clone of *Actinobacillus actinomycetemcomitans*. *J Dent Res* 2001; **80**: 1580–3.
6 Alpha CX, Guthmiller JM, Cummings HE, Schomberg LL, Noorani SM. Molecular analysis of *Peptostreptococcus micros* isolates from patients with periodontitis. *J Periodontol* 2001; **72**: 877–82.
7 Yoshihara A, Sugita N, Yamamoto K *et al.* Analysis of vitamin D and Fcgamma receptor polymorphisms in Japanese patients with generalized early-onset periodontitis. *J Dent Res* 2001; **80**: 2051–4.
8 Kubota T, Morozumi T, Shimizu K *et al.* Differential gene expression in neutrophils from patients with generalized aggressive periodontitis. *J Periodontal Res* 2001; **36**: 390–7.
9 Endo M, Tai H, Tabeta K *et al.* Analysis of single nucleotide polymorphisms in the 5′-flanking region of tumor necrosis factor-alpha gene in Japanese patients with early-onset periodontitis. *J Periodontol* 2001; **72**: 1554–9.
10 Albandar JM, DeNardin AM, Adesanya MR, Diehl SR, Winn DM. Associations between serum antibody levels to periodontal pathogens and early-onset periodontitis. *J Periodontol* 2001; **72**: 1463–9.

Diabetes

Uncontrolled diabetes can lead to accelerated periodontitis [1].

REFERENCE

1 Emingil G, Darcan S, Keskinoglu A, Kutukculer N, Atilla G. Localized aggressive periodontitis in a patient with type 1 diabetes mellitus: a case report. *J Periodontol* 2001; **72**: 1265–70.

HIV infection

HIV disease can be complicated by necrotizing ulcerative gingivitis (see p. 66.74), periodontitis, candidiasis, herpetic ulceration, Kaposi's sarcoma, lymphomas and other gingival lesions [1].

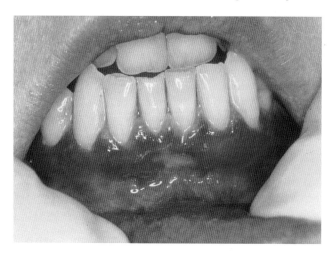

Fig. 66.15 Desquamative gingivitis.

REFERENCE

1 Laskaris G, Scully C, eds. *Periodontal Manifestations of Local and Systemic Disease*. Berlin: Springer, 2003.

Desquamative gingivitis

In this fairly common condition, the labial gingiva are persistently glazed, red and sometimes sore but the gingival margins may be spared, differentiating desquamative gingivitis from chronic marginal gingivitis (Fig. 66.15).

Desquamative gingivitis typically affects middle-aged or elderly women and is usually a manifestation of mucous membrane pemphigoid or lichen planus [1–5]. Rarely, it may be seen in pemphigus, dermatitis herpetiformis, linear IgA disease, chronic ulcerative stomatitis with epithelial antinuclear antibodies or other dermatoses [4,5].

Desquamative gingivitis tends to be chronic and recalcitrant. The underlying condition should be treated where possible. Improved oral hygiene and topical corticosteroids in a nocturnally worn polythene splint may help. Dapsone or topical ciclosporin or tacrolimus may be beneficial in severe cases.

REFERENCES

1 Nisengard RJ, Nieders M. Desquamative lesions of the gingiva. *J Periodontol* 1981; **52**: 500–10.
2 Nisengard RJ, Levine RA. Diagnosis and management of desquamative gingivitis. *Periodontol Insights* 1995; **2**: 4–10.
3 Rees TD. Vesiculo-ulcerative diseases and periodontal practice. *J Periodontol* 1995; **66**: 747–8.
4 Scully C, Laskaris G. Mucocutaneous disorders. In: Scully C, ed. *Oral Pathology and Medicine in Periodontics*. Copenhagen: Munksgaard, 1998: 81–94.
5 Scully C, Porter SR. The clinical spectrum of desquamative gingivitis. *Semin Cutan Med Surg* 1997; **16**: 308–13.

Allergic gingivostomatitis
SYN. ATYPICAL OR PLASMA-CELL GINGIVOSTOMATITIS

Diffusely red, swollen gingivae with or without oral ulceration may occasionally follow exposure to various allergens and other substances. Such reactions have followed the use of certain chewing gums, confectionery such as mints, and dentifrices [1–7] and dental materials [8], particularly 'tartar control' dentifrices containing cinnamon or cinnamaldehyde [2].

Biopsy is usually not indicated and is fairly non-specific with epithelial atrophy, oedema and a variable cellular infiltrate in the lamina propria which, in the earlier reported cases due to chewing gum, was often predominantly plasmacytic [1,3,5–7]. The lesions resolve on withdrawal of the causal agent and reappear on rechallenge. Patch testing may be of value in diagnosis.

REFERENCES

1 Kerr DA, McClarchey KD, Regezi JA. Allergic gingivostomatitis (due to gum chewing). *J Periodontol* 1971; **42**: 709–12.
2 Lamey PJ, Lewis MAO, Rees TD *et al.* Sensitivity reaction to the cinnamaldehyde component of toothpaste. *Br Dent J* 1990; **168**: 115–8.
3 Lubow RM, Cooley RL, Hartman KJ *et al.* Plasma cell gingivitis: report of a case. *J Periodontol* 1984; **55**: 234–41.
4 MacLeod FI, Ellis JE. Plasma cell gingivitis related to the use of herbal toothpaste. *Br Dent J* 1989; **166**: 375–6.
5 Owings JR. An atypical gingivostomatitis: a report of four cases. *J Periodontol* 1969; **40**: 538–42.
6 Palmer RM, Eveson JW. Plasma cell gingivitis. *Oral Surg* 1981; **51**: 187–9.
7 Perry HO. Idiopathic gingivostomatitis. *Dermatol Clin* 1987; **5**: 719–22.
8 Izumi AK. Allergic contact gingivostomatitis due to gold. *Arch Dermatol Res* 1982; **272**: 387–91.

Idiopathic plasmacytosis (see also Plasma-cell balanitis, Chapter 68)

This term refers to red, velvety gingival lesions associated with a plasmacytic infiltrate. Most cases are restricted to the gingiva (atypical gingivostomatitis, plasmacyte gingivitis, allergic gingivostomatitis) [1], while a few have supraglottic laryngeal lesions [2]. Corticosteroids are the main treatment but irradiation may be required [3].

REFERENCES

1 White JW, Olsen KD, Banks PM. Plasma cell orofacial mucositis. *Arch Dermatol* 1986; **122**: 1321–4.
2 Timms M, Sloan P. Association of supraglottic and gingival idiopathic plasmacytosis. *Oral Surg* 1991; **71**: 451–3.
3 Fogarty G, Turner H, Corry J. Plasma cell infiltration of the upper aerodigestive tract treated with radiation therapy. *J Laryngol Otol* 2001; **115**: 928–30.

Fibroepithelial polyp
SYN. FIBROUS LUMP

Fibrous lumps are common in the mouth and are seen

mainly in adults. They appear to be purely reparative in nature. They may attain their full size (which rarely exceeds 2.5 cm diameter) quite rapidly, and then stop growing. Fibrous lumps should not be confused with the true fibroma, a benign neoplasm derived from fibroblasts, which is rare in the mouth (see below).

The variable inflammatory changes account for the different clinical presentations of fibrous lumps from red, shiny, soft lumps to those which are pale, stippled and firm [1]. Commonly, they are round pedunculated swellings arising from the marginal or papillary gingiva (epulides), sometimes adjacent to sites of irritation (e.g. a carious cavity). They are usually painless. They may reach quite a large size, but the prognosis is good.

Fibrous epulides should be removed down to the periosteum, which should be curetted thoroughly.

Fibroma [1]

The true fibroma, a benign neoplasm of fibroblastic origin, is rare in the oral cavity and many lesions in the past called fibromas were probably fibroepithelial polyps.

Histology shows marked proliferation of fibroblasts, with nuclei of uniform shape, size and staining characteristics.

The true fibroma is a continuously enlarging new growth, not necessarily arising at a site of potential trauma. It is a pedunculated growth with a smooth, non-ulcerated, pink surface.

Removal should be total, deep and wide.

REFERENCE

1 Lee KW. The fibrous epulis and related lesions. *Periodontics* 1986; **6**: 277–99.

Pyogenic granuloma (see Chapter 53)

Pyogenic granuloma commonly affects the gingiva, the lip or the tongue [1]. In these sites, the lesion should be excised completely. It will readily recur if excision is not adequate.

REFERENCE

1 Vilmann A, Vilmann P, Vilmann H. Pyogenic granuloma: evaluation of oral conditions. *Br J Oral Surg* 1986; **24**: 376–82.

Giant cell epulis
SYN. PERIPHERAL GIANT CELL GRANULOMA

The giant cell epulis probably arises because chronic irritation triggers a reactionary hyperplasia of muco-periosteum and excessive production of granulation tissue.

Giant cell granulomas are occasionally a feature of hyper-parathyroidism.

The giant cell epulis characteristically arises interdentally, adjacent to permanent teeth that have had deciduous predecessors [1], i.e. not the permanent molars. Classically, the most notable feature is the deep-red colour, although older lesions tend to be paler.

This is a benign lesion which is cured by excision.

REFERENCE

1 Giansanti JS, Waldron CA. Peripheral giant cell granuloma: review of 720 cases. *J Oral Surg* 1969; **27**: 787–91.

Pregnancy gingivitis and epulis

There can be an exaggerated inflammatory reaction to dental bacterial plaque in pregnancy, and chronic gingivitis may therefore be aggravated giving rise to 'pregnancy gingivitis' [1,2] and, occasionally, a pyogenic granuloma (pregnancy epulis).

Pregnancy gingivitis is characterized by soft reddish enlargements, usually of the gingival papillae, varying from small smooth enlargements to more extensive, ragged, granular lumps resembling the surface of a strawberry. Changes of pregnancy gingivitis usually appear about the second month of pregnancy, and reach a peak at the eighth month. Poor oral hygiene predisposes to these changes. A similar appearance may occur with oral contraceptives.

Sometimes there is a localized epulis (pregnancy epulis) that, although unsightly, is usually painless. Occasionally it ulcerates or interferes with eating. Despite the vascularity, the immaturity of the vessels may lead to superficial ischaemia and ulceration. Larger lesions are prone to trauma, which may contribute to the ulceration.

Oral hygiene should be improved. Most lesions tend to resolve on parturition. There is one report of a beneficial effect of folic acid on pregnancy gingivitis [3]. An epulis requires excision only if it is being traumatized or is grossly unaesthetic [2].

REFERENCES

1 Amar S, Chung KM. Influence of hormonal variation on the periodontium in women. *Periodontology* 1994; **6**: 79–87.
2 Chiodo GT, Rosenstein DI. Dental treatment during pregnancy: a preventive approach. *J Am Dent Assoc* 1985; **110**: 365–8.
3 Pack ARC, Thomson ME. Effect of topical and systemic folic acid supplementation on gingivitis of pregnancy. *J Clin Periodontol* 1980; **7**: 402–14.

Drug-induced gingival swelling

Gingival swelling is a recognized adverse effect of medication, especially following use of phenytoin, calcium-channel blockers and ciclosporin.

Phenytoin

Phenytoin induces gingival swelling presumably by an effect on fibroblast activity. There is no correlation between the extent of overgrowth and the dose of phenytoin, its serum level, or the age and sex of the patient. Rather, the hyperplasia is aggravated by poor oral hygiene.

Phenytoin can produce a variable degree of gingival enlargement, which characteristically affects the interdental papillae first but which may later involve the marginal and even attached gingiva. The palatal and lingual gingivae are usually involved less than the buccal and labial gingivae [1–4].

The enlargement is characteristically firm, pale and tough, with coarse stippling, although these features may take several years to develop, and earlier lesions may be softer and redder (see Fig. 66.12).

The patient's level of plaque control should be improved [5] and a 0.2% aqueous chlorhexidine mouthwash may be helpful. Excision of the enlarged tissue may be indicated but the swelling unfortunately readily recurs, although this is less likely with meticulous oral hygiene, particularly if the phenytoin can be stopped. Folic acid may improve the condition and systemic isotretinoin may be of some value [2].

Calcium-channel blockers

Nifedipine can cause gingival swelling, typically affecting the papillae in a similar fashion to phenytoin [3,6]. Several other calcium-channel blockers have a similar effect [7].

Improved oral hygiene may reduce the hyperplasia [8]. Excision of the enlarged tissue may be followed by recurrence, and patients should be warned accordingly. If possible the medication should be changed.

Ciclosporin

Ciclosporin also causes gingival hyperplasia, initially of papillae [3,9]. Only about one-third of patients are affected, more commonly children, and this change may be lessened by meticulous removal of plaque before the drug is introduced.

REFERENCES

1 Hassell TM. *Epilepsy and the Oral Manifestations of Phenytoin Therapy*. In: Myers HM, eds. *Monographs in Oral Science*. Basel: Karger, 1981: 9–12.
2 Norris JF, Cunliffe WJ. Phenytoin-induced gum hypertrophy improved by isotretinoin. *Int J Dermatol* 1987; **26**: 602–3.
3 Slavin J, Taylor J. Cyclosporin, nifedipine and gingival hyperplasia. *Lancet* 1987; ii: 739.
4 Stinnett E, Rodu B, Grizzle WE. New developments in understanding phenytoin-induced gingival hyperplasia. *J Am Dent Assoc* 1987; **114**: 814–6.
5 Modeer T, Dahllof G. Development of phenytoin-induced gingival overgrowth in non-institutionalised epileptic children subjected to different plaque control programs. *Acta Odontol Scand* 1987; **45**: 81–5.
6 Shaftic AA, Widdup LL, Abate MA *et al.* Nifedipine-induced gingival hyperplasia. *Drug Intell Clin Pharm* 1986; **20**: 602–5.
7 Steele RM, Schuna AA, Schreiber RT. Calcium antagonist-induced gingival hyperplasia. *Ann Intern Med* 1994; **120**: 663–4.
8 Hancock RH, Swan RH. Nifedipine-induced gingival overgrowth: report of a case treated by controlling plaque. *J Clin Periodontol* 1992; **19**: 12–4.
9 Daley TD, Wysocki GP, Day C. Clinical and pharmacological correlations in cyclosporin-induced gingival hyperplasia. *Oral Surg* 1986; **62**: 417–21.

Scurvy (see Chapter 57)

Scurvy (vitamin C deficiency) causes gingival swelling, bleeding and oral purpura, but is now rare in the West.

Disorders affecting the oral mucosa or lips

Swellings

Mucosal swelling may be seen after trauma and in angio-oedema, Crohn's disease, orofacial granulomatosis, sarcoidosis, Wegener's granulomatosis, amyloidosis and other disorders. Localized swellings may be of local aetiology or can be manifestations of neoplasia or systemic disease.

Pigmentation

Mucosal pigmentation is usually seen in dark-skinned races (but may be seen even in white people) (see Fig. 66.13). Other common causes include amalgam tattoo and melanotic macules.

Addison's disease, Kaposi's sarcoma, melanoma, Laugier–Hunziker syndrome, pigmentary incontinence and other causes must be excluded. Peutz–Jeghers disease is the association of circumoral and sometimes intraoral melanosis with small-intestinal polyposis (see Chapter 59). Oral petechiae are usually caused by trauma or suction. More widespread purpura is most frequently a manifestation of a bleeding tendency caused by thrombocytopenia and may also be seen in infectious mononucleosis, rubella, HIV infection, leukaemia or scurvy. Petechiae may also occur in amyloidosis.

Redness

Red lesions may be inflammatory, or represent erythroplasia, haemangiomas or neoplasms such as carcinoma, Wegener's granulomatosis or Kaposi's sarcoma [1,2].

Candidiasis is a common cause of red lesions, which may be sore. Widespread erythema, particularly if associated with soreness, is usually caused by primary herpes simplex stomatitis or a mucocutaneous disorder such as lichen planus or mucous membrane pemphigoid, rarely by pemphigus or other dermatoses and occasionally by allergic responses.

Localized red areas may represent erythroplasia, carcinoma, candidiasis, lichen planus or lupus erythematosus. Kaposi's sarcoma may present as a red, purple, brown or bluish macule or nodule as may epithelioid angiomatosis. Hereditary mucoepithelial dysplasia is a rare cause of oral erythema.

Telangiectasia may be a manifestation of hereditary haemorrhagic telangiectasia, primary biliary cirrhosis or systemic sclerosis, or may follow radiotherapy. Haemangiomas are usually isolated but may occasionally extend deeply and rarely involve the ipsilateral meninges, producing a facial angioma and epilepsy, sometimes with learning disability (Sturge–Weber syndrome). Intraoral haemangiomas may be seen in Maffucci's syndrome.

Lingual depapillation in deficiencies of iron, folate or vitamin B_{12} may produce the red tongue termed 'glossitis'. Geographical tongue may also produce red patches.

Mucositis can readily be induced by irradiation or chemotherapy.

Ulcers

Oral ulcers are often caused by trauma or recurrent aphthae (see p. 66.43). Malignant neoplasms may present as ulcers. Various infections or systemic disorders, particularly those of blood, gastrointestinal tract or skin, also produce mouth ulcers, as may drugs and irradiation (see Table 66.10).

Blisters

Blisters may be seen as a result of burns but the most important vesiculobullous disorders affecting the oral mucosa are pemphigoid (including cicatricial pemphigoid) and pemphigus (see Table 66.10). The bullae of mucous membrane pemphigoid may or may not be blood-filled and, in the former case, a bleeding tendency must be excluded. Blood-filled blisters may also be caused by localized oral purpura (angina bullosa haemorrhagica) or amyloidosis. The bullae of pemphigus are rarely seen as they break down rapidly to produce ulcers. Epidermolysis bullosa and erythema multiforme may present with oral bullae or vesicles, although ulcers are more common. Vesicles may be seen in viral infections, especially in herpes simplex stomatitis, chickenpox, herpangina and hand, foot and mouth disease.

Mucoceles, caused by extravasation of mucus from minor salivary glands, produce isolated blisters, typically in the lower labial mucosa.

White patches (see Table 66.9)

Thrush (acute candidiasis) is a 'disease of the diseased' and produces oral white patches.

HIV infection causes hairy leukoplakia, a white lesion on the tongue (see p. 66.89).

Leukoplakia is often associated with friction or smoking, occasionally with syphilis, candidiasis or chronic renal failure, but most cases are idiopathic. Lichen planus and lupus erythematosus may present as white lesions. Rarely, lichenoid lesions are associated with various drugs, liver disease or GVHD. Carcinoma may present as a white lesion.

Inherited causes of white patches, such as white sponge naevus and dyskeratosis congenita, are rare [1–5].

REFERENCES

1 Scully C, Porter SR. Diseases of the oral mucosa. *Med Int* 1990; **76**: 3154–62.
2 Scully C, Porter SR. Oral medicine 2. Disorders affecting the oral mucosa. *Postgrad Dent* 1992; **2**: 109–13.
3 Scully C. *ABC of Oral Health.* London: BMJ Books, 2000.
4 Scully C. *Handbook of Oral Disease: Diagnosis and Management.* London: Martin Dunitz, 1999.
5 Scully C, Flint S, Porter SR, Moos K. *Oral and Maxillofacial Diseases.* London: Martin Dunitz, 2004.

Genetic disorders affecting the oral mucosa or lips

This section discusses the main congenital causes of white or whitish lesions, pigmented lesions, red lesions, vesiculoerosive lesions, lumps and swellings, and some orocutaneous disorders.

White or whitish lesions

Sebaceous glands

Fordyce spots
SYN. FORDYCE'S GRANULES

Fordyce spots are yellowish small grains seen beneath the buccal or labial mucosa. Fordyce spots are sebaceous glands containing neutral lipids similar to those found in skin sebaceous glands [1] but are not associated with hair follicles.

Fordyce spots are extremely common: probably 80% of the population have them. They are usually seen in the buccal mucosa, particularly inside the commissures (Fig. 66.16), and sometimes in the retromolar regions and upper lip [1–5]. Fordyce spots are often not noticeable in children until after puberty (although they are present histologically), and they seem to be more obvious in males, patients with greasy skin and the elderly, and they may be increased in some rheumatic disorders [6].

Fordyce spots are totally benign, although the occasional patient or physician becomes concerned about them or misdiagnoses them as thrush or lichen planus. Occasionally they may be mistaken for leukoplakia [7].

No treatment is indicated, other than reassurance. The spots may become less prominent if isotretinoin is given [8].

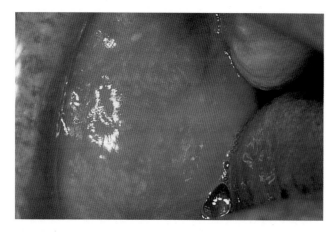

Fig. 66.16 Fordyce spots: sebaceous glands in the buccal mucosa.

REFERENCES

1 Nordstrom KM, McGinley KJ, Lessin SR *et al.* Neutral lipid composition of Fordyce's granules. *Br J Dermatol* 1989; **121**: 669–70.
2 Batsakis JG, el-Naggar AK. Sebaceous lesions of salivary glands and oral cavity. *Ann Otol Rhinol Laryngol* 1990; **99**: 416–8.
3 Dreher A, Grevers G. Fordyce spots. A little regarded finding in the area of lip pigmentation and mouth mucosa. *Laryngorhinootologie* 1995; **74**: 390–2.
4 Sewerein I. The sebaceous glands in the vermilion border of the lips and the oral mucosa of man. *Acta Odontol Scand* 1975; **33** (Suppl. 68): 13–226.
5 Daley TD. Pathology of intraoral sebaceous glands. *J Oral Pathol Med* 1993; **22**: 241.
6 Vilpoula AH, Vli-kerttula UI, Terho PE *et al.* Sebaceous glands in the buccal mucosa in patients with rheumatic disorders. *Scand J Rheumatol* 1983; **12**: 337–42.
7 Sengupta P, Haldar B. Fordyce disease resembling leukoplakia. Report of a case. *Indian J Dermatol* 1982; **27**: 149–52.
8 Monk BE. Fordyce spots responding to isotretinoin therapy. *Br J Dermatol* 1994; **131**: 335.

Sebaceous adenoma

Sebaceous adenomas are exceedingly rare in the mouth, except in association with salivary glands but have been described in the buccal mucosa [1–5].

REFERENCES

1 Daley TD. Pathology of intraoral sebaceous glands. *J Oral Pathol Med* 1993; **22**: 241.
2 Batsakis JG, el-Naggar AK. Sebaceous lesions of salivary glands and oral cavity. *Ann Otol Rhinol Laryngol* 1990; **99**: 416–8.
3 Miller AS, McCrea MW. Sebaceous gland adenoma of the buccal mucosa. *J Oral Surg* 1968; **26**: 593–5.
4 Orlian AI, Salman L, Reddi T, Yamane GM, Chaudhry AP. Sebaceous adenoma of the oral mucosa. *J Oral Med* 1987; **42**: 38–9.
5 Iezzi G, Rubini C, Fioroni M, Piattelli A. Sebaceous adenoma of the cheek. *Oral Oncol* 2002; **38**: 111–3.

Nevus sebaceus of Jadassohn
SYN. LINEAR NAEVUS SYNDROME

Oral manifestations may rarely occur as fibroepitheliomatous nodules in patients with a sebaceous naevus of the skin but are extremely rarely seen in isolation [1–3].

REFERENCES

1 Kelley JE, Hibbard E, Giansanti J. Epidermal nevus syndrome: report of a case with unusual oral manifestations. *Oral Surg* 1972; **34**: 774–80.
2 Morency R, Labelle H. Nevus sebaceus of Jadassohn: a rare oral presentation. *Oral Surg* 1987; **64**: 460–2.
3 Reichart PA, Lubach D, Becker J. Gingival manifestation in linear nevus sebaceus syndrome. *Int J Oral Surg* 1983; **12**: 437–43.

Epithelium

Leukoedema

Leukoedema is not a mucosal disease but simply the name given to the faint whitish lines seen in some normal buccal mucosae, often prominent in black people. The whitish lines disappear if the mucosa is stretched—a diagnostic test [1–3]. Confusion with lichen planus should thereby be avoided.

REFERENCES

1 Axell T, Henricsson V. Leukoedema: an epidemiologic study with special reference to the influence of tobacco habits. *Community Dent Oral Epidemiol* 1981; **9**: 142–6.
2 Duncan SC, Su WPD. Leukoedema of the oral mucosa (possibly an acquired white sponge naevus). *Arch Dermatol* 1980; **116**: 906–8.
3 Van Wyk CW, Ambrosio SC. Leukoedema: ultrastructural and histochemical observations. *J Oral Pathol* 1983; **12**: 29–35.

Clouston syndrome (see above)

See also Chapter 12.

White-sponge naevus
SYN. CANNON'S DISEASE; PACHYDERMIA ORALIS;
WHITE FOLDED GINGIVOSTOMATOSIS

Aetiology. A rare familial disorder usually first seen in childhood and inherited as an autosomal dominant trait [1,2]; there appear to be defects in keratins 4 and 13 with abnormal tonofilament aggregation [3–6].

Pathology. There is hyperplastic acanthotic epithelium in which gross oedema causes a basket-weave appearance. The superficial epithelium has a 'washed-out' appearance as it stains only very lightly.

Clinical features. The oral mucosa is almost invariably involved in white-sponge naevus. Painless shaggy or folded white lesions typically affect the buccal mucosa bilaterally but may also involve other areas, although rarely the gingival margins.

Similar lesions may also affect the upper respiratory tract, genitalia and anus [1,2].

Diagnosis. The family history and clinical examination are usually adequate to differentiate this from other more common causes of white lesions such as cheek biting, burns, lichen planus and candidiasis.

Treatment. This is a benign condition with an excellent prognosis. Reassurance is all that is required, although some have suggested that tetracyclines clear the lesions [7,8].

REFERENCES

1 Jorgenson RJ, Levin LS. White sponge naevus. *Arch Dermatol* 1981; **117**: 73–6.
2 Hernandez-Martin A, Fernandez-Lopez E, de Unamuno P, Armijo M. Diffuse whitening of the oral mucosa in a child. *Pediatr Dermatol* 1997; **14**: 316–20.
3 Terrinoni A, Rugg EL, Lane EB et al. A novel mutation in the keratin 13 gene causing oral white sponge nevus. *J Dent Res* 2001; **80**: 919–23.
4 Terrinoni A, Candi E, Oddi S et al. A glutamine insertion in the 1A alpha helical domain of the keratin 4 gene in a familial case of white sponge nevus. *J Invest Dermatol* 2000; **114**: 388–91.
5 Richard G, De Laurenzi V, Didona B, Bale SJ, Compton JG. Keratin 13 point mutation underlies the hereditary mucosal epithelial disorder white sponge nevus. *Nat Genet* 1995; **11**: 453–5.
6 Rugg EL, McLean WH, Allison WE et al. A mutation in the mucosal keratin K4 is associated with oral white sponge nevus. *Nat Genet* 1995; **11**: 450–2.
7 McDonagh AJG, Gawkrodger DJ, Walker AE. White sponge naevus successfully treated with tetracycline. *Clin Exp Dermatol* 1990; **15**: 152–3.
8 Lim J, Keting S. Oral tetracycline rinse improves symptoms of white sponge naevus. *J Am Acad Dermatol* 1992; **26**: 1003–5.

Dyskeratosis congenita (see Chapter 12)
SYN. ZINSSER–ENGMAN–COLE SYNDROME

Dyskeratosis congenita usually presents with oral lesions between the ages of 5 and 10 years, when the tongue and sometimes the buccal mucosa and palate develop diffuse white lesions with a malignant potential [1,2]. The lesions resemble leukoplakia or lichen planus and show nonspecific hyperkeratosis, a prominent granular cell layer and mild acanthosis [1–5].

Other manifestations include lesions of other mucosae, skin and appendages, and bone marrow dysfunction. Other rare oral features include taurodont or hypocalcified teeth and mucosal hyperpigmentation.

REFERENCES

1 Cannell H. Dyskeratosis congenita. *Br J Oral Surg* 1971; **9**: 8–10.
2 Moretti S, Spallanzani A, Chiarugi A, Muscarella G, Battini ML. Oral carcinoma in a young man: a case of dyskeratosis congenita. *J Eur Acad Dermatol Venereol* 2000; **14**: 123–5.
3 Loh HS, Koh ML, Giam YC. Dyskeratosis congenita in two male cousins. *Br J Oral Surg* 1987; **25**: 492–9.
4 Ogden GR, Connor E, Chisholm D. Dyskeratosis congenita: report of a case and review of the literature. *Oral Surg* 1988; **65**: 586–91.
5 Brown CJ. Dyskeratosis congenita: report of a case. *Int J Paediatr Dent* 2000; **10**: 328–34.

Pachyonychia congenita (see Chapter 62)
SYN. JADASSOHN–LEWANDOWSKY SYNDROME

Pachyonychia congenita is a benign disorder associated with mutations in keratin 16 [1,2]. About 60% of patients have oral keratosis, 16% have natal or neonatal teeth, and 10% have angular stomatitis. Some patients also develop chronic intraoral candidiasis [3–5].

The keratosis requires no treatment. Dental advice should be sought regarding natal or neonatal teeth.

REFERENCES

1 Swensson O. Pachyonychia congenita. Keratin gene mutations with pleiotropic effect. *Hautarzt* 1999; **50**: 483–90.
2 Smith FJ, Fisher MP, Healy E et al. Novel keratin 16 mutations and protein expression studies in pachyonychia congenita type 1 and focal palmoplantar keratoderma. *Exp Dermatol* 2000; **9**: 170–7.
3 Feinstein A, Friedman J, Schewach-Millet M. Pachyonychia congenita. *J Am Acad Dermatol* 1988; **19**: 705–11.
4 Lim TW, Paik JH, Kim NI. A case of pachyonychia congenita with oral leukoplakia and steatocystoma multiplex. *J Dermatol* 1999; **26**: 677–81.
5 Wimmershoff MB, Stolz W, Schiffner R, Landthaler M. Type I pachyonychia congenita (Jadassohn–Lewandowsky). *Klin Pediatr* 1999; **211**: 179–83.

Tylosis [1–4] (see Chapter 34)

Tylosis is an autosomal dominant syndrome of palmoplantar hyperkeratosis that may predispose to oesophageal carcinoma but although oral white lesions have also been described, there is little evidence that these are premalignant.

REFERENCES

1 O'Mahoney MY, Ellis JP, Hellier M. Familial tylosis and carcinoma of the oesophagus. *J R Soc Med* 1984; **77**: 514–7.
2 Tyldesley WR, Osborne-Hughes R. Tylosis, leukoplakia and oesophageal carcinoma. *BMJ* 1973; **4**: 427.
3 Tyldesley WR. Oral leukoplakia associated with tylosis and esophageal carcinoma. *J Oral Pathol* 1974; **3**: 62–70.
4 Ellis A, Field JK, Field EA et al. Tylosis associated with carcinoma of the oesophagus and oral leukoplakia in a large Liverpool family: a review of six generations. *Oral Oncol* 1994; **30B**: 102–12.

Focal palmoplantar and oral hyperkeratosis syndrome (keratosis palmaris et plantaris)

Focal hyperkeratosis at weight-bearing areas of the palms and soles, with hyperkeratosis of the attached gingiva and occasionally other sites, is an autosomal dominant trait [1–3].

REFERENCES

1 Fred HL, Gieser RG, Berry WR, Eiband JM. Keratosis palmaris et plantaris. *Arch Intern Med* 1964; **113**: 866–87.
2 Laskaris G, Vareltzidis H, Augernou G. Focal palmoplantar and oral mucosa hyperkeratosis syndrome. *Oral Surg* 1980; **50**: 250.
3 Bethke G, Kolde G, Bethke G, Reichart PA. Focal palmoplantar and oral mucosa hyperkeratosis syndrome. *Mund Kiefer Gesichtschir* 2001; **5**: 202–5.

Olmsted's syndrome [1–3] (see Chapter 34)

SYN. CONGENITAL PALMOPLANTAR AND PERIORIFICIAL KERATODERMA WITH CORNEAL EPITHELIAL DYSPLASIA

Perioral keratoderma may be seen associated with palmoplantar keratoderma and corneal epithelial dysplasia.

REFERENCES

1 Judge MR, Misch K, Wright P, Harper JI. Palmoplantar and periorificial keratoderma with corneal epithelial dysplasia: a new syndrome. *Br J Dermatol* 1991; **125**: 186–8.
2 Poulin Y, Perry HO, Muller SA. Olmsted syndrome: congenital palmoplantar and periorificial keratoderma. *J Am Acad Dermatol* 1984; **10**: 600–10.
3 Fonseca E, Pena C, Del Pozo J *et al.* Olmsted syndrome. *J Cutan Pathol* 2001; **28**: 271–5.

Hereditary benign intraepithelial dyskeratosis [1–3]

SYN. WITKOP–VON SALLMANN SYNDROME

Aetiology. Hereditary benign intraepithelial dyskeratosis is a rare, benign, autosomal dominant condition associated with chromosome 4 anomalies, seen mainly in some groups of mixed ethnic origin, predominantly in North Carolina, USA.

Pathology. There is pronounced epithelial acanthosis, vacuolization in the stratum spinosum and eosinophilic cells apparently engulfed by normal squamous cells ('tobacco cells').

Clinical features. Oral milky white, smooth, somewhat translucent plaques appear in childhood and become more obvious by adolescence. These lesions affect predominantly the buccal mucosae, lips and ventrum of the tongue.

Ocular lesions include conjunctivitis with gelatinous conjunctival plaques, which become evident in infancy. There may be photophobia and eventual corneal involvement.

Oral biopsy is usually indicated for diagnosis.

Treatment. No treatment is required.

REFERENCES

1 Witkop CJ, Shankle CM, Graham JB. Hereditary benign intraepithelial dyskeratosis. II. Oral manifestations and hereditary transmission. *Arch Pathol* 1960; **70**: 696–711.
2 Haisley-Royster CA, Allingham RR, Klintworth GK, Prose NS. Hereditary benign intraepithelial dyskeratosis: report of two cases with prominent oral lesions. *J Am Acad Dermatol* 2001; **45**: 634–6.
3 Allingham RR, Seo B, Rampersaud E *et al.* A duplication in chromosome 4q35 is associated with hereditary benign intraepithelial dyskeratosis. *Am J Hum Genet* 2001; **68**: 491–4.

Darier's disease (see Chapter 40)

Oral lesions are seen in up to 50% of patients with skin

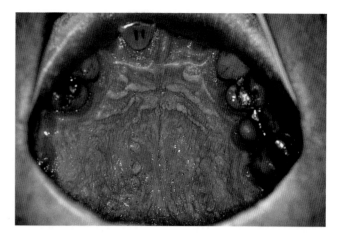

Fig. 66.17 Darier's disease: oral white lesions resemble those of nicotinic stomatitis.

lesions of Darier's disease. The oral changes are most marked in patients with the most severe skin changes and are typically flattish, coalescing, red plaques that eventually turn white and affect the keratinized mucosa of the dorsum of the tongue, palate and gingiva (Fig. 66.17) and then may resemble nicotinic stomatitis clinically [1–3].

Salivary duct anomalies, including dilatations with periodic strictures and indentations, may affect the main ducts [4,5].

REFERENCES

1 Ferris T, Lamey PJ, Rennie JS. Darier's disease: oral features and genetic aspects. *Br Dent J* 1990; **168**: 71–3.
2 Macleod RI, Munro CS. The incidence and distribution of the oral lesions in patients with Darier's disease. *Br Dent J* 1991; **171**: 133–6.
3 Spouge JD, Trott JR, Chesko G. Darier–White's disease: a cause of white lesions of the oral mucosa. Report of four cases. *Oral Surg* 1966; **21**: 441–57.
4 Tegner E, Jonsson N. Darier's disease with involvement of both submandibular glands. *Acta Derm Venereol (Stockh)* 1990; **70**: 451–2.
5 Adams AM, Macleod RI, Munro CS. Symptomatic and asymptomatic salivary duct abnormalities in Darier's disease: a sialographic study. *Dentomaxillofac Radiol* 1994; **23**: 25–8.

Warty dyskeratoma [1–4] (see Chapter 34)

SYN. FOCAL ACANTHOLYTIC DYSKERATOSIS

Warty dyskeratoma, oral warty dyskeratoma or focal acantholytic dyskeratosis is rare in the oral cavity but typically presents as a nodule or papule on the gingiva, palate or alveolar ridge. The histology is similar to that of Darier's disease and transient acantholytic dermatosis, with suprabasal epithelial splits and corps ronds.

REFERENCES

1 Laskaris G, Sklavounou A. Warty dyskeratoma of the oral mucosa. *Br J Oral Surg* 1985; **23**: 371–5.
2 Leider AS, Eversole LR. Focal acantholytic dyskeratosis of the oral mucosa. *Oral Surg* 1984; **58**: 64–70.

3 Chau MN, Radden BG. Oral warty dyskeratoma. *J Oral Pathol* 1984; **13**: 546–56.
4 Neville BW, Coleman PJ, Richardson MS. Verruciform xanthoma associated with an intraoral warty dyskeratoma. *Oral Surg Oral Med Oral Pathol Oral Radiol Endod* 1996; **81**: 3–4.

Keratitis, ichthyosis and deafness syndrome
(see Chapter 34)
SYN. KID SYNDROME

Dental dysplasia, persistent oral ulceration, chronic muco-cutaneous candidiasis and occasional carcinoma may be seen in the KID syndrome of keratitis, ichthyosiform dermatosis and deafness [1,2].

REFERENCES

1 Baden HP, Alper JC. Ichthyosiform dermatosis, keratitis and deafness. *Arch Dermatol* 1977; **113**: 1701–4.
2 Cremers CWRJ, Philipsen VMJG, Mali JWH. Deafness, ichthyosiform erythroderma, cornea involvement, photophobia and dental dysplasia. *J Laryngol Otol* 1977; **91**: 585–7.

Chronic mucocutaneous candidiasis (see Chapter 31)

Chronic mucocutaneous candidiasis includes a range of congenital disorders characterized by chronic candidiasis involving mouth, nails and other sites. Persistent adherent white lesions are seen in the mouth, often with angular stomatitis [1–4]; in candidiasis–endocrinopathy syndrome, there may also be enamel hypoplasia [5,6] and, rarely, oral carcinoma [7].

REFERENCES

1 Scully C, El-Kabir M, Samaranayake LP. *Candida* and oral candidiasis. *Crit Rev Oral Biol Med* 1994; **5**: 124–58.
2 Challacombe SJ. Immunologic aspects of oral candidiasis. *Oral Surg Oral Med Oral Pathol* 1994; **78**: 202–10.
3 Fotos PG, Ray TL. Oral and perioral candidiasis. *Semin Dermatol* 1994; **13**: 118–24.
4 Nielson H, Dangaard K, Schiodt M. Chronic mucocutaneous candidiasis: a review. *Tandlaegkbladet* 1985; **89**: 667–73.
5 Porter SR, Scully C. Candidiasis endocrinopathy syndrome. *Oral Surg* 1986; **61**: 573–8.
6 Porter SR, Eveson JW, Scully C. Enamel hypoplasia secondary to candidiasis endocrinopathy syndrome. *Pediatr Dent* 1995; **17**: 216–9.
7 Firth NA, O'Grady JF, Reade PC. Oral squamous cell carcinoma in a young person with candidiasis endocrinopathy syndrome: a case report. *Int J Oral Maxillofac Surg* 1997; **26**: 42–4.

Pigmented lesions

Most oral hyperpigmentation is racial in origin (see Fig. 66.13). Seen mainly in blacks and Asians it can also be noted in patients of Mediterranean descent, sometimes even in some fairly light-skinned people. It is most obvious in the anterior labial gingivae and palatal mucosa and pigmentation is usually symmetrically distributed. Patches may be seen elsewhere. Pigmentation may be first noted by the patient in adult life and then incorrectly assumed to be acquired rather than congenital in origin.

Melanotic macule

The melanotic macule is an acquired, small, flat, brown to brown-black, asymptomatic, benign lesion, unchanging in character [1,2]. Oral melanotic macule is similar to the ephelis and lentigo.

Melanotic macules may be seen in up to 3% of normal persons, at any age. Melanotic macules are usually solitary, discrete, pigmented brown collections of melanin-containing cells. The macules are less than 2 cm in diameter, seen especially on the vermilion of the lips, gingiva, buccal mucosa or palate. Most on the lips are seen near the midline, on the lower lip vermilion. Most are solitary and seen in white adults and their colour ranges from brown to black [1,3,4]. Occasional cases are seen in HIV infection [5].

Clinically, the melanotic macule may resemble other lesions such as early melanoma and ephelides, although the latter tend to fade in winter and darken in summer. Histopathologically, the mucosal epithelium is normal apart from increased pigmentation of the basal layer, accentuated at the tips of rete ridges. There are no naevus cells or elongated rete ridges [3]. There is melanin in the epithelial basal layer and/or upper lamina propria. Occasionally they are seen along with melanonychia striata (Laugier–Hunziker syndrome, see below).

Melanotic macules can be excised to exclude melanoma or for cosmetic reasons, or hidden by lipstick.

REFERENCES

1 Weathers DR, Corio RL, Crawford BE. The labial melanotic macule. *Oral Surg Oral Med Oral Pathol* 1976; **42**: 192–205.
2 Wescott WB, Correll RW, Friedlander AH. Pigmented macules on the lower lip. *J Am Dent Assoc* 1983; **107**: 100–1.
3 Spann CR, Owen LG, Hodge SJ. The labial melanotic macule. *Arch Dermatol* 1987; **123**: 1029–31.
4 Ho KL, Dervan P, O'Loughlin S, Powell FC. Labial melanotic macule: a clinical, histopathologic and ultrastructural study. *J Am Acad Dermatol* 1993; **28**: 33–9.
5 Ficarra G, Shillitoe EJ, Adler-Storthz K. Oral melanotic macules in patients infected with human immunodeficiency virus. *Oral Surg Oral Med Oral Pathol* 1990; **70**: 748–55.

Peutz–Jeghers syndrome (see Chapter 39)

Peutz–Jeghers syndrome is as an autosomal dominant trait characterized by hamartomatous intestinal polyposis and mucocutaneous melanotic pigmentation, especially circumorally. Those affected have discrete, brown to bluish black macules mainly around the oral, nasal and ocular orifices. The lips, especially the lower, have pigmented macules in about 98% of patients (Fig. 66.18). Oral brown or black macules, unlike the circumoral lesions, do not

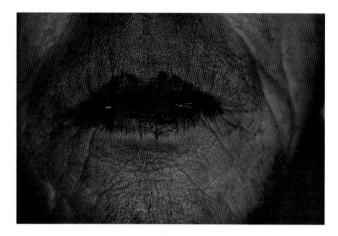

Fig. 66.18 Peutz–Jeghers syndrome.

fade after puberty. Mucosal and facial hyperpigmentation may also be seen in relatives [1–3].

Intestinal polyps are found mainly in the small intestine in Peutz–Jeghers syndrome. They rarely undergo malignant change but if they produce intussusception, surgical intervention is required. There is a slightly increased risk of gastrointestinal carcinoma and carcinomas of the pancreas, breast and reproductive organs [4–7].

Ruby and argon lasers have been used to treat the pigmentation of the lips and oral mucosa [8] (see Chapter 77).

REFERENCES

1 Marlette RH. Generalized melanoses and nonmelanotic pigmentations of the head and neck. *J Am Dent Assoc* 1975; **90**: 141–7.
2 Wesley RK, Delaney JR, Pensler L. Mucocutaneous melanosis and gastrointestinal polyposis (Peutz–Jeghers syndrome): clinical considerations and report of case. *J Dent Child* 1977; **44**: 131–4.
3 Wescott WB, Correll RW. Oral and perioral pigmented macules in a patient with gastric and intestinal polyposis. *J Am Dent Assoc* 1984; **108**: 385–6.
4 Burdick D, Prior JT. Peutz–Jeghers syndrome: a clinicopathological study of a large family with a 27 year follow-up. *Cancer* 1982; **50**: 2139–46.
5 Boardman LA, Pittelkow MR, Couch FJ et al. Association of Peutz–Jeghers-like mucocutaneous pigmentation with breast and gynecologic carcinomas in women. *Medicine (Baltimore)* 2000; **79**: 293–8.
6 Buck JL, Harned RK, Lichtenstein JE, Sobin LH. Peutz–Jeghers syndrome. *Radiographics* 1992; **12**: 365–78.
7 Gardiello FM, Welsh SB, Hamilton SR et al. Increased risk of cancer in the Peutz–Jeghers syndrome. *N Engl J Med* 1987; **316**: 1511–4.
8 Ohshiro T, Maruyama Y, Nakajima H, Mima M. Treatment of pigmentation of the lips and oral mucosa in Peutz–Jeghers' syndrome using ruby and argon lasers. *Br J Plast Surg* 1980; **33**: 346–9.

Laugier–Hunziker syndrome

SYN. LAUGIER–HUNZIKER–BARAN SYNDROME [1–4]

Laugier–Hunziker syndrome presents with labial, oral mucosal and nail hyperpigmentation. A possible variant of this or Peutz–Jeghers syndrome has been termed *idiopathic lenticular pigmentation* [5], in which there are oral, labial, perianal and digital hyperpigmented lenticular macules. Similar patients have been reported previously [6–8].

REFERENCES

1 Haneke E. Laugier–Hunziker–Baran syndrome. *Hautarzt* 1991; **42**: 512–5.
2 Lamey PJ, Nolan A, Thomson E, Lewis MA, Rademaker M. Oral presentation of the Laugier–Hunziker syndrome. *Br Dent J* 1991; **171**: 59–60.
3 Mowad CM, Shrager J, Elenitsas R. Oral pigmentation representing Laugier–Hunziker syndrome. *Cutis* 1997; **60**: 37–9.
4 Mignogna MD, Lo Muzio L, Ruoppo E et al. Oral manifestations of idiopathic lenticular mucocutaneous pigmentation (Laugier–Hunziker syndrome): a clinical, histopathological and ultrastructural review of 12 cases. *Oral Dis* 1999; **5**: 80–6.
5 Gerbig AW, Hunziker T. Idiopathic lenticular mucocutaneous pigmentation or Laugier–Hunziker syndrome with atypical features. *Arch Dermatol* 1996; **132**: 844–5.
6 Calnan CD. The Peutz–Jeghers syndrome. *Trans St John's Hosp Dermatol Soc* 1960; **44**: 58–64.
7 Bologa EI, Bene M, Pasztor P. Considerations sur la lentiginose eruptive de la face. *Ann Dermatol Syphiligr* 1965; **92**: 277–86.
8 Dupre A, Viraben R. Laugier's disease. *Dermatologica* 1990; **181**: 183–6.

Pseudoxanthoma elasticum

See Chapter 46.

Lentiginoses

The lentiginoses (or lentigenoses) include Peutz–Jeghers syndrome (Chapter 39) and the LEOPARD syndrome, which comprises:
- *l*entigines (multiple);
- *e*lectrocardiographic conduction abnormalities;
- *o*cular hypertelorism;
- *p*ulmonary stenosis;
- *a*bnormalities of genitalia;
- *r*etardation of growth; and
- *d*eafness.

The lentiginoses also include the syndrome of arterial dissections with lentiginosis, Laugier–Hunziker syndrome, Cowden disease, Ruvalcaba–Myhre–Smith (Bannayan–Zonana) syndrome, and the centrofacial, benign patterned and segmental lentiginoses, all of which can be associated with a variety of developmental defects.

Centrofacial lentiginosis syndrome

SYN. TOURAINE'S CENTROFACIAL LENTIGINOSIS

Centrofacial lentiginosis [1] is associated with bone abnormalities, malformations due to dysraphia, endocrine dysfunctions and neurological diseases.

REFERENCE

1 Dociu I, Galaction-Nitelea O, Sirjita N, Murgu V. Centrofacial lentiginosis. A survey of 40 cases. *Br J Dermatol* 1976; **94**: 39–43.

Complex of myxomas, spotty pigmentation and endocrine overactivity

SYN. CARNEY'S SYNDROME; CARNEY COMPLEX

This autosomal dominant trait causes cardiac and cutaneous myxomas, with mammary myxoid fibroadenomas, spotty cutaneous hyperpigmentation, primary pigmented nodular adrenocortical disease, testicular Sertoli cell tumours and growth hormone-secreting pituitary adenoma. It may present with oral hyperpigmentation and myxomas [1–4]. The hyperpigmentation in Carney complex is facial and occurs on the vermilion of the lips in about 35%, although about 8% have pigmented lesions on the oral mucosa and about 2% have oral myxomas, usually on the palate or tongue [2]. Carney complex differs clinically from Peutz–Jeghers syndrome in that hyperpigmentation is less common intraorally but more common on the conjunctiva, and other manifestations are also present.

Cases previously described as NAME syndrome (*n*aevi, *a*trial myxoma, *m*yxoid neurofibromas, *e*phelides) and LAMB syndrome (*l*entigines, *a*trial myxoma, *m*ucocutaneous myxoma, *b*lue naevi) may represent this complex, which also has close similarities to LEOPARD syndrome and the syndrome of arterial dissections with lentiginosis (see Chapter 39).

REFERENCES

1 Carney JA, Gordon H, Carpenter PC *et al*. The complex of myxomas, spotty pigmentation and endocrine overactivity. *Medicine (Baltimore)* 1985; **64**: 270–83.
2 Cook CA, Lund BA, Carney JA. Mucocutaneous pigmented spots and oral myxomas: the oral manifestations of the complex of myxomas, spotty pigmentation and endocrine overactivity. *Oral Surg* 1987; **63**: 175–83.
3 Ohara N, Takasu N, Komiya I *et al*. Case of Carney's syndrome with primary pigment nodular adrenocortical disease (PPNAD) and pigmented spots of the lips. *Nippon Naika Gakkai Zasshi* 1993; **82**: 1718–9.
4 Stratakis CA, Carney JA, Lin J-P *et al*. Carney complex, a familial multiple neoplasia and lentiginosis syndrome. *J Clin Invest* 1996; **97**: 699–705.

Inherited patterned lentiginosis in black people

This autosomal dominant condition is characterized by small, discrete, hyperpigmented macules on the face, lips, extremities, buttocks and palmoplantar areas [1]. No patients have been reported with oral mucosal lesions or internal organ system abnormalities.

This condition can resemble other lentiginosis syndromes, especially Peutz–Jeghers syndrome, centrofacial lentiginosis syndrome and Carney complex.

REFERENCE

1 O'Neill JF, James WD. Inherited patterned lentiginosis in blacks. *Arch Dermatol* 1989; **125**: 1231–5.

Naevi

Pigmented naevi are much less common in the oral mucosa than in skin. Approximately half of naevi are histologically of the intradermal (intramucosal) type; one-third are blue naevi, many others are compound naevi and some are junctional naevi.

Pathology. They are formed from increased melanin-containing cells, are flat or raised, do not change rapidly in size or colour, are painless and are seen particularly on the palate. The intramucosal type of naevus is most common (about 60%), while another 25% are blue naevi. Compound and junctional naevi and combined naevi are rare in the mouth. The intramucosal naevus consists of a collection of melanocytic cells in the lamina propria without involvement of the epithelium. The blue naevus consists of spindle cells at any level in the lamina propria. The junctional naevus consists of clusters of benign naevus cells at the epithelio-mesenchymal junction and the lamina propria is otherwise not involved.

Clinical features. Pigmented naevi are seen particularly on the vermilion border of the lip and on the palate or buccal mucosa [1]. These lesions are usually brown, macular, do not change rapidly in size or colour and are painless. The prognosis is good.

Treatment. There is no evidence that most naevi, except junctional naevi, progress to melanoma. However, they may resemble melanomas. If early detection of oral melanomas is to be achieved, all pigmented oral cavity lesions should be viewed with suspicion. Therefore, excision biopsy is recommended to exclude malignancy, because of the premalignant potential of some, particularly the junctional naevus, and for cosmetic reasons (Table 66.11). This is particularly important if the lesions are raised or nodular [2].

REFERENCES

1 Buchner A, Hansen LS. Pigmented nevi of the oral mucosa. *Oral Surg Oral Med Oral Pathol* 1980; **49**: 55–62.
2 Hansen LS, Buchner A. Changing concepts of the junctional naevus and melanoma. Review of the literature and report of a case. *J Oral Surg* 1981; **39**: 961–5.

Red lesions

Vascular anomalies

Hereditary haemorrhagic telangiectasia (see Chapter 51)

SYN. OSLER–RENDU–WEBER SYNDROME

This syndrome is characterized by multiple telangiectasia on the lips, perioral skin, oral and nasal mucosae [1,2] as

Table 66.11 Causes of mucosal pigmentation.

Localized
Amalgam tattoo
Ephelis (freckle)
Naevus
Malignant melanoma
Kaposi's sarcoma
Peutz–Jegher syndrome
Laugier–Hunziker syndrome
Melanotic macules
Complex of myxomas, spotty pigmentation and endocrine
    overactivity

Generalized
Racial
Localized irritation, e.g. smoking
Drugs, e.g. phenothiazines, antimalarials, minocycline,
    contraceptives, mephenytoin
Addison's disease
Nelson's syndrome
Ectopic adrenocorticotrophic hormone (e.g. bronchogenic
    carcinoma)
Heavy metals
Albright's syndrome
Other rare causes, e.g. haemochromatosis, generalized
    neurofibromatosis, incontinentia pigmenti
Malignant acanthosis nigricans

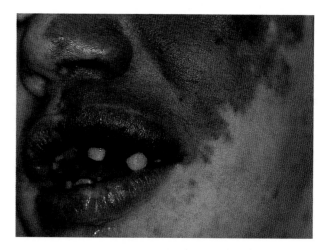

Fig. 66.19 Haemangioma affecting the lip in Sturge–Weber syndrome.

well as the gastrointestinal tract. Occasionally there are colonic or hepatic complications [3,4]. Oral haemorrhage can be controlled by cryotherapy, cautery, infrared coagulation or Nd-Yag laser [5,6].

REFERENCES

1 Flint SR, Keith O, Scully C. Hereditary haemorrhagic telangiectasia: family study and review. *Oral Surg* 1988; **66**: 440–4.
2 Christensen GJ. Nosebleeds may mean something much more serious: an introduction to HHT. *J Am Dent Assoc* 1998; **129**: 635–7.
3 Hisamura M, Akita K, Ide H. A case of Rendu–Osler–Weber disease associated with simultaneous, multiple advanced cancers in the colon. *Hokkaido Igaku Zasshi* 1994; **69**: 1468–75.
4 Selmaier M, Cidlinsky K, Ell C, Hahn EG. Liver hemangiomatosis in Osler's disease. *Dtsch Med Wochenschr* 1993; **118**: 1015–9.
5 Colver GB, Davies S, Bullock J. Infra red coagulation for bleeding mucosal telangiectasia. *J Laryngol Otol* 1992; **106**: 992–3.
6 Galletta A, Amato G. Hereditary hemorrhagic telangiectasia (Osler–Rendu–Weber disease). Management of epistaxis and oral hemorrhage by Nd-Yag laser. *Minerva Stomatol* 1998; **47**: 283–6.

Haemangioma

Haemangiomas are usually deep red or blue–purple, blanch on pressure, are fluctuant to palpation, and are level with the mucosa or have a lobulated or raised surface [2]. Most are small and of no consequence [1,2].

Most haemangiomas are seen in isolation but a few may be multiple and/or part of a wider syndrome such as Maffucci syndrome [3]. Large facial haemangiomas, which can involve the lips, may be associated with Sturge–Weber syndrome (Fig. 66.19) [3] or Dandy–Walker

syndrome, or other posterior cranial fossa malformations [4].

Haemangiomas are at risk from trauma and prone to excessive bleeding if damaged (e.g. during tooth extraction). Occasionally, oral haemangiomas develop phlebolithiasis.

Oral lesions suspected of being haemangiomatous should not be routinely biopsied; aspiration is far safer. Kaposi's sarcoma and epithelioid angiomatosis should be excluded. After intravenous administration of contrast medium, enhancement is observed in haemangiomas in areas corresponding to those with high signal on T_2-weighted magnetic resonance imaging (MRI).

Oral haemangiomas are left alone unless causing symptoms, when they are best treated with cryosurgery or laser if small, or by ligation or embolization of feeding vessels if large.

REFERENCES

1 Kaban LB, Mulliken JB. Vascular anomalies of the maxillofacial region. *J Oral Maxillofac Surg* 1986; **44**: 203–13.
2 Stal S, Hamilton S, Spira M. Haemangioma, lymphangioma and vascular malformations of the head and neck. *Otolaryngol Clin North Am* 1986; **19**: 769–96.
3 Scully C. Orofacial manifestations of the neurodermatoses. *J Dent Child* 1980; **47**: 255–60.
4 Reese V, Frieden IJ, Paller AS. Association of facial hemangiomas with Dandy–Walker and other posterior fossa malformations. *J Pediatr* 1993; **122**: 379–84.

Sturge–Weber–Krabbe syndrome [1–5] (see Chapter 15)

The haemangioma in the trigeminal area in Sturge–Weber syndrome is usually unilateral, may involve the mouth but fortunately rarely involves bone. It may be associated with hypertrophy of affected tissues and, if the patient is treated with phenytoin, with gingival hyperplasia [3].

REFERENCES

1 Uram M, Zubillaga C. The cutaneous manifestations of Sturge–Weber syndrome. *J Clin Neuro Ophthalmol* 1982; **2**: 245–8.
2 Scully C. Orofacial manifestations of the neurodermatoses. *J Dent Child* 1980; **47**: 255–60.
3 Huang JS, Chen CC, Wu YM *et al.* Periodontal manifestations and treatment of Sturge–Weber syndrome: report of two cases. *Kaohsiung J Med Sci* 1997; **13**: 127–35.
4 Ahluwalia TP, Lata J, Kanwa P. Sturge Weber syndrome with intraoral manifestations. A case report. *Indian J Dent Res* 1998; **9**: 140–4.
5 Terezhalmy GT, Riley CK. Clinical images in oral medicine. Encephalo-trigeminal syndrome (Sturge–Weber disease). *Quintessence Int* 2000; **31**: 62–3.

Klippel–Trenaunay–Weber syndrome (see Chapter 15)

Haemangiomas of the buccal mucosa and tongue, macroglossia, maxillary hyperplasia and an anterior open bite have been recorded in this syndrome [1–5]. Post-extraction bleeding can be a problem [6].

REFERENCES

1 Sciubba JJ, Brown AM. Oral–facial manifestations of Klippel–Trenaunay–Weber syndrome. *Oral Surg* 1977; **43**: 227–32.
2 Steiner M, Gould AR, Graves SM *et al.* Klippel–Trenaunay–Weber syndrome. *Oral Surg* 1987; **63**: 208–15.
3 Hallett KB, Bankier A, Chow CW, Bateman J, Hall RK. Gingival fibromatosis and Klippel–Trenaunay–Weber syndrome. Case report. *Oral Surg Oral Med Oral Pathol Oral Radiol Endod* 1995; **79**: 578–82.
4 Miteva LG, Dourmishev AI, Schwartz RA, Mitev VI. Oral vascular manifestations of Klippel–Trenaunay syndrome. *Cutis* 1998; **62**: 171–4.
5 Mueller-Lessmann V, Behrendt A, Wetzel WE, Petersen K, Anders D. Orofacial findings in the Klippel–Trenaunay syndrome. *Int J Paediatr Dent* 2001; **11**: 225–9.
6 Ita M, Okafuji M, Maruoka Y, Shinozaki F. An unusual postextraction hemorrhage associated with Klippel–Trenaunay–Weber syndrome. *J Oral Maxillofac Surg* 2001; **59**: 205–7.

Blue rubber–bleb naevus syndrome (see Chapter 15)
SYN. BEAN'S SYNDROME

Oral haemangiomas may be seen [1–3].

REFERENCES

1 Crosher RF, Blackburn CW, Dinsdale RCW. Blue rubber-bleb naevus syndrome. *Br J Oral Surg* 1988; **26**: 160–4.
2 Sumi Y, Taguchi N, Kaneda T. Blue rubber bleb nevus syndrome with oral hemangiomas. *Oral Surg Oral Med Oral Pathol* 1991; **71**: 84–6.
3 McKinlay JR, Kaiser J, Barrett TL, Graham B. Blue rubber bleb nevus syndrome. *Cutis* 1998; **62**: 97–8.

Maffucci's syndrome (see Chapter 15)

Oral haemangiomas may be seen [1–4].

REFERENCES

1 Laskaris G, Skouteris C. Maffucci syndrome: report of a case with oral haemangiomas. *Oral Surg* 1984; **57**: 263–6.
2 Yavuzyilmaz E, Yamalik N, Eratalay K, Atakan N. Oral–dental findings in a case of Maffucci's syndrome. *J Periodontol* 1993; **64**: 673–7.
3 Skouteris CA. More on hemangiomas in patients with Maffucci's syndrome. *J Oral Maxillofac Surg* 1994; **52**: 205.
4 Lee NH, Choi EH, Choi WK, Lee SH, Ahn SK. Maffucci's syndrome with oral and intestinal haemangioma. *Br J Dermatol* 1999; **140**: 968–9.

Hereditary mucoepithelial dysplasia

Hereditary mucoepithelial dysplasia is an autosomal dominant dyskeratotic epithelial syndrome affecting oral, nasal, vaginal, urethral, anal, bladder and conjunctival mucosae, causing cataracts, follicular keratosis, non-scarring alopecia and terminal lung disease [1–4].

Pathology. The condition is probably a pan-epithelial cell defect of desmosomal and gap junction structure. Histochemically there is a lack of cornification and keratinization. Electron microscopy shows an abnormality in desmosomes and gap junctions, with a lack of keratohyalin granules, a paucity of desmosomes, intercellular accumulations, cytoplasmic vacuolization, and formation of bands and aggregates of filamentous fibres and structures in the cytoplasm resembling desmosomes and gap junctions. There is some acantholysis as well as benign dyskeratosis of individual cells [1,2]. Histologically the mucosal epithelium shows dyshesion, thinning of the epithelial layer and dyskeratosis. Mucosal Papanicolaou smears show lack of epithelial maturation, cytoplasmic vacuoles and inclusions, and individual cell dyskeratosis.

Clinical features. Red, periorificial mucosal lesions are typically noted during infancy and may persist throughout life. The oral lesions are painless red macules or maculopapules and are seen predominantly on the palate and gingiva.

Severe photophobia, tearing and nystagmus in infancy herald the development of keratitis, corneal vascularization and lens cataracts.

In addition there may be various cardiorespiratory complications, especially potentially lethal bullous lung disease—spontaneous pneumothorax and bullous emphysema, terminating in cor pulmonale. Chronic rhinorrhoea and repeated upper respiratory infections frequently progress to bilateral pneumonia. Loss of hair, diarrhoea, melaena, enuresis, pyuria and haematuria may also be seen.

REFERENCES

1 Witkop CJ, White JG, Sank JJ *et al.* Clinical, histologic, cytologic and ultrastructural characteristics of the oral lesions from hereditary mucoepithelial dysplasia. *Oral Surg* 1978; **46**: 645–57.
2 Witkop CJ Jr, White JG, King RA *et al.* Hereditary mucoepithelial dysplasia: a disease apparently of desmosome and gap junction formation. *Am J Hum Genet* 1979; **31**: 414–27.
3 Scheman AJ, Ray DJ, Witkop CJ *et al.* Hereditary mucoepithelial dysplasia. *J Am Acad Dermatol* 1989; **21**: 351–7.
4 Rogers M, Kourt G, Cameron A. Hereditary mucoepithelial dysplasia. *Pediatr Dermatol* 1994; **11**: 133–8.

Wiskott–Aldrich syndrome (see Chapter 14)

Oral petechiae and infections such as candidiasis may occur in the Wiskott–Aldrich syndrome of thrombocytopenia, immune deficiency and eczema [1–3].

REFERENCES

1 Porter SR, Sugermann PB, Scully C et al. Orofacial manifestations in the Wiskott–Aldrich syndrome. J Dent Child 1994; **61**: 404–7.
2 Boraz RA. Dental considerations in the treatment of Wiskott–Aldrich syndrome: report of case. ASDC J Dent Child 1989; **56**: 225–7.
3 Walcott DW, Linehan T 4th, Hilman BC, Hershfield MS, el Dahr J. Failure to thrive, diarrhea, cough, and oral candidiasis in a three-month-old boy. Ann Allergy 1994; **72**: 408–14.

Vesiculoerosive disorders

Acrodermatitis enteropathica

Acrodermatitis enteropathica is an inborn error of metabolism resulting in zinc malabsorption and severe zinc deficiency [1–4].

Clinical features. Diarrhoea, mood changes, anorexia and neurological disturbance are reported most frequently in infancy. Growth retardation, alopecia, weight loss and recurrent infections are prevalent in affected toddlers and schoolchildren. A vesiculobullous dermatitis with perioral involvement may be seen, often sparing the vermilion [2]. Zinc deficiency during growth periods results in growth failure and lack of gonadal development in males. Other effects of zinc deficiency include skin changes, poor appetite, mental lethargy, delayed wound healing, neurosensory disorders and cell-mediated immune disorders. Skin lesions and poor wound healing are observed in severe forms and the disorder can be lethal.

Diagnosis. Assays of zinc in granulocytes and lymphocytes provide better diagnostic criteria for marginal zinc deficiency than plasma zinc assays. In cases of doubt, zinc absorption tests using radioisotopes (^{65}Zn or ^{69m}Zn) may be performed. Levels of alkaline phosphatase are reduced.

Management. Management includes zinc sulphate 2 mg/kg daily, at least until adult life.

REFERENCES

1 Van Wouwe JP. Clinical and laboratory diagnosis of acrodermatitis enteropathica. Eur J Pediatr 1989; **149**: 2–8.
2 Carr PM, Wilkin JK, Rosen T. Sparing of the vermilion border in an acrodermatitis enteropathica-like syndrome. Cutis 1983; **31**: 82–3.
3 Goskowicz M, Eichenfield LF. Cutaneous findings of nutritional deficiencies in children. Curr Opin Pediatr 1993; **5**: 441–5.
4 Prasad AS. Zinc: an overview. Nutrition 1995; **11** (Suppl.): 93–9.

Epidermolysis bullosa (see Chapter 40)

Epidermolysis bullosa is characterized by blisters, sometimes preceded by white patches, which develop rapidly, particularly where there is trauma. Blisters rupture to produce ulcers, often with eventual scarring, particularly in the recessive dystrophic types [1–5]. Oral lesions are fairly common in dystrophic and lethal forms of epidermolysis bullosa but are rare in most simplex types except the superficial type, where they are found in 70% of patients [2,6–8]. Overall, oral mucosal lesions are found in about 30% of patients with epidermolysis bullosa [1–5]. There is a predisposition to oral squamous cell carcinoma, mainly in the Hallopeau–Siemens type.

Dental hypoplasia and other defects and delayed tooth eruption may also be a feature, especially in junctional epidermolysis bullosa (Table 66.12) and, with the difficulty in maintaining adequate oral hygiene, there is a predisposition to caries [4].

Patients with recessive dystrophic epidermolysis bullosa suffer from severe growth inhibition due to reduced food intake as a result of severe oropharyngeal and oesophageal blistering or scarring, with smaller maxillae and smaller mandibles than normal [9–11]. Treatment is improved with modalities such as implants [12–14].

The oral manifestations in the various inherited forms of this condition are summarized in Table 66.12 and epidermolysis bullosa acquisita is discussed in Chapter 41.

REFERENCES

1 Album MM, Gaisin A, Leek WT et al. Epidermolysis bullosa dystrophica polydysplastica. Oral Surg 1977; **43**: 859–72.
2 Fine JD, Johnson L, Wright T. Epidermolysis bullosa simplex superficialis. Arch Dermatol 1989; **125**: 633–8.
3 Sedano HO, Gorlin RJ. Epidermolysis bullosa. Oral Surg 1989; **67**: 555–63.
4 Wright JT, Capps J, Johnson LB et al. Oral and ultrastructural dental manifestations of epidermolysis bullosa. J Dent Res 1988; **67**: 249.
5 Wright JT, Fine JD, Johnson L. Hereditary epidermolysis bullosa: oral manifestations and dental management. Pediatr Dent 1993; **15**: 242–7.
6 Pearson RW. Clinicopathologic types of epidermolysis bullosa and their non-dermatological complications. Arch Dermatol 1988; **124**: 718–25.
7 Rubenstein R, Esterly NB, Fine JD. Childhood epidermolysis bullosa acquisita. Arch Dermatol 1987; **123**: 772–6.
8 Nowak AJ. Oropharyngeal lesions and their management in epidermolysis bullosa. Arch Dermatol 1988; **124**: 742–5.
9 Kostara A, Roberts GJ, Gelbier M. Dental maturity in children with dystrophic epidermolysis bullosa. Pediatr Dent 2000; **22**: 385–8.
10 Shah H, McDonald F, Lucas V, Ashley P, Roberts G. A cephalometric analysis of patients with recessive dystrophic epidermolysis bullosa. Angle Orthod 2002; **72**: 55–60.
11 Harris JC, Bryan RA, Lucas VS, Roberts GJ. Dental disease and caries related microflora in children with dystrophic epidermolysis bullosa. Pediatr Dent 2001; **23**: 438–43.
12 Serrano Martinez C, Silvestre Donat FJ, Bagan Sebastian JV, Penarrocha Diago M, Alio Sanz JJ. Hereditary epidermolysis bullosa. Dental management of three cases. Med Oral 2001; **6**: 48–56.
13 Engineer L, Ahmed AR. Emerging treatment for epidermolysis bullosa acquisita. J Am Acad Dermatol 2001; **44**: 818–28.
14 Penarrocha-Diago M, Serrano C, Sanchis JM, Silvestre FJ, Bagan JV. Placement of endosseous implants in patients with oral epidermolysis bullosa. Oral Surg Oral Med Oral Pathol Oral Radiol Endod 2000; **90**: 587–90.

Table 66.12 Oral manifestations in epidermolysis bullosa (EB).

Type	EB subtype	Mucosal lesions	Dental hypoplasia
I Epidermolytic (simplex); autosomal dominant	Generalized (Koebner)	±	–
	Localized (Weber–Cockayne)	–	–
	Localized (Kallin)	–	Anodontia
	With mottled pigmentation and punctate keratoderma	+	–
	With bruising (Ogna)	–	±
	Herpetiform (Dowling–Meara)	+	–
	Superficial	+	–
II Junctional; autosomal recessive	Generalized, severe (Herlitz)	+	++
	Generalized, mild	+	+
	Localized	±	+
	Inverse	±	+
	Progressive	+	–
III Dermolytic (dystrophic) Autosomal dominant	Hyperplastic (Cockayne–Touraine)	±	–
	Albopapuloid (Pasini)	+	–
	Pretibial (Kuske–Portugal)	–	–
Autosomal recessive (Hallopeau-Siemens)	Localized	+	±
	Generalized	++	++
	Mutilating	+++	+++
	Inverse	+	–
VI Acquired type	Adult form	±	–
	Child form	+	–

–, absent; +, mild; ++, moderate; +++, severe.

Felty's syndrome

Oral ulceration may be seen in Felty's syndrome [1–3].

REFERENCES

1 Freeman NS, Plezia RA. Felty's syndrome. *Oral Surg Oral Med Oral Pathol* 1975; **40**: 409–13.
2 Holbrook WP, Turner EP, MacIver JE. Felty's syndrome. *Br J Oral Surg* 1979; **17**: 157–60.
3 Stanworth SJ, Bhavnani M, Chattopadhya C, Miller H, Swinson DR. Treatment of Felty's syndrome with the haemopoietic growth factor granulocyte colony-stimulating factor (G-CSF). *Q J Med* 1998; **91**: 49–56.

Immune defects

Mouth ulcers (and early-onset periodontitis) feature in congenital immune defects [1–7], including Chédiak–Higashi syndrome, Papillon–Lefèvre syndrome, familial neutropenia, cyclic neutropenia, Job's syndrome, chronic granulomatous disease and glycogen storage disease type 1b.

REFERENCES

1 Dougherty N, Gataletto MA. Oral sequelae of chronic neutrophil defects: case report of a child with glycogen storage disease type 1b. *Pediatr Dent* 1995; **17**: 224–9.
2 Porter SR, Scully C. Orofacial manifestations in primary immunodeficiencies: polymorphonuclear leukocyte defects. *J Oral Pathol Med* 1993; **22**: 310–1.
3 Porter SR, Scully C. Orofacial manifestations in primary immunodeficiencies: T lymphocyte defects. *J Oral Pathol Med* 1993; **22**: 308–9.
4 Porter SR, Scully C. Orofacial manifestations in primary immunodeficiencies involving IgA deficiency. *J Oral Pathol Med* 1993; **22**: 117–9.
5 Scully C. Orofacial manifestations in chronic granulomatous disease of childhood. *Oral Surg* 1981; **51**: 148–51.
6 Scully C, Macfadyen E, Campbell A. Oral manifestations in cyclic neutropenia. *Br J Oral Surg* 1982; **20**: 96–101.
7 Scully C, Porter SR. Orofacial manifestations in primary immunodeficiencies: common variable immunodeficiencies. *J Oral Pathol Med* 1993; **22**: 157–8.

Lumps and swellings

Hereditary angio-oedema (C1 esterase inhibitor deficiency)

Hereditary angio-oedema mimics allergic angio-oedema (see Chapter 47), although it produces a more severe reaction, with oedema affecting the lips, mouth, face and neck region, the extremities and gastrointestinal tract after minor trauma [1,2].

Blunt injury is the most consistent precipitating event. The trauma of dental treatment is a potent trigger, and some attacks even follow emotional stress. Oedema may persist for many hours and even up to 4 days. Involvement of the airway is a constant threat. The mortality may be as high as 30% in some families but the disease is compatible with prolonged survival if emergencies are avoided or effectively treated.

Diagnosis. In 85% of cases plasma C1 esterase levels are reduced (type 1 hereditary angio-oedema) but in 15% the enzyme is present but dysfunctional (type 2 hereditary angio-oedema). In both types, plasma C4 levels fall but C3 levels are normal.

Management. C1 esterase concentrates are available for treatment [3]. Plasminogen inhibitors such as tranexamic acid can be used to mitigate attacks [4], although more effective agents are the androgenic steroids danazol and stanozolol, which raise plasma C1 esterase inhibitor levels to normal [1,2].

REFERENCES

1 Cicardi M, Agostoni A. Hereditary angioedema. *N Engl J Med* 1996; **334**: 1666–7.
2 McCarthy NR. Diagnosis and management of hereditary angioedema. *Br J Oral Maxillofac Surg* 1985; **23**: 123–7.
3 Waytes AT, Rosen FS, Frank MM. Management of hereditary angioedema with a vapor heated C1 inhibitor concentrate. *N Engl J Med* 1996; **334**: 1630–4.
4 Crosher R. Intravenous tranexamic acid in the management of hereditary angio-oedema. *Br J Oral Maxillofac Surg* 1987; **25**: 500–6.

Focal dermal hypoplasia (see Chapter 12)
SYN. GOLTZ–GORLIN SYNDROME

Focal dermal hypoplasia is a rare, presumably X-linked, genodermatosis [1] involving developmental anomalies of tissues and organs of mesoectodermal origin. Thus there are abnormalities of the eyes, skin, musculoskeletal system, central nervous system (CNS) and oral structures.

Papillomas, usually of the oral mucosae and lips, dental anomalies and occasional cleft lip and palate are the main oral features [2,3]. The dental anomalies, seen in about half of affected individuals, include hypodontia, enamel defects and taurodontism [4–6].

REFERENCES

1 Greer RO, Reissner MW. Focal dermal hypoplasia: current concepts and differential diagnosis. *J Periodontol* 1989; **60**: 330–5.
2 Ishibashi A, Kurihara Y. Goltz's syndrome: focal dermal dysplasia syndrome (focal dermal hypoplasia). Report of a case and its etiology and pathogenesis. *Dermatologica* 1972; **144**: 156–60.
3 Valerius NH. A case of focal dermal hypoplasia syndrome (Goltz) with bilateral cheilo-gnatho-palatoschisis. *Acta Paediatr Scand* 1984; **63**: 287–90.
4 Stephen LX, Behardien N, Beighton P. Focal dermal hypoplasia: management of complex dental features. *J Clin Pediatr Dent* 2001; **25**: 259–61.
5 Baxter AM, Shaw MJ, Warren K. Dental and oral lesions in two patients with focal dermal hypoplasia (Goltz syndrome). *Br Dent J* 2000; **189**: 550–3.
6 McNamara T, Trotman CA, Hahessy AM, Kavanagh P. Focal dermal hypoplasia (Goltz–Gorlin) syndrome with taurodontism. *Spec Care Dent* 1996; **16**: 26–8.

Acanthosis nigricans (see Chapter 34)

Oral papilliferous lesions may be a feature of both familial [1,2] and malignant [1,3–6] acanthosis nigricans. Between 30 and 50% of patients with acanthosis nigricans secondary to neoplasia (malignant acanthosis nigricans) have oral lesions, which involve the tongue and lips predominantly.

REFERENCES

1 Sedano HO, Gorlin RJ. Acanthosis nigricans. *Oral Surg* 1987; **68**: 74–9.
2 Bazopoulou E, Laskaris G, Katsabas A *et al.* Familial benign acanthosis nigricans with predominant early oral manifestations. *Clin Genet* 1991; **50**: 160.
3 Mostofi RS, Hayden NP, Soltani K. Oral malignant acanthosis nigricans. *Oral Surg* 1983; **56**: 372–4.
4 Nomachi K, Mori M, Matsuda N. Improvement of oral lesions associated with malignant acanthosis nigricans after treatment of lung cancer. *Oral Surg* 1989; **68**: 74–9.
5 Cairo F, Rubino I, Rotundo R, Prato GP, Ficarra G. Oral acanthosis nigricans as a marker of internal malignancy. A case report. *J Periodontol* 2001; **72**: 1271–5.
6 Scully C, Barrett WA, Gilkes J, Rees M, Sarner M, Southcott RJ. Oral acanthosis nigricans, the sign of Leser-Trelat and cholangiocarcinoma. *Br J Dermatol* 2001; **145**: 506–7.

Lymphangioma (see Chapter 51)

Lymphangioma is uncommon in the mouth. At least some are hamartomas and many are of similar structure to haemangiomas and can clinically resemble them, with a 'frog-spawn' appearance, but they contain lymph rather than blood (Fig. 66.20).

Lymphangiomas are usually solitary and affect the tongue predominantly. They are occasionally associated with cystic hygroma [1–5].

Small lymphangiomas need no treatment. Larger lesions may require excision, although cryotherapy can be useful. Contrast-enhanced T_1-weighted MRI can be used to differentiate between lymphangiomas and deep haemangiomas [6]. One study has found blue, domed lymphangiomas on the alveolar ridges of about 4% of newborn black children [3]. These lesions, which were usually bilateral, often regressed spontaneously.

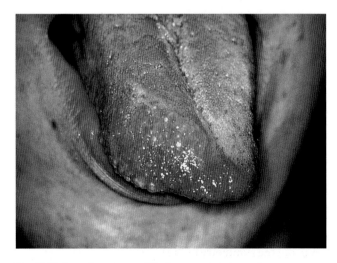

Fig. 66.20 Lymphangioma of the tongue: a common site.

REFERENCES

1 Karmody CS, Fortson JK, Calcaterra VE. Lymphangiomas of the head and neck in adults. *Otolaryngol Head Neck Surg* 1982; **90**: 283.
2 Tanaka N, Murata A, Yamaguchi A, Kohama G. Clinical features and management of oral and maxillofacial tumors in children. *Oral Surg Oral Med Oral Pathol Oral Radiol Endod* 1999; **88**: 11–5.
3 Levin LS, Jorgenson RJ, Jarvey BA. Lymphangiomas of the alveolar ridge in neonates. *Pediatrics* 1976; **56**: 881.
4 Flaitz CM. Oral and maxillofacial pathology case of the month. Lymphangioma. *Tex Dent J* 2000; **117**: 65, 112–3.
5 Schwab J, Baroody F. Lymphangioma circumscriptum: an unusual oral presentation. *Clin Pediatr* 1999; **38**: 619–20.
6 Yonetsu K, Nakayama E, Kawazu T *et al.* Value of contrast-enhanced magnetic resonance imaging in differentiation of hemangiomas from lymphangiomas in the oral and maxillofacial region. *Oral Surg Oral Med Oral Pathol Oral Radiol Endod* 1999; **88**: 496–500.

Dermoid cyst (see Chapter 15)

Dermoid cyst is a hamartoma, a developmental lesion commonly arising in the midline of the neck, above the mylohyoid muscle, occasionally elsewhere, even in the tongue or antrum [1–4]. It usually becomes clinically obvious in the second decade of life and causes elevation of the tongue.

Occasionally dermoid cysts become infected and then painful. Treatment is by surgical excision.

REFERENCES

1 Naritomi K. Oral dermoids. *Ryoikibetsu Shokogun Shirizu* 2001; **34**: 390–1.
2 Garcia Callejo FJ, Rosello Millat P, Alpera Lacruz R, Platero Zamarreno A, Jubert A. True double dermoid cyst of the tongue. *Acta Otorrinolaringol Esp* 2001; **52**: 626–32.
3 Halfpenny W, Odell EW, Robinson PD. Cystic and glial mixed hamartoma of the tongue. *J Oral Pathol Med* 2001; **30**: 368–71.
4 Torske KR, Benson GS, Warnock G. Dermoid cyst of the maxillary sinus. *Ann Diagn Pathol* 2001; **5**: 172–6.

Lingual tonsil

The lingual tonsil is a mass of lymphoid tissue in the posterior third of the tongue, between the epiglottis posteriorly and the circumvallate papillae anteriorly [1,2]. It is usually divided in the midline by a ligament (Fig. 66.21). Although usually small and asymptomatic, it may become enlarged, especially in atopic individuals, in patients taking phenytoin or in some infections. It may be so prominent that it fills the vallecula and impinges against the epiglottis. If the lingual tonsil is large, it may cause a globus sensation, alteration of the voice, obstructive sleep apnoea or airways obstruction [3–6]. It tends to involute with increasing age.

Occasionally, there may be lingual tonsillitis with a red, swollen, painful tongue, fever and neutrophilia [7].

The condition must be distinguished from benign and malignant tumours of the tongue, including lingual thyroid, but the symmetry of the lingual tonsil and its midline division are helpful diagnostic pointers.

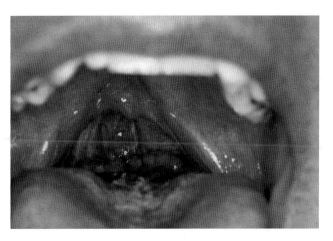

Fig. 66.21 Lingual tonsil showing a well-demarcated midline groove. (Courtesy of Dr C.T.C. Kennedy, Bristol Royal Infirmary, Bristol, UK.)

Treatment may be required if the enlarged tonsil causes symptoms. Surgery may be hazardous because of the copious blood supply to the tongue base. Electrocautery and cryotherapy are generally regarded as the safer procedures [1].

REFERENCES

1 Golding-Wood DG, Whittet HB. The lingual tonsil. A neglected symptomatic structure? *J Laryngol Otol* 1989; **103**: 922–5.
2 Hellings P, Jorissen M, Ceuppens JL. The Waldeyer's ring. *Acta Otorhinolaryngol Belg* 2000; **54**: 237–41.
3 Ralph WM Jr, Huh SK, Kim H. Phenytoin-induced lingual tonsil hyperplasia causing laryngeal obstruction. *Ann Otol Rhinol Laryngol* 2001; **110**: 790–3.
4 Salvi L, Juliano G, Zucchetti M, Sisillo E. Hypertrophy of the lingual tonsil and difficulty in airway control. A clinical case. *Minerva Anestesiol* 1999; **65**: 549–53.
5 Dell RG. Upper airway obstruction secondary to a lingual tonsil. *Anaesthesia* 2000; **55**: 393.
6 Marcos Ordonez M, Benito Orejas JI, Blasco Gutierrez MJ, Morais Perez D, Ramirez Cano B. Oropharyngeal tuberculosis. Report of a case in a lingual tonsil. *Acta Otorrinolaringol Esp* 1999; **50**: 575–8.
7 Joseph M, Reardon E, Goodman M. Lingual tonsillectomy: a treatment for inflammatory lesions of the lingual tonsil. *Laryngoscope* 1984; **94**: 179–84.

Lingual thyroid

Ectopic thyroid tissue may rarely present in the mouth. Some 10% of cadaver tongues contain thyroid tissue, although clinical presentation is much less common. Typically, there is an asymptomatic smooth-surfaced lump in the midline of the base of the tongue, between the sulcus terminalis and epiglottis at the site of the foramen caecum [1–4]. Occasionally, a lingual thyroid may produce dysphagia, cough, pain or, rarely, airways obstruction [1–10].

Not all lingual thyroid tissue is functional, and function tends to decline with age. Where thyroid-stimulating hormone levels are high, thyroid hormone supplements are indicated [1]. Malignant change is rare in lingual thyroid, although follicular carcinomas have been recorded. MRI and ^{99m}Tc pertechnetate scintiscanning is important to ensure the presence of normal thyroid tissue in the neck [11,12] before considering treatment of a lingual thyroid by surgery or radioiodine [1,2,13].

REFERENCES

1 Weider DJ, Parker W. Lingual thyroid. Review, case reports and therapeutic guidelines. *Ann Otol Rhinolaryngol* 1977; **86**: 841–5.
2 Jones JAH. Lingual thyroid. *Br J Oral Surg* 1986; **24**: 58–62.
3 Scott PM, Soo G, van Hasselt CA, Kew J. Lingual thyroid in a young woman. *Hong Kong Med J* 1997; **3**: 111.
4 Andrieux S, Douillard C, Nocaudie M *et al.* Lingual thyroid. A case report. *Ann Endocrinol* 2001; **62**: 538–41.
5 Oppenheimer R. Lingual thyroid associated with chronic cough. *Otolaryngol Head Neck Surg* 2001; **125**: 433–4.
6 Buckland RW, Pedley J. Lingual thyroid: a threat to the airway. *Anaesthesia* 2000; **55**: 1103–5.
7 Palmer JH, Ball DR. Lingual thyroid: another potential airway threat. *Anaesthesia* 2001; **56**: 386.
8 Koch CA, Picken C, Clement SC, Azumi N, Sarlis NJ. Ectopic lingual thyroid: an otolaryngologic emergency beyond childhood. *Thyroid* 2000; **10**: 511–4.
9 Gallo A, Leonetti F, Torri E *et al.* Ectopic lingual thyroid as unusual cause of severe dysphagia. *Dysphagia* 2001; **16**: 220–3.
10 Basaria S, Westra WH, Cooper DS. Ectopic lingual thyroid masquerading as thyroid cancer metastases. *J Clin Endocrinol Metab* 2001; **86**: 392–5.
11 Takashima S, Ueda M, Shibata A *et al.* MR imaging of the lingual thyroid. Comparison to other submucosal lesions. *Acta Radiol* 2001; **42**: 376–82.
12 Aktolun C, Demir H, Berk F, Metin Kir K. Diagnosis of complete ectopic lingual thyroid with Tc-99m pertechnetate scintigraphy. *Clin Nucl Med* 2001; **26**: 933–5.
13 Danner C, Bodenner D, Breau R. Lingual thyroid: iodine 131: a viable treatment modality revisited. *Am J Otolaryngol* 2001; **22**: 276–81.

Multiple mucosal neuroma syndrome

The syndrome of multiple endocrine neoplasia (MEN) type 2b (also called type 3) is inherited as an autosomal dominant, although new cases often arise sporadically. The gene locus is on chromosome 10.

MEN2b is characterized by medullary carcinoma of the thyroid and phaeochromocytoma, in association with multiple mucosal neuromas and an abnormal phenotype—a striking facial appearance, with thick, slightly everted lips that usually have a slightly bumpy surface due to multiple neuromas [1,2]. These are actually mucosal and submucosal hamartomatous proliferations of nerve axons, Schwann cells and ganglion cells.

Lesions may also involve the tongue and commissures but are less frequent on the buccal mucosa, gingivae, palate, pharynx or larynx (Fig. 66.22). Ganglioneuromatosis may also occur throughout the gastrointestinal tract, and this may result in constipation or megacolon [3]. Ocular changes include yellowish masses on the conjunctivae, thickened corneal nerves and keratitis due to decreased tear production [4].

Most patients have an asthenic marfanoid habitus, with high arched palate, pectus excavatum, arachnodactyly and kyphoscoliosis, but the lens subluxation and cardio-

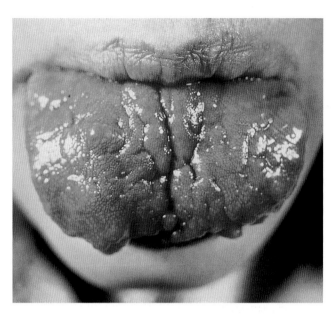

Fig. 66.22 Multiple neuromas of the lips and tongue in a patient with multiple endocrine neoplasia syndrome (type 2). (Courtesy of Dr M. Hartog, Bristol Royal Infirmary, Bristol, UK.)

vascular abnormalities of Marfan's syndrome are not present [5–8].

REFERENCES

1 Brown RS, Colle F, Tashjian AH. The syndrome of multiple endocrine neoplasia and medullary thyroid carcinoma in childhood: importance of recognition of the phenotype. *J Pediatr* 1975; **86**: 77–83.
2 Casino AJ, Sciubba J, Ohri JL *et al.* Oral–facial manifestations of the multiple endocrine neoplasia syndrome. *Oral Surg* 1981; **51**: 516–23.
3 Carney JA, Go VLW, Sizemore GW *et al.* Alimentary tract ganglioneuromatosis: a major component of the syndrome of multiple endocrine neoplasia. *N Engl J Med* 1976; **295**: 1287–91.
4 Colombo CD, Watson AG. Ophthalmological manifestations of the multiple endocrine neoplasia type 3 syndrome. *Can J Ophthalmol* 1976; **11**: 290–4.
5 Montgomery TB, Mandelstam P, Tachman ML. Multiple endocrine neoplasia type IIB: a description of several patients and review of the literature. *J Clin Hypertens* 1987; **3**: 31–49.
6 Ohishi M, Ishii T, Shiratsychi H, Tashiro H. Mucosal endocrine neoplasia type 3: three cases with mucosal neuromata. *Br J Oral Maxillofac Surg* 1990; **28**: 317–21.
7 Rashid R, Khairi MRA, Dexter RN. Mucosal neuroma pheochromocytoma and medullary thyroid carcinoma: multiple endocrine neoplasia Type III. *Medicine* 1975; **54**: 89–112.
8 Schimke RN. Multiple endocrine adenomatosis syndromes. *Adv Intern Med* 1976; **21**: 249–65.

Other congenital anomalies

Ankyloglossia

Ankyloglossia, or tongue-tie, is an uncommon and typically isolated anomaly in which the lingual fraenum is tight and the tongue cannot be fully protruded [1].

There may be a family history and sometimes deviation of the epiglottis or larynx [2]. The association of cleft palate with ankyloglossia is inherited as a semi-dominant

X-linked disorder previously described in several large families of different ethnic origins and related to chromosome Xq21: the T-box transcription factor gene *TBX22* is mutated [3,4].

Speech is not usually affected in patients with ankyloglossia but the ability to suckle [5] and to cleanse the buccal sulcus with the tongue may be, and there can be effects on jaw development [6]. If necessary, surgery to the fraenum will relieve ankyloglossia [7,8].

REFERENCES

1 Kern I. Tongue tie. *Med J Aust* 1991; **155**: 33–4.
2 Mukai S, Mukai C, Asaoka K. Ankyloglossia with deviation of the epiglottis and larynx. *Ann Otol Rhinol Laryngol* 1991; **100**: 3–19.
3 Braybrook C, Doudney K, Marcano AC *et al*. The T-box transcription factor gene TBX22 is mutated in X-linked cleft palate and ankyloglossia. *Nat Genet* 2001; **29**: 179–83.
4 Braybrook C, Warry G, Howell G *et al*. Physical and transcriptional mapping of the X-linked cleft palate and ankyloglossia (CPX) critical region. *Hum Genet* 2001; **108**: 537–45.
5 Notestine GE. The importance of the identification of ankyloglossia (short lingual frenulum) as a cause of breast feeding problems. *J Hum Lact* 1990; **6**: 113–5.
6 Defabianis P. Ankyloglossia and its influence on maxillary and mandibular development. (A seven year follow-up case report.) *Funct Orthod* 2000; **17**: 25–33.
7 Messner AH, Lalakea ML. Ankyloglossia: controversies in management. *Int J Pediatr Otorhinolaryngol* 2000; **54**: 123–31.
8 Kotlow LA. Ankyloglossia (tongue-tie): a diagnostic and treatment quandary. *Quintessence Int* 1999; **30**: 259–62.

Fissured tongue

Fissured tongue (plicated or scrotal tongue) is a common condition affecting more than 5% of the population [1]. The cause is unclear, but it is often accompanied by geographical tongue (Fig. 66.23).

Patients with Down's syndrome often have a fissured tongue and it is a feature of the rare Melkersson–Rosenthal syndrome.

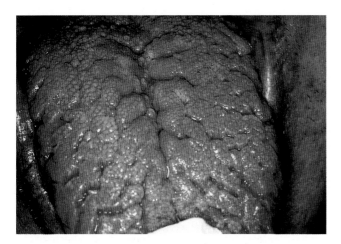

Fig. 66.23 Fissured or scrotal tongue.

REFERENCE

1 Kullaa-Mikkonen A, Sorvari T, Kotilainen R *et al*. Morphological variations on the dorsal surface of the human tongue. *Proc Finn Dent Soc* 1985; **81**: 104–10.

Oral hair

Oral hair is a rare innocuous anomaly [1], not to be confused with hairy tongue (see p. 66.90).

REFERENCE

1 Baughman RA, Heidrich PD. The oral hair: an extremely rare phenomenon. *Oral Surg* 1980; **49**: 530–1.

Various orocutaneous syndromes

Cleft lip

Cleft lip and/or palate are the most common congenital craniofacial abnormalities. Cleft lip occurs in about 1 per 1000 white-skinned neonates. The prevalence is higher in oriental neonates (about 1.7 per 1000 births) and lower in black neonates (approximately 1 per 2500 births) and appears reduced if women take multivitamins containing folic acid early in pregnancy [1]. Clefts are often accompanied by impaired facial growth, dental anomalies, speech disorders, poor hearing and psychosocial problems [2]. Clefts can be seen in over 300 different syndromes [3].

Cleft lip is not always complete (i.e. extending into the nostril). A cleft may involve only the upper lip or may extend to involve the nostril and the hard and soft palates. In about 9% of the cases, the cleft is associated with skin bridges or Simonart's bands.

Isolated cleft lip may be unilateral or bilateral (approximately 20%). When unilateral, the cleft is more common on the left side (about 70%).

Lips are more frequently cleft bilaterally (approximately 25%) when combined with cleft palate. Cleft lip and palate is more common in men. Cleft lip and palate comprises about 50% of the cases, with cleft lip and isolated cleft palate each comprising about 25%. About 85% of bilateral cleft lips and 70% of unilateral cleft lips are associated with cleft palate. One subgroup have cleft lip and palate with median facial dysplasia and cerebrofacial malformations [4], others with laryngotracheal oesophageal clefts (Opitz–Firas or G syndrome) or cranial asymmetry (Opitz or B syndrome) [5].

Clefts in the middle of the upper lip may be true or false. True median clefts have been described in association with bifid nose and ocular hypertelorism. Other cases of true median labial cleft are associated with polydactyly or other digital anomalies, constituting an autosomal recessive trait called *orofaciodigital syndrome II*.

Pseudocleft of the middle of the upper lip may occur in *orofaciodigital syndrome I*. A somewhat similar central defect, but of mild degree, is seen in chondroectodermal dysplasia (Ellis–van Creveld syndrome). Clefts in the lower lip are rare and usually median but may involve the mandible and sometimes the tongue. Management of cleft lip is discussed elsewhere [6,7].

REFERENCES

1 Shaw GM, Lammer EJ, Wasserman CR *et al.* Risks of orofacial clefts in children born to women using multivitamins containing folic acid periconceptionally. *Lancet* 1995; **346**: 393–6.
2 Habel A, Sell D, Mars M. Management of cleft lip and palate. *Arch Dis Child* 1996; **74**: 360–6.
3 Cohen MM, Bankier A. Syndrome delineation involving orofacial clefting. *Cleft Palate J* 1991; **28**: 119–20.
4 Noordhoff MS, Huang C-S, Lo L-J. Median facial dysplasia in unilateral and bilateral cleft lip and palate: a subgroup of median cerebrofacial malformations. *Plast Reconstr Surg* 1993; **91**: 966–1005.
5 Bershof JF, Guyuron B, Olsen MM. G syndrome: a review of the literature and a case report. *J Craniomaxillofac Surg* 1992; **20**: 24–7.
6 Kaufman FL. Managing the cleft lip and palate patient. *Pediatr Clin North Am* 1991; **38**: 1127–47.
7 Melnick J. Cleft lip with or without cleft palate. *Can Dent Assoc J* 1986; **14**: 92–8.

Cowden's syndrome (see Chapter 12)
SYN. MULTIPLE HAMARTOMA SYNDROME

Cowden's syndrome may be associated with the *PTEN* gene [1] and multiple hamartomas [2]. Oral mucosal lesions may be found in the presence or absence of cutaneous stigma [3–7]. The oral lesions are typically smooth, pink or whitish benign fibromas found especially on the palatal, gingival and labial mucosae. Oral squamous carcinoma is a rare complication [8]. There may be overlap with Bannayan–Riley–Ruvalcaba syndrome [9,10].

Treatment with acitretin may lead to regression of the hypertrophic lesions of the lip and mouth [11].

REFERENCES

1 Kato N, Kimura K, Sugawara H *et al.* Germline mutation of the PTEN gene in a Japanese patient with Cowden's disease. *Int J Oncol* 2001; **18**: 1017–22.
2 Cohen MM Jr. Some neoplasms and some hamartomatous syndromes: genetic considerations. *Int J Oral Maxillofac Surg* 1998; **27**: 363–9.
3 Rosenberg-Gertzman CB, Clark M, Gaston B. Multiple hamartoma and neoplasia syndrome (Cowden's syndrome). *Oral Surg* 1980; **49**: 314–6.
4 Swart JGN, Lekkas C, Allard RHB. Oral manifestations in Cowden's syndrome. *Oral Surg* 1985; **59**: 264–8.
5 Porter SR, Cawson RA, Scully C, Eveson JW. Multiple hamartoma syndromes presenting with oral lesions. *Oral Surg* 1996; **82**: 295–301.
6 Almenar Beso R, Bagan Sebastian JV, Milian Masanet MA, Jimenez Soriano Y. Cowden syndrome: clinical case presentation with oral lesions. *An Med Interna* 2001; **18**: 426–8.
7 Chaudhry SI, Shirlaw PJ, Morgan PR, Challacombe SJ. Cowden's syndrome (multiple hamartoma and neoplasia syndrome): diagnostic dilemmas in three cases. *Oral Dis* 2000; **6**: 248–52.
8 Shapiro SD, Lambert WC, Schwartz RA. Cowden's disease: a marker for malignancy. *Int J Dermatol* 1988; **27**: 232–7.
9 Starink TM, van Der Veen JP, Arwert F. The Cowden syndrome: a clinical and genetic study in 21 patients. *Clin Genet* 1986; **29**: 222–33.
10 Perriard J, Saurat JH, Harms M. An overlap of Cowden's disease and Bannayan–Riley–Ruvalcaba syndrome in the same family. *J Am Acad Dermatol* 2000; **42**: 348–50.
11 Cnudde F, Boulard F, Muller P, Chevallier J, Teron-Abou B. Cowden disease: treatment with acitretine. *Ann Dermatol Vénéréol* 1996; **123**: 739–41.

De Lange syndrome
SYN. AMSTERDAM DWARF

Classical Brachmann or Cornelia de Lange syndrome presents with a striking face, pronounced growth and learning disability, and variable limb deficiencies. Most cases are sporadic [1]. A long philtrum and crescent-shaped mouth with down-turned corners is typical [2,3].

The characteristic face of classical de Lange syndrome is present at birth and changes little throughout life, although there is some lengthening of the face with age and the jaw becomes squared.

REFERENCES

1 Allanson JE, Hennekam RC, Ireland M. De Lange syndrome: subjective and objective comparison of the classical and mild phenotypes. *J Med Genet* 1997; **34**: 645–50.
2 Scully C. The de Lange syndrome. *J Oral Med* 1980; **35**: 32–4.
3 Barrett AW, Griffiths MJ, Scully C. The Cornelia de Lange syndrome in association with a bleeding tendency. *Int J Oral Maxillofac Surg* 1993; **22**: 171–2.

Double lip

Double lip is a developmental anomaly usually involving the upper lip. A fold of redundant tissue is found on the inner aspect of the involved lip [1]. It is reported to be common among some groups of Africans [2].

Double lip may occur alone or in association with other anomalies. The association with blepharochalasis (laxity of the upper eyelid skin) and sometimes non-toxic thyroid enlargement is known as *Ascher's syndrome* [3] (see Chapter 46).

Double lip requires no treatment except for cosmetic purposes.

REFERENCES

1 Beumeir P, Weinberg A, Neuman A *et al.* Congenital double lip: report of five cases and a review of the literature. *Ann Plast Surg* 1992; **28**: 180–2.
2 Sawyer DR, Taiwo EO, Mosadomi A. Oral anomalies in Nigerian children. *Community Dent Oral Epidemiol* 1984; **12**: 269–33.
3 Halling F, Sandrock D, Merten HA *et al.* Das Ascher Syndrom. *Dtsch Z Mund Kiefer Gesichtschrift* 1991; **15**: 440–4.

Down's syndrome

The incidence of angular cheilitis is increased in people with Down's syndrome, caused by an increased level of *Staphylococcus aureus* and *Candida albicans*, possibly because of the immune defects [1–3]. Lip fissures may appear intermittently over a period of years or be intractable and long-standing (see p. 66.120).

REFERENCES

1 Butterworth T, Leoni EP, Beerman H. Cheilitis of mongolism. *J Invest Dermatol* 1960; **35**: 347–52.
2 Scully C, Van Bruggen W, Dios P, Porter S, Davison MF. Down syndrome: lip lesions (angular stomatitis and fissures) and *Candida albicans*. *Br J Dermatol* 2002; **147**: 37–40.
3 Carlstedt K, Krekmanova L, Dahllof G et al. Oral carriage of *Candida* species in children and adolescents with Down syndrome. *Int J Paediatr Dent* 1996; **6**: 95–100.

Erythropoietic protoporphyria

Erythropoietic protoporphyria is an autosomal dominant disorder of ferrochelatase, resulting in inhibition of the conversion of protoporphyrin to haem.

Shallow elliptical or linear scars around the lips and linear perioral furrowing (pseudorhagades) are subtle changes that are pathognomonic when observed in children [1,2].

REFERENCES

1 Gross U, Frank M, Doss MO. Hepatic complications of erythropoietic protoporphyria. *Photodermatol Photoimmunol Photomed* 1998; **14**: 52–7.
2 Lim HW, Murphy GM. The porphyrias. *Clin Dermatol* 1996; **14**: 375–87.

Focal mucinosis

Oral focal mucinosis is an uncommon clinicopathological entity considered to be the oral counterpart of cutaneous focal mucinosis and/or cutaneous myxoid cyst. The nature of the lesion is unclear but may be the result of fibroblastic overproduction of hyaluronic acid. It comprises a clinically elevated mass with a histological picture of localized areas of myxomatous connective tissue. Most of the lesions affect the gingiva and alveolar mucosa [1–3].

All these diseases share distinct histological features. There is an increased number of fibroblast-like cells in early lesions, whereas these are diminished or predominantly at the margin in advanced ones. The myxomatous areas show slight to absent reticulum and elastic fibres, and collagen fibres are fragmented and replaced by variable amounts of mucin. Vimentin is consistently present and correlates with the number of fibroblast-like cells, these being negative for S-100 protein, Leu7, desmin and α-SMA [4].

REFERENCES

1 Saito I, Ide F, Enomoto T, Kudo I. Oral focal mucinosis. *J Oral Maxillofac Surg* 1985; **43**: 372–4.
2 Buchner A, Merrell PW, Leider AS, Hansen LS. Oral focal mucinosis. *Int J Oral Maxillofac Surg* 1990; **19**: 337–40.
3 Soda G, Baiocchini A, Bosco D, Nardoni S, Melis M. Oral focal mucinosis of the tongue. *Pathol Oncol Res* 1998; **4**: 304–7.
4 Wilk M, Schmoeckel C. Cutaneous focal mucinosis: a histopathological and immunohistochemical analysis of 11 cases. *J Cutan Pathol* 1994; **21**: 446–52.

Gardner's syndrome (see Chapter 12)

Multiple jaw osteomas are a feature of Gardner's syndrome of familial adenomatous polyposis coli [1,2]. Some 80% of patients with familial adenomatosis coli have osteomas and 30% have dental anomalies such as supernumerary or impacted teeth, or odontomes [3–9].

REFERENCES

1 Gardner EJ. Familial polyposis coli and Gardner's syndrome: is there a difference? *Prog Clin Biol Res* 1983; **115**: 39–43.
2 Perniciaro C. Gardner's syndrome. *Dermatol Clin* 1995; **13**: 51–6.
3 Sondergaard JO, Bulow S, Jarvinen H et al. Dental anomalies in familial adenomatous polyposis coli. *Acta Odontol Scand* 1987; **45**: 61–3.
4 Wolfe J, Jarvinen HJ, Hietanen J. Gardner's dento-maxillary stigmas in patients with familial adenomatosis coli. *Br J Oral Maxillofac Surg* 1986; **24**: 410–6.
5 Cohen MM Jr. Perspectives on craniofacial asymmetry. VI. The hamartoses. *Int J Oral Maxillofac Surg* 1995; **24**: 195–200.
6 Takeuchi T, Takenoshita Y, Kubo K, Iida M. Natural course of jaw lesions in patients with familial adenomatosis coli (Gardner's syndrome). *Int J Oral Maxillofac Surg* 1993; **22**: 226–30.
7 Lew D, DeWitt A, Hicks RJ, Cavalcanti MG. Osteomas of the condyle associated with Gardner's syndrome causing limited mandibular movement. *J Oral Maxillofac Surg* 1999; **57**: 1004–9.
8 Yuasa K, Yonetsu K, Kanda S et al. Computed tomography of the jaws in familial adenomatosis coli. *Oral Surg Oral Med Oral Pathol* 1993; **76**: 251–5.
9 Jones K, Korzcak P. The diagnostic significance and management of Gardner's syndrome. *Br J Oral Maxillofac Surg* 1990; **28**: 80–4.

Gorlin's syndrome (naevoid basal cell carcinoma syndrome) (see Chapter 36)

Odontogenic keratocysts (primordial cysts) of the jaws are a prominent feature of Gorlin's syndrome [1–3]. The syndrome is caused by mutations in the Sonic Hedgehog *patched* gene, a tumour-suppressor gene [4]. A single point mutation in one *patched* allele may be responsible for the various malformations found in the syndrome [5–10]. Inactivation of both *patched* alleles results in the formation of tumours and cysts (basal cell carcinomas, odontogenic keratocysts and medulloblastomas) [4].

The keratocysts should be surgically removed but have a tendency to recur. There are also occasional reports of oral neoplasms, notably fibrosarcoma, ameloblastoma and squamous carcinoma [5–10].

REFERENCES

1 Gorlin RJ. Nevoid basal-cell carcinoma syndrome. *Medicine* 1987; **66**: 98–113.
2 Mirowski GW, Liu AA, Parks ET, Caldemeyer KS. Nevoid basal cell carcinoma syndrome. *J Am Acad Dermatol* 2000; **43**: 1092–3.
3 Cohen MM. Nevoid basal cell carcinoma syndrome: molecular biology and new hypotheses. *Int J Oral Maxillofac Surg* 1999; **28**: 216–23.
4 Zedan W, Robinson PA, Markham AF, High AS. Expression of the Sonic Hedgehog receptor 'PATCHED' in basal cell carcinomas and odontogenic keratocysts. *J Pathol* 2001; **194**: 473–7.
5 MacIntyre DR, Hislop SWG, Ross JW et al. The basal cell naevus syndrome. *Dental Update* 1985; **12**: 630–5.
6 Myoung H, Hong SP, Hong SD et al. Odontogenic keratocyst: review of 256 cases for recurrence and clinicopathologic parameters. *Oral Surg Oral Med Oral Pathol Oral Radiol Endod* 2001; **91**: 328–33.

7 Lo Muzio L, Nocini PF, Savoia A *et al.* Nevoid basal cell carcinoma syndrome. Clinical findings in 37 Italian affected individuals. *Clin Genet* 1999; **55**: 34–40.
8 Moos KF, Rennie JS. Squamous cell carcinoma arising in a mandibular keratocyst in a patient with Gorlin's syndrome. *Br J Oral Surg* 1987; **25**: 280–4.
9 Lo Muzio L, Nocini P, Bucci P *et al.* Early diagnosis of nevoid basal cell carcinoma syndrome. *J Am Dent Assoc* 1999; **130**: 669–74.
10 Maroto MR, Porras JL, Saez RS, de los Rios MH, Gonzalez LB. The role of the orthodontist in the diagnosis of Gorlin's syndrome. *Am J Orthod Dentofacial Orthop* 1999; **115**: 89–98.

Jacob's disease

Jacob's disease is a rare condition consisting of new joint formation between the coronoid process of the mandible and the inner aspect of the zygomatic arch [1].

REFERENCE

1 de la Torre OE, Klok EV, Roig AM, Mommaerts MY, Ayats JP. Jacob's disease: report of two cases and review of the literature. *J Craniomaxillofac Surg* 2001; **29**: 372–6.

Kindler syndrome

Kindler syndrome is characterized by bulla formation, which starts at birth on areas of the skin that receive pressure and may lead to bilateral incomplete syndactylies involving all web spaces [1].

Oral lesions may include atrophy of the buccal mucosa, trismus (an inability to fully open the mouth) and a form of desquamative gingivitis [2].

Histology shows classical features of poikiloderma, namely epidermal atrophy with flattening of the rete ridges, vacuolization of basal keratinocytes, pigmentary incontinence and mild dermal perivascularization. Ultrastructural studies demonstrate reduplication of the basal lamina with branching structures within the upper dermis and cleavage between the lamina densa and the cell membrane of the keratinocytes. Antibody against type VII collagen shows extensive broad bands with intermittently discontinuous and reticular staining at the dermal–epidermal junction.

REFERENCES

1 Suga Y, Tsuboi R, Hashimoto Y, Yaguchi H, Ogawa H. Japanese case of Kindler syndrome. *Int J Dermatol* 2000; **39**: 284–6.
2 Ricketts DNJ, Morgan CL, McGregor JM, Morgan PR. Kindler syndrome: a rare cause of desquamative lesions of the gingiva. *Oral Surg Oral Med Oral Pathol* 1997; **84**: 488–91.

Lip pits and sinuses

Dimples are common at the commissures. They should be distinguished from *commissural pits*, which are distinct definite pits ranging from 1 to 4 mm in diameter and depth [1,2] present from infancy, often showing a familial tendency and probably determined by a dominant gene

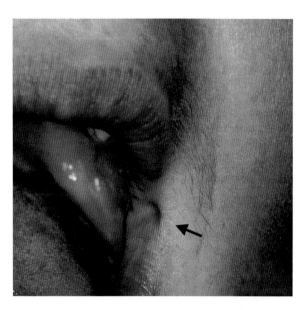

Fig. 66.24 Angular sinus (lip-pit), a congenital anomaly.

(Fig. 66.24). Their incidence is 1–20% in various population groups [2,3]; for example, in one series they were found in 12% of white people and 20% of black people [4]. Commissural pits are sometimes associated with aural sinuses or pits. Rarely, they may be infected and present as recurrent or refractory angular cheilitis.

Congenital lip pits or sinuses are small blind fistulae on the vermilion border [5]. They are usually bilateral and symmetrical, often just to one side of the philtrum. The pits may be up to 3–4 mm in diameter and up to 2 cm deep. They may communicate with underlying minor salivary glands. They may appear as isolated findings, but are often (67%) associated with cleft lip and/or palate (Van der Woude syndrome) [6–9]. This autosomal dominant syndrome [10,11] has a frequency of 1 in 75 000 to 1 in 100 000 in white populations (see Chapter 12).

Surgical removal may be indicated for cosmetic purposes.

REFERENCES

1 Witkop CJ, Barros L. Oral and genetic studies of Chileans, 1960. I. Oral anomalies. *Am J Phys Anthropol* 1963; **21**: 15–24.
2 Sedano HO. Congenital oral anomalies in Argentinian children. *Community Dent Oral Epidemiol* 1975; **3**: 61–3.
3 Everett FG, Wescott WB. Commissural lip pits. *Oral Surg Oral Med Oral Pathol* 1961; **14**: 202–9.
4 Baker B. Commissural lip pits. *Oral Surg* 1966; **21**: 56.
5 Watanabe Y, Igaku-Hakushi K, Otake K *et al.* Congenital fistulas of the lower lip. *Oral Surg Oral Med Oral Pathol* 1951; **4**: 709–22.
6 Van der Woude A. Fistula labii inferius congenita and its association with cleft lip and palate. *Am J Hum Genet* 1954; **6**: 244–56.
7 Gordon H, Davis D, Friedberg S. Congenital pits of the lower lip with cleft lip and palate. *S Afr Med J* 1969; **43**: 1275–9.
8 Rintala AE, Lahti AY, Gylling US. Congenital sinuses of the lower lip in connection with cleft lip and palate. *Cleft Palate J* 1970; **7**: 336–46.
9 Tan KL, Wong TT, Ong ES, Chiang SP. Congenital lip pits with cleft lip or palate. *J Singapore Paediatr Soc* 1971; **13**: 75–8.

10 Cervenka J, Gorlin RJ, Anderson VE. The syndrome of pits of the lower lip and cleft lip and/or palate. Genetic considerations. *Am J Hum Genet* 1967; **19**: 416–32.
11 Wang MK, Macomber WB. Congenital deformities of the lips. In: Converse MA, ed. *Reconstructive Plastic Surgery*. Philadelphia: Saunders, 1977: 1540–1.

Noonan's syndrome
SYN. ULLRICH–TURNER SYNDROME

Ullrich–Turner syndrome is caused by monosomy X or a structural abnormality of the second X chromosome. It is seen in females with a syndrome of short stature, sexual infantilism and a pattern of characteristic minor anomalies including pterygium colli. This syndrome was later called Noonan's syndrome, and it was shown that central giant cell lesions or cherubism of the jaws may be present [1–7]. Oral keratosis is sometimes seen [8].

REFERENCES

1 Nirmal T, Muthu MS, Arranganal P. Noonan syndrome: a case report. *J Indian Soc Pedod Prev Dent* 2001; **19**: 77–9.
2 Betts NJ, Stewart JC, Fonseca RJ, Scott RF. Multiple central giant cell lesions with a Noonan-like phenotype. *Oral Surg Oral Med Oral Pathol* 1993; **76**: 601–7.
3 Addante RR, Breen GH. Cherubism in a patient with Noonan's syndrome. *J Oral Maxillofac Surg* 1996; **54**: 210–3.
4 van Damme PA, Mooren RE. Differentiation of multiple giant cell lesions, Noonan-like syndrome, and (occult) hyperparathyroidism. Case report and review of the literature. *Int J Oral Maxillofac Surg* 1994; **23**: 32–6.
5 Levine B, Skope L, Parker R. Cherubism in a patient with Noonan syndrome: report of a case. *J Oral Maxillofac Surg* 1991; **49**: 1014–8.
6 Cohen MM Jr, Gorlin RJ. Noonan-like/multiple giant cell lesion syndrome. *Am J Med Genet* 1991; **40**: 159–66.
7 Dunlap C, Neville B, Vickers RA, O'Neil D, Barker B. The Noonan syndrome/cherubism association. *Oral Surg Oral Med Oral Pathol* 1989; **67**: 698–705.
8 Lucker GP, Steijlen PM. Widespread leucokeratosis in Noonan's syndrome. *Clin Exp Dermatol* 1994; **19**: 414–7.

Tuberous sclerosis (see Chapter 12)
SYN. EPILOIA; BOURNEVILLE DISEASE

Oral manifestations in tuberous sclerosis include pit-shaped enamel defects in both dentitions, and gingival fibromatosis [1–6] and rare instances of myxoma or desmoplastic fibroma [7,8].

REFERENCES

1 Lygidakis NA, Lindenbaum RH. Oral fibromatosis in tuberous sclerosis. *Oral Surg* 1989; **68**: 725–8.
2 Scully C. The orofacial manifestations of tuberous sclerosis. *Oral Surg* 1977; **44**: 706–16.
3 Smith D, Porter SR, Scully C. Gingival and other oral manifestations in tuberous sclerosis. *Periodont Clin Invest* 1993; **15**: 13–8.
4 Weits-Binnerts JJ, Hoff M, van Grunsven MF. Dental pits in deciduous teeth: an early sign in tuberous sclerosis. *Lancet* 1982; **ii**: 1344–5.
5 Cutando A, Gil JA, Lopez J. Oral health management implications in patients with tuberous sclerosis. *Oral Surg Oral Med Oral Pathol Oral Radiol Endod* 2000; **90**: 430–5.
6 Helling K, Flottmann T, Schmitt-Graff A, Scherer H. Manifestation of tuberous sclerosis in the ENT area. *HNO* 1996; **44**: 264–6.
7 Harrison MG, O'Neill ID, Chadwick BL. Odontogenic myxoma in an adolescent with tuberous sclerosis. *J Oral Pathol Med* 1997; **26**: 339–41.
8 Miyamoto Y, Satomura K, Rikimaru K, Hayashi Y. Desmoplastic fibroma of the mandible associated with tuberous sclerosis. *J Oral Pathol Med* 1995; **24**: 93–6.

Van der Woude syndrome

Van der Woude syndrome is a rare autosomal dominant syndrome [1] in which lower lip pits are associated with cleft lip and/or palate [2–5], sometimes seen with syndactyly or talipes equinovarus.

REFERENCES

1 Cervenka J, Gorlin RJ, Anderson VE. The syndrome of pits of the lower lip and cleft lip and/or palate. Genetic considerations. *Am J Hum Genet* 1967; **19**: 416–32.
2 Van der Woude A. Fistula labii inferius congenita and its association with cleft lip and palate. *Am J Hum Genet* 1954; **6**: 244–56.
3 Gordon H, Davis D, Friedberg S. Congenital pits of the lower lip with cleft lip and palate. *S Afr Med J* 1969; **43**: 1275–9.
4 Rintala AE, Lahti AY, Gylling US. Congenital sinuses of the lower lip in connection with cleft lip and palate. *Cleft Palate J* 1970; **7**: 336–46.
5 Vignale R, Araujo J, Pascal G et al. Van der Woude syndrome: a case report. *Pediatr Dermatol* 1998; **15**: 459–63.

Von Recklinghausen's neurofibromatosis

Neurofibromatosis (NF) consists of distinct variants due to *NF* gene mutations [1]: type I (NF-I), often referred to as von Recklinghausen's disease or generalized neurofibromatosis; and type II (NF-II), a much less common disorder of bilateral acoustic schwannomas. The incidence of head and neck manifestations in patients with NF varies between 14 and 37%. Cosmetic lesions include pigmentary changes (café-au-lait spots) and prominent neurofibromas [2–6].

Neurofibromas may be seen mainly in NF-I. Neurofibromas may also be seen in NF-II, but bilateral acoustic neuromas are the hallmark of this disease and neurilemmomas and acoustic neuromas are this predominant neural tumours. Neurofibromas may also be part of the MEN syndrome (see Chapter 59).

Oral lesions are not uncommon in von Recklinghausen's generalized NF [7–14]. About two-thirds of patients have intraoral neurofibromas affecting predominantly the tongue, lips, buccal mucosa or palate. Neurofibroma represents a benign overgrowth of all elements of a peripheral nerve (axon cylinder, Schwann cells and fibrous connective tissue), arranged in a variety of patterns. Enlarged fungiform papillae are found in about 50% of patients. About 60% of patients have radiographic evidence of disease, especially enlargement of the inferior alveolar canal or foramen, or branching of the canal.

Neurofibromas may occur multiply as a feature of NF but only rarely undergo sarcomatous change [15]. Other rare malignant tumours include nerve sheath tumour [16], triton tumour [17] and Merkel cell carcinoma [18].

REFERENCES

1 Buske A, Gewies A, Lehmann R *et al.* Recurrent NF1 gene mutation in a patient with oligosymptomatic neurofibromatosis type 1 (NF1). *Am J Med Genet* 1999; **86**: 328–30.

2 Scully C. Orofacial manifestations of the neurodermatoses. *J Dent Child* 1980; **47**: 255–60.

3 Keutel C, Vees B, Krimmel M, Cornelius CP, Schwenzer N. Oral, facial and cranial manifestations of von Recklinghausen neurofibromatosis (NF). *Mund Kiefer Gesichtschir* 1997; **1**: 268–71.

4 Sobol SE, Tewfik TL, Ortenberg J. Otolaryngologic manifestations of neurofibromatosis in children. *J Otolaryngol* 1997; **26**: 13–9.

5 Baart JA, van Hagen JM. Syndromes 18. Von Recklinghausen's disease. *Ned Tijdschr Tandheelkd* 2000; **107**: 57–9.

6 D'Ambroso JA, Langlais RP, Young RS. Jaw and skull changes in neurofibromatosis. *Oral Surg* 1988; **66**: 391–6.

7 Zuccoli G, Ferrozzi F, Tognini G, Troiso A. Enlarging tongue masses in neurofibromatosis type 1: MR findings of two cases. *Clin Imaging* 2001; **25**: 268–71.

8 Bekisz O, Darimont F, Rompen EH. Diffuse but unilateral gingival enlargement associated with von Recklinghausen neurofibromatosis: a case report. *J Clin Periodontol* 2000; **27**: 361–5.

9 Holtzman L. Radiographic manifestation and treatment considerations in a case of multiple neurofibromatosis. *J Endod* 1998; **24**: 442–3.

10 Allen CM, Miloro M. Gingival lesion of recent onset in a patient with neurofibromatosis. *Oral Surg Oral Med Oral Pathol Oral Radiol Endod* 1997; **84**: 595–7.

11 Curtin JP, McCarthy SW. Perineural fibrous thickening within the dental pulp in type 1 neurofibromatosis: a case report. *Oral Surg Oral Med Oral Pathol Oral Radiol Endod* 1997; **84**: 400–3.

12 Van Damme PA, Freihofer HP, De Wilde PC. Neurofibroma in the articular disc of the temporomandibular joint: a case report. *J Craniomaxillofac Surg* 1996; **24**: 310–3.

13 Geist JR, Gander DL, Stefanac SJ. Oral manifestations of neurofibromatosis types I and II. *Oral Surg Oral Med Oral Pathol* 1992; **73**: 376–82.

14 Gutteridge DL Neurofibromatosis: an unusual oral manifestation. *Br Dent J* 1991; **170**: 303–4.

15 Neville BW, Hann J, Narang R, Garen P. Oral neurofibrosarcoma associated with neurofibromatosis type I. *Oral Surg Oral Med Oral Pathol* 1991; **72**: 456–61.

16 Muraki Y, Tateishi A, Tominaga K *et al.* Malignant peripheral nerve sheath tumour in the maxilla associated with von Recklinghausen's disease. *Oral Dis* 1999; **5**: 250–2.

17 Shotton JC, Stafford ND, Breach NJ. Malignant triton tumour of the palate: a case report. *Br J Oral Surg* 1988; **26**: 120–3.

18 Antoniades K, Giannouli T, Kaisaridou D. Merkel cell carcinoma in a patient with Recklinghausen neurofibromatosis. *Int J Oral Maxillofac Surg* 1998; **27**: 213–4.

Xeroderma pigmentosum

Squamous cell carcinoma of the lip may arise in patients with xeroderma pigmentosum [1,2] and therefore it is crucial to institute sun protection. Oral retinoids such as etretinate or isotretinoin may be of prophylactic value [3,4]. Topical 5-fluorouracil or surgery may be used to treat potentially malignant lesions (see Actinic cheilitis, p. 66.115).

REFERENCES

1 Yagi KI, Prabhu S. Carcinoma of the lip in xeroderma pigmentosum. A case report. *J Oral Med* 1983; **38**: 97–8.

2 Laskaris G, Stavrou A. [Xeroderma pigmentosum with carcinoma of the lower lip.] *Hell Stomatol Chron* 1984; **28**: 107–9.

3 Berth-Jones J, Graham-Brown RAC. Xeroderma pigmentosum variant: response to etretinate. *Br J Dermatol* 1990; **122**: 559–61.

4 Kraemer KH, DiGiovanna JJ, Moshell AN. Prevention of skin cancer in xeroderma pigmentosum with the use of oral isotretinoin. *N Engl J Med* 1988; **318**: 1630–7.

Acquired disorders of the oral mucosa or lips

This section discusses the main acquired causes of mouth ulcers, other causes of oral soreness, white, pigmented or red lesions, and lumps and swellings. Further detail is available elsewhere [1–5].

REFERENCES

1 Neville BW, Damm DD, Allen CM, Bouquot JE. *Oral and Maxillofacial Pathology*. Philadelphia: Saunders, 1995.

2 Millard HD, Mason DK, eds. *Perspectives on 1998 World Workshop on Oral Medicine*. Michigan: University of Michigan, 2000.

3 Scully C. *ABC of Oral Health*. London: BMJ Books, 2000.

4 Scully C. *Handbook of Oral Disease: Diagnosis and Management*. London: Martin Dunitz, 1999.

5 Scully C, Flint S, Porter SR, Moos K. *Oral and Maxillofacial Diseases*. London: Martin Dunitz, 2004.

Mouth ulcers

The causes of mouth ulcers are diverse (Tables 66.10 & 66.13), partly because lesions such as vesicles rapidly break down in the mouth as a result of trauma, moisture and infection. Ulcers are usually caused by the following.

1 Local factors
2 Recurrent aphthous stomatitis
3 Neoplasms
4 Systemic conditions
   (a) Hematological
   (b) Gastroenterological
   (c) Dermatological
   (d) Infective
   (e) Vasculitis
   (f) Iatrogenic
   (g) Uncertain causes
5 Drugs.

Mouth ulcers of local aetiology

It is surprising that oral ulceration due to local factors is not more frequent. Accidental cheek biting or facial trauma may cause ulceration in any individual; the his-

Table 66.13 Causes of mouth ulcers (see also Table 66.10).

Local causes (e.g. trauma)
Recurrent aphthae (and Behçet's syndrome)
Malignant neoplasms
Ulcers associated with systemic disease
Drugs
Irradiation of the oral mucosa
Disorders of uncertain pathogenesis

tory is usually quite clear and a single ulcer of short duration (5–10 days) is present. Ulceration due to biting an anaesthetized lower lip or tongue following a dental local analgesic injection is a fairly common problem in young children.

Orthodontic appliances or, more commonly, dentures (especially if new) are responsible for many traumatic oral ulcers. These ulcers are usually clearly related to the appliance and have been a problem in the care of cleft-palate patients [1]. Chronic trauma may cause a well-defined ulcer with a whitish keratotic halo [2].

The possibility of some other aetiology for ulcers of apparently local cause should always be borne in mind. Child abuse may cause ulcers, especially over the upper labial fraena. Self-mutilation may be seen in some psychologically disturbed patients [3,4], patients with learning disability, individuals with sensory impairment, and in Lesch–Nyhan syndrome [5–9]. Oral purpura or ulceration may be seen on the lingual fraenum or palate due to cunnilingus or fellatio respectively [10]. Other local causes of ulceration include thermal burns, especially of the tongue and palate (e.g. 'pizza burn—now more common with microwave oven use'), chemical burns from the holding of medicaments or drugs (e.g. aspirin or cocaine) against the mucosa [11], and irradiation mucositis.

Prognosis. Most ulcers of local cause heal spontaneously within 7–14 days if the cause is removed.

Treatment. Maintenance of good oral hygiene and the use of hot saline mouthbaths and 0.2% aqueous chlorhexidine gluconate mouthwash aid healing. A 0.1% benzydamine mouthwash may help give relief. Occasionally, mechanical protection with a plastic guard may help [7].

Patients should be reviewed within 3 weeks to ensure healing has occurred. Any patient with a single ulcer lasting more than 2–3 weeks should be regarded with suspicion and investigated further, usually by biopsy—it may be a neoplasm or other serious disorder.

REFERENCES

1 Bacher M, Goz G, Pham T *et al*. Congenital palatal ulcers in newborn infants with cleft lip and palate: diagnosis, frequency and significance. *Cleft Palate J* 1996; **33**: 37–42.
2 Reade PC, Rich AM, Steidler NE. Peripheral keratosis on oral mucosal ulcers: a clinical sign of non-neoplastic disease. *Br J Oral Surg* 1984; **22**: 372–7.
3 Kotansky K, Goldberg M, Tenenbaum HC, Mock D. Factitious injury of the oral mucosa: a case series. *J Periodontol* 1995; **66**: 241–5.
4 Lamey PJ, McNab L, Lewis MAO, Gibb R. Oral artefactual disease. *Oral Surg* 1994; **77**: 131–4.
5 Scully C. The orofacial manifestations of the Lesch–Nyhan syndrome. *Int J Oral Surg* 1981; **10**: 380–3.
6 Stewart DJ, Kernohan DC. Self-inflicted gingival injuries: gingivitis artefacta, factitial gingivitis. *Dent Pract Dent Rec* 1972; **22**: 418–26.
7 Sugahara T, Mishima K, Mori Y. Lesch–Nyhan syndrome: successful prevention of lower lip ulceration caused by self-mutilation by use of mouth guard. *Int J Oral Maxillofac Surg* 1994; **23**: 37–8.
8 Cusumano FJ, Penna KJ, Panossian G. Prevention of self-mutilation in patients with Lesch–Nyhan syndrome: review of literature. *ASDC J Dent Child* 2001; **68**: 175–8.
9 Symons AL, Rowe PV, Romanink K. Dental aspects of child abuse. *Aust Dent J* 1987; **32**: 42–7.
10 Van Wyk CW. An oral lesion caused by fellatio. *Am J Forensic Med Pathol* 1981; **2**: 217–9.
11 Gendeh BS, Ferguson BJ, Johnson JT, Kapadia S. Progressive septal and palatal perforation secondary to intranasal cocaine abuse. *Med J Malaysia* 1998; **53**: 435–8.

Eosinophilic ulcer [1–4]

SYN. TRAUMATIC EOSINOPHILIC GRANULOMA

Eosinophilic ulcer is a rare self-limiting disease that often appears on the tongue in older adults or children. Its aetiology remains obscure and may be associated with traumatic factors. Eosinophilic ulcers are unifocal, with a benign course. Pathological features show an extensive inflammatory cell infiltration, with predominantly eosinophilic cells throughout the submucosa. The peripheral blood eosinophil count is normal. Diagnosis and treatment is with either conservative excision or incisional biopsy.

REFERENCES

1 Gao S, Wang Y, Liu N, Du Li S, J. Eosinophilic ulcer of the oral mucosa: a clinicopathological analysis. *Chin J Dent Res* 2000; **3**: 47–50.
2 El-Mofty SK, Swanson PE, Wick MR, Miller AS. Eosinophilic ulcer of the oral mucosa: report of 38 new cases with immunohistochemical observations. *Oral Surg* 1993; **75**: 716–22.
3 Elzay RP. Traumatic ulcerative granuloma with stromal eosinophilia (Riga–Fede disease and traumatic eosinophilic granuloma). *Oral Surg* 1983; **55**: 497–506.
4 Sklavounou A, Laskaris G. Eosinophilic ulcer of the oral mucosa. *Oral Surg* 1984; **58**: 431–6.

Recurrent aphthous stomatitis

SYN. APHTHAE; CANKER SORES

Recurrent aphthous stomatitis (RAS) is characterized by recurring episodes of ulcers, typically from childhood or adolescence, each lasting from 1 to about 4 weeks before healing. Aphthae typically are multiple round or ovoid ulcers with a circumscribed margin, erythematous halo and a yellow or grey floor (Fig. 66.25). The term 'recurrent oral ulcer' is rather imprecise and should be avoided [1–4].

Aetiology. The aetiology of RAS is not clear. A positive family history is found with about one-third of patients and there is an increased frequency of human leukocyte antigens (HLA)-A2, HLA-A11, HLA-B12 and HLA-DR2, supporting a genetic basis for susceptibility in some patients [1–4].

There are identifiable predisposing factors in some patients (Table 66.14). A minority (about 10–20%) of patients attending outpatient clinics with RAS have an

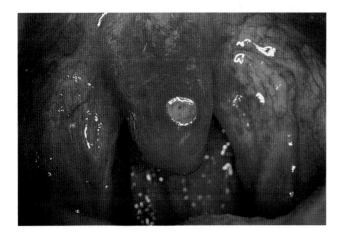

Fig. 66.25 Recurrent aphthae.

underlying haematological abnormality, usually a low serum iron or ferritin, or deficiency of folate or vitamin B_{12}. A few have multiple deficiencies [5,6]. Up to 3% of RAS patients have coeliac disease but in others a gluten-free diet is of no value [7]. Patients with deficiency states often, but not always, have gastrointestinal symptoms, and their RAS is often of recent onset. Other aetiological factors in RAS can include stress, trauma and cessation of tobacco smoking. Ulcers similar to aphthae are also seen in Behçet's syndrome; Sweet's syndrome; HIV infection, cyclic neutropenia and other immunodeficiencies; and, rarely, in children in association with fever and pharyngitis (periodic fever, aphthous stomatitis, pharyngitis and cervical adenitis; PFAPA) [8,9]. Orogenital ulceration with aphthae is probably a forme fruste of Behçet's syndrome.

There is no evidence that RAS is an autoimmune disease [1–4]. There is no known association with systemic autoimmune disorders, none of the common autoantibodies are found, and RAS tends to resolve or decrease spontaneously with increasing age. The serum immunoglobulin levels are usually normal, although IgA and IgG may be increased, and immune complexes may be found.

It now seems likely that there is a minor degree of immunological dysregulation underlying aphthae. Attempts to implicate a variety of viruses or bacteria in the aetiology of RAS have largely been unsuccessful, but there may be cross-reacting antigens between the oral mucosa and microorganisms such as *Streptococcus sanguis* or its L form, or heat-shock protein [10].

Cell-mediated immune mechanisms appear to be involved in the pathogenesis of RAS. In the lesions, helper T cells predominate early on, with some natural killer cells. Cytotoxic cells then appear and there is evidence for an antibody-dependent cellular cytotoxicity reaction [1–4].

Clinical features. RAS is a common disease that probably afflicts at least 20% of the population. There is a high prevalence in higher socio-economic classes.

There are three main clinical types of RAS. Most common are minor aphthous ulcers, which account for 80% of all RAS. Some 10% of patients with RAS have major aphthous ulcers, and a further 10% suffer from a herpetiform type of ulceration (Table 66.15).

Table 66.14 Systemic and other factors that may occasionally underlie or be associated with recurrent aphthous stomatitis (RAS).

	Comments
Behçet's syndrome	Association of RAS with ocular lesions, genital ulcers and multisystem disease
Sweet's syndrome	See Chapter 49
Haematinic deficiency	In some studies, 10–20% of patients with RAS have deficiencies of iron, folic acid or vitamin B_{12}
Gastrointestinal disease	Malabsorption states (pernicious anaemia, coeliac disease and Crohn's disease) may precipitate RAS in a small minority
Endocrine factors	In some women, RAS is clearly related to a fall in progestogens in the luteal phase of the menstrual cycle; hormone therapy may be beneficial
Immunodeficiency	A few patients with RAS have an immune defect such as human immunodeficiency virus disease
Other factors	Trauma, certain foods, stress and cessation of smoking may play a part

Table 66.15 Main features of recurrent aphthous stomatitis.

	Minor aphthae	Major aphthae	Herpetiform ulcers
Age of onset	Childhood or adolescence	Childhood or adolescence	Young adult
Ulcer size	2–4 mm	May be 10 mm or larger	Initially tiny but ulcers coalesce
Number of ulcers	Up to about 6	Up to about 6	10–100
Sites affected	Mainly vestibule, labial, buccal mucosa and floor of mouth; rarely dorsum of tongue, gingiva or palate	Any site	Any site but often on ventrum of tongue
Duration of each ulcer	Up to 10 days	Up to 1 month	Up to 1 month
Other comments	Most common type of aphthae	May heal with scarring	Affects females predominantly

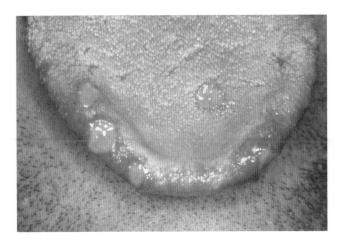

Fig. 66.26 Major aphthous ulcers.

Minor aphthous ulcers (syn. Mikulicz ulcers). Minor RAS (MiRAS) occur mainly in the 10–40-year age group, and often cause minimal symptoms. MiRAS are usually 2–4 mm in diameter and found mainly on the non-keratinized mobile mucosa of the lips, cheeks and floor of the mouth, sulci or ventrum of the tongue. They are uncommon on the gingiva, palate or dorsum of the tongue. Only a few ulcers (one to six) appear at a time; they heal in 7–10 days and recur at variable intervals. MiRAS are usually round or ovoid, but are often more linear when in the buccal sulcus, a common site. The ulcer floor is initially yellowish but becomes greyish as epithelialization proceeds. There is an erythematous halo and some oedema but MiRAS heal with little or no evidence of scarring.

Major aphthous ulcers (syn. Sutton's ulcers). Previously known as periadenitis mucosa necrotica recurrens (PMNR), major RAS (MaRAS) are larger, recur more frequently, last longer and are more painful than MiRAS. They may reach a large size, even more than 1 cm in diameter. MaRAS are found on any area of the oral mucosa, including the dorsum of the tongue or palate. Usually only a few ulcers (one to six) occur at one time; they heal slowly over 10–40 days, and recur frequently. MaRAS are round or ovoid with an inflammatory halo, and may heal with scarring (Fig. 66.26). Occasionally, a raised erythrocyte sedimentation rate or plasma viscosity is found.

Herpetiform ulceration. Herpetiform ulceration (HU) is found in a slightly older age group and there is a female predominance. Herpetiform ulcers are often extremely painful and recur so frequently that ulceration may be virtually continuous. HU begins with vesiculation, which passes rapidly into multiple, minute (2 mm), discrete ulcers at any oral site. The ulcers increase in size and coalesce to leave large ragged ulcers that heal in 10 days or longer. Their similarity to herpetic stomatitis gives her-

petiform ulcers their name, but there is no evidence that herpes simplex virus is involved.

Prognosis. RAS in most patients resolves or abates spontaneously with age. An underlying identifiable predisposing cause is particularly likely where RAS commences or worsens in adult life.

Diagnosis. Diagnosis is based on history and clinical features, since specific tests are unavailable. Biopsy is indicated only where some other cause of ulceration is suspected. To exclude relevant systemic predisposing factors it is often useful to perform:
• full blood count;
• haemoglobin assay;
• white cell count and differential;
• red cell indices;
• iron studies;
• red cell folate level;
• serum vitamin B_{12} measurements;
• serum antiendomysial antibodies.
The relevance of HLA studies for differentiating RAS from Behcet's syndrome is discussed on p. 66.46.

Management. Few patients have spontaneous remission until after several years and thus treatment is often indicated [11]. Fortunately, the natural history of RAS is one of eventual remission in most cases.

Predisposing factors should be corrected. If there is an obvious relationship to certain foods, the causal food should be excluded from the diet [12]. Good oral hygiene should be maintained: chlorhexidine or triclosan mouthwashes help achieve this and may help reduce ulcer duration [1–4].

Ulcer pain can usually be reduced, and the time to healing reduced, with hydrocortisone hemisuccinate pellets (Corlan) 2.5 mg or triamcinolone acetonide in carboxymethylcellulose paste (Adcortyl in Orabase) used four times daily; failing the success of these, a stronger topical corticosteroid (e.g. betamethasone, beclomethasone, fluticasone, mometasone) [13] or systemic corticosteroid (e.g. prednisolone) may be required (see Chapter 49).

Other therapies for RAS, such as sucralfate [14], colchicine and pentoxifylline (oxpentifylline), may have a role in individual cases but are not generally very effective or have adverse effects [3,15,16].

Thalidomide, in doses from 50 mg up to 300 mg daily, can frequently induce remission, especially in major aphthae, but its important teratogenic effects and the risk of neuropathy must be considered [17]. Topical tacrolimus may be effective but randomized trials are awaited.

There are multiple other therapies available for RAS, including carbenoxolone, benzydamine, dapsone, cromoglicate, levamisole and many others, but generally their

Features		Incidence (%)
Major criteria		
Oral	Aphthae	90–100
Genital	Ulcers	64–88
Neuro-ocular	Iridocyclitis	10–90
	Retinal vasculitis	
	Optic atrophy	
	Syndromes resembling disseminated sclerosis, pseudobulbar palsy or neurosyphilis	
	Meningoencephalitis	
	Others	
Dermatological	Pustules	48–88
	Erythema nodosum	
	Pathergy	
Minor criteria	Proteinuria and haematuria	
	Thrombophlebitis	
	Aneurysms	
	Arthralgias	

Table 66.16 Behçet's syndrome.

efficacy has not been well proven or they have unacceptable adverse effects [3].

REFERENCES

1 Eversole LR. Immunopathology of oral mucosal ulcerative, desquamative and bullous diseases. *Oral Surg* 1994; **77**: 555–71.
2 Porter SR, Hegarty A, Kaliakatsou F, Hodgson TA, Scully C. Recurrent aphthous stomatitis. *Clin Dermatol* 2000; **18**: 569–78.
3 Porter SR, Scully C. Aphthous ulcers: recurrent. *Clin Evidence* 2001; **6**: 1037–41.
4 Porter SR, Scully C, Pedersen A. Recurrent aphthous stomatitis. *Crit Rev Oral Biol Med* 1998; **9**: 306–21.
5 Porter SR, Flint S, Scully C, Keith O. Recurrent aphthous stomatitis: the efficacy of replacement therapy in patients with underlying haematinic deficiencies. *Ann Dent* 1992; **L1**: 14–6.
6 Porter SR, Scully C, Flint SR. Haematological status in recurrent aphthous stomatitis compared with other oral disease. *Oral Surg* 1988; **66**: 41–4.
7 Hunter IP, Ferguson MM, Scully C *et al*. Effects of dietary gluten elimination in patients with recurrent minor aphthous stomatitis and no detectable gluten enteropathy. *Oral Surg* 1993; **75**: 595–8.
8 Rogers RS. Recurrent aphthous stomatitis and Behçet's syndrome. In: Safai R, Good RA, eds. *Immunodermatology*. New York: Plenum Press, 1981: 345.
9 Marshall GS, Edwards KM, Butler J *et al*. Syndrome of periodic fever, pharyngitis and aphthous stomatitis. *J Pediatr* 1987; **110**: 43–6.
10 Hasan A, Childerstone A, Pervink T *et al*. Recognition of a unique peptide epitope of the mycobacterial and human heat shock protein 65–60 antigen by T cells of patients with recurrent oral ulcers. *Clin Exp Immunol* 1995; **99**: 392–7.
11 McBride DR. Management of aphthous ulcers. *Am Fam Physician* 2000; **62**: 149–54, 160.
12 Hay KD, Reade PC. The use of an elimination diet in the treatment of recurrent aphthous ulceration of the oral cavity. *Oral Surg* 1984; **57**: 504–7.
13 Teixeira F, Mosqueda-Taylor A, Montano S, Dominguez-Soto L. Treatment of recurrent oral ulcers with mometasone furoate lotion. *Postgrad Med J* 1999; **75**: 574.
14 Rattan J, Schneider M, Arber N *et al*. Sucralfate suspension as a treatment of recurrent aphthous stomatitis. *J Intern Med* 1994; **236**: 341–3.
15 Katz J, Langevitz P, Shemer J *et al*. Prevention of recurrent aphthous stomatitis with colchicine: an open trial. *J Am Acad Dermatol* 1994; **31**: 459–61.
16 Wahba-Yahav AV. Severe idiopathic recurrent aphthous stomatitis: treatment with pentoxifylline. *Acta Derm Venereol (Stockh)* 1995; **75**: 157.
17 Grinspan D, Blanco GF, Aguero S. Treatment of aphthae with thalidomide. *J Am Acad Dermatol* 1989; **20**: 1060–3.

Behçet's syndrome
SYN. ADAMANTIADES SYNDROME

Definition. Behçet's syndrome (BS) is the association of RAS with genital ulceration and eye disease (especially iridocyclitis and retinal vasculitis) [1–5]. There may be a number of other systemic or cutaneous manifestations (Table 66.16).

Aetiology. The aetiology of BS is uncertain but it appears to be becoming more common. There is a genetic background and, as in RAS, there are occasional familial cases and associations with HLA types, in BS particularly with HLA-B5 (Bw51 split). HLA-B51 or its B101 allele is significantly associated with BS in Japan, Korea, Turkey and France, as well as with the ocular manifestations in Britain. The MICA6 allele, a member of the polymorphic MHC class I-related gene A (MICA) family, is thought to be in linkage disequilibrium with HLA-B51 and has been shown to be significantly associated with BS in Japan and France [6]. HLA-DR/DQ haplotypes are more important than individual HLA-DR and HLA-DQ phenotypes for the development of mucocutaneous type of BS and for disease shift from RAS to mucocutaneous type of BS [7].

The aetiopathogenesis of BS is still unclear [8,9]. It does not appear to be infectious, contagious or sexually transmitted. The disease is found worldwide but is most common in the eastern Mediterranean countries and eastern Asia, along the Silk Road taken by Marco Polo. In these countries, it is a leading cause of blindness though this is not the case in the Western world.

There are many immunological findings in BS:
• circulating autoantibodies against a number of components, including intermediate filaments found in mucous membranes, cardiolipin and neutrophil cytoplasm;

Table 66.17 Oculomucocutaneous syndromes.*

| Disease | Main lesions | | |
	Oral and genital	Ocular	Skin
Behçet's syndrome	Aphthae	Uveitis	Erythema nodosum
Sweet's syndrome	Aphthae	Conjunctivitis, episcleritis	Inflamed papule or nodule
Erythema multiforme	Erosions	Erosions	Target lesions
Cicatricial pemphigoid	Bullae	Erosions	Occasional dome-shaped bullae
	Erosions	Scarring	
Pemphigus	Erosions	Erosions	Multiple, flaccid bullae
Reiter's syndrome	Ulcers	Conjunctivitis	Keratoderma blenorrhagica

* Ulcerative colitis, herpes simplex, syphilis, lupus erythematosus, mixed connective tissue disease and other disorders may also cause oral, cutaneous and ocular lesions.

- circulating immune complexes and changed levels of complement;
- immunoglobulins and complement deposition within and around blood vessel walls;
- decreased ratio of T-helper (CD4) cells to T-suppressor (CD8) cells.

These immunological changes mimic those seen in patients with RAS—various T-lymphocyte abnormalities (especially T-suppressor cell dysfunction), changes in serum complement and increased polymorphonuclear leukocyte motility. There is also evidence that mononuclear cells may initiate antibody-dependent cellular cytotoxicity to oral epithelial cells, and evidence of disturbance of natural killer cell activity.

The common denominator in all systems is vasculitis, usually leukocytoclastic vasculitis. Many of the features of BS (erythema nodosum, arthralgia, uveitis) are common to established immune complex disease and, indeed, immune complexes (usually antigen–antibody complexes) are found in the sera. The antigen responsible has not been reliably identified but may include herpes simplex virus or streptococcal antigens [10–12]. As in RAS, heat-shock proteins have been implicated.

Clinical features. BS is a chronic multisystem disorder, most patients being male, usually in their third or fourth decade.

Because BS is rare and symptoms of the disease overlap symptoms of other diseases, it can be very difficult to diagnose. Spontaneous remission is common for patients with BS; this can add to the difficulty in diagnosis.

BS is characterized mainly by a triad of RAS [13,14], genital ulcers [15,16] and ocular lesions. The CNS, heart and intestinal tract may be involved.

One variant of BS (MAGIC syndrome) is associated with mouth and genital ulcers and inflamed cartilage [17]. Other oculomucocutaneous syndromes (Table 66.17) may cause similar manifestations [18,19].

Diagnosis. BS is usually diagnosed on clinical grounds,

although findings of HLA-B5101 and pathergy are supportive, as are antibodies to cardiolipin and neutrophil cytoplasm. Disease activity may be assessed by serum levels of acute phase proteins or antibodies to intermediate filaments, or by erythrocyte sedimentation rate; all are raised in active BS.

Differential diagnosis is mainly from the following.
- Sweet's syndrome: aphthae, conjunctivitis, episcleritis, inflamed tender papule or nodule.
- Erythema multiforme: erosions, target (iris) lesions.
- Pemphigoid: bullae, erosions.
- Pemphigus: erosions, multiple flaccid bullae.
- Reiter's syndrome: ulcers, conjunctivitis, keratoderma blenorrhagica.
- Ulcerative colitis.
- Herpes simplex.
- Syphilis.
- Lupus erythematosus.
- Mixed connective tissue disease.

The diagnosis is often made on the basis of RAS plus two or more of recurrent genital ulceration, eye lesions, skin lesions and pathergy [20,21].

Major criteria include:

1 RAS: in 90–100% of cases.

2 Recurrent painful genital ulcers that tend to heal with scars in 64–88% of cases. Genital ulcers are especially common in females with BS, and resemble RAS.

3 Ocular lesions: uveitis with conjunctivitis (early) and hypopyon (late), retinal vasculitis (posterior uveitis), iridocyclitis and optic atrophy. The most common ocular manifestation is relapsing iridocyclitis but uveitis, retinal vascular changes and optic atrophy may occur. Both eyes are eventually involved and blindness may result.

4 CNS lesions: meningoencephalitis, cerebral infarction, psychosis, cranial nerve palsies, cerebellar and spinal cord lesions, hemiparesis and quadriparesis.

5 Skin lesions: erythema nodosum, papulopustular lesions and acneform nodules. Venepuncture is, in some patients, followed by pustulation (pathergy).

Minor criteria are:

1 Arthralgia: large joint arthropathies that are subacute, non-migratory, self-limiting and non-deforming.
2 Superficial or deep migratory thrombophlebitis, especially of lower limbs.
3 Intestinal lesions: inflammatory bowel disease with discrete ulcerations.
4 Lung involvement: pneumonitis.
5 Haematuria and proteinuria.

However, very non-specific signs and symptoms, which may be recurrent, may precede the onset of the mucosal membrane ulceration by 6 months to 5 years. These include malaise, anorexia, weight loss, generalized weakness, headache, perspiration, decreased or elevated temperature, lymphadenopathy and pain in the substernal and temporal regions.

A history of repeated sore throats, tonsillitis, myalgias and migratory erythralgias without overt arthritis is also common.

Management. Unlike RAS, BS is not self-limiting. It causes morbidity (especially in terms of ocular and neurological disease) and mortality. Most patients present with oral and ocular disease but there follows a relapsing and remitting but variable course. CNS involvement, thromboses of major vessels and gastrointestinal perforation result in a poor prognosis. Few patients with BS have spontaneous remission and thus treatment is indicated [22,23].

Chronic morbidity is usual; the leading cause is ophthalmic involvement, which can result in blindness. The effects of the disease may be cumulative, especially with neurological, vascular and ocular involvement. Mortality is low but can occur from neurological involvement, vascular disease, bowel perforation, cardiopulmonary disease or as a complication of immunosuppressive therapy. In the face of the serious potential complications, patients with suspected BS should be referred early for specialist advice.

Topical treatment for RAS (see p. 66.45). Oral ulcers may respond to topical corticosteroids or 5-aminosalicylic acid [24]. Even nicotine patches may have some success [25].

Systemic treatment includes mainly colchicine 0.5–1.5 mg daily.

Other systemic treatments include corticosteroids, azathioprine, ciclosporin, chlorambucil, cyclophosphamide, dapsone, interferon-alpha, levamisole or thalidomide. Ocular lesions usually respond to ciclosporin, but tend to relapse when treatment is stopped. Thalidomide at a dose of up to 400 mg daily may be of value in recalcitrant orogenital ulceration, although it must be used with caution as it is teratogenic and carries a risk of neuropathy [26,27].

REFERENCES

1 Ghate JV, Jorizzo JL. Behcet's disease and complex aphthosis. *J Am Acad Dermatol* 1999; **40**: 1–18.
2 Kaklamani VG, Vaiopoulos G, Kaklamanis PG. Behcet's disease. *Semin Arthritis Rheum* 1998; **27**: 197–217.
3 Sakane T, Takeno M, Suzuki N, Inaba G. Behcet's disease. *N Engl J Med* 1999; **341**: 1284–91.
4 Lee LA. Behcet disease. *Semin Cutan Med Surg* 2001; **20**: 53–7.
5 Yazici H, Yurdakul S, Hamuryudan V. Behcet's syndrome. *Curr Opin Rheumatol* 1999; **11**: 53–7.
6 Mizuki N, Inoko H, Ohno S. Molecular genetics (HLA) of Behcet's disease. *Yonsei Med J* 1997; **38**: 333–49.
7 Sun A, Hsieh RP, Chu CT *et al.* Some specific human leukocyte antigen (HLA)-DR/DQ haplotypes are more important than individual HLA-DR and -DQ phenotypes for the development of mucocutaneous type of Behcet's disease and for disease shift from recurrent aphthous stomatitis to mucocutaneous type of Behcet's disease. *J Oral Pathol Med* 2001; **30**: 402–7.
8 Inoue C, Itoh R, Kawa Y, Mizoguchi M. Pathogenesis of mucocutaneous lesions in Behcet's disease. *J Dermatol* 1994; **21**: 474–80.
9 Sakane T, Suzuki N, Nagafuchi H. Etiopathology of Behcet's disease: immunological aspects. *Yonsei Med J* 1997; **38**: 350–8.
10 Narikawa S, Suzuki Y, Takahashi M *et al. Streptococcus oralis* previously identified as uncommon '*Streptococcus sanguis*' in Behcet's disease *Arch Oral Biol* 1995; **40**: 685–90.
11 Lehner T, Lavery E, Smith R *et al.* Association between the 65-kilodalton heat shock protein, *Streptococcus sanguis*, and the corresponding antibodies in Behcet's syndrome. *Infect Immunol* 1991; **59**: 1434–41.
12 Pervin K, Childerston A, Shinnick T *et al.* T cell epitope expression of mycobacterial and homologous human 65-kilodalton heat shock protein peptides in short-term lines from patients with Behcet's disease. *J Immunol* 1993; **151**: 2273–82.
13 Krause I, Rosen Y, Kaplan I *et al.* Recurrent aphthous stomatitis in Behcet's disease: clinical features and correlation with systemic disease expression and severity. *J Oral Pathol Med* 1999; **28**: 193–6.
14 Verpilleux MP, Bastuji-Garin S, Revuz J. Comparative analysis of severe aphthosis and Behcet's disease: 104 cases. *Dermatology* 1999; **198**: 247–51.
15 Krause I, Uziel Y, Guedj D *et al.* Mode of presentation and multisystem involvement in Behcet's disease: the influence of sex and age of disease onset. *J Rheumatol* 1998; **25**: 1566–9.
16 Gharibdoost F, Davatchi F, Shahram F *et al.* Clinical manifestations of Behcet's disease in Iran. Analysis of 2176 cases. In: Godeau P, Wechsler B, eds. *Proceedings of the 6th International Conference on Behcet's Disease.* Amsterdam: Elsevier, 1993: 153–8.
17 Firestein GS, Gruber HC, Weisman MH *et al.* Mouth and genital ulcers with inflamed cartilage: MAGIC syndrome. *Am J Med* 1985; **79**: 65–72.
18 Grattan CEH, Scully C. Oral ulceration: a diagnostic problem. *BMJ* 1986; **292**: 1093–4.
19 Hamza M. Orogenital ulcerations in mixed connective tissue disease. *J Rheumatol* 1985; **12**: 643–4.
20 International Study Group for Behcet's Disease. Criteria for diagnosis of Behcet's disease. *Lancet* 1990; **i**: 1078–80.
21 Lee S. Diagnostic criteria of Behcet's disease: problems and suggestions. *Yonsei Med J* 1997; **38**: 365–9.
22 Sakane T, Takeno M. Current therapy in Behcet's disease. *Skin Ther Lett* 2000; **5**: 3–5.
23 Fresko I, Yurdakul S, Hamuryudan V *et al.* The management of Behcet's syndrome. *Ann Med Interne (Paris)* 1999; **150**: 576–81.
24 Ranzi T, Campanini M, Bianchi RA. Successful treatment of genital and oral ulceration in Behçet's disease with topical 5-aminosalicylic acid. *Br J Dermatol* 1989; **120**: 471–2.
25 Scheid P, Bohadana A, Martinet Y. Nicotine patches for aphthous ulcers due to Behcet's syndrome. *N Engl J Med* 2000; **343**: 1816–7.
26 Bowers PW, Powell RJ. Effect of thalidomide on oral ulceration. *BMJ* 1983; **287**: 799–800.
27 Jenkins JS, Powell RJ, Allen BR *et al.* Thalidomide in severe orogenital ulceration. *Lancet* 1984; **ii**: 1424–6.

Sweet's syndrome (see Chapter 49)

Pustular lesions leading to aphthous-like ulcers may be

found in Sweet's syndrome and there are occasional associations with BS and Sjögren's syndrome, each of which has oral manifestations. About 5% of patients in the UK with Sweet's syndrome have oral aphthae, although up to 30% of Japanese patients suffer aphthae [1–3].

REFERENCES

1 Driban NE, Alvarez MA. Oral manifestations of Sweet's syndrome. *Dermatologica* 1984; **169**: 102–3.
2 Mizoguchi M, Chikakane K, Goh K *et al.* Acute febrile neutrophilic dermatosis (Sweet's syndrome) in Behçet's disease. *Br J Dermatol* 1987; **116**: 727–34.
3 Femiano F, Gombos F, Scully C. Sweet's syndrome: recurrent oral ulceration, pyrexia, thrombophlebitis, and cutaneous lesions. *Oral Surg Oral Med Oral Pathol Oral Radiol Endod* 2003; **95**:324–7.

Malignant neoplasms

More than 90% of malignant neoplasms in the mouth are squamous cell carcinomas. Nearly 30% of all squamous cell carcinomas affect the lip; some 25% affect the tongue, the most common intraoral site [1–5]. Most intraoral cancers involve the posterolateral border of the tongue and/or the floor of the mouth (the 'graveyard' area).

Oral cancer is a significant world health problem, being overall the sixth most common malignant neoplasm. In parts of South-East Asia for example, particularly India, some 40% of all malignancy is oral cancer. High levels are also seen in other parts of the developing world such as Brazil, but also in parts of Europe such as areas of northern France and eastern Europe.

Oral squamous cell carcinoma

Cancer of the oral cavity is classified according to site:
- lip (International Classification of Diseases [ICD] 140);
- tongue (ICD 141);
- gum (ICD 143);
- floor of the mouth (ICD 144); and
- unspecified parts of the mouth (ICD 145).

Carcinoma of the lip

Squamous carcinoma is the commonest malignancy to affect the vermilion zone and, as with squamous carcinoma of the glabrous skin, it is usually due to actinic damage [1]. Like actinic cheilitis it is most common on the lower lip of fair-skinned, outdoor workers in sunny climates, and is relatively rare in pigmented skin [2–4]. Lip cancer is common in certain population groups in the UK, Romania, Hungary, Poland, Spain, Finland, Israel, Canada, the USA and Australia, but in most areas reported the incidence is falling [4–7].

Lip cancer generally occurs in men who are employed in outdoor activities such as farming and fishing [8]. Squamous cell carcinomas occur on the lower lip in 89%,

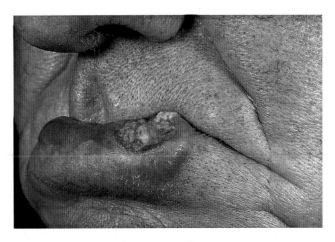

Fig. 66.27 Squamous cell carcinoma of lip.

with 3% on the upper lip and 8% at the commissures [9]. Although sunlight is accepted as the major aetiological factor, some studies have shown a poor correlation between the incidence of lip cancer and the rate of annual solar radiation [10]. *Actinic radiation* may predispose to lip cancer. Facts that support such a relationship include the following.
- Lip cancer involves the more exposed lower lip, rather than the upper lip.
- There is a higher incidence of lip cancer in outdoor workers and rural populations than in office workers or urban populations.
- Fair-skinned more than dark-skinned people tend to develop lip cancer (as well as skin cancer and melanoma) in sunny climates.

Other risk factors may include low social class, tobacco smoking, syphilis, poor dentition, infection with herpes simplex virus [3,5,8] and immune suppression [11]; for example lip cancer is increased in immunosuppressed renal transplant recipients.

The initial features are a keratinous growth or swelling of the lip (Fig. 66.27), soreness and ulceration. Most lesions are amenable to surgical excision, with more than 70% surviving for 5 years.

REFERENCES

1 Zitsch RP. Carcinoma of the lip. *Otolaryngol Clin North Am* 1993; **26**: 265–77.
2 Keller AZ. Cellular types, survival, race, nativity, occupations, habits and associated diseases in the pathogenesis of lip cancers. *Am J Epidemiol* 1970; **91**: 486–99.
3 Picascia DD, Robinson JK. Actinic cheilitis: a review. *J Am Acad Dermatol* 1987; **17**: 255–64.
4 Szpak CA, Stone MJ, Frenkel EP. Some observations concerning the demographic and geographic incidence of carcinoma of the lip and buccal cavity. *Cancer* 1977; **40**: 343–8.
5 Keller AZ. The epidemiology of lip, oral and pharyngeal cancers, and the association with selected systemic diseases. *Am J Public Health* 1963; **53**: 1214–28.

6 MacFarlane GJ, Boyle P, Evstifeeva T, Scully C. Epidemiological aspects of lip cancer in Scotland. *Community Dent Oral Epidemiol* 1993; **21**: 279–82.

7 Scully C, Cawson RA. Potentially malignant oral lesions. *J Epidemiol Biostat* 1996; **1**: 3–12.

8 Pukkala E, Soderholm A-L, Linqvist C. Cancers of the lip and oropharynx in different social and occupational groups in Finland. *Oral Oncol* 1994; **30B**: 209–15.

9 del Regato JA. Cancer of the respiratory system and upper digestive tract. In: del Regato JA, ed. *Ackerman and Del Regato's Cancer*, 6th edn. St Louis: Mosby, 1985: 248–72.

10 Lindqvist C. Risk factors of lip cancer: a critical evaluation based on epidemiological comparisons. *Am J Public Health* 1979; **69**: 256–60.

11 King GN, Healy C, Glover MT et al. Increased prevalence of dysplastic and malignant lip lesions in renal transplant recipients. *N Engl J Med* 1995; **332**: 1052–7.

Intraoral carcinoma

Most intraoral carcinoma is squamous cell carcinoma [1–3]. In many countries there is evidence for an increase in oral squamous cell carcinoma (OSCC) over recent years [4–7], especially in young persons. There is marked inter-country variation in both the incidence of, and mortality from, OSCC [8]. In addition, there is also growing evidence of intra-country ethnic differences in incidence and mortality, especially in the UK and USA.

In the developing world, particularly South-East Asia and Brazil, the incidence of OSCC varies widely in different areas and there are ethnic differences in incidence, often attributed to lifestyle habits.

In the developed world OSCC is uncommon. The incidence varies between countries and between different regions of the same country. For example, parts of France and Newfoundland have the highest incidence in the West, with about 10 times the incidence of oral carcinoma in the UK. Oral cancer is more than twice as common in Scotland than in England and Wales and, for example, even within Scotland there are regional differences.

Potentially malignant states. Some potentially malignant (precancerous) lesions that can progress to OSCC include especially [9] *erythroplasia* (erythroplakia), the most likely lesion to progress to severe dysplasia or carcinoma (see p. 66.96); and *leukoplakia* (see p. 66.85), particularly proliferative verrucous leukoplakia, sublingual leukoplakia, candidal leukoplakia and syphilitic leukoplakia.

Some other potentially malignant (precancerous) conditions include:
• lichen planus—there are also cases of dysplasia with a lichenoid appearance (lichenoid dysplasia);
• discoid lupus erythematosus;
• submucous fibrosis;
• atypia in immunocompromised patients;
• dyskeratosis congenita;
• Paterson–Kelly syndrome (sideropenic dysphagia, Plummer–Vinson syndrome).
One of the main features that appears to precede the onset of malignancy is epithelial dysplasia, although dysplasia can also be seen in regenerating tissue and some non-precancerous lesions such as ulcers, viral infections, candidal infections and granular cell tumours.

Dysplasia varies in severity, and it is the more severe grades that are associated with higher malignant potential.

Predisposing factors (risk factors) [1–3,10–13]. In the developed world, OSCC is seen especially in tobacco users, alcohol users, lower socio-economic groups and ethnic minority groups.

In the developing world, OSCC is seen especially in tobacco users, alcohol users, 'betel quid' users (some 20% of the world's population use betel) and lower socio-economic groups. In peoples from parts of Asia, tobacco-chewing, along with a variety of ingredients in 'betel quid' (betel vine leaf, betel [areca] nut, catechu, slaked lime, together with tobacco), appears to predispose to OSCC, particularly when it is started early in life and is used frequently and for prolonged periods. Various other risky chewing habits, usually containing tobacco, are used in different cultures (e.g. khat, shammah, toombak).

Microorganisms such as *Candida* and human papillomavirus (HPV) have been detected in some potentially malignant lesions and some OSCC, where they may play a role. HPV is especially implicated in tonsillar carcinoma; HPV-16 is particularly implicated.

In contrast, diets rich in fresh fruits and vegetables and vitamin A may have a protective effect.

Clinical features. OSCC may present as the following [1–3] (Fig. 66.28).

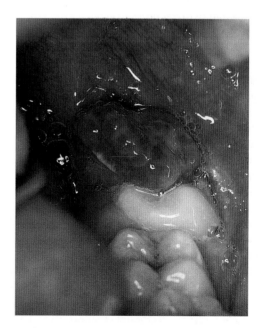

Fig. 66.28 Oral squamous cell carcinoma.

Table 66.18 TNM classification of malignant neoplasms.*

Primary tumour size (T)

Tx	No available information
T_0	No evidence of primary tumour
T_{is}	Only carcinoma *in situ*
T_1, T_2, T_3, T_4	Increasing size of tumour†

Regional lymph node involvement (N)

Nx	Nodes could not or were not assessed
N_0	No clinically positive nodes
N_1	Single clinically positive homolateral node less than 3 cm in diameter
N_2	Single clinically positive homolateral node 3–6 cm in diameter, or multiple clinically positive homolateral nodes, none more than 6 cm in diameter
N_{2a}	Single clinically positive homolateral node 3–6 cm in diameter
N_{2b}	Multiple clinically positive homolateral nodes, none more than 6 cm in diameter
N_3	Massive homolateral node(s), bilateral nodes, or contralateral node(s)
N_{3a}	Clinically positive homolateral node(s), one more than 6 cm in diameter
N_{3b}	Bilateral clinically positive nodes
N_{3c}	Contralateral clinically positive node(s)

Involvement by distant metastases (M)

Mx	Distant metastasis was not assessed
M_0	No evidence of distant metastasis
M_1, M_2, M_3	Distant metastasis is present. Increasing degrees of metastatic involvement, including distant nodes

* Several other classifications are available, e.g. STNM (S, site).
† T_1, maximum diameter 2 cm; T_2, maximum diameter 4 cm; T_3, maximum diameter > 4 cm; T_4, massive tumour > 4 cm diameter, with involvement of antrum, pterygoid muscles, base of tongue or skin.

- A red lesion (erythroplasia).
- A granular ulcer with fissuring or raised exophytic margins.
- A white or mixed white and red lesion.
- A lump sometimes with abnormal supplying blood vessels.
- An indurated lump/ulcer, i.e. a firm infiltration beneath the mucosa.
- A non-healing extraction socket.
- A lesion fixed to deeper tissues or to overlying skin or mucosa.
- Cervical lymph node enlargement, especially if there is hardness in a lymph node or fixation.

Enlarged nodes in a patient with oral carcinoma may be caused by infection, reactive hyperplasia secondary to the tumour, or metastatic disease. Occasionally, a swollen lymph node is detected in the absence of any obvious primary tumour.

In patients with OSCC for over 3 years, second primary neoplasms in the aerodigestive tract may be seen in up to 25% and in up to 40% of those who continue to smoke.

Diagnosis. Early diagnosis is important since it improves prognosis and minimizes the extent of interventions [14–16]. There should be a high index of suspicion, especially of a solitary lesion present for over 3 weeks: biopsy is invariably indicated. Clinicians should be aware that single ulcers, lumps, red patches or white patches, particularly if any of these persist for more than 3 weeks, may be manifestations of frank malignancy. Scalpel biopsy is required and toluidine blue staining may help highlight the most appropriate area for biopsy [17–19].

The whole oral mucosa should be examined as there may be widespread dysplastic mucosa ('field change') or even a second neoplasm and the cervical lymph nodes must be examined. Frank tumours should be inspected and palpated to determine extent of spread; for tumours in the posterior tongue, examination under general anaesthesia may facilitate this.

OSCC should be staged according to the TNM classification of the International Union against Cancer, where T represents tumour size, N nodal metastases and M distant metastases (Table 66.18), since this classification relates well to overall survival rate, i.e. the earlier the tumour, the better the prognosis and the less complicated the treatment.

Investigations. The principles include the following.
1 Confirm the diagnosis histopathologically and determine the presence of malignant disease elsewhere.
   (a) Are bone, muscles or cervical lymph nodes involved?
   (b) Are there other primary tumours (typically in the upper aerodigestive tract—mouth, nares, pharynx, larynx, oesophagus)? There is controversy as to the need for endoscopy in all cases to detect such tumours.
   (c) Are there metastases, initially to regional lymph nodes and later to liver, bone and brain? Imaging may detect abnormalities that escape clinical examination.

2 Ensure that the patient is as prepared as possible for the major surgery required, particularly in terms of general anaesthesia, potential blood loss and ability to metabolize drugs.

3 Address any potential dental or oral problems pre-operatively, to avoid later complications such as osteora-dionecrosis.

The following investigations are therefore almost invariably indicated.

• Lesional biopsy. Incisional biopsy, which is invariably required, should be sufficiently large to include enough suspect and apparently normal tissue. Red, rather than white, areas are most likely to show dysplasia, and hence should be biopsied. Attempts to highlight probable dysplastic areas before biopsy, for example by using toluidine blue dye, are unfortunately not reliable, but may be of some help in deciding which area is best to biopsy where there is widespread 'field change'. An excisional biopsy should be avoided unless the lesion is extremely small, since this is unlikely to have excised an adequately wide margin of tissue if the lesion is malignant, but will have destroyed for the surgeon or radiotherapist clinical evidence of the site and character of the lesion.

• Biopsy of equivocal neck lymph nodes.

• Jaw radiography (often rotating pantomography), although this is inadequate to exclude bone invasion.

• Chest radiography: important as a pre-anaesthetic check, especially in patients with known pulmonary or airways disease, and to demonstrate metastasis to lungs or hilar lymph nodes, ribs or vertebrae.

• MRI or computed tomography (CT) of the primary site, head and neck, and suspected sites of distant metastases, and MRI of the neck to delineate the extent of cervical node metastases. Some units routinely examine chest and abdomen. MRI is particularly useful for determining tumour spread, bone involvement and nodal metastases.

• Electrocardiography.

• Blood tests.

• Full blood picture and haemoglobin.

• Blood for grouping and cross-matching.

• Urea and electrolytes.

• Liver function tests.

In selected cases, the following may also be useful.

• Bronchoscopy: if chest radiography reveals any lesions.

• Endoscopy of the upper aerodigestive tract: especially if there is a history of tobacco use.

• Gastroscopy: if a per-endoscopic gastrostomy is to be used for feeding.

• Liver ultrasound: if there is hepatomegaly or abnormal liver function.

• Doppler duplex flow studies: in planning radial free forearm flaps.

• Angiography: in planning lower limb free flaps.

Treatment. The prognosis of OSCC is around 30% sur-vival at 5 years [20]. The major impact that treatment has had on the prognosis of oral cancer has been in relation to improved anaesthetic and medical care. Surgical reconstruction has also been markedly improved [21] and there are fewer side effects from modern radiotherapy.

The treatment of oral cancer involves one or a combination of radiotherapy, surgery and, very occasionally, chemotherapy. Serious consideration must be given to the complications of the various modalities [22,23] and the quality of life achieved [24,25].

There is now evidence that vitamin A derivatives may be of benefit in patients with premalignant lesions, and in preventing second primary neoplasms [26–27].

REFERENCES

1 Silverman S. Oral cancer. *Semin Dermatol* 1994; **13**: 132–7.
2 Prince S, Bailey BM. Squamous carcinoma of the tongue: review. *Br J Oral Maxillofac Surg* 1999; **37**: 164–74.
3 Renaud-Salis JL, Blanc-Vincent MP, Brugere J *et al.* Epidermoid cancers of the oropharynx. *Br J Cancer* 2001; **84** (Suppl. 2): 37–41.
4 Boyle P, MacFarlane GJ, Zheng T *et al.* Recent advances in the epidemiology of head and neck cancer. *Curr Opin Oncol* 1992; **4**: 471–7.
5 MacFarlane GJ, Boyle P, Evstifeeva T, Robertson C, Scully C. Rising trends of oral cancer mortality in males worldwide: the return of an old public health problem. *Cancer Causes Control* 1994; **5**: 259–65.
6 MacFarlane GJ, Evstifeeva TV, Robertson C, Boyle P, Scully C. Trends of oral cancer mortality among females worldwide. *Cancer Causes Control* 1994; **5**: 255–8.
7 Mackenzie J, Ah-See K, Thakker N *et al.* Increasing incidence of oral cancer amongst young persons: what is the aetiology? *Oral Oncol* 2000; **36**: 387–9.
8 Scully C, Bedi R. Ethnicity and oral cancer. *Lancet Oncol* 2000; **1**: 37–42.
9 Scully C, Cawson RA. Oral potentially malignant lesions. *J Epidemiol Biostat* 1996; **1**: 3–12.
10 Hashibe M, Mathew B, Kuruvilla B *et al.* Chewing tobacco, alcohol, and the risk of erythroplakia. *Cancer Epidemiol Biomarkers Prev* 2000; **9**: 639–45.
11 Bedi R, Jones P, eds. *Betel-quid and Tobacco Chewing Among the Bangladeshi Community in the United Kingdom: Usage and Health Issues.* London: Centre for Transcultural Oral Health, 1995.
12 Jaber MA, Porter SR, Scully C, Gilthorpe MS, Bedi R. Role of alcohol in non-smokers and tobacco in non-drinkers in the aetiology of oral epithelial dysplasia. *Int J Cancer* 1998; **77**: 333–6.
13 Jaber MA, Porter SR, Gilthorpe MS, Bedi R, Scully C. Risk factors for oral epithelial dysplasia: the role of smoking and alcohol. *Oral Oncol* 1999; **35**: 151–6.
14 Mashberg A, Samit A. Early diagnosis of asymptomatic oral and oropharyngeal squamous cancers. *CA Cancer J Clin* 1995; **45**: 328–51.
15 Scully C, Ward-Booth P. Detection and treatment of early cancers of the oral cavity. *Crit Rev Oncol Hematol* 1995; **21**: 63–75.
16 Sciubba JJ. Oral cancer. The importance of early diagnosis and treatment. *Am J Clin Dermatol* 2001; **2**: 239–51.
17 Scully C. Clinical diagnostic methods for the detection of premalignant and early malignant oral lesions. *Community Dent Health* 1993; **1** (Suppl. 1): 43–52.
18 Sciubba JJ. Improving detection of precancerous and cancerous oral lesions. Computer-assisted analysis of the oral brush biopsy. U.S. Collaborative Oral CDx Study Group. *J Am Dent Assoc* 1999; **130**: 1445–57.
19 Epstein JB, Scully C, Spinelli JJ. Toluidine blue and Lugol's iodine application in the assessment of oral malignant disease and lesions at risk of malignancy. *J Oral Pathol Med* 1992; **21**: 160–3.
20 Chiesa F, Mauri S, Tradati N *et al.* Surfing prognostic factors in head and neck cancer at the Millenium. *Oral Oncol* 1999; **35**: 590–6.
21 Langdon JD, Patel MF. *Operative Maxillofacial Surgery.* London: Chapman & Hall, 1998.
22 de Graeff A, de Leeuw JR, Ros WJ *et al.* A prospective study on quality of life of patients with cancer of the oral cavity or oropharynx treated with surgery with or without radiotherapy. *Oral Oncol* 1999; **35**: 27–32.

23 Rogers SN, Hannah L, Lowe D, Magennis P. Quality of life 5–10 years after primary surgery for oral and oro-pharyngeal cancer. *J Craniomaxillofac Surg* 1999; **27**: 187–91.
24 Singh N, Scully C, Joyston-Bechal S. Oral complications of cancer therapies: prevention and management. *Clin Oncol* 1996; **8**: 15–24.
25 Scully C, Epstein JB. Oral health care in the cancer patient. *Oral Oncol* 1996; **32B**: 281–92.
26 Scully C. Oral precancer: preventive and medical approaches to management. *Oral Oncol* 1995; **31B**: 16–26.
27 Scully C. Chemoprevention in oral cancer. *J Managed Care* 1997; **1**: 116–22.

Verrucous carcinoma

Verrucous carcinoma is an uncommon, warty, white neoplasm that is rarely ulcerated [1–4]. It may develop from proliferative verrucous leukoplakia (see p. 66.86). Risk factors include a possible association with HPV and some verrucous carcinoma develops as a result of the local use of snuff or tobacco. Confirmation of diagnosis by biopsy is particularly important because verrucous carcinoma responds well to excision but, if irradiated, may undergo anaplastic change, with subsequent acceleration of growth and invasiveness [5]. Methisoprinol may be of value [6].

REFERENCES

1 Koch BB, Trask DK, Hoffman HT *et al.* National survey of head and neck verrucous carcinoma: patterns of presentation, care, and outcome. *Cancer* 2001; **92**: 110–20.
2 Hume WJ, Quayle AA. An unusual epithelial neoplasm of gingiva resembling the keratoacanthoma. *Br J Oral Surg* 1985; **23**: 366–70.
3 McDonald JS, Crissman JD, Gluckman JL. Verrucous carcinoma of the oral cavity. *Head Neck Surg* 1982; **5**: 22–8.
4 Firth NA. Oral lesions with a papillary surface texture: clinical and pathological correlations. *Ann R Australas Coll Dent Surg* 2000; **15**: 111–5.
5 Yoshimura Y, Mishima K, Obara S *et al.* Treatment modalities for oral verrucous carcinomas and their outcomes: contribution of radiotherapy and chemotherapy. *Int J Clin Oncol* 2001; **6**: 192–200.
6 Femiano F, Gombos F, Scully C. Oral proliferative verrucous leukoplakia: open trial of surgery compared with combined therapy using surgery and methisoprinol. *Int J Oral Maxillofac Surg* 2001; **30**: 318–22.

Florid oral papillomatosis

Florid oral papillomatosis is a rare but well-defined clinical entity of unknown pathogenesis. Risk factors include possible association with HPV, tobacco, and chronic inflammation or irritation.

Florid oral papillomatosis is essentially a verrucous carcinoma, a clinicopathological variant of squamous cell carcinoma also known by a confusing array of names such as Ackerman's tumour, Buschke–Loewenstein tumour, epithelioma cuniculatum, carcinoma cuniculatum and cutis papillomatosis carcinoides of Gottron.

Clinical features. The lesions are exuberant, warty or verrucous, and characterized by their benign appearance on histology, although this is usually associated with a marked capacity for recurrence and and a tendency for carcinomatous change. Its apparent clinical benignity may lead to lengthy periods of misdiagnosis, during which it slowly but relentlessly destroys and extends into underlying tissue but rarely metastasizes to lymph nodes [1–3].

Diagnosis. Biopsy is required, although to those unfamiliar with the diagnosis the relatively bland histological features are often more suggestive of verruca vulgaris or pseudoepitheliomatous hyperplasia than of squamous cell carcinoma. Alternatively, when it extends into underlying tissues, it may be mistaken for a benign adnexal tumour or even a cyst.

Management. Treatment in the early stage of the disease is usually successful. Etretinate therapy (200 mg/day) or chemotherapy with bleomycin may reduce the lesion bulk [4–6]. Surgical or laser excision is favoured. The use of radiotherapy is controversial since in numerous reported cases this has produced an anaplastic squamous cell carcinoma.

REFERENCES

1 Schwartz RA. Verrucous carcinoma of the skin and mucosa. *J Am Acad Dermatol* 1995; **32**: 1–21.
2 Tyler MT, Ficarra G, Silverman S Jr, Odom RB, Regezi JA. Malignant acanthosis nigricans with florid papillary oral lesions. *Oral Surg Oral Med Oral Pathol Oral Radiol Endod* 1996; **81**: 445–9.
3 Cannon CR, Hayne ST. Concurrent verrucous carcinomas of the lip and buccal mucosa. *South Med J* 1993; **86**: 691–3.
4 Burg G, Sobetzko R. Florid oral papillomatosis: an indication for etretinate? *Hautarzt* 1990; **41**: 314–6.
5 Gaillard A, Hofmann B, Sapanet M, Gaillard F. Treatment of florid oral papillomatosis. Apropos of 10 cases. *Rev Stomatol Chir Maxillofac* 1983; **84**: 363–7.
6 Wienert V, Grussendorf EI. Treatment of florid oral papillomatosis with bleomycin. *Z Hautkr* 1978; **53**: 781–6.

Basal cell carcinoma

Actinic radiation is a major aetiological factor in the development of basal cell carcinoma (BCC), greater than 85% occurring on the sun-exposed areas of the head and neck [1]. Fair-skinned individuals who burn and those whose occupations require excessive exposure to sunshine are at greatest risk; the tumour is rare in dark-skinned persons, and 95% occur after the age of 40 years [2].

Other significant risk factors for the development of BCC include prior burns, vaccinations, irradiation, exposure to inorganic arsenic, genetic syndromes (e.g. xeroderma pigmentosum, naevoid BCC syndrome, albinism and Bazex's syndrome) and immunosuppression [3–8].

Clinical features. On the lip these manifest as a pearly, sometimes ulcerated, nodule or papule. Unlike squamous cell carcinomas, BCCs only rarely originate on the vermilion but commonly occur periorally [9–11]. In contrast to squamous cell carcinomas, BCCs more commonly arise on the upper than the lower lip. The lesions can also arise *de novo* on the vermilion [12] or occasionally the mucosa of the lip, although spread of a tumour from an adjacent site may rarely occur.

BCC has multiple forms that can be simplistically divided as follows.

• Nodular: the most frequent type around the lips presents as a waxy translucent nodule with fine telangiectasias, often ulcerated.

• Morphoeic: an atrophic plaque resembling a scar, with an aggressive infiltrative growth pattern and high rate of recurrence after excision.

• Superficial: appears as an erythematous plaque with elevated borders and central atrophy or ulceration. It is rare around the lips.

Although the tumour rarely metastasizes, it is responsible for considerable functional and cosmetic morbidity.

Multiple lesions are commonly encountered and the various forms have overlapping clinical features. BCC can be frequently pigmented, resembling melanomas and other melanocytic lesions. BCC may of course be a feature of naevoid BCC syndrome (Gorlin–Goltz syndrome, see p. 66.39). Furthermore, in addition to having a significantly increased risk for new skin cancers, patients with BCC have been shown to have an increased risk of developing non-cutaneous cancers, including respiratory cancers, testicular cancer, breast cancer and non-Hodgkin's lymphoma [13,14].

Diagnosis. BCC of the lips must be differentiated from other nodules, including squamous cell carcinoma, keratoacanthoma, trichoepithelioma and sebaceous adenoma. Since lesions that arise periorally are often aggressive, and early detection and confirmation by biopsy will prevent infiltration and destruction of the underlying structures.

Management. Various treatment modalities for BCC include scalpel, electrosurgery, cryosurgery and laser surgery, radiation, curettage and intralesional chemotherapy. Selection of the treatment modality depends on size, site and histological pattern of the tumour as well as the age of the patient. Since lip lesions are often of the nodular or morphoeic types, Mohs' micrographic surgery, utilizing microscopically controlled excision, potentially offers the highest cure rate with the greatest preservation of tissue. The cure rate for BCC is over 90% [15].

REFERENCES

1 Lear JT, Smith AG. Basal cell carcinoma. *Postgrad Med J* 1997; **73**: 538–42.
2 Miller SJ. Biology of basal cell carcinoma (Part 1). *J Am Acad Dermatol* 1991; **24**: 1–13.
3 Allison JR. Radiation-induced basal-cell carcinoma. *J Dermatol Surg Oncol* 1984; **10**: 200–3.
4 Di Tondo U, Berloco P, Trombetta G *et al*. Incidence of tumors in organ transplants. *Transplant Proc* 1997; **29**: 3623–4.
5 Goldberg LH. Basal cell carcinoma. *Lancet* 1996; **347**: 663–7.
6 Kimonis VE, Goldstein AM, Pastakia R *et al*. Clinical manifestations in 105 persons with naevoid basal cell carcinoma syndrome. *Am J Med Genet* 1997; **31**: 299–308.
7 Noodleman RF, Pollack SV. Trauma as a possible etiologic factor in basal cell carcinoma. *J Dermatol Surg Oncol* 1986; **12**: 841–6.
8 Schoolmaster WL, White DR. Arsenic poisoning. *South Med J* 1980; **73**: 198–207.
9 Bussani R, Grandi G, Cosatti C, Silvestri F. Basal cell epithelioma of the lip. Analysis of 42 cases. *Pathologica* 1989; **81**: 499–504.
10 Weitzner S, Heutel W. Multicentric basal cell carcinoma of the vermilion mucosa and skin of lower lip: report of a case. *Oral Surg* 1968; **26**: 269–72.
11 Weitzner S. Basal-cell carcinoma of the vermilion mucosa and skin of the lip. *Oral Surg Oral Med Oral Pathol* 1975; **39**: 634–7.
12 Oriba HA, Sandermann S, Kircik L, Snow SN. Basal cell carcinoma of the vermilion zone of the lower lip: a report of 3 cases. *Oral Oncol* 1998; **34B**: 309–12.
13 Karagas MR, Greenberg ER, Mott LA, Baron JA, Ernster VL. Occurrence of other cancers among patients with prior basal cell and squamous cell skin cancer. *Cancer Epidemiol Biomarkers Prev* 1998; **7**: 157–61.
14 Frisch M, Hjalgrim H, Olsen JH, Melbye M. Risk for subsequent cancer after diagnosis of basal-cell carcinoma. A population-based epidemiologic study. *Ann Intern Med* 1996; **125**: 815–21.
15 Rowe DE, Carroll RJ, Day CL Jr. Long term recurrence rates in previously untreated (primary) basal cell carcinoma: implications for patient follow-up. *J Dermatol Surg Oncol* 1989; **15**: 315–27.

Keratoacanthoma

Keratoacanthoma is a benign, often rapidly growing lesion that probably arises from the supraseboglandular part of a sebaceous gland. Keratoacanthomas are common, self-limiting, proliferative tumours that arise most frequently in men after the sixth decade of life [1,2].

The lesions mimic squamous cell carcinoma both clinically and microscopically. Although some believe keratoacanthomas represent well-differentiated squamous cell carcinomas, significant differences between the two entities have been demonstrated [3]. A number of well-documented variants, many with generally distributed eruptive keratoacanthomas, have been described. One variant, Ferguson–Smith syndrome, is a familial trait.

Aetiology. The role of actinic damage is strongly supported by the fact that the majority of lesions occur on sun-exposed skin (90%), with up to 10% occurring periorally or on the vermilion border of the lips. HPV has also been suggested as an aetiological agent [4], and increased numbers of keratoacanthomas have been reported in immunocompromised patients.

Clinical features. Keratoacanthomas often manifest at the vermilion border, as indurated dome-shaped nodules displaying a characteristic central, keratin-filled, crusted and frequently darkened crater. Cutaneous lesions are asymptomatic but oral and lip lesions are frequently painful [5–7]. Intraoral keratoacanthomas are rare [8,9]. They usually appear as an ulcer with a rolled margin, clinically indistinguishable from squamous cell carcinoma, usually on the anterior or maxillary gingiva. It is unclear whether intraoral keratoacanthomas regress spontaneously, as all have been excised for diagnosis. Keratoacanthomas grow rapidly, attaining a size typically greater than 1 cm, may be locally invasive and result in significant tissue damage but, if left untreated, many undergo spontaneous involution after 1–2 months.

Diagnosis. Keratoacanthomas require differentiation from squamous cell carcinoma. When lesions develop intraorally or on the lips, they should immediately be subjected to biopsy for confirmation, since squamous cell carcinomas at these sites frequently metastasize.

Management. Management is often by surgical excision. Intralesional therapy with methotrexate or 5-fluorouracil can also be employed with excellent results. Other suggested medical therapies include intralesional interferon alpha-2a and systemic isotretinoin [10–12].

REFERENCES

1 Kingman J, Callen JP. Keratoacanthoma: a clinical study. *Arch Dermatol* 1984; **120**: 736–40.
2 Schwartz RA. Keratoacanthoma. *J Am Acad Dermatol* 1994; **30**: 1–19.
3 Waring AJ, Takata M, Rehman I, Rees JL. Loss of heterozygosity analysis of keratoacanthoma reveals multiple differences from cutaneous squamous cell carcinoma. *Br J Cancer* 1996; **73**: 649–53.
4 Hsi ED, Svoboda-Newman SM, Stern RA, Nickoloff BJ, Frank TS. Detection of human papillomavirus DNA in keratoacanthomas by polymerase chain reaction. *Am J Dermatopathol* 1997; **19**: 10–5.
5 Berrone S, De Gioanni PP, Gallesio C. Keratoacanthoma of the lower lip. A review of the literature and clinical case report. *Minerva Stomatol* 1992; **41**: 597–601.
6 de Visscher JGAM, van der Wal JE, Starink ThM, Tiwari RM, van der Waal I. Giant keratoacanthoma of the lower lip. Report of a case of spontaneous regression. *Oral Surg* 1996; **81**: 193–6.
7 Azaz B, Lustmann J. Keratoacanthoma of the lower lip. Review of the literature and report of a case. *Oral Surg Oral Med Oral Pathol* 1974; **38**: 918–27.
8 Eversole LR, Leider AS, Alexander G. Intraoral and labial keratoacanthomas. *Oral Surg* 1982; **54**: 663–7.
9 Whyte AM, Hansen LS, Lee C. The intraoral keratoacanthoma: a diagnostic problem. *Br J Oral Surg* 1986; **24**: 438–41.
10 Melton JR, Nelson BR, Stough DB *et al.* Treatment of keraotoacanthoma with intralesional methotrexate. *J Am Acad Dermatol* 1991; **25**: 1017–23.
11 Grobb JJ, Suzini F, Richard MA *et al.* Large keratoacanthomas treated with intralesional interferon alpha-2a. *J Am Acad Dermatol* 1993; **29**: 237–41.
12 Schaller M, Korting HC, Wolff H, Schirren CG, Burgdorf W. Multiple keratoacanthomas, giant keratoacanthoma and keratoacanthoma centrifugum marginatum: development in a single patient and treatment with oral isotretinoin. *Acta Derm Venereol (Stockh)* 1996; **76**: 40–2.

Other oral malignant primary neoplasms

The following comprise up to 10% of all oral malignant tumours.

1 Salivary gland tumours.
2 Malignant melanoma.
3 Lymphomas: non-Hodgkin's lymphomas are increasingly seen in the fauces in HIV disease and immunocompromised persons.
4 Sarcomas.

5 Kaposi's sarcoma: oral Kaposi's sarcoma is typically seen in HIV disease or other immunocompromised persons and especially in the posterior palate as a brown or purple macule that becomes nodular and ulcerates.
6 Some odontogenic tumours.
7 Maxillary antral carcinoma (or other neoplasms).
8 Langerhans' cell histiocytosis.
9 Neoplasms of bone and connective tissue.
10 Other neoplasms.

Abrikossoff's tumour

Abrikossoff's tumour is a disease that develops between the second and sixth decades of life, more frequently among women and blacks. The head and neck area is affected in 45–65% of cases and, of these, 70% are located intraorally (tongue, oral mucosa, hard palate) [1].

The benign form shows polygonal cells with granular eosinophilic cytoplasm and small nuclei. The malignant form, however, is associated with a high mitotic index and pleomorphic cellular tissue.

The clinical feature of either is a swelling covered by mucosa of normal clinical appearance. Histological examination is required. The treatment is surgery.

REFERENCE

1 Becelli R, Perugini M, Gasparini G, Cassoni A, Fabiani F. Abrikossoff's tumor. *J Craniofac Surg* 2001; **12**: 78–81.

Metastatic oral neoplasms

Metastases to the oral tissues are rare, accounting for only 1% of all oral tumours and most appear in bone, especially the mandibular premolar or molar area or condyle. Most oral metastases originate from carcinomas of breast, lung, kidney, thyroid, stomach, liver, colon or prostate [1–10].

Metastases may present with pain, paraesthesia, sensory loss, loosening of teeth, delayed healing of an extraction wound or pathological fracture. Metastases may occasionally appear as an alveolar or gingival swelling or ulcer.

Tumour deposits arise from lymphatic or haematogenous spread.

Clinical features. Metastases usually present as a lesion arising in the jaw, sometimes only revealed coincidentally by imaging, at other times causing symptoms. In up to one-third of patients the jaw lesions are the first manifestation of the tumour. Non-Hodgkin's lymphomas are frequently gingival or faucial in location.

Many metastases are asymptomatic but others manifest with:

• pain;
• paraesthesia or hypoaesthesia;
• swelling;

- tooth mobility;
- non-healing extraction sockets;
- pathological fracture;
- radiolucency or radio-opacity.

Diagnosis. Diagnosis is from history and clinical features supplemented by radiography and histopathology.

Treatment. Radiotherapy, surgery or chemotherapy.

REFERENCES

1 Abdullah BH, Yahya HI, Talabani NA, Alash NI, Mirza KB. Gingival and cutaneous angiosarcoma. *J Oral Pathol Med* 2000; **29**: 410–2.
2 Alandez J, Llanes F, Herrera JI, Carasol M, Bascones A. Metastatic lung carcinoma involving the periodontium. Report of a case. *J Periodontol* 1995; **66**: 896–8.
3 Ardekian L, Rosen DJ, Peled M *et al.* Primary gingival malignant melanoma. Report of 3 cases. *J Periodontol* 2000; **71**: 117–20.
4 Bschorer R, Lingenfelser T, Kaiserling E, Schwenzer N. Malignant lymphoma of the mucosa-associated lymphoid tissue (MALT): consecutive unusual manifestation in the rectum and gingiva. *J Oral Pathol Med* 1993; **22**: 190–2.
5 Ellis GL, Jensen JL, Reingold IM, Barr RJ. Malignant neoplasms metastatic to gingivae. *Oral Surg Oral Med Oral Pathol* 1977; **44**: 238–45.
6 Horie Y, Suou T, Hirayama C *et al.* Hepatocellular carcinoma metastatic to the oral cavity including the maxilla and the mandible: report of two cases and review of the literature. *Gastroenterol Jpn* 1985; **20**: 604–10.
7 Keller EE, Gunderson LL. Bone disease metastatic to the jaw. *J Am Dent Assoc* 1987; **115**: 697–701.
8 Margiotta V, Franco V, Rizzo A *et al.* Gastric and gingival localization of mucosa-associated lymphoid tissue (MALT) lymphoma. An immunohistochemical, virological and clinical case report. *J Periodontol* 1999; **70**: 914–8.
9 Medina BR, Barba EM, Torres AV, Trujillo SM. Gingival metastases as first sign of a primary uterine angiosarcoma. *J Oral Maxillofac Surg* 2001; **59**: 467–71.
10 Nishimura Y, Yakata H, Kawasaki T *et al.* Metastatic tumours of the mouth and jaws: a review of the Japanese literature. *J Maxillofac Surg* 1982; **10**: 253–8.

Ulcers in association with systemic disease

Aphthae (see p. 66.43) are occasionally associated with systemic disease. However, a wide range of systemic diseases, especially haematological, gastrointestinal and dermatological disorders, may cause other oral lesions which, because of the moisture, trauma and infection in the mouth, tend to break down to leave ulcers or erosions. Oral ulceration is also frequently caused by infections and can be caused by iatrogenic problems such as drugs or irradiation (see Table 66.13).

Haematological diseases

Deficiency states

Low iron, folate or vitamin B$_{12}$ levels may predispose to aphthae. A few of these patients also have anaemia, sometimes with other oral features such as glossitis or angular stomatitis, but many have a deficiency state with no established anaemia [1,2]. Occasionally, patients with deficiency of B vitamins may develop other types of oral ulcer, and sometimes epithelial dysplasia [3].

REFERENCES

1 Field EA, Speechley JA, Rugman FR *et al.* Oral signs and symptoms in patients with undiagnosed vitamin B12 deficiency. *J Oral Pathol Med* 1995; **24**: 468–70.
2 Tyldesley WR. Oral signs and symptoms in anaemias. *Br Dent J* 1985; **139**: 232–6.
3 Theaker JM, Porter SR, Fleming KA. Oral epithelial dysplasia in vitamin B12 deficiency. *Oral Surg* 1989; **67**: 81–3.

Leukopenias and agranulocytosis

White cell dyscrasias and HIV infection are also often complicated by oral ulceration (Fig. 66.29). Oral ulceration may be a major symptom in patients with leukopenias, and may be the first manifestation of drug-induced agranulocytosis. Painful, deep, irregular ulcers, often with only a minimal inflammatory halo, involve the mouth and/or pharynx and tend to extend and penetrate slowly. In cyclic neutropenia, ulcers appear episodically at 21-day intervals in association with the neutropenic episodes. Severe periodontitis is often also a feature of leukocyte and other immune defects and the patients may suffer from recurrent infections elsewhere [1–3]. Methotrexate can cause oral ulceration in the absence of leukopenia.

REFERENCES

1 Baehni PC, Payot P, Tsai CC *et al.* Periodontal status associated with chronic neutropenia. *J Clin Periodontol* 1983; **10**: 222–30.
2 Porter SR, Scully C, Standen G. Autoimmune neutropenia manifesting as recurrent oral ulceration. *Oral Surg* 1994; **78**: 178–80.
3 Scully C, Gilmour G. Neutropenia and dental patients. *Br Dent J* 1986; **160**: 43–6.

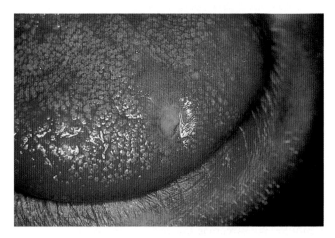

Fig. 66.29 Aphthous-like ulceration in HIV disease.

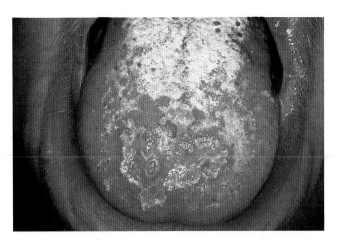

Fig. 66.30 Herpes simplex lingual recurrence, and candidiasis in leukaemia: similar lesions may be seen in HIV infection.

Leukaemias

Oral ulceration may be a prominent feature, especially in the acute leukaemias. Other oral manifestations of leukaemia include mucosal pallor, gingival haemorrhage, gingival swelling, petechiae and ecchymoses [1–4]. Oral infections with *Candida albicans* and Gram-negative bacteria including *Pseudomonas* species, *Escherichia coli*, *Proteus*, *Klebsiella* and *Serratia* species are common, especially in acute leukaemias, and may act as a portal for septicaemia [5]. Herpes simplex or zoster–varicella virus ulcers are also common (Fig. 66.30). Chemotherapy complicates the situation because it too can produce oral ulceration [1,6].

Other findings include paraesthesia (particularly of the lower lip), extrusion of teeth or bone, painful swellings over the mandible and parotid swelling (Mikulicz's syndrome) [7].

REFERENCES

1 Barrett AP. A long term prospective clinical study of oral complications during conventional chemotherapy for acute leukemia. *Oral Surg* 1987; **63**: 313–6.
2 Dreizen S, McCredie KB, Body GP *et al.* Quantitative analysis of the oral complications of anti-leukemia chemotherapy. *Oral Surg* 1986; **62**: 650–3.
3 Dreizen S, McCredie KB, Keating MJ *et al.* Malignant gingival and skin infiltrates in adult leukemia. *Oral Surg* 1983; **55**: 572–8.
4 Scully C, MacFarlane TW. Orofacial manifestations in childhood malignancy: clinical and microbiological findings during remission. *ASDC J Dent Child* 1983; **50**: 121–5.
5 Dreizen S, McCredie KB, Bodey GP *et al.* Microbial mucocutaneous infections in acute adult leukaemia. *Postgrad Med* 1986; **79**: 107–18.
6 Dreizen S, McCredie KB, Keating MJ. Chemotherapy-associated oral hemorrhages in adults with acute leukemia. *Oral Surg* 1984; **57**: 494–8.
7 Filippi A, Dreyer T, Bohle RM, Pohl Y, Rosseau S. Sequestration of the alveolar bone by invasive aspergillosis in acute myeloid leukemia. *J Oral Pathol Med* 1997; **26**: 437–40.

Granulocytic sarcoma
SYN. CHLOROMA

Granulocytic sarcomas are rare in the oral cavity. Most present with swelling or symptoms related to skeletal involvement [1–3]. The maxilla is particularly involved [1,4].

REFERENCES

1 Barker GR, Sloan P. Maxillary chloroma: a myeloid leukaemic deposit. *Br J Oral Surg* 1988; **26**: 124–8.
2 Ficarra G, Silverman S, Quivey JM *et al.* Granulocytic sarcoma (chloroma) of the oral cavity: a case with aleukaemic presentation. *Oral Surg* 1987; **63**: 709–14.
3 Hansen LS, Merrell PW, Bainton DF, Taylor KL. Granulocytic sarcoma: an aleukemic oral presentation. *Can Dent Assoc J* 1982; **10**: 41–6.
4 Castella A, Davey FR, Elbadawi A, Gordon GB. Granulocytic sarcoma of the hard palate: report of the first case. *Hum Pathol* 1984; **15**: 1190–2.

Myelodysplastic syndrome

Oral manifestations in myelodysplastic syndrome include particularly ulceration but also paraesthesiae, petechiae, burning mouth, gingival swelling, xerostomia and herpes labialis [1–4].

REFERENCES

1 Epstein JB, Priddy RW, Sparling T *et al.* Oral manifestations in myelodysplastic syndrome. *Oral Surg* 1986; **61**: 466–70.
2 Flint SR, Sugerman P, Scully C *et al.* The myelodysplastic syndromes: case report and review. *Oral Surg* 1990; **70**: 579–83.
3 Gibson J, Lamey P-J, Watson WH *et al.* The myelodysplastic syndrome presenting with oral symptoms. *Br Dent J* 1987; **163**: 234–5.
4 Porter SR, Scully C. Gingival and oral mucosal ulceration associated with the myelodysplastic syndrome. *Oral Oncol* 1994; **30B**: 346–50.

Lymphomas

Some 2–10% of lymphomas present first in the oral cavity. Of these oral lymphomas, 80% are composed of follicular centre cells or post-follicular cells [1–5]. Lymphomas usually occur on the pharynx or palate, but occasionally on the tongue, gingivae or lips; they may appear as oral swellings, which sometimes ulcerate and may cause pain or sensory disturbance. Oral herpes zoster and herpes simplex infections are common in patients with lymphomas.

There is an increased incidence of oral lymphomas in HIV disease [6] including oral plasmablastic lymphomas [7,8].

Lethal midline granuloma. Lethal midline granuloma is the term sometimes used to include a spectrum of conditions including Wegener's granulomatosis, polymorphic reticulosis (lymphomatoid granulomatosis) and idiopathic midline destructive disease.

Wegener's granulomatosis. Although not a lymphoma, Wegener's granulomatosis is discussed here. Oral manifestations are common and may be the first sign of Wegener's granulomatosis [9–20]. A painless progressive swelling of the gingiva in a previously healthy mouth, particularly associated with swollen inflamed papillae, should arouse suspicion of Wegener's granulomatosis. The gingival enlargement may have a fairly characteristic 'strawberry-like' appearance. Wegener's granulomatosis may also present with oral ulceration, failure of an extraction socket to heal or occasionally swelling of the lip or salivary gland.

Polymorphic reticulosis (syn. lymphomatoid granulomatosis). The most common oral presentation of polymorphic reticulosis is palatal ulceration but ulceration may occur elsewhere [17].

Idiopathic midline destructive disease [21–23]. Downward spread from nasal disease can lead to palatal necrosis and ulceration in idiopathic midline destructive disease. Occasionally the disease presents with delayed healing of an extraction socket.

REFERENCES

1 Epstein JB, Epstein JD, Le ND, Gorsky M. Characteristics of oral and paraoral malignant lymphoma: a population-based review of 361 cases. *Oral Surg Oral Med Oral Pathol Oral Radiol Endod* 2001; **92**: 519–25.
2 Baden E, Carter R. Intraoral presentation of American Burkitt's lymphoma after extraction of a mandibular left third molar. *J Oral Maxillofac Surg* 1987; **45**: 689–93.
3 Savarrio L, Gibson J, Dunlop DJ, O'Rourke N, Fitzsimons EJ. Spontaneous regression of an anaplastic large cell lymphoma in the oral cavity: first reported case and review of the literature. *Oral Oncol* 1999; **35**: 609–13.
4 Born S, Gaber G, Willgeroth K *et al.* Metastasising malignant lymphoma mimicking necrotising and hyperplastic gingivostomatitis. *Eur J Dermatol* 1999; **9**: 569–73.
5 Eisenbud L, Sciubba JJ, Mir R *et al.* Oral presentations in non-Hodgkins lymphoma: a review of thirty one cases. *Oral Surg* 1983; **56**: 151–6.
6 Ioachim HL, Cooper MC, Hellman GC. Lymphomas in men at high risk for acquired immune deficiency syndrome (AIDS): a study of 21 cases. *Cancer* 1985; **56**: 2831–42.
7 Porter SR, Diz Dios P, Kumar N *et al.* Oral plasmablastic lymphoma in previously undiagnosed HIV disease. *Oral Surg Oral Med Oral Pathol* 1999; **87**: 730–4.
8 Flaitz CM, Nichols CM, Walling DM, Hicks MJ. Plasmablastic lymphoma: an HIV-associated entity with primary oral manifestations. *Oral Oncol* 2002; **38**: 96–102.
9 Lilly J, Juhlin T, Lew D, Vincent S, Lilly G. Wegener's granulomatosis presenting as oral lesions: a case report. *Oral Surg Oral Med Oral Pathol Oral Radiol Endod* 1998; **85**: 153–7.
10 Abraham-Inpijn L. Oral and otal manifestations as the primary symptoms in Wegener's granulomatosis. *J Head Neck Pathol* 1983; **2**: 20–2.
11 Allen CM, Canisa C, Salewski C, Weiland JE. Wegeners granulomatosis: report of three cases with oral lesions. *J Oral Maxillofac Surg* 1991; **49**: 294–8.
12 Israelson H, Binnie WH, Hurt WC. The hyperplastic gingivitis of Wegener's granulomatosis. *J Periodontol* 1981; **52**: 81–7.
13 Lutcavage GJ, Schaberg SJ, Arendt DA, Malmquist JP. Gingival mass with massive soft-tissue necrosis. *J Oral Maxillofac Surg* 1991; **49**: 1332–8.
14 Parsons E, Seymour RA, MacLeod RI *et al.* Wegener's granulomatosis: distinct gingival lesion. *J Clin Periodontol* 1992; **19**: 64–6.
15 Patten SF, Tomecki KJ. Wegeners granulomatosis: cutaneous and oral mucosal disease. *J Am Acad Dermatol* 1993; **28**: 710–8.
16 Hansen LS, Silverman S, Pons VG *et al.* Limited Wegener's granulomatosis. Report of a case with oral, renal and skin involvement. *Oral Surg* 1985; **60**: 524–30.
17 McDonald TJ, De Remee RA, Weiland LH. Wegener's granulomatosis and polymorphic reticulosis: two diseases or one? Experience with 90 patients. *Arch Otolaryngol* 1981; **107**: 141–6.
18 Fauci AS, Haynes BF, Katz P *et al.* Wegener's granulomatosis: prospective clinical and therapeutic experience with 85 patients for 21 years. *Ann Intern Med* 1983; **98**: 76–85.
19 Rahilly G, Rahilly M. A case of palatal Wegener's granulomatosis. *Oral Dis* 2000; **6**: 259–61.
20 Rasmussen N. Management of the ear, nose, and throat manifestations of Wegener granulomatosis: an otorhinolaryngologist's perspective. *Curr Opin Rheumatol* 2001; **13**: 3–11.
21 Crissman JD, Weiss MA, Gluckman J. Midline granuloma syndrome. A clinicopathologic study of 13 patients. *Am J Surg Pathol* 1982; **6**: 335–8.
22 Nelson JF, Finkelstein MW, Acevedo A *et al.* Midline 'non-healing' granuloma. *Oral Surg* 1984; **58**: 554–60.
23 Tsokos M, Fauci AS, Costa J. Idiopathic midline destructive disease (IMDD). A subgroup of patients with the midline granuloma syndrome. *Am J Clin Pathol* 1982; **77**: 162–7.

Mycosis fungoides

Oral lesions in mycosis fungoides typically are red or white areas on the tongue but are usually late manifestations of this disease [1–6].

REFERENCES

1 Barnett ML, Cole RJ. Mycosis fungoides with multiple oral mucosal lesions. *J Periodontol* 1985; **56**: 690–3.
2 Evans GE, Dalziel KL. Mycosis fungoides with oral involvement. *Int J Oral Maxillofac Surg* 1987; **16**: 634–7.
3 Patel SP, Hotterman OA. Mycosis fungoides: an overview. *J Surg Oncol* 1983; **22**: 221–6.
4 de la Fuente EG, Rodriguez-Peralto JL, Ortiz PL *et al.* Oral involvement in mycosis fungoides: report of two cases and a literature review. *Acta Derm Venereol (Stockh)* 2000; **80**: 299–301.
5 Harman M, Akdeniz S, Arslan A, Koyoglu S. Mycosis fungoides with involvement of the oral cavity. *J Eur Acad Dermatol Venereol* 1998; **10**: 253–6.
6 Hata T, Aikoh T, Hirokawa M, Hosoda M. Mycosis fungoides with involvement of the oral mucosa. *Int J Oral Maxillofac Surg* 1998; **27**: 127–8.

Pseudolymphoma

Rare tumour-like lymphoproliferative infiltrates that lack the malignant potential of lymphomas may be seen intraorally, notably in the palate [1].

REFERENCE

1 Wright JM, Dunsworth AR. Follicular lymphoid hyperplasia of the hard palate: a benign lymphoproliferative process. *Oral Surg* 1983; **55**: 162–8.

Histiocytoses

The histiocytoses typically produce lytic bone lesions but gingival swelling, periodontal destruction with loosening of teeth, non-healing extraction sockets and mouth ulceration may be seen. ^{111}In-pentetreotide imaging may be useful in diagnosis of Langerhans' cell histiocytosis [1–7].

REFERENCES

1 Broadbent V, Pritchard J. Histiocytosis X: current controversies. *Arch Dis Child* 1985; **60**: 605–8.
2 Favera BE, McCarthy RC, Mieran GW. Histiocytosis X. *Hum Pathol* 1983; **14**: 663–76.
3 Hartman KS. Histiocytosis X. A review of 114 cases with oral involvement. *Oral Surg* 1980; **49**: 38–54.
4 Langowska-Adamczyk H, Jedrusik-Pawlowska M. Disseminated form of Langerhans cell histiocytosis discovered in stomatological examination: a case report. *Med Sci Monit* 2000; **6**: 1174–8.
5 Shirley JC, Thornton JB. Oral manifestations of Langerhans' cell histiocytosis: review and report of case. *ASDC J Dent Child* 2000; **67**: 293–6.
6 Chen N, Peron JM. The nonhealing of the buccal mucosa after tooth extraction. Apropos a case of histiocytosis X. *Rev Stomatol Chir Maxillofac* 2000; **101**: 33–5.
7 Milian MA, Bagan JV, Jimenez Y *et al.* Langerhans' cell histiocytosis restricted to the oral mucosa. *Oral Surg Oral Med Oral Pathol Oral Radiol Endod* 2001; **91**: 76–9.

Multicentric reticulohistiocytosis

Oral lesions are seen in up to 50% of patients with multicentric reticulohistiocytosis [1]. Lesions are collections of histiocytes that form nodular or granular lesions, particularly in the labial or buccal mucosa. The temporomandibular joint may also be involved as part of the polyarthropathy.

REFERENCE

1 Katz RW, Anderson KF. Multicentric reticulohistiocytosis. *Oral Surg* 1988; **65**: 721–5.

Hypereosinophilic syndrome

Oral erosions affecting buccal, gingival or labial mucosae may be a feature of the hypereosinophilic syndrome [1–4] and may herald cardiac involvement [2]. Etoposide therapy may be effective [4].

REFERENCES

1 Aractingi S, Janin A, Zini JM *et al.* Specific mucosal erosions in hypereosinophilic syndrome. *Arch Dermatol* 1996; **132**: 535–41.
2 Leiferman KM, O'Duffy D, Perry HO *et al.* Recurrent incapacitating mucosal ulcerations: a prodrome of the hypereosinophilic syndrome. *Am J Med* 1982; **247**: 1018–20.
3 Billon C, Gautier C, Villaret E *et al.* Isolated mucosal ulcers disclosing idiopathic hypereosinophilic syndrome. *Ann Dermatol Vénéréol* 1997; **124**: 248–50.
4 Smit AJ, van Essen LH, de Vries EG. Successful long-term control of idiopathic hypereosinophilic syndrome with etoposide. *Cancer* 1991; **67**: 2826–7.

Hypoplasminogenaemia

Gingival swelling and ulceration are features of hypoplasminogenaemia [1].

REFERENCE

1 Scully C, Gokbuget AY, Allen C *et al.* Oral lesions indicative of plasminogen deficiency (hypoplasminogenemia). *Oral Surg Oral Med Oral Pathol Oral Radiol Endod* 2001; **91**: 334–7.

Gastrointestinal diseases

Aphthae in gastrointestinal diseases are discussed on p. 66.45. Other types of mouth ulcer are also sometimes found in ulcerative colitis and Crohn's disease.

Pyostomatitis vegetans

The oral lesions termed pyostomatitis vegetans are deep fissures, pustules and papillary projections. Less than 50 cases have been recorded and most patients have had inflammatory bowel disease, i.e. ulcerative colitis or Crohn's disease [1–12]. The course of these lesions tends to follow that of the associated bowel disease [1–5].

Although the oral lesions may respond at least partially to topical therapy (e.g. corticosteroids), systemic treatment is often needed [1–5,12].

REFERENCES

1 Ballo FS, Camisa C, Allen CM. Pyostomatitis vegetans. *J Am Acad Dermatol* 1989; **21**: 381–7.
2 Basu MK, Asquith P. Oral manifestations of inflammatory bowel disease. *Clin Gastroenterol* 1980; **9**: 307.
3 Chan S, Scully C, Prime SS *et al.* Pyostomatitis vegetans: oral manifestation of ulcerative colitis. *Oral Surg* 1991; **27**: 689–92.
4 Neville B, Laden SA, Smith SE *et al.* Pyostomatitis vegetans. *Am J Dermatopathol* 1985; **7**: 69–77.
5 Thornhill MH, Zakrzewska JM, Gilkes JJH. Pyostomatitis vegetans: report of three cases and review of the literature. *J Oral Pathol Med* 1992; **21**: 128–33.
6 Van Hale HM, Rogers RS, Zone JJ. Pyostomatitis vegetans: a reactive mucosal marker for inflammatory disease of the gut. *Arch Dermatol* 1985; **121**: 94–8.
7 Chaudhry SI, Philpot NS, Odell EW, Challacombe SJ, Shirlaw PJ. Pyostomatitis vegetans associated with asymptomatic ulcerative colitis: a case report. *Oral Surg Oral Med Oral Pathol Oral Radiol Endod* 1999; **87**: 327–30.
8 Al-Rimawi HS, Hammad MM, Raweily EA, Hammad HM. Pyostomatitis vegetans in childhood. *Eur J Pediatr* 1998; **157**: 402–5.
9 Oettinger R, Gerner P, Borner N, Schopf RE. Pyostomatitis vegetans and Crohn's disease. A specific association of 2 diseases. *Dtsch Med Wochenschr* 1998; **123**: 285–8.
10 Healy CM, Farthing PM, Williams DM, Thornhill MH. Pyostomatitis vegetans and associated systemic disease. A review and two case reports. *Oral Surg Oral Med Oral Pathol* 1994; **78**: 323–8.
11 Prendiville JS, Israel DM, Wood WS, Dimmick JE. Oral pemphigus vulgaris associated with inflammatory bowel disease and herpetic gingivostomatitis in an 11-year-old girl. *Pediatr Dermatol* 1994; **11**: 145–50.
12 Calobrisi SD, Mutasim DF, McDonald JS. Pyostomatitis vegetans associated with ulcerative colitis. Temporary clearance with fluocinonide gel and complete remission after colectomy. *Oral Surg Oral Med Oral Pathol Oral Radiol Endod* 1995; **79**: 452–4.

Orofacial granulomatosis (OFG)

Aetiology. Crohn's disease can affect the mouth but some patients appear to develop similar oral lesions because of an adverse reaction to various food additives, such as cinnamaldehyde or benzoates, butylated hydroxyanisole or dodecyl gallate (in margarine), or to menthol (in peppermint oil) or cobalt, although these reactions are by no means always relevant [1–15]. For example, the lesions in only one of nine patients in one study had any relationship to food intake [15]. The genetic background [16], any role of allergy [17] and diverse possible other aetiological factors such as *Mycobacterium paratuberculosis* [18] is unclear.

The term 'orofacial granulomatosis' is preferred in some centres since it is unclear where in the spectrum of Crohn's disease/sarcoidosis/allergy/infection these lesions (and related conditions such as Melkersson–Rosenthal syndrome and granulomatous cheilitis) lie [8,19–21].

Pathology. Non-caseating granulomas and lympho-edema may be seen but the granulomas tend to be sparse and deep, close to the muscle.

Clinical features. Ulcers classically involve the buccal sulcus where they appear as linear ulcers, often with granulomatous masses flanking them.

Mucosal lesions also include thickening and folding of the mucosa to produce a 'cobblestone' type of appearance and mucosal tags. Purple granulomatous enlargements may appear on the gingiva. The lips or face may swell and there may be splitting of the lips and angular stomatitis [22,23].

Diagnosis. The oral history is not specific, and investigation of the gastrointestinal tract is mandatory. Investigations such as chest radiography, serum angiotensin-converting enzyme and a gallium scan may be required to exclude sarcoidosis. Patch tests may be indicated to exclude reactions to various foodstuffs or additives.

Treatment. Elimination diets may be warranted in patients with OFG if allergy is suspected [11]. Topical or intralesional corticosteroids may effectively control the oral lesions [6]. Intralesional corticosteroid injections may also reduce the swelling. The injection of up to 10 mL triamcinolone (10 mg/L) into the lips after local analgesia may be effective [15,24–26]. The injections may have to be repeated every 4–6 months once a response plateau has been reached. Systemic corticosteroids are rarely indicated and in any event not all patients respond [26]. Metronidazole may be of value in some cases [3].

Clofazimine in a dose of 100 mg twice daily for 10 days, then twice weekly for 4 months appears to help the majority of patients [27,28]. Clofazimine appears to be most effective during the early stages and works by clearing granulomas.

REFERENCES

1 Field EA, Tyldesley WR. Oral Crohn's disease revisited: a 10 year review. *Br J Oral Maxillofac Surg* 1989; **27**: 114–23.
2 Halme L, Meurman JH, Laine P et al. Oral findings in patients with active or inactive Crohn's disease. *Oral Surg* 1993; **76**: 175–81.
3 Kano Y, Shiohara T, Yagita A. Treatment of recalcitrant cheilitis granulomatosa with metronidazole. *J Am Acad Dermatol* 1992; **27**: 629–30.
4 Patton DW, Ferguson MM, Forsyth A et al. Orofacial granulomatosis: a possible allergic basis. *Br J Oral Maxillofac Surg* 1985; **23**: 235–42.
5 Ronney T. Dental caries prevalence in patients with Crohn's disease. *Oral Surg* 1984; **57**: 623–4.
6 Sakuntabhai A, MacLeod RI, Lawrence CM. Intralesional steroid injection after nerve block anesthesia in the treatment of orofacial granulomatosis. *Arch Dermatol* 1993; **129**: 477–80.
7 Scully C, Cochran KM, Russell RI et al. Crohn's disease of the mouth: an indication of intestinal involvement. *Gut* 1982; **23**: 198–201.
8 Scully C, Eveson JW. Orofacial granulomatosis. *Lancet* 1991; **338**: 20–1.
9 Shehade SA, Foulds IS. Granulomatous cheilitis and a positive Kveim test. *Br J Dermatol* 1986; **115**: 619–22.
10 Sundh B, Emilson CG. Salivary and microbial conditions and dental health in patients with Crohn's disease: a 3-year study. *Oral Surg* 1989; **67**: 286–90.
11 Sweatman MC, Tasker R, Warner JO et al. Orofacial granulomatosis. Response to elimination diet and provocation by food additives. *Clin Allergy* 1986; **16**: 331–7.
12 Pryce DW, King CM. Orofacial granulomatosis associated with delayed hypersensitivity to cobalt. *Clin Exp Dermatol* 1990; **15**: 384–96.
13 Lewis FM, Shah M, Gawkrodger DJ. Contact sensitivity to food additives can cause oral and perioral symptoms. *Contact Dermatitis* 1995; **33**: 429–30.
14 McKenna KE, Walsh MY, Burrows D. The Melkersson–Rosenthal syndrome and food additive hypersensitivity. *Br J Dermatol* 1994; **131**: 921–2.
15 Pemberton M, Yeoman CM, Clark A et al. Allergy to octyl gallate causing stomatitis. *Br Dent J* 1993; **175**: 106–8.
16 Gibson J, Wray D. Human leucocyte antigen (HLA) typing in orofacial granulomatosis. *Br J Dermatol* 2000; **143**: 1119–21.
17 Wray D, Rees S, Gibson J, Forsyth A. The role of allergy in oral mucosal diseases. *Q J Med* 2000; **93**: 507–11.
18 Riggio MP, Gibson J, Lennon A, Wray D, MacDonald DG. Search for *Mycobacterium paratuberculosis* DNA in orofacial granulomatosis and oral Crohn's disease tissue by polymerase chain reaction. *Gut* 1997; **41**: 646–50.
19 Worsaae N, Pindborg JJ. Granulomatous gingival manifestations of Melkersson–Rosenthal syndrome. *Oral Surg* 1980; **49**: 131–8.
20 Worsaae N, Christensen KO, Bondesen S et al. Melkersson–Rosenthal syndrome and Crohn's disease. *Br J Oral Surg* 1980; **18**: 254–8.
21 Zimmer WM, Rogers RS, Reeve CM, Sheridan PJ. Orofacial manifestations of Melkersson–Rosenthal syndrome. *Oral Surg* 1992; **74**: 610–9.
22 Wiesenfield DW, Ferguson MM, Mitchell D et al. Orofacial granulomatosis: a clinical and pathological analysis. *Q J Med* 1985; **54**: 101–13.
23 Williams AJK, Wray D, Ferguson A. The clinical entity of orofacial Crohn's disease. *Q J Med* 1991; **79**: 451–8.
24 Cermale D, Serri F. Intralesional injection of triamcinolone in the treatment of cheilitis granulomatosa. *Arch Dermatol* 1963; **72**: 695–6.
25 Williams PM, Greenberg MS. Management of cheilitis granulomatosa. *Oral Surg* 1991; **72**: 436–9.
26 Krutchkoff D, James R. Cheilitis granulomatosa: successful treatment with combined local triamcinolone injections and surgery. *Arch Dermatol* 1978; **114**: 1203–6.
27 Neuhofer J, Fritsch P. Cheilitis granulomatosa: therapy with clofazimine. *Hautarzt* 1984; **35**: 459–63.
28 Podmore P, Burrows D. Clofazimine: an effective treatment for Melkersson–Rosenthal syndrome or Miescher's cheilitis. *Clin Exp Dermatol* 1986; **11**: 173–8.

Crohn's disease

Crohn's disease lesions are indistinguishable from OFG.

Dermatological diseases

Several dermatoses can be associated with oral ulcers or erosions; lichen planus (LP) is the most common, pemphigus the most serious and pemphgoid is intermediate.

Lichen planus (see Chapter 42)

Oral LP may affect up to 1–2% of the population and is probably about eight times more common than cutaneous LP. The oral mucosa may be involved alone or in association with lesions on skin or other mucosa, and oral lesions may precede, accompany or follow lesions elsewhere [1–4]. The association of oral LP with gingival involvement, together with vulvovaginal lesions, has been termed the *vulvovaginal–gingival syndrome*.

Aetiology. Most oral LP is idiopathic but significantly greater anxiety and depression are observed among patients with oral LP compared with controls [5].

Some lichenoid lesions may be related to dental materials: the prevalence of positive reactions to potential allergens in the North American Contact Dermatitis Group (NACDG) is higher in oral LP for chromate, gold and thimerosal [6]. Other lichenoid reactions may be caused by GVHD, drug use (e.g. non-steroidal anti-inflammatory agents), diabetes [7] or liver disease. Chronic liver disease, especially chronic active hepatitis and hepatitis C virus (HCV) infection, may be associated with erosive LP in persons of southern European, Japanese or some other extractions [8] and there may be anticardiolipin antibodies [9]. In persons of northern European extraction, oral LP is only rarely associated with liver disease or with hepatitis C, hepatitis G or transfusion-transmitted virus [10–12].

Pathology. The pathology is similar to that of cutaneous LP, although sawtooth rete ridges are rarely seen in oral biopsies, and other epithelial changes may be less distinct.

Clinical features. The common oral lesions of LP are bilateral white lesions in the buccal and/or lingual mucosa. They may be reticular, papular or plaque-like (Figs 66.31–66.35). They are often symptomless but may cause soreness [1–4].

Erosive LP, which frequently affects the dorsum and lateral borders of the tongue or the buccal mucosae on both sides, is uncommon. The erosions are often large, slightly depressed or raised with a yellow slough, and have an irregular outline (Fig. 66.34), but they are not always as painful as might be imagined. The surrounding mucosa is often erythematous and glazed in appearance, with loss of filiform papillae of the tongue, and there are often pathognomonic whitish striae. LP may also produce

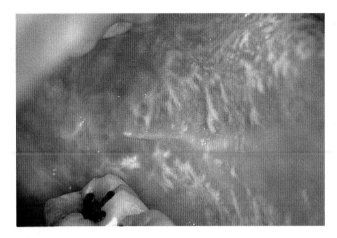

Fig. 66.31 Lichen planus: reticulopapular lesions in the common oral site, the buccal mucosa.

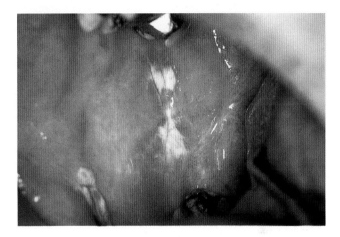

Fig. 66.32 Lichen planus: plaque-like lesions resemble leukoplakia.

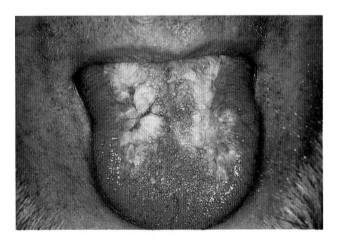

Fig. 66.33 Lichen planus on the tongue.

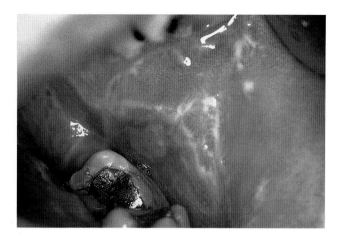

Fig. 66.34 Erosive lichen planus.

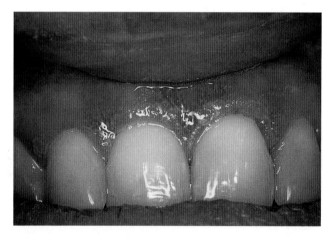

Fig. 66.35 Lichen planus on the gingivae: white and desquamative lesions.

a desquamative gingivitis (see p. 66.100). Candidiasis may complicate oral LP.

Reticular LP is the most frequent clinical presentation in both HCV-positive and HCV-negative patients. HCV-positive patients particularly have lip, tongue and gingival lesions [13].

Prognosis. There appears to be a predisposition for some oral LP, particularly the non-reticular forms, to develop carcinoma—possibly a risk of up to 5% over 10 years [1–4].

Diagnosis. Biopsy with immunofluorescence is often indicated to exclude keratosis, chronic ulcerative stomatitis with stratified epithelium-specific antinuclear antibodies, lichen sclerosus, lupus erythematosus, malignancy and other disorders.

Management. Treatment is not always necessary, unless there are symptoms. Unfortunately, although the natural

history of cutaneous LP is one of remission in most cases, in few patients with oral LP does the disorder remit, and thus treatment is indicated for symptomatic oral LP [1–4,14].
• Predisposing factors should be corrected. It may be wise to consider removal of dental amalgams if the lesions are closely related to these, or are unilateral, but there are no tests (e.g. patch tests) that will reliably indicate which patients will benefit from this.

If drugs are implicated, the physician should be consulted as to possible changes in therapy. If there is diabetes or HCV infection, this should be treated by a physician.
• Improvement in oral hygiene may result in some subjective benefit. Thus good oral hygiene should be maintained. Chlorhexidine or triclosan mouthwashes may help.
• Symptoms can often be controlled with topical medication: topical corticosteroids, such as betamethasone valerate aerosol or pastes containing fluocinonide, fluocinolone, triamcinolone, betamethasone valerate or clobetasol [15,16]; or topical tacrolimus [17,18]. Antifungals may help, especially where there is candidal superinfection.
1 *Mild LP.* Topical corticosteroids are the mainstay of therapy (e.g. triamcinolone acetate, betamethasone or fluocinolone). Erosive and gingival lesions are often recalcitrant. Next, high-potency corticosteroids such as clobetasol, fluocinonide or fluticasone may be employed initially and then changed to a lower potency drug.
2 *Moderate LP.* If there is severe or extensive oral involvement, topical ciclosporin or tacrolimus may be of significant benefit, often being used with a high-potency or super-potent topical steroid such as clobetasol, fluticasone or mometasone. Topical creams or pastes can be applied in a suitable customized tray or veneer to be worn at night. This regimen is useful in the management of LP-related desquamative gingivitis recalcitrant to other therapies.
3 *Severe LP.* In severe LP in multiple sites, patients may require systemic corticosteroids, azathioprine, cyclophosphamide, hydroxychloroquine, acitretin, thalidomide or ciclosporin. Dapsone is occasionally effective.
• Other therapies for LP include retinoids, dapsone, low-molecular-weight heparin [19] and many others, but either their efficacy has not been well proven or they have unacceptable adverse effects.
• Patients with non-reticular LP should be monitored to exclude development of carcinoma. Tobacco and alcohol use should be minimized.

REFERENCES

1 Scully C, Beyli M, Feirrero M *et al.* Update on oral lichen planus: aetiopathogenesis and management. *Crit Rev Oral Biol Med* 1998; **9**: 86–122.
2 Wright JM. A review and update of intraoral lichen planus. *Tex Dent J* 2001; **118**: 450–4.
3 Chainani-Wu N, Silverman S Jr, Lozada-Nur F, Mayer P, Watson JJ. Oral

lichen planus: patient profile, disease progression and treatment responses. *J Am Dent Assoc* 2001; **132**: 901–9.

4 Eisen D. The clinical features, malignant potential, and systemic associations of oral lichen planus: a study of 723 patients. *J Am Acad Dermatol* 2002; **46**: 207–14.

5 Vallejo MJ, Huerta G, Cerero R, Seoane JM. Anxiety and depression as risk factors for oral lichen planus. *Dermatology* 2001; **203**: 303–7.

6 Scalf LA, Fowler JF Jr, Morgan KW, Looney SW. Dental metal allergy in patients with oral, cutaneous, and genital lichenoid reactions. *Am J Contact Dermatitis* 2001; **12**: 146–50.

7 Romero MA, Seoane J, Varela-Centelles P, Diz-Dios P, Garcia-Pola MJ. Prevalence of diabetes mellitus amongst oral lichen planus patients. Clinical and pathological characteristics. *Med Oral* 2002; **7**: 121–9.

8 Carrozzo M, Gandolfo S, Lodi G *et al.* Oral lichen planus patients infected or non-infected with hepatitis C virus: the role of autoimmunity. *J Oral Pathol Med* 1999; **28**: 16–9.

9 Nagao Y, Tsubone K, Kimura R *et al.* High prevalence of anticardiolipin antibodies in patients with HCV-associated oral lichen planus. *Int J Mol Med* 2002; **9**: 293–7.

10 Ingafou M, Porter SR, Scully C, Teo CG. No evidence for HCV infection or liver disease in British patients with lichen planus. *Int J Oral Maxillofac Surg* 1998; **27**: 65–6.

11 Lodi G, Carrozzo M, Harris K *et al.* Hepatitis G virus-associated oral lichen planus: no influence from hepatitis G virus co-infection. *J Oral Pathol Med* 2000; **29**: 39–42.

12 Bez C, Hallet R, Carrozzo M *et al.* Lack of association between hepatotropic transfusion transmitted virus infection and oral lichen planus in British and Italian populations. *Br J Dermatol* 2001; **145**: 990–3.

13 Romero MA, Seoane J, Varela-Centelles P, Diz-Dios P, Otero XL. Clinical and pathological characteristics of oral lichen planus in hepatitis C-positive and -negative patients. *Clin Otolaryngol* 2002; **27**: 22–6.

14 Scully C, Eisen D, Carrozzo M. Management of oral lichen planus. *Am J Clin Dermatol* 2000; **1**: 287–306.

15 Carbone M, Conrotto D, Carrozzo M *et al.* Topical corticosteroids in association with miconazole and chlorhexidine in the long-term management of atrophic-erosive lichen planus: a placebo-controlled and comparative study between clobetasol and fluocinonide. *Oral Dis* 1999; **5**: 44–9.

16 Muzio LL, della Valle A, Mignogna MD *et al.* The treatment of oral aphthous ulceration or erosive lichen planus with topical clobetasol propionate in three preparations: a clinical and pilot study on 54 patients. *J Oral Pathol Med* 2001; **30**: 611–7.

17 Kaliakatsou F, Hodgson TA, Lewsey JD *et al.* Management of recalcitrant ulcerative oral lichen planus with topical tacrolimus. *J Am Acad Dermatol* 2002; **46**: 35–41.

18 Rozycki TW, Rogers RS 3rd, Pittelkow MR *et al.* Topical tacrolimus in the treatment of symptomatic oral lichen planus: a series of 13 patients. *J Am Acad Dermatol* 2002; **46**: 27–34.

19 Femiano F, Gombos F, Scully C. Oral erosive/ulcerative lichen planus: preliminary findings in an open trial of sulodexide compared with cyclosporine (ciclosporin) therapy. *Int J Dermatol* 2001; **42**: 308–11.

Overlap syndromes

Lichen planus pemphigoides. Oral lesions in LP pemphigoides may be similar to those of LP or pemphigoid, clinically and histologically [1,2].

Lichen planus/lichen sclerosus overlap syndrome. This may involve the oral and/or vulval mucosae [3].

REFERENCES

1 Allen CM, Camisa C, Grinwood R. Lichen planus pemphigoides: report of a case with oral lesions. *Oral Surg* 1987; **63**: 184–8.

2 Maceyko RF, Camisa C, Bergfeld WF, Valenzuela R. Oral and cutaneous lichen planus pemphigoides. *J Am Acad Dermatol* 1992; **27**: 889–92.

3 Marren P, Millard P, Chia Y, Wojnarowska F. Mucosal lichen sclerosus/lichen planus overlap syndromes. *Br J Dermatol* 1994; **131**: 118–23.

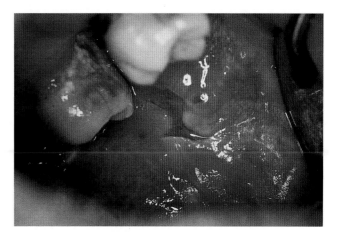

Fig. 66.36 Pemphigus vulgaris: irregular persistent oral erosions.

Pemphigus (see Chapter 41)

Oral lesions are the rule in pemphigus vulgaris (PV), but rare in the superficial forms of pemphigus [1].

Pemphigus vulgaris. The main antigen in PV is desmoglein (Dsg) 3. However, 50% of patients with PV also have autoantibodies to Dsg1 (the main antigen in pemphigus foliaceus) and the proportion of Dsg1 and Dsg3 antibodies appears to be related to clinical severity. Those cases of PV which are predominantly oral have only Dsg3 antibodies. Dsg1 autoantibodies are found in over 50% of cases of PV, and the frequency may differ with race since they are found in a significantly greater proportion of patients of Indian origin than white northern Europeans [1–4]; such variations may be HLA-related [5].

Typically, an individual patient develops a single variant of pemphigus, although cases have been described of transition to another variant, presumably through epitope spread, and the clinical manifestations of a single variant can change over time, possibly related to changes in the proportions of Dsg1 and Dsg3 autoantibodies.

The oral mucosa is almost invariably involved in PV and oral lesions are commonly the presenting feature (Fig. 66.36). Bullae appear on any part of the oral mucosa including the palate, but break so rapidly that they are rarely seen [1,6–12]. Usually, the patient presents with large, painful, irregular and persistent red lesions which, by the time they become secondarily infected, can be difficult to differentiate clinically from those of other erosive conditions, such as pemphigoid and other immune blistering disorders, although intact bullae are more commonly seen in these, whereas the Nikolsky sign is more often positive in pemphigus. Oral lesions of PV are typically seen in adults, rarely in childhood.

The prevalence of oral involvement varies: one multicentre study involving patients from several countries showed that Bulgarian patients with PV had oral mucous

Table 66.19 Immunostaining in oral mucosal vesiculobullous disorders.

Disease	DIF	Oral mucosal deposits mainly:	Pattern of IF	IIF	Autoantibodies against:
Pemphigus	+	IgG C3	Epithelial intercellular	+	Epithelial intercellular cement
Mucous membrane pemphigoid	+	C3 IgG	Linear epithelial basement membrane	±	Epithelial basement membrane
Bullous pemphigoid	+	IgG C3	Linear epithelial basement membrane	+	Epithelial basement membrane
Dermatitis herpetiformis	+	IgA C3	Granular epithelial basement membrane	–	Reticulin
Linear IgA disease	+	IgA C3	Linear epithelial basement membrane	–	–
Erythema multiforme	±	C3 IgM	Vessel walls in lamina propria	–	–
Lichen planus*	±	Fibrin† IgM, IgG, IgA, C3	Globular epithelial or lamina propria and in Civatte bodies	–	–
Discoid lupus erythematosus*	+	IgG, IgA IgM, C3	Granular epithelial basement membrane	±	None, or antinuclear
Angina bullosa haemorrhagica	–	–	–	–	–
Superficial mucoceles	–	–	–	–	–

DIF, direct immunofluorescence (biopsy); IF, immunofluorescence; IIF, indirect immunofluorescence (serology); +, present; –, absent; ±, sometimes.
* Rarely vesiculobullous.
† Non-specific deposits.

membrane lesions less frequently (66%) than Italian (83%) or Israeli (92%) patients [8]. Rarely in PV there can be an acquired macroglossia [11] or desquamative gingivitis [12].

Diagnosis should be confirmed by biopsy and immune studies. A biopsy of perilesional mucosa should be taken for H+E sections and immunostaining (Table 66.19) and serum collected for autoantibody titres, which can help diagnosis and monitoring of disease activity. Differential binding of anti-Dsg antibodies suggests that both human skin and monkey oesophagus should be used in the diagnosis of PV, since patients with predominantly oral disease may only have Dsg3 antibodies, which are not always detectable using human skin [13]. Oral smears for cytology are of little practical value.

Treatment is largely based on systemic immunosuppression using corticosteroids, with azathioprine, dapsone, methotrexate, cyclophosphamide, gold or ciclosporin as adjuvants or alternatives; this has significantly reduced the mortality [1,14]. Adverse effects of these drugs are common, though deflazacort may have slightly fewer effects [15]. Mycophenolate mofetil offers the hope of relatively safer immunosuppression with no nephrotoxicity or hepatotoxicity [16,17].

Mucosal lesions are recalcitrant, often only healing after skin lesions have resolved when immunosuppressive therapy is given, and they may persist even though skin lesions are controlled. Topical corticosteroids may then help, or possibly prostaglandin E_2 [18]. Tacrolimus may

well prove to have a place in the control of oral lesions [19].

REFERENCES

1 Scully C, Challacombe SJ. Pemphigus vulgaris: update on etiopathogenesis, oral manifestations and management. *Crit Rev Oral Biol Med* 2002; **13**: 397–408.
2 Harman KE, Gratian MJ, Seed PT *et al.* Diagnosis of pemphigus by ELISA: a critical evaluation of two ELISAs for the detection of antibodies to the major pemphigus antigens, desmoglein 1 and 3. *Clin Exp Dermatol* 2000; **25**: 236–40.
3 Harman KE, Gratian MJ, Bhogal BS, Challacombe SJ, Black MM. A study of desmoglein 1 autoantibodies in pemphigus vulgaris: racial differences in frequency and the association with a more severe phenotype. *Br J Dermatol* 2000; **143**: 343–8.
4 Harman KE, Seed PT, Gratian MJ *et al.* The severity of cutaneous and oral pemphigus is related to desmoglein 1 and 3 antibody levels. *Br J Dermatol* 2001; **144**: 775–80.
5 Loiseau P, Lecleach L, Prost C *et al.* HLA class II polymorphism contributes to specify desmoglein derived peptides in pemphigus vulgaris and pemphigus foliaceus. *J Autoimmun* 2000; **15**: 67–73.
6 Davenport S, Chen SY, Miller AS. Pemphigus vulgaris: clinicopathologic review of 33 cases in the oral cavity. *Int J Periodont Restorative Dent* 2001; **21**: 85–90.
7 Casiglia J, Woo SB, Ahmed AR. Oral involvement in autoimmune blistering diseases. *Clin Dermatol* 2001; **19**: 737–41.
8 Brenner S, Tur E, Shapiro J *et al.* Pemphigus vulgaris: environmental factors. Occupational, behavioral, medical, and qualitative food frequency questionnaire. *Int J Dermatol* 2001; **40**: 562–9.
9 Mignogna MD, Lo Muzio L, Galloro G *et al.* Oral pemphigus: clinical significance of esophageal involvement: report of eight cases. *Oral Surg Oral Med Oral Pathol Oral Radiol Endod* 1997; **84**: 179–84.
10 Scully C, Almeida OPD, Porter SR, Gilkes J. Pemphigus vulgaris: the manifestations and long-term management of 55 patients with oral lesions. *Br J Dermatol* 1999; **140**: 84–9.

11 Milgraum SS, Kanzler MH, Waldinger TP et al. Macroglossia: an unusual presentation of pemphigus vulgaris. Arch Dermatol 1985; 121: 1328–9.
12 Navarro CM, Sposto MR, Onofre MA, Scully C. Gingival lesions diagnosed as pemphigus vulgaris in an adolescent. J Periodontol 1999; 70: 808–12.
13 Challacombe SJ, Setterfield J, Shirlaw P et al. Immunodiagnosis of pemphigus and mucous membrane pemphigoid. Acta Odontol Scand 2001; 59: 226–34.
14 Lamey PJ, Rees TD, Binnie WH et al. Oral presentation of pemphigus vulgaris and its response to systemic steroid therapy. Oral Surg 1992; 74: 54–7.
15 Mignogna MD, Lo Muzio L, Mignogna RE et al. Oral pemphigus: long term behaviour and clinical response to treatment with deflazacort in sixteen cases. J Oral Pathol Med 2000; 29: 145–52.
16 Bredlich RO, Grundmann-Kollmann M, Behrens S, Kerscher M, Peter RU. Mycophenolate mofetil monotherapy for pemphigus vulgaris. Br J Dermatol 1999; 141: 934.
17 Enk AH, Knop J. Mycophenolate is effective in the treatment of pemphigus vulgaris. Arch Dermatol 1999; 135: 54–6.
18 Morita H, Morisaki S, Kitano Y. Clinical trial of prostaglandin E2 on the oral lesions of pemphigus vulgaris. Br J Dermatol 1995; 132: 165–6.
19 Wu SJ, Tanphaichitr A, Ly M. Recent advances in dermatology. Clin Podiatr Med Surg 2002; 19: 65–78.

Paraneoplastic pemphigus. Apart from PV, the other important pemphigus variant affecting the mouth is paraneoplastic pemphigus, usually associated with lymphoproliferative disease or thymoma [1], although one case associated with OSCC has been reported [2]. Oral lesions may be the sole manifestation [3] and have also been seen in all reported cases of paraneoplastic pemphigus [4–8]. Oral lesions may be seen in isolation [1].

Painful extensive stomatitis, painful paronychia and lichenoid papules may be seen, and histology may show lichenoid changes, acantholytic blister formation and apoptotic keratinocytes. Direct immunofluorescence is positive for IgG both in the epidermal intercellular spaces and along the basement membrane zone. Indirect immunofluorescence is similarly positive in a PV pattern.

There is often only a partial response to intravenous corticosteroids. Recent therapeutic advances include the use of anti-CD20 monoclonal antibody (rituximab) [9] and mycophenolate [10].

REFERENCES

1 Allen CM, Camisa C. Paraneoplastic pemphigus: a review of the literature. Oral Dis 2000; 6: 208–14.
2 Wong KC, Ho KK. Pemphigus with pemphigoid-like presentation, associated with squamous cell carcinoma of the tongue. Australas J Dermatol 2000; 41: 178–80.
3 Bialy-Golan A, Brenner S, Anhalt GJ. Paraneoplastic pemphigus: oral involvement as the sole manifestation. Acta Derm Venereol (Stockh) 1996; 76: 253–4.
4 Anhalt GJ, Kim SC, Stanley JR et al. Paraneoplastic pemphigus. An autoimmune mucocutaneous disease associated with neoplasia. N Engl J Med 1990; 323: 1729–35.
5 Laskaris GC, Papavasiliou SS, Bovopoulou OD, Nicolis GD. Association of oral pemphigus with chronic lymphocytic leukemia. Oral Surg Oral Med Oral Pathol 1980; 50: 244–9.
6 Fullerton SH, Woodley DT, Smoller BR, Anhalt GJ. Paraneoplastic pemphigus with autoantibody deposition in bronchial epithelium after autologous bone marrow transplantation. JAMA 1992; 267: 1500–2.
7 Camisa C, Helm TN, Liu YC et al. Paraneoplastic pemphigus: a report of three cases including one long-term survivor. J Am Acad Dermatol 1992; 27: 547–53.

8 Favia GF, Di Alberti L, Piattelli A. Paraneoplastic pemphigus: a report of two cases. Oral Oncol 1998; 34: 571–5.
9 Borradori L, Lombardi T, Samson J et al. Anti-CD20 monoclonal antibody (rituximab) for refractory erosive stomatitis secondary to CD20(+) follicular lymphoma-associated paraneoplastic pemphigus. Arch Dermatol 2001; 137: 269–72.
10 Williams JV, Marks JG Jr, Billingsley EM. Use of mycophenolate mofetil in the treatment of paraneoplastic pemphigus. Br J Dermatol 2000; 142: 506–8.

Pemphigus vegetans. Oral lesions in pemphigus vegetans are hyperplastic masses which, on the tongue, can give a cerebriform appearance [1,2].

REFERENCES

1 Ahmed AR, Blose DA. Pemphigus vegetans: Neumann type and Hallopeau type. Int J Dermatol 1984; 23: 135–41.
2 Premalatha S, Jayakumar S, Yesudian P et al. Cerebriform tongue: a clinical sign in pemphigus vegetans. Br J Dermatol 1981; 104: 587–91.

Other pemphigus variants. Oral lesions may be seen in less common pemphigus variants, especially in most cases with IgA pemphigus (intraepithelial IgA pustulosis or intraepidermal neutrophilic IgA dermatosis) [1–3], and in some cases of pemphigus associated with inflammatory bowel disease [4–9].

REFERENCES

1 Beutner EH, Chorzelski TP, Wilson RM et al. IgA pemphigus foliaceus: report of two cases and a review of the literature. J Am Acad Dermatol 1989; 20: 89–97.
2 Borradori L, Saada V, Rybojad M et al. Oral intraepidermal IgA pustulosis and Crohn's disease. Br J Dermatol 1992; 126: 383–6.
3 Teraki Y, Amagou N, Hashimoto T. Intracellular IgA dermatosis of childhood. Selective deposition of monomer IgA1 in the intercellular space of the epidermis. Arch Dermatol 1991; 127: 221–4.
4 Stone DD. Rectal lesions and toxic dilatation of the colon in a case of pemphigus vulgaris. Am J Dig Dis 1971; 16: 163–6.
5 Lubach D, Reichart P, Wellman W. Oral manifestations during the concurrent appearance of pemphigus and ulcerative colitis. Dtsch Z Mund Kiefer Gesichtschir 1984; 8: 308–12.
6 Fabbri P, Emmi L, Vignoli L et al. Chronic pemphigus vulgaris associated with ulcerative rectocolitis. Apropos of a clinical case. G Ital Dermatol Venereol 1986; 21: 355–9.
7 Delfino M, Suppa F, Piccirillo A. Pemphigus vulgaris and ulcerative colitis. Dermatologica 1986; 172: 230.
8 Schwermann M, Lechner W, Elsner C, Kirchner T. Pemphigus vulgaris involving duodenum and colon. Z Hautkr 1988; 63: 101–4.
9 Prendiville JS, Israel DM, Wood WS, Dimmick JE. Oral pemphigus vulgaris associated with inflammatory bowel disease and herpetic gingivostomatitis in an 11-year old girl. Pediatr Dermatol 1994; 11: 145–50.

Subepithelial immune bullous diseases

A spectrum of immune-mediated subepithelial bullous diseases can present with oral blisters and/or erosions, and with immune deposits at the epithelial basement membrane zone. Several distinct groups, and probably several overlap syndromes, are now recognized to exist.

Mucous membrane pemphigoid (see Chapter 41). Mucous membrane pemphigoid is a mucocutaneous, immune-mediated,

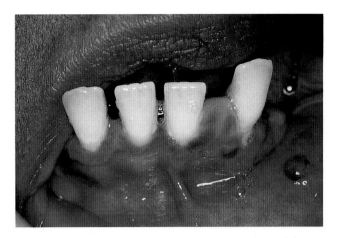

Fig. 66.37 Pemphigoid: vesicles and desquamative gingivitis.

subepithelial blistering disease characterized by autoantibodies to different molecules in the basement membrane zone [1,2]. The mouth may be involved as part of a wider disease, though in many patients only oral lesions are seen. Sera of oral pemphigoid patients selectively and specifically bind to human α6 integrin, a 120-kDa protein that appears to be a target antigen in this particular variant [3].

Mucous membrane pemphigoid involves the oral mucosa in more than one-third of cases, commonly causing gingival lesions [1,2,4,5]. The usual lesion, desquamative gingivitis, is characterized by erythematous, glazed, sore gingivae (Fig. 66.37). Bullae are less common, and are seen particularly on the soft palate. They rupture to form erosions [1–5].

The bullae in mucous membrane pemphigoid are subepithelial and tend to persist for longer than those of pemphigus. Oral lesions may scar but this is uncommon. The bullae are typically filled with serous fluid and should be distinguished from superficial mucoceles (see p. 66.81), epidermolysis bullosa acquisita, dermatitis herpetiformis and linear IgA disease. Occasionally blisters are blood-filled, and then must be differentiated from angina bullosa haemorrhagica (see p. 66.80).

A biopsy is required for diagnosis [5]. Serum autoantibodies to epithelial basement membrane may be detected in a few patients (see Table 66.19) but many have immune deposits at the epithelial and mucous gland basement membrane zone. A very small minority of patients have an associated internal malignancy which should be excluded.

Topical corticosteroids usually help if the lesions are restricted to the oral mucosa; azathioprine may be an alternative [6]. Systemic corticosteroids may occasionally be required but tetracyclines with or without nicotinamide may help [7,8]. Dapsone may be useful, especially in the treatment of desquamative gingivitis [9,10]. The evidence for efficacy of tacrolimus or mycophenolate mofetil is weak [11,12].

REFERENCES

1 Scully C, Carrozzo M, Gandolfo S, Puiatti P, Monteil R. Update on mucous membrane pemphigoid (an immune mediated sub-epithelial blistering disease): a heterogeneous entity. *Oral Surg Oral Med Oral Pathol* 1999; **88**: 56–68.
2 Chan LS, Ahmed AR, Anhalt GJ *et al.* The first international consensus on mucous membrane pemphigoid: definition, diagnostic criteria, pathogenic factors, medical treatment, and prognostic indicators. *Arch Dermatol* 2002; **138**: 370–9.
3 Bhol KC, Goss L, Kumari S, Colon JE, Ahmed AR. Autoantibodies to human alpha6 integrin in patients with oral pemphigoid. *J Dent Res* 2001; **80**: 1711–5.
4 Venning VA, Frith PA, Bron AJ *et al.* Mucosal involvement in bullous and cicatricial pemphigoid. A clinical and immunopathological study. *Br J Dermatol* 1988; **118**: 7–15.
5 Challacombe SJ, Setterfield J, Shirlaw P *et al.* Immunodiagnosis of pemphigus and mucous membrane pemphigoid. *Acta Odontol Scand* 2001; **59**: 226–34.
6 Epstein JB, Gorsky M, Epstein MS, Nantel S. Topical azathioprine in the treatment of immune-mediated chronic oral inflammatory conditions: a series of cases. *Oral Surg Oral Med Oral Pathol Oral Radiol Endod* 2001; **91**: 56–61.
7 Poskitt L, Wojnarowska F. Minimizing cicatricial pemphigoid orodynia with minocycline. *Br J Dermatol* 1995; **132**: 784–9.
8 Poskitt L, Wojnarowska F. Treatment of cicatricial pemphigoid with tetracycline and nicotinamide. *Clin Exp Dermatol* 1995; **20**: 258–9.
9 Rogers RS, Seehafer JR, Perry H. Treatment of cicatricial (benign mucous membrane) pemphigoid with dapsone. *J Am Acad Dermatol* 1982; **6**: 215–23.
10 Matthews RW, Pinkney RC, Scully C. The management of desquamative gingivitis with dapsone. *Ann Dent* 1981; **48**: 41–3.
11 Letko E, Ahmed AR, Foster CS. Treatment of ocular cicatricial pemphigoid with tacrolimus (FK 506). *Graefes Arch Clin Exp Ophthalmol* 2001; **239**: 441–4.
12 Nousari HC, Sragovich A, Kimyai-Asadi A, Orlinsky D, Anhalt GJ. Mycophenolate mofetil in autoimmune and inflammatory skin disorders. *J Am Acad Dermatol* 1999; **40**: 265–8.

Vegetating cicatricial pemphigoid (syn. pemphigoid vegetans). A subset of bullous pemphigoid, although clinically indistinguishable from pemphigus vegetans and sometimes producing oral blisters and erosions, vegetating cicatricial pemphigoid shows linear deposits of IgG and C3 at the epithelial basement membrane zone on oral biopsy but no circulating basement membrane antibodies [1].

Palate and gingiva have been especially involved in the rare cases described [2,3].

REFERENCES

1 Vincent SD, Lilly GE, Baker KA. Clinical, historic and therapeutic features of cicatricial pemphigoid. *Oral Surg* 1993; **76**: 453–9.
2 Liu HN, Su WP, Rogers RS *et al.* Clinical variants of pemphigoid. *Int J Dermatol* 1986; **25**: 17–27.
3 Wolf K, Rappersberger K, Steiner A *et al.* Vegetating cicatricial pemphigoid. *Arch Dermatol Res* 1987; **279**: S30–S37.

Epidermolysis bullosa acquisita (see Chapter 41). Blisters or ulcers may be seen in the oral mucosa in epidermolysis bullosa acquisita, with antibodies directed against collagen VII. Lesional biopsy shows IgG and C3 in the sublamina densa zone of the epithelial basement membrane using immunoelectron microscopy [1–3].

REFERENCES

1 Prost C, Labeille B, Chanssade V *et al.* Immunoelectron microscopy in subepidermal autoimmune bullous diseases: a prospective study of IgG and C3 bound *in vivo* in 32 patients. *J Invest Dermatol* 1987; **89**: 567–73.
2 Rubenstein R, Sterley NB, Fine JD. Childhood epidermolysis bullosa acquisita. *Arch Dermatol* 1987; **123**: 772–6.
3 Tokuda Y, Amagai M, Yaoita H *et al.* A case of an inflammatory variant of epidermolysis bullosa acquisita: chronic bullous dermatosis associated with nonscarring mucosal blisters and circulating IgG anti-type-VII-collagen antibody. *Dermatology* 1998; **197**: 58–61.

Dermatitis herpetiformis and adult linear IgA disease. Oral lesions may occur in dermatitis herpetiformis and in most patients with linear IgA disease. Macules, papules, petechiae, vesicles, bullae and erosions are the usual manifestations [1–10]. These disorders must be differentiated, especially from pemphigoid, angina bullosa haemorrhagica, superficial mucoceles and LP.

Salivary IgA antigliadin antibodies may be found but this is not useful diagnostically. Dapsone and sulfapyridine are the most effective therapeutic agents along with a gluten-free diet in dermatitis herpetiformis.

REFERENCES

1 Chan LS, Regezi JA, Cooper KD. Oral manifestations of linear IgA disease. *J Am Acad Dermatol* 1990; **22**: 362–5.
2 Cowan CG, Lamey PJ, Walsh M *et al.* Linear IgA disease (LAD): immunoglobulin deposition in oral and colonic lesions. *J Oral Pathol Med* 1995; **24**: 374–8.
3 Economopoulou P, Laskaris G. Dermatitis herpetiformis: oral lesions as an early manifestation. *Oral Surg* 1986; **62**: 77–80.
4 Hall RP, Waldbauer GV. Characterisation of the mucosal immune response to dietary antigens in patients with dermatitis herpetiformis. *J Invest Dermatol* 1988; **90**: 658–63.
5 Kelly SE, Frith PA, Millard PR *et al.* A clinopathological study of mucosal involvement in linear IgA disease. *Br J Dermatol* 1988; **119**: 161–70.
6 Porter SR, Bain SE, Scully C. Linear IgA disease manifesting as recalcitrant desquamative gingivitis. *Oral Surg* 1992; **74**: 179–82.
7 Porter SR, Scully C, Midda M *et al.* Adult linear IgA disease manifesting as desquamative gingivitis. *Oral Surg* 1990; **70**: 450–3.
8 Wiesenfeld D, Martin A, Scully C *et al.* Oral manifestations in linear IgA disease. *Br Dent J* 1982; **153**: 389–9.
9 Cohen DM, Bhattacharyya I, Zunt SL, Tomich CE. Linear IgA disease histopathologically and clinically masquerading as lichen planus. *Oral Surg Oral Med Oral Pathol Oral Radiol Endod* 1999; **88**: 196–201.
10 Femiano F, Scully C, Gombos F. Linear IgA dermatosis induced by a new angiotensin-converting enzyme inhibitor. *Oral Surg Oral Med Oral Pathol Oral Radiol Endod* 2003; **95**: 169–73.

Chronic bullous dermatosis of childhood (see Chapter 41). Oral ulceration has been reported [1,2].

REFERENCES

1 Wojnarowska F, Marsden RA, Bhogal B, Black MM. Chronic bullous disease of childhood, childhood cicatricial pemphigoid and linear IgA disease of adults: a comparative study demonstrating clinical and immunopathological overlap. *J Am Acad Dermatol* 1988; **19**: 792–805.
2 Casiglia J, Woo SB, Ahmed AR. Oral involvement in autoimmune blistering diseases. *Clin Dermatol* 2001; **19**: 737–41.

Erythema multiforme (see Chapter 74). The aetiology of erythema multiforme (EM) is unclear in most patients, but appears to be an immunological hypersensitivity reaction with the appearance of cytotoxic effector cells (CD8$^+$ T lymphocytes) in the epithelium, inducing apoptosis of scattered keratinocytes and leading to satellite cell necrosis.

Predisposing factors. There may be a genetic predisposition, with associations of recurrent EM with HLA-B15(B62), HLA-B35, HLA-A33, HLA-DR53 and HLA-DQB1*0301. HLA-DQ3 has been proven to be especially related to recurrent EM and may be a helpful marker for distinguishing this herpes-associated EM from other diseases with EM-like lesions. Patients with extensive mucosal involvement may have the rare HLA allele DQB1*0402 [1].

The reaction is triggered by the following.
• *Infective agents*, particularly herpes simplex virus (herpes-associated EM), which is implicated in 70% of recurrent EM. Bacteria (*Mycoplasma pneumoniae*, and many others), other viruses, fungi or parasites are less commonly implicated [2,3].
• *Drugs* such as sulphonamides (e.g. co-trimoxazole), cephalosporins, aminopenicillins, quinolones, barbiturates, oxicam non-steroidal anti-inflammatory drugs, anticonvulsants, protease inhibitors, allopurinol and many others may trigger severe EM or toxic epidermal necrolysis in particular [4,5].
• *Food additives or chemicals* such as benzoates, nitrobenzene, perfumes, terpenes.
• *Immune conditions* such as BCG or hepatitis B immunization, sarcoidosis, GVHD, inflammatory bowel disease, polyarteritis nodosa or systemic lupus erythematosus (SLE).

Clinical features. Most patients with EM (70%), of either minor or major forms, have oral lesions. The oral mucosa may be involved alone or in association with skin lesions. Mucosal lesions begin as erythematous areas that blister and break down to irregular, extensive, painful erosions with extensive surrounding erythema. The labial mucosa is often involved, and a serosanguinous exudate leads to crusting of the swollen lips [6–11].

Mucosal erosions plus typical or raised atypical targets and epidermal detachment involving less than 10% of the body surface and usually located on the extremities and/or the face characterize herpes simplex-induced EM major.

Mucosal erosions plus widespread distribution of flat atypical targets or purpuric macules and epithelial detachment involving less than 10% of body surface on the trunk, face and extremities are characteristic of drug-induced Stevens–Johnson syndrome [12].

Diagnosis. A diagnosis of EM can be difficult to readily establish, and there may be a need to differentiate from viral stomatitides, pemphigus, toxic epidermal necrolysis and the subepithelial immune blistering disorders (pemphigoid and others). There are no specific diagnostic tests.

The diagnosis is mainly clinical; the Nikolsky sign is negative. It may be helpful to undertake serology for *Mycoplasma pneumoniae* or herpes simplex virus, or other microorganisms. Biopsy of perilesional tissue with immunostaining and histological examination may help, although pathology can be variable and immunostaining is not specific.

Management. Spontaneous healing can be slow, up to 2–3 weeks in EM minor and up to 6 weeks in EM major. Treatment is thus indicated but controversial. No specific treatment is available but supportive care is important; a liquid diet and intravenous fluid therapy may be necessary. Electrolytes and nutritional support should be started as soon as possible. Oral hygiene should be improved with 0.2% aqueous chlorhexidine mouthbaths.

The use of corticosteroids is controversial [13–14].

• EM minor may respond to topical corticosteroids, although systemic corticosteroids may still be required.

• EM major should be treated with systemic corticosteroids (prednisolone 0.5–1 mg/kg/day tapered over 7–10 days) and/or azathioprine or other immunomodulatory drugs. Levamisole [15] and thalidomide have occasionally been used to some effect. Plasmapheresis possibly has a place in the management of severe disease.

Antimicrobials may be indicated [16,17].

• Aciclovir in EM related to herpes simplex virus (HSV). Give a 5-day course at the first sign of lesions, or give 400 mg four times daily for 6 months for prophylaxis in EM related to HSV. Continuous therapy with valaciclovir 500 mg twice a day has also been reported to be effective [17].

• Tetracycline is indicated in EM related to *Mycoplasma pneumoniae*.

REFERENCES

1 Malo A, Kampgen E, Wank R. Recurrent herpes simplex virus-induced erythema multiforme: different HLA-DQB1 alleles associate with severe mucous membrane versus skin attacks. *Scand J Immunol* 1998; **47**: 408–11.

2 Aslanzadeh J, Helm KF, Espy MJ, Muller SA, Smith TF. Detection of HSV-specific DNA in biopsy tissue of patients with erythema multiforme by polymerase chain reaction. *Br J Dermatol* 1992; **126**: 19–23.

3 Weston WL, Morelli JG. Herpes simplex virus-associated erythema multiforme in prepubertal children. *Arch Pediatr Adolesc Med* 1997; **151**: 1014–6.

4 Roujeau JC, Kelly JP, Naldi L *et al.* Medication use and the risk of Stevens–Johnson syndrome or toxic epidermal necrolysis. *N Engl J Med* 1995; **333**: 1600–7.

5 Scully C, Diz Dios P. Orofacial effects of antiretroviral therapies. *Oral Dis* 2001; **7**: 205–10.

6 Cote B, Wechsler J, Bastuji-Garin S. Clinicopathologic correlation in erythema multiforme and Stevens–Johnson syndrome. *Arch Dermatol* 1995; **131**: 1268–72.

7 Eversole LR. Immunopathology of oral mucosal ulcerative, desquamative, and bullous diseases. Selective review of the literature. *Oral Surg Oral Med Oral Pathol* 1994; **77**: 555–71.

8 Silverman S. The bullous desquamative lesions of oral mucosa. *J Calif Dent Assoc* 2000; **28**: 928–32.

9 Stewart MG, Duncan NO 3rd, Franklin DJ, Friedman EM, Sulek M. Head and neck manifestations of erythema multiforme in children. *Otolaryngol Head Neck Surg* 1994; **111**: 236–42.

10 Siegel MA, Balciunas BA. Oral presentation and management of vesiculobullous disorders. *Semin Dermatol* 1994; **13**: 78–86.

11 Farthing PM, Maragou P, Coates M *et al.* Characteristics of the oral lesions in patients with cutaneous recurrent erythema multiforme. *J Oral Pathol Med* 1995; **24**: 9–13.

12 Assier H, Bastuji-Garin S, Revuz J. Erythema multiforme with mucous membrane involvement and Stevens–Johnson syndrome are clinically different disorders with distinct causes. *Arch Dermatol* 1995; **131**: 539–43.

13 Tripathi A, Ditto AM, Grammer LC *et al.* Corticosteroid therapy in an additional 13 cases of Stevens–Johnson syndrome: a total series of 67 cases. *Allergy Asthma Proc* 2000; **21**: 101–5.

14 Eastham JH, Segal JL, Gomez MF, Cole GW. Reversal of erythema multiforme major with cyclophosphamide and prednisone. *Ann Pharmacother* 1996; **30**: 606–7.

15 Lozada-Nur F, Cram D, Gorsky M. Clinical response to levamisole in thirty-nine patients with erythema multiforme. An open prospective study. *Oral Surg Oral Med Oral Pathol* 1992; **74**: 294–8.

16 Katz J, Livneh A, Shemer J, Danon YL, Peretz B. Herpes simplex-associated erythema multiforme (HAEM): a clinical therapeutic dilemma. *Pediatr Dent* 1999; **21**: 359–62.

17 Kerob D, Assier-Bonnet H, Esnault-Gelly P. Recurrent erythema multiforme unresponsive to acyclovir prophylaxis and responsive to valaciclovir continuous therapy. *Arch Dermatol* 1998; **134**: 876–7.

Toxic epidermal necrolysis
SYN. LYELL'S DISEASE

Toxic epidermal necrolysis is a rare clinicopathological entity, with a high mortality, characterized by extensive detachment of full-thickness epithelium. Toxic epidermal necrolysis and Stevens–Johnson syndrome appear to be severity variants of the same disease, which differs from EM. The distinction from EM is unclear, however, but most cases of toxic epidermal necrolysis are drug-induced and the lesions are extremely widespread [1,2].

Recently, an increased number of cases in patients with HIV/acquired immune deficiency syndrome (AIDS) has been recorded [3].

Clinical features. Toxic epidermal necrolysis presents with cough, sore throat, burning eyes, malaise and low fever, followed after about 1–2 days by skin and mucous membrane lesions. Oral lesions can be seen in over 95% of patients with toxic epidermal necrolysis. The entire skin surface and oral mucosa may be involved, with up to 100% sloughing off. Gingival lesions are common and clinically are inflamed, with blister formation leading to painful widespread erosions. The blisters and erosions may precede the skin lesions by a day or so and may persist [3–6].

Diagnosis. Sheet-like loss of the epithelium and a positive Nikolsky sign are characteristic. Biopsy of perilesional tissue with immunostaining and histological examination are essential to the diagnosis. Histopathological examination is characteristic, showing necrosis of the whole epithelium detached from the lamina propria.

Management. Patients must be admitted to an intensive care unit as soon as possible for management [7]. There is no specific therapy for oral lesions but 2% lidocaine (lignocaine) and 0.2% aqueous chlorhexidine mouthbaths may provide symptomatic relief.

REFERENCES

1 Roujeau JC. Stevens–Johnson syndrome and toxic epidermal necrolysis are severity variants of the same disease which differs from erythema multiforme. *J Dermatol* 1997; **24**: 726–9.
2 Bastuji-Garin S, Rzany B, Stern RS. Clinical classification of cases of toxic epidermal necrolysis, Stevens–Johnson syndrome, and erythema multiforme. *Arch Dermatol* 1993; **129**: 92–6.
3 Schmidt-Westhausen A, Grunewald T, Reichart PA, Pohle HD. Oral manifestations of toxic epidermal necrolysis (TEN) in patients with AIDS: report of five cases. *Oral Dis* 1998; **4**: 90–4.
4 Marra LM, Wunderlee RC. Oral presentation of toxic epidermal necrolysis. *J Oral Maxillofac Surg* 1982; **40**: 59–61.
5 Revuz J, Penso D, Roujeau JC. Toxic epidermal necrolysis: clinical findings and prognostic factors in 87 patients. *Arch Dermatol* 1987; **123**: 1160–5.
6 Barrera JE, Meyers AD, Hartford EC. Hypopharyngeal stenosis and dysphagia complicating toxic epidermal necrolysis. *Arch Otolaryngol Head Neck Surg* 1998; **124**: 1375–6.
7 Roujeau JC. Treatment of severe drug eruptions. *J Dermatol* 1999; **26**: 718–22.

Lichen sclerosus (see Chapter 56). Oral lichen sclerosus et atrophicus is uncommon but since it presents with whitish plaques, papules or a reticular pattern, or erosions, all features of LP [1–8], it may be underdiagnosed. Histologically, however, lichen sclerosus has epithelial atrophy with hyperkeratosis, oedema in the papillary corium and the lymphocytic infiltrate is less close to the epithelium than in LP. It has been suggested that mucosal lichen sclerosus is more common than formerly thought and may even cause dysplasia [5].

REFERENCES

1 MacLeod RI, Soames JV. Lichen sclerosus et atrophicus of the oral mucosa. *Br J Oral Maxillofac Surg* 1991; **89**: 64–5.
2 Ravits HG, Welsh AL. Lichen sclerosus et atrophicus of the mouth. *Arch Dermatol* 1957; **76**: 56–8.
3 De Araujo VC, Orsini SC, Marcucci G *et al.* Lichen sclerosus et atrophicus. *Oral Surg* 1985; **60**: 655–7.
4 Miller RF. Lichen sclerosus et atrophicus with oral involvement. *Arch Dermatol* 1957; **76**: 43–55.
5 Maren P, Millard P, Chia Y, Wojnarowska F. Mucosal lichen sclerosus/lichen planus overlap syndromes. *Br J Dermatol* 1994; **131**: 118–23.
6 Schulten EA, Starink TM, van der Waal I. Lichen sclerosus et atrophicus involving the oral mucosa: report of two cases. *J Oral Pathol Med* 1993; **22**: 374–7.
7 Brown AR, Dunlap CL, Bussard DA, Lask JT. Lichen sclerosus et atrophicus of the oral cavity: report of two cases. *Oral Surg Oral Med Oral Pathol Oral Radiol Endod* 1997; **84**: 165–70.
8 Buajeeb W, Kraivaphan P, Punyasingh J, Laohapand P. Oral lichen sclerosus et atrophicus. A case report. *Oral Surg Oral Med Oral Pathol Oral Radiol Endod* 1999; **88**: 702–6.

Chronic ulcerative stomatitis with epithelial antinuclear antibodies. Chronic erosive or ulcerative stomatitis often presents as desquamative gingivitis with or without lesions on buccal or lingual mucosa and sometimes resembles LP,

and may be associated with lichenoid histology, but is associated with antinuclear antibodies directed against stratified squamous epithelia [1–3]. These autoantibodies are directed against a 70-kDa epithelial nuclear protein homologous to the p53 tumour suppressor and the p73 putative tumour suppressor, and shown to be a splicing variant of the *KET* gene [4,5].

The lesions may respond to hydroxychloroquine [1–3].

REFERENCES

1 Jarenko WM, Beutner EH, Kumar V *et al.* Chronic ulcerative stomatitis associated with a specific immunologic marker. *J Am Acad Dermatol* 1990; **22**: 215–20.
2 Beutner EH, Chorzelski TP, Parodi A *et al.* Ten cases of chronic ulcerative stomatitis with stratified epithelium-specific antinuclear antibody. *J Am Acad Dermatol* 1991; **24**: 781–2.
3 Church LF, Schosser RH. Chronic ulcerative stomatitis associated with stratified epithelial specific antinuclear antibody. *Oral Surg* 1992; **73**: 579–82.
4 Parodi A, Cozzani E, Cacciapuoti M, Rebora A. Chronic ulcerative stomatitis: antibodies reacting with the 70-kDa molecule react with epithelial nuclei. *Br J Dermatol* 2000; **143**: 671–2.
5 Lee LA, Walsh P, Prater CA *et al.* Characterization of an autoantigen associated with chronic ulcerative stomatitis: the CUSP autoantigen is a member of the p53 family. *J Invest Dermatol* 1999; **113**: 146–51.

Lupus erythematosus (see Chapter 56)

Almost half of the patients with SLE suffer from oral lesions, which begin as red patches that break down to irregular slit-like ulcers which often heal with scarring [1]. Lesions particularly affect the palate. Sjögren's syndrome may occur in SLE. Oral petechiae and herpetic infections are also common. Rarely, dental surgery has been followed by facial swelling [2].

Similar erosions, with a white border, occur in discoid lupus erythematosus (Fig. 66.38). Discoid lupus erythematosus may predispose to oral carcinoma [3]. Oral ulceration has also been described in drug-induced lupus.

Systemic corticosteroids, often with an immunosuppressant, may be required in severe cases.

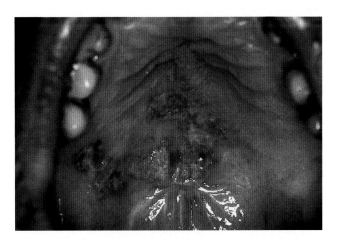

Fig. 66.38 Chronic oral lesions in discoid lupus erythematosus.

Other collagen–vascular diseases

Dermatomyositis and mixed connective tissue disease may be associated with non-specific mucosal erosions [4].

Oral involvement in Reiter's syndrome may include red patches or superficial painless mucosal erosions which may resemble erythema migrans (geographical tongue) both clinically and histologically.

REFERENCES

1 Schiodt M. Oral manifestations of lupus erythematosus. *Int J Oral Surg* 1984; **13**: 101–47.
2 Loescher A, Edmondson HD. Lupus erythematosus: a case of facial swelling. *Br J Oral Surg* 1988; **26**: 129–32.
3 Handlers JP, Abrams AM, Aberle AM *et al*. Squamous cell carcinoma of the lip developing in discoid lupus erythematosus. *Oral Surg* 1985; **60**: 382–6.
4 Porter SR, Malamos D, Scully C. Mouth–skin interface: 2. Connective tissue and metabolic disorders. *Update* 1986; **33**: 94–6.

Infective diseases

Oral ulceration is common worldwide in some viral infections, typically in the herpesvirus or enterovirus infections seen in childhood. It can also be seen in several bacterial diseases, notably acute necrotizing gingivitis (but also in tuberculosis and syphilis), but is rare in fungal infections in the developed world, although the deep mycoses may be responsible for infection in the developing world, in travellers or in the immunocompromised.

Herpesviruses

Oral infection is common with the herpesviruses, which thereafter remain latent, are often excreted in saliva (especially in immunocompromised persons), and are sometimes implicated in clinical recurrences and malignant complications.

Herpes simplex stomatitis

Aetiology. HSV infection is a very common oral infection. In general, HSV-1 causes primary herpetic stomatitis (and the secondary infection of recurrent herpes labialis). There are no precise distinctions nowadays, presumably with more frequent orogenital and oroanal sexual practices, and oral infection with HSV-2 is also frequently seen [1,2].

With improving socio-economic circumstances and standards of hygiene, a larger number of children are not exposed to HSV and enter adult life without immunity. Cases of primary herpetic stomatitis are therefore now seen occasionally in adults, and the manifestations can be severe. HSV is usually transmitted in saliva and can be shed in asymptomatic individuals [3,4].

Clinical features. The incubation period is 3–7 days. Many infections with HSV occur in childhood and are subclin-

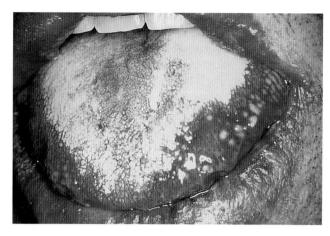

Fig. 66.39 Scattered ulcers and a furred tongue in primary herpetic stomatitis.

ical and, where there is disease, it varies greatly in severity. In many it is trivial and misdiagnosed or passed off as 'teething' [5,6].

Primary herpetic stomatitis typically presents with malaise, anorexia, irritability, fever, enlarged and tender anterior cervical lymph nodes, and a diffuse, purple, boggy gingivitis (hence the alternative term *herpetic gingivostomatitis*), especially anteriorly, with multiple vesicles followed by round or ovoid ulcers 1–3 mm in diameter scattered across the oral mucosa and gingiva (Fig. 66.39) in an acute illness lasting only up to about 14 days [1,2]. In immunocompromised persons, diagnosis can be difficult since herpes may manifest with chronic ulcers [7–11].

Prognosis. Herpetic stomatitis resolves spontaneously in 7–14 days but HSV remains latent in the trigeminal ganglion. The most obvious sequel is that about one-third of patients are thereafter predisposed to recurrences. HSV is shed intermittently into the saliva [3,4]. HSV is implicated in many instances of EM (see p. 66.67) and may cause chronic ulcers in the immunocompromised (see below).

Diagnosis. The main differential diagnoses of herpetic stomatitis in otherwise healthy persons are chickenpox and other viral causes of mouth ulcers, and acute leukaemia. In immunocopromised persons, the differential is wider. A full blood picture, white-cell count and differential, and viral studies may therefore be required [1,2,12,13]. The latter include the following:
• Culture: this takes days to give a result.
• Electron microscopy: this is not always available.
• Polymerase chain reaction (PCR) detection of HSV DNA: this is sensitive but expensive.
• Immunodetection: detection of HSV antigens is of some value. Conventional enzyme-linked immunosorbent assays (ELISA) for serum antibodies have poor sensitivity and specificity; newer assays based on HSV glycoproteins

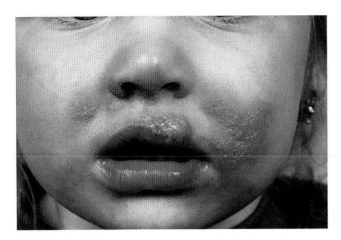

Fig. 66.40 Primary herpetic stomatitis with extraoral lesions.

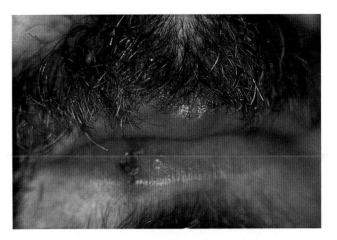

Fig. 66.41 Herpes labialis.

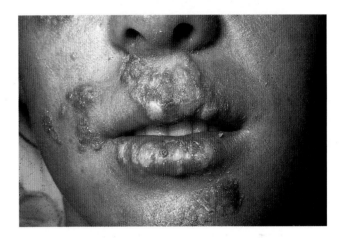

Fig. 66.42 Impetigo.

are comparable with Western blot assays. A rising titre of serum antibodies is confirmatory but only gives the diagnosis retrospectively.

- Smears for viral-damaged cells: now rarely used.

Treatment. Specific antiviral agents are most useful in the very early stages of disease (though most patients present later) and for immunocompromised patients who may otherwise suffer severe infection. Both oral and intravenous aciclovir appear to be effective, as are the newer antivirals [14,15].

For most, however, management is supportive with antipyretic analgesics (e.g. acetaminophen/paracetamol), sponging with tepid water and a high fluid intake. Analgesics (as elixirs or syrups for children) and, in adults, lidocaine mouthbaths help ease discomfort and 0.2% aqueous chlorhexidine mouthbaths aid resolution.

An antihistamine such as promethazine may help sedate an irritable child.

Recurrent labial HSV infection. Primary oral infection by HSV may produce perioral lesions (Fig. 66.40). However, recurrent herpes labialis involving the lip is the more common cause of blisters at the mucocutaneous junction (Fig. 66.41) [1,2]. The lesions arise at the mucocutaneous junction as itching papules which progress to vesicles, pustules and then scab. They are unsightly and occasionally become infected with *Staphylococcus* or *Streptococcus*, resulting in impetigo (Fig. 66.42). In immunocompromised persons, extensive and persistent lesions may result. In atopic persons, the lesions may spread to produce eczema herpeticum (Fig. 66.43). Aciclovir has been the standard treatment used as a 5% cream, although penciclovir 1% is more effective [16].

Recurrent intraoral HSV infection. Chronic oral herpetic ulcers, often with a raised white border and sometimes with a dendritic appearance, may occasionally affect

apparently healthy individuals, especially at sites of trauma, for example following palatal infiltration of a local anaesthetic. Chronic indolent lesions, usually ulcerative or nodular, may be seen in patients with neutropenia or chronic leukaemia; in patients with more severe immunosuppression, such as acute leukaemia or HIV infection, more aggressive chronic ulcers may be seen [7–11]. Aciclovir may be indicated systemically [8].

REFERENCES

1 Whitley RJ, Roizman B. Herpes simplex virus infections. *Lancet* 2001; **357**: 1513–8.
2 Scully C. Orofacial herpes simplex virus infections: current concepts in the epidemiology, pathogenesis and treatment, and disorders in which the virus may be implicated. *Oral Surg* 1989; **68**: 701–10.
3 Yoshida M, Amatsu A. Asymptomatic shedding of herpes simplex virus into the oral cavity of patients with atopic dermatitis. *J Clin Virol* 2000; **16**: 65–9.
4 Knaup B, Schunemann S, Wolff MH. Subclinical reactivation of herpes simplex virus type 1 in the oral cavity. *Oral Microbiol Immunol* 2000; **15**: 281–3.
5 Kimberlin DW, Lin CY, Jacobs RF *et al.* Natural history of neonatal herpes simplex virus infections in the acyclovir era. *Pediatrics* 2001; **108**: 223–9.

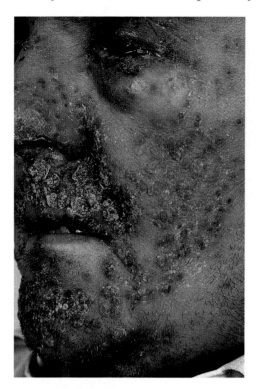

Fig. 66.43 Eczema herpeticum.

6 Scully C. Ulcerative stomatitis gingivitis and rash: a diagnostic dilemma. *Oral Surg* 1985; **59**: 261–3.

7 Samonis G, Mantadakis E, Maraki S. Orofacial viral infections in the immunocompromised host. *Oncol Report* 2000; **7**: 1389–94.

8 Cohen SG, Greenberg MS. Chronic oral herpes simplex virus infection in immunocompromised patients. *Oral Surg* 1985; **59**: 465–71.

9 Bergmann OJ, Mogensen SC, Ellegaard J. Herpes simplex virus and intra-oral ulcers in immunocompromised patients with haematologic malignancies. *Eur J Clin Microbiol Infect Dis* 1990; **9**: 184–90.

10 Greenberg MS, Cohen SG, Boosz B *et al.* Oral herpes simplex infections in patients with leukaemia. *J Am Dent Assoc* 1987; **114**: 483–6.

11 Grossman ME, Stevens AW, Cohen PR. Herpetic geometric glossitis. *N Engl J Med* 1993; **329**: 1859–60.

12 Bezold G, Volkenandt M, Gottlober P, Peter RU. Detection of herpes simplex virus and varicella-zoster virus in clinical swabs: frequent inhibition of PCR as determined by internal controls. *Mol Diagn* 2000; **5**: 279–84.

13 Goldman BD. Herpes serology for dermatologists. *Arch Dermatol* 2000; **136**: 1158–61.

14 Birek C. Herpesvirus-induced diseases: oral manifestations and current treatment options. *J Calif Dent Assoc* 2000; **28**: 911–21.

15 Flaitz CM, Baker KA. Treatment approaches to common symptomatic oral lesions in children. *Dent Clin North Am* 2000; **44**: 671–96.

16 Femiano F, Gombos S, Scully C. Recurrent herpes labialis: efficacy of topical therapy with penciclovir compared with acyclovir (aciclovir). *Oral Dis* 2001; **7**: 31–2.

Chickenpox

SYN. VARICELLA (see Chapter 25)

Chickenpox affects children predominantly and may present with mouth ulcers that resemble those of herpetic stomatitis, but there is no gingivitis [1]. There may be a contact history. Many primary infections with varicella-zoster virus are subclinical or produce so few lesions as to pass almost unnoticed. Varicella-zoster virus remains latent in sensory ganglia and may be reactivated to produce shingles.

Herpes zoster

SYN. SHINGLES

If shingles affects the maxillary or mandibular divisions of the trigeminal nerve, mouth ulcers are usually seen [2,3].

Clinical features. The pain of trigeminal zoster may simulate toothache. Severe pain often precedes, accompanies and follows the rash, and post-herpetic neuralgia may persist for months or years.

The rash is restricted to a dermatome and is unilateral, but sometimes a few chickenpox-type lesions can be found elsewhere. Oral ulcers appear in the distribution of the involved nerve division [3]. There is ulceration of one side of the tongue, floor of mouth and lower labial and buccal mucosa if the mandibular division of the trigeminal nerve is involved. One side of the palate, the upper gingiva and buccal sulcus are involved in maxillary zoster. Rarely, mandibular or maxillary zoster may disturb the formation of developing teeth [4] or cause jaw necrosis [5].

If the geniculate ganglion of the facial nerve is affected, there may be unilateral facial palsy, with vesicles in the ipsilateral ear and ulcers in the soft palate ipsilaterally (Ramsay–Hunt syndrome) [6].

Occasionally there is misdiagnosis of toothache, leading to extraction, the true diagnosis becoming apparent only when the rash appears. Zoster resolves spontaneously but post-herpetic neuralgia can be distressing.

Management. An underlying immune defect, such as AIDS or malignancy, should be excluded in patients with zoster, although most zoster is related simply to lesser problems in advanced age.

Treatment is mainly supportive but antivirals such as aciclovir can be useful. Analgesics are indicated in zoster, although the pain may prove refractory to even potent analgesics [7], when antidepressants such as amitriptyline and fluphenazine may have a place [8].

REFERENCES

1 Kolokotronis A, Louloudiadis K, Fotiou G, Matiais A. Oral manifestations of infections due to varicella zoster virus in otherwise healthy children. *J Clin Pediatr Dent* 2001; **25**: 107–12.

2 Braverman I, Uri N, Greenberg E. Trigeminal herpes zoster/chocolate-vanilla tongue. *Otolaryngol Head Neck Surg* 2000; **122**: 463.

3 Scully C, Samaranayake LP. *Clinical Oral Virology*. Cambridge: Cambridge University Press, 1992.

4 Smith S, Ross JR, Scully C. An unusual oral complication of herpes zoster infection. *Oral Surg* 1984; **57**: 388–9.

5 Wright WE, Davis ML, Geffen DB *et al.* Alveolar bone necrosis and tooth loss: a rare complication associated with herpes zoster infection of the fifth cranial nerve. *Oral Surg* 1983; **56**: 39–46.

6 Sweeney CJ, Gilden DH. Ramsay Hunt syndrome. *J Neurol Neurosurg Psychiatry* 2001; **71**: 149–54.
7 Birek C. Herpesvirus-induced diseases: oral manifestations and current treatment options. *J Calif Dent Assoc* 2000; **28**: 911–21.
8 Graff-Radford SB, Shaw LR, Naliboff BN. Amitriptyline and fluphenazine in the treatment of postherpetic neuralgia. *Clin J Pain* 2000; **16**: 188–92.

Epstein–Barr virus infections (see Chapter 25)

Epstein–Barr virus (EBV) is responsible for infectious mononucleosis and is found in pharyngeal epithelium and appears in the saliva of patients and for several months after clinical recovery. Infection appears to be spread by close oral contact, especially kissing. It is typically a disease of the student population.

Infection is often subclinical. Infectious mononucleosis is also protean in its clinical manifestations, which include particularly lymphadenopathy, sore throat, fever, malaise and rashes. In the anginose type (sore-throat type), the throat is sore with soft-palate petechiae and a whitish exudate on oedematous tonsils. There may be non-specific oral ulceration or pericoronitis [1]. The glandular type of infectious mononucleosis is characterized by generalized lymph node enlargement and splenomegaly; the febrile type is characterized by fever.

Similar syndromes may be caused by cytomegalovirus (CMV), human herpesvirus (HHV)-6, toxoplasmosis and HIV. Characteristic of infectious mononucleosis are large numbers of atypical mononuclear cells in the blood and a wide variety of serological changes, particularly heterophil antibodies, which are detectable by the Paul–Bunnell or Monospot tests, usually during the first or second week of illness. Several other antibodies against EBV appear during the course of infectious mononucleosis, but the most frequent is the antibody to viral capsid antigen, the titre of which reaches a peak at about 4 weeks.

No specific treatment is available for infectious mononucleosis, but supportive care is important, not only because of the potential for airways obstruction but also because of the associated lassitude. Systemic corticosteroids are required if there is pharyngeal oedema severe enough to hazard the airway.

EBV is also commonly found in the mouths of immunocompromised patients [2–5], and is implicated in oral hairy leukoplakia (see p. 66.89), oral ulceration [6] and some oral lymphomas, although any relationship with other malignancies such as OSCC is controversial [7,8].

REFERENCES

1 Scully C, Samaranayake LP. *Clinical Oral Virology*. Cambridge: Cambridge University Press, 1992.
2 Ammatuna P, Campisi G, Giovannelli L et al. Presence of Epstein–Barr virus, cytomegalovirus and human papillomavirus in normal oral mucosa of HIV-infected and renal transplant patients. *Oral Dis* 2001; **7**: 34–40.
3 Ammatuna P, Capone F, Giambelluca D et al. Detection of Epstein–Barr virus (EBV) DNA and antigens in oral mucosa of renal transplant patients without

clinical evidence of oral hairy leukoplakia (OHL). *J Oral Pathol Med* 1998; **27**: 420–7.
4 Triantos D, Boulter AW, Leao JC et al. Diversity of naturally-occuring Epstein–Barr virus revealed by nucleotide sequence polymorphism in hypervariable domains in the BamH1 K and N subgenomic regions. *J Gen Virol* 1998; **79**: 2809–17.
5 Triantos D, Leao JC, Porter SR, Scully CM, Teo CG. Tissue distribution of Epstein–Barr virus genotypes in hosts coinfected by HIV. *AIDS* 1998; **12**: 2141–6.
6 Syrjanen S, Leimola-Virtanen R, Schmidt-Westhausen A, Reichart PA. Oral ulcers in AIDS patients frequently associated with cytomegalovirus (CMV) and Epstein–Barr virus (EBV) infections. *J Oral Pathol Med* 1999; **28**: 204–9.
7 Gonzalez-Moles M, Gutierrez J, Ruiz I et al. Epstein–Barr virus and oral squamous cell carcinoma in patients without HIV infection: viral detection by polymerase chain reaction. *Microbios* 1998; **96**: 23–31.
8 Goldenberg D, Golz A, Netzer A et al. Epstein–Barr virus and cancers of the head and neck. *Am J Otolaryngol* 2001; **22**: 197–205.

Cytomegalovirus infection

CMV may cause a glandular fever type of syndrome, and rarely causes oral ulceration. Indolent CMV-induced oral ulcers may be seen in immunosuppressed patients and in AIDS [1–4].

REFERENCES

1 Epstein JB, Scully C. Cytomegalovirus: a virus of increasing relevance to oral medicine and pathology. *J Oral Pathol Med* 1993; **22**: 348–53.
2 Kanas RJ, Jensen JL, Abrams AM et al. Oral mucosal cytomegalovirus as a manifestation of the acquired immune deficiency syndrome. *Oral Surg* 1987; **64**: 183–9.
3 Myerson D, Hackman RC, Nelson JA et al. Widespread evidence of histologically occult cytomegalovirus. *Hum Pathol* 1984; **15**: 430–9.
4 Syrjanen S, Leimola-Virtanen R, Schmidt-Westhausen A, Reichart PA. Oral ulcers in AIDS patients frequently associated with cytomegalovirus (CMV) and Epstein–Barr virus (EBV) infections. *J Oral Pathol Med* 1999; **28**: 204–9.

Herpesviruses 6, 7 and 8

Oral lesions have yet to be demonstrated in infections with HHV-6 or HHV-7. However, HHV-8 is implicated in oral Kaposi's sarcoma [1–4]. Treatment with highly active antiretroviral therapy (HAART) may reduce HHV-8 infection [5].

REFERENCES

1 Di Alberti L, Porter SR, Scully C et al. Genetic polymorphism of, and new diseases associated with, Kaposi's sarcoma herpes virus (KSHV). *J Oral Pathol Med* 1996; **25**: 282. 66.
2 DiAlberti L, Ngui SL, Porter SR et al. Presence of human herpesvirus-8 variants in the oral ulcer tissues of human immunodeficiency virus-infected persons. *J Infect Dis* 1997; **175**: 703–7.
3 DiAlberti L, Porter SR, Speight P et al. Detection of human herpesvirus 8 DNA in oral ulcer tissues of HIV-infected individuals. *Oral Dis* 1997; **3** (Suppl. 1): S133–S134.
4 Leao JC, Porter SR, Scully C. Human herpesvirus 8 and oral health care: an update. *Oral Surg Oral Med Oral Pathol Oral Radiol Endod* 2000; **90**: 694–704.
5 Leao JC, Kumar N, McLean KA et al. Effect of human immunodeficiency virus-1 protease inhibitors on the clearance of human herpesvirus 8 from blood of human immunodeficiency virus-1-infected patients. *J Med Virol* 2000; **62**: 416–20.

Enteroviruses

Herpangina

Aetiology. Herpangina is caused by Coxsackieviruses mainly. The incubation period is 3–7 days and young children are predominantly affected.

Clinical features. Many infections are subclinical but features of the clinical syndrome include malaise, anorexia, irritability, low fever, slightly enlarged and tender anterior cervical lymph nodes and mouth ulcers, predominantly on the soft palate [1].

Diagnosis. There may be a contact history. It is possible to culture Coxsackieviruses in suckling mice if absolutely necessary.

The main differential diagnosis is primary herpetic stomatitis, but in herpangina there is less fever, no acute gingivitis and ulceration is mainly restricted to the soft palate.

Treatment. The condition is self-limiting and treatment is supportive only.

REFERENCE

1 Bell EJ, Williams GR, Grist NR *et al.* Enterovirus infections. *Update* 1983; **26**: 967–78.

Hand, foot and mouth disease (see Chapter 25)

Aetiology. Hand, foot and mouth disease is caused particularly by Coxsackie A viruses but sometimes by Coxsackie B viruses or enteroviruses.

Clinical features. The incubation period is 3–10 days and, although young children are predominantly infected, there are occasional outbreaks in adults. Many infections are subclinical but features of the clinical syndrome include the following.
• General features: malaise, anorexia, irritability and fever may be present but usually only in severe cases.
• Anterior cervical lymph nodes may occasionally be slightly enlarged and tender.
• Mouth ulcers are round or ovoid, usually sparse and may affect any site [1–3].
• Rash: painful, sometimes deep-seated vesicles may appear, usually on the hand and/or feet, particularly on digits or at the base of the phalanges.

Hand, foot and mouth disease is self-limiting and only rarely complicated by systemic illness such as encephalitis. The condition tends to be more severe when it occurs in adults.

Diagnosis and management are as for herpangina.

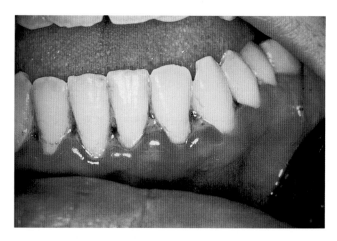

Fig. 66.44 Acute necrotizing gingivitis showing typical ulceration of interdental gingival papillae. This was in HIV infection.

REFERENCES

1 Conway SP. Coxsackie B2 virus causing simultaneous hand, foot and mouth disease and encephalitis. *J Infect* 1987; **15**: 191.
2 Goh KT, Doraisingham S, Tan JC *et al.* An outbreak of hand, foot and mouth disease in Singapore. *Bull WHO* 1982; **60**: 965–9.
3 Ishimaru Y, Nakano S, Yamaoka K *et al.* Outbreak of hand, foot and mouth disease caused by Enterovirus 71. *Arch Dis Child* 1980; **55**: 583–8.

Bacterial infections

Acute necrotizing (ulcerative) gingivitis and noma

Aetiology. There is no firm evidence of communicability of acute necrotizing gingivitis, although it may occur in epidemic form, especially in institutions or in the military (trench mouth). Viral respiratory infections, overwork and fatigue, smoking or immune defects may precede the onset of disease, suggesting depression of immunity as a predisposing cause. A similar lesion may be a feature of HIV infection and related diseases.

A mixed, mostly anaerobic, flora (the fusospirochaetal complex), consisting mainly of *Fusobacterium nucleatum* (*F. fusiformis* or *Bacillus fusiformis*) and *Borrelia vincentii*, is associated with this infection [1,2].

Clinical features. The mouth ulceration is usually restricted to the gingiva, specifically the interdental papillae, which appear blunted (Figs 66.44 & 66.45). The history is characteristic, with an acute onset of gingival soreness, bleeding and halitosis. Acute necrotizing gingivitis occurs especially in the anterior part of the mouth where the affected gingiva are extremely tender to touch and readily bleed on minimal pressure. Occasionally the ulceration extends elsewhere on the gingiva, or onto the adjacent mucosa. There is often enlargement of the cervical lymph nodes and there may be pyrexia and malaise.

Prognosis. Failure to adequately treat acute necrotizing gingivitis may predispose to recurrence and, in malnour-

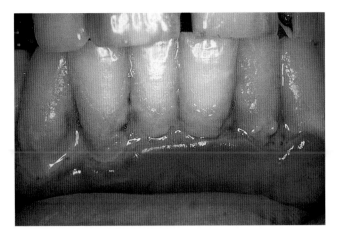

Fig. 66.45 Untreated acute necrotizing gingivitis can lead to extensive gingival ulceration and irreparable damage.

ished or immunocompromised individuals, may lead to noma (cancrum oris) [3–7]. Similar lesions of gangrenous stomatitis are increasingly reported in HIV disease.

Diagnosis. Diagnosis is mainly from gingival lesions in primary herpetic stomatitis, leukaemias and HIV disease. A bacteriological smear may be helpful.

Treatment. Gentle cleansing with a hydrogen peroxide mouthwash and a soft toothbrush is remarkably effective. Oral metronidazole 200 mg should be given three times daily for 3–7 days to limit the tissue destruction. Penicillin is equally effective. The patient should also be referred for dental advice [1].

REFERENCES

1 Johnson BD, Engel D. Acute necrotising ulcerative gingivitis: a review of diagnosis, etiology and treatment. *J Periodontol* 1986; **57**: 141–50.
2 Osuji OO. Necrotizing ulcerative gingivitis and cancrum oris (noma) in Ibadan, Nigeria. *J Periodontol* 1990; **61**: 769–72.
3 Enwonwu CO. Infectious oral necrosis (cancrum oris) in Nigerian children. *Community Dent Oral Epidemiol* 1985; **13**: 190–4.
4 Madden N. An interesting case of facial gangrene (from Papua, New Guinea). *Oral Surg* 1985; **59**: 279.
5 Sabiston CB. A review and proposal for the etiology of acute necrotizing gingivitis. *J Clin Periodontol* 1986; **13**: 727–34.
6 Sawyer D, Nwoku AJ. Cancrum oris (noma): past and present. *J Dent Child* 1981; **48**: 138–41.
7 Stassen LFA, Batchelor AGG, Rennie JS *et al.* Cancrum oris in an adult Caucasian female. *Br J Oral Maxillofac Surg* 1989; **27**: 417–22.

Syphilis

Oral ulcers may be seen at any stage but particularly in secondary syphilis [1–3]. In primary syphilis, a primary chancre (hard or Hunterian chancre) may involve the lips, tongue or palate. A small, firm, pink macule changes to a papule which ulcerates to form a painless round ulcer with a raised margin and indurated base [4]. Chancres heal spontaneously in 3–8 weeks but are highly infectious

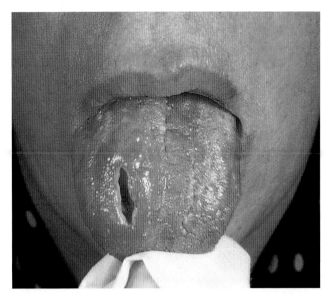

Fig. 66.46 Gumma.

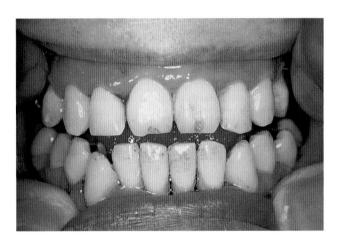

Fig. 66.47 Hutchinson's maxillary central incisors.

and are associated with enlarged, painless regional lymph nodes.

Secondary syphilis follows after 6–8 weeks, with oral lesions in about one-third of patients [1,3]. These are highly infectious and are usually fairly painless ulcers (mucous patches and snail-track ulcers).

The most characteristic oral lesion of tertiary syphilis is a localized granuloma (gumma) that varies in size from a pinhead to several centimetres, affecting particularly the palate, or the tongue. Gummas break down to form deep chronic punched-out ulcers that are not infectious (Fig. 66.46). However, the most common oral manifestation of tertiary syphilis is leukoplakia, which particularly affects the dorsum of the tongue and has a high potential for malignant change.

Congenital syphilis may, when the permanent teeth erupt, present with dental anomalies such as Hutchinson's teeth (Fig. 66.47). Oral ulcers are rare.

Exudate from a suspected oral lesion of syphilis should be examined for treponemes by dark-ground microscopy; however, since the diagnosis can be confused by oral commensal treponemes, lesions should first be thoroughly swabbed with a sterile gauze or cotton-wool and then gently scraped with a sterile spatula, the scraping being examined immediately by dark-ground microscopy. Serology is indicated. Biopsy is not usually indicated, but lesions are characterized by a dense plasma cell infiltrate.

REFERENCES

1 Manton SL, Eggleston SI, Alexander I *et al.* Oral presentation of secondary syphilis. *Br Dent J* 1986; **160**: 237–8.
2 Samaranayake LP, Scully C. Oral disease and sexual medicine. *Br J Sex Med* 1988; **15**: 138–43, 174–80.
3 Terezhalmy GT. Oral manifestations of sexually-related diseases. *Ear Nose Throat J* 1983; **62**: 287–96.
4 Cousteau C, Leyder P, Laufer J. Syphilis primaire buccale: un diagnostic parfois difficile. *Rev Stomatol Chir Maxillofac* 1984; **85**: 391–8.

Gonorrhoea

Oral mucosal erythema, sometimes with oedema and ulceration, is occasionally seen in oropharyngeal gonorrhoea. Oropharyngeal asymptomatic carriage of gonococci is more common, found in around 4% of those attending clinics for sexually transmitted diseases [1,2].

REFERENCES

1 Brown RT, Lossick JG, Mosure DJ *et al.* Pharyngeal gonorrhoea screening in adolescents: is it necessary? *Pediatrics* 1989; **84**: 623–5.
2 Guinta JL, Fiumara NJ. Facts about gonorrhoea and dentistry. *Oral Surg* 1986; **62**: 529.

Tuberculosis

Oral lesions can develop in pulmonary tuberculosis but are not common. A chronic ulcer, usually of the dorsum of the tongue, is the most common oral presentation but jaw lesions or cervical lymph node involvement may be seen [1–4]. Atypical mycobacteria are not uncommonly involved.

Mycobacterial oral ulcers, particularly caused by *Mycobacterium avium–intracellulare*, have been reported as a complication of AIDS and occasionally in apparently healthy individuals [5]. Cervicofacial infection is occasionally caused by *M. chelonei*, usually in the form of lymph node abscesses, or occasionally as intraoral swellings [6–9].

REFERENCES

1 Dimitrakopoulos I, Zouloumis L, Lazaridis N *et al.* Primary tuberculosis of the oral cavity. *Oral Surg* 1991; **72**: 712–5.
2 Haddad NM, Zaytoun GM, Hadi U. Tuberculosis of the soft palate: an unusual presentation of oral tuberculosis. *Otolaryngol Head Neck Surg* 1987; **97**: 91–9.
3 Michaud M, Blanchette G, Tomich CF. Chronic ulceration of the hard palate: first clinical sign of undiagnosed pulmonary tuberculosis. *Oral Surg* 1984; **57**: 63–7.
4 Waldman RH. Tuberculosis and the atypical mycobacteria. *Otolaryngol Clin North Am* 1982; **15**: 581–96.
5 Morris CA, Grant GH, Everall PH *et al.* Tuberculoid lymphadenitis due to *Mycobacterium chelonei. J Clin Pathol* 1973; **26**: 422–6.
6 Blake GC, Murray JJ, Lee KW. Cervicofacial infection with *Mycobacterium chelonei. Br J Oral Surg* 1976; **13**: 278–81.
7 Boyd BW. Oral infection with associated lymphadenopathy due to *Mycobacterium chelonei. Ala Med* 1984; **54**: 9–10.
8 Pedersen A, Reibel J. Intraoral infection with *Mycobacterium chelonei. Oral Surg* 1989; **67**: 262–5.
9 Volpe F, Schwimmer A, Barr C. Oral manifestations of disseminated *Mycobacterium avium-intracellulare* in a patient with AIDS. *Oral Surg* 1985; **60**: 567–70.

Epithelioid (bacillary) angiomatosis (see Chapter 27)

Oral lesions clinically and, to some extent, histologically reminiscent of Kaposi's sarcoma have been seen in HIV disease [1–3], sometimes as the first manifestation of HIV infection [3].

REFERENCES

1 Glick M, Cleveland DB. Oral mucosal bacillary epithelioid angiomatosis in a patient with AIDS associated with rapid alveolar bone loss. *J Oral Pathol Med* 1993; **22**: 235–9.
2 Levell NJ, Bewley AP, Chopra S *et al.* Bacillary angiomatosis with cutaneous and oral lesions in an HIV-infected patient from the UK. *Br J Dermatol* 1995; **132**: 113–5.
3 Speight PM, Zakrzewska J, Fletcher CDM. Epithelioid angiomatosis affecting the oral cavity as the first sign of HIV infection. *Br Dent J* 1991; **171**: 367–70.

Fungal infections

Oral fungal infections, apart from candidiasis, which rarely causes mouth ulcers in Western societies, are usually seen in the West only in immunocompromised or debilitated patients, including those with AIDS. However, they may be seen occasionally in otherwise healthy persons from the tropics (Table 66.20).

Aspergillosis. Rhinocerebral aspergillosis may ulcerate through to the mouth. This is a rare event, except in the severely immunocompromised [1]. Occasionally, solitary aspergillosis arises as a consequence of endodontic treatment where root canal filling material enters the antrum [2] but this does not cause oral ulceration. Surgical débridement is usually indicated.

REFERENCES

1 Schubert MM. Head and neck aspergillosis in patients undergoing bone-marrow transplantation. *Cancer* 1986; **57**: 1092–6.
2 Beck-Mannagetta J, Necek D, Grasserbauer M. Solitary aspergillosis of maxillary sinus, a complication of dental treatment. *Lancet* 1983; **ii**: 1260.

Table 66.20 Rare orofacial fungal infections.

Infection	Oral manifestations
Aspergillosis	Aspergilloma
	Rhinocerebral type causes palatal necrosis
	Disseminated in immunocompromised patients
Blastomycosis	
North American	Oral ulcers or suppurating granulomas
South American (paracoccidioidomycosis)	Oral ulcers and lymphadenopathy
Coccidioidomycosis	Rarely oral ulcers
Cryptococcosis	Oral ulcers
Histoplasmosis	Lumps or ulcers in mouth
Phycomycosis (mucormycosis, zygomycosis)	Antral involvement with palatal ulceration in immunocompromised patients, especially diabetics
Sporotrichosis	Oral lesions rare

Blastomycoses. Blastomycoses may produce oral lesions which are typically mulberry-like, ulcerated swellings especially seen on the gingiva and alveolus [1,2].

REFERENCES

1 Almeida OP, Jacks J, Scully C *et al.* Orofacial manifestations of paracoccidioidomycosis (South American blastomycosis). *Oral Surg* 1991; **72**: 430–5.
2 Sposto MR, Scully C, Almeida OPD *et al.* Oral paracoccidioidomycosis: a study of 36 South American patients. *Oral Surg* 1993; **75**: 461–5.

Cryptococcosis. *Cryptococcus neoformans* may occasionally produce indolent oral ulcers in immunocomprised patients [1,2].

REFERENCES

1 Glick M, Cohen SG, Cheney RT *et al.* Oral manifestations of disseminated *Cryptococcus neoformans* in a patient with acquired immunodeficiency syndrome. *Oral Surg* 1987; **64**: 454–9.
2 Lynch DP, Naftolin LZ. Oral *Cryptococcus neoformans* infection in AIDS. *Oral Surg* 1987; **64**: 449–53.

Geotrichosis. Geotrichosis is a rare, livid, sharply defined enanthema of the oral mucosa with ulcerations seen in immunocompromised persons, such as those with leukaemia or HIV infection. *Geotrichum capitatum* is responsible and there may also be pneumonic lung infiltrates [1].

Treatment includes amphotericin, 5-fluorocytosine and itraconazole.

REFERENCE

1 Listemann H, Schonrock-Nabulsi P, Kuse R, Meigel W. Geotrichosis of oral mucosa. *Mycoses* 1996; **39**: 289–91.

Histoplasmosis. Oral lesions of histoplasmosis are uncommon. They are typically seen in chronic disseminated histoplasmosis, usually as a non-specific lump or ulcer on the tongue, palate, buccal mucosa or gingiva [1–5], sometimes in AIDS [6–8].

REFERENCES

1 Adekeye EO, Edwards MB, Williams HK. Mandibular African histoplasmosis: imitation of neoplasia or giant cell granuloma. *Oral Surg* 1988; **65**: 81–4.
2 Cobb CM, Shultz RE, Brewer JH *et al.* Chronic pulmonary histoplasmosis with an oral lesion. *Oral Surg* 1989; **67**: 73–6.
3 Goodwin RA, Shapiro JL, Thurman GH *et al.* Disseminated histoplasmosis: clinical and pathologic correlations. *Medicine* 1980; **59**: 93–100.
4 Miller RL, Gould AR, Skolnick JL *et al.* Localised oral histoplasmosis. *Oral Surg* 1982; **53**: 367–74.
5 Scully C, Almeida O. Orofacial manifestations of the systemic mycoses. *J Oral Pathol Med* 1992; **21**: 289–94.
6 Filho FJS, Lopes M, Almeida OPD, Scully C. Mucocutaneous histoplasmosis in AIDS. *Br J Dermatol* 1995; **133**: 472–4.
7 Scully C, Almeida OPD, Sposto MR. Deep mycoses in HIV infection. *Oral Dis* 1997; **3** (Suppl. 1): 200–7.
8 Casariego Z, Rey Kelly G, Perez H *et al.* Disseminated histoplasmosis with orofacial involvement in HIV-1-infected patients with AIDS: manifestations and treatment. *Oral Dis* 1997; **3**: 184–7.

Mucormycosis. Rhinocerebral mucormycosis typically commences in the nasal cavity or paranasal sinuses and invades the palate to produce a black necrotic ulcer, although it might occasionally commence in the palate [1–3]. Most cases are seen in diabetics or in immunocompromised patients such as those with AIDS [4]. Biopsy and radiography are required for diagnosis. Treatment is surgical débridement together with amphotericin intravenously and/or azoles.

REFERENCES

1 Forteza G, Burgeno M, Martorell V, Sierra I. Rhinocerebral mucormycosis. *J Craniomaxillofac Surg* 1988; **16**: 80–4.
2 Hauman CHJ, Raubenheimer EJ. Orofacial mucormycosis. *Oral Surg* 1989; **68**: 624–7.
3 Jones AC, Bentsen TY, Freedman PD. Mucor in the oral cavity. *Oral Surg* 1993; **75**: 455–60.
4 Moraru RA, Grossman ME. Palatal necrosis in an AIDS patient: a case of mucormycosis. *Cutis* 2000; **66**: 15–8.

Protozoal infestations

Leishmaniasis is rare in northern Europe and the USA; it is not uncommon, however, in hotter climes and may cause ulcers in the mouth or more commonly on the lips [1–4], and is seen increasingly in HIV disease [5–9] or in other immunocompromised persons.

REFERENCES

1 Abbas K, El Toumn IA, El Hassan AM. Oral leishmaniasis associated with kala-azar. *Oral Surg* 1992; **73**: 583–4.
2 Baily GG, Pitt MA, Cury A *et al.* Leishmaniasis of the tongue treated with liposomal amphotericin B. *J Infect* 1994; **28**: 327–31.
3 Kerdel-Vegas F. American leishmaniasis. *Int J Dermatol* 1982; **21**: 291–303.
4 Marsden PD, Sampaio RN, Rocha R *et al.* Mucocutaneous leishmaniasis: an unsolved clinical problem. *Trop Doct* 1977; **7**: 7–11.
5 Imhof M, Schofer H, Milbradt R, Lutz T. Mucocutaneous leishmaniasis in a European HIV-positive patient. *Eur J Dermatol* 1995; **5**: 594–6.
6 Michiels JF, Monteil RA, Hofman P *et al.* Oral leishmaniasis and Kaposi's sarcoma in an AIDS patient. *J Oral Pathol Med* 1994; **23**: 45–6.
7 Miralles ES, Nunez M, Hilara Y *et al.* Mucocutaneous leishmaniasis and HIV. *Dermatology* 1994; **189**: 275–7.
8 Montalban C, Calleja JL, Erice A. Visceral leishmaniasis in patients infected with human immunodeficiency virus. *J Infect* 1990; **21**: 261–70.
9 Milian MA, Bagan JV, Jimenez Y, Perez A, Scully C. Oral leishmaniasis in a HIV-positive patient. Report of a case involving the palate. *Oral Dis* 2002; **8**: 59–61.

Immune defects

Human immunodeficiency virus infection [1–5]
(see Chapter 26)

Oral ulceration in patients infected with HIV may be due to any of the causes of mouth ulceration (see p. 66.42), and aphthous-like ulcers are also seen. However, it is important to exclude infections, mainly herpesviruses. There are also occasional examples of mouth ulcers due to mycobacteria, *Rochalimaea*, syphilis, *Histoplasma*, *Cryptococcus*, leishmaniasis and others. Malignant disease (mainly Kaposi's sarcoma or non-Hodgkin's lymphoma) may result in lumps that can ulcerate.

Aphthous-like ulcers in HIV may respond to local treatment or, failing that, 100 mg thalidomide at night for 2 weeks and then 100 mg every fifth day may prove effective [5].

Other mouth ulcers should be treated as appropriate.

REFERENCES

1 Scully C, Laskaris G, Pindborg J *et al.* Oral manifestations of HIV infection and their management. *Oral Surg* 1991; **71**: 158–71.
2 Porter SR, Scully C. HIV: the surgeon's perspective. 1: Update of pathogenesis, epidemiology, management and risk of nosocomial transmission. *Br J Oral Maxillofac Surg* 1994; **32**: 222–30.
3 Porter SR, Scully C. HIV: the surgeon's perspective. 2: Diagnosis and management of non-malignant oral manifestations. *Br J Oral Maxillofac Surg* 1994; **32**: 231–40.
4 Porter SR, Scully C. HIV: the surgeon's perspective. 3: Diagnosis and management of malignant neoplasms. *Br J Oral Maxillofac Surg* 1994; **32**: 241–7.
5 Youle M, Clarbour J, Farthing C *et al.* Treatment of resistant aphthous ulceration with thalidomide in patients positive for HIV antibody. *BMJ* 1989; **298**: 432.

Vasculitides

Periarteritis nodosa

Transient submucosal oral nodules may occur singly or in crops along the path of vessels and especially in the tongue. Other mucosal lesions include erythema, papules, haemorrhages, ulceration or necrosis [1–4].

REFERENCES

1 Cowpe JG, Hislop WS. Oral presentation of polyarteritis nodosa. *Oral Surg* 1983; **56**: 597–601.
2 Standefer JA Jr, Mattox DE. Head and neck manifestations of collagen vascular diseases. *Otolaryngol Clin North Am* 1986; **19**: 181–210.
3 Ekman-Joelsson BM, Kjellman B, Hattevig G. Tongue necrosis due to vasculitis. *Acta Paediatr* 1995; **84**: 1333–6.
4 Taillandier J, Taillandier-Heriche E, Alemann M, Emile JF. Polyarteritis nodosa with temporal and oral involvement. *Rev Rhum Engl Ed* 1999; **66**: 523–4.

Giant cell arteritis
SYN. HORTON'S DISEASE

Patients may suffer ischaemic pain during mastication, intermittent claudication of the tongue [1] or, rarely, facial palsy [2] or lumps [3,4]. Ulceration and necrosis of the tongue [5–11] or occasionally the lip [12] have also been observed [2,3].

REFERENCES

1 Lamey P-J, Taylor JA, Devine J. Giant cell arteritis: a forgotten diagnosis. *Br Dent J* 1988; **164**: 48–50.
2 Sadzot B, Branas C. Neurovascular facial pain. *Rev Med Liege* 1995; **50**: 472–6.
3 Kannan R, Allen CM, Ockner SA, Schneider KE. Intraoral lesion in giant cell arteritis. *Oral Surg Oral Med Oral Pathol Oral Radiol Endod* 1996; **82**: 473–4.
4 Ruiz-Masera JJ, Alamillos-Granados FJ, Dean-Ferrer A *et al.* Submandibular swelling as the first manifestation of giant cell arteritis. Report of a case. *J Craniomaxillofac Surg* 1995; **23**: 119–21.
5 Patterson A, Barnard N, Scully C *et al.* Necrosis of the tongue in a patient with intestinal infarction. *Oral Surg* 1992; **74**: 582–6.
6 Cikes A, Depairon M, Jolidon RM, Wyss P, Lang HJ. Necrosis of the tongue and unilateral blindness in temporal arteritis. *Vasa* 2001; **30**: 222–4.
7 Kleinjung T, Strutz J. Spontaneous, unilateral necrosis of the tongue. Temporal arteritis. *HNO* 1998; **46**: 274–5.
8 Crevits I, Hermans R, Wilms G, Baert AL. Tongue necrosis as a complication of temporal arteritis: CT and angiographic findings. *J Belge Radiol* 1996; **79**: 258–9.
9 Navarro M, Niembro E, Scola B, Scola E, del Pozo A. Necrosis of the tongue secondary to Horton's disease. *Acta Otorrinolaringol Esp* 1995; **46**: 227–9.
10 Llorente Pendas S, De Vicente Rodriguez JC, Gonzalez Garcia M, Junquera Gutierrez LM, Lopez Arranz JS. Tongue necrosis as a complication of temporal arteritis. *Oral Surg Oral Med Oral Pathol* 1994; **78**: 448–51.
11 McRorie ER, Chalmers J, Campbell IW. Lingual infarction in cranial arteritis. *Br J Clin Pract* 1994; **48**: 280.
12 Scully C, Eveson JW, Barrett AW *et al.* Necrosis of the lip in giant cell arteritis. *J Oral Maxillofac Surg* 1993; **51**: 581–3.

Iatrogenic conditions

Mucositis

Mucositis, sometimes called *mucosal barrier injury*, is the term given to the widespread oral erythema, ulceration and soreness that is a common complication of a number of therapeutic procedures involving chemotherapy, radiotherapy or chemoradiotherapy, used largely in the treatment of cancer but also in the conditioning prior to bone marrow transplantation (i.e. haematopoietic stem cell transplantation). Mucositis appears 3–15 days after cancer treatment, earlier after chemotherapy than after radiotherapy.

Mucositis invariably follows external beam radiotherapy involving the orofacial tissues, and is also common in upper mantle head and neck radiation, and particularly in total body irradiation.

Some 40–90% of patients on chemotherapy develop mucositis. Patients on fluorouracil and cisplatin in particular develop mucositis, while etoposide and melphalan cause particularly severe mucositis. Oral mucositis is particularly severe after haemopoietic stem cell transplantation, because of radiation damage and myeloablation, and the course follows the polymorphonuclear leukocyte count.

The impaired mucosal barrier in mucositis predisposes to life-threatening septic complications; the prevalence of an oral focus in febrile neutropenia has been reported in up to 30% of cases [1–4].

Mucositis typically presents with pain (which can be so intense as to interfere with eating and significantly affect the quality of life), erythema, ulceration and sometimes bleeding.

Diagnosis is clinical and it is helpful to score the degree of mucositis in order to monitor progression and therapy.

Management. The basic strategies in management of mucositis aim at pain relief, efforts to hasten healing and prevention of infectious complications. However, prophylaxis is the goal.

Pain relief is usually achieved with opioids given by patient-controlled analgesia and benzydamine can aid relief. Oral cooling with ice chips ameliorates chemotherapy-induced mucositis [5,6].

Other treatments currently used but for which hard data for reliable efficacy are unavailable include the following.
• Medications to reduce salivation and thus exposure of the mucosa to chemotherapeutic drugs that are secreted in saliva.
• Anti-inflammatory medications.
• Cytokines such as interleukin (IL)-1, IL-11, TGF-beta3 and keratinocyte growth factor.
• Granulocyte–macrophage colony-stimulating factor (GM-CSF) and granulocyte colony-stimulating factor (G-CSF).
• Thalidomide: an angiogenesis-inhibiting drug.
• Amifostine: a cytoprotector.
• Melatonin: the pineal hormone.
• Protegrin antimicrobial peptides, which possess activity against Gram-positive and Gram-negative bacteria and yeasts.
• Low-energy lasers.
• Other agents such as sucralfate, tretinoin, glutamine and misoprostol [1–4,6].

Monitoring microbial colonization and the institution of antiviral prophylaxis and antifungal prophylaxis, to avoid colonization and superinfection, is particularly important in patients with low neutrophil counts.

Invasive fungal infections of the oral cavity can be associated with systemic fungal infection and are indications for the use of liposomal amphotericin.

REFERENCES

1 Sonis ST, Clark J. Prevention and management of oral mucositis induced by antineoplastic therapy. *Oncology* 1991; **5**: 11–6.
2 Blijlevens NM, Donnelly JP, De Pauw BE. Mucosal barrier injury: biology, pathology, clinical counterparts and consequences of intensive treatment for haematological malignancy: an overview. *Bone Marrow Transplant* 2000; **25**: 1269–78.
3 Stiff P. Mucositis associated with stem cell transplantation: current status and innovative approaches to management. *Bone Marrow Transplant* 2001; **27** (Suppl. 2): S3–S11.
4 Scully C, Epstein JB. Oral healthcare for the cancer patient. *Oral Oncol* 1996; **32**: 281–92.
5 Epstein JB, Stevenson-Moore P, Jackson S, Mohammed JH, Spinelli JJ. Prevention of oral mucositis in radiation therapy: a controlled study with benzydamine hydrochloride rinse. *Int J Radiat Oncol Biol Phys* 1989; **16**: 1571–5.
6 Clarkson JE, Worthington HV, Eden OB. Prevention of oral mucositis or oral candidiasis for patients with cancer receiving chemotherapy (excluding head and neck cancer). *Cochrane Database Syst Rev* 2000; CD000978.

Bone marrow transplantation (haematopoietic stem cell transplantation)

Oral complications are common and can be a major cause of morbidity following bone marrow transplantation. Mucositis, infections, bleeding, xerostomia and loss of taste result from the effects of the underlying disease, chemotherapy or radiotherapy, and GVHD. The ventrum of the tongue, buccal and labial mucosa and gingiva may be affected by ulceration or mucositis [1–6].

REFERENCES

1 Barrett AP. Oral complications of bone marrow transplantation. *Aust N Z J Med* 1986; **16**: 239–40.
2 Berkowitz RJ, Strandford S, Jones P et al. Stomatologic complications of bone marrow transplantation in a pediatric population. *Pediatr Dent* 1987; **9**: 105–10.
3 Dahllof G, Heimdahl A, Modeer T et al. Oral mucous membrane lesions in children treated with bone marrow transplantation. *Scand J Dent Res* 1989; **97**: 268–77.

4 Dreizen S, McCredie KB, Dicke KA *et al.* Oral complications of bone marrow transplantation in adults with acute leukaemia. *Postgrad Med* 1979; **66**: 187–93.
5 Seto BG. Oral mucositis in patients undergoing bone-marrow transplantation. *Oral Surg* 1985; **60**: 493–7.
6 Kolbinson DA, Schubert MM, Flourney N *et al.* Early oral changes following bone marrow transplantation. *Oral Surg* 1988; **66**: 130–8.

Graft-versus-host disease

The oral manifestations of acute GVHD consist of painful mucosal desquamation and ulceration, and/or cheilitis, and the presence of lichenoid plaques or striae. Small white lesions affect the buccal and lingual mucosa early on, but clear by day 14. Erythema and ulceration are most pronounced at 7–11 days, and may be associated with obvious infection. Candidiasis is common, as is herpes simplex stomatitis (occasionally zoster) and there may be oral purpura, especially in adults [1,2].

The oral lesions in chronic GVHD are coincident with skin lesions, and include generalized mucosal erythema, lichenoid lesions, mainly in the buccal mucosa, and xerostomia. There may be depressed salivary IgA levels in minor gland saliva [3]. Xerostomia is most significant in the first 14 days after transplant and is a consequence of drug treatment, irradiation and/or GVHD.

Lip biopsy is useful in the diagnosis of chronic GVHD and should include both mucosa and underlying minor salivary glands [4]. Histology shows changes similar to those seen in Sjögren's syndrome.

REFERENCES

1 Dreizen S, McCredie KB, Dicke KA *et al.* Oral complications of bone marrow transplantation in adults with acute leukaemia. *Postgrad Med* 1979; **66**: 187–93.
2 Graham-Brown RAG, Jones JAG, Shaw PV *et al.* A graft-versus-host disease-like syndrome with carcinomatosis. *Br J Dermatol* 1987; **116**: 249–52.
3 Izutsu KT, Menard TW, Schubert MM. Graft versus host disease-related secretory immunoglobulin A deficiency in bone marrow transplant recipients: findings in labial saliva. *Lab Invest* 1985; **52**: 292–7.
4 Sale GE, Shulman HM, Schubert MM. Oral and ophthalmic pathology of graft-versus-host disease in man: predictive value of the lip biopsy. *Hum Pathol* 1981; **12**: 1022–30.

Drugs

A wide range of drugs can occasionally induce mouth ulcers, by a variety of effects [1]. Oral use of caustics or agents such as cocaine can cause erosions or ulcers [2]. Oral ulcers are regularly produced by cytotoxic agents [3] (see Mucositis above). Aphthous-like ulcers may follow the use of the potassium channel blocking cardioactive agent nicorandil [4].

Drugs may also cause mucocutaneous lesions. Oral ulcers of a lichenoid type may follow exposure to non-steroidal anti-inflammatory drugs and other agents (see p. 66.61). Erythema multiforme may follow the use of a range of drugs (see p. 66.67). Drug-induced mouth ulcers may also resemble toxic epidermal necrolysis (see p. 66.68) or may have features reminiscent of other dermatological disorders.

The ulcers usually resolve in 10–14 days if the offending drug can be identified and withdrawn.

REFERENCES

1 Porter SR, Scully C. Adverse drug reactions in the mouth. *Clin Dermatol* 2000; **18**: 525–32.
2 Parry J, Porter SR, Scully C *et al.* Mucosal lesions due to oral cocaine use. *Br Dent J* 1996; **180**: 462–4.
3 Berkowitz RJ, Jones P, Barsetti J *et al.* Stomatologic complications of bone marrow transplantation in a pediatric population. *Paediatr Dent* 1987; **9**: 105–10.
4 Scully C, Azul A, Crighton A *et al.* Nicorandil can induce severe oral ulceration. *Oral Surg Oral Med Oral Pathol Oral Radiol Endod* 2001; **91**: 189–93.

Acrodynia
SYN. PINK DISEASE

Oral and perioral ulceration, hypersalivation, gingivitis and early tooth loss are features of acrodynia caused by mercury poisoning, now rarely seen [1].

REFERENCE

1 Dinehart SM, Dillard R, Rainer SS *et al.* Cutaneous manifestations of acrodynia (Pink disease). *Arch Dermatol* 1988; **124**: 107–9.

Disorders of uncertain pathogenesis

Angina bullosa haemorrhagica
SYN. LOCALIZED ORAL PURPURA

This is the term given to a benign, fairly common condition of unknown aetiology that usually presents in the elderly with oral blood blisters. These subepithelial blisters are seen mainly in the soft palate and after a few hours rupture to leave ulcers (Fig. 66.48). The patients appear well otherwise, with no detectable immunological or bleeding disorder [1–3]. Occasional cases are related to the use of corticosteroid inhalers. Only symptomatic care is available.

REFERENCES

1 Hopkins R, Walker DM. Oral blood blisters: angina bullosa haemorrhagica. *Br J Oral Surg* 1985; **23**: 9–16.
2 Stephenson P, Lamey P-J, Scully C *et al.* Angina bullosa haemorrhagica: clinical and laboratory features in 30 patients. *Oral Surg* 1987; **63**: 560–5.
3 Stephenson P, Scully C, Prime SS *et al.* Angina bullosa haemorrhagica: lesional immunostaining and haematological findings. *Br J Oral Surg* 1987; **25**: 488–91.

Monoclonal plasmacytic ulcerative stomatitis

Ulcerative stomatitis may occasionally appear with a lichenoid rash, related to a plasmacytic infiltrate [1,2].

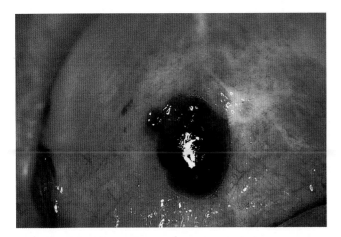

Fig. 66.48 Angina bullosa haemorrhagica: a large blood blister in a typical site on the soft palate. The adjacent whitish lesions are from scarring after a previous biopsy.

REFERENCES

1 Bowden JR, Scully C, Eveson JW *et al.* Multiple myeloma and bullous lichenoid lesions: an unusual association. *Oral Surg* 1990; **70**: 587–9.
2 Layton SA, Cook JN, Henry JA. Monoclonal plasmacytic ulcerative stomatitis. *Oral Surg* 1993; **75**: 483–7.

Mucocutaneous lymph node syndrome
SYN. KAWASAKI DISEASE (see Chapter 27)

Mucocutaneous lymph node syndrome is a disorder of uncertain, but possibly infectious, aetiology. Male children are predominantly affected.

At least one oral feature should be present for the diagnosis to be made. The oral and pharyngeal mucosa become generally red and sore and the lips dry and fissured. There may be oral ulceration and a 'strawberry tongue' appearance [1,2].

Cervical lymphadenopathy, conjunctivitis and fever also occur, followed later by the characteristic desquamation of the skin of the hands and feet.

Early therapy with immunoglobulin is essential to avoid cardiac complications.

REFERENCES

1 Ogden GR, Kerr M. Mucocutaneous lymph node syndrome (Kawasaki disease). *Oral Surg* 1989; **67**: 569–72.
2 Terezhalmy GT. Mucocutaneous lymph node syndrome. *Oral Surg* 1979; **47**: 26–30.

Superficial mucoceles

Superficial extravasation mucoceles of the intraoral minor salivary glands in the palate, buccal mucosa or labial mucosa are not uncommon, especially associated with oral LP in middle-aged or elderly women. This is a benign self-limiting condition that may cause confusion with vesiculobullous disorders [1].

REFERENCE

1 Eveson JW. Superficial mucoceles: pitfall in clinical and microscopic diagnosis. *Oral Surg* 1988; **66**: 318–22.

Necrotizing sialometaplasia

Necrotizing sialometaplasia is an uncommon, benign, self-limiting condition seen predominantly in the posterior hard palate of young adult males, most of whom smoke tobacco [1]. A painless deep ulcer persists for several weeks before spontaneously healing. Biopsy reveals necrosis and pseudoepitheliomatous changes probably resulting from squamous metaplasia following infarction of minor salivary glands. This benign lesion must be differentiated from malignancy.

REFERENCE

1 Kinney RB, Burton CS, Vollmer RT. Necrotizing sialometaplasia: a sheep in wolf's clothing. *Arch Dermatol* 1986; **12**: 208–10.

Mucha–Haberman disease

Erythematous and ulcerative oral lesions have been reported in pityriasis lichenoides et varioliformis acuta (Mucha–Haberman disease) [1,2].

REFERENCES

1 Burke DP, Adams RM, Arundell FD. Ulceronecrotic Mucha–Haberman's disease. *Arch Dermatol* 1969; **100**: 201–6.
2 McDaniel RK, White JW, Edwards PA. Mucha–Haberman's disease with oral lesions. *Oral Surg* 1982; **53**: 596–601.

Metabolic disorders

Glucagonoma

Oral ulceration can be a severe manifestation in glucagonoma [1].

REFERENCE

1 Ditty FR, Lang PG. Cutaneous and oral changes as the only manifestations of the glucagonoma syndrome. *South Med J* 1982; **75**: 222–4.

Oral soreness

Most oral pain is of local aetiology, usually resulting from odontogenic infections. Neurological, vascular and referred causes are less common, but must also be excluded. Psychogenic pain is all too frequent and this is discussed below.

Chronic oral soreness may be particularly caused by ulceration, or by mucosal lesions in geographical tongue,

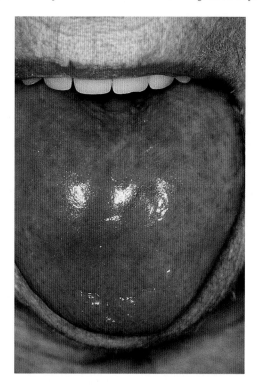

Fig. 66.49 Atrophic glossitis in vitamin B$_{12}$ deficiency.

LP or deficiency states. Geographical tongue and burning mouth syndrome are the common causes of a sore tongue. LP is the most common cause of chronic soreness in the buccal mucosae. Desquamative gingivitis is the common cause of persistently sore gingivae.

Geographical tongue (see p. 66.94)

Lichen planus (see p. 66.61)

Deficiency glossitis

Aetiology. Deficiency glossitis may be related particularly to deficiency of iron, folate or vitamin B$_{12}$, and may then be associated with angular stomatitis and/or mouth ulcers. Deficiencies of other B-group vitamins occasionally cause glossitis, usually in chronic alcoholics or in those with malabsorption [1–3].

Pathology. Epithelial atrophy, rarely with some dysplasia, is seen.

Clinical features. In anaemic glossitis the tongue is red, sore and smooth (Fig. 66.49). Occasionally pernicious anaemia can also produce red areas or patterns of red lines.

In many other patients the tongue can become sore but appear clinically completely normal and such patients' complaints are liable to be mislabelled as psychogenic.

Diagnosis. A full blood picture and assays of iron, folate and vitamin B$_{12}$ are essential in management, as sore tongue can be the initial symptom of a deficiency and can precede any fall in the haemoglobin level.

Treatment. The cause of the deficiency should be sought before replacement treatment is given.

REFERENCES

1 Drummond JF, White DK, Damin DD. Megaloblastic anaemia with oral lesions: a consequence of gastric bypass surgery. *Oral Surg* 1985; **59**: 149–53.
2 Greenberg MS. Clinical and histologic changes of the oral mucosa in pernicious anaemia. *Oral Surg* 1981; **52**: 38–42.
3 Ramasinghe AW, Warnakulasuriya KAAS, Tennekoon GE *et al*. Oral mucosal changes in iron deficiency anaemia in a Sri Lankan female population. *Oral Surg* 1983; **55**: 29–32.

Burning mouth syndrome

SYN. ORAL DYSAESTHESIA; GLOSSOPYROSIS; GLOSSODYNIA

Burning mouth syndrome (BMS) most frequently affects middle-aged and elderly females [1–4].

Aetiology. Several organic lesions, for example haematinic deficiency states, erythema migrans, ulcers, mucositis, LP and candidiasis, can cause oral soreness or burning sensation.

BMS with a tongue of normal clinical appearance may be seen in deficiency states, and with psychogenic causes, drugs (e.g. angiotensin-converting enzyme inhibitors such as captopril, enalapril, lisinopril; protease inhibitors; cytotoxic agents; clonazepam) and diabetes mellitus. A monosymptomatic hypochondriasis or an underlying anxiety about cancer or venereal disease with perhaps excessive tongue activity appear to be the basis for the complaint of BMS in many patients (Table 66.21) [1–8].

Uncommon causes that may need to be considered include hypothyroidism, lupus erythematosus, hypersensitivity (to sodium metabisulphite, nuts, dental materials and other substances) and galvanic reactions to metals in the mouth [9–12]. However, BMS is often a medically unexplained symptom.

Clinical features. Although the tongue is most frequently involved, the patient may also occasionally complain of burning lips, gums or palate. The burning sensation is usually bilateral and often relieved by eating and drinking [1]. In contrast, oral discomfort associated with inflammatory lesions is typically aggravated by eating.

Diagnosis. Oral examination very occasionally reveals an organic cause. Xerostomia should be excluded as this may predispose to candidiasis. Laboratory screening for anaemia, diabetes, a deficiency state or candidiasis should be undertaken.

Table 66.21 Causes of burning mouth.

Local
Candidiasis
Other infections
Geographical tongue
Lichen planus
Oral submucous fibrosis
Dentures

Systemic
Psychogenic
  Cancerophobia
  Depression
  Anxiety states
  Hypochondriasis
Deficiency states
  Pernicious anaemia and other vitamin B deficiencies
  Folate deficiency
  Iron deficiency
Diabetes
Drugs (captopril)

Management. Few patients with BMS have spontaneous remission in the short term, and thus an attempt at treatment is indicated. Reassurance, treatment of any defined underlying organic abnormality and, occasionally, psychological treatment, antidepressants or psychiatric care are indicated, but active dental or oral surgical treatment, or attempts at 'hormone replacement', in the absence of any specific indication, should be avoided. However, treatment is rarely completely successful, although the condition only infrequently becomes severe. Fortunately, about 50% remit spontaneously over 6 or 7 years.

• Patients should avoid anything that aggravates symptoms, such as sparkling wines, citrus drinks and spices.

• Reassurance and attention to any factors such as dentures or haematinic deficiencies may be indicated. There are few treatments of proven benefit [13]. Cognitive–behavioural therapy or a specialist referral may be indicated [14].

• Some patients respond to medication:
  (a) effects of vitamin B are controversial [15,16];
  (b) topical benzydamine 0.01% rinse or spray [17];
  (c) although antidepressants must be given for at least 2–3 weeks to achieve any antidepressive effect, most patients with medically unexplained symptoms show benefit within 1 week [18–20];
  (d) topical capsaicin cream 0.025% (Zacin) or 0.075% (Axsain);
  (e) clonazepam tablet sucked locally;
  (f) α-lipoic acid systemically [21].

REFERENCES

1 Van der Waal I. *The Burning Mouth Syndrome.* Copenhagen: Munksgaard, 1990.
2 Marbach JJ. Medically unexplained chronic orofacial pain. Temporomandibular pain and dysfunction syndrome, orofacial phantom pain, burning mouth syndrome, and trigeminal neuralgia. *Med Clin North Am* 1999; **83**: 691–710.
3 Silvestre FJ, Serrano C. Burning mouth syndrome: concepts review and update. *Med Oral* 1997; **2**: 30–8.
4 Muzyka BC, De Rossi SS. A review of burning mouth syndrome. *Cutis* 1999; **64**: 29–35.
5 Bergdahl M, Bergdahl J. Burning mouth syndrome: prevalence and associated factors. *J Oral Pathol Med* 1999; **28**: 350–4.
6 Maresky LS, Van der Bijl P, Gird I. Burning mouth syndrome. Evaluation of multiple variables among 85 patients. *Oral Surg* 1993; **75**: 303–7.
7 Bogetto F, Maina G, Ferro G, Carbone M, Gandolfo S. Psychiatric comorbidity in patients with burning mouth syndrome. *Psychosom Med* 1998; **60**: 378–85.
8 Rojo L, Silvestre FJ, Bagan JV, de Vincente T. Psychiatric morbidity in burning mouth syndrome. Psychiatric interview versus depression and anxiety scales. *Oral Surg* 1993; **75**: 308–11.
9 Van Joost TH, Van Ulsen J, Van Loon LAJ. Contact allergy to denture materials in the burning mouth syndrome. *Contact Dermatitis* 1988; **18**: 97–9.
10 Wardrop RW, Hailes J, Burger H *et al.* Oral discomfort at menopause. *Oral Surg* 1989; **67**: 535–40.
11 Dutree-Meulenberg ROGM, Kozel MMA, van Joost TH. Burning mouth syndrome: a possible etiologic role for local contact hypersensitivity. *J Am Acad Dermatol* 1992; **26**: 935–40.
12 Helton J, Storrs F. The burning mouth syndrome: lack of a role for contact urticaria and contact dermatitis. *J Am Acad Dermatol* 1994; **31**: 201–5.
13 Buchanan J, Zakrzewska J. Burning mouth syndrome. *Clin Evidence* 2003; 1239–43.
14 Bergdahl J, Anneroth G, Perris H. Cognitive therapy in the treatment of patients with burning mouth syndrome: a controlled study. *J Oral Pathol Med* 1995; **24**: 213–5.
15 Lamey PJ, Allam BF. Vitamin status of patients with burning mouth syndrome and the response to replacement therapy. *Br Dent J* 1986; **168**: 81–4.
16 Hugoson A, Thorstensson B. Vitamin B status and response to replacement therapy in patients with burning mouth syndrome. *Acta Odontol Scand* 1991; **49**: 367–75.
17 Sardella A, Uglietti D, Demarosi F *et al.* Benzydamine hydrochloride oral rinses in management of burning mouth syndrome. A clinical trial. *Oral Surg Oral Med Oral Pathol Oral Radiol Endod* 1999; **88**: 683–6.
18 Tammiala-Salonen T, Forssell H. Trazodone in burning mouth pain: placebo-controlled, double-blind study. *J Orofac Pain* 1999; **13**: 83–8.
19 Woda A, Navez ML, Picard P, Gremeau C, Picard-Leandri E. A possible therapeutic solution for stomatodynia (burning mouth syndrome). *J Orofac Pain* 1998; **12**: 272–8.
20 Loldrup D, Langemark M, Hansen HJ, Olesen J, Bech P. Clomipramine and mianserin in chronic idiopathic pain syndrome. A placebo controlled study. *Psychopharmacology* 1989; **99**: 1–7.
21 Femiano F, Gombos F, Scully C, Busciolano M, Luca PD. Burning mouth syndrome (BMS): controlled open trial of the efficacy of alpha-lipoic acid (thioctic acid) on symptomatology. *Oral Dis* 2000; **6**: 274–7.

White lesions

Acquired white lesions in the mouth are usually innocuous keratoses or caused by cheek biting or chemical burns, but infections, dermatoses (usually LP), neoplastic disorders and other conditions must be excluded (see Table 66.9). Congenital lesions are discussed on p. 66.24.

Cheek biting
SYN. MORSICATIO BUCCARUM

Cheek biting causes a whitish shredded appearance usually of the buccal or lower labial mucosa at the occlusal line (adjacent to where the teeth meet) (Fig. 66.50) [1–3]. The habit is most common in tense or anxious individuals who may also show bruxism, mandibular pain dysfunction or other oral features of psychogenic disorders. The

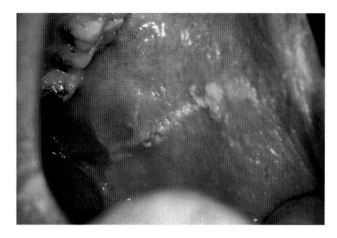

Fig. 66.50 Frictional keratosis and cheek biting (morsicatio buccarum) at the occlusal line.

lesion is benign but may simulate white-sponge naevus (see p. 66.24).

REFERENCES

1 Precheur I. Morsicatio buccarum: cytological study of 29 cases. *Inf Dent* 1983; **65**: 2935–9.
2 Schulten EA, Jovanovic A, van der Waal I. Prevalence study of oral mucosal lesions in 300 patients. *Ned Tijdschr Tandheelkd* 1989; **96**: 538–9.
3 Glass LF, Maize JC. Morsicatio buccarum et labiorum (excessive cheek and lip biting). *Am J Dermatopathol* 1991; **13**: 271–4.

Burns

Chemical burns (due, for example, to holding mouthwashes in the mouth or drugs against the buccal mucosa) or burns caused by heat, cold or irradiation can cause white sloughing lesions of the mucosa [1–8]. Such lesions typically heal spontaneously within 1–3 weeks.

REFERENCES

1 Bernstein ML. Oral mucosal white lesions associated with excessive use of Listerine mouthwash. *Oral Surg* 1978; **46**: 781.
2 Sapir S, Bimstein E. Cholinsalicylate gel induced oral lesion: report of case. *J Clin Pediatr Dent* 2000; **24**: 103–6.
3 Parry J, Porter SR, Scully C et al. Mucosal lesions due to oral cocaine use. *Br Dent J* 1996; **180**: 462–4.
4 Flaitz CM. Chemical burn of the labial mucosa and gingiva. *Am J Dent* 2001; **14**: 259–60.
5 Ameneiros Lago E, Marino Callejo A, Echarri Piudo A, Sesma Sanchez P. [Burns in the oral mucosa and skin erosions.] *An Med Interna* 2001; **18**: 448.
6 Kerekhanjanarong V, Supiyaphun P, Saengpanich S. Upper aerodigestive tract burn: a case report of firework injury. *J Med Assoc Thai* 2001; **84**: 294–8.
7 Nahlieli O, Shapira Y, Yoffe B, Baruchin AM. An unusual iatrogenic burn from a heated dental instrument. *Burns* 2000; **26**: 676–8.
8 Shimoyama T, Kaneko T, Nasu D, Suzuki T, Horie N. A case of an electrical burn in the oral cavity of an adult. *J Oral Sci* 1999; **41**: 127–8.

Lichen planus

See Chapter 42.

Candidiasis

Up to 50% of the healthy population harbour *Candida albicans* as an oral commensal. Carriage is more common in cigarette smokers. *Candida* resides particularly on the posterior dorsum of the tongue [1–5].

Infection is likely to result from xerostomia, local disturbances in salivary flora such as occurs during broad-spectrum antimicrobial treatment, or depressed immune responses [1–4]. Of the several clinical presentations of oral candidiasis, only thrush, candidal leukoplakia and chronic mucocutaneous candidiasis present as white lesions; the other types, acute and chronic atrophic candidiasis, are red (Table 66.22).

Table 66.22 Intraoral candidiasis.

Type of candidiasis	Usual age at onset	Predisposing factors*
Acute pseudomembranous candidiasis (thrush)†	Any	Local: dry mouth, antimicrobials General: corticosteroids, leukaemia, HIV
Acute atrophic candidiasis ('antibiotic mouth'; antibiotic sore mouth)	Any	Broad-spectrum antibiotics or corticosteroids
Erythematous candidiasis	Any	HIV especially
Chronic atrophic candidiasis (denture-induced stomatitis)	Adults	Denture wearing, especially at night
Chronic hyperplastic candidiasis (candidal leukoplakia)†	Usually middle-aged or elderly	Tobacco smoking, denture wearing, immune defect
Median rhomboid glossitis	Third or later decades	Tobacco smoking, denture wearing, HIV
Chronic mucocutaneous candidiasis†	Usually first decade	Often immune defect; rarely endocrinopathy

HIV, human immunodeficiency virus.
* Immune defects can predispose to any form.
† White lesions.

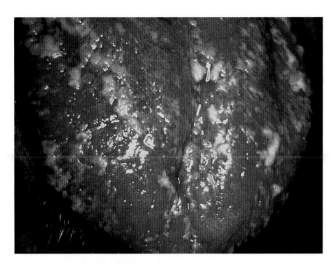

Fig. 66.51 Thrush: scattered white lesions on an erythematous background.

Thrush
SYN. ACUTE PSEUDOMEMBRANOUS CANDIDIASIS

Healthy neonates, who have yet to develop immunity to *Candida* species, may develop thrush. In other patients, predisposing factors include antibiotic or corticosteroid use, xerostomia and severe T-cell immune defects associated with immunosuppression (e.g. given to prevent graft rejection in organ transplantation) or immunodeficiencies such as leukaemia or HIV disease. Oral candidiasis is a common and early feature of HIV infection and may be a portent of developing AIDS [1–4].

The soft creamy patches of thrush, which resemble milk curds, can be wiped off the oral mucosa with gauze, leaving an area of erythema (Fig. 66.51).

Chronic candidiasis

Long-standing oral candidiasis may produce tough, adherent white patches (chronic hyperplastic candidiasis or candidal leukoplakias) which can have a premalignant potential, and may be indistinguishable from other leukoplakias except by biopsy. Candidal leukoplakias may, however, be speckled. In only a few patients with this type of chronic oral candidiasis can either a local cause or underlying immune defect be identified [1–3]. Chronic mucocutaneous candidiasis syndromes are rare (see Chapter 31).

Diagnosis. The diagnosis of oral thrush is usually clinical but it tends to be overdiagnosed by physicians. In contrast, erythematous candidiasis is probably underdiagnosed. In immunosuppressed patients, a Gram-stained smear should be taken to distinguish thrush from the plaques produced by opportunistic bacteria. Hyphae seem to indicate that the *Candida* organisms are acting as pathogens and not simple commensals.

Suspected candidal leukoplakia should be biopsied, both to distinguish it from other non-candidal plaques and also because of possible dysplasia. Although candidal hyphae and a neutrophil infiltrate may be seen on haematoxylin and eosin staining, PAS will demonstrate the purple staining of the hyphae.

Treatment

Acute candidiasis. Except in healthy neonates, possible predisposing causes should be looked for and treated. Topical polyenes such as nystatin or amphotericin, or imidazoles such as miconazole are often indicated but, in HIV infection, fluconazole may be required.

Chronic hyperplastic candidiasis. The oral lesions of chronic hyperplastic candidiasis may respond poorly to the polyenes. These cases, and some cases of chronic mucocutaneous candidiasis, may respond only to flucytosine, ketoconazole, fluconazole or itraconazole [1,6–8].

REFERENCES

1 Scully C, El-Kabir M, Samaranayake LP. Candida and oral candidiasis. *Crit Rev Oral Biol Med* 1994; **5**: 124–58.
2 Smith CB. Candidiasis: pathogenesis, host resistance and predisposing factors. In: Bodey GP, Feinstein V, eds. *Candidiasis.* New York: Raven Press, 1985: 53–72.
3 Epstein JB, Truelove EL, Izutzu KT. Oral candidiasis: pathogenesis and host defence. *Rev Infect Dis* 1984; **6**: 96–106.
4 Odds FC. *Candida* infections: an overview. *CRC Crit Rev Microbiol* 1987; **15**: 1–5.
5 Al-Karaawi ZM, Manfredi M, Waugh ACW *et al.* Molecular characterization of *Candida* spp. isolated from the oral cavity of patients from diverse clinical settings. *Oral Microbiol Immunol* 2002; **17**: 44–9.
6 Hay RJ, Clayton YM. Fluconazole in the management of patients with chronic mucocutaneous candidiasis. *Br J Dermatol* 1988; **119**: 683–5.
7 Nielson H, Dangaard K, Schiodt M. Chronic mucocutaneous candidiasis: a review. *Tandlaegkbladet* 1985; **89**: 667–73.
8 Porter SR, Scully C. Candidiasis endocrinopathy syndrome. *Oral Surg* 1986; **61**: 573–8.

Leukoplakia

The World Health Organization defines leukoplakia as a white patch or plaque on the mucosa that cannot be rubbed off and that is not recognized as a specific disease entity [1], which implies a diagnosis of exclusion (e.g. of LP, candidiasis). The term is also used irrespective of the presence or absence of epithelial dysplasia, although there is a small premalignant potential to some keratoses [1–3].

Leukoplakia is common in adults: around 1% are affected, although some populations show higher prevalences. Most cases are seen in the 50–70 age group [4–9].

Leukoplakia can be totally benign or sometimes can be precancerous or a marker for cancer elsewhere in the upper aerodigestive tract.

Oral keratoses

Aetiology. The cause of most keratoses is unknown (idiopathic keratoses or leukoplakia) but some are caused by chronic irritation, particular lifestyle habits or infective agents [10–17].

Tobacco-induced keratoses. Consumption of tobacco products has long been causally connected with oral cancer and is a common cause of keratosis. Tobacco use also predisposes to cancers elsewhere in the upper aerodigestive tract, bladder and other sites. Tobacco use should thus be discouraged; the drug amfebutamone (Zyban) may help users break the habit.

Tobacco chewing. Tobacco is chewed in many parts of the world and may induce keratosis. In many communities from the developing world, tobacco is a component of betel quid, along with areca nut and betel leaf, and sometimes slaked lime and spices. Sometimes betel is used without tobacco (pan or paan), though others use paan with tobacco. Oral carcinoma can result.

Reverse smoking (bidi). In some communities, especially in Asia, cigarettes are smoked with the lit end within the mouth. Palatal or other oral carcinoma can result.

Cigarette-induced keratoses. Mild keratosis may be seen especially on the palate, lip (occasionally nicotine-stained) and at the commissures, along with nicotine-stained teeth. Malignant change is uncommon.

Pipe smoking. Diffuse whiteness over the palate is termed 'smoker's keratosis' or 'stomatitis nicotina'. The palatal minor salivary gland orifices appear red against this white background. Malignant change is uncommon.

Cigar smoking. Cigar smokers may develop stomatitis nicotina and nicotine-stained teeth. Malignant change is uncommon.

Snuff dipper's keratosis and other smokeless tobacco lesions. Snuff may produce keratosis—white hyperkeratotic lesions caused by snuff-dipping (holding flavoured tobacco powder in the oral sulcus or vestibule), together with gingival recession at the site of use, often the buccal sulcus. Malignant change is rare.

Other aetiological factors
• Proliferative verrucous leukoplakia is often associated with HPV. Malignant change is uncommon.
• Candidal leukoplakias may be associated with an increased risk of malignant change, although it is uncommon.

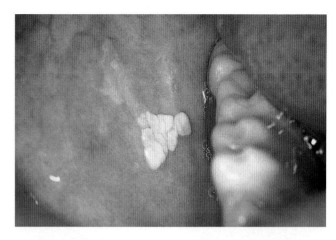

Fig. 66.52 Homogeneous leukoplakia in the buccal mucosa.

• Syphilitic leukoplakia is rarely seen now. Malignant change is uncommon.
• Hairy leukoplakia is caused by EBV and seen especially in HIV disease. Malignant change is not recorded.

Clinical features. Leukoplakias vary in size: some are small and focal, others more widespread, occasionally involving very large areas of the oral mucosa; in other patients several discrete separate areas of leukoplakia can be seen. Leukoplakia has a wide range of clinical presentations, from homogeneous white plaques that can be faintly white or very thick and opaque, to nodular white lesions or lesions admixed with red lesions [1–4]. The malignant potential depends on the following.

Appearance. Homogeneous leukoplakia, the most common, presents with uniformly white plaques, common in the buccal (cheek) mucosa and usually of low premalignant potential (Fig. 66.52).

Non-homogeneous or heterogeneous leukoplakias are nodular, verrucous and speckled leukoplakias that consist of white patches or nodules in a red, often eroded, area of mucosa (Fig. 66.53). They have a high risk of malignant transformation and are therefore far more serious.

Site. High-risk sites for malignant transformation include the soft palate complex and ventrolateral tongue and floor of the mouth (where sublingual keratosis has a particularly high risk of malignant change; Fig. 66.54). Sublingual keratosis is more common in women than men, has a typical 'ebbing-tide' appearance clinically and has a high malignant potential.

Aetiological factors
• Proliferative verrucous leukoplakia is a diffuse white and/or papillary lesion seen in elderly patients, often associated with HPV, and shows an inexorable slow progression over one or two decades to verrucous or squamous cell carcinoma.

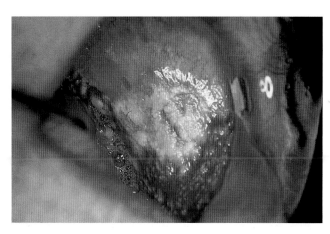

Fig. 66.53 Speckled leukoplakia.

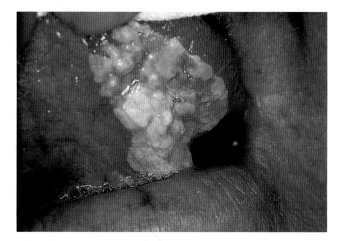

Fig. 66.54 Sublingual keratosis.

• Candidal leukoplakias may be associated with an increased risk of malignant change. Chronic candidal infection is common in speckled leukoplakias and *C. albicans* can cause or colonize other keratoses, particularly in smokers, and is especially likely to form speckled leukokplakias at commissures. It may be dysplastic and have higher malignant potential than some other keratoses. Candidal leukoplakias may respond to antifungals and cessation of smoking.

• Syphilitic leukoplakia, especially of the dorsum of tongue, is a feature of tertiary syphilis rarely seen now, although the malignant potential is high.

• Hairy leukoplakia is caused by EBV. It usually has a corrugated surface and mainly affects margins of the tongue almost exclusively. It is seen in the immuno-compromised and is a complication of HIV infection. It is seen in all groups at risk of HIV infection. The condition appears to be benign and self-limiting. Leukoplakia in chronic renal failure causes similar symmetrical soft keratoses, and may be caused by EBV.

Diagnosis. There are no signs or symptoms which reliably predict whether a leukoplakia will undergo malignant change, and thus histology must be used to detect dysplasia. Scalpel or punch biopsy is therefore generally indicated. Biopsy is mandatory for those leukoplakias that exhibit the following characteristics:

• found in patients with previous or concurrent head and neck cancer;
• are non-homogeneous, i.e. have red areas and/or are verrucous and/or are indurated;
• in a high-risk site such as floor of mouth or tongue;
• focal;
• with symptoms;
• without obvious aetiological factors.

Pathology. Keratoses show, to a varying degree, increased keratin production, change in epithelial thickness and disordered epithelial maturation. Mild dysplasia is not usually regarded as of serious significance. The presence of severe epithelial dysplasia is thought to indicate a considerable risk of malignant development [18]. Pagetoid dyskeratosis is considered a selective keratinocytic response in which a small part of the normal population of keratinocytes is induced to proliferate in response to friction [19]. Pagetoid dyskeratosis has been found in 42.2% of lip biopsies, more frequent in younger patients and in women. Pagetoid cells are more common in suprabasal location and in the labial mucosa. These cells show positivity for high-molecular-weight cytokeratin and negative reaction for low-molecular-weight cytokeratin, epithelial membrane antigen, carcinoembryonic antigen and HPV. The immunohistochemical profile is different from the surrounding keratinocytes, indicating premature keratinization. The morphological features of dyskeratotic pagetoid cells are distinctive and easily recognized as an incidental finding, thus preventing confusion with other important entities including an intraepidermal tumour.

The main differential diagnoses include white-sponge naevus, leukoedema, oral koilocytoses, hairy leukoplakia, pagetoid squamous cell carcinoma *in situ* and extramammary Paget's disease of the oral mucosa.

Prognosis. Overall, around 2–5% of leukoplakias become malignant in 10 years and 5–20% of leukoplakias are dysplastic. Of leukoplakias with dysplasia, 10–35% proceed to carcinoma. There is thus clear evidence of the malignant potential of some oral leukoplakias, although some leukoplakias (15–30%) regress clinically, not only when supposed aetiological factors have been removed but also sometimes spontaneously. Malignant change to carcinoma is most frequent in women older than 50 years and in large lesions. Interestingly, leukoplakias developing in non-smokers have a higher rather than lower risk of malignant change.

At present, it is not possible to reliably predict which dysplastic lesions will progress to carcinoma and which will regress, and there is concern over observer and inter-observer variation in diagnosis of dysplasia [20,21]. Over the recent past, much effort has gone into identifying tissue markers of malignant potential [22], in particular the genetic changes that underlie oral carcinoma, resulting in the identification of biomarkers such as DNA ploidy, p53, and chromosome 3 and 9 changes that might predict neoplastic change in potentially malignant lesions [23–30].

Management. Management can be difficult, not least because of the wide extent of some lesions, their frequent admixture with areas of erythroplasia (speckled leukoplakias), and controversy as to the prognosis and long-term benefit and effects of various therapies. Indeed, no controlled studies are available [31]. Treatment therefore is empirical [32,33].

Removal of known risk factors (tobacco, alcohol and trauma) is a mandatory first step. The patient should be re-examined 3 months after instituting this. If the lesion persists, it should be removed [33–36].

Surgery (scalpel or laser excision) is an obvious option for the management of leukoplakias with a high predisposition to malignant transformation, such as leukoplakias that are:

- speckled;
- verrucous;
- from high-risk sites (e.g. floor of mouth/ventrum of tongue, or soft palate/fauces);
- in a patient with previous cancer of the upper aerodigestive tract;
- dysplastic;
- polysomic (aneuploidy or tetraploidy);
- positive for genetic markers such as mutated tumour-suppressor factor p53, or for loss of heterozygosity on chromosomes 3p or 9p—such advances in molecular biology mean that it should soon be possible to ascertain the malignant potential of leukoplakia from genetic and DNA studies.

Chemotherapy and chemoprevention are attractive possibilities [37]. Topical 0.5% bleomycin in dimethyl sulfoxide (dimethyl sulphoxide) is being evaluated [13]. Although they may induce regression of some leukoplakias and may inhibit their development, topical or systemic vitamin A derivatives, methisoprinol and calcipotriol have not been widely used because of adverse effects or their uncertain long-term consequences [38–42].

REFERENCES

1 World Health Organization Collaborating Centre for Oral Precancerous Lesions. Definitions of leucoplakia and related lesions. *Oral Surg* 1978; **45**: 518–39.

2 Axell T, Holmstrup P, Kramer IRH *et al.* International seminar on oral leucoplakia and associated lesions related to tobacco habits. *Community Dent Oral Epidemiol* 1984; **12**: 145–54.

3 van der Waal I, Schepman KP, van der Meij EH. A modified classification and staging system for oral leukoplakia. *Oral Oncol* 2000; **36**: 264–6.

4 Wright JM. Oral precancerous lesions and conditions. *Semin Dermatol* 1994; **13**: 125–31.

5 Sciubba JJ. Oral leukoplakia. *Crit Rev Oral Biol Med* 1995; **6**: 147–60.

6 Scully C, Cawson RA. Potentially malignant oral lesions. *J Epidemiol Biostat* 1996; **1**: 3–12.

7 Bouquot J, Weiland L, Ballard D, Kurland L. Leukoplakia of the mouth and pharynx in Rochester, MN 1935–1984: incidence, clinical features and follow-up of 463 patients from a relatively unbiased patient pool. *J Oral Pathol* 1988; **17**: 436.

8 Bouquot JE, Gorlin RJ. Leukoplakia, lichen planus and other oral keratoses in 23616 white Americans over the age of 35 years. *Oral Surg Oral Med Oral Pathol* 1986; **61**: 373–81.

9 Bouquot JE, Weiland LH, Kurland LT. Leukoplakia and carcinoma in situ synchronously associated with invasive oral/oropharyngeal carcinoma in Rochester, Minn, 1975–1984. *Oral Surg Oral Med Oral Pathol* 1988; **65**: 199–207.

10 Jaber MA, Porter SR, Scully C, Gilthorpe MS, Bedi R. Role of alcohol in non-smokers and tobacco in non-drinkers in the aetiology of oral epithelial dysplasia. *Int J Cancer* 1998; **77**: 333–6.

11 Jaber MA, Porter SR, Gilthorpe MS, Bedi R, Scully C. Risk factors for oral epithelial dysplasia: the role of smoking and alcohol. *Oral Oncol* 1999; **35**: 151–6.

12 Shiu MN, Chen TH, Chang SH, Hahn LJ. Risk factors for leukoplakia and malignant transformation to oral carcinoma: a leukoplakia cohort in Taiwan. *Br J Cancer* 2000; **82**: 1871–4.

13 Hashibe M, Sankaranarayanan R, Thomas G *et al.* Alcohol drinking, body mass index and the risk of oral leukoplakia in an Indian population. *Int J Cancer* 2000; **88**: 129–34.

14 Larsson A, Axell T, Andersson G. Reversibility of snuff dippers' lesion in Swedish moist snuff users: a clinical and histologic follow-up study. *J Oral Pathol Med* 1991; **20**: 258–64.

15 Kaugars GE, Riley WT, Brandt RB *et al.* The prevalence of oral lesions in smokeless tobacco users and an evaluation of risk factors. *Cancer* 1992; **70**: 2579–85.

16 Field EA, Field JK, Martin MV. Does *Candida* have a role in oral epithelial neoplasia? *J Med Vet Mycol* 1989; **27**: 277–94.

17 Krogh P. The role of yeasts in oral cancer by means of endogenous nitrosation. *Acta Odontol Scand* 1990; **48**: 85–8.

18 Lumerman H, Freedman P, Kerpel S. Oral epithelial dysplasia and the development of invasive squamous cell carcinoma. *Oral Surg Oral Med Oral Pathol* 1995; **79**: 321–9.

19 Garijo MF, Val D, Val-Bernal JF. Pagetoid dyskeratosis of the lips. *Am J Dermatopathol* 2001; **23**: 329–33.

20 Abbey LM, Kaugars GE, Gunsolley JC *et al.* Interexaminer and intra-examiner reliability in the diagnosis of oral epithelial dysplasia. *Oral Surg Oral Med Oral Pathol Oral Radiol Endod* 1995; **80**: 188–91.

21 Karabulut A, Reibel J, Therkildsen MH *et al.* Observer variability in the histologic assessment of oral premalignant lesions. *J Oral Pathol Med* 1995; **24**: 198–200.

22 Scully C, Burkhardt A. Tissue markers of potentially malignant oral epithelial lesions. *J Oral Pathol Med* 1993; **22**: 246–56.

23 Saito T, Yamashita T, Notani K *et al.* Flow cytometric analysis of nuclear DNA content in oral leukoplakia: relation to clinicopathologic findings. *Int J Oral Maxillofac Surg* 1995; **24**: 44–7.

24 Lee JJ, Hong WK, Hittelman WN *et al.* Predicting cancer development in oral leukoplakia: ten years of translational research. *Clin Cancer Res* 2000; **6**: 1702–10.

25 Lippman SM, Hong WK. Molecular markers of the risk of oral cancer. *N Engl J Med* 2001; **344**: 1323–6.

26 Mao L. Can molecular assessment improve classification of head and neck premalignancy? *Clin Cancer Res* 2000; **6**: 321–2.

27 Kim J, Shin DM, El-Naggar A *et al.* Chromosome polysomy and histological characteristics in oral premalignant lesions. *Cancer Epidemiol* 2001; **10**: 319–25.

28 Sudbo J, Kildal W, Risberg B *et al.* DNA content as a prognostic marker in patients with oral leukoplakia. *N Engl J Med* 2001; **344**: 1270–8.

29 Zhang L, Cheung KJ, Lam WL *et al.* Increased genetic damage in oral leukoplakia from high risk sites. *Cancer* 2001; **91**: 2148–55.

30 Poh CF, Zhang L, Lam WL *et al.* A high frequency of allelic loss in oral verrucous lesions may explain malignant risk. *Lab Invest* 2001; **81**: 629–34.

31 Lodi G, Sardella A, Bez C, Demarosi F, Carrassi A. Interventions for treating oral leukoplakia (Cochrane Review). In: *The Cochrane Library, Issue 1.* Oxford: Update Software, 2002.

32 Alexander RE, Wright JM, Thiebaud S. Evaluating, documenting and following up oral pathological conditions. A suggested protocol. *J Am Dent Assoc* 2001; **132**: 329–35.

33 Tradati N, Grigolat R, Calabrese L *et al*. Oral leukoplakias: to treat or not? *Oral Oncol* 1997; **33**: 317–22.

34 Schoelch ML, Sekandari N, Regezi JA, Silverman S Jr. Laser management of oral leukoplakias: a follow-up study of 70 patients. *Laryngoscope* 1999; **109**: 949–53.

35 Gooris PJ, Roodenburg JL, Vermey A, Nauta JM. Carbon dioxide laser evaporation of leukoplakia of the lower lip: a retrospective evaluation. *Oral Oncol* 1999; **35**: 490–5.

36 Pandey M, Thomas G, Somanathan T *et al*. Evaluation of surgical excision of non-homogeneous oral leukoplakia in a screening intervention trial, Kerala, India. *Oral Oncol* 2001; **37**: 103–9.

37 Lippman SM. Head and neck chemoprevention: recent advances. *Cancer Control* 1997; **4**: 128–35.

38 Leunig A, Betz CS, Baumgartner R, Grevers G, Issing WJ. Initial experience in the treatment of oral leukoplakia with high-dose vitamin A and follow-up 5-aminolevulinic acid induced protoporphyrin IX fluorescence. *Eur Arch Otorhinolaryngol* 2000; **257**: 327–31.

39 Femiano F, Gombos F, Scully C. Oral proliferative verrucous leukoplakia: open trial of surgery compared with combined therapy using surgery and methisoprinol. *Int J Oral Maxillofac Surg* 2001; **30**: 318–22.

40 Femiano F, Gombos F, Scully C *et al*. Oral leukoplakia: open trial of topical therapy with calcipotriol compared with tretinoin. *Int J Oral Maxillofac Surg* 2001; **30**: 402–6.

41 Malmstrom M, Hietanen J, Sane J *et al*. Topical treatment of oral leucoplakia with bleomycin. *Br J Oral Surg* 1988; **26**: 491–8.

42 Scully C. Oral precancer: preventive and medical approaches to management. *Oral Oncol* 1995; **31B**: 16–26.

Actinic cheilitis (see p. 66.115)

Hairy leukoplakia

Aetiology. Hairy leukoplakia (HL) is seen in severe immune defects, especially HIV infection, and occasionally in the apparently immunocompetent [1,2]. HIV is not found within the genome of epithelial cells in HL and it is more likely that the features are a consequence of an opportunistic infection with EBV. It is now clear that normal human oral mucosa from HIV-negative and HIV-positive individuals may contain latent EBV [3,4].

EBV has been shown to be present in HL, especially in the upper layers of the epithelium. The oral site of predilection for HL appears to relate to the presence of EBV receptors only on the parakeratinized mucosae such as the lateral margin of the tongue. HL regresses on treatment with antivirals but fails to resolve with antifungals, despite the frequent presence of *Candida* species.

Pathology. Histological features of HL include hyperparakeratosis, hyperplasia and ballooning of prickle cells, few or absent Langerhans' cells, and only a sparse inflammatory cell infiltrate in the lamina propria.

Clinical features. HL is a white patch, usually seen on the parakeratinized mucosa of the tongue, frequently bilaterally (Fig. 66.55). The lesions are corrugated or have a shaggy or hairy appearance, are mostly symptomless and, unlike some oral keratoses, have no known premalignant potential [1,5]. The majority of the affected patients who

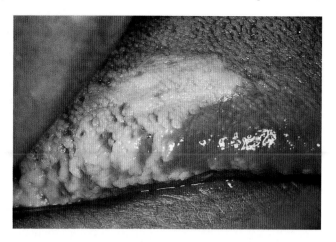

Fig. 66.55 Hairy leukoplakia. Found mainly in HIV infection, vertical white ridges on the lateral margin of the tongue.

are HIV positive appear eventually to develop AIDS. HL also occurs in HIV-negative persons [6–12].

Diagnosis. Some of the histological features typical of HL, especially the hyperparakeratosis, can be seen in oral white lesions other than HL in HIV-infected persons [13]. Not only are there oral lesions that mimic HL in HIV infection, but lesions similar to HL can be seen in other immunocompromised persons and even in some apparently healthy individuals.

However, most cases can be distinguished from the HL of HIV infection by the absence of EBV DNA on histology and, of course, by examination for HIV serum antibody.

Treatment. HL really needs no treatment but in HIV-infected individuals may occasionally improve spontaneously or with the antiretroviral agents aciclovir or ganciclovir.

REFERENCES

1 Schiodt M, Greenspan D, Daniels TE *et al*. Clinical and histologic spectrum of oral hairy leucoplakia. *Oral Surg* 1987; **64**: 716–20.

2 Scully C, Laskaris G, Pindborg J *et al*. Oral manifestations of HIV infection and their management. *Oral Surg* 1991; **71**: 158–66, 167–71.

3 Triantos D, Leao JR, Porter SR, Scully C, Teo CG. Tissue distribution of Epstein–Barr virus genotypes in hosts co-infected by HIV. *AIDS* 1998; **12**: 2141–6.

4 Scully C, Porter SR, Di Alberti L, Jalal M, Maitland N. Detection of Epstein–Barr virus in oral scrapes in HIV infection, in hairy leukoplakia, and in healthy non-HIV-infected people. *J Oral Pathol Med* 1998; **27**: 480–2.

5 Shiboski CH, Neuhaus JM, Greenspan D, Greenspan JS. Effect of receptive oral sex and smoking on the incidence of hairy leukoplakia in HIV-positive gay men. *J Acquir Immune Defic Syndr* 1999; **21**: 236–42.

6 King GN, Healy CM, Glover T *et al*. Prevalence and risk factors associated with leukoplakia, hairy leukoplakia, erythematous candidiasis and gingival hyperplasia in renal transplant recipients. *Oral Surg* 1994; **78**: 718–21.

7 Euvrard S, Kanitakis J, Puteil-Nobel C *et al*. Pseudo-oral hairy leukoplakia in a renal allograft recipient. *J Am Acad Dermatol* 1994; **30**: 300–3.

8 Itin P, Rufli T, Rudlinger R *et al*. Oral hairy leukoplakia in an HIV-negative renal transplant patient: a marker for immunosuppression? *Dermatologica* 1988; **177**: 126–8.

9 Syrjanen S, Laine P, Happonen R *et al.* Oral hairy leukoplakia is not a specific sign of HIV-infection but related to immunodepression in general. *J Oral Pathol Med* 1989; **18**: 28–31.
10 Greenspan D, Greenspan JS, De Souza YG *et al.* Oral hairy leukoplakia in an HIV-negative renal transplant recipient. *J Oral Pathol Med* 1989; **18**: 32–4.
11 Kanitakis J, Euvrard S, Lefrancois N *et al.* Oral hairy leukoplakia in a HIV-negative renal graft recipient. *Br J Dermatol* 1991; **124**: 483–6.
12 Eisenberg E, Krutchkoff D, Yamase H. Incidental oral hairy leukoplakia in immunocompetent persons. *Oral Surg Oral Med Oral Pathol* 1992; **74**: 563–6.
13 Green TL, Greenspan JS, Greenspan D *et al.* Oral lesions mimicking hairy leukoplakia: a diagnostic dilemma. *Oral Surg Oral Med Oral Pathol* 1989; **67**: 422–6.

Psoriasis (see Chapter 35)

The oral mucosa appears to be rarely involved in psoriasis, with less than 100 cases reported, although there are occasionally lip lesions or white oral lesions, especially in the buccal mucosa, or lesions clinically indistinguishable from geographical tongue (sometimes termed 'annulus migrans' or 'erythema circinatum'), particularly in generalized pustular psoriasis [1–12].

REFERENCES

1 Heitanen J, Salo OP, Kanerva L *et al.* Study of the oral mucosa in 250 consecutive patients with psoriasis. *Scand J Dent Res* 1984; **92**: 50–4.
2 O'Keefe E, Braverman IM, Cohen T. Annulus migrans: identical lesions in pustular psoriasis, Reiter's syndrome, and geographic tongue. *Arch Dermatol* 1973; **107**: 240–4.
3 Morris LF, Phillips CM, Binnie WH *et al.* Oral lesions in patients with psoriasis: a controlled study. *Cutis* 1992; **49**: 339–44.
4 Pogrel MA, Cram D. Intraoral findings in patients with psoriasis with a special reference to ectopic geographic tongue. *Oral Surg* 1988; **66**: 184–9.
5 Wagner G, Luckasen J, Goltz R. Mucous membrane involvement in generalised pustular psoriasis. *Arch Dermatol* 1976; **112**: 1010–4.
6 White DK, Leis HJ, Miller AS. Intraoral psoriasis associated with widespread dermal psoriasis. *Oral Surg* 1976; **41**: 174–81.
7 Zhu JF, Kaminski MJ, Pulitzer DR, Hu J, Thomas HF. Psoriasis: pathophysiology and oral manifestations. *Oral Dis* 1996; **2**: 135–44.
8 Younai FS, Phelan JA. Oral mucositis with features of psoriasis: report of a case and review of the literature. *Oral Surg Oral Med Oral Pathol Oral Radiol Endod* 1997; **84**: 61–7.
9 Kaur I, Handa S, Kumar B. Oral lesions in psoriasis. *Int J Dermatol* 1997; **36**: 78–9.
10 Brice DM, Danesh-Meyer MJ. Oral lesions in patients with psoriasis: clinical presentation and management. *J Periodontol* 2000; **71**: 1896–903.
11 Richardson LJ, Kratochvil FJ, Zieper MB. Unusual palatal presentation of oral psoriasis. *J Can Dent Assoc* 2000; **66**: 80–2.
12 Tosti A, Misciali C, Cameli N, Vincenzi C. Guess what! Psoriasis of the lips. *Eur J Dermatol* 2001; **11**: 589–90.

Koplik's spots (see Chapter 25)

White specks may be seen in the buccal mucosa in early measles.

Pigmented lesions

Congenital lesions are described on p. 66.27. The tongue is often discoloured due to superficial staining from foods, drinks or habits such as tobacco or betel use. Localized hyperpigmented lesions are usually due to pigmentary incontinence, amalgam tattoos, melanotic macule or naevi,

although melanomas, Kaposi's sarcoma and epithelioid angiomatosis must be excluded. Generalized oral mucosal hyperpigmentation is usually racial in origin and only occasionally has a systemic cause such as Addison's disease.

Furred, brown and black hairy tongue

Aetiology and pathology. Children rarely have a furred tongue in health but it may be coated with off-white debris in febrile and other illnesses.

Adults, however, not infrequently have a coating on the tongue in health, particularly if they are edentulous, are on a soft non-abrasive diet, have poor oral hygiene or are fasting. The coating appears more obvious in xerostomic and in ill patients, especially those who cannot maintain oral hygiene.

The coating in most cases appears to be of epithelial, food and microbial debris; indeed, the tongue is the main oral reservoir of some microorganisms, such as *Candida albicans* and viridans streptococci. The filiform papillae are excessively long and stained by the accumulation of squames and chromogenic microorganisms.

Habits such as tobacco and betel use, and various medicaments such as chlorhexidine or iron, can cause a black or brown superficial staining of the tongue (and teeth).

Occasionally, a brown hairy tongue may be caused by drugs that induce xerostomia, lansoprazole or antimicrobial therapy, when it may be related to overgrowth of microorganisms such as *Candida* species and may respond to withdrawal of the drug [1,2].

Clinical features. Black hairy tongue affects mainly the posterior part of the dorsum of the tongue, especially centrally (Fig. 66.56) [3,4].

Treatment. Patients with black hairy tongue may find the condition improves if they avoid habits or drugs that stain the tongue, increase their standard of oral hygiene, brush the tongue with a hard toothbrush, use sodium bicarbonate mouthwashes, chew gum or suck a peach stone. Topical tretinoin may be effective [5].

REFERENCES

1 Heymann WR. Psychotropic agent-induced black hairy tongue. *Cutis* 2000; **66**: 25–6.
2 Scully C. Discoloured tongue: a new cause? *Br J Dermatol* 2001; **144**: 1293–4.
3 Winer LH. Black hairy tongue. *Arch Dermatol* 1958; **77**: 97–103.
4 Boni R. What is your diagnosis? Hairy tongue (lingua villosa nigra). *Schweiz Rundsch Med Prax* 2000; **89**: 1543–4.
5 Langtry JAA, Carr MM, Steele MC, Ive FA. Topical tretinoin: a new treatment for black hairy tongue (lingua villosa nigra). *Clin Exp Dermatol* 1992; **17**: 163–4.

Pigmentary incontinence

Melanin pigment ingested by macrophages in the upper

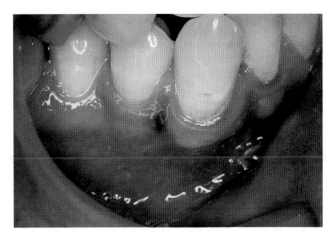

Fig. 66.57 Amalgam tattoo in a common site. This was presumably related to filling of the deciduous predecessor.

2 Dummett CO. Pertinent considerations in oral pigmentation. *Br Dent J* 1985; **158**: 9–12.
3 Owens BM, Johnson WW, Schuman NJ. Oral amalgam pigmentations (tattoos): a retrospective study. *Quintessence Int* 1992; **23**: 805–10.
4 Mohr W, Gorz E. Association of silver granules with elastic fibers in amalgam reaction of mouth mucosa. *HNO* 2001; **49**: 454–7.
5 Peters E, Gardner DG. A method of distinguishing between amalgam and graphite in tissue. *Oral Surg* 1986; **62**: 73–6.
6 Schawaf M. Gingival tattoo: an unusual gingival pigmentation. *J Oral Med* 1986; **41**: 130–3.
7 Telang GH, Ditre CM. Blue gingiva, an unusual oral pigmentation resulting from gingival tattoo. *J Am Acad Dermatol* 1994; **30**: 125–6.

Body art

Tattooing of the lower lip may occasionally be seen. A tattooed lower lip in a Sudanese woman, for example, signifies that she is married [1]. The Wodaabe people of Nigeria and Cameroon may tattoo on the skin surface at the angle of the mouth, a practice which has its basis in ritual warding-off of the 'evil eye'. Similar tattoos may be seen on Bedouin women of North Africa. Tattooing of the chin is seen increasingly in Maoris ('Moki') and tattooing inside the lip may now be seen in developed countries. Mathur and Sahoo [2] reported an instance of fatal septicaemia following the placement of tribal tattoo marks at the angle of the mouth in a Nigerian infant.

The practice of piercing oral and facial soft tissues and then placing foreign objects in the defects on a more or less permanent basis is one which has also been largely confined until recently to certain tribal groups in continental Africa and isolated Amazon regions of South America, for example the Suia and Txukahameis tribes of Brazil, but it is now not uncommon in developed countries.

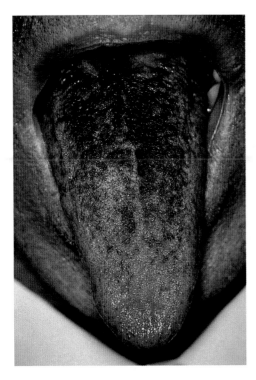

Fig. 66.56 Black hairy tongue.

lamina propria (pigmentary incontinence) may give rise to hyperpigmentation in LP, especially in dark-skinned people [1].

REFERENCE

1 Cawson RA, Binnie WH, Eveson JW. *Colour Atlas of Oral Disease: Clinical and Pathologic Correlations*. London: Heinemann, 1994: 1515.

Tattoos

Amalgam tattoos are common causes of blue-black pigmentation, usually seen in the mandibular gingiva or at least close to the teeth (Fig. 66.57), or in the scar of an apicectomy where there has been a retrograde root-filling [1–3]. The amalgam associates with elastin fibres [4]. Radio-opacities may or may not be seen on radiography. Similar lesions can result if for some reason pencil lead or other similar foreign bodies become embedded in the oral tissues [5].

Radiography may help to confirm the diagnosis. Biopsy may be indicated to exclude a melanoma but otherwise these innocuous lesions can be left alone.

Deliberate tattooing is a rare cause of oral pigmentation [6,7].

REFERENCES

1 Buchner A, Hansen LS. Amalgam pigmentation (amalgam tattoo) of the oral mucosa: a clinicopathological study of 268 cases. *Oral Surg* 1980; **49**: 139–47.

REFERENCES

1 Wilson DF, Grappin G, Miquel JL. Traditional, cultural, and ritual practices involving the teeth and orofacial soft tissues. In: Prabhu SR, Wilson DS,

Daftary DK, Johnson NW, eds. *Oral Diseases in the Tropics*. Oxford: Oxford University Press, 1992: 91–124.
2 Mathur DR, Sahoo A. *Pseudomonas* septicaemia following tribal tattoo marks. *Trop Geogr Med* 1984; **36**: 301–2.

Food, habits, heavy metal and drug-induced hyperpigmentation

Causes (see Table 66.11) [1–4] include:
- Foods and beverages (such as beetroot, red wine, coffee and tea) cause superficial staining.
- Confectionery (such as liquorice) causes superficial staining.
- Smoking tobacco is now a fairly common cause (smoker's melanosis) and may produce extrinsic discoloration but also intrinsic pigmentary incontinence, with pigment cells increasing and appearing in the lamina propria. This is especially likely in persons who smoke with the lighted end of the cigarette within the mouth (reverse smoking), as practised mainly in some Asian communities [5,6].
- Chewing betel may cause superficial brownish-red discoloration mainly in the buccal mucosa (and on the teeth), with an irregular epithelial surface that has a tendency to desquamate, seen mainly in women from South and South-East Asia. The epithelium in betel chewer's mucosa is often hyperplastic, and brownish amorphous material from the betel quid may be seen on the epithelial surface and intracellularly and intercellularly, with ballooning of epithelial cells [7]. Betel chewer's mucosa is not known to be precancerous but betel use predisposes to submucous fibrosis and cancer.
- Drugs such as chlorhexidine, iron salts, griseofulvin, crack cocaine, minocycline, bismuth subsalicylate, lansoprazole and hormone replacement therapy. Chlorhexidine and iron salts cause superficial staining. Drugs that cause intrinsic staining include the following [8–16].
  - Antimalarials produce a variety of colours in the mucosa, ranging from yellow with mepacrine to blue–black with amodiaquine.
  - Minocycline may cause blackish discoloration of teeth, gingivae and bone, skin, sclera and even breast milk. Minocycline can, in a minority of patients, produce blue–grey gingival pigmentation caused by staining of the underlying bone, and some intrinsic faint bluish-grey staining, mainly at the anterior teeth.
  - Busulphan, some other cytotoxic drugs, oral contraceptives, phenothiazines and anticonvulsants may also occasionally produce, or increase, brown pigmentation. Adrenocorticotrophic hormone (ACTH) therapy may also produce brown pigmentation, as may zidovudine and clofazimine.
  - Gold may produce purplish gingival discoloration. Many of the heavy metals formerly implicated in producing oral hyperpigmentation (such as mercury, lead and bismuth) are not used therapeutically now, although industrial or accidental exposure is still occa-

sionally seen [17]. Metallic sulphides deposited in the tissues were seen especially where oral hygiene was poor, with bacteria producing sulphides that resulted in pigmentation at the gingival margin (e.g. lead line).

Management. Some drug-induced hyperpigmentation resolves on cessation of exposure to the drug and improved oral hygiene, although resolution can take months or years.

REFERENCES

1 Seoane Leston JM, Vazquez Garcia J, Aguado Santos A, Varela-Centelles PI, Romero MA. Dark oral lesions: differential diagnosis with oral melanoma. *Cutis* 1998; **61**: 279–82.
2 Lenane P, Powell FC. Oral pigmentation. *J Eur Acad Dermatol Venereol* 2000; **14**: 448–65.
3 Eisen D. Disorders of pigmentation in the oral cavity. *Clin Dermatol* 2000; **18**: 579–87.
4 Dereure O. Drug-induced skin pigmentation. Epidemiology, diagnosis and treatment. *Am J Clin Dermatol* 2001; **2**: 253–62.
5 Axell A, Hedin A. Epidemiologic study of excessive oral melanin pigmentation with special reference to the influence of tobacco habits. *Scand J Dent Res* 1982; **90**: 432–42.
6 Mercado-Ortiz G, Wilson D, Jiang DJ. Reverse smoking and palatal mucosal changes in Filipino women. Epidemiological features. *Aust Dent J* 1996; **41**: 300–3.
7 Reichart PA, Phillipsen HP. Betel chewer's mucosa: a review. *J Oral Pathol Med* 1998; **27**: 239–42.
8 Birek C, Main JHP. Two cases of oral pigmentation associated with quinidine therapy. *Oral Surg* 1988; **66**: 59–61.
9 Hertz RS, Beckstead PC, Brown WJ. Epithelial melanosis possibly resulting from the use of oral contraceptives. *J Am Dent Assoc* 1980; **100**: 713–4.
10 Berger RS, Mandel EB, Hayes TJ *et al*. Minocycline staining of the oral cavity. *J Am Acad Dermatol* 1989; **21**: 1300–1.
11 Siller GM, Tod MA, Savage NW. Minocycline-induced oral pigmentation. *J Am Acad Dermatol* 1994; **30**: 350–4.
12 Patel K, Cheshire D, Vance A. Oral and systemic effects of prolonged minocycline therapy. *Br Dent J* 1998; **185**: 560–2.
13 Ozog DM, Gogstetter DS, Scott G, Gaspari AA. Minocycline-induced hyperpigmentation in patients with pemphigus and pemphigoid. *Arch Dermatol* 2000; **136**: 1133–8.
14 Cheek CC, Heymann HO. Dental and oral discolorations associated with minocycline and other tetracycline analogs. *J Esthetic Dent* 1999; **11**: 43–8.
15 Scully C. Drug induced oral mucosal hyperpigmentation. *Prim Dent Care* 1997; **4**: 35–6.
16 Scully C. Discoloured tongue: a new cause? *Br J Dermatol* 2001; **144**: 1293–4.
17 Lockhart PB. Gingival pigmentation as the sole presenting sign of chronic lead poisoning in a mentally retarded adult. *Oral Surg* 1981; **52**: 143–9.

ACTH-induced hyperpigmentation

Oral hyperpigmentation may be seen in ACTH therapy, Addison's disease, Nelson's syndrome or ectopic ACTH production (e.g. by bronchogenic carcinoma). The brown or black pigmentation is variable in distribution but is seen typically on the soft palate, buccal mucosa and at sites of trauma [1–7].

REFERENCES

1 Scully C. Drug-induced oral mucosal hyperpigmentation. *Prim Dent Care* 1997; **4**: 35–6.
2 Chuong R, Goldberg MH. Case 47, part II: oral hyperpigmentation associated with Addison's disease. *J Oral Maxillofac Surg* 1983; **41**: 680–2.

3 Zain RB, Ling KC. Oral and laryngeal histoplasmosis in a patient with Addison's disease. *Ann Dent* 1988; **47**: 31–3.
4 Kim HW. Generalized oral and cutaneous hyperpigmentation in Addison's disease. *Odontostomatol Trop* 1988; **11**: 87–90.
5 Lamey PJ, Carmichael F, Scully C. Oral pigmentation, Addison's disease and results of screening. *Br Dent J* 1985; **158**: 297–305.
6 Moyer GN, Terezhalmy GT, O'Brien JT. Nelson's syndrome: another condition associated with mucocutaneous hyperpigmentation. *J Oral Med* 1982; **1**: 13–7.
7 Merchant HW, Hayes LE, Ellison LT. Soft palate pigmentation in lung disease, including cancer. *Oral Surg* 1976; **41**: 726–33.

HIV infection

Oral hyperpigmentation may be seen in HIV infection, sometimes related to adrenal hypofunction or drug use [1,2].

REFERENCES

1 Porter SR, Glover S, Scully C. Oral hyperpigmentation and adrenocortical hypofunction in a patient with AIDS. *Oral Surg Oral Med Oral Pathol* 1990; **67**: 301–2.
2 Granel F, Truchetet F, Grandidier M. Diffuse pigmentation (nail, mouth and skin) associated with HIV infection. *Ann Dermatol Vénéréol* 1997; **124**: 460–2.

Oral mucosal melanotic macule, reactive type
SYN. MELANOACANTHOMA; MELANOACANTHOSIS

Melanotic macules occasionally appear suddenly as reactive lesions following trauma [1–9]. Melanoacanthoma is a misnomer: most reported cases have been in black people as reactive lesions [4]. A hyperpigmented symptomless macule appears over a course of days or weeks. The course is benign, and some cases resolve spontaneously within 6 months.

Pigment-filled dendritic cells that appear to be melanocytes are found in the stratum malpighii but, in contrast to melanoma, basal layer melanocytes are not increased.

Excision biopsy may be indicated to exclude melanoma.

REFERENCES

1 Buchner A, Hansen LS. Melanotic macule of the oral mucosa. *Oral Surg* 1979; **48**: 244–9.
2 Lamey PJ, Nolan A, Thomson E *et al.* Oral presentation of the Laugier–Hunziker syndrome. *Br Dent J* 1991; **171**: 59–60.
3 Laugier P, Hunziker N. Pigmentation melanique lenticulaire essentielle de la muquese jugale et des lèvres. *Arch Belg Dermatol Syphilol* 1970; **26**: 391–9.
4 Horlick HP, Wather RR, Zegarelli DJ *et al.* Mucosal melanotic macule, reactive type. A simulation of melanoma. *J Am Acad Dermatol* 1988; **19**: 786–91.
5 Maize JC. Mucosal melanosis. *Dermatol Clin* 1988; **6**: 283–93.
6 Zemtsov A, Bergfeld WF. Oral melanoacanthoma with prominent spongiotic intraepithelial vesicles. *J Cutan Pathol* 1989; **16**: 365–9.
7 Tomich CE, Zunt SL. Melanoacanthosis (melanoacanthoma) of the oral mucosa. *J Dermatol Surg Oncol* 1990; **16**: 231–6.
8 Eisen D, Voorhees JJ. Oral melanoma and other pigmented lesions of the oral cavity. *J Am Acad Dermatol* 1991; **24**: 527–37.
9 Heine BT, Drummond JF, Damm DD, Heine RD 2nd. Bilateral oral melanoacanthoma. *Gen Dent* 1996; **44**: 451–2.

Malignant melanoma (see Chapter 38)

Oral malignant melanoma is rare. Most patients are over 50 years of age and there is a male preponderance.

Malignant melanoma may arise in apparently normal oral mucosa or in a pre-existent pigmented naevus, most commonly in the palate or maxillary alveolus [1–5]. Metastatic melanoma is rare [4]. Features suggestive of malignancy include a rapid increase in size, change in colour, ulceration, pain, bleeding, the occurrence of satellite pigmented spots, or regional lymph node enlargement. The prognosis is poor unless detected very early [2,3]. The histology may show anaplastic spindle-shaped or squamoid cells. However, the histology is quite varied and staining with dopa or antibodies may be required to help the diagnosis. Most cases are positive for S-100, tyrosinase, and Mart-1/melana-A. Lesions suspected to be malignant melanoma should not be biopsied until the time of definitive surgical excision [6–10].

REFERENCES

1 Batsakis JG, Regezi JA, Solomon AR *et al.* The pathology of head and neck tumours: mucosal melanomas. *Head Neck Surg* 1982; **4**: 404–18.
2 Eisen D, Voorhees JJ. Oral melanoma and other pigmented lesions of the oral cavity. *J Am Acad Dermatol* 1991; **24**: 527–37.
3 Hoyt DJ, Jordan T, Fisher SR. Mucosal melanoma of the head and neck. *Arch Otolaryngol Head Neck Surg* 1989; **115**: 1096–9.
4 Patton LL, Brahim JS, Baker AR. Metastatic malignant melanoma of the oral cavity. *Oral Surg* 1994; **78**: 51–6.
5 Rapini RP, Golitz LE, Greer RO *et al.* Primary malignant melanoma of the oral cavity. *Cancer* 1985; **55**: 1543–51.
6 Sooknundun M, Kacker SK, Kapila K *et al.* Oral malignant melanoma (a case report and review of the literature). *J Laryngol Otol* 1986; **100**: 371–5.
7 Tanaka N, Mimura M, Ichinose S, Odajima T. Malignant melanoma in the oral region: ultrastructural and immunohistochemical studies. *Med Electron Microsc* 2001; **34**: 198–205.
8 Owens JM, Gomez JA, Byers RM. Malignant melanoma in the palate of a 3-month-old child. *Head Neck* 2002; **24**: 91–4.
9 Prasad ML, Jungbluth AA, Iversen K, Huvos AG, Busam KJ. Expression of melanocytic differentiation markers in malignant melanomas of the oral and sinonasal mucosa. *Am J Surg Pathol* 2001; **25**: 782–7.
10 Gorsky M, Epstein JB. Melanoma arising from the mucosal surfaces of the head and neck. *Oral Surg Oral Med Oral Pathol Oral Radiol Endod* 1998; **86**: 715–9.

Kaposi's sarcoma (see Chapter 53)

Kaposi's sarcoma (KS) is seen predominantly as a consequence of HIV infection, mainly in men who have sex with men. It appears to be associated with HHV-8 [1,2]. Up to 50% of male homosexual AIDS patients have developed oral KS, although it appears to be declining in frequency and is rare in other HIV-infected patients.

Oral KS is the first presentation of HIV in 20–60% of affected patients, often associated with oral candidiasis. KS affects the hard-palate mucosa in particular (Fig. 66.58). Up to 95% of lesions are seen in the palate, 23% in the gingiva and others on the tongue or buccal mucosa. A red-purple macule is the early lesion, progressing to a purple nodular swelling that may be extensive and ulcerated.

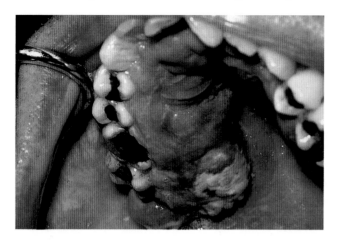

Fig. 66.58 Kaposi's sarcoma in a typical site with a characteristic purplish appearance. (Courtesy of Dr J.B. Epstein, Cancer Control Agency, Vancouver, Canada.)

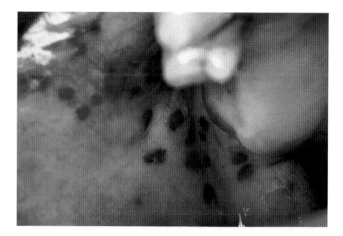

Fig. 66.59 Oral purpura in thrombocytopenia.

Multiple lesions are common [3–6]. Lesions are often asymptomatic but more than 25% are painful and about 8% bleed. Oral KS is also occasionally seen in other non-HIV-infected immunocompromised patients.

Oral KS may regress occasionally spontaneously, or with HAART, zidovudine or systemic vinca alkaloids, etoposide or interferon, but the more usual treatment is local radiotherapy, laser removal or intralesional vinblastine. The latter produces fewer adverse effects than radiotherapy [4,7–9].

REFERENCES

1 Chang Y, Cesarman E, Pessin MS *et al.* Identification of herpesvirus-like DNA sequences in AIDS-associated Kaposi's sarcoma. *Science* 1994; **266**: 1865–9.
2 DiAlberti L, Teo CG, Porter S *et al.* Kaposi's sarcoma herpesvirus in oral Kaposi's sarcoma. *Oral Oncol* 1996; **32B**: 68–9.
3 Epstein JB, Scully C. HIV infection: clinical oral features and management in 33 homosexual males referred with Kaposi's sarcoma. *Oral Surg* 1991; **71**: 38–41.
4 Epstein J, Scully C. Neoplastic disease in the head and neck of patients with AIDS. *Int J Oral Maxillofac Surg* 1992; **2**: 219–26.
5 Ficarra G, Berson AM, Silverman S *et al.* Kaposi's sarcoma of the oral cavity: a study of 134 patients with a review of the pathogenesis, epidemiology, clinical aspects and treatment. *Oral Surg* 1988; **66**: 543–50.
6 Lumerman H, Freedman PD, Kerpel SM *et al.* Oral Kaposi's sarcoma: a clinicopathologic study of 23 homosexual and bisexual men from the New York metropolitan area. *Oral Surg* 1988; **65**: 711–6.
7 Scully C, Porter SR. An ABC of oral health care in HIV infection. *Br Dent J* 1990; **170**: 149–50.
8 Scully C, Spittle M. Malignant tumours of the oral cavity in HIV disease. In: Langdon J, Henk JM, eds. *Malignant Tumours of the Mouth, Jaws and Salivary Glands.* London: Arnold, 1995: 246–57.
9 Porter SR, Scully C, eds. *Oral Health Care for Those with HIV Infection and Other Special Needs.* Northwood: Science Reviews, 1995: 51–61.

Purpura

Petechiae are usually caused by trauma, often from suction, but a bleeding tendency (as in infectious mononucleosis or HIV infection) or leukaemias must be excluded (Fig. 66.59). Blood-filled blisters may be seen in localized oral purpura (angina bullosa haemorrhagica) and pemphigoid, and occasionally in amyloidosis. Rarely a purpuric lesion may be seen in pigmented purpuric stomatitis [1].

REFERENCE

1 Scully C, Eveson JW. Pigmented purpuric stomatitis. *Oral Surg* 1992; **74**: 780–2.

Red lesions

Many oral red lesions are inflammatory in nature, although epithelial thinning (in geographical tongue) and desquamation (in desquamative gingivitis) are fairly common, and epithelial atrophy is an important cause, especially in deficiency glossitis and erythroplasia. Telangiectases are usually red and haemangiomas purplish in colour.

Benign migratory glossitis
SYN. LINGUAL ERYTHEMA MIGRANS;
GEOGRAPHICAL TONGUE

Definition. A benign inflammatory condition of the tongue with map-like areas of erythema which are not constant in size, shape or location. Lingual erythema migrans is unrelated to cutaneous erythema migrans.

Aetiology. Unknown, but many patients with a fissured tongue (scrotal tongue) also have lingual erythema migrans. It is a common condition, affecting about 1–2% of the population [1,2]. A positive family history may be obtainable. HLA findings have been equivocal, with reports of associations with B15 and DR7 [3].

Some patients with lingual erythema migrans have atopic allergies such as hay fever and a few relate the oral

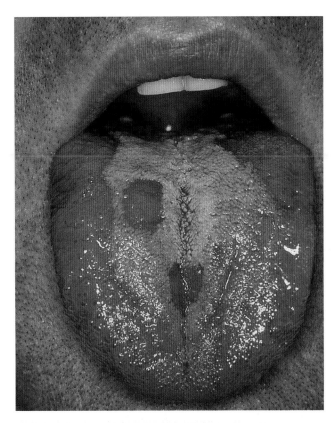

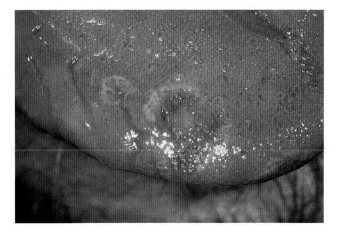

Fig. 66.61 Somewhat less obvious signs of lingual erythema migrans.

Fig. 66.60 Classical geographical tongue (lingual erythema migrans).

lesions to a particular food, for example cheese, or to stress. Similar oral lesions may be seen in Reiter's syndrome, generalized pustular psoriasis and acrodermatitis continua of Hallopeau [4]. Purported associations with diabetes [5] may be coincidental.

Pathology. There is epithelial thinning at the centre of the lesion with an inflammatory infiltrate mainly of polymorphonuclear leukocytes [1,2].

Clinical features. Geographical tongue may be asymptomatic or cause a sore tongue. Patients of any age may be affected but why the condition sometimes gives rise to symptoms after it has been present asymptomatically for decades is unclear [6–8].

Geographical tongue is characterized by map-like red areas with increased thickness of intervening filiform papillae. Alternatively, there are rounded, sometimes scalloped, reddish areas with a white margin (Figs 66.60 & 66.61). These patterns change from day to day and even within a few hours.

Rarely, other sites, such as the labial or palatal mucosa, are affected. The tongue is usually, but not invariably, affected simultaneously with the other sites [9].

There are no complications.

Diagnosis. Clinical examination usually suffices to differentiate the condition from LP, candidiasis, psoriasis, larva migrans or deficiency glossitis.

Treatment. Blood and urine examination may be necessary to exclude anaemia and diabetes. In those with no systemic disorder, no effective treatment is available except reassurance.

REFERENCES

1 Drezner DA, Schaffer SR. Geographic tongue. *Otolaryngol Head Neck Surg* 1997; **117**: 291.
2 Marks R, Radden BG. Geographic tongue: a clinicopathological review. *Aust J Dermatol* 1981; **22**: 75–9.
3 Marks R, Tait B. HLA antigens in geographical tongue. *Tissue Antigens* 1980; **15**: 60–2.
4 Casper U, Seiffert K, Dippel E, Zouboulis CC. Exfoliatio areata linguae et mucosae oris: a mucous membrane manifestation of psoriasis pustulosa? *Hautarzt* 1998; **49**: 850–4.
5 Wysocki GP, Daley T. Benign migratory glossitis in patients with juvenile diabetes. *Oral Surg* 1987; **63**: 68–70.
6 Brooks JK, Balciunas BA. Geographic stomatitis: review of the literature and report of five cases. *J Am Dent Assoc* 1987; **115**: 421–4.
7 Kullaa-Mikkonen A. Geographic tongue, a scanning electron microscope study. *J Cutan Pathol* 1986; **13**: 154–62.
8 Correll RW, Wescott WB, Jenson JL. Non-painful, erythematous circinate lesions of a protean nature on a fissured tongue. *J Am Dent Assoc* 1984; **109**: 90–1.
9 Luker J, Scully C. Erythema migrans affecting the palate. *Br Dent J* 1983; **155**: 385.

Larva migrans (see Chapter 32)

Cutaneous larva migrans is rarely seen in the mouth, where it presents as irregular linear lesions with an inflammatory border resembling erythema migrans [1].

REFERENCE

1 Lopes MA, Zaia AA, Almeida OPD, Scully C. Larva migrans affecting the mouth. *Oral Surg* 1994; **77**: 362–7.

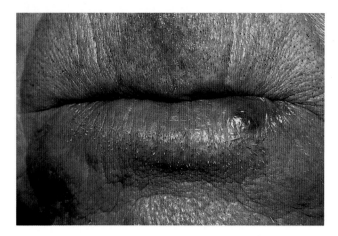

Fig. 66.62 Venous lake of the lip. (Courtesy of Addenbrooke's Hospital, Cambridge, UK.)

Glossitis (see p. 66.82)

Strawberry tongue

Prominence of the lingual papillae may be seen in scarlet fever, Kawasaki disease and Riley–Day syndrome (familial dysautonomia), giving rise to an appearance similar to a strawberry.

Telangiectasia (see Chapter 51)

Oral telangiectases occur mainly in hereditary haemorrhagic telangiectasia, CREST (calcinosis, Raynaud's, esophageal, sclerodactyly, telangiectasia) syndrome [1] (see Chapter 56), chronic liver disease, pregnancy and after irradiation.

REFERENCE

1 Ueda M, Abe Y, Fujiwara H et al. Prominent telangiectasia associated with marked bleeding in CREST syndrome. *J Dermatol* 1993; **20**: 180–4.

Venous lake

SYN. VENOUS VARIX; SENILE HAEMANGIOMA OF LIP

This is a bluish-purple soft swelling, 2–10 mm in diameter, usually seen on the lower lip of an elderly person, due to a venous dilatation (Fig. 66.62). The lesion is lined by a single layer of flattened endothelial cells with a thick wall of fibrous tissue. The lesion empties on prolonged pressure [1,2].

A venous lake may be only a trivial cosmetic problem or it can bleed severely after trauma. It can be excised, but careful cryotherapy, electrocautery or treatment with an argon laser [2] can also give good results.

REFERENCES

1 Alcalay J, Sandbank M. The ultrastructure of cutaneous venous lakes. *Int J Dermatol* 1987; **26**: 645–6.
2 Neumann RA, Knobler RM. Venous lakes (Bean–Walsh) of the lips: treatment experience with the argon laser and 18 months follow-up. *Clin Exp Dermatol* 1990; **15**: 115–8.

Proliferative vascular lesions

Benign atypical vascular lesions may exhibit cytological or architectural features that simulate angiosarcoma such that considerable caution is required in diagnosis [1]. The head and neck region is a common location particularly for lobular capillary haemangioma (pyogenic granuloma), while the lip is an especially common site for lobular capillary haemangioma [2] and intravascular papillary endothelial hyperplasia (Masson's haemangioma or pseudoangiosarcoma) [3,4]. Intravascular papillary endothelial hyperplasia is a benign, non-neoplastic, vascular lesion characterized histologically by papillary fronds lined by proliferating endothelium and probably represents an organizing thrombus. Seen mainly in the lip or tongue in females, it may simulate angiosarcoma histologically [5]. Excision suffices.

Vascular lesions such as epithelioid haemangioma, epithelioid haemangioendothelioma, spindle-cell haemangioendothelioma, acquired progressive lymphangioma, or angiosarcoma and KS may also occasionally be seen.

REFERENCES

1 Renshaw AA, Rosai J. Benign atypical vascular lesions of the lip. *Am J Surg Pathol* 1993; **17**: 557–65.
2 Kerr DA. Granuloma pyogenicum. *Oral Surg Oral Med Oral Pathol* 1951; **4**: 158–76.
3 Kuo TT, Sayers CP, Rosai J. Masson's 'Vegetant intravascular hemangioendothelioma': a lesion often mistaken for angiosarcoma. Study of 17 cases located in the skin and soft tissues. *Cancer* 1976; **38**: 1227–36.
4 Mills SE, Cooper PH, Fechner RE. Lobular capillary hemangioma: the underlying lesion of pyogenic granuloma. A study of 73 cases from the oral and nasal mucous membranes. *Am J Surg Pathol* 1980; **4**: 471–9.
5 Tosios K, Koutlas IG, Papanicolaou SI. Intravascular papillary endothelial hyperplasia of the oral soft tissues. *J Oral Maxillofac Surg* 1994; **52**: 1263–8.

Varicosities

Bluish oral varicosities may often be seen in elderly patients, particularly in the ventrum and lateral margin of the tongue. They are benign and inconsequential.

Erythroplasia

Erythroplasia (erythroplakia) is a red velvety lesion level with, or depressed below, the surrounding mucosa. It is uncommon and affects patients of either sex in their sixth and seventh decades [1–3]. Erythroplasia usually involves the floor of the mouth, the ventrum of the tongue, or the

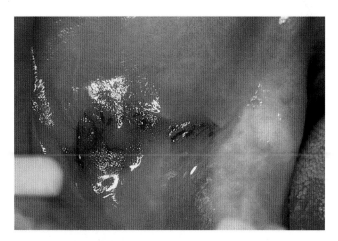

Fig. 66.63 Erythroplasia. (Courtesy of Professor R.A. Cawson, Eastman Dental Institute, London, UK.)

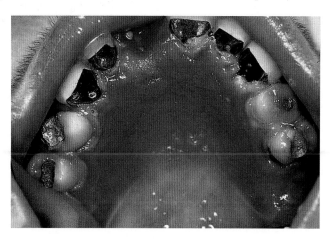

Fig. 66.64 Denture-induced stomatitis showing diffuse erythema in the denture-bearing area.

soft palate (Fig. 66.63) [1–4]. With regard to the risk of erythroplasia, a more than additive interaction has been found between tobacco chewing and low vegetable intake, whereas a more than multiplicative interaction has been found between alcohol drinking and low vegetable intake, and between drinking and low fruit intake [5].

Some 75–90% of cases of erythroplasia prove to be carcinoma or carcinoma *in situ* or show severe dysplasia. The incidence of malignant change in erythroplasia is 17 times higher than in leukoplakia.

Areas of erythroplasia should be excised and sent for histological examination.

REFERENCES

1 Eveson JW. Oral premalignancy. *Cancer Surv* 1983; **2**: 403–24.
2 Scully C, Cawson RA. Oral potentially malignant lesions. *J Epidemiol Biostat* 1996; **1**: 3–12.
3 Melrose RJ. Premalignant oral mucosal diseases. *J Calif Dent Assoc* 2001; **29**: 593–600.
4 Mashberg A. Diagnosis of early oral and oropharyngeal squamous carcinoma: obstacles and their amelioration. *Oral Oncol* 2000; **36**: 253–5.
5 Hashibe M, Mathew B, Kuruvilla B *et al.* Chewing tobacco, alcohol, and the risk of erythroplakia. *Cancer Epidemiol Biomarkers Prev* 2000; **9**: 639–45.

Erythematous candidiasis

Oral candidiasis can cause erythema and soreness of the oral mucosa, with or without the more usual thrush.

Denture-related stomatitis
SYN. DENTURE SORE MOUTH

This common form of mild, chronic, atrophic oral candidiasis occurs only beneath a denture, usually a complete upper denture, and is not often sore despite its name [1,2]. Dentures worn throughout the night, or with a dry mouth, favour development of this infection with *Candida* species. It is not caused by allergy to the denture material and it is

not clear why only some denture wearers develop the condition. It is a disease mainly of the middle-aged or elderly and is more prevalent in women than men. Patients appear otherwise healthy. In some studies of institutionalized elderly patients, as many as 70% have been found to have denture-related stomatitis but overall it is considerably less common, particularly in normal healthy subjects.

Denture-related stomatitis consists of mild inflammation and erythema of the mucosa beneath a denture (Fig. 66.64).

Aetiopathogenesis [5–8]. Dentures can produce a number of ecological changes, including the following:
• Changes in the oral flora.
• Plaque accumulation between the mucosal surface of the denture and the palate.
• Saliva present between the maxillary denture and the mucosa may have a lower pH than usual.
• Accumulation of microbial plaque (bacteria and/or yeasts) on and in the fitting surface of the denture and the underlying mucosa.

In some persons, the cause appears to be related to a non-specific plaque [1–4]. This plaque undergoes sequential development, and is colonized by *Candida* organisms. Although there is no increased aspartyl proteinase production from the *Candida* involved, the decreased salivary flow and a low pH under the denture probably results in a high *Candida* enzymatic activity, which can cause inflammation.

Yeasts such as *Candida* are isolated in up to 90% of persons with denture-related stomatitis but even 66% of denture wearers have them. The most frequently isolated species is *Candida albicans*. Of the *C. albicans* isolates, 75% are serotype A and 25% serotype B, a significant increase in serotype B compared with a control group of non-denture-wearing HIV-seronegative individuals with oral candidiasis. Resistogram strain-C is the most predominant (24% of total isolates), while strain A-CDE is the least (1.5% of total isolates). Adherence of *C. albicans* to denture-base materials *in vitro* is related to the hydrophobicity of the organism. When *Candida* is involved in denture-related stomatitis, the more common terms 'Candida-associated denture stomatitis', 'denture-induced candidiasis' or 'chronic atrophic candidiasis' are used. However, denture-induced stomatitis is not exclusively associated with *Candida* and, occasionally, other factors such as bacterial infection or mechanical irritation are at play.

Histological examination of the soft tissue beneath dentures has shown proliferative or degenerative responses with reduced keratinization and thinner epithelium.

However, it not clear why only some denture wearers develop denture-related stomatitis, since most patients appear otherwise healthy. There have been few studies. Patients with denture-related stomatitis have no serious cell-mediated immune defects but they may sometimes be deficient in migration inhibition factor and may have overactive suppressor T cells or other T-lymphocyte/ phagocyte defects. Mean concentrations of serum IL-6 and tumour necrosis factor (TNF)-α are statistically significantly higher and soluble TNF receptors lower in denture wearers compared with controls but there are no differences when stomatitis is present [9].

Predisposing factors. Dental appliances (mainly maxillary dentures), especially when worn throughout the night, or with a dry mouth, are the major predisposing factor. Diabetes or a high-carbohydrate diet occasionally predispose [10–12] and HIV is a rare underlying factor.

Factors that are usually *not* significant include allergy to the dental material (if it were, denture-related stomatitis would affect mucosae other than just that beneath the appliance), trauma (the condition is more common beneath maxillary dentures than mandibular dentures, yet trauma is more common with the latter), pharmacological agents and smoking.

Clinical features. The characteristic presenting features of denture-related stomatitis are:
• chronic erythema and oedema of the mucosa that contacts the fitting surface of the denture (usually a complete upper denture);
• the mucosa below lower dentures is rarely involved;
• erythema is restricted to the denture-bearing area;
• usually there are no symptoms;
• uncommon complications include angular stomatitis, and papillary hyperplasia in the vault of the palate.

Diagnosis. Denture-related stomatitis is a clinical diagnosis; the lesions have been classified into three clinical types (Newton's types), increasing in severity.

• Type 1: a localized simple inflammation or a pinpoint hyperaemia.
• Type 2: an erythematous or generalized simple type presenting as more diffuse erythema involving a part of, or the entire, denture-covered mucosa.
• Type 3: a granular type (inflammatory papillary hyperplasia) commonly involving the central part of the hard palate and the alveolar ridge.

Management. Any underlying systemic disease should be treated where possible.

The denture plaque and fitting surface is infested, usually with *C. albicans*. This must be removed regularly. Therefore, to treat and prevent recurrence of denture-related stomatitis, dentures should be removed from the mouth at night, cleaned and disinfected, and stored in an antiseptic. Cleansing is crucial to therapeutic success [13]. Denture cleansers can be divided into groups according to their main components: alkaline peroxides, alkaline hypochlorites, acids, yeast lytic enzymes, proteolytic enzymes and disinfectants such as hypochlorite. Denture soak solution containing benzoic acid completely eradicates *C. albicans* from the denture surface as it is taken up into the acrylic resin. An oral rinse containing chlorhexidine gluconate also results in complete elimination of *C. albicans* on the acrylic resin surface of the denture, and in reduction of palatal inflammation. A protease-containing denture soak (Alcalase) is also an effective way of removing denture plaque, especially when combined with brushing. Hypochlorite is an effective anticandidal but can turn chrome cobalt dentures black.

The mucosal infection is eradicated by brushing the palate and using antifungals for at least 4 weeks. Effective agents include nystatin pastilles or suspension, amphotericin lozenges, miconazole gel or fluconazole suspension or tablets, administered concurrently with an oral antiseptic such as chlorhexidine, which itself has antifungal activity. Isolates are usually sensitive to amphotericin and nystatin but less sensitive to miconazole. Fluconazole is as effective as newer agents such as itraconazole. The cyclodextrin solution and the capsule preparations of itraconazole are equally effective adjuncts in the treatment but, because of side effects, the capsules are preferred. Miconazole lacquer or fluconazole in tissue conditioners applied to the denture fitting surface are also effective [14–16].

Surgery may be needed to excise papillary hyperplasia [17].

REFERENCES

1 Wilson J. The aetiology, diagnosis and management of denture stomatitis. *Br Dent J* 1998; **185**: 380–4.
2 Nikawa H, Hamada T, Yamamoto T. Denture plaque: past and recent concerns. *J Dent* 1998; **26**: 299–304.

3 Fenlon MR, Sherriff M, Walter JD. Factors associated with the presence of denture related stomatitis in complete denture wearers: a preliminary investigation. *Eur J Prosthodont Restorative Dent* 1998; **6**: 145–7.

4 Monsenego P. Presence of microorganisms on the fitting denture complete surface: study 'in vivo'. *J Oral Rehabil* 2000; **27**: 708–13.

5 Webb BC, Thomas CJ, Willcox MD, Harty DW, Knox KW. *Candida*-associated denture stomatitis. Aetiology and management: a review. Part 3. Treatment of oral candidiasis. *Aust Dent J* 1998; **43**: 244–9.

6 Webb BC, Thomas CJ, Willcox MD, Harty DW, Knox KW. *Candida*-associated denture stomatitis. Aetiology and management: a review. Part 2. Oral diseases caused by *Candida* species. *Aust Dent J* 1998; **43**: 160–6.

7 Radford DR, Challacombe SJ, Walter JD. Denture plaque and adherence of *Candida albicans* to denture-base materials *in vivo* and *in vitro*. *Crit Rev Oral Biol Med* 1999; **10**: 99–116.

8 McMullan-Vogel CG, Jude HD, Ollert MW, Vogel CW. Serotype distribution and secretory acid proteinase activity of *Candida albicans* isolated from the oral mucosa of patients with denture stomatitis. *Oral Microbiol Immunol* 1999; **14**: 183–9.

9 Pietruski JK, Pietruska MD, Jablonska E *et al*. Interleukin 6, tumor necrosis factor alpha and their soluble receptors in the blood serum of patients with denture stomatitis and fungal infection. *Arch Immunol Ther Exp (Warsz)* 2000; **48**: 101–5.

10 Vitkov L, Weitgasser R, Lugstein A *et al*. Glycaemic disorders in denture stomatitis. *J Oral Pathol Med* 1999; **28**: 406–9.

11 Guggenheimer J, Moore PA, Rossie K *et al*. Insulin-dependent diabetes mellitus and oral soft tissue pathologies. II. Prevalence and characteristics of *Candida* and candidal lesions. *Oral Surg Oral Med Oral Pathol Oral Radiol Endod* 2000; **89**: 570–6.

12 Maruo Y, Sato T, Hara T, Shirai H. The effect of diabetes mellitus on histopathological changes in the tissues under denture base bearing masticatory pressure. *J Oral Rehabil* 1999; **26**: 345–55.

13 Markovic D, Puskar T, Tesic D. Denture cleaning techniques in the elderly affecting the occurrence of denture-induced stomatitis. *Med Pregl* 1999; **52**: 57–61.

14 Chow CK, Matear DW, Lawrence HP. Efficacy of antifungal agents in tissue conditioners in treating candidiasis. *Gerodontology* 1999; **16**: 110–8.

15 Cross LJ, Bagg J, Wray D, Aitchison T. A comparison of fluconazole and itraconazole in the management of denture stomatitis: a pilot study. *J Dent* 1998; **26**: 657–64.

16 Cross LJ, Bagg J, Aitchison TC. Efficacy of the cyclodextrin liquid preparation of itraconazole in treatment of denture stomatitis: comparison with itraconazole capsules. *Antimicrob Agents Chemother* 2000; **44**: 425–7.

17 Antonelli JR, Panno FV, Witko A. Inflammatory papillary hyperplasia: supraperiosteal excision by the blade-loop technique. *Gen Dent* 1998; **46**: 390–7.

Acute candidiasis

Acute oral candidiasis may complicate corticosteroid or antibiotic therapy, particularly with long-term broad-spectrum antimicrobials such as used in transplant or terminally ill patients [1–3]. There is widespread erythema and soreness of the oral mucosa, sometimes with thrush, particularly noticeable on the tongue.

REFERENCES

1 Wright BA, Fenwick F. Candidiasis and atrophic tongue lesions. *Oral Surg Oral Med Oral Pathol* 1981; **51**: 55–61.

2 Sweeney MP, Bagg J, Baxter WP, Aitchison TC. Oral disease in terminally ill cancer patients with xerostomia. *Oral Oncol* 1998; **34**: 123–6.

3 Bengtsson L, Ransjo U. Acute atrophic glossitis after open-heart surgery. *Scand J Thorac Cardiovasc Surg* 1988; **22**: 143–4.

HIV-associated candidiasis

Candida infections in and around the mouth have increased greatly, particularly as the HIV epidemic has spread, and now other species (especially *C. krusei*) and antifungal resistance are serious clinical realities [1–4]. There may be transmission of *Candida* species from HIV-infected persons [5] and new species and clades are being recognized [6]. The most dominant oral species, in decreasing order of frequency, are:

- *C. albicans*;
- *C. tropicalis*;
- *C. glabrata*;
- *C. parapsilosis*;
- *C. krusei*;
- other *Candida* species such as *C. dubliniensis, C. africanus* and *C. inconspicua*;
- other genera (*Rhodotorula, Saccharomyces*, etc.), which are rare and transient.

Erythematous or atrophic candidiasis may arise as a consequence of persistent acute pseudomembranous candidiasis when the pseudomembranes are shed, may develop *de novo*, or in HIV infection may precede pseudomembranous candidosis. The clinical presentation is of erythematous areas generally on the dorsum of the tongue, palate or buccal mucosa. Lesions on the dorsum of the tongue present as depapillated areas. Red areas are often seen in the palate in HIV disease. There can be an associated angular stomatitis and/or thrush.

Thrush is a well-recognized feature of T-cell immunodeficiencies, particularly after the severe T-cell immunosuppression necessary for organ transplantation and in other secondary immunodeficiencies, such as leukaemia, diabetes or HIV/AIDS. It is a common and early feature of AIDS.

Furthermore, with increasing use of antimycotic therapy, especially in HIV disease, there is a shift towards not only resistant *C. albicans*, as well as the appearance of novel species, but also other species such as *C. glabrata* and *C. krusei*. Thrush is characterized by white patches on the surface of the oral mucosa, tongue and elsewhere. The lesions develop to form confluent plaques that resemble milk curds, and can be wiped off to reveal a raw, erythematous and sometimes bleeding base. Complications of oropharyngeal thrush may sometimes present as lesions of the adjacent mucosa, particularly in the upper respiratory tract and the oesophagus. The combination of oral and oesophageal candidiasis is particularly prevalent in HIV-infected patients. Antifungal therapy is indicated.

REFERENCES

1 Korting HC. Clinical spectrum of oral candidosis and its role in HIV-infected patients. *Mycoses* 1989; **32** (Suppl. 2): 123–9.

2 Scully C, El-Kabir M, Samaranayake LP. *Candida* and oral candidosis. *Crit Rev Oral Biol Med* 1994; **5**: 124–58.

3 Odds FC. Mycology in oral pathology. *Acta Stomatol Belg* 1997; **94**: 75–80.

4 Campisi G, Pizzo G, Milici ME, Mancuso S, Margiotta V. Candidal carriage in the oral cavity of human immunodeficiency virus-infected subjects. *Oral Surg Oral Med Oral Pathol Oral Radiol Endod* 2002; **93**: 281–6.

5 Milan EP, Kallas EG, Costa PR, da Matta DA, Lopes Colombo A. Oral colonization by *Candida* spp. among AIDS household contacts. *Mycoses* 2001; **44**: 273–7.

6 Blignaut E, Pujol C, Lockhart S, Joly S, Soll DR. Ca3 fingerprinting of *Candida albicans* isolates from human immunodeficiency virus-positive and healthy individuals reveals a new clade in South Africa. *J Clin Microbiol* 2002; **40**: 826–36.

Median rhomboid glossitis

SYN. CENTRAL PAPILLARY ATROPHY OF
THE TONGUE

Aetiology. This red, depapillated, rhomboidal area in the centre line of the dorsum of the tongue, just anterior to the sulcus terminalis, was formerly thought to be caused by persistence of the tuberculum impar. However, it is now thought to be associated with candidiasis [1–3]. Multiple oral lesions may occasionally be present, especially a 'kissing' lesion in the palatal vault [4,5]. Smoking, denture wearing and, occasionally, immune defects (including HIV) and diabetes predispose to this lesion [6,7].

Pathology. Histology shows irregular pseudoepitheliomatous epithelial hyperplasia that may resemble a carcinoma but it is not a malignant condition.

Clinical features. There is typically a red central lesion of somewhat rhomboidal shape anterior to the sulcus terminalis on the dorsum of the tongue (Fig. 66.65). Occasionally, there is a nodular component.

There may also sometimes be a coexistent erythematous candidiasis in the palate [4,5], which some have termed 'chronic oral multifocal candidiasis'.

Diagnosis and management. Median rhomboid glossitis is usually diagnosed on clinical grounds, although biopsy may be indicated, since some lesions are nodular and may simulate a neoplasm. It may respond to the use of antifungals and to cessation of smoking.

REFERENCES

1 Touyz LZG, Peters E. Candidal infection of the tongue with non-specific inflammation of the palate. *Oral Surg* 1987; **63**: 304–8.

2 van der Waal I. *Candida albicans* in median rhomboid glossitis: a post-mortem study. *Int J Oral Maxillofac Surg* 1986; **15**: 322–5.

3 Barrett AW, Kingsmill VJ, Speight PM. The frequency of fungal infection in biopsies of oral mucosal lesions. *Oral Dis* 1998; **4**: 26–31.

4 Holmstrup P, Besserman M. Clinical, therapeutic and pathogenic aspects of chronic oral multifocal candidiasis. *Oral Surg* 1984; **56**: 388–95.

5 Brown RS, Krakow AM. Median rhomboid glossitis and a 'kissing' lesion of the palate. *Oral Surg Oral Med Oral Pathol Oral Radiol Endod* 1996; **82**: 472–3.

6 Barasch A, Safford MM, Catalanotto FA, Fine DH, Katz RV. Oral soft tissue manifestations in HIV-positive vs. HIV-negative children from an inner city population: a two-year observational study. *Pediatr Dent* 2000; **22**: 215–20.

7 Guggenheimer J, Moore PA, Rossie K *et al.* Insulin-dependent diabetes mellitus and oral soft tissue pathologies. II. Prevalence and characteristics of *Candida* and candidal lesions. *Oral Surg Oral Med Oral Pathol Oral Radiol Endod* 2000; **89**: 570–6.

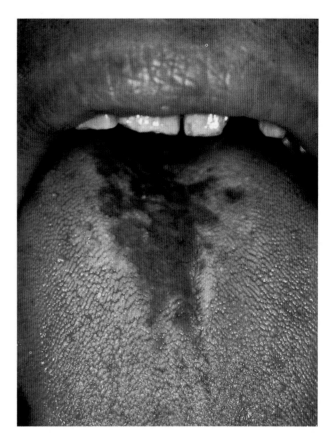

Fig. 66.65 Median rhomboid glossitis.

Desquamative gingivitis

This is usually caused by pemphigoid or lichen planus.

Loss of elasticity of oral tissues

Fibrosis of oral tissues can follow burns or irradiation. It may also be associated with habits such as the chewing of betel nut (areca), which predisposes to oral submucous fibrosis (see below) and may be caused by a connective tissue disorder such as scleroderma. Rarely it is occupational (polyvinylchloride workers). Epidermolysis bullosa and mucous membrane pemphigoid may cause scarring and the orofacial region is occasionally involved in multiple idiopathic fibrosis [1].

REFERENCE

1 Lewin IG, Carter JLB, Evans N *et al*. Multiple idiopathic fibrosis presenting as facial pain and trismus. *Br J Oral Surg* 1985; **23**: 135–9.

Oral submucous fibrosis

Aetiology. Oral submucous fibrosis is a chronic disease of the oral mucosa that appears to be caused by exposure to constituents of the areca nut. It is found virtually exclusively in persons from the Indian subcontinent; most of those affected chew areca nut with tobacco, betel leaf and lime [1,2].

Pathology. There is a subepithelial chronic inflammatory reaction with fibrosis extending to the submucosa and muscle. Epithelial changes range from atrophy to keratosis and there may be dysplasia.

Clinical features. Oral submucous fibrosis develops insidiously, often initially presenting with oral dysaesthesia and a non-specific vesicular stomatitis [3]. Later there may be symmetrical fibrosis of the cheeks, lips or palate, which may be symptomless and noted only as bands running through the mucosa. This can, however, become so severe that the affected site becomes white and firm, with severely restricted opening of the mouth.

Oral submucous fibrosis appears to be restricted to the mouth, although many patients are also anaemic. Oral submucous fibrosis may predispose to the development of oral carcinoma, which occurs in 2–10% of patients over a period of 10 years [4,5].

The diagnosis can be confirmed by biopsy.

Treatment. Management is difficult. Intralesional corticosteroids and jaw exercises may be useful in the early stages, but surgery may be needed to relieve the fibrosis [1,6].

REFERENCES

1 Caniff JP. Mucosal diseases of uncertain etiology. III. Oral submucous fibrosis. In: Mackenzie IC, Squier CA, Dabelsteen E, eds. *Oral Mucosal Diseases: Biology, Etiology and Therapy.* Copenhagen: Laegeforeningen Forlag, 1987: 87–91.
2 Caniff JP, Harvey W. The aetiology of oral submucous fibrosis: the stimulation of collagen synthesis by extracts of areca nut. *Int J Oral Surg* 1981; **10**: 163–7.
3 Pindborg JJ, Bhonsle RB, Murti PR *et al.* Incidence and early forms of oral submucous fibrosis. *Oral Surg* 1980; **50**: 40–4.
4 Gupta PC, Bhonsle RB, Murti PR *et al.* An epidemiologic assessment of cancer risk in oral precancerous lesions in India with special reference to nodular leukoplakia. *Cancer* 1989; **63**: 2247–52.
5 Pindborg JJ, Murti PR, Bhonsle RB *et al.* Oral submucous fibrosis as a precancerous condition. *Scand J Dent Res* 1984; **92**: 224–9.
6 Yen DJ. Surgical treatment of submucous fibrosis. *Oral Surg* 1982; **54**: 269–72.

Systemic sclerosis (see Chapter 56)

Oral features are common in systemic sclerosis and are generally more obvious in those with diffuse than localized scleroderma. About 70% of patients have xerostomia, and there is an increase in both caries and periodontal disease. A characteristic finding is of increased width of the periodontal ligament space of all teeth on radiography [1]. There are mandibular erosions in the angle particularly, but also in the condyle, coronoid or digastric regions. Telangiectasia may be seen and most patients have restricted oral opening with linear wrinkles of the lips [2,3].

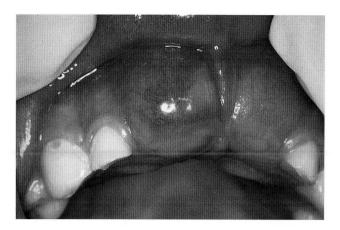

Fig. 66.66 Bluish, fluctuant swelling of an oral cyst, in this case an eruption cyst over an erupting maxillary permanent incisor. (The lesion on the maxillary canine is early dental caries.)

REFERENCES

1 Alexandridis C, White SC. Periodontal ligament changes in patients with progressive systemic sclerosis. *Oral Surg* 1984; **58**: 113–8.
2 Masmary Y, Glais R, Pisanty S. Scleroderma: oral manifestations. *Oral Surg* 1981; **52**: 32–7.
3 Wood RE, Lee P. Analysis of the oral manifestations of systemic sclerosis (scleroderma). *Oral Surg* 1988; **65**: 172–8.

Lumps and swellings

Lumps in the mouth range from simple anatomical variants, which can cause the patient considerable concern, to lumps caused by inflammatory, cystic (Fig. 66.66), neoplastic and other disorders (Table 66.23).

Foliate papillitis

The foliate lingual papillae may become inflamed and swell. Because of their location on the posterolateral tongue this may give undue concern about malignancy. The condition resolves spontaneously.

Angio-oedema

Oral swelling may be a feature of acquired angio-oedema. The swelling is of acute onset, may affect the lips, tongue or other areas, and is often only mild and transient, although there is always the potential for obstruction of the airway. Local anaesthetics [1] or more commonly angiotensin-converting enzyme inhibitors [2–6] may cause angio-oedema, which can occasionally be lethal [4].

It may respond to a sympathomimetic agent such as epinephrine (adrenaline) or to antihistamines.

REFERENCES

1 Yaman Z, Kisnisci RS. Idiopathic swelling of the lower lip associated with topical anaesthesia. Report of three cases. *Aust Dent J* 1998; **43**: 324–7.

Table 66.23 Lesions that may cause the complaint of lumps or swellings in the mouth.

Normal anatomical features
Pterygoid hamulus
Parotid papillae
Foliate or other lingual papillae
Unerupted teeth

Developmental
Haemangioma
Lymphangioma
Maxillary and mandibular tori
Hereditary gingival fibromatosis
Von Recklinghausen's neurofibromatosis
Cysts of developmental origin
Odontomes

Inflammatory
Abscess
Pyogenic granuloma
Oral Crohn's disease
Orofacial granulomatosis
Pulse granuloma
Sarcoidosis
Wegener's granuloma
Others

Traumatic
Epulis
Fibroepithelial polyp
Denture-induced granuloma
Mucocele
Herniation of buccal fat pad

Infective
Various papillomatous lesions

Cystic
Cysts of odontogenic origin (e.g. dental cysts)

Drug therapy (gingival swelling only)
Oral contraceptive (pill gingivitis)
Phenytoin
Calcium-channel blockers
Ciclosporin

Hormonal
Pubertal gingivitis
Pregnancy epulis/gingivitis

Blood dyscrasias
Leukaemia, lymphoma and myeloma

Benign neoplasms
Various

Malignant neoplasms
Primary and secondary

Others
Angio-oedema
Amyloidosis
Fibro-osseous diseases
Acanthosis nigricans

2 Ebo DG, Steven WJ. Angioedema of ACE inhibitors. *Allergy* 1997; **52**: 354–5.
3 Lapostolle F, Borron SW, Bekka R, Baud FJ. Lingual angioedema after perindopril use. *Am J Cardiol* 1998; **81**: 523.
4 Seymour RA, Thomason JM, Nolan A. Angiotensin converting enzyme (ACE) inhibitors and their implications for the dental surgeon. *Br Dent J* 1997; **183**: 214–8.

5 Ulmer JL, Garvey MJ. Fatal angioedema associated with lisinopril. *Ann Pharmacother* 1992; **26**: 1245–56.
6 Vleeming W, van Amstedam JG, Stricker BH, de Widt DJ. ACE inhibitor-induced angioedema. Incidence, prevention and management. *Drug Saf* 1998; **18**: 171–88.

Oral allergy syndrome

Oral allergy syndrome is the combination of oral pruritus, irritation and swelling of the lips, tongue, palate and throat, sometimes associated with other allergic features such as rhinoconjunctivitis, asthma, urticaria–angio-oedema, and anaphylactic shock, precipitated mainly by fresh foods such as fruits and vegetables, sometimes by pollens because of cross-reacting allergens [1,2]. Cooking often destroys the allergens.

It may respond to antihistamines or to a sympathomimetic agent such as ephedrine which can be taken by mouth.

REFERENCES

1 Escribano MM, Serrano P, Munoz-Bellido FJ, De la Calle A, Coude J. Oral allergy syndrome to bird meat associated with egg intolerance. *Allergy* 1998; **53**: 903–4.
2 Liccardi G, D'Amato M, D'Amato G. Oral allergy syndrome after ingestion of salami in a subject with monosensitisation to mite allergens. *J Allergy Clin Immunol* 1996; **98**: 850–2.

Osteoma mucosae
SYN. OSSEOUS CHORISTOMA

There are rare cases of osteoma of the oral mucosa, usually in the tongue. Most have been in females in the third and fourth decades and have arisen as pedunculated, hard, painless lumps on the dorsum of the tongue immediately posterior to the foramen caecum [1–3]. They may arise from thyroid anlages. Simple excision suffices.

REFERENCES

1 Busuttil A. An osteoma of the tongue. *J Laryngol* 1977; **91**: 259–61.
2 Markaki S, Gearty J, Markakis P. Osteoma of the tongue. *Br J Oral Surg* 1987; **25**: 79–82.
3 Sheridan SM. Osseous choristoma: a report of two cases. *Br J Oral Surg* 1984; **22**: 99–102.

Abscesses

Most intraoral abscesses are odontogenic in origin, as a final consequence of dental caries. Most abscesses discharge in the mouth on the buccal gingiva but occasionally discharge palatally, lingually, on the chin or submental region (Fig. 66.67), or elsewhere. Very occasionally abscesses follow trauma or a foreign body, or rarely are related to unusual oral infections such as actinomycosis [1], nocardiosis or botryomycosis [2]. Drainage and appropriate antimicrobials are indicated [3]. Dental

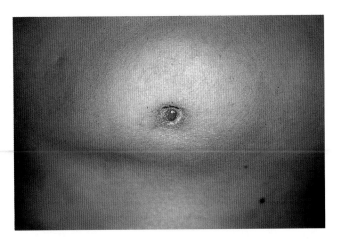

Fig. 66.67 Sinus on chin related to a dental abscess on a mandibular incisor tooth.

attention is required; dental abscesses are drained by tooth extraction, incision and drainage, or through the root canal (endodontics).

REFERENCES

1 Brignall ID, Gilhooly M. Actinomycosis of the tongue: a diagnostic dilemma. *Br J Oral Surg* 1989; **27**: 249–53.
2 Small IA, Kobernick S. Botryomycosis of the tongue. *Oral Surg* 1967; **24**: 503–9.
3 Luker J. A case of lingual abscess. *Br Dent J* 1985; **159**: 300.

Sarcoidosis

Isolated nodules [1,2], gingival lesions [3], facial or labial swelling [4] and salivary gland involvement are the main oral or perioral lesions of sarcoidosis, but are uncommon. However, even where the mucosa is clinically normal, patients with sarcoidosis may have characteristic changes in palatal or labial salivary gland biopsies [5].

REFERENCES

1 Mendelsohn SS, Field EA, Woolgar J. Sarcoidosis of the tongue. *Clin Exp Dermatol* 1992; **17**: 47–8.
2 Tillman HH, Taylor RG, Carchidi JE. Sarcoidosis of the tongue. *Oral Surg* 1968; **21**: 190–5.
3 Hayter JP, Robertson JM. Sarcoidosis presenting as gingivitis. *BMJ* 1988; **296**: 1504.
4 Gold RS, Sager E. Oral sarcoidosis: review of the literature. *J Oral Surg* 1976; **34**: 237–44.
5 Van Maarsseveen ACMTH, Van der Waal I, Stam J *et al*. Oral involvement in sarcoidosis. *Int J Oral Surg* 1982; **11**: 21–9.

Pulse granuloma

SYN. LEWAR'S DISEASE

Chronic mandibular periostitis caused by embedded vegetable matter of dietary origin is uncommon but typic-ally presents as a submucosal lump over the lower alveolus. Histology shows amorphous hyaline material and a granulomatous inflammatory reaction [1]. Excision suffices.

REFERENCE

1 Keirby FAR, Soames JV. Periostitis and osteitis associated with hyaline bodies. *Br J Oral Surg* 1985; **23**: 346–50.

Denture-induced hyperplasia

SYN. DENTURE GRANULOMA; EPULIS FISSURATUM

Where a denture flange is overextended and irritates the vestibular mucosa, a linear reparative process may result, eventually producing an elongated fibroepithelial enlargement known as denture-induced hyperplasia [1]. The pathology is that of a fibrous lump (see p. 66.20).

Firm, leaf-like, painless swellings are seen, usually in the buccal or labial vestibule.

A denture-induced granuloma should be excised and examined histologically, if modification of the denture does not induce regression. Rarely, a denture granuloma arises because some other lesion develops beneath a denture and causes the mucosa to be irritated.

REFERENCE

1 Budzt-Jorgensen E. Oral mucosal lesions associated with the wearing of removable dentures. *J Oral Pathol* 1981; **10**: 65–80.

Mucocele (mucous cyst)

SYN. MUCOUS RETENTION CYST; RANULA; MUCOCELE; MYXOID CYST OF LIP

Superficial mucoceles are seen mainly in lichen planus. Deeper mucoceles are more common and are usually seen in the lower labial mucosa (Fig. 66.68), usually resulting from the escape of mucus into the lamina propria from a damaged minor salivary gland duct.

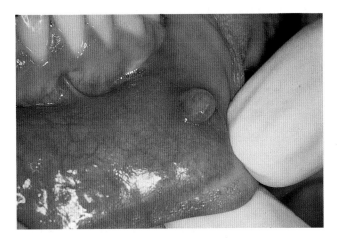

Fig. 66.68 Mucocele in a typical site.

They appear as painless dome-shaped, translucent, whitish blue papules or nodules [1].

Care should be taken to ensure that the lesion is not a salivary gland tumour with cystic change, especially when dealing with an apparent mucous cyst in the upper lip. The cysts can be excised but they also respond well to cryosurgery, using a single freeze–thaw cycle [2].

REFERENCES

1 Lattanand A, Johnson WC. Mucous cyst (mucocele): a clinico-pathologic and histochemical study. *Arch Dermatol* 1970; **101**: 673–8.
2 Bohler-Sommeregger K. Cryosurgical management of myxoid cysts. *J Dermatol Surg Oncol* 1988; **14**: 1405–8.

Buccal fat-pad herniation

Trauma may rarely cause the buccal pad of fat to herniate through the buccinator muscle, producing an intraoral swelling [1]. This usually occurs in males under the age of 4 years. Surgery is indicated.

REFERENCE

1 Fleming P. Traumatic herniation of buccal fat pad: a report of two cases. *J Oral Surg* 1986; **24**: 265–8.

Oral papilloma

Aetiology. These are caused by HPV [1].

Pathology. Histology includes acanthotic and sometimes hyperkeratotic epithelium with occasional koilocytosis.

Clinical features. Papillomas can appear anywhere in the mouth, but are most common at the junction of the hard and soft palate. The papilloma is a white or pink, cauliflower-like lesion that may resemble a wart. Papillomas of normal colour may be confused with the commoner fibroepithelial polyps, although the latter are commonest at sites of potential trauma.

Prognosis. Unlike some papillomas of the larynx or bowel, oral papillomas remain benign.

Diagnosis. Oral papillomas should be examined histologically to establish a correct diagnosis.

Treatment. Excision must be total, deep and wide enough to include any abnormal cells beyond the zone of the pedicle.

REFERENCE

1 Scully C, Cox MF, Prime SS et al. Papillomaviruses: the current status in relation to oral disease. *Oral Surg* 1988; **65**: 526–32.

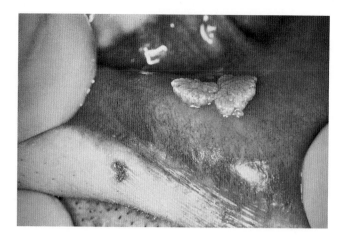

Fig. 66.69 Genital warts on the lower lip in HIV infection. (There is also a healing herpes simplex lesion on the lip.)

Warts (see Chapter 25)

Common warts (verrucae vulgaris) and venereal warts (condyloma acuminatum) are both caused by papillomaviruses [1–3]. They are rare in the mouth (Fig. 66.69) but are more common in HIV disease. None is known to be premalignant. Most can be removed by excision, cryosurgery or laser, or podophyllum or imiquimod.

REFERENCES

1 Green TL, Eversole LP, Leider AS. Oral and labial verruca vulgaris: clinical, histologic and immunohistochemical evaluation. *Oral Surg* 1986; **62**: 410–6.
2 Scully C, Cox M, Maitland N et al. Papillomaviruses: their current status in relation to oral disease. *Oral Surg* 1988; **65**: 526–32.
3 Scully C, Prime S, Maitland N. Papillomaviruses: their possible role in oral disease. *Oral Surg* 1985; **60**: 166–74.

Focal epithelial hyperplasia
SYN. HECK'S DISEASE

Focal epithelial hyperplasia is a rare, benign, familial disorder with no sex predisposition, characterized by multiple, soft, circumscribed, sessile, nodular elevations of the oral mucosa [1,2].

Heck's disease occurs particularly in native Americans and in Inuits in Greenland but has been reported rarely from many other countries. The prevalence in Greenland and Venezuela approaches 35% [1,3,4].

Aetiology. The papillomaviruses HPV-13 and HPV-32 appear to be causal in patients with the genetic predisposition to focal epithelial hyperplasia [5–8].

Pathology. The characteristics of focal epithelial hyperplasia are local epithelial hyperplasia, acanthosis and elongated 'Bronze Age axe' rete ridges, together with a ballooning type of nuclear degeneration. Epithelial cells have a pseudomitotic appearance.

Clinical features. Among native Americans, focal epithelial hyperplasia mainly affects children and usually involves the lower lip, whereas in the Inuit and in white people the lesions are found mainly in the fourth decade and later and often affect the tongue. This is a benign asymptomatic condition, requiring only reassurance.

REFERENCES

1 Axell T, Hammarstrom L, Larsson A. Focal epithelial hyperplasia in Sweden. *Acta Odontol Scand* 1981; **39**: 201–8.
2 Starink TM, Woerdeman MJ. Focal epithelial hyperplasia of the oral mucosa. *Br J Dermatol* 1977; **96**: 375–80.
3 Praetorius-Clausen F, Mogeltoft M, Roed-Petersen B *et al.* Focal epithelial hyperplasia of the oral mucosa in a South-West Greenlandic population. *Scand J Dent Res* 1970; **78**: 287–94.
4 Scully C, Cox M, Prime SS *et al.* Papillomaviruses: the current status in relation to oral disease. *Oral Surg* 1988; **65**: 526–32.
5 Beaudenon S, Praetorius F, Kremsdorf D *et al.* A new type of human papillomavirus associated with oral focal epithelial hyperplasia. *J Invest Dermatol* 1987; **88**: 130–5.
6 Garlick JA, Calderon S, Buchner A *et al.* Detection of human papillomavirus in focal epithelial hyperplasia. *J Oral Pathol Med* 1989; **18**: 172–7.
7 Henke RP, Guerin-Reverschon I, Milde-Langosch K *et al.* In situ detection of human papillomavirus types 13 and 32 in focal epithelial hyperplasia of the oral mucosa. *J Oral Pathol Med* 1989; **18**: 419–21.
8 Hernandes-Juaregui P, Eriksonn A, Tamayo-Perez R *et al.* Human papillomavirus type 13 DNA in focal epithelial hyperplasia among Mexicans. *Arch Virol* 1987; **93**: 131–7.

Papillary hyperplasia

Papillary hyperplasia may be seen in the vault of the palate, typically in persons with chronic denture-related stomatitis and occasionally in its absence [1,2]. It may require excision or laser removal.

REFERENCES

1 O'Driscoll PM. Papillary hyperplasia of the palate. *Br Dent J* 1965; **118**: 77–80.
2 Schmitz JF. A clinical study of inflammatory papillary hyperplasia. *J Prosthet Dent* 1964; **14**: 1034–9.

Rhabdomyoma

Rhabdomyomas are rare but most extracardiac rhabdomyomas present in the mouth, typically as lumps in the floor of mouth, tongue or soft palate [1,2]. Most are seen in the sixth decade, predominantly in males. Surgery is effective provided total excision is achieved.

REFERENCES

1 Corio RL, Lewis DM. Intraoral rhabdomyomas. *Oral Surg* 1979; **48**: 525–31.
2 Reid CO, Smith CJ. Rhabdomyoma of the floor of the mouth: a new case and review of recently reported intraoral rhabdomyomas. *Br J Oral Surg* 1985; **23**: 284–91.

Rhabdomyosarcoma

Some 45% of soft-tissue sarcomas in the head and neck region are rhabdomyosarcomas. The most common oral presentation is a progressively enlarging mass; some 20% have enlarged regional lymph nodes [1]. In advanced disease there may be pain, paraesthesia, trismus or loosening of teeth.

The prognosis is poor. Treatment includes cytotoxic chemotherapy, surgery and radiotherapy.

REFERENCE

1 Bras J, Batsakis JG, Luna MA. Rhabdomyosarcoma of the oral soft tissues. *Oral Surg* 1987; **64**: 585–96.

Nodular fasciitis (see Chapter 53)

Nodular (pseudosarcomatous) fasciitis affects the head and neck in 20% of cases but rarely involves the mouth [1,2].

REFERENCES

1 Davies HT, Bradley N, Bowerman JE. Oral nodular fasciitis. *Br J Oral Surg* 1989; **27**: 147–51.
2 Kawana T, Yamamoto H, Deguchi A *et al.* Nodular fasciitis of the upper labial fascia. Cytometric and ultrastructural studies. *Int J Oral Surg* 1986; **15**: 464–8.

Verruciform xanthoma

Although verruciform xanthoma was originally described as a distinct oral entity, it is now also known occasionally to affect the skin and non-oral mucosae [1]. The aetiology is unknown but may be a reaction to some irritant.

The lesions consist of parakeratotic verruciform epithelium, with large foamy xanthoma cells containing slightly PAS-positive granules and abundant lipid in the lamina propria between the epithelial pegs [2].

Verruciform xanthoma is usually a solitary symptomless lesion, typically on the gingiva, with a normal, pale, reddish or keratotic surface [1,2]. Excision is only rarely followed by recurrence.

REFERENCES

1 Neville BW, Weathers DR. Verruciform xanthoma. *Oral Surg* 1980; **49**: 429–34.
2 Nowparast B, Howell FV, Rick GM. Verruciform xanthoma: a clinicopathologic review and report of fifty-four cases. *Oral Surg* 1981; **51**: 619–25.

Lipoma (see Chapter 55)

Lipomas are uncommon in the mouth, comprising less than 5% of oral benign tumours [1]. They present as slow-growing, spherical, smooth and soft semi-fluctuant lumps with a characteristic yellowish colour. Most involve the buccal mucosa or floor of mouth. Occasionally, although benign, they infiltrate. Histology shows adult fat cells gathered into lobules by vascular septa of fibrous connective tissue. Surgery is rarely indicated except for infiltrating lipomas.

REFERENCE

1 Batsakis JG, Regezi JA, Rice DH. The pathology of head and neck tumors: part 8. *Head Neck Surg* 1980; **3**: 145–68.

Myxoma

Myxomas are rare in the oral cavity. They can arise in bone or soft tissue and, although benign, are aggressive and difficult to eradicate because of the tendency to infiltrate normal tissue.

Leiomyoma

This benign tumour of smooth muscle is rare in the oral cavity but usually affects the tongue or palate.

Macroglossia

The tongue may be congenitally enlarged (macroglossia) in Down's syndrome or Beckwith–Wiedemann syndrome or where there is an angioma. It may also enlarge in angio-oedema, gigantism, acromegaly or amyloidosis.

Myeloma and paraproteinaemias

Multiple myeloma very occasionally presents with an intraoral mass or oral bleeding. Bone lesions are more common. Solitary plasmacytomas may also be seen; indeed, some 80% of these rare tumours are found in the head and neck region but typically in the nasal cavity or pharynx rather than in the mouth [1,2].

Waldenström's macroglobulinaemia

Oral manifestations in Waldenström's macroglobulinaemia include purpura, ulceration and occasional mental nerve anaesthesia [3–5].

REFERENCES

1 Epstein JB, Boss NJS, Stevenson-Moore P. Maxillofacial manifestations of multiple myeloma. *Oral Surg* 1984; **57**: 267–71.
2 Woodruff RK, Whittle JM, Malpas JS. Solitary plasmacytoma. 1. Extramedullary soft tissue plasmacytoma. *Cancer* 1979; **43**: 2340–3.
3 Gamble JW, Driscoll EJ. Oral manifestations of macroglobulinaemia of Waldenstrom. *Oral Surg* 1960; **13**: 104–10.
4 Klokkevold PR, Miller DA, Friedlander AH. Mental nerve neuropathy: a symptom of Waldenstrom's macroglobulinaemia. *Oral Surg* 1989; **67**: 689–93.
5 Zulian M, Bellome J, DeBoom GW. Multiple linear ulcers on the dorsum of the tongue in a patient with Waldenstrom's macroglobulinaemia. *J Am Dent Assoc* 1987; **114**: 79–80.

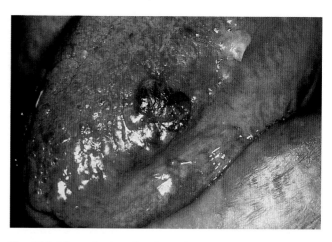

Fig. 66.70 Macroglossia and oral petechiae in amyloidosis.

Franklin's disease
SYN. HEAVY-CHAIN DISEASE

Palatal oedema and oral ulceration have been described in a few patients with heavy-chain disease, but the former feature is not as invariable as initially described [1,2].

REFERENCES

1 Kanoch T, Takigawa M, Niwa Y. Cutaneous lesions in heavy chain disease. *Arch Dermatol* 1988; **124**: 1538–40.
2 Seligmann M. Heavy chain diseases. In: Delamore IW, ed. *Multiple Myeloma and Other Paraproteinaemias*. Edinburgh: Churchill Livingstone, 1986: 263–85.

Thrombotic thrombocytopenic purpura

This may present with oral purpura and/or spontaneous gingival haemorrhage [1,2]. Gingival biopsy is a recommended investigation [3,4].

REFERENCES

1 Fox P, Gordon RE, Williams AC. Thrombotic thrombocytopenic purpura: report of a case. *J Oral Surg* 1977; **35**: 921–3.
2 Ridolfi R, Bell W. Thrombotic thrombocytopenic purpura: report of 25 cases and review of the literature. *Medicine* 1981; **60**: 413–28.
3 Goodman A, Ramos P, Petrelli M *et al*. Gingival biopsy in thrombotic thrombocytopenic purpura. *Ann Intern Med* 1978; **89**: 501–4.
4 Nishioka GJ, Chilcoat CC, Aufdenorte TB *et al*. The gingival biopsy in the diagnosis of thrombotic thrombocytopenic purpura. *Oral Surg* 1988; **65**: 580–5.

Amyloidosis (see Chapter 57)

In primary amyloidosis the tongue is enlarged and hard. There may also be yellowish submucosal nodules, lumps or petechiae (Fig. 66.70). Rarely, there are similar deposits elsewhere (e.g. in the soft palate), jaw claudication, salivary gland swelling or xerostomia [1–5].

Secondary amyloidoses rarely involve the mouth except in the case of multiple myeloma or haemodialysis-associated amyloid, which may occasionally produce oral nodules [6,7].

Some 10% of patients with oral amyloidosis have amyloid in their submandibular glands. Solitary intraoral amyloid is rare [8].

Congo red or thioflavine T staining of a biopsy usually confirms the diagnosis, although in extreme cases the deposits are seen on haematoxylin and eosin staining. Treatment is unsatisfactory but the underlying disease, where present, should be treated.

REFERENCES

1 Al-Hashimi I, Drinnan AJ, Uthman AA et al. Oral amyloidosis: two unusual case presentations. Oral Surg 1987; **63**: 586–91.
2 Babejews A. Occult multiple myeloma associated with amyloid of the tongue. Br J Oral Maxillofac Surg 1985; **23**: 298–303.
3 Gertz MA, Kyle RA, Griffing WL et al. Jaw claudication in primary systemic amyloidosis. Medicine 1986; **65**: 173–9.
4 Salisbury PS, Jacoway JR. Oral amyloidosis: a late complication of multiple myeloma. Oral Surg 1983; **56**: 48–50.
5 Van der Waal I, Fehmers MCO, Kraal ER. Amyloidosis: its significance in oral surgery. Oral Surg 1973; **36**: 469–81.
6 Reinish EI, Raviv M, Srolovitz H, Gornitsky M. Tongue, primary amyloidosis, and multiple myeloma. Oral Surg 1994; **77**: 121–5.
7 Guccion JG, Redman RS, Winne CE. Hemodialysis-associated amyloidosis presenting as lingual nodules. Oral Surg 1989; **68**: 618–23.
8 Raymond AK, Sneige N, Batsakis JG. Amyloidosis in the upper aerodigestive tracts. Ann Otol Rhinol Laryngol 1992; **101**: 794–6.

Oral manifestations of systemic diseases

Oral manifestations can occasionally occur in many systemic diseases (Tables 66.24–66.38). Space precludes all but a brief tabular synopsis here. Further details can be found elsewhere [1–10].

REFERENCES

1 Jones JH, Mason DK, eds. Oral Manifestations of Systemic Disease, 2nd edn. London: Baillière-Tindall, 1990.

Table 66.25 Liver diseases.

Disease	Oral manifestations
Most liver diseases with jaundice	Bleeding tendency
	Jaundice
Alcoholic cirrhosis	Bleeding tendency
	Sialosis
Chronic active hepatitis	Lichen planus
Primary biliary cirrhosis	Sjögren's syndrome
	Lichen planus
Hepatitis C	Lichen planus
	Sjögren's syndrome

Table 66.26 Psychiatric disease.

Disease	Oral manifestations
Depression, hypochondriasis and various psychoses	Various complaints such as dry mouth, discharges, pain, disturbed taste and sensation
	Drug reactions
	Often multiple complaints
	Artefactual ulcers
Anxiety states	Cheek biting
	Bruxism (teeth grinding)
Bulimia	Tooth erosion

Table 66.24 Endocrine disorders.

Disease	Oral manifestations
Pituitary dwarfism	Microdontia
	Retarded tooth eruption
Congenital hypothyroidism	Macroglossia
	Retarded tooth eruption
Congenital hypoparathyroidism	Dental hypoplasia
	May be chronic candidiasis if associated immune defect
Gigantism/acromegaly	Spaced teeth
	Mandibular prognathism
	Macroglossia
	Megadontia (in gigantism)
Hyperparathyroidism	Bone rarefaction
	Brown tumours
Addison's disease	Mucosal hyperpigmentation
Diabetes mellitus	Periodontal disease
	Xerostomia
	Candidiasis
	Sialosis
	Lichen planus
Pregnancy	Gingivitis
	Epulis
Precocious puberty	Accelerated tooth eruption (fibrous dysplasia in Albright's syndrome)

Table 66.27 Drug effects.

Tissue	Drug effect	Drugs commonly implicated
Teeth	Discoloration	Tetracyclines
		Chlorhexidine
	Root anomalies	Phenytoin
		Cytotoxic drugs
Gingiva	Swelling	Phenytoin
		Ciclosporin
		Nifedipine
		Diltiazem
Salivary glands	Dry mouth	Tricyclic antidepressants
		Phenothiazines
		Antihypertensives
		Lithium
Taste	Disturbed	Metronidazole
		Penicillamine
Facial movements	Dyskinesias	Phenothiazines
		Metoclopramide
Mucosa	Thrush	Broad-spectrum antimicrobials
		Corticosteroids
		Cytotoxic drugs
	Ulcers	Cytotoxic drugs
		Non-steroidal anti-inflammatory agents
	Lichenoid lesions	Non-steroidal anti-inflammatory agents
	Erythema multiforme	Barbiturates
		Sulphonamides

Table 66.28 Gastrointestinal diseases.

Disease	Oral manifestations
Pernicious anaemia	Ulcers
	Glossitis
	Angular stomatitis
	Red lesions
Any cause of malabsorption	Ulcers
	Glossitis
	Angular stomatitis
Any cause of regurgitation	Tooth erosion
	Halitosis
Tylosis	Leukoplakia
Crohn's disease (and orofacial granulomatosis)	Facial swelling
	Mucosal tags
	Gingival hyperplasia
	Cobblestoning of mucosa
	Ulcers
	Glossitis
	Angular stomatitis
Coeliac disease	Ulcers
	Glossitis
	Angular stomatitis
	Dental hypoplasia
Peutz–Jegher syndrome (small intestinal polyps)	Melanosis
Chronic pancreatitis	Sialosis (rarely)
Cystic fibrosis	Salivary gland swelling
Gardner's syndrome (familial colonic polyposis)	Osteomas

Table 66.29 Renal diseases.

Disease	Oral manifestations
Chronic renal failure of any cause	Xerostomia
	Halitosis/taste disturbance
	Leukoplakia
	Dental hypoplasia in children
	Renal osteodystrophy
	Bleeding tendency (especially if anticoagulated)
Post renal transplant (immunosuppressed)	Infections, particularly herpetic and candidal
	Bleeding tendency if anticoagulated
	Gingival hyperplasia if on ciclosporin
	Kaposi's sarcoma (rarely)
	Hairy leukoplakia (rarely)
Nephrotic syndrome	Dental hypoplasia
Renal rickets (vitamin D resistant)	Delayed tooth eruption
	Dental hypoplasia (rarely)
	Enlarged pulp

2 Scully C, Flint S, Porter SR. *Colour Atlas of Oral Diseases*. London: Martin Dunitz, 1996.

3 Millard HD, Mason DK. *1998 World Workshop on Oral Medicine*. Michigan: University of Michigan, 2000.

4 Scully C, Cawson RA. Oral medicine. *Med Int* 1986; **28**: 1129–51.

5 Scully C, Cawson RA. *Medical Problems in Dentistry*, 4th edn. Oxford: Wright, 1998.

6 Scully C, Cawson RA. *Colour Aids to Oral Medicine*. Edinburgh: Churchill Livingstone, 1988.

7 Scully C, Porter SR. Oral medicine. *Med Int* 1990; **76**: 3145–74.

8 Porter SR, Scully C. HIV: the surgeon's perspective. *Br J Oral Maxillofac Surg* 1994; **32**: 222–47 (3 parts).

Table 66.30 Haematological diseases.

Disease	Oral manifestations
Deficiency of the haematinics (iron, folic acid or vitamin B_{12})	Burning mouth sensation Ulcers Glossitis Angular stomatitis
Sickle-cell anaemia	Jaw deformities Osteomyelitis or pain
Thalassaemia major	Jaw deformities
Aplastic anaemia	Ulcers Bleeding tendency
Haemolytic disease of newborn	Tooth pigmentation Enamel defects
Any leukocyte defect	Infections, especially herpetic and candidal Ulcers
Any cause of purpura	Bleeding tendency Purpura
Leukaemia/lymphoma	Infections Ulcers Bleeding tendency and purpura (in leukaemias only) Gingival swelling in myelomonocytic leukaemia
Multiple myeloma	Bone pain Tooth mobility Amyloidosis
Amyloid disease	Enlarged tongue Purpura

Table 66.31 Cardiovascular diseases.

Disease	Oral manifestations
Any disorder causing right-to-left shunt, e.g. Fallot's tetralogy	Cyanosis Delayed tooth eruption
Angina pectoris	Pain referred to jaw
Hereditary haemorrhagic telangiectasia	Telangiectasis
Giant cell arteritis (cranial or temporal arteritis)	Tongue pain or necrosis
Polyarteritis nodosa	Ulcers
Any disorder in which anticoagulants are used	Bleeding tendency
Hypertension	Dry mouth and other problems caused by some antihypertensives, e.g. gingival hyperplasia (nifedipine or diltiazem), lichenoid lesions (methyldopa and others)

9 Scully C, Welbury RA, Flaitz C, Almeida ODP. *A Colour Atlas of Orofacial Diseases in Children and Adolescents*. London: Martin Dunitz, 2001.
10 Scully C, Samaranayake LP. *Clinical Virology in Oral Medicine and Dentistry*. Cambridge: Cambridge University Press, 1992.

Acquired lip lesions

Cheilitis

SYN. INFLAMMATION OF THE LIPS

Cheilitis may arise as a primary disorder of the vermilion zone or the inflammation may extend from nearby skin or, less often, from the oral mucosa (Table 66.39) [1].

REFERENCE

1 Scully C, Bagan JV, Eisen D, Porter S, Rogers RS. *Dermatology of the Lips*. Oxford: Isis Medical Media, 2000.

'Chapping' of the lips

Chapping is a reaction to adverse environmental conditions usually caused by exposure to freezing cold or to hot dry winds. The keratin of the vermilion loses its plasticity, so that the lips become sore, cracked and scaly. The affected person tends to lick the lips, or to pick at the scales, which may aggravate the condition.

Table 66.32 Primary and secondary immunodeficiencies.

Disease	Oral manifestations
Severe combined immunodeficiency	Candidiasis
	Viral infections
	Ulcers
	Absent tonsils
	Recurrent sinusitis
Sex-linked agammaglobulinaemia	Ulcers
	Recurrent sinusitis
	Absent tonsils
Common variable immunodeficiency	Recurrent sinusitis
	Candidiasis
Selective IgA deficiency	Tonsillar hyperplasia
	Ulcers
	Viral infections
	Parotitis
DiGeorge's syndrome	Abnormal facies
	Candidiasis
	Viral infections
	Bifid uvula
Ataxia-telangiectasia	Recurrent sinusitis
	Ulcers
	Telangiectasia
Wiskott–Aldrich syndrome	Candidiasis
	Viral infections
	Purpura
Hereditary angio-oedema	Swellings
Chronic benign neutropenia	Ulcers
	Severe periodontitis
Cyclic neutropenia	Ulcers
	Severe periodontitis
	Eczematous lesions of the face
Chronic granulomatous disease	Candidiasis
	Enamel hypoplasia
	Acute gingivitis
	Ulcers
Myeloperoxidase deficiency	Candidiasis
Chédiak–Higashi syndrome	Ulcers
	Periodontitis
Job's syndrome	Abnormal facies
Secondary immune defects	Ulcers
	Periodontitis
	Candidiasis
	Viral infections
	Malignant neoplasms
	Hairy leukoplakia

Table 66.33 Metabolic disorders.

Disease	Oral manifestations
Congenital hyperuricaemia (Lesch–Nyhan syndrome)	Self-mutilation
Mucopolysaccharidoses	Spaced teeth
	Retarded tooth eruption
	Cystic radiolucencies
	Temporomandibular joint anomalies
	Enamel defects
	Gingival hyperplasia
Niemann–Pick disease	Retarded tooth eruption
	Loosening of teeth
	Mucosal pigmentation
Mucolipidoses	Gingival hyperplasia
Hypophosphatasia	Loosening and loss of teeth
Erythropoietic porphyria	Reddish teeth
	Bullae/erosions
	Dental hypoplasia
Amyloidosis	Macroglossia
	Purpura
Vitamin B_{12} or folic acid deficiency	Ulcers
	Glossitis
	Angular stomatitis
Scurvy	Gingival swelling
	Purpura
	Ulcers
Rickets (vitamin D dependent)	Dental hypoplasia
	Large pulp chambers
	Large tooth eruption

Table 66.34 Collagen–vascular diseases.

Disease	Oral manifestations
Any collagen–vascular disease	Sjögren's syndrome
Rheumatoid arthritis	Temporomandibular arthritis
	Drug reaction (e.g. lichenoid)
	Ulcers in Felty's syndrome
	Temporomandibular ankylosis in juvenile arthritides
Lupus erythematosus	White lesions
	Ulcers
Systemic sclerosis	Stiffness of lips, tongue, etc.
	Trismus
	Telangiectasia
	Mandibular condylar resorption
	Periodontal ligament widened on X-ray

Treatment is by application of petroleum jelly and avoidance of the adverse environmental conditions.

Eczematous cheilitis

The lips are often involved secondarily to atopic eczema (see Chapter 18). The treatment is with emollients and topical corticosteroids. A potent steroid such as fludrocortisone may be required to bring the condition under control.

Contact cheilitis

Contact cheilitis is an inflammatory reaction provoked by the irritant or sensitizing action of chemicals. Many cases are caused by lipsticks or lipsalves but a large number of substances have been incriminated.

Lipsticks and lipsalves (Table 66.40). Lipsticks are composed of mineral oils and wax (which form the stick), castor oil as a solvent for the dyes, lanolin as an emollient, preservatives, perfumes and colours [1]. The dyes may include azo dyes and eosin, a bromofluorescein derivative. An eosin

Table 66.35 Miscellaneous disorders.

Disease	Oral manifestations
Sarcoidosis	Xerostomia
	Salivary gland swelling
	Heerfordt's syndrome (parotid swelling, lacrimal swelling, facial palsy)
	Gingival swelling
Behçet's syndrome	Ulcers like aphthae
Sweet's syndrome	Ulcers like aphthae
Reiter's syndrome	Ulcers
Langerhans' cell histiocytosis	Loosening of teeth
	Jaw radiolucencies
Wegener's granulomatosis	Gingival swellings
	Ulcers
Kawasaki disease (mucocutaneous lymph node syndrome)	Sore tongue
	Cheilitis
Ellis–van Creveld syndrome (chondroectodermal dysplasia)	Multiple fraena
	Short roots
	Hypodontia
Tuberous sclerosis	Enamel defects
	Gingival fibromatosis

Table 66.36 Other infections.

Disease	Oral manifestations
Syphilis	Chancre
	Mucous patches
	Ulcers
	Gumma
	Pain from neurosyphilis
	Leukoplakia
	Lymph node enlargement
	Hutchinson's teeth in congenital syphilis
Gonorrhoea	Pharyngitis (occasionally)
	Gingivitis (occasionally)
	Temporomandibular arthritis (rarely)
Tuberculosis (including atypical mycobacteria)	Ulcers (rarely)
Leprosy	Cranial nerve palsies (rarely)
Lyme disease	Facial palsy
Candidiasis	White lesions
	Red lesions
	Angular stomatitis
Cryptococcosis	Ulcers
Coccidioidomycosis	Ulcers
Histoplasmosis	Ulcers (especially in immune defects)
Blastomycosis	Ulcers
Paracoccidioidomycosis	Ulcers
Mucormycosis, aspergillosis	Antral infections or ulcers (especially in immune defects)

Table 66.37 Viral infections.

Disease	Oral manifestations
Herpes simplex	Ulcers in primary infection
	Gingivitis in primary infection
	Vesicles on lips in recurrence (rarely oral ulcers)
Herpes zoster–varicella	Ulcers in chickenpox, or in zoster of maxillary or mandibular divisions of the trigeminal nerve
	Pain in maxillary or mandibular zoster
Coxsackieviruses and echoviruses	Ulcers in herpangina and hand, foot and mouth disease
Epstein–Barr virus (in infectious mononucleosis)	Sore throat
	Tonsillar exudate
	Palatal petechiae
	Recurrent parotitis (possibly)
	Hairy leukoplakia
Measles	Koplik's spots
Mumps	Salivary gland swelling
Papillomaviruses	Warts
	Papillomas
	Focal epithelial hyperplasia
Human immunodeficiency virus	
Common	Candidiasis
	Hairy leukoplakia
	Gingival and periodontal disease
	Herpes simplex infection
	Herpes zoster infection
	Papillomavirus infection
	Kaposi's sarcoma
	Aphthous-like ulcers
	Xerostomia
Uncommon	Infections
	Cryptococcus
	Mycobacteria
	Histoplasma
	Cytomegalovirus
	Others
	Salivary gland swelling
	Sjögren's syndrome-like disease
	Cranial neuropathies
	Fetal AIDS syndrome

impurity used to be an important sensitizer [2] but is now rarely if ever used. Other ingredients occasionally incriminated include azo dyes, carmine, oleyl alcohol [3], lanolin, perfumes, azulene, propyl gallate, sesame oil [4], stearates [5], shellac and colophony [6]. Sunscreens in lip-stick or lipsalve (e.g. cinnamic aldehyde) can also cause contact cheilitis [7]. Phenyl salicylate and antibiotics have also been incriminated [8,9]. Petrolatum chapsticks may cause an unusual form of acne with a single row of large open comedones along the cutaneous margin of the upper lip [10].

Mouthwashes and dentrifices [11]. Sensitizers used in some toothpastes include essential oils, such as peppermint, cinnamon, clove and spearmint; carvone along with imonene, pinene, phellandrene, dipentene, cineole, linalool, and esters of dihydrocuminyl alcohol and dehydrocarveol; bactericidal agents; propolis, derived from resin collected by bees [12,13]; and tartar-control dentifrices, which contain pyrophosphate compounds [14].

Table 66.38 Neurological disorders.

Disease	Oral manifestations
Facial palsy of any cause	Palsy and poor natural cleansing of mouth on same side
Trigeminal neuralgia	Pain
Bulbar palsy	Fasciculation of tongue
Parkinsonism	Drooling
	Tremor of tongue
	Dysarthria
Neurosyphilis	Pain (rarely)
	Dysarthria
	Tremor of tongue
Cerebral palsy	Spastic tongue
	Dysarthria
	Attrition
	Periodontal disease
Choreoathetosis	Green staining of teeth in kernicterus
	Hypoplasia of deciduous dentition in congenital rubella
Epilepsy	Trauma to teeth/jaws/mucosa
	Gingival hyperplasia if taking phenytoin
Down's syndrome	Delayed tooth eruption
	Macroglossia
	Scrotal tongue
	Maxillary hypoplasia
	Anterior open bite
	Hypodontia
	Periodontal disease
	Cleft lip or palate in some

Table 66.39 Causes of cheilitis.

Chapping due to cold and wind
Eczematous cheilitis
Contact cheilitis
Drug-induced cheilitis
Infective cheilitis
Angular cheilitis
Ultraviolet irradiation
   Actinic cheilitis
   Actinic prurigo of the lip
Glandular cheilitis
Granulomatous cheilitis
Exfoliative (factitious) cheilitis
Plasma cell cheilitis
Nutritional cheilitis
Dermatoses
Trauma

Table 66.40 Possible allergens in lipsticks and lipsalves.

Azo dyes
Azulene
Benzoic acid
Carmine
Castor oil
Cinnamon
Colophony
Eosin
Ester gum
Eusolex
Lanolin
Oleyl alcohol
Oxybenzone p-tertiary-butylphenol
Phenyl salicylate
Propolis
Propyl gallate
Ricinoleic acid
Salol
Sesame oil
Shellac
Vanilla
Wax

Table 66.41 Possible fruit and vegetable allergens.

Apple
Artichoke
Asparagus
Banana
Carrot
Celery
Cherry
Fennel
Garlic
Kiwi fruit
Lemon
Lime
Mango
Onion
Orange
Parsley
Parsnip
Peach
Pear
Pineapple
Plum
Potato
Tomato

Dental preparations. Mercury, eugenol, and plastics including epimine-containing materials can cause cheilitis [15–17].

Foods (Table 66.41). Peppermint, carvone, spearmint [18], citrus fruits [19], artichokes [20], nuts [21], pineapple [22], mangoes [23–25], asparagus [26] and cinnamon oil [27,28] occasionally cause allergic cheilitis and perioral dermatitis. The oil on the peel of citrus fruits is irritant to the skin; in addition, some sweet oranges contain a weakly phototoxic agent that can cause a reaction in pale-skinned people [29].

Miscellaneous objects. Metal hair clips, metal pencils, the cobalt paint on blue pencils [30], nail varnish [31], and the metal, wooden, nickel and reed mouthpieces of musical instruments [32–34] may cause cheilitis.

Clinical features. Lipstick cheilitis is sometimes confined to the vermilion but more often extends beyond. There may be persistent irritation and scaling or a more acute reaction with oedema and vesiculation.

The other forms of cheilitis vary greatly in their clinical appearance. Those caused by foods commonly also involve the skin around the mouth. If a small, sucked object is responsible, the reaction may be confined to one part of the lips.

Diagnosis. If acute eczematous changes are obviously present, the diagnosis of contact cheilitis presents no difficulty. If the changes are confined to irritation and scaling, the various forms of exfoliative cheilitis must be excluded.

If an allergic reaction is suspected, patch tests should be carried out.

Treatment. Topical corticosteroids will give symptomatic relief but the offending substance must be identified and avoided.

REFERENCES

1 Cronin E. *Contact Dermatitis.* Edinburgh: Churchill Livingstone, 1980: 141.
2 Calnan CD, Sarkany I. Studies in contact dermatitis II. Lipstick cheilitis. *Trans Rep St John's Hosp Derm Soc Lond* 1957; **39**: 28–36.
3 Calnan CD, Sarkany I. Studies in contact dermatitis XII. Sensitivity to oleyl alcohol. *Trans Rep St John's Hosp Derm Soc Lond* 1960; **44**: 47–50.
4 Hayakawa R, Matsunaga K, Suzuki M *et al.* Is sesamol present in sesame oil? *Contact Dermatitis* 1987; **17**: 133–5.
5 Hayakawa R, Matsunaga K, Suzuki M *et al.* Lipstick dermatitis due to C_{18} aliphatic compounds. *Contact Dermatitis* 1987; **16**: 215–9.
6 Rademaker M, Kirby JD, White IR. Contact cheilitis to shellac, Lampol 5 and colophony. *Contact Dermatitis* 1987; **15**: 307–8.
7 Maibach HJ. Cheilitis: occult allergy to cinnamic aldehyde. *Contact Dermatitis* 1986; **15**: 106–7.
8 Hindson C. Phenyl salicylate in a lip salve. *Contact Dermatitis* 1980; **6**: 216.
9 Marchand B, Barbier P, Ducombs G *et al.* Allergic contact dermatitis to various salols (phenyl salicylates). A study in man and guinea-pig. *Arch Dermatol Res* 1982; **272**: 61–6.
10 Shelley WB, Shelley ED. Chapstick acne. *Cutis* 1986; **37**: 459–60.
11 Fisher AA. *Contact Dermatitis,* 2nd edn. Philadelphia: Lea & Febiger, 1973: 320.
12 Trevisar G, Kokelj F. Contact dermatitis from propolis: role of gastrointestinal absorption. *Contact Dermatitis* 1987; **16**: 48.
13 Young E. Contact dermatitis from sensitivity to propolis. *Contact Dermatitis* 1987; **16**: 49.
14 Beacham BE, Kurgansky D, Gould WM. Circumoral dermatitis and cheilitis caused by tartar control dentifrices. *J Am Acad Dermatol* 1990; **22**: 1029–32.
15 Duxbury AJ, Turner EP, Watts DC. Hypersensitivity to epimine containing dental materials. *Br Dent J* 1979; **147**: 331–3.
16 Kulenkamp D, Hausen BM, Schulz KH. Kontakt Allergie durch neuartige, zahnartzlich verwendete Abdruckmaterialien. *Hautarzt* 1977; **28**: 353–8.
17 Maurice PD, Hopper C, Punnia-Moorthy A *et al.* Allergic contact stomatitis and cheilitis from iodoform used in a dental dressing. *Contact Dermatitis* 1988; **18**: 114–6.
18 Hjorth N, Jervoe P. Allergies to essential oils. *Tandlaegeblader* 1967; **71**: 937.
19 Schur A. Dermatitis venenata: report of a case due to the osage orange. *Arch Dermatol Syphil* 1932; **26**: 312–3.
20 Pindborg JJ. Disorders of the oral cavity and lips. In: Rook AJ, Wilkinson DS, Ebling FJ, eds. *Textbook of Dermatology,* 2nd edn. Oxford: Blackwell Scientific Publications, 1972: 1672–721.
21 Siegal S. Local allergic oedema induced by procaine. *J Allergy* 1958; **29**: 329–35.
22 Polunin J. Pineapple dermatosis. *Br J Dermatol* 1951; **63**: 441–55.
23 Kirby-Smith JL. Mango dermatitis. *Am J Trop Med* 1938; **18**: 373–84.
24 Asai T. About mango-dermatitis. *Jpn J Dermatol Urol* 1939; **46**: 44–5.
25 Brown A, Brown FR. Mango dermatitis. *J Allergy* 1941; **12**: 310–1.
26 Halberg V. Tilfaetden af aspargedermatitis. *Hospitalstid* 1932; **75**: 1235–41.
27 Leifer W. Contact dermatitis due to cinnamon. *Arch Dermatol Syphil* 1951; **64**: 52–5.
28 Miller J. Cheilitis from sensitivity to oil of cinnamon present in bubble gum. *JAMA* 1941; **116**: 131–2.
29 Volden G, Krokan H, Kavli G. Phototoxic and contact toxic reactions of the exocarp of sweet oranges: a common cause of cheilitis? *Contact Dermatitis* 1983; **9**: 201–4.
30 Bruynzeel DP. A child with perioral eczema. *Contact Dermatitis* 1987; **16**: 43.
31 Cronin E. *Contact Dermatitis.* Edinburgh: Churchill Livingstone, 1980: 154.
32 Hausen BM, Bruhn G, Koenig WA. New hydroxyisoflavans as contact sensitizers in cocus wood *Brya ebenus* DC (Fabaceae). *Contact Dermatitis* 1991; **25**: 149–55.
33 Friedman SJ, Connolly SM. Clarinettists' cheilitis. *Cutis* 1986; **38**: 183–4.
34 Bischof RD. Drum and bugle corps: medical issues and problems. *Med Prob Perform Art* 1994; **9**: 131–6.

Drug-induced cheilitis

Haemorrhagic crusting of the lips (Fig. 66.71) is a feature of erythema multiforme (particularly in Stevens–Johnson syndrome) (see p. 66.67), but cheilitis can also occur as an isolated feature of a drug reaction.

Aromatic retinoids such as etretinate and isotretinoin cause cheilitis, dryness and cracking of the lips in many patients.

Infective cheilitis

Viral. Rare viral infections such as orf [1,2] and vaccinia [3] can affect the lips.

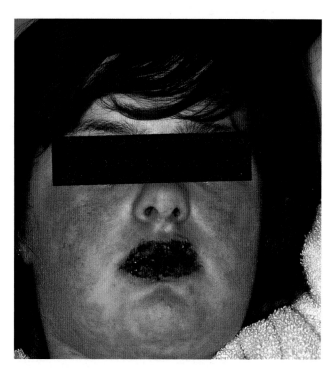

Fig. 66.71 Haemorrhagic crusting of the lips in Stevens–Johnson syndrome.

Bacterial. Dental infection or occasionally a furuncle or carbuncle may cause swelling of the lip. Impetigo may mimic herpes labialis (see Chapter 27). Cancrum oris (fusospirochaetal infection) may cause labial and buccal necrosis [4,5].

The lip is the most common extragenital site for a primary syphilitic lesion. Most lip chancres in males tend to occur on the upper lip, in females on the lower lip. In secondary syphilis, moist, flat, papulonodular lesions (condylomata lata) often appear at the mucocutaneous junctions and on mucosal surfaces especially at the commissures [6]. The tropical treponematoses may present similarly to syphilis.

Rhinoscleroma initially affects the nasal mucosa but may spread slowly to the upper lip, producing plaques or nodules with sunken centres. The extreme hardness of the infiltrations is characteristic. The lip can appear to fuse to the alveolar process but the overlying skin and mucosa remain normal.

Protozoal. Cutaneous or mucocutaneous leishmaniasis typically causes swellings on the upper lip with later enlargement and destruction of the lip [7–10], reflecting the three stages of oedema, granulomatous proliferation and then necrosis.

Fungal. Blastomycosis and paracoccidioidomycosis are uncommon causes of chronic ulceration affecting the lip, producing very similar clinical lesions to leishmaniasis [11].

Others. Red swollen lips with fissuring and exfoliation are prominent in mucocutaneous lymph node syndrome (Kawasaki disease).

REFERENCES

1 Parnell AG. Ecthyma contagiosum (orf). *Br J Oral Surg* 1965; **3**: 128–35.
2 Meechan JG, MacLeod RI. Human labial orf: a case report. *Br Dent J* 1992; **173**: 343–4.
3 Scully C. Vaccinia of the lip. *Br Dent J* 1977; **143**: 57–9.
4 Enwonwu CO. Infectious oral necrosis (cancrum oris) in Nigerian children. *Community Dent Oral Epidemiol* 1985; **13**: 190–4.
5 Sawyer D, Nwoku AJ. Cancrum oris (noma): past and present. *J Dent Child* 1981; **48**: 138–41.
6 Manton SL, Eggleston SI, Alexander I, Scully C. Oral presentation of secondary syphilis. *Br Dent J* 1986; **160**: 237–8.
7 Sitheeque MA, Quazi AA, Ahmed GA. A study of cutaneous leishmaniasis: involvement of the lips and perioral tissues. *Br J Oral Maxillofac Surg* 1990; **28**: 43–6.
8 Asvesti C, Anastassiadis G, Kolokotronis A, Zographakis I. Oriental sore: a case report. *Oral Surg* 1992; **73**: 56–8.
9 Sangueza OP, Sangueza JM, Stiller MJ, Sangueza P. Mucocutaneous leishmaniasis: a clinicopathological classification. *J Am Acad Dermatol* 1993; **28**: 927–32.
10 Ramesh V, Mirra RS, Saxena U, Mukherjee A. Post-kala-azar dermal leishmaniasis: a clinical and therapeutic study. *Int J Dermatol* 1993; **32**: 272–5.
11 Spostos R, Scully C, Almeida OPD *et al.* Oral paracoccidioidomycosis: a study of 36 South American patients. *Oral Surg Oral Med Oral Pathol* 1993; **75**: 461–5.

Angular cheilitis
SYN. ANGULAR STOMATITIS

Angular cheilitis is an acute or chronic inflammation of the skin and contiguous labial mucous membrane at the angles of the mouth [1].

Aetiology. Most cases in adults are due to mechanical and/or infective causes, but in children nutritional or immune defects are more prominent causes.

Infective agents. These are the major cause. *Candida* or staphylococci are isolated from most patients [2–4]. Permanent cure can be achieved only by eliminating the *Candida* beneath the upper denture [5]. Candidiasis was probably responsible for some of the cases of cheilitis attributed to allergy to denture materials, since contamination of denture material by *Candida* may cause false-positive patch-test reactions [6].

Immune deficiency, such as diabetes and HIV infection, may present with angular stomatitis. Outbreaks of acute pustular and fissured cheilitis may occur in children, particularly if they are malnourished, and in some cases streptococci or staphylococci have appeared to be causative [7].

Mechanical factors in edentulous patients who do not wear a denture or who have inadequate dentures, and also as a normal consequence of the ageing process, produce an oblique curved fold and keep the small area of skin constantly macerated. The recurrent trauma of dental flossing is a very rare cause of angular cheilitis [8].

Nutritional deficiencies, particularly deficiencies of riboflavin, folate, iron and general protein malnutrition, may produce smooth, shiny, red lips associated with angular stomatitis, a combination called *cheilosis* [1,9–11]. Crohn's disease or orofacial granulomatosis may be found in some [12].

Clinical features. Angular cheilitis presents as a roughly triangular area of erythema and oedema at one, or more commonly both, angles of the mouth (Fig. 66.72). Linear furrows or fissures radiating from the angle of the mouth (rhagades) are seen in the more severe forms, especially in denture wearers.

Diagnosis. This is usually obvious. *Candida* should be sought not only in the lesions but also beneath the denture.

Treatment. Dentures should be removed from the mouth at night and stored in a candidacidal solution such as hypochlorite. Denture-related stomatitis should be treated with an antifungal. Miconazole may be preferable

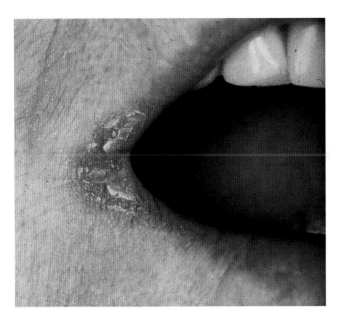

Fig. 66.72 Angular cheilitis.

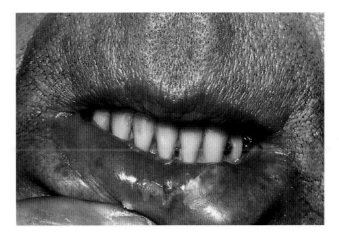

Fig. 66.73 Chronic actinic cheilitis with leukoplakia. (Courtesy of Addenbrooke's Hospital, Cambridge, UK.)

treatment for candidiasis (cream applied locally, together with the oral gel) as it has some Gram-positive bacteriostatic action. New dentures that restore facial contour may help. The skin lesions should be swabbed and staphylococcal infection treated with fusidic acid ointment or cream at least four times daily.

REFERENCES

1 Schoenfeld RJ, Schoenfeld FI. Angular cheilitis. *Cutis* 1977; **19**: 213–6.
2 Ohman SC, Dahlen G, Moller A *et al.* Angular cheilitis: a clinical and microbial study. *J Oral Pathol* 1986; **15**: 213–7.
3 MacFarlane TW, Helnarska SJ. The microbiology of angular cheilitis. *Br Dent J* 1976; **140**: 403.
4 Dahlen G. A retrospective study of microbiologic samples from oral mucosal lesions. *Oral Surg* 1982; **53**: 350–4.
5 Scully C. Chronic atrophic candidiasis. *Lancet* 1986; **ii**: 437–8.
6 Salo OP, Hirvonen ML. Yeasts as a cause of false-positive reactions in patch-tests for allergy to dental materials. *Br J Dermatol* 1969; **81**: 338–41.
7 MacFarlane TW, McGill JC, Samaranayake LB. Antibiotic testing and phage typing of *Staphylococcus aureus* isolated from non-hospitalized patients with angular cheilitis. *J Hosp Infect* 1984; **5**: 444–6.
8 Kahana M, Yakalom M, Yakalom R *et al.* Recurrent angular cheilitis caused by dental flossing. *J Am Acad Dermatol* 1986; **15**: 113–4.
9 Murphy NC, Bissada NF. Iron deficiency: an overlooked predisposing factor in angular cheilitis. *J Am Dent Assoc* 1979; **99**: 640–1.
10 Rose JA. Aetiology of angular cheilosis: iron metabolism. *Br Dent J* 1968; **125**: 67–72.
11 Parodi A, Priano L, Rebora A. Chronic zinc deficiency in a patient with psoriasis and alcoholic liver cirrhosis. *Int J Dermatol* 1991; **30**: 45–7.
12 Wiesenfeld D, Ferguson MM, Mitchell DN *et al.* Orofacial granulomatosis: clinical and pathological analysis. *Q J Med* 1985; **213**: 101–13.

Actinic cheilitis

SYN. ACTINIC KERATOSIS OF LIP; SOLAR CHEILOSIS

This is a premalignant keratosis of the lip caused by exposure to solar irradiation.

Aetiology. Actinic cheilitis is most common in hot dry regions, in outdoor workers and in fair-skinned people (skin types I and II). The vermilion of the lower lip receives a high dose of UV irradiation because it is almost at right angles to the rays of the midday sun and is poorly protected by keratin and melanocytes. Most actinic cheilitis is seen on the lower lip of fair-skinned men in their fourth to eighth decade of life.

Pathology. Histology shows a flattened or atrophic epithelium, beneath which is a band of inflammatory infiltrate in which plasma cells may predominate [1]. Nuclear atypia and abnormal mitoses may be seen in the more severe cases, and some develop into invasive squamous carcinoma [2]. The collagen generally shows basophilic (elastotic) degeneration [3].

Clinical features (Fig. 66.73). Actinic cheilitis tends to affect the lower lip of adults who have had prolonged exposure to sunlight [4]. In the early stages there may be redness and oedema, but later the lips become dry and scaly. Later still, the epithelium becomes palpably thickened with small greyish-white plaques and, eventually, warty nodules may form. Eventually these may undergo malignant change, the possibility of which must always be considered when ulceration develops or when there are other suspect features such as:
• a red and white, blotchy appearance with an indistinct vermilion border;
• generalized atrophy with focal areas of whitish thickening;
• persistent flaking and crusting [5,6].

Diagnosis. This is clinical.

Treatment. Treatment of actinic cheilitis is required to relieve symptoms and to prevent development of squamous carcinoma.

- Topical agents: 5% fluorouracil three times daily for 10 days is suitable [7]. Topical tretinoin [8] or trichloracetic acid [9] may also be effective.
- Vermilionectomy (lip shave) [10–12].
- Laser ablation [13–16].

Following treatment, prevention of recurrence by the regular use of a sunscreen lipsalve containing *p*-aminobenzoic acid probably gives the best protection [17,18].

Particular care should be taken to protect the vermilion of the lips with adequate sunscreens in patients with photosensitivity disorders, such as xeroderma pigmentosum, and in those whose exposure to UVB is high, such as mountaineers, windsurfers and skiers.

REFERENCES

1 Koten JW. Histopathology of actinic cheilitis. *Dermatologica* 1967; **135**: 465–71.
2 Picascia DD, Robinson JK. Actinic cheilitis, a review of the aetiology, differential diagnosis and treatment. *J Am Acad Dermatol* 1987; **17**: 255–64.
3 Schmitt CK. Histologic evaluation of degenerative changes of the lower lip. *J Oral Surg* 1968; **26**: 51–6.
4 Cotaldo E. Solar cheilitis. *J Dermatol Surg Oncol* 1981; **7**: 289–95.
5 La Riviere W, Pickett AB. Clinical criteria in diagnosis of early squamous carcinoma of the lower lip. *J Am Dent Assoc* 1979; **99**: 972–7.
6 Birt AR, Hogg GR. The actinic cheilitis of hereditary polymorphic light eruption. *Arch Dermatol* 1979; **115**: 699–702.
7 Epstein E. Treatment of actinic cheilitis with topical fluorouracil. *Arch Dermatol* 1977; **113**: 906–8.
8 Kligman A. Topical tretinoin: indications, safety and effectiveness. *Cutis* 1987; **39**: 486–8.
9 Turk LL, Winder PR. Carcinomas of the skin and their treatment. *Semin Oncol* 1980; **7**: 376–84.
10 Birt BD. The lip-shave operation for premalignant conditions of the lower lip. *Otolaryngology* 1977; **6**: 407–11.
11 Robinson JK. Actinic cheilitis: a prospective study comparing four treatment methods. *Arch Otolaryngol Head Neck Surg* 1989; **115**: 848–52.
12 Sanchez-Conejo-Mir J, Perez-Bernal AM, Mormo-Jiminez JC *et al.* Follow-up of vermilionectomies. *J Dermatol Surg Oncol* 1986; **12**: 180–4.
13 David LM. Laser vermilion ablation for actinic cheilitis. *J Dermatol Surg Oncol* 1984; **11**: 605–8.
14 Dufresne RG, Garrett AB, Bailin PL, Ratz JL. Carbon dioxide laser treatment of chronic actinic cheilitis. *J Am Acad Dermatol* 1988; **19**: 876–8.
15 Stanley RJ. Actinic cheilitis: treatment with the carbon dioxide laser. *Mayo Clin Proc* 1988; **63**: 230–5.
16 Zelickson BD, Roenigk RK. Actinic cheilitis: treatment with the carbon dioxide laser. *Cancer* 1990; **65**: 1307–11.
17 Lundeen RC, Langlais RP. Sunscreen protection for lip mucosa. A review and update. *J Am Dent Assoc* 1985; **11**: 617–21.
18 Payne TE. An evaluation of actinic blocking agents for the protection of lip mucosa. *J Am Dent Assoc* 1976; **92**: 409–11.

Actinic prurigo (see Chapter 24)

Actinic prurigo is a type of familial photodermatitis, seen mainly in native Americans living at high altitudes [1,2] especially in Latin America, and in China [3]. It usually presents in young women as a photosensitive facial rash with pruritic lower lip cheilitis, and it may be associated with conjunctivitis, eyebrow alopecia and pterygia.

Actinic prurigo is due to enhanced sensitivity to sunlight and is distinguished from actinic cheilitis, which is due to prolonged and excessive exposure to UV irradiation, by the relative absence of epidermal dysplasia and solar elastosis [4]. Polymorphous light eruption is almost invariably present in the actinic prurigo of native Americans [5,6].

Treatment is with sunscreens, β-carotene, psoralen and UVA (PUVA), and antihistamines. Oral thalidomide may be tried [7].

REFERENCES

1 Birt AR, Davis RA. Hereditary polymorphic light eruption of American Indians. *Int J Dermatol* 1975; **14**: 105–11.
2 Scheen SR, Connolly SM, Dicken CH. Actinic prurigo. *J Am Acad Dermatol* 1981; **5**: 183–90.
3 Guogi X, Yiming H, Huibao S *et al.* Pruritic cheilitis: six cases. *Oral Surg* 1983; **55**: 359–62.
4 Herrera-Goepfert R, Magana M. Follicular cheilitis. *Am J Dermatopathol* 1995; **17**: 357–61.
5 Calnan CD, Meara RH. Actinic prurigo (Hutchinson's summer prurigo). *Clin Exp Dermatol* 1977; **2**: 365–77.
6 Mounsden T, Kratochvil T, Auclair P *et al.* Actinic prurigo of the lower lip. Review of the literature and report of 5 cases. *Oral Surg Oral Med Oral Pathol* 1988; **65**: 327–32.
7 Londono F. Thalidomide in the treatment of actinic prurigo. *Int J Dermatol* 1973; **12**: 323–8.

Glandular cheilitis

Definition. Glandular cheilitis is characterized by inflammatory changes and swelling of salivary glands in the lips [1–3].

Aetiology. This is an uncommon idiopathic condition which in a few cases has apparently been familial [4]. Although it was originally thought that the condition was due to inflammation of enlarged heterotopic salivary glands, the glands are often normal in size, depth and histology [5]. It is possible that the excessive salivary secretion from minor salivary glands in this condition might be an unusual clinical response to irritation of the lip from some other cause such as actinic damage or repeated licking.

Pathology. In the milder forms there is some fibrosis surrounding the salivary glands, while in the more severe forms there may be a dense chronic inflammatory infiltrate. Only rarely do patients show genuine hyperplasia of the salivary glands or duct ectasia.

Clinical features. The onset is at any age from childhood onwards. In simple glandular cheilitis, the lower lip is slightly thickened and bears numerous pinhead-sized orifices, from which mucous saliva can readily be squeezed. The upper lip is rarely involved [6].

In the more severe suppurative form (*Volkmann's cheilitis*) the lip is considerably and permanently enlarged, and subject to episodes of pain, tenderness and increased enlargement. The surface is covered by crusts and scales, beneath which the salivary duct orifices may be discovered. In the most severe forms there may be deep-seated infection with abscess formation and fistulous tracts.

The condition can evidently be premalignant; in some series 20–30% of cases progress to squamous cancer. This does, of course, support the suggestion that in many cases glandular cheilitis is a consequence of actinic cheilitis [5].

Treatment. Actinic cheilitis, if identified, should be treated appropriately. If the lips are grossly enlarged, excision of an elongated ellipse of tissue may be required; in other cases shave vermilionectomy may be all that is necessary. Other conditions such as atopic disease or factitial cheilitis would require different treatment.

REFERENCES

1 Rada DC. Cheilitis glandularis. A disorder of ductal ectasia. *J Dermatol Surg Oncol* 1985; **1**: 372–5.
2 Stuller CB, Schaberg SJ, Stokos J. Cheilitis glandularis. *Oral Surg* 1982; **53**: 602–5.
3 Thiele B, Mahrle G, Ippen H. Cheilitis glandularis simplex. *Hautarzt* 1983; **34**: 232–4.
4 Weir TW, Johnson WC. Cheilitis glandularis. *Arch Dermatol* 1971; **103**: 433–7.
5 Swerlick RA, Cooper PH. Cheilitis glandularis: a re-evaluation. *J Am Acad Dermatol* 1984; **10**: 466–72.
6 Winchester L, Scully C, Prime SS, Eveson JW. Cheilitis glandularis: a case affecting the upper lip. *Oral Surg Oral Med Oral Pathol* 1986; **62**: 654–6.

Granulomatous cheilitis

SYN. MIESCHER'S CHEILITIS

Definition. A chronic swelling of the lip due to granulomatous inflammation of unknown cause.

Nomenclature. Melkersson in 1928 [1] described labial oedema in association with recurrent facial palsy. Rosenthal in 1930 emphasized the role of genetic factors and added scrotal tongue to the syndrome. The full syndrome has since been called Melkersson–Rosenthal syndrome [2].

In Miescher's cheilitis the granulomatous changes are confined to the lip, and this is generally regarded as a monosymptomatic form of Melkersson–Rosenthal syndrome, although the possibility remains that these may be two separate diseases.

Aetiology. The cause is unknown, but there may be a genetic predisposition to Melkersson–Rosenthal syndrome [3]; siblings have been affected and a scrotal tongue may be present in otherwise normal relatives.

There is no convincing evidence that granulomatous cheilitis is due to an infective agent. Some cases may represent a localized form of sarcoidosis [4] or ectopic Crohn's disease [5,6] or orofacial granulomatosis. There is increasing evidence that some patients with granulomat-

ous cheilitis are predisposed to Crohn's disease [6]. In some cases, granulomatous cheilitis is followed some years later by regional ileitis [7–10]. A few patients react to cobalt [11] or to food additives such as cinnamic aldehyde [12–14] and have no extra oral lesions, although these reactions are by no means always relevant; for example, in one study only one of nine patients had a relationship between cheilitis and food intake [15].

Pathology. Biopsy of the swollen lip or facial tissues during the early stages of the disease shows only oedema and perivascular lymphocytic infiltration. In some cases of long duration no other changes are seen, but in others the infiltrate becomes more dense and pleomorphic and small focal granulomas are formed, indistinguishable from sarcoidosis or Crohn's disease. Similar changes may be present in cervical lymph nodes [16–19]. In some cases, small granulomas occur in the lymphatic walls [20].

Clinical features. The condition affects the sexes equally. The earliest manifestations usually develop in childhood or adolescence but may be delayed until middle or old age. The earliest cutaneous manifestation is sudden diffuse or nodular swellings [21] involving the upper lip, the lower lip and one or both cheeks in decreasing order of frequency [5,19]. Labial swelling occurs in about 75% and facial swelling in 50% of patients [22]. Less commonly, the forehead, eyelids or one side of the scalp may be involved. The attacks are sometimes accompanied by fever and mild constitutional symptoms, including headache and even visual disturbance. At the first episode the oedema typically subsides completely in hours or days, but after recurrent attacks the swelling may persist, and slowly increases in degree (Fig. 66.74). It gradually becomes firmer and eventually acquires the consistency of firm rubber. After some years, the swelling may very slowly regress.

A fissured or scrotal tongue is seen in 20–40% of cases. It is present from birth in some, which may indicate genetic susceptibility. There may be loss of sense of taste and decreased salivary gland secretion [19].

The regional lymph nodes are enlarged in 50% of cases [3] but not usually very greatly.

Facial palsy of the lower motor neurone type occurs in some 30% of cases. It may precede the attacks of oedema by months or years, but more commonly develops later. Although intermittent at first, the palsy may become permanent. It may be unilateral or bilateral, and partial or complete [19]. Other cranial nerves (olfactory, auditory, glossopharyngeal and hypoglossal) may occasionally be involved. Involvement of the CNS has also been reported, but the significance of the resulting symptoms is easily overlooked as they are very variable, sometimes simulating disseminated sclerosis but often with a poorly defined association of psychotic and neurological features. Autonomic disturbances may occur.

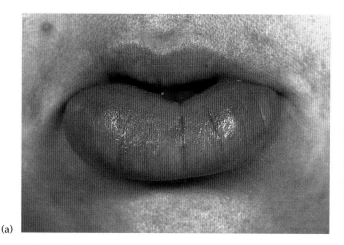

(a)

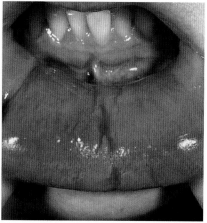

(b)

Fig. 66.74 Granulomatous cheilitis of the lower lip. (Courtesy of Addenbrooke's Hospital, Cambridge, UK.)

Diagnosis. The essential feature of the syndrome is the granulomatous swelling of lip or face. In the early attacks clinical differentiation from angio-oedema may be impossible in the absence of either scrotal tongue or facial palsy. Persistence of the swelling between attacks should suggest the diagnosis, which can sometimes be confirmed by biopsy. However, the histological changes are not always conspicuous or specific.

In established cases, other causes of macrocheilia (Table 66.42) must be excluded. Ascher's syndrome associated with blepharochalasia is likely to cause confusion, although the swelling of the lip is caused by redundant salivary tissue and is present from childhood. Lymphoma is a rare differential diagnosis [23].

Treatment. Reactions to dietary components should be sought and possible antigens avoided. The injection of up to 10 mL triamcinolone (10 mg/L) into the lips after local analgesia may be effective [15,24,25]. The injections may have to be repeated every 4–6 months once a response plateau has been reached. This treatment has also been successfully combined with surgical reduction (cheiloplasty) [26,27]. The injections must be continued periodically after the surgery or there may be an exaggerated recurrence of the condition. Surgery alone is relatively unsuccessful [28].

Systemic corticosteroids are rarely indicated [29]. Not all respond [27,30] and adverse effects may be a problem. Clofazimine appears to help the majority of patients [31,32], in a dose of 100 mg twice daily for 10 days, then twice weekly for 4 months. Metronidazole may also produce resolution in granulomatous cheilitis [33,34].

Other treatments which have occasionally been helpful include long-term penicillin, erythromycin, sulfasalazine (sulphasalazine) or ketotifen.

Table 66.42 Macrocheilia: acute or chronic enlargement of one or both lips.

Acute	Chronic
Traumatic	Developmental
Infective	Familial idiopathic
Pyococcal	Double lip
Anthrax	Ascher's syndrome
Diphtheria	Lymphangioma
Primary syphilis	Haemangioma
Trichophytosis	Neurofibroma
Leishmaniasis	Mucopolysaccharidoses
Herpes simplex	Fucosidosis
Trichiniasis	Coffin–Siris syndrome
Angio-oedema	Acquired
Erythema multiforme	Post-traumatic
Actinic cheilitis	Post-infective on basis of developmental
Other forms of cheilitis	lymphatic defect
	Infective
	Tuberculosis
	Leprosy
	Rhinoscleroma
	Leishmaniasis
	Neoplastic
	Melkersson–Rosenthal syndrome
	Cheilitis glandularis
	Sarcoidosis
	Crohn's disease
	Orofacial granulomatosis

REFERENCES

1 Melkersson E. Case of recurrent facial paralysis with angio-neurotic edema. *Hygien* 1928; **90**: 737–41.

2 Wadlington WB, Riley HD, Lowbeer I. The Melkersson–Rosenthal syndrome. *Pediatrics* 1984; **73**: 502–6.

3 Hornstein OP. Melkersson–Rosenthal syndrome: a neuro-mucocutaneous disease of complex origin. *Curr Probl Dermatol* 1973; **5**: 117–56.

4 Shedade SA, Foulds IS. Granulomatous cheilitis and a positive Kveim test. *Br J Dermatol* 1986; **115**: 619–22.

5 Tatnall FM, Dodd HJ, Sarkany I. Crohn's disease with metastatic cutaneous involvement and granulomatous cheilitis. *J R Soc Med* 1987; **80**: 49–50.

6 Kano Y, Shiohara T, Yagita A, Nagashima M. Association between cheilitis granulomatosa and Crohn's disease. *J Am Acad Dermatol* 1993; **28**: 801.

7 Carr D. Granulomatous cheilitis in Crohn's disease. *BMJ* 1974; **iv**: 636.

8 Talbot T, Jewell L, Schloss E *et al*. Cheilitis antedating Crohn's disease. Case report and literature review. *J Clin Gastroenterol* 1984; **6**: 349–54.
9 Verbov JL. The skin in patients with Crohn's disease and ulcerative colitis. *Trans Rep St John's Hosp Derm Soc Lond* 1973; **59**: 30–8.
10 Wiesenfeld D, Ferguson MM, Mitchell DN *et al*. Orofacial granulomatosis: a clinical and pathological analysis. *Q J Med* 1985; **54**: 101–13.
11 Pryce DW, King CM. Orofacial granulomatosis associated with delayed hypersensitivity to cobalt. *Clin Exp Dermatol* 1990; **15**: 384–96.
12 McKenna KE, Walsh MY, Burrows D. The Melkersson–Rosenthal syndrome and food additive hypersensitivity. *Br J Dermatol* 1994; **131**: 921–2.
13 Patton DW, Ferguson MM, Forsyth A, James J. Orofacial granulomatosis: a possible allergic basis. *Br J Oral Maxillofac Surg* 1985; **23**: 235–42.
14 Sweatman MC, Tasker R, Warner JO *et al*. Orofacial granulomatosis response to elemental diet and provocation by food additives. *Clin Allergy* 1986; **16**: 331–8.
15 Sakuntabhai A, MacLeod RI, Lawrence CM. Intralesional steroid injection after nerve block anaesthesia in the treatment of orofacial granulomatosis. *Arch Dermatol* 1993; **129**: 477–80.
16 Hernandez G, Hernandez F, Lucas M. Miescher's granulomatous cheilitis: literature review. *J Oral Maxillofac Surg* 1986; **44**: 474–8.
17 Kint A, De Brauwere D. Cheilitis granulomatosa und Crohnsche Krankheit. *Hautarzt* 1977; **28**: 319–21.
18 Rhodes EL, Stirling GA. Granulomatous cheilitis. *Arch Dermatol* 1965; **92**: 40–4.
19 Worsaae N, Christensen KC, Schiodt M. Melkersson–Rosenthal syndrome and cheilitis granulomatosa. *Oral Surg* 1982; **54**: 404–13.
20 Nozicka Z. Endovasal granulomatous lymphangitis as a pathogenetic factor in cheilitis granulomatosa. *J Oral Pathol* 1985; **14**: 363–5.
21 Ficarra G, Cicchi P, Amorosi A, Piluso S. Oral Crohn's disease and pyostomatitis vegetans. *Oral Surg Oral Med Oral Pathol* 1993; **75**: 220–4.
22 Zimmer WM, Rogers RS, Reeve CM, Sheridan PJ. Orofacial manifestations of Melkersson–Rosenthal syndrome. *Oral Surg* 1992; **74**: 610–9.
23 Scully C, Eveson JW, Witherow H *et al*. Oral presentation of lymphoma: case report of T-cell lymphoma masquerading as oral Crohn's disease, and review of the literature. *Oral Oncol* 1993; **29B**: 225–30.
24 Cermale D, Serri F. Intralesional injection of triamcinolone in the treatment of cheilitis granulomatosa. *Arch Dermatol* 1963; **72**: 695–6.
25 Williams AJK, Wray D, Ferguson A. The clinical entity of orofacial Crohn's disease. *Q J Med* 1991; **79**: 451–8.
26 Eisenbud L, Hymowitz S, Shapiro R. Cheilitis granulomatosa. *Oral Surg Oral Med Oral Pathol* 1971; **32**: 384–9.
27 Krutchkoff D, James R. Cheilitis granulomatosa: successful treatment with combined local triamcinolone injections and surgery. *Arch Dermatol* 1978; **114**: 1203–6.
28 Scully C, Cochran KM, Russell RI *et al*. Oral Crohn's disease as an indicator of intestinal involvement. *Gut* 1982; **23**: 198–201.
29 Williams PM, Greenberg MS. Management of cheilitis granulomatosa. *Oral Surg* 1991; **72**: 436–9.
30 Allen CM, Camisa C, Hamzeh S, Stephens L. Cheilitis granulomatosa: report of six cases and review of the literature. *J Am Acad Dermatol* 1990; **23**: 444–50.
31 Neuhofer J, Fritsch P. Cheilitis granulomatosa: therapy with clofazimine. *Hautarzt* 1984; **35**: 459–63.
32 Podmore P, Burrows D. Clofazimine: an effective treatment for Melkersson–Rosenthal syndrome or Miescher's cheilitis. *Clin Exp Dermatol* 1986; **11**: 173–8.
33 Kano Y, Shiohara T, Yagita A. Treatment of recalcitrant cheilitis granulomatosa with metronidazole. *J Am Acad Dermatol* 1992; **27**: 629–30.
34 Scully C, Eveson JW. Oral granulomatosis. *Lancet* 1991; **338**: 20–1.

Exfoliative cheilitis
SYN. FACTITIOUS CHEILITIS; LE TIC DE LÈVRES

Exfoliative cheilitis is a chronic superficial inflammatory disorder of the vermilion borders of the lips characterized by persistent scaling (Fig. 66.75). The diagnosis is now restricted to those few patients whose lesions cannot be attributed to other causes, such as contact sensitization or light (see actinic cheilitis, p. 66.115). Many of these cases

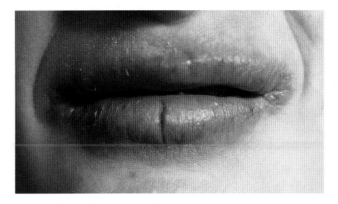

Fig. 66.75 Factitious cheilitis due to repeated lip sucking.

are now thought to be factitious, owing to repeated lip sucking, chewing or other manipulation of the lips [1,2]. There is no association with dermatological or systemic disease, although rare cases are seen in HIV infection. Some are infected with *Candida* species [3].

Most cases occur in girls or young women, and the majority have a personality disorder [4,5]. The process, which often starts in the middle of the lower lip and spreads to involve the whole of the lower or both lips, consists of scaling and crusting, more or less confined to the vermilion border, and persisting in varying severity for months or years. The patient often complains of irritation or burning, and can be observed frequently biting or sucking the lips. In some cases the condition appears to start with chapping or with atopic eczema, and develops into a habit tic.

In a large Russian series, almost half the cases had associated thyroid disease [6], but this observation has not been confirmed.

Diagnosis. Contact and active cheilitis must be carefully excluded. Chronic exfoliative cheilitis is readily contaminated by *Candida*. In such cases the clinical features are variable and may simulate carcinoma, LP or lupus erythematosus.

Treatment. Some cases resolve spontaneously [2,7] or with improved oral hygiene [8]. Reassurance and topical corticosteroids may be helpful in some cases [1], but others require psychotherapy or tranquillizers [7,9].

REFERENCES

1 Thomas JR, Greene SL, Dicken CH. Factitious cheilitis. *J Am Acad Dermatol* 1983; **8**: 368–72.
2 Daley TD, Gupta AK. Exfoliative cheilitis. *J Oral Pathol Med* 1995; **24**: 177–9.
3 Reade PC, Rich AM, Hay KD, Radden BG. Cheilo-candidiasis: a possible clinical entity. *Br Dent J* 1982; **152**: 305–8.
4 Jeanmougin M, Civatte J, Bertail MA. Cheilites squamo-crouteuses factices. *Ann Dermatol Vénéréol* 1984; **111**: 1007–11.
5 Reade PC, Sim R. Exfoliative cheilitis: a factitious disorder? *Int J Oral Maxillofac Surg* 1986; **15**: 313–7.

6 Kutin SA. Clinical aspects and pathogenesis of exfoliative cheilitis. *Vestn Dermatol Venerol* 1970; **44**: 39–43.

7 Postlethwaite KR, Hendrickse MA. A case of exfoliative cheilitis. *Br Dent J* 1988; **165**: 23.

8 Brooke RI. Exfoliative cheilitis. *Oral Surg* 1978; **45**: 52–5.

9 Crotty CP, Dicken CH. Factitious lip crusting. *Arch Dermatol* 1981; **117**: 338–40.

Plasma cell cheilitis

SYN. PLASMA CELL ORIFICIAL MUCOSITIS

Plasma cell cheilitis is an idiopathic benign inflammatory condition, characterized by dense plasma cell infiltrates in the lips and other mucosae close to body orifices [1–3]. The condition has been reported (under a wide variety of names) to affect the penis, vulva, lips, buccal mucosa, palate, gingiva, tongue, epiglottis and larynx.

Plasma cell cheilitis is the counterpart of Zoon's plasma cell balanitis (see Chapter 68). It presents as circumscribed flat or elevated patches of erythema, usually on the lower lip in an elderly person. The cause is unknown, but it responds to the application of powerful topical cortico-steroids such as clobetasol, or to the intradermal injection of triamcinolone [4], or to systemic griseofulvin [5].

A similar lesion, which tends to form a tumorous mass with a hyperkeratotic surface and needs to be differentiated from extramedullary plasmacytoma [6], has been called *plasma-acanthoma* [7,8].

REFERENCES

1 Baughman RD. Plasma cell cheilitis. *Arch Dermatol* 1974; **110**: 725–6.

2 Luders G. Plasmacytosis mucosae: Ein oft verkanntes neues Krankheitsbild. *Munch Med Wochenschr* 1972; **114**: 8–12.

3 White JW, Olsen KD, Banks PM. Plasma cell orificial mucositis. Report of a case and review of the literature. *Arch Dermatol* 1986; **122**: 1321–4.

4 Jones SK, Kennedy CTC. Response of plasma cell orificial mucositis to topically applied steroids. *Arch Dermatol* 1988; **124**: 1871–2.

5 Tamaki K, Osada A, Tsukamato K, Ohtake N, Furue M. Treatment of plasma cell cheilitis with griseofulvin. *J Am Acad Dermatol* 1994; **30**: 789–90.

6 Burke WA, Merritt CC, Briggaman RA. Disseminated extramedullary plasmacytomas. *J Am Acad Dermatol* 1986; **14**: 335–9.

7 Ferreira-Marques J. Beitrag zur Kenntnis der Plasmocytosis circumorificialis (Scheuermann) 'Plasmoakanthoma'. *Arch Klin Exp Dermatol* 1962; **215**: 151–64.

8 Ramos E, Silva J. Das Plasmoakanthom. *Hautarzt* 1965; **16**: 7–11.

Lupus erythematosus

Involvement of the vermilion zone is quite common in both discoid erythematosus and SLE [1]. Discoid lupus can be premalignant, and should be treated vigorously with topical steroid ointments and sunscreens [2,3]. The cheilitis of SLE tends to be more severe, with erosions and haemorrhagic crusts.

Lupus erythematosus can be very difficult to distinguish from LP of the lips, both clinically and by histology (Fig. 66.76).

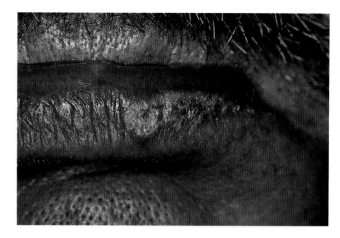

Fig. 66.76 Discoid lupus erythematosus of the lower lip.

REFERENCES

1 Coulson IH, Marsden RA. Lupus erythematosus cheilitis. *Clin Exp Dermatol* 1986; **11**: 309–13.

2 Martin S, Rosen T, Locker E. Metastatic squamous cancer of lips. Occurrence in Blacks with discoid lupus erythematosus. *Arch Dermatol* 1979; **115**: 1214.

3 Fotos PG, Finkelstein MW. Discoid lupus erythematosus of the lip and face. *J Oral Maxillofac Surg* 1992; **50**: 642–5.

Sarcoidosis (see Chapter 58)

Sarcoidosis may cause chronic violaceous lesions on, or swelling of, the lips [1].

REFERENCE

1 James DG. Lupus pernio. *Lupus* 1992; **1**: 129–31.

Lip fissure

A lip fissure may develop when a patient, typically a child, is mouth-breathing (Fig. 66.77). Otherwise the aetiology may be obscure, though sun, wind, cold weather and smoking are thought to predispose. A hereditary predisposition for weakness in the first branchial arch fusion seems to exist.

Lip fissures are common in Down's syndrome and the lips may also crack in this way if swollen, for example in cheilitis granulomatosa [1–4].

Clinical features. Most lip fissures are seen in males, typically median in the lower lip and chronic, causing discomfort and possibly bleeding from time to time. Contrary to the clinical impression that fissures are seen only in the lower lip, there is also a high prevalence in the upper lip.

Diagnosis. The diagnosis is clinical.

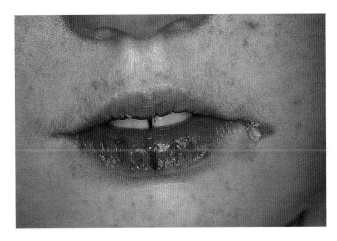

Fig. 66.77 Lip fissure.

Management. Predisposing factors should be managed. Bland creams may help the lesion heal spontaneously. Otherwise, local applications of 1–2% silver nitrate, 0.5% balsam of Peru, salicylic acid and topical antimicrobials seem less effective than excision, preferably with a Z-plasty [5–7] or cryosurgery [8].

REFERENCES

1 Axell T, Skoglund A. Chronic lip fissures. *Int J Oral Surg* 1981; **10**: 354–8.
2 Ball G, Barnard D. The treatment of chronic lip fissures with cryotherapy. *Br Dent J* 1984; **157**: 64–6.
3 Dingman RO. Chronic fissure of the lower lip. *Plast Reconstr Surg* 1948; **3**: 613.
4 Ecker H. Medial clefts of the lips. *Am J Surg* 1958; **96**: 815.
5 Scully C, Van Bruggen W, Dios PD, Porter SR, Davison M. Down syndrome: lip lesions and *Candida albicans*. *Br J Dermatol* 2002; **147**: 37–40.
6 Maisels DO. Chronic lip fissures. *Br J Dermatol* 1969; **81**: 621–2.

7 Rashid N, Yusuf H. Median lip fissures and their management. *Int J Oral Maxillofac Surg* 1997; **26**: 299–300.
8 Rosenquist B. Median lip fissure: etiology and suggested treatment. *Oral Surg* 1991; **72**: 10–4.

Lip ulcer due to calibre-persistent artery

A calibre-persistent artery is defined as an artery with a diameter larger than normal near a mucosal or external surface. When such arteries occur in the gut wall (Dieulafoy malformation) they may bleed, but in the lip they tend to cause chronic ulceration that can be mistaken for a squamous cancer. The ulcer is attributed to continual pulsation from the large artery running parallel to the surface, although the exact mechanism is obscure [1,2].

Ligation of the artery appears successful [3].

REFERENCES

1 Mike T, Adler P, Endes P. Simulated cancer of lower lip attributed to a 'calibre-persistent artery'. *J Oral Pathol* 1980; **9**: 137–44.
2 Marshall RI, Leppard BJ. Ulceration of the lip associated with a 'calibre-persistent artery'. *Br J Dermatol* 1985; **113**: 757–60.
3 Lovas JGL, Goodday RHB. Clinical diagnosis of calibre-persistent labial artery of the lower lip. *Oral Surg* 1993; **76**: 480–3.

Reactive perforating collagenosis (see Chapter 46)

Crateriform papules of the lower lip have been reported in reactive perforating collagenosis [1].

REFERENCE

1 Trattner A, Lueber A, Sandbank M. Mucosal involvement in reactive perforating collagenosis. *J Am Acad Dermatol* 1991; **25**: 1079–81.

Chapter 67

The Breast

D.A. Burns

The terms 'breasts' and 'mammary glands' are often accepted as equivalent, but they are not strictly synonymous, because the breasts contain tissues (fat, vessels, nerves, etc.) other than the glandular elements.

In the evolutionary sense, the mammary glands are believed to be related to the apocrine sweat glands. They develop from ectodermal mammary ridges ('milk lines'). The classical view, derived from comparative anatomy, that the mammary ridges extend from the base of the upper limb bud to the base of the lower limb bud, is now questioned. It is considered that the mammary ridge extends only over the axillopectoral area [1].

The skin of the breast does not differ structurally from that of the neighbouring chest wall, but the skin of the nipple and areola is very highly specialized. There are individual and racial variations in the size, shape and colour of the nipple and areola. The periphery of the areola contains hair follicles, and the development of coarse terminal hairs in this site may be a cosmetic problem for some women.

The nipple is glabrous. Lactiferous ducts and sebaceous glands open only at its tip. Sensory nerve end organs are also confined to the tip of the nipple. The areola has clusters of large sebaceous glands [2] and the so-called tubercles of Montgomery. These elevations on the areola are produced by the glands of Montgomery [3]. Each of these is a combined sebaceous unit and lactiferous gland, with the lactiferous duct opening into the sebaceous duct close to the areola or occasionally directly onto the areola [1]. The glands of Montgomery are an integral part of the lactiferous apparatus, secreting milk during lactation.

The development of the breasts at puberty requires oestrogens and progesterone, and, in a more minor role, insulin, growth hormone, corticosteroids and prolactin. The adult breast consists of several lobes, each of which is drained by a ductal system ending in a lactiferous duct which opens at the nipple. Each lobe contains up to 40 lobules, and each lobule 10–100 alveoli, the basic secretory units [1].

The breasts enlarge during pregnancy, and the veins become prominent. The areolae also enlarge and become darker. This pigmentation decreases after parturition but does not fade completely.

Although most of the more serious diseases of the breast come within the province of the surgeon, the gynaecologist or the endocrinologist, there are some diseases which affect only the breast skin and are wholly the concern of the dermatologist, and others which may involve the skin and present difficult problems in differential diagnosis.

REFERENCES

1 Hughes LE, Mansel RE, Webster DJT. *Benign Disorders and Diseases of the Breast*, 2nd edn. London: Saunders, 2000.
2 Montagna W. Histology and cytochemistry of human skin, 35: the nipple and areola. *Br J Dermatol* 1970; **83**: 2–13.
3 Montagna W, Yun JS. The glands of Montgomery. *Br J Dermatol* 1972; **86**: 126–33.

Supernumerary breasts or nipples [1,2]

Supernumerary (accessory) breasts (polymastia) and the far more common supernumerary nipples (polythelia) usually develop along the course of the milk lines. Accessory glandular tissue most frequently occurs in the axillae [3], but rarely breast components occur in other sites [4–6].

Accessory breast tissue may consist of nipple, areola or glandular tissue singly, or in any combination (Fig. 67.1). The condition is very common in women, with an incidence of around 2–4%, although in the majority of cases the accessory nipple is insignificant, appearing as a small brown papule, usually on the chest wall, just below the breast. Much more rarely, the condition occurs in men, and in one case a fully developed breast was located on the posterior aspect of the thigh of a male [7]. A familial incidence is sometimes noted [8,9].

Polythelia has been found in association with various rare genodermatoses [10–17]. A suggested association between the presence of supernumerary nipples and urinary tract anomalies in children [18–20] prompted debate about whether to investigate the renal tract in children

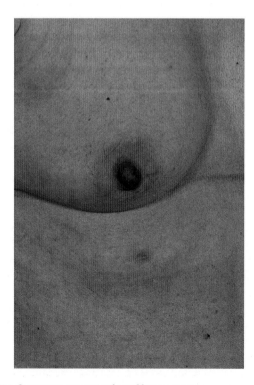

Fig. 67.1 Supernumerary nipple and breast tissue.

with supernumerary nipples and no other obvious anomaly [21,22]. However, more recent publications have not demonstrated an association between supernumerary nipples and urinary tract malformations [23,24].

The Simpson–Golabi–Behmel syndrome is an X-linked overgrowth syndrome caused by deletions in glypican 3. It is characterized by a specific facial appearance, supernumerary nipples, polydactyly, midline defects and mild mental retardation [25].

An accessory nipple is usually recognized if the diagnosis is considered, but is often otherwise confused with a pigmented naevus. If functional breast tissue is present, enlargement at puberty or in pregnancy may be embarrassing or painful. Simple excision is advisable, as carcinoma may occur.

REFERENCES

1 Grossl NA. Supernumerary breast tissue: historical perspectives and clinical features. *South Med J* 2000; **93**: 29–32.
2 Velanovich V. Ectopic breast tissue, supernumerary breasts, and supernumerary nipples. *South Med J* 1995; **88**: 903–6.
3 Jordan K, Laumann A, Conrad S, Medenica M. Axillary mass in a 20-year-old woman. *Arch Dermatol* 2001; **137**: 1367–72.
4 Tow SH, Shanmugaratnam K. Supernumerary mammary gland in the vulva. *BMJ* 1962; **ii**: 1234–6.
5 Shewmake SW, Izuno GT. Supernumerary areolae. *Arch Dermatol* 1977; **113**: 823–5.
6 Leung W, Heaton JPW, Morales A. An uncommon urologic presentation of a supernumerary breast. *Urology* 1997; **50**: 122–4.
7 Camisa C. Accessory breast on the posterior thigh of a man. *J Am Acad Dermatol* 1980; **3**: 467–9.
8 Cellini A, Offidani A. Familial supernumerary nipples and breasts. *Dermatology* 1992; **185**: 56–8.
9 Galli-Tsinopoulou A, Krohn C, Schmidt H. Familial polythelia over three generations with polymastia in the youngest girl. *Eur J Pediatr* 2001; **160**: 375–7.
10 Hay RJ, Wells RS. The syndrome of ankyloblepharon, ectodermal defects and cleft lip and palate: an autosomal dominant condition. *Br J Dermatol* 1976; **94**: 277–89.
11 Wittebol-Post D, Hennekam RC. Blepharophimosis, ptosis, polythelia and brachydactyly (BPPB): a new autosomal dominant syndrome? *Clin Dysmorphol* 1993; **2**: 346–50.
12 Halper S, Rubenstein D. Aplasia cutis congenita associated with syndactyly and supernumerary nipples; report of a second family. *Pediatr Dermatol* 1991; **8**: 32–4.
13 Bonnekoh B, Wevers A, Spangenberger H *et al.* Keratin pattern of acanthosis nigricans in syndrome-like association with polythelia, polycystic kidneys and syndactyly. *Arch Dermatol* 1993; **129**: 117–82.
14 Sabry MA, Al-Saleh Q, Al-Saw'an R *et al.* Right upper limb bud triplication and polythelia, left sided hemihypertrophy and congenital hip dislocation, facial dysmorphism, congenital heart disease, and scoliosis: disorganization-like spectrum or patterning gene defect? *J Med Genet* 1995; **32**: 555–6.
15 Zannolli R, Mostardini R, Metera M *et al.* Char syndrome: an additional family with polythelia, a new finding. *Am J Med Genet* 2000; **95**: 201–3.
16 Marble M, Pridjian G. Scalp defects, polythelia, microcephaly, and developmental delay: a new syndrome with apparent autosomal dominant inheritance. *Am J Med Genet* 2002; **108**: 327–32.
17 Shafeghati Y, Karimi-Nejad A, Karimi-Nejad R. Supernumerary nipples in a Bartsocas–Papas patient in a consanguineous Iranian family. *Clin Dysmorphol* 1999; **8**: 155–6.
18 Varsano IB, Jaber L, Garty B-Z *et al.* Urinary tract abnormalities in children with supernumerary nipples. *Pediatrics* 1984; **73**: 103–5.
19 Méhes K, Pintér A. Minor morphological aberrations in children with isolated urinary tract malformations. *Eur J Pediatr* 1990; **149**: 339–402.
20 Meggyessy V, Méhes K. Association of supernumerary nipples with renal anomalies. *J Pediatr* 1987; **111**: 412–3.

21 Hersh J. Association of supernumerary nipples and renal anomalies. *Am J Dis Child* 1988; **142**: 591–2.
22 Mimouni F. Association of supernumerary nipples and renal anomalies. *Am J Dis Child* 1988; **142**: 591.
23 Jójárt G, Seres E. Supernumerary nipples and renal anomalies. *Int Urol Nephrol* 1994; **26**: 141–4.
24 Grotto I, Browner-Elhanan K, Mimouni D *et al.* Occurrence of supernumerary nipples in children with kidney and urinary tract malformations. *Pediatr Dermatol* 2001; **18**: 291–4.
25 Li M, Shuman C, Fei YL *et al.* GPC3 mutation analysis in a spectrum of patients with overgrowth expands the phenotype of Simpson–Golabi–Behmel syndrome. *Am J Med Genet* 2001; **102**: 161–8.

Breast hypertrophy

Unusually large breasts may be problematic for a number of reasons, and postural abnormalities, backache and psychological disturbance may prompt referral to a plastic surgeon for a reduction mammaplasty. A dermatologist may be consulted about associated problems such as submammary intertrigo.

Breast enlargement in the setting of human immunodeficiency virus (HIV) infection is a relatively recently described phenomenon. It may be a component of the lipodystrophy syndrome (lipomastia), or there may be true gynaecomastia (see below). Breast ultrasonography allows these two states to be differentiated [1].

REFERENCE

1 Qazi NA, Morlese JF, King DM *et al.* Gynaecomastia without lipodystrophy in HIV-1-seropositive patients on efavirenz: an alternative hypothesis. *AIDS* 2002; **16**: 506–7.

Gigantomastia (macromastia)

Gigantomastia is a condition in which the female breasts enlarge rapidly until they reach a tremendous size. The overlying skin may become inflamed, oedematous and tender, and there may be striae or even severe ulceration [1]. The condition may occur at puberty [2–4] or during pregnancy [1,5]. The aetiology is obscure, but a suggested cause is increased sensitivity of the breast tissue to normal levels of circulating hormones.

The condition is occasionally familial [6].

Penicillamine therapy can also cause gigantomastia [7,8].

Bromocriptine may be of benefit in patients in whom the condition occurs during pregnancy, but in many patients, and certainly in pubertal cases, reduction mammaplasty is usually required.

REFERENCES

1 Gargan TJ, Goldwyn RM. Gigantomastia complicating pregnancy. *Plast Reconstr Surg* 1987; **80**: 121–4.
2 Hollingsworth DR, Archer R. Massive virginal breast hypertrophy at puberty. *Am J Dis Child* 1973; **125**: 293–5.
3 O'Hare PM, Frieden IJ. Virginal breast hypertrophy. *Pediatr Dermatol* 2000; **17**: 277–81.
4 Arscott GDL, Craig HR, Gabay L. Failure of bromocriptine therapy to control juvenile mammary hypertrophy. *Br J Plast Surg* 2001; **54**: 720–3.
5 Stavrides S, Hacking A, Tiltman A, Dent DM. Gigantomastia in pregnancy. *Br J Surg* 1987; **74**: 585–6.
6 Kupfer D, Dingman D, Broadbent R. Juvenile breast hypertrophy: report of a familial pattern and review of the literature. *Plast Reconstr Surg* 1992; **90**: 303–9.
7 Passas C, Weinstein A. Breast gigantism with penicillamine therapy. *Arthritis Rheum* 1978; **21**: 167–8.
8 Kahl LE, Medsger TA Jr, Klein I. Massive breast enlargement in a patient receiving d-penicillamine for systemic sclerosis. *J Rheumatol* 1985; **12**: 990–1.

Gynaecomastia [1–4]

Gynaecomastia, which may be defined as benign enlargement of the male breast caused by proliferation of the glandular components, can occur as an isolated defect or as a manifestation of a wide range of different pathological states in which it may be a valuable diagnostic sign. The multiplicity of syndromes associated with gynaecomastia reflects the complexity of the hormonal mechanisms concerned in breast enlargement. The patient complains of enlargement of the breast, which may be unilateral or bilateral, and is often tender.

Gynaecomastia can be distinguished from fatty enlargement of the breast in obesity (pseudogynaecomastia) by grasping the breast between thumb and forefinger and moving the digits up towards the nipple with the patient supine. In gynaecomastia a rubbery, mobile, disc-like mound will be felt beneath the areola.

Oestrogens stimulate and androgens inhibit development of breast tissue, and gynaecomastia occurs as a result of a disturbance of the ratio of free androgen to free oestrogen, with a relative increase in oestrogen levels. Peripheral conversion of androgens to oestrogen by aromatization contributes to oestrogen production. Local susceptibility of hormone receptors or local hormone conversion presumably play a role in unilateral gynaecomastia.

The histopathological changes [5] are related to the duration of gynaecomastia and not to its cause. At early stages, there are active proliferating ducts in a vascular fibroblastic stroma. Later, there is progressive fibrosis and hyalinization, and the number of ducts is reduced.

Gynaecomastia may be either physiological or pathological. Some of the causes are listed in Table 67.1.

Physiological gynaecomastia

There are three peaks in the age distribution of physiological gynaecomastia. It occurs in most male neonates due to transplacental passage of oestrogen from the mother. It is usually bilateral, but may be unilateral, and it regresses spontaneously. Some enlargement of the breast occurs at puberty in about 38% of normal boys [6]. The peak incidence is around the age of 14 years. It is unilateral in about 25% of cases. The degree of enlargement is usually slight, but may be sufficient to cause embarrassment and

Table 67.1 Causes of gynaecomastia.

Physiological
  Neonatal
  Adolescent
  Old age
Endocrine disorders
  Hypogonadism, e.g. Klinefelter's syndrome
  Excess oestrogen or chorionic gonadotrophin, e.g. from testicular
    tumour
  Hyperthyroidism
Other diseases
  Starvation, cachexia or refeeding
  Renal disease and haemodialysis
  Liver disease
  Paraplegia
  Erythroderma
Idiopathic
Drugs (see Table 67.2)

Table 67.2 Drugs which may produce gynaecomastia.

Amiloride
Anabolic steroids
Antiandrogens, e.g. cyproterone acetate
Amiodarone
Amphetamines
Androgens
Busulphan
Cannabis
Captopril
Chorionic gonadotrophin
Cimetidine
Cytotoxic agents
Diazepam
Diethylpropion
Digitalis
Domperidone
Finasteride
Highly active antiretroviral therapy (HAART)
Isoniazid
Ketoconazole
Melatonin
Methyldopa
Metoclopramide
Methotrexate
Nifedipine
Nitrosoureas
Oestrogens
Omeprazole
Penicillamine
Phenothiazines
Phenytoin
Reserpine
Spironolactone
Tricyclic antidepressants
Vincristine

anxiety. Spontaneous regression usually takes place within a few months, but the enlargement occasionally persists for 2–3 years.

Gynaecomastia also appears to be frequent over the age of 65 years, increasing with age.

Gynaecomastia in endocrine disorders

Gynaecomastia occurs in a very wide range of endocrine disorders. Primary or secondary reduction of testicular androgen production is of special importance. Some tumours of the testis are associated with gynaecomastia, notably seminoma, Leydig cell tumour, Sertoli cell tumour and certain teratomas.

Gynaecomastia occurs in most men with Klinefelter's syndrome, and there is an increased risk of breast cancer in this syndrome [7,8], although other causes of gynaecomastia are not associated with an increased risk of cancer [1].

In other endocrine disorders, gynaecomastia is less common, but may occur in association with tumours or hyperplasia of the adrenal gland, pituitary tumours and hyperthyroidism [9].

Gynaecomastia in nutritional, metabolic, renal and hepatic disease

Gynaecomastia may occur during starvation or on resumption of a more adequate diet after prolonged starvation [10].

Chronic renal failure and haemodialysis may also be associated with gynaecomastia [11–13], although the incidence of gynaecomastia in dialysis patients has decreased in recent years.

Hepatic cirrhosis is usually listed as a cause of gynaecomastia, but one study found that palpable gynaecomastia was not a uniform feature in advanced cirrhosis, and that its prevalence was similar to that in a non-obese, non-cirrhotic, age-matched control population [14].

Gynaecomastia occasionally occurs in association with erythroderma [15].

Drug-induced gynaecomastia [16–33]

Drugs which may produce gynaecomastia are listed in Table 67.2.

They produce their effect by different mechanisms, for example spironolactone and cimetidine are antiandrogens, and neuroleptic drugs produce hyperprolactinaemia (Fig. 67.2). Testosterone might act by peripheral aromatization to oestrogens.

True gynaecomastia, as opposed to breast hypertrophy secondary to lipodystrophy syndrome, can occur with all currently available classes of antiretroviral agents. The mechanism responsible is unclear, but it has been proposed that it may be related to improvement in the T-helper cytokine response after starting highly active antiretroviral therapy (HAART) [28]. Cytokines produced

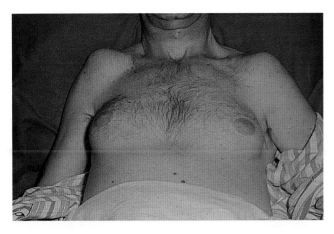

Fig. 67.2 Gynaecomastia in a man taking stilboestrol for carcinoma of the prostate.

during the immune restoration process have an effect on breast tissue, resulting in gynaecomastia. Once immune restoration has occurred, the cytokine levels fall, and the gynaecomastia resolves spontaneously.

Finasteride treatment of male androgenetic alopecia may be associated with gynaecomastia [29,30], and it has also been recorded in individuals who have used oestrogen-containing hair preparations [31,32] and in a men's hairdresser who had massaged the scalps of his balding customers with an oestrogen-containing lotion [33].

Management of gynaecomastia [3]

In the majority of patients, history and examination will suggest the likely cause of the gynaecomastia. Careful examination for underlying disease and a full drug history are required, particularly if the gynaecomastia is symptomatic, progressive or of recent onset in an adult, but it should be remembered that a large proportion of otherwise normal men have some slight gynaecomastia.

In unilateral disease, particularly in older men, breast cancer should be excluded.

Spontaneous resolution occurs in many 'physiological' cases, or following cessation of the causative drug when it is drug related.

For patients with considerable breast discomfort, or if the condition is severe enough to cause embarrassment, treatment with tamoxifen, clomiphene or danazol has been employed.

In extreme cases, subcutaneous mastectomy or liposuction may be performed by a plastic surgeon.

REFERENCES

1 Braunstein GD. Gynaecomastia. *N Engl J Med* 1993; **328**: 490–5.
2 Sizonenko PC. Gynaecomastia. In: Grossman A, ed. *Clinical Endocrinology*, 2nd edn. Oxford: Blackwell Science, 1998: 761–8.
3 Hughes LE, Mansel RE, Webster DJT. *Benign Disorders and Diseases of the Breast*, 2nd edn. London: Saunders, 2000.
4 Ismail AA, Barth JH. Endocrinology of gynaecomastia. *Ann Clin Biochem* 2001; **38**: 596–607.
5 Nicolis GL, Modlinger RS, Gabrilove JL. A study of the histopathology of human gynaecomastia. *J Clin Endocrinol Metab* 1971; **32**: 173–8.
6 Nydick M, Bustos J, Dale JH Jr, Rawson RW. Gynecomastia in adolescent boys. *JAMA* 1961; **178**: 449–54.
7 Scheike O, Visfeldt J, Peterson B. Male breast cancer: breast carcinoma in association with Klinefelter syndrome. *Acta Pathol Microbiol Scand* 1973; **81**: 352–8.
8 Smyth CM, Bremner WJ. Klinefelter syndrome. *Arch Intern Med* 1998; **158**: 1309–14.
9 Tan YK, Birch CR, Valerio D. Bilateral gynaecomastia as the primary complaint in hyperthyroidism. *J R Coll Surg Edin* 2001; **46**: 176–7.
10 Smith SR, Chhetri MK, Johanson AJ et al. The pituitary–gonadal axis in men with protein-calorie malnutrition. *J Clin Endocrinol Metab* 1975; **41**: 60–9.
11 Sawin CT, Longcope C, Schmitt GW, Ryan RJ. Blood levels of gonadotrophin and gonadal hormones in gynaecomastia associated with chronic haemodialysis. *J Clin Endocrinol Metab* 1973; **36**: 988–90.
12 Distiller LA, Morley JE, Sagel J et al. Pituitary–gonadal function in chronic renal failure: the effect of luteinizing hormone-releasing hormone and the influence of dialysis. *Metabolism* 1975; **24**: 711–20.
13 Davison AM, Cameron JS, Grünfeld JP et al., eds. *Oxford Textbook of Clinical Nephrology*, 2nd edn. Vol. 3. Oxford: Oxford University Press, 1998: 1874.
14 Cavanaugh J, Niewoehner CB, Nuttall FQ. Gynaecomastia and cirrhosis of the liver. *Arch Intern Med* 1990; **150**: 563–5.
15 Shuster S, Brown JB. Gynaecomastia and urinary oestrogens in patients with generalized skin disease. *Lancet* 1962; **ii**: 1358.
16 Dukes MNG, Aronson JK, eds. *Meyler's Side Effects of Drugs*. Amsterdam: Elsevier, 2000.
17 Antonelli D, Luboshitzky R, Gelbendorf A. Amiodarone-induced gynecomastia. *N Engl J Med* 1986; **315**: 1553.
18 Markusse HM, Meyboom RHB. Gynaecomastia associated with captopril. *BMJ* 1988; **296**: 1262–3.
19 Clyne CAC. Unilateral gynaecomastia and nifedipine. *BMJ* 1986; **292**: 380.
20 Tanner LA, Bosco LA. Gynecomastia associated with calcium channel blocker therapy. *Arch Intern Med* 1988; **148**: 379–80.
21 Reid DM, Martynoga AG, Nuki G. Reversible gynaecomastia associated with D-penicillamine in a man with rheumatoid arthritis. *BMJ* 1982; **285**: 1083–4.
22 Monson JP, Scott DF. Gynaecomastia induced by phenytoin in men with epilepsy. *BMJ* 1987; **294**: 612.
23 Trump DL, Pavy MD, Staal S. Gynecomastia in men following antineoplastic therapy. *Arch Intern Med* 1982; **142**: 511–3.
24 Turner AR, Morrish DW, Berry J, Macdonald N. Gynecomastia after cytotoxic therapy for metastatic testicular cancer. *Arch Intern Med* 1982; **142**: 896–7.
25 Del Paine DW, Leek JC, Jakle C, Robbins DL. Gynecomastia associated with low dose methotrexate therapy. *Arthritis Rheum* 1983; **26**: 691–2.
26 Thomas E, Leroux JL, Blotman F. Gynecomastia in patients with rheumatoid arthritis treated with methotrexate. *J Rheumatol* 1994; **21**: 1777–8.
27 De Bleecker JL, Lamont BH, Verstraete AG, Schelfhout VJ. Melatonin and painful gynaecomastia. *Neurology* 1999; **53**: 435–6.
28 Qazi NA, Morlese JF, King DM et al. Gynaecomastia without lipodystrophy in HIV-1-seropositive patients on efavirenz: an alternative hypothesis. *AIDS* 2002; **16**: 506–7.
29 Wade MS, Sinclair RD. Reversible painful gynaecomastia induced by low-dose finasteride. *Australas J Dermatol* 2000; **41**: 55.
30 Ferrando J, Grimalt R, Alsina M, Manasievska E. Unilateral gynecomastia induced by treatment with 1 mg of oral finasteride. *Arch Dermatol* 2002; **138**: 543–4.
31 Edidin DV, Levitsky LL. Prepubertal gynecomastia associated with estrogen-containing hair cream. *Am J Dis Child* 1982; **136**: 587–8.
32 Gabrilove JL, Luria M. Persistent gynecomastia resulting from scalp inunction of estradiol. *Arch Dermatol* 1978; **114**: 1672–3.
33 Cimorra GA, Gonzalez-Peirona E, Ferrandez A. Percutaneous oestrogen-induced gynaecomastia: a case report. *Br J Plast Surg* 1982; **35**: 209–10.

Black galactorrhoea

Galactorrhoea is sometimes caused by drugs such as phenothiazines. In one patient taking perphenazine, the droplets of milk were stained black, due to the concomitant administration of minocycline for acne [1]. The pigment which produces the black discoloration of breast milk in women taking minocycline is thought to be due to an iron chelate of minocycline within macrophages [2].

REFERENCES

1 Basler RSW, Lynch PJ. Black galactorrhea as a consequence of minocycline and phenothiazine therapy. *Arch Dermatol* 1985; **121**: 417–8.
2 Hunt MJ, Salisbury ELC, Grace J, Armati R. Black breast milk due to minocycline therapy. *Br J Dermatol* 1996; **134**: 943–4.

Hypomastia or amastia [1]

Very small breasts are fairly common in otherwise normal women, in whom they may cause considerable psychological distress. There is some evidence of an association between hypoplastic breasts (defined as a breast size of 200 mL or less) and mitral valve prolapse [1].

Becker's naevus is occasionally associated with unilateral breast hypoplasia [2,3], possibly as a result of high androgen-receptor activity on the affected side, and with areolar hypoplasia in males [4,5].

Unilateral symbrachydactyly and ipsilateral aplasia of the sternal head of the pectoralis major muscle, aplasia of the breast and absence of axillary hair, are features of the *Poland syndrome* [6].

Breast hypoplasia or aplasia is a feature of the *AREDYLD* (acrorenal field defect, ectodermal dysplasia, and lipoatrophic diabetes) *syndrome* [7].

REFERENCES

1 Rosenberg CA, Derman GH, Grabb WC, Buda AJ. Hypomastia and mitral-valve prolapse. *N Engl J Med* 1983; **309**: 1230–2.
2 Formigón M, Alsina MM, Mascaró JM, Rivera F. Becker's nevus and ipsilateral breast hypoplasia. Androgen-receptor study in two patients. *Arch Dermatol* 1992; **128**: 992–3.
3 Van Gerwen HJL, Koopman RJJ, Steijlen PM, Happle R. Becker's naevus with localized lipoatrophy and ipsilateral breast hypoplasia. *Br J Dermatol* 1993; **129**: 213.
4 Sharma R, Mishra A. Becker's naevus with ipsilateral areolar hypoplasia in three males. *Br J Dermatol* 1997; **136**: 471–2.
5 Crone AM, James MP. Giant Becker's naevus with ipsilateral areolar hypoplasia and limb asymmetry. *Clin Exp Dermatol* 1997; **22**: 240–1.
6 McKusick VA, ed. *Mendelian Inheritance in Man*, 11th edn, Vol. 2. Baltimore: Johns Hopkins University Press, 1994: 1168–9.
7 McKusick VA, ed. *Mendelian Inheritance in Man*, 11th edn, Vol. 2. Baltimore: Johns Hopkins University Press, 1994: 1634–5.

Morphoea [1]

If morphoea occurs on the chest wall prior to or during breast development, severe hypoplasia of the breast may result [2,3] (Fig. 67.3).

A feature of generalized morphoea is sparing of the nipples and areolae. Christianson *et al.* [4] noted that the skin was pinched or squeezed like 'rising biscuits on a platter' (Fig. 67.4).

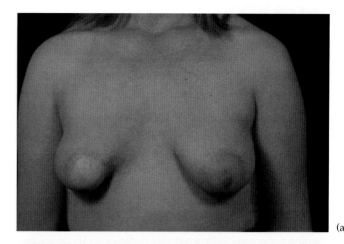

(a)

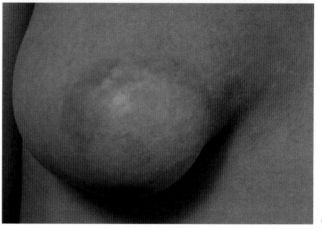

(b)

Fig. 67.3 (a, b) Breast hypoplasia associated with a plaque of morphoea which occurred during breast development.

There is a well-described occurrence of localized morphoea at the site of radiotherapy for breast cancer [5–9].

REFERENCES

1 Whitaker-Worth DL, Carlone V, Susser WS *et al.* Dermatologic diseases of the breast and nipple. *J Am Acad Dermatol* 2000; **43**: 733–51.
2 Treiber ES, Goldberg NS, Levy H. Breast deformity produced by morphoea in a young girl. *Cutis* 1994; **54**: 267–8.
3 Slavin SA, Gupta S. Reconstruction of scleroderma of the breast. *Plast Reconstr Surg* 1997; **99**: 1736–41.
4 Christianson HB, Dorsey CS, O'Leary PA, Kierland RR. Localized scleroderma: a clinical study of two hundred thirty-five cases. *Arch Dermatol* 1956; **74**: 629–39.
5 Neill SM, Nicholl JJ, Hanham IWF, Staughton RCD. Localized morphoea at site of previous radiotherapy. *Br J Dermatol* 1988; **119** (Suppl. 33): 110–1.
6 Colver GB, Rodger A, Mortimer PS *et al.* Post-irradiation morphoea. *Br J Dermatol* 1989; **120**: 831–5.
7 Verbov J. Post-irradiation morphoea. *Br J Dermatol* 1989; **121**: 819–20.
8 Trattner A, Figer A, David M *et al.* Circumscribed scleroderma induced by postlumpectomy radiation therapy. *Cancer* 1991; **68**: 2131–3.
9 Davis DA, Cohen PR, McNeese MD, Duvic M. Localized scleroderma in breast cancer patients treated with supervoltage external beam radiation: radiation port scleroderma. *J Am Acad Dermatol* 1996; **35**: 923–7.

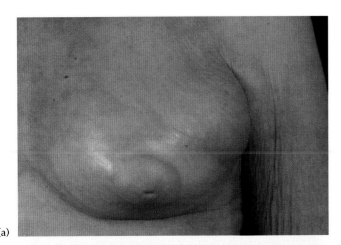

(a)

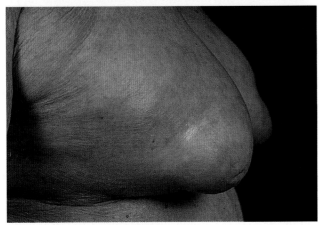

(b)

Fig. 67.4 (a, b) A patient with generalized morphoea, showing sparing of the nipple and areola.

Silicone breast implants and autoimmune disease

In the early 1990s, a major controversy arose about a possible relationship between silicone gel breast implants and subsequent development of connective tissue disease. Although the most common specific disease was scleroderma, many cases had a non-specific syndrome. Because of safety concerns, the US Food and Drug Administration imposed a moratorium on the use of such implants in 1992. The UK Medical Devices Directorate reviewed the scientific evidence relating to connective tissue disease and silicone gel breast implants, and in April 1992 presented a report to an independent Expert Advisory Group. The Group concluded that, on the basis of all available data, there was no evidence of an increased incidence of connective tissue disease associated with silicone gel breast implants [1]. An Independent Advisory Committee in Canada concluded that there was an absence of evidence establishing that women with silicone gel implants were more likely than those without such implants to have autoimmune disorders [2]. The issue provoked intense medicolegal activity.

Although a retrospective cohort study of 395 542 female health professionals, involving self-reported data, suggested a small increased risk of connective tissue diseases among women with breast implants [3], numerous controlled epidemiological studies did not demonstrate any statistically significant association between a recognized connective tissue disease and silicone breast implants [4], and three meta-analyses of the data failed to show an association [5–7]. However, the controversy continued [8,9]. Further studies showed no evidence of an association [10,11], and the UK Independent Review Group on Silicone Gel Breast Implants concluded that these implants were not associated with any greater health risk than other surgical implants, and that if there was any risk of connective tissue disease it was too small to be quantified [12]. At about the same time as this report was issued, a settlement of the medicolegal issues was proposed [13].

REFERENCES

1 Tinkler J, Gott D, Ludgate S. Breast implants: is there an association with connective tissue disease? *Health Trends* 1994; **26**: 25–6.
2 Independent Advisory Committee on Silicone-Gel-filled Breast Implants. Summary of the report on silicone-gel-filled breast implants. *Can Med Assoc J* 1992; **147**: 1141–6.
3 Hennekens CH, Lee I-M, Cook NR *et al.* Self-reported breast implants and connective-tissue diseases in female health professionals. *JAMA* 1996; **275**: 616–21.
4 Rose NR. The silicone breast implant controversy: the other courtroom. *Arthritis Rheum* 1996; **39**: 1615–8.
5 Hochberg MC, Perlmutter D. The association of augmentation mammoplasty with connective tissue disease, including systemic sclerosis (scleroderma): a meta-analysis. *Curr Top Microbiol Immunol* 1995; **210**: 411–7.
6 Perkins LL, Clark BD, Klein PJ, Cook RR. A meta-analysis of breast implants and connective tissue disease. *Ann Plast Surg* 1995; **35**: 561–70.
7 Wong O. A critical assessment of the relationship between silicone breast implants and connective tissue disease. *Regul Toxicol Pharmacol* 1996; **23**: 74–85.
8 Ault A. US Institute of Medicine panel deliberates on breast-implant safety. *Lancet* 1998; **352**: 380.
9 Cooper C, Dennison E. Do silicone breast implants cause connective tissue disease? *BMJ* 1998; **316**: 403–4.
10 Nyrén O, Yin L, Josefsson S *et al.* Risk of connective tissue disease and related disorders among women with breast implants: a nation-wide retrospective cohort study in Sweden. *BMJ* 1998; **316**: 417–22.
11 Edworthy SM, Martin L, Barr SG *et al.* A clinical study of the relationship between silicone breast implants and connective tissue disease. *J Rheumatol* 1998; **25**: 254–60.
12 McMenemy MC. UK review group gives silicone implants all clear. *Lancet* 1998; **352**: 211.
13 Rovner J. Breast-implant settlement reached in USA. *Lancet* 1998; **352**: 211.

Rudimentary nipples

The association of absent or rudimentary nipples with abnormalities of the scalp and ears has been reported as an autosomal-dominant trait [1–3].

Rudimentary nipples are also a feature of the ablepharon–macrostomia and Barber–Say syndromes, whose other features include absence of the eyelids or ectropion, macrostomia, ear anomalies, redundant skin, abnormal genitalia and hypertrichosis in the Barber–Say syndrome [4,5].

REFERENCES

1 Finlay AY, Marks R. An hereditary syndrome of lumpy scalp, odd ears and rudimentary nipples. *Br J Dermatol* 1978; **99**: 423–30.
2 Le Merrer M, Renier D, Briard ML. Scalp defect, nipples absence and ears abnormalities: another case of Finlay syndrome. *Genet Couns* 1991; **2**: 233–6.
3 Edwards MJ, McDonald D, Moore P, Rae J. Scalp–ear–nipple syndrome: additional manifestations. *Am J Med Genet* 1994; **50**: 247–50.
4 Stevens CA, Sargent LA. Ablepharon–macrostomia syndrome. *Am J Med Genet* 2002; **107**: 30–7.
5 Dinulos MB, Pagon RA. Autosomal dominant inheritance of Barber–Say syndrome. *Am J Med Genet* 1999; **86**: 54–6.

Adnexal polyp of neonatal skin [1,2]

This is a small, usually solitary, tumour which occurs mainly on the areola of the neonate. It is firm and pink, but becomes dry and brown and falls off within a few days of birth. Histologically, it contains hair follicles, eccrine glands and vestigial sebaceous glands. A survey in Tokyo showed that the condition occurred in 4% of 3257 newborn infants.

REFERENCES

1 Hidano A, Kobayashi T. Adnexal polyp of neonatal skin. *Br J Dermatol* 1975; **92**: 659–62.
2 Koizumi H, Itoh E, Ohkawara A. Adnexal polyp of neonatal skin observed beyond the neonatal period. *Acta Derm Venereol (Stockh)* 1998; **78**: 391–2.

Inverted nipple

Inverted nipple is common, affecting up to 10% of adult females [1], and potentially leading to functional problems with breastfeeding, and psychological distress. There are three main causes: congenital, periductal inflammation and tumour infiltration. It is also important to remember that in postmenopausal women it may result from the involutional process of periductal fibrosis. In most cases, the abnormality is congenital, and the fault lies in failure of the normal eversion process [2]. The lactiferous ducts are shortened and there is a reduction in the amount of dense connective tissue which is present beneath a normal nipple [3]. The abnormality is usually bilateral, but may affect only one nipple.

Many women with inverted nipples are able to breastfeed without difficulty, probably because the nipple itself plays a relatively small part in the anatomical aspects of suckling, as the infant makes a 'teat' from the surrounding breast tissue as well as the nipple [2].

If inverted nipples pose a cosmetic problem, surgical correction may be considered. Numerous techniques have been described, suggesting that none is ideal. Procedures which involve division of the lactiferous ducts are probably more effective, but breast function is destroyed. One of the more recent suggestions, which preserves breast function, involves piercing the base of the nipple and inserting a stainless steel barbell of a type employed in decorative body piercing [4].

REFERENCES

1 Alexander JM, Campbell MJ. Prevalence of inverted and non-protractile nipples in antenatal women who intend to breast feed. *Breast* 1997; **5**: 88–9.
2 Hughes LE, Mansel RE, Webster DJT. *Benign Disorders and Diseases of the Breast*, 2nd edn. London: Saunders, 2000.
3 Schwager RG, Smith JW, Gray GF, Goulian D Jr. Inversion of the human female nipple, with a simple method of treatment. *Plast Reconstr Surg* 1974; **54**: 564–9.
4 Scholten E. A contemporary correction of inverted nipple. *Plast Reconstr Surg* 2001; **107**: 511–3.

The duct ectasia/periductal mastitis complex [1]

A number of pathological processes contribute to the clinical features of this complex. These features include nipple discharge, subareolar abscess, mammary duct fistula and nipple retraction. It is a rare occurrence in males, but has been described in association with HIV infection [2].

REFERENCES

1 Hughes LE, Mansel RE, Webster DJT. *Benign Disorders and Diseases of the Breast*, 2nd edn. London: Saunders, 2000.
2 Downs AMR, Fisher M, Tomlinson D, Tanner A. Male duct ectasia associated with HIV infection. *Genitourin Med* 1996; **72**: 65–6.

Hyperkeratosis of the nipple and areola

On the basis of reported cases, hyperkeratosis of the nipple and areola is considered to be a rare condition. The classical Levy-Franckel classification includes three categories [1,2]: as an extension of an epidermal naevus, in which involvement tends to be unilateral and both sexes may be affected; in association with ichthyosis, in which involvement is bilateral and both sexes are affected; a naevoid type, usually bilateral, and occurring predominantly in women in the second or third decade of life. Pérez-Izquierdo *et al.* [3] suggested an alternative classification of two types: (i) idiopathic or naevoid (unilateral or bilateral); and (ii) secondary, local (unilateral or bilateral)—acanthosis nigricans, verrucous naevus or seborrhoeic keratosis; systemic (bilateral)—dermatosis, ichthyosis, malignant lymphomas, Darier's disease, chronic eczemas; or drug-related—diethylstilboestrol, spironolactone. Another classification, proposed by Mehanna *et al.* [4], includes a suggestion that the term 'naevoid' should be replaced by 'idiopathic'.

Whether described as naevoid or idiopathic, there is a distinct entity of verrucous thickening and brownish discoloration of the nipples and areolae which occurs predominantly in women in the second or third decade of life [5], in the absence of associated skin disease. It is usually bilateral, although unilateral involvement has been described [6,7], and it occasionally occurs in men [8]. Histology shows hyperkeratosis, filiform acanthosis and papillomatosis and keratin plugging.

Hyperkeratosis of the nipples may also occur in association with ichthyosis, ichthyosiform erythroderma, acanthosis nigricans, Darier's disease (in association with other skin lesions, but also described as an isolated presenting phenomenon [9]), and T-cell lymphoma [10,11]. It has also been described in men with carcinoma of the prostate treated with oestrogens [12,13].

An appearance resembling verrucous naevi around both areolae has been described as a manifestation of inadequate hygiene [14].

Suggested treatments for naevoid hyperkeratosis include topical retinoic acid [3], topical calcipotriol [15], cryotherapy [6] and the carbon dioxide laser [16].

REFERENCES

1 Levy-Franckel A. Les hyperkératoses de l'aréole et du mamelon. *Paris Med* 1938; **28**: 63–6.
2 Whitaker-Worth DL, Carlone V, Susser WS *et al.* Dermatologic diseases of the breast and nipple. *J Am Acad Dermatol* 2000; **43**: 733–51.
3 Pérez-Izquierdo JM, Vilata JJ, Sánchez JL *et al.* Retinoic acid treatment of nipple hyperkeratosis. *Arch Dermatol* 1990; **126**: 687–8.
4 Mehanna A, Malak JA, Kibbi A-G. Hyperkeratosis of the nipple and areola. *Arch Dermatol* 2001; **137**: 1327–8.
5 Baykal C, Büyükbabani N, Kavak A, Alper M. Nevoid hyperkeratosis of the nipple and areola: a distinct entity. *J Am Acad Dermatol* 2002; **46**: 414–8.
6 Vestey JP, Bunney MH. Unilateral hyperkeratosis of the nipple: the response to cryotherapy. *Arch Dermatol* 1986; **122**: 1360–1.
7 Revert A, Bañuls J, Montesinos E *et al.* Nevoid hyperkeratosis of the areola. *Int J Dermatol* 1993; **32**: 745–6.
8 Kubota Y, Koga T, Nakayama J, Kiryu H. Naevoid hyperkeratosis of the nipple and areola in a man. *Br J Dermatol* 2000; **142**: 382–4.
9 Fitzgerald DA, Lewis-Jones MS. Darier's disease presenting as isolated hyperkeratosis of the breasts. *Br J Dermatol* 1997; **136**: 290.
10 Allegue F, Soria C, Rocamora A *et al.* Hyperkeratosis of the nipple and areola in a patient with cutaneous T-cell lymphoma. *Int J Dermatol* 1990; **29**: 519–20.
11 Ahn SK, Chung J, Lee WS *et al.* Hyperkeratosis of the nipple and areola simultaneously developing with cutaneous T-cell lymphoma. *J Am Acad Dermatol* 1995; **32**: 124–5.
12 Schwartz RA. Hyperkeratosis of nipple and areola. *Arch Dermatol* 1978; **114**: 1844–5.
13 Mold DE, Jegasothy BV. Estrogen-induced hyperkeratosis of the nipple. *Cutis* 1980; **26**: 95–6.
14 Ruiz-Maldonado R, Durán-McKinster C, Tamayo-Sánchez L, de la Luz Orozco-Covarrubias M. Dermatitis neglecta: dirt crusts simulating verrucous nevi. *Arch Dermatol* 1999; **135**: 728–9.
15 Bayramgürler D, Bilen N, Apaydin R, Erçin C. Nevoid hyperkeratosis of the nipple and areola: treatment of two patients with topical calcipotriol. *J Am Acad Dermatol* 2002; **46**: 131–3.
16 Busse A, Peschen M, Schöpf E, Vanscheidt W. Treatment of hyperkeratosis areolae mammae naeviformis with the carbon dioxide laser. *J Am Acad Dermatol* 1999; **41**: 274–6.

Eczema of the nipple and areola

Although eczema of the nipple and areola occurs mainly in women (Fig. 67.5), it is an occasional occurrence in men (Fig. 67.6); it may be unilateral or bilateral [1,2]. Often no cause can be established, although there is an association with atopy [3].

Contact dermatitis is a possibility, and allergic contact dermatitis of the nipples has been reported in a breast-feeding woman using a beeswax nipple protector [4], and two others applying Roman chamomile ointment [5].

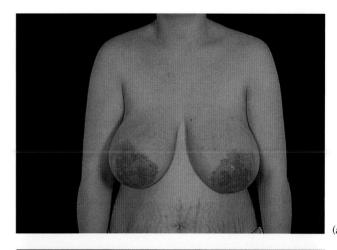
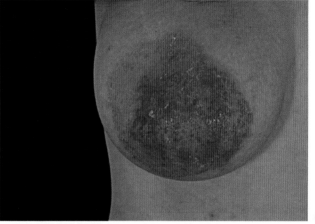

(a)

(b)

Fig. 67.5 (a, b) Severe bilateral nipple eczema in a young woman.

Irritation from friction must also be considered (see the section on jogger's and cyclist's nipple, below), and unilateral nipple dermatitis in three women with large asymmetrical breasts was attributed to friction between the larger breast and the seam of the brassiere cup [6].

Treatment of nipple eczema is with mild to moderate potency topical steroids.

The intermittent course, more severe itching, indefinite margin and lack of distortion of the nipple help to distinguish eczema from Paget's disease (Chapter 36, Fig. 67.7). Erosive adenomatosis of the nipple (see p. 67.11) may have an eczematous appearance, and a case of clear cell acanthoma presenting as nipple eczema has been described [7]. If the diagnosis is at all doubtful, biopsy should be performed, particularly if there has been no response to topical steroids.

REFERENCES

1 Graham DF. Eczema of the nipple. *Trans St John's Hosp Dermatol Soc* 1972; **58**: 98–9.
2 Topham EJ, Mortimer PS. Nipple eczema as a presenting complaint to the dermatology clinic: a 16 patient series [abstract]. *Br J Dermatol* 2002; **147** (Suppl. 62): 27.

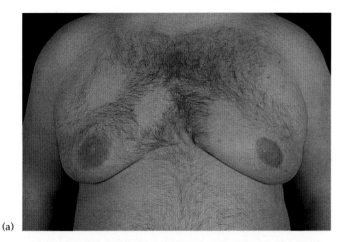

(a)

(b)

Fig. 67.6 (a, b) Bilateral nipple eczema in a man.

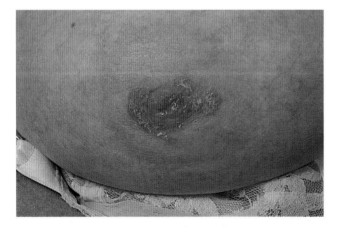

Fig. 67.7 Paget's disease of the nipple.

3 Mevorah B, Frenk E, Wietlisbach V, Carrel CF. Minor clinical features of atopic dermatitis: evaluation of their diagnostic significance. *Dermatologica* 1988; **177**: 360–4.
4 García M, del Pozo MD, Díez J *et al.* Allergic contact dermatitis from a beeswax nipple-protective. *Contact Dermatitis* 1995; **33**: 440–1.
5 McGeorge BCL, Steele MC. Allergic contact dermatitis of the nipple from Roman chamomile ointment. *Contact Dermatitis* 1991; **24**: 139–40.
6 Kapur N, Goldsmith PC. Nipple dermatitis: not all what it 'seams'. *Contact Dermatitis* 2001; **45**: 44–5.

7 Kim DH, Kim CW, Kang SJ, Kim TY. A case of clear cell acanthoma presenting as nipple eczema. *Br J Dermatol* 1999; **141**: 950–1.

'Cracked' nipples in lactation

Many women experience discomfort, irritation and fissuring of the nipples early in the puerperium when they are trying to establish breastfeeding. Anatomical features, such as relatively flat nipples, contribute to the development of this problem. Mastitis and deep abscesses may occur due to penetration of the broken skin by pyogenic bacteria. The problem is, in essence, one of friction and irritancy resulting from vigorous suckling, and can be eased considerably by the judicious use of gentle cleansing and emollients such as white soft paraffin.

Jogger's and cyclist's nipples [1,2]

Long-distance runners of either sex may suffer from irritation of the nipples caused by prolonged friction against a shirt. The problem is more pronounced in women who do not wear a brassiere. The condition is self-healing; prevention includes the application of petrolatum or powder to the nipples to reduce friction, and the use of a sports brassiere.

Cyclists may suffer from cold injury to the nipple as evaporation of perspiration and wind chill combine to lower the temperature of the nipple on a cold day [3]. Pain, which may last for several days, soreness and tenderness are the result. Cycling jackets made of wind-resistant fabric offer a solution.

REFERENCES

1 Levit F. Jogger's nipples. *N Engl J Med* 1977; **297**: 1127.
2 Adams BB. Dermatologic disorders of the athlete. *Sports Med* 2002; **32**: 309–21.
3 Powell B. Bicyclist's nipples. *JAMA* 1983; **249**: 2457.

Nipple piercings

Body piercing has been practised in some societies since antiquity, but it has usually been confined to the ears and nose. In recent years it has become 'fashionable' in Western countries, and devotees indulge not only in piercings on the face and ears, but also the genitalia and nipples. In a recent study of American undergraduates, 3% of males and 6% of females had pierced nipples [1]. Of these, 21% had experienced trauma or bleeding and the piercing had been removed in a third (mainly male).

Nipple piercings may cause problems either due to trauma or infection [2,3] or the development of allergy to the metal. Lactiferous ducts may be damaged when the nipple is pierced, but this does not appear to lead to problems with breastfeeding [4].

Tassel ornaments suspended from the breasts have

been popular in some cultures, particularly in the Middle East, for many generations. Some dancers have their nipples pierced to accommodate a ring from which ornaments are suspended and this can cause breast duct ectasia [5].

REFERENCES

1 Mayers LB, Judelson DA, Moriarty BW, Rundell KW. Prevalence of body art (body piercing and tattooing) in university undergraduates and incidence of medical complications. *Mayo Clin Proc* 2002; **77**: 29–34.
2 Ochsenfahrt C, Friedl R, Hannekum A, Schumacher BA. Endocarditis after nipple piercing in a patient with a bicuspid aortic valve. *Ann Thorac Surg* 2001; **71**: 1365–6.
3 Javaid M, Shibu M. Breast implant infection following nipple piercing. *Br J Plast Surg* 1999; **52**: 676–7.
4 Ferguson H. Body piercing. *BMJ* 1999; **319**: 1627–9.
5 Collins REC. Breast disease associated with tassel dancing. *BMJ* 1981; **283**: 1660.

Artefactual breast disease

There are relatively few reports of artefactual breast disease, but the features of reported cases are as varied and bizarre as factitial lesions elsewhere on the body [1–6].

REFERENCES

1 Schwartz DL, So HB, Schneider KM, Becker JM. Chronic insertion of foreign bodies into the mature breast. *J Pediatr Surg* 1977; **12**: 743–4.
2 Rosenberg MW, Hughes LE. Artefactual breast disease: a report of three cases. *Br J Surg* 1985; **72**: 539–41.
3 Benson EA. Artefactual breast disease. *Br J Surg* 1986; **73**: 163.
4 Mudan SS, Ibrahim AEK, Wise M, Perry PM. Nipple discharge in a teenager. *J R Soc Med* 1998; **91**: 490–1.
5 Sampson D. An unusual self-inflicted injury of the breast. *Postgrad Med J* 1975; **51**: 116–8.
6 Whitaker-Worth DL, Carlone V, Susser WS *et al.* Dermatologic disease of the breast and nipple. *J Am Acad Dermatol* 2000; **43**: 733–51.

Vasculitis of the breast

Vasculitis affecting breast tissue is rare. It may occur as part of a systemic vasculitis, or as localized disease.

There are several reported cases of polyarteritis nodosa presenting as tender breast nodules [1,2], and breast lesions may also be a feature of Wegener's granulomatosis, sometimes as an initial manifestation [3,4].

REFERENCES

1 Ng WF, Chow LTC, Lam PWY. Localized polyarteritis nodosa of breast: report of two cases and a review of the literature. *Histopathology* 1993; **23**: 535–9.
2 Trüeb RM, Scheidegger EP, Pericin M *et al.* Periarteritis nodosa presenting as a breast lesion: report of a case and review of the literature. *Br J Dermatol* 1999; **141**: 1117–21.
3 Jordan JM, Rowe WT, Allen NB. Wegener's granulomatosis involving the breast: report of three cases and review of the literature. *Am J Med* 1987; **83**: 159–64.
4 Trüeb RM, Pericin M, Kohler E *et al.* Necrotizing granulomatosis of the breast. *Br J Dermatol* 1997; **137**: 799–803.

Lupus panniculitis
SYN. LUPUS ERYTHEMATOSUS PROFUNDUS; LUPUS MASTITIS [1–4]

Lupus panniculitis can result in breast nodules, which may be mistaken for carcinoma. Lesions are usually chronic and disfiguring. The treatment of choice is antimalarial therapy.

REFERENCES

1 Whitaker-Worth DL, Carlone V, Susser WS *et al.* Dermatologic diseases of the breast and nipple. *J Am Acad Dermatol* 2000; **43**: 733–51.
2 Harris RB, Winkelmann RK. Lupus mastitis. *Arch Dermatol* 1978; **114**: 410–2.
3 Cernea SS, Kihara SM, Sotto MN, Vilela MAC. Lupus mastitis. *J Am Acad Dermatol* 1993; **29**: 343–6.
4 Holland NW, Mcnight K, Challa VR, Agudelo CA. Lupus panniculitis (profundus) involving the breast: report of 2 cases and review of the literature. *J Rheumatol* 1995; **22**: 344–6.

Sarcoidosis of the breast [1–5]

Although involvement of the breast with sarcoidosis is rare, it is important to be aware of its occurrence, as it mimics breast carcinoma. It can present as solitary or multiple, unilateral or bilateral subcutaneous masses, which may be associated with other manifestations of the disease or occur as an isolated phenomenon. Lesions may be fixed or mobile, tender or non-tender, and with or without palpable axillary lymphadenopathy.

REFERENCES

1 Mingins C, Williams MR, Cox NH. Subcutaneous sarcoidosis mimicking breast carcinoma. *Br J Dermatol* 2002; **146**: 924–5.
2 Gansler TS, Wheeler JE. Mammary sarcoidosis. Two cases and literature review. *Arch Pathol Lab Med* 1984; **108**: 673–5.
3 Harris KP, Faliakou EC, Exon DJ *et al.* Isolated sarcoidosis of the breast. *J R Soc Med* 2000; **93**: 196–7.
4 Banik S, Bishop PW, Ormerod LP, O'Brien TEB. Sarcoidosis of the breast. *J Clin Pathol* 1986; **39**: 446–8.
5 Fitzgibbons PL, Smiley DF, Kern WH. Sarcoidosis presenting initially as breast mass: report of two cases. *Hum Pathol* 1985; **16**: 851–2.

Erosive adenomatosis of the nipple [1–5]
SYN. BENIGN PAPILLOMATOSIS OF THE NIPPLE; FLORID PAPILLOMATOSIS OF THE NIPPLE DUCTS; PAPILLARY ADENOMA OF THE NIPPLE; SUBAREOLAR DUCT PAPILLOMATOSIS; SUPERFICIAL PAPILLARY ADENOMATOSIS

Definition. A complex benign tumour arising from the lactiferous ducts of the nipple.

Incidence. This is an uncommon tumour, which occurs mainly in middle-aged women, but it can occur at any age [6], and occasionally in males [7–9]. In one case, the lesion developed 10 years after treatment for carcinoma of the prostate by bilateral orchidectomy and diethylstilbestrol [10].

Pathology [1,4,11–14]. The lesion consists of tubules, with an inner layer of columnar cells and an outer layer of cuboidal myoepithelial cells. A major feature is the presence of superficial keratocysts lined by both squamous and columnar epithelium, and filled with keratin flakes and an eosinophilic material, apparently secreted by the columnar cells. The cysts seem to reproduce the terminal portion of the nipple duct system. Within some of the superficial cysts or ducts, foreign-body giant cells may be seen. Some degree of intraluminal growth (intraductal papillomatosis) is present in many cases. This ranges from small papillary epithelial tufts to almost complete occlusion of the lumina by solid epithelial plugs, and there may be evidence of apocrine decapitation secretion. The overlying epidermis may show acanthosis and hyperkeratosis.

The major histopathological diagnostic pitfall is confusing erosive adenomatosis with sweat gland tumours, and as it may also be difficult to differentiate from papillary breast carcinoma, immunohistological techniques are of value in demonstrating the layer of myoepithelial cells [12,13].

Clinical features. These are variable. The condition may start with a blood-stained or serous discharge, and the nipple may be enlarged, eroded, crusted or eczematous. There may be a small nodule on the nipple, and the symptoms may be worse in the premenstrual phase. The condition is commonly misdiagnosed as Paget's disease or eczema. It is usually unilateral, but bilateral involvement has been reported [15,16], and it has been described in an accessory nipple [17].

Treatment. Excision is curative—either simple local excision, or partial or complete resection of the nipple, depending on the size of the tumour [18]. There are reports of successful treatment by cryosurgery [19] and Mohs surgery [20].

REFERENCES

1 Brownstein MH, Phelps RG, Magnin PH. Papillary adenoma of the nipple: analysis of fifteen new cases. *J Am Acad Dermatol* 1985; **12**: 707–15.
2 Lewis HM, Ovitz ML, Golitz LE. Erosive adenomatosis of the nipple. *Arch Dermatol* 1976; **112**: 1427–8.
3 Bourlond J, Bourlond-Rinert L. Erosive adenomatosis of the nipple. *Dermatology* 1992; **185**: 319–24.
4 Moulin G, Darbon P, Balme B, Frappart L. Adénomatose érosive du mamelon. A propos de 10 cas avec étude histochimique. *Ann Dermatol Venereol* 1990; **117**: 537–45.
5 Montemarano AD, Sau P, James WD. Superficial papillary adenomatosis of the nipple: a case report and review of the literature. *J Am Acad Dermatol* 1995; **33**: 871–5.
6 Albers SE, Barnard M, Thorner P, Krafchick BR. Erosive adenomatosis of the nipple in an eight-year-old girl. *J Am Acad Dermatol* 1999; **40**: 834–7.
7 Miller G, Bernier L. Adénomatose érosive du mamelon. *Can J Surg* 1965; **8**: 261–6.
8 Taylor HB, Robertson AG. Adenomas of the nipple. *Cancer* 1965; **18**: 995–1002.
9 Richards AT, Jaffe A, Hunt JA. Adenoma of the nipple in a male. *S Afr Med J* 1973; **47**: 581–3.
10 Waldo ED, Sidhu GS, Hu AW. Florid papillomatosis of male nipple after diethylstilbestrol therapy. *Arch Pathol* 1975; **99**: 364–6.
11 Perzin KH, Lattes R. Papillary adenoma of the nipple (florid papillomatosis): a clinico-pathologic study. *Cancer* 1972; **29**: 996–1009.
12 Smith NP, Wilson-Jones E. Erosive adenomatosis of the nipple. *Clin Exp Dermatol* 1977; **2**: 79–84.
13 Diaz NM, Palmer JO, Wick MR. Erosive adenomatosis of the nipple: histology, immunohistology and differential diagnosis. *Mod Pathol* 1992; **5**: 179–84.
14 Moulin G. Superficial papillary adenomatosis of the nipple. *J Am Acad Dermatol* 1997; **36**: 133.
15 Handley RS, Thackray AC. Adenoma of nipple. *Br J Cancer* 1962; **16**: 187–94.
16 Bergdahl L, Bergman F, Rais O, Westling P. Bilateral adenoma of nipple. *Acta Chir Scand* 1971; **137**: 583–6.
17 Civatte J, Restout S, Delomenie DC. Adénomatose érosive sur mamelon surnuméraire. *Ann Dermatol Venereol* 1977; **104**: 777–9.
18 Vianna LL, Millis RR, Fentiman IS. Adenoma of the nipple: a diagnostic dilemma. *Br J Hosp Med* 1993; **50**: 639–42.
19 Kuflik EG. Erosive adenomatosis of the nipple treated with cryosurgery. *J Am Acad Dermatol* 1998; **38**: 270–1.
20 Van Mierlo PL, Geelen GM, Neumann HA. Mohs micrographic surgery for an erosive adenomatosis of the nipple. *Dermatol Surg* 1998; **24**: 681–3.

Sebaceous hyperplasia of the areolae

This is a rare abnormality characterized clinically by yellowish thickening of the areolae, and histologically by large numbers of hyperplastic sebaceous lobules [1–3].

REFERENCES

1 Hammerton MD, Shrank AB. Superficial sebaceous hyperplasia of the areolae. *Br J Dermatol* 1993; **129**: 649–50.
2 Belinchón I, Aguilar A, Tardío J, Gallego MA. Areolar sebaceous hyperplasia: a case report. *Cutis* 1996; **58**: 63–5.
3 Fariña MC, Soriano ML, Escalonilla P *et al.* Unilateral areolar sebaceous hyperplasia in a male. *Am J Dermatopathol* 1996; **18**: 417–9.

Breast telangiectasia

White [1] described a 77-year-old man with bilateral patches of perfectly circular, symmetrical telangiectasia of the areolae. The condition had been present for as long as he could remember, with no associated abnormalities.

Blue areolae were one feature of a familial disorder named 'hereditary acrolabial telangiectasia' [2], and Schlappner and Shelley reported a 35-year-old woman with symmetrical essential telangiectasis of the breasts, recurrent aphthous stomatitis and hypersplenism [3].

REFERENCES

1 White GM, Jeffes EWB. Congenital circumareolar telangiectasia. *Arch Dermatol* 1990; **126**: 1656.
2 Millns JL, Dicken CH. Hereditary acrolabial telangiectasia: a report of familial blue lips, nails and nipples. *Arch Dermatol* 1979; **115**: 474–8.
3 Schlappner OLA, Shelley WB. Telangiectasia, aphthous stomatitis and hypersplenism. *Arch Dermatol* 1971; **104**: 668.

Mammary duct fistula [1]

SYN. RECURRENT SUBAREOLAR ABSCESS

This condition typically occurs in a young adult woman who has a history of recurrent abscesses in a breast which have been treated by surgical drainage or have discharged spontaneously. There is typically partial inversion of the nipple and a scar or scars at the edge of the areola.

The condition is treated by passing a probe into the opening of the discharging sinus, along the track of the fistula, and out of the nipple. The fistula is then laid open (fistulotomy) and left to heal by granulation, or the whole tract is excised (fistulectomy) and the wound allowed to granulate.

REFERENCE

1 Hughes LE, Mansel RE, Webster DJT. *Benign Disorders and Diseases of the Breast*, 2nd edn. London: Saunders, 2000.

Breast abscess [1]

Breast abscesses may be classified as lactational (occurring in the puerperium) and non-lactational. The majority of lactational abscesses are caused by *Staphylococcus aureus*, and present as a painful, red, swollen breast, associated with fever.

Non-lactational abscesses include subareolar abscess, which is seen mainly in women in their reproductive years in association with the duct ectasia/periductal mastitis complex, and peripheral abscess, which occurs as a typical inflammatory breast abscess in postmenopausal women. The former is associated with a mixed bacterial spectrum, and the latter with *S. aureus*. Lactational abscesses are now uncommon in comparison with the frequency of non-lactational lesions [2].

REFERENCES

1 Hughes LE, Mansel RE, Webster DJT. *Benign Disorders and Diseases of the Breast*, 2nd edn. London: Saunders, 2000.
2 Schofield JH, Duncan JL, Rogers K. Review of a hospital experience of breast abscesses. *Br J Surg* 1987; **74**: 469–70.

Breast cancer (Fig. 67.8)

This common and important condition lies in the province of the surgeon rather than the dermatologist, but all physicians have a duty to detect and diagnose early breast cancer, which can sometimes be discovered on routine examination. Inspection and palpation of the breasts should be included in any full examination. The breasts should be inspected with the arms by the side, above the head and pressing on the hips, because in some cases these manoeuvres will demonstrate a visible mass, or a change in contour of the breast, or early retraction or dimpling of the skin caused by a breast cancer. The dermatologist should also remember that redness or oedema of the breast skin can be due to underlying cancer. Breast cancer can also cause flattening, broadening or inversion of the nipple. It is important that all four quadrants of the breast,

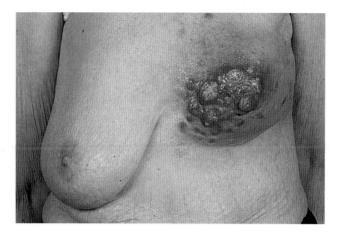

Fig. 67.8 Advanced carcinoma of the breast.

including the axillary tail and axillary lymph nodes, should be palpated.

The dermatologist should examine the breasts carefully in all patients presenting with skin disease which may be associated with systemic malignancy, for example acanthosis nigricans or dermatomyositis.

The term *peau d'orange* is applied to dimpled oedematous or indurated skin resembling the surface of an orange. The finding of peau d'orange should lead to an intensive search for underlying carcinoma. Rarely, it occurs in the absence of any clinically palpable tumour. It has also been reported as a complication of anasarca, nephrotic syndrome and cardiac failure [1].

Breast cancer frequently involves the skin, and there are several different clinicopathological types of cutaneous involvement [2]. These include Paget's disease of the nipple, inflammatory metastatic carcinoma (carcinoma erysipeloides), carcinoma en cuirasse, telangiectatic metastatic carcinoma, nodular metastatic carcinoma, alopecia neoplastica, carcinoma of the inframammary crease and metastatic mammary carcinoma of the eyelid. Carcinoma metastatic to the eyelids is a rare phenomenon, and breast carcinoma is responsible for a sizeable proportion of these cases. Involvement may be unilateral, with the right eyelids affected more frequently than the left [3], or bilateral [4,5]. In many of the reported cases, the histology has shown prominent histiocytoid features [2].

Pigmented primary carcinoma of the breast is rare, and may mimic malignant melanoma clinically and histologically [6,7]. Metastatic melanoma may be responsible for inflammatory changes in breast skin [8].

Other conditions which may mimic breast carcinoma include postsurgical lymphoedema [9] and sarcoidosis [10].

Virgili *et al.* [11] described four patients with what were thought to represent cutaneous tumour-related granulomatous lesions following mastectomy for carcinoma of the breast. The lesions developed on the arm on the same side as the previous mastectomy.

REFERENCES

1 McElligott G, Harrington MG. Heart failure and breast enlargement suggesting cancer. *BMJ* 1986; **292**: 446.
2 Schwartz RA. Cutaneous metastatic disease. *J Am Acad Dermatol* 1995; **33**: 161–82.
3 Rubio FA, Pizarro A, Robano G *et al.* Eyelid metastasis as the presenting sign of recurrent carcinoma of the breast. *Br J Dermatol* 1997; **137**: 1026–7.
4 Grinspan D, Abulafia J, Abbruzzese M. Metastatic involvement of four eyelids. *J Am Acad Dermatol* 1997; **37**: 362–4.
5 Zimmerman T, Jappe U, Hausser I *et al.* Persistent erythematous eyelid swelling due to metastatic lobular carcinoma of the breast. *Br J Dermatol* 2002; **146**: 919.
6 Sau P, Solis J, Lupton GP, James WD. Pigmented breast carcinoma. A clinical and histopathologic simulator of malignant melanoma. *Arch Dermatol* 1989; **125**: 536–9.
7 Saitoh K, Saga K, Okazaki M, Maeda K. Pigmented primary carcinoma of the breast: a clinical mimic of malignant melanoma. *Br J Dermatol* 1998; **139**: 287–90.
8 Tan BB, Marsden JR, Sanders DSA. Melanoma erysipeloides: inflammatory metastatic melanoma of the skin. *Br J Dermatol* 1993; **129**: 327–9.
9 King R, Duncan L, Shupp DL, Googe PB. Postsurgical dermal lymphedema clinically mimicking inflammatory breast carcinoma. *Arch Dermatol* 2001; **137**: 969–70.
10 Mingins C, Williams MR, Cox NH. Subcutaneous sarcoidosis mimicking breast carcinoma. *Br J Dermatol* 2002; **146**: 924–5.
11 Virgili A, Maranini C, Califano A. Granulomatous lesions of the homolateral limb after previous mastectomy. *Br J Dermatol* 2002; **146**: 891–4.

Breast cancer in men

Breast cancer in men is relatively rare, accounting for around 0.2% of all cancers in men in the USA and less than 1% of all cases of breast cancer [1].

Risk factors include conditions associated with reduced testicular function, excess oestrogen exposure, Klinefelter's syndrome [2], and a family history of breast carcinoma. Case–control studies indicate that the disease is commoner in black men and in those who have never married [3].

The mean age of presentation is 60–65 years, and is approximately 5 years older than that for breast carcinoma in women.

As in women, the clinical features include a breast mass, which is typically subareolar, nipple inversion and nipple discharge (Fig. 67.9). Infiltrating ductal carcinoma is the predominant histological type. Paget's disease may be the presenting feature [4,5].

REFERENCES

1 Donegan WL, Redlich PN. Breast cancer in men. *Surg Clin North Am* 1996; **76**: 343–63.
2 Scheike O, Visfeldt J, Peterson B. Male breast cancer: breast carcinoma in association with Klinefelter syndrome. *Acta Pathol Microbiol Scand* 1973; **81**: 352–8.
3 Sasco AJ, Lowenfels AB, Pasker de-Jong P. Epidemiology of male breast cancer: a meta-analysis of published case control studies and discussion of selected aetiological factors. *Int J Cancer* 1993; **53**: 538–49.
4 Ratón JA, Bilbao I, Gardeazábal J *et al.* Skin involvement in male breast carcinoma. *Arch Dermatol* 1998; **134**: 517–8.
5 Bodnar M, Miller F, Tyler W. Paget's disease of the male breast associated with intraductal carcinoma. *J Am Acad Dermatol* 1999; **40**: 829–31.

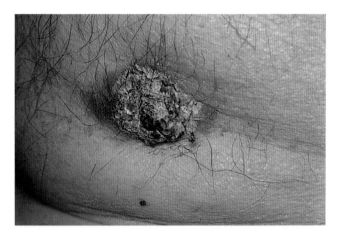

Fig. 67.9 Breast carcinoma in a man, showing destruction of the nipple and areola.

Basal cell carcinoma of the nipple [1–4]

This is a very rare lesion. It can occur in either men or women, usually in old age. It usually presents as a red, eczema-like patch of the nipple or areola and runs a long, indolent course. Biopsy is essential to differentiate it from Paget's disease.

Paget's disease, which is a marker of an underlying breast carcinoma, is discussed in Chapter 36.

REFERENCES

1 Cain RJ, Sau P, Benson PM. Basal cell carcinoma of the nipple: report of two cases. *J Am Acad Dermatol* 1990; **22**: 207–10.
2 Benharroch D, Geffen DB, Peiser J, Rosenberg L. Basal cell carcinoma of the male nipple: case report and review of the literature. *J Dermatol Surg Oncol* 1993; **19**: 137–9.
3 Zhu YI, Ratner D. Basal cell carcinoma of the nipple: a case report and review of the literature. *Dermatol Surg* 2001; **27**: 971–4.
4 Yamamoto H, Ito Y, Hayashi T *et al.* A case of basal cell carcinoma of the nipple and areola with intraductal spread. *Breast Cancer* 2001; **8**: 229–33.

Hair sinus of the breast

Hair sinus of the periareolar area of the breast has been observed in women engaged in sheep shearing (roustabout's breast) and hairdressing [1] (Fig. 67.10), and in canine beauticians whose work leaves them covered in dog hairs [2]. The lesions are similar to the interdigital pilonidal sinuses which may occur in barbers and dog groomers [3]. The histology shows a granulomatous reaction. Repeated breast abscesses in female sheep shearers may provoke concern about the ability to breastfeed or even lead to women contemplating mastectomy. This problem prompted the manufacture, in New Zealand, of a protective brassiere, the Baa Bra [4].

REFERENCES

1 Bowers PW. Roustabouts' and barbers' breasts. *Clin Exp Dermatol* 1982; **7**: 445–7.

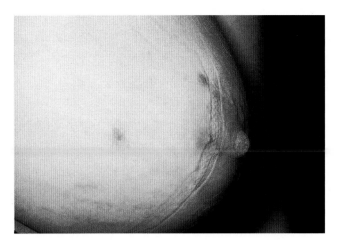

Fig. 67.10 Hair sinuses in a sheep-shearer. (Courtesy of Dr W. Bowers, Treliske Hospital, Truro, UK.)

2 Banerjee A. Pilonidal sinus of the nipple in a canine beautician. *BMJ* 1985; **291**: 1787.
3 Price SM, Popkin GL. Barbers' interdigital hair sinus. *Arch Dermatol* 1976; **112**: 523–4.
4 Gardiner G. Breast infections due to wool. *N Z Med J* 1994; **107**: 494.

Seborrhoeic warts

SYN. BASAL CELL PAPILLOMAS (Chapter 36)

These are particularly common in the submammary creases in middle-aged or elderly women, often in association with intertrigo (Fig. 67.11). Seborrhoeic warts may also occur as sharply demarcated papules or plaques on the nipple and areola [1].

REFERENCE

1 Baykal C, Büyükbabani N, Kavak A, Alper M. Nevoid hyperkeratosis of the nipple and areola: a distinct entity. *J Am Acad Dermatol* 2002; **46**: 414–8.

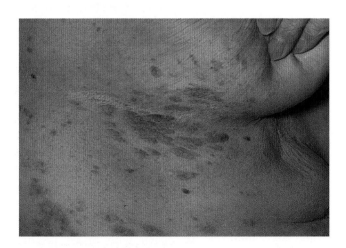

Fig. 67.11 Submammary seborrhoeic warts.

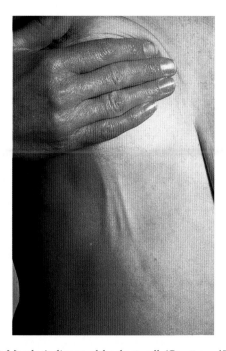

Fig. 67.12 Mondor's disease of the chest wall. (Courtesy of Professor A.Y. Finlay, University of Wales College of Medicine, Cardiff, UK.)

Mondor's disease (Fig. 67.12)

SYN. SCLEROSING PERIPHLEBITIS OF THE CHEST WALL

Mondor's disease is usually regarded as an obliterative phlebitis affecting the thoracoepigastric, lateral thoracic or superior epigastric vein. It occurs mainly between the ages of 30 and 60 years and affects women much more frequently than men [1,2]. Risk factors cited for the development of the condition include large, pendulous breasts, strenuous physical activity, direct trauma, breast surgery and infection near the affected vessels. Breast cancer is an occasional cause [3], and mammography is recommended even when no mass is palpable [4–6]. Mondor's disease has characteristic mammographic and sonographic features [5,6]. It has also been described in association with metastatic axillary adenopathy 2 years after radical mastectomy for breast carcinoma [7], and in a patient with metastatic lung cancer in the breast [8].

In a case of recurrent Mondor's disease of the thoraco-epigastric vein, resolution occurred after excision of a lipoma which was in close proximity to the vein [9]. It is a rare occurrence in pregnancy [10,11].

Other rare causes include intravenous drug abuse, following use of the breasts as injection sites [12], jellyfish stings [13] and a lupus erythematosus-like syndrome probably induced by procainamide [14]. However, often no cause is apparent.

Rarely, the condition is bilateral [14], and in one such case potential aetiological factors included breast surgery, the use of oral contraceptives, hereditary protein C deficiency and anticardiolipin antibodies [15].

There may be some tenderness or discomfort, but there are often no symptoms until the patient discovers a red linear cord running from the lateral margin of the breast, crossing the costal margin and extending to the abdominal wall. The cord is 2–3 mm in diameter and is attached to the skin but not to the deep fascia. It is usually only a few centimetres long, but may extend to 30–40 cm. The symptoms subside in a few weeks and there are no known complications.

REFERENCES

1 Farrow JH. Thrombophlebitis of the superficial veins of the breast and anterior chest wall (Mondor's disease). *Surg Gynecol Obstet* 1955; **101**: 63–8.
2 Bejanga BI. Mondor's disease: analysis of thirty cases. *J R Coll Surg Edin* 1992; **37**: 322–4.
3 Levi I, Baum M. Mondor's disease as a presenting symptom of breast cancer. *Br J Surg* 1987; **74**: 700.
4 Catania S, Zurrida S, Veronesi P *et al.* Mondor's disease and breast cancer. *Cancer* 1992; **69**: 2267–70.
5 Conant EF, Wilkes AN, Mendelson EB, Feig SA. Superficial thrombophlebitis of the breast: mammographic findings. *Am J Roentgenol* 1993; **160**: 1201–3.
6 Shetty MK, Watson AB. Mondor's disease of the breast: sonographic and mammographic findings. *Am J Roentgenol* 2001; **177**: 893–6.
7 Miller DR, Cesario TC, Slater LM. Mondor's disease associated with metastatic axillary nodes. *Cancer* 1985; **56**: 903–4.
8 Courtney SP, Polacarz S, Raftery AT. Mondor's disease associated with metastatic lung cancer in the breast. *Postgrad Med J* 1989; **65**: 779–80.
9 Rubegni P, De Aloe G, Biagioli M *et al.* Recurrent Mondor's disease resolved after exeresis of abdominal lipoma. *Dermatol Surg* 1999; **25**: 563–5.
10 Duff P. Mondor disease in pregnancy. *Obstet Gynecol* 1981; **58**: 117–20.
11 Hacker SM. Axillary string phlebitis in pregnancy: a variant of Mondor's disease. *J Am Acad Dermatol* 1994; **30**: 636–8.
12 Cooper RA. Mondor's disease secondary to intravenous drug abuse. *Arch Surg* 1990; **125**: 807–8.
13 Ingram DM, Sheiner HJ, Ginsberg A. Mondor's disease of breast resulting from jellyfish sting. *Med J Aust* 1992; **157**: 836–7.
14 Skipworth GB, Morris JB, Goldstein N. Bilateral Mondor's disease. *Arch Dermatol* 1967; **95**: 95–7.
15 Wester JP, Kuenen BC, Meuwissen OJ, de Maat CE. Mondor's disease as first thrombotic event in hereditary protein C deficiency and anticardiolipin antibodies. *Neth J Med* 1997; **50**: 85–7.

Other conditions which may involve the breast

Vitiligo sometimes shows a striking symmetrical involvement of the breasts.

Psoriasis may be provoked by the trauma of suckling.

Pityriasis rosea commonly presents with a herald patch on the breast, and has been reported as a localized eruption on one breast [1].

REFERENCE

1 Ahmed I, Charles-Holmes R. Localized pityriasis rosea. *Clin Exp Dermatol* 2000; **25**: 624–6.

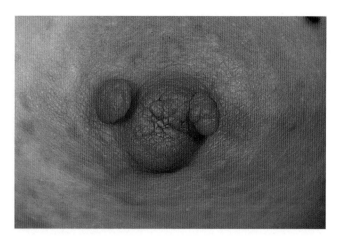

Fig. 67.13 Neurofibromatosis, showing the predilection of this condition for the nipple.

Cutaneous larva migrans may occur on the breast when women have lain 'topless' on a tropical beach in the prone position.

Neurofibromas have a predilection for the areola (Fig. 67.13) [1].

REFERENCE

1 Riccardi VM. Neurofibromatosis: an overview and new directions in clinical investigations. In: Riccardi VM, Mulvihill JJ, eds. *Advances in Neurology*, Vol. 29: *Neurofibromatosis (von Recklinghausen's Disease), Genetics, Cell Biology, & Biochemistry*. New York: Raven Press, 1981: 1–9.

Scabies often produces papules around the nipple, which may persist after treatment.

Granular parakeratosis of the submammary regions has been described [1].

REFERENCE

1 Wohlrab J, Lüftl M, Wolter M, Marsch WCH. Submammary granular parakeratosis: an acquired punctate hyperkeratosis of exogenous origin. *J Am Acad Dermatol* 1999; **40**: 813–4.

Lichen sclerosus et atrophicus confined to the areola has been reported [1].

REFERENCE

1 Starzycki Z. Lichen sclerosus et atrophicus confined to the areolae. *Br J Dermatol* 1993; **129**: 748–9.

Fox–Fordyce disease (Chapter 45) may produce intensely irritable papules on the areolae.

Carney complex (myxomas, spotty pigmentation and endocrine overactivity) is associated with breast myxoid fibroadenomas and ductal adenomas [1,2].

REFERENCES

1 Armstrong DKB, Irvine AD, Handley JM *et al*. Carney complex: report of a kindred with predominantly cutaneous manifestations. *Br J Dermatol* 1997; **136**: 578–82.
2 Courcoutsakis NA, Chow CK, Shawker TH *et al*. Syndrome of spotty skin pigmentation, myxomas, endocrine overactivity, and Schwannomas (Carney complex): breast imaging findings. *Radiology* 1997; **205**: 221–7.

Cowden's syndrome (multiple hamartoma syndrome) [1] is an autosomal-dominant disorder associated with hamartomas of various tissues and an increased risk of breast cancer, usually ductal carcinoma.

REFERENCE

1 Schrager CA, Schneider D, Gruener AC *et al*. Clinical and pathological features of breast disease in Cowden's syndrome: an underrecognized syndrome with an increased risk of breast cancer. *Hum Pathol* 1998; **29**: 47–53.

Hidradenitis suppurativa of the breasts tends to affect the inter- and inframammary folds [1].

REFERENCE

1 Hughes LE, Mansel RE, Webster DJT. *Benign Disorders and Diseases of the Breast*, 2nd edn. London: Saunders, 2000: 242–4.

Diffuse dermal angiomatosis of the breast, responding to isotretinoin, has been reported by McLaughlin *et al*. [1].

REFERENCE

1 McLaughlin ER, Morris R, Weiss SW, Arbiser JL. Diffuse dermal angiomatosis of the breast: response to isotretinoin. *J Am Acad Dermatol* 2001; **45**: 462–5.

Mucinosis of the areolae has been described as a presenting feature of mycosis fungoides [1].

REFERENCE

1 Vásquez-Doval FJ, Sola MA. Mucinosis of the mammary areolae and mycosis fungoides. *Clin Exp Dermatol* 1996; **21**: 374–6.

Chapter 68

The Genital, Perianal and Umbilical Regions

C.B. Bunker & S.M. Neill

Introduction

A number of common skin diseases affect the umbilical, perianal, genital and genitocrural skin only incidentally, and may present in these areas with unusual features. These will be dealt with briefly or by cross-reference to their full description elsewhere. However, those conditions that are entirely or predominantly confined to these regions are discussed in detail.

General approach to the patient and the problem

Clinical assessment begins with the history and examination. Patients with anogenital symptoms may be embarrassed and present late, or present to specialties (urology, gynaecology, general or colorectal surgery, genitourinary medicine) where training and experience are not focused on dermatological diagnosis and management.

Itching, rashes and tumours are the major components of general dermatology and the anogenital area is not spared. The pruritic diseases that may affect the anogenital region are listed in Tables 68.1–68.3. Itch occurring in the absence of specific diagnostic skin lesions is not usually confined to the anogenital area, but if so it should not be labelled as psychogenic until all possible causes have

Table 68.1 Common causes of anogenital pruritus. (After Bunker [1]. © 2004, with permission from Elsevier.)

Pruritus ani
Eczema/dermatitis
   Exogenous
      Contact
         irritant
         allergic
   Endogenous
      Atopic
      Seborrhoeic
      Lichen simplex
Psoriasis
Lichen sclerosus
Lichen planus
Perianal streptococcal dermatitis
Erythrasma
Herpes simplex
Candidosis
Tinea
Onchocerciasis (in developing countries)
Phthiriasis
Scabies

been excluded. The intensity with which itch can be perceived in the anogenital area may be a result of the vagaries of cortical representation afforded the region in the sensorium as well as anxiety about exposure to sexually transmitted disease and anogenital cleanliness.

Table 68.2 Rare causes of anogenital pruritus. (After Bunker [1]. © 2004, with permission from Elsevier.)

Insect bites/papular urticaria
Radiodermatitis
Hirsutism
Hyperhidrosis
Fox–Fordyce disease
Urticaria and dermographism [2]
Dermatitis herpetiformis
Chlamydia
Gonorrhoea
Syphilis
Other sexually transmitted diseases
Trichosporosis
Larva currens
Cutaneous larva migrans
Onchocerciasis (in Western practice)
Bowen's disease
Extramammary Paget's disease
Langerhans' cell histiocytosis
Drugs
Foods
Senile pruritus
Dysaesthesia syndromes

Table 68.3 Causes of genital itching in the absence of fixed clinical findings. (After Bunker [1]. © 2004, with permission from Elsevier.)

Symptomatic dermatographism
Contact urticaria
  Non-immunological (e.g. mechanical friction of pubic hair, topical substances)
  Immunological (latex, body fluids)
Contact dermatitis
Incognito disease
  Psoriasis
  Candidosis
  Scabies
Drugs and foods
Senile pruritus
Delusions of parasitosis
Dermatological non-disease
Dysaesthesia syndromes
Psychosexual

Table 68.4 Common causes of anogenital intertrigo.

Eczema
  Exogenous
    irritant contact
  Endogenous
    seborrhoeic
Psoriasis (inverse pattern/flexural)
Erythrasma
Candidosis
Tinea
Trichosporosis (in India)
Pseudoacanthosis nigricans

Table 68.5 Rare causes of anogenital intertrigo. (After Bunker [1]. © 2004, with permission from Elsevier.)

Eczema
  Exogenous
    allergic contact
  Endogenous
    atopic
Reiter's syndrome
Lichen sclerosus
Hailey–Hailey disease
Darier's disease
Streptococcal dermatitis
Gonorrhoea
Secondary syphilis
  Part of a syphilide
  Mucous patch
Congenital syphilis (in the infant)
Trichosporosis (in industrialized countries)
Extramammary Paget's disease
Kaposi's sarcoma
Langerhans' cell histiocytosis
Carcinoma erysipeloides

The symptomatology of anogenital dermatology is more extensive than the standard symptomatic presentation of skin disease. This obliges the clinician to elicit symptoms resulting from sexual dysfunction (e.g. preputial dysfunction—soreness, pain, bleeding or tearing on intercourse) and the components of sexual function (erection, lubrication, libido, ejaculation, orgasm, fertility), urinary dysfunction (frequency, discharge, dysuria) or colorectal symptomatology (pain, bleeding, discharge).

History taking must involve attention to the sexual history (orientation, marital status, last sexual activity (when; how—vaginal, oral, anal; contraception), regular partner(s), partner symptomatology) and drug history (topical and systemic, prescribed and over-the-counter). The personal

and family history of atopy, psoriasis and seborrhoeic dermatitis is often relevant. Smoking habits should be documented; smoking is a risk factor for anogenital cancer.

Complete examination is mandatory because common diagnoses will be reached with the assistance of important signs at extragenital sites. Often the patient will not have had his/her genitalia or perineum examined. The practice of anogenital dermatology demands careful inspection and often requires internal examination and urinalysis. Drawings are made and photographs obtained. Signs are described in conventional and specific terms (e.g. posthitis, phimosis).

Intertrigo describes any dermatosis occurring in skinfolds; frictional abrasion and a degree of epithelial loss may result in erosion that renders the site especially susceptible to secondary infection (e.g. with *Candida*). Causes are listed in Tables 68.4 and 68.5.

Pigmentary change is common. Causes of anogenital hypopigmentation and leukoderma include striae, vitiligo, lichen sclerosus, viral warts, leukoplakia and post-inflammatory changes (Table 68.6). Rarer causes include

Table 68.6 Causes of anogenital post-inflammatory hypopigmentation. (After Bunker [1]. © 2004, with permission from Elsevier.)

Following cryotherapy
  Electrotherapy
  Chemocautery
  Laser surgery
Contact dermatitis
Lichen sclerosus
Systemic sclerosis
Lichen planus
Cicatricial pemphigoid
Gonococcal dermatitis
Syphilis
  Leukoderma—post-secondary syphilide
  Gumma
  Post-gummatous atrophic scar
Herpes simplex
Pityriasis versicolor
Onchocerciasis 'leopard skin'
Peyronie's disease
Pseudoepitheliomatous micaceous and keratotic balanitis (PEMKB)

Table 68.7 Causes of anogenital post-inflammatory hyperpigmentation. (After Bunker [1]. © 2004, with permission from Elsevier.)

Post-traumatic
Lichen planus
Herpes simplex
Fixed drug eruption

Table 68.8 Causes of white patches and plaques. (After Bunker [1]. © 2004, with permission from Elsevier.)

Post-traumatic or surgical scar
Lichen simplex
Lichen sclerosus
Vitiligo
Mucous membrane (cicatricial) pemphigoid
Peyronie's disease
Syphilis
  Leukoderma—post-secondary syphilide
  Gumma
  Post-gummatous atrophic scar
Viral warts
Pityriasis versicolor
Pseudoepitheliomatous micaceous and keratotic balanitis (PEMKB)
Intraepithelial neoplasia
Squamous cell carcinoma

Table 68.9 Common causes of anogenital ulcers. (After Bunker [1]. © 2004, with permission from Elsevier.)

Trauma
Pressure sores
Aphthae
Pilonidal sinus
Anal fistula
Anal fissure
Erythema multiforme/Stevens–Johnson syndrome
Hidradenitis suppurativa
Crohn's disease
Chancroid
Donovanosis/granuloma inguinale
Lymphogranuloma venereum
Syphilis—primary chancre
Squamous carcinoma

Candida, extramammary Paget's disease, mycosis fungoides and melanoma. Common causes of anogenital hyperpigmentation include tattoos, purpura, lentigines, naevi, pseudoacanthosis nigricans and post-inflammatory changes (Table 68.7). Rarer or potential causes include Addison's disease, Nelson's syndrome, genital melanosis, Laugier–Hunziker syndrome [3], Peutz–Jeghers syndrome [4,5], LAMB syndrome (lentigines, atrial myxoma, mucocutaneous myxoma, blue naevi) [6,7], LEOPARD syndrome, Ruvalcaba–Myhre–Smith syndrome [8,9], acanthosis nigricans, acral lentiginous melanoma, drugs and metals. Both post-inflammatory hypo- and hyperpigmentation are possible after acute and chronic inflammation from diverse causes; both may be more pronounced in ethnically darker skin. Lichen planus, fixed drug eruptions and recurrent herpes simplex are the common causes of post-inflammatory hyperpigmentation. Genital trauma from a zipper injury can lead to macular pseudolentiginous lesions on the glans and shaft of the penis.

A mucosal white patch or plaque is sometimes called leukoplakia (Table 68.8). This is not a diagnostic term, and it is unhelpful as it evokes connotations from oral medicine of premalignancy or even frank neoplasia.

Anogenital ulceration requires meticulous elucidation. The principal causes are benign aphthae, sexually transmitted and non-sexually transmitted infection, cancer and artefact. Tables 68.9 and 68.10 list all the causes. Several causes can co-present, especially in HIV/AIDS.

Commonly required investigations include microbiology or virology of a swab or smear, scrapings for fungal microscopy and culture, scrapings for mite identification, skin biopsy, Wood's light to demonstrate vitiligo and erythrasma, and blood tests (e.g. ASOT, HLA B27, HIV). Investigations pertinent to the evaluation of sexually transmitted diseases are not discussed further, but it bears re-emphasis that if a diagnosis of a potentially sexually transmitted disease is reached (warts, molluscum contagiosum, herpes simplex, scabies, pediculosis) then the patient should be referred for a genitourinary opinion and advised to inform their partner(s) so that they may be screened also.

The opinion of another specialist may be necessary and should be sought as dictated by the urological, gynaecological, colorectal or genitourinary situation. Combined clinics are the ideal.

Table 68.10 Rare causes of anogenital ulcers. (After Bunker [1]. © 2004, with permission from Elsevier.)

Extrusion of testicular prosthesis
Embolization
Dermatitis artefacta
Penile necrosis
Spontaneous scrotal ulceration
Sarcoid
Autoimmune bullous diseases
 Bullous pemphigoid
 Mucous membrane (cicatricial) pemphigoid
 Linear IgA disease
Necrobiosis lipoidica
Pyoderma gangrenosum
Necrotizing vasculitis
Degos' malignant atrophic papulosis
Calciphylaxis
Hypereosinophilic syndrome
Pseudomonas
 Ecthyma gangrenosum
 Necrotizing anorectal ulcer in leukaemia
Gonorrhoea
Chancroid
Donovanosis (granuloma inguinale)
Lymphogranuloma venereum
Fournier's gangrene
Tuberculosis and tuberculides
Syphilis—snail track ulcers
Yaws
Non-syphilitic spirochaetal ulcerative balanoposthitis
Herpes simplex
HIV
Deep fungal infections
 Histoplasmosis
 Blastomycosis
 Cryptococcosis
Actinomycosis
Paracoccidioidomycosis
Leishmaniasis
Amoebiasis
Filariasis
Langerhans' cell histiocytosis
Extramammary Paget's disease
Basal cell carcinoma
Squamous carcinoma
Verrucous carcinoma
Sweat gland carcinoma
Melanoma
Kaposi's sarcoma
Leukaemia
Lymphoma
Drug reaction

REFERENCES

1 Bunker CB. *Male Genital Skin Disease*. London: Saunders, 2004 (in press).
2 Shertertz EF. Symptomatic dermographism as a cause of genital pruritus. *J Am Acad Dermatol* 1994; **31**: 1040–1.
3 Began D, Mirowski G. Perioral and acral lentigines in an African American man. *Arch Dermatol* 2000; **136**: 419–22.
4 Gass JDM, Glatzer RJ. Acquired pigmentation simulating Peutz–Jeghers syndrome: initial manifestation of diffuse uveal melanocytic proliferation. *Br J Ophthalmol* 1991; **75**: 693–5.
5 Eng A, Armin A, Massa M, Gradini R. Peutz-Jeghers -like melanotic macules associated with oesophageal adenocarcinoma. *Am J Dermatopathol* 1991; **13**: 152–7.
6 Voron DA, Hatfield HH, Kalkhoff RK. Multiple lentigines syndrome. *Am J Med* 1976; **60**: 447–56.
7 Rhodes AR, Silverman RA, Harrist TJ, Perez-Atayde AR. Mucocutaneous lentigines, cardiomucocutaneous myxomas, and multiple blue nevi: the 'LAMB' syndrome. *J Am Acad Dermatol* 1984; **10**: 72–82.
8 Gretzula JC, Hevia O, Schachner LS *et al.* Ruvalcaba–Myhre–Smith syndrome. *Pediatr Dermatol* 1988; **5**: 28–32.
9 Perriard J, Saurat JH, Harms M. An overlap of Cowden's disease and Bannayan–Riley–Ruvalcaba syndrome in the same family. *J Am Acad Dermatol* 2000; **42**: 348–50.

Genitocrural dermatology

Introduction

The genitocrural folds represent a region of the body that is particularly prone to intertrigo and flexural forms of common dermatoses, probably because of koebnerization. Moisture and friction also lead to maceration and fissuring, and secondary infections readily supervene. Vegetating reactions can prove resistant to treatment. Itch may be prominent in psoriasis, infections and infestations of the area. Crab louse and *Oxyuris* infestation must be excluded as primary causes of rash. Lichenification occurs readily.

Inflammatory dermatoses

Intertrigo

Intertrigo is a generic name for an inflammatory dermatosis involving the body folds, notably those of the submammary and genitocrural regions. There may be no clear distinction between constitutional and infective causes (listed in Tables 68.4 & 68.5). Physical factors such as obesity, sweating, friction, incontinence and faecal soiling may cause erythema or fissuring, and render the skin vulnerable to the effects of other agents. Initially, it is marked by soreness or slight itching, and a superficial mild erythema of the apposed surfaces. Secondary infection occurs rapidly, and the condition is then perpetuated as an infective dermatitis. In eczematous subjects this will take on the physical characteristics of eczema; in others, the infection may progress to crusting, pustular or vegetating lesions. The organisms concerned are *Staphylococcus aureus*, rarely the haemolytic streptococcus, *Escherichia coli*, *Proteus* spp. and, occasionally, *Pseudomonas aeruginosa*. In infants, diabetics and the obese, yeasts are often present. Latent diabetes should be borne in mind when the disease is refractory to treatment. Overtreatment may compound the irritation or lead to a sensitization dermatitis.

Candidosis and contact dermatitis are differentiated by the history, the appearance and microscopic examination. The diffuse macerated erythema, often with fissures at the apex of the fold and without a sharply defined edge, distinguishes intertrigo from psoriasis and dermatophytosis, although scrapings and culture should always be undetaken. Mistakes in diagnosis arise from failure to recognize that two or more aetiological factors may co-exist [1]. In India, *Trichosporon* species, which normally cause white piedra trichomycosis, have been implicated in causing cutaneous lesions resembling genitocrural intertrigo [2]. Langerhans' cell histiocytosis (see Chapter 52) has a predilection for the perineum or inguinal regions [3] and is a rare cause of genitocrural intertrigo; likewise extramammary Paget's disease. Congenital syphilis may present as intertrigo in an infant.

In the early stages, the condition can be controlled by avoidance of friction and tight clothing. Driving or sitting for long periods should be avoided. In severe cases, the patient must rest in bed, preferably with groins unclothed and bedclothes lifted by a cradle, the apposed skin surfaces being kept apart with appropriate dressings. Obesity, diabetes and incontinence should receive attention. Wet dressings are often useful initially in acute cases, and may be followed by bland or mild antibacterial creams or lotions. The aniline dyes and magenta paints still have a place in therapy. In general, lotions, paints and powders are more acceptable than creams. Nystatin, hydroxyquinoline and imidazoles can be applied alone or with topical steroids for a few days.

Genitocrural dermatitis

Lichen simplex is a result and/or cause of severe and spasmodic itch; the psychological mechanisms involved are similar to those discussed in relation to pruritus vulvae and pruritus ani. The 'giant' form of lichenification described by Pautrier [4] may be extremely resistant to treatment. Local treatment with corticosteroid applications is supplemented by reassurance, rest and sedation. All factors provoking local itching must, as far as possible, be removed.

Contact dermatitis (see Chapters 19–21) may present suddenly with pruritus, oedema and erythema, or insidiously as a gradual intensification of a pre-existing dermatitis. Sensitization to applied medicaments, contraceptives or, in men, industrial or other contact agents transferred by hand may be responsible for allergic contact dermatitis, especially if the scrotum and thighs are also affected. Irritant contact dermatitis is common and caused by excessive or exuberant use of soap and toiletries. A good example is nappy (diaper) rash where urine, occlusion, friction and *Candida* contribute to the clinical presentation. Classically, the convex surfaces are affected and the flexures are spared, distinguishing it from psoriasis [5]. Nappy rash has become much less common with the availability of absorbent disposable paper napkins. A severe erosive form (Jacquet's dermatitis) is still occasionally seen in children with urinary or faecal incontinence.

Constitutional eczema should be considered in the differential diagnosis of napkin erythema in an infant (see Chapter 14). In adults, the genitocrural and lower abdominal folds are likely to be involved in seborrhoeic or intertriginous dermatitis.

Miscellaneous

Psoriasis and lichen planus are recognized by their special characteristics, although the diagnosis may be difficult when they arise in an exclusively flexural distribution. In the flexures and at anogenital sites, seborrhoeic dermatitis and psoriasis may be indistinguishable.

Impetigo herpetiformis frequently starts in the groin with small inflammatory yellowish green pustules, which rupture to produce scabs and crusts. Acrodermatitis enteropathica and the acquired zinc deficiency syndrome may well be overlooked as causes of genitocrural dermatitis. The distinction of Jacquet's eruption from congenital syphilis and from the exuberant plaques and nodules of infantile gluteal granuloma [5,6] is important. Hidradenitis suppurativa usually involves the area widely, although localized lesions are sometimes seen.

All forms of pemphigus and pemphigoid (especially pemphigus vegetans [7] and pyodermite végétante [8]) affect this region, and juvenile pemphigoid and pemphigoid gestationis affect it selectively and sometimes exclusively. Pemphigus vegetans must be distinguished from vegetating forms of pyoderma, which are not uncommon in the groins, and from blastomycosis and other mycoses, verrucoid forms of tuberculosis and granuloma inguinale. Mucous membrane (cicatricial) pemphigoid [9] may affect the groin. Benign familial pemphigoid (Hailey–Hailey disease) affected the groins or genitalia in 14 out of 21 patients in one series [10]. It can involve the groins in isolation. Secondary infection with herpes simplex has been reported after treatment with retinoids [11]. Very rarely, papular plaques similar in appearance to genital warts have been reported. Darier's disease (see Chapter 34) involving the flexures is mild in most patients but does occur in the vast majority. It can be very sore and malodorous. The intertriginous features are similar to those of Hailey–Hailey disease. There have been several reports of a genital, inguinal and perineal eruption, with clinical and histological similarity to Darier's disease and Hailey–Hailey disease, called genitocrural papular acantholytic dermatosis. The patients had no rash elsewhere, no family history and negative immunofluorescence [12]. Subcorneal pustular dermatosis extends outwards from the inguinal folds as flaccid pustules, rapidly rupturing to form gyrate and circinate crusted lesions. Dystrophic forms of epidermolysis bullosa may cause separation of the skin during delivery or, if less severe, bullae and erosions at these sites of friction.

Epidermal necrolysis may present as desquamation, sometimes involving the whole region. Severe erythema multiforme involves the genital or anal mucosa in half of the cases. Necrolytic migratory erythema also extends in waves from this area [13].

REFERENCES

1 Schlappner OLA, Rosenblum GA, Rowden G *et al*. Concomitant erythrasma and dermatophytosis of the groin. *Br J Dermatol* 1970; **100**: 147–51.
2 Kamalam A, Senthamilselvi A, Ajuthades K *et al*. Cutaneous trichosporosis. *Mycopathologia* 1988; **101**: 167–75.
3 Chu T. Langerhans' cell histiocytosis. *Australas J Dermatol* 2001; **42**: 237–42.
4 Pautrier LM. In: Darier J, ed. *Nouvelle Pratique Dermatologique*, Vol. 7. Paris: Masson, 1936: 497.
5 Hamado T. Granuloma intertriginosum infantum. *Arch Dermatol* 1975; **111**: 1072–3.
6 Tappeiner J, Pfleger L. Granuloma gluteale infantum. *Hautarzt* 1971; **22**: 383–8.
7 Winkelmann RK, Su WP. Pemphigoid vegetans. *Arch Dermatol* 1979; **115**: 446–8.
8 Neuman HAM, Faber WR. Pyodermite vegetante of Hallopeau: immunofluorescence studies performed in an early disease stage. *Arch Dermatol* 1980; **116**: 1169–71.
9 Lever WF, ed. *Pemphigus and Pemphigoid*. Springfield: Thomas, 1965.
10 Raaschou-Nielsen W, Reymann F. Familial benign chronic pemphigus. *Acta Derm Venereol (Stockh)* 1959; **39**: 280–91.
11 Stallman D, Schmoeckel C. Morbos Hailey–Hailey mit dissemination und eczema herpeticum unter Etretinat therapie. *Hautartz* 1988; **39**: 454–6.
12 Wong TY, Milm MC Jr. Acantholytic dermatosis localized to genitalia and crural areas of male patients: a report of three cases. *J Cutan Pathol* 1994; **21**: 27–32.
13 Wilkinson DS. Necrolytic migratory erythema with carcinoma of the pancreas. *Trans St John's Hosp Dermatol Soc* 1973; **59**: 244–50.

Infections

Erythrasma

Erythrasma (see Chapter 27) is a common genitocrural infection, especially of the male. It is caused by *Corynebacterium minutissimum*, an organism that is normally a commensal but which in warmer climates may become pathogenic. Tawny, slightly scaly plaques are seen on the upper inner thighs. In the inguinal folds, erythrasma may present as an intertrigo and can be macerated and eroded. It is not usually very itchy, but can be slightly sore. Lesions are usually also found in the axillae or toe webs. It may coexist with *Trichophyton rubrum* [1] and candidosis. Pruritus ani has also been reported [2]. Erythrasma is a clinical diagnosis confirmed by demonstration of coral pink fluorescence under Wood's light (resulting from a porphyrin elaborated by the bacterium). Treatment is with topical clindamycin, erythromycin or an imidazole, or with oral erythromycin. It is prone to recur.

Candidosis

Candidosis (thrush) presents as an intertrigo. Symptoms of burning and soreness are more common than itch. Coalescent red patches or plaques involve the folds, often with superficial erosions. Pustulosis extends out onto the skin of the abdomen, buttocks or thighs from the irregularly marginated intertriginous lesions. It can be a primary infection, particularly in infants, and in pregnancy and diabetes, but *Candida* may be more often a secondary pathogen in anogenital dermatoses. Observing the signs of candidosis or demonstrating the presence of the organism does not prove that it is the cause of all the symptoms and signs. *Candida albicans* is such a ready opportunist because it is a part of the resident flora of the gastrointestinal tract and may be retrieved from intertriginous areas, including the preputial folds, in the absence of symptoms and signs. A search for an underlying dermatological or medical cause should be undertaken. The symptoms and signs of *Candida* may be more florid than the underlying predisposing cause. Obesity predisposes to candidal intertrigo but medical causes include diabetes mellitus, iatrogenic immunosuppression and systemic antibiotic treatment. Although oropharyngeal candidosis is almost invariably found in HIV infection, anogenital candidosis is not generally associated, perhaps because it is overlooked or because many patients take long-term imidazole antifungals orally.

Underlying disease should be identified and treated, and predisposing factors rectified. Treatment includes topical nystatin, clioquinol or an imidazole, often very usefully combined with hydrocortisone or a moderately potent corticosteroid. If the infection is severe, an oral imidazole may be indicated.

Tinea cruris

Tinea (see Chapter 31) is a common disease of the groins and is usually caused by *Trichophyton rubrum*. It is generally rare in women, but occurs more frequently in hot climates. Spread occurs onto the thighs, buttocks and pubis. Many patients have been previously misdiagnosed and/or partially treated with topical corticosteroids and/or topical antifungal agents. Tinea and *Candida* may complicate other dermatoses such as psoriasis. Tinea incognito/occulta is therefore common. There is a fine peripheral scaling (eczema marginé of Hebra). Cases have been described in infants [3].

Microscopy will confirm the clinical diagnosis, and in tinea incognito/occulta there are numerous fungal elements.

Dermatophyte infection of the anogenital skin usually requires oral treatment with griseofulvin, terbinafine or itraconazole. Topical treatments often fail because the anatomical complexity of the area makes topical treatment difficult, and there may be reinfection from concomitant involvement of feet or hands, toe or finger nails.

Miscellaneous

Bacterial or candidal infections complicate intertrigo, eczema, napkin erythema, scabies and many tropical diseases. Vincent's organism, *Pseudomonas aeruginosa* and a wide variety of Gram-negative organisms are commonly found. Gangrenous ecthyma of infants may, very rarely, affect the inguinocrural area. Bullous impetigo occurs in childhood, often secondary to scabies. Giant condylomata acuminata may infiltrate the groin [4]. Gangrene has followed operations for inguinal hernia [5]. Sacral herpes zoster may present with groin lesions and retention of urine or constipation.

Phthiriasis pubis is sometimes overlooked as a cause of pruritus in the female. In the hirsute male, the infestation may be widespread. Oxyuriasis can cause localized urticaria as well as pruritus. Scabies in children is diffuse, and the inguinal glands are often enlarged from secondary infection. Seabather's eruption and 'seaweed dermatitis' affect the bathing trunk area.

Schistosomiasis and amoebiasis cause phagedenic necrosis, fistulae and pseudoelephantiasis, and may also give rise to granulomas and condylomatous masses [6]. Onchocerciasis causes depigmentation, nodules, atrophy, lymphadenopathy and a 'hanging groin' [7]. Trichosporosis is a common cause of genitocrural intertrigo in India, with symptoms of itching or burning. Scaly papules may accompany the intertrigo. Coexisting dermatophyte, *Candida*, trichomycosis and erythrasma infection may be found. Dequalinium chloride is applied topically for treatment [8]. Trichomycosis presents with malodour and discolored broken hairs [9], which should be distinguished from those of trichorrhexis nodosa, caused by repeated scratching [10]. Blastomycosis, actinomycosis and other deep fungal infections (see Chapter 31) simulate tuberculosis, but are more prone to form fissures, sinuses and vegetating or exuberant granulomatous lesions. They are distinguished by histological and bacteriological examination.

Among chronic infections, tuberculosis, tertiary syphilis and leishmaniasis are diagnosed by their characteristic features, which are described elsewhere. Congenital syphilis can be overlooked as a cause of genitocrural intertrigo in an infant. In tropical countries, tuberculous inguinal lymphadenopathy may be a cause of genitocrural lymphoedema. Amoebiasis involves the groins and perineum by extension from the anus.

Sexually transmitted diseases are fully discussed in Chapters 27 and 30. Granuloma inguinale affects the genitalia in less than half of cases, causing coalescing nodules, serpiginous ulcers and fungating masses. The buboes and fistulae of lymphogranuloma venereum are characteristic. Vulval (rarely scrotal) lymphoedema and elephantiasis may occur in both diseases.

REFERENCES

1 Schlappner OLA, Rosenblum GA, Rowden G *et al.* Concomitant erythrasma and dermatophytosis of the groin. *Br J Dermatol* 1979; **100**: 147–51.
2 Bowyer A, McColl I. Erythrasma and pruritus ani. *Acta Derm Venereol* 1971; **51**: 444–7.
3 Parry EL, Foshee WS, Hall W *et al.* Diaper dermatophytosis. *Am J Dis Child* 1982; **136**: 273–4.
4 Eng AM, Morgan NE, Blekys I. Giant condyloma acuminatum. *Cutis* 1979; **24**: 203–6.
5 Audebert C. La gangrene post-operatoire progressive de la peau. *Ann Dermatol Vénéréol* 1981; **108**: 451–5.
6 Biagi FF, Martuscelli QA. Cutaneous amebiasis in Mexico. *Dermatol Trop* 1963; **2**: 129–36.
7 Nelson GS. 'Hanging groin' and hernia, complications of onchocerciasis. *Trans R Soc Trop Med Hyg* 1958; **52**: 272–5.
8 Kamalam A, Senthamilselvi G, Ajithadas K, Thambiah AS. Cutaneous trichosporosis. *Mycopathologia* 1988; **101**: 167–75.
9 White SW, Smith J. Trichomycosis pubis. *Arch Dermatol* 1979; **115**: 444–5.
10 Chernosky ME, Owen DW. Trichorrhexis nodosa: clinical and investigative studies. *Arch Dermatol* 1966; **94**: 577–85.

Miscellaneous

In the 'short bowel syndrome', kwashiorkor-like changes include an 'enamel paint skin' [1]. Dowling–Degos disease (reticulate pigmented anomaly of the flexures) involved the flexures in eight out of 10 patients [2], but may be restricted entirely to the vulval skin [3].

Acanthosis nigricans almost invariably affects the groins. Pseudoacanthosis nigricans can present as a macerated intertrigo and with secondary infection. These can be distinguished from each other and from lichenification in pigmented skins by a rubber silicone impression technique [4]. Calcinosis involving the upper inner thighs may resemble pseudoxanthoma elasticum [5].

The following entities are encountered in the genitocrural area. Angiomas and angiokeratomas—diffuse angiomas or lymphangiomas may cause irregular subcutaneous swellings; angiokeratoma corporis diffusum may be a feature of several very rare congenital diseases affecting lysosomes, with the pinhead-sized lesions of Anderson–Fabry disease (α-galactosidase deficiency) occurring around the lower limb girdle and upper thighs from the navel to the knees. Epidermal naevi are not uncommon. Seborrhoeic warts may be mistaken for viral warts [6] or Bowenoid papulosis, as may melanocytic naevi or acrochordons. Papilliferous naevi and skin tags often become large and pedunculated on the inner aspect of the thighs. Inguinogenital epidermoid cysts may become infected; lesions containing molluscum contagiosum have been described [7]. Pilar cyst, including giant forms, is much rarer [8].

Pubic hair problems are relatively rare in men, whereas women may be troubled by hirsutism or pili incarnati. Alopecia areata rarely affects this region alone. Vitiligo is common in the groins.

Extramammary Paget's disease can involve the genitocrural folds and present as an intertrigo.

Carcinoma erysipeloides (from anogenital disease) [9] is probably more common in the genitocrural area than reports would suggest. Carcinoma of the cervix, bladder and prostate may be the cause [10].

REFERENCES

1 Smith SR. Skin changes in short bowel syndrome. *Ann Dermatol Vénéréol* 1977; **113**: 657–9.

2 Wilson Jones E, Grice K. Reticulate pigmented anomaly of the flexures: Dowling–Degos disease, a new genodermatosis. *Arch Dermatol* 1976; **114**: 1150–7.

3 Milde P, Goerz G, Plewig G. Morbus Dowling–Degos mit ausschliesslich genitaler Manifestation. *Hautartz* 1992; **43**: 369–72.

4 Sarkany I. A method of studying the microtopography of the skin. *Br J Dermatol* 1962; **74**: 254–9.

5 Cochran RJ, Wilkin JK. An unusual case of calcinosis cutis. *J Am Acad Dermatol* 1983; **8**: 103–6.

6 Friedman SJ, Fox BJ, Albert HL. Seborrhoeic keratoses of the penis. *Urology* 1987; **29**: 204–6.

7 Park SK, Lee JY, Kim YH *et al*. Molluscum contagiosum occurring in an epidermal cyst: report of three cases. *J Dermatol* 1992; **19**: 119–21.

8 Shah SS, Varea EG, Farsaii A *et al*. Giant epidermoid cyst of the penis. *Urology* 1979; **14**: 389–91.

9 Cohen EL, Kim SW. Cutaneous manifestation of carcinoma of urinary bladder: carcinoma erysipeloides. *Urology* 1980; **16**: 410–2.

10 Ng CS. Carcinoma erysipeloides from prostate cancer presenting as cellulitis. *Cutis* 2000; **65**: 215–6.

Male genital dermatology

Introduction

Male patients with non-venereological and non-urological skin problems commonly present to genitourinary or urology clinics where the training and expertise are not orientated to adequate dermatological diagnosis and treatment [1].

Careful dermatological evaluation, including a full history and complete examination, usually allows confident clinical differential diagnosis. A biopsy and other investigations are sometimes indicated. It is important to consider the possibility of sexually transmitted disease or a urological disorder and refer accordingly; combined clinics are useful.

History taking and the primary symptomatology of anogenital dermatology are discussed on pp. 68.1–68.4. It may be necessary actively to elicit symptoms caused by sexual dysfunction, and it should be remembered that male sexual function amounts to more than erectile potency; libido, ejaculation and orgasm are the other components [2].

Complete examination is mandatory to elicit important signs at extragenital sites. The physical examination of the male at any age is incomplete without examination of the genitals and scrotum (but this is frequently not carried out in general clinical settings) and urologists teach that there are three primary reasons for careful examination of the scrotum: pain, swelling and absence of contents. The presence or absence of the prepuce, phimosis or paraphimosis should be sought and the foreskin retracted gently (if present). The gluteal and crural folds should be parted to allow adequate inspection. Sometimes it is useful to elicit dermatographism of the inner thighs. Urinalysis completes the physical examination.

Findings specific to the male genitalia include phimosis, paraphimosis, balanitis and posthitis. Phimosis ('muzzling') refers to a non-retractable foreskin. The literature can be confusing; Rickwood [3] has defined it as scarring

Table 68.11 Causes of phimosis. (After Bunker [7]. © 2004, with permission from Elsevier.)

Non-specific balanoposthitis (e.g. in diabetes)
Lichen sclerosus
Lichen planus
Hidradenitis suppurativa
Crohn's disease
Cicatricial pemphigoid
Chronic penile lymphoedema
Kaposi's sarcoma

Table 68.12 Causes of paraphimosis. (After Bunker [7]. © 2004, with permission from Elsevier.)

Acute contact urticaria
Acute allergic contact dermatitis
Lichen sclerosus

of the tip of the foreskin. There are several possible causes of phimosis (Table 68.11). In adults, phimosis is usually the consequence of disease processes. It has also been attributed to titanium formulated in proprietary topical preparations [4]. Diabetes was diagnosed in 36% of men between 17 and 59 years of age presenting with phimosis of less than 2 years' duration, with no specific preputial pathology identified histologically [5]. In boys, the histological findings may be normal in nearly half of those circumcised [6].

Paraphimosis refers to a foreskin fixed in retraction. Although some authors have used the term to describe a foreskin that is tight in retraction around the flaccid penile shaft, 'waisting' may be a better term [7]. Rickwood [8] has said that paraphimosis results from abuse not disease of the foreskin, but some medical causes can be identified (Table 68.12).

Balanitis is inflammation of the glans penis; posthitis is inflammation of the prepuce [9]. Balanoposthitis means inflammation of the glans and prepuce and can be regarded as a special form of intertrigo (Tables 68.13 & 68.14). By definition therefore, balanoposthitis cannot occur in the circumcised male. Generally, dermatologists feel that balanitis, posthitis and balanoposthitis are probably more commonly caused by inflammatory and precancerous dermatoses than do genitourinary physicians, who teach that most cases are caused by infection, usually with *Candida* [10,11]. However, the evidence for *Candida* as a cause for balanoposthitis is not strong [12].

General aspects of anogenital ulceration are discussed on pp. 68.3–68.4 and in Tables 68.9 and 68.10. The principal causes of male genital ulceration are sexually transmitted and non-sexually transmitted infection, cancer and artefact [13]. Several causes can co-present, especially in HIV/AIDS. Dorsal perforation of the prepuce is a recently highlighted complication of several ulcerative penile diseases, sexually and non-sexually acquired, as listed in

Table 68.13 Common causes of balanoposthitis. (After Bunker [7]. © 2004, with permission from Elsevier.)

Eczema
    Exogenous
        allergic contact
        irritant contact
    Endogenous
        seborrhoeic
Psoriasis
Reiter's disease
Zoon's plasma cell balanitis
Lichen sclerosus
Gonorrhoea
Human papillomavirus
Herpes simplex
Candidosis

Table 68.14 Rare causes of balanoposthitis. (After Bunker [7]. © 2004, with permission from Elsevier.)

Crohn's disease
Streptococcal dermatitis
Staphylococcal cellulitis
Gonorrhoea
Syphilis
    Chancre with balanitis of Follman
    Mucous patch
Mycoplasma
Trichomonas vaginalis
Lymphogranuloma venereum
Non-syphilitic spirochaetal ulcerative balanoposthitis
Tinea
Amoebiasis
Myiasis
Scabies
Eccrine syringofibroadenomatosis
Erythroplasia of Queyrat
Kaposi's sarcoma
Chronic lymphatic leukaemia
Fixed drug eruption

Table 68.15 Causes of dorsal perforation of the prepuce.

Hidradenitis suppurativa
Pyoderma gangrenosum
Florid condylomata
Podophyllin
Chancroid
Herpes simplex

Table 68.15 [14,15]. Penile necrosis is a rare but devastating presentation with an important differential diagnosis.

Special investigations appropriate to anogenital cases are discussed on p. 68.3. In genitourinary clinics, application of 3–5% acetic acid to the penis is used as an aid to the clinical diagnosis of viral warts and is held to reveal subclinical infection [16], but is not in routine use in dermatological practice. Human papillomavirus (HPV) polymerase chain reaction (PCR) screening suggests that the acetowhite test is not very specific [17–19]. A penis biopsy can be highly informative in selected cases [20]. It is safe to use small amounts of adrenaline in the local anaesthetic. Beware of the distal ventral midline area where the urethra is very close to the skin surface. It is often not necessary to suture a punch biopsy site.

Structure and function of the male genitalia

The penis is the male organ of urinary elimination and sexual function for the insemination of the female. The prepuce and its secretions provide physical and immunological protective functions, and it has erogenous properties (e.g. the penile dartos muscle and the corpuscular receptor-rich ridged band), but none of these is indispensible for erogenous function in copulation [21]. The scrotum maintains the testes at the ideal temperature for spermatogenesis. The male genital structures are illustrated in Fig. 68.1. The anatomical position is that of full penile erection.

The anatomy is explained by the embryology [22]. At about the third week of fetal development, mesenchymal tissue from the primitive streak forms cloacal folds

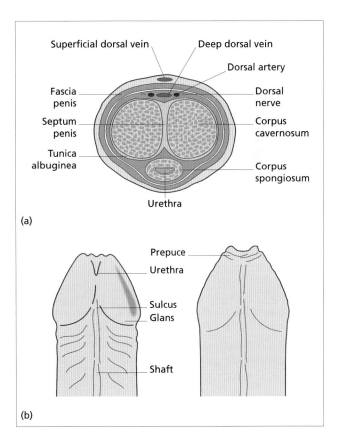

Fig. 68.1 (a) Cross section of the body of the penis. (b) Circumcised and uncircumcised glans penis. (Adapted from *Last's Anatomy*, 9th edn. Reproduced from Bunker CB. *Male Genital Skin Disease*, © 2004, with permission from Elsevier.)

around the cloacal membrane, joined anteriorly and cranially to form the genital tubercle, posteriorly and caudally to form an annulus. The cloacal membrane is thus divided into urogenital and anal membranes craniocaudally, and lateral genital swellings appear as precursors of either the scrotum or labia majora.

Fetal and testicular androgens then induce lengthening of the genital tubercle to form first an urethral groove and then the urethral canal. The urethral epithelium of the penis is therefore derived from endoderm. Initially, it is incomplete cranially where the glans has developed from the genital tubercle. The glandular urethra and the meatus form from an invading canalizing cord of ectoderm. The scrotal swellings fuse posteriorly at about 14 weeks but are empty until birth.

The prepuce [21] is formed by a midline fusion of ectoderm, neuroectoderm and mesenchyme, resulting in a pentalaminar structure consisting of (from the inner layer outwards) squamous mucosal epithelium, lamina propria, dartos muscle, dermis and glabrous skin. The preputial fold progressively extends, but there is also an ingrowth of a cellular lamella. It then fuses with the mucosa of the glans. The female analogue is the clitoral hood.

The anogenital area is densely endowed with eccrine and apocrine sweat glands. Also in plentiful number are holocrine sebaceous glands, usually in association with hair follicles but also occurring as free glands at some sites such as the anal rim or around the coronal sulcus (Tyson's glands). These secretions exist to lubricate hair, lubricate the mucocutaneous junctions to assist in the voiding of excreta and protect the epithelia from irritation and to lubricate the penis for sexual activity (probably mainly the retraction of the foreskin rather than the penetration of the vagina).

Pubic hair appears in puberty as vellus hair that is focally replaced by terminal hair. The pattern of pubic hair in men is different from that in woman, and its distribution varies widely between men. McGregor [23] defined three patterns (Fig. 68.2). Generally, the abdominal wall, pubic mound, groins, scrotum and perineum are hairy but the natal cleft, perianal skin, distal penile shaft, prepuce and glans are hairless.

The pattern of keratinization of the epithelium is different throughout the anogenital area, particularly at the mucosal junctions, the prepuce and distal penile shaft and the glans in the circumcised male. The spectrum of differentiation of the male urogenital tract is manifest in the expression of differing epithelial cytokeratins [24].

Normal variants

Normal male genital variants include pigmentary variation, hair variation as above, skin tags, pearly penile papules, sebaceous prominence (Fig. 68.3), melanocytic naevi, prominent veins, angiomas and angiokeratomas, common congenital abnormalities and circumcision.

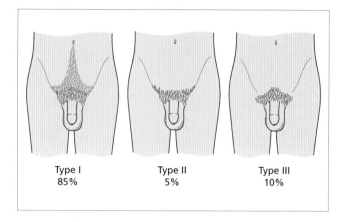

Fig. 68.2 Normal distribution of pubic hair in men. (After McGregor [23]. Reproduced from Bunker CB. *Male Genital Skin Disease*, © 2004, with permission from Elsevier.)

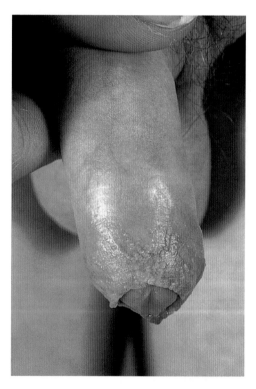

Fig. 68.3 Prominent sebaceous glands on the penis. (Courtesy of Dr F.A. Ive, Durham, UK.)

Skin tags are common in the groins, especially of obese men. They may catch on clothing, bleed and become infected. Treatment is by electrocautery or scissor amputation and cautery. Fibrosed haemorrhoids result in perianal skin tags. Larger, fleshier, more oedematous skin tags should arouse the suspicion of Crohn's disease. They can predate gastrointestinal disease by several years. Sigmoidoscopy and biopsy should be considered [25].

Pearly pink penile papules [26] are common; they may be found in up to 50% of men [27]. They present as flesh-coloured smooth rounded 1–3 mm papules, occurring predominantly around the coronal margin of the glans,

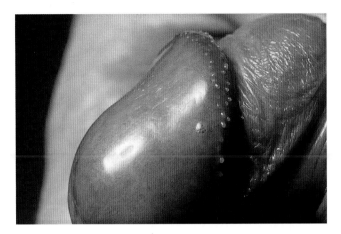

Fig. 68.4 Pearly penile papules. (Courtesy of Dr D.A. Burns, Leicester, UK.)

rarely on the glans, in rows or rings (Fig. 68.4). Ectopic lesions on the penile shaft have been reported [28]. They are frequently mistaken for warts and misdiagnosed as Tyson's or ectopic sebaceous glands of Fordyce. The patient is often an anxious adolescent. The histology is that of angiofibroma. The lesion is analogous to other acral angiofibromas such as adenoma sebaceum, subungual and periungual fibromas, fibrous papule of the nose, acquired acral angiofibroma and oral fibroma [29]. Reassurance is usually sufficient but cryotherapy and laser treatment can be effective [30, 31].

Sebaceous gland prominence, Tyson's glands, sebaceous hyperplasia and ectopic sebaceous glands of Fordyce are all virtually synonymous, common, normal variants of the skin of the scrotal sac and penile shaft, but they may cause concern to the patient. Fordyce's condition also commonly affects the vermilion border of the lips. Naevoid linear lesions on the penile shaft have been seen [32]. The glans can be affected [33]. Reassurance is usually all that is required, but dysmorphophobia can occur.

Congenital and acquired melanocytic naevi are common. It is possible that naevi on the penis occur more frequently in patients with the atypical naevus syndrome, but this has not been formally documented. Genital epithelioid blue naevus is very rare [34]. Divided or 'kissing' naevus (analogous to the entity recognized on the eyelids) has been reported, with one component located on the glans and the other on the distal penile shaft or prepuce, separated by uninvolved skin across the coronal sulcus [35]. Large 'bathing trunk' naevi frequently involve the anogenital area and pose significant management problems (see Chapter 38).

Prominent veins are common, if not universal, and occasionally give rise to concern. Vascular white spots are sometimes seen on the glans, and are possibly analogous to Bier's spots seen on the palms and forearms.

Cherry Campbell de Morgan angiomas may, unusually, be confined to the genitalia. Angiokeratomas on the

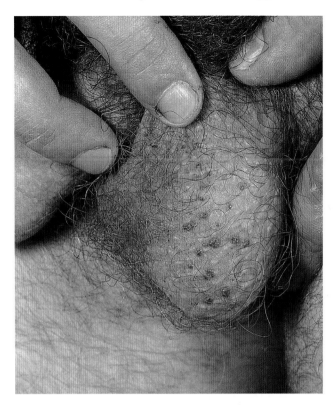

Fig. 68.5 Scrotal angiokeratoma of Fordyce (Courtesy of Dr D.A. Burns, Leicester, UK.)

genitalia have also confusingly been given the Fordyce eponym (Fig. 68.5). They are multiple, rarely solitary, blue to purple, smooth, 2–5 mm papules on the scrotum or penile shaft, rarely the glans. Angiomas and angiokeratomas may bleed following trauma. The differential diagnosis includes angiokeratoma corporis diffusum, acquired capillary and cavernous haemangiomas, Masson's tumour, glomus tumour, epithelioid haemangioma, bacillary angiomatosis, Kaposi's sarcoma and epithelioid haemangioendothelioma. Hyfrecation, electrocautery or laser ablation [36] can be offered, but lesions recur. Many patients are content with reassurance and a biopsy is not usually necessary.

The foreskin

The prepuce has been present in primates for 65–100 million years. It is usual for it to be adherent to the glans at birth. Four per cent of boys have a retractable foreskin at birth, 15% at 6 months, 50% at 1 year and 80–90% at 3 years; the process should be complete by 17 years [21]. The foreskin varies in length and retractability: 'short' and 'long' variants are seen.

Circumcision

Circumcision has been performed for religious, cultural or medical reasons throughout history [37]. Worldwide, it has been estimated that approximately 25% of men have been circumcised [38]. Routine neonatal circumcision is controversial [39]. The UK General Medical Council (GMC) undertook a review of infantile circumcision in 1997, which 'demonstrated widely conflicting views in society that neither doctors nor the GMC can resolve' [40].

During infancy, circumcised boys have a higher incidence of penile problems than the uncircumcised, but after infancy the situation is significantly reversed [41,42]. Many have concluded that circumcision protects men from cancer of the penis and urinary tract, and sexually transmitted infections including HIV [43]. However, the incidence of penis cancer is low in countries where circumcision is uncommon [44], so other factors are important in penile carcinogenesis (see pp. 68.36–68.38). Also, the effects of circumcision on the other outcomes may be small [45] (e.g. urethritis may be more common in the circumcised, whereas ulcerative disease is more common in the uncircumcised). Circumcision protects men from inflammatory genital dermatoses including psoriasis, seborrhoeic dermatitis, lichen planus and lichen sclerosus [46].

Circumcision is important in the management of disorders of the penis and the foreskin, including dermatological disease. However, variability exists between clinicians in the indications for circumcision, especially in children. They include true phimosis, recurrent balanoposthitis, lichen sclerosus, penile lymphoedema, intraepithelial neoplasia and carcinoma.

The consensus is that circumcision has insignificant adverse effects on health, but it is not risk or complication free: bleeding, infection, adhesions, fistula, keloid, concealed or buried penis, amputation, excision of excessive penile skin, meatal stenosis, meatitis and meatal ulcer, cysts, chordee, hypospadias and epispadias, amputation neuromas, abnormal sexual behaviour, psychological distress and dysmorphophobia [47–53]. 'Uncircumcision' describes preputial restoration performed throughout history for various reasons [54,55].

Congenital and developmental abnormalities

Congenital and developmental anomalies are common because of the complicated embryogenesis and subsequent sexual differentiation of the anogenital region. The dermatologist may not be called upon to make a primary diagnosis, but needs to be aware of anatomical and functional abnormalities because these additionally predispose the area to dermatoses and infections.

Naevi are discussed above. Other common abnormalities include meatal pit, sacral pit, hypospadias [56], median raphe cysts, canals and sinuses, and ambiguous genitalia.

Other rare anomalies include hypospadias variants, epispadias, penile hypoplasia, mucoid or urethral cysts, dermoid cyst, juvenile xanthogranuloma, buried penis, urethral atresia, penoscrotal transposition, congenital lymphoedema, giant prepucial sac, megaprepuce, accessory scrotum, haemangiomas, strawberry naevus, os penis, true aposthia and faun tail [7].

REFERENCES

1 Hillman RJ, Walker MM, Harris JRW, Taylor-Robinson D. Penile dermatoses: a clinical and histopathgological study. *Genitourin Med* 1992; **68**: 166–9.
2 Gasser TC, Lehmann K. Male sexual function is more than erection. *Lancet* 1995; **346**: 706.
3 Rickwood AM, Hemalatha V, Batcup G, Spitz L. Phimosis in boys. *Br J Urol* 1980; **52**: 147–50.
4 Dundas SAC, Laing RW. Titanium balanitis with phimosis. *Dermatologica* 1988; **176**: 305–7.
5 Chopra R, Fisher RD, Fencel R. Phimosis and diabetes mellitus. *J Urol* 1982; **127**: 1101–2.
6 Clemmensen OJ, Krogh J, Petri M. The histologic spectrum of prepuces from patients with phimosis. *Am J Dermatopathol* 1988; **10**: 104–8.
7 Bunker CB. *Male Genital Skin Disease.* London: Saunders, 2004 (in press).
8 Rickwood AM. Medical indications for circumcision. *BJU Int* 1999; **83** (Suppl. 1): 45–51.
9 Waugh MA. Balanitis. *Dermatol Clin* 1998; **16**: 757–62.
10 Edwards S. Balanitis and balanoposthitis: a review. *Genitourin Med* 1996; **72**: 155–9.
11 English JC III, Laws RA, Keough GC *et al.* Dermatoses of the glans penis and prepuce. *J Am Acad Dermatol* 1997; **37**: 1–24.
12 Birley HDL, Walker MM, Luzzi GA *et al.* Clinical features and management of recurrent balanitis: association with atopy and genital washing. *Genitourin Med* 1993; **69**: 400–3.
13 Rosen T, Brown TJ. Genital ulcers: evaluation and treatment. *Dermatol Clin* 1998; **16**: 673–85.
14 Gupta S, Kumar B. Dorsal perforation of prepuce: a common end point of severe ulcerative genital diseases? *Sex Transm Infect* 2000; **76**: 210–2.
15 Gupta S, Kumar B. Dorsal perforation of prepuce due to locally erosive condylomata acuminata. *Sex Transm Infect* 2001; **77**: 77–8.
16 Steinberg JL, Cibley LJ, Rice PA. Genital warts: diagnosis, treatment, and counselling for the patient. *Curr Clin Top Infect Dis* 1993; **13**: 99–122.
17 Mazzatenta C, Andreassi L, Biagioli M, Ricci S, Ratti G. Detection and typing of genital papillomaviruses in men with a single polymerase chain reaction and type specific DNA probes. *J Am Acad Dermatol* 1993; **28**: 704–10.
18 Wikström A, Hedblad MA, Johansson B *et al.* The acetic acid test in evaluation of subclinical genital papillomavirus infection: a comparative study on penoscopy, histopathology, virology and scanning electron microscopy findings. *Genitourin Med* 1992; **68**: 90–9.
19 Voog E, Ricksten A, Olofsson S *et al.* Demonstration of Epstein–Barr virus DNA and human papillomavirus DNA in acetowhite lesions of the penile skin and the oral mucosa. *Int J STD AIDS* 1997; **8**: 772–5.
20 Mallon E, Ross JS, Hawkins DA *et al.* Biopsy of male genital dermatosis. *Genitourin Med* 1997; **73**: 421.
21 Cold CJ, Taylor JR. The prepuce. *BJU Int* 1999; **83** (Suppl. 1): 34–44.
22 Ammini AC, Sabherwal U, Mukhopadhyay C, Vijayaraghavan M, Pandey J. Morphogenesis of the human external male genitalia. *Pediatr Surg Int* 1997; **12**: 401–6.
23 McGregor D. Distribution of pubic hair in sample of fit men. *Br J Dermatol* 1961; **73**: 61–4.
24 Achtstätter T, Moll R, Moore B, Franke WW. Cytokeratin polypeptide patterns of different epithelia of the human male urogenital tract: immunofluorescence and gel electrophoretic studies. *J Histochem Cytochem* 1985; **33**: 415–26.
25 Alexander-Williams J, Buchmann P. Perianal Crohn's disease. *World J Surg* 1980; **4**: 203–8.
26 Oates JK. Pearly penile papules. *Genitourin Med* 1997; **73**: 137–8.
27 Sonnex C, Dockerty WG. Pearly penile papules: a common cause of concern. *Int J STD AIDS* 1999; **10**: 726–7.
28 Neri I, Bardazzi F, Raone B, Negosanti M, Patrizi A. Ectopic pearly penile papules: a paediatric case. *Genitourin Med* 1997; **73**: 136.
29 Ackerman AD, Kornberg R. Pearly penile papules. *Arch Dermatol* 1973; **108**: 673–5.
30 Porter W, Bunker CB. Treatment of pearly penile papules with cryotherapy. *Br J Dermatol* 2000; **142**: 847–8.

31 McKinlay JR, Graham BS, Ross EV. The clinical superiority of continuous exposure versus short-pulsed carbon dioxide laser exposures for the treatment of pearly penile papules. *Dermatol Surg* 1999; **25**: 124–6.

32 Kumar A, Kossard S. Band-like sebaceous hyperplasia over the penis. *Australas J Dermatol* 1999; **40**: 47–8.

33 Massmanian A, Valis GS, Sempere FJV. Fordyce spots on the glans penis. *Br J Dermatol* 1995; **133**: 498–9.

34 Izquierdo MJ, Pastor MA, Carrasco L *et al*. Epithelioid blue naevus of the genital mucosa: report of four cases. *Br J Dermatol* 2001; **145**: 496–501.

35 Choi GS, Won DH, Lee SJ, Lee JH, Kim YG. Divided naevus on the penis. *Br J Dermatol* 2000; **143**: 1126–7.

36 Occella C, Bleidl D, Rampini P, Schiazza L, Rampini E. Argon laser treatment of cutaneous multiple angiokeratomas. *Dermatol Surg* 1995; **21**: 170–2.

37 Dunsmuir WD, Gordon EM. The history of circumcision. *BJU Int* 1999; **83** (Suppl. 1): 1–12.

38 Moses S, Bailey RC, Ronald AR. Male circumcision: assessment of health benefits and risks. *Sex Transm Infect* 1998; **74**: 368–73.

39 Whitfield H. Circumcision. *BJU Int* 1999; **83** (Suppl. 1): 1–113.

40 Anonymous. *Guidance for Doctors who are Asked to Circumcise Male Children.* London: General Medical Council, 1997.

41 Fergusson DM, Lawton JM, Shannon FT. Neonatal circumcision and penile problems: an 8 year longitudinal study. *Pediatrics* 1988; **81**: 537–41.

42 Van Howe RS. Variability in penile appearance and penile findings: a prospective study. *Br J Urol* 1997; **80**: 776–82.

43 O'Farrell N, Egger M. Circumcision in men and the prevention of HIV infection: a 'meta-analysis' revisited. *Int J STD AIDS* 2000; **11**: 137–42.

44 Frisch M, Friis S, Kjaer SK, Melbye M. Falling incidence of penis cancer in an uncircumcised population (Denmark 1943–90). *BMJ* 1995; **311**: 1471.

45 Laumann EO, Masi CM, Zuckerman EW. Circumcision in the United States: prevalence, prophylactic effects, and sexual practice. *JAMA* 1997; **277**: 1052–7.

46 Mallon E, Hawkins D, Dinneen M *et al*. Circumcision and genital dermatoses. *Arch Dermatol* 2000; **136**: 350–4.

47 Williams N, Kapila L. Complications of circumcision. *Br J Surg* 1993; **80**: 1231–6.

48 Gürünlüoğlu R, Bayramicli M, Dogan T, Numanoglu A. Unusual complications of circumcision. *Plast Reconstr Surg* 1999; **104**: 1938–9.

49 Esen AA, Aslan G, Kazimoğlu H, Arslan D, Çelebi I. Concealed penis: rare complication of circumcision. *Urol Int* 2001; **66**: 117–8.

50 Coskunfirat OK, Sayilkan S, Velidedeoğlu H. Glans and penile skin amputation as a complication of circumcision. *Ann Plast Surg* 1999; **43**: 457.

51 Quintela R, Delmas V, Cannistra C, Boccon-Gibod L. Plastic surgery of the penis after circumcision. *Prog Urol* 2000; **10**: 476–8 [in French].

52 Kaplan GW: Complications of circumcision. *Urol Clin North Am* 1983; **10**: 543–9.

53 Goldman R. The psychological impact of circumcision. *BJU Int* 1999; **83** (Suppl. 1): 93–102.

54 Schultheiss D, Truss MC, Stief CG, Jonas U. Uncircumcision: a historical review of preputial restoration. *Plast Reconstr Surg* 1998; **101**: 1990–8.

55 Brandes SB, McAninch JW. Surgical methods of restoring the prepuce: a critical review. *BJU Int* 1999; **83** (Suppl. 1): 109–13.

56 Ellsworth P, Cendron M, Ritland D, McCullough M. Hypospadias repair in the 1990s. *AORN J* 1999; **69**: 148–53, 155–6, 159–61.

Trauma and artefact

Penile haematoma and rupture

The genitals may be readily traumatized by sexual activity. The penis is very vascular but haematoma formation and 'fracture' (penile rupture) are quite rare [1]. Pain, swelling and deformity associated with the history of a cracking noise during strenuous or contorted intercourse characterize the diagnosis. Splitting of the tunica albuginea of the corpus cavernosum can result in urethral damage, haematoma and retention. The prognosis is generally good but Peyronie's disease can occur [2]. Injection of drugs for erectile dysfunction can be complicated by haematoma.

Sclerosing lymphangitis

Non-venereal sclerosing lymphangitis/penile venereal oedema/Mondor's phlebitis/localized penile (venereal) lymphoedema/penile lymphocoele presents with a serpiginous mass in the coronal sulcus. The lesion usually arises after prolonged or frequent sexual intercourse with a passive or unenthusiastic partner; subsequent sexual activity may result in tenderness and enlargement. The circumferential scar left by circumcision may be a predisposing factor. There may be spontaneous resolution, or surgical excision may be needed [3]. It is not known whether lymphangitis or phlebitis is the cause [4]. True phlebitis of penile and scrotal veins has been reported in three patients, one of whom had been injured by a golf ball but the others were idiopathic [5]. Thrombophlebitis of superficial penile and scrotal veins is analogous to Mondor's phlebitis of the chest wall (see Chapter 67), but it may be associated with polyarteritis nodosa and thromboangiitis obliterans [6]. Penile thrombophlebitis has been misdiagnosed as Peyronie's disease, and has also been the initial manifestation of a paraneoplastic migratory thrombophlebitis resulting from pancreatic cancer [7].

Strangulation of the penis

The penis may be strangulated by ring devices [8] , including vacuum erection equipment [9], condom rings [10], rubber bands, string, rings (washers), nuts, bushes and sprockets, which are placed deliberately on the penis by the patient for masturbation or by his partner to prolong erection [11,12]. In boys, strangulation can occur following experimental use of rubber bands or string or thread to control enuresis, or resulting from encoiled hair after circumcision [13]. Penile strangulation—the tourniquet syndrome—causes pain, swelling, urethral fistula, pseudoainhum, gangrene and amputation.

Foreign body

Self-instrumentation of the external genitalia may have an autoerotic, psychiatric, therapeutic (relief of itch [14], aiding voiding, cleaning) or accidental aetiology [15]. Complications include frequency, haematuria, abscess, retention, fistulae and calculi. The diagnosis is made by palpation and radiography. Endoscopic removal is usually possible for foreign bodies below the urogenital diaphragm.

Glass beads, spheres of plastic or small round smooth stones (even pearls) may be introduced under the skin of the penis for erotic reasons, causing clinical and radiographical confusion. If oil, petroleum jelly or silicone is used then a paraffinoma, silicone granuloma or (sclerosing) lipogranuloma can result. In the Philippines, this practice is called 'bulleetus', in Sumatra 'persimbraon', in Korea 'chagan ball' and in Thailand it is called 'mukhsa' or 'tancho' [16].

Extrusion of a testicular prosthesis has been reported to cause scrotal ulceration because of a sinus tract [17].

Lipogranuloma

Mineral oil, petroleum jelly and silicone introduced into the genital skin can elicit lipogranuloma. Most cases are self-induced, either to create testicular prostheses or to increase penile size, enhance sexual pleasure, mutilate or malinger, although some may be accidental [18,19]. One patient injected his penis with an industrial high-pressure pneumatic grease-gun [20]. Endogenous fat liberation is a possible mechanism and idiopathic cases have been reported, predominantly from Japan [21].

Dermatitis artefacta

Dermatitis artefacta on the genitalia does occur. Lesions are typically geometrical, angulated and rectilinear. Sometimes they are induced by needles, knives or cigarette burns, and extraneous foreign material may be introduced into the skin (lipogranuloma and silicone granuloma are discussed above).

Psychotic patients may mutilate their genitalia, as can transvestites [22], but non-psychotic genital self-mutilation can also occur. Australian aborigines slit the penis—open the urethra ventrally, creating hypospadias—and this is called subincision [23]. Ritual female circumcision in Islam, and male circumcision in the Jewish culture, Islam and Western society may be perceived as similar practices.

Biopsy and other investigations may be necessary to exclude penile cancer. It is important also to consider pyoderma gangrenosum, which is rare but frequently omitted from the differential diagnosis of penile ulceration by non-dermatologists.

Child abuse

Physical and sexual child abuse should be suspected in the differential diagnosis of cutaneous disease of the anogenital area in children (Table 68.16), but signs should be interpreted with caution and re-examination should be avoided [25–29]. Child abuse may be erroneously suspected (Table 68.17) when the anogenital area is involved by a dermatosis or a diarrhoeal illness [30].

The significance of anogenital warts in suggesting possible child sexual abuse is controversial. However, early recognition as a marker for child sexual abuse is in the child's long-term best interest [31].

Table 68.16 Anogenital signs of child abuse. (After Bunker [24].)

Overall context
Emotional disturbance
Passivity on anogenital examination
Anal relaxation/dilatation
Purpura, bruising, tearing
Signs of sexually transmitted disease

Table 68.17 Anogenital mimics of child abuse. (After Bunker [24].)

Nappy rash
Innocent skin tags and fissures
Threadworms
Eczema
Phytophotodermatitis
Lichen sclerosus
Henoch–Schönlein purpura
Acute haemorrhagic oedema of childhood
Anogenital streptococcal dermatitis
Causes of diarrhoea
Haemolytic–uraemic syndrome
Crohn's disease
Causes of constipation
Hirschsprung's disease

Miscellaneous

Sometimes the penis is bitten by another individual or an animal [32]. Purpura and ecchymoses may develop after oral sex ('love bites') or the use of vacuum erection devices [33]. Degloving injuries can occur in accidents with industrial or agricultural equipment [34]. Electric burns are rare [35]. Sex aids can result in abrasions, eczema and ulceration. Anogenital tattoos are commonplace [36].

Localized gangrene of the scrotum and penis resulting from arterial embolization with particulate matter complicating accidental femoral self-injection of heroin in an addict has been reported [37].

REFERENCES

1 Nouri M, Koutani A, Tazi K *et al.* Fractures of the penis: apropos of 56 cases. *Prog Urol* 1998; **8**: 542–7.
2 Goh SH, Trapnell IE. Fracture of the penis. *Br J Surg* 1980; **67**: 680–1.
3 Kraus S, Lüdecke G, Weidner W. Mondor's disease of the penis. *Urol Int* 2000; **64**: 99–100.
4 Tanii T, Hamada T, Asai Y, Yorifuji T. Mondor's phlebitis of the penis: a study with factor VIII related antigen. *Acta Derm Venereol* 1984; **64**: 337–40.
5 Harrow BR, Sloane IA. Thrombophlebitis of superficial penile and scrotal veins. *J Urol* 1963; **89**: 841–2.
6 Coldiron B, Jacobson C. Common penile lesions. *Urol Clin North Am* 1988; **15**: 671–85.
7 Horn AS, Pecora A, Chiesa JC, Alloy A. Penile thrombophlebitis as a presenting manifestation of pancreatic carcinoma. *Am J Gastroenterol* 1985; **80**: 463–5.
8 Wasadikar PP. Incarceration of the penis by a metallic ring. *Postgrad Med J* 1997; **73**: 255.
9 Ganem JP, Lucey DT, Janosko EO, Carson CC. Unusual complications of the vacuum erection device. *Urology* 1998; **51**: 627–31.
10 Tash JA, Eid JF. Urethrocutaneous fistula due to a retained ring of condom. *Urology* 2000; **56**: 508.

11 Snoy FJ, Wagner SA, Woodside JR, Orgel MG, Borden TA. Management of penile incarceration. *Urology* 1984; **24**: 18–20.

12 Bhat AL, Kumar A, Mathur SC, Gangwal KC. Penile strangulation. *Br J Urol* 1991; **68**: 618–21.

13 Pohlman RB. Photo quiz: a lesion that should raise suspicion. *Am Fam Physician* 2000; **62**: 2095–6.

14 Al-Durazi M, Saleem I, Mohammed AA. Urethral foreign body. *Br J Urol* 1992; **69**: 434.

15 Aliabadi H, Cass AS, Gleich P, Johnson CF. Self-inflicted foreign bodies involving the lower urinary tract and male genitals. *Urology* 1985; **26**: 12–6.

16 George WM. Papular pearly penile pearls. *J Am Acad Dermatol* 1989; **20**: 852.

17 Gordon JA, Schwartz BB. Delayed extrusion of testicular prosthesis. *Urology* 1979; **14**: 59–60.

18 Coldiron B, Jacobson C. Common penile lesions. *Urol Clin North Am* 1988; **15**: 671–85.

19 Santucci RA, Zehring RD, McClure D. Petroleum jelly lipogranuloma of the penis treated with excision and native skin coverage. *Urology* 2000; **56**: 331.

20 Kalsi JS, Arya M, Peters J, Minhas S, Ralph DJ. Grease-gun injury to the penis. *J R Soc Med* 2002; **95**: 254.

21 Matsuda T, Shichiri Y, Hida S *et al.* Eosinophilic sclerosing lipogranuloma of the male genitalia not caused by exogenous lipids. *J Urol* 1988; **140**: 1021.

22 Greilsheimer H, Groves JE. Male genital self-mutilation. *Arch Gen Psychiatry* 1979; **36**: 441–6.

23 Pounder DJ. Ritual mutilation: subincision of the penis among Australian aborigines. *Am J Forensic Med Pathol* 1983; **4**: 227–9.

24 Bunker CB. *Male Genital Skin Disease.* London: Saunders, 2004 (in press).

25 McCann J, Voris J. Perianal injuries resulting from sexual abuse: a longitudinal study. *Pediatrics* 1993; **91**: 390–3.

26 Clayden G. Anal appearances and child sex abuse. *Lancet* 1987; **1**: 620–1.

27 Priestley BL, Bamford FN, Miles VM *et al. Physical Signs of Sexual Abuse in Children*, 2nd edn. Report of a working party of the Royal College of Physicians. London: Royal College of Physicians, 1997.

28 Hobbs CJ, Wynne JM. Physical signs of sexual abuse in children. *J R Coll Phys Lond* 1997; **31**: 580–1.

29 Wynne JM, Hobbs CJ. Examination of children who may have been sexually abused. *Arch Dis Child* 2000; **82**: 268.

30 Vickers D, Morris K, Coulthard MG, Eastham EJ. Anal signs in haemolytic uraemic syndrome. *Lancet* 1998; **1**: 998.

31 Hobbs CJ, Wynne JM. How to manage warts. *Arch Dis Child* 1999; **81**: 460.

32 Gomes CM, Ribeiro-Filho L, Giron AM *et al.* Genital trauma due to animal bites. *J Urol* 2001; **165**: 80–3.

33 Ganem JP, Lucey DT, Janosko EO, Carson CC. Unusual complications of the vacuum erection device. *Urology* 1998; **51**: 627–31.

34 Hrbatý J, Molitor M. Traumatic skin loss from the male genitalia. *Acta Chir Plast* 2001; **43**: 17–20.

35 Xu X, Zhu W, Wu Y. Experience of the treatment of severe electric burns on special parts of the body. *Ann N Y Acad Sci* 1999; **888**: 121–30.

36 Goldstein N. Psychological implications of tattoos. *J Dermatol Surg Oncol* 1979; **5**: 883.

37 Somers WJ, Lowe FC. Localized gangrene of the scrotum and penis: a complication of heroin injection into the femoral vessels. *J Urol* 1986; **136**: 111–3.

Inflammatory dermatoses

Urticaria and dermographism

These are usually generalized eruptions (see Chapter 47) but it has been proposed that they may account for some of the symptomatology in some patients with unexplained genital itching (and pruritus ani—see below). Stroking the inside of the thigh might induce a weal; indeed, stroking can cause itching without any discernible redness or wealing [1,2]. Contact urticaria is discussed below. Lisinopril has been reported to cause genital angio-oedema [3].

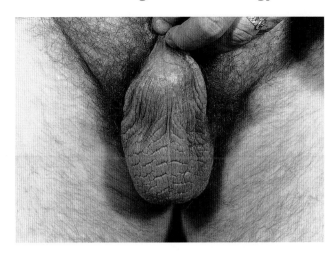

Fig. 68.6 Scrotal lichen simplex. (Courtesy of Dr F.A. Ive, Durham, UK.)

Eczematous dermatoses

Itching and lichenification, particularly around the scrotum, are common presenting problems. Contributory factors include pre-existing dermatoses such as xerosis, atopy and psoriasis, sedentary occupations, motor car and aeroplane travel, and tight underclothing and trousers.

Irritation is a key adverse exogenous influence to which anogenital sites are vulnerable, and sweat, sebum, desquamated corneocytes, dirt, excreta, sexual secretions, clothing, detergents, toiletries, cosmetics, contraceptives and some therapeutic topical treatments are all potential irritants.

Frequently underrated are the effects of overwashing and the excessive use of soap and toiletries, especially in the presence of skin symptoms or urinary or bowel problems, and particularly if patients feel that they might have been exposed to a sexually transmitted disease.

Lichen simplex

Lichen simplex is common around the male genitalia. It is not usually a flexural condition but can be seen on the penile shaft and scrotum (Fig. 68.6). Giant forms (of Pautrier) occur, giving a pineapple appearance [4]. The skin may be broken by excoriations and become secondarily impetiginized or colonized by *Candida*.

Treatment follows the lines of management above and below relating to irritants. There is emphasis on the relief of scratching, soap substitution and moisturization are recommended and the area occluded if possible with a bland dressing—wet if the skin is fiercely eczematized. A potent topical corticosteroid ointment can be used for a few days and then tailed off. Preparations containing tar or combinations of antibacterial and anticandidal and antifungal agents are also useful. Two cases of extensive

Table 68.18 Anogenital irritants. (After Bunker [5]. © 2004, with permission from Elsevier.)

Sweat
Sebum
Desquamated corneocytes
Dirt
Excreta
Sexual secretions
Clothing
Soap and detergents
Toiletries
Toilet paper
Cosmetics
Contraceptives
Therapeutic
Friction
Maceration

Table 68.19 Allergens of particular relevance to anogenital contact dermatitis. (After Bunker [5]. © 2004, with permission from Elsevier.)

Euxyl K 400 (methyldibromoglutaronitrile)
Kathon CG (isothiazolinones)
Lidocaine (lignocaine) and other topical anaesthetics
Neomycin
Nystatin
Steroid moieties
Thiuramdisulphide—rubber
Latex condoms
Spermicides
Mitomycin C

giant lichen simplex of the scrotum have been successfully treated by hemiscrotectomy [4].

Irritant contact dermatitis

Anogenital irritants are discussed above and listed in Table 68.18. Friction [6], maceration, overwashing, concomitant anorectal or urological disease are the chief influences. There may be an association with atopy; Birley [7] diagnosed irritant dermatitis in 72% of patients presenting to a genitourinary clinic with 'balanitis' (probably meaning balanoposthitis) of whom a possible 67% had a history of atopy, but none of these patients was patch tested. An irritant scrotal dermatitis in cellists has been described [8]. Topical 5-fluorouracil used to treat keratoses at extragenital sites has caused genital irritant dermatitis [9]. Acute or chronic, sterile or superinfected (with staphylococci or *Candida*, or both), eroded or hyperkeratotic presentations are seen, depending on the scenario. A good example is nappy (diaper) rash (see Chapter 14).

Management follows lines similar to those for pruritus ani (see p. 68.87). Irritants should be identified and eliminated or reduced. Advice is given about soap substitutes, moisturizers, towels and toilet paper. Topical corticosteroid ointments, with or without antibiotic and anticandidal agents, are employed to control the dermatitis. Oral antihistamines are useful. Topical local anaesthetics should be avoided because of the risk of sensitization. Occasionally, secondary infection may be severe; a swab should be taken and oral antibiotics and oral antifungals prescribed.

A more acute picture (itch, burning or pain, swelling, erythema, vesiculation) may occur if highly irritant chemicals in high concentration are accidentally or deliberately used on the genitalia. Patients with a genital rash who are frightened that it may have been sexually acquired will sometimes self-treat with unsuitable preparations and in the process increase their morbidity and conceal an underlying sexually transmitted disease or dermatosis. Treatment is with potassium permanganate soaks, very potent topical corticosteroid creams (sometimes systemic corticosteroids) and systemic antibiotics.

Allergic contact dermatitis

The risks of allergic contact dermatitis of the genital skin come about from: (i) direct contact with the allergen (e.g. medicaments—even coal tar allergy has been reported [10]), contraceptive usage and prosthetic limbs in amputees [11]; or, very rarely, (ii) transfer of allergen (e.g. urushiol as in poison oak, poison ivy and poison sumac dermatitis) to the genitalia [12] and possibly subsequent exposure to sunlight (e.g. psoralens from fig or citrus plants, as in phytodermatitis); and (iii) involvement in a more generalized eczematous response (e.g. to a medicament or dressing used on venous eczema or ulceration, as in the autosensitization/secondary spread/secondary generalization syndrome).

Acute or chronic eczematous symptomatology appears approximately 1 week after first contact with the allergen if previously unsensitized, or within a few hours if already allergic. The patient may present with pruritus ani [13] or paraphimosis [14]. More immediate symptomatology and acute erythema and angio-oedema suggest a contact urticaria, which can occur with some of the rubber constituents of condoms and gloves [15].

The principles of management are the identification of the potential allergen (Table 68.19) and its likely source, and then its elimination. There may be clues to these factors at presentation but subsequent patch testing is often required. Following patch testing, Bauer *et al.* [16] made a final diagnosis of allergic contact dermatitis in 35% of patients with anogenital skin problems. Allergic contact dermatitis can persist even with the withdrawal of the trigger allergen. Management is otherwise as for irritant contact dermatitis, lichen simplex and pruritus ani (see above and p. 68.87).

The most common relevant sensitivities are to rubber, contraceptives, preservatives and fragrances in toiletries and medicaments, and the active agents (antibiotics, steroids, anaesthetics) in medicaments.

Genital rubber dermatitis is not confined to young sexually active male condom users and their partners [17–20]. Incontinent men who use external urinary collection devices (Paul's tubing) are also at risk. Latex allergy may be a problem in patients with spinal cord injury using rubber products for the management of urinary difficulties; life-threatening anaphylactic reactions have occurred [19]. Condoms made from lamb caecum are available for rubberallergic patients but they may provide less protection against sexually transmitted disease than latex. Creating hypoallergenic condoms by washing in an ammonium solution to remove the residues of the accelerator chemicals that actually cause the hypersensitivity has proved unsuccessful [21]. Patients may become sensitized to the spermicide [17].

Celandine juice [14] and clothing dye dermatitis of the scrotum [22] have been reported.

Atopic dermatitis

Genital skin disease caused by atopic dermatis (AD) is not uncommon but rarely occurs in isolation, unlike other common chronic dermatoses such as seborrhoeic dermatitis and psoriasis. It is not known how genital AD is related to circumcision, sexual activity and sexually transmitted disease. Evidence of atopy was found in a possible 67% of a total of 72% of patients diagnosed as having irritant dermatitis from a consecutive series of men presenting to a genitourinary clinic with 'balanitis'—probably balanoposthitis [6]. AD in HIV/AIDS is discussed in Chapter 26.

Radiodermatitis

Radiodermatitis (see Chapter 76) is not usually a diagnostic challenge or a therapeutic problem in the acute stage after radiotherapy to the anogenital skin for skin disease or internal cancer. In the chronic state, there may be pruritus together with the typical poikiloderma. Radiotherapy confers a long-term increased risk of skin cancer, especially basal cell carcinoma. There is concern that radiotherapy for Bowen's disease or erythroplasia of Queyrat may increase the subsequent risk of invasive carcinoma.

Seborrhoeic dermatitis

Genital involvement is frequent with this common dermatosis. The groins and penis may be the only sites involved. A good history (including family history) and careful examination of other sites typically affected aid the diagnosis. On the scalp, the face, in the flexures and at anogenital sites seborrhoeic dermatitis and psoriasis may be indistinguishable. Seborrhoeic dermatitis in HIV/AIDS is discussed in Chapter 26.

Diagnosis is established on clinical grounds, including response to therapy, and it is not usually necessary to perform a biopsy.

No treatment may be required other than reassurance that it is not sexually transmitted or related to poor hygiene. However, treatments that diminish the *Malassezia* load and reduce irritation and eczematization can be successfully and safely used long term. These include topical antifungals (such as clioquinol, nystatin and imidazoles) as ointments, creams, lotions or shampoos, and mixtures of the same agents with mild and moderately potent topical corticosteroids used alongside emollients and soap substitutes. In severe cases, patients with concomitant seborrhoeic folliculitis, or in patients with HIV/AIDS, treatment with an oral imidazole and/or an oral tetracycline may be suitable.

Psoriasis

Approximately 2% of the population are said to have psoriasis but it is possible that many more than 2% of men may have or have had anogenital psoriasis at some time; it is certainly a common anogenital diagnosis in isolation.

Psoriasis and its clinical manifestations are discussed in Chapter 35; the relationship of psoriasis with HIV/AIDS is discussed in Chapter 26. Anogenital presentations of psoriasis may be vague in symptomatology and nonspecific on examination. It is not usually itchy; significant itch should arouse suspicions of another dermatosis such as an eczematous dermatitis or tinea. Soreness occurs with superinfection, especially with *Candida*. Other typically affected sites should be examined for signs of the disease. Genital appearances may be challenging to interpret, especially in the uncircumcised patient, because a mucosal site is affected rather than keratinized skin. The diagnosis is usually easier in the circumcised male where the morphology is similar to extragenital lesions.

Inverse pattern psoriasis refers to the manifestation of the disease on intertriginous skin in the axillae, natal cleft, gluteal folds, groins and in the preputial sac and on the glans of the uncircumcised male, where its occurrence is probably brought about by the Koebner phenomenon.

Usually, the diagnosis of psoriasis is clinical, but a biopsy may be necessary (e.g. of a solitary mucosal lesion in an uncircumcised individual) to distinguish psoriasis from Zoon's balanitis, lichen planus, erythroplasia of Queyrat or Kaposi's sarcoma. Bowen's disease and extramammary Paget's disease may be misdiagnosed as psoriasis when there are single or several foci on the penile shaft and/or in the groins.

Topical treatment includes emollients, soap substitutes, corticosteroids combined with antibiotic and antifungal agents or weak tar solutions. Strong crude tar preparations should be avoided at this site given that anogenital skin has a propensity to increased absorption of topical agents and because of the risk of genital cancer; one of the first occupational diseases described was scrotal carcinoma in chimney sweeps. Dithranol is usually avoided in this region. The vitamin D analogue calcipotriol can be helpful. Topical ciclosporin (100 mg/mL in wet dressings three times daily) has been advocated [23]. Phototherapy is contraindicated because of the risk of anogenital cancer. Severe anogenital psoriasis can be an indication for systemic treatment.

Reiter's disease or syndrome (part of the same continuum as psoriasis in genetically predisposed individuals) is discussed in Chapter 35. Characteristic, sometimes severe, involvement of the penis (circinate balanitis) occurs. The penile lesions have the same histopathology as psoriasis [24].

REFERENCES

1 Sherertz EF. Symptomatic dermographism as a cause of genital pruritus. *J Am Acad Dermatol* 1994; **31**: 1040–1.
2 Bernhard JD. Dermographic pruritus: invisible dermographism. *J Am Acad Dermatol* 1995; **33**: 322.
3 Henson EB, Bess DT, Abraham L, Bracikowski JP. Penile angioedema possibly related to lisinopril. *Am J Health Syst Pharm* 1999; **56**: 1773–4.
4 Porter WM, Bewley A, Dinneen M *et al.* Nodular lichen simplex of the scrotum treated by surgical excision. *Br J Dermatol* 2001; **144**: 915–6.
5 Bunker CB. *Male Genital Skin Disease.* London: Saunders, 2004 (in press).
6 Ramam M, Khaitan BK, Singh MK, Gupta SD. Frictional sweat dermatitis. *Contact Dermatitis* 1998; **38**: 49.
7 Birley HDL, Walker MM, Luzzi GA *et al.* Clinical features and management of recurrent balanitis; association with atopy and genital washing. *Genitourin Med* 1993; **69**: 400–3.
8 Shapiro PE. 'Cello scrotum' questioned. *J Am Acad Dermatol* 1991; **24**: 665.
9 Shelley WB, Shelley ED. Scrotal dermatitis caused by 5-fluorouracil (Efudex). *J Am Acad Dermatol* 1988; **19**: 929–31.
10 Cusano F, Capozzi M. Photocontact dermatitis from ketoprofen with cross-reactivity to ibuproxam. *Contact Dermatitis* 1992; **27**: 50–9.
11 Lyon CC, Kulkarni J, Zimerson E *et al.* Skin disorders in amputees. *J Am Acad Dermatol* 2000; **42**: 501–7.
12 Gamulka BD. Index of suspicion. Case No 1. Diagnosis: allergic contact dermatitis. *Pediatr Rev* 2000; **21**: 421–6.
13 Harrington CI, Lewis FM, McDonagh AJ, Gawkrodger DJ. Dermatological causes of pruritus ani. *BMJ* 1992; **305**: 955.
14 Fariña LA, Alonso MV, Horjales M, Zungri ER. Contact-derived allergic balanoposthitis and paraphimosis through topical application of celandine juice. *Actas Urol Esp* 1999; **23**: 554–5.
15 Turjanmaa K, Alenius H, Makinen-Kiljunen S, Reunala T, Palosuo T. Natural rubber latex allergy. *Allergy* 1996; **51**: 593–602.
16 Bauer A, Geier J, Elsner P. Allergic contact dermatitis in patients with anogenital complaints. *J Reprod Med* 2000; **45**: 649–54.
17 Hindson TC. Studies in contact dermatitis. *Trans St. John's Hosp Dermatol Soc* 1966; **52**: 1–9.
18 Bircher AJ, Hirsbrunner P, Langauer S. Allergic contact dermatitis of the genitals from rubber additives in condoms. *Contact Dermatitis* 1993; **28**: 125–6.
19 Shenot P, Rivas DA, Kalman DD, Staas WE. Latex allergy manifested in urological surgery and care of adult spinal cord injured patients. *Arch Phys Med Rehabil* 1994; **75**: 1263–5.
20 Harmon CB, Connolly SM, Larson TR. Condom-related allergic contact dermatitis. *J Urol* 1995; **153**: 1227–8.
21 Rademaker M, Forsyth A. Allergic reactions to rubber condoms. *Genitourin Med* 1989; **65**: 194–5.
22 Lucke TW, Fleming CJ, McHenry P. Clothing dye dermatitis of the scrotum. *Contact Dermatitis* 1998; **38**: 224.
23 Jemec GBE, Baadsgaard O. Effect of cyclosporin on genital psoriasis and lichen planus. *J Am Acad Dermatol* 1993; **29**: 1048–9.
24 Kanerva L, Kousa M, Niemi KM *et al.* Ultrahistology of balanitis circinata. *Br J Vener Dis* 1982; **58**: 188–95.

Zoon's balanitis

Aetiology. Zoon's plasma cell balanitis (ZB) is a disorder of the middle-aged and older uncircumcised male [1,2], although an analogous condition has been reported to afflict the vulva (see p. 68.59), mouth, lips [3] and epiglottis [3,4]. Since Zoon's original reports there have been many accounts in the literature but the aetiology remains uncertain.

The evidence suggests that ZB is a chronic, reactive, principally irritant mucositis brought about by a dysfunctional prepuce. Retention of urine and squames between two tightly apposed and infrequently and inadequately separated and/or inappropriately bathed, commensally hypercolonized, desquamative, secretory epithelial surfaces leads to a disturbed 'preputial ecology' and excessive frictional trauma (ZB is often located on the dorsal aspect of the glans and/or the adjacent prepuce, sites of maximal friction on foreskin retraction) and irritation by urine [5–7]. There is no evidence of an infectious cause, and immunohistochemical findings suggest that ZB represents a non-specific polyclonal tissue reaction [8,9], consistent with an irritant mucositis.

Clinical features. The presentation is classically indolent and asymptomatic, although staining of the underclothes with blood has been reported [10]. Well-demarcated, glistening, moist, bright red or autumn brown patches involve the glans and mucosal prepuce [7], with sparing of the keratinized penile shaft and foreskin (Fig. 68.7). The urethra (fossa navicularis) may be involved. Other signs include dark red stippling—'cayenne pepper spots'—and purpura with haemosiderin, solitary or multiple lesions of differing sizes (guttate or nummular), characteristically symmetrical about the axis of the coronal sulcus and 'kissing'. Although vegetative and nodular presentations have been recorded, atypical or unusual morphology should be viewed with great suspicion and biopsied.

Histopathology. The classic histology is of epidermal attenuation with absent granular and horny layers, and diamond- or lozenge-shaped basal cell keratinocytes with sparse dyskeratosis and spongiosis. There is a band of dermal infiltration with plasma cells of variable density. Extravasated erythrocytes, haemosiderin and vascular proliferation are also seen. Although Zoon stressed the presence of the plasma cell infiltrate in this condition, the plasma cell numbers can be very variable [7,11].

Differential diagnosis. The differential diagnosis includes erosive lichen planus, psoriasis, seborrhoeic dermatitis, contact dermatitis, fixed drug eruption, secondary syphilis, histoplasmosis [12], erythroplasia of Queyrat [13] and Kaposi's sarcoma. A confident clinical diagnosis is not always possible or safe [6], so a biopsy is advisable and the

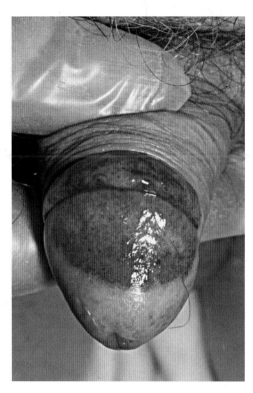

Fig. 68.7 Zoon's balanitis. Symmetrical moist erythema of glans and prepuce. (Courtesy of Dr C.B. Bunker, with permission from Medical Illustration UK, Chelsea & Westminster Hospital, London, UK.)

pathologist should be asked to look for concomitant disease. Frank cases of lichen sclerosus, lichen planus, Bowenoid papulosis and penile cancer often appear to have ZB-like changes on clinical examination and on histology. In other words, the signs of ZB may be secondary to underlying preputial disease. It is likely that some of the clinical and histological variants that have been reported [14–16], and a recent claim that ZB *per se* is a premalignant condition in a single case report [17], are a consequence of this phenomenon. ZB indicates a dysfunctional foreskin and a more sinister dermatosis may be concealed.

Treatment. Although ZB can improve with altered washing habits and the intermittent application of a mild or potent topical corticosteroid (with or without an antibiotic and anticandidal agent), it usually persists or relapses. Definitive curative treatment is circumcision [7]. Again, the pathologist should be asked to examine the whole specimen for signs of another underlying dermatosis. It has been claimed that the carbon dioxide laser is effective [18].

REFERENCES

1 Zoon JJ. Verenigingsverslagen. *Ned Tijdschr Geneeskd* 1950; **94**: 1528–30.
2 Zoon JJ. Balanoposthite chronique circonscrite benigne a plasmocytes. *Dermatologica* 1952; **105**: 1–7.
3 Baughman RD, Berger P, Pringle WM. Plasma cell cheilitis. *Arch Dermatol* 1974; **110**: 725–6.
4 White JW Jr, Olsen KD, Banks PM. Plasma cell orificial mucositis. *Arch Dermatol* 1986; **122**: 1321–4.
5 Yoganathan S, Bohl TG, Mason G. Plasma cell balanitis and vulvitis (of Zoon). *J Reprod Med* 1994; **39**: 939–44.
6 Altmeyer P, Kastner U, Luther H. Balanitis/balanoposthitis chronica circumscripta benigna plasmacellularis: entity or fiction? *Hautarzt* 1998; **49**: 552–5.
7 Bunker CB. Topics in penile dermatology. *Clin Exp Dermatol* 2001; **26**: 469–79.
8 Nishimura M, Matsuda T, Muto M, Hori Y. Balanitis of Zoon. *Int J Dermatol* 1990; **29**: 421–3.
9 Farrell AM, Francis N, Bunker CB. Zoon's balanitis: an immunohistochemical study. *Br J Dermatol* 1996; **135** (Suppl. 47): 57.
10 Jolly BB, Krishnamurty S, Vaidyanathan S. Zoon's balanitis. *Urol Int* 1993; **50**: 182–4.
11 Souteyrand P, Wong E, MacDonald DM. Zoon's balanitis (balanitis circumscripta plasmacellularis). *Br J Dermatol* 1981; **105**: 195–9.
12 Shelley WB, Shelley ED. *Advanced Dermatologic Diagnosis*. Philadelphia: Saunders, 1992: 609.
13 Davis-Daneshfar A, Trueb RM. Bowen's disease of the glans penis (erythroplasia of Queyrat) in plasma cell balanitis. *Cutis* 2000; **65**: 395–8.
14 Bureau Y, Barriere H, Evin Y-P. Les erythroplasies benignes a plasmocytes. *Ann Dermatol Syphiligr* 1962; **89**: 271–84.
15 Jonquières EDL. Balanitis pseudoeritroplasicas. *Arch Argentinos Dermatol* 1971; **21**: 85–95.
16 Dupré A, Schnitzler L. Plasmocytic proliferative lesions of the foreskin: a variety of Zoon's benign circumscribed balanitis. *Ann Dermatol Vénéréol* 1977; **104**: 127–31 [in French].
17 Joshi UY. Carcinoma of the penis preceded by Zoon's balanitis. *Int J STD AIDS* 1999; **10**: 823–5.
18 Aynaud O, Casanova JM, Tranbaloc P. CO_2 laser for therapeutic circumcision in adults. *Eur Urol* 1995; **28**: 74–6.

Lichen sclerosus

Aetiology. Lichen sclerosus is discussed in Chapter 56. The aetiopathogenesis is not known. Poorly understood are the predilection for the genitalia generally (in males, particularly the uncircumcised [1]), the association with organ-specific autoimmune disease and the propensity to progress to squamous carcinoma [2–5]. HPV (types 6, 16 and 18) is present in 70% of cases of childhood penile lichen sclerosus [6,7], but the epidemiology and clinical tenor of lichen sclerosus is not that of an infectious or sexually transmitted disease [5,8]. Anatomical abnormality and trauma seem to be contributing factors [5,9]. Specifically, lichen sclerosus has been related to hypospadias and its repair [10]. The presence of the histopathological features of lichen sclerosus in a percentage of acrochordons (skin tags) has led to the suggestion that occlusion of flaccid skin is a pathogenic factor [11].

Clinical features. Lichen sclerosus of the penis may be asymptomatic, but diverse, often vague, symptomatology is usually encountered [12]. Patients may describe itching, burning, bleeding, tearing, splitting, haemorrhagic blisters, any manner of symptoms signifying sexual dysfunction or dyspareunia, discomfort with urination and narrowing of the urinary stream, and/or be concerned about the changing anatomy of their genitalia [5]. Other presentations are non-retractile foreskin (phimosis)

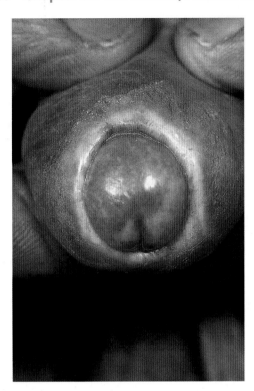

Fig. 68.8 Lichen sclerosus causing phimosis. (Courtesy of Dr D.A. Burns, Leicester, UK.)

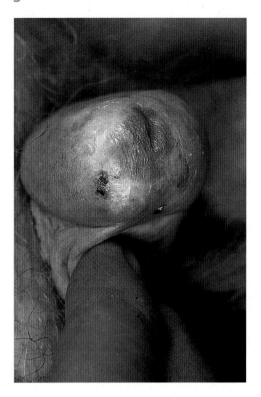

Fig. 68.9 Lichen sclerosus. White plaques and haemorrhagic areas on the glans. (Courtesy of Dr D.A. Burns, Leicester, UK.)

(Fig. 68.8), foreskin fixed in retraction (paraphimosis) and urinary retention, even renal failure.

Genital, like extragenital, lichen sclerosus can manifest as atrophic leukodermic patches or plaques, or lilac, slightly scaly patches with telangiectasia and sparse purpura (Fig. 68.9). Predominant purpura, bullae, erosions and ulceration may be encountered [5,13,14]. The signs may be subtle, with meatal 'pin hole' narrowing, slight tightening of the retracted prepuce because of sclerotic plaques and bands, with or without difficulty in retraction—incomplete paraphimosis or 'waisting' (Fig. 68.10) or they may be florid, with severe changes caused both by the lichen sclerosus and by associated Zoon's balanoposthitis-like changes: adhesions, loss of anatomical definition and dissolution or effacement of the normally sharply defined architectural features, especially of the frenulum and the coronal sulcus. Changes resulting from ZB may be more florid than the underlying lichen sclerosus. Post-inflammatory hyper- and hypopigmentation are occasionally seen.

Whereas posthitis xerotica obliterans refers to chronic damage to the prepuce by lichen sclerosus, balanitis xerotica obliterans (BXO) properly describes involvement of the glans penis (although the term has been used imprecisely). BXO can be a consequence of other scarring dermatoses such as lichen planus and cicatricial pemphigoid [15].

Genital lichen sclerosus is more common than extragen-

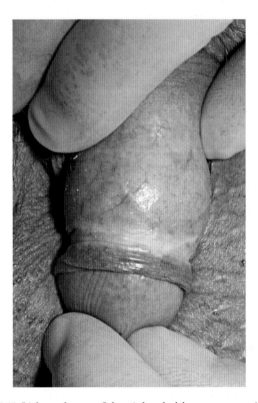

Fig. 68.10 Lichen sclerosus. Sclerotic band of the prepuce causing 'waisting'. (Courtesy of Dr C.B. Bunker, with permission from Medical Illustration UK, Chelsea & Westminster Hospital, London, UK.)

ital or oral disease, but there may (rarely) be concomitant involvement of these sites. In adults, anogenital lichen sclerosus is said to be about 10 times more common in women than men. Perianal disease seems rare in the male. The involvement of the anterior urethra can be serious: 29% of patients undergoing urethroplasty for urethral stricture had pathological evidence of lichen sclerosus [16].

The first report of genital lichen sclerosus in boys appeared only in 1977 [17], and lichen sclerosus may be much more frequent than is generally supposed in young boys. The development of secondary phimosis in school-age boys is highly suggestive of lichen sclerosus [18]. In the older male, persistent primary phimosis or the secondary development of phimosis in a previously retractable foreskin may be related to lichen sclerosus [5].

Most cases of genital lichen sclerosus can be diagnosed clinically. Lichen planus and the much rarer mucous membrane pemphigoid are in the differential diagnosis. A biopsy should be performed if there is clinical doubt or if the lesion is eroded or verrucous.

Histopathology. The histology is classic (see Chapter 56). The occasional association of endarteritis led originally to the usage of the term 'obliterans' [19]. In two cases in boys, a dermal lymphohistiocytic and granulomatous phlebitis has been found, and one also had evidence of HPV [20]. A garland-like basal lamina has been found ultrastructurally [21]. Sometimes, lichen sclerosus may be difficult to differentiate from lichen planus, and criteria to assist, in the vulva, have been proposed by Fung and LeBoit [22].

Treatment. Guidelines for the management of lichen sclerosus have been published by the British Association of Dermatologists [23]. A very potent topical corticosteroid (used under supervision) is effective [24]. The plasticity of the epithelium at this site seems to allow significant remodelling, with the relief of phimosis, improvement of incomplete phimosis or waisting, improvement in the histological changes and avoidance of circumcision [5,12]. Secondary candidal and bacterial infection should be treated. There are reports of the efficacy of long-term systemic antibiotic therapy (penicillin and azithromycin) in cases of lichen sclerosus thought to be associated with *Borrelia* infection [25,26]. Testosterone propionate ointment, oral stanozolol, freezing with ethyl chloride, liquid nitrogen cryotherapy, carbon dioxide laser and adrenocorticotrophic hormone (ACTH) have been used with variable success [5].

If medical treatment is not possible or fails, then surgery may be indicated. Circumcision, frenuloplasty, meatotomy and sophisticated plastic repair, depending upon the clinical presentation, can be offered. In boys, complete circumcision is the treatment of choice because all affected tissue is removed and any secondary involvement of the glans probably regresses or resolves [18]; it is the unproven impression that this phenomenon also occurs in most adult patients. Lichen sclerosus can recur in donor grafts from unrelated sites [13,27]. Carbon dioxide laser circumcision has been advocated [28].

Squamous carcinoma of the penis is the most serious potential complication of lichen sclerosus; *in situ* change can occur often after long periods [5,29]. A risk of 4–9.5% has been claimed, depending on length of follow-up; the latent period may be one to three decades [30–32]. Verrucous carcinoma (Buschke–Löwenstein tumour) has been associated with previous lichen sclerosus [33,34]. Carcinoma complicating lichen sclerosus constituted one-third of all cases of penile cancer seen by Campus *et al.* [35] and, of 20 patients with penile squamous cell carcinoma (SCC) studied by Powell *et al.* [36], 11 had a clinical history and/or histological evidence of lichen sclerosus. Involvement of the glans penis confers a greater risk [32].

The effect of medical and surgical treatment on the subsequent incidence of penile cancer is not known [37,38]. Liatsikos *et al.* [39] report SCC of the glans developing in one of eight patients followed-up after circumcision for lichen sclerosus. Patients should be followed-up long term, especially if circumcision has not been performed or if symptoms persist or recur after any form of treatment.

REFERENCES

1 Ledwig PA, Weigand DA. Late circumcision and lichen sclerosus et atrophicus of the penis. *J Am Acad Dermatol* 1989; **20**: 211–4.
2 Ridley CM. Lichen sclerosus et atrophicus. *BMJ* 1987; **295**: 1295–6.
3 Meffert JJ, Davis BM, Grimwood RE. Lichen sclerosus. *J Am Acad Dermatol* 1995; **32**: 393–416.
4 Powell JJ, Wojnarowska F. Lichen sclerosus. *Lancet* 1999; **353**: 1777–83.
5 Bunker CB. Topics in penile dermatology. *Clin Exp Dermatol* 2001; **26**: 469–79.
6 Ansink AC, Krul MRL, de Weger RA *et al.* Human papillomavirus, lichen sclerosus, and squamous cell carcinoma of the vulva: detection and prognostic significance. *Gynecol Oncol* 1994; **52**: 180–4.
7 Drut RM, Gómez MA, Drut R, Lojo MM. Human papillomavirus is present in some cases of childhood penile lichen sclerosus: an *in situ* hybridization and SP-PCR study. *Pediatr Dermatol* 1998; **15**: 85–90.
8 Farrell AM, Millard PR, Schomberg KH, Wojnarowska F. An infective aetiology for lichen sclerosus re-addressed. *Clin Exp Dermatol* 1999; **24**: 479–83.
9 English JC III, King DH, Foley JP. Penile shaft hypopigmentation: lichen sclerosus occurring after the initiation of alprostadil intracavernous injections for erectile dysfunction. *J Am Acad Dermatol* 1998; **39**: 801–3.
10 Uemura S, Hutson JM, Woodward AA, Kelly JH, Chow CW. Balanitis xerotica obliterans with urethral stricture after hypospadias repair. *Pediatr Surg Int* 2000; **16**: 144–5.
11 Weigand DA. Microscopic features of lichen sclerosus et atrophicus in acrochordons: a clue to the cause of lichen sclerosus et atrophicus? *J Am Acad Dermatol* 1993; **28**: 751–4.
12 Riddell L, Edwards A, Sherrard J. Clinical features of lichen sclerosus in men attending a department of genitourinary medicine. *Sex Transm Infect* 2000; **76**: 311–3.
13 Wallace HJ. Lichen sclerosus et atrophicus. *Trans St John's Hosp Dermatol Soc* 1971; **57**: 9–30.
14 Lipscombe TK, Wayte J, Wojnarowska F, Marren P, Luzzi G. A study of clinical and aetiological factors and possible associations of lichen sclerosus in males. *Australas J Dermatol* 1997; **38**: 132–6.
15 Ridley CM, Neill SM. Circumcision. *BMJ* 1993; **306**: 583–4.
16 Barbagli G, Lazzeri M, Palminteri E, Turini D. Lichen sclerosis [sic] of male genitalia involving anterior urethra. *Lancet* 1999; **354**: 429.

17 Götz H, Zabel M, Patiri C. Lichen sclerosus at atrophicus: first observation on a boy's genitalia. *Hautarzt* 1977; **28**: 235–8.

18 Meuli M, Brinker J, Hanimann B, Sacher P. Lichen sclerosus et atrophicus causing phimosis in boys: a prospective study with 5-year follow-up after complete circumcision. *J Urol* 1994; **152**: 987–9.

19 Das S, Tunuguntla HSGR. Balanitis xerotica obliterans: a review. *World J Urol* 2000; **18**: 382–7.

20 Cabaleiro P, Drut RM, Drut R. Lymphohistiocytic and granulomatous phlebitis in penile lichen sclerosus. *Am J Dermatopathol* 2000; **22**: 316–20.

21 Dupré A, Viraben R. Basal lamina with a garland-like pattern in a case of sclero-atrophic lichen: ultrastructural study. *Ann Dermatol Vénéréol* 1988; **115**: 19–26 [in French].

22 Fung MA, LeBoit PE. Light microscopic criteria for the diagnosis of early vulvar lichen sclerosus: a comparison with lichen planus. *Am J Surg Pathol* 1998; **22**: 473–8.

23 Neill SM, Tatnall FM, Cox NH. Guidelines for the management of lichen sclerosus. *Br J Dermatol* 2002; **147**: 640–9.

24 Tremaine RDL, Miller RAW. Lichen sclerosus et atrophicus. *Int J Dermatol* 1989; **28**: 10–6.

25 Schempp C, Bocklage H, Lange R, Kölmel HW, Orfanos CE. Further evidence for *Borrelia burgdorferi* infection in morphoea and lichen sclerosus et atrophicus confirmed by DNA amplification. *J Invest Dermatol* 1993; **100**: 717–20.

26 Shelley WB, Shelley ED, Grunenwald MA, Anders TJ, Ramnath A. Long-term antibiotic therapy for balanitis xerotica obliterans. *J Am Acad Dermatol* 1999; **40**: 69–72.

27 Lee SJ, Phillips SMA. Recurrent lichen sclerosus et atrophicus in urethroplasties from multiple skin grafts. *Br J Urol* 1994; **74**: 802–3.

28 Kartamaa M, Reitamo S. Treatment of lichen sclerosus with carbon dioxide laser vaporization. *Br J Dermatol* 1997; **136**: 356–9.

29 Simonart T, Noël JC, De Dobbeleer G, Simonart JM. Carcinoma of the glans penis arising 20 years after lichen sclerosus. *Dermatology* 1998; **196**: 337–8.

30 Bouyssou-Gauthier ML, Boulinguez S, Dumas JP, Bedane C, Bonnetblanc JM. Penile lichen sclerosus: follow-up study. *Ann Dermatol Vénéréol* 1999; **126**: 804–7.

31 Nasca MR, Innocenzi D, Micali G. Penile cancer among patients with genital lichen sclerosus. *J Am Acad Dermatol* 1999; **41**: 911–4.

32 Micali G, Nasca MR, Innocenzi D. Lichen sclerosus of the glans is significantly associated with penile carcinoma. *Sex Transm Infect* 2001; **77**: 226.

33 Weber P, Rabinovitz H, Garland L. Verrucous carcinoma in penile lichen sclerosus et atrophicus. *J Dermatol Surg Oncol* 1987; **13**: 529.

34 O'Gorman-Lalor O, Walker NPJ, Matthews S *et al.* Successful treatment of Buschke-Löwenstein tumour of the penis with carbon dioxide laser vaporisation. *Clin Exp Dermatol* (in press).

35 Campus GV, Alia F, Bosincu L. Squamous cell carcinoma and lichen sclerosus et atrophicus of the prepuce. *Plast Reconstr Surg* 1992; **89**: 962–4.

36 Powell J, Robson A, Cranston D, Wojnarowska, F, Turner R. High incidence of lichen sclerosus in patients with squamous cell carcinoma of the penis. *Br J Dermatol* 2001; **145**: 85–9.

37 Maden C, Sherman KJ, Beckmann AM *et al.* History of circumcision, medical conditions, and sexual activity and the risk of penile cancer. *J Natl Cancer Inst* 1993; **85**: 19–24.

38 Holly EA, Palefsky JM. Factors related to risk of penile cancer: new evidence from a study in the Pacific Northwest. *J Natl Cancer Inst* 1993; **85**: 2–3.

39 Liatsikos EN, Perimenis P, Dandinis K *et al.* Lichen sclerosus et atrophicus: findings after complete circumcision. *Scand J Urol Nephrol* 1997; **31**: 453–6.

Lichen planus

Aetiology. Lichen planus is discussed in Chapter 42. It is a common inflammatory dermatosis with a particular predilection for the mucosae [1]. The aetiopathogenesis of lichen planus is not known. Drugs can cause a generalized lichenoid eruption; a case of a lichenoid drug eruption confined to the penis resulting from propranolol has been reported [2].

Clinical features. Lichen planus can present in, and remain localized to the anogenital area, including the

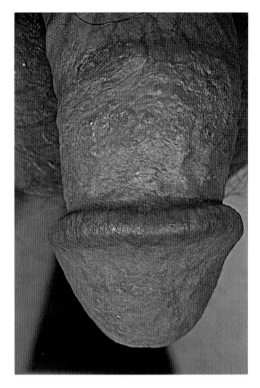

Fig. 68.11 Lichen planus. Papules and annular lesions with Wickham's striae on the glans and shaft. (Courtesy of Dr C.B. Bunker, with permission from Medical Illustration UK, Chelsea & Westminster Hospital, London, UK.)

groins and perianal skin. Like the classical disease at other sites, it presents as itchy red–purple papules, also as patches or plaques and annular lesions (Fig. 68.11) or as phimosis [3]. The Koebner phenomenon may partly explain the orogenital predilection [4].

Occasionally, an erosive form is encountered. There is a male equivalent of the vulvovaginal syndrome of Hewitt —the genito-gingival syndrome—with chronic erosive gingival and genital lesions [5]. In most cases, anogenital lichen planus is self-limiting, although some patients relapse and remit. Adhesions can form. Post-inflammatory hyperpigmentation can persist for months or years. A case of paraneoplastic lichen planus with orogenital and cicatrizing conjunctival involvement in a patient with thymoma has been reported [6].

Chronic mucosal erosive lichen planus is associated with a risk of progression to SCC but most reports concern oral lichen planus. SCC may complicate hypertrophic lichen planus of the glans penis [7,8].

Lichen nitidus has an affinity for the penis. It can be difficult to diagnose because the signs may be subtle, even when the lesions are widespread.

The differential diagnosis of anogenital lichen planus includes psoriasis, ZB, lichen sclerosus, viral warts, Bowenoid papulosis and porokeratosis. A biopsy is frequently necessary for diagnostic purposes and in the follow-up of cases of chronic anogenital disease if erosive, ulcerative or verrucous features arouse concern about the development of SCC.

Treatment. Potent and ultrapotent topical corticosteroids usually suffice for treatment. Patients are told to continue with the treatment until the lesions are non-itchy and flat; they are warned about post-inflammatory hyperpigmentation. Topical and oral ciclosporin have been used [9,10]. Circumcision may be necessary for phimosis [11] and should be considered in refractory erosive disease [12]. The rationale being that the abolition of koebnerization influences and facilitates resolution of the lichen planus. Photodynamic therapy was used inadvertently in one patient with lichen planus of the glans penis, to good effect [13].

REFERENCES

1 Barnette DJ Jr, Curtin TJ, Yeager JK, Corbett DW. Asymptomatic penile lesions. *Cutis* 1993; **51**: 116–8.
2 Massa MC, Jason SM, Gradini R, Welykyj S. Lichenoid drug eruption secondary to propanolol. *Cutis* 1991; **48**: 41–3.
3 Bunker CB. Topics in penile dermatology. *Clin Exp Dermatol* 2001; **26**: 469–79.
4 El-Gadi S. Biopsy before excision. *J Eur Acad Dermatol Venereol* 1996; **7**: 87–90.
5 Cribier B, Ndiaye I, Grosshans E. Peno-gingival syndrome: a male equivalent of vulvo-vagino-gingival syndrome. *Rev Stomatol Chir Maxillofac* 1993; **94**: 148–51.
6 Hahn JM, Meisler DM, Lowder CY, Tung RC, Camisa C. Cicatrizing conjunctivitis associated with paraneoplastic lichen planus. *Am J Ophthalmol* 2000; **129**: 98–9.
7 Worheide J, Bonsmann G, Kolde G, Hamm H. Plattenepithyelkarzinom auf dem Boden eines lichen ruber hypertrophicus an der glans penis. *Hautarzt* 1991; **42**: 112–5.
8 Leal-Khouri S, Hruza GJ. Squamous cell carcinoma developing within lichen planus of the penis: treatment with Mohs micrographic surgery. *J Dermatol Surg Oncol* 1994; **20**: 272–6.
9 Jemec GBE, Baadsgaard O. Effect of cyclosporin on genital psoriasis and lichen planus. *J Am Acad Dermatol* 1993; **29**: 1048–9.
10 Schmitt EC, Pigatto PD, Boneschi V, Bigardi AS, Finzi AF. Erosiver lichen planus der glans penis: behandlung mit cyclosporin A. *Hautarzt* 1993; **44**: 43–5.
11 Aste N, Pau M, Ferreli C, Biggio P. Lichen planus in a child requiring circumcision. *Pediatr Dermatol* 1997; **14**: 129–30.
12 Porter WM, Bewley A, Dinneen M *et al.* Nodular lichen simplex of the scrotum treated by surgical excision. *Br J Dermatol* 2001; **144**: 915–6.
13 Kirby B, Whitehurst C, Moore JV, Yates VM. Treatment of lichen planus of the penis with photodynamic therapy. *Br J Dermatol* 1999; **141**: 765–6.

Ulcerative disease and penile necrosis

Aphthous ulceration of the penis and scrotum can occur, including in HIV/AIDS (see Chapter 26), but specific exclusion of sexually transmitted diseases and consideration of other causes of genital ulceration, especially Behçet's syndrome, is necessary. The causes are obscure and the histology is non-specific.

Five cases of spontaneous scrotal ulceration in young, previously fit men have been described [1]. Histology showed non-specific vasculitis, and spontaneous resolution occurred. This entity may be related to idiopathic scrotal panniculitis and fat necrosis. This condition is distinct from other causes of the acute scrotum in prepubertal boys. It presents as acute tender, sometimes painful, swelling (classically, but not always, after swimming in cold water). Masses may be palpable in the scrotal wall. Otherwise, the boy is well, with no fever or leukocytosis. Idiopathic scrotal necrosis in a 2-month-old boy has been documented by Sarihan [2], where trauma, extreme cold and Fournier's gangrene were excluded. Management is expectant and conservative [3,4]. In adults, one case of idiopathic scrotal panniculitis has been reported [5] and another associated with pancreatitis [6].

Subtle or severe orogenital ulceration can occur in erythema multiforme or the Stevens–Johnson syndrome (see Chapter 74).

Behçet's disease is discussed in Chapter 66. Recurrent genital ulceration is not mandatory for the diagnosis; if patients do not have genital ulceration then they must have ophthalmic and dermatological involvement or a positive pathergy test [7]. In practice, there are many patients who have an incomplete syndrome. Other anogenital manifestations include epididymitis and urethritis [8], spontaneous haematocoele from venous rupture resulting from lymphocytic venulitis [9] and erectile dysfunction [10]. The genital ulcers in men can be very painful and occur anywhere on the anogenital area, including the perianal skin. Generally, they are larger, deeper, fewer and less recurrent than those in the mouth. Patients with relapsing polychondritis and Behçet's disease have been reported, and the acronym MAGIC (mouth and genital ulcers with inflamed cartilage) syndrome has been proposed [11,12]. The histology of Behçet's disease is usually non-specific and does not enable it to be distinguished from idiopathic aphthae, although sometimes necrotizing vasculitis can be present.

Degos' malignant atrophic papulosis (see Chapter 48) has caused penile ulceration, which preceded the development of the rash and eventual fatal involvement of other organs, despite aggressive treatment [13].

The hypereosinophilic syndrome involves the skin in up to 50% of cases, with orogenital ulceration, erythroderma and urticaria [14]. It may occur in HIV infection.

Penile necrosis has a wide differential diagnosis (Table 68.20). Many of the causes are discussed in this or other sections.

Two cases of necrobiosis have been reported presenting as erythematous ulcerated lesions of the glans penis. One patient was diabetic and had lesions on the legs [22]; the other had penile lesions only and was treated with oral pentoxifylline [23].

There are a number of case reports of pyoderma gangrenosum (see Chapter 49), including the variant superficial granulomatous pyoderma, involving the penis and scrotum in adults and children (where the anogenital area is a site of predilection as well as the head and neck)

Table 68.20 Causes of penile necrosis. (After Bunker [15]. © 2004, with permission from Elsevier.)

Decubitus ulcer
Spider bite
Priapism
Embolism
Strangulation and tourniquet syndromes
Vacuum erection device
Vasculitis [16]
Diabetes mellitus [17,18]
Chronic renal failure [19]
Thrombocytopenia
Polycythaemia
Cryoglobulinaemia
Coagulopathy [20]
Pyoderma gangrenosum
Calciphylaxis
Ecthyma gangrenosum
Fournier's gangrene
Herpes simplex
Leukaemia
Mucormycosis (in acute myeloblastic leukaemia) [21]
Warfarin
Fixed drug eruption

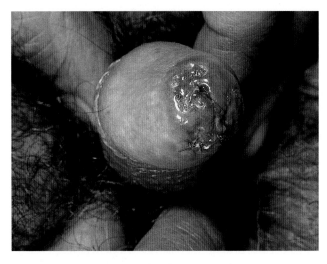

Fig. 68.12 Pyoderma gangrenosum in a patient with severe seronegative arthropathy. (Courtesy of Dr F.A. Ive, Durham, UK.)

(Fig. 68.12) [24,25]. Genital pyoderma gangrenosum may occur following local trauma such as urological surgery [26], or complicate ulcerative colitis [27] or chronic lymphocytic leukaemia, or it may be idiopathic [28–31]. Pyoderma gangrenosum is a diagnosis made when other causes of purulent ulceration, such as infection (sexually acquired and exotic), malignancy and artefact have been excluded.

Calciphylaxis (see Chapter 59) is a rare and serious complication of chronic renal failure in which extending ischaemic gangrenous necrosis affects acral tissues and sometimes the thighs, buttocks and genitals [32–34].

REFERENCES

1 Piñol Aguade J. XIVe congres de l'association des dermatologistes et syphiligraphers de langue francaise, Geneve, 1973. II. Vascularites. Geneva: Medecine et Hygiene, 1974: 112.
2 Sarihan H. Idiopathic scrotal necrosis. *Br J Urol* 1994; **74**: 259.
3 Koster LH, Antoon SJ. Fat necrosis in the scrotum. *J Urol* 1980; **123**: 599–600.
4 Hollander JB, Begun FP, Lee RD. Scrotal fat necrosis. *J Urol* 1985; **134**: 150–1.
5 Tsurusaki T, Maruta N, Iwasaki S, Iwasaki K, Saito Y. Idiopathic bilateral panniculitis of the spermatic cord in an elderly male patient. *J Urol* 2000; **164**: 1657–8.
6 Lin Y, Lin M, Huang G *et al.* Acute pancreatitis masquerading as testicular torsion. *Am J Emerg Med* 1996; **14**: 654–5.
7 International Study Group for Behçet's disease. Criteria for diagnosis of Behçet's disease. *Lancet* 1990; **335**: 1078–80.
8 Kirkali Z, Yigitbasi O, Sasmaz R. Urological aspects of Behçet's disease. *Br J Urol* 1991; **67**: 638–9.
9 Orhan I, Onur R, Ardicoglu A, Salatan Y. Behçet's disease and spontaneous haematocoele: an unusual complication. *BJU Int* 1999; **84**: 739–40.
10 Aksu K, Keser G, Gunaydin G *et al.* Erectile dysfunction in Behçet's disease without neurological involvement: two case reports. *Rheumatology (Oxford)* 2000; **39**: 1429–31.
11 Firestein GS, Gruber HE, Weisman MH *et al.* Mouth and genital and inflamed cartilage. MAGIC syndrome. *Am J Med* 1985; **79**: 65–72.
12 Orme RL, Nordlund JJ, Barich L, Brown T. The MAGIC syndrome (mouth and genital ulcers with inflamed cartilage). *Arch Dermatol* 1990; **126**: 940–4.
13 Thomson KF, Highet AS. Penile ulceration in fatal malignant atrophic papulosis (Degos' disease). *Br J Dermatol* 2000; **143**: 1320–2.
14 Morgan MB, Viloria J, Morgan JD, Suarez-Hoyos J. Human immunodeficiency virus infection and hypereosinophilic syndrome. *J Florida Med Assoc* 1994; **81**: 401–2.
15 Bunker CB. *Male Genital Skin Disease*. London: Saunders, 2004 (in press).
16 Rubio FA, Robayna G, Herranz P *et al.* Necrotizing vasculitis of the glans penis. *Br J Dermatol* 1999; **40**: 756–7.
17 Bour J, Steinhardt G. Penile necrosis in diabetes mellitus and end stage renal disease. *J Urol* 1984; **132**: 560–2.
18 Frydenberg M. Penile gangrene: a separate entity from Fournier's syndrome? *Br J Urol* 1988; **61**: 532–3.
19 Lowe FC, Brendler CB. Penile gangrene: a complication of secondary hyperparathyroidism from chronic renal failure. *J Urol* 1984; **132**: 1189–91.
20 Sodal G, Ly B, Borchgrevink HH. Thrombosis of the inferior vena cava, disseminated intravascular coagulation and gangrene of the penis. *Acta Med Scand* 1978; **203**: 535–8.
21 Grossklaus DJ, Dutta SC, Shappel S, Kirchner FK. Cutaneous mucormycosis presenting as a penile lesion in a patient with acute myeloblastic leukaemia. *J Urol* 1999; **161**: 1906–7.
22 Lecroq C, Thomine E, Bouillie MC, Lauret P. Necrobiose lipoidique atypique genitale. *Ann Dermatol Vénéréol* 1984; **111**: 717–8.
23 Espana A, Sanchez-Yus E, Serna MJ *et al.* Chronic balanitis with palisading granuloma: an atypical genital localization of necrobiosis lipoidica responsive to pentoxifylline. *Dermatology* 1994; **188**: 222–5.
24 Bigler LR, Flint ID, Davis LS. Painful ulcers of the scrotum. *Arch Dermatol* 1995; **31**: 609–14.
25 Çalikoğlu E. Superficial granulomatous pyoderma of the scrotum: an extremely rare cause of genital ulcer. *Acta Dermatol Venereol* 2000; **80**: 311–2.
26 Farrell AM, Black MM, Bracka A, Bunker CB. Pyoderma gangrenosum of the penis. *Br J Dermatol* 1998; **138**: 337–40.
27 Sanusi ID, Gonzalez E, Venable DD. Pyoderma gangrenosum of penile and scrotal skin. *J Urol* 1982; **127**: 547–9.
28 Harto A, Gutiérrez Sanz-Gadea C, Vives R, Romero Maroto J, Ledo A. Pioderma gangrenoso en pene. *Acta Urol Esp* 1985; **9**: 263–6.
29 Sánchez MH, Sánchez SR, del Cerro Heredero M *et al.* Pyoderma gangrenosum of penile skin. *Int J Dermatol* 1997; **36**: 638–9.
30 Güngör E, Karakayali G, Alli N, Artuz F, Lenk N. Penile pyoderma gangrenosum. *J Eur Acad Dermatol Venereol* 1999; **12**: 59–62.
31 Park HJ, Kim YC, Cinn YW, Yoon TY. Granulomatous pyoderma gangrenosum: two unusual cases showing necrotizing granulomatous inflammation. *Clin Exp Dermatol* 2000; **25**: 617–20.
32 Ivker RA, Woosley J, Briggaman R. Calciphylaxis in three patients with end-stage renal disease. *Arch Dermatol* 1995; **131**: 63–8.

33 Siami GA, Siami FS. Intensive tandem cryofiltration apheresis and haemodialysis to treat a patient with severe calciphylaxis, cryoglobulinemia, and end-stage renal disease. *ASAIO J* 1999; **45**: 229–33.
34 Boccaletti VP, Ricci R, Sebastio N, Cortellini P, Alinovi A. Penile necrosis. *Arch Dermatol* 2000; **136**: 261, 264.

Pilonidal sinus

Pilonidal sinus very rarely affects the penis, but when it does it is usually in the coronal sulcus. Some of the reported cases have been complicated by actinomycosis [1,2] and another has been associated with a dermoid cyst [3].

REFERENCES

1 Rashid AMH, Menai Williams R, Parry D, Malone PR. Actinomycosis associated with pilonidal sinus of the penis. *J Urol* 1992; **148**: 405–6.
2 Val-Bernal JF, Azcarretazabal T, Garijo MF. Pilonidal sinus of the penis: a report of two cases, one of them associated with actinomycosis. *J Cutan Pathol* 1999; **26**: 155–8.
3 Tomasini C, Aloi F, Puiatti P, Caliendo V. Dermoid cyst of the penis. *Dermatology* 1997; **194**: 188–90.

Penile acne

There is no literature on this condition but it is occasionally encountered. Patients have comedones, papules, pustules and inflammatory nodules of the proximal shaft of the penis. The differential diagnosis should include chloracne (see Chapter 43). Patients respond to conventional treatment for acne.

Peyronie's disease

Peyronie's disease [1,2], which affects middle-aged and older men, is a localized fibrotic disorder involving tissue immediately adjacent to the erectile tissues. It presents with pain and curvature on erection, a sensation of a cord within the penis, palpation of a lump or knot, decreased erection distal to the plaque, interference with intercourse and progressive impotence. It may be subclinical in many men, given that 23% of autopsies have shown histological evidence of the condition [1]. Psychological complications and marital difficulties occur. The penis curves towards the lesion, with dorsal curvature being most common. Peyronie (a physician to Louis XIV) described nodules as 'rosary beads' but plaques vary in size. It has been associated with systemic sclerosis [3], and such patients may have penile Raynaud's phenomenon [4]. It has occurred as a complication of the use of a vacuum erection device [5], but in most men the cause is unknown. Some evidence has been advanced for an autoimmune pathogenesis [6].

The differential diagnosis includes congenital curvature, fibrosis secondary to trauma or urethritis and abscess, syphilitic gumma, lymphogranuloma venereum, and infiltrative tumours (e.g. lipogranuloma). Penile thrombophlebitis as the initial presentation of a paraneoplastic migratory thrombophlebitis resulting from pancreatic cancer has been misdiagnosed as Peyronie's disease [7].

In some men there may be spontaneous regression. Treatments include intralesional corticosteroid injection [8], including delivery by Dermojet [9]. Surgery is avoided, but some specialized techniques are available [10]. Symptomatic relief has been claimed following iontophoresis of drugs such as dexamethasone, lidocaine (lignocaine) and verapamil [11].

REFERENCES

1 Smith BH. Subclinical Peyronie's disease. *Am J Clin Pathol* 1969; **52**: 385–90.
2 Billig R, Baker R, Immergut M, Maxted W. Peyronie's disease. *Urology* 1975; **6**: 409–18.
3 Simeon CP, Fonollosa V, Vilardell M *et al.* Impotence and Peyronie's disease in systemic sclerosis. *Clin Exp Rheumatol* 1994; **12**: 464.
4 Mooradian AD, Viosca SP, Kaiser FE *et al.* Penile Raynaud's phenomenon: a possible cause of erectile failure. *Am J Med* 1988; **85**: 748–50.
5 Ganem JP, Lucey DT, Janosko EO, Carson CC. Unusual complications of the vacuum erection device. *Urology* 1998; **51**: 627–31.
6 Schiavino D, Sasso F, Nucera E *et al.* Immunologic findings in Peyronie's disease: a controlled study. *Urology* 1997; **50**: 764–8.
7 Horn AS, Pecora A, Chiesa JC, Alloy A. Penile thrombophlebitis as a presenting manifestation of pancreatic carcinoma. *Am J Gastroenterol* 1985; **80**: 463–5.
8 Desanctis PN, Furey CA Jr. Steroid injection therapy for Peyronie's disease: a 10-year summary and review of 38 cases. *J Urol* 1967; **97**: 114–6.
9 Winter CC, Khanna R. Peyronie's disease: results with dermo-jet injection of dexamethasone. *J Urol* 1975; **114**: 898–900.
10 Chun JL, McGregor A, Krishnan R, Carson CC. A comparison of dermal and cadaveric pericardial grafts in the modified Horton–Devine procedure for Peyronie's disease. *J Urol* 2001; **166**: 185–8.
11 Riedl CR, Plas E, Engelhardt P, Daha K, Pfluger H. Iontophoresis for treatment of Peyronie's disease. *J Urol* 2000; **163**: 95–9.

Drug reactions

The penis is a site of predilection for fixed drug eruption, like the face and extremities (see Chapter 73). The symptoms are itch or burning. The eruption is acute with a swollen plaque, sometimes with central blister formation, erosion and ulceration. Gruber *et al.* [1] describe the case of a man with known sensitivity to co-trimoxazole who developed a penile fixed drug eruption after intercourse with his wife while she was taking the drug for a sore throat. The differential diagnosis includes herpes simplex and erythema multiforme.

Ulceration has been reported following the inadvertent subcutaneous injection of papaverine for the treatment of erectile impotence [2]. Dequalinium is a topical antibacterial that was used for the treatment of impetigo and moniliasis in the 1950s and 1960s, but it caused a necrotizing balanitis with ulceration when used for the treatment of balanitis in uncircumcised men [3]. Warfarin necrosis can affect the genitalia [4]. All-*trans*-retinoic acid has been reported to induce scrotal ulceration in a patient with acute promyelocytic leukaemia [5]. Foscarnet is a recognized cause of genital ulceration in HIV-infected patients [6–8]. Erosion following the use of topical steroids has been seen.

REFERENCES

1 Gruber F, Stasic A, Lenkovic M, Brajac I. Postcoital fixed drug eruption in a man sensitive to trimethoprim-sulphamethoxazole. *Clin Exp Dermatol* 1997; **22**: 144–5.
2 Borgstrom E. Penile ulcer as complication in self-induced papaverine erections. *Urology* 1988; **32**: 416–7.
3 Coles RB, Wilkinson DS. Necrosis and dequalinium. I. Balanitis. *Trans St John's Hosp Dermatol Soc* 1965; **51**: 46–8.
4 Harmanyeri Y, Taskapan O, Dogan B, Baloglu H, Basak M. A case of coumarin necrosis with penile and pedal involvement. *J Eur Acad Dermatol Venereol* 1998; **10**: 248–52.
5 Esser AC, Nossa R, Shoji T, Sapadin AN. All-*trans*-retinoic acid-induced scrotal ulcerations in a patient with acute promyelocytic leukaemia. *J Am Acad Dermatol* 2000; **43**: 316–7.
6 Evans LM, Grossman ME. Foscarnet-induced penile ulcer. *J Am Acad Dermatol* 1992; **27**: 124–6.
7 Gross AS, Dretler RH. Foscarnet-induced penile ulcer in an uncircumcised patient with AIDS. *Clin Infect Dis* 1993; **17**: 1076–7.
8 Moyle G, Gazzard BG. Opportunistic infections and tumours: cytomegalovirus infection. In: Gazzard BG, ed. *AIDS Care Handbook*. London: Mediscript, 2002.

Miscellaneous

It is not unusual for the herald patch of pityriasis rosea to appear on suprapubic skin or in the groin. Incomplete or limited presentations (e.g. affecting the pelvic girdle) are not rare, although careful examination may elicit another patch on the neck or in the axilla.

Bottomley and Cotterill [1] have described an acutely tender erythematous scrotum associated with zinc deficiency in a patient with Crohn's disease. Necrolytic migratory erythema can be localized to the genitalia [2].

Autoimmune bullous diseases such as pemphigus can involve the penis (the glans is the usual site) (Fig. 68.13), but very rarely in isolation [3]. Pemphigus vegetans presenting with a 4-year history of indolent tender balanitis, where the glans penis was involved with a moist vegetative plaque with beefy red erosions separating irregular hyperkeratotic mounds, has been reported [4]. Linear immunoglobulin A (IgA) disease commonly involves the mucosae. Mucosal lesions of bullous pemphigoid are uncommon; their presence suggests another diagnosis or an underlying neoplasm. Pelvic girdle lesions are often seen, but rarely in isolation.

Cicatricial pemphigoid or (benign) mucous membrane pemphigoid is a rare variant of bullous pemphigoid in which blisters affect the skin and the mucous membranes. Skin lesions are usually less widespread than in bullous pemphigoid and they may heal with scarring. Oral lesions predominantly involve the palate and gingivae, but there may be oesophageal involvement with dysphagia, and conjunctival disease can lead to blindness. Involvement of the penis may be with blisters, erosions, ulcers, transcoronal adhesions, scarring and phimosis [5,6]. Although direct immunofluorescence is usually positive, circulating antibodies to the basement membrane zone are rarely found. The disease often responds poorly to oral steroids,

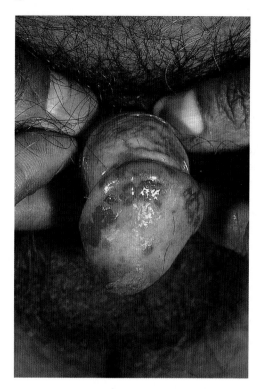

Fig. 68.13 Pemphigus of the penis. (Courtesy of Dr F.A. Ive, Durham, UK.)

but dapsone or other sulpha drugs such as sulphamethoxypyridazine can be effective. Regular haematology screening is mandatory with dapsone because of the risk of agranulocytosis.

One patient with Darier's disease developed an HPV 16-associated squamous carcinoma of the scrotum during oral isotretinoin treatment; he had not previously had radiotherapy to the genitocrural area [7]. Genitocrural papular acantholytic dermatosis can involve the penis, as can granuloma annulare. Erythematous smooth, round and linear nodules are described in the latter. Most patients are uncircumcised. Extragenital granuloma annulare is uncommon in these patients.

Occasionally, patients with generalized cutaneous sarcoid present with genital lesions [8]. Tender erythematous induration of the distal shaft of the penis and several yellowish subcutaneous nodules on the glans have been described [9]. A case presenting with penile ulceration has been reported [10]. Importantly, sarcoid can masquerade as testicular malignancy [11–13].

A granulomatous lymphangitis may be found histologically in the investigation of penile lymphoedema [14]. It can be a rare feature of the Melkersson–Rosenthal syndrome. Crohn's disease can involve the penis and scrotum [15–20].

A soft-tissue mass in the penis associated with systemic amyloid has been reported [21]. Primary amyloid of the urethra is very rare indeed, but accurate diagnosis is essential, as its presentation simulates carcinoma, with dysuria, bloody discharge and tender induration of the penis [22], or as an obstructive voiding syndrome, with tender periurethral masses and irregular urethral strictures [23].

One case each of eccrine syringofibroadenomatosis with penile involvement manifesting as a balanoposthitis [24], benign mucinous metaplasia with a prepucial 0.6 cm papule replacing the superficial epidermis [25], and mucinous syringometaplasia with an ulcerated papule on the shaft of the penis [26] have been reported.

Acute scrotum is a clinical syndrome defined as acute painful swelling of the scrotum or its contents, usually in boys, accompanied by local signs and general symptoms [27]. The critical differential diagnosis is torsion of the testis or spermatic cord. Other causes include idiopathic scrotal oedema, epididymitis, orchitis, hernia and haematocoele. Thromboangiitis obliterans has been found in two cases [28]. Acute scrotal swelling may be a physical sign of primary peritonitis in children and infants [29] or secondary peritonitis resulting from appendicitis, healed meconium peritonitis in the neonate, haemoperitonitis (ruptured spleen) and pseudotorsion resulting from ventriculoperitoneal shunts inserted for hydrocephalus that have migrated into the scrotum from the peritoneum. Acute idiopathic scrotal oedema usually affects children aged 4–12 years old. Allergy, infection (umbilical sepsis), trauma, insect bites, urinary extravasation and Henoch–Schönlein purpura have all been considered as causes. It is rare in adults, but cases in association with septic diabetic foot have been reported [30].

Henoch–Schönlein purpura/anaphylactoid purpura may affect the genitalia. Ureteritis, renal pelvic haemorrhage and pain and swelling of the spermatic cord have been reported. The incidence of scrotal involvement ranges from 2 to 38%. In some cases, the presentation has masqueraded as testicular torsion, resulting in unnecessary surgical exploration. Ultrasonography can help to distinguish between them [31]. However, testicular torsion can also be a serious complication of Henoch–Schönlein purpura [31].

Acute haemorrhagic oedema of childhood may present as tenderness, redness and swelling of the penis and scrotum with the development of more widespread haemorrhagic lesions [32]. The differential diagnosis includes acute febrile neutrophilic dermatosis, erythema multiforme, Henoch–Schönlein purpura and child abuse. The prognosis for complete recovery is excellent. Acute inflammation of the scrotum in patients with familial Mediterranean fever can occur [33]. It is manifested by pain, erythema and swelling, fever, leukocytosis and elevated erythrocyte sedimentation rate (ESR). It may occur in isolation or accompanying peritonitis. The differential diagnosis includes torsion, orchitis and epididymitis in boys.

Polyarteritis nodosa may be associated with testicular and epididymal involvement, with scrotal pain and swelling. In one case these were the sole presenting features and testicular biopsy provided the diagnosis [34–36].

REFERENCES

1 Bottomley WW, Cotterill JA. Acquired zinc deficiency presenting with an acutely tender erythematous scrotum. *Br J Dermatol* 1993; **129**: 501–2.
2 Bewley AP, Ross JS, Bunker CB, Staughton RC. Successful treatment of a patient with octreotide-resistant necrolytic migratory erythema. *Br J Dermatol* 1996; **134**: 1101–4.
3 Sami N, Ahmed AR. Penile pemphigus. *Arch Dermatol* 2001; **137**: 756–8.
4 Castle WN, Wentzell JM, Schwartz BK *et al.* Chronic balanitis due to pemphigus vegetans. *J Urol* 1987; **137**: 289–91.
5 Kirtschig G, Mengel R, Mittag H, Flores-De-Jacoby L, Happle R. Desquamative gingivitis and balanitis: linear IgA disease or cicatricial pemphigoid? *Clin Exp Dermatol* 1998; **23**: 173–7.
6 Ramlogan D, Coulsom IH, McGeorge A. Cicatricial pemphigoid: a diagnostic problem for the urologist. *J R Coll Surg Edinb* 2000; **45**: 62–3.
7 Orihuela E, Tyring SK, Pow-Sang M *et al.* Development of human papillomavirus type 16-asssociated squamous cell carcinoma of the scrotum in a patient with Darier's disease treated with systemic isotreinoin. *J Urol* 1995; **153**: 1940–3.
8 Wei H, Friedman KA, Rudikoff D. Multiple indurated papules on penis and scrotum. *J Cutan Med Surg* 2000; **4**: 202–4.
9 Rubinstein I, Baum GL, Hiss Y. Sarcoidosis of the penis: report of a case. *J Urol* 1986; **135**: 1016–7.
10 Mahmood N, Afzal N, Joyce A. Sarcoidosis of the penis. *Br J Urol* 1997; **80**: 155.
11 Turk CO, Schacht M, Ross L. Diagnosis and management of testicular sarcoidosis. *J Urol* 1986; **135**: 380–1.
12 Sieber PR, Duggan FE. Sarcoidosis and testicular tumors. *Urology* 1988; **31**: 140–1.
13 Gross AJ, Heinzer H, Loy V, Dieckmann K-P. Unusual differential diagnosis of testis tumor: intrascrotal sarcoidosis. *J Urol* 1992; **147**: 1112–4.
14 Mor Y, Zaidi SZ, Rose DS, Ransley PG, Mouriquand PD. Granulomatous lymphangitis of the penile skin as a cause of penile swelling in children. *J Urol* 1997; **158**: 591–2.
15 Goh CL, Ang CB, Chan RK, Cheong WK. Comparing treatment response and complications between podophyllin 0.5–0.25% in ethanol vs. podophyllin 25% in tincture benzoin for penile warts. *Singapore Med J* 1998; **39**: 17–9.
16 Corazza M, Ughi G, Spisani L, Virgili A. Metastatic ulcerative penile Crohn's disease. *J Eur Acad Dermatol Venereol* 1999; **13**: 224–6.
17 Lehrnbecher T, Kontny HU, Jeschke R. Metastatic Crohn's disease in a 9-year-old boy. *J Pediatr Gastroenterol Nutr* 1999; **28**: 321–3.
18 Acker SM, Sahn EE, Rogers HC *et al.* Genital cutaneous Crohn disease: two cases with unusual clinical and histopathologic features in young men. *Am J Dermatopathol* 2000; **22**: 443–6.
19 Slaney G, Muller S, Clay J *et al.* Crohn's disease involving the penis. *Gut* 1986; **27**: 329–33.
20 Phillips SS, Baird DB, Joshi VV, Rosenberg AJ, Janosko EO. Crohn's disease of the prepuce in a 12-year-old boy: a case report and review of the literature. *Pediatr Pathol Lab Med* 1997; **17**: 497–502.
21 Leal SM, Novsam N, Kacks SI. Case report: amyloidosis presenting as a penile mass. 1988; **140**: 830–1.
22 Provet JA, Rakham J, Mennen J, Golimbu M, Sabatini M. Primary amyloidosis of urethra. *Urology* 1989; **34**: 106–8.
23 Noone TC, Clark RL. Primary isolated urethral amyloidosis. *Abdom Imaging* 1997; **22**: 448–9.
24 Ochonisky S, Wechsler J, Marinho E, Revuz J. Eccrine syringofibroadenomatosis (Mascaro) with mucous involvement. *Arch Dermatol* 1994; **130**: 933–4.
25 Val-Bernal JF, Hernandez-Nieto E. Benign mucinous metaplasia of the penis: a lesion resembling extramammary Paget's disease. *J Cutan Pathol* 2000; **27**: 76–9.
26 Kappel TJ, Abenoza P. Mucinous syringometaplasia. *Am J Dermatopathol* 1993; **15**: 562–7.
27 Melekos MD, Asbach HW, Markou SA. Aetiology of acute scrotum in 100 boys with regard to age distribution. *J Urol* 1988; **139**: 1023.

28 Nesbit RM, Hodgson NB. Thromboangutis obliterans of the spermatic cord. *Trans Am Assoc Genitourin Surg* 1959; **51**: 92–4.

29 Udall DA, Drake DJ, Rosenberg RS. Acute scrotal swelling: a physical sign of primary peritonitis. *J Urol* 1981; **125**: 750–1.

30 Fahal AH, Suliman SH, Sharfi AR, el Mahadi EM. Acute idiopathic scrotal oedema in association with diabetic septic foot. *Diabetes Res Clin Pract* 1993; **21**: 197–200.

31 Laor T, Atala A, Teele RL. Scrotal ultrasonography in Henoch–Schönlein purpura. *Pediatr Radiol* 1992; **22**: 505–6.

32 Dubin BA, Bronson DM, Eng AM. Acute hemorrhagic oedema of childhood: an unusual variant of leukocytoclastic vasculitis. *J Am Acad Dermatol* 1990; **23**: 347–50.

33 Gedalia A, Adar A, Gorodischer R. Familial Mediterranean fever in children. *J Rheumatol* 1992; **19** (Suppl. 35): 1–9.

34 Dahl EV, Baggenstoss AH, deWeerd JH. Testicular lesions of periarteritis nodosa, with special reference to diagnosis. *Am J Med* 1960; **28**: 222–8.

35 Lee LM, Moloney PJ, Wong HCG, Magil AB, McLoughlin MG. Testicular pain: an unusual presentation of polyarteritis nodosa. 1983; **129**: 1243–4.

36 Wright LF, Bicknell SL. Systemic necrotizing vasculitis presenting as epididymitis. *J Urol* 1986; **136**: 1094.

Non-sexually transmitted infections

Staphylococcal cellulitis

Cellulitis may affect the penis. Piercing and genital jewellery predispose to infection. Cellulitis and abscess formation can complicate cysts, sinuses and fistulae and sexually transmitted infections. The exact relationship between episodes of acute infection and chronic penile oedema (CPL; see below), which often is complicated by cellulitis, is uncertain.

Anogenital infection in patients with malignant disease is serious, and potentially life-threatening necrotizing fasciitis and Fournier's gangrene may occur.

Streptococcal dermatitis/perianal cellulitis

This syndrome in children [1] probably also has a corollary in adults [2], but it is much more common in boys in whom, if the penis is involved, there may be dysuria, erythema and swelling of the penis and balanoposthitis.

Chronic idiopathic penile oedema

Chronic penile lymphoedema (CPL) is a relatively rare, reactive, disfiguring condition that causes sexual dysfunction and phimosis [3]. It has previously been called tumorous lymphoedema or elephantiasis verrucosa nostra [4]. Evidence of streptococcal infection may be present, and this could lead to irreversible lymphatic damage, whereas other cases seem idiopathic, and are perhaps brought about by primary hypoplastic lymphatics. Some patients have another penile dermatosis. Few cases of CPL have been reported before [3,5,6], and the aetiopathogenesis may have been misunderstood. Penoscrotal oedema has also been attributed to continuous ambulatory peritoneal dialysis [7], amputation of septic limbs in diabetes [8], acute necrotizing pancreatitis [9] and streptococcal infections [10]. Penile venereal oedema has been associated with gonococcal and herpes infection, and scabies infestation, and resolves after treatment of the underlying disease [11]. Similarly childhood penile oedema is self-limiting [12].

Filariasis and pelvic mass lesions should be excluded. Imaging of lymphatic channels is not particularly helpful [13]. It is possible that cases of CPL are related to any of the above factors and/or temporally unrelated but repetitive sexually transmitted disease. Persistent lymphatic insult from whatever cause could result in an inflammatory process affecting genital and pelvic vessels and nodes. Therefore all cases of penoscrotal oedema should be treated aggressively at first presentation, because the more chronic the genital lymphoedema the more difficult it is to treat, both medically and surgically [14]. The aim of treatment of CPL must be prophylaxis against further infective episodes and aggressive treatment of relapses.

Patients with CPL present with chronic swelling of the penis, foreskin, scrotum, pubic mound, buttocks and thighs, which may be warm and red. There may be intercurrent attacks of cellulitis and/or erysipelas with systemic upset.

Acute attacks require admission to hospital and treatment with systemic broad-spectrum antibiotics; a short course of prednisolone may also be helpful. Long-term treatment with erythromycin, clarithromycin or ciprofloxacin appears to improve and stabilize the process, and improves the appearance and function of the penis. The success of this approach argues the importance of infection as a factor in the perpetuation if not initiation of the process. Medical control with antibiotics then allows surgical intervention in the form of circumcision. Plastic repair may be necessary after excision of affected tissue [15,16].

Ecthyma gangrenosum

Ecthyma gangrenosum has a predilection for the acral and anogenital regions, and may affect the penis in isolation, leading to gangrene [17]. The prognosis is poor. A case has been reported that was probably caused by direct arterial septic embolization of the penis from femoral heroin injection [18].

Fournier's gangrene

Fournier's gangrene is analogous to necrotizing fasciitis and Meleney's gangrene. In 1883, the Parisian dermatologist Alfred Fournier described five cases of spontaneous genital gangrene and ulceration, but Baurienne (1764) probably first reported this condition [19]. The disease begins with urethral or appendageal polybacterial infection. Most of the organisms isolated are resident urethral or lower gastrointestinal flora, and most patients have mixed infections. In children, staphylococci and strepto-

Table 68.21 Risk factors for Fournier's gangrene.

Diabetes mellitus
Alcoholism
Anogenital infection
Chemotherapy
HIV
Post-instrumentation in the immunocompromised
Postoperative (urological and colorectal)
Heroin addiction
Trauma
Unconventional sexual practices

Table 68.22 Differential diagnosis of Fournier's gangrene. (After Bunker [25]. © 2004, with permission from Elsevier.)

Trauma
Herpes simplex
Cellulitis (streptococcal, staphylococcal)
Streptococcal necrotizing fasciitis
Gonococcal balanitis and oedema
Ecthyma gangrenosum
Allergic vasculitis
Polyarteritis nodosa
Necrolytic migratory erythema
Vascular occlusion syndromes
Warfarin necrosis

cocci are most commonly isolated [20]. A necrotizing vasculitis, possibly exotoxin-mediated, ensues with devastating consequences for involved skin, subcutis, fascia and muscle. It is held to be the human counterpart of the local Shwartzman phenomenon [21,22]. Painful erythematous swelling of the genitals (a black spot may appear on the scrotum [23]), perianal or lower abdominal skin with no suppuration but marked systemic toxicity (may be absent in children [20]), and urinary retention, is a typical presentation. Necrosis of skin and deeper tissues can occur rapidly, and there is a very high mortality unless the diagnosis is made promptly and radical mangement undertaken. Plain X-rays may show soft-tissue gas [24]. Predisposing factors are listed in Table 68.21. Preceding surgery, including vasectomy and instrumentation, especially in patients with the listed risk factors, is particularly important. The differential diagnosis is given in Table 68.22.

If a diagnosis of Fournier's gangrene is made, radical surgical débridement of all affected tissue is undertaken and broad-spectrum systemic antibiotic therapy initiated. Plastic repair can be undertaken if the patient survives. Hyperbaric oxgen and high-dose systemic steroid treatment have been used [22,26,27]. Children can be treated with more conservative surgery, and the mortality rate is lower [20,28]. In adults, the mortality is approximately 25%.

Trichomycosis pubis

Trichomycosis pubis causes asymptomatic yellow, red or black micronodules around hair shafts [29]. Pubic and axillary hair may be involved. The skin is normal but the sweat may be discolored. Trichomycosis pubis is rare in Western dermatological practice but is common in the Middle East [30], and may occur concomitantly with trichosporosis in India [31]. It is caused by *Corynebacterium* spp. The differential diagnosis includes true mycoses such as white or black piedra. Treatment is with topical benzoic acid, salicylic acid, clindamycin or naftifine [29].

Tuberculosis

Tuberculosis of the penis is rare [32] but important given the resurgence of the disease. Primary penile ulceration (solitary and multiple), with or without inguinal lymphadenopathy, caused by sexual infection or contact with infected clothing may occur [33], or the ulceration may be secondary to tuberculosis elsewhere (e.g. the lung) [34]. A cold abscess (presenting as erectile impotence) has been reported [35]. Tuberculides have involved the penis, including in isolation [36].

Non-syphilitic spirochaetal ulcerative balanoposthitis

This condition is recognized in the Tropics and South Africa, presenting as large serpiginous foul-smelling ulcers in uncircumcised men, associated in some with non-tender inguinal lymphadenopathy. Treatment is with penicillin or metronidazole [37].

Yaws

An ulcerated, crusted and papillomatous lesion has been reported on the prepuce as part of disseminated early yaws (with other skin lesions elsewhere) in a patient in an endemic region. Several family members were also infected. The genital lesion probably arose from auto-innoculation [38].

Candidosis

Genitourinary physicians maintain that *Candida* can be the cause of urethritis and balanoposthitis [39]. The glans penis and prepuce may be eroded. *Candida* of the penis (with a prevalence of approximately 10% of that of vaginal candidosis) has attracted very little research interest [40].

Candida may be more often a secondary pathogen than a sexually acquired infection. Observing the signs of candidosis, or demonstrating the presence of the organism, does not prove that it is the cause of all the symptoms and signs. An underlying dermatological or medical cause should be excluded. The symptoms and signs of *Candida* may be more florid than the underlying predisposing cause. Medical causes include diabetes mellitus, iatrogenic immunosuppression and systemic antibiotic treatment. Although oropharyngeal candidosis is almost invariably found in HIV infection, candidal balanoposthitis is not generally associated, perhaps because it is overlooked or because many patients take long-term imidazole antifungals orally.

Candida albicans is such a ready opportunist organism because it is a part of the resident flora of the gastrointestinal tract and may be retrieved from intertriginous areas, including the preputial folds, in the absence of symptoms and signs. Candidal balanoposthitis could be a sexually transmitted disease that may have an affinity for the anatomically or physiologically abnormal penis, or in individuals predisposed by other factors or disease, and where there is chronic vaginal or anal carriage in a partner. Screening should be performed for other sexually transmitted diseases.

Diagnosis is discussed in Chapter 31. Underlying disease should be identified and treated, and predisposing factors rectified. Treatment includes topical nystatin, clioquinol or an imidazole, often very usefully combined with hydrocortisone or a moderately potent corticosteroid. In severe disease, an oral imidazole may be indicated.

Tinea

Tinea of the penis or scrotum is uncommon and when it occurs it is usually associated with crural disease. Rarely encountered is the occurrence of tinea on the glans penis as a seat of itch or pain, and producing an erythematous patch or a crop of scaly papules [41–46]. Penile tinea in India has been associated with occlusion resulting from the wearing of a langota—a T-shaped piece of cloth tied over the genitalia [43].

Deep fungal infections

Although histoplasmosis is a common cause of disseminated fungal infection in the USA, urological and anogenital disease, usually ulceration and adenopathy in an ill patient, is rare [47,48]. An otherwise well man with a small warty nodule on the glans penis has been reported [49]. One patient with a penile ulcer transmitted the disease venereally to his wife [50].

In blastomycosis, although the genitourinary (prostate and epididymis) tract is involved in 20–30% of cases [51], involvement of the genital skin is rare. However, lesions of the prepuce and perianal skin have been recorded [52,53].

Paracoccidioidomycosis can be the cause of scrotal swelling and genital nodules and erosions [54].

Miscellaneous

Bacillary angiomatosis (see Chapter 26) is important in the differential diagnosis of AIDS-related Kaposi's sarcoma. A case in which the presenting tender red nodules affected the scrotum and groins has been published [55].

The penis is rarely affected by pityriasis versicolor and probably almost never in isolation [56,57]. Occasionally, the anterior pelvic girdle is the site involved.

One case only of superficial phaeohyphomycosis manifesting as multiple, 1–3 mm, pigmented papules, resembling seborrhoeic keratoses, on the scrotum of an HIV-positive patient has been described. Microscopy showed a mass of mycelia, and two dematiaceous fungi were cultured [58].

Occasionally, genital herpes simplex may be acquired non-sexually (e.g. during contact sports such as rugby football [59]). A phenomemenon of chronic erosive and verrucous herpes as part of immunoreconstitution disease has been described in HIV infection [60].

Sacral herpes zoster is discussed in Chapter 25. Lesions may be found on the scrotum and penis, and urinary retention and constipation can occur.

Amoebiasis can rarely present as a painful ulcerative balanitis, with swelling, frequency, dysuria and retention in tropical countries [61]. Self-inoculation from concomitant intestinal infection, by heterosexual intercourse where the female partner has amoebic vaginitis, or by sodomy, are the putative mechanisms. Amoebiasis as the cause of genital ulceration should lead to the suspicion of underlying HIV infection [62].

Cutaneous leishmaniasis can affect the genitalia [63,64]. An erythematous scaly plaque on the glans has been reported [65] and post-kala-azar dermal leishmaniasis of the penis and scrotum is encountered. Rarely, genital skin lesions may lead to the diagnosis of schistosomiasis. They occur because ova shed by worms enter the perineal vessels [66]. The papules and nodules may be skin-coloured, pink or brown, scattered or grouped, affecting the penis and scrotum. They can spread onto the perineum and around the anus, and may develop into soft warty vegetating lesions. Ulceration is rare and, even more rarely, concomitant carcinoma has been reported [67].

The anogenital consequences of onchocerciasis are 'leopard skin' hypopigmentation (the scrotum is commonly involved), ileal crest and scrotal nodules, 'hanging groin', and scrotal enlargement [68,69]. The differential diagnosis of the scrotal enlargement includes bancroftian filariasis [68]. Other filarial infections can lead to mild hydrocoele or gross elephantiasis. Filariasis can cause secondary lymphangiectasis. Excision, grafting and genital reconstruction can be undertaken [70].

REFERENCES

1 Peltola H. Images in clinical medicine: bacterial perianal dermatitis. *N Engl J Med* 2000; **342**: 1877.

2 Neri I, Bardazzi F, Marzaduri S, Patrizi A. Perianal streptococcal dermatitis in adults. *Br J Dermatol* 1996; **135**: 796–8.

3 Porter WM, Dinneen M, Bunker C. Chronic penile lymphoedema. *Arch Dermatol* 2001; **137**: 1108–10.

4 Luelmo J, Tolosa C, Prats J *et al.* Tumorous lymphoedema of the penis: report of verrucous elephantiasis—a brief case. Preliminary note. *Actas Urol Esp* 1995; **19**: 585–7.

5 Thomas JA, Matanhelia SS, Rees RWM. Recurrent adult idiopathic penile oedema: a new clinical entity? *Hosp Update* 1993; **Dec**: 667–8.

6 Geyer H, Geyer A, Schubert J. Erysipelas and elephantiasis of the scrotum: surgical and drug therapy. *Urologe A* 1995; **34**: 59–61.

7 Abraham G, Blake PG, Mathews R *et al.* Genital swelling as a surgical complication of continuous ambulatory peritoneal dialysis. *Surg Gynecol Obstet* 1990; **170**: 306–8.

8 Fahal AH, Suliman SH, Sharfi AR, el Mahadi EM. Acute idiopathic scrotal oedema in association with diabetic septic foot. *Diabetes Res Clin Pract* 1993; **21**: 197–200.

9 Choong KK. Acute penoscrotal oedema due to acute necrotizing pancreatitis. *J Ultrasound Med* 1996; **15**: 247–8.

10 Mendelson J, Miller M. Streptococcal venereal edema of the penis. *Clin Infect Dis* 1997; **24**: 516–7.

11 Wright RA, Judson FN. Penile venereal edema. *JAMA* 1979; **241**: 157–8.

12 Brandes SB, Chelsky MJ, Hanno PM. Adult acute idiopathic scrotal oedema. *Urology* 1994; **44**: 602–5.

13 Samsoen M, Deschler JM, Servelle M *et al.* Le lymphoedeme penoscrotal: two observations. *Ann Dermatol Vénéréol* 1981; **108**: 541–6.

14 Malloy TR, Wein AJ, Gross P. Scrotal and penile lymphedema: surgical considerations and management. *J Urol* 1983; **130**: 263–5.

15 Morey AF, Meng MV, McAninch JW. Skin graft reconstruction of chronic genital lymphoedema. *Urology* 1997; **50**: 423–6.

16 Muehlberger T, Homann HH, Kuhnen C, Vogt PM, Steinau HU. Aetiology, clinical aspects and therapy of penoscrotal lymphoedema. *Chirurg* 2001; **72**: 414–8 [in German].

17 Rabinowitz R, Lewin EB. Gangrene of the genitalia in children with *Pseudomonas* sepsis. *J Urol* 1980; **124**: 431–2.

18 Cunningham DL, Persky L. Penile ecthyma gangrenosum. *Urology* 1989; **34**: 109–12.

19 Smith GL, Bunker CB, Dineen MD. Fournier's gangrene. *Br J Urol* 1998; **81**: 347–55.

20 Adams JR Jr, Mata JA, Venable DD, Culkin DJ, Bocchini JA Jr. Fournier's gangrene in children. *Urology* 1990; **35**: 439–41.

21 van der Meer JB, de Jong MCJM. Recent aspects of pathogenesis and therapy of fulminant elapsing necrosis. *Neth J Med* 1992; **40**: 244–53.

22 Schultz ES, Diepgen TL, von den Driesch P, Hornstein OP. Systemic corticosteriods are important in the treatment of Fournier's gangrene: a case report. *J Dermatol* 1995; **133**: 633–5.

23 Bubrick MP, Hitchcock CR. Necrotizing anorectal and perineal infection. *Surgery* 1979; **86**: 655–62.

24 Fisher JR, Conway Ml, Takeshita RT *et al.* Necrotizing fasciitis: importance of roentgenographic studies for soft-tissue gas. *JAMA* 1979; **241**: 803–6.

25 Bunker 2003 Bunker CB. *Male Genital Skin Disease*. London: Saunders, 2004 (in press).

26 Chantarasak ND, Basu PK. Fournier's gangrene following vasectomy. *Br J Urol* 1988; **61**: 538–9.

27 van der Meer JB, van der Wal T, Bos WH *et al.* Fournier's gangrene: the human counterpart of the local Shwartzman phenomenon? *Arch Dermatol* 1990; **126**: 1376–7.

28 Sussman SJ, Schiller RP, Shashikumar VL. Fournier's syndrome: report of three cases and a review of the literature. *Am J Dis Child* 1978; **132**: 1189–91.

29 Rosen T, Krawczynska AM, McBride ME, Ellner K. Naftifine treatment of trichomycosis pubis. *Int J Dermatol* 1991; **30**: 667–9.

30 Lestringant GG, Khalil I, Fletcher S. Is the incidence of trichomycosis of genital hair underestimated? *J Am Acad Dermatol* 1991; **24**: 297–8.

31 Kamalam A, Senthamilselvi G, Ajithadas K, Thambiah AS. Cutaneous trichosporosis. *Mycopathologia* 1988; **101**: 167–75.

32 Minkin W, Frank SB, Cohen HJ. Penile granuloma. *Arch Dermatol* 1972; **106**: 756.

33 Rossi R, Urbano F, Tortoli E *et al.* Primary tuberculosis of the penis. *J Eur Acad Dermatol Venereol* 1999; **12**: 174–6.

34 Burns DA, Sarkany I. Tuberculous ulceration of the penis. *Proc R Soc Med* 1976; **69**: 883–4.

35 Murali TR, Raja NS. Cavernosal cold abscess: a rare cause of impotence. *Br J Urol* 1998; **82**: 929–30.

36 Kashima M, Mori K, Kadono T *et al.* Tuberculide of the penis without ulceration. *Br J Dermatol* 1999; **140**: 757–9.

37 Piot P, Duncan M, van Dyck E *et al.* Ulcerative balanoposthitis associated with non-syphilitic spirochaetal infection. *Genitourin Med* 1986; **62**: 44–6.

38 Engelkens HJ, Judanarso J, van der Sluis JJ, van der Stek J, Stolz E. Disseminated early yaws: report of a child with a remarkable genital lesion mimicking venereal syphilis. *Pediatr Dermatol* 1990; **7**: 60–2.

39 Wisdom A, Hawkins DA. *Diagnosis in Color. Sexually Transmitted Diseases*, 2nd edn. London: Mosby-Wolfe, 1997: 154–6.

40 Odds FC. Genital candidiasis. *Clin Exp Dermatol* 1982; **7**: 345–54.

41 Pillai KG, Singh G, Sharma BM. Trichophyton rubrum: infection of the penis. *Dermatologica* 1975; **100**: 252–4.

42 Kumar B, Talwar P, Kaur S. Penile tinea. *Mycopathologia* 1981; **75**: 169–72.

43 Pandey SS, Chandra S, Guha PK, Kaur P, Singh G. Dermatophyte infection of the penis: association with a particular undergarment. *Int J Dermatol* 1981; **20**: 112–4.

44 Dekio S, Jidio J. Tinea of the glans penis. *Dermatologica* 1989; **178**: 112–4.

45 Dekio S, Qin LM, Jidio J. Tinea of the glans penis: report of a case presenting a crop of papules. *J Dermatol* 1991; **18**: 52–5.

46 Pielop J, Rosen T. Penile dermatophytosis. *J Am Acad Dermatol* 2001; **44**: 864–7.

47 Jayalakshmi P, Goh KL. Disseminated histoplasmosis presenting as penile ulcer. *Aust NZ J Med* 1990; **20**: 175–6.

48 Preminger B, Gerard PS, Lutwick L *et al.* Histoplasmosis of the penis. *J Urol* 1993; **149**: 848–50.

49 Mankodi RC, Kanvinde MS, Mohapatra LN. Penile histoplasmosis: a case report. *Indian J Med Sci* 1970; **24**: 354–6.

50 Sills M, Schwartz A, Weg JG, Arbor A. Conjugal histoplasmosis: a consequence of progressive dissemination in the index case after steroid therapy. *Ann Intern Med* 1973; **79**: 221–4.

51 Craig MW, Davey WN, Green RA. Conjugal blastomycosis. *Am Rev Respir Dis* 1970; **102**: 86–90.

52 Eickenberg H, Amin M, Lich R. Blastomycosis of the genitourinary tract. *J Urol* 1975; **113**: 650–2.

53 English JC III, Laws RA, Keough GC *et al.* Dermatoses of the glans penis and prepuce. *J Am Acad Dermatol* 1997; **37**: 1–24; quiz 25–6.

54 Severo LC, Kauer CL, Oliveira F *et al.* Paracoccidioidomycosis of the male genital tract: report of 11 cases and a review of Brazilian literature. *Rev Inst Med Trop Sao Paulo* 2000; **42**: 37–40.

55 Fagan WA, Skinner SM, Ondo A *et al.* Bacillary angiomatosis of the skin and bone marrow in a patient with HIV infection. *J Am Acad Dermatol* 1995; **32**: 510–2.

56 Avram A, Rousselet G, Benazeraf C, Grupper C. 'Pityriasis versicolor' de la verge. *Bull Soc Francaise Dermatol Syphiligr* 1973; **80**: 607–8.

57 Aljabre SHM, Sheikh YH. Penile involvement in pityriasis versicolor. *Trop Geogr Med* 1994; **46**: 184–7.

58 Duvic M, Lowe L. Superficial phaeohyphomycosis of the scrotum in a patient with the acquired immunodeficiency syndrome. *Arch Dermatol* 1987; **123**: 1597–9.

59 Estéve E, Gironet N, Barthez JP, Maitre F. Case for diagnosis: herpes rugbiorum. *Ann Dermatol Vénéréol* 1998; **125**: 527–8.

60 Fox PA, Barton SE, Francis N *et al.* Chronic erosive herpes simplex virus infection of the penis: a possible immune reconstitution disease. *HIV Med* 1999; **1**: 10–8.

61 Cooke RA, Rodriguez RB. Amoebic balanitis. *Med J Aust* 1964; **5**: 114–7.

62 Gbery IP, Dheja D, Kacou DE *et al.* Chronic genital ulcerations and HIV infection: 29 cases. *Med Trop* 1999; **59**: 279–82.

63 Cain C, Seabury-Stone M, Thieburg M, Wilson ME. Non-healing genital ulcers. *Arch Dermatol* 1994; **130**: 1311–6.

64 Schubach A, Cuzzi-Maya T, Goncalves-Costa SC, Pirmez C, Oliveira-Neto MP. Leishmaniasis of glans penis. *J Eur Acad Dermatol Venereol* 1998; **10**: 226–8.

65 Grunwald MH, Amichai B, Trau H. Cutaneous leishmaniasis on an unusual site: the glans penis. *Br J Urol* 1998; **82**: 928.

66 Adeyemi-Doru FAB, Osoba OA, Junaid TA. Perigenital cutaneous schistosomiasis. *Br J Vener Dis* 1979; **55**: 446–9.

67 Zawahry ME. Cutaneous amoebiasis. *Indian J Dermatol* 1966; **11**: 77–8.

68 Akogun OB, Akoh JI, Hellandendu H. Non-ocular clinical onchocerciasis in relation to skin microfilaria in the Taraba River Valley, Nigeria. *J Hyg Epidemiol Microbiol Immunol* 1992; **36**: 368–83.

69 McMahon JE, Simonsen PE. Filariases: onchocerciasis. In: Cook GC, ed. *Manson's Tropical Diseases*, 20th edn. London: Saunders, 1996: 1338–51.

70 Das S, Tuerk D, Amar AD, Sommer J. Surgery of male genital lymphedema. *J Urol* 1983; **129**: 1240–2.

Dermatological aspects of sexually transmitted disease

Syphilis

Syphilis (see Chapter 30) is endemic throughout the world. It is enjoying a resurgence in homosexual men. All manifestations of syphilis can affect the genital region [1]. Balanoposthitis can complicate and obscure penile chancre. The granulomatous gumma may affect the genital area as an ulcer, a white plaque or as an atrophic scar. Pseudochancre redux describes gummatous (tertiary stage) recurrence at the site of the primary chancre [2]; it is very rare.

Viral warts

Circumcised men are more likely to have genital warts than the uncircumcised [3]. The risk of acquiring genital warts is significantly reduced by using condoms [4]. Clinically inapparent disease may present as balanoposthitis [5]. Subclinical or latent genital HPV infection may be 100 times more common than classical condylomas [6]. The 5% acetic acid test is not a very specific aid to the identification of warts or dysplastic lesions [7]. Congenital and acquired immunosuppression increases the susceptibility of the anogenital region to HPV infection and progression to dysplasia and frank malignancy [8].

The clinical diagnosis of HPV infection is usually certain but condylomata lata (secondary syphilis), lichen planus, molluscum contagiosum, Bowenoid papulosis and pearly penile papules enter the differential diagnosis. Solitary lesions have a wider differential diagnosis, including giant condyloma, squamous carcinoma and transitional cell carcinoma of the distal urethra, which can present as a warty lesion at the urethral meatus [9]. Biopsy should be performed if there is diagnostic doubt or dysplasia. Patients with anogenital warts and their partners may require full sexually transmitted disease and sometimes colorectal assessment.

Molluscum contagiosum

Molluscum contagiosum is discussed in Chapter 25. Young men are commonly seen with penile and pubic lesions and it is assumed that this is a sexually transmitted infection, but this may not always be the case.

Table 68.23 Causes of penile and scrotal ulcers in HIV infection.

Pseudomonas
Syphilis
Chancroid
Herpes simplex
Penicilliosis
Amoebiasis
Fournier's gangrene
Squamous cell carcinoma
Kaposi's sarcoma
Drugs (e.g. foscarnet)

Human immunodeficiency virus infection

Ulcerative genital disease is a risk factor for HIV [10], but anogenital ulceration may be a consequence of HIV infection (see Chapter 26) [11]. Table 68.23 lists the main causes. Biopsy, with special stains and culture, is mandatory. Other genital problems in HIV, such as psoriasis, warts, intraepithelial neoplasia, squamous carcinoma and Kaposi's sarcoma, are discussed elsewhere.

Phthiriasis

Phthiriasis (see Chapter 33) can present with marked genital and pubic itching with few overt physical signs, or as an infected genitocrural and pubic eczema that conceals the underlying primary signs. In hirsute men, the abdomen, chest, axillae and thighs may also be involved. Screening for other sexually transmitted diseases should be offered to the patient and partner(s).

Scabies

Scabies may present with anogenital itch, 'folliculitis' (including of the buttocks) and penile, scrotal and pubic nodules (Fig. 68.14). The patient must be told to advise close physical contacts and family to be treated simultaneously.

Benign tumours

The following entities are all encountered in the male genital area: angiomas and angiokeratomas, and angiokeratoma corporis diffusum; basal cell papillomas may be mistaken for viral warts [12] or Bowenoid papulosis, as may melanocytic naevi; inguinogenital epidermoid cysts may become infected: lesions containing molluscum contagiosum have been described [13]; pilar cyst, including giant forms, is much rarer [14].

Median raphe cysts

Congenital cystic median raphe anomalies may remain unobtrusive until adulthood. Cystic or nodular and linear

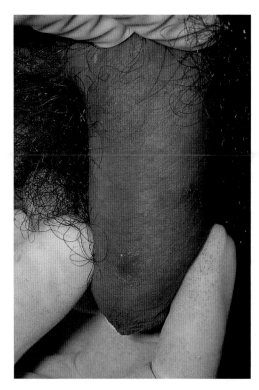

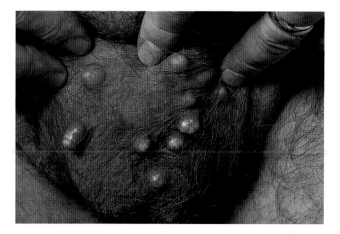

Fig. 68.15 Scrotal calcinosis. (Courtesy of Dr D.A. Burns, Leicester, UK.)

Fig. 68.14 Papules on the penis in scabies. (Courtesy of Dr C. White, University Hospital of North Durham, Durham, UK.)

swellings of the ventral penis occur near the glans. In adolescence or adulthood they may become traumatized or infected with staphylococci, gonococci or *Trichomonas* and present as tender erythematous purulent nodules [1]. Histologically, they are either dermoid or mucoid, depending on their embryology or epithelial lining [15]. Very rarely, the basal epithelial lining of the cysts may contain melanocytes, imparting a brown-black pigment to the lesion [16].

Mucoid cysts

These are rare lesions that present from birth or childhood as small flesh-coloured mobile cystic papules or nodules with no punctum, commonly on the ventral glans or foreskin, rarely in the perineum. They can be asymptomatic, become infected or interfere with intercourse. The histological features suggest that they arise from ectopic urethral tissue during embryological development [17].

Scrotal calcinosis

Scrotal calcinosis is a relatively common benign idiopathic disorder presenting as solitary or multiple, hard, smooth, white papules or nodules on the scrotum, rarely the penis (Fig. 68.15). Interestingly, these lesions are much rarer on the vulva [18]. Occasionally, they may become secondarily inflamed or infected following trauma.

Their occurrence was first described by Hutchinson [19]. Their origin has been debated: they have been said to arise from epidermoid cysts, eccrine duct milia, eccrine epithelial cysts, dystrophy of the dartos muscle, trauma and the presence of foreign bodies [1,20–30]. Scrotal calcinosis may occur after meconium peritonitis, with leakage of meconium through the processus vaginalis, and in testicular tumours such as teratomas, gonadoblastomas and Leydig cell tumours [27]. In endemic areas of onchocerciasis, calcified scrotal cysts may be caused by the living or dead nematodes, and patients have evidence of the disease elsewhere [31,32]. Onchocercal nodules are more common on the iliac crests and the rib cage (see Chapter 32).

The unsightly and embarrassing lesions can be treated by incision and eventration under local anaesthesia.

Verruciform xanthoma

Verruciform xanthoma mainly affects the mouth (see Chapter 66). The genitalia are the next most frequently involved, where it presents as a painless, yellow-brown or red, verrucous, sessile or papillary plaque. Fewer than 20 cases have been reported [33]. The histological findings are hyperkeratosis, focal parakeratosis, acanthosis and fat-filled foam cells in the papillary dermis. Verrucous xanthoma is thought to represent epidermal degeneration, with keratinocyte lipid then taken up by dermal macrophages [34] or fibroblasts to form the foam cells. HPV 6 has been implicated in one case [35]. Treatment is by surgical excision.

Miscellaneous

Naevus comedonicus of the glans penis, generally devoid of pilosebaceous structures, has been reported [36].

Keloid is rare, but can complicate circumcision [37,38], and other surgery and trauma [39,40]. Keloid has been simulated on the dorsum of the penis by chronic oedema caused by a condom catheter [41].

Dermoid cyst affecting the penis, presenting with pain, swelling and suppuration from abscess formation, has been reported [42].

Acanthosis nigricans almost always affects the groins. In pseudoacanthosis nigricans, the associated obesity is almost always responsible for associated intertrigo and skin tags.

Some cases of multiple syringoma localized to the penis have been described, mimicking genital warts or lichen planus [43–46].

Other benign tumours that have been reported rarely to affect the anogenital area include apocrine cystadenoma [47,48], mixed syringocystadenoma papilliferum and papillary eccrine adenoma occurring in a scrotal condyloma [49], dermatofibroma [50], giant cell fibroblastoma (scrotum) [51], connective tissue naevi (scrotum) [52], fibrous hamartoma of infancy (scrotum) [53], leiomyoma [50,54], genital smooth muscle hamartoma (scrotum) [55], neurofibroma, neurilemoma, granular cell myoblastoma [50,56–58], varicosities (venous lakes), acquired capillary and cavernous haemangioma of the penis have been described [50] (other angiomatous lesions are very much rarer, and controversy exists as to whether they represent a true neoplasm, herniation of the corpus spongiosum or vascularization of a haematoma or thrombus [59]), Masson's vegetant intravascular haemangioendothelioma [60], angiokeratoma circumscriptum of Mibelli [61], glomus tumour [50,62], port-wine stain, strawberry naevus [63–65], epithelioid haemangioma [66], epithelioid haemangioendothelioma [50,67], angiolymphoid hyperplasia with eosinophilia/Kimura's disease (penis and spermatic cord) [68,69] and lymphangioma circumscriptum [70,71].

REFERENCES

1 Bunker CB. *Male Genital Skin Disease*. London: Saunders, 2004 (in press).
2 Evans AL, Summerly R. Pseudo-chancre redux with negative serology: a case report. *Br J Vener Dis* 1964; **40**: 222–4.
3 Cook LS, Koutsky LA, Holmes KK. Clinical presentation of genital warts among circumcised and uncircumcised heterosexual men attending an urban STD clinic. *Genitourin Med* 1993; **69**: 262–4.
4 Wen LM, Estcourt CS, Simpson JM, Mindel A. Risk factors for the acquisition of genital warts: are condoms protective? *Sex Transm Infect* 1999; **75**: 312–6.
5 Lowhagen GB, Bolmstedt A, Ryd W, Voog E. The prevalence of the 'high risk' HPV types in penile condylomata-like lesions: correlation between HPV type and morphology. *Genitourin Med* 1993; **69**: 87–90.
6 von Krogh G. Clinical relevance and evaluation of genitoanal papilloma virus infection in the male. *Semin Dermatol* 1992; **11**: 229–40.
7 Voog E, Ricksten A, Olofsson S *et al*. Demonstration of Epstein–Barr virus DNA and human papillomavirus DNA in acetowhite lesions of the penile skin and the oral mucosa. *Int J STD AIDS* 1997; **8**: 772–5.
8 Daneshpouy M, Socic G, Clavel C *et al*. Human papillomavirus infection and anogenital condyloma in bone marrow transplant recipients. *Transplantation* 2001; **71**: 167–9.
9 Langlois NEI, McClinton S, Miller ID. An unusual presentation of transitional cell carcinoma of the distal urethra. *Histopathology* 1992; **21**: 482–4.
10 Stamm WE, Handsfield HH, Rompalo AM *et al*. The association between genital ulcer disease and acquisition of HIV infection in homosexual men. *JAMA* 1988; **260**: 1429–33.
11 Cope R, Debou JM. AIDS and anorectal pathology. *Ann Chirurg* 1995; **49**: 310–6.
12 Friedman SJ, Fox BJ, Albert HL. Seborrhoeic keratoses of the penis. *Urology* 1987; **29**: 204–6.
13 Park SK, Lee JY, Kim YH *et al*. Molluscum contagiosum occurring in an epidermal cyst: report of three cases. *J Dermatol* 1992; **19**: 119–21.
14 Shah SS, Varea EG, Farsaii A *et al*. Giant epidermoid cyst of the penis. *Urology* 1979; **14**: 389–91.
15 Oshin DR, Bowles WT. Congenital cysts and canals of the scrotal and perineal raphe. *J Urol* 1962; **88**: 406–8.
16 Urahashi J, Hara H, Yamaguchi Z, Morishima T. Pigmented median raphe cysts of the penis. *Acta Dermatol Venereol* 2000; **80**: 297–8.
17 Cole LA, Helwig EB. Mucoid cysts of the penile skin. *J Urol* 1976; **115**: 397–400.
18 Jamaleddine FN, Salman SM, Shbaklo Z, Kibbi AG, Zaynoun S. Idiopathic vulvar calcinosis: the counterpart of idiopathic scrotal calcinosis. *Cutis* 1988; **41**: 273–5.
19 Hutchinson J. Sebaceous gland tumours in the scrotum. Plate LXVIII. *Illustrations of Clinical Surgery*, Vol 2. Philadelphia: Blakiston, 1888.
20 King DT, Brosman S, Hirose FM, Gillespie LM. Idiopathic calcinosis of scrotum. *Urology* 1979; **14**: 92–4.
21 Shapiro L, Platt N, Torres-Rodriguez VM. Idiopathic calcinosis of the scrotum. *Arch Dermatol* 1970; **102**: 199–204.
22 Veress B, Malik MAO. Idiopathic scrotal calcinosis: a report of six cases from the Sudan. *East Afr Med J* 1975; **52**: 705–10.
23 Fisher BK, Dvoretsky I. Idiopathic calcinosis of the scrotum. *Arch Dermatol* 1978; **114**: 957.
24 Takayama H, Pak K, Tomoyoshi T. Electron microscopic study of mineral deposits in idiopathic calcinosis of the scrotum. *J Urol* 1982; **127**: 915–8.
25 Dare AJ, Axelsen RA. Scrotal calcinosis: origin from dystrophic calcification of eccrine duct milia. *J Cutan Pathol* 1988; **15**: 142–9.
26 Ito A, Sakamoto F, Ito M. Dystrophic scrotal calcinosis originating from benign eccrine epithelial cysts. *Br J Dermatol* 2001; **144**: 146–50.
27 Swinehart JM, Golitz LE. Scrotal calcinosis. *Arch Dermatol* 1982; **118**: 985–8.
28 Sarma DP, Weilbaecher TG. Scrotal calcinosis: calcification of epidermal cysts. *J Surg Oncol* 1984; **27**: 76–9.
29 Song DH, Lee KH, Kang WH. Idiopathic calcinosis of the scrotum: histopathologic observations of 51 nodules. *J Am Acad Dermatol* 1988; **19**: 1095–101.
30 Wright S, Navsaria H, Leigh IM. Idiopathic scrotal calcinosis is idiopathic. *J Am Acad Dermatol* 1991; **24**: 727–30.
31 Browne SG. Calcinosis circumscripta of the scrotal wall: the aetiological role of *Onchocerca volvulus*. *Br J Dermatol* 1962; **74**: 136–40.
32 Akogun OB, Akoh JI, Hellandendu H. Non-ocular clinical onchocerciasis in relation to skin microfilaria in the Taraba River Valley, Nigeria. *J Hyg Epidemiol Microbiol Immunol* 1992; **36**: 368–83.
33 Mohsin SK, Lee MW, Amin MB *et al*. Cutaneous verruciform xanthoma: a report of five cases investigating the aetiology and nature of xanthomatous cells. *Am J Surg Pathol* 1998; **22**: 479–87.
34 Orchard GE, Jones EW, Jones RR. Verruciform xanthoma: an immunocytochemical study. *Br J Biomed Sci* 1994; **51**: 28–34.
35 Khaskhely NM, Uezato H, Kamiyama T *et al*. Association of human papillomavirus type 6 with a verruciform xanthoma. *Am J Dermatopathol* 2000; **22**: 447–52.
36 Abdel-Aal H, Abdel-Aziz AM. Naevus comedonicus: report of three cases localized on glans penis. *Acta Dermatol Venereol* 1975; **55**: 78–80.
37 Warwick DJ, Dickson WA. Keloid of the penis after circumcision. *Postgrad Med J* 1993; **69**: 236–7.
38 Gürünlüoğlu R, Bayramicli M, Dogan T, Numanoglu A. Unusual complications of circumcision. *Plast Reconstr Surg* 1999; **104**: 1938–9.
39 Parsons RW. A case of keloid of the penis. *Plast Reconstr Surg* 1966; **37**: 431–2.
40 Kormoczy I. Enormous keloid (?) on a penis. *Br J Plast Surg* 1978; **31**: 268–9.
41 Bang RL. Penile oedema induced by continuous condom catheter use and mimicking keloid scar. *Scand J Urol Nephrol* 1994; **28**: 333–5.
42 Tomasini C, Aloi F, Puiatti P, Caliendo V. Dermoid cyst of the penis. *Dermatology* 1997; **194**: 188–90.
43 Lo JS, Dijkstra JW, Bergfeld WF. Syringomas on the penis. *Int J Dermatol* 1990; **29**: 309–10.
44 Sola Casas MA, de Delas JS, Bellon PR, Gutierrez EQ. Syringomas localized to the penis. *Clin Exp Dermatol* 1993; **18**: 384–5.

45 Zalla JA, Perry HO. An unusual case of syringoma. *Arch Dermatol* 1971; **103**: 215–7.
46 Lipshultz RL, Kantor GR, Vonderheid EC. Multiple penile syringomas mimicking verrucae. *Int J Dermatol* 1991; **30**: 69.
47 de Dulanto F, Armijo-Moreno M, Camacho Martinez F. Nodular hidradenoma (apocrine cystadenoma) of the penis. *Ann Dermatol Syphiligr (Paris)* 1973; **100**: 417–22.
48 Flessati P, Camoglio FN, Bianchi S, Fasoli L, Menghi A. An apocrine hidrocystoma of the scrotum: a case report. *Minerva Chir* 1999; **54**: 87–9.
49 Coyne JD, Fitzgibbon JF. Mixed syringocystadenoma papilliferum and papillary eccrine adenoma occurring in a scrotal condyloma. *J Cutan Pathol* 2000; **27**: 199–201.
50 Dehner LP, Smith BH. Soft tissue tumours of the penis. *Cancer* 1970; **25**: 1431–47.
51 DeSanctis DP, Maglietta R, Miranda R, Betta PG. Giant cell fibroblastoma of the scrotum: a case report. *Tumori* 1993; **79**: 367–9.
52 Fork HE, Sanchez RL, Wagner RF Jr, Raimer SS. A new type of connective tissue nevus: isolated exophytic elastoma. *J Cutan Pathol* 1991; **18**: 457–63.
53 Thami GP, Jaswal R, Kanwar AJ. Fibrous hamartoma of infancy in the scrotum. *Pediatr Dermatol* 1998; **15**: 326.
54 Ohtake N, Maeda S, Kanzaki T, Shimoinaba K. Leiomyoma of the scrotum. *Dermatology* 1997; **194**: 299–301.
55 Hsiao GH, Chen JS. Acquired genital smooth-muscle hamartoma: a case report. *Am J Dermatopathol* 1995; **17**: 67–70.
56 Chan WP, Chiang SS, Huang AH, Lin CN. Penile frenulum neurilemoma: a rare and unusual genitourinary tract tumor. *J Urol* 1990; **144**: 136–7.
57 Littlejohn JO, Belman AB, Selby D. Plexiform neurofibroma of the penis in a child. *Urology* 2000; **56**: 669.
58 Fernandez MJ, Martino A, Khan H, Considine TJ, Burden J. Giant neurilemoma: unusual scrotal mass. *Urology* 1987; **30**: 74–6.
59 Senoh K, Miyazaki T, Kikuchi I, Sumiyoshi A, Kohga A. Angiomatous lesions of the glans penis. *Urology* 1981; **17**: 194–6.
60 Paul AB, Johnston CAB, Nawroz I. Masson's tumour of the penis. *Br J Urol* 1994; **74**: 261–2.
61 Bruce DH. Angiokeratoma circumscriptum and angiokeratoma scroti. *Arch Dermatol* 1960; **81**: 388–93.
62 Macaluso JN, Sullivan JW, Tomberlin S. Glomus tumor of the glans penis. *Urology* 1985; **25**: 409–10.
63 Eastridge RR, Carrion HM, Politano VA. Hemangioma of the scrotum perineum and buttocks. *Urology* 1979; **14**: 61–3.
64 Gotoh M, Tsai S, Sugiyama T, Miyake K, Mitsuya H. Giant scrotal hemangioma with azoospermia. *Urology* 1983; **22**: 637–9.
65 Achauer BM, Vander Kam VC. Ulcerated anogenital hemangioma of infancy. *Plast Reconstr Surg* 1991; **87**: 861–8.
66 Srigley JR, Ayala AG, Ordóñez NG, van Nostrand AW. Epithelioid hemangioma of the penis: a rare and distinctive vascular lesion. *Arch Pathol Lab Med* 1985; **109**: 51–4.
67 Quante M, Patel NK, Hill S *et al*. Epithelioid hemangioendothelioma presenting in the skin: a clinicopathologic study of eight cases. *Am J Dermatopathol* 1998; **20**: 541–6.
68 Rao RN, Spurlock BO, Witherington R. Angiolymphoid hyperplasia with eosinophilia: report of a case with penile lesions. *Cancer* 1981; **47**: 944–9.
69 Van Gulik TM, Jansen JW, Taat CW. Kimura's disease in the spermatic cord: an unusual site of a rare tumor. *Neth J Surg* 1986; **38**: 93–5.
70 Osborne GE, Chinn RJ, Francis ND, Bunker CB. Magnetic resonance imaging in the investigation of penile lymphangioma circumscriptum. *Br J Dermatol* 2000; **143**: 467–8.
71 Sadikoğlu B, Kuran I, Özcan H, Gözü A. Cutaneous lymphatic malformation of the penis and scrotum. *J Urol* 1999; **162**: 1445–6.

Precancerous dermatoses

Squamous hyperplasia

Such lesions consist of white patches or plaques. Although it is the most common epithelial abnormality found in association with invasive squamous carcinoma of the penis, histologically there is *no* cytological atypia; acanthosis and orthokeratotic hyperkeratosis are found [1].

Penile horn

It is rare for cutaneous horn to affect the penis [2]. The underlying causes include pseudoepitheliomatous micaceous and keratotic balanitis [3], verrucous carcinoma [4–6] and squamous carcinoma [7]. Chronic inflammation and recent circumcision for long-standing phimosis are said to be important predisposing factors. The lesion is premalignant or, in one-third of cases, malignant at presentation, with squamous carcinoma the underlying pathology. Treatment should be dictated by precise diagnosis achieved by adequate excision and histology of the whole lesion. Follow-up is mandatory because recurrence may occur.

Porokeratosis

Genital porokeratosis of Mibelli is rare, but classical lesions have been found on the penis and scrotum. Ulceration may occur [8]. Porokeratosis may be confused with psoriasis, Bowen's disease, granuloma annulare or lichen planus; biopsy differentiates these conditions [9]. Topical 5-fluorouracil can be used [10].

Pseudoepitheliomatous micaceous and keratotic balanitis

Pseudoepitheliomatous micaceous and keratotic balanitis (PEMKB) is a rare penile condition. It presents as thick scaly micaceous patches (possibly a cutaneous horn) on the glans penis in older uncircumcised men [3,11]. Histological examination shows hyperkeratosis, parakeratosis, acanthosis, prolongation of the rete ridges and mild lower epidermal dysplasia, with a non-specific dermal inflammatory infiltrate of eosinophils and lymphocytes. Some consider that PEMKB is a form of locally invasive verrucous carcinoma [12], others that it is a variant of lichen sclerosus [13]. Metastatic spread has not occurred except where there was a penile horn [14], and in one patient who developed an aggressive soft-tissue sarcoma of the penis [15]. Recurrence is common. Topical 5-fluorouracil, radiotherapy and surgery are the principal treatment choices [3].

Erythroplasia of Queyrat, Bowen's disease of the penis and bowenoid papulosis

Erythroplasia of Queyrat (EQ), Bowen's disease of the penis (BDP) and bowenoid papulosis (BP) are three clinical variants of carcinoma *in situ* of the penis [16–18]. Penile intraepithelial neoplasia (PIN—corresponding to cervical, vulval and anal intraepithelial neoplasia; CIN, VIN and AIN) is the term favoured by some, and may be a convenient umbrella term, but there is no formal consensus on clinicopathological classification (particularly

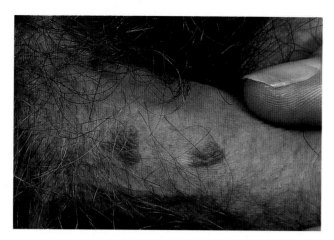

Fig. 68.16 Bowenoid papulosis. (Courtesy of Dr D.A. Burns, Leicester, UK.)

'grade') and clinical utility. An alternative expression 'squamous intraepithelial lesion' (SIL) has been proposed, and qualified by the descriptor 'high-' or 'low-grade' [19]. EQ, BDP and BP all describe disorders of the penis predominantly in uncircumcised white men, although EQ has been recorded in a circumcised man [20]. CIN, VIN and AIN are terms analogous to PIN.

Although EQ and BDP are synonymous in describing carcinoma *in situ* of the penis, BD is used to refer to squamous carcinoma *in situ* at other cutaneous sites. EQ should be used to describe red shiny patches or plaques of the mucosal penis (glans and prepuce of the uncircumcised). BDP should be used to describe red, sometimes slightly pigmented, scaly patches and plaques of the keratinized penis. This distinction has not always been made in the literature. BP is analogous to, but clinically different from, EQ and BDP. The term should be used to describe multiple warty lesions, which are often pigmented in keratinized sites, and more numerous and more inflamed at mucosal sites (Fig. 68.16). BP lesions are less papillomatous, smoother topped, more polymorphic and more coalescent than common genital viral condylomata acuminata, and occur in younger, sexually active men, as opposed to the patches or scaly plaques of EQ and BDP, respectively, seen in older men. BP may be associated with a lesser risk of squamous carcinoma than EQ and BDP. It is associated with HPV infection (especially HPV 16) and HIV infection. Voltz *et al.* [21] found anogenital warts in 16% of all HIV-positive males, nearly half of whom showed histological signs of intraepithelial neoplasia.

The aetiology of EQ, BDP and BP is unknown. Local carcinogenic influences in uncircumcised men such as poor hygiene, smegma, trauma, friction, heat, maceration, inflammation, phimosis, dermatoses such as lichen sclerosus and smoking (tar metabolites in urine) have been proposed [22], as have HPV, particularly in BP [23]. BP is probably virus-induced epithelial dysplasia associated mainly with HPV 16, but other types have been found [24,25]. Recently, EQ has been shown to be associated with co-infection with the rare epidermodysplasia verruciformis-associated HPV 8 and the genital high-risk HPV 16 [26]. There is a high prevalence of PIN in male sexual partners of women with CIN [27,28], but many patients with PIN have consorts with no evidence of warts or CIN. Immunosuppression is important: 50% of HIV patients with anogenital warts had squamous carcinoma *in situ* on histology [21]. Nothing is known about the influence of immunogenotype. The evidence confirming that EQ/BDP may result in squamous carcinoma has been reviewed comprehensively [22,29]. The risk of progression of BP to invasive squamous carcinoma is not known, but is probably low in the absence of other risk factors, especially immunocompromise. The grade of the intraepithelial neoplasia and the development of invasive carcinoma are related to age [30]. *p53* mutations do not appear to be important in male genital carcinogenesis [31].

Some patients with these lesions may be quite young [32]. There may be several foci of BDP or EQ and they may occur concomitantly. The non-specificity of the clinical appearances makes for an important differential diagnosis, which includes psoriasis, lichen sclerosus, erosive lichen planus, ZB and extramammary Paget's disease. The differential diagnosis of BP includes lichen planus, common warts, seborrhoeic warts, naevi and condylomata lata. A biopsy is indicated in instances where the clinical diagnosis is uncertain. Aynaud *et al.* [33] have suggested that shrewd clinical interpretation predicts which lesions will show squamous carcinoma histologically and which will contain oncogenic HPV. Occasionally, it may be necessary to perform a second biopsy if the initial histology is inconclusive. It has been suggested that, where glans and shaft are both involved, the glans may be the preferential biopsy site. On histological examination, there are the features of an intraepithelial carcinoma.

Treatment. Treatment depends on many factors. Circumcision removes a major risk factor for cancer and provides extensive tissue for histology. Topical 5-fluorouracil as a 5% cream is a well-established conventional option for the treatment of BD, EQ and BP [17] but there have been no clinical trials.

Other treatments include cryosurgery, curettage and electrocautery, excisional surgery, radiotherapy (controversial), Mohs' micrographic surgery, laser and photodynamic therapy. Topical imiquimod is under evaluation [34,35]. Patients presenting with these conditions should be counselled and screened for HPV and other sexually transmitted diseases, including HIV infection. This advice should be extended to sexual partners. Follow-up should be long term [17,30].

REFERENCES

1 Cubilla AL, Meijer CJLM, Young RH. Morphological features of epithelial abnormalities and precancerous lesions of the penis. *Scand J Urol Nephrol* 2000; **205** (Suppl.): 215–9.

2 Garcia Panos JM, Buendia Gonzalez E, Jimenez Leiro F *et al.* Penile cutaneous horn: report of a case and review of the literature. *Arch Esp Urol* 1999; **52**: 173–4.

3 Bart RS, Kopf AW. Tumor conference No. 14: on a dilemma of penile horns—pseudoepitheliomatous, hyperkeratotic and micaceous balanitis. *J Dermatol Surg Oncol* 1977; **3**: 580.

4 Willsher MK, Daley KJ, Conway JF *et al.* Penile horns. *J Urol* 1984; **132**: 1192–3.

5 Yeager JK, Findlay RF, McAleer IM. Penile verrucous carcinoma. *Arch Dermatol* 1990; **126**: 1208–10.

6 Karthikeyan, Thappa DM, Jaisankar TJ *et al.* Cutaneous horn of glans penis. *Sex Transm Infect* 1998; **74**: 456–7.

7 Ponce De Leon J, Algaba F, Salvador J. Cutaneous horn of the glans penis. *Br J Urol* 1994; **74**: 257–8.

8 Watanabe T, Murakami T, Okochi H, Kikuchi K, Furue M. Ulcerative porokeratosis. *Dermatology* 1998; **196**: 256–9.

9 Levell NJ, Bewley AP, Levene GM. Porokeratosis of Mibelli on the penis, scrotum and natal cleft. *Clin Exp Dermatol* 1994; **19**: 77–8.

10 Porter WM, Du P Menagé H, Philip G, Bunker CB. Porokeratosis of the penis. *Br J Dermatol* 2001; **144**: 643–4.

11 Ganem JP, Steele BW, Creager AJ, Carson CC. Pseudo-epitheliomatous keratotic and micaceous balanitis. *J Urol* 1999; **161**: 217–8.

12 Beljaards RC, van Dijk E, Hausman R. Is pseudoepitheliomatous, micaceous and keratotic balanitis synonymous with verrucous carcinoma? *Br J Dermatol* 1987; **117**: 641–6.

13 Ridley CM. Lichen sclerosus et atrophicus. *BMJ* 1987; **295**: 1295–6.

14 Goldstein, HH. Cutaneous horn of penis. *J Urol* 1933; **30**: 367–74.

15 Irvine C, Anderson JR, Pye RJ. Micaceous and keratotic pseudoepitheliomatous balanitis and rapidly fatal fibrosarcoma occuring in the same patient. *Br J Urol* 1987; **116**: 719–25.

16 Porter W, Bunker CB. Treatment of pearly penile papules with cryotherapy. *Br J Dermatol* 2000; **142**: 847–8.

17 Bunker CB. Topics in penile dermatology. *Clin Exp Dermatol* 2001; **26**: 469–79.

18 Bunker CB. *Male Genital Skin Disease*. London: Saunders, 2004 (in press).

19 Cubilla AL, Velazques EF, Reuter VE *et al.* Warty (condylomatous) squamous cell carcinoma of the penis: a report of 11 cases and proposed classification of 'verruciform' penile tumors. *Am J Surg Pathol* 2000; **24**: 505–12.

20 Milstein HG. Erythroplasia of Queyrat in a partially circumcised man. *J Am Acad Dermatol* 1982; **10**: 398.

21 Voltz JM, Drobacheff C, Derancourt C *et al.* Papillomavirus-induced anogenital lesions in 121 HIV seropositive men: clinical, histological, viral study, and evolution. *Ann Dermatol Vénéréol* 1999; **126**: 424–9.

22 Graham JH, Helwig EB. Erythroplasia of Queyrat: a clinicopathologic and histochemical study. *Cancer* 1973; **32**: 1396–414.

23 Griffiths TRL, Mellon JK. Human papillomavirus and urological tumours: basic science and role in penile cancer. *BJU Int* 1999; **84**: 579–86.

24 Guerin-Reverchon I, Chardonnet Y, Viac J *et al.* Human papillomavirus infection and filaggrin expression in paraffin-embedded biopsy specimens of extragenital Bowen's disease and genital bowenoid papulosis. *J Cancer Res Clin Oncol* 1990; **116**: 295–300.

25 Yoneta A, Yamashita T, Jin HY *et al.* Development of squamous cell carcinoma by two high-risk human papillomaviruses (HPVs), a novel HPV-67 and HPV-31 from bowenoid papulosis. *Br J Dermatol* 2000; **143**: 604–8.

26 Wieland U, Jurk S, Weissenborn S *et al.* Erythroplasia of Queyrat: co-infection with cutaneous carcinogenic human papillomavirus type 8 and genital papillomaviruses in a carcinoma *in situ*. *J Invest Dermatol* 2000; **115**: 396–401.

27 Barrasso R, De Brux J, Croissant O, Orth G. High prevalence of papillomavirus associated penile intraepithelial neoplasia in partners of women with cervical intraepithelial neoplasia. *N Engl J Med* 1987; **317**: 916–23.

28 Kennedy L, Buntine DW, O'Connor D, Frazer IH. Human papillomavirus: a study of male sexual partners. *Med J Aust* 1988; **149**: 309–11.

29 Blau S, Hyman AB. Erythroplasia of Queyrat. *Acta Derm Venereol* 1955; **35**: 341–78.

30 Aynaud O, Asselain B, Bergeron C *et al.* Carcinomes intraépithéliaux et carcinomes invasifs de la vulve, du vagin et du pénis en Ile-de-France: enquête PETRI portant sur 423 cas. *Ann Dermatol Vénéréol* 2000; **127**: 479–83.

31 Castren K, Vähäkangas K, Heikkinen E, Ranki A. Absence of *p53* mutations in benign and pre-malignant male genital lesions with over-expressed p53 protein. *Int J Cancer* 1998; **77**: 674–8.

32 McAninch JW, Moore CA. Precancerous penile lesions in young men. *J Urol* 1970; **104**: 287–90.

33 Aynaud O, Ionesco M, Barrasso R. Penile intraepithelial neoplasia: specific clinical features correlate with histologic and virologic findings. *Cancer* 1994; **74**: 1762–7.

34 Wigbels B, Luger T, Metze D. Imiquimod: a new treatment possibility in bowenoid papulosis? *Hautarzt* 2001; **52**: 128–31.

35 Pehoushek J Smith KJ. Imiquimod and 5% fluorouracil therapy for anal and perianal squamous cell carcinoma *in situ* in an HIV-1 positive man. *Arch Dermatol* 2001; **137**: 14–6.

Squamous carcinoma

Genital squamous carcinoma is sometimes called epidermoid carcinoma. The aetiology is not clearly understood but HPV is implicated [1,2]. Diagnosis and management can present difficulties. Squamous carcinoma should be suspected in all nodulo-ulcerative genital disease, especially in the context of lichen sclerosus, lichen planus, hidradenitis suppurativa, intraepithelial neoplasia and immunocompromise. Genitourinary and urological assessment should be sought. Proctoscopy and sigmoidoscopy are necessary to exclude anorectal cancer. Suspect lesions should be biopsied.

Carcinoma of the penis

Incidence and aetiology. Carcinoma of the penis accounts for less than 1% of deaths from cancer in the USA (100 per year in the UK, and unchanged over several decades) but constitutes 10–20% of tumours seen in males in either underdeveloped countries or in areas where early circumcision is not routinely practised [3–6].

The earliest stages of penis cancer and precancer form a spectrum of disease [7]. Although some penile cancers arise *de novo*, others develop from premalignant states, which may be misdiagnosed or may be difficult to diagnose [8], and there are the issues of multifocality and field change [9] to acknowledge.

The precise aetiology of the types of PIN, verrucous carcinoma and frank invasive squamous carcinoma of the penis is unknown, as is their precise relationship to the various types of precursor lesion. However, Cubilla *et al.* [10] have defined several types of preceding epithelial abnormality: squamous hyperplasia and SIL (squamous, basaloid or warty, high or low grade).

The presence of a foreskin confers cancer risk (Table 68.24). Circumcision appears to protect against penile carcinoma [11–13], unless the circumcision was performed for penile disease [14,15]. However, there have been very rare cases in Jews and others circumcised at birth [16–18].

Carcinoma of the penis is more common in males in either underdeveloped countries or in areas where early circumcision is not routinely practised [4,19], but the incidence of penis cancer is low in Japan and Denmark,

Table 68.24 Risk factors for squamous carcinoma of the penis.

Uncircumcised
Phimosis
Poor hygiene
Chronic irritation, inflammation, scarring
Smoking
Lichen sclerosus
Lichen planus
Human papillomavirus
HIV
Squamous hyperplasia
Bowen's disease
Erythroplasia of Queyrat
Bowenoid papulosis
Giant condyloma/verrucous carcinoma
Photochemotherapy
Iatrogenic immunosuppression
   Renal transplantation
   Systemic lupus erythematosus

where circumcision is rare [20,21], so other factors are important in carcinogenesis.

Phimosis and balanitis are known risk factors for penile cancer [3,11,22–24]. Poor personal and sexual hygiene [12] and phimosis may lead to the retention of smegma and development of balanitis. However, the carcinogenicity of human smegma has not been ascertained [25] and it is not widely appreciated that phimosis is a physical sign and not a diagnosis. Hence, there may be more in the carcinogenic propensity of phimosis than simply physical retention of smegma.

Lichen sclerosus is a common cause of phimosis in males and it predisposes to penile carcinoma [26–30]. Powell *et al.* [31] found that half of patients with penis cancer had a clinical history and/or histological evidence of lichen sclerosus. Chronic erosive and hypertrophic lichen planus are premalignant conditions, and lichen planus is a cause of phimosis [32,33]. An underlying skin disorder was found in 22 out of 23 patients with vulval squamous carcinoma [34].

Chronic irritation and inflammation or scarring are all risk factors for squamous carcinoma of the skin generally and the penis is no exception; penis cancer complicating a burn scar has been reported [35]. Quantifying the malignant potential of the precancerous dermatoses, BDP, EQ and PIN, is not possible, but they are acknowledged risks for penile cancer [36–38].

Smoking is a risk factor, independent of phimosis, for penile carcinoma [23], and is also a recognized risk factor for anal [39] and cervical cancer [3]. Smoking may cause squamoepithelial cancer, not only in parts of the body in contact with smoke but also at distant sites by dissemination of carcinogens in the circulation or in secretions [40,41]. The presence of tobacco-specific nitrosamines in the preputial secretions of rats has been demonstrated [42].

Penile carcinoma is a complication of psoralens and UVA therapy (PUVA) [43,44], and posssibly other treatments for psoriasis [45,46]. The photodye treatment of genital herpes simplex ceased in the 1970s because of the occurrence of BDP in young men who did not have other risk factors for erythroplasia [47]. However, increased UV exposure of the genitals from sunlamps and sunbeds had not led to an increase in genital skin cancer in the USA by 1986 [48].

Although penile cancer is associated with multiple sexual partners and previous sexually transmitted disease, including HIV, the epidemiological features are not those characteristic of a sexually transmitted disease [25]— unlike carcinoma of the cervix and, to a lesser extent, anal carcinoma [49]. In cervical cancer, the evidence is that it is a sexually transmitted disease and that HPV is the aetiological agent [50–52]. Yet penile cancer puts wives and consorts at risk of cervical cancer [53], there is a high prevalence of PIN in sexual partners of women with CIN [54,55] and PIN can be found in men being screened for HPV infection [56].

HPV is implicated [1,2], but its role is still uncertain, as many patients with penis cancer have no evidence of infection. Oncogenic HPV types 16 and 18 have been incriminated [24,57–65]. In Brazil, Villa and Lopes [59] found HPV 18 in seven out of 18 penile squamous carcinomas and, in Argentina, Picconi *et al.* [65] found HPV DNA in 71% of 65 penis cancers, 81% of which were 'high-risk' HPV with predominance of HPV 18. Gregoire *et al.* [66] associated HPV with higher grade, more aggressive squamous carcinomas of predominantly the glans penis showing basaloid changes. The overall frequency of HPV in penile squamous carcinoma suggests [10,66] that a proportion of these cancers can arise from HPV-associated SIL. As in vulval cancer [67,68], a bimodal hypothesis of HPV-related and non-HPV-related causation has evolved [10,69].

Penis cancer has been reported to complicate immunosuppression in renal transplantation [70] and HIV infection [71].

Clinical features. Itch, irritation, pain, bleeding, discharge, ulceration or the discovery of a mass are the presenting symptoms of squamous carcinoma. There is often a long history of preceding problems with the penis and foreskin manifest as dyspareunia, balanoposthitis or phimosis and dysuria. Irregular nodular and ulcerative morphology is found on examination (Figs 68.17 & 68.18) and there may be background BDP, EQ and BP, lichen sclerosus or lichen planus. Phimosis should be regarded as a sinister situation, not least because it does not allow complete inspection and palpation of the glans and coronal sulcus. The inguinal lymph glands must be palpated, although in penile cancer only 50% of enlarged glands will be found to contain tumour [4]. The concomitant presence of sexually

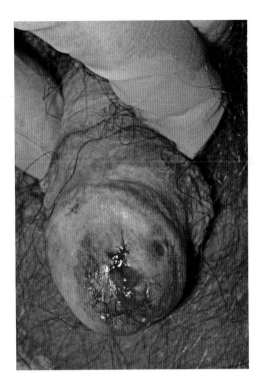

Fig. 68.17 High-grade dysplasia and invasive squamous carcinoma. (Courtesy of Dr C.B. Bunker, with permission from Medical Illustration UK, Chelsea & Westminster Hospital, London, UK.)

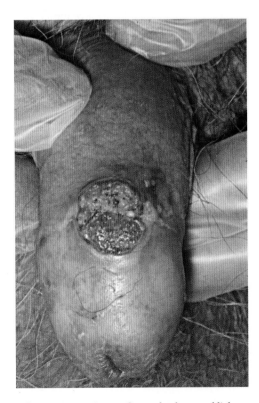

Fig. 68.18 Squamous carcinoma. Severe background lichen sclerosus. (Reproduced from Bunker CB. Skin conditions of the male genitalia. *Medicine* 2001; **29**: 9–13, by kind permission of The Medicine Publishing Company.)

transmitted diseases and immunocompromise should be excluded [72]. The differential diagnosis includes the manifestations of intraepithelial neoplasia (and the differential diagnosis of these), erosive or ulcerative sexually transmitted disease, basal cell carcinoma, Kaposi's sarcoma, pyoderma gangrenosum and artefact. Genitourinary and urological assessment should be sought.

Histopathology. Diagnosis is confirmed histologically. A biopsy should be of adequate size and depth, and it may be necessary to sample several sites. The biopsy(ies) may need to be performed by a urologist under general anaesthesia. Patients who have negative or equivocal biopsies, but who have risk factors or in whom there is a high index of suspicion, should be followed-up closely and rebiopsied if indicated.

Histologically, squamous carcinoma manifests tongues of invasive atypical keratinocytes penetrating the dermis, and contains foci of aberrant and ectopic keratinization called squamous pearls [23]. Background histological signs of lichen sclerosus are commonly found in penile cancer in men, as in vulvar cancer [73]. Verrucous carcinoma is discussed below. Spindle cell carcinoma of the penis is a very rare variant [74]. Telomerase activity is high in penis cancer [75].

Cubilla *et al.* [9] have identified four histological types of squamous carcinoma of the penis:

1 *Superficial spreading* (42%): a biphasic infiltrative and radially extensive carcinoma *in situ* contiguously involving several anatomical sites or compartments (glans, coronal sulcus, foreskin, even urethra)

2 *Vertical growth* (32%): unifocal high-grade deeply invasive, unassociated with carcinoma *in situ*

3 *Verrucous* (18%): low-grade, papillary or endophytic (see below)

4 *Multicentric* (8%): two or more independent primary tumours without contiguous field change.

These observations have implications for the pathogenesis of the different types, and in determining management in individual cases.

REFERENCES

1 McDougall JK. Immortalization and transformation of human cells by human papillomavirus. *Curr Top Microbiol Immunol* 1994; **186**: 101–19.
2 Kadish AS. Biology of anogenital neoplasia. *Cancer Treat Res* 2001; **104**: 267–86.
3 Muir CS, Nectoux J. Epidemiology of carcinoma of the testis and penis. *Natl Cancer Inst Monogr* 1979; **53**: 157–64.
4 Droller MJ. Carcinoma of the penis: an overview. *Urol Clin North Am* 1980; **7**: 783–4.
5 Micali G, Innocenzi D, Nasca MR *et al.* Squamous cell carcinoma of the penis. *J Am Acad Dermatol* 1996; **35**: 432–51.
6 Soria J-C, Théodore C, Gerbaulet A. Carcinome épidermoïde de la verge (squamous cell carcinoma of the penis). *Bull Cancer* 1998; **85**: 773–84.
7 Grossman HB. Premalignant and early carcinomas of the penis and scrotum. *Urol Clin North Am* 1992; **19**: 221–6.
8 von Krogh G, Horenblas S. Diagnosis and clinical presentation of premalignant lesions of the penis. *Scand J Urol Nephrol* 2000; **205** (Suppl.): 201–4.

9 Cubilla AL, Barreto J, Caballero C, Ayala G, Riveros M. Pathologic features of epidermoid carcinoma of the penis: a prospective study of 66 cases. *Am J Surg Pathol* 1993; **17**: 753–63.

10 Cubilla AL, Meijer CJLM, Young RH. Morphological features of epithelial abnormalities and precancerous lesions of the penis. *Scand J Urol Nephrol* 2000; **205** (Suppl.): 215–9.

11 Wolbarst AL. Circumcision and penile cancer. *Lancet* 1932; **1**: 150–3.

12 Schrek R, Lenowitz H. Aetiological factors in carcinoma of the penis. *Cancer Res* 1947; **7**: 180–7.

13 Schoen EJ, Oehrli M, Colby CJ, Machin G. The highly protective effect of newborn circumcision against invasive penile cancer. *Pediatrics* 2000; **105**: E36.

14 Maden C, Sherman KJ, Beckmann AM et al. History of circumcision, medical conditions, and sexual activity and the risk of penile cancer. *J Natl Cancer Inst* 1993; **85**: 19–24.

15 Holly EA, Palefsky JM. Factors related to risk of penile cancer: new evidence from a study in the Pacific northwest. *J Natl Cancer Inst* 1993; **85**: 2–3.

16 Melmed EP, Payne JR. Carcinoma of the penis in a Jew circumcised in infancy. *Br J Surg* 1967; **54**: 729–31.

17 Boczko S, Freed S. Penile carcinoma in circumcised males. *NY State J Med* 1979; **79**: 1903–4.

18 Rogus BJ. Squamous cell carcinoma in a young circumcised man. *J Urol* 1987; **138**: 861–2.

19 Schoeneich G, Perabo FG, Muller SC. Squamous cell carcinoma of the penis. *Andrologia* 1999; **31** (Suppl. 1): 17–20.

20 Williams N, Kapila L. Complications of circumcision. *Br J Surg* 1993; **80**: 1231–6.

21 Frisch M, Friis S, Krüger Kjaer S, Melbye M. Falling incidence of penis cancer in an uncircumcised population (Denmark 1943–90). *BMJ* 1995; **311**: 1471.

22 Reddy CRRM, Devendranath V, Pratap S. Carcinoma of the penis: role of phimosis. *Urology* 1984; **24**: 85–8.

23 Lucia MS, Miller GJ. Histopathology of malignant lesions of the penis. *Urol Clin North Am* 1992; **19**: 227–46.

24 Maiche AG. Epidemiological aspects of cancer of the penis in Finland. *Eur J Cancer Prev* 1992; **1**: 153–8.

25 Hellberg D, Valentin J, Eklund T et al. Penile cancer: is there an epidemiological role for smoking and sexual behaviour? *BMJ* 1987; **295**: 1306–8.

26 Bart RS, Kopf AW. Tumor conference No 18: squamous cell carcinoma arising in balanitis xerotica. *J Dermatol Surg Oncol* 1978; **4**: 556–8.

27 Bingham JS. Carcinoma of the penis developing in lichen sclerosus et atrophicus. *Br J Vener Dis* 1978; **54**: 350–1.

28 Schnitzler L, Sayag J, Sayag J, Roux G. Épithélioma spino-cellulaire aigu de la verge et lichen scléro-atrophique. *Ann Dermatol Vénéréol* 1987; **114**: 979–81.

29 Pride HB, Miller OF, Tyler WB. Penile squamous cell carcinoma arising from balanitis xerotica obliterans. *J Am Acad Dermatol* 1993; **29**: 469–73.

30 Bunker CB. Topics in penile dermatology. *Clin Exp Dermatol* 2001; **26**: 469–79.

31 Powell J, Robson A, Cranston D, Wojnarowska, F, Turner R. High incidence of lichen sclerosus in patients with squamous cell carcinoma of the penis. *Br J Dermatol* 2001; **145**: 85–9.

32 Worheide J, Bonsmann G, Kolde G, Hamm H. Plattenepithyelkarzinom auf dem Boden eines lichen ruber hypertrophicus an der glans penis. *Hautarzt* 1991; **42**: 112–5.

33 Itin PH, Hirsbrunner P, Buchner S. Lichen planus: an unusual cause of phimosis. *Acta Dermatol Venereol* 1992; **72**: 41–2.

34 Derrick EK, Ridley CM, Kobza-Black A, McKee PH, Neill SM. A clinical study of 23 cases of female anogenital carcinoma. *Br J Dermatol* 2000; **143**: 1217–23.

35 Selli C, Scott CA, De Antoni P et al. Squamous cell carcinoma arising at the base of the penis in a burn scar. *Urology* 1999; **54**: 923.

36 Blau S, Hyman AB. Erythroplasia of Queyrat. *Acta Dermatol Venereol* 1955; **35**: 341–78.

37 Graham JH, Helwig EB. Erythroplasia of Queyrat: a clinicopathologic and histochemical study. *Cancer* 1973; **32**: 1396–414.

38 Gerber GS. Carcinoma *in situ* of the penis. *J Urol* 1994; **151**: 829–33.

39 Moore TO, Moore AY, Carrasco D et al. Human papillomavirus, smoking and cancer. *J Cutan Med Surg* 2001; **5**: 323–8.

40 Winkelstein W. Smoking and cancer of the uterine cervix: hypothesis. *Am J Epidemiol* 1977; **106**: 257–9.

41 Sasson I, Haley N, Hoffmann D, Wynder E. Cigarette smoking and neoplasia of the uterine cervix: smoke constituents in cervical mucus. *N Engl J Med* 1985; **31**: 315–6.

42 Castonguay A, Tjalve H, Hecht SS. Tissue distribution of the the tobacco specific carcinogen 4-(methylnitrosamino)-1-(3-pyridyl)-1-butanone and its metabolites in F344 rats. *Cancer Res* 1983; **43**: 630–8.

43 Stern RS. Genital tumours among men with psoriasis exposed to psoralens and ultraviolet A radiation (PUVA) and ultraviolet B radiation. *N Engl J Med* 1990; **322**: 1093–7.

44 Perkins W, Lamont, MacKie RM. Cutaneous malignancy in males treated with photochemotherapy. *Lancet* 1990; **336**: 1248.

45 Brassinne de la M, Richert B. Genital squamous-cell carcinoma after PUVA therapy. *Dermatology* 1992; **185**: 316–8.

46 Loughlin KR. Psoriasis: association with two rare cutaneous urological malignancies. *J Urol* 1997; **157**: 622–3.

47 Berger RS, Papa CM. Photodye herpes therapy: Cassandra confirmed? *JAMA* 1977; **238**: 133–4.

48 Goldoft MJ, Weiss NS. Incidence of male genital skin tumours: lack of increase in the United States. *Cancer Causes Control* 1992; **3**: 91–3.

49 Xavier Bosch F, Michele Manos M, Muñoz N et al. International Biological Study on Cervical Cancer (IBSCC) Study Group. Prevalence of human papillomavirus in cervical cancer: a worldwide perspective. *J Natl Cancer Inst* 1995; **87**: 796–802.

50 zur Hausen H. Genital papillomavirus infections. *Prog Med Virol* 1985; **32**: 15–21.

51 Keerti VS. Human papillomaviruses and anogenital cancers. *N Engl J Med* 1997; **337**: 1386–7.

52 Walboomers JMM, Meijer CJLM. Do HPV-negative cervical carcinomas exist? *J Pathol* 1997; **181**: 253–4.

53 Smith PG, Kinlen LJ, White GC et al. Mortality of wives of men dying with cancer of the penis. *Br J Cancer* 1980; **41**: 422–8.

54 Barrasso R, De Brux J, Croissant O, Orth G. High prevalence of papillomavirus associated penile intraepithelial neoplasia in partners of women with cervical intraepithelial neoplasia. *N Engl J Med* 1987; **317**: 916–23.

55 Kennedy L, Buntine DW, O'Connor D, Frazer IH. Human papillomavirus: a study of male sexual partners. *Med J Aust* 1988; **149**: 309–11.

56 Zabbo A, Stein BS. Penile intraepithelial neoplasia in patients examined for exposure to human papilloma virus. *Urology* 1993; **41**: 24–6.

57 Dürst M, Kleinheinz A, Hotz M, Gissmann L. The physical state of human papillomavirus type 16 DNA in benign and malignant genital tumours. *DHJJ Gen Virol* 1985; **6**: 1515–22.

58 Boshart M, Gissmann L, Ikenberg H et al. A new type of papillomavirus DNA, its presence in genital cancer biopsies and in cell lines derived from cervical cancer. *EMBO J* 1984; **3**: 1151–7.

59 Villa LL, Lopes A. Human papillomavirus DNA sequences in penile carcinomas in Brazil. *Int J Cancer* 1986; **37**: 853–5.

60 Löning T, Riviere A, Henke RP, von Preyss S, Dorner A. Penile/anal condylomas and squamous cell cancer: a HPV DNA hybridization study. *Virchows Arch A Pathol Anat Histopathol* 1988; **413**: 491–8.

61 Strickler HD, Schiffman MH, Shah KV et al. A survey of human papillomavirus 16 antibodies in patients with epithelial cancers. *Eur J Cancer Prev* 1998; **7**: 305–13.

62 Cupp MR, Malek RS, Goellner JR, Smith TF, Espy MJ. The detection of human papillomavirus deoxyribonucleic acid in intraepithelial, *in situ*, verrucous and invasive carcinoma of the penis. *J Urol* 1995; **154**: 1024–9.

63 Majewski S, Jablonska S. Human papillomavirus-associated tumors of the skin and mucosa. *J Am Acad Dermatol* 1997; **36**: 659–85.

64 Griffiths TRL, Mellon JK. Human papillomavirus and urological tumours: basic science and role in penile cancer. *BJU Int* 1999; **84**: 579–86.

65 Picconi MA, Eijan AM, Distefano AL et al. Human papillomavirus (HPV) DNA in penile carcinomas in Argentina: analysis of primary tumors and lymph nodes. *J Med Virol* 2000; **61**: 65–9.

66 Gregoire L, Cubilla AL, Reuter VE, Haas GP, Lancaster WD. Preferential association of human papillomavirus with high-grade histologic variants of penile-invasive squamous cell carcinoma. *J Natl Cancer Inst* 1995; **87**: 1705–9.

67 Leibowitch M, Neill S, Pelisse M, Moyal-Baracco M. The epithelial changes associated with squamous cell carcinoma of the vulva: a review of the clinical, histological and viral findings in 78 women. *Br J Obstet Gynaecol* 1990; **97**: 1135–9.

68 Jones RW, Baranyai J, Stables S. Trends in squamous cell carcinoma of the vulva: the influence of vulvar intraepithelial neoplasia. *Obstet Gynecol* 1997; **90**: 448–52.

69 Horenblas S, von Krogh G, Cubilla AL et al. Squamous cell carcinoma of the penis: premalignant lesions. *Scand J Urol Nephrol* 2000; **205** (Suppl.): 187–8.

70 Previte SR, Karian S, Cho SI, Austen G. Penile carcinoma in renal transplant recipient. *Urology* 1979; **13**: 298–9.

71 Poblet E, Alfaro L, Fernander-Segoviano P, Jimenez-Reyes J, Salido EC. Human papillomavirus-associated penile squamous cell carcinoma in HIV-positive patients. *Am J Surg Pathol* 1999; **23**: 1119–23.

72 Heyns CF, van Vollenhoven P, Steenkamp JW, Allen FJ. Cancer of the penis: a review of 50 patients. *S Afr J Surg* 1997; **35**: 120–4.

73 Powell J, Robson A, Cranston D, Wojnarowska, F, Turner R. High incidence of lichen sclerosus in patients with squamous cell carcinoma of the penis. *Br J Dermatol* 2001; **145**: 85–9.

74 Patel B, Hashmat A, Reddy V, Angkustsiri K. Spindle cell carcinoma of the penis. *Urology* 1982; **19**: 93–5.

75 Alves G, Fiedler W, Guenther E *et al.* Determination of telomerase activity in squamous cell carcinoma of the penis. *Int J Oncol* 2001; **18**: 67–70.

Carcinoma of the scrotum

Squamous carcinoma of the scrotum has been recognized in chimney sweeps (exposed to carcinogens in soot) [1], mule spinners (exposed to carcinogens in lubricating oils for the spinning jenny in the cloth industry), Persian nomads (who travelled with pots of burning charcoal between their legs) and Indian jute oil processors [2–6]. Oil-mist exposure in industry continues to be widespread and, apart from scrotal cancer, has been associated with other cutaneous problems (such as contact dermatitis and oil acne) and respiratory diseases, including cancer [7].

Other individuals at risk of scrotal squamous carcinoma include those with a history of psoriasis treated with arsenic, coal tar, UVB and PUVA [8–13], previous radiotherapy treatment [8], scrotal HPV infection, hidradenitis suppurativa and multiple cutaneous keratoses and epitheliomas [14–17]. Rarely, black men may be affected [18].

The presentation of scrotal carcinoma is similar to that of penis cancer, with itch, irritation, pain, bleeding, discharge, ulceration or the discovery of a lump, and irregular nodular and ulcerative clinical features. A pigmented squamous carcinoma of the scrotum has been reported [19]. The differential diagnosis includes the manifestations of intraepithelial neoplasia (and the differential diagnosis of these), erosive or ulcerative sexually transmitted disease, basal cell carcinoma, Kaposi's sarcoma, pyoderma gangrenosum and artefact. The diagnosis is confirmed by biopsy.

Treatment of squamous carcinoma

The treatment of anogenital squamous carcinoma is not generally the province of the dermatologist. The overriding general principle is to offer adequate surgical excision, including circumcision, for disease of the penis. The penile surgery may need to be radical, total or partial, depending on location and extent [20–22]. To minimize residual sexual dysfunction, conservative plastic techniques are increasingly used [23], as are laser treatment [24] and Mohs' micrographic surgery [25–28] for squamous carcinoma of the penis, but the concepts of field change and the implications of infection by HPV and multifocality must be considered. Combination chemotherapy has been used for palliation and proposed for adjuvant treatment of carcinoma of the penis, but remains under evaluation [29].

Lymphatic or haematogenous dissemination of genital cancer dictates individualized multidisciplinary treatment. The management of ilioinguinal lymphadenopathy is controversial [20,22,30].

The prognosis of penis cancer relates to the extent of inguinal lymphadenopathy [31,32] and involvement of the corpus [33]. It does not correlate with HPV status [34]. The prognosis for scrotal carcinoma is not good, despite apparently adequate primary surgical treatment: the 5-year mortality is 50–60% [3,4].

Penile cancer puts wives and consorts at risk of cervical cancer [35]. In black men who develop penile cancer there is a substantial risk (18%) of the later development of a second primary malignancy [36].

REFERENCES

1 Potts P. Cancer scroti. *Chirurgical Works* 1779; **3**: 225–9.

2 Graves RC, Flo S. Carcinoma of the scrotum. *J Urol* 1940; **43**: 309–32.

3 Lowe FC. Squamous cell carcinoma of the scrotum. *J Urol* 1983; **130**: 423–7.

4 Gerber WL. Scrotal malignancies: the University of Iowa experience and a review of the literature. *Urology* 1985; **26**: 337–42.

5 Grossman HB. Premalignant and early carcinomas of the penis and scrotum. *Urol Clin North Am* 1992; **19**: 221–6.

6 Murthy KVN. Primary cutaneous carcinoma of the scrotum. *J Occup Med* 1993; **35**: 888–9.

7 Karube H, Aizawa Y, Nakamura K *et al.* Oil mist exposure in industrial health: a review. *Sangyo Eiseigaku Zasshi* 1995; **37**: 113–22.

8 Ray B, Whitmore WF Jr. Experience with carcinoma of the scrotum. *J Urol* 1977; **117**: 741–5.

9 McGarry GW, Robertson JR. Scrotal carcinoma following prolonged use of crude coal tar ointment. *Br J Urol* 1989; **63**: 211–9.

10 Stern RS. Genital tumours among men with psoriasis exposed to psoralens and ultraviolet A radiation (PUVA) and ultraviolet B radiation. *N Engl J Med* 1990; **322**: 1093–7.

11 Perkins W, Lamont D, MacKie RM. Cutaneous malignancy in males treated with photochemotherapy. *Lancet* 1990; **336**: 1248.

12 Gross DJ, Schosser RH. Squamous cell carcinoma of the scrotum. *Cutis* 1991; **47**: 402–4.

13 Loughlin KR. Psoriasis: association with two rare cutaneous urological malignancies. *J Urol* 1997; **157**: 622–3.

14 Dean AL. Epithelioma of the scrotum. *J Urol* 1948; **60**: 508–18.

15 Black SB, Woods JE. Squamous cell carcinoma complicating hidradenitis suppurativa. *J Surg Oncol* 1982; **19**: 25–6.

16 Andrews PE, Farrow GM, Oesterling JE. Squamous cell carcinoma of the scrotum: long-term follow-up of 14 patients. *J Urol* 1991; **146**: 1299–304.

17 Burmer GC, True LD, Krieger JN. Squamous cell carcinoma of the scrotum associated with human papillomaviruses. *J Urol* 1993; **149**: 374–7.

18 Lowe FC. Squamous cell carcinoma of scrotum. *Urology* 1985; **25**: 63–5.

19 Matsumoto M, Sonobe H, Takeuchi T *et al.* Pigmented squamous cell carcinoma of the scrotum associated with a lentigo. *Br J Dermatol* 1999; **141**: 132–6.

20 Heyns CF, van Vollenhoven P, Steenkamp JW, Allen FJ. Cancer of the penis: a review of 50 patients. *S Afr J Surg* 1997; **35**: 120–4.

21 Prošvic P, Morávek P, Stefan H, Veselský Z. Uncommon finding of penile carcinoma: case record. *Rozhl Chir* 1997; **76**: 454–7.

22 Schoeneich G, Perabo FG, Muller SC. Squamous cell carcinoma of the penis. *Andrologia* 1999; **31** (Suppl. 1): 17–20.

23 Donnellan SM, Webb DR. Management of invasive penile cancer by synchronous penile lengthening and radical tumour excision to avoid perineal urethrostomy. *Aust NZ J Surg* 1998; **68**: 369–70.

24 Tietjen DN, Malek RS. Laser therapy of squamous cell dysplasia and carcinoma of the penis. *Urology* 1998; **52**: 559–65.

25 Mohs FE, Snow SN, Messing EM, Kuglitsch ME. Microscopically controlled surgery in the treatment of carcinoma of the penis. *J Urol* 1985; **133**: 961–6.

26 Bernstein G, Forgaard DM, Miller JE. Carcinoma of the glans penis and distal urethra. *J Dermatol Surg Oncol* 1986; **12**: 450.

27 Brown MD, Zachary CB, Grekin RC *et al.* Penile tumours: their management by Mohs micrographic surgery. *J Dermatol Surg Oncol* 1987; **13**: 1163–7.

28 Brown MD, Zachary CB, Grekin RC, Swanson NA. Genital tumours: their management by micrographic surgery. *J Am Acad Dermatol* 1988; **18**: 115–22.

29 Roth AD, Berney CR, Rohner S *et al.* Intra-arterial chemotherapy in locally advanced or recurrent carcinomas of the penis and anal canal: an active treatment modality with curative potential. *Br J Cancer* 2000; **83**: 1637–42.

30 McDougal WS, Kirchner FR, Edwards RH, Killion LZ. Treatment of carcinoma of the penis: case for primary lymphadenectomy. *J Urol* 1986; **136**: 38–41.

31 Droller MJ. Carcinoma of the penis: an overview. *Urol Clin North Am* 1980; **7**: 783–4.

32 Srinivas V, Morse MJ, Herr HW, Sogani PC, Whitmore WF. Penile cancer: relation of extent of nodal metastasis and survival. *J Urol* 1987; **137**: 880.

33 Soria J-C, Fizazi K, Piron D *et al.* Squamous cell carcinoma of the penis: multivariate analysis of prognostic factors and natural history in a monocentric study with a conservative policy. *Ann Oncol* 1997; **8**: 1089–98.

34 Bezerra ALR, Lopes A, Santiago GH *et al.* Human papillomavirus as a prognostic factor in carcinoma of the penis: analysis of 82 patients treated with amputation and bilateral lymphadenectomy. *Cancer* 2001; **91**: 2315–21.

35 Smith PG, Kinlen LJ, White GC *et al.* Mortality of wives of men dying with cancer of the penis. *Br J Cancer* 1980; **41**: 422–8.

36 Hubbell CR, Rabin VR, Mora RG. Cancer of the skin in blacks. V. A review of 175 black patients with squamous cell carcinoma of the penis. *J Am Acad Dermatol* 1988; **18**: 292–8.

Verrucous carcinoma/giant condyloma/Buschke–Löwenstein tumour

Buschke–Löwenstein tumour and verrucous carcinoma can probably be regarded as synonymous. They represent verrucous low-grade well-differentiated squamous carcinoma. It is perhaps more accurate and more clinically useful to consider giant condyloma as a separate HPV-related entity with a better prognosis, but controversy exists [1–7].

Verrucous carcinoma is rare. It produces dramatic polypoid or cauliflower-like clinical lesions (Fig. 68.19). Presentation as a penile cutaneous horn has been described

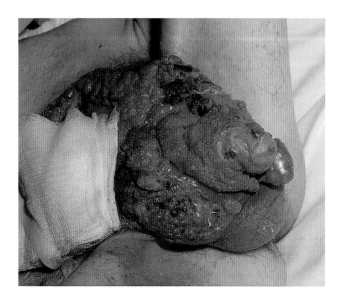

Fig. 68.19 Gross condylomas of Buschke–Löwenstein of the penis. (Courtesy of Professor R.M. MacKie, Glasgow University, Glasgow, UK.)

[8,9]. Although locally deeply invasive, the tumour is well demarcated from surrounding tissue and is unlikely to metastasize. Both sexes can be affected.

A specific aetiology for verrucous carcinoma of Buschke–Löwenstein has not been unequivocally identified, but an origin from genital warts is likely. HPV types 6 and 11 are the most commonly associated [1,3,4,10–16]. A patient taking ciclosporin for psoriasis developed a verrucous carcinoma containing HPV 6 and 16 [17]. Multiple HPV types were found in a transplant patient [18]. Tumours containing several HPV types may be mixed, containing verrucous carcinoma adjacent to squamous carcinoma [19]. Cases emanating from background lichen sclerosus have occurred [20,21]. Chronic hidradenitis suppurativa may rarely be a predisposing factor [22].

If verrucous carcinoma is suspected, then a deep surgical biopsy must be planned. The tumour has a different histology from squamous carcinoma, showing deep lobular invaginations of well-defined proliferative epithelium consisting of typical clear pale keratinocytes [23]. Frank squamous carcinoma [24] and foci of invasive squamous carcinoma [25] have been reported in some cases of anogenital verrucous carcinoma. Ultrastructurally, verrucous carcinoma is distinct from condyloma acuminatum but similar to SCC [26].

Clinical, histological and virological differences may distinguish verrucous carcinoma (potential for aggressive lethal behaviour) from Buschke–Löwenstein tumour and giant condyloma (no malignant potential) and this distinction should direct treatment [3,4,11,13,16].

Surgical excision is the treatment usually recommended (e.g. glansectomy [27] or penectomy). Mohs' micrographic surgery [28–30], cryotherapy [31], laser treatment [32], interferon-α [33–36], radiotherapy [37] or bleomycin [38] are alternatives.

The prognosis is poor because the tumour can continue to grow and invade locally, causing death by exsanguination from femoral arterial invasion or cachexia [39]. Even with treatment, recurrence and progressive malignant transformation do occur [40,41], so follow-up is necessary.

REFERENCES

1 Schwartz RA, Janniger CK. Bowenoid papulosis. *J Am Acad Dermatol* 1991; **24**: 261–3.

2 Schwartz RA. Buschke–Loewenstein tumor: verrucous carcinoma of the penis. *J Am Acad Dermatol* 1993; **23**: 723–7.

3 Niederauer HH, Weindorf N, Schultz-Ehrenburg U. Ein fall von condyloma acuminatum giganteum. *Hautarzt* 1993; **44**: 795–9.

4 Anadolu R, Boyvat A, Calikoglu E, Gurler A. Buschke–Loewenstein tumour is not a low-grade carcinoma but a giant verruca. *Acta Dermatol Venereol* 1999; **79**: 253–4.

5 Dogan G, Oram Y, Hazneci E *et al.* Three cases of verrucous carcinoma. *J Dermatol* 1998; **39**: 251–4.

6 Codina I, Muniz C, Beyrie W, Goza F, Iturralde Y. Giant condyloma of the penis. *Arch Esp Urol* 1999; **52**: 1090–2.

7 Cubilla AL, Velazques EF, Reuter VE *et al.* Warty (condylomatous) squamous cell carcinoma of the penis: a report of 11 cases and proposed classification of 'verruciform' penile tumors. *Am J Surg Pathol* 2000; **24**: 505–12.

8 Yeager JK, Findlay RF, McAleer IM. Penile verrucous carcinoma. *Arch Dermatol* 1990; **126**: 1208–10.

9 Karthikeyan K, Thappa DM, Jaisankar TJ *et al.* Cutaneous horn of glans penis. *Sex Transm Infect* 1998; **74**: 456–7.

10 Boshart M, zur Hausen H. Human papillomaviruses in Buschke–Löwenstein tumours: physical state of the DNA and identification of a tandem duplication in the non-coding region of a human papillomavirus 6 subtype. *J Virol* 1986; **58**: 963–6.

11 Noel JC, Vandenbossche M, Peny MO *et al.* Verrucous carcinoma of the penis: importance of human papillomavirus typing for diagnosis and therapeutic decision. *Eur Urol* 1992; **22**: 83–5.

12 Grassegger A, Hopfl R, Hussl H, Wicke K, Fritsch P. Buschke–Loewenstein tumour infiltrating pelvic organs. *Br J Dermatol* 1994; **130**: 221–5.

13 Gonzalez-Lopez A, Esquivias JI, Miranda-Romero A *et al.* Buschke–Löwenstein tumor and immunity. *Cutis* 1997; **59**: 119–22.

14 Dianzani C, Bucci M, Pierangeli A, Calvieri S, Degener AM. Association of human papilloma virus type 11 with carcinoma of the penis. *Urology* 1998; **51**: 1046–8.

15 Yagi H, Igawa M, Shiina H *et al.* A study of growth pattern in giant condyloma acuminatum. *Urol Int* 1998; **61**: 188–91.

16 Haycox CL, Kuypers J, Krieger JN. Role of human papillomavirus typing in diagnosis and clinical decision making for a giant verrucous genital lesion. *Urology* 1999; **53**: 627–30.

17 Piepkorn M, Kumasaka B, Krieger JN, Burmer GC. Development of human papillomavirus-associated Buschke–Löwenstein penile carcinoma during cyclosporine therapy for generalized pustular psoriasis. *J Am Acad Dermatol* 1993; **29**: 321–5.

18 Soler C, Chardonnet Y, Allibert P *et al.* Detection of multiple types of human papillomavirus in a giant condyloma from a grafted patient: analysis by immunohistochemistry, *in situ* hybridization, Southern blot and polymerase reaction. *Virus Res* 1992; **23**: 193–208.

19 Noel JC, de Dobbeleer G. Development of human papillomavirus-associated Buschke–Löwenstein penile carcinoma during cyclosporine therapy for generalized pustular psoriasis. *J Am Acad Dermatol* 1994; **31**: 299–300.

20 Weber P, Rabinovitz H, Garland L. Verrucous carcinoma in penile lichen sclerosus et atrophicus. *J Dermatol Surg Oncol* 1987; **13**: 529.

21 Micali G, Nasca MR, Innocenzi D. Lichen sclerosus of the glans is significantly associated with penile carcinoma. *Sex Transm Infect* 2001; **77**: 226.

22 Cosman BC, O'Grady TC, Pekarske S. Verrucous carcinoma arising in hidradenitis suppurativa. *Int J Colorectal Dis* 2000; **15**: 342–6.

23 Lucia MS, Miller GJ. Histopathology of malignant lesions of the penis. *Urol Clin North Am* 1992; **19**: 227–46.

24 Sturm JT, Christenson CE, Vecker JH *et al.* Squamous cell carcinoma of the anus arising in a giant condyloma acuminatum. *Dis Colon Rectum* 1975; **18**: 147–51.

25 Johnson DE, Lo RK, Srigley J, Ayala AG. Verrucous carcinoma of the penis. *J Urol* 1985; **133**: 216–8.

26 Hull MT, Eble JN, Priest JB, Mulcahy JJ. Ultrastructure of Buschke–Loewenstein tumor. *J Urol* 1981; **126**: 485–9.

27 Hatzichristou DG, Apostolidis A, Tzortzis V *et al.* Glansectomy: an alternative surgical treatment for Buschke–Löwenstein tumors of the penis. *Urology* 2001; **57**: 966–9.

28 Mohs FE, Sahl WJ. Chemosurgery for verrucous carcinoma. *J Dermatol Surg Oncol* 1979; **5**: 302.

29 Brown MD, Zachary CB, Grekin RC *et al.* Penile tumours: their management by Mohs micrographic surgery. *J Dermatol Surg Oncol* 1987; **13**: 1163–7.

30 Brown MD, Zachary CB, Grekin RC, Swanson NA. Genital tumours: their management by micrographic surgery. *J Am Acad Dermatol* 1988; **18**: 115–22.

31 Hughes PSH. Cryosurgery of verrucous carcinoma of the penis (Buschke–Löwenstein tumor). *Cutis* 1979; **24**: 43–5.

32 Lenk S, Oesterwitz H, Audring H. Laser surgery in superficial penile tumours. *Int Urol Nephrol* 1991; **23**: 357–63.

33 Zachariae H, Larsen PM, Sogaard H. Recombinant interferon-α2A (Roferon-A) in a case of Buschke–Löwenstein giant condyloma. *Dermatologica* 1988; **177**: 175–9.

34 Risse L, Négrier P, Dang PM *et al.* Treatment of verrucous carcinoma with recombinant alfa-interferon. *Dermatology* 1995; **190**: 142–4.

35 Geusau A, Heinz-Peer G, Volc-Platzer B, Stingl G, Kirnbauer R. Regression of deeply infiltrating giant condyloma (Buschke–Löwenstein tumor) following long-term intralesional interferon alfa therapy. *Arch Dermatol* 2000; **136**: 707–10.

36 Gomez De La Fuente E, Castano Suarez E, Vanaclocha Sebastian F, Rodriguez-Peralto JL, Iglesias Diez L. Verrucous carcinoma of the penis

completely cured with shaving and intralesional interferon. *Dermatology* 2000; **200**: 152.

37 Sobrado CW, Mester M, Nadalin W *et al.* Radiation-induced total regression of a highly recurrent giant perianal condyloma: report of case. *Dis Colon Rectum* 2000; **43**: 257–60.

38 Puissant A, Pringuet R, Noory JY *et al.* Condylome acumine geant (syndrome de Buschke–Löwenstein): action de la bleomycine. *Bull Soc Francaise Dermatol Syphiligr* 1972; **79**: 9–12.

39 South LM, O'Sullivan JP, Gazet JC. Giant condylomata of Buschke and Löwenstein. *Clin Oncol* 1977; **3**: 107–15.

40 Tessler AN, Applebaum SM. The Buschke–Löwenstein tumor. *Urology* 1982; **20**: 36–9.

41 Creasman C, Haas PA, Fox TA Jr, Balazs M. Malignant transformation of anorectal giant condyloma acuminatum (Buschke–Loewenstein tumour). *Dis Colon Rectum* 1989; **32**: 481–7.

Other malignant neoplasms

Extramammary Paget's disease

Extramammary Paget's disease (EMPD) presents as irritating, itchy, burning, red scaly patches or plaques that may be solitary or multifocal. EMPD can occur anywhere in the anogenital area, including the glans penis, and may be multicentric [1–3]. An 'underpants' pattern of erythema has been reported in a number of patients [4]. EMPD is frequently misdiagnosed as psoriasis or eczema [5], or Bowen's disease. Subclinical EMPD has been documented, where the skin looks normal macroscopically but is involved microscopically. EMPD behaves indolently, spreading by local extension and metastasis [6,7].

The concurrence of genital and extragenital EMPD is extremely rare, but overt and latent axillary EMPD can coexist and change daily in association with penile and pubic EMPD [8]. Also very rare is depigmented EMPD of the genitalia, evoking the differential diagnosis of vitiligo, hypopigmented mycosis fungoides and lichen sclerosus [9]. A focus of cutaneous squamous carcinoma has been reported complicating genital EMPD [10].

Diagnosis is by biopsy. Histological examination shows nests of large vacuolated cells with circular nuclei and foamy pale cytoplasm in the epidermis (Paget's cells). Dermal involvement signifies a poor prognosis. Pagetoid dyskeratosis can be found in a number of benign lesions such as naevi, skin tags and lentigines [11]. Pale cells resembling Paget's cells can be seen incidentally in benign papular intertriginous conditions, and in nearly 40% of prepuces sent for histological examination following circumcision for phimosis [11–13]. Anogenital Paget's disease can be accompanied by epidermal hyperplasia similar to fibroepithelioma of Pinkus [14]. Immunohistochemical and enzyme histochemical evidence points to sweat gland epithelium as the source of Paget's cells in EMPD [15]. The distribution along the 'milk line' has led to the suggestion that the 'clear cells of Toker' are the histogenic precursors of both clear cell papulosis and mammary and extramammary Paget's disease, respectively [9]. HPV is not present [16], but the c-erbB-2 oncoprotein may have a role in the pathogenesis of EMPD [17].

Mammary Paget's disease is an epidermal manifestation of an underlying breast adenocarcinoma [18]. EMPD is found in areas rich in apocrine sweat glands, such as the axillae and anogenital region. EMPD can also be associated with an underlying malignancy [6]. In a large series, 24% of patients had a proximate cutaneous adnexal adenocarcinoma, 12% were found to have a concurrent, and another 17% to have a non-concurrent internal malignancy [19].

Although properly regarded as a type of carcinoma *in situ*, EMPD may itself become invasive and metastatic [20–22]. There may be subjacent carcinoma (e.g. in periurethral glands) [23] or distant carcinoma (e.g. prostate [24] or bladder [25]), or both (e.g. periurethral glands and bladder [26]). Pagetoid epidermal invasion of inguinal cutaneous metastatic mesothelioma of the tunica vaginalis of the testis has been reported [27].

Treatments used for EMPD include cryotherapy and topical 5-fluorouracil [28], wide excisional surgery [20], micrographic surgery [29,30], radiotherapy [7,31] and photodynamic therapy [32].

REFERENCES

1 Metcalf JS, Lee RE, Maize JC. Epidermotropic urothelial carcinoma involving the glans penis. *Arch Dermatol* 1985; **121**: 532–4.
2 Redondo P, Idoate M, España A, Quintanilla E. Pruritus ani in an elderly man: extramammary Paget's disease. *Arch Dermatol* 1995; **131**: 952–3.
3 Butler JD, Hersham MJ, Wilson CA, Bryson JR. Perianal Paget's disease. *J R Soc Med* 1997; **90**: 688–9.
4 Murata Y, Kumano K, Tani M. Underpants-pattern erythema: a previously unrecognized cutaneous manifestation of extramammary Paget's disease of the genitalia with advanced metastatic spread. *J Am Acad Dermatol* 1999; **40**: 949–56.
5 Aldeen T, Lau RK. Genital eczema in an elderly man. *Int J STD AIDS* 1999; **10**: 124–6.
6 Helwig EB, Graham IH. Anogenital (extramammary) Paget's disease: a clinicopathological study. *Cancer* 1963; **16**: 387–403.
7 Gerber WL. Scrotal malignancies: the University of Iowa experience and a review of the literature. *Urology* 1985; **26**: 337–42.
8 Imakado S, Abe M, Okuno T *et al.* Two cases of genital Paget's disease with bilateral axillary involvement: mutability of axillary lesions. *Arch Dermatol* 1991; **127**: 1243.
9 Chen YH, Wong TW, Lee JY. Depigmented genital extramammary Paget's disease: a possible histogenetic link to Toker's clear cells and clear cell papulosis. *J Cutan Pathol* 2001; **28**: 105–8.
10 Tanabe H, Kishigawa T, Sayama S, Tanaka T. A case of giant extramammary Paget's disease of the genital area with squamous cell carcinoma. *Dermatology* 2001; **202**: 249–51.
11 Tschen JA, McGavran MH, Kettler AH. Pagetoid dyskeratosis: a selective keratinocytic response. *J Am Acad Dermatol* 1988; **19**: 891–4.
12 Val-Bernal JF, Garijo MF. Pagetoid dyskeratosis of the prepuce: an incidental histologic finding resembling extramammary Paget's disease. *J Cutan Pathol* 2000; **27**: 387–91.
13 Kohler S, Rouse RV, Smoller BR. The differential diagnosis of Pagetoid cells in the epidermis. *Mod Pathol* 1998; **11**: 79–92.
14 Ishida-Yamamoto A, Sato K, Wada T *et al.* Fibroepithelioma-like changes occurring in perianal Paget's disease with rectal mucinous carcinoma: case report and review of 49 cases of extramammary Paget's disease. *J Cutan Pathol* 2002; **29**: 185–9.
15 Hamm H, Vroom TM, Czametski BM. Extramammary Paget's cells: further evidence of sweat gland derivation. *J Am Acad Dermatol* 1986; **15**: 1275–81.
16 Snow SN, Desouky S, Lo JS, Kurtycz D. Failure to detect human papillomavirus DNA in extramammary Paget's disease 1992; **69**: 249–51.

17 Wolber RA, Dupuis BA, Wick MR. Expression of C-erb-2 oncoprotein in mammary and extramammary Paget's disease. *Am J Clin Pathol* 1991; **96**: 243–7.
18 Paget J. On disease of the mammary areola preceding carcinoma of the mammary gland. *St Bart's Hosp Rep* 1874; **10**: 87–9.
19 Chanda JJ. Extramammary Paget's disease: prognosis and relationship to internal malignancy. *J Am Acad Dermatol* 1985; **13**: 1009–14.
20 Jensen SL. A randomized trial of simple excision of non-specific hypertrophied anal papillae versus expectant management in patients with chronic pruritus ani. *Ann R Coll Surg Engl* 1988; **70**: 348–9.
21 Iwamura H, Horri Y, Tokuchi H, Arai E. A case of genital Paget's disease with severe dermal invasion and early dissemination. *Acta Urol Jap* 1999; **45**: 281–4.
22 Khoubehi B, Schofield A, Leslie M *et al.* Metastatic *in situ* perianal Paget's disease. *J R Soc Med* 2001; **94**: 137–8.
23 Jenkins IL. Extra-mammary Paget's disease of the penis. *Br J Urol* 1989; **63**: 103–4.
24 Koh FBH, Nazarina AR. Paget's disease of the scrotum: report of a case with underlying carcinoma of the prostate. *Br J Dermatol* 1995; **133**: 306–7.
25 Turner AG. Pagetoid lesions associated with carcinoma of the bladder. *J Urol* 1980; **123**: 124–6.
26 Tomaszewski JE, Korat OC, LiVolsi VA, Connor AM, Wein A. Paget's disease of the urethral meatus following transitional cell carcinoma of the bladder. *J Urol* 1986; **135**: 368–70.
27 Cartwright LE, Steinman HK. Malignant papillary mesothelioma of the tunica vaginalis testes: cutaneous metastases showing epidermal invasion. *J Am Acad Dermatol* 1987; **17**: 887–90.
28 Arensmeier M, Theuring U, Franke I, Willgeroth C, Kuhne KH. Topical therapy of extramammary Paget's disease. *Hautarzt* 1994; **45**: 780–2.
29 Mohs FE, Blanchard I. Microscopically controlled surgery for extramammary Paget's disease. *Arch Dermatol* 1979; **115**: 706–8.
30 Brown MD, Zachary CB, Grekin RC, Swanson NA. Genital tumours: their management by micrographic surgery. *J Am Acad Dermatol* 1988; **18**: 115–22.
31 Rosin RD. Paget's disease of the anus. *J R Soc Med* 1991; **84**: 112–3.
32 Petrelli NJ, Cebollero JA, Rodriguez-Bigas M, Mang T. Photodynamic therapy in the management of neoplasms of the perianal skin. *Arch Dermatol* 1992; **127**: 1436–8.

Malignant melanoma

This is a very rare condition of the penis (fewer than 100 cases reported). It is estimated to account for 1–1.5% of all malignancies of the penis [1,2] and less than 0.15% of all melanomas [3]. Melanoma is even rarer on the scrotum, with only four cases appearing in the literature [4,5].

Genital melanoma presents as a pigmented macule or as a pigmented or amelanotic papule or nodule (possibly developing from a lentiginous area or pre-existing dysplastic naevus), which may ulcerate or bleed [1,2,6–14]. Patients are usually middle-aged or older, although it has been reported in a boy [15]. It is exceedingly rare in Asians and has not been reported in black people (although a case of melanoma of the urethra has been seen) [16].

Sixty to 70% of lesions occur on the glans. There may be a family history of melanoma and other atypical or 'dysplastic' naevi on examination. The inguinal and other nodes, as well as the abdomen, should be palpated. Forty to 50% of patients have lymphatic or other metastatic dissemination at the time of presentation. Clinically atypical lesions should be biopsied and the histology critically reviewed [7,11]. Malignant melanoma of any histological subtype may be encountered [17].

Treatment is by primary excision. Subsequent management depends on the Breslow thickness of the lesion and complete clinical staging. Radical surgery and chemotherapy may be needed, but the prognosis is poor for all melanomas that have already metastasized [1,15,18].

Kaposi's sarcoma

Solitary Kaposi's sarcoma (KS) of the penis was very rarely seen before the HIV epidemic and cases are still occasionally seen in HIV-negative patients [19,20], but genital KS is essentially an HIV-associated problem. It presents as a dull red patch or plaque of the glans or prepuce, or anywhere else on the penis or scrotum, perineum or perianal skin in one of its classic forms: purple, slightly scaly patches or plaques, nodules or ulcerative lesions [21]. More atypical presentations that have been seen include engorgement with hypervascularity [22], penile lymphoedema [23] and phimosis. The differential diagnosis includes cellular naevus, histiocytoma, angioma, angiokeratoma, pseudo-Kaposi's sarcoma [24], bacillary angiomatosis and melanoma.

Miscellaneous

Although basal cell carcinoma is the most common type of skin cancer, it is rare in the anogenital area, although over 100 cases have been reported [25], including one case report of fibroepithelioma of Pinkus affecting the base of the penis [26]. A case of multiple erosive scrotal basal cell carcinomas with metastasis has been described [27].

Fibrosarcoma, haemangiopericytoma, leiomyosarcoma, malignant fibrous histiocytoma, epithelioid sarcoma, dermatofibrosarcoma protuberans and spindle cell sarcoma may occur, presenting as painful or painless nodules, masses or swelling with dysuria and erectile difficulties (e.g. masquerading as Peyronie's disease) [19,28]. Other rarities include Merkel cell carcinoma [29], malignant eccrine poroma [30], malignant schwannoma [19,31] and solitary reticulohistiocytic granuloma of the scrotum [32].

Involvement of the penis with Langerhans' cell histiocytosis is very rare; a fleshy papule on the dorsal penis and primary penile ulceration have been reported [33].

Mycosis fungoides can be confined to or concentrated in the genital region. Localized perianal involvement has been described [34].

Although lymphoma is the most frequent secondary tumour of the testis, it is rare in other parts of the male urogenital tract [19]. Penile lymphoma can present as painless subcutaneous nodules, erythematous swelling and ulceration [35–37]. There may be no evidence of systemic lymphoma. A fungating nodular scrotal lymphoma has been reported [38], as have scrotal and penile ulceration resulting from leukaemic infiltration [39,40].

Metastases to the penis are rare, but several hundred cases have been reported [41]. They are usually secondary to cancer of the urogenital tract [42] or gastrointestinal system, or other common cancers such as of the lung [43], and present with pain, swelling, priapism, urinary symptoms or haematuria. A very rare cause is secondary melanoma [41].

REFERENCES

1 Johnson DE, Ayala AG. Primary melanoma of the penis. *Urology* 1973; **2**: 174–7.
2 Stillwell TJ, Zincke H, Gaffey TA, Woods JE. Malignant melanoma of the penis. 1988; **140**: 72–5.
3 Cascinelli N. Melanoma maligno del pene. *Tumori* 1969; **55**: 313–5.
4 Gerber WL. Scrotal malignancies: the University of Iowa experience and a review of the literature. *Urology* 1985; **26**: 337–42.
5 Davis NS, Kim CA, Dever DP. Primary malignant melanoma of the scrotum: case report and literature review. *J Urol* 1991; **145**: 1056–7.
6 Bracken RB, Diokno AC. Melanoma of the penis and the urethra: two case reports and review of the literature. *J Urol* 1974; **111**: 198–200.
7 Jaeger N, Wirler H, Tschubel K. Acral lentiginous melanoma of the penis. *Eur J Urol* 1982; **8**: 182–4.
8 Jorda E, Verdeger JM, Moragon M *et al.* Desmoplastic melanoma of the penis. *J Am Acad Dermatol* 1987; **16**: 619–20.
9 Oldbring J, Mikulowski P. Malignant melanoma of the penis and male urethra: report of nine cases and review of the literature. *Cancer* 1987; **59**: 581–7.
10 Manivel JC, Fraley EE. Malignant melanoma of the penis and male urethra: four case reports and literature review. *J Urol* 1988; **139**: 813.
11 Weiss J, Elder D, Hamilton R. Melanoma of the male urethra: surgical approach and pathological analysis. *J Urol* 1982; **128**: 382–5.
12 de Bree E, Sanidas E, Tzardi M, Gaki B, Tsiftsis D. Malignant melanoma of the penis. *Eur J Surg Oncol* 1997; **23**: 277–9.
13 Demitsu T, Nagato H, Nishimaki K *et al.* Melanoma *in situ* of the penis. *J Am Acad Dermatol* 2000; **42**: 386–8.
14 Honda S, Yamamoto O, Suenaga Y, Asahi M, Nakayama K. Six cases of metastatic malignant melanoma with apparently occult primary lesions. *J Dermatol* 2001; **28**: 265–71.
15 Begun FP, Grossman HB, Dionko AC *et al.* Malignant melanoma of the penis and male urethra. *J Urol* 1984; **132**: 123–5.
16 Sanders TJ, Venable DD, Sanusi ID. Primary malignant melanoma of the urethra in a black man: a case report. *J Urol* 1986; **135**: 1012–4.
17 Lucia MS, Miller GJ. Histopathology of malignant lesions of the penis. *Urol Clin North Am* 1992; **19**: 227–46.
18 Bundrick WS, Culkin DJ, Mata JH *et al.* Penile malignant melanoma in association with squamous carcinoma of the penis 1991; **146**: 1364–5.
19 Dehner LP, Smith BH. Soft tissue tumours of the penis. *Cancer* 1970; **25**: 1431–7
20 Kavak A, Akman RY, Alper M, Büyükbabani N. Penile Kaposi's sarcoma in a human immunodeficiency virus-seronegative patient. *Br J Dermatol* 2001; **144**: 207–8.
21 Schwartz JJ, Dias BM, Safari B. HIV-related malignancies. *Dermatol Clin* 1991; **9**: 503–15.
22 Bayne D, Wise GJ. Kaposi sarcoma of the penis and genitalia: a disease of our times. *Urology* 1988; **31**: 22–5.
23 Schwartz RA, Cohen JB, Watson RA *et al.* Penile Kaposi's sarcoma preceded by chronic penile lymphoedema. *Br J Dermatol* 2000; **142**: 153–6.
24 Kapdağli H, Gunduz K, Ozturk G, Kandiloglu G. Pseudo-Kaposi's sarcoma (Mali type). *Int J Dermatol* 1998; **37**: 223–5.
25 Gibson GE, Ahmed I. Perianal and genital basal cell carcinoma: a clinicopathologic review of 51 cases. *J Am Acad Dermatol* 2001; **45**: 68–71.
26 Heymann WR, Soifer I, Burk PG. Penile premalignant fibroepithelioma of Pinkus. *Cutis* 1983; **31**: 519–21.
27 Staley TE, Nieh PT, Ciesielski TE, Cieplinski W. Metastatic basal cell carcinoma of the scrotum. *J Urol* 1983; **130**: 792–4.
28 Moore SW, Wheeler JE, Hefter LG. Epithelioid sarcoma masquerading as Peyronie's disease. *Cancer* 1975; **35**: 1706–10.
29 Best TJ, Metcalfe JB, Moore RB, Nguyen GK. Merkel cell carcinoma of the scrotum. *Ann Plast Surg* 1994; **33**: 83–5.

30 Werdin R, Kupczyk-Joeris D, Schumpelick V. Malignant eccrine poroma: case report of a rare tumour of the skin. *Chirurg* 1991; **62**: 350–2.

31 Marsidi PJ, Winter CC. Schwannoma of penis. *Urology* 1980; **16**: 303.

32 Anaguchi S, Sinomiya S, Kinebuchi S, Kumakiri M. Solitary reticulohistiocytic granuloma: a report of three cases and a review of the literature. *Nippon Hifuka Gakkai Zasshi* 1991; **101**: 735–42.

33 Seseke F, Kugler A, Hermanns M et al. Langerhans' cell histiocytosis of the penis. *Urologe A* 1999; **38**: 42–5 [in German].

34 Hill VA, Hall-Smith P, Smith NP. Cutaneous T-cell lymphoma presenting with atypical perianal lesions. *Dermatology* 1995; **190**: 313–6.

35 Gonzalez-Campora R, Nogales FF Jr, Lerma E, Navarro A, Matilla A. Lymphoma of the penis. *J Urol* 1981; **126**: 270–1.

36 Marks D, Crosthwaite A, Varigos G et al. Therapy of primary diffuse large cell lymphoma of the penis with preservation of function. *J Urol* 1988; **139**: 1057.

37 Cribier B, Lipsker D, Grosshans E et al. Genital ulceration revealing a primary cutaneous anaplastic lymphoma. *Genitourin Med* 1997; **73**: 325.

38 Doll DC, Diaz-Arias AA. Peripheral T-cell lymphoma of the scrotum. *Acta Haematologica* 1994; **91**: 77–9.

39 Gatto-Weis C, Topolsky D, Sloane B et al. Ulcerative balanoposthitis of the foreskin as a manifestation of chronic lymphocytic leukemia: case report and review of the literature. *Urology* 2000; **56**: 669.

40 Zax RH, Kulp-Shorten CL, Callen JP. Leukaemia cutis presenting as a scrotal ulcer. *J Am Acad Dermatol* 1989; **21**: 410–3.

41 Sagar SM, Retsas S. Metastasis of the penis from malignant melanoma: case report and review of the literature. *Clin Oncol* 1992; **4**: 130–1.

42 Miyamoto T, Ikehara A, Araki M, Akaeda T, Mihara M. Cutaneous metastatic carcinoma of the penis: suspected metastasis implantation from a bladder tumor. *J Urol* 2000; **163**: 1519.

43 Ortiz de Saracho J, Castrodeza Sanz R, Guzmán Dávila G. Penile metastasis and pulmonary carcinoma. *Arch Bronconeumol* 1998; **34**: 226–7 [in Spanish].

Miscellaneous

Pigmentary change is dealt with in the general introduction on pp. 68.2–68.3, and causes of anogenital hypo- and hyperpigmentation are listed in Tables 68.6 and 68.7.

Penile melanosis

Pigmented macules are not uncommon on the glans and shaft of the penis [1]. They are benign but, because they may be large or enlarging, with irregular edges and multifocal and variegated pigmentary patterns, they arouse concern about atypical melanocytic proliferation and acral lentiginous melanoma. Such clinical concerns should lead to biopsy [2]. Post-inflammmatory hyperpigmentation (e.g. lichen sclerosus, lichen planus) may be the cause in many patients. Some cases have been associated with previous treatment with anthralin, or PUVA therapy for psoriasis, or diabetes [3,4]. On histological examination there may be increased basal epidermal pigmentation, with or without benign lentiginous melanocytic hyperplasia, or an increase in basal melanocyte number. Breathnach et al. [5] have proposed that depigmentation is an essential element of penile melanosis and demonstrated melanocytic hyperplasia in areas of hyperpigmentation.

Penile melanosis is the term for lesions without lentiginous hyperplasia [4,6]. Revuz and Clerici [6] proposed the grouping of penile melanosis, vulvovaginal melanosis and the predominantly oral mucosal hyperpigmentation of the Laugier–Hunziker syndrome under the umbrella of essential melanotic hyperpigmentation of the mucosa. Lenane et al. [7] used the term genital melanotic macules.

Patients ask for treatment of penile melanosis as it is unsightly and embarrassing. Laser treatment may help [8].

Hypopigmentation

Striae as a consequence of growth or weight surges are common around the pelvic girdle or represent a complication of topical corticosteroid application [9]. Initially, they are often purple-red in colour. Vitiligo is a commonly observed affliction of the male genitalia, although patients may be unaware of it and clinicians might not always observe it [10].

Acral lentiginous melanoma is very rare but important [11,12].

REFERENCES

1 Kaporis A, Lynfield Y. Penile lentiginosis. *J Am Acad Dermatol* 1998; **38**: 781.

2 Kopf AW, Bart RS. Tumor conference 43: penile lentigo. *J Dermatol Surg Oncol* 1982; **8**: 637–9.

3 Rhodes AR, Harrist TJ, Momtaz TK. The PUVA-induced pigmented macule: a lentiginous proliferation of large, sometimes cytologically atypical, melanocytes. *J Am Acad Dermatol* 1983; **9**: 47–58.

4 Barnhill RL, Albert LS, Sharma SK et al. Genital lentiginosis: a clinical and histopathologic study. *J Am Acad Dermatol* 1990; **22**: 453–60.

5 Breathnach AS, Balus L, Amantea A. Penile lentiginosis: an ultrastructural study. *Pigment Cell Res* 1992; **5**: 404–13.

6 Revuz J, Clerici T. Penile melanosis. *J Am Acad Dermatol* 1989; **20**: 567–70.

7 Lenane P, Keane CO, Connell BO, Loughlin SO, Powell FC. Genital melanotic macules: clinical, histologic, immunohistochemical, and ultrastructural features. *J Am Acad Dermatol* 2000; **42**: 640–4.

8 Delaney TA, Walker NPJ. Penile melanosis successfully treated with the Q-switched ruby laser. *Br J Dermatol* 1994; **130**: 663–4.

9 Stankler L. Striae of the penis. *Br J Dermatol* 1982; **107**: 371–2.

10 Moss JR, Stevenson CJ. Incidence of male genital vitiligo: report of a screening programme. *Br J Vener Dis* 1981; **57**: 145–6.

11 Jaeger N, Wirler H, Tschubel K. Acral lentiginous melanoma of the penis. *Eur J Urol* 1982; **8**: 182–4.

12 Weiss J, Elder D, Hamilton R. Melanoma of the male urethra: surgical approach and pathological analysis. *J Urol* 1982; **128**: 382–5.

Pain and swelling

Some presentations of many entities can be painful but generally pain is an unusual presentation for a dermatosis. Swelling is more common and may be painful or not. A common factor in many but not all causes of swelling may be oedema or lymphoedema. Causes of anogenital lymphoedema and penoscrotal swelling are listed in Tables 68.25–68.27.

Iatrogenic swellings and lymphoedema

Congenital defects of the inguinal canal and other non-inguinal peritoneal leaks can lead to scrotal and penile swelling as a manifestation of dialysate oedema in patients with end-stage renal failure treated by continuous ambulatory peritoneal dialysis [7]. Genital oedema is

Table 68.25 Causes of anogenital lymphoedema. (After Bunker [6].)

Idiopathic congenital lymphoedema (Milroy's disease)
Lipogranuloma and silicone granuloma
Strangulation of the penis
Iatrogenic
Radical abdominopelvic surgery
Radiotherapy
Granulomatous lymphangitis
Post-infectious
    Cellulitis and erysipelas
    Chancroid
    Lymphogranuloma venereum
    Tuberculosis
    Leprosy
    Syphilis
    Filariasis/onchocerciasis
Carcinomatosis
    Lymphatic involvement
    Lymphatic blockage
Lymphoma

Table 68.26 Commoner causes of penoscrotal swelling. (After Bunker [6]. © 2004, with permission from Elsevier.)

Paraphimosis
Foreign body
Strangulation of the penis
Iatrogenic
    Continuous ambulatory peritoneal dialysis
    Genital oedema resulting from raised right heart filling pressure
      in ITU
    Postoperative
    Post-radiotherapy
Varicocoele
Hydrocoele
Priapism
Peyronie's disease
Epididymitis and orchitis
Cellulitis
Idiopathic penile oedema
Testicular tumours

Table 68.27 Rarer causes of penoscrotal swelling. (After Bunker [6]. © 2004, with permission from Elsevier.)

Idiopathic congenital lymphoedema [1]
Giant haemangioma
Urethral diverticulum
Segmental urethral hypospadias
Accessory scrotum [2,3]
Herniation of scrotal contents into penile shaft
Foreign body
Lipogranuloma and silicone granuloma
Aortic aneurysm [4]
Scrotal fat necrosis
Henoch–Schönlein purpura
Familial Mediterranean fever
Acute haemorrhagic oedema of childhood
Granulomatous lymphangitis
Sarcoid
Infected cyst
Abscess of corpus cavernosum [5]
Tuberculosis
Paracoccidioidomycosis
Giant scrotal tumours (e.g. neurilemoma)
Epithelioid haemangioma
Kaposi's sarcoma
Epithelioid haemangioendothelioma
Lymphoma
Sarcoma
Drugs (e.g. angio-oedema caused by lisinopril)

Table 68.28 Complications of plastic surgery to the penis. (After Bunker [6] (© 2004, with permission from Elsevier) and Alter [11].)

Hypertrophic scars
Wide scars
Proximal penile hump (thick hair-bearing Y flap)
Low-hanging penis
Loss of fat
Nodules
Deformed shaft

commonplace in intensive care units, because of the practice of maintaining a raised right heart filling pressure. Radical cancer surgery and/or radiotherapy to the anogenital area and the lymphatics can cause swelling because of lymphoedema, early or delayed [8]. Chronic oedema, resembling keloid, of the penis has been caused by a condom catheter for neurogenic bladder [9].

Increasingly, patients seek plastic surgery to the penis [10] for psychosexual reasons (e.g. dysmorphophobia) but surgery can result in significant complications (Table 68.28).

Idiopathic lipogranuloma

Cases of characteristic, spontaneously resolving, painless, Y-shaped swelling of the scrotum embracing the penile root, with sclerosing eosinophilic lipogranuloma on histology and electron microscopy (but no exogenous lipids) and associated with blood eosinophilia (one patient had arthralgia), have been reported from Japan [12].

REFERENCES

1 Bolt RJ, Peelen W, Nikkels PG, de Jong TP. Congenital lymphoedema of the genitalia. *Eur J Pediatr* 1998; **157**: 943–6.
2 Szylit J-A, Grossman ME, Luyando Y, Olarte MR, Nagler H. Becker's nevus and an accessory scrotum. *J Am Acad Dermatol* 1986; **14**: 905–7.
3 Yokokawa K, Nakano E, Takaha M. Accessory scrotum: a case report. *J Urol* 1986; **135**: 593–4.
4 Ward CS, Dundas DD, Dow J, Shearer RJ. Scrotal swelling due to perianeurysmal fibrosis. *Br J Urol* 1988; **61**: 536–8.
5 Kameda K, Hayashi N, Arima K *et al.* Abscess of corpus cavernosum: a case report. *Hinyokika Kiyo* 1998; **44**: 893–5 [in Japanese].
6 Bunker CB. *Male Genital Skin Disease*. London: Saunders, 2004 (in press).
7 Kopecky RT, Funk MM, Kreitzer PR. Localized genital oedema in patients undergoing continuous ambulatory peritoneal dialysis. *J Urol* 1985; **134**: 880–4.
8 Horinaga M, Masuda T, Jitsukawa S. A case of scrotal elephantiasis 30 years after treatment of penile carcinoma. *Hinyokika Kiyo* 1998; 44: 839–41.
9 Bang RL. Penile oedema induced by continuous condom catheter use and mimicking keloid scar. *Scand J Urol Nephrol* 1994; **28**: 333–5.

10 Austoni E, Guarneri A, Gatti G. Penile elongation and thickening: a myth? Is there a cosmetic or medical indication? *Andrologia* 1999; **31** (Suppl. 1): 45–51.
11 Alter GJ. Reconstruction of deformities resulting from penile enlargement surgery. *J Urol* 1997; **158**: 2153–7.
12 Matsuda T, Shichiri Y, Hida S *et al*. Eosinophilic sclerosing lipogranuloma of the male genitalia not caused by exogenous lipids. *J Urol* 1988; **140**: 1021.

Priapism

Priapism is defined as the prolonged painful erection of the penis, unassociated with sexual desire and not relieved by ejaculation. Although not predominantly a dermatological concern, it has an important differential diagnosis. The principal causes are listed in Table 68.29. It results in impotence in more than 50% of those affected [3,4] and can lead to gangrenous penile necrosis [5].

Levine *et al.* [1] distinguish veno-occlusive priapism from arterial priapism. Veno-occlusive priapism results from persistent obstruction to venous outflow from the lacunar spaces. It is a potential vascular emergency because, as the corporeal bodies expand to maximal volume, an obstructed outflow causes decreased arterial inflow, with the potential for ischaemia, pain, fibrosis and hence impotence. Arterial priapism is usually secondary

Table 68.29 Causes of priapism. (After Levine *et al.* [1] and Bunker [2]. © 2004, with permission from Elsevier.)

Idiopathic
Os penis
    Congenital
    Acquired—ageing, trauma, metabolic disorder
Perineal trauma
Strangulation
Hypertension
Nephrotic syndrome
Neurological causes
Quadriplegia
Spinal canal stenosis
Cauda equina compression
Sickle cell disease
Coagulopathy
    Protein C deficiency
    Factor V Leiden
    Warfarin necrosis
Peyronie's disease
Rheumatoid arthritis
Vasculitis
Tuberculosis
Pelvic tumours
Leukaemia
Lymphoma
Penile metastases
Drugs
    Papaverine
    Antipsychotics—chlorpromazine, trazodone
    Antihypertensives—hydralazine, guanethidine, prazosin
    Marijuana
    Adrenal corticosteroids
    Warfarin necrosis

to trauma, such that a damaged cavernosal artery causes unregulated blood flow to the lacunar spaces; it is thus non-ischaemic [1].

REFERENCES

1 Levine FJ, de Tejada IS, Payton TR, Goldstein I. Recurrent prolonged erections and priapism as a sequela of priapism: pathophysiology and management. *J Urol* 1991; **145**: 764–7.
2 Bunker CB. *Male Genital Skin Disease*. London: Saunders, 2004 (in press).
3 Nelson JH III, Winter CC. Priapism: evolution of management in 48 patients in a 22-year series. *J Urol* 1977; **117**: 455–8.
4 O'Brien WM, O'Connor KP, Lynch JH. Priapism: current concepts. *Ann Emerg Med* 1989; **18**: 980–3.
5 Khoriaty N, Schick E. Penile gangrene: an unusual complictaion of priapism. How to avoid it. *Urology* 1980; **16**: 280.

Dermatological non-disease, dysaesthesia and chronic pain syndromes

'Dermatological non-disease' may be the diagnosis where there is a paucity or even absence of primary dermatological signs to account for florid symptomatology. Genital symptoms include itching, excessive redness, burning and discomfort—in some cases so severe that it prevents the patient from sitting down. Dysmorphophobia, depression and psychosis may be present, and attempted suicide is a real risk in such patients [1,2].

Itching of the urethra may lead to insertion of a foreign body into the urethra in an attempt to relieve the sensation [3], or this might be done for sexual gratification.

Patients with symptoms of itching, burning and pain localized to the penis or scrotum are not uncommonly encountered. The skin is usually completely normal. The situation is analogous to vulvodynia in women, and terms such as penodynia and scrotodynia have been coined to describe the syndrome in men. Doxepin, amitriptyline and paroxetine can afford some relief.

Fisher [4] has defined the red, burning scrotum syndrome as 'persistent redness of the anterior half of the scrotum that may involve the base of the penis . . . usually accompanied by a persistent itching or burning sensation and hyperalgesia'. It is a chronic condition that is resistant to treatment and its cause is unknown [4,5]. Accompanying the erythema there may be telangiectasia. It is related to idiopathic penile and scrotal pain syndromes [6]. Prednisolone and antidepressants have given some relief to some patients.

Localized dermatographism should be sought by stroking the inside of the thigh, because such patients may be helped by oral antihistamine treatment.

The possibilities of zinc deficiency and necrolytic migratory erythema should be entertained.

Chronic urogenital and rectal pain syndromes include penile pain (penodynia), scrotodynia, orchialgia, prostatodynia, coccygodynia, proctalgia fugax, perineal pain, the descending perineum syndrome and vulvodynia

[7–9]. The neuroanatomy of the pelvis is complicated and the neurophysiological basis of the pathogenesis of these syndromes is poorly understood, but their clinical presentations are well recognized. The differential diagnosis is addressed above.

A diagnosis of a chronic pain syndrome implies the prospect of considerable psychological morbidity. Treatment is challenging and only empirical at best. Most agree that invasive and irreversible procedures should be avoided if at all possible. Multidisciplinary management is recommended [6].

REFERENCES

1 Cotterill JA. A dermatological non-disease: a common and potentially fatal disturbance of cutaneous body image. *Br J Dermatol* 1981; **104**: 611–9.
2 Bunker CB, Bridgett CK. Depression and the skin. In: Robertson MM, Katona CLE, eds. *Depression and Physical Illness*. London: John Wiley, 1997.
3 Al-Durazi M, Saleem I, Mohammed AA. Urethral foreign body. *Br J Urol* 1992; **69**: 434.
4 Fisher BK. The red scrotum syndrome. *Cutis* 1997; **60**: 139–41.
5 Markos AR. The male genital skin burning syndrome (dysaesthetic peno/scroto-dynia). *Int J STD AIDS* 2002; **13**: 271–2.
6 Wesselmann U, Burnett AL, Heinberg LJ. The urogenital and rectal pain syndromes. *Pain* 1997; **73**: 269–94.
7 Parks AG, Porter NH, Hardcastle J. The syndrome of descending perineum. *Proc R Soc Med* 1966; **59**: 477–82.
8 Lask B. Chronic perianal pain. *J R Soc Med* 1982; **75**: 370.
9 Neill ME, Swash M. Chronic perianal pain: an unsolved problem. *J R Soc Med* 1982; **75**: 96–101.

Hair disorders

Alopecia areata can affect the pubic hair, but usually as part of more widespread involvement as in alopecia universalis. Loss of pubic hair occurs in secondary syphilis and has been reported in primary systemic amyloid [1]. Trichotillomania of the pubic hair has been described [2,3].

REFERENCES

1 Brownstein MH, Helwig EB. The cutaneous amyloidoses. II. Systemic forms. *Arch Dermatol* 1970; **102**: 20–8.
2 Davis-Daneshfar A, Trüeb RM. Tonsur-Trichotillomanie. *Hautartz* 1995; **46**: 804–7.
3 Cohen LJ, Stein DJ, Simeon D *et al*. Clinical profile, comorbidity, and treatment history in 123 hair pullers: a survey study. *J Clin Psychiatry* 1995; **56**: 319–26.

Female genital dermatology

Introduction

Disorders of the vulval epithelium have proved confusing to the many and varied specialists who have been involved in their diagnosis and treatment. The difficulty has arisen because the majority of the problems are dermatological and the specialists—gynaecologists, urologists, paediatricians and genitourinary physicians—have had little or no training in dermatology. The problem is compounded by the fact that the normal characteristics of common diseases at this flexural site are lost or modified, making the diagnosis difficult even for an experienced dermatologist. Over the years, classifications of vulval disorders have been devised to help, but unfortunately these have only resulted in further confusion. There is no need for a separate classification for vulval disorders, as the current classifications that exist for dermatology and pathology can be used [1,2].

Dystrophy, leukoplakia and kraurosis vulvae have all now been abandoned as diagnostic terms [3]. Over the years, the term leukoplakia has unfortunately had the sinister implication that it always represented a premalignant condition [4], but now leukoplakia is used as a descriptive term only and may represent anything from a patch of lichen simplex to an SCC. Similarly, squamous cell hyperplasia is not a diagnosis but a histological description, and can be seen in many disorders including psoriasis, candidosis and hypertrophic lichen planus.

Vulval clinics have been an important step forward in the diagnosis and management of women with vulval problems [5,6]. These clinics ideally should be multidisciplinary with input from dermatology, gynaecology, genitourinary medicine and pathology. It is important that there are links with other specialists including paediatricians and plastic surgeons, as well as psychologists and psychosexual therapists.

The development of these clinics has been extremely important, not only for improved patient care but also for the valuable interdisciplinary education of the doctors involved.

An accurate diagnosis depends on a thorough history, examination of the affected skin and skin at extragenital sites, and pertinent investigations. The history must include the chief complaint, how long it has been present, how the problem changes in certain circumstances (e.g. variation with the menstrual cycle), what treatment has been prescribed and what were the effects of the treatment. A drug history is important, and should include direct questioning about over-the-counter oral and topical medications, oral contraceptives and hormone replacement therapy (HRT). The latter two are included in this direct questioning as patients do not always consider these as medications, particularly if the HRT is in a topical formulation. A personal and family history of autoimmune disease, atopy or psoriasis should be established, and any known skin sensitivities. The patient should also be asked about vaginal discharge, urinary symptoms and bowel function. Finally, as the vulva is important for normal sexual function, it is important to include relevant questions on problems with intercourse where appropriate.

The complaint of irritation has many meanings and it is sometimes helpful to ask the patient exactly what they mean by the term. It may be the sensation of itch, dryness, pain, burning or rawness. This point is important as a patient with itch will scratch or rub the skin, and the response will be lichen simplex or lichenification, whereas with discomfort or pain there will be no such change as the patient avoids touching the area.

Lichen simplex and lichenification. Lichen simplex and lichenification are terms used to describe the exaggerated normal rhomboidal patterning of the skin surface. Lichen simplex is used to describe the changes seen on apparently normal skin secondary to itching and rubbing, although the provoking symptom of itch may be initiated by a low-grade dermatosis such as psoriasis or seborrhoeic eczema. The term lichenification is used for similar changes arising on a background of a visible dermatosis.

The lesions of lichen simplex tend to be in one isolated area, usually on the labia majora or mons pubis. They are well defined, with a pale grey or white surface.

The histological changes of lichen simplex and lichenification are similar, except that there are the changes of the background dermatosis in the latter. There is hyperkeratosis, acanthosis, a prominent granular layer, lengthened rete ridges and a chronic inflammatory dermal infiltrate. In addition, lamellar thickening of the papillary dermis and perineural fibrosis can be seen. Twelve cases of what was termed multinucleated atypia of the vulva have been reported [7], but this is thought to be a non-specific change found in lichenified skin [8,9].

Treatment of the underlying dermatosis will usually resolve the lichenification. In cases of lichen simplex with no underlying dermatosis, the treatment is the application of a potent topical steroid to encourage a disruption of the itch–scratch cycle. A soap substitute should be introduced and possible irritants avoided. If these measures are unsuccessful, patch testing should be performed to exclude the possibility of an unsuspected allergen.

The examination is often very embarrassing for the patient, so it must be carried out sympathetically to ease any tension. It is important that there is good lighting, and a means of magnification. The skin and the mucosae are examined in the anogenital area for changes in colour, epithelial integrity and texture. If there is scarring this will be seen in loss of characteristic features (e.g. introital narrowing, loss of the labia minora or sealing of the clitoral hood). The examination must also include examination of other flexural sites and mucosae, the scalp and nails. It is also useful to determine if the patient exhibits dermographism [10]. The vagina and cervix should be examined in patients who have dermatoses that affect mucosal surfaces and in patients with symptoms of dyspareunia, vaginal discharge or postcoital bleeding. Investigations are determined by the specific problem and include microbiological assessment. The investigation of the common bacterial or fungal problems can be easily performed by a dermatologist but if an exotic bacterial or sexually transmitted infection is high on the differential diagnosis, it is important to involve a genitourinary physi-

Table 68.30 Causes of vaginal discharge.

Physiological
Ovulation

Iatrogenic
Medications (e.g. tamoxifen, oral contraceptive pill)

Infective
Candidosis
Bacterial vaginosis
Cervicitis

Inflammatory
Lichen planus
Mucous membrane pemphigoid
Pemphigus
Erythema multiforme
Stevens–Johnson syndrome
Vaginal adenosis
Cervical erosion

Neoplastic
Langerhans' cell histiocytosis
Vaginal, uterine or fallopian tube tumours

cian in the investigation and work-up of these patients and their partners. A biopsy is important, particularly in cases where there is no response to treatment. If a biopsy is performed, it is important to let the pathologist know what area has been biopsied, as the vulva is a mucocutaneous junction and the normal histological changes of a mucosal epithelium differ significantly from those of cornified epithelium and may be misinterpreted as pathological changes. Other investigations include those performed routinely for skin problems elsewhere (e.g. patch testing, examination with Wood's light, Tzanck smears). Some investigations are not the usual remit of the dermatologist but are necessary in patients with anogenital dermatoses, and will include a cervical smear and proctoscopy.

On occasions, the vulval changes are not caused by a primary problem of the vulval skin but are the secondary consequences of pathology at another site (e.g. an irritant vulval dermatitis resulting from a vaginal discharge because of cervical, uterine or vaginal pathology).

Diagnosis and management of vaginal discharge

The diagnosis usually falls into one of the following categories: physiological, iatrogenic, infective, inflammatory or neoplastic (Table 68.30).

Physiological

Between 5 and 10% of women complaining of vaginal discharge do not have an infection. The discharge may be caused by an excess physiological secretion of mucus, usually resulting from a cervical erosion or an increase in the amount of vaginal transudate. The discharge is thick, with a grey-white appearance, and is odourless and non-irritant. Vaginal pH is normal.

Iatrogenic

This is usually secondary to medications that have an effect on the vaginal epithelium (e.g. tamoxifen, which has an oestrogenic effect on the vagina); oral contraceptive pills can cause a cervical erosion and an increase in vaginal discharge.

Infective

This is the most common cause of a vaginal discharge, and a pH greater than 6 is highly predictive of an infectious cause [11]. Bacterial vaginosis is the usual diagnosis [12]. The patient complains of excessive grey watery discharge, associated with a 'fishy' malodour, which is worsened with intercourse. Vulval irritation is slight or absent in this group, and the smell is the most distressing symptom. The condition is invariably associated with infection by a small aerobic Gram-negative rod known as *Gardnerella vaginalis*, after its discoverer Gardner [13]. It would appear that this organism alone is incapable of causing infection, and non-specific vaginitis is now regarded as a complex interrelationship between *Gardnerella* and anaerobic species of bacteria [14], two of which belong to the genus *Mobiluncus*. The fishy odour of the discharge can be accentuated by the addition of an alkali such as 10% potassium hydroxide (the Whiff test). A wet mount of a vaginal smear in saline will identify 'clue cells'. These are vaginal epithelial cells with a granular cytoplasmic appearance and indistinct cellular outlines. This indistinct border is caused by the attachment of the small Gram-negative rods to the cell [15]. Bacterial vaginosis is not always sexually acquired—its incidence is equal in virginal and sexually active groups [16,17]. This type of abnormal bacterial colonization may be associated with preterm delivery and late miscarriage in pregnant patients [18]. Treatment is with metronidazole 400 mg twice daily for 5 days or 2 g as a single dose.

Patients with infective cervicitis will also present with an increased vaginal discharge. The four most common pathogens involved are *Neisseria gonorrhoeae*, *Chlamydia trachomatis*, *Trichomonas vaginalis* and herpes virus hominis. *Chlamydia trachomatis* has been grown from the cervices of 50% of women with mucopurulent cervicitis [19]. The main symptoms are discharge, deep pelvic pain and dyspareunia.

Infestation with thread worms, *Enterobius vermicularis*, has also been recorded as a cause of a vulvovaginitis [20].

Inflammatory

Vaginal or cervical ulceration and erosion resulting from inflammatory conditions can give rise to an increased vaginal discharge. The most common inflammatory conditions are lichen planus and pemphigus [21]. The diagnosis is often missed, particularly if these sites are affected in isolation. There is a chronic odourless discharge, which may be blood-tinged. The patient will also complain of postcoital bleeding if she is sexually active. An accurate diagnosis requires a biopsy, and immunofluorescence studies should be performed both on tissue and serum. Examination of eyes and mouth may help if the patient also has disease at these sites. Treatment requires topical steroids in the form of foams or pessaries that are currently used for inflammatory bowel disease.

Neoplastic

Tumours of the fallopian tubes, uterus, cervix and vagina may all cause an increased vaginal discharge. Rarer causes of a chronic vaginal discharge include Langerhans' cell histiocytosis.

Management of vulval disorders depends upon the diagnosis, but general measures include the use of a soap substitute and avoidance of irritants (e.g. bubble baths, shampooing hair in the bath). If there is an incontinence problem, a barrier ointment helps to protect the skin. Weak potassium permanganate solution or Burow's solution can be used when there is erosive disease. Topical steroids are best used in an ointment formulation to avoid the irritant effect of preservatives and alcohol. Many of the patients are elderly and may have difficulty treating themselves. It is often helpful to take time in the clinic, using a mirror, to explain exactly where the treatment should be applied.

REFERENCES

1 Kiryu H Ackerman AB. A critique of current classifications of vulval disease. *Am J Dermatopathol* 1990; **12**: 377–92.
2 Wilkinson EJ, Kneale B, Lynch PJ. Report of the ISSVD terminology committee. *J Reprod Med* 1986; **31**: 973–4.
3 Ridley CM, Frankman O, Jones ISC *et al*. New nomenclature for vulval disease: report of the committee on terminology. *Am J Obstet Gynecol* 1989; **160**: 769.
4 Wallace HJ, Whimster IW. Vulval atrophy and leukoplakia. *Br J Dermatol* 1951; **63**: 241–57.
5 Weisfogel E. Aims of joint gynecologic, dermatologic and pathologic vulval clinics. *N Y State J Med* 1969; **69**: 1184–6.
6 Heller DS, Randolph P, Young A, Tancer ML, Fromer D. The cutaneous–vulvar clinic revisited: a 5-year experience of the Columbia Presbyterian Medical Center cutaneous vulvar service. *Dermatology* 1997; **195**: 26–9.
7 McLachlin CM, Mutter GL, Crum CP. Multinucleated atypia of the vulva: report of a distinct entity not associated with human papillomavirus. *Am J Surg Pathol* 1994; **18**: 1233–9.
8 LeBoit PE. Multinucleated atypia. *Am J Surg Pathol* 1996; **20**: 507.
9 Tagamai H, Uehara M. Multinucleated epidermal giant cells in inflammatory skin diseases. *Arch Dermatol* 1981; **117**: 23–5.
10 Shenertz EF. Clinical pearl: symptomatic dermographism as a cause of genital pruritus. *J Am Acad Dermatol* 1994; **31**: 1040–1.
11 Hanna NF, Taylor-Robinson D, Kalodikki-Karamanoli M *et al*. The relation between vaginal pH and the microbiological status in vaginitis. *Br J Obstet Gynaecol* 1985; **92**: 1267–71.
12 Vontver LA, Eschenbach DA. The role of *Gardnerella vaginalis* in non-specific vaginitis. *Clin Obstet Gynecol* 1981; **24**: 439–60.

13 Gardner HL. *Haemophilus vaginalis* vaginitis after 25 years. *Am J Obstet Gynecol* 1980; **137**: 385–91.

14 Speigel CA, Amsel R, Eschenbach D *et al*. Anaerobic bacteria in non-specific vaginitis. *N Engl J Med* 1980; **303**: 601–7.

15 De Boer JM, Plantema FHF. Ultrastructure of the *in situ* adherence of *Mobiluncus* to vaginal epithelial cells. *Can J Microbiol* 1988; **34**: 757–66.

16 Holst E. Reservoir of four organisms associated with bacterial vaginosis suggests lack of sexual transmission. *J Clin Microbiol* 1990; **28**: 2033–9.

17 Bump RC, Buesching WJ. Bacterial vaginosis in virginal and sexually active adolescent females: evidence against sexual transmission. *Am J Obstet Gynecol* 1988; **158**: 935–9.

18 Hay PE, Lamont RF, Taylor-Robinson D *et al*. Abnormal bacterial colonization of the genital tract and subsequent preterm delivery and late miscarriage. *BMJ* 1994; **308**: 295–8.

19 Brunham RC, Paavonen J, Stevens CE *et al*. Mucopurulent cervicitis: the ignored counterpart in women of urethritis in men. *N Engl J Med* 1984; **311**: 1–6.

20 Kacker TP. Vulvovaginitis in an adult with threadworms in the vagina. *Br J Vener Dis* 1973; **49**: 314–5.

21 Batta K, Munday PE, Tatnall FM. Pemphigus vulgaris localized to the vagina and presenting as a chronic vaginal discharge. *Br J Dermatol* 1999; **140**: 945–7.

Structure and function of the female genitalia

The vulva is the collective term for the structures that comprise the female external genitalia. Anatomically, it is the region known as the urogenital triangle, bounded anteriorly by the symphysis pubis, the pubic rami laterally and the transverse perineal body posteriorly. The vulval structures included within this area are the mons pubis, paired labia majora and labia minora, clitoris and vulval vestibule. The epithelia that cover the vulva change from skin on the outer aspects to mucosa on the innermost region.

The mons pubis lies in front of and above the upper part of the symphysis pubis. It is softly rounded because of a thick cushion of subcutaneous fat. The epithelium is densely covered in hairs and possesses all the adnexal structures usually found in skin.

The labia majora are paired rounded folds of skin and are the homologue of the scrotum. They extend downwards and backwards from the mons pubis and meet posteriorly in the midline to form the posterior commissure, which lies approximately 2 cm anterior to the anus. The epithelium is similar in structure to that on the mons pubis in that there is a thick layer of adipose tissue and a dense distribution of hair on the outer surfaces of the labia. Hair is absent from the inner surfaces but numerous sebaceous glands remain. The inner aspects of the labia majora fuse into the outer aspects of the labia minora laterally, forming the interlabial sulci. The labia majora enclose an elliptical fissure which is known as the pudendal cleft—this contains the vestibule with the openings of the vagina and urethra.

The labia minora are the equivalent of the prepuce, and part of the ventral portion of the penis and the floor of the spongy part of the male urethra. They are paired pendulous folds, which lie between the labia majora and the vulval vestibule. Anteriorly they split into two folds on each side, which fuse in the midline. The superior folds cover the clitoris like a hood, forming the prepuce of the clitoris, and the lower folds fuse on the inferior aspect of the clitoris, forming the clitoral frenulum. Posteriorly, the labia minora fuse to form the fourchette, and sometimes form a depression in the midline, the fossa navicularis. The labia minora possess little subcutaneous fat. Their epithelium lacks hair but there are numerous sebaceous glands and sweat glands. The epithelium is cornified but its barrier function is not as effective as skin elsewhere.

The clitoris is the homologue of the penis and contains all the vascular and muscular structures found in its male counterpart. The end of the clitoris is surmounted by a small rounded tubercle, the glans clitoris.

The vestibule is usually considered as part of the vulva, although many anatomy books refer to it as the vestibule of the vagina. It is the area that lies between the labia minora and contains the openings of the urethra and vagina. The vaginal opening is partially closed by the hymen. When the hymen is ruptured, its remnants form rounded crenulations, the hymenal caruncle. The fold between the hymenal caruncle and the vestibular floor is the nymphohymenal sulcus. Sometimes a clear line of demarcation between the labia minora and the epithelium of the vestibule can be seen, Hart's line. The vestibule is a mucosal epithelium and lacks hairs and sebaceous glands. On each side, the duct of the major vestibular gland, Bartholin's gland, can be seen sited between the hymenal ring and posterior part of the labium minus. The ducts of the minor vestibular glands, Skene's glands, open on either side of the urethral orifice. The epithelial surface is usually smooth, but occasionally tiny frond-like papillae may be seen distributed symmetrically laterally and posteriorly on the vestibule (Fig. 68.20). These vestibular papillae are a variant of normal and not related to HPV infection.

Normal flora

The skin of the perineal area has a higher pH, temperature and degree of humidity than skin elsewhere and, because of its proximity to the vagina and rectum, harbours many of the flora from these sites [1,2]. The main resident organisms are micrococci, diphtheroids and lactobacilli. Lactobacilli are probably the most common organisms, particularly on the labial mucosa, as the glycogenated epithelium of the vagina, under the influence of oestrogen, encourages colonization by them. The lactobacilli in turn metabolize the glycogen to lactic acid, which keeps the vaginal pH at approximately 4.5, restricting the growth of many organisms.

REFERENCES

1 Aly R. Microbial flora of the vulva. In: Elsner P, Martius J, eds. *Vulvovaginitis*. New York: Marcel Dekker, 1993: 19–28.

2 Mårdh P-A. The vaginal ecosystem. *Am J Obstet Gynecol* 1991; **165**: 1163–8.

tosis [6]. The last two suggest that HPV is implicated but the evidence now suggests that the known HPV types are not associated with these papillae [7–9]. Clinically, vestibular papillae are unlike the lesions induced by HPV as they are symmetrically arranged and each papilla has a solitary base. Histologically, problems arise if the pathologist is unaware that the tissue is the vestibule, which has heavily glycogenated epithelial cells that become vacuolated on processing and may resemble koilocytes. The problem is also compounded by the fact that koilocyte-like lesions can be found on vulval biopsies but these are not necessarily associated with HPV infection [10]. Currently, it is believed that this entity is a normal variant and the female equivalent of pearly penile papules.

Varicosities of the labial veins may occur unilaterally in association with limb varicosities, or appear in pregnancy. The other changes in pregnancy include a fall in the pH and increased pigmentation. At the menopause, vascularity decreases and the sebaceous glands become less active.

REFERENCES

1 Blair C. Angiokeratoma of the vulva. *Br J Dermatol* 1970; **83**: 409–11.
2 Rocamora A, Santonja C, Vives R *et al.* Sebaceous gland hyperplasia of the vulva: a case report. *Obstet Gynecol* 1986; **68** (Suppl.): 63–5.
3 Altmeyer P, Cliff GN, Holzmann H. Hirsutes papillaris vulvae (pseudokondylome der vulva). *Hautarzt* 1982; **33**: 281–3.
4 Khoda H, Hino Y, Fukuda H. Hirsutoid papillomas of vulva. *J Dermatol* 1986; **13**: 154–6.
5 Friedrich EG Jr. The vulvar vestibule. *J Reprod Med* 1983; **28**: 773–7.
6 Manoharon V, Somerville JM. Benign squamous papillomatosis: case report. *Genitourin Med* 1987; **63**: 393–5.
7 Bergeron C, Ferenczy A, Richart RM *et al.* Micropapillomatosis labialis appears unrelated to human papilloma virus. *Obstet Gynecol* 1990; **76**: 281–6.
8 Moyal-Barracco M, Leibowitch M, Orth G. Vestibular papillae of the vulva: lack of evidence for human papilloma virus aetiology. *Arch Dermatol* 1990; **126**: 1594–8.
9 Wilkinson EJ, Guerrero E, Daniel R *et al.* Vulvar vestibulitis is rarely associated with human papilloma virus infection types 6, 11, 16, or 18. *Int J Gynecol Pathol* 1993; **12**: 344–9.
10 Dennerstein GJ, Scurry JP, Garland SM *et al.* Human papilloma virus vulvitis: a new disease or an unfortunate mistake? *Br J Obstet Gynaecol* 1994; **101**: 992–8.

Congenital and developmental abnormalities [1]

Ambiguous external genitalia

In some individuals, the external genitalia are not phenotypically characteristic of either male or female. An attempt at classification of these abnormalities is based on aetiology and clinical syndromes; there are three main groups [2,3]:
1 Female hermaphroditism
2 Male pseudohermaphroditism
3 Abnormal external genitalia in females may also be associated with abnormalities of the upper reproductive tract or urinary system [4].

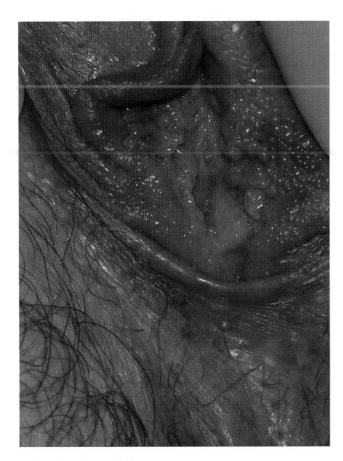

Fig. 68.20 Vestibular papillae.

Normal variants

Angiokeratomas are small vascular 1–4 mm papules found on the labia majora [1]. They vary in colour from red to blue-black and are normally asymptomatic, but can become quite large and bleed if traumatized, particularly in pregnancy.

Sebaceous gland hyperplasia is seen on the inner aspects of the labia majora and labia minora where the glands do not usually have an associated hair unit. The glands open directly onto the surface, and may be very prominent and numerous. The yellow uniform papules are often best seen when the skin is stretched. Prominent and numerous glands may be associated with pruritus. Occasionally, they can become very large and be mistaken for a sebaceous gland adenoma [2].

Vestibular papillomatosis is the term used to describe the occasional normal finding of myriad tiny filiform or soft frond-like projections on the vestibular epithelium and inner aspects of the labia minora. These lesions have had various names in the past, including papillomatosis labialis, hirsuties papillaris [3], hirsutoid papillomas of the vulva [4], vestibular papillae [5], pseudocondylomas, vestibular microwarts and vulval squamous papilloma-

Labial problems

There may be persistence of most caudal elements of the milk line in the labia majora, and there is great variation in the size and symmetry of normal labia minora. There may be very marked hypertrophy of the labia minora, some cases of which are examples of neurofibromatosis [5].

Labial adhesions may occur as an inherited familial trait [6] or in association with abnormal sexual differentiation. In general, most occur in the neonatal period and early infancy, and usually divide spontaneously by the time the child is 6 years old. No intervention is necessary unless there is a problem with urination. Some cases of labial adhesions result from lichen sclerosus.

Accessory labioscrotal folds are rare in women and are divided into two types, depending on whether or not there is an associated perineal lipoma [7].

The clitoris may be absent because of a failure of the genital tubercle to fuse, remain hypoplastic [8] or be enlarged because of congenital adrenal hyperplasia. The Lawrence–Seip syndrome, which is a congenital generalized lipodystrophy with the onset of insulin-resistant diabetes around the time of puberty, may also result in clitoral hypertrophy. There are clitoral tumours that may mimic genital sexual ambiguity (e.g. haemangioma, neurofibroma, lipoma [5,9–11]).

Virilization of the external genitalia may also occur with maternal ingestion of testosterone or synthetic progestogens in the first trimester, and if taken later in pregnancy there may be clitoral hypertrophy alone.

An imperforate hymen is usually discovered at puberty and is caused either by failure of the epithelial cells of the hymen to degenerate or by scarring after an inflammatory reaction in the hymen at birth.

REFERENCES

1 McLean JM. Embryology and congenital anomalies of the vulva. In: Ridley CM, Neill SM, eds. *The Vulva*, 2nd edn. Oxford: Blackwell Science, 1999: 1–36.
2 Grumbach MM, Conte FA. Disorders of sex differentiation. In: Wilson JD, Foster DW, eds. *Williams' Textbook of Endocrinology*, 8th edn. Philadelphia: Saunders, 1992: 853–951.
3 Simpson JL. Abnormal sexual differentiation in humans. *Ann Rev Genet* 1982; **16**: 193–224.
4 Warkany J. *Congenital Malformations*. Chicago: Year Book Medical, 1971.
5 Labardini MM, Kallet HA, Cerny JC. Urogenital neurofibromatosis simulating an intersex problem. *J Urol* 1968; **98**: 627–32.
6 Klein VR, Willman SP, Carr BR. Familial posterior labial fusion. *Obstet Gynecol* 1989; **73**: 500–2.
7 Sule JD, Skoog SJ, Tank ES. Perineal lipoma and the accessory labioscrotal fold: an aetiological relationship. *J Urol* 1994; **151**: 475–7.
8 Falk HC, Hyman AB. Congenital absence of clitoris: a case report. *Obstet Gynecol* 1971; **38**: 269–71.
9 Gersell DJ, Fulling KH. Localized neurofibromatosis of the female genitourinary tract. *Am J Surg Pathol* 1989; **13**: 873–8.
10 Kauffmann-Friedman K. Hemangioma of clitoris: confused with adrenogenital syndrome—a case report. *Plast Reconstr Surg* 1978; **62**: 452–4.
11 Haddad HM, Jones WH. Clitoral enlargement simulating pseudohermaphroditism. *Am J Dis Child* 1960; **99**: 282–7.

Trauma and artefact

Factitial dermatitis

There are various causes of vulval trauma, including accidental injury, obstetrical tears, damage at the time of surgery in a nearby site and coital and sexual mutilation, both cultural and self-induced [1–3].

Nymphohymenal tears induced by sexual intercourse are not uncommon and may mimic the symptoms of vulval vestibulodynia (see p. 68.82).

Sclerosing lipogranuloma [4] is a granulomatous response induced artefactually.

REFERENCES

1 Wilson KFG. Lower genital tract trauma. *Aust NZ J Obstet Gynecol* 1966; **6**: 291–3.
2 Reich LH, Wehr T. Female genital self-mutilation. *Obstet Gynecol* 1973; **41**: 239–42.
3 French AP, Nelson HL. Genital self-mutilation in women. *Arch Gen Psychiatry* 1972; **27**: 618–21.
4 Kempson RL, Sherman AI. Sclerosing lipogranuloma of the vulva. *Am J Obstet Gynecol* 1968; **101**: 854–6.

Female genital mutilation [1]

Ritual and cultural female genital mutilation (FGM), although banned in most European countries, is still forced on millions of women worldwide [2,3], particularly in Africa and in some countries where there is a large Muslim population. However, it is not practised in certain Muslim countries, including Saudi Arabia [4]. Although it is unusual in Western society, many cases are now being seen in the UK because of the rise in immigration of women who have had previous FGM.

There are four types of operation performed, which vary according to the country and culture:
1 *Circumcision*: removal of the clitoris or the clitoral hood (Sunna circumcision).
2 *Excision*: removal of the clitoris and part or all of the labia minora.
3 *Infibulation*: removal of the clitoris, labia minora and partial removal of the labia majora. The introitus is then sutured leaving a tiny opening for urination and menstruation.
4 Another type includes a variety of different practices. It might involve cauterization, applying corrosive material, piercing or cutting of the clitoris, surrounding skin or vagina.

FGM may be carried out at any age from the neonate to the adolescent. It is often performed without an anaesthetic in unhygienic circumstances. There may be damage to the urethra and vagina at the time of the operation, and later there may be severe damage to the urethra, bladder or anal sphincter during delivery in those that have had infibulation. Many of the women who have had FGM experience difficulties with sexual intercourse, urination and pregnancy and seek help in the clinics of their new country of residence, where unfortunately many of the health care professionals have not encountered their specific problem [5]. There are now a number of clinics being set up to deal specifically with these patients. The initial findings of a specialized clinic set up by a central London maternity unit found that many of the patients referred to them for problems in pregnancy were reluctant to volunteer the fact that they had been circumcised, and less than 10% refused to continue the tradition of FGM [6].

REFERENCES

1 Morrone A, Hercogova J, Lotti T. Stop female genital mutilation: appeal to the international dermatologic community. *Int J Dermatol* 2002; **41**: 253–63.
2 Macready N. Female genital mutilation outlawed in the United States. *BMJ* 1996; **313**: 1103.
3 Gallard C. Female genital mutilation in France. *BMJ* 1995; **310**: 1592–3.
4 Weins J. Female circumcision is curbed in Egypt. *BMJ* 1996; **313**: 249.
5 Chalmers B, Hashi KO. 432 Somali women's birth experiences in Canada after earlier female genital mutilation. *Birth* 2000; **27**: 227–34.
6 Momoh C, Ladhani S, Lochrie DP *et al.* Female genital mutilation: analysis of the first 12 months of a southeast London specialist clinic. *Br J Obstet Gynaecol* 2001; **108**: 186–91.

Dermatological manifestations of sexual abuse of children

Childhood sexual abuse is not the usual domain of the dermatologist, but occasionally it can be encountered when a dermatological opinion is sought on a genital skin problem. Lichen sclerosus and other dermatoses can be mistaken for sexual abuse [1–4], but sometimes the sexual abuse may be the initiating or exacerbating factor of the dermatological condition [5]. The possibility of sexual abuse sometimes has to be considered in a child whose lichen sclerosus, despite appropriate treatment and compliance, has not responded as expected. Sexual abuse always has to be excluded in the child who presents with a sexually transmitted disease [6,7], but conditions such as molluscum contagiosum, bacterial vaginosis [8] and genital warts are not necessarily indicative of sexual activity, and can be acquired by non-sexual means [9,10]. Genital warts in children may carry both genital and skin-type viruses [11]. If gonorrhoea or semen is found the situation is clear-cut, with the exception of neonatal infection and gonococcal eye disease [12]. Herpes simplex of the prepubertal genitalia is relatively uncommon [13] and sexual transmission may be implicated in both HSV-1 and -2 infections [14]. In a review of six cases, sexual abuse was proved in four. In the two innocently acquired cases, HSV-1 infection of the oral cavity immediately preceded the genital signs [15].

There are strict protocols for the examination and assessment of a child who is suspected to be a victim of sexual abuse [16]. It is important that this evaluation is carried out by a skilled specialist, usually a paediatrician [17].

HIV has rarely been reported as being transmitted by sexual abuse of children [18,19], but direct transmission is possible, and sexual abuse may be a risk factor for HIV in later life [20–22].

REFERENCES

1 Handfield Jones SE, Hinde FJR, Kennedy CTC. Lichen sclerosus et atrophicus in children misdiagnosed as sexual abuse. *BMJ* 1987; **294**: 1404–5.
2 Jenny C, Kirbu P, Furquay D. Genital lichen sclerosus mistaken for child sexual abuse. *Pediatrics* 1989; **83**: 597–9.
3 Hey F, Bucham PC, Littlewood JM, Hall RI. Differential diagnosis in child sexual abuse. *Lancet* 1986; **ii**; 792–6.
4 Levine V, Sanchez M, Nestor M. Localized vulvar pemphigoid in a child misdiagnosed as sexual abuse. *Arch Dermatol* 1992; **128**: 804–6.
5 Warrington SA, San Lazaro C. Lichen sclerosus et atrophicus and sexual abuse. *Arch Dis Child* 1996; **75**: 512–6.
6 Dattell BJ, Landers DV, Coulter K *et al.* Isolation of *Chlamydia trachomatis* from sexually abused female adolescents. *Obstet Gynecol* 1988; **72**: 240–2.
7 Herman-Giddens ME, Gutman LT, Berson N. Association of coexisting vaginal infections and multiple abusers in female children with genital warts. *Sex Transm Dis* 1988; **15**: 63–7.
8 Bump RC, Buesching WJ. Bacterial vaginosis in virginal and sexually active adolescent females: evidence against exclusive sexual transmission. *Am J Obstet Gynecol* 1988; **158**: 935–9.
9 Cohen BA, Honig P, Andophy E. Anogenital warts in children. *Arch Dermatol* 1990; **126**: 1575–80.
10 Obalek S, Misiewicz J, Jablonska S, Favre M, Orth G. Childhood condyloma acuminatum: association with genital and cutaneous infection with human papilloma viruses. *Pediatr Dermatol* 1993; **10**: 101–6.
11 Padel AF, Venning VA, Evans MF *et al.* Human papillomavirus in anogenital warts in children: typing by *in situ* hybridization. *BMJ* 1990; **300**: 1491–4.
12 Sgroi SM. Pediatric gonorrhoea and child sex abuse: the venereal disease connection. *Sex Transm Dis* 1982; **9**: 154–6.
13 Stumpf P. Increasing occurrence of condylomata acuminata in premenarchal children. *Obstet Gynecol* 1979; **56**: 562–4.
14 Gardner M, Jones JG. Genital herpes acquired by sexual abuse of children. *J Pediatr* 1984 ; **104**: 243–4.
15 Kaplan KM, Fleischer GP, Paradise JE *et al.* Social tolerance of genital herpes simplex in children. *Am J Dis Child* 1984; **138**: 872–4.
16 Royal College of Physicians of London. *Physical Signs of Sexual Abuse in Children*, 2nd edn. London: Royal College of Physicians, 1997.
17 Makoroff KL, Brauley JL, Brandner AM, Myers PA, Shapiro RA. Genital examinations for alleged sexual abuse of prepubertal girls: findings by pediatric emergency medicine physicians compared with child abuse trained physicians. *Child Abuse Negl* 2002; **26**: 1235–42.
18 Liedermann BA, Grimm KT. A child with HIV infection. *JAMA* 1986; **256**: 3904.
19 Straka BF, Whitaker DL, Morrison SH *et al.* Cutaneous manifestations of acquired immunodeficiency syndrome in children. *J Am Acad Dermatol* 1988; **18**: 1089–102.
20 Lindegren ML, Hanson IC, Hammett TA *et al.* Sexual abuse of children: intersection with the HIV epidemic. *Pediatrics* 1998; **102**: 967–8.
21 Allers CT, Benjack KJ, White J, Rousey JT. HIV vulnerability and the adult survivor of childhood sexual abuse. *Child Abuse Negl* 1993; **17**: 291–8.
22 Lyon ME, Richmond D, D'Angelo LJ. Is sexual abuse in childhood or adolescence a predisposing factor for HIV infection during adolescence? *Pediatr AIDS HIV Infect* 1995; **6**: 271–5.

Inflammatory dermatoses

Eczema

Atopic eczema can involve the vulva but the eczematous dermatoses affecting the vulva in isolation are seborrhoeic eczema, irritant contact dermatitis and allergic contact dermatitis.

Seborrhoeic eczema

This condition has both eczematous and psoriasiform features, sometimes making differentiation between it and psoriasis difficult. The inguinal and genitocrural folds, labia majora, mons pubis, perineal body and perianal skin are the usual sites involved. Vulval involvement may be associated with skin changes on the scalp and changes at other flexural sites. Histological examination is not always helpful, as there may be features of both eczema and psoriasis. There is moderate acanthosis with slight spongiosis and a mild dermal inflammatory infiltrate.

Irritant contact dermatitis

The barrier function of the vulval skin is impaired, as measured by transepidermal water loss [1], and there is an increased susceptibility to irritant contact eczema [2,3]. The problem may occur because of the dampness and maceration secondary to a heavy vaginal discharge, or increased contact with urine in the incontinent patient. Contact with irritant chemicals in topical agents, particularly cleansing agents, bubble baths, disinfectants, lubricants, perfumed products, deodorants and medicaments (e.g. 5-fluorouracil, podophyllotoxin and dequalinium), may all be responsible for an irritant dermatitis.

Allergic contact dermatitis

In spite of the frequent use of topical agents in the vulval area, allergic contact dermatitis is extremely rare in clinical practice. However, high incidences of contact dermatitis in vulval dermatoses have been reported [4,5]. An explanation for these unexpected high incidences may be that the patients in the studies had perianal skin involvement as well as vulval involvement, and allergic contact dermatitis to topical medicaments is more frequently encountered in perianal skin. One study has shown a higher incidence of positive patch tests in patients with anogenital dermatoses if both the genital and perianal areas are involved, compared with dermatoses affecting the genital skin alone [6].

There are reports of allergy to vaginal preparations and an intrauterine device [7–9], sanitary wear [10] and condoms [11]. Oestradiol may rarely cause a localized allergic contact dermatitis at a transdermal patch site, or generalized contact dermatitis with oral therapy [12].

Allergic contact urticaria

The two most common causes of contact urticaria in the vulvovaginal area are latex and semen [13], and there is usually a history of atopy [14]. Seminal fluid usually induces an urticarial immediate type I reaction and rarely produces a type IV contact allergy. There are reports of mixed sensitivities: one patient was allergic to semen and latex and another to her husband's semen and sweat [15,16]. However, semen itself may not be the responsible allergen, the problem being caused by a medication or other allergen carried in the seminal fluid [17–19]. Specific immunotherapy against semen has been successfully employed on occasion [20]. A fixed eruption to seminal fluid has been reported [21], and familial allergy to semen [22].

REFERENCES

1 Elsner P, Wilhelm D, Maibach HI. Physiological skin surface water loss dynamics of human vulvar and forearm skin. *Acta Derm Venereol (Stockh)* 1990; **70**: 141–4.
2 Britz MB, Maibach HI. Human cutaneous vulvar reactivity to irritants. *Contact Dermatitis* 1979; **5**: 375–7.
3 Elsner P, Wilhelm D, Maibach HI. Multiple paramater assessment of vulvar irritant contact dermatitis. *Contact Dermatitis* 1990; **23**: 20–6.
4 Marren P, Wojnarowska F, Powell S. Allergic contact dermatitis and vulvar dermatoses. *Br J Dermatol* 1992; **126**: 52–6.
5 Lewis FM, Harrington CI, Gawkrodger DJ. Contact sensitivity in pruritus vulvae: a common and manageable problem. *Contact Dermatitis* 1994; **31**: 264–5.
6 Goldsmith PC, Rycroft RJ, White IR et al. Contact sensitivity in women with anogenital dermatoses. *Contact Dermatitis* 1997; **36**: 174–5.
7 Robin J. Contact dermatitis to acetarsol. *Contact Dermatitis* 1978; **4**: 309–10.
8 Romaguera C, Grimalt F. Contact dermatitis from a copper-containing IUD. *Contact Dermatitis* 1981; **7**: 163–4.
9 Corazza M, Vigili A, Mantovani L. Vulval contact dermatitis to nifuratel. *Contact Dermatitis* 1992; **27**: 273–7.
10 Sterry W, Schmoll M. Contact urticaria and dermatitis from self-adhesive pads. *Contact Dermatitis* 1985; **13**: 284–8.
11 Bircher AJ, Hirsbrunner P, Langauer S. Allergic contact dermatitis of the genitals to additives in condoms. *Contact Dermatitis* 1993; **28**: 125–6.
12 Corazza M, Mantovani L, Montanari A Virgili A. Allergic contact dermatitis from transdermal estradiol and systemic contact dermatitis from oral estradiol. *J Reprod Med* 2002; **47**: 507–9.
13 Schimkat H-G, Meynadier JM, Meynadier J. Contact urticaria. In: Elsner P, Martius J, eds. *Vulvovaginitis*. New York: Marcel Dekker, 1993: 85–110.
14 Mathias CGT, Frick OL, Caldwell TM et al. Immediate hypersensitivity to seminal fluid and atopic dermatitis. *Arch Dermatol* 1980; **116**: 209–12.
15 Kint B, Degreef H, Dooms-Goossens A. Combined allergy to human seminal plasma and latex: case report and review of the literature. *Contact Dermatitis* 1994; **30**: 7–11.
16 Freeman S. Woman allergic to husband's sweat and semen. *Contact Dermatitis* 1986; **14**: 110–2.
17 Green RL, Green MA. Post-coital urticaria in a penicillin-sensitive patient: possible seminal transfer of penicillin. *JAMA* 1985; **254**: 531.
18 Sell MB. Sensitization to thioridazine through sexual intercourse. *Am J Psychiatry* 1985; **142**: 271–2.
19 Paladine WJ, Cunningham TJ, Donovan MA, Dumper CW. Possible sensitivity to vinblastine in prostatic or seminal fluid [Letter]. *N Engl J Med* 1975; **292**: 52.
20 Boom BW, van Toorenenbergen AW, Nierop G et al. A case of seminal fluid allergy successfully treated with immunotherapy in a one day rush procedure. *J Dermatol* 1991; **18**: 206–10.
21 Best CL, Waters C, Adelman DC. Fixed cutaneous eruption to seminal plasma challenge. *Fertil Steril* 1988; **50**: 532–4.
22 Chang T. Familial allergic seminal vulvovaginitis. *Am J Obstet Gynecol* 1976; **126**: 442–4.

Psoriasis

The pattern of psoriasis affecting the anogenital skin is

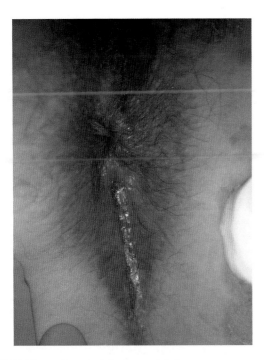

Fig. 68.21 Fissured psoriasis in the natal cleft.

most frequently flexural. The areas involved include the genitocrural folds, mons pubis, outer aspects of the labia majora, the perianal skin and the natal cleft (Fig. 68.21). The characteristic silvery scaling is absent in these occluded sites and the main clinical picture is intense erythema with a well-defined margin. Rarely, there may be some scarring associated with vulval psoriasis with loss of the labia minora and fusion of the clitoral hood.

The histology is not always typical, and there may be marked spongiosis and papillary oedema.

Reiter's disease (circinate ulcerative vulvitis)

Circinate balanitis is well recognized but the corresponding vulvitis is much rarer [1–4]. The lesions may be eroded, ulcerative or scaly. Histologically, the changes are of those seen in pustular psoriasis [5], with hyperkeratosis, parakeratosis, psoriasiform hyperplasia, an absent granular layer and collections of polymorphs in the epidermis.

REFERENCES

1 Thambar IV, Dunlop R, Thin RN *et al.* Circinate vulvitis in Reiter's syndrome. *Br J Vener Dis* 1977; **53**: 260–2.
2 Daunt O'N, Kotowski KE, O'Reilly AP *et al.* Ulcerative vulvitis in Reiter's syndrome: a case report. *Br J Vener Dis* 1982; **58**: 405–7.
3 Haake N, Altmeyer P. Vulvovaginitis circinata bei morbus Reiter. *Hautarzt* 1988; **39**: 748–9.
4 Edwards L, Hansen RC. Reiter's syndrome of the vulva. *Arch Dermatol* 1992; **128**: 811–4.
5 Kanerva L, Kouse M, Niema KM *et al.* Ultrahistopathology of balanitis circinate. *Br J Vener Dis* 1982; **58**: 185–95.

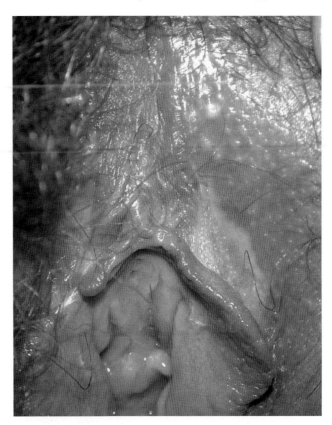

Fig. 68.22 White patches of lichen planus in the interlabial sulci.

Lichen planus [1–3]

Lichen planus (LP) can affect the vulva in isolation or at the same time as a generalized outbreak, when approximately 20% of patients will have genital lesions. The vulval lesions are similar to those seen at other sites and may be violaceous or erythematous papules, white (Fig. 68.22) or annular plaques, and erosions with or without a lacy white border. These lesions may all ulcerate. Wickham's striae occur infrequently (Fig. 68.23). If the vulva is affected in isolation, the disease is more often erosive, with most of the lesions around the labia minora, clitoris and clitoral hood. Confluent white and red patches will also be seen in this variant. A careful examination of the oral mucosae is helpful, as LP be may found on the tongue, palate, gingivae and lateral buccal mucosae.

The other clinical forms of vulval LP include the following.
1 *Pigmented flexural lichen planus* (Fig. 68.24). This variant of LP can affect the vulval area, particularly the mons pubis, the inguinal and genitocrural folds. The characteristic and striking finding is brown pigmented patches, some so deeply pigmented that they resemble melanocytic naevi. If the disease is seen in the early stages, a violaceous erythema is also observed. This form of LP is also found in the inframammary areas and axillae.

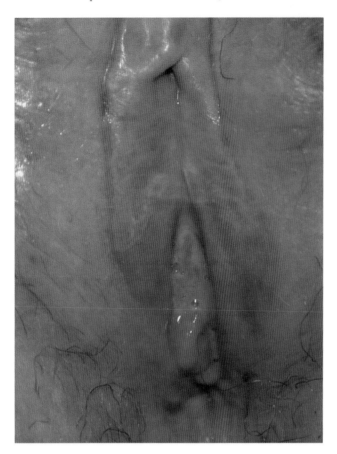

Fig. 68.23 Delicate white striae of lichen planus, with the labia minora flattening and fusing into the surrounding skin.

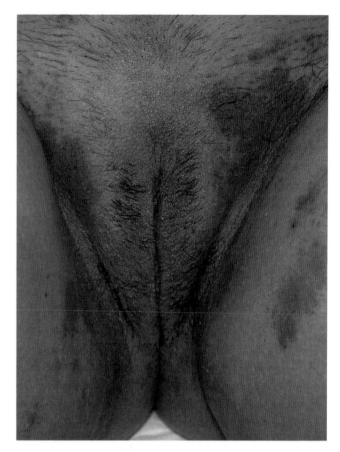

Fig. 68.24 Patches of pigmented flexural lichen planus.

2 *Vulvovaginal–gingival lichen planus* (VVG-LP) (syndrome of Hewitt and Pelisse; desquamative vaginitis). This distinctive erosive form of LP is clinically very similar to mucous membrane pemphigoid [4,5]. In the past, many cases labelled desquamative vaginitis were probably this entity [6,7]. VVG-LP principally affects the inner aspects of the labia minora, vestibule and vagina. The condition is chronic and painful, and there is an increase in vaginal discharge, dysuria, dyspareunia and postcoital bleeding. Clinically, the epithelia are eroded and often there is a distinctive fine white lacy border. There may be marked loss of architecture (Fig. 68.25). The anal margin may also be involved. The vaginal lesions are velvety red erosions or bright red, glazed erythema, which is friable and bleeds when touched. Vaginal synechiae and adhesions develop, leading in some cases to vaginal stenosis. The cervix may also be involved [5,8,9]. Oral LP lesions can occur at any site, but the characteristic finding is an intense erythema of the gingivae, which may be asymptomatic (Fig. 68.26). Unusual extragenital lesions have been described on the conjunctiva [10], lachrymal gland canal [11], oesophagus [12–15] and the auditory canal [16]. The manifestations of this syndrome do not necessarily all occur synchronously. 3 *Lichen planopilaris* has been described on the vulva [17].

Histopathology. On cornified epithelium there is hyperkeratosis, irregular acanthosis with a typical saw-tooth appearance of the rete pegs, an increased granular layer, and disruption of the basal layer with a closely apposed dermal band-like lymphocytic infiltrate. The acanthosis and hyperkeratosis are marked in the hypertrophic form and, because of the chronicity of this form, the characteristic band-like infiltrate is not obvious but will be found focally. Eosinophilic colloid bodies may be seen. Immunofluorescence studies reveal uneven staining of the basement membrane zone for fibrinogen and IgM, cytoid bodies and, on occasion, IgG or IgA.

Differential diagnosis. The main differential diagnosis is usually lichen sclerosus, but mucous membrane pemphigoid and morphoea could also be included. In some cases, the differentiation between lichen sclerosus (LS) and LP can be extremely difficult, even impossible, as the two diseases share so many features in common [18,19]. If a definite diagnosis cannot be made on a combination of clinical, histological and immunofluorescence findings and response to treatment, it is perhaps best to allocate the case as an overlap of the two disorders. Frequently, there are cases of LP misdiagnosed as Zoon's vulvitis.

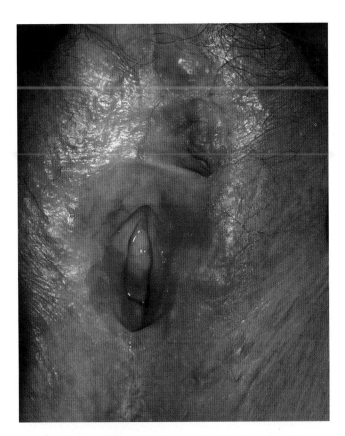

Fig. 68.25 Lichen planus: vulval aspect showing glazed erythema and distortion of the architecture, with a remnant of the left labium minus and buried clitoris above it.

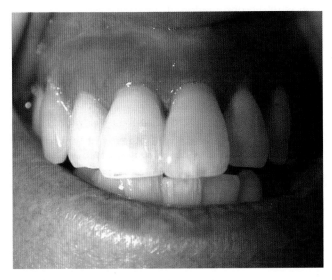

Fig. 68.26 Lichen planus. Intense glazed erythema of gingiva.

Treatment. First-line treatment is with potent topical steroids. If the vagina is involved, a topical steroid can be introduced with a vaginal applicator, or steroid foams or suppositories that are available for inflammatory bowel

conditions can be used [20,21]. Topical retinoids are useful for hyperkeratotic and hypertrophic LP, and recently topical tacrolimus has been used [22]. Other treatments tried with variable success include oral steroids, oral and topical retinoids, methotrexate [23], ciclosporin [24] and azathioprine.

REFERENCES

1 Edwards L. Vulvar lichen planus. *Arch Dermatol* 1989; **125**: 1677–80.
2 Lewis FM, Shah M, Harrington CI. Vulval involvement in lichen planus: a study of 37 women *Br J Dermatol* 1996; **135**: 89–91.
3 Ridley CM, Neill SM. Non-infective cutaneous conditions of the vulva. In: Ridley CM, Neill SM, eds. *The Vulva*. Oxford: Blackwell Science, 1999: 164–8.
4 Pelisse M, Leibowitch M, Sedel D *et al.* Un nouveau syndrome vulvo-vagino-gingival: lichen plan erosif plurimuqueux. *Ann Dermatol Vénéréol* 1982; **109**: 797–8.
5 Eisen D. The vulvovaginal–gingival syndrome: the clinical characteristics of 22 patients. *Arch Dermatol* 1994; **130**: 1379–82.
6 Edwards L, Friedrich EG. Desquamative vaginitis: lichen planus in disguise. *Obstet Gynecol* 1988; **71**: 32–6.
7 Ridley CM. Chronic erosive vulval disease. *Clin Exp Dermatol* 1990; **15**: 245–52.
8 Gougerot H, Burnier R. Lichen plan du col uterin, accompagnant un lichen plan jugalet un lichen plan stomacal: lichen plurimuqueux sans lichen cutane. *Bull Soc Francaise Dermatol Syphiligr* 1937; **44**: 637–40.
9 Pelisse M. Erosive vulvar lichen planus and desquamative vaginitis. *Semin Dermatol* 1996; **15**: 47–50.
10 Moyal-Barracco M, Lautier-Frau M, Bechéral PA *et al.* Lichen plan conjunctival: une observation. *Ann Dermatol Vénéréol* 1993; **120**: 857–9.
11 McNab AA. Lacrimal gland canalicular obstruction in lichen planus. *Orbit* 1998; **17**: 201–2.
12 Sheehan-Dare RA, Cotterill JA, Simmons AV. Oesophageal lichen planus. *Br J Dermatol* 1986; **115**: 729–30.
13 Dickens CM, Hesletine D, Walton S *et al.* The oesophagus in lichen planus: an endoscopic study. *BMJ* 1990; **300**: 84.
14 Bobadilla J, van der Hulst RW, ten Kate FJ. Oesophageal lichen planus. *Gastrointest Endosc* 1999; **50**: 268–71.
15 Menges M, Hohloch K, Pueschel W, Stallmach A. Lichen planus with oesophageal involvement: a case report and review of the literature. *Digestion* 2002; **65**: 184–9.
16 Martin L, Moriniere S, Machet M-C. Bilateral conductive deafness related to erosive lichen planus. *J Laryngol Otol* 1998; **112**: 365–6.
17 Grunald MH, Zvulunov A, Halevy S. Lichen planopilaris of the vulva. *Br J Dermatol* 1998; **136**: 477–8.
18 Marren P, Millard P, Chia Y, Wojnarowska F. Mucosal lichen sclerosus/lichen planus overlap syndromes. *Br J Dermatol* 1994; **131**: 118–23.
19 Fung MA, LeBoit PE. Light microscopic criteria for the diagnosis of early vulvar lichen sclerosus: a comparison with lichen planus. *Am J Surg Pathol* 1998; **22**: 473–8.
20 Anderson M, Kutzner S, Kaufman R. Treatment of vulvovaginal lichen planus with vaginal hydrocortisone suppositories. *Obstet Gynecol* 2002; **100**: 359–62.
21 Sobel JD. Treatment of vulvovaginal lichen planus with hydrocortisone suppositories. *Curr Infect Dis Rep* 2002; **4**: 507–8.
22 Kirtschig G, Van Der Meulen AJ, Ion Lipan JW, Stoof TJ. Successful treatment of erosive vulvovaginal lichen planus with topical tacrolimus [Letter]. *Br J Dermatol* 2002; **147**: 625–6.
23 Nylander-Lunqvist E, Wahlin YB, Hofer PA. Methotrexate supplemented with steroid ointments for the treatment of severe erosive lichen ruber. *Acta Dermatol Venereol* 2002; **82**: 63–4.
24 Borrego L, Ruiz-Rodriguez R, Ortiz de Frutos J. Vulvar lichen planus treated with topical cyclosporin. *Arch Dermatol* 1993; **129**: 794.

Zoon's vulvitis

It is likely that plasma cell vulvitis (PCV; vulvitis

circumscripta plasmacellularis) is not a single disease entity but represents a reaction pattern to another inflammatory condition. A plasma cell-rich infiltrate in a vestibular biopsy may be a misleading finding, because plasma cells are commonly found in inflammatory conditions of the vestibule as it is a mucosal epithelium.

Many of the cases are examples of unrecognized dermatoses such as LP, and in others the persistent change may represent a chronic post-inflammatory phenomenon.

The first descriptions of the female equivalent of ZB were by Garnier and Zoon [1–3]. The lesions described in these reports were erythematous patches with a glazed appearance, with the histological findings of a plasma cell-rich dermal infiltrate and no cytological atypia. The disorder followed a chronic but benign course. The disorder appears to be less common in women, and in one series of 20 cases there was only one female [4].

Most of the reports of this condition in women describe the lesions in the vestibule and labia minora, whereas the typical site in men is the glans and prepuce. The glans clitoris is rarely, if ever, affected.

Histology. The criteria needed to make the diagnosis have varied in the literature, and there is some doubt whether PCV is a distinct clinicopathological entity, as many of the reports of vestibular Zoon's are probably LP [5].

The essential features are epidermal thinning, absent horny and granular layers and distinctive lozenge-shaped keratinocytes with widened intercellular spaces; in the dermis there is a dense inflammatory infiltrate composed largely of plasma cells, with dilated blood vessels and usually much haemosiderin. Russell bodies and dermal–epidermal splitting have also been described [6].

Treatment. Treatment depends on the underlying inflammatory dermatosis responsible for this histological change. In the majority of cases this is LP, and a potent topical steroid should be tried. If the inflammatory phase of disease has resolved and the patient is complaining of a sensation of rawness or burning, then topical 5% lidocaine can be effective. Finally, a barrier ointment such as Vaseline petroleum jelly may offer some relief if there is an irritant component to the problem.

Chronic vulval purpura

It is not uncommon to find patients with purpuric patches, often at the vestibule, in which haemosiderin and plasma cells are found without any specific epidermal change, and the term chronic vulval purpura may be a more accurate description [7]. An association with lichen aureus has been suggested, as pressure factors are thought to be relevant in the extravasation of blood [8].

REFERENCES

1 Garnier G. Vulvite erythemateuse circonscrite benigne a type erythroplasique. *Bull Soc Francaise Dermatol Syphilogr* 1954; **61**: 102–3.
2 Zoon JJ. Balanitis and vulvitis plasma cellularis. *Dermatologica* 1955; **111**: 157.
3 Garnier G. Benign plasma cell erythroplasia. *Br J Dermatol* 1957; **69**: 77–81.
4 Souteyrand P, Wong E, MacDonald DM. Zoon's balanitis (balanitis circumscripta plasmacellularis). *Br J Dermatol* 1981; **105**: 195–9.
5 Scurry J, Dennerstein G, Brennan J et al. Vulvitis circumscripta plasmacellularis: a clinicopathologic entity? *J Reprod Med* 1993; **38**: 14–8.
6 Woodruff JD, Sussman J, Shakfeh S. Vulvitis circumscripta plasmacellularis: a report of four cases. *J Reprod Med* 1989; **34**: 369–72.
7 Kato T, Kuramoto Y, Tadaki T et al. Chronic vulvar purpura. *Dermatologica* 1990; **180**: 174–6.
8 Kossard S, Shumack S. Lichen aureus of the glans penis as an expression of Zoon's balanitis. *J Am Acad Dermatol* 1989; **21**: 804–6.

Lichen sclerosus [1–6]

Lichen sclerosus (LS) was first described as a variant of LP with a tendency to affect the genital area. The old terms leukoplakia, leukoplakic vulvitis and kraurosis vulvae were clearly applied to examples of LS or LP, and the use of these terms led to confusion. The term vulval dystrophy was introduced in the 1960s in an attempt to overcome the problems in distinguishing and classifying vulval dermatoses characterized by pallor and scarring [7]. This terminology unfortunately proved unsuccessful in its objectives, as its use discouraged attempts to differentiate between disorders such as LS, LP and mucous membrane pemphigoid. In 1983, the Terminology Committee of the International Society for the Study of Vulvovaginal Dermatoses recommended a new classification with discontinuation of the term dystrophy [8]. The term vulval squamous cell hyperplasia was introduced with this classification (see p. 68.49).

Aetiology and pathogenesis. The aetiology is still unknown but there is mounting evidence that LS is a genetically determined autoimmune disorder. A positive family history is recognized [9] and the disorder has been described in twins, both identical [10] and non-identical [11]. An association of LS in females with other autoimmune disease has been noted [12–14]. Attempts to establish a specific HLA linkage in patients with LS were initially inconclusive [15] but a later study has shown an increased incidence of DQ7 [16]. Similar findings have been reported in LS in girls [17].

The role of *Borrelia burgdorferi* as an aetiological trigger is controversial. A study in the UK showed no evidence histologically of spirochaetes but did show 'cocci' with a Fite stain, which later proved to be mast cells when stained with toluidine blue [18].

Clinical features. LS can affect females of any age, but the majority of patients are either prepubertal or menopausal. There is still uncertainty whether LS in prepubertal girls

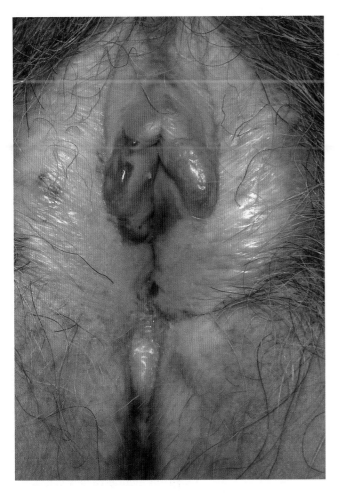

Fig. 68.27 Oedema and ecchymosis of lichen sclerosus.

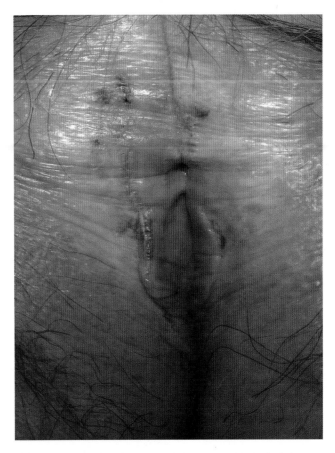

Fig. 68.28 Lichen sclerosus. Pallor and atrophy of the vulval skin with loss of the labia minora and burying of the clitoris.

remits spontaneously at puberty. The presenting symptom is usually itching, which is often severe and distressing.

The classical lesions seen on the extragenital skin are ivory white papules and plaques with follicular delling. Anogenital disease tends to be characterized by flatter lesions of atrophic whitened epithelium, which may become confluent, extending around the vulval and perianal skin in a figure-of-eight configuration. There may also be oedema, ecchymosis, bullae, erosions and ulceration (Fig. 68.27). The sites most commonly affected are the genito-crural folds, the inner aspects of the labia majora, labia minora, clitoris and clitoral hood. Vestibular involvement is rare and vaginal lesions do not occur, as LS seems to spare non-cornified stratified squamous epithelia (mucosal epithelium). Perianal lesions occur in approximately 30% of female patients, in contrast with men who do not seem to develop perianal involvement. Extragenital lesions occur in 10% of women with vulval disease. The extragenital areas may be truncal, at sites of pressure, upper back, wrists, buttocks and thighs. The Koebner phenomenon has also been reported at sites of

radiotherapy [19], scar tissue [20], vaccination [21] and congenital haemangioma [22]. Facial [23], scalp [24] and nail involvement [25,26] have been recorded.

Lesions of LS in the oral cavity are extremely rare. Many of the reports of oral involvement in the literature have often not been confirmed histologically [27] and may have been examples of LP. It is not uncommon for patients with vulval LS to have coexistent oral LP [28].

The author (SMN) has seen two cases of oral LS, confirmed histologically, and both were on the tongue. This is one of the few sites in the mouth that has cornified stratified squamous epithelium.

LS is a scarring dermatosis and the changes that can occur on the vulva include loss of the labia minora, and sealing over of the clitoral hood, burying the clitoris (Fig. 68.28). Introital narrowing resulting from anterior and posterior labial fusion sometimes results in a tiny opening into the vestibule. Milia may occur [29].

Histology. The classic histology is a thinned epidermis with flattening of the rete pegs. The underlying dermis is hyalinized and there are often extravasated red cells. Below the hyalinized area is a band-like zone of chronic inflammatory cells. There is an absence of elastic fibres in the upper dermis. There have been attempts to grade the histological appearances [30] but there is probably little correlation between the timing of a lesion and its histological appearance [31].

In some cases the epidermis is thickened, and this is LS with squamous cell hyperplasia. It is found in approximately 30% of cases of LS in association with vulval SCC [32].

There are abnormalities of the basement membrane, but it is uncertain whether these are a primary or secondary event [33]. Immunofluorescence studies are usually negative or demonstrate non-specific fibrin deposition at the dermal–epidermal junction. There is also an alteration of the elastin and fibrillin in the affected dermis [34].

Differential diagnosis. Vitiligo, mucous membrane pemphigoid, LP and morphoea may present with a similar clinical appearance. There can be clinical and histological overlap between morphoea, LP and LS, and they may represent a spectrum of disease rather than three distinct conditions [35,36].

Lichen sclerosus and vulval malignancy

There is undoubtedly an association between vulval SCC and LS that was probably underestimated in the past (Fig. 68.29) [37]. The incidence of SCC developing on LS in clinical practice is of the order of 4% or less [1]. However, in retrospective reviews of pathological specimens of vulval carcinoma, histological evidence of LS is found in approximately half of the cases [37–40]. These series included patients presenting with SCC as well as those on long-term follow-up. A longitudinal cohort study of 211 patients showed that the number of invasive SCCs significantly exceeded that in an age-matched group [41]. It is not known whether good control of LS reduces this risk.

There appears to be a bimodal pattern for vulval SCC. In younger women the tumour is associated as a rule with oncogenic types of HPV and intraepithelial neoplasia, and in the older woman with a chronic dermatosis without evidence of HPV infection [42–44].

The histological patterns associated with SCC arising on LS include epithelial hyperplasia and differentiated intraepithelial neoplasia (dysplastic changes that are confined to the basal layers) [45].

LS has been reported in association with verrucous carcinoma [46,47], basal cell carcinoma [48] and melanoma [49]. However, malignant melanoma is known to be difficult to diagnose in the presence of LS [50], and the validity of the case report of an association between malignant melanoma and LS was questioned [51]. However, the original authors upheld their view.

Treatment [52,53]. The current and recommended treat-

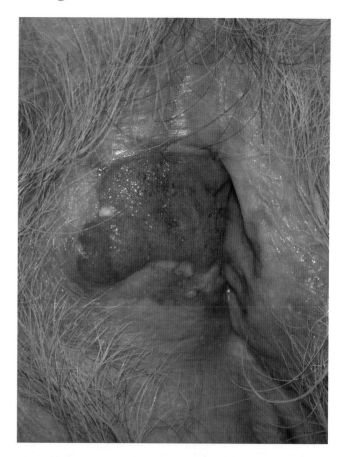

Fig. 68.29 Squamous cell carcinoma arising on a background of lichen sclerosus.

ment for uncomplicated LS is the potent topical corticosteroid, clobetasol propionate. There are no randomized controlled trials providing evidence for any particular corticosteroid or treatment regimen being more effective than any other. The regimen recommended by the author (SMN) for a newly diagnosed case is initially clobetasol propionate once nightly for 4 weeks, then alternate nights for 4 weeks, and twice a week for a further month. A 30-g tube of clobetasol propionate should last 12 weeks, and the patient is then reviewed. The clobetasol propionate is then used as and when required to control itching. Most patients seem to require 30–60 g annually. A proportion of patients go into complete remission and do not require further treatment. Others will continue to have flares and remissions and they are advised to use clobetasol propionate as required. A soap substitute is also recommended and an information sheet on LS, including instructions for the use of the topical steroid, is provided.

Topical testosterone currently has no role in the management of LS. It is expensive and is not as effective as clobetasol propionate [54].

Surgical excision is not necessary in the management of most cases of LS and it should be used exclusively for the management of functional problems caused by post-inflammatory scarring [55,56], premalignant lesions and malignancy.

REFERENCES

1 Wallace HJ. Lichen sclerosus et atrophicus. *Trans St John's Hosp Dermatol Soc* 1971; **57**: 9–30.

2 Tremaine RDL, Miller RAW. Lichen sclerosus et atrophicus. *Int J Dermatol* 1989; **28**: 10–6.

3 Meffert JJ, Davis BM, Grimwood RE. Lichen sclerosus. *J Am Acad Dermatol* 1995; **32**: 393–416.

4 Ridley CM, Neill SM. Non-infective cutaneous conditions of the vulva. In: Ridley CM, Neill SM, eds. *The Vulva*. Oxford: Blackwell Science, 1999: 154–6.

5 Powell JJ, Wojnarowska F. Lichen sclerosus. *Lancet* 1999; **353**: 1777–83.

6 Ridley CM. Genital lichen sclerosus (lichen sclerosus et atrophicus) in childhood and adolescence. *J R Soc Med* 1993; **86**: 69–75.

7 Jeffcoate TNA, Woodcock AS. Premalignant conditions of the vulva, with particular reference to chronic epithelial dystrophies. *BMJ* 1961; **ii**: 127–34.

8 Wilkinson EJ, Kneale B, Lynch PJ. Report of the ISSVD terminology committee. *J Reprod Med* 1986; **31**: 973–4.

9 Friedrich EG Jr, MacLaren NK. Genetic aspects of vulvar lichen sclerosus. *Am J Obstet Gynecol* 1984; **150**: 161–6.

10 Meyrick-Thomas RH, Meyrick-Thomas RH, Kennedy CTC. The development of lichen sclerosus et atrophicus in monozygotic twin girls. *Br J Dermatol* 1986; **114**: 377–9.

11 Cox NH, Mitchell JNS, Morley WN. Lichen sclerosus et atrophicus in non-identical female twins. *Br J Dermatol* 1986; **115**: 743.

12 Goolamali SK, Barnes EW, Irvine WJ *et al.* Organ-specific antibodies in patients with lichen sclerosus. *BMJ* 1974; **iv**: 78–9.

13 Harrington CI, Dunsmore IR. An investigation into the incidence of auto-immune disorders in patients with lichen sclerosus et atrophicus. *Br J Dermatol* 1981; **104**: 563–6.

14 Meyrick Thomas RH, Ridley CM, McGibbon DH *et al.* Lichen sclerosus et atrophicus and autoimmunity. *Br J Dermatol* 1988; **118**: 41–6.

15 Purcell KG, Spencer LV, Simpson PM *et al.* HLA antigens in lichen sclerosus et atrophicus. *Arch Dermatol* 1990; **126**: 1043–5.

16 Marren P, Yell J, Charnock FM *et al.* The association between lichen sclerosus and antigens of the HLA system. *Br J Dermatol* 1995; **132**: 197–203.

17 Powell J, Wojnarowska F, Winsey S *et al.* Lichen sclerosus premenarche: autoimmunity and immunogenetics. *Br J Dermatol* 2000; **142**: 481–4.

18 Farrell AM, Millard PR, Schomberg KH, Wojnarowska F. An infective aeti-ology for vulval lichen sclerosus re-addressed. *Clin Exp Dermatol* 1999; **24**: 479–83.

19 Yates VM, King CM, Dave VK. Lichen sclerosus et atrophicus following radiation therapy. *Arch Dermatol* 1985; **121**: 1044–7.

20 Pass CJ. An unusual variant of lichen sclerosus et atrophicus: delayed appearance in a surgical scar. *Cutis* 1984; **33**: 405–8.

21 Anderton RL, Abele DC. Lichen sclerosus et atrophicus in a vaccination site. *Arch Dermatol* 1976; **112**: 1787.

22 Ostlere LS, Tildsley G, Holden CA. Lichen sclerosus over a strawberry naevus: a new example of the Koebner phenomenon? [Letter]. *Clin Exp Dermatol* 1996; **21**: 394–5.

23 Dalziel K, Reynolds AJ, Holt PJA. Lichen sclerosus et atrophicus with ocular and maxillary complications. *Br J Dermatol* 1983; **116**: 735–7.

24 Foulds IS. Lichen sclerosus et atrophicus of the scalp. *Br J Dermatol* 1980; **103**: 197–200.

25 Kossard S, Cornish N. Localized lichen sclerosus with nail loss. *Australas J Dermatol* 1998; **39**: 119–20.

26 Noda Cabrera A, Saez Rodriguea M, Garcia-Bustinduy M *et al.* Localized lichen sclerosus of the finger without nail dystrophy. *Dermatology* 2002; **205**: 303–4.

27 Brown AR, Dunlap CL, Bussard DA *et al.* Lichen sclerosus of the oral cavity: a report of two cases. *Oral Surg Oral Med Oral Pathol Oral Radiol Endod* 1997; **84**: 165–70.

28 Marren P, Millard P, Chia Y *et al.* Mucosal lichen sclerosus/lichen planus overlap. *Br J Dermatol* 1994; **131**: 118–23.

29 Leppard B, Sneddon IB. Milia occurring in lichen sclerosus et atrophicus. *Br J Dermatol* 1975; **92**: 711–4.

30 Hewitt J. Histologic criteria for lichen sclerosus of the vulva. *J Reprod Med* 1986; **31**: 781–7.

31 Marren P, Millard PR, Wojnarowska F. Vulval lichen sclerosus: lack of correlation between duration of clinical symptoms and histological appearances. *J Eur Acad Dermatol Venereol* 1997; **8**: 212–6.

32 Hart WR, Norris HJ, Helwig EB. Relation of lichen sclerosus et atrophicus of the vulva to development of squamous cell carcinoma. *Obstet Gynecol* 1975; **45**: 369–77.

33 Marren P, Dean D, Charnock M *et al.* Basement membrane zone in lichen sclerosus: an immunohistological study. *Br J Dermatol* 1997; **136**: 508–14.

34 Farrell AM, Dean D, Millard PR, Charnock FM, Wojnarowska F. Alterations in fibrillin as well as collagens I and III and elastin occur in vulval lichen sclerosus. *J Eur Acad Dermatol Venereol* 2001; **15**: 212–7.

35 Shono S, Imura M, Ota M *et al.* Lichen sclerosus et atrophicus, morphea, and coexistence of both diseases. *Arch Dermatol* 1991; **127**: 1352–6.

36 Connelly MG, Winkelmann RK. Coexistence of lichen sclerosus, morphea and lichen planus: report of 4 cases and review of the literature. *J Am Acad Dermatol* 1985; **12**: 844–51.

37 Zaki I, Dalziel KL, Solomons FA *et al.* The under-reporting of skin disease in association with squamous cell carcinoma of the vulva. *Clin Exp Dermatol* 1997; **21**: 334–7.

38 Walkden V, Chia Y, Wojnarowska F. The association of squamous cell car-cinoma of the vulva and lichen sclerosus: implications for management and follow-up. *J Obstet Gynecol* 1997; **17**: 551–3.

39 Leibowitch M, Neill S, Pelisse M, Moyal-Barracco M. The epithelial changes associated with squamous cell carcinoma of the vulva: a review of the clin-ical, histological and viral findings in 78 women. *Br J Obstet Gynaecol* 1990; **97**: 1135–9.

40 Vilmer C, Cavelier-Balloy B, Nogues C, Trassard M, Le Doussal V. Analysis of alterations adjacent to invasive vulvar cancer and their relationship with the associated carcinoma: a study of 67 cases. *Eur J Gynecol Oncol* 1998; **19**: 25–31.

41 Carli P, Cattaneo A, de Magnis A *et al.* Squamous cell carcinoma arising in lichen sclerosus: a longitudinal cohort study. *Eur J Cancer Prev* 1995; **4**: 491–5.

42 Crum CP. Carcinoma of the vulva: epidemiology and pathogenesis. *Obstet Gynecol* 1992; **79**: 428–58.

43 Carlson JA, Ambros R, Malfetano J *et al.* Vulval lichen sclerosus and squam-ous cell carcinoma: a cohort, case control, and investigational study with histologic perspective—implications for chronic inflammation and scler-osis in the development of neoplasia. *Hum Pathol* 1998; **29**: 932–48.

44 Toki T, Kurman, RJ, Park JS *et al.* Probable non-papillomavirus aetiology of squamous cell carcinoma of the vulva in older women: a clinicopathologic study using *in situ* hybridization and polymerase chain reaction. *Int J Gynecol Pathol* 1991; **10**: 107–25.

45 Crum CP, McLachlin CM, Tate JE, Mutter GL. Pathobiology of vulval squamous neoplasia. *Curr Opin Obstet Gynecol* 1997; **9**: 63–9.

46 Brisigotti M, Moreno A, Murcia C *et al.* Verrucous carcinoma of the vulva: a clinopathologic and immunohistochemical study of five cases. *Int J Gynecol Pathol* 1989; **8**: 1–7.

47 Derrick EK, Ridley CM, Kobza-Black A, McKee PH, Neill SM. A clinical study of 23 cases of female anogenital carcinoma. *Br J Dermatol* 2000; **143**: 1217–23.

48 Meyrick-Thomas RH, McGibbon DH, Munro DD. Basal cell carcinoma of the vulva in association with vulval lichen sclerosus et atrophicus. *J R Soc Med* 1985; **78**: 16–8.

49 Friedman RJ, Kopf AW, Jones WB. Malignant melanoma in association with lichen sclerosus on the vulva of a 14-year-old. *Am J Dermatopathol* 1984; **6** (Suppl. 1): 253–6.

50 Ackerman AB. Melanocytic proliferation that simulates malignant mela-noma histopathologically. In: Mihm MC, Murphy GF, Kaufman N, eds. *Pathology and Recognition of Malignant Melanoma*. Baltimore: Williams and Wilkins, 1988: 166–7.

51 Carlson JA, Mihm MC. Vulvar naevi, lichen sclerosus and vitiligo. *Arch Dermatol* 1997; **133**: 1314–5.

52 Neill SM, Ridley CM. Management of anogenital lichen sclerosus. *Clin Exp Dermatol* 2001; **26**: 637–43.

53 Neill SM, Tatnall FM, Cox NH. Guidelines on the management of lichen sclerosus. *Br J Dermatol* 2002; **147**: 640–9.

54 Bornstein J, Heifetz S, Kellner Y, Stolar Z, Abramovici H. Clobetasol dipro-pionate 0.05% versus testosterone 2% topical application for severe vulvar lichen sclerosus. *Am J Obstet Gynecol* 1998; **178**: 80–4.

55 Paniel B. Surgical procedures in benign vulval disease. In: Ridley CM, Neill SM, eds. *The Vulva*. Oxford: Blackwell Science, 1999: 288–90.

56 Rouzier R, Haddad B, Deyrolle C *et al.* Perineoplasty for the treatment of introital stenosis related to vulval lichen sclerosus. *Am J Obstet Gynecol* 2002; **186**: 49–52.

Crohn's disease

Anogenital lesions occur in approximately 30% of patients with intestinal Crohn's disease, either as a direct extension of active intestinal disease or as metastatic disease. Vulval disease may present many years before intestinal involvement, and in some cases there is vulval oedema only, with no evidence of granulomatous inflammation [1,2]. The more usual presentation is ulceration, abscess, sinus and fistula formation, with a granulomatous histology. There may be deep linear fissures (knife cut sign) along the skin creases.

A separate form of vulval granuloma akin to the orofacial lesions seen in Melkersson–Rosenthal syndrome has been described [3,4].

REFERENCES

1 Urbanek M, McKee PH, Neill SM. Vulval Crohn's: difficulties in diagnosis. *Clin Exp Dermatol* 1996; **21**: 211–4.
2 Martin J, Holdstock G. Isolated vulval oedema as a feature of Crohn's disease. *J Obstet Gynecol* 1997; **17**: 92–3.
3 Hackel H, Hartmann AA, Burg G. Vulvitis granulomatosa and anoperineitis granulomatosa. *Dermatologica* 1991; **182**: 128–31.
4 Knopf B, Schaarschmidt H, Wollina U. Monosymptomatisches Melkersson–Rosenthal syndrom mit nachfolgender vulvitis und perivulvitis granulomatosa. *Hautartz* 1992; **43**: 711–3.

Ulcerative and bullous disorders

Any of the blistering disorders of the skin can occur on the vulva and vagina, either as part of the generalized disease or in isolation. Diagnosis can be more difficult in the latter case.

There are many causes of vulval ulceration and some features are important in narrowing down the differential diagnosis. It is helpful to divide them into acute and chronic types.

Acute genital ulceration

Benign aphthae

Many eponymous names have been assigned to acute vulval ulcers and several of these disorders are probably examples of benign aphthae. Reiter's syndrome may be associated with an ulcerative vulvitis [1].

Benign aphthae of the vulva may or may not occur with concomitant oral lesions. The age of onset is in childhood, about the age of 6 years, and there may be a family history. The lesions are usually multiple and small, and less commonly solitary or few and larger—referred to as giant aphthae. Herpetic infection should be excluded. There are often premenstrual exacerbations once the menarche is reached. The aetiology remains unknown.

The lesions are superficial and painful, with a yellow base surrounded by a red areola. They are distributed

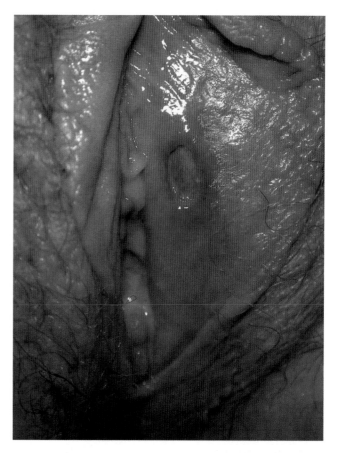

Fig. 68.30 Solitary benign aphthous ulcer of the left labium minus.

most frequently on the labia minora, and heal quickly (Fig. 68.30).

Sutton's ulcer (periadenitis mucosa necrotica recurrens) was originally reported in the mouth [2] but vulval lesions have also been given this label. The ulcer is characterized as being solitary, painful and recurring [2]. This type of ulceration, in the light of today's knowledge, would now be regarded as an example of benign aphthosis or a manifestation of Behçet's syndrome. Lipschutz's ulcer, described 2 years after Sutton's report, encompassed three types of ulcer (ulcus vulvae acutum), two of which today would be assigned to either aphthous ulceration or Behçet's syndrome. Only one is still regarded as being a separate entity [3]. This remaining form of ulceration is sometimes associated with a systemic infection such as infectious mononucleosis [4,5], typhoid or paratyphoid fever. Epstein–Barr virus (EBV) has been isolated from the ulcers [6], and there is one case of a mistaken diagnosis of lymphoma [7]. The Lipschutz-type ulcer usually affects adolescent girls and has a rapid onset. The ulcer may be very deep and large, and has a surrounding red areola and a thick adherent slough. It is most often solitary on one side of the vulva, usually the inner aspect of the labium minus, but lesions may occur bilaterally. Healing is spontaneous, but may take several weeks and leaves some scarring.

Treatment includes analgesics, potassium permanganate soaks and the application of a topical steroid with or without a topical tetracycline. In very severe ulceration, a short course of oral steroids may be required.

Erythema multiforme

The pattern of recurrent acral erythema multiforme is rarely associated with genital lesions, whereas oral lesions are nearly always present. The vulva is affected in Stevens–Johnson syndrome, often with erosions.

Bullous fixed drug eruptions

These are less common (or less commonly recognized) on the vulva than on the penis, where the commonly implicated medications include paracetemol and tetracycline. It is now rare to see cases involving phenolphthalein, sulphonamides and barbiturates.

Chronic genital ulceration

Any chronic ulcer of the genital mucosa must be considered malignant until proved otherwise. The differential diagnosis of chronic ulceration includes the diseases listed below, which are discussed fully in the relevant sections of this and other chapters.

1 *Genetic.* Epidermolysis bullosa, Hailey–Hailey disease and Darier's disease may all be responsible for chronic recurring ulceration. Exacerbations may follow friction, infection, irritants and herpes simplex infections.

2 *External trauma.* Nymphohymenal tears, dermatitis artefacta and radiation damage. Nymphohymenal tears may occur with sexual intercourse but most heal spontaneously. They tend to occur around the nymphohymenal sulcus, usually in the inferior segment at the 5 and 7 o'clock positions (Fig. 68.31). Those that do not heal can be excised radially.

3 *Malignancy.* The two most common malignant ulcers of the vulva are squamous cell carcinoma and basal cell carcinoma. Melanoma may also present as an amelanotic ulcerating nodule. Langerhans' cell histiocytosis may present with vulval and vaginal ulceration.

4 *Infection.* Chronic infective ulcers occur in tuberculosis, actinomycosis and other deep mycoses. The late stages of lymphogranuloma venereum cause ulceration and scarring.

5 *Inflammatory.* LS, LP and lupus erythematosus can all cause chronic ulceration. Pyoderma gangrenosum may be mistaken for malignancy on the vulva [8]. Hidradenitis suppurativa and Crohn's disease can sometimes be difficult to distinguish, particularly if they occur together. Pilonidal sinuses have been recorded on the vulva and clitoris [9].

Several of the autoimmune bullous diseases affect the

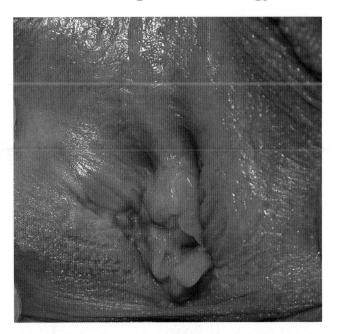

Fig. 68.31 Tear of the right inferior aspect of the nymphohymenal sulcus.

vulva. Juvenile pemphigoid, mucous membrane pemphigoid (Fig. 68.32), pemphigus vulgaris and vegetans may all present with vulval and vaginal ulceration.

REFERENCES

1 Daunt SO, Kotowski KE, O'Reilly AP, Richardson AT. Ulcerative vulvitis in Reiter's syndrome. *Br J Vener Dis* 1982; **58**: 405–7.
2 Sutton RL. Periadenitis mucosa necrotica recurrens. *J Cutan Dis* 1911; **29**: 65–71.
3 Lipschutz B. Über eine eigenartige Geschwüursform des weiblichen Genitales (ulcus vulvae acutum). *Arch Dermatol Syphilis (Berlin)* 1913; **114**: 363–96.
4 Brown ZA, Stenchever MA. Genital ulceration and infectious mononucleosis. *Am J Obstet Gynecol* 1977; **127**: 673–4.
5 Lampert A, Assier-Bonnet H, Chevallier B *et al.* Lipschutz's genital ulceration: a manifestation of Epstein–Barr virus primary infection. *Br J Dermatol* 1996; **135**: 663–5.
6 Portnoy J, Arontheim GA, Ghibu F *et al.* Recovery of Epstein–Barr virus from genital ulcers. *N Engl J Med* 1984; **311**: 966–8.
7 Eghbali H, Lacut JY, Hoernie B. Genital infectious mononucleosis mimicking high grade non-Hodgkin's lymphoma. *Med Mal Infect* 1989; **19**: 83–6.
8 McCalmont CS, Leshin B, White WL, Greiss FC Jr, Jorizzo JL. Vulvar pyoderma gangrenosum. *Int J Gynaecol Obstet* 1991; **35**: 175–8.
9 Radman HM, Bhagavan BS. Pilonidal disease of the female genitals. *Am J Obstet Gynecol* 1972; **114**: 271–3.

Non-sexually transmitted infections

Bacterial infections

Staphylococci

Staphylococcus aureus is usually the causative agent in infective folliculitis, boils and abscesses of the vulva. It is often associated with an underlying problem (e.g.

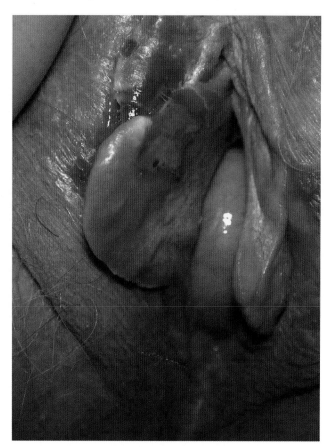

Fig. 68.32 Erosions in vulval mucous membrane pemphigoid.

diabetes, immunosuppression). Pseudofolliculitis is a sterile folliculitis that may follow shaving and is caused by the newly regrowing hairs inducing an inflammatory reaction. It is a foreign body reaction and results in changes from mild inflammation to the formation of abscesses and sinuses. A staphylococcal folliculitis on the buttocks may occur secondary to the pruritus induced by intestinal infestation with pin worm.

An exotoxin associated with phage group 1 staphylococci has been implicated in production of the collapse, fever and morbilliform rash seen in the toxic shock syndrome. Although the syndrome occurs most commonly in menstruating women who use tampons, the association is not exclusive.

Histology. The impetiginous lesion shows subcorneal pustules filled with neutrophils and some spongiosis, with a moderate inflammatory response in the papillary dermis.

The acute folliculitis may be superficial with a subcorneal pustule present at the follicular opening, or deep and associated with a perifollicular abscess, and destruction of the follicle wall and sebaceous gland. Chronic deep intrafollicular abscesses may have the additional features of fibrosis and foreign body giant cells.

Streptococcal infections

Beta-haemolytic Lancefield group A bacteria may be the cause of vulval cellulitis. The erythema and oedema may be extreme, and vesicles and bullae develop. There are usually associated systemic signs. The infection arises at sites of trauma where there is a wound and it is commonly seen following a vulvectomy with lymphadenectomy. If there is residual lymphoedema then further attacks of cellulitis are more common. Streptococcal dermatitis usually affects the anogenital area of children [1].

Synergistic bacterial gangrene

This severe and rapidly extending disease is caused by the synergistic effect of a microaerophilic streptococcus and *Staphylococcus aureus* (see Chapter 27).

Hidradenitis suppurativa

This is dealt with fully in Chapter 27, but mention is made here as staphylococcal and streptococcal infection have a secondary role. The primary problem is an abnormality of the follicular epithelium of the apocrine gland ducts, which starts with a spongiform infundibular folliculitis [2]. *Streptococcus milleri* is often found as a secondary pathogen [3].

Histology. This is characterized by distension and inflammation of apocrine ducts, with polymorphs in and around the ducts. The apocrine glands may become necrotic, with an infiltrate of lymphocytes, plasma cells and macrophages. Sinuses are lined by keratinized epithelium. Fibrosis and a foreign body reaction with granulomatous changes are common. Pseudoepitheliomatous hyperplasia may be seen, and at least nine cases of SCC have been reported—two of these were in females with buttock lesions [4].

Treatment is with long-term antibiotics, and in some cases oral isotretinoin may be helpful. The important differential diagnosis is Crohn's disease, but hidradenitis suppurativa and Crohn's disease may coexist [5,6].

Gram-negative bacilli

Pseudomonas aeruginosa is a common problem in patients with bladder problems but it is not a cause of vulvovaginitis. There has been a report of blue staining of napkins in infants with this infection [7].

Despite its name, *Trichomycosis* is caused by species of corynebacteria, which lead to red, yellow or black nodules on the shafts of the axillary and pubic hairs (see Chapter 27). Histological examination shows that these nodules consist of concretions of bacteria. The hair shafts may be damaged [8].

Diphtheria, caused by *Corynebacterium diphtheriae*, is rare in developed countries. Vulval infection takes the form of ulcers, often with a greyish membrane. It has been described in children [9,10] and in adults [11,12].

Mycobacterial infections

Vulval tuberculosis, caused by *Mycobacterium tuberculosis*, is uncommon in the UK. It may occur by means of haematogenous spread from foci outside the genital tract, by distal spread from the upper genital tract, or as a primary exogenous infection contracted from sputum or sexual intercourse. Vulval tuberculosis has been reported in a renal transplant patient [13], and three cases were described in a series of 26 patients with genital tuberculosis [14]. Genitourinary tuberculous infection is more common in HIV-positive subjects. In a primary infection the initial lesion may be inconspicuous, the main feature being a caseating lymphadenopathy. In other cases the lesions are masses or nodules that may ulcerate and lead to lymphoedema [15]. Bartholin's gland may be involved [16].

Leprosy (see Chapter 29)

The female genital tract may be involved in infection by *Mycobacterium leprae* [17], but vulval lesions are rare [18]. Pubic hair may be lost [19].

Higher bacterial infection

Higher bacteria is the name assigned to those bacteria that, like filamentous fungi, are capable of forming true branches. They include the genera *Streptomyces*, *Actinomyces* and *Nocardia*.

Actinomycosis

The Gram-positive acid-fast organisms responsible for actinomycosis are predominantly *Actinomyces israelii* and *Actinomyces gerencseriae*. They may colonize intrauterine devices and are usually asymptomatic, but invasion of the genital tract can occur [20,21]. Genital infection usually arises from bowel disease [22]. Lesions of the vulva alone have been reported [23].

Mycoplasmas

Mycoplasma hominis and *Ureaplasma urealyticum* are found in the vagina and rarely cause disease. There are rare reports of *M. hominis* being isolated from cases of Bartholin's abscess [24,25].

Abscesses of Bartholin's gland may be caused by pyococcal organisms, gonococcus and *Chlamydia trachomatis* [26]. In one study, only 21 of 109 cases were caused by staphylococci, whereas 50 were caused by *Escherichia coli* and 46 by *Streptococcus faecalis* [27]. The abscess results from distal blockage of the duct. The patient presents with fever, malaise and a tender swelling arising posterior to the origin of the labium minus. Episodes of bartholinitis may be mild and recurrent until fibrosis supervenes.

REFERENCES

1 Krol AL. Perianal streptococcal dermatitis. *Pediatr Dermatol* 1990; **7**: 97–100.
2 Boer J, Weltevreden EF. Hidradenitis suppurativa or acne inversa: a clinico-pathological study of early lesions. *Br J Dermatol* 1996; **135**: 721–5.
3 Highet AS, Warren RE, Staughton RCD *et al.* *Streptococcus milleri* causing treatable infection in perineal hidradenitis suppurativa. *Br J Dermatol* 1980; **103**: 375–82.
4 Sparks MK, Kuhlmann DS, Pietro A *et al.* Hypercalcaemia in association with cutaneous squamous cell carcinoma: occurrence as a late complication of hidradenitis suppurativa. *Arch Dermatol* 1985; **12**: 243–6.
5 Ostlere LS, Langtry JAA, Mortimer PS, Staughton RCD. Hidradenitis suppurativa in Crohn's syndrome. *Br J Dermatol* 1991; **125**: 384–6.
6 Burrows NP, Russell-Jones R. Crohn's disease in association with hidradenitis suppurativa. *Br J Dermatol* 1992; **126**: 523–9.
7 Thearle MJ, Wise R, Allen JT. Blue nappies [Letter]. *Lancet* 1973; **ii**: 499–500.
8 Orfanos CE, Schloesser E, Mahrie G. Hair destroying growth of *Corynebacterium tenuis* in the so-called trichomycosis axillaris. *Arch Dermatol* 1971; **103**: 632–6.
9 Barabe P, Delpe P, Vedy J *et al.* Primary vulvovaginal diphtheria (apropos of a case in Chad). *Med Trop* 1972; **32**: 637–9.
10 Charles V, Charles SX. A case of vulvovaginal diphtheria in a girl of 7 years. *Indian J Pediatr* 1978; **15**: 257–8.
11 Parks J. Diphtheric vaginitis in the adult. *Am J Obstet Gynecol* 1941; **41**: 714–8.
12 Machnicki S. Diphtheria of the vulva and vagina. *Z Haut Geschlechtskr* 1953; **86**: 386.
13 Tham SN, Choong HL. Primary tuberculous chancre in a renal transplant patient. *J Am Acad Dermatol* 1992; **26**: 342–4.
14 Moore D. Genito-peritoneal tuberculosis: a review of 26 cases. *S Afr Med J* 1954; **28**: 666–70.
15 Millar JW, Holt S, Gilmour HM, Robertson DHH. Vulval tuberculosis. *Tubercle* 1979; **60**: 173–6.
16 Schaefer G. Diagnosis and treatment of female genital tuberculosis. *Clin Obstet Gynecol* 1959; **2**: 530–5.
17 Bonar E, Rabson AS. Gynaecological aspects of leprosy. *Obstet Gynecol* 1957; **9**: 33–8.
18 Grabstold H, Swan L. Genitourinary lesions in leprosy with special reference to atrophy of the testis. *JAMA* 1952; **149**: 1287–91.
19 Klostermann GF. *Handbuch der speziellen pathologischen Anatomie und Histologie Weibliche Geschelentsorgave*. Berlin: Springer-Verlag, 1972.
20 Purdie DW, Cartie MJ, McLeod TIF. Tubo-ovarian actinomycosis and the intrauterine contraceptive device. *BMJ* 1977; **ii**: 1392.
21 Lomax CW, Harbert GM, Thornton WN. Actinomycosis of the genital tract. *Obstet Gynecol* 1976; **48**: 341–6.
22 Wagman H. Genital actinomycosis. *Proc R Soc Med* 1975; **68**: 228–30.
23 Daniel C, Mavrodin A. L'actinomycose genitale de la femme. *Rev Francaise Gynecol Obstet* 1954; **29**: 1–11.
24 Dienes L, Edsall G. Observations on the L-organisim of Kleinberger. *Proc Soc Exp Biol Med* 1937; **36**: 740–5.
25 Davies JA, Rees E, Jobson D *et al.* Isolation of *Chlamydia trachomatis* from Bartholin's ducts. *Br J Vener Dis* 1978; **54**: 409–13.
26 Mayer HGK. Pathogénie et traitement des pretendus abcés et kystes de la glande de Bartholin. *J Gynecol Obstet Biol Reprod* 1972; **1**: 71–6.
27 Lee Y-H, Rankin JS, Alpert S *et al.* Microbiological investigation of Bartholin's gland abscesses and cysts. *Am J Obstet Gynecol* 1977; **129**: 150–3.

Fungal infections

Candidal vulvovaginitis

Candida and *Torulopsis* are both yeasts that can infect the vulva and vagina. *Torulopsis* accounts for very few infections, whereas *Candida albicans* is the most frequently isolated.

Candida albicans is dimorphic, with both yeast and mycelial forms. It is a non-pathogenic commensal in the intestinal tract in 30% of the normal population. Infection in women is usually a vulvovaginitis. Changes in host factors are probably responsible for transition to pathogenicity, and are generally not directly associated with sexual contact. Factors related to cell-mediated immunity are doubtless important, but as yet are ill-understood. Pregnancy, diabetes, possibly oral antibiotics, high-dose oestrogen oral contraceptive pills and immunosuppression may all be predisposing factors. The primary infection arises in the vagina, causing inflammation and a heavy white curdy discharge, which then leads to a secondary vulvitis with well-demarcated sheets of erythema on the outer aspects of the vulva, sometimes extending on occasions into the genitocrural folds and perianally. There may be a scaly or vesiculopustular edge. Beyond this edge lie grouped or isolated superficial small pustules, which rupture rapidly, leaving a slightly scaly periphery. In all cases of candidal vulvovaginitis, but particularly in the middle-aged patient, late-onset diabetes should be considered, and appropriate tests carried out.

Diagnosis is confirmed by direct microscopy and culture.

Treatment of vulvovaginal candidiasis requires vaginal pessaries or creams and/or oral imidazoles.

In some cases of vulval eczema and psoriasis, *Candida* is cultured from skin swabs, but the candidal overgrowth is a secondary problem arising on a background of an inflamed epithelium. Treating the dermatosis alone with a topical steroid will usually resolve the problem, without the addition of anticandidal agents.

Dermatophyte fungi

Dermatophyte infections of the vulval skin are uncommon in cooler climates. The sites affected are usually the inguinal folds and perianal area. The causative agents are *Trichophyton rubrum* or *Epidermophyton floccosum*. The vulval epithelium in the adult seems to be relatively immune to dermatophyte infections. The lesions are erythematous and scaly, with a spreading raised circinate edge. Folliculitis is also seen, particularly in the perianal area. Tinea incognito may also occur perianally following the injudicious use of a topical steroid in the presence of an unrecognized dermatophyte infection. The diagnosis is usually made by direct microscopy and culture of skin scrapings, and treatment is usually oral terbinafine or griseofulvin because the skin is hair-bearing.

Miscellaneous

Pityriasis versicolor classically occurs on the trunk, but in

severe widespread infection there may be vulval involvement [1,2].

The black and white forms of piedra (trichosporosis) are caused by *Piedraia hortai* and *Trichosporon beigelii*, respectively, the latter acting synergistically with a corynebacterium. The hair-bearing parts of the vulva can be affected with black and white nodules along the hair shafts [3]. The diagnosis is made by microscopy and culture.

Vulval phycomycosis has been described [4]. Subcutaneous infections occur in children and young adults. Histologically, the epidermis is unremarkable but subcutaneously there are deep granulomatous masses containing hyphae.

There is one case report of chromomycosis (chromoblastomycosis) affecting the vulva [5].

Cryptococcus neoformans can induce painless ulceration of the vulva in the immunosuppressed patient [6].

REFERENCES

1 Bumgarner FE, Burke RC. Pityriaisis versicolor: atypical clinical and mycological variants. *Arch Dermatol* 1949; **59**: 192–4.
2 Jelliffe DB, Jacobson FW. The clinical picture of tinea versicolor in negro infants. *J Trop Med Hygiene* 1954; **57**: 290–2.
3 Kalter DC, Tschen JA, Cernoch PK. Genital white piedra: epidemiology, microbiology and therapy. *J Am Acad Dermatol* 1986; **14**: 982–93.
4 Scott RA, Gallis HA, Livengood CH. Phycomycosis of the vulva. *Am J Obstet Gynecol* 1985; **153**: 675–6.
5 Kakoti LM, Dey NC. Chronic blastomycosis in India. *J Indian Med Assoc* 1957; **28**: 351.
6 Blocher KS, Weeks JA, Noble RC. Cutaneous cryptococcal infection presenting as vulval lesion. *Genitourin Med* 1987; **63**: 341–3.

Infections with protozoa

Infection with *Trichomonas vaginalis* causes a frothy malodorous greyish green watery discharge, and a bright red vaginal mucosa studded with petechiae. The vaginal discharge may cause a secondary vulvitis, with erythema and swelling of the vestibule and labia minora. Colonization of the urethra and paraurethral glands often occurs. The diagnosis is made by microscopic examination of wet preparations and culture.

Treatment is with metronidazole 400 mg twice daily for 5 days or 2 g in a single dose.

The flagellate protozoan *Leishmania tropica* causes cutaneous, mucocutaneous and visceral forms of leishmaniasis. The vulva is mainly affected by the cutaneous form, which is endemic in areas of the eastern Mediterranean, Asia Minor and India; and to a lesser extent by the mucocutaneous form, found in Central and South America. An example of sexual transmission from post-kala-azar dermal leishmaniasis has been reported [1]. Transmission of infection is usually by sandflies. The lesions are nodular or ulcerative.

Entamoeba histolytica is found worldwide and intestinal amoebiasis may be transmitted from the bowel to other areas including the genital tract, although such involvement is rare [2]. It appears as warty or ulcerative masses of the vulva, perineum and cervix. Live amoebae may be recovered from scrapings, or the organism seen as a small eosinophilic body in an inflammatory histological reaction.

Vulval schistosomiasis is usually caused by *Schistosoma haematobium*. The lesions are chronic, scarring and granulomatous, and may ulcerate and calcify [3–5].

Histologically, there is inflammation surrounding the organisms and their remains, with granuloma formation and many eosinophils. Ova may be found in the vagina, urine and faeces.

REFERENCES

1 Symmers WS. Leishmaniasis acquired by contagion: a case of marital infection in Britain. *Lancet* 1960; **i**: 127–32.
2 Majmudar B, Chaikaen MC, Lee KU. Amoebiasis of the clitoris mimicking carcinoma. *JAMA* 1976; **236**: 1145–6.
3 McKee PH, Wright E, Hutt MSR. Vulval schistosomiasis. *Clin Exp Dermatol* 1983; **8**: 189–94.
4 Friedberg D, Berry AV, Schneider J. Schistosomiasis of the female genital tract. *S Afr Med J* 1991; **80**: 2–15.
5 Goldsmith PC, Leslie TA, Sams V *et al.* Lesions of schistosomiasis mimicking warts on the vulva. *BMJ* 1993; **307**: 556–7.

Viruses

Three groups of viruses are important causes of infection in the genital area: the poxviruses, papillomaviruses and herpesviruses. Other viruses seldom give rise to distinctive clinical pictures, although vulval lesions may occur as part of a generalized viral infection.

Genital HPV infection and herpes simplex are discussed later in the section on sexually transmitted infections (see p. 68.70).

The most common poxvirus is mollusum contagiosum virus, two types of which have been identified. There is no relationship between virus type and anatomical distribution of lesions [1]. Vulval lesions in childhood are common and usually acquired innocently, but they are more likely to be acquired sexually in adults. Lesions are often found on the mons pubis and labia majora, and if inflamed they may mimic folliculitis. The clinical diagnosis is straightforward when there are multiple pearly lesions with an umbilicated centre, but solitary large lesions can cause diagnostic problems. It is the solitary giant lesion that may miss immediate diagnosis until it is biopsied. Lesions of molluscum contagiosum can be profuse and large in immunosuppressed women, especially in those with AIDS. The condition is more fully described in Chapter 26.

Other poxvirus infections of the vulva are rare, but there are isolated reports of orf [2] and cowpox [3].

Herpes simplex (see below).

Varicella-zoster virus. This may also affect the vulva if the

third sacral dermatome is involved. It may be accompanied by bowel and bladder dysfunction [4].

Epstein–Barr virus. This has been found rarely in genital ulcers at the time of infectious mononucleosis [5–7]. EBV may also be shed from the cervix [8] but there is no link with vulval malignancy [9].

Cytomegalovirus (CMV). CMV inclusions were seen in a biopsy and a positive culture for CMV was obtained in an infant with congenital HIV disease who presented with pustular and ulcerative lesions on the perineum [10].

REFERENCES

1 Porter CD, Blake NW, Archard LC *et al.* Molluscum contagiosum: virus types in genital and non-genital lesions. *Br J Dermatol* 1989; **121**: 37–41.
2 James JRE. Orf in man. *BMJ* 1968; **iii**: 804–6.
3 Claudy AL, Gaudin OG, Granovillet R. Pox virus infection in Darier's disease. *Clin Exp Dermatol* 1982; **7**: 260–5.
4 Fugelso PD, Newman SB, Beamer JE. Herpes zoster of the anogenital area affecting urination and defaecation. *Br J Dermatol* 1973; **89**: 285–8.
5 Portnoy J, Ahronheim GA, Ghibu F *et al.* Recovery of Epstein–Barr virus from genital ulcers. *N Engl J Med* 1984; **311**: 966–8.
6 McKenna G, Edwards S, Cleland H. Genital ulceration secondary to Epstein–Barr virus infection. *Genitourin Med* 1994; **70**: 356–67.
7 Lampert A, Assier-Bonnet H, Chevalier B *et al.* Lipschutz's genital ulceration: a manifestation of Epstein–Barr virus primary infection. *Br J Dermatol* 1996; **135**: 663–5.
8 Naher H, Gissman L, Freese UK *et al.* Subclinical Epstein–Barr virus infection of both the male and female genital tracts: indication of sexual transmission. *J Invest Dermatol* 1992; **98**: 791–3.
9 Cheung ANY, Khoo VS, Kwong KY *et al.* Epstein–Barr virus in carcinoma of the vulva. *J Clin Pathol* 1993; **46**: 849–51.
10 Thiboutot DM, Beckford A, Mart CA *et al.* Cytomegalovirus diaper dermatitis. *Arch Dermatol* 1991; **127**: 396–8.

Malakoplakia of the vulva [1–4]

Malakoplakia (meaning 'soft plaque') is a granulomatous response to infection. It is not usually caused by one specific agent but the organisms involved include *Escherichia coli*, *Pseudomonas* and *Staphylococcus aureus*. Malakoplakia most often affects the urinary or gastrointestinal tract but cutaneous lesions may occur on the vagina, vulva and perineum. Involvement of Bartholin's gland has been described [5]. The lesions include persistent plaques, ulcers, nodules and sinuses. There is often underlying immunosuppression, the aetiology of which may include malignancy, dermatomyositis [6], lupus erythematosus, rheumatoid arthritis and organ transplantation [7].

Histopathology. There are confluent sheets of histiocytes with eosinophilic granular cytoplasm and small eccentric nuclei. Round, sometimes laminated structures are found with these cells and are known as Michaelis–Gutmann bodies. The histiocytic infiltrate may be mixed with neutrophils, lymphocytes and plasma cells, with associated granulation tissue. Electron microscopy of malakoplakia shows that the histiocytes contain numerous phagolysosomes within which there may be occasional intact and partly digested bacteria.

REFERENCES

1 McClure J. Malakoplakia. *J Pathol* 1983; **140**: 275–330.
2 Remond B, Dompmartin A, Moreau A *et al.* Cutaneous malakoplakia. *Int J Dermatol* 1994; **33**: 538–42.
3 Sarkell B, Dannenberg M, Blaylock WK, Patterson JW. Cutaneous malakoplakia. *J Am Acad Dermatol* 1994; **30**: 834–6.
4 Lowitt MH, Kariniemi A-L, Niemi KM, Kao GF. Cutaneous malakoplakia: a report of two cases and review of the literature. *J Am Acad Dermatol* 1996; **34**: 325–32.
5 Paquin ML, Davis JR, Weiner S. Malakoplakia of Bartholin's gland. *Arch Pathol Lab Med* 1986; **110**: 757–8.
6 Singh M, Kaur S, Vijpayer BK, Banerjee AK. Cutaneous malakoplakia with dermatomyositis. *Int J Dermatol* 1987; **26**: 190–1.
7 Sian CS, McCabe RE, Lattes CG. Malakoplakia of skin and subcutaneous tissue in a renal transplant recipient. *Arch Dermatol* 1981; **117**: 654–5.

Sexually transmitted disease

A brief outline of the main sexually transmitted diseases that can affect the vulval skin is given below. Fuller descriptions of the individual diseases are given elsewhere (see Chapters 25–27 and 30).

Herpes simplex virus

Once this sexually transmitted DNA virus is acquired it lies dormant in dorsal root ganglia and can give rise to recurrent symptomatic lesions. It exists in two types: I and II. Type I usually affects non-genital sites and type II is responsible for 50–80% of genital infections. Ninety-five per cent of infections are acquired sexually and the rest are cases of autoinoculation or non-sexual contact. The lesions are typically painful vesicles or ulcers, which are often multiple in primary infection but are fewer and usually localized to one side with recurrences. There may be prodromal symptoms of tingling or tender enlarged inguinal nodes. Paraesthesiae may occur, affecting S2–4, which may lead to urinary retention. Pain and oedema may also lead to retention, particularly in primary infections. It is important to obtain a definite diagnosis with a positive culture of HSV and it is necessary to perform the test as soon as the blisters arise, as the virus is harder to culture from older lesions. However, a negative test does not exclude an infection with HSV.

The treatment is either oral aciclovir 200 mg five times daily for 5 days, valaciclovir 500 mg twice daily for 5 days or famciclovir 250 mg three times daily for 5 days.

Suppressant therapy is sometimes required for patients with frequent recurrences (six or more in a year).

Human papillomavirus infection

HPV is a small DNA virus, and is discussed in more detail in Chapter 25. Those that most commonly infect the vulval skin are HPV 6, 11, 16 and 18. The warty lesions are known as condylomata acuminata. Extensive vegetating masses can cover the vulva and perianal area, particularly in diabetes, pregnancy and immunocompromised patients. Patients with genital warts should be screened for other sexually transmitted diseases. Secondary syphilis may also present with extensive papulosquamous lesions and has to be considered in the differential diagnosis.

Types 16 and 18 are linked with cervical and anogenital intraepithelial neoplasia and SCC.

The histology of genital warts is characterized by the koilocyte, a vacuolated squamous cell with a basophilic and pyknotic nucleus in the upper part of the epidermis; it is important not to confuse it with the heavily glycogenated clear cells of vestibular epithelium. Other histological features are elongated dermal papillae, acanthosis, a prominent granular layer often containing koilocytes, and a stratum corneum of variable thickness.

Treatment. Podophyllotoxin is the recommended initial treatment. It is applied twice daily for 3 consecutive days each week for 4 weeks. This treatment is contraindicated in pregnancy because of the theoretical risk of teratogenicity. Diathermy, hyfrecation, topical trichloroacetic acid, cryotherapy and carbon dioxide laser have been used with variable success. These treatments are successful in patients where the lesions are few or filiform in morphology.

The new immune response modulating cream, imiquimod, is now used for resistant cases or patients with extensive lesions. This has to be used with care as it also induces an inflammatory response in patients who have a background dermatitis. It should not be used in patients who have benign vulval aphthous ulcers.

In pregnancy, only cryotherapy or destructive techniques with cautery or hyfrecation can be used safely.

Gonorrhoea

The urethra, cervix and rectum may be infected by *Neisseria gonorrhoea* and spread occurs to the endometrium and fallopian tubes. Vulval involvement is rare in adults, and infection is sited in the paraurethral and Bartholin's glands, resulting in painful abscess formation. In children, the infection is usually a result of sexual abuse, and an acute vulvitis may develop [1].

Syphilis

The causative organism is *Treponema pallidum* and vulval lesions may occur in both early and late syphilis. The primary chancre is an ulcerative lesion and is usually accompanied by unilateral or bilateral lymphadenopathy. In secondary syphilis, condylomata lata, flat-topped warty papules, affect the vulva, as may also mucous patches, which are greyish white moist-looking lesions. Gummas, which are a manifestation of tertiary syphilis, are extremely rare on the vulva, and clinically they occur as either single or multiple swellings or nodules.

Bullous, papular, papulosquamous lesions and mucous patches occur on the vulva in early congenital syphilis and condylomata lata may develop later.

The diagnosis of syphilis is made by dark ground microscopy, immunofluorescence of scrapings or serology.

Histologically, the findings are very variable but, typically, early lesions show inflammation with perivascular plasma cells and lymphocytes together with an endarteritis. There is marked epithelial hyperplasia in lesions of condylomata lata, with a prominent perivascular lymphocytic and plasma cell infiltrate.

Chancroid [2]

This sexually transmitted disease, caused by *Haemophilus ducreyi*, is rare in the UK [2] as it is normally found in tropical and semitropical countries, although the incidence is falling in Africa [3]. Single or multiple small tender ulcers appear on the labia majora, perineum and perianal area, and may also affect the vagina and cervix. The inguinal lymph glands are involved in half of cases and the adenitis is unilateral in most. Buboes develop, which are fluctuant, and rupture leaving extensive ulceration. Co-infections with *Treponema pallidum* or HSV are frequent [4].

Diagnosis may be confirmed by culture of scrapings from the ulcer base or aspirated pus. Microscopy of scrapings or pus will show Gram-negative coccobacilli. PCR may also be used. The histological features include epithelial hyperplasia adjacent to the ulceration, with three relatively distinct zones at the base of the ulcer. The superficial zone consists of a thin band of neutrophils, fibrin and necrotic debris; the middle zone of oedema with thin-walled, dilated and vertically orientated blood vessels; and the deep zone of a dense perivascular infiltrate of lymphocytes and plasma cells. A Giemsa or Brown–Brenn stain may reveal organisms in the superficial zone staining blue or red, respectively.

Treatment. Azithromycin, ceftriaxone, ciprofloxacin or erythromycin can be used. The recent guidelines issued by the Communicable Disease Centre (CDC) should be consulted (http://www.cdc.gov/std). Special considerations should be given to patients with HIV infection.

Donovanosis [5]
SYN. GRANULOMA VENEREUM; GRANULOMA INGUINALE

The causative organism is *Calymmatobacterium granulomatis*, formerly known as *Donovania granulomatis*. The disease is sexually transmitted and found in New Guinea,

India, South Africa and Brazil. Papules or nodules break down to form ulcers with a rolled edge. Large areas are involved, and granulomatous masses may involve any part of the genitocrural area, although the lymph nodes themselves are not affected. The vagina and cervix may be involved. Scarring and lymphoedema may ensue.

Histopathology shows epithelial hyperplasia adjacent to the ulcer, sometimes with spongiosis and intraepithelial neutrophilic abscesses, and a dense dermal or submucosal infiltrate with neutrophilic abscesses surrounded by plasma cells, histiocytes and lymphocytes. The organisms occasionally are visible with silver stains, which show intracytoplasmic inclusions (Donovan bodies), seen as black oval or rod-shaped structures in the cytoplasm of histiocytes. The organisms are more reliably demonstrated on smear preparations than tissue sections.

Chlamydia (lymphogranuloma venereum)

Chlamydia trachomatis is a Gram-negative intracellular bacterium that is an obligatory parasite. The serovars L1–3 cause lymphogranuloma venereum, which occurs in tropical and subtropical countries. The incubation period varies from a few days to a few weeks. A small papule develops on the vulva, usually at the fourchette, heals quickly and is followed weeks later by striking lymphadenopathy. The nodes may form a suppurative mass that heals with scarring, leading to lymphoedema, which may be gross. Generalized chronic infection leads to abscess and fistula formation, and finally genital and anal strictures and elephantiasis.

Rectal lesions present as a proctocolitis with subsequent stricture formation.

The histology of the vulval ulcers is non-specific, but the affected nodes show epithelioid cells and giant cells, and later stellate abscesses develop that are surrounded by epithelioid cells, granulomatous tissue and plasma cells. Fibrosis and necrosis are seen in chronic lesions.

REFERENCES

1 Barlow D, Phillips I. Gonorrhoea in women: diagnostic, clinical and laboratory aspects. *Lancet* 1978; **i**: 761–3.
2 Langley C. Update on chancroid: an important cause of genital ulcer disease. *J Am Acad Dermatol* 1999; **41**: 511–32.
3 Douglas CP. Lymphogranuloma venereum and granuloma inguinale of the vulva. *Am J Obstet Gynecol* 1962; **69**: 871–80.
4 Editorial. Chancroid. *Lancet* 1982; **ii**: 747–8.
5 Richens J. The diagnosis and treatment of donovanosis (granuloma inguinale). *Genitourin Med* 1991: **67**: 441–52.

Benign tumours and tumour-like lesions of the vulva [1,2]

Most of the tumours that arise on the anogenital skin are similar to those that occur on the skin elsewhere. Fibromas arise from deeper connective tissue structures, particularly those surrounding the introitus and perineal body. They usually occur on the labia majora, are often pedunculated or pendulous, and can attain a very large size. Fibroepitheliomatous polyps (skin tags) are usually solitary and appear as soft wrinkled polypoidal nodules. There is a fibrovascular connective tissue core covered by squamous epithelium, which may be atrophic or, more commonly, mildly acanthotic and hyperkeratotic. Cellular atypia is occasionally seen in the stromal cells. Lipomas develop from the fatty tissue of the labia majora, but there have been reports of localization to the clitoris [3], as has also been reported with haemangiomas [3,4,].

Two types of lymphangioma may occur on the vulva: lymphangioma circumscriptum, which are localized thin-walled vesicles [5], and cavernous lymphangioma, which arise in childhood and present as a soft compressible mass, which, although usually located in the labia minora, can involve the whole of the vulva [6]. Acquired lymphangiectasia is discussed on p. 68.81.

Melanocytic naevi include junctional, intradermal and compound types, which generally share the same clinical and histological features as naevi at other sites of the body, with the exception that in premenopausal women vulval naevi sometimes have atypical histological features [7]. The atypia may extend into the adnexal structures, but the overall symmetry of the lesion, with cellular maturation in the deeper dermis, should help to distinguish it from a truly malignant lesion. Sometimes, differentiation from melanoma can be difficult and evaluation by an experienced dermatopathologist may be necessary.

Epidermal cysts of the vulva may develop from epithelial implants following surgical trauma, from epidermal inclusions occurring at fusion sites during embryogenesis, or from obstructed sebaceous gland ducts that have undergone squamous metaplasia. They may be single or multiple, and occur most commonly in the labia majora. Steatocystoma may present as a solitary cyst in the vulval region [8]. Calcified nodules have been recorded [9].

Syringomas

These are considered to be adenomas of the intraepidermal eccrine sweat gland ducts. They do not require treatment as they are usually asymptomatic, although there may be pruritus [10]. Vulval syringomas are multiple, bilateral and symmetrical, although a solitary lesion may occur. One case was reported that had the typical histological features of a syringoma mixed with pilosebaceous elements [11].

Papillary hidradenoma

This sweat gland adenoma with apocrine differentiation occurs almost exclusively in the anogenital region of middle-aged white women. It has been associated with anogenital glands [12]. It is a firm asymptomatic papule or nodule, which can occasionally be painful, and occurs most commonly on the labia majora, interlabial sulcus, lateral surfaces of the labia minora or perineal region [13]. Although usually single, there are occasionally multiple lesions. Curiously, when they are multiple all the lesions tend to develop on one side of the vulva. In most patients, the covering epidermis remains intact, but in a proportion the elevated epithelium may become ulcerated [14].

Malignant change within a papillary hidradenoma has been reported: apocrine carcinoma [15] and adenosquamous carcinoma [16].

Fox–Fordyce disease

In this condition, described in detail in Chapter 45, the apocrine ducts become blocked, with retention of sweat. Itchy skin-coloured papules appear on the mons pubis, labia majora, axillae and on the breast. They develop around the time of puberty and there are menstrual exacerbations. There is some improvement in pregnancy and after the menopause.

REFERENCES

1 Fox H, Buckley CD. Neoplastic disease of the vulva and associated structures. In: Fox H, Wells M, eds. *Haines and Taylor Obstetrical and Gynaecological Pathology*, 5th edn. Edinburgh: Churchill Livingstone, 2003: 95–145.
2 Nucci MR, Fletcher CDM. Vulvovaginal soft tissue tumours: update and review. *Histopathology* 2000; **36**: 97–100.
3 Haddad HM, Jones WH. Clitoral enlargement simulating pseudohermaphroditism. *Am J Dis Child* 1960; **99**: 282–7.
4 Kaufmann-Friedman K. Hemangioma of clitoris: confused with adrenogenital syndrome—a case report. *Plast Reconstr Surg* 1978; **62**: 452–4.
5 Abu-Hamad A, Provencher D, Ganjei P Penalver M *et al.* Lymphangioma circumscriptum of the vulva: case report and review of the literature. *Obstet Gynecol* 1989; **73**: 496–9.
6 Brown JV, Stenchever MA. Cavernous lymphangioma of the vulva. *Obstet Gynecol* 1989; **73**: 877–9.
7 Christensen WN, Friedman KJ, Woodruff JD, Hood AF. Histological characteristics of vulval naevocellular naevi. *J Cutan Pathol* 1987; **14**: 87–91.
8 Brownstein MH. Steatocystoma simplex. *Arch Dermatol* 1982; **118**: 409–11.
9 Jameleddine FN, Salmon SM, Shbaklo Z *et al.* Vulvar calcinosis, the counterpart of idiopathic scrotal calcinosis. *Cutis* 1988; **41**: 273–5.
10 Carter J, Elliott P. Syringoma: an unusual cause of pruritus vulvae. *Aust NZ J Obstet Gynaecol* 1990; **30**: 382–3.
11 Guindi SF, Silverberg BK, Evans TL. Multifocal mixed adenoid tumors of the vulva. *Int J Gynaecol Obstet* 1974; **12**: 138–40.
12 van der Putte SCJ. Anogenital 'sweat' glands: histology and pathology of a gland that may mimic mammary glands. *Am J Dermatopathol* 1991; **13**: 557–65.
13 Basta A, Madej JG. Hydradenoma of the vulva: incidence and clinical observations. *Eur J Gynaecol Oncol* 1990; **11**: 185–9.
14 Veraldi S, Schianchi-Veraldi R, Marini D. Hidradenoma papilliferum of the vulva: report of a case characterized by unusual clinical behaviour. *J Dermatol Surg Oncol* 1990; **16**: 674–6.
15 Pelosi G, Martignoni, G, Bonetti F. Intraductal carcinoma of mammary-type apocrine epithelium arising within a papillary hydradenoma of the vulva: report of a case and review of the literature. *Arch Pathol Lab Med* 1991; **115**: 1249–54.
16 Bannatyne P, Elliott P, Russell P. Vulvar adenosquamous carcinoma arising in a hidradenoma papilliferum with rapidly fatal outcome: a case report. *Gynecol Oncol* 1989; **35**: 395–8.

Mucinous cysts

Mucinous cysts of the vulva are not uncommon. They are usually found in the vestibule where they develop secondary to obstruction of the duct of one of the many minor vestibular mucus-secreting glands. The cysts are of urogenital sinus origin and not, as was once thought, of Müllerian origin [1,2].

REFERENCES

1 Robboy SJ, Ross JS, Prat J et al. Urogenital sinus origin of mucinous and ciliated cysts of the vulva. Obstet Gynecol 1978; **51**: 347–51.
2 Oi RH, Munn R. Mucous cysts of the vulvar vestibule. Hum Pathol 1982; **13**: 584–6.

Bartholin's duct tumours

These are very rare and there is debate as to whether they are true neoplasms or better regarded as examples of hyperplasia or hamartoma [1,2].

REFERENCES

1 Koenig C, Tavassoli FA. Nodular hyperplasia adenoma, and adenomyoma of Bartholin's gland. Int J Dermatol 1998; **17**: 289–94.
2 Argenta PA, Bell K, Reynolds C, Weinstein R. Bartholin's gland hyperplasia in a postmenopausal woman. Obstet Gynecol 1997; **90**: 695–7.

Neurofibroma and neurofibromatosis

Vulval neurofibromas may occur either as solitary lesions with no other features of neurofibromatosis, or as part of generalized neurofibromatosis. In one series, 18% had vulval lesions [1]. Vulval neurofibromas have also been described as one component of a localized neurofibromatosis of the female genitourinary tract [2,3]. Some cases have led to confusion by mimicking an intersex problem [4–7].

REFERENCES

1 Schreiber MM. Vulval von Recklinghausen's disease. Arch Dermatol 1963; **88**: 320–1.
2 Gersell DJ, Fulling KH. Localized neurofibromatosis of the female genitourinary tract. Am J Surg Pathol 1989; **13**: 873–8.
3 Lewis FM, Lewis-Jones MS, Toon PG et al. Neurofibromatosis of the vulva. Br J Dermatol 1992; **127**: 540–1.
4 Kenny FM, Fetterman GH, Preeyasombat C. Neurofibromata simulating a penis and labioscrotal gonads in a girl with von Recklinghausen's disease. Pediatrics 1966; **37**: 956–9.
5 Labardini MM, Kallet HA, Cerny JC. Urogenital neurofibromatosis simulating an intersex problem. J Urol 1968; **98**: 627–32.
6 Schepel SJ, Tolhurst DE. Neurofibromata of clitoris and labium majus simulating a penis and testicle. Br J Plast Surg 1981; **34**: 221–3.
7 Ravikumar VR, Lakshmanan DA. Solitary neurofibroma of the clitoris masquerading as an intersex. J Pediatr Surg 1983; **18**: 617.

Glomus tumour

There are rare reports of this tumour on the labia minora giving rise to dyspareunia [1,2].

REFERENCES

1 Kohorn EI, Merino MJ, Goldenhersh M. Vulvar pain and dyspareunia due to a glomus tumor. Obstet Gynecol 1986; **67**: 41–42S.
2 Katz VL, Askin FB, Bosch BD. Glomus tumor of the vulva: a case report. Obstet Gynecol 1986; **67**: 43–45S.

Leiomyoma

Vulval leiomyomas are uncommon [1,2], and there is no association with uterine leiomyomas. It is unclear whether these tumours originate from the smooth muscle of the vulval erectile tissue, from the muscular elements of the round ligament, or from the myoepithelial cells of Bartholin's gland.

Vulval leiomyomas occur during the reproductive years and usually present as well-circumscribed painless non-tender nodules or swellings in the labia. Lesions may enlarge in pregnancy. A clitoral leiomyoma can cause a mistaken diagnosis of an intersex disorder. A clitoral leiomyoma associated with a leiomyoma of the oesophagus has been reported [3].

REFERENCES

1 Neri A, Peled Y, Braslavski D. Vulvar leiomyoma. Acta Obstet Gynecol Scand 1993; **72**: 221–2.
2 Nielsen GP, Rosenberg AE, Koerner FC, Young RH, Scully RE. Smooth muscle tumours of the vulva: a clinicopathological study of 25 cases and a review of the literature. Am J Surg Pathol 1996; **20**: 779–93.
3 Stenchever MA, McDivett RW, Fisher JA. Leiomyoma of the clitoris. J Reprod Med 1973; **2**: 75–6.

Rarer tumours include granular cell myoblastoma [1,2], which present as flesh-coloured, occasionally pedunculated or ulcerated lesions. Verruciform xanthomas have a predilection for the oral mucosa and the genital skin. They are rare on the vulva [3,4]. Clinically, they present as solitary plaques or warty lesions and vary in colour from yellow to grey or pink. There is acanthosis, papillomatosis and parakeratosis, and the presence of foamy macrophages in the papillary dermis and tips of the elongated rete ridges distinguishes this entity from a viral wart. Nodular fasciitis presents as a painless mass and has rarely been reported on the vulva [5].

Urethral caruncle and urethral prolapse, which are common, can sometimes be mistaken for neoplasms. A urethral caruncle occurs in postmenopausal women as a red fleshy lesion around the urethral meatus and is a chronically inflamed eversion of the urethral mucosa. It may measure from a few millimetres to a few centimetres in diameter and is usually asymptomatic; it may cause dysuria or bleeding if ulcerated. Histologically, it is essentially the same as a pyogenic granuloma, showing a highly vascular connective tissue with a heavy inflammatory infiltrate of lymphocytes and plasma cells. Enmeshed in this inflamed stroma are varying quantities of glandular structures or solid islands of urethral epithelium.

Prolapse of the urethra may occur at any age. Histologically, there is marked oedema of the underlying connective tissue, and the overlying urethral mucosa may be focally ulcerated. The underlying stroma shows marked vascular distension and engorgement, often with thrombosis. The epithelial inclusions typically seen in a urethral caruncle are not present.

REFERENCES

1 Gifford RRM, Birch HW. Granular cell myoblastoma of multicentric origin involving the vulva: a case report. *Am J Obstet Gynecol* 1973; **117**: 184–7.
2 Sadler WP, Docherty MB. Malignant myoblastoma vulvae. *Am J Obstet Gynecol* 1951; **61**: 1047–55.
3 Santa Cruz DJ, Martin SA. Verruciform xanthoma of the vulva. *Am J Clin Pathol* 1979; **71**: 224–8.
4 De Rosa G, Barra E. Verruciform xanthoma of the vulva: case report. *Genitourin Med* 1989; **65**: 252–4.
5 O'Connell JX, Young RH, Nielsen GP *et al*. Nodular fasciitis of the vulva: a study of six cases and a review of the literature. *Int J Gynecol Pathol* 1997; **16**: 117–23.

Precancerous dermatoses

Vulval intraepithelial neoplasia

This term was introduced by the International Society for the Study of Vulvovaginal Diseases (ISSVD) to replace the previous terms dystrophy with atypia, Bowen's disease, bowenoid papulosis, erythroplasia of Queyrat and squamous carcinoma *in situ* [1–3]. It is defined as loss of the normal orientation and architecture of the epithelium with cellular atypia. It was also graded into VIN1–3, according to the percentage of the epithelium involved. This classification also included EMPD and melanoma *in situ*. There are now proposals to change this classification, reserving the term VIN exclusively for squamous cell dysplasia that has a risk of malignant transformation. This would not include Paget's disease or melanoma *in situ*. The newer terminology for VIN also recommends abolishing the current grading system. The three tier grading of VIN is often misleading [4,5], as many cases of VIN1 with basal atypia are not truly premalignant but reparative (e.g. LP). The important VIN with malignant potential is that with atypia involving two-thirds to full thickness of the epithelium (undifferentiated VIN [VIN2 and VIN3]), or severe atypia confined to the basal layers with fairly normal differentiation of the upper layers (differentiated VIN). The rete ridges may be long and forked, with keratin pearls. This change on a background of LS/LP represents either very early invasive disease or heralds its imminent onset.

Undifferentiated vulval intraepithelial neoplasia
SYN. BOWEN'S DISEASE; BOWENOID PAPULOSIS; CARCINOMA IN SITU; CARCINOMA SIMPLEX

There is a complete loss of cellular stratification throughout the epidermis, with large hyperchromatic cells, dyskeratosis, multinucleated cells and numerous typical and atypical mitoses. Originally, two distinct histological types of VIN were described: bowenoid, characterized by individual cell keratinization and abnormal cellular differentiation; and basaloid, with atypical parabasal cells extending throughout the full thickness of the epithelium. However, both types can sometimes be found in the same histological section so it is no longer considered helpful to distinguish the two.

Multifocal anogenital disease is strongly associated with the oncogenic papillomaviruses, particularly HPV 16 and 18, and almost exclusively occurs in smokers [6,7]. The condition is caused by a failure of the host to mount an immune response to the HPV. Patients who are immunocompromised have a higher incidence of this problem, but the majority of young women with this problem do not have an identifiable immunodeficiency. In addition to being multifocal, VIN may be associated with multicentric disease, with lesions of intraepithelial neoplasia involving the cervix, vagina and perianal skin. Up to two-thirds of patients with VIN have a current or past history of CIN [8].

Clinically, the lesions of intraepithelial neoplasia can be solitary or multiple. The morphology of the lesions is also very diverse, with lesions that resemble viral warts, plaques that may be shiny and smooth, skin-coloured, red or white, or others that are warty and pigmented and resemble seborrhoeic keratoses [9,10]. Less commonly, the lesions may be large and papillomatous, particularly perianally, where they may be polypoid. The main symptom is pruritus, which can be severe and troublesome (Figs 68.33–68.35).

Vaginal involvement is uncommon. Initially, it was felt that BP could be distinguished histologically from Bowen's disease but time has proved this not to be the case.

The risk of progression to invasive disease is estimated as 10% or less in multifocal disease, but this risk is higher in immunocompromised patients, particularly with perianal disease [11] and in the older woman with a solitary plaque [12].

There also have been reports of vulval cancer in patients with Fanconi's anaemia [13,14].

Treatment. This is tailored to the individual patient's needs. In the case of a solitary lesion that is amenable to simple excision, this is the treatment of choice. In the woman with extensive disease, surgery would be mutilating physically and distressing psychologically, and does not guarantee a cure as the risk of recurrence is significant

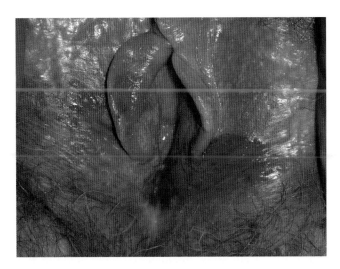

Fig. 68.33 Vulval intraepithelial neoplasia. Erythematous patches with one warty plaque inferiorly on the inner aspect of the right labium minus.

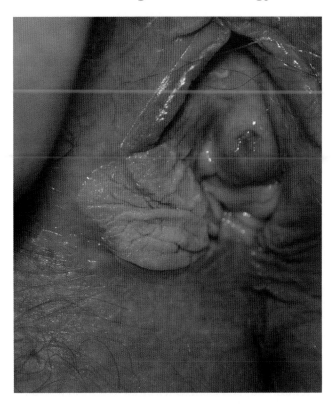

Fig. 68.34 Vulval intraepithelial neoplasia. Solitary warty plaque.

[15,16]. Such patients require regular and long-term follow-up, with biopsies of suspicious areas. Thick or polypoid lesions should be excised, as early invasive changes are difficult to detect in these areas [17]. Cryotherapy is not effective, but 5-fluorouracil can be used successfully for lesions of the labia minora, vestibule and clitoral area [16]. It is not effective on the hair-bearing parts of the vulva, probably because of the deep adnexal structures, which can all be involved. Laser vaporization has a high recurrence rate, particularly if the hair-bearing parts of the vulva are involved, and there is the additional danger that early invasive disease may be missed and therefore inappropriately treated. It is also extremely painful postoperatively.

As VIN is a multicentric problem, the other sites that need to be monitored are the cervix, vagina and perianal area. If there is perianal disease, anoscopy should be performed to exclude involvement of the anal canal.

REFERENCES

1 Wilkinson EJ, Kneale B, Lynch P. Report of the ISSVD Terminology Committee. *J Reprod Med* 1986; **31**: 973–4.
2 Wilkinson EJ. Normal histology and nomenclature of the vulva and malignant neoplasms including VIN. *Dermatol Clin* 1992; **10**: 283–96.
3 Hart WR. Vulvar intraepithelial neoplasia: historical aspects and current status. *Int J Gynecol Pathol* 2001; **20**: 16–30.
4 Preti M, Mezzetti M, Robertson C, Sideri M. Interobserver variation in histopathological diagnosis and grading of vulvar intraepithelial neoplasia: results of a European collaborative study. *Br J Obstet Gynaecol* 2000; **107**: 594–9.
5 van Beurden M, deCraen AJ, deVet HC *et al.* The contribution of MIB1 in the accurate grading of vulvar intraepithelial neoplasia. *J Clin Pathol* 1999; **52**: 820–4.
6 Lookingbill DP, Kreider JW, Howett MK, Olmstrad PM, Conner GH. Human papilloma virus type 16 in Bowenoid papulosis, intraoral papillomas and squamous cell carcinoma of the tongue. *Arch Dermatol* 1987; **123**: 363–8.

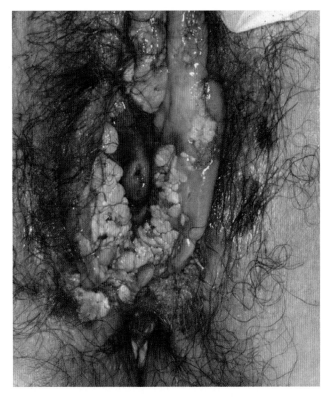

Fig. 68.35 Vulval intraepithelial neoplasia. Pigmented seborrhoeic keratosis-like lesions.

7 Buscema J, Naghashfar AZ, Sawada E *et al.* The predominance of human papilloma virus 16 in vulvar neoplasia. *Obstet Gynecol* 1988; **71**: 601–6.

8 Obalek S, Jablonska S, Beauderron Walcsak L, Orth G. Bowenoid papulosis of the male and female genitalia: risk of cervical neoplasia. *J Am Acad Dermatol* 1986; **14**: 433–44.

9 Wade TR, Kopf AW, Ackerman AB. Bowenoid papulosis of the genitalia. *Arch Dermatol* 1979; **115**: 306–8.

10 Patterson JW, Kao GF, Graham JH *et al.* Bowenoid papulosis: a clinico-pathologic study with ultrastructural observations. *Cancer* 1986; **83**: 738–58.

11 Rudlinger R, Buchmann P. HPV 16-positive Bowenoid papulosis and squa-mous cell carcinoma of the anus in an HIV-positive man. *Dis Colon Rectum* 1989; **32**: 1042–5.

12 Belilovsky C de, Leibowitch M. Maladie de Bowen et papulose bowenoide: donnees cliniques virologiques et evolutives comparatives. *Contracep Fertil Sex* 1993; **21**: 231–6.

13 Kennedy AW, Hart WR. Multiple squamous cell carcinomas in Fanconi's anaemia. *Cancer* 1982; **50**: 811–4.

14 Wilkinson EJ, Morgan LS, Friedrich EG. Association of Fanconi's anaemia and squamous cell carcinoma of the lower female genital tract with condy-lomata acuminata: a report of two cases. *J Reprod Med* 1984; **29**: 447–53.

15 Powell LC, Dinh TV, Rajaraman S *et al.* Carcinoma *in situ* of the vulva: a clinicopathologic study of 50 cases. *J Reprod Med* 1986; **31**: 808–14.

16 Shafi MI, Luesley DM, Byrne P *et al.* Vulval intraepithelial neoplasia: man-agement and outcome. *Br J Obstet Gynaecol* 1989; **96**: 1339–44.

17 Chafe W, Richards A, Morgan L, Wilkinson E. Unrecognized invasive carcinoma in vulval intraepithelial neoplasia (VIN). *Gynecol Oncol* 1988; **31**: 154–62.

Vulval malignancy [1]

The most common malignancy by far is SCC, followed by basal cell carcinoma, adenocarcinoma, melanoma and verrucous carcinoma.

Squamous cell carcinoma

Aetiologically, there appear to be two types of vulval squamous cell carcinoma [2–5]. The first and largest group occurs in elderly women on a background of a chronic dermatosis such as LS or LP. The second type, which accounts for approximately 40% of cases, occurs in younger women and is associated with intraepithelial neoplasia associated with oncogenic-type HPV infection. A link with HPV has not yet been established with the first group [6].

In the 1990s, the staging of vulval cancer was replaced by a combined clinical and surgical staging [7]. One of the reasons for this change was to remove the term microinvas-ive carcinoma of the vulva, as at that time its definition was misleading. In this new classification, stage I tumours are less than 2 cm diameter and are further subdivided into Ia and Ib. Ia are lesions with less than 1 mm depth of invasion. There are some difficulties as to how this meas-urement should be made. The most recent recommenda-tion is to measure from the dermal–epidermal junction of the nearest dermal papilla to the deepest point of invasion [8]. Lymph node dissection is mandatory for all lesions greater than 1 mm but can be avoided in those with stage Ia. There are three histological types of SCC: keratinizing, basaloid and warty carcinomas.

Keratinizing tumours are those seen in the older women, which are not HPV-related, and the basaloid and warty tumours are those found in younger women with HPV-related VIN.

There is also an adenoid variant of SCC with acantho-lysis in the centres of some of the infiltrating nests, pro-ducing cystic spaces lined by cubocolumnar nests. These pseudocysts do not contain mucin, which differentiates them from adenosquamous cell carcinoma.

Treatment. Surgical excision is tailored to the individual, and is determined by the size and site of the tumour.

The overall 5-year survival is approximately 75%, which rises to 90% or greater in those with no nodal meta-stases. The main reason for failure of treatment is the inability to control lymphatic and distant metastases, lym-phatic spread being the most important factor. The vulval lymphatics drain to the inguinal and femoral nodes and from there to the pelvic nodes. Central lesions (those placed near the clitoris, urethra, vagina, fourchette and perianal area) have a bilateral lymphatic drainage, and it is import-ant in these cases that the inguinofemoral nodes on both sides are excised. Radiotherapy is used as an adjuvant in patients with positive nodes and in those with inoperable tumours. It is also sometimes used as a primary treatment in tumours of the anus and urethra, to reduce their size before surgery and to try to preserve sphincter function.

REFERENCES

1 Fox H, Buckley CH. Neoplastic disease of the vulva and associated struc-tures. In: Fox H, Wells M, eds. *Haines and Taylor Obstetrical and Gynaecological Pathology*, 5th edn. London: Churchill Livingstone, 2003: 95–145.

2 Anderson WA, Franquemont DW, Williams J, Taylor PT, Crum CP. Vulval squamous cell carcinoma and papillomavirus: two separate entities? *Am J Obstet Gynecol* 1991; **165**: 329–36.

3 Crum C. Carcinoma of the vulva: epidemiology and pathogenesis. *Obstet Gynecol* 1992; **79**: 448–58.

4 Hording U, Junge J, Daugaard S *et al.* Vulval squamous cell carcinoma and papilloma viruses: indications for two different aetiologies. *Gynecol Oncol* 1994; **52**: 241–6.

5 Trimble CL, Hildesheim A, Brinton LA, Shah KV, Kurman RJ. Heterogene-ous aetiology of squamous cell carcinoma of the vulva. *Obstet Gynecol* 1996; **87**: 59–64.

6 Toki T, Kurma RJ, Park JS *et al.* Probable non-papillomavirus etiology of squamous cell carcinoma of the vulva in older women: a clinicopathologic study using *in situ* hybridization and polymerase chain reaction. *Int J Gynecol Pathol* 1991; **10**: 107–25.

7 Shepherd JH. Staging announcement FIGO staging of gynecologic cancers: cervical and vulva. *Int J Gynecol Cancer* 1995; **5**: 319.

8 Wilkinson EJ. Superficially invasive carcinoma of the vulva. In: Wilkinson EJ, ed. *Pathology of the Vulva and Vagina*. New York: Churchill Livingstone, 1987: 103–17.

Verrucous carcinoma

SYN. GIANT CONDYLOMA OF BUSCHKE–LÖWENSTEIN

This tumour occurs in older women, and many arise on a background of LS [1]. There is also a strong relationship to vulval condylomas. Clinically, the lesions appear as a warty plaque or cauliflower-like tumour, which can ulcer-ate and become extremely large (Fig. 68.36).

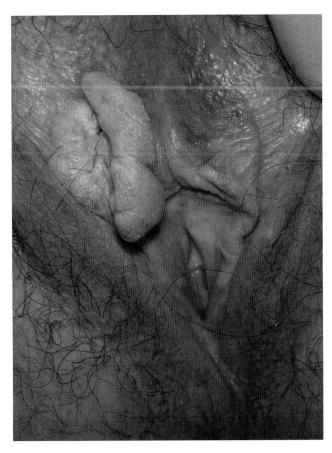

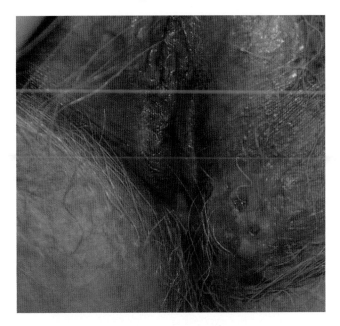

Fig. 68.37 Basal cell carcinoma: lower left labium majus.

Fig. 68.36 Verrucous carcinoma on a background of lichen sclerosus.

The histological changes include epidermal acanthosis, with large bulbous rete ridges which compress and push down the underlying stroma. There is very little cellular atypia and the few, if any, mitoses are confined to the basal layers. Koilocytes are usually present. Lymph node and distant metastases occur rarely.

Treatment is wide local excision. Radiotherapy is not used as it is associated with a worse prognosis, probably because it can induce anaplastic transformation [2]. Oral retinoids may also be helpful [3].

REFERENCES

1 Japaze H, Dinh TV, Woodruff JD. Verrucous carcinoma of the vulva. *Obstet Gynecol* 1982; **60**: 462–6.
2 Kraus FT, Perez-Mesa C. Verrucous carcinoma: clinical and pathologic study of 105 cases including oral cavity, larynx and genitalia. *Cancer* 1966; **19**: 26–38.
3 Mehta RK, Rytina E, Sterling JC. Treatment of verrucous carcinoma of vulva with acetretin. *Br J Dermatol* 2000; **142**: 1195–8.

Basal cell carcinoma

Vulval basal cell carcomas are not uncommon and present as an eroded plaque, which may be pigmented. Less com-monly, the tumour may form a nodule or ulcer. They occur most frequently on the labia majora (Fig. 68.37) [1].

Histologically, the appearances are identical to BCCs seen elsewhere. Inadequate excision accounts for a high recurrence rate and metastases to regional lymph nodes [2]. Mohs' surgery is often recommended to ensure ade-quate local excision [3,4].

REFERENCES

1 Feakins RM, Lowe DG. Basal cell carcinoma of the vulva: a clinicopathologic study of 45 cases. *Int J Gynecol Pathol* 1997; **16**: 319–24.
2 Mizushima J, Ohara K. Basal cell carcinoma of the vulva with lymph node metastasis: report of a case and review of 20 Japanese cases. *J Dermatol* 1995; **22**: 36–42.
3 Mohs FE. Carcinoma of the vulva. In: *Chemosurgery, Microscopically Controlled Surgery of Skin Cancer*. Springfield: Charles C Thomas, 1978: 215–9.
4 Brown MD, Zachary CB, Grekin RC, Swanson N. Genital tumors: their management by micrographic surgery. *J Am Acad Dermatol* 1998; **18**: 115–22.

Adenocarcinoma

Primary adenocarcinoma unrelated to underlying glan-dular adnexae is exceedingly rare. The lesion usually presents as a painless subcutaneous nodule which, as it expands, becomes fixed and painful. The tumour can invade deeply into fat, muscle or bone and may be asso-ciated with a Bartholin's gland abscess. Adenocarcinoma may be associated with EMPD.

Many of the mucinous carcinomas that arise are pos-sibly of cloacal origin [1].

There is one report of a mucinous carcinoma with neuro-endocrine differentiation [2].

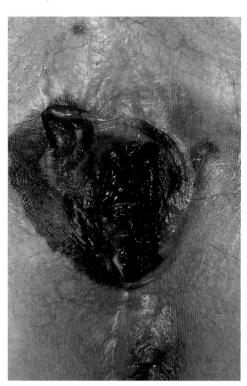

Fig. 68.38 Melanoma of the vulva. (Courtesy of Dr F.A. Ive, Durham, UK.)

REFERENCES

1 Willen R, Bekassy D, Carlen B, Bozoky B, Cajander S. Cloacogenic adenocarcinoma of the vulva. *Gynecol Oncol* 1999; **74**: 298–301.
2 Graf AH, Su HC, Tubbs RR *et al.* Primary neuroendocrine differentiated mucinous adenocarcinoma of the vulva: case report and review of the literature. *Anticancer Res* 1998; **18**: 2041–5.

Melanoma

Vulval melanomas account for approximately 5% of vulval malignancy. Any of the variants of melanoma may occur on the vulva, and the clinical and histological features are the same as for melanomas elsewhere (Fig. 68.38). However, in one cohort of 219 patients, 27% of lesions were amelanotic [1,2]. Melanomas at this site carry the same prognosis according to the Clarke level of invasion, the Breslow thickness and the presence or absence of a vertical growth phase. They may be mistakenly diagnosed as EMPD.

REFERENCES

1 Ragnarsson-Olding BK, Kanter-Lewensohn LR, Lagerlöf B *et al.* Malignant melanoma of the vulva in a nationwide, 25-year study of 219 Swedish females: clinical observations and pathological features. *Cancer* 1999; **86**: 1273–84.
2 Ragnarsson-Olding BK, Nilsson BR, Kanter-Lewensohn LR *et al.* Malignant melanoma of the vulva in a nationwide, 25-year study of 219 Swedish females: predictors of survival. *Cancer* 1999; **86**: 1285–93.

Vulval extramammary Paget's disease

EMPD is fully discussed in Chapter 36. EMPD is a rare dermatosis, and is distinct from Paget's disease of the nipple, which is always associated with underlying breast neoplasia. The vulva is the most common site for EMPD, which is subdivided into primary and secondary disease. Primary, or cutaneous EMPD, is an intraepithelial adenocarcinoma arising in the epidermis or the epithelia of the local skin appendages. Secondary EMPD is epidermal involvement from a non-cutaneous internal neoplasm, either by direct extension or metastasis. The two most common tumours associated with secondary vulval EMPD are anorectal adenocarcinoma and urothelial carcinoma of the bladder or urethra. Other associated tumours reported include cervix, endometrium and ovary [1,2].

The differentiation between primary and secondary disease is not always straightforward clinically and sometimes relies on immunohistological investigations [3,4].

Additional changes to the vulval EMPD classification have been proposed, based on aetiology [5]. The primary and secondary categories are retained, but each is divided into three types. The primary intraepithelial disease, primary with invasion, and EMPD as a manifestation of an underlying primary adenocarcinoma of a vulval skin appendage or subcutaneous vulval gland. The secondary category has three groups according to the tumour from which it arises: EMPD secondary to anorectal adenocarcinoma, EMPD secondary to urothelial carcinoma and EMPD secondary to an adenocarcinoma or related tumour at other sites.

It is important to distinguish primary from secondary EMPD as management depends on the correct diagnosis.

Clinical features. Clinically, the lesion is typically a moist red oozing plaque, which looks like impetiginized eczema or psoriasis. The associated symptoms include pruritus and burning (Fig. 68.39).

Histopathology. There is frequently epidermal hyperplasia. The epidermis is infiltrated with pale-staining Paget's cells. The Paget's cells are PAS-positive and diastase-resistant, and stain with Alcian blue and markers for the simple keratins. In the lower epidermis, the tumour cells may compress the basal cells.

Treatment. In primary EMPD, excision of visible disease is often recommended for treatment and to exclude underlying appendageal adenocarcinoma. Sometimes in the very elderly, with extensive disease or recurrence after vulvectomy, this is not always an option that the patient wishes to accept. Patients should be regularly monitored, and topical steroids can be used if there is troublesome pruritus. Topical 5-fluorouracil, bleomycin and imiquimod have been used, as well as oral retinoids, with some

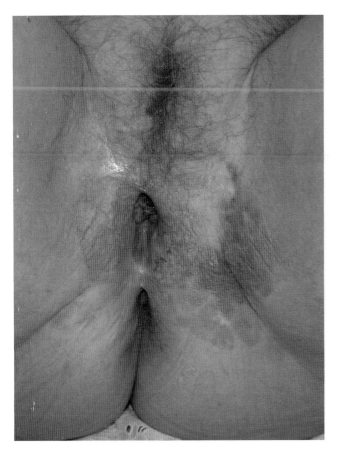

Fig. 68.39 Extramammary Paget's disease.

success. The recurrence rates are high after carbon dioxide laser and radiotherapy.

In secondary disease, the treatment is directed predominantly at the associated carcinoma.

REFERENCES

1 Parker L-P, Parker JR, Bodurka-Bevers D *et al.* Paget's disease of the vulva: pathology, pattern of involvement and prognosis. *Gynecol Oncol* 2000; **77**: 183–9.
2 Kodama S, Kaneko T, Saito M, Yoshiya N *et al.* A clinicopathologic study of 30 patients with Paget's disease of the vulva. *Gynecol Oncol* 1997; **56**: 63–70.
3 Brown HM, Wilkinson EJ. Uroplakin-III to distinguish primary vulvar Paget disease from Paget disease secondary to urothelial carcinoma. *Hum Pathol* 2002; **33**: 545–8.
4 Goldblum JR, Hart WR. Vulvar Paget's disease: a clinicopathologic and immunohistochemical study of 19 cases. *Am J Surg Pathol* 1997; **21**: 1178–1187.
5 Wilkinson EJ, Brown HM. Vulvar Paget disease of urothelial origin: a report of three cases and a proposed classification of vulval Paget disease. *Hum Pathol* 2002; **33**: 549–54.

Other malignancies

Langerhans' cell histiocytosis

The anogenital skin may be one of the sites involved in disseminated Langerhans' cell histiocytosis (LCH), but lesions may occur at this site only. Perianal ulceration is the most common presentation in adults and children [1,2], and genital involvement is more common in women [3,4]. The lesions may be plaques, nodules, erosions, ulcers or pustules. The Letterer–Siwe form consists of a seborrhoeic dermatitis-like eruption on the intertriginous zones and scalp. Some of the lesions may be purpuric.

REFERENCES

1 Rivera-Luna R, Martinez-Guerra G, Altamirano-Awarez E *et al.* Langerhans' cell histiocytosis: clinical experience with 124 patients. *Pediatr Dermatol* 1988; **5**: 145–50.
2 Stein SL, Paller AS, Haut PR, Mancini AJ. Langerhans' cell histiocytosis presenting in the neonatal period: a retrospective case series. *Arch Pediatr Adolesc Med* 2001; **155**: 778–83.
3 Axiotis CA, Merino MJ, Duray PH. Langerhans' cell histiocytosis of the female genital tract. *Cancer* 1991; **67**: 1650–60.
4 Hoang MP, Owen SA, Haisley-Royster C *et al.* Papular eruption of the scalp accompanied by axillary and vulvar ulcerations. *Arch Dermatol* 2001; **137**: 1241–6.

Lymphomas

Non-Hodgkin's lymphoma of the vulva is more frequently reported [1,2] than Hodgkin's lymphoma [3]. Non-Hodgkin's lymphoma has also been reported post-transplantation [4] and in association with HIV infection [5].

REFERENCES

1 Vang R, Medeiros J, Fuller GN *et al.* Non-Hodgkin's lymphoma involving the gynaecologic tract: a review of 88 cases. *Adv Anat Pathol* 2001; **8**: 200–17.
2 Vang R, Medeiros J, Malpica A *et al.* Non-Hodgkin's lymphoma involving the vulva. *Int J Gynecol Pathol* 2000; **19**: 236–42.
3 Hahn GA. Gynecologic considerations in malignant lymphoma. *Am J Obstet Gynecol* 1958; **75**: 673–83.
4 Kaplan MA, Jacobson MO, Ferry JA, Harris NL. T-cell lymphoma of the vulva in a renal allograft recipient with associated hemophagocytosis. *Am J Surg Pathol* 1993; **17**: 842–9.
5 Kaplan EG, Chadburn A, Caputo TA. HIV-related primary non-Hodgkin's lymphoma of the vulva. *Gynecol Oncol* 1996; **61**: 131–8.

Miscellaneous tumours

There are a few reports of vulval dermatofibrosarcoma protuberans on the labia majora [1], slow-growing liposarcoma [2], epithelioid sarcoma [3], Merkel cell carcinoma [4] and Bartholin's gland carcinoma [5].

REFERENCES

1 Moodley M, Moodley J. Dermatofibrosarcoma protuberans of the vulva: case report and review of the literature. *Gynecol Oncol* 2000; **78**: 74–6.
2 Nucci MR, Fletcher CDM. Liposarcoma (atypical lipomatous tumors) of the vulva: a clinicopathologic study of 6 cases. *Int J Gynecol Pathol* 1998; **17**: 17–23.
3 Ulbright TM, Brokaw SA, Stehman FB *et al.* Epithelioid sarcoma of vulva. *Cancer* 1983; **52**: 1462–9.
4 Gil-Moreno A, Garcia-Jiminez A, Gonzalea-Bosquet J *et al.* Merkel cell tumour of the vulva. *Gynecol Oncol* 1997; **64**: 526–32.
5 Felix JC, Cote RJ, Kramer EE, Saigo P, Goldman GH. Carcinoma of Bartholin's gland: histogenesis and the aetiological role of human papilloma virus. *Am J Pathol* 1993; **142**: 925–33.

Metastatic tumours

These are uncommon and may be from malignancies of the cervix, endometrium, vagina, ovary, urethra, kidney, breast and lung, in descending order of frequency [1].

REFERENCE

1 Dehner IP. Metastatic and secondary tumours of the vulva. *Obstet Gynecol* 1973; **42**: 47–57.

Miscellaneous

Pigmentary disorders

Hypopigmentation

As at other sites, this can be naevoid, a post-inflammatory problem or vitiligo.

Hyperpigmentation

The increased pigmentation may be caused by haemosiderin, which results in a reddish brown discoloration. It is the result of extravasation of red blood cells and is seen in capillaritis, urethral caruncle, lichen sclerosus, Zoon's vulvitis and chronic vulval purpura. However, increased pigmentation is more commonly related to melanin. There is considerable variation in the distribution and amount of melanocytes and melanin in the normal vulva, depending on site, age, ethnicity and hormonal status.

Post-inflammatory pigmentation may follow any inflammatory dermatosis, particularly if there has been a disruption of the dermal–epidermal junction and in darker skins. It is a common sequela of LP and sometimes LS.

Vulval melanosis. Intense macular hyperpigmentation of vulval skin can be difficult to categorize, and a biopsy is essential for an accurate diagnosis and to exclude malignant melanoma (Fig. 68.40a) [1]. If the lesions are widespread and accompanied by oral pigmentation, they may be considered as examples of Laugier–Hunziker syndrome [2,3]. The term vulval melanosis is used for those cases where there is extensive macular pigmentation affecting the vulval skin, with the histological changes of basal hypermelanosis and a slight increase in the number of melanocytes. There may also be some pigmentary incontinence, but there is no abnormal junctional melanocytic proliferation (Fig. 68.40b) [4–8]. There have been other suggested terms: idiopathic lenticular mucocutaneous pigmentation [9] and genital lentiginosis, particularly if there is melanocytic hyperplasia [10].

The accepted view is that vulval melanosis is a benign condition, but there are no long-term follow-up studies reported. Therefore, most clinicians advise continuing observation, using photographs or diagrams as an aid.

Lentigines. Vulval lentigines may be sporadic or part of a syndrome (e.g. LAMB syndrome) [11,12]. There is an increase in the number of basal melanocytes, with increased melanin in the epidermis and stratum corneum. Pigment-laden macrophages are found in the papillary dermis, and the rete ridges are elongated.

Acanthosis nigricans. This condition is usually associated with insulin resistance and rarely with malignancy. Initially, the appearance is of a dark and velvety thickening of

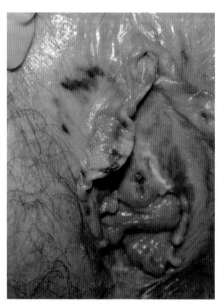 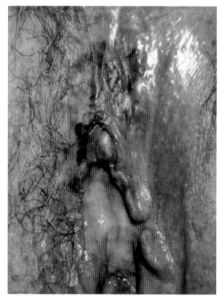

(a)   (b)

Fig. 68.40 (a) *In situ* melanoma. (b) Vulval melanosis.

the skin in the genitocrual folds and upper inner thighs, which later becomes warty. Skin tags may also occur.

A fixed drug eruption leaves behind residual hyperpigmentation. Some laxatives are reduced in the bowel to dithranol and this may stain the skin in contact with faeces and lead to a reddish brown discoloration of the urine and vaginal secretions [13,14]. Trichomycosis and chromidrosis may cause some discoloration.

REFERENCES

1 Carli P, De Giorgi V, Nardini P et al. Vulvar melanosis mimicking melanoma: a cause for concern in patients and clinicians. G Ital Dermatol Venereol 1994; **129**: 143–6.
2 Laugier P, Hunziker N, Olmos L. Pigmentation melanique lenticulaire essentielle de la muqueuse jugale et des levres. Ann Dermatol Vénéréol 1977; **104**: 181–4.
3 Dupré A, Viraben R. Laugier's disease. Dermatologica 1990; **181**: 183–6.
4 Rudolph RI. Vulvar melanosis. J Am Acad Dermatol 1990; **23**: 982–4.
5 Sisson-Torre EQ, Ackerman AB. Melanosis of the vulva: a clinical simulator of malignant melanoma. Am J Dermatopathol 1985; **7**: 51–60.
6 Kanj LF, Rubeiz NG, Mrouett AM et al. Vulvar melanosis and lentiginosis: a case report. J Am Acad Dermatol 1992; **27**: 777–8.
7 Jackson R. Melanosis of the vulva. J Dermatol Surg Oncol 1984; **10**: 119–21.
8 Estrada R, Kaufman R. Benign vulvar melanosis. J Reprod Med 1993; **38**: 5–8.
9 Gerbig AW, Hunziker T. Idiopathic lenticular mucocutaneous pigmentation or Laugier–Hunziker syndrome with atypical features. Arch Dermatol 1996; **32**: 844–5.
10 Barnhill RL, Albert LS, Shama SK et al. Genital lentiginosis: a clinical and histopathologic study. J Am Acad Dermatol 1990; **22**: 453–60.
11 Rhodes AR, Silverman RA, Harrist TJ et al. Mucocutaneous lentigines, cardiomucocutaneous myxomas and multiple blue naevi: the LAMB syndrome. J Am Acad Dermatol 1984; **10**: 72–82.
12 Reed OM, Mellette JR, Fitzpatrick JE. Cutaneous lentiginosis with atrial myxomas. J Am Acad Dermatol 1986; **15**: 398–402.
13 Barth JH, Reshad H, Darley CR, Gibson JR. A cutaneous complication of Dorbanex therapy. Clin Exp Dermatol 1984; **9**: 95–6.
14 Greer IA. Orange periods. BMJ 1984; **289**: 323.

Necrolytic migratory erythema

This rare dermatosis occurs on the genital skin and lower abdomen and is almost always associated with an underlying pancreatic glucagonoma, although there are exceptional cases where it is not [1].

REFERENCE

1 Masri-Fridling GD, Turner MLC. Necrolytic migratory erythema without glucagonoma. J Am Acad Dermatol 1992; **27**: 486.

Vulval oedema, lymphoedema and lymphangiectasia

Oedema, hereditary angio-oedema [1] and dermographism [2] may all involve the vulva. Vulval oedema may be the only manifestation of Crohn's disease [3].

Lymphoedema occurs when there is impairment of the lymph drainage and it is a frequent complication following surgery and lymphadenectomy for vulval carcinoma. Lymphangiectasia is acquired dilatation of the skin lymphatics secondary to obstruction of the lymphatic vessels.

It is most frequently reported following treatment of cervical carcinoma with surgery and/or radiotherapy [4–6]. Lymphangiectasia may be very profuse in Crohn's disease and carbon dioxide laser treatment can be used in patients with troublesome lymphorrhoea [7]. Repeated episodes of cellulitis may also result in lymphangiectasia, but there may be an underlying abnormality of the lymphatics that predisposed the patient to the cellulitis initially. Lymphangiectasia may be mistaken clinically for viral warts [8].

Endometriosis

Endometriosis occasionally occurs on the vulva or in the vagina as a direct implantation. The condition may follow a previous surgical procedure [9,10], and in episiotomy scars after delivery [11,12]. It presents as firm bluish nodules, which become tender or bleed during menstruation. Clear cell adenocarcinoma has arisen in vulval endometriosis [13].

Genital papular acantholytic dyskeratosis

This was first described in 1984 [14], and is characterized by the presence of multiple papules or, less frequently, a single papule or plaque-like lesions on genital skin [15–18]. Cases with disseminated lesions have been described [19]. The histological changes are similar to those seen in Darier's disease or Hailey–Hailey disease, but there is no positive family history or evidence of these diseases at other sites. It is considered a distinct entity, although it may represent a forme fruste of Hailey–Hailey or Darier's disease.

REFERENCES

1 Warin RP, Champion RH. Urticaria. London: Saunders, 1974: 114.
2 Lambiris A, Greaves MW. Dyspareunia and vulvodynia are probably common manifestations of facticious urticaria. Br J Dermatol 1997; **136**: 140–1.
3 Martin J, Holdstock G. Isolated vulval oedema as a feature of Crohn's disease. J Obstet Gynecol 1997; **17**: 92–3.
4 LaPolla J, Foucar E, Leshin B, Whitaker D, Anderson B. Vulvar lymphangioma circumscriptum: a rare complication of therapy for squamous cell carcinoma of the cervix. Gynecol Oncol 1985; **22**: 363–6.
5 Handfield-Jones SE, Prendeville WL, Norman S. Vulval lymphangiectasia. Genitourin Med 1989; **65**: 335–7.
6 Fisher I, Orkin M. Acquired lymphangioma (lymphangiectasia). Arch Dermatol 1970; **102**: 230–4.
7 Landthaler M, Hohenleutner U, Braun-Falco O. Acquired lymphangioma of the vulva: palliative treatment by means of laser vaporization carbon dioxide. Arch Dermatol 1990; **126**: 967–8.
8 Harwood CA, Mortimer PS. Acquired lymphangiomata mimicking genital warts. Br J Dermatol 1993; **129**: 334–6.
9 Duson CK, Zelenik JS. Vulvar endometriosis apparently produced by menstrual blood. Obstet Gynecol 1954; **3**: 76–9.
10 Dutta P. Vulval endometriosis. J Indian Med Assoc 1987; **85**: 237–8.
11 Catherwood AE, Cohen ES. Endometriosis with decidual reaction in episiotomy scar. Am J Obstet Gynecol 1951; **62**: 1364–6.
12 Brougher JC. Endometrial cyst in an episiotomy scar. Am J Obstet Gynecol 1947; **54**: 127–8.
13 Mesko JD, Gates H, McDonald TW, Youmans R, Lewis J. Clear cell (mesonephroid) adenocarcinoma of the vulva arising in endometriosis: a case report. Gynecol Oncol 1988; **29**: 385–91.

14 Chorzelski TP, Kudejko J, Jablonska S. Is papular acantholytic dyskeratosis of the vulva a new entity? *Am J Dermatopathol* 1984; **6**: 557–60.
15 Cooper PH. Acantholytic dermatosis localized to the vulvocrural area. *J Cutan Pathol* 1989; **16**: 81–4.
16 Lee SH, Jang JG. Papular acantholytic dyskeratosis of the genitalia. *J Dermatol* 1989; **16**: 312–4.
17 Pestereli HE, Karaveli S, Oztekin S, Zorlu G. Benign persistent acantholytic and dyskeratotic eruption of the vulva: a case report. *Int J Gynecol Pathol* 2000; **19**: 374–6.
18 Bell HK, Farrar CW, Curley RK. Papular acantholytic dyskeratosis of the vulva. *Clin Exp Dermatol* 2001; **26**: 386–8.
19 Ciupinska M, Kalbarczyk K, Jablonska S. Disseminated papular acantholytic dyskeratosis. *J Eur Acad Dermatol Venereol* 1998; **11**: 55–8.

Vulval pain syndromes

Vulvodynia

The term vulvodynia was first introduced in 1983 by the ISSVD to categorize those patients who complained of a chronic sensation of burning or rawness of the vulval skin [1]. Initially, vulvodynia included several subcategories [2], but these proved unsatisfactory in the light of further experience [3].

A diagnosis of vulvodynia should be strictly reserved for those patients who have the symptoms of pain or discomfort for 3 months or more in the absence of any visible abnormality or explanation that would account for their symptoms. If any active dermatosis or dermographism is found that could account for the symptoms then that condition is the diagnosis rather than vulvodynia.

Advances in the last decade have improved our knowledge and understanding of pain in general, and the existence of complex regional pain syndromes is now well recognized. Chronic pain syndromes are rarely caused by primary psychiatric disorders as originally thought, but are the result of peripheral and/or central neuronal sensitization.

In the 1990s it was felt that vulvodynia fulfilled many of the criteria of a complex regional pain syndrome. In clinical practice there appeared to be two major types of vulvodynia: vestibulitis and dysaesthetic vulvodynia. The main differentiation between the two was that vestibulitis was characterized by pain localized to the vulval vestibule that was precipitated by touch alone, whereas dysaesthetic vulvodynia was diffuse vulval pain that occurred spontaneously and which might or might not be aggravated by touch. The term vestibulitis was unfortunate and misleading as it suggested an inflammatory condition.

The 1999 meeting of the ISSVD recognized that there was a need for further changes in the nomenclature to fit in with the classification used for chronic pain syndromes elsewhere. It was suggested that the term dysaesthetic vulvodynia be retained for vulval pain that was diffuse, constant and spontaneous. Localized pain triggered by touch alone, previously termed vestibulitis, would be referred to by the newer and more accurate term vestibu-lodynia. It was also proposed that in those cases where the pain is localized at another site that this should be specified (e.g. clitorodynia if the pain is localized to the clitoris). There will probably be further terminology as our knowledge about these chronic pain syndromes increases.

Vestibulodynia
SYN. VESTIBULITIS

The term vulval vestibulitis was first defined as a triad of clinical signs and symptoms that included dyspareunia, vestibular tenderness to light touch and erythema of the vestibular epithelium [4]. This syndrome was certainly recognized earlier and terms such as focal vulvitis, hyperaesthesia of the vulva and vestibular adenitis had been used to describe the condition. It is usually a disorder of younger women, who present with the complaint of secondary dyspareunia. Most patients give a history of a precipitating event and some recall that it started during a particularly stressful time. Vestibulitis it is not an inflammatory condition [5], and for this reason alone vestibulodynia is a better term. There is no evidence to support an association with chronic infection with either *Candida* or HPV. The aetiology remains unknown and it is currently best categorized as a chronic pain syndrome [6]. The majority of patients affected by vestibulodynia are psychologically normal but they do have higher anxiety and somatization scores [7,8]. Patients also seem more susceptible to irritants, not only on the vulval skin but also at other sites (e.g. hand dermatitis, poor tolerance to earrings if made of base metals). However, patch testing is usually negative [9]. It is important to assess if the patient is dermographic, as dermographism may mimic or exacerbate vulvodynia. Sometimes it is helpful to perform an examination after recent intercourse as nymphohymenal tears, fourchette fissuring and herpes simplex infection can all be overlooked as the cause of recurrent vulval pain precipitated or exacerbated by intercourse.

Dysaesthetic vulvodynia

Dysaesthetic vulvodynia is most frequently seen in older, postmenopausal women who are often not sexually active and there is usually no precipitating event. The pain is spontaneous and often occurs independently of touch. Many of these patients are depressed, but it is difficult to establish whether this is a primary phenomenon or secondary to chronic pain. Much of the literature on the psychological profiles of patients with vulvodynia is difficult to interpret, as very often the distinction between vestibulitis and dysaesthetic vulvodynia is unclear. Dysaesthetic vulvodynia is a frequent problem following inflammatory conditions of the vulva, particularly the vestibule. It is seen most frequently following LP, when the patient still has symptoms despite the fact that the dermatitis has responded to treatment. The use of 5% lidocaine ointment usually resolves this problem.

Some of the younger patients who develop dysaesthetic vulvodynia initially had vestibulodynia.

Treatment. Management requires an unrushed and sympathetic consultation, with time spent explaining the problem of pain syndromes and the rationale for the planned treatment. Initially, topical agents are used, which include a soap substitute, avoidance of irritants and regular application of the local anaesthetic 5% lidocaine ointment. The other topical 'caine' anaesthetics should be avoided because of the risk of contact sensitivity, which is rare with lidocaine. If the patient is dermographic, an oral antihistamine should be added. If the topical measures are of no benefit or only partially effective, a tricyclic antidepressant may be used for its central action on pain. Alternative medications include gabapentin and carbamazepine. If there are secondary psychological or sexual issues, the input from a specialist in this field will be important. Biofeedback may improve some patients, particularly if there is associated vaginismus [10]. The patients may also wish to join a self-support group; in the UK this is the Vulval Pain Society.

REFERENCES

1 McKay M. Burning vulva syndrome. Report of the ISSVD taskforce. *J Reprod Med* 1984; **29**: 457.
2 McKay M, Frankman O, Benson JH *et al.* Vulvar vestibulitis and vestibular papillomatosis. Report of the ISSVD Committee on Vulvodynia. *J Reprod Med* 1991; **36**: 413–5.
3 Ridley CM. Vulvodynia: evolution of classification and management. *J Eur Acad Dermatol Venereol* 1996; **7**: 129–34.
4 Friedrich EG. Vulvar vestibulitis syndrome. *J Reprod Med* 1987; **32**: 110–4.
5 Nylander Lundquist E, Hofer PA, Olofsson JI, Sjoberg I. Is vulvar vestibulitis an inflammatory condition? A comparison of histological findings in affected and healthy women. *Acta Derm Venereol (Stockh)* 1997; **77**: 319–22.
6 Bergeron S, Binik YM, Khalife S, Pagidas K. Vulvar vestibulitis syndrome: a critical review. *Clin J Pain* 1997; **13**: 27–42.
7 van Lankveld JJDM, Weijenborg PTM, Ter Kuile MM. Psychologic profiles of and sexual function in women with vulvar vestibulitis and their partners. *Obstetrics* 1996; **88**: 65–70.
8 Danielsson I, Sjöberg I, Wikman M. Vulvar vestibulitis: medical, psychosexual and psychosocial aspects, a case–control study. *Acta Obstet Gynecol Scand* 2000; **79**: 872–8.
9 Nunns D, Ferguson J, Beck M, Mandal D. Is patch testing necessary in vulval vestibulitis? *Contact Dermatitis* 1997; **37**: 87–9.
10 Bergeron S, Binik Y, Khalife S *et al.* A randomized comparison of group cognitive–behavioural therapy, surface electromyographic biofeedback, and vestibulectomy in the treatment of dyspareunia resulting from vulvar vestibulitis. *Pain* 2001; **91**: 297–306.

Perineal and perianal dermatology

Introduction

Dermatologists should be able to assess the area competently and know when to involve colleagues in other disciplines. The perineum involves the perianal skin, groins and scrotum or vulva.

Pruritus ani is a symptom, not a diagnosis, unless qualified as constitutional or idiopathic, and, in roughly half of patients with pruritus ani, a cause will be established after dermatological evaluation [1–6]. The topic is discussed at length below (see p. 68.85).

Inflammatory and infectious disorders of the area may be difficult to differentiate. The presence of an infective condition in this area may overlie and disguise a more important lesion of the colon or rectum [7].

The differential diagnosis of anogenital ulceration is addressed on p. 68.3 and in Tables 68.9 and 68.10. Many banal conditions take on a vegetating appearance in this area, especially in hot humid climates and in the presence of infection. For these, the term dermatitis vegetans can be used.

Elephantiasis forms of progressive tuberculosis [8] and syphilis are now seldom seen, but deep fungal infections must not be overlooked.

Anal and perianal symptoms and signs in homosexual males [9] have become of greater significance because of the increasing prevalence of AIDS [10–12]. Whatever the presentation of the patient, it is important to look for infective conditions and suspect the possibility of two or more concomitant diseases. Painful lesions of the anus in homosexual men are common [13], and may include traumatic lesions and herpes genitalis. Anorectal sepsis, including chronic intersphincteric abscesses, anal fistulae, fissures and ulcerated haemorrhoids were seen more frequently in a group of male homosexuals than in heterosexuals [14]. Anal intraepithelial neoplasia may be clinically subtle and invasive carcinoma is not rare. The dermatology of HIV infection is discussed generally in Chapter 26, and of the perineal and anal area below.

REFERENCES

1 Smith LE, Henrichs D, McCullah RD. Prospective studies on the aetiology and treatment of pruritus ani. *Dis Colon Rectum* 1982; **25**: 358–63.
2 Alexander-Williams J. Pruritus ani. *BMJ* 1983; **287**: 159–60.
3 Verbov J. Pruritus ani and its management: a study and reappraisal. *Clin Exp Dermatol* 1984; **9**: 46–52.
4 Hanno R, Murphy P. Pruritus ani: classification and management. *Dermatol Clin* 1987; **5**: 811–6.
5 Jones DJ. Pruritus ani. *BMJ* 1992; **305**: 575–7.
6 Rohde H. Routine anal cleansing, so-called hemorrhoids, and perianal dermatitis: cause and effect? *Dis Colon Rectum* 2000; **43**: 561–3.
7 Grosshans E, Jenn P, Baumann R *et al.* Manifestations anales des maladies du tube digestif. *Ann Dermatol Vénéréol* 1979; **106**: 25–30.
8 Delacrétaz J, Christeler A. Demonstrations. *Dermatologica* 1969; **139**: 313–9.
9 Felman YM, Nikitas JA. Sexually transmitted diseases in the male homosexual. *Cutis* 1982; **30**: 706–24.
10 Penneys NS, ed. *Skin Manifestations of AIDS*. London: Martin Dunitz, 1990.
11 Cope R. Mise au point sur les lesions anoperineals et rectales observees au cours du SIDA. *Contracep Fertil Sex* 1994; **22**: 187–94.
12 Matis WL, Triana A, Shapiro R *et al.* Dermatologic findings associated with the human immunodeficiency virus. *J Am Acad Dermatol* 1987; **17**: 746–51.
13 McMillan A, Smith IW. Painful anal ulceration in homosexual men. *Br J Surg* 1984; **71**: 215–6.
14 Carr ND, Mercey D, Slack WW. Non-condylomatous perianal skin disease in homosexual men. *Br J Surg* 1989; **76**: 1064–6.

Structure and function

The anus is principally for the evacuation of faeces from the gastrointestinal tract [1], but may also be an organ of sexual utility.

The deep natal cleft, the inguinal (crural) folds and the infragluteal folds are special sites because they are areas where two layers of skin come into close apposition. Together these sites function as part of the hinge between the lower limbs and the trunk, as well as abutting the mucocutaneous junctions of anus and genitalia. The natal cleft is deep and firmly fixed to underlying fibrous and fascial tissues, and its sides are steep and closely apposed. Mucous discharges, excreta and moisture are retained easily within it. Proximity to the genital organs and anus give it a special physical and psychological importance.

The perineum is endowed with numerous eccrine sweat glands whose function is retained after lumbar and thoracolumbar sympathectomies. Sweating may be caused by an alternative parasympathetic sudomotor pathway from the fourth sacral anterior root. Apocrine glands are present but many are functionless. A variable number of sebaceous glands are present both in pilosebaceous units and as individual 'free' sebaceous glands at the transitional part of the anal canal.

The cloacal membrane is where ectodermal and endodermal tissues are in direct apposition caudally in the embryo. The separation into urogenital membrane and anal membrane with the formation of the perineum at about 7 weeks of gestation is brought about by the separation of the cloacal portion of the hindgut by the urorectal septum growing caudally between the allantois anteriorly and the hindgut posteriorly, thus partitioning the cloaca into the urogenital sinus anteriorly and the anorectal canal posteriorly. The anal membrane disintegrates at about 9 weeks to open into an ectodermal anal pit formed in the posterior cloacal folds.

Congenital and developmental abnormalities

Gross anomalies will be seen only incidentally by the dermatologist because of skin complications. Minor abnormalities such as haemangiomas, skin tags and papilliferous acanthomas are common on the inner sides of the thighs and infragluteal region. Pigmented, hairy naevi may involve one or both buttocks. Involvement of the buttocks with atypical naevi is a feature of the dysplastic naevus syndrome.

Developmental cysts, fistulae, sinuses and tumours

These are not uncommon, and frequently become infected. They may be mistaken for hidradenitis suppurativa or furuncles. Dermoid cysts occur on or adjacent to the perineal raphe and scrotum. Cloacal sinuses form fistulae from the anus to the adjoining skin; others involve the urethra and perineum.

Chordoma cutis

Chordomas [2] arise from the embryonic precursor of the axial skeleton, the notochord. They can involve the skin of the perineum, sacral area and buttocks by direct extension, recurrence or metastasis. They present as single or multiple, smooth, skin-coloured, non-tender nodules. Sacrococcygeal pain of a persistent nature may precede the diagnosis for years, in a manner that may mimic the presentation of sacral cysts [3], and require scanning procedures to differentiate between them.

Miscellaneous

Congenital hypertrichosis over the midline in the lumbosacral area—faun tail—is a sign of underlying spinal dysraphism (e.g. spina bifida occulta). Pilonidal sinus is discussed on p. 68.88.

REFERENCES

1 Leiberman DA. Common anorectal disorders. *Ann Intern Med* 1984; **101**: 837–46.
2 Su WPD, Louback JB, Gagne EJ, Scheithauer BW. Cutaneous chordoma: a report of 19 patients with cutaneous involvement of chordoma. *J Am Acad Dermatol* 1993; **29**: 63–6.
3 Van Kleft E, Van Vyve M. Chronic perineal pain related to meningeal cysts. *Neurosurgery* 1991; **29**: 223–31.

Trauma and artefact

Anal trauma is not uncommon. The two most common causes of acute painful anal ulceration in homosexual men are trauma and herpes simplex. Primary syphilis, chancroid, lymphogranuloma venereum, granuloma inguinale and amoebiasis, in decreasing order of frequency, are much less common [1]. Foreign bodies are occasionally inserted into the rectum. Anogenital tattoos have become commonplace [2].

Pressure sore

Pressure sores (decubitus ulcers) in the sacral area are common. In elderly, debilitated or bedridden patients, a persistent patch of erythema on the sacral or ischial region is a sign of impending ulceration. Squamous carcinoma is a potential complication, as with all chronic ulceration.

Umbilical artery catheterization

Unilateral skin necrosis of the buttock has been reported following indwelling umbilical artery catheterization [3–5], probably resulting from thrombosis leading to occlusion of the inferior gluteal artery. A similar case was caused by misdirection of the tip of the arterial catheter [6].

Child sexual abuse

The significance of anogenital warts in suggesting possible child sexual abuse is controversial. However, early recognition as a marker for child sexual abuse is in the child's long-term best interest [7].

REFERENCES

1 McMillan A, Smith IW. Painful anal ulceration in homosexual men. *Br J Surg* 1984; **71**: 215–6.
2 Goldstein N. Psychological implications of tattoos. *J Dermatol Surg Oncol* 1979; **5**: 883–8.
3 Bonifazi E, Meneghini C. Perianal gangrene of the buttock: an iatrogenic or spontaneous condition? *J Am Acad Dermatol* 1980; **3**: 596–8.
4 Cutler VE, Stretcher GS. Cutaneous complications of central umbilical artery catheterization. *Arch Dermatol* 1977; **113**: 61–3.
5 Mann PN. Gluteal skin necrosis after umbilical artery catheterization. *Arch Dis Child* 1980; **55**: 815–7.
6 Rudolph N, Wang HH, Dragutsky D. Gangrene of the buttock: a complication of umbilical artery catheterization. *Pediatrics* 1974; **53**: 106–9.
7 Hobbs CJ, Wynne JM. How to manage warts. *Arch Dis Child* 1999; **81**: 460.

Inflammatory dermatoses

The causes of perianal inflammation in infants are dealt with in Chapter 14. In adults, inflammation may result from the coexistence of several factors: haemorrhoids, anal discharge, proctitis, the presence of fissures or the effect of scratching. Five common conditions cause diagnostic difficulties: seborrhoeic dermatitis, psoriasis, contact dermatitis, lichen simplex and mycotic infections. *Oxyuris* infestation is sometimes postulated but seldom confirmed in adults. Phthiriasis pubis must be excluded.

The lesions of seborrhoeic dermatitis are brownish red, with branny or large, greasy scales towards the edge, extending beyond and outside the fold, and involving other areas of the body.

Psoriasis has a smooth glazed surface and a dull red hue, and is often fissured; other signs of the disease are nearly always present.

Contact dermatitis is markedly inflamed, and has an ill-defined spreading border. Irritant dermatitis results mainly from detergents; allergic dermatitis can have many causes (Table 68.19). In 43 suspected cases, neomycin (27%) and 'caine mix' (24%) were the most frequent offenders; quinolines (7%), lanolin (7%) and ethylenediamine (5%) were less common [1]. When resulting from a medicament, the hands may be involved. Other reports concern biocide preservatives and fragrances in moistened toilet tissue [2–5], lidocaine [6,7] and tetracaine (amethocaine) hydrochloride [8] used in topical antipruritics for piles, and Mitomycin C [9]. The role of food allergy in causing perianal symptoms is debatable [10].

Anoreceptive homosexual men may be susceptible to condom hypersensitivity.

Gross lichenification (lichen simplex) simulates psoriasis but is usually unilateral, except when it involves the perianal area. It may occur as a small, intensely irritable area, localized to the edge of the anus in one site, which is indicated exactly by the patient.

Tinea corporis presents classical signs unless there has been prior use of topical corticosteroids, which modify the features and thus create diagnostic confusion.

In all cases of perianal and perineal inflammation, the urine should be tested for sugar, and swabs and scrapings examined for organisms. A vaginal or rectal examination is mandatory. Any irregularity of the bowels that causes straining or soiling should be corrected.

REFERENCES

1 Wilkinson JD, Hambly EM, Wilkinson DS. Comparison of patch test results in two adjacent areas in England. *Acta Dermatol Venereol (Stockh)* 1980; **60**: 245–9.
2 Swinyer LJ. Connubial contact dermatitis from perfumes. *Contact Dermatitis* 1980; **6**: 226.
3 Van Ginkel CJ, Rundervoort GJ. Increasing incidence of contact allergy to the new preservative: 1,2-dibromo-2,4-dicyanobutane (methyldibromoglutaronitril). *Br J Dermatol* 1995; **132**: 918–20.
4 De Groot AC, Toon J, Baar M, Terpstra H, Weyland JW. Contact allergy to moist toilet paper. *Contact Dermatitis* 1991; **24**: 135–6.
5 Lucker GPH, Hulsmans R-FHJ, van der Kley AMJ, van de Staak WJBM. Evaluation of the frequency of contact allergic reactions to kathon CG in the Maastricht area, 1987–90. *Dermatology* 1992; **184**: 90–3.
6 Handfield-Jones SE, Cronin E. Contact sensitivity to lignocaine. *Clin Exp Dermatol* 1993; **18**: 342–3.
7 Hardwick N, King CM. Contact allergy to lignocaine with cross-reaction to bupivacaine. *Contact Dermatitis* 1994; **30**: 245–6.
8 Sanchez-Perez J, Cordoba S, Cortizas CF, Garcia-Diez A. Allergic contact balanitis due to tetracaine (amethocaine) hydrochloride. *Contact Dermatitis* 1998; **39**: 268.
9 Fisher AA. Allergic contact dermatitis to mitomycin C. *Cutis* 1991; **47**: 225.
10 Sapan N. Food induced pruritus ani: a variation of allergic target organ? *Eur J Pediatr* 1993; **152**: 701–2.

Pruritus ani

The symptom complex of pruritus ani has many causes: it is not a diagnosis unless qualified as constitutional or idiopathic. Fifty per cent of patients with pruritus ani will have a cause after dermatological evaluation [1–6]. Pruritus ani is seen especially in middle-class middle-aged white males [7]. It occurs less frequently in females, either alone or with pruritus vulvae. It can be associated with most forms of anal disease and with skin conditions involving the perianal area. The contributory factors are complex and may complement or perpetuate each other. Anal itching occurs to a variable degree with any inflammatory or eczematous condition of the skin of that area, with anal fissures, whatever their aetiology, and with malignant tumours. Mycotic infection often causes intense pruritus, and diabetes must be excluded in all severe or persistent candidal infections. Threadworm infestation is a well-recognized cause in childhood and occasionally in adults. Idiopathic anal itching, in which there is no obvious primary dermatological cause, is discussed further here. Lichenification, excoriation and secondary bacterial and candidal infection (induced by scratching) can supervene, and a contact dermatitis can be caused by overwashing and treatment, both self-directed and physician-prescribed.

The common factor linking most cases of pruritus ani is faecal contamination [2,8]. Faeces are themselves irritant and may generate perianal itch [8,9]. The itch may be triggered by a bowel movement or wiping with toilet paper, but often occurs at night, waking the patient from sleep. Faeces also contain potential allergens and endopeptidases of bacterial origin [10,11]. In the presence of pre-existing skin disease (e.g. seborrhoeic dermatitis or flexural psoriasis), or even in the absence of visible disease, these enzymes are capable of inducing both itching and inflammation [12].

Pruritus ani may be associated with anal leakage resulting from coexisting anal disease or an exaggerated recto-anal inhibitory reflex [13] and anal sphincter dysfunction [14], or be precipitated by broad-spectrum antibiotics and diarrhoea. Hypertrophy of anal papillae is probably not relevant [15]. Many patients have a dermatosis and some will have irritant or allergic contact dermatitis [16–18].

Psychological factors often contribute to pruritus ani, particularly when the itching appears to be out of proportion to the changes observed. However, as Whitlock [19] points out in a careful review, the evidence is unsatisfactory, except perhaps in primary lichen simplex. Psychosexual connotations of suppressed homosexuality do not withstand critical assessment. It is quite understandable, however, that prolonged pruritus ani can lead to tension, irritability or depression, and the treatment of this is an important part of the management of the condition. Idiopathic pruritus ani has been attributed to stress and anxiety and sedentary occupations.

The causes of faecal contamination are as follows (more than one factor may be operative).

Difficulty in cleansing the area. This may be caused by the following factors:
1 *Simple obesity*: poor ventilation and maceration have an additional role.
2 *Frequency of defaecation*: patients with a colostomy never suffer from perianal itching. Patients with pruritus ani are rarely constipated, although they may sit long at stool owing to faulty training techniques, with resultant prolapse or haemorrhoids and soiling [2,14,20]. Patients frequently admit to two or more motions a day. They are often tense individuals in whom everyday problems induce a profound colonic reflex, resulting in defaecation and soiling.

3 *Anatomical factors*: it is often noted that the anus is deeply placed. The association of this 'funnel anus' with marked hirsutism causes mechanical problems in the maintenance of hygiene.

Anal leakage. This may result from the following factors:
1 *Local causes*: such as haemorrhoids, perianal tags or fissures, which interfere with the efficient functions of the anus.
2 *Primary anal sphincter dysfunction*: anal canal manometry studies have shown that leakage of infused saline occurs early [13], and in one common group of patients the sphincter relaxes in response to rectal distension in a more rapid and profound manner than in a control group [14]. The arrival of faeces or flatus in the rectum may then regularly result in reflex faecal soiling.

Bacterial contamination. This is frequently a secondary cause, but rarely a primary cause alone. However, cross-infection of staphylococci may occur (e.g. between the ears and the anus).

Food and drink. The role of ingested metabolites or food chemicals in inducing pruritus ani is still uncertain and virtually unexplored, but anecdotal evidence in individual cases is sometimes compelling [21].

Clinical features. Clinical features vary somewhat, with possible contributions from the effects of rubbing, secondary infection, contact dermatitis or an underlying psoriatic diathesis.
1 Lichen simplex may be present in a 'pure' form, often localized to a small area at the edge of the anus or slightly away from it. The perception of itch from 'easily alerted' nerve endings is more acute in those of anxious temperament or at times of psychic trauma or fatigue.
2 A more general area of maceration, lichenification and fissuring—the 'mossy bank' anus—may be present. The architecture of the anal margin may be distorted by haemorrhoids, tags, oedema and infection. There is usually a gross degree of discharge [14].
3 Features of acute eczema may be caused by secondary infection of possibly minimal seborrhoeic dermatitis or psoriasis, or by contact dermatitis. The last mentioned should always be suspected when there has been any sudden change of pattern or intensity of a rash. The fingers may also be involved. One of the most common offenders is the 'caine' group of drugs [22], often self-prescribed.
4 Intense erythema with no obvious features of eczema may occur. This tends to vary in intensity over short periods, and probably represents the pruritic stage of the next group.
5 There may be no visible abnormality at the time of examination. These patients may have noticed erythema at times, or intense itching, and commonly give a story of

an intermittent sensation of wet anal margins and slight faecal soiling. It is in this group that dyskinesia of the sphincter appears to be a primary factor.

Diagnosis. A full history is essential and a search for underlying disease must be carried out. It is important to exclude staphylococcal infection, folliculitis, erythrasma, *Candida*, tinea, warts and thread/pinworms, and to establish whether there are other underlying skin diseases such as psoriasis [23], atopic dermatitis, LP, LS or EMPD [15]. Anal fistulae are particularly prevalent in chronic pruritus ani [24]. However, the majority of patients with piles, skin tags, fissures, warts, diarrhoea or faecal soiling do not itch [3]. Systemic diseases that have been associated with pruritus ani include lymphoma, pellagra, hypovitaminosis A and D and diabetes mellitus [4].

A rectal examination and referral for proctoscopy and sigmoidoscopy may be indicated [25]. In the young, threadworms should be sought with the Sellotape test or by stool examination for parasites. Patch testing is helpful to explore sensitivity to lanolin, medicaments, rubber, perfumed paper, etc.

Treatment. Management [2] begins with attention to the patient's washing habits. Soap is replaced with a suitable substitute and a moisturizer prescribed. A moisturizer (others recommend talcum powder) should be applied after each wash. A barrier preparation can be pre-applied to the perianal skin before the bowels are opened. Washing after defaecation in a bidet is preferable to wiping with toilet paper, if possible. Rubbing with toilet paper should be discouraged and dabbing recommended. Premoistened toilet papers should be avoided because of the potential irritancy of the moisturizing agent, which may be alcohol, and the risk of developing allergic sensitivity to fragrance or preservative components. Underwear should be loose and preferably made of cotton. Patients are best advised not to use topical anaesthetics in order to avoid sensitization to their constituents [26].

Coffee consumption might be curtailed [21]. Any other foods, such as nuts, that provoke the pruritus should be excluded from the diet, and a high-fibre diet should be encouraged if there is any history of constipation or haemorrhoids [27].

Local applications should be mild and soothing. A topical corticosteroid/antibiotic/antifungal preparation is useful for acute episodes. A wick of bandage impregnated with hydrocortisone 1% and silicone 10% inserted in the natal cleft is anti-inflammatory and lubricating. Other treatments that have been advocated include zinc paste with 1–2% phenol, St Mark's lotion, half-strength Castellani's paint, weak (0.05–0.25%) silver nitrate solution (if wet), cryotherapy, oral antihistamines, corticosteroid suppositories, intralesional triamcinolone, a 10-day tapering course of prednisolone, and intralesional methy-

lene blue, with or without marcaine/epinephrine/xylocaine [3,4,28,29]. Caution should be exercised with topical steroid treatment because the anal skin is 'quasi-occluded' and is easily damaged by fluorinated corticosteroids.

Concomitant proctological disease (haemorrhoids, fissures, anal spasm and occult mucosal prolapse) should be treated, if found [30]. When active pathology such as fissures, haemorrhoids or anal spasm are present, surgery will be needed. Lord's stretch procedure [31] has proved helpful. The long-term results are particularly satisfactory in those patients with strong ultra-low-pressure waves [27]. However, it may not always relieve the pruritus [32]. Simple excision of anal tags is unhelpful in relieving symptoms [15].

Some authorities see a psychosexual significance in pruritus ani in men [19], and this may rarely require attention. Patients should be reassured that they do not have cancer [1].

REFERENCES

1 Smith LE, Henrichs D, McCullah RD. Prospective studies on the etiology and treatment of pruritus ani. *Dis Colon Rectum* 1982; **25**: 358–63.
2 Alexander-Williams J. Pruritus ani. *BMJ* 1983; **287**: 159–60.
3 Verbov J. Pruritus ani and its management: a study and reappraisal. *Clin Exp Dermatol* 1984; **9**: 46–52.
4 Hanno R, Murphy P. Pruritus ani: classification and management. *Dermatol Clin* 1987; **5**: 811–6.
5 Jones DJ. Pruritus ani. *BMJ* 1992; **305**: 575–7.
6 Rohde H. Routine anal cleansing, so-called hemorrhoids, and perianal dermatitis: cause and effect? *Dis Colon Rectum* 2000; **43**: 561–3.
7 Leiberman DA. Common anorectal disorders. *Ann Intern Med* 1984; **101**: 837–46.
8 Kocsard E. Pruritus ani: a symptom of fecal contamination. *Cutis* 1981; **27**: 518.
9 Caplan RM. The irritant role of faeces in the genesis of perianal itch. *Gastroenterology* 1966; **50**: 19–23.
10 Keele CA. Chemical causes of pain and itch. *Proc R Soc Med* 1957; **50**: 477–84.
11 Shelley WB, Arthur RP. The neurohistology and neurophysiology of the itch sensation in man. *Arch Dermatol* 1957; **76**: 296–323.
12 Andersen PH, Bucher AP, Saeed I *et al.* Faecal enzymes: *in vivo* skin irritation. *Contact Dermatitis* 1994; **30**: 152–8.
13 Allan A, Ambrose NS, Silverman S *et al.* Physiological study of pruritus ani. *Br J Surg* 1987; **74**: 576–9.
14 Eyers AA, Thompson JPS. Pruritus ani: is anal sphincter dysfunction important in aetiology? *BMJ* 1979; **ii**: 1549–51.
15 Jensen SL. A randomized trial of simple excision of non-specific hypertrophied anal papillae versus expectant management in patients with chronic pruritus ani. *Ann R Coll Surg Engl* 1988; **70**: 348–9.
16 Harrington CI, Lewis FM, McDonagh AJ, Gawkrodger DJ. Dermatological causes of pruritus ani. *BMJ* 1992; **305**: 955.
17 Dasan S, Neill SM, Donaldson DR, Scott HJ. Treatment of persistent pruritus ani in a combined colorectal and dermatological clinic. *Br J Surg* 1999; **86**: 1337–40.
18 Bauer A, Geier J, Elsner P. Allergic contact dermatitis in patients with anogenital complaints. *J Reprod Med* 2000; **45**: 649–54.
19 Whitlock FA, ed. *Psychophysiological Aspects of Skin Disease.* London: Saunders, 1976: 118–21.
20 Kaufman HD, ed. In: *The Haemorrhoid Syndrome.* Tunbridge Wells: Abacus, 1981: 61.
21 Veien NK, Hattel T, Justesen O *et al.* Dermatoses in coffee drinkers. *Cutis* 1987; **40**: 421–2.
22 Wilkinson JD, Hambly EM, Wilkinson DS. Comparison of patch test results in two adjacent areas of England. II. Medicaments. *Acta Derm Venereol (Stockh)* 1980; **60**: 245–9.
23 Farber EM, Nall L. Perianal and intergluteal psoriasis. *Cutis* 1992; **50**: 336–8.

24 Petros JG, Rimm EB, Robillard RJ. Clinical presentation of chronic anal fissures. *Am Surg* 1993; **59**: 666–8.
25 Daniel GL, Longo WE, Vernava III AM. Pruritus ani: causes and concerns. *Dis Colon Rectum* 1994: **37**: 670–4.
26 Handfield-Jones SE, Cronin E. Contact sensitivity to lignocaine. *Clin Exp Dermatol* 1993; **18**: 342–3.
27 Hancock BD. In: Kaufman HD, ed. *The Haemorrhoid Syndrome*. Tunbridge Wells: Abacus, 1981: 93–104.
28 Minvielle L, Hernandez VL. The use of intralesional triamcinolone hexacetonide in treatment of idiopathic pruritus ani. *Dis Colon Rectum* 1969; **12**: 340–3.
29 Eusebio EB. New treatment of intractable pruritus ani. *Dis Colon Rectum* 1991; **34**: 289.
30 Pirone E, Infantin A, Masin A *et al*. Can proctological procedures resolve perianal pruritus and mycosis? *Int J Colorectal Dis* 1992; **7**: 18–20.
31 Lord PH. Diverse methods of managing haemorrhoids: dilatation. *Dis Colon Rectum* 1973; **16**: 180–92.
32 Ortiza H, Marti J, Jaurieta E *et al*. Lord's procedure: a critical study of its basic principle. *Br J Surg* 1978; **65**: 281–4.

Danthron erythema

This form of irritant contact dermatitis per rectum is caused by the use of a laxative containing danthron [1,2]. It is seen in those with Hirschsprung's disease or encopresis, and sometimes in elderly incontinent patients [2–4]. Danthron (1,8-dihydroxyanthroquinone) is reduced in the large bowel to 1,8-dihydroxyanthron, which is the active agent [2]. This is chemically identical to dithranol, and the lesions produced by faecal incontinence are equivalent to dithranol 'burns'. A bizarre livid erythema in the perianal area, groins, thighs and buttocks, with sharp outlines, corresponds to the area of contact with the faeces. Danthron erythema is easily differentiated from other causes of perianal or inguino-crural lesions.

Lichen sclerosus et atrophicus

The perianal skin is rarely affected alone, but is involved in up to two-thirds of the cases in which the vulva is affected [5], forming a characteristic figure-of-eight distribution. One case of carcinoma has been reported [6]. Perianal LS is rare in males.

Anal fissure

Small erosions and fissures may occur in the sulcus beneath oedematous haemorrhoids or in any area of dermatitis. The presence of even a small fissure in an area of dermatitis maintains the pruritus and prolongs the course.

A true anal fissure is a midline linear perianal ulcer; 90% posteriorly, 10% anteriorly. Many are idiopathic; the cause is probably related to defaecation of hard stool causing pressure trauma and necrosis, or it may be a postoperative complication. Sexually transmitted diseases and Crohn's disease should be excluded. Intense pruritus, pain, bleeding, mucous discharge and constipation constitute the symptomatology. On examination there may be a 'sentinel pile' at the anal pole of the ulcer. Management is

surgical: proctoscopy is mandatory if the aetiology is in doubt, and especially if the fissure extends to the anal margin or within. Benign fissures are superficial and not indurated, but when persistent they may be painful and cause bleeding, especially in the elderly. Unless they heal quickly under treatment, a biopsy should always be performed to exclude malignancy.

Small erosions and excoriations frequently heal with treatment for anogenital pruritus. If they are hidden between haemorrhoids or anal tags, protective pastes are helpful. Fissures in psoriasis and seborrhoeic dermatitis are difficult to heal, particularly in the natal cleft. If the underlying disease is satisfactorily controlled, the lesion will heal without special attention. Intralesional corticosteroids may be effective in non-infective inflammatory conditions.

Anal fistula

A perianal fistula is a communication between the anal canal and the perianal skin. Most are on the midline posteriorly, but there may be multiple openings. The origin is from infection and abscesses within the anal glands, but Crohn's disease, foreign body and tuberculosis are classic causes and hidradenitis suppurativa is an important differential diagnosis. Squamous carcinoma is a rare complication. The presentation is usually of pruritus ani related to seropurulent discharge but there may be pain resulting from abscess formation. Surrounding skin may be indurated. Management is surgical.

Pilonidal cyst/sinus

Pilonidal sinus probably derives from the perineal pilosebaceous unit and precursor pits (not the common congenital sacral pits) associated with trapped hairs [7,8]. Clinically, pilonidal sinus constitutes part of the 'follicular–occlusion tetrad' alongside hidradenitis suppurativa, acne conglobata and dissecting cellulitis of the scalp. Symptoms include itch, pain, recurrent abscess, purulent discharge and persistent nodule. Pilonidal sinus occurs in the midline. The sacrococcygeal location is the most common site but it can occur on the pubis, anterior perineum and, very rarely, the penis. It may present as a nodule or cyst, often with a pigmented or hairy surface, which ruptures and quickly becomes infected (Fig. 68.41). The sinus usually extends to the sacrum and causes sacrococcygeal fistulae with deep ramifications. This heals if the track is thoroughly cleaned. Treatment is surgical [8,9]. Squamous carcinoma can supervene [10].

REFERENCES

1 Bunney MH, Noble IM. Red skin and Dorbanex. *BMJ* 1974; **ii**: 731.
2 Ippen H. Toxizität und stoffwechsel des cignolins (Wz). *Dermatologica* 1959; **119**: 211–20.

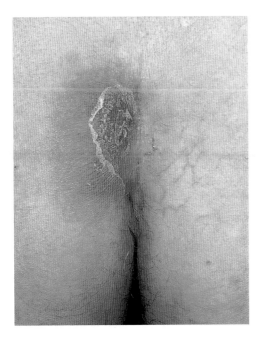

Fig. 68.41 Pilonidal sinus. (Courtesy of Dr D.A. Burns, Leicester, UK.)

3 Barth JH, Reshad H, Darley CR *et al*. A cutaneous complication of Dorbanex therapy. *Clin Exp Dermatol* 1984; **9**: 95–6.

4 Broholm KA. A controlled trial of a new combined preparation for the treatment of constipation in geriatric patients. *Gerontol Clin (Basel)* 1973; **15**: 25–31.

5 Wallace HJ. Lichen sclerosus et atrophicus. *Trans St John's Hosp Dermatol Soc* 1971; **57**: 9–30.

6 Sloan PJM, Goepel J. Lichen sclerosus et atrophicus and perianal carcinoma. *Clin Exp Dermatol* 1981; **6**: 399–402.

7 Millar DM. Aetiology of post-anal pilonidal disease. *Proc R Soc Med* 1970; **63**: 1263–4.

8 Allen-Mersh TG. Pilonidal sinus: finding the right track for treatment. *Br J Surg* 1990; **77**: 123–32.

9 Lord PH, Millar DM. Pilonidal sinus: a simple treatment. *Br J Surg* 1965; **52**: 298–300.

10 Sagi A, Rosenberg L, Grief M *et al*. Squamous cell carcinoma arising in a pilonidal sinus: a case report and review of the literature. *J Dermatol Surg Oncol* 1984; **10**: 210–2.

Hidradenitis suppurativa

Hidradenitis suppurativa ('chronic perianal pyoderma' in Japan) (see Chapter 27) can give rise to all degrees of inflammation and scarring. Friction and pressure accentuate the inflammatory changes that invade the fat and cause further granulomatous change extending widely over the buttocks and thighs. Persistent perineal sinuses are frequent, and deep lesions cause anal fistulae. In mild cases, only a few isolated lesions are present. Secondary bacterial invasion, often from the gut [1], is an important complicating factor. Seven cases have been associated with an oestrogen–progesterone contraceptive pill [2].

There is a clinical spectrum overlapping with chronic folliculitis (e.g. of the buttocks and 'penile acne'). In established hidradenitis, bridged comedones, folliculitis and furunculosis, deep burrowing discharging sinuses, nodules, cysts, fluctuant abscesses, scarring and fibrosis in the groins and axillae, the natal cleft and buttocks [3] may all be present. Some patients may also have conglobate acne, dissecting cellulitis and pilonidal sinus. Hidradenitis is more common in black and Mediterranean individuals. It affects the axillae preferentially in women and the perineum in men. A urethral–cutaneous fistula and phimosis have been reported [4]. Scarring from the disease and its treatment can be extensive. The morbidity of hidradenitis may be severe, interfering with sitting, sleeping, walking, defaecation and sexual activity, and responsible for depression. Disease that has persisted for more than 20 years carries a significant risk of progression to SCC [5–7] and rarely verrucous carcinoma [8].

Differential diagnosis. Hidradenitis is usually a clinical diagnosis. Swabs should be taken for bacteriological evaluation and to guide therapy, but the patient should be fully evaluated for sexually transmitted diseases should the presentation be in any way suspicious. An important differential diagnosis of acneiform disease presenting at any site is chloracne (see Chapter 43). A biopsy may be necessary to exclude carcinoma or Crohn's disease. Perineal Crohn's disease mimics hidradenitis, with its granulomatous inflammation, ulceration and fistula formation, but it is less painful. Also, the disease is absent from the axillae and it is rare for patients to be free of overt gastrointestinal symptoms. Very florid perianal disease can be seen in myeloma and leukaemia [9], and in homosexual men and in AIDS [10].

Mild or localized forms are frequently misdiagnosed as furunculosis or 'infected cysts', and confusion occurs with severe acne, developmental fistulae and lymphogranuloma venereum. The relatively painless recurrences in the same or other sites, and oblique sinuses that end in soft swollen inflamed nodules, are characteristic.

Treatment. This is challenging [11]. Small localized sinuses may be phenolized successfully, and early lesions may respond to intralesional corticosteroids. However, this treatment may have to be repeated, and recurrent or extensive lesions may require a more radical approach. Marsupialization (as with pilonidal sinuses) [12] and diathermy destruction of the affected tissue have been very successful in some cases, even those involving the scrotum. Treatment with carbon dioxide laser, with secondary intention healing, is very effective [13,14]. The use of Silastic foam dressing may facilitate healing [15]. Otherwise, plastic surgery with complete excision of all the involved skin may be required [16]. Long-term antibiotic therapy (erythromycin, flucloxacillin, ciprofloxacin, metronidazole) is often given 'blind', but is seldom of lasting value, although elimination of specific secondary invaders such as *Streptococcus milleri* [1] has given good results. Oral prednisolone can be used alongside antibiotics to control intercurrent exacerbations. More recently, isotretinoin (1 mg/kg) for 6–8 months has been used with mixed results, but is occasionally helpful in difficult cases [17,18]. Antiandrogen therapy has yet to be evaluated.

REFERENCES

1 Highet AS, Warren RE, Weekes AJ. Bacteriology and antibiotic treatment of perineal suppurative hidradenitis. *Arch Dermatol* 1988; **124**: 1047–51.
2 Stellon AJ, Wakeling M. Hidradenitis suppurativa associated with use of oral contraceptives. *BMJ* 1989; **298**: 28–9.
3 Coda A, Ferri F. Perianal Verneuil's disease. *Minerva Chir* 1991; 46: 465–7.
4 Chaikin DC, Volz LR, Broderick G. An unusual presentation of hidradenitis suppurativa: case report and review of the literature. *Urology* 1994; **44**: 606–8.
5 Black SB, Woods JE. Squamous cell carcinoma complicating hidradenitis suppurativa. *J Surg Oncol* 1982; **19**: 25–6.
6 Shukla VK, Hughes LE. A case of squamous cell carcinoma complicating hidradenitis suppurativa. *Eur J Surg Oncol* 1995; **21**: 106–9.
7 Ishizawa T, Koseki S, Mitsuhashi Y, Kondo S. Squamous cell carcinoma arising in chronic perianal pyoderma: a case report and review of Japanese literature. *J Dermatol* 2000; **27**: 734–9.
8 Cosman BC, O'Grady TC, Pekarske S. Verrucous carcinoma arising in hidradenitis suppurativa. *Int J Colorectal Dis* 2000; **15**: 342–6.
9 Alexander-Williams J, Buchmann P. Perianal Crohn's disease. *World J Surg* 1980; **4**: 203–8.
10 Carr ND, Mercey D, Slack WW. Non-condylomatous perianal skin disease in homosexual men. *Br J Surg* 1989; **76**: 1064–6.
11 Mouly MR. A propos des suppurations périnéo-fessieres chroniques et de leur traitement chirurgical. *Bull Soc Fr Dermatol Syphiligr* 1969; **76**: 23–7.
12 Brown SCW, Kazzasi N, Lord PH. Surgical treatment of perineal hidradenitis suppurativa with special reference to recognition of the perianal form. *Br J Surg* 1986; **73**: 978–80.
13 Lapins J, Marcusson JA, Emtestam L. Surgical treatment of chronic hidradenitis suppurativa: CO₂ laser stripping—secondary intention technique. *Br J Dermatol* 1994; **131**: 551–6.
14 Finley EM, Ratz JL. Treatment of hidradenitis suppurativa with carbon dioxide laser excision and second-intention healing. *J Am Acad Dermatol* 1996; **34**: 465–9.
15 Morgan WP, Harding KG, Richardson G *et al.* The use of Silastic foam dressing in the treatment of advanced hidradenitis suppurativa. *Br J Surg* 1980; **67**: 277–80.
16 Šlauf P, Antoš F, Novák J, Beneš J, Kálal J. Perianal pyoderma. *Rozhl Chir* 1993; **72**: 331–3.
17 Brown CF, Gallup DG, Brown VM. Hidradenitis suppurativa of the anogenital region: response to isotretinoin. *Am J Obstet Gynecol* 1988; **158**: 13–5.
18 Jones DH, Cunliffe W, King K. Hidradenitis suppurativa: lack of success with *cis*-retinoic acid. *Br J Dermatol* 1982; **107**: 252.

Crohn's disease

SYN. REGIONAL ILEITIS

It is a well-known aphorism that Crohn's disease can affect any part of the gut and its cutaneous borders from the mouth to the anus. The cutaneous manifestations of Crohn's disease are listed in Table 68.31. Perianal disease may occur in up to 75–90% of patients [7,8]. Table 68.32 lists the perianal features of Crohn's disease [9]; it includes those common to most chronic diarrhoeal illnesses such as pruritus ani, skin maceration, and erosions with secondary infection. Perianal manifestations of Crohn's disease in childhood are a major cause of morbidity, but only rarely progress in a destructive manner (Fig. 68.42) [9].

Table 68.31 The cutaneous manifestations of Crohn's disease [1–6].

Erythema nodosum
Anal and perianal lesions
Spreading ulceration of perineum and buttocks after colectomy
Skin changes around ileostomies and colostomies
Genital lesions
Balanitis, posthitis and granulomatous lymphangitis
Vulval lesions
    'Sarcoid' type lesions in remote sites
    Pyoderma gangrenosum
Granulomatous cheilitis
Epidermolysis bullosa acquisita
Non-specific changes resulting from malabsorption

Table 68.32 Perianal features of Crohn's disease.

Pruritus ani
Maceration
Erosion
Secondary infection
Skin tags
Fissures
Anal stenosis
Fistula-*in-ano*
Abscess
'Metastatic' granulomatous plaques

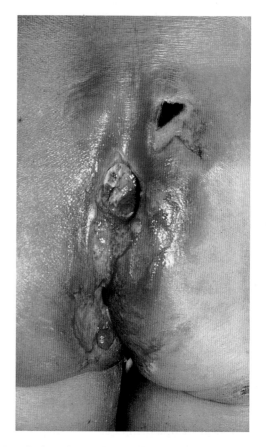

Fig. 68.42 Crohn's disease: perianal lesions. (Courtesy of Dr D.I. McCallum, Inverness, UK.)

Clinical features. The skin tags of Crohn's disease are larger, thicker and harder than ordinary tags. Deep undermined angulated fissures with cyanotic edges may fuse to form 'flying buttress' skin bridges, characterized by relative lack of pain. Fistulae are less common than fissures; they may be asymptomatic even when multiple. Pain usually means that an abscess has formed because of blockage of a fistula. Multiple external openings can be encountered all over the buttock, on the scrotum and on the thigh; a distinctive sign is the cyanotic hue of the indurated skin. Anal stenosis, faecal incontinence and carcinoma are complications [10].

Clinical diagnosis may be achieved based on symptoms, signs and investigation results (e.g. radiography and gut biopsy) consistent with Crohn's disease. Any anal lesion in a patient who is known to be suffering from Crohn's disease is likely to be perianal Crohn's [11]. Difficulty arises when the anogenital disease represents the first manifestation. Histologically positive perianal disease of all clinical types may predate frank gastrointestinal Crohn's disease by several years [12], including in children [9]. The relative lack of pain, multiplicity of lesions, oedema of skin tags and eccentricity of fissures are important pointers [11]. Biopsy of skin lesions is helpful, and sigmoidoscopy and biopsy of intestinal mucosal lesions is mandatory. Swabs should be taken and the patient fully evaluated for sexually transmitted diseases should the presentation be in any way atypical.

Differential diagnosis. The differential diagnosis includes the causes of pruritus ani and non-specific anal fissures and fistulae. Similar, although less extensive, lesions occur, but much less commonly, in ulcerative colitis, and only very rarely in diverticulitis [2]. Hidradenitis suppurativa presents with nodules, sinuses and purulence but is more painful; other sites may be involved and severe acne is often present. Similarily florid perianal disease can be seen in myeloma and leukaemia [11]. Proctitis, perianal ulceration, abscess, fissure and fistula are prevalent in homosexual men and those with HIV/AIDS [13,14]. Perineal pyoderma gangrenosum has been misdiagnosed as Crohn's disease. A solitary granulomatous nodule, with or without ulceration, carries a differential diagnosis that includes sarcoid, schistosomiasis, leishmaniasis, tuberculosis, atypical mycobacterial infection, deep fungal infection, granuloma inguinale, lymphogranuloma venereum, chancroid, amoebiasis and syphilis. Florid condylomata acuminata [15], anorectal carcinoma presenting with an ischiorectal abscess [16] and other mucocutaneous malignancies (basal cell carcinoma, Kaposi's sarcoma and amelanotic malignant melanoma) may rarely be encountered.

Treatment. The treatment of the anogenital manifestations of Crohn's disease depends to some extent on the treatment of active intestinal disease. Local measures include soaks with potassium permanganate and aluminium acetate, potent or very potent topical corticosteroid/antibiotic combinations and oral antibiotics (as for hidradenitis). A role has been advocated for long-term oral metronidazole (20 mg/kg/day in divided doses) [17,18]. Perianal abscess may respond to sulfasalazine and anal fissure to prednisolone and azathioprine [5]. The surgical philosophy is conservative [3,9]. Resection of the affected segment of bowel does not always cure the lesions or prevent their recurrence, especially at ileostomy or colostomy sites.

REFERENCES

1 Markowitz J, Davim F, Aiges H *et al.* Perianal disease in children and adolescents with Crohn's disease. *Gastroenterology* 1984; **86**: 829–33.
2 Crohn NN, Yarnis H, eds. *Regional Ileitis*, 2nd edn. New York: Grune & Stratton, 1958.
3 Hibbiss JH, Schofield PF. Management of perianal Crohn's disease. *J R Soc Med* 1982; **75**: 414–7.
4 Lockhart-Mummery HE. Non-venereal lesions of the anal region. *Br J Vener Dis* 1963; **39**: 15–7.
5 Rankin GB. National co-operative Crohn's disease study. *Gastroenterology* 1979; **77**: 914–20.
6 Smith JN, Winship DH. Complications and extraintestinal problems in inflammatory bowel disease. *Med Clin North Am* 1980; **64**: 1161–71.
7 Fielding JF. Perianal lesions in Crohn's disease. *J R Coll Surg Edinb* 1972; **17**: 32–7.
8 Gruwez JA, Christiaens MR, Laquet A. La maladie de Crohn de l'anus. *Acta Endoscop* 1983; **13**: 285–92.
9 Palder SB, Shandling B, Bilik R, Griffiths AM, Sherman P. Perianal complications of pediatric Crohn's disease. *J Pediatr Surg* 1991; **26**: 513–5.
10 Slater G, Greenstein A, Aufses A. Anal carcinoma in patients with Crohn's disease. *Ann Surg* 1984; **199**: 348–50.
11 Alexander-Williams J, Buchmann P. Perianal Crohn's disease. *World J Surg* 1980; **4**: 203–8.
12 Baker WN, Milton-Thompson GJ. The anal lesion as the sole presenting symptom of intestinal Crohn's disease. *Gut* 1971; **12**: 865.
13 Carr ND, Mercey D, Slack WW. Non-condylomatous perianal skin disease in homosexual men. *Br J Surg* 1989; **76**: 1064–6.
14 Denis BJ, May T, Bigard MA, Canton P. Anal and perianal lesions in symptomatic HIV infections: prospective study of a series of 190 patients. *Gastroenterol Clin Biol* 1992; **16**: 148–54.
15 Thomson JPS, Grace RH. The treatment of perianal and anal condylomata accuminata: a new operative technique. *J R Soc Med* 1978; **71**: 180–5.
16 Tait WF, Sykes PA. Unusual presentation of anorectal carcinoma. *BMJ* 1982; **285**: 1742.
17 Bernstein LH, Frank MS, Brant LJ, Boley SJ. Healing of perineal Crohn's disease with metronidazole. *Gastroenterology* 1980; **79**: 357–65.
18 Brandt LJ, Bernstein LH, Boley SJ *et al.* Metronidazole therapy for perianal Crohn's disease: a follow-up study. *Gastroenterology* 1982; **83**: 383–7.

Miscellaneous

Radiodermatitis is occasionally encountered following previous treatment for *in situ* or frank carcinoma or, decades ago, pruritus ani. LP involving the buttocks and perianal region is extremely irritable and may become excoriated or hypertrophic; LP must be considered in the differential diagnosis of pruritus ani and perianal fissures. Solitary involvement of the perianal skin may occur (Fig. 68.43).

Behçet's disease occasionally presents with multiple shallow ulcers and fissures of the anal margin.

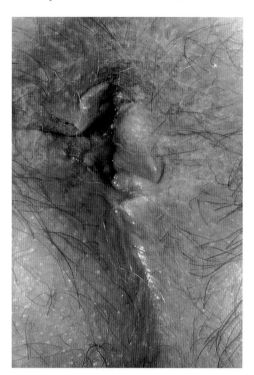

Fig. 68.43 Perianal lichen planus. (Courtesy of Dr F.A. Ive, Durham, UK.)

Calciphylaxis sometimes affects the thighs and buttocks [1–3].

Acrodermatitis enteropathica should be considered in the differential diagnosis of perianal eczema, psoriasis or candidosis in the paediatric setting, or in the presence of gastrointestinal disease causing malabsorption syndromes (e.g. Crohn's disease), extensive gastrointestinal surgery such as small intestinal bypass, malnutrition in alcoholism and recent prolonged parenteral nutrition where zinc supplementation may not have been optimal. A reticulate eczematous eruption may be found on the extensor aspects of the limbs in alcoholics but has also been reported to affect the perianal and scrotal skin [4,5]. Other deficiency diseases with some similarity to acrodermatitis enteropathica are pellagra, maple syrup urine disease and neonatal citrullinaemia.

Benign mucosal pemphigoid (cicatricial pemphigoid) [6] may affect the groin, perineum and perianal skin, and may cause anal stenosis. The drug clonidine may have been responsible in one case [7]. Pyodermite végétante can be distinguished by the histology and by immunofluorescence studies. Ulcerative colitis may be present [8].

The anus is involved in about 5% of cases of Stevens–Johnson syndrome. A connection has been recognized between epidermolysis bullosa acquisita [9] and inflammatory bowel disease, particularly Crohn's disease [10–12].

Fixed drug eruption may produce striking pigmentation. Prolonged use of potent topical corticosteroids causes a dusky erythema, atrophy or induration.

REFERENCES

1 Ivker RA, Woosley J, Briggaman R. Calciphylaxis in three patients with end-stage renal disease. *Arch Dermatol* 1995; **131**: 63–8.
2 Siami GA, Siami FS. Intensive tandem cryofiltration apheresis and hemodialysis to treat a patient with severe calciphylaxis, cryoglobulinemia, and end-stage renal disease. *ASAIO J* 1999; **45**: 229–33.
3 Boccaletti VP, Ricci R, Sebastio N, Cortellini P, Alinovi A. Penile necrosis. *Arch Dermatol* 2000; **136**: 261, 264.
4 Ecker RI, Schroeter AL. Acrodermatitis and acquired zinc deficiency. *Arch Dermatol* 1978; **114**: 937–9.
5 Gaveau D, Piette F, Cortot A *et al.* Cutaneous manifestations of zinc deficiency in ethylic cirrhosis. *Ann Dermatol Vénéréol* 1987; **114**: 39–53 [in French].
6 Lever WF, ed. *Pemphigus and Pemphigoid.* Springfield: Thomas, 1965.
7 Van Joost TH, Faber WR, Manuel HR. Drug-induced anogenital cicatricial pemphigoid. *Br J Dermatol* 1980; **102**: 715–8.
8 Forman L. The skin and colon. *Trans St John's Hosp Dermatol Soc* 1966; **52**: 139–62.
9 Ray TL, Levine JB, Weiss W *et al.* Epidermolysis bullosa acquisita and inflammatory bowel disease. *J Am Acad Dermatol* 1982; **6**: 242–52.
10 Chouvet B, Guillet G, Perrot H *et al.* L'epidermolyse bulleuse acquise: association a la maladie de Crohn. Revue generale a propos de deux observations. *Ann Dermatol Vénéréol* 1982; **109**: 53–63.
11 Livden JK, Thunold S, Schsonsby H. Epidermolysis bullosa acquisita and Crohn's disease. *Acta Derm Venereol (Stockh)* 1978; **58**: 241–4.
12 Pegum JS, Wright JT. Epidermolysis bullosa acquisita and Crohn's disease. *Proc R Soc Med* 1973; **66**: 234–5.

Primary systemic cutaneous anosacral amyloid

This has a predilection for the anogenital region, particularly the sacrum, in elderly Japanese people [1–3]. Moderately pruritic pigmented macules and glossy hyperkeratotic lesions fan out in lines from the anus. There are no systemic changes. Amyloid deposits are seen in the upper reticular dermis and around hair follicles. It is thought to represent an ageing process.

REFERENCES

1 Yamamoto T, Mukai H. Amyloidosis of the ano-sacral skin. *Jpn J Dermatol* 1981; **91**: 398–443.
2 Yanaghihara M, Fukishima N, Mori S. Anosacral amyloidosis. *Proceedings of 16th Congress on Dermatology.* Tokyo: Tokyo University Press, 1982: 922.
3 Mukai H, Eto H, Yamamoto T. Ano-sacral cutaneous amyloidosis. *Jpn J Dermatol* 1986; **96**: 1247–51.

Infections

Folliculitis and furunculosis

The anogenital area, particularly the buttocks and thighs of men, can be susceptible to infection with *Staphylococcus aureus*. Severe involvement with furunculosis and abscesses suggests an overlap with hidradenitis suppurativa. Although the high temperature and humidity of this area, combined with pressure [1] and friction, encourage colonization by staphylococci, primary pyococcal infections are now uncommon in countries with cultural or acquired habits of cleanliness. The perineal carriage of staphylococci [2] may not cause local lesions in the host, but is especially important in acting as a reservoir from which

Table 68.33 Differential diagnosis of anogenital cellulitis. (After Bunker [5]. © 2004, with permission from Elsevier.)

Hidradenitis suppurativa
Crohn's disease
Staphylococcal cellulitis
Streptococcal cellulitis
Gonococcal cellulitis
Fournier's gangrene and necrotizing fasciitis
Extramammary Paget's disease
Carcinoma erysipeloides (bladder and prostate)

S. aureus may be disseminated to other sites or to eczematous lesions elsewhere. In adults, the carriage rate is of the order of 13–22%; in neonates it may be higher. Some persons are better 'dispersers' of staphylococci than others, and the organisms may remain (and even increase) after washing. The risk of dispersion of staphylococci from this site is of obvious importance in hospital operating theatres, where attempts have been made to minimize it by the provision of special clothing [3]. Nasal carriage, diabetes and immunodeficiency should be considered. Bacterial perianal infection is commonly seen in leukaemic patients [4].

Staphylococcal cellulitis

Cellulitis and abscess formation can complicate cysts, sinuses and fistulae. The differential diagnosis is given in Table 68.33.

Anorectal infection in patients with malignant disease is serious and potentially life-threatening [6]. Although some cases of anorectal cellulitis will respond to antibiotics alone, necrotizing fasciitis and Fournier's gangrene are risks. Swelling and fluctuance signifying abscess formation may develop late. It is difficult to decide on the timing of surgery. Perianal infiltration, ulceration or abscess occurs in 5% of haematological malignancies and may rarely be the presenting feature [7].

Streptococcal dermatitis/perianal cellulitis

This syndrome in children [8] probably has a corollary in adults [9]. A child may present with pruritus, painful defaecation, anal soreness and redness (without nappy/diaper rash) and satellite pustulosis of the buttocks. Examination of the anus shows a pronounced, sharply demarcated, boggy erythema and causes discomfort to the child. Rarely, there may be a systemic presentation with fever and rash [10]. It is much more common in boys, and the penis may be involved. An association with acute guttate psoriasis has been reported [11,12]. Group A β-haemolytic streptococci is the usual cause, although *S. aureus* has been retrieved from one child who also had satellite pustules on the buttocks [13]. Proctocolitis has

occurred [14]. Perianal disease may be misinterpreted as sexual abuse [15]. Streptococcal infection of the upper respiratory tract in other members of the family may be found. Communal bathing has been blamed for outbreaks. Treatment is generally with systemic penicillin or topical mupirocin, or erythromycin if clinically less acute [16].

REFERENCES

1 Felman YM, Kikitas JA. Non-venereal anogenital lesions. *Cutis* 1980; **26**: 347, 351, 354, 357.
2 Noble WC, Somerville DA. In: Rook AJ, ed. *Microbiology of Human Skin*, Vol. 2. *Major Problems in Dermatology*. London: Saunders, 1974.
3 Mitchell NJ, Gamble DR. Clothing design for operating room personnel. *Lancet* 1974; ii: 1133–6.
4 Carlson GW, Ferguson CM, Amerson JR. Perianal infections in acute leukaemia. *Am Surg* 1988; **54**: 693–5.
5 Bunker CB. *Male Genital Skin Disease*. London: Saunders, 2004 (in press).
6 Glenn J, Cotton D, Wesley R, Pizzo P. Anorectal infections in patients with malignant diseases. *Rev Infect Dis* 1988; **10**: 42–52.
7 Vanheuverzwyn R, Delannoy A, Michaux JL, Dive C. Anal lesions in haematologic disorders. *Dis Colon Rectum* 1980; **23**: 310–2.
8 Peltola H. Images in clinical medicine: bacterial perianal dermatitis. *N Engl J Med* 2000; **342**: 1877.
9 Neri I, Bardazzi F, Maraduri S, Patrizi A. Perianal streptococcal dermatitis in adults. *Br J Dermatol* 1996; **135**: 796–52.
10 Vélez A, Moreno JC. Febrile perianal streptococcal dermatitis. *Pediatr Dermatol* 1999; **16**: 23–4.
11 Rehder PA, Eliezer ET, Lane AT. Perianal cellulitis. *Arch Dermatol* 1988; **124**: 702–4.
12 Patrizi A, Costa AM, Fiorillo L *et al*. Perianal streptococcal dermatitis associated with guttate psoriasis and/or balanoposthitis: a study of five cases. *Pediatr Dermatol* 1994; **11**: 168–71.
13 Montemarano AD, James WD. *Staphylococcus aureus* as a cause of perianal dermatitis. *Pediatr Dermatol* 1993; **10**: 259–62.
14 Guss C, Larsen JG. Group A beta-hemolytic streptococcal proctocolitis. *Pediatr Infect Dis* 1984; **3**: 442.
15 Duhra P, Ilchyshyn A. Perianal streptococcal cellulitis with penile involvement. *Br J Dermatol* 1990; **123**: 793–6.
16 Paradisi M, Cianchini G, Angelo C, Conti G, Puddu P. Efficacy of topical erythromycin in treatment of perianal streptococcal dermatitis. *Pediatr Dermatol* 1993; **10**: 297–8.

Perianal abscess

Perianal/anorectal/ischiorectal abscess presents with painful swelling and suppuration and is commonly complicated by anal fistula. The likeliest cause of perianal abscess is infection of the anal glands but trauma (e.g. impacted fish bone), diabetes and anal cancer predispose to its development. Crohn's disease, hidradenitis, tuberculosis and *Enterobius vermicularis* [1] should be considered.

Ecthyma gangrenosum

Gram-negative organisms are seldom pathogenic unless the balance of the skin flora is grossly disturbed. *Pseudomonas aeruginosa* may be found in deep ulcers and fissures. Ecthyma gangrenosum has a predilection for the anogenital (and acral) extremities. The prognosis is poor. Ill patients with leukaemia may develop a necrotizing anorectal ulcer caused by *Pseudomonas*, presenting with severe anal pain, anorectal ulceration and septicaemia. Anorectal ulceration may be the portal of entry of the infection or a consequence of it [2]. The mortality is high.

Thread/pinworms

Thread/pinworms can cause pruritus ani. Excoriations, eczematization and impetiginization may be present, sometimes away from the site of infestation on the buttocks and upper thighs, particularly in the younger child. However, often there are few physical signs. Perianal abscess may occur very rarely [1].

Common mycoses

Candidosis causes a bright red, glazed area, often with outlying small pustules, and may spread to the groins or natal cleft. Microscopy and culture distinguish it from other fungal infections, and from psoriasis and pyococcal infections.

The well-defined scaly circinate edge, the spread and the chronicity of *Trichophyton rubrum* infection offer clues to diagnosis, which can be confirmed by microscopy and culture. However, prior treatment with corticosteroids may disguise the appearance. The possibility of fungal infection should therefore be considered in all unusual forms of perianal dermatitis.

Necrotizing infections

A number of overlapping severe gangrenous and necrotizing diseases may affect the anorectal and perineal (and genital) skin and subcutaneous tissues. Although they may often be a complication of surgery or trauma, they are mentioned here because of the crucial importance of their early recognition and treatment (see also Chapter 27). These conditions are described under several names [3]:
1 Clostridial and non-clostridial gangrene [3–5]
2 Streptococcal cellulitis and myositis
3 Synergistic necrotizing cellulitis
4 Necrotizing fasciitis [6–8]
5 Meleney's progressive bacterial synergistic gangrene [9]
6 Synergistic gangrene [10]
7 Fournier's gangrene, etc.

Clinical features. Although middle-aged and elderly subjects are most often affected, the conditions can follow trauma in young adults, and the prognosis in the latter, given vigorous early treatment, is good [3]. They have also been described in children [11], particularly following circumcision or scalds, but sometimes after a bout of severe diarrhoea [12], or even spontaneously [13]. The problem may present as a primary perirectal abscess in the perineum (or on the scrotum or labia). Pain is generally the

first symptom, and may be severe. A distinct dusky red to black spot may appear in affected tissue and is of ominous significance. Tenderness and a dusky erythema extend with extreme rapidity to involve wide areas, and all the perirectal and perineal spaces (hence the terms fasciitis and myositis). Crepitus is an important feature, as is the presence of a dark brown, turbid fluid without pus. Many patients are diabetic [3,7] or leukaemic; in these, the mortality is much higher than the overall rate of 12–25% [7]. A perianal distribution, old age and delay in treatment also greatly reduce the survival rate.

Bacteriology. Swabs should be taken from the margin of the lesion [10]. An immediate Gram stain will distinguish clostridial infections by the finding of large Gram-positive rods. *Clostridium perfringens* was the most common organism in one series [3], but other clostridia, aerobic and anaerobic streptococci, and *Pseudomonas* species [11] have all been isolated. Anaerobes may easily be missed. A wide variety of secondary organisms are commonly cultured.

Treatment. Early recognition and immediate and aggressive treatment are essential in this devastating condition. Electrolyte and fluid balance must be established, and high-dosage antibiotic therapy started without waiting for the result of culture. This will normally consist of intravenous penicillin (24–30 million units/day [3]) together with a broad-spectrum antibiotic, usually an aminoglycoside or a cephalosporin; this regimen can be modified later.

The most important single therapeutic manoeuvre is rapid and extensive débridement of all affected tissue. Other surgical procedures, such as colostomy, may also be necessary. The value of hyperbaric oxygen [14] is disputed.

REFERENCES

1 Mortensen NJ, Thomson JP. Perianal abscess due to *Enterobius vermicularis*: report of a case. *Dis Colon Rectum* 1984; **27**: 677–8.
2 Givler RL. Necrotizing lesions associated with *Pseudomonas* infection in leukaemia. *Dis Colon Rectum* 1969; **12**: 438–40.
3 Bubrick MP, Hitchcock CR. Necrotizing anorectal and perineal infection. *Surgery* 1979; **86**: 655–62.
4 Bessman AN, Wagner W. Non-clostridial gas gangrene: report of 48 cases and a review of the literature. *JAMA* 1975; **233**: 958–63.
5 Skiles MS, Covert GK, Fletcher HS. Gas producing clostridial and non-clostridial infections. *Surg Gynecol Obstet* 1978; **147**: 65–7.
6 Fisher JR, Conway MJ, Takeshita RT *et al*. Necrotizing fasciitis: importance of roentgenographic studies for soft tissue gas. *JAMA* 1979; **241**: 803–6.
7 Oh C, Lee C, Jacobson JH. Necrotizing fasciitis of the perineum. *Surgery* 1982; **91**: 49–51.
8 Rosenberg PH, Shuck JM, Tempest BD *et al*. Diagnosis and therapy of necrotizing soft tissue infections of the perineum. *Ann Surg* 1978; **187**: 430–4.
9 Meleney FL. Hemolytic streptococcus gangrene. *Arch Surg* 1924; **9**: 317–64.
10 Flanigan RC, Kursh FD, McDougal WS *et al*. Synergistic gangrene of the scrotum and penis secondary to colorectal disease. *J Urol* 1978; **119**: 369–71.
11 Rabinowitz R, Lewin EB. Gangrene of the genitalia in children with *Pseudomonas* sepsis. *J Urol* 1980; **124**: 431–2.

12 Chuang JH, Wong KS. Necrotizing perianal infection in children. *J Pediatr Gastroenterol Nutr* 1990; **10**: 409–12.

13 Boisseau AM, Sarlangue J, Perel Y *et al.* Perineal ecthyma gangrenosum in infancy and early childhood: septicaemic and non-septicaemic forms. *J Am Acad Dermatol* 1992; **27**: 415–8.

14 Schweigel JF, Shim SS. A comparison of the treatment of gas gangrene with and without hyperbaric oxygen. *Surg Gynecol Obstet* 1973; **136**: 969–70.

Dermatological aspects of sexually transmitted disease

Gonorrhoea can result in anal inflammation and discharge, or an oedematous perianal dermatitis with multiple fissures and erosions.

Chancroid can cause extremely painful anal lesions instead of the classic multiple soft chancres. The initial rapidly ulcerating papule of granuloma inguinale (see Chapter 27) may occur in the perianal region in homosexual males. It is soft, painless and bleeds easily on trauma. It may be hypertrophic, sclerotic or phagedenic. There is normally no regional adenopathy, but a 'pseudobubo' may be present. In the anal canal, the lesion never extends beyond the stratified epithelium and strictures do not occur, but anal stenosis or, rarely, epitheliomatous change can supervene. If undiagnosed, lymphogranuloma venereum causes widespread vegetating and scarring lesions of the genitoperineal area. The Frei and complement fixation tests distinguish it from hidradenitis suppurativa.

Syphilis (see Chapter 30) [1] is becoming more common in homosexual men. It should never be forgotten as a possible cause of anal ulceration. Anal chancres are often mistaken for fissures; at the anal margin their significance may not be appreciated. Pain on defaecation or at night may be severe if there is secondary infection of the chancre, but is often absent. The posterior midline is the site of election. Bilateral lymphadenopathy is extremely rare with other perianal ulcers. Dark-ground examination may not be diagnostic if lubricants or ointments have been used. Discharge and bleeding, fissures (especially laterally) and fistulae should also arouse suspicion of anorectal primary syphilis. Painful syphilitic proctitis in the absence of anal lesions can occur [2,3]. Moist flat condylomata lata (Fig. 68.44) can affect all anogenital intertriginous sites and the differential diagnosis includes intertrigo as well as warts, lichen planus and bowenoid papulosis. The granulomatous gumma may affect the anal area as an ulcer, a white plaque or as an atrophic scar.

Perianal viral warts (condylomata acuminata) (Fig. 68.45) occasionally occur in infants and young children, but they are normally seen in young adults, and are not always sexually transmitted. They may be extraordinarily profuse, extending into the anal canal, especially in homosexuals or in immunodeficient (congenital or acquired) subjects in whom there is also a higher risk of progression to dysplasia and frank malignancy [4]. For example, anogenital warts are common in HIV-positive males,

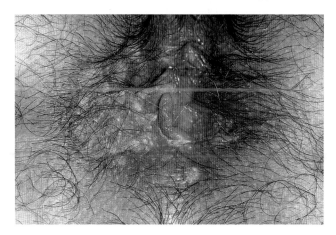

Fig. 68.44 Condylomata lata. (Courtesy of Dr S.C. Gold, London, UK.)

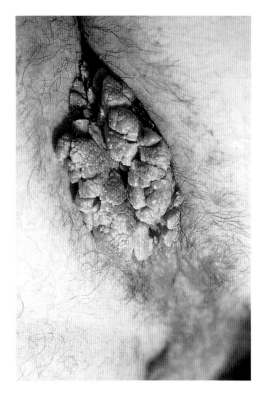

Fig. 68.45 Perianal condylomata acuminata. (Courtesy of Dr F.A. Ive, Durham, UK.)

nearly half of whom show histological signs of intraepithelial neoplasia. The clinical diagnosis of HPV is usually certain but condylomata lata (secondary syphilis), LP, molluscum contagiosum and BP enter the differential diagnosis. Solitary lesions have a wider differential diagnosis, including giant condyloma and squamous carcinoma. Biopsy should be performed if there is diagnostic doubt or if dysplasia or worse is suspected. Morphology and histology cannot distinguish virus-associated from non-virus-associated lesions; molecular techniques may be preferable but are not yet routinely available [5].

Table 68.34 Causes of anal ulceration in HIV infection.

Idiopathic
Haemorrhoids
Fissures
Sepsis
Syphilis (chancre)
Herpes simplex
Cytomegalovirus
Kaposi's sarcoma
Non-Hodgkin's lymphoma
Squamous carcinoma

Patients with anogenital warts, and their partners, may require full STD and sometimes colorecral assessment. Anogenital HPV can be very difficult to treat.

A phenomenon of chronic erosive and verrucous herpes simplex as part of immunoreconstitution disease has been described in HIV infection [6].

Human immunodeficiency virus infection

Anal ulceration may be a feature of HIV infection; Table 68.34 lists the main causes. Biopsy with special stains and culture is mandatory.

Other problems in HIV infection, including psoriasis, warts, intraepithelial neoplasia, squamous carcinoma and KS are discussed elsewhere.

CMV has been recorded in persistent perineal ulcers in immunosuppressed patients [7]. EBV DNA has been found in epithelial cells from the anal canals of asymptomatic HIV-positive male homosexuals, indicating possible sexual transmissibility [8]. Herpes simplex, gonorrhoea and anal condylomas were commonly associated in a US study on early HIV positivity [9]. Similar findings relate to a central African group with more advanced disease [10]. The importance of primary rectal syphilis has been emphasized [2]. Amoebiasis [11] may be overlooked. Dark-ground examination, and culture and microscopy for ova, should be obligatory [12]. In the absence of organisms, if pus cells are found, a rectal biopsy is indicated. KS of the rectum has been recorded in HIV-positive males [13]. The relationship of KS to anoreceptive anal intercourse and HHV 8 is discussed in Chapter 26 [14,15].

REFERENCES

1 McMillan A, Smith IW. Painful anal ulceration in homosexual men. *Br J Surg* 1984; **71**: 215–6.
2 Gluckman JB, Kleinman MS, May AG. Primary syphilis of rectum. *NY State J Med* 1974; **74**: 2210–1.
3 Akdamar K, Martin RJ, Ichinose H. Syphilitic proctitis. *Am J Dig Dis* 1977; **22**: 701.
4 Daneshpouy M, Socie G, Clavel C *et al.* Human papillomavirus infection and anogenital condyloma in bone marrow transplant recipients. *Transplantation* 2001; **71**: 167–9.
5 Strand A, Andersson S, Zehbe I, Wilander E. HPV prevalence in anal warts tested with the MY09/MY11 SHARP signal system. *Acta Dermatol Venereol* 1999; **79**: 226–9.
6 Fox PA, Barton SE, Francis N *et al.* Chronic erosive herpes simplex virus infection of the penis: a possible immune reconstitution disease. *HIV Med* 1999; **1**: 10–8.
7 Horn TD, Hood AF. Cytomegalovirus is predictably present in perineal ulcers of immunosuppressed patients. *Arch Dermatol* 1990; **126**: 642–4.
8 Naher H, Lenhard B, Wilms J, Nickel P. Detection of Epstein–Barr virus DNA in anal scrapings from HIV-positive homosexual men. *Arch Dermatol Res* 1995; **287**: 608–11.
9 Berger RS, Stoner MF, Hobbs ER *et al.* Cutaneous manifestations of early human immunodeficiency virus exposure. *J Am Acad Dermatol* 1988; **19**: 298–303.
10 Hira SK, Wadhawam D, Kamanga J *et al.* Cutaneous manifestations of human immunodeficiency virus in Lusaka, Zambia. *J Am Acad Dermatol* 1988; **19**: 451–7.
11 Robertson DHH, McMillan A, Young H. Homosexual transmission of amoebiasis. *J R Soc Med* 1982; **75**: 564.
12 Felman YM, Nikitas JA. Sexually transmitted diseases in the male homosexual. *Cutis* 1982; **30**: 706–24.
13 Lorenz HP, Wilson W, Leigh B, Schecter WP. Kaposi's sarcoma of the rectum in patients with the acquired immune deficiency syndrome. *Am J Surg* 1990; **160**: 681–2.
14 Chang Y, Cesarman E, Pessin MS *et al.* Identification of herpes virus-like DNA sequences in AIDS-associated Kaposi's sarcoma. *Science* 1994; **266**: 1865–9.
15 Lin JC, Lin SC, Mar EC *et al.* Is Kaposi's sarcoma-associated herpes virus detectable in semen in HIV infected homosexual men? *Lancet* 1995; **346**: 1601–2.

Miscellaneous

Pruritus ani has been attributed to erythrasma [1]. Erythrasma, present also at other sites, was found in 15 of 81 patients examined using Wood's light [1]; all were males. In infants, coxsackie A infections can cause a transient papular or papulovesicular eruption of the perianal area and buttocks. An erythematous desquamating perineal eruption occurring in the first week of the disease may be the first cutaneous feature in up to two-thirds of children with Kawasaki disease [2].

Fournier's gangrene and its differential diagnosis (Table 68.22) is discussed on pp. 68.28–68.29. Anorectal presentation is more serious than urogenital disease because the presentation may be more cryptic and there may be a longer delay in diagnosis [3].

Perianal tuberculosis (see Chapter 28) [4] is still seen where tuberculosis is common, but must always be considered, even in western Europe [5]. A primary lesion is exceptional; the accompanying unilateral lymphadenopathy is an important feature. Indolent, irregular, painful ulcers, fistulae and abscesses may be difficult to distinguish from those accompanying Crohn's disease [6]. Lupus vulgaris and verrucous tuberculosis may spread widely over the buttocks and postanal region, or assume a fungating and vegetating appearance. Tuberculosis cutis orificialis is thought to arise from autoinoculation of organisms contained in swallowed sputum from pulmonary lesions. It may occur in the immunocompromised and has been reported in association with Evans' syndrome (autoimmune haemolytic anaemia and immune thrombocytopenia) [7]. Perineal scrofuloderma (secondary skin involvement from underlying lymph node disease) may cause diagnostic confusion [8]. Pyoderma gangrenosum, Crohn's disease, hidradenitis, neoplasia, artefact, sexually transmitted diseases, amoebiasis and deep mycoses appear in the differential diagnosis [9].

Daughter yaws (see Chapter 30), initially papules but rapidly becoming ulcerated crusted plaques, have a predilection for periorificial sites on the face and around the perineum.

The giant condyloma of Buschke–Löwenstein (see p. 68.42) is rare. It is probably HPV-related [10].

Non-genital herpes simplex (see Chapter 25) occurs frequently around the pelvic girdle. Vaccinia, usually acquired by indirect transmission [11], is now never seen, but orf still occurs occasionally [12].

Sacral herpes zoster [11] is rare but can be cryptic in presentation; when involving S2–S4 or, less commonly, the ileoinguinal segment of L1–L2, it may cause significant morbidity from acute cystitis or urinary or faecal retention [13–15]. Hospitalization and urological and colorectal assessment are required, and treatment should be with intravenous aciclovir. AIDS has presented as anogenital herpes zoster [16].

Trichosporosis is a common cause of genito-crural and perianal intertrigo in India. Symptoms are itching or burning. Accompanying the intertrigo may be scaly papules. Coexisting dermatophyte, *Candida*, trichomycosis and erythrasma infection may be found. Topical dequalinium chloride is used for treatment in India [17].

Amoebiasis (see Chapter 32) of the perianal skin [18] is usually associated with bowel infections but, where the disease is endemic, direct inoculation of abraded skin or operation wounds can occur. Abscesses and fistulae may at first be indolent and symptomless. Ulcers typically extend slowly, with serpiginous outlines, firm cord-like edges and a whitish slough [19]. Sometimes, however, progression is rapid and remorseless, until a phagedenic ulcer completely destroys the perianal and sacral tissues [20]. A black foul-smelling eschar is surrounded by a violaceous edge, resembling pyoderma gangrenosum. The patient is extremely ill. Vegetating or condyloma-like lesions of intermediate severity occur less frequently. Amoebiasis should be suspected when such a lesion occurs unexpectedly in the course of 'ulcerative colitis' or in a prolonged mild undiagnosed colitis. Cases have been described in infants [21]. Destructive [21] perianal and buttock ulceration may masquerade as squamous carcinoma; however, very rarely, concomitant carcinoma has been reported [22]. The diagnosis is made by finding the *Entamoeba* species in a biopsy specimen from the edge of a lesion (which is always secondarily infected) or by examination, while warm, of a fresh high sigmoidoscopy swab. Treatment with metronidazole may be dramatically effective, but in severe cases surgery may also be required.

Perineal granulomatous lesions are a rare manifestation of schistosomiasis (bilharziasis), which may present as pruritic papules in the genital, umbilical and perineal regions in countries where it is endemic [23,24]. It is usually preceded by rectal or intestinal symptoms. The papules and nodules may be skin-coloured, pink or brown, scattered or grouped, affecting the penis, scrotum and vulva. They can spread onto the perineum and around the anus, and may develop into soft warty vegetating lesions, but remain relatively asymptomatic. Genital lesions simulating warts have been seen in travellers returning from endemic areas [25]. Ulceration is rare and, even more rarely, concomitant carcinoma has been reported [22]. The unusual occurrence of anogenital lesions results from ova shed by worms that have entered the perineal vessels [23]. Viable or calcified ova are found in the dermis.

Larva currens caused by *Strongyloides stercoralis* commonly occurs around the anus and on the buttocks. Likewise, cutaneous larva migrans resulting from the dog hookworm *Ancylostoma brasiliense* may occur around the pelvic girdle.

Perianal histoplasmosis and blastomycosis have also been recorded. Actinomycosis has resulted in multifocal perineal and buttock ulceration in G6PD deficiency [26]. Ulcerating and vegetating lesions, often unrecognized and of long duration, have followed trauma in patients with actinomycosis [27]. Correct diagnosis depends on histological confirmation, but the yellow or red granular pus should arouse suspicion [26].

Classic lesions of scabies commonly involve the buttocks, and nodules are sometimes seen in the perineum.

REFERENCES

1 Bowyer A, McColl I. Erythrasma and pruritus ani. *Acta Derm Venereol (Stockh)* 1971; **51**: 444–7.

2 Friter BS, Lucky AW. The perineal eruption of Kawasaki syndrome. *Arch Dermatol* 1988; **124**: 1805–10.

3 Enriquez JM, Moreno S, Devesa M *et al.* Fournier's syndrome of urogenital and anogenital origin: a retrospective, comparative study. *Dis Colon Rectum* 1987; **36**: 33–7.

4 Strescobich D, Donadio R, Aguilar OG *et al.* Fistulas anales de etiología poco frecuente. *Prensa Med Argent* 1969; **56**: 622–3.

5 Lé Bourgeois PC, Poynard T, Modai J *et al.* Ulceration perianale: ne pas oublier la tuberculose. *Presse Med* 1984; **13**: 2507–9.

6 Morson BC. Histopathology of Crohn's disease. *Proc R Soc Med* 1968; **61**: 79–81.

7 Kim SW, Choi SW, Cho BK, Houh W, Lee JW. Tuberculosis cutis orificialis: an association with Evan's syndrome. *Acta Dermatol Venereol* 1995; **75**: 84–5.

8 Poláková K. Atypically localized scrofuloderma. *Bratisl Lek Listy* 1993; **94**: 536–8.

9 Betlloch I, Bañuls J, Sevila A *et al.* Perianal tuberculosis. *Int J Dermatol* 1994; **33**: 270–1.

10 Alexander RM, Kaminsky DB. Giant condyloma acuminatum (Buschke–Löwenstein tumour) of the anus. *Dis Colon Rectum* 1979; **22**: 561–5.

11 Bessiere L, Allain D, Meleville J. La vaccine ano-genitale. *Ann Dermatol Vénéréol* 1979; **105**: 339–41.

12 Kennedy CTC, Lyell A. Perianal orf. *J Am Acad Dermatol* 1984; **11**: 72–4.

13 Fugelso PD, Reed WB, Newman SB, Beamer JE. Herpes zoster of the anogenital area affecting urination and defaecation. *Br J Dermatol* 1973; **89**: 285–8.

14 Waugh MA. Herpes zoster of the anogenital area affecting urination and defaecation [Letter]. *Br J Dermatol* 1974; **90**: 235.

15 Weaver SM, Keely AP. Herpes zoster as a cause of neurogenic bladder. *Cutis* 1982; **29**: 611–2.

16 Thune P, Andersson T, Skjorten F. AIDS manifesting as anogenital herpes zoster eruption: demonstration of virus-like particles in lymphocytes. *Acta Derm Venereol (Stockh)* 1983; **63**: 540–3.

17 Kamalam A, Senthamilselvi A, Ajuthades K *et al*. Cutaneous trichosporosis. *Mycopathologia* 1988; **101**: 167–75.

18 Lord PH, Sakellariades P. Perianal skin gangrene due to amoebic infection in a diabetic. *Proc R Soc Med* 1973; **66**: 677–8.

19 Smith JN, Winship DH. Complications and extraintestinal problems in inflammatory bowel disease. *Med Clin North Am* 1980; **64**: 1161–71.

20 Venkataramaiah NR, Reinaerta HHM, Van Roalte JE *et al*. Pseudomalignant cutaneous amoebiasis. *Trop Doctor* 1982; **12**: 162–3.

21 Wynne JM. Perineal amoebiasis. *Arch Dis Child* 1980; **55**: 234–6.

22 Zawahry ME. Cutaneous amoebiasis. *Indian J Dermatol* 1966; **11**: 77–8.

23 Adeyemi-Doru FAB, Osoba OA, Junaid TA. Perigenital cutaneous schistosomiasis. *Br J Vener Dis* 1979; **55**: 446–9.

24 Cohn R, Loubiere R, Guillaume A *et al*. Les lesions cutanées de bilharziose: a propos de 14 observations. *Ann Dermatol Vénéréol* 1980; **107**: 759–67.

25 Goldsmith PC, Leslie TA, Sams V *et al*. Lesions of schistosomiasis mimicking warts on the vulva. *BMJ* 1993; **307**: 556–7.

26 Millet P, Sonneck J-M, Lanternier G *et al*. Actinomycose perineofessiere et deficit en G6PD. *Ann Dermatol Vénéréol* 1982; **109**: 789–90.

27 Grigoriu D, Delecretaz J. Actinomyocose peri-anale pruritive. *Ann Dermatol Vénéréol* 1981; **108**: 159–61.

Benign tumours

The following entities are encountered in the perineal/perianal area: angiomas and angiokeratomas; basal cell papillomas may be mistaken for viral warts or BP, as may melanocytic naevi; inguinogenital epidermoid cysts may become infected; lesions containing molluscum contagiosum have been described; pilar cyst, including giant forms, is much rarer.

Haemorrhoids

Haemorrhoids/piles (Latin *pila*, a ball) are dilatations in the venous system draining the anus, mucosal prolapse or loose tethering of mucosa to the anal wall [1]. Symptoms are rectal bleeding, mucous discharge, pruritus ani and prolapse. The complications of piles are thrombosis, strangulation, ulceration, fibrosis, infection and abscess, which give rise to pain. Patients presenting with these symptoms should be assessed by a proctologist, and by proctoscopy and sigmoidoscopy. Signs depend on the presentation. Perianal skin tags from fibrosed piles are extremely common. The differential diagnosis includes distal bowel cancer, as well as naevi, Crohn's disease, KS and perianal metastases. Treatment is the domain of the colorectal surgeon and gastroenterologist.

Premalignant dermatoses and frank malignancies

The anogenital area is not exposed to solar radiation, the principal cutaneous carcinogen. Treatment of pruritus in the past with radiotherapy or tar preparations, and the use of radiotherapy for gynaecological malignancy, carry theoretical hazards and can occasionally be incriminated in carcinogenesis. However, they do not appear to have influenced greatly the frequency of perineal tumours. Post-granulomatous scarring is an important background to perianal malignancy in some parts of the world, and other chronic inflammatory processes, such as LS, are a potential hazard. There are cases where condylomata acuminata have preceded SCC of the anal or perianal skin [2,3] and HPV has become a major suspect in the precancerous process.

Porokeratosis

Genital porokeratosis of Mibelli is rare but classic lesions have been found on the penis, scrotum and in the natal cleft. Ulceration may occur [4]. Porokeratosis may be confused with psoriasis, Bowen's disease, granuloma annulare or LP. Histopathology of a biopsy confirms the diagnosis [5]. Topical 5-fluorouracil can be used [6].

Anal intraepithelial neoplasia

Anal intraepithelial neoplasia (AIN) describes full-thickness dysplasia of the anus and perianal skin [7]. It can present relatively asymptomatically as red, shiny or scaly patches like Bowen's disease, or as warty lesions like BP. AIN is frequently associated with homosexuality, anal warts, HPV and HIV, although it is not a prominent feature of other conditions involving immunosuppression. Women with anogenital Bowen's disease have an increased risk of intraepithelial neoplasia or invasive malignancy elsewhere in the genital tract [8,9], and a full gynaecological examination is thus obligatory in such cases. In AIDS, the overall risk of progression of AIN associated with HPV to invasive squamous carcinoma is low [10]. Immunoreconstitution with highly active antiretroviral treatment (HAART) may not achieve regression of AIN [11]. Routine screening of the HIV-positive patient with anal cytology is advocated [11]. Treatment options are similar to those for PIN. Relapse is common. Expert proctological advice should be sought.

Carcinoma of the anus

Anogenital squamous carcinoma is sometimes called epidermoid carcinoma. Fifty-six per cent of all anal carcinomas are of the squamous variety [12]. They are slightly more common in women, but seem to be more aggressive in men [13]. In Denmark, the incidence of anal carcinoma has tripled since 1960 to 0.74 cases per 100 000 population [14].

Although associations with smoking, cervical intraepithelial dysplasia and changing sexual habits, including homosexual anal intercourse, have been postulated

[14,15] and coexistent Crohn's disease has been said to be associated with a 10-fold increase in anal carcinoma [16], the aetiology is not clearly understood. HPV is implicated [17,18], especially in verrucous carcinoma (see below) [19]. Anal carcinoma is often associated with a history of anogenital warts. More than 90% of anogenital condylomata contain HPV 6 or 11, although these subtypes are not associated with cancer, and it is rare for condylomata to contain HPV 16, which has a well-documented association with anal carcinoma. Homosexual men have a higher incidence of both perianal warts and anal carcinoma (both *in situ* and invasive), and this may be related to receptive anal intercourse [15], and HPV as well as other sexually transmitted diseases such as gonorrhoea, herpes simplex and *Chlamydia trachomatis* infection [20]. These infections are also risk factors for anal carcinoma in heterosexual men and women, as is cigarette smoking [21]. A role for seminal fluid prostaglandins in homosexual anal cancer has been proposed [22]. Immunosuppression, including by HIV infection, is a risk factor for AIN and anal cancer [23]. A case of Peutz–Jeghers syndrome associated with anal squamous carcinoma has been reported [24].

Diagnosis can present difficulties. Symptoms may include bleeding, pain, presence of a mass and change in bowel habit. Examination will reveal a hard mass that may be flat, raised or polypoid [25]. Squamous carcinoma should be suspected in all nodulo-ulcerative anal and perianal disease, especially in the context of LS, LP, hidradenitis suppurativa, intraepithelial neoplasia and immunocompromise.

Regarding the differential diagnosis [26], it must be appreciated that anal carcinoma often presents with similar symptoms to benign anal lesions such as piles and fissures (pruritus, discomfort or pain, and bleeding). The most common tumours of the anal margin are viral warts, which are distinguished by their multiplicity, their lack of induration and ulceration, and their rapid evolution. Rarely, these may give rise to anal carcinoma [27]. Syphilitic condylomas are also multiple and not indurated. A syphilitic chancre of the anal margin or canal may be more easily mistaken for carcinoma. Amoebiasis and tuberculosis must also be considered. The differential diagnosis includes the manifestations of intraepithelial neoplasia (and the differential diagnosis of these), erosive or ulcerative sexually transmitted disease, basal cell carcinoma, KS, hidradenitis suppurativa, Crohn's disease, pyoderma gangrenosum and artefact. The differential diagnosis also includes ischiorectal or perianal abscess [28–30]. Colorectal assessment should be sought. Proctoscopy and sigmoidoscopy are necessary to exclude anorectal cancer [28–30].

An important consideration in the management of anal carcinoma is the preservation of sphincter function, and this frequently involves combined radiotherapy and chemotherapy [31,32]. Surgical excision of the tumour, and of the inguinal lymph nodes when these are involved,

is the treatment of choice. For small well-differentiated tumours, particularly adenocarcinomas, a local excision and repair is ideal. Small squamous carcinomas may respond well to radiotherapy.

Lymphatic or haematogenous dissemination of anogenital cancer dictates individualized multidisciplinary management. The management of ilioinguinal lymphadenopathy is controversial [33–35].

The prognosis for anal carcinoma is variable [32].

REFERENCES

1 Nisar PJ, Scholefield JH. Clinical review: managing haemorrhoids. *BMJ* 2003; **327**: 847–51.
2 South LM, O'Sullivan JP, Gazet JC. Giant condylomata of Buschke and Löwenstein. *Clin Oncol* 1977; **3**: 107–15.
3 Sturm JT, Christenson CE, Vecker JH *et al.* Squamous cell carcinoma of the anus arising in a giant condyloma acuminatum. *Dis Colon Rectum* 1975; **18**: 147–51.
4 Watanabe T, Murakami T, Okochi H, Kikuchi K, Furue M. Ulcerative porokeratosis. *Dermatology* 1998; **196**: 256–9.
5 Levell NJ, Bewley AP, Levene GM. Porokeratosis of Mibelli on the penis, scrotum and natal cleft. *Clin Exp Dermatol* 1994; **19**: 77–8.
6 Porter WM, Menage H du P, Philip G, Bunker CB. Porokeratosis of the penis. *Br J Dermatol* 2001; **144**: 643–4.
7 Zbar AP, Fenger C, Efron J, Beer-Gabel M, Wexner SD. The pathology and molecular biology of anal intraepithelial neoplasia: comparisons with cervical and vulvar intraepithelial carcinoma. *Int J Colorectal Dis* 2002; **17**: 203–15.
8 Franklin EW, Rutledge FD. Epidemiology of epidermoid carcinoma of the vulva. *Obstet Gynecol* 1972; **39**: 165–72.
9 Reynolds VH, Madden JJ, Franlin JD *et al.* Preservation of anal function after total excision of the anal mucosa for Bowen's disease. *Ann Surg* 1984; **199**: 563–8.
10 Morgan AR, Miles AJ, Wastell C. Anal warts and squamous carcinoma *in situ* of the anal canal. *J R Soc Med* 1994; **87**: 15.
11 Martin F, Bower M. Anal intraepithelial neoplasia in HIV-positive people. *Sex Transm Infect* 2001; **77**: 327–31.
12 Boman B, Moertel CG, O'Connell MJ. Carcinoma of the anal canal. *Cancer* 1984; **54**: 114–25.
13 Serota AI, Weil M, Williams RA. Anal cloacogenic carcinoma. *Arch Surg* 1981; **116**: 456–9.
14 Frisch M, Melbye M, Moller H. Trends in incidence of anal cancer in Denmark. *BMJ* 1993; **306**: 419–22.
15 Cantril ST, Green JP, Schall GL. Primary radiation therapy in the treatment of anal carcinoma. *Radiol Oncol Biol Physiol* 1983; **9**: 1271–8.
16 Slater G, Greenstein A, Aufses A. Anal carcinoma in patients with Crohn's disease. *Ann Surg* 1984; **199**: 348–50.
17 McDougall JK. Immortalization and transformation of human cells by human papillomavirus. *Curr Topics Microbiol Immunol* 1994; **186**: 101–19.
18 Kadish AS. Biology of anogenital neoplasia. *Cancer Treat Res* 2001; **104**: 267–86.
19 Chang F, Kosunen O, Kosma VM *et al.* Verrucous carcinoma of the anus containing human papilloma virus type 16 DNA detected by *in situ* hybridization. *Genitourin Med* 1990; **66**: 342–5.
20 Gal AA, Meyer PR, Taylor CR. Papillomavirus antigens in anorectal condyloma and carcinoma in homosexual men. *JAMA* 1987; **257**: 337–40.
21 Daling JR, Sherman KJ, Hislop TG *et al.* Cigarette smoking and the risk of anogenital cancer. *Am J Epidemiol* 1992; **135**: 180–9.
22 Kondlapoodi P. Anorectal cancer and homosexuality. *JAMA* 1982; **248**: 2114–5.
23 Gibbs SJ, Spittle MF. Seminoma and squamous cell carcinomas in association with lymphopenia. *Clin Oncol* 1995; **7**: 46–7.
24 Mullhaupt B, Bauerfeind P, Kurrer MO, Fried M. Anal squamous cell carcinoma in a patient with Peutz–Jeghers syndrome. *Dig Dis Sci* 2001; **46**: 273–7.
25 Stearns MW, Urmacher C, Sternberg SS. Cancer of the anal canal. *Curr Probl Cancer* 1980; **4**: 1–44.
26 Fenger C. Anal neoplasia and its precursors: facts and controversies. *Semin Diagn Pathol* 1991; **8**: 190–201.

27 Goodman P, Halpert RD. Invasive squamous cell carcinoma of the anus arising in condyloma acuminatum: CT demonstration. *Gastrointest Radiol* 1991; **16**: 267–70.

28 Drumm J, Donovan IA, Clain A. Unusual presentation of anorectal carcinoma. *BMJ* 1982; **285**: 1393.

29 McConnell EM. Squamous carcinoma of the anus: a review of 96 cases. *Br J Surg* 1970; **57**: 89–92.

30 Tait WF, Sykes PA, Taylor GM, Galland RB, Ross HB. Unusual presentation of anorectal carcinoma. *BMJ* 1982; **285**: 1742.

31 Chawla AK, Willett CG. Squamous cell carcinoma of the anal canal and anal margin. *Hematol Oncol Clin North Am* 2001; **15**: 321–44.

32 Esiashvili N, Landry J, Matthews RH. Carcinoma of the anus: strategies in management. *Oncologist* 2002; **7**: 188–99.

33 McDougal WS, Kirchner FR, Edwards RH, Killion LZ. Treatment of carcinoma of the penis: the case for primary lymphadenectomy. *J Urol* 1986; **136**: 38–41.

34 Heyns CF, van Vollenhoven P, Steenkamp JW, Allen FJ. Cancer of the penis: a review of 50 patients. *S Afr J Surg* 1997; **35**: 120–4.

35 Schoeneich G, Perabo FG, Muller SC. Squamous cell carcinoma of the penis. *Andrologia* 1999; **31** (Suppl. 1): 17–20.

Extramammary Paget's disease (see Chapter 36)

Seventy-three per cent of cases of extramammary Paget's disease (EMPD) present as pruritus ani [1]. The association with an underlying malignancy is variable. Two reviews of the literature revealed only a 25% association [2,3]. Despite this, a search for a primary adenocarcinoma of underlying secretory glands should be carried out in perianal EMPD [4]. In some cases, the primary tumour is an anorectal, or even more distant, carcinoma [5,6]. The primary tumour and the Paget's cells in the epidermis are usually mucus secreting. Electron microscopy has shown the Paget's cells to be squamous in character in some patients, but more recent immunohistochemical and enzyme histochemical methods have demonstrated a close relationship between Paget's cells and sweat gland epithelial cells [7]. Anorectal carcinomas may arise from rectal mucosa or from the intramuscular glands. In the latter case, the malignant cells may track to the buttock through the ischiorectal fossa, and the Paget's plaque may begin at a distance from the anal margin, rather like an ischiorectal abscess. Topographical studies have shown that the plaque of Paget's disease is much larger than the visible lesion [8]. Any attempt at removal must be radical and histologically controlled [9].

Extensive surgery in conjunction with photodynamic therapy involving infusion of dihaematoporphyrin and an argon pumped dye laser has been effective in curing a patient with previous postoperative recurrences [10].

The pattern of the intramuscular glands and of the wide range of tumours that arise from them ('cloacogenic' carcinoma) resembles genitourinary rather than intestinal endothelium [11]. The carcinoma may spread, either to involve the anorectal mucosa, or through the perianal tissue to produce a chronic fistula-*in-ano* [12]. It may on occasion mimic a basal cell carcinoma both in clinical and histological appearance [13].

REFERENCES

1 Jensen SL, Sjolin KE, Shokouh-Amiri MH. Paget's disease of the anal margin. *Br J Surg* 1988; **75**: 1089–92.

2 Mohs FE, Blanchard I. Microscopically controlled surgery for extramammary Paget's disease. *Arch Dermatol* 1979; **115**: 706–8.

3 Breen JL, Smith CI, Gregori CA. Extramammary Paget's disease. *Clin Obstet Gynecol* 1978; **21**: 1107–15.

4 van der Putte SCK, van Gorp LHM. Adenocarcinoma of the mammary-like glands of the vulva: a unifying concept. *J Cutan Pathol* 1994; **21**: 157–63.

5 Fetherston WC, Friedrich EG. The origin and significance of vulvar Paget's disease. *Obstet Gynecol* 1972; **39**: 735–44.

6 Helwig EB, Graham JH. Anogenital (extramammary) Paget's disease: a clinicopathological study. *Cancer* 1963; **16**: 387–403.

7 Hamm H, Vroom TM, Czarnetski BM. Extramammary Paget's cells: further evidence of sweat gland derivation. *J Am Acad Dermatol* 1986; **15**: 1275–81.

8 Gunn RA, Gallagher S. Vulvar Paget's disease: a topographic study. *Cancer* 1980; **46**: 590–4.

9 Coldiron BM, Goldsmith BA, Robinson JK. Surgical treatment of extramammary Paget's disease. *Cancer* 1991; **67**: 933–8.

10 Petrelli NJ, Cebollero JA, Rodriguez-Bigas M *et al*. Photodynamic therapy in the management of neoplasms of the perianal skin. *Arch Surg* 1992; **127**: 1436–8.

11 Grenvalsky HT, Helwig EB. Carcinoma of the anorectal junction. I. Histological considerations. *Cancer* 1956; **19**: 480–8.

12 Zeinberg VH, Kays S. Anorectal carcinomas of extramucosal origin. *Ann Surg* 1957; **145**: 344–54.

13 Espana A, Redondo P, Idoate MA *et al*. Perianal basal cell carcinoma. *Clin Exp Dermatol* 1992; **17**: 360–2.

Miscellaneous

Extramucosal anorectal carcinoma presents as an inflammatory rather than a malignant condition and so is not biopsied (or not biopsied deeply) and the diagnosis is missed or delayed; there are many cases in the literature of cancers arising from anal glands adjacent to the anorectal wall and not emergent from the mucosa [1]. Cloacogenic carcinoma constitutes only 2–3% of anorectal cancer, but may behave aggressively [2]. It derives from remnants of the cloacal membrane proximal to the pectinate line where there is an area of transitional mucosa (between keratinized and non-keratinized squamous epithelium) penetrated by the anal glands. Most rectal cancer is adenocarcinoma (columnar epithelium).

Although basal cell carcinoma is the most common type of skin cancer, it is rare in the anogenital area, but over 100 cases have been reported [3,4]. Small basal cell carcinomas may respond well to irradiation.

Anorectal melanoma accounts for only 1% of all tumours of this area [5]; it may occur concomitantly with melanosis of the gastrointestinal tract [6].

Anogenital KS is essentially an HIV-related problem.

Fibrosarcoma, haemangiopericytoma, leiomyosarcoma, malignant fibrous histiocytoma, epithelioid sarcoma, dermatofibrosarcoma protuberans and spindle cell sarcoma may occur, presenting as painful or painless nodules, masses or swellings [7]. Other rarities include Merkel cell carcinoma [8], malignant eccrine poroma [9] and malignant schwannoma [7,10].

Non-Hodgkin's lymphoma of the perianal area has been described in HIV/AIDS [11].

Perianal infiltration, ulceration or abscess occurs in 5% of haematological malignancies [12]. Chronic lymphocytic leukaemia has presented as a painless firm white mass at the anal orifice, associated with weight loss and inguinal lymphadenopathy [13]. Perianal ulceration and suppuration have been reported as the presenting manifestations of primary lymphoma of the anus [14].

Perineal/perianal metastases from transitional cell carcinoma of the distal urethra [15], from rectal carcinoma [16] and from epidermoid anal canal carcinoma [17] have occurred. Carcinoma erysipeloides has been observed in the perineum and on the thigh in carcinoma of the bladder and prostate [18].

A periorificial form of Langerhans' cell histiocytosis/ eosinophilic granuloma may cause ulcerating and vegetating lesions within the anal canal and in the perianal skin [19].

REFERENCES

1 Zimberg YH, Kay S. Anorectal carcinomas of extra-mucosal origin. *Ann Surg* 1957; **145**: 344.
2 Serota AI, Weil M, Williams RA. Anal cloacogenic carcinoma. *Arch Surg* 1981; **116**: 456–9.
3 Espana A, Redondo P, Idoate MA *et al.* Perianal basal cell carcinoma. *Clin Exp Dermatol* 1992; **17**: 360–2.
4 Gibson GE, Ahmed I. Perianal and genital basal cell carcinoma: a clinico-pathologic review of 51 cases. *J Am Acad Dermatol* 2001; **45**: 68–71.
5 Johnson A, Mathai G, Robinson WA. Malignant melanoma of the perineum. *J Surg Oncol* 1993; **54**: 185–9.
6 Horowitz M, Nobrega MM. Primary anal melanoma associated with melanosis of the upper gastrointestinal tract. *Endoscopy* 1998; **30**: 662–5.
7 Dehner LP, Smith BH. Soft tissue tumours of the penis. *Cancer* 1970; **25**: 1431–47.
8 Best TJ, Metcalfe JB, Moore RB, Nguyen GK. Merkel cell carcinoma of the scrotum. *Ann Plast Surg* 1994; **33**: 83–5.
9 Werdin R, Kupczyk-Joeris D, Schumpelick V. Malignant eccrine poroma: case report of a rare tumour of the skin. *Chirurg* 1991; **62**: 350–2.
10 Marsidi PJ, Winter CC. Schwannoma of penis. *Urology* 1980; **16**: 303.
11 Denis BJ, May T, Bigard MA, Canton P. Anal and perianal lesions in symptomatic HIV infections: prospective study of a series of 190 patients. *Gastroenterol Clin Biol* 1992; **16**: 148–54.
12 Vanheuverzwyn R, Delannoy A, Michaex JL, Dive C. Anal lesions in haematological disorders. *Dis Colon Rectum* 1980; **23**: 310–2.
13 Cresson DH, Siegal GP. Chronic lymphocytic leukaemia presenting as an anal mass. *J Clin Gastroenterol* 1985; **7**: 83–7.
14 Steele RJ, Eremin O, Krajewski AS, Ritchie GL. Primary lymphoma of the anal canal presenting as perianal suppuration. *BMJ* 1985; **291**: 311.
15 Langlois NEI, McClinton S, Miller ID. An unusual presentation of transitional cell carcinoma of the distal urethra. *Histopathology* 1992; **21**: 482–4.
16 García-Armengol J, Roig JV, Alós R, Solana A. Perianal cutaneous metastasis of rectal adenocarcinoma. *Rev Esp Enferm Dig* 1995; **87**: 342–3.
17 Nazzari G, Drago F, Malatto, M, Crovato F. Epidermoid anal canal carcinoma metastic to the skin: a clinical mimic of prostate adenocarcinoma metastases. *J Dermatol Surg Oncol* 1994; **20**: 765–6.
18 Cohen EL, Kim SW. Cutaneous manifestation of carcinoma of urinary bladder: carcinoma erysipelatodes. *Urology* 1980; **16**: 410–2.
19 Tait WF, Sykes PA. Unusual presentation of anorectal carcinoma. *BMJ* 1982; **285**: 1742.

Anal manifestations of intestinal disease

These have been well documented [1]. Although they are usually non-specific, the particular skin manifestations of tuberculosis, amoebiasis, schistosomiasis and Crohn's disease may lead to diagnosis of the underlying disease by their typical histology.

REFERENCE

1 Grosshans E, Jenn P, Baumann R *et al.* Manifestations anales de maladies du tube digestif. *Ann Dermatol Vénéréol* 1979; **106**: 25–30.

Miscellaneous

Effects of topical corticosteroids

The prolonged use of potent topical corticosteroids for inflammatory conditions of the groins or perianal area can produce misleading appearances. Tinea incognito [1] is well recognized, but a persistent, deep, livid erythema of the perianal skin may not be regarded as primarily infective. Striae occur readily on the thighs. Multiple perianal comedones followed the application of a topical corticosteroid for 3 years [2]. 'Infantile gluteal granuloma' [3] (see Chapter 14), usually affecting infants of 4–6 months, may also occur in incontinent elderly patients [4].

Chronic perianal pain and the 'perineal syndrome'

A number of names have been given to sensations of pain localized to the anogenital region in the absence of evident organic cause [5,6]. Proctalgia fugax affects young adult males, and occurs chiefly at night in the form of a sudden cramp-like pain, which resolves in a few minutes. 'Coccygodynia', 'descending perineum syndrome' and 'chronic idiopathic anal pain' chiefly affect females. The pain is described as dull and throbbing. In 35 such patients, it was noted that the pain was precipitated by sitting, and that these three conditions differed from proctalgia fugax [5]. Electrophysiological studies gave variable results. There was a high incidence of previous sciatica and damage to the pelvic floor musculature. Treatment was disappointing. Rarely, sacral cysts and even chordoma can present with this symptomatology.

Such patients will present to surgeons or gynaecologists; however, dermatologists may be confronted by a similar problem in which a patient complains of short-lived episodes of intense burning, which may be accompanied by sweating, limited to the perineum or occasionally the scrotum. Attacks occur without warning, but may be brought about by a full rectum. In one patient, the attacks were severe enough to cause him to stop walking for some minutes. The patients tend to be stressed individuals, as are those with proctalgia fugax [6]. The skin is entirely normal.

The mechanism is unknown. Two patients appeared to have been helped by propantheline, suggesting a cholinergic mechanism [7]. However, the condition may also fall into the group of 'dermatological non-disease' [8], in which the perineum was affected in eight out of 24 patients. The condition has also been reported in children suffering from intrafamilial stresses [9] (see also pp. 68.48 and 68.82).

REFERENCES

1 Ive FA, Marks R. Tinea incognito. *BMJ* 1968; **iii**: 149–52.
2 Oliet EJ, Estes SA. Perianal comedones associated with chronic topical fluorinated steroid use. *J Am Acad Dermatol* 1982; **7**: 405–7.
3 Ortonne JP, Perrot H, Thivolet J. Granulome gluteal infantile (GGI): étude ultrastructurale. *Ann Dermatol Vénéréol* 1980; **107**: 631–4.
4 Maekawa Y, Sakazaki Y, Hayashibara T. Diaper area granuloma of the aged. *Arch Dermatol* 1978; **114**: 382–3.
5 Neill ME, Swash M. Chronic perianal pain: an unsolved problem. *J R Soc Med* 1982; **75**: 96–101.
6 Parks AG, Porter NH, Hardcastle J. The syndrome of descending perineum. *Proc R Soc Med* 1966; **59**: 477–82.
7 Monro PAG, ed. *Sympathectomy.* Oxford: Clarendon Press, 1959: 146.
8 Cotterill JA. A dermatological non-disease: a common and potentially fatal disturbance of cutaneous body image. *Br J Dermatol* 1980; **103** (Suppl. 18): 13.
9 Lask B. Chronic perianal pain. *J R Soc Med* 1982; **75**: 370.

Umbilical dermatology

Introduction

The umbilicus is considered here for convenience. Although the umbilicus is not strictly part of the genital apparatus, its evolution and connections link it to the pelvic region.

Structure and function

At birth, the umbilical cord contains two arteries and a vein, the rudimentary arachus (allantois) and the vitelline (omphalomesenteric) duct, enveloped in Wharton's jelly. After separation and retraction of the stump, an umbilicus of variable depth is formed. Persistence of the urachal or vitelline ducts at this 'carrefour embryologique' may cause trouble in early or later life. A deeply retracted umbilicus may be the site of infection or foreign bodies.

Congenital and developmental abnormalities [1]

These are all rare, more common in males, and usually brought about by failure of obliteration of the omphalomesenteric duct or urachus. They present as fistulae, cysts or polypoid tumours.

Patent urachal duct

The umbilical opening is lined by skin or a pouting mucous membrane. Urine may be seen to escape from it, particularly in the elderly, when an obstruction to micturition exists. The condition is rare.

Persistent vitelline duct and polyp

If a connection with the intestine persists, it may become inflamed or cause a faecal umbilical discharge. More commonly, the remains of the duct give rise to a polyp in later life [2]. This may be accompanied by intermittent bleeding or a more persistent mucoid discharge, sometimes profuse. A symptomless sterile umbilical discharge should always arouse suspicion. The histopathological features are those of intestinal mucosa. It may be mistaken for a pyogenic granuloma [3].

Periumbilical 'choristia'

Under this title (meaning dysgenetic translocation of tissue), Bellone *et al.* [4] described extending crusted erythematous periumbilical plaques, in which islands of intestinal mucosal cells were found in the epidermis.

Omphalocele

This form of abdominal hernia appears to be more common in African people. In 5 years in Ibadan, 33 cases were seen [5]. The minor form is caused by herniation of the umbilical cord; a major form is probably because of a fault of embryonic folding of the fetus.

REFERENCES

1 Nix TE, Young CJ. Congenital umbilical anomalies. *Arch Dermatol* 1964; **90**: 160–5.
2 Hejazi N. Umbilical polyp: a report of two cases. *Dermatologica* 1975; **150**: 111–5.
3 Laradle De Luna M, Gcioni V, Herrara A *et al.* Umbilical polyps. *Pediatr Dermatol* 1987; **4**: 341–3.
4 Bellone AG, Raimondi L, Gasparini G *et al.* Choristia intestinale périumbilicale en plaques. *Ann Dermatol Vénéréol* 1978; **105**: 601–6.
5 Nivabueze I, Hekwaba F. Omphalocele: experience in the African tropics. *Postgrad Med J* 1981; **57**: 635–9.

Trauma and artefact

The umbilicus in the newborn

Haemorrhages may occur from slipped ligatures. The cord normally separates within a week of birth, and the raw surface is epithelialized by day 15. During this time, the umbilicus is prone to infection, especially in maternity hospitals and nurseries. Impetigo (pemphigus neonatorum) or, rarely, more severe bacterial infections may occur (see below). The 'absent navel' syndrome has been described as a sign of dystrophic epidermolysis bullosa [1].

Talc granuloma

This lesion, which is probably more frequent than is recognized, occurs in infants and very young children. It is distinguished histologically from a pyogenic granuloma (on which it may supervene) by the doubly refractile talc crystals [2].

Pyogenic granuloma

This is a dull-red fleshy polypoid lesion, often pedunculated. Bleeding readily takes place from trauma. If it occurs early in life, it may be confused with a capillary haemangioma.

Ileo-umbilical fistula

This may follow laparotomy for Crohn's disease, or may rarely occur spontaneously [3].

Omphalith

In deeply set umbilici, an accumulation of sebum and keratin may lead to the gradual formation of a hard stone-like mass, which may remain unnoticed for many years until discovered accidentally or revealed by secondary infection or ulceration.

'Spontaneous gangrene'

This can occur without catheterization, possibly owing to minor trauma to the umbilicus [4]. Very rarely, the bladder and kidney may also be involved.

Unilateral skin necrosis of the buttock has been reported following indwelling umbilical artery catheterization [4–6], probably caused by thrombosis leading to occlusion of the inferior gluteal artery. A similar case was caused by misdirection of the tip of the arterial catheter [7].

REFERENCES

1 Paslin D. People without navels. *Br J Dermatol* 1978; **98**: 584.
2 McCallum DJ, Hall GFM. Umbilical granulomata: with particular reference to talc granuloma. *Br J Dermatol* 1970; **83**: 151–6.
3 Reutz TW Jr, Warden CS, Garcia FJ. Crohn's disease with spontaneous ileo-umbilical and ileo-vesical fistulae. *Dig Dis Sci* 1979; **24**: 316–8.
4 Bonifazi E, Meneghini C. Perianal gangrene of the buttock: an iatrogenic or spontaneous condition? *J Am Acad Dermatol* 1980; **3**: 596–8.
5 Cutler VE, Stretcher GS. Cutaneous complications of central umbilical artery catheterization. *Arch Dermatol* 1977; **113**: 61–3.
6 Mann PN. Gluteal skin necrosis after umbilical artery catheterization. *Arch Dis Child* 1980; **55**: 815–17.
7 Rudolph N, Wang HH, Dragutsky D. Gangrene of the buttock: a complication of umbilical artery catheterization. *Pediatrics* 1974; **53**: 106–9.

Inflammatory dermatoses

Eczematous conditions and psoriasis

Allergic contact dermatitis is usually brought about by medicaments. Irritant dermatitis from soap and quaternary ammonium compounds also occurs. Psoriasis commonly involves the umbilicus.

Miscellaneous

A pilonidal sinus may occur [1]. Granulomas [2] may present as such, or with an associated discharge, infection, bleeding or profuse sterile purulent exudate. The umbilicus is not infrequently involved in bullous and cicatricial pemphigoid; it may be the site of presentation of the latter (see Chapter 41).

Perforating pseudoxanthoma elasticum occurs in the umbilicus, and was the only site involved in six obese multiparous American black females [3]. It is only rarely associated with systemic problems [4,5].

Pregnancy, Addison's disease and other pigmentary disorders increase the pre-existing pigmentation. Acanthosis nigricans causes acanthotic and papillomatous lesions in the perineum. Periumbilical staining (Cullen's sign) occurs in acute pancreatitis, and occasionally in ruptured ectopic pregnancy or with duodenal ulcer perforation [6].

Umbilical haemorrhage has been described as a complication of cirrhosis following gross ulceration of the umbilical vein [7].

Infections

Infection of the umbilicus in the newborn used to carry a high mortality. It still occurs in some countries. A number of bacterial organisms may be responsible, but staphylococcal, *Pseudomonas* and clostridial species [8] are the most important. Minor forms consist of oozing, crusting and cellulitis, but a spreading oedematous erythema, progressing to necrotizing fasciitis, is of very serious import. Septicaemia and its complications may supervene [9]. At any time in later life, but usually after middle age, the umbilicus may be the seat of intertrigo or candidosis. This is more common in the obese or in those with poor personal hygiene. Genital and perianal warts can occasionally be associated with similar lesions within the umbilicus [10]. Foreign bodies, inserted by children or psychotics, may be overlooked as a cause of purulent infection in a deeply set umbilicus. The periumbilical skin is a common site of schistosomiasis when it affects the skin [11]. Disseminated strongyloidiasis has presented as periumbilical purpura [12].

Tumours and implantations

The umbilicus is a site of implantation of endometriomas [13], which may clinically resemble melanomas. A unique case of postoperative endosalpingosis has also been reported [14]. Colonic mucosa was implanted in an infant, after colostomy for Hirschsprung's disease [15]. A single case of carcinoid of the umbilicus has been noted [16]. Paget's disease has also been recorded [17,18]. Skin metastases from neoplasms of the digestive tract occurred in

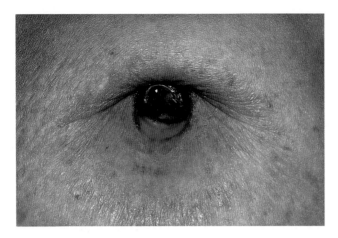

Fig. 68.46 'Sister Joseph's nodule'. (Courtesy of Dr J. Marks, Newcastle-upon-Tyne, UK.)

only 3% of 2187 cases [19], but the umbilicus is a characteristic site, especially for cancer of the stomach (Sister Joseph's nodule) (Fig. 68.46) [20], which was the primary source in 33 out of 40 cases [20]. The ovary, uterus and colon are responsible for most of the others [21–23], although the pancreas has also been a rare primary site [24]. A leiomyosarcoma of the small intestinal wall has presented in this way, as has a malignant peritoneal mesothelioma [25,26]. The lesions usually present as firm irregular nodules, but can occasionally infiltrate diffusely, or ulcerate and produce a fetid discharge. Such metastases were the presenting sign in 18 out of 40 cases, and were a major diagnostic feature in 28 cases [27]. The prognosis is always poor, but not entirely hopeless [28]. Histological identification of the site of the primary tumour may be difficult, and proved possible in only 21 of 85 cases [29,30]. Fine-needle aspiration of the nodule is not particularly helpful in reaching a diagnosis [30]. CT and surgical intervention are obligatory, because it may represent the earliest and only metastasis [23].

REFERENCES

1 Eby CS, Jetton RL. Umbilical pilonidal sinus. *Arch Dermatol* 1972; **106**: 893.

2 Laradle De Luna M, Gcioni V, Herrara A *et al.* Umbilical polyps. *Pediatr Dermatol* 1987; **4**: 341–3.

3 Hicks J, Carpenter CL, Reed RJ. Periumbilical perforating pseudoxanthoma elasticum. *Arch Dermatol* 1979; **115**: 300–3.

4 Goldstein BG, Lesher JL. Periumbilical pseudoxanthoma elasticum with systemic manifestations. *South Med J* 1991; **84**: 788–9.

5 Kim YH, Yoon JS, Lee JH *et al.* Periumbilical pseudoxanthoma elasticum. *Ann Dermatol* 1994; **6**: 49–51.

6 Evans DM. Cullen's sign in perforated duodenal ulcer. *BMJ* 1971; **i**: 154.

7 Douglas JG. Umbilical haemorrhage: an unusual complication of cirrhosis. *Postgrad Med J* 1981; **57**: 461–2.

8 Gormley D. Neonatal anaerobic (clostridial) cellulitis and omphalitis. *Arch Dermatol* 1977; **113**: 683–4.

9 Oranje AP, van Gysel D, van Praag MCG. Acquired neonatal infections. In: Harper J, Oranje A, Prose N, eds. *Textbook of Pediatric Dermatology*. Oxford: Blackwell Science, 2000: 73–7.

10 Nathan M. Umbilical warts: a new entity? *Genitourin Med* 1994; **70**: 49–50.

11 Colin M, Loubiere R, Guillaume A *et al.* Les lesions cutanées de bilharziose: a propos de 14 observations. *Ann Dermatol Vénéréol* 1980; **107**: 759–67.

12 Kalb R, Grossman ME. Periumbilical purpura in disseminated strongyloidiasis. *J Am Acad Dermatol* 1986; **256**: 1170–1.

13 Williams HE, Barsky S, Storino W. Umbilical endometrioma (silent type). *Arch Dermatol* 1976; **112**: 1435–6.

14 Dore N, Landry M, Cadotte M *et al.* Cutaneous endosalpingosis. *Arch Dermatol* 1980; **116**: 909–12.

15 Peachey RDG. Implantation of colonic mucosa in skin around colostomy. *Br J Dermatol* 1974; **90**: 108.

16 Brody HJ, Stallings WP, Fine RM *et al.* Carcinoid in an umbilical nodule. *Arch Dermatol* 1978; **114**: 570–2.

17 Ueki H, Kohda M. Multilokulärer extramammärer morbus Paget. *Hautarzt* 1979; **30**: 267–70.

18 Remond B, Aractingi S, Blanc F *et al.* Umbilical Paget's disease and prostatic carcinoma. *Br J Dermatol* 1993; **128**: 448–50.

19 Texier L, Geniaux M, Tamisier JM *et al.* Métastases cutanées des cancers digestifs. *Ann Dermatol Vénéréol* 1978; **105**: 913–9.

20 Samitz MH. Umbilical metastasis from carcinoma of the stomach. *Arch Dermatol* 1975; **111**: 1478–9.

21 Patel KS, Watkins RM. Recurrent endometrial adenocarcinoma presenting as an umbilical metastasis. *Br J Clin Pract* 1992; **46**: 69–70.

22 Brustman L, Seltzer V. Sister Joseph's nodule: seven cases of umbilical metastases from gynecologic malignancies. *Gynecol Oncol* 1984; **19**: 155–62.

23 Sharaki M, Abdel-Kader M. Umbilical deposits from internal malignancy (the Sister Joseph's nodule). *Clin Oncol* 1981; **7**: 351–5.

24 Shvili D, Halevy S, Sandbank M. Umbilical metastasis as the presenting sign of pancreatic adenocarcinoma. *Cutis* 1983; **31**: 555–8.

25 Powell FC, Cooper AJ, Massa MC *et al.* Leiomyosarcoma of the small intestine: metastatic to the umbilicus. *Arch Dermatol* 1984; **120**: 402–3.

26 Chen KTK. Malignant mesothelioma presenting as a Sister Joseph's nodule. *Am J Dermatopathol* 1991; **13**: 300–3.

27 Steck WD, Helwig EB. Tumors of the umbilicus. *Cancer* 1965; **18**: 907–15.

28 Chatterjee SN, Bauer HM. Umbilical metastasis from carcinoma of the pancreas. *Arch Dermatol* 1980; **116**: 954–5.

29 Powell FC, Cooper AJ, Massa MC *et al.* Sister Mary Joseph's nodule: a clinical and histologic study. *J Am Acad Dermatol* 1984; **10**: 610–5.

30 Schneider V, Smyczek B. Sister Mary Joseph's nodule. *Acta Cytol* 1990; **34**: 555–8.

Chapter 69

Racial Influences on Skin Disease

D.J. Gawkrodger

Definition and classification of race

The concept of race was first developed in the 18th century as an arbitrary classification to help understand evolution and human variation [1]. The division of our species *Homo sapiens* into 'races' is to some extent artificial, given that the species shows a continuous variability of characteristics and all humans are apparently derived from common ancestors (see Chapter 2). However, there are obviously differences between groups of humans that, in the present context, have an influence on the appearance and susceptibility to disease. The classification into racial groups therefore allows an examination of the genetic and environmental influences on human morphology and on disease.

Definitions

Many definitions are unsatisfactory. A race has been defined as 'a group united by heredity', or 'a major segment of a species' or 'a breeding population' [2]. It can also be regarded as 'one of the divisions of humankind as differentiated by physical characteristics' [1].

Scientifically, race is a matter of genetic variation. A definition that takes this into account is that of Boyd, who defined race as 'a population which differs significantly from other populations in regard to the frequency of one or more of the genes it possesses' [3]. Even this gives considerable latitude to defining quite a small subgroup as a 'race'.

Ethnicity

Another concept to consider is that of ethnicity. This is different from race, but equally difficult to define. Ethnicity can be regarded as a 'people or tribe' and implies shared origins or social background, shared cultural traditions that are maintained between generations and, often, a common language or religion [1,4,5]. One or more of these things leads to a sense of identity as a group.

Racial origins

Little is known about how the races originally differentiated and why they assumed their own characteristics. Conventional theory outlines that a change in gene frequency can occur due to mixture (with other races), mutation, natural selection and genetic drift (i.e. the accidental loss of a gene from the communal pool) [6]. It is assumed that some differences, such as skin pigmentation, are an adaptation to environmental conditions, although often it is still unclear as to exactly what advantage is conferred. Migrations of populations over the last few thousand years have meant that in certain places there has long been an admixture of genes. For example, many invaders who have swept over Europe in the last 2000 years, including Romans, Celts, Slavs and Moors, have left a genetic legacy behind them. In view of this, it is difficult to accept the concept of a 'pure' race. Isolated groups such as the Australian aborigines, who are thought to have migrated from the South Pacific Islands, may not have had much intermixture of genes from other races until recent times.

No racial group is characterized by a completely distinctive genetic make-up [7]. There is considerable genetic variation within racial groups and sharing of genetic characteristics between them.

Classification of races

In the past, classifications have relied on various physical characteristics such as stature, cephalic index, nasal index, prognathism, capacity of the skull, hair texture, hairiness, skin colour, hair and eye colour, and other special traits such as the epicanthic fold of the eyelid (a Mongoloid feature) or steatopygia (a heavy deposit of fat in the buttocks, seen in Bushmen and Hottentot women) [8]. A satisfactory classification must take most of these factors into account. There are three main divisions—namely, Mongoloid, black African and Caucasoid—which account for over 90% of the world's population [8]. The remaining groups, grouped together by Coon [9] as the Australoid and Capoid races, occupy a doubtful position, as they frequently show some features of the other races. These main races broadly show a geographical grouping. Within each 'geographical' race, it is possible to define 'local' races and so on. A convenient division of the geographical races, albeit with some reservations, is as follows [8–10]:

1 Australoid: Australian aborigines, Melanesians, Papuans and Negritos.
2 Capoid: Bushmen and Hottentots.
3 Caucasoids: Europeans, peoples of the Mediterranean, Middle East and most of the Indian subcontinent, and the Ainu of Japan.
4 Mongoloids: peoples of East Asia, Indonesia and Polynesia, native Americans and Eskimos.
5 Negroids: black people and pygmies of Africa.

REFERENCES

1 Senior PA, Bhopal R. Ethnicity as a variable in epidemiological research. *BMJ* 1994; **309**: 327–30.
2 Garn SM. *Human Races*. Springfield, IL: Thomas, 1961.
3 Boyd WC. *Genetics and the Races of Man*. Oxford: Blackwell, 1950.
4 Marmot MG. General approaches to migrant studies: the relation between disease, social class and ethnic origin. In: Cruickshank JK, Beevers DG, eds. *Ethnic Factors in Health and Disease*. London: Wright, 1989: 12–7.
5 Bhopal RS, Phillimore P, Kohli HS. Inappropriate use of the term 'Asian': an obstacle to ethnicity and health research. *J Public Health Med* 1991; **13**: 244–6.
6 Rife DC. Race and heredity. In: Kuttner RE, ed. *Race and Modern Science*. New York: Social Science Press, 1967: 141–68.
7 Cooper R. A note to the biological concept of race and its application in epidemiological research. *Am Heart J* 1984; **108**: 715–23.
8 Kroeber AL. *Anthropology: Biology and Race*. New York: Harcourt Brace and World, 1963.
9 Coon CS. *The Living Races of Man*. New York: Knopf, 1965.
10 Baker JR. *Race*. London: Oxford University Press, 1974.

Characteristics and variations between racial groups

There is a considerable overlap of features between the racial groups; for example, not all black Africans have tightly curled hair and not all Caucasoids have a lightly pigmented skin. Some characteristics may show considerable variation within a race—for example, head shape for Caucasoids is very variable, but other features are much more constant; for example, straight, black hair is almost universal in Mongoloids.

Australoids. Australian aborigines show some black African features such as black skin, a broad nose and prognathism, but their hirsutism, full beards and wavy hair are more Caucasoid. In addition, they have heavy eyebrow ridges [1–3].

Capoids. Bushmen and Hottentots show mainly black African characteristics, but some of their features are possibly Caucasoid (e.g. thin lips) or Mongoloid (e.g. a type of epicanthic fold) [1,4,5].

Caucasoids. There are at least four Caucasoid subraces extending from Europe, the Mediterranean and North Africa across to the Indian subcontinent. All show wavy hair and abundant facial and body hair. The skin colour is fair to brown and the nose is usually narrow. The Ainu of Japan are classified as Caucasoids, mainly because of their heavy body hair, curly scalp and beard hair and European-like facial features [1,4,5].

Mongoloids. This group extends through the extremes of climatic conditions, from the extreme north (Eskimos) to the equator (Malaysian types) and includes the Chinese and the native Americans in North and South America. Body hair is scanty and scalp hair is straight and black [2,3].

Negroids. Originally confined to Africa. The main characteristics are dark pigmentation, tightly curled hair and a broad nose [4,5].

Jews. Jews, on the whole, are not a race but a cultural community. They usually approximate genetically to the community in which they live [2,5]. However, certain genes are more frequent in certain Jewish communities than in the surrounding population.

The black people of North America are regarded by some as a local race [6]. A study of blood groups in American blacks has revealed the following admixture of Caucasoid genes: in Oakland (California) 22%, in Detroit 26%, in New York 19%, in Charleston 4% [3]. Some also may have native American genes [4]. Many of the studies on dermatology in 'Negroids' have been done on black Americans and hence may not be strictly applicable for all black Africans.

There is now a tendency in the USA and elsewhere for individuals with any degree of black African descent to adopt the term 'black'. This has come about because of a new consciousness by this group of a shared identity. In some places, the term 'black' has been more widely used and may be implied to include some darkly skinned Caucasoids, such as Mediterranean or Indian people [7]. Quite often, the description 'Afro-Caribbean' is used and, in North America, recently there has been a tendency to use 'African American'. The term 'black African' will therefore often be used to avoid any confusion about which group is being referred to. The terms Australoid, Mongoloid and Caucasoid will also be used to describe racial groups.

REFERENCES

1 Baker JR. *Race*. London: Oxford University Press, 1974.
2 Dunn LC. *Heredity and Evolution in Human Populations*. Cambridge, MA: Harvard University Press, 1959.
3 Reed TE. Caucasian genes in American negroes. *Science* 1969; **165**: 762–8.
4 Coon CS. *The Living Races of Man*. New York: Knopf, 1965.
5 Kroeber AL. *Anthropology: Biology and Race*. New York: Harcourt Brace and World, 1963.
6 Cobb WM. Physical anthropology of the American Negro. *Am J Phys Anthropol* 1942; **29**: 113–223.
7 Banton M. *The Idea of Race*. Cambridge: Tavistock, 1977.

Ethnic groups

Some groups of humans do not fit easily into a race, for example pygmies, but ethnicity creates a new category for each group [1,2]. Ethnicity is a social phenomenon with imprecise and fluid boundaries. It is often used, incorrectly, as interchangeable with 'race' [3]. Broad ethnic divisions, for instance into Asian or Afro-Caribbean, may have limited value due to the great diversity of cultural and other variations within the groups. Nonetheless, because of the association with social and cultural factors, ethnicity often has a bearing on disease.

A current recommendation is that, in describing disease or characteristics in a racial or ethnic group, the most precise description possible is given for that group [4]. This will be followed when appropriate, but where it seems desirable to look at racial characteristics more generally, the broad racial groupings will be applied.

REFERENCES

1 Cooper R. A note on the biological concept of race and its application in epidemiological research. *Am Heart J* 1984; **108**: 715–23.
2 Senior PA, Bhopal R. Ethnicity as a variable in epidemiological research. *BMJ* 1994; **309**: 327–30.
3 Sheldon TA, Parker H. Race and ethnicity in health research. *J Public Health Med* 1992; **14**: 104–10.
4 McKenzie K, Crowcroft NS. Describing race, ethnicity, and culture in medical research. *BMJ* 1996; **312**: 1054.

Racial variations in the structure and function of the skin

The degree of pigmentation is one of the most obvious and immediate factors in distinguishing the main geographical races. Other differences in the structure and function of the skin are less obvious and not so well studied, but are of some importance [1].

REFERENCE

1 Taylor SC. Skin of color: biology, structure, function, and implications for dermatologic disease. *J Am Acad Dermatol* 2002; **46**: S41–S62.

Pigmentation

Variation

Skin colour depends largely on the content and distribution of melanin in the epidermis. In Caucasoids, the constitutive skin colour (i.e. the amount of melanin pigmentation in the absence of sun exposure) is darkest on the upper thigh and lightest on the lumbar area, whereas in black Africans the abdomen is darkest, although the lumbar area is also the lightest [1]. Males are normally darker than females. In general, the geographical distribution of the intensity of racial pigmentation correlates with the areas of greatest sun exposure, although there are anomalies such as the Tasmanian Australoids, who were dark although they lived in a temperate latitude, and native Americans (Mongoloids), who have a similar pigmentation across the whole continent of North America.

Melanosomes

The density of melanocytes differs between various parts of the body [2] and is similar in most races, although melanocytes may be more numerous in the Australian aborigine [3]. There are differences in the size, distribution and shape of melanosomes. In Caucasoids, the melanosomes are small and aggregated in groups of three or more within a membrane in the keratinocyte [4] and are broken up by lysosomal enzymes before reaching the stratum corneum [5]. In black Africans and Australoids, the melanosomes are larger, distributed singly within keratinocytes, and persist up to the stratum corneum.

Inheritance

Skin colour is continuously variable and its inheritance is

complex. Over the last few years, mutations have been found in redheaded people, in the melanocortin 1 receptor (MCR1), for which the ligand is α-melanocyte-stimulating hormone, that lead to a shift from eumelanin to phaeomelanin production [6]. Between races, there is allelic diversity at the MCR1 and this is greater in pale non-African populations [7]. The exact interpretation of this is still to be resolved.

Physiological effects of skin pigmentation

The minimal erythema dose in black African skin is about 33 times that for Caucasoid [4]. Obviously, a pigmented skin protects against sunlight and particularly against sunburn and skin cancer. However, it seems doubtful that protection against skin cancer conveys an evolutionary advantage, as under 'natural' conditions survival is unlikely to be affected. According to Wasserman [8,9], racial pigmentation is a secondary phenomenon, related to resistance to infection. The disadvantages of a pigmented skin are increased heat absorption and reduced vitamin D synthesis. Black Africans absorb 30% more heat than Caucasoids, although this is partially offset by more efficient sweating [10,11]. Ultraviolet B radiation at low dose enhances natural killer cell activity in black individuals but not in white subjects, suggesting increased immunological resistance to disorders such as photoinduced skin cancer [12].

REFERENCES

1 Selmanowitz VJ, Krivo JM. Pigmentary demarcation lines. *Br J Dermatol* 1975; **93**: 371–7.
2 Szabo G. Quantitative histological investigations on the melanocyte system of the human epidermis. In: Gordon M, ed. *Pigment Cell Biology*. New York: Academic Press, 1959: 99–125.
3 Mitchell RE. The skin of the Australian aborigine: a light and electron-microscopical study. *Aust J Dermatol* 1968; **9**: 314–28.
4 Olson RL, Gaylor J, Everett MA. Skin color, melanin and erythema. *Arch Dermatol* 1973; **108**: 541–4.
5 Hori Y, Toda K, Pathak MA. A fine structure study of the human epidermal melanosome complex and its acid phosphate activity. *J Ultrastruct Res* 1968; **25**: 109–20.
6 Valverde P, Healy E, Jackson I *et al*. Variations of the melanocyte-stimulating hormone receptor gene are associated with red hair and fair skin in humans. *Nature Genet* 1995; **11**: 328–30.
7 Harding RM, Healy E, Ray AJ *et al*. Evidence for variable selection at the human pigmentation locus MCR1. *Am J Hum Genet* 2000; **66**: 1351–61.
8 Wasserman HP. Melanokinetics and the biological significance of melanin. *Br J Dermatol* 1970; **82**: 530–4.
9 Wasserman HP. *Ethnic Pigmentation*. Amsterdam: Excerpta Medica, 1974.
10 Blum HF. Physiological effects of sunlight on man. *Physiol Rev* 1945; **25**: 483–530.
11 Blum HF. Does the melanin pigment of human skin have adaptive value? *Q Rev Biol* 1961; **36**: 50–63.
12 Matsuoka LY, McConnachie P, Wortsman J, Holick MF. Immunological responses to ultraviolet light B radiation in Black individuals. *Life Sci* 1999; **64**: 1563–9.

Hair

Variations in hair depend on a wide range of genetically controlled factors, both between and within races [1]. Hair form is inherited separately from skin colour, and of the two is the more dominant.

Hair forms

Hair form depends on the three-dimensional structure of the hair shaft. There are broadly four hair types—straight, wavy, helical and spiral [2,3]. The helical forms coil with a constant diameter. Spiral forms coil with a decreasing diameter outwards; the extreme of this is 'peppercorn' hair, which is tightly curled and shows multiple kinks [4]. Hair that is elliptical in cross-section is curly, whereas round hair is straight.

Mongoloid hair is usually straight, circular in diameter, and with the largest diameter of all the races. The hair in black Africans and Capoids tends to be short, helical or spiral, flattened or elliptical in cross-section, and midway between the Mongoloid and Caucasoid in thickness. Spiral hair is produced by hair follicles that are curved and upwardly convex towards the epidermis. Black African hair tends to be drier and more brittle than the hair of other races, probably due in part to its intrinsic properties [5]. Hair density in black Africans is less than in Caucasoids (mean ± SD 190 ± 40; 227 ± 55 hairs/cm^2) and hair growth is slower (256 ± 44; 396 ± 55 μm/day) [6]. Telogen counts are higher in black Africans than in Caucasoids, although this contrasts with the lesser degree and later onset of androgenetic hair loss observed [6].

In Caucasoids, the hair is variable and may be straight, wavy, or helical and round or oval in cross-section. It tends to be the thinnest in diameter of all the races. Despite these variations for scalp hair, beard, pubic and eyelash hair is elliptical in all races. The morphology and chemical composition of hair is similar in all races [7].

Hair colour

Mongoloids, black Africans, Capoids and Australoids have hair that is predominantly black, although it may be red in colour. Caucasoid hair is widely variable: in northern Europe it tends to be blond, in southern and eastern Europe it is commonly black [8]. However, blond hair may be found in North Africa and the Middle East, and is even seen in some Australoids. Greying of the hair starts on average in the third decade in Caucasoids, and in the fourth decade in black Africans. Caucasoids show more balding over the vertex than do black Africans [9].

Body hair

Caucasoids have earlier and greater axillary and beard growth than Mongoloids [10] and more extensive male secondary sexual hair. In general, Mongoloids have less body hair than Caucasoids, with black Africans and Capoids occupying an intermediate position.

Selective advantage of hair forms

Any evolutionary advantage conferred by the different hair forms is unclear. Short, curly hair facilitates evaporation of sweat, but thick wavy hair provides a greater degree of physical protection. Hair, especially on the scalp, protects against ultraviolet radiation.

REFERENCES

1 Baden HP. Chemistry, structure and function of hair. In: Baden HP, ed. *Symposium on Alopecia*. New York: HP Publishing, 1987: 3–10.
2 Steggerda M, Seibert HC. Size and shape of head hairs from 6 racial groups. *J Hered* 1942; **32**: 315–8.
3 Vernall DG. Study of the size and shape of hair from 4 races of man. *Am J Phys Anthropol* 1961; **19**: 345–50.
4 Hrdy D. Quantitative hair form variation in 7 populations. *Am J Phys Anthropol* 1973; **39**: 7–17.
5 Halder RM. Hair and scalp disorders in blacks. *Cutis* 1983; **32**: 378–80.
6 Loussouarn G. African hair growth parameters. *Br J Dermatol* 2001; **145**: 294–7.
7 Hrdy D, Baden HP. Biochemical variations of hair keratins in man and non-human primates. *Am J Phys Anthropol* 1973; **39**: 19–24.
8 Sunderland E. Hair colour variation in the United Kingdom. *Ann Hum Genet* 1955; **20**: 312–3.
9 Setty LR. Hair patterns of the scalp in white and negro males. *Am J Phys Anthropol* 1970; **33**: 49–55.
10 Hamilton JB. Age, sex and genetic factors in the regulation of hair growth in man: a comparison of Caucasian and Japanese populations. In: Montagna W, Ellis RA, eds. *The Biology of Hair Growth*. New York: Academic Press, 1958: 399–433.

Sweat glands

Eccrine glands

There is little or no difference in the sweating ability of black Africans in comparison with Caucasoids [1]. A study in the Bantu did show a greater number of sweat glands per unit area than in European Caucasoids [2], but such changes are now thought to be due to adaptation to climatic factors [3]. Increased sweating is known to be accompanied by hypertrophy of the sweat glands [4]. Indeed, in Australoids, sweat glands were noted to be larger but not more numerous than in Caucasoids [1].

Keratosis punctata, a hyperkeratosis of the acrosyringeal orifice seen on the palmar creases, is found in 1–2% of black Africans and in less than 0.1% of Latin Americans, but it is not seen in European or Middle Eastern Caucasoids [5].

Apocrine glands

An early paper mentions that apocrine glands are more numerous in black African skin than in Caucasoid skin [6], but the variation in the distribution of apocrine glands between individuals is so great [7] that it is difficult to place much emphasis on this report.

REFERENCES

1 Green LMA. The distribution of eccrine sweat glands of Australian aborigines. *Aust J Dermatol* 1971; **12**: 143–8.
2 Glaser S. Sweat glands in Negro and European. *Am J Phys Anthropol* 1934; **18**: 371–6.
3 Kawahata A, Sakamoto H. Some observations on sweating of the Aino. *Jpn J Physiol* 1951; **2**: 166–9.
4 Warter G, Diolombi G. Sweat gland tumours in Niger. *Ann Dermatol Vénéréol* 1989; **116**: 621–7.
5 Pierard-Franchimont C, Pierard GE, Melotte P et al. Keratosis punctata of the palmar creases. *Ann Soc Belg Med Trop* 1989; **69**: 257–61.
6 Homma H. On apocrine sweat glands in white and negro men and women. *Bull Johns Hopkins Hosp* 1926; **38**: 365–71.
7 Woollard HH. The cutaneous glands of man. *J Anat* 1930; **64**: 415–21.

Sebaceous glands

Black African skin showed no consistent difference in sebaceous gland activity as compared with Caucasoid skin [1]. There have been no substantial studies on the comparative number of sebaceous glands in the different races.

REFERENCE

1 Pochi PE, Strauss JS. Sebaceous gland activity in black skin. *Dermatol Clin* 1988; **6**: 349–51.

The epidermis

Comparative studies have been performed on black African and Caucasoid epidermis. The stratum corneum in both has an equal thickness, although in black skin there are more cell layers and it requires more tape strips to remove it than Caucasoid stratum corneum [1]. The stratum corneum in black subjects seems to show greater intracellular cohesion than in Caucasoids. It has a higher lipid content [2] and an increased electrical resistance [3]. There is no difference in corneocyte surface area between Caucasoids, Mongoloids and black Africans, but desquamation was up to 2.5 times greater from black skin, compared with the other two races [4]. Recently, it has been found that quantities of cerumides in the stratum corneum are lower in black Africans than in Caucasoids [5]. The composition of ear wax (cerumen) varies between different races: in black Africans and Caucasoids, it is honey-coloured, wet and sticky; in Mongoloids, it is grey, dry and brittle [6].

Not surprisingly, black African epidermis is more effective at blocking the transmission of ultraviolet radiation, transmitting only 7.4% of UVB as compared to 29.4% for Caucasoid epidermis [7]. Black African skin shows a higher transepidermal water loss than Caucasoid [8]; this is thought to be due to differences in thermoregulation and in the stratum corneum lipids. Some substances do not penetrate black skin as well as Caucasoid, but this is not universally the case [9].

REFERENCES

1 Weigand DA, Haygood C, Gaylor JR. Cell layers and density of Negro and Caucasian stratum corneum. *J Invest Dermatol* 1974; **62**: 563–8.
2 Rienertson RP, Wheatley VR. Studies on the chemical composition of human epidermal lipids. *J Invest Dermatol* 1959; **32**: 49–59.
3 Johnson LC, Corah NL. Racial differences in skin resistance. *Science* 1963; **139**: 766–7.
4 Corcuff P, Lotte C, Rougier A, Maibach HI. Racial differences in corneocytes. *Acta Derm Venereol (Stockh)* 1991; **71**: 146–8.
5 Sugino K, Imokawa G, Maibach HI. Ethnic difference of stratum corneum lipid in relation to stratum corneum function. *J Invest Dermatol* 1993; **100**: 597–9.
6 Hanger HC, Mulley GP. Cerumen: its fascination and clinical importance. *J R Soc Med* 1992; **85**: 346–9.
7 Kaidbey KH, Agin PP, Sayre RM *et al.* Photoprotection by melanin: a comparison of black and caucasian skin. *J Am Acad Dermatol* 1979; **1**: 249–60.
8 Wilson D, Berardesca E, Maibach HI. *In vitro* transepidermal water loss: differences between black and white human skin. *Br J Dermatol* 1988; **119**: 647–52.
9 Wedig JH, Maibach HI. Percutaneous penetration of dipyrithione in man: effect of skin color (race). *J Am Acad Dermatol* 1981; **5**: 433–8.

The dermis

Black African skin may be slightly more extensible than Caucasoid [1], although the difference is small. The vasodilatory response after exposure to nicotinate is reduced in black Africans compared with Caucasoids, and hyperaemia after vasoconstrictive stimuli may be different [1,2].

REFERENCES

1 Berardesca E. Racial differences in skin function. *Acta Derm Venereol (Stockh)* 1994; **185** (Suppl.): 44–6.
2 Berardesca E, de Rigal J, Leveque JL, Maibach HI. *In vivo* biophysical characterization of skin physiological differences in races. *Dermatologica* 1991; **182**: 89–93.

Peripheral vascular responses to cold

Eskimos (Mongoloids) are able to maintain a higher hand blood flow than Caucasoids under identically cold conditions [1]. At −12°C, the finger temperature in black Africans fell more rapidly (and the metabolic rate rose less rapidly) than in Caucasoids under similar conditions [2]. The extent to which these observations represent physiological adaptations, rather than significant interracial differences, is not known.

REFERENCES

1 Brown GM, Page J. Effect of chronic exposure to cold on temperature and blood flow of hand. *J Appl Physiol* 1952; **5**: 221–7.
2 Rennie DW, Adams T. Comparative thermoregulatory responses of negroes and white persons to acute cold stress. *J Appl Physiol* 1957; **11**: 201–4.

Common diseases that show racially dependent variations

Many dermatoses manifest themselves similarly in the different races, but not infrequently—due to differences in pigmentation, hair or other factors—the appearance of a disorder varies depending on the racial constitution of the individual. It is not intended here to provide a comprehensive list of every possible racially influenced dermatosis, but rather to select the most important differences, especially for the commonest conditions.

Dermatoses that in white Caucasoid skin appear red or brown appear black, grey or purple in pigmented skin. Furthermore, any pigmentation may mask an erythematous reaction. Inflammation in pigmented skin may provoke reactions of a hyperpigmentary or hypopigmentary nature that persist after the initiating eruption has faded [1]. These pigmentary reactions may be of greater concern to the patient than the eruption itself and are often the reason why medical help is sought. Pigmented skin may have an inherent tendency to show reaction patterns that are different from those seen in white Caucasoid skin. For example, follicular, papular and annular patterns are seen more frequently in Afro-Caribbean skin than in Caucasoid [1].

There are few data on the frequency with which people of different races attend a dermatologist. In an office-based study in the USA, patients classified as 'white' or 'Asian or Pacific Islander' attended a dermatologist proportionally more than 'black' people or 'native Americans or Eskimos', but this may well have been because of economic or social reasons [2].

Some general texts give a useful overview of this topic [3,4].

REFERENCES

1 McLaurin CI. Unusual patterns of common dermatoses in blacks. *Cutis* 1983; **32**: 352–60.
2 Fletcher AB, Feldman SR, Bradham DD. Office-based physician services provided by dermatologists in the United States in 1990. *J Invest Dermatol* 1994; **102**: 93–7.
3 Johnson BL, Moy RL, White GM. *Ethnic Skin: Medical and Surgical.* St Louis: Mosby, 1998.
4 Archer CB, Robertson SJ. *Black and White Skin: an Atlas and Text.* Oxford: Blackwell Scientific Publications, 1995.

Acne

The prevalence of acne seems to be similar in both North American black Africans and Caucasoids [1], although it may be more severe in the latter [2]. However, acne is less common in the Mongoloid Japanese [3]. In pigmented skin, acne lesions may become hyperpigmented (Fig. 69.1).

'Pomade' acne is seen in certain Afro-Caribbean groups, due to the custom of anointing the scalp hair with pomades, oils and creams. Up to 70% of long-term users of pomades suffer from this complication [4]. It may be seen in children as well as adults. There is some evidence that black Africans react to comedogenic substances in a different way from Caucasoids. Kaidbey and Kligman studied the comedogenic effects of coal tar in Caucasoids and

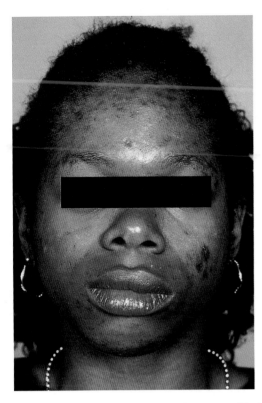

Fig. 69.1 Pigmentation associated with acne. (Courtesy of Dr A.G. Messenger, Royal Hallamshire Hospital, Sheffield, UK.)

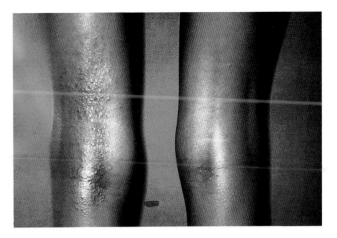

Fig. 69.2 Hyperpigmentation associated with atopic eczema.

black Africans and found that whereas Caucasoids produced an inflammatory response with papules and pustules, black Africans did not usually show this but rather developed small comedones [5].

REFERENCES

1 Pochi PE, Strauss JS. Sebaceous gland activity in black skin. *Dermatol Clin* 1988; **6**: 349–51.
2 Wilkins JW Jr, Voorhees JJ. Prevalence of nodulocystic acne in white and negro males. *Arch Dermatol* 1970; **102**: 631–4.
3 Hamilton JB, Terada H, Mestler GE. Greater tendency to acne in white Americans than Japanese populations. *J Clin Endocrinol* 1964; **24**: 267–72.
4 Verhagen AR. Pomade acne in black skin. *Arch Dermatol* 1974; **110**: 465.
5 Kaidbey KH, Kligman AM. A human model of coal tar acne. *Arch Dermatol* 1974; **109**: 212–5.

Atopic eczema

The inheritance of atopic eczema is 'polygenic'. It is a disease that is seen worldwide and in all races. Comparative figures are not generally available. There was an impression in the UK that atopic eczema may be more common in Caucasoids from the Indian subcontinent [1], but a subsequent cohort study has not confirmed this [2]. It may be that over-representation of Asian children with atopic eczema in dermatology clinics results from a lower level of familiarity with the disease in this community. In another study, from London, UK, it was suggested that

atopic eczema is more prevalent in 'black Caribbean' children than in other ethnic groups, including Asians [3]. In India, it is suggested that atopic eczema is not as severe as in Western countries [4].

In black Africans, there is a tendency towards the development of follicular lesions in atopic eczema, and a micropapular follicular form of lichenification resembling lichen nitidus is common [1,5,6]. The follicular eruption may predate the onset of other features of the disease [5,6]. Flexural involvement may be less common than in other races, but the severity of the eczema seems to be no different [3].

Lichenification is seen in all races, but is particularly pronounced in Mongoloids. Postinflammatory hyperpigmentation is a problem in black skin (Fig. 69.2).

REFERENCES

1 Graham-Brown RAC, Berth-Jones J, Dure-Smith B *et al*. Dermatologic problems for immigrant communities in a Western environment. *Int J Dermatol* 1990; **29**: 94–101.
2 Berth-Jones J, George S, Graham-Brown RAC. A birth cohort study on prevalence of atopic dermatitis. *Br J Dermatol* 1994; **131** (Suppl. 44): 24–5.
3 Williams HC, Pembroke AC, Fordyke H *et al*. London-born black Caribbean children are at increased risk of atopic dermatitis. *J Am Acad Dermatol* 1995; **32**: 212–7.
4 Kanwar AJ, Dhar S. Severity of atopic dermatitis in India. *Br J Dermatol* 1994; **131**: 733–4.
5 McLaurin CI. Unusual patterns of common dermatoses in blacks. *Cutis* 1983; **32**: 352–60.
6 Rosen T, Martin S. *Atlas of Black Dermatology*. Boston: Little, Brown, 1981.

Contact dermatitis

Studies using irritants suggest that black African skin is less susceptible to irritants than Caucasoid skin [1], although the difference is not detectable when the stratum corneum has been removed. A comparison of the susceptibility of the skin of Japanese and Caucasoid women revealed that for acute and—to a lesser extent—cumulative irritant exposures, Japanese skin was more easily irritated than was Caucasoid [2].

There is little evidence that there is any racial predisposition for the development of allergic contact dermatitis. A comparative study of Caucasoids and African Americans found similar rates of sensitization to common allergens, the only differences being higher frequency of contact allergy to *para*-phenylenediamine (PPD, e.g. in hair dye) and imidazolidinyl urea (a preservative) in African Americans [3]. The differences are probably due to increased use of hair dyes and hair-care products in African Americans, although racial differences in N-acetylation in the skin may also explain the PPD finding [3]. Others have confirmed few differences between races in contact sensitization [4]. A study from Singapore of contact allergy to topical medicaments showed no differences between Chinese, Malays and Indians [5]. Overall rates for a 'sensitive skin', as judged by telephone interview, did not differ between Afro-American, Asian, Euro-American or Hispanic women, but Afro-Americans had less reactivity to environmental factors, Asians complained more of itch and reacted more to temperature and wind, Euro-Americans had less reactivity to cosmetics but reacted more to wind, whilst Hispanics had lower skin reactivity to alcohol [6].

However, certain patterns of contact dermatitis are recognized in specific groups due to the use of traditional or ethnic preparations. Indian women may develop an allergic contact dermatitis to materials in 'Bindi', a pigment applied as a paste or powder to the central forehead for religious and social reasons [7].

Some reported differences in the prevalence of contact allergy to certain allergens are likely to represent a difference in exposure. The equal sex incidence of nickel allergy in Nigeria [8], distinct from the female preponderance in most Western countries [9], is probably due to the equal popularity of the wearing of jewellery by both men and women in Nigeria. Clinically, contact dermatitis appears different in black skin as compared with Caucasoid. In the latter, acute contact dermatitis produces vesiculation and exudation, whereas in black skin, lichenification and disordered pigmentation are more common. Hyperpigmentation occurs after contact with mild irritants [10], and certain chemicals—for example, phenolic detergents [11]—cause hypopigmentation.

REFERENCES

1 Weigand DA, Gaylor JR. Irritant reaction in negro and caucasian skin. *South Med J* 1974; **67**: 548–51.
2 Foy V, Weinkauf R, Whittle E, Basketter DA. Ethnic variation in the skin irritation response. *Contact Dermatitis* 2001; **45**: 346–9.
3 Dickel H, Taylor JS, Evey P, Merk HF. Comparison of patch test results with a standard series among white and black racial groups. *Am J Contact Dermatitis* 2001; **12**: 77–82.
4 Kligman AM, Epstein W. Updating the maximization test for identifying contact allergens. *Contact Dermatitis* 1975; **1**: 231–9.
5 Goh CL. Contact sensitivity to topical medicaments. *Int J Dermatol* 1989; **28**: 25–8.

6 Jourdain R, de Lacharriere O, Bastien P, Maibach HI. Ethnic variations in self-perceived sensitive skin: epidemiological survey. *Contact Dermatitis* 2002; **46**: 162–9.
7 Kumar AS, Pandhi RK, Bhutani LK. Bindi dermatoses. *Int J Dermatol* 1986; **25**: 434–5.
8 Olumide YM. Contact dermatitis in Nigeria. *Contact Dermatitis* 1975; **12**: 241–6.
9 Gawkrodger DJ, Vestey JP, Wong WK, Buxton PK. Contact clinic survey of nickel-sensitive subjects. *Contact Dermatitis* 1986; **14**: 165–9.
10 Berardesca E, Maibach HI. Contact dermatitis in blacks. *Dermatol Clin* 1988; **6**: 363–8.
11 Fisher AA. Vitiligo due to contactants. *Cutis* 1976; **17**: 431–7.

Kaposi's sarcoma

The appearance of the lesions of acquired immune deficiency syndrome (AIDS)-related Kaposi's sarcoma can show variation between the different races. In black Africans, lesions may vary from being slightly hyperpigmented to being a deep purple in colour [1]. The classical form of Kaposi's sarcoma is commonest in mid-European Caucasoids of Jewish lineage, and occurs 10 times more frequently in males than in females [2]. Another, more rapidly progressive form, affects black Africans in central Africa [3].

REFERENCES

1 Penneys NS. AIDS in black patients. *Dermatol Clin* 1988; **6**: 435–42.
2 Friedman-Birnbaum R, Weltfriend S, Katz I. Kaposi's sarcoma: retrospective study of 67 cases with the classical form. *Dermatologica* 1990; **180**: 13–7.
3 Oluwasanmi JO, Williams AO, Alli AF. Superficial cancer in Nigeria. *Br J Cancer* 1969; **23**: 714–28.

Keloid formation

Keloids occur in all races, but are more common in black Africans and Mongoloids than in Caucasoids. The exact incidence ratio for black Africans over Caucasoids varies from twice to 19 times, according to the study consulted [1]. In Malaysia, Chinese are more prone to keloids than Indians or Malays [2]. In Hawaii, keloids are five times more common in the Japanese, and three times more frequent in the Chinese, than in Caucasoids [3]. Keloids can occur anywhere on the body, but have a predilection for the shoulders, ears, upper back and anterior chest (Fig. 69.3). They usually follow trauma to the skin, but can arise spontaneously. In black Africans, they may develop in areas of scarification. Treatment options have been reviewed in detail recently [4].

REFERENCES

1 Kelly AP. Keloids. *Dermatol Clin* 1988; **6**: 413–24.
2 Alhady SM, Sivanantharajah K. Keloids in various races: a review of 175 cases. *Plast Reconstr Surg* 1969; **44**: 564–6.
3 Arnold HL Jr, Grauer FH. Keloids: etiology and management by excision and intensive prophylactic radiation. *Arch Dermatol* 1959; **80**: 772–7.
4 Shaffer JJ, Taylor SC, Cook-Bolden F. Keloidal scars: a review with a critical look at therapeutic options. *J Am Acad Dermatol* 2002; **46**: S63–S97.

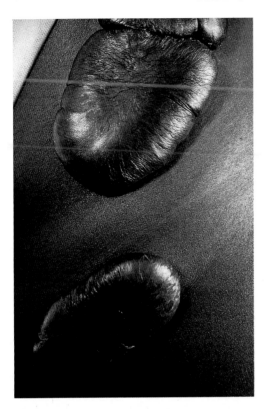

Fig. 69.3 Huge spontaneous keloids in an African. (Courtesy of Professor J.L. Burton, Bristol Royal Infirmary, Bristol, UK.)

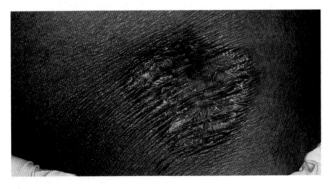

Fig. 69.4 Hyperpigmented lichen planus.

Lichen planus

Lichen planus is a worldwide problem and occurs in all races. In Singapore, lichen planus was proportionally more common in Indians and less common in Chinese and Malays than would be expected, given the composition of the local population [1]. There are no other studies to suggest a racial predisposition, although the appearances may differ between races. In darkly pigmented patients, papules of lichen planus typically are purple in colour (Fig. 69.4). Oral lesions are said to be uncommon in black Africans but frequent in Caucasoids, while the hypertrophic variant, and possibly the erosive type, are more often seen in black Africans [2]. In black Africans,

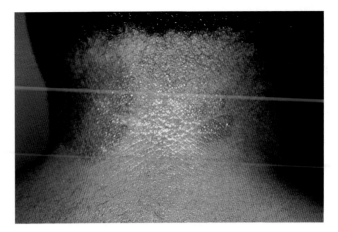

Fig. 69.5 Hyperpigmented lichen simplex chronicus.

postinflammatory hyperpigmentation may be prolonged [3]. In Asian Caucasoids, itching is often not prominent and hyperpigmentation is a more common presentation [4]. Histologically, Asian Caucasoids show less inflammation and basal cell degeneration than black Africans or European Caucasoids [4].

REFERENCES

1 Vijayasingham SM, Lim KB, Yeoh KH *et al.* Lichen planus: a study of 72 cases in Singapore. *Ann Acad Med Singapore* 1988; **17**: 541–4.
2 Rosen T, Martin S. *Atlas of Black Dermatology.* Boston: Little, Brown, 1981.
3 McLaurin CI. Unusual patterns of common dermatoses in blacks. *Cutis* 1983; **32**: 352–60.
4 Fallowfield ME, Harwood C, Cook MG, Marsden RA. Lichen planus in Asians? *Br J Dermatol* 1993; **129** (Suppl. 42): 59.

Lichen simplex chronicus

Lichenification is particularly readily induced in Mongoloid and black African skin (Fig. 69.5). Lichen simplex chronicus may affect the neck, forearms and lower legs, and be associated with hyperpigmentation [1]. A common variant is lichen simplex chronicus of the scrotum in elderly black African males.

REFERENCE

1 Rosen T, Martin S. *Atlas of Black Dermatology.* Boston: Little, Brown, 1981.

Lupus erythematosus

It used to be said that lupus erythematosus was uncommon in black Africans, but this is no longer believed to be the case. Indeed, the black populations of North America and North Africa seem to develop severe forms of the disease [1]. In New Zealand, systemic lupus erythematosus was found to be three times as common in Mongoloids as in Caucasoids [2].

Lupus erythematosus is closely associated with certain genetic and human leukocyte antigen (HLA) markers. North American and European Caucasoids with systemic lupus erythematosus show an increased frequency of a C4A, CYP21A gene deletion, often in association with the HLA-B8, -DR3, C4A*Q0 extended haplotype [3]. In African Americans, a large C4A, CYP21A gene deletion, particularly associated with HLA-B44, -DR2 and -DR3 alleles, is a strong genetic risk factor for the development of systemic lupus erythematosus [3]. Complete or partial deficiency of C4A allele has also been identified as a genetic determinant of systemic lupus erythematosus in Chinese and Japanese Mongoloids [4]. West Indian, and to a lesser extent North African, black people have a more severe form of systemic lupus erythematosus than European Caucasoids, mainly due to a higher prevalence of renal disease [1]. The mortality from systemic lupus erythematosus in African Americans is higher than in Caucasoids [5]. Discoid lupus erythematosus also seems to have a nearly similar incidence in all races. In those with a dark skin, the face, scalp and—commonly—the lower lip tend to be affected. Hypopigmentation and gross scarring may result.

Although the difference in prevalence of lupus erythematosus and other autoimmune diseases in Africans in West Africa compared with American Africans may be due to genetic admixture, exposure to malaria has also been proposed as being important [6–9]. Whilst on the one hand scanty congenital *Plasmodium* parasites have been proposed as a cause of autoimmune disease [8], several studies have suggested that malaria may induce a form of tolerance against autoimmune disease; altered macrophage function, tumour necrosis factor levels and nitric oxide production have been suggested to be protective. Antinuclear antibodies and antiphospholipid antibodies occurring in patients with malaria have different specificities compared with those in autoimmune disease [7]. Experimentally, serum from mice infected with *Plasmodium chabaudi* slows development of autoimmune disease when injected into a strain of lupus-prone mice [9].

REFERENCES

1 Gioud-Paquet M, Chamot AM, Bourgeois P *et al.* Différences symptomatiques et pronostiques selon la communauté ethnique dans le lupus érythémateux systémique. Etude contrôlée sur 3 populations. *Presse Méd* 1988; **17**: 103–6.
2 Hart HH, Grigor RR, Caughey DE. Ethnic differences in the prevalence of systemic lupus erythematosus. *Ann Rheum Dis* 1983; **42**: 529–32.
3 Olsen ML, Goldstein R, Arnett FC *et al.* C4A gene deletion and HLA associations in black Americans with systemic lupus erythematosus. *Immunogenetics* 1989; **30**: 27–33.
4 Dunkley H, Gatenby PA, Hawkins B *et al.* Deficiency of C4A is a genetic determinant of systemic lupus erythematosus in three ethnic groups. *J Immunogenet* 1987; **14**: 209–18.
5 Reveille JD, Bartolucci A, Alarcon GS. Prognosis in systemic lupus erythematosus: negative impact of increasing age at onset, black race, and

thrombocytopenia, as well as causes of death. *Arthritis Rheum* 1990; **33**: 37–48.
6 Symmons DP. Frequency of lupus in people of African origin. *Lupus* 1995; **4**: 176–8.
7 Daniel-Ribeiro CT, Zanini G. Autoimmunity and malaria: what are they doing together? *Acta Tropica* 2000; **76**: 205–21.
8 Yaffe I. Scanty congenital *Plasmodium* parasites as a possible cause for several autoimmune diseases. *Med Hypotheses* 2001; **56**: 335–8.
9 Hentati B, Sato MN, Payelle-Brogard B, Avrameas S, Ternynck T. Beneficial effect of polyclonal immunoglobulins from malaria-infected BALB/c mice on the lupus-like syndrome of (NZBxNZW) F1 mice. *Eur J Immunol* 1994; **24**: 8–15.

Melanocytic naevi

Caucasoids have more melanocytic naevi than other races. Black Africans have the fewest naevi, with Mongoloids occupying an intermediate position [1]. Caucasoid children had a median total number of 17 naevi, compared with 2.5 in non-Caucasoids [1]. Young Caucasoid adults had a median of 61 naevi, compared with 16 for non-Caucasoids [1]. A study of schoolchildren in Queensland, Australia, confirmed these findings, but found an even higher prevalence of naevi [2]. Children less than 12 years old had a mean of 28 naevi, with boys having significantly more than girls, and those with a pale skin and light-coloured hair having the highest prevalence [2]. Non-Caucasoid heritage has a protective effect for naevus development, independent of pigmentary characteristics [2].

REFERENCES

1 Rampen FH, de Wit PE. Racial differences in mole proneness. *Acta Derm Venereol (Stockh)* 1989; **69**: 234–6.
2 Green A, Siskind V, Hansen ME *et al.* Melanocytic nevi in school-children in Queensland. *J Am Acad Dermatol* 1989; **20**: 1054–60.

Palmoplantar keratodermas (Chapter 34)

Some palmoplantar keratodermas are said to be seen more often in black Africans than in other races [1]. One example is keratosis punctata of the palmar creases [2], in which small crateriform pits are visible on the palmar creases (Fig. 69.6). *Focal acral hyperkeratosis* is a type of papular keratoderma, dominantly inherited in familial cases, that occurs almost exclusively in black Africans [3]. It is characterized by oval or polygonal papules, which may show central pigmented pits, situated on the borders of the palms and soles.

REFERENCES

1 Shrank AB, Harman RRH. The incidence of skin disease in a Nigerian teaching hospital dermatological clinic. *Br J Dermatol* 1966; **78**: 235–41.
2 Penas PF, Rois-Buceta L, Sanchez-Perez J *et al.* Keratosis punctata of the palmar creases: case report and prevalence study in caucasians. *Dermatology* 1994; **188**: 200–2.
3 Lucker GPH, van der Kerkhof PCM, Steijlen PM. The hereditary palmoplantar keratoses: an updated review and classification. *Br J Dermatol* 1994; **131**: 1–14.

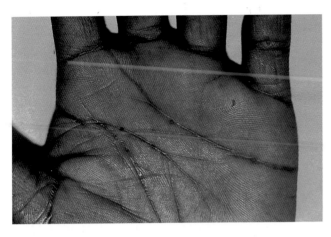

Fig. 69.6 Keratosis punctata of the palmar creases with hyperpigmentation. (Courtesy of Dr D.J. Barker, Bradford Royal Infirmary, Bradford, UK.)

Photodermatoses

Racial pigmentation protects from some of the immediate and long-term adverse effects of sunlight. However, even a pigmented skin may be sunburnt, although it may be difficult to see the erythema because of the pigmentation [1]. Conditions such as polymorphic light eruption occur in all races, but some have a particular presentation depending on the race of the individual. In black Africans or Australoids, for example, an actinic cheilitis (or discoid lupus erythematosus) may affect the lower lip, which may not be protected by the same amount of pigment as on other sites of the body.

One photodermatosis that seems to have a racial predilection is actinic prurigo of native Americans [2], although it may be a form of polymorphic light eruption [3] (Chapter 24). It may present as a lower lip cheilitis, but also produces a conjunctivitis, pterygium and eyebrow alopecia [2]. Actinic prurigo has a female : male ratio of 3 : 1 and usually has an onset in the first two decades of life [4]. Those with an early onset tend to have cheilitis and may improve; those with a later onset have a milder disease, which may be more persistent [4].

REFERENCES

1 Willis I. Photosensitivity reactions in black skin. *Dermatol Clin* 1988; **6**: 369–75.
2 Mounsdon T, Kratochvil F, Auclair P *et al.* Actinic prurigo of the lower lip: review of the literature and report of five cases. *Oral Surg Oral Med Oral Pathol* 1988; **65**: 327–32.
3 Fletcher DC, Romanchuk KG, Lane PR. Conjunctivitis and pterygium associated with the American Indian type of polymorphous light eruption. *Can J Ophthalmol* 1988; **23**: 30–3.
4 Lane PR, Hogan DJ, Martel MJ *et al.* Actinic prurigo: clinical features and prognosis. *J Am Acad Dermatol* 1992; **26**: 683–92.

Pityriasis rosea

In black Africans, this eruption shows several unusual features. It shows an 'inverse' pattern, with lesions on the face, neck, extremities and lower abdomen, rather than on the trunk as is usual [1]. In addition, it may be papular, may affect the palms and soles, and shows a brown-grey or even purple pigmentation [2,3]. The recurrence rate seems to be higher in black Africans than in other races [4] and the hyperpigmentation that may follow can persist for some months.

REFERENCES

1 McLaurin CI. Unusual patterns of common dermatoses in blacks. *Cutis* 1983; **32**: 352–60.
2 Hendricks AA, Lohr JA. Pityriasis in infancy. *Arch Dermatol* 1979; **115**: 896–7.
3 Jacyk WK. Pityriasis rosea in Nigerians. *Int J Dermatol* 1980; **19**: 397–9.
4 Chuang TY, Illstrup DM, Perry HO *et al.* Pityriasis rosea in Rochester, Minnesota, 1969–78. *J Am Acad Dermatol* 1982; **7**: 80–9.

Postinflammatory pigmentary changes

Pigmented skin shows more of a pigmentary reaction following trauma or inflammation than non-pigmented or lightly pigmented skin. In black Africans, it is also not uncommon to see secondary hypopigmentation after eczema, pityriasis alba, sarcoidosis, leprosy, herpes zoster, pityriasis versicolor or other common eruptions [1,2]. It may also follow cryotherapy and the topical use or intralesional injection of corticosteroids. Table 69.1 lists causes of hypopigmentation in a pigmented skin [1–3]. Sometimes unusual patterns of pigmentation are found; for example, black Africans with systemic sclerosis may develop a

Table 69.1 Causes of hypopigmentation in a pigmented skin.

Division	Disorders
Congenital or genetic	Albinism, piebaldness
Infections	Leprosy, onchocerciasis, pinta, pityriasis versicolor, herpes zoster
Papulosquamous disorders	Pityriasis alba, pityriasis rosea, pityriasis lichenoides chronica, psoriasis, seborrhoeic dermatitis
Physical or chemical agents	Burns, cryotherapy, ammoniated mercury, hydroquinone products, fluorinated corticosteroids
Postinflammatory	Discoid lupus erythematosus, systemic sclerosis, sarcoidosis, some eczematous eruptions
Miscellaneous	Vitiligo, idiopathic guttate hypomelanosis

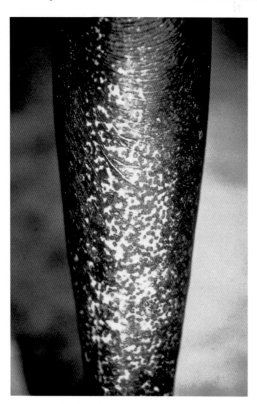

Fig. 69.7 Onchocerciasis showing 'leopard skin' depigmentation. (Courtesy of Dr M.E. Murdoch, Watford District General Hospital, Watford, UK.)

mottled and vitiligo-like hypopigmentation [3] (Chapter 56). Complete or patchy 'leopard skin' depigmentation may be seen with onchocerciasis (Fig. 69.7). On the other hand, some dermatoses result in hyperpigmentation, and it is not unusual to find both hyper- and hypopigmentation coexisting in the same individual.

Hyperpigmentation may occur in black African skin with acne, eczema, sarcoidosis, psoriasis, mycosis fungoides, lichen planus, fixed drug eruption and lupus erythematosus, and frequently is seen when the skin is lichenified, as in chronic eczema [2]. Hyperpigmentation, particularly of the face, may also be acquired due to exposure to a variety of agents. These include exogenous ochronosis from hydroquinone-containing skin-bleaching creams, and mercury deposition from skin-lightening creams containing mercury, and also from exposure to photosensitizing drugs and herbal potions [4].

REFERENCES

1 Olumide YM, Odunowo BD, Odiase AO. Depigmentation in black African patients. *Int J Dermatol* 1990; **29**: 166–74.
2 McLaurin CI. Unusual patterns of common dermatoses in blacks. *Cutis* 1983; **32**: 352–60.
3 Kenney JA Jr. Pigmentary disorders in black skin. *Clin Dermatol* 1989; **7**: 1–10.
4 Olumide YM, Odunowo BD, Odiase AO. Regional dermatoses in the African, 1: facial hypermelanosis. *Int J Dermatol* 1991; **30**: 186–9.

Psoriasis

The genetic basis for psoriasis is well established, although not well understood. It is relatively common in European Caucasoids (prevalence about 2%), although within the Caucasoid group it is said to vary, being more common in Parsees than in Hindus or Moslems [1]. A high prevalence is reported in East Africans [2] and a low prevalence in West Africans [3–5], which may explain the low prevalence in African Americans. Psoriasis is almost unknown in the Mongoloid native Americans [3] and Eskimos [6], and in Australian aborigines [7]. It is rare in the Japanese (Mongoloid), although the prevalence in the latter is increasing [8]. The prevalence in Mongoloids in Hong Kong, mainland China and Japan was estimated to be 0.3% [9].

In black skin, psoriatic plaques may appear violaceous or bluish black due to pigmentary incontinence. Grey, silvery scales may be seen. Postinflammatory hyperpigmentation may be left after clearing of the lesions [10]. This may be a persistent cosmetic disability.

REFERENCES

1 Gans O. Some observations on the pathogenesis of psoriasis. *Arch Dermatol* 1952; **66**: 598–611.
2 Verhagen AR, Koten JW. Psoriasis in Kenya. *Arch Dermatol* 1967; **96**: 39–41.
3 Kerdel-Vegas F. The challenge of tropical dermatology. *Trans St John's Hosp Dermatol Soc* 1973; **59**: 1–9.
4 Lomholt G. Psoriasis in Uganda: a comparative study with other parts of Africa. In: Farber EM, Cox AJ, eds. *Psoriasis: Proceedings of the First International Symposium*. Stanford: Stanford University Press, 1971: 41.
5 Obasi OE. Psoriasis vulgaris in the Guinea Savannah region of Nigeria. *Int J Dermatol* 1986; **25**: 181–3.
6 Horrobin DF. Low prevalence of coronary heart disease, psoriasis, asthma and rheumatoid arthritis in Eskimos: are they caused by high dietary intake of eicosapentaenoic acid, a genetic variation of essential fatty acid metabolism or both? *Med Hypotheses* 1987; **22**: 421–8.
7 Green AC. Australian aborigines and psoriasis. *Aust J Dermatol* 1984; **25**: 18–24.
8 Yasudo T, Ishikawa E, Mori S. Psoriasis in the Japanese. In: Farber EM, Cox AJ, eds. *Psoriasis: Proceedings of the First International Symposium*. Stanford: Stanford University Press, 1971: 25–34.
9 Yip SY. The prevalence of psoriasis in the mongoloid race. *J Am Acad Dermatol* 1984; **10**: 965–8.
10 Rosen T, Martin S. *Atlas of Black Dermatology*. Boston: Little, Brown, 1981.

Sarcoidosis

In the USA, sarcoidosis is 10 times more common in African Americans than in Caucasoids [1]. Skin signs are seen in between one-tenth and one-third of patients with sarcoidosis [2]. Erythema nodosum is the commonest non-specific lesion of sarcoidosis, but is much more frequent in Caucasoids than in black Africans [3,4]. In Africans, the commonest sarcoidal skin lesions are flesh-coloured or slightly hypopigmented papules which tend to occur around the nose, mouth and occiput [2]. Hypopigmented macules, violaceous plaques (often on the face or arms) and subcutaneous nodules are also seen.

Ulceration may occur. Lupus pernio is apparently infrequent in black Africans [2].

In contrast to the American experience, sarcoidosis was said to be uncommon in West Africans, but this may not be the case [5]. It has a very low reported prevalence in the Far East.

REFERENCES

1 Abeles H, Robins AB, Chaves AD. Sarcoidosis in New York City. *Am Rev Respir Dis* 1961; **84**: 120–1.
2 Minus HR, Grimes PE. Cutaneous manifestations of sarcoidosis in blacks. *Cutis* 1983; **32**: 361–8.
3 Caruthers B, Day TB, Minus HR *et al.* Sarcoidosis: a comparison of cutaneous manifestations with chest radiographic changes. *J Natl Med Assoc* 1975; **67**: 364–7.
4 James DG. Dermatological aspects of sarcoidosis. *QJM* 1959; **28**: 108–24.
5 Alabi GO, George AO. Cutaneous sarcoidosis and tribal scarifications in West Africa. *Int J Dermatol* 1989; **28**: 29–31.

Skin cancer

Most forms of skin malignancy and sun-induced degenerative change are more common in North European Caucasoids than in other racial groups. Black Africans have the lowest incidence (1/70 that of Caucasoids) of non-melanoma skin cancer [1], with Mongoloids occupying an intermediate position. Genetic variations that have a racial aspect, e.g. the allelic diversity seen in pale non-Africans for the MC1R locus, will have a bearing on racial susceptibility to skin cancer [2]. In black people, squamous cell carcinoma is the commonest skin tumour [3], as opposed to basal cell carcinoma in Caucasoids. Scarring—for example, from burns or discoid lupus erythematosus—is a predisposing factor in squamous cell carcinoma in Africans [4]. The prognosis in black Africans in the USA is generally worse than in Caucasoids, because of later presentation or more aggressive disease [5]. Basal cell carcinoma is often pigmented in non-Caucasoids.

Malignant melanoma is 10 times more common in North American 'European' Caucasoids than in African Americans, with an incidence in New Mexican Hispanic Caucasoids and Puerto Rico Hispanic Caucasoids of 3.7 and 1.6 times that of African Americans [6]. Puerto Rico Hispanics have more admixture of African genes than Hispanics from New Mexico. In black Africans, malignant melanoma mostly affects the soles or palms [3]. Presentation may be delayed. Malignant melanoma of the sole of the foot, in North America, has a similar incidence in black people as in Caucasoids [7]. Extradermal acrolentiginous tumours with a poor prognosis—e.g. those involving the vulva, cervix, vagina or the anorectal area—made up 44% of new primary malignant melanomas in a study of black American women [8]. In the Mongoloid Japanese, the acral lentiginous type of malignant melanomas makes up a large proportion of cases and the incidence at this site is similar to that for Caucasoids in other sites [9].

Japanese residents in Hawaii had a rate for non-melanoma skin cancer that was 88 times higher than that reported in Japan [10]. This higher rate was attributed to increased sun exposure, and possibly to arsenic exposure. The incidence of basal cell carcinoma in Hong Kong Chinese trebled between 1990 and 1999 (0.32–9.2/100 000/year) and that of squamous cell carcinoma doubled (0.16–0.34) [11].

REFERENCES

1 Scotto J, Fraumeni JF Jr. Skin-cancer other than melanoma. In: Scottenfeld D, Fraumeni JF Jr, eds. *Cancer Epidemiology and Prevention.* Philadelphia: Saunders, 1982: 996–1011.
2 Harding RM, Healy E, Ray AJ *et al.* Evidence for variable selection at the human pigmentation locus MCR1. *Am J Hum Genet* 2000; **66**: 1351–61.
3 Halder RM, Bang KM. Skin cancer in blacks in the United States. *Dermatol Clin* 1988; **6**: 397–405.
4 Mora RG, Perniciaro C. Cancer of the skin in blacks: a review of 163 patients with cutaneous squamous cell carcinoma. *J Am Acad Dermatol* 1981; **5**: 535–43.
5 Halder RM, Bridgeman-Shah S. Skin cancer in African Americans. *Cancer* 1995; **75**: 667–73.
6 Bergfelt L, Newell GR, Sider JG *et al.* Incidence and anatomical distribution of cutaneous melanoma among United States Hispanics. *J Surg Oncol* 1989; **40**: 222–6.
7 Stevens NG, Liff JM, Weiss NS. Plantar melanoma: is the incidence of melanoma of the sole of the foot really higher in blacks than in whites? *Int J Cancer* 1990; **45**: 691–3.
8 Muchmore JH, Mizuguchi RS, Lee C. Malignant melanoma in American black females: an unusual distribution of primary sites. *J Am Coll Surg* 1996; **183**: 457–65.
9 Elwood JM. Epidemiology and control of melanoma in white populations and in Japan. *J Invest Dermatol* 1989; **92**: 214S–21S.
10 Leong GK, Stone JL, Farmer ER *et al.* Nonmelanoma skin cancer in Japanese residents of Kauai, Hawaii. *J Am Acad Dermatol* 1987; **17**: 233–8.
11 Cheng SY, Luk NM, Chong LY. Special features of non-melanoma skin cancer in Hong Kong Chinese patients: 10-year retrospective study. *Hong Kong Med J* 2001; **7**: 22–8.

Syphilis

The primary chancre is similar in Caucasoids and black Africans, but the manifestations of secondary syphilis can be different. In Caucasoids, macular lesions are common, but in black Africans, follicular and papular forms are more frequent and may be hyperpigmented [1]. Annular secondary syphilis is almost unique to Negroids [2]; corymbose forms (a central lesion with surrounding small satellites) are also seen [1]. Palmoplantar lesions in black Africans may be keratotic. The non-venereal treponematoses yaws, pinta and bejel are endemic in certain parts of the world. No racial predilection exists, although the appearances may be modified in different races.

REFERENCES

1 Rosen T, Martin S. *Atlas of Black Dermatology.* Boston: Little, Brown, 1981.
2 McLaurin CI. Annular facial dermatoses in blacks. *Cutis* 1983; **32**: 369–70.

Systemic sclerosis

There are racial differences in the patterns of disease for

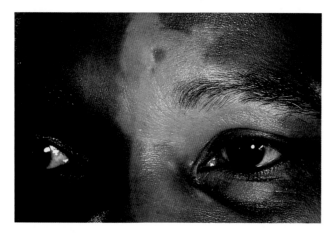

Fig. 69.8 Vitiligo. (Courtesy of Dr A.G. Messenger, Royal Hallamshire Hospital, Sheffield, UK.)

people affected by systemic sclerosis (scleroderma). African Americans and Hispanics (who often have inherited some black African genes) are more likely to have diffuse skin involvement, pigmentary change, digital ulceration and pulmonary hypertension than Caucasoids, who exhibit more facial telangiectasia and associated hypothyroidism [1]. The Choctaw Native American Indians (Mongoloids) have a high prevalence of systemic sclerosis that has been identified as being due to a defect in a gene for fibrillin 1 on chromosome 15q, dating from 10 generations ago ('founder effect') [2].

REFERENCES

1 Reveille JD, Fischbach M, McNearney T *et al.* Systemic sclerosis in 3 US ethnic groups: a comparison of clinical, socioeconomic, serological and immunogenetic determinants. *Semin Arthritis Rheum* 2001; **30**: 332–46.
2 Tan FK, Stivers DN, Foster MW *et al.* Association of microsatellite markers near the fibrillin 1 gene on human chromosome 15q with scleroderma in a Native American Indian population. *Arthritis Rheum* 1998; **41**: 1729–37.

Vitiligo

Vitiligo has the same incidence in all races [1] but its manifestations are much more significant in those with a dark skin than in lightly pigmented individuals (Fig. 69.8). In Afro-Caribbeans, vitiligo may show a 'trichrome' pattern, with hypopigmented as well as depigmented areas.

REFERENCE

1 Kenney JA. Vitiligo. *Dermatol Clin* 1988; **6**: 425–34.

Diseases with a distinct racial or ethnic predisposition

Several disorders have a significant racial predisposition as discussed below and in general reference texts [1,2].

REFERENCES

1 Johnson BL, Moy RL, White GM. *Ethnic Skin. Medical and Surgical.* St Louis: Mosby, 1998.
2 Archer CB, Robertson SJ. *Black and White Skin. An Atlas and Text.* Oxford: Blackwell Scientific Publications, 1995.

Hair disorders

Dissecting folliculitis (Chapter 63)
SYN. DISSECTING CELLULITIS; PERIFOLLICULITIS CAPITIS ABSCEDENS ET SUFFODIENS

This is an uncommon, chronic, progressive and suppurative scalp disorder that almost exclusively affects Afro-Caribbean males. Painful, boggy, sterile abscesses form on the scalp (Fig. 69.9) and are connected by sinus tracts [1]. As the disease progresses, scarring and alopecia are seen, and keloids may form [2]. The cause is unknown. Treatment has been difficult in the past as intralesional steroids and systemic antibiotics provide only partial relief, but it is now known that isotretinoin is effective in this condition, although it needs to be continued for 4 months after clinical control is achieved to prevent relapse [3]. Resistant cases may require surgical excision and grafting [4]. Dissecting folliculitis may be associated with acne conglobata and hidradenitis suppurativa, to form the so-called 'follicular occlusion' triad, in which abnormal follicular keratinization and occlusion occur [5].

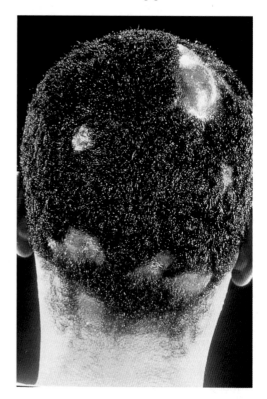

Fig. 69.9 Dissecting cellulitis of the scalp. (Courtesy of Professor H.C. Williams, Queen's Medical Centre, Nottingham, UK.)

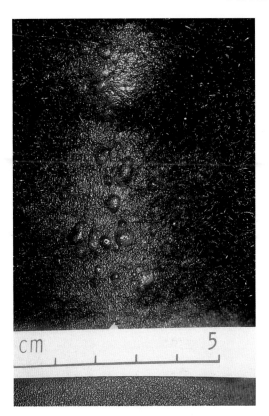

Fig. 69.10 Folliculitis keloidalis. (Courtesy of Dr A.G. Messenger, Royal Hallamshire Hospital, Sheffield, UK.)

REFERENCES

1 Halder RM. Hair and scalp disorders in blacks. *Cutis* 1983; **32**: 378–80.
2 Scott DA. Disorders of the hair and scalp in blacks. *Dermatol Clin* 1988; **6**: 387–95.
3 Scerri L, Williams HC, Speight EL, Allen BR. Dissecting cellulitis of the scalp: response to isotretinoin. *Br J Dermatol* 1995; **133** (Suppl. 45): 41.
4 Dellon AL, Orlando JC. Perifolliculitis capitis. surgical treatment for the resistant case. *Ann Plast Surg* 1982; **9**: 254–9.
5 Baden HP. *Diseases of the Hair and Nails*. Chicago: Year Book Medical Publishing, 1987.

Folliculitis keloidalis (Chapter 27)

SYN. ACNE KELOIDALIS NUCHAE

This condition is seen almost exclusively in black Africans, with males being mostly affected [1]. Firm, discrete, follicular and perifollicular papules develop, usually on the nape of the neck, but often extending into the occipital scalp or beyond (Fig. 69.10). Complications include pustule formation, hypertrophic scars, keloids and alopecia [2]. The aetiology is unknown, but probably related to the curved shape of the hair follicle. Treatment includes intralesional steroid injection and topical and systemic antibiotics [1].

REFERENCES

1 Halder RM. Hair and scalp disorders in blacks. *Cutis* 1983; **32**: 378–80.
2 Rosen T, Martin S. *Atlas of Black Dermatology*. Boston: Little, Brown, 1981.

Hot-comb alopecia (Chapter 63)

Hot combing is a method of straightening curly black hair, although it has to a large extent been replaced by chemical methods [1]. Oil is applied to the hair and acts as a lubricant and heat conductor. A metal comb, heated to 150–260°C, is applied to the hair, re-arranging the hydrogen and disulphide bonds and straightening the hair [2]. The hot comb and oil may break the hair and a traction alopecia may also result. Repeated contact of the hot oil with the scalp can produce a scarring alopecia [3]. Recent evidence suggests that hot combing may not be the reason for the hair loss, which is usually seen in young adult women, and that the histological end-result, follicular degeneration, may have some other cause [4].

Hair-shaft breakage may also be seen with the inappropriate use of chemical relaxers and straighteners [1]. A scarring alopecia may also be seen, again in young women, following the use of hair-straightening chemicals [5].

REFERENCES

1 Scott DA. Disorders of the hair and scalp in blacks. *Dermatol Clin* 1988; **6**: 387–95.
2 Halder RM. Hair and scalp disorders in blacks. *Cutis* 1983; **32**: 378–80.
3 LoPresti P, Papa CM, Kligman AM. Hot comb alopecia. *Arch Dermatol* 1968; **98**: 234–8.
4 Sperling LC, Sau P. The follicular degeneration syndrome in black patients: 'hot comb alopecia' revisited and revised. *Arch Dermatol* 1992; **128**: 68–74.
5 Nicholson AG, Harland CC, Ball RH *et al*. Chemically induced cosmetic alopecia. *Br J Dermatol* 1993; **128**: 537–41.

Pseudofolliculitis barbae (Chapter 22)

This is a disorder common in black African males who shave and is related to the curved hair follicles found in such individuals [1]. Once shaved, the cut hair retracts beneath the skin surface into the curved follicle and grows in a circular direction. The sharpened hair end either penetrates the wall of the follicle, causing a foreign-body reaction, or grows out of the follicle but re-enters the skin and penetrates the dermis, again setting up an inflammatory reaction [1]. Perifollicular papules and pustules develop and scarring may result (Fig. 69.11). The beard area is usually affected, but pseudofolliculitis may involve any site that is shaved, including the pubic area and the scalp [2]. Recommended treatment is to grow a beard, use electric clippers, depilatory creams or a manual razor, sometimes with topical or systemic antibiotics [3].

REFERENCES

1 Scott DA. Disorders of the hair and scalp in blacks. *Dermatol Clin* 1988; **6**: 387–95.
2 Smith JD, Odom RB. Pseudofolliculitis capitis. *Arch Dermatol* 1977; **113**: 328–9.
3 Brown LA. Pathogenesis and treatment of pseudofolliculitis barbae. *Cutis* 1983; **32**: 373–5.

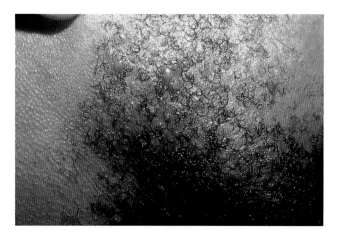

Fig. 69.11 Pseudofolliculitis barbae. (Courtesy of Dr C. St J. O'Doherty, Queen Elizabeth II Hospital, Welwyn Garden City, London, UK.)

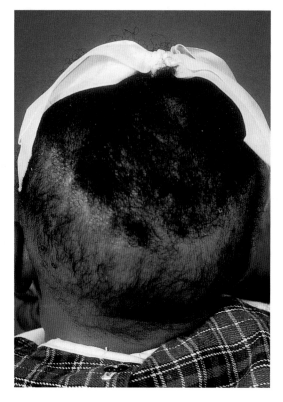

Fig. 69.12 Traction alopecia. (Courtesy of Dr A.G. Messenger, Royal Hallamshire Hospital, Sheffield, UK.)

Traction alopecia (Chapter 63)

Traction alopecia (Fig. 69.12) is mainly seen in black Africans, because of the practices of plaiting or tightly braiding the hair into multiple braids (corn rowing), although it is not entirely confined to this group [1]. It may also follow the use of tight rollers or 'picking out' the hair with a hard comb to create the 'Afro' hairstyle [2]. Hairs are loosened from their follicles and inflammation and

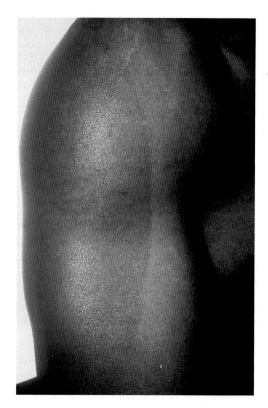

Fig. 69.13 Futcher's lines. (Courtesy of the late Dr R.R.M. Harman, Bristol Royal Infirmary, Bristol, UK.)

atrophy may result. The distribution depends on the pattern of braiding, but often involves the temporal regions. Treatment consists of persuading the patient to discontinue the offending practice. In long-standing cases, alopecia may be permanent.

REFERENCES

1 Scott DA. Disorders of the hair and scalp in blacks. *Dermatol Clin* 1988; **6**: 387–95.
2 Halder RM. Hair and scalp disorders in blacks. *Cutis* 1983; **32**: 378–80.

Variations of normal pigmentation

Futcher's or Voigt's lines

These are sharply demarcated bilateral lines of pigmentation (Fig. 69.13) that are seen at the anterolateral junction usually of the upper arms, where there is a transition from extensor to flexor surface and from darker to lighter pigmentation [1]. The lines correspond to a dermatome [2]. A second hyperpigmented line may occur on the posteromedial part of the lower aspect of the limbs [3]. The presence of Futcher's lines is proportional to the degree of pigmentation of the individual; they are present in 25% of black Africans [3]. Overall, about 75% of black people have at least one hypo- or hyperpigmented line [3]. These lines may be seen to a lesser extent in other races.

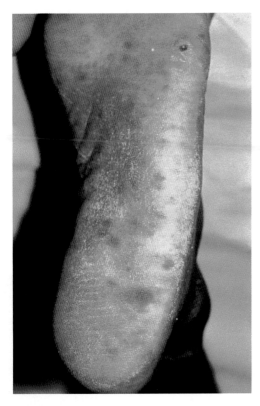

Fig. 69.14 Mottled macular pigmentation on the soles. (Courtesy of Dr D.J. Barker, Bradford Royal Infirmary, Bradford, UK.)

REFERENCES

1 Henderson AL. Skin variations in blacks. *Cutis* 1983; **32**: 376–7.
2 Futcher PH. A peculiarity of pigmentation of the upper arms of negroes. *Science* 1938; **88**: 570–1.
3 McLaurin CI. Cutaneous reaction patterns in blacks. *Dermatol Clin* 1988; **6**: 353–62.

Hyperpigmentation of the palms and soles

Discrete, ill-defined or mottled macular pigmentation is frequently seen on the palms and soles (Fig. 69.14) of African patients, especially those with a darker skin colour [1].

REFERENCE

1 Chapel TA, Taylor RM, Pinkus H. Volar melanotic macules. *Int J Dermatol* 1979; **18**: 222–5.

Midline hypopigmentation

This appears as a line or band of hypopigmentation, or as discrete oval macules, on the anterior chest and mid-sternal area. Lesions sometimes extend down to the abdomen or up to the neck, where lines of hypopigmentation may radiate out to the clavicles [1,2]. It is commonly seen in black African males, but may occur in other races.

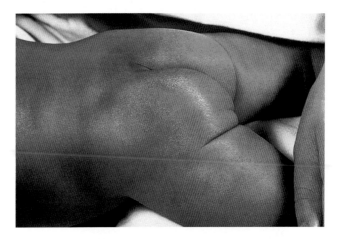

Fig. 69.15 Mongolian spot. (Courtesy of Professor S.S. Bleehen, Royal Hallamshire Hospital, Sheffield, UK.)

REFERENCES

1 Selmanowitz V, Krivo JM. Hypopigmented markings in negroes. *Int J Dermatol* 1973; **12**: 229–35.
2 Weary PE, Behlen CH. Unusual familial hypopigmentary anomaly. *Arch Dermatol* 1965; **92**: 54–5.

Mongolian spot (Chapter 39)

SYN. CONGENITAL DERMAL MELANOCYTOSIS

Mongolian spot refers to a slatey brown or blue-grey macular pigmentation observed at birth or in the neonatal period (Fig. 69.15). It is present in 100% of Mongoloid babies [1], between 70 and 96% of black Africans, and in up to 10% of Caucasoids [2,3]. The pigmentation is usually faint, round or oval in shape, and ranges in size from a few millimetres to greater than 10 cm in diameter. Mongolian spots are normally located over the sacral area, but the buttocks, flank or shoulders may be involved. Occasionally, multiple or extensive lesions are seen. The pigmentation generally reaches its peak at 2 years and fades by the age of 6 or 7 years.

REFERENCES

1 Leung AK. Mongolian spots in Chinese children. *Int J Dermatol* 1988; **27**: 106–8.
2 Cordova A. The Mongolian spot: a study of ethnic differences and a literature review. *Clin Pediatr* 1981; **20**: 714–9.
3 Osburn K, Schosser RH, Everett MA. Congenital pigmented and vascular lesions in newborn infants. *J Am Acad Dermatol* 1987; **16**: 788–92.

Nail pigmentation

Longitudinal bands of brown or black pigmentation may be seen (Fig. 69.16); they occur with a higher frequency on the thumb and index fingernails [1,2]. They are present in more than 50% of black Africans, are more common in those with heavy pigmentation, and increase with advancing age.

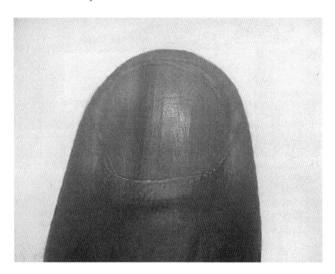

Fig. 69.16 Nail pigmentation.

REFERENCES

1 Leyden JJ, Spott D, Goldschmidt H. Diffuse and banded melanin pigmentation in nails. *Arch Dermatol* 1972; **105**: 548–50.
2 Monash S. Normal pigmentation in the nails of the negro. *Arch Dermatol* 1932; **25**: 876–81.

Oral pigmentation

Oral macular pigmentation is seen in black Africans. It most often affects the gingivae, but may also involve the hard palate, buccal mucosa and tongue [1].

REFERENCE

1 Dummett CO, Sakumura JS, Barens G. The relationship of facial skin complexion to oral mucosal pigmentation and tooth color. *J Prosthet Dent* 1980; **4**: 392–6.

Pigmentary disorders

Acanthosis nigricans (Chapter 34)

In some Mongoloid native American tribes, acanthosis nigricans is very common [1]. It may indicate a high risk of diabetes mellitus.

REFERENCE

1 Stuart CA, Smith MM, Gilkison CR *et al.* Acanthosis nigricans among Native Americans: an indicator of high diabetes risk. *Am J Public Health* 1994; **84**: 1839–42.

Dermatosis papulosa nigra (Chapter 36)

This condition is characterized by hyperpigmented, smooth-surfaced, round or filiform papules usually on the face (Fig. 69.17), but sometimes on the neck or upper trunk

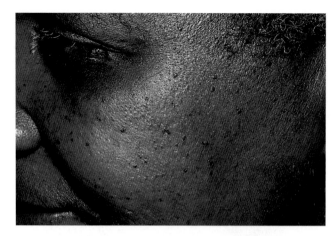

Fig. 69.17 Dermatosis papulosa nigra.

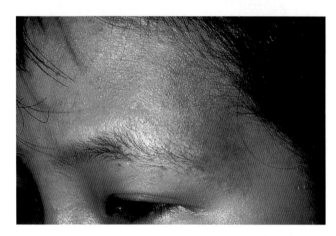

Fig. 69.18 Naevus of Ota.

[1,2]. The papules measure 1–5 mm in diameter. It is most common in black Africans, affecting up to three-quarters of adults (the majority being women), but is occasionally found in Caucasoids and Mongoloids [1]. The cause is unknown.

REFERENCES

1 Grimes PE, Arora S, Minus HR *et al.* Dermatosis papulosa nigra. *Cutis* 1983; **32**: 385–92.
2 Hairston N, Reed R, Derbes V. Dermatosis papulosa nigra. *Arch Dermatol* 1964; **89**: 655–8.

Naevus of Ota (Chapter 38)

Macular pigmentation, due to dermal melanocytes, is seen adjacent to the eye and also involves the sclera (Fig. 69.18). The pigmentation in naevus of Ota is variable and may be blue, slatey blue or brown. The naevus is usually unilateral and affects the eyelid, maxillary and zygomatic areas—regions that are innervated by the first and second branches of the trigeminal nerve [1]. It is most common in Mongoloids, but may occur in other racial groups. The prevalence in the Japanese is 0.4–0.8% [2]. Over 80% of cases appear in women. About two-thirds of patients have ocular involvement, commonly of the sclera, but also of the cornea, conjunctiva and retina [1]. Malignant melanoma may develop in the naevus of Ota, more frequently in Caucasoid than Mongoloid patients [3].

REFERENCES

1 Kopf AW, Weidman AI. Nevus of Ota. *Arch Dermatol* 1962; **85**: 195–208.
2 Jimbow M, Jimbow K. Pigmentary disorders in oriental skin. *Clin Dermatol* 1989; **7**: 11–27.
3 Jay B. Malignant melanoma of the orbit in a case of oculodermal melanocytosis (naevus of Ota). *Br J Ophthalmol* 1965; **49**: 359–63.

Naevus of Ito (Chapter 38)

This is a variant of the naevus of Ota, and is characterized by macular pigmentation involving the shoulder, supraclavicular area, sides of the neck and upper arm—the areas supplied by the posterior supraclavicular and lateral brachial nerves [1,2]. It is more common in the Japanese and may occur alone or associated with a naevus of Ota.

REFERENCES

1 Ito M. Studies on melanin: nevus fusco-caeruleus acromiodeltoideus. *Tohoku J Exp Med* 1954; **60**: 10.
2 Mishima Y, Mevorah B. Nevus Ota and nevus Ito in American negroes. *J Invest Dermatol* 1961; **36**: 133–54.

Other conditions

Ainhum (Chapter 46)

Ainhum is characterized by the development of a constricting band around a digit (often the fifth toe) which may progress to spontaneous amputation of the digit [1]. It is generally found in black inhabitants of tropical countries, but has been described in African Americans [2]. The trauma and infection associated with walking barefoot may stimulate fibrosis. Pseudo-ainhum occurs in all races as a feature of mutilating keratoderma.

REFERENCES

1 Browne S. Ainhum: a clinical and etiological study of 83 cases. *Ann Trop Med Parasitol* 1961; **55**: 314–20.
2 Hucherson DC. Ainhum (dactylolysis spontanea): review of 10 cases. *Ann Surg* 1950; **132**: 312–4.

Cutaneous amyloidosis (Chapter 57)

Both the lichenoid type and the macular type are more common in Mongoloid subjects, but may be seen in any racial group [1–3]. Lichen amyloidosis consists of discrete, firm papules which often involve the lower leg, extensor aspect of the arms and lower back. The pigmented macular variant commonly affects the scapular region and shows a rippled pattern of pigmentation.

REFERENCES

1 Black MM, Wilson-Jones E. Macular amyloidosis: a study of 21 cases with special reference to the role of the epidermis and its histogenesis. *Br J Dermatol* 1971; **84**: 199–209.
2 Tay CH, DaCosta JL. Lichen amyloidosis: clinical study of 40 cases. *Br J Dermatol* 1970; **82**: 129–36.
3 Looi LM. Primary localised cutaneous amyloidosis in Malaysians. *Aust J Dermatol* 1991; **32**: 39–44.

Disseminate and recurrent infundibulofolliculitis (Chapter 27)

This is a type of follicular eczema mainly seen in black Africans [1,2]. Pruritic, follicle-based papules are present on the neck, trunk or limbs. Juxtaclavicular beaded lines are a somewhat similar condition. They consist of asymptomatic parallel rows of skin-coloured papules on the neck and overlying the clavicles [1]. They are also seen in Caucasoids.

REFERENCES

1 McLaurin CI. Cutaneous reaction patterns in blacks. *Dermatol Clin* 1988; **6**: 353–62.
2 Rosen T, Martin S. *Atlas of Black Dermatology*. Boston: Little, Brown, 1981.

Facial Afro-Caribbean childhood eruption

In facial Afro-Caribbean childhood eruption (FACE), monomorphic flesh-coloured or hypopigmented papules are seen on the face, particularly around the mouth (Fig. 69.19), eyelids and ears, in Afro-Caribbean children [1,2]. The eruption persists for several months, but resolves spontaneously without scarring. The cause is unknown.

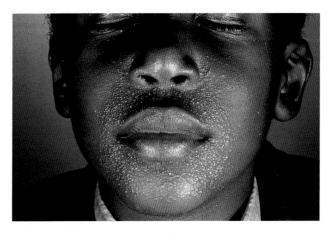

Fig. 69.19 Facial Afro-Caribbean childhood eruption. (Courtesy of Professor H.C. Williams, Queen's Medical Centre, Nottingham, UK.)

REFERENCES

1 Marten RH, Presbury DGC, Adamson JE *et al*. An unusual papular and acneiform facial eruption in the negro child. *Br J Dermatol* 1976; **91**: 435–8.
2 Williams HC, Ashworth J, Pembroke AC *et al*. FACE: facial Afro-Caribbean childhood eruption. *Clin Exp Dermatol* 1990; **15**: 163–6.

Fogo selvagem (endemic pemphigus foliaceus)
(Chapter 41)

One report suggests this type of pemphigus, seen in clusters in jungle areas of South America, is more common in Native Indians (Mongoloids), who may be genetically predisposed to develop the disorder [1].

REFERENCE

1 Friedman H, Campbell I, Rocha-Alvarez R *et al*. Endemic pemphigus foliaceus (fogo selvagem) in native Americans from Brazil. *J Am Acad Dermatol* 1995; **32**: 949–56.

Hamartoma moniliformis (Chapter 15)

An asymptomatic disorder of small, discrete, flesh-coloured papules seen over the face and neck [1]. Histology reveals an increase in collagen and elastic fibres, capillary endothelial hyperplasia and proliferation of dermal nerves. The condition was first recognized in mentally retarded black children [1], but may occur in Caucasoid children and in mentally normal children.

REFERENCE

1 Butterworth T, Graham JH. Linear papular ectodermal–mesodermal hamartoma (hamartoma moniliformis). *Arch Dermatol* 1970; **101**: 191–205.

Infantile acropustulosis (Chapter 14)

Crops of small, intensely itchy papules appear between 2 and 10 months of age. The papules evolve into pustules and are mostly found on the palms, soles, wrists and ankles [1,2]. Lesions clear within 3 weeks, but recur until the disease resolves spontaneously at the age of about 2 or 3 years. It occurs predominantly in black African infants and the cause is unknown.

REFERENCES

1 Jarratt M, Ramsdell W. Infantile acropustulosis. *Arch Dermatol* 1979; **115**: 834–6.
2 Kahn G, Rywlin AM. Acropustulosis of infancy. *Arch Dermatol* 1979; **115**: 831–3.

Mudi-chood

A papular eruption with a firm adherent scale, known as mudi-chood, is seen on the nape of the neck and upper

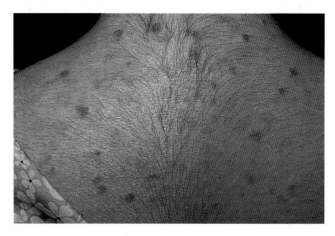

Fig. 69.20 Mudi-chood. (Courtesy of Dr P. Sugathan, Baby Memorial Hospital, Calicut, India.)

back in young Dravidian women in Kerala State, south India. It seems to be due to the effects of oils applied to the hair [1,2]. The early lesions are follicular pustules, although later, flat-topped brownish black papules, with a keratinous rim, are seen (Fig. 69.20). Histologically, there is parakeratosis and acanthosis [1]. The Dravidians were the original inhabitants of India. Their racial origin is not quite clear, but they differ from the Caucasoid peoples of central and northern India, e.g. the Punjabis and Rajasthanis (who are descended from invaders from Persia and Central Asia). Dravidians have a darker skin colour and are shorter than their compatriots from north India: they have a prominent premaxilla, black hair and dark irises (P. Sugathan, personal communication). Mudi-chood can be improved by the application of 5% salicylic acid ointment, which removes the scales to leave hyperpigmented macules. Reducing the use of oils or cutting the hair shorter results in cure.

REFERENCES

1 Sugathan P, Balaraman Nair M. Mudi-chood: a new dermatosis. In: Marshall J, ed. *Essays on Tropical Dermatology*, Vol. 2. Amsterdam: Exerpta Medica, 1972: 183.
2 Gharpuray MB, Kulkarni V, Tolat S. Mudi-chood: an unusual tropical dermatosis. *Int J Dermatol* 1992; **31**: 396–7.

Papular eruption in black males

Described in young African American males, this monomorphic eruption consists of pruritic dermal papules with a predilection for the trunk, upper arms and postauricular area [1]. The condition may be persistent and resistant to treatment. The cause is not known.

REFERENCE

1 Rosen T, Algra RJ. Papular eruption in black men. *Arch Dermatol* 1980; **116**: 416–8.

Papuloerythroderma of Ofuji (Chapter 17)

The unusual eruption, characterized by solid papules coalescing into erythroderma with sparing of the body folds, was first described in elderly Mongoloid Japanese men, but has since also been reported in Caucasoids [1]. The cause is unknown.

REFERENCE

1 Nazzari G, Crovato F, Nigro A. Papuloerythroderma (Ofuji): two additional cases and a review of the literature. *J Am Acad Dermatol* 1992; **26**: 499–501.

Pityriasis rotunda (Chapter 34)

An eruption of asymptomatic discrete, large, scaly, oval or circular plaques on the trunk, mostly reported in Mongoloid or black African individuals [1,2]. It is a type of acquired ichthyosis and in some cases is associated with serious disease such as tuberculosis, leprosy, cirrhosis or underlying malignancy.

REFERENCES

1 Pinto GM, Tapadinhas C, Moura C, Afonso A. Pityriasis rotunda. *Cutis* 1996; **58**: 406–8.
2 Grimalt R, Gelmetti C, Brusasco A *et al*. Pityriasis rotunda: report of a familial occurrence and review of the literature. *J Am Acad Dermatol* 1994; **31**: 866–71.

Sickle cell disease (Chapter 50)

Sickle cell disease occurs in black African races. The main cutaneous findings are the hand–foot syndrome and leg ulceration. The hand–foot syndrome is the most common and often the initial manifestation of the disease in children and consists of painful, non-pitting oedema of the hands and feet, caused by infarction of the small bones [1]. Ischaemic leg ulcers are, overall, the most frequent skin complication of sickle cell disease, but are rare under the age of 15 years [2].

REFERENCES

1 Stevens MC, Padwick M, Serjeant GR. Observations on the natural history of dactylitis in homozygous sickle cell disease. *Clin Pediatr* 1981; **20**: 311–7.
2 Morgan AG. Proteinuria and leg ulcers in homozygous sickle cell disease. *J Trop Med Hyg* 1982; **85**: 205–8.

Transient neonatal pustular melanosis (Chapter 14)

A transient eruption of sterile vesicles and pustules, with surrounding erythema, which is present at birth. The vesicles rupture easily and leave pigmented macules that fade within the first few weeks of life [1,2]. It affects 4.4% of black Africans and 0.2% of Caucasoid neonates and tends to involve the face, neck, lower back and shins.

REFERENCES

1 Barr RJ, Globerman LM, Werber FA. Transient neonatal pustular melanosis. *Int J Dermatol* 1979; **18**: 636–8.
2 Ramamurthy RS, Reveri M, Esterly NB *et al*. Transient neonatal pustular melanosis. *J Pediatr* 1976; **88**: 831–5.

Vascular naevi (Chapter 15)

Vascular birthmarks, such as the naevus flammeus usually seen on the neck (the 'stork mark') or sometimes on the forehead or eyelids, or the port-wine stain naevus, are more common in Caucasoids than in black Africans or, to a lesser extent, in Mongoloids [1]. Naevus flammeus is seen in 30% of Caucasoid newborns and in 22% of black newborns [1]. Port-wine stain naevi are found in 1% of Caucasoid infants, but are rarer in other races [1].

REFERENCE

1 Osburn K, Schosser RH, Everett MA. Congenital pigmented and vascular lesions in newborn infants. *J Am Acad Dermatol* 1987; **16**: 788–92.

Chapter 70

The Ages of Man and their Dermatoses

R.A.C. Graham-Brown

Introduction

Human life is a continuum, but within the continuum there are several identifiable phases, which we (the present and previous authors and editors) have called, after Shakespeare, the 'Ages of Man' [1]. We all begin by passing through a period of development to the point of 'maturity', which is then followed by a process of intrinsic ageing leading inexorably to senescence. During these ages, alterations take place in the structure and function of the skin, and there are important differences in the range, presentation, prognosis and treatment of skin disorders at various points in life. Indeed, some of the physiological events that accompany puberty, pregnancy, the menopause and old age can, of themselves, be sufficient reason for the patient to seek specialist dermatological advice.

This chapter aims to provide an overview of these stages in the life of the skin. The dermatological problems of the neonatal period and infancy have been dealt with elsewhere (see Chapter 14). This chapter deals principally with the skin and skin disorders of puberty, the menstrual cycle, pregnancy, childbirth and the puerperium, the menopause and old age.

REFERENCE

1 Shakespeare W. *As You Like It* II. vii. 139.

Birth to puberty

Somatic growth

Growth, defined as an increase in size, occurs in most tissues, including the reproductive system. In particular, the changes in the skeleton, which can be monitored radiologically, and in the visible teeth, have been used as indices of maturity [1].

Between birth and maturity the skeleton and body keep in step with increases in weight of 20–25-fold, whereas the somatic muscles increase by 30–40-fold, and the nervous system by less than fivefold. The surface area of the skin increases sevenfold. In the first year after birth the body length increases by approximately 50% to around 75 cm, and another 12–13 cm are added in the second year. Subsequently, growth remains steady at 6 cm/year until the spurt associated with puberty. Weight follows a similar pattern.

Postnatal growth is dependent on growth hormone, or somatotrophin, secreted by the anterior pituitary, although other hormonal interactions may also be involved [2,3]. Human growth hormone is a protein with 191 amino acids. It exerts an effect on a number of tissues including the viscera and bone. In particular, it affects stature by stimulating proliferation of cartilage cells at the epiphyseal plates until the point when the epiphyses of the long bones have fused. Growth hormone also antagonizes the

70.1

actions of insulin, possibly by reducing the binding of insulin at its target sites, or by interacting with a second-messenger system.

Some of the effects of growth hormone are indirect, in the sense that they are mediated through the production of polypeptide growth factors in the target tissue. The most important of these, which affects the uptake of sulphate into cartilage, is somatomedin C, initially called 'sulphation factor' but now known to be identical with insulin-like growth factor 1 (IGF-1) and closely similar to IGF-2. Somatomedins have also been shown to stimulate incorporation of $[^{14}C]$ leucine into glycosaminoglycans in cartilage and of $[^{14}C]$ proline into collagen.

The secretion of growth hormone from the pituitary is mediated primarily by the interaction between hypothalamic growth hormone-releasing hormone and somatostatin, a 14-amino acid polypeptide that has numerous regulatory and neuromodulatory effects [4]. Negative feedback by both somatomedin C and growth hormone itself may also be involved. The basal concentration of growth hormone in the plasma is below 1 mIU/L, but it can reach peaks of up to 60 times this amount in adolescence. Bursts of secretion occur every 1–2 h during sleep, but can also be produced by physiological and psychological stresses.

Excessive secretion before puberty gives rise to gigantism, but once the epiphyses of the long bones have fused it results in thickening of the bones and enlargement of the hands and feet, known as acromegaly. Acromegalics also have, on average, abnormally high sebum secretion.

Deficiency of growth hormone, either in isolation or as a component of general hypopituitarism, is one cause of short stature.

REFERENCES

1 Sinclair D. *Human Growth After Birth*, 5th edn. Oxford: Oxford University Press, 1989.
2 O'Riordan JLO, Malan PG, Gould RP, eds. *Essentials of Endocrinology*, 2nd edn. Oxford: Blackwell Scientific Publications, 1988.
3 Underwood LE, Van Wyk JJ. Normal and aberrant growth. In: Wilson JD, Foster DW, eds. *Textbook of Endocrinology*. Philadelphia: Saunders, 1985: 155–205.
4 Reisine T, Bell GI. Molecular biology of somatostatin receptors. *Endocr Rev* 1995; **16**: 427–42.

Sexual development

The period between infancy and puberty that we call childhood is, in relation to sexual development, a hiatus in hormonally controlled events that have already been initiated in the fetus. While the dermatological problems of the neonatal period are so distinctive and of such practical importance as to merit a separate chapter, an understanding of the hormonal status of the fetus and the neonate, and of the cutaneous implications, is an essential starting point for a journey through the 'Ages of Man'.

Males become differentiated from females by their possession of a Y chromosome, which causes the indifferent gonads to become testes [1,2]. The fetal testis secretes a factor known as anti-Müllerian hormone, which induces regression of the Müllerian ducts between the seventh and eighth weeks of gestation, and testosterone, which causes virilization of the Wolffian duct to form most of the male system. Conversion of testosterone to 5α-dihydrotestosterone (see Chapter 4) is necessary for the development of the prostate from the urinogenital sinus, and of the external genitalia. In the latter trimesters of intrauterine life, the testicles descend to their position in the scrotum in response to gonadotrophin from the fetal pituitary, in addition to testosterone.

In females, where testicular secretions are lacking, the Müllerian ducts persist and give rise to the female reproductive tract.

The fetal testis continues to secrete testosterone even after birth [3]. At 50 days of age the level of plasma testosterone (250 ng/100 mL) is more than seven times that in umbilical cord blood (35 ng/100 mL), and is unlikely to be of maternal origin. It falls to the low level of the rest of childhood by about the age of 6 months.

In males, this production of testosterone appears at first sight to be related to the activity of the sebaceous glands, which become functional by 17 weeks of gestation. The glands are large at birth and the skin surface lipid is high, approximately 400 g/cm², remaining so for approximately 3 months [4,5]. The level throughout the rest of childhood is maintained at approximately 100 g/cm².

Neonatal skin-surface lipid is, however, as high in females as in males, although the hormonal pattern is quite different; the maximum plasma testosterone occurs immediately after birth and falls very rapidly [3]. The pattern of dehydroepiandrosterone, however, very closely follows that of the casual sebum levels in both sexes [6]. For these reasons, it seems possible that the production of sebum in the neonatal period and the occurrence of acne in prepubertal children may be related to adrenal activity.

Sebaceous activity starts to increase again towards the end of childhood, in advance of other signs of approaching puberty [7,8]. Dramatic changes take place between the ages of 8 and 9 years, in both males and females [9], and it seems possible that these are related to an increase in output of adrenal androgens. Comedones start to increase around this period [10].

REFERENCES

1 Grumbach MM, Conte FA. Disorders of sexual differentiation. In: Wilson JD, Foster DW, eds. *Textbook of Endocrinology*. Philadelphia: Saunders, 1985: 312–401.
2 O'Riordan JLH, Malan PG, Gould RP, eds. *Essentials of Endocrinology*. Oxford: Blackwell Scientific Publications, 1988.
3 Forest MG, Cathiard AM, Bertrand JA. Evidence of testicular activity in early infancy. *J Clin Endocrinol Metab* 1973; **37**: 148–51.

4 Agache P, Blanc D, Barrand C et al. Sebum levels during the first year of life. Br J Dermatol 1980; **103**: 643–9.
5 Emanuel SV. Quantitative determination of the sebaceous gland's function, with particular mention of the method employed. Acta Derm Venereol (Stockh) 1936; **17**: 444.
6 de Peretti D, Forest MG. Unconjugated DHEA plasma levels in normal subjects from birth to adolescence in humans: the use of a sensitive radioimmunoassay. J Clin Endocrinol Metab 1976; **43**: 982–91.
7 Constans S, Makki S, Petiot F et al. Sebaceous levels from 6 to 15 years: comparison with pubertal events. J Invest Dermatol 1985; **84**: 454–5.
8 Pochi PE, Strauss JS, Downing DT. Age-related changes in sebaceous gland activity. J Invest Dermatol 1979; **73**: 108–11.
9 Ramasastry P, Downing DT, Pochi PE et al. Chemical composition of human skin surface lipids from birth to puberty. J Invest Dermatol 1970; **54**: 139–44.
10 Burton JL, Cunliffe WJ, Stafford I et al. The prevalence of acne vulgaris in adolescence. Br J Dermatol 1971; **85**: 119–26.

The skin in childhood

The skin, along with other organ systems, undergoes some degree of maturation during the hiatus of childhood, before the resumption of sexual development at puberty and the transition to adulthood. The skin disorders seen in children in part reflect these physiological changes, but many of the most troublesome cutaneous problems encountered result from intrinsic genetic abnormalities conditioned by environmental influences. Perhaps the best example is atopic dermatitis (see Chapter 18), which has now reached very high levels of prevalence in some societies [1]. The ways in which the environment affects the child changes as he or she becomes more mobile and travels further and further afield.

School years bring exposure to a wide variety of infections and contagions, such as measles, chickenpox, impetigo, warts, molluscum contagiosum, scabies and head lice. There is also a gradual increase in contact with potential irritants: at school during lessons, in sporting activities such as swimming and team games, and in hobbies. The wearing of jewellery and cosmetics, and exposure to sensitizers such as rubber chemicals in footwear and preservatives in medicaments, bring a further range of dermatological problems in the form of allergic contact dermatitis, which is not as rare before puberty as is often suggested [2]. One disorder that seems to have a definite predilection for the prepubertal period in girls is lichen sclerosus et atrophicus [3], which may improve and disappear as puberty approaches, although this is not always the case [4]. In boys, the same pathological changes are frequently found in prepuces removed to relieve phimosis.

There has also been an increasing awareness in recent years that both girls and boys may present to the dermatologist with symptoms and signs that indicate sexual abuse [5]. Vulval or perianal soreness and inflammation for which no other cause can be found should be considered suspicious, as should the presence of anogenital warts [6], although some are undoubtedly acquired innocently. Proof of sexual abuse is always difficult unless there has been disclosure or confession from within the family

unit. Furthermore, the social and legal implications of formal investigations for the child and his or her family are enormous. Inquiries must therefore be undertaken with care, although there is a well-established framework in many countries to deal with the problem, generally involving paediatricians, social workers and the police [5]. It is important to note that the changes associated with lichen sclerosus and Crohn's disease in childhood can be mistaken, by non-dermatologists, for evidence of sexual abuse [2], although their presence does not exclude it.

Syndromes of short stature

There is no uniformly agreed definition of short stature, although a reasonable cut-off would seem to be below the third centile for the child's community [7]. There are several disorders in which abnormal or delayed growth and development are accompanied by cutaneous changes. Some lead to short stature (a term preferred to 'dwarfism'), which is a common feature of chromosomal abnormalities. In others, delayed sexual development (infantilism) is also present, and this will be discussed briefly in relation to premature and delayed puberty. It is important to note that due allowance must be made for parental height in assessing possible delayed growth in a child [8].

Some of the more important of the disorders in which skin changes accompany short stature are listed in Table 70.1.

Furthermore, it is well known that severe skin disease of any kind in childhood can have a considerable impact on general physical development. Atopic dermatitis is a good example, short stature being very common in severely affected individuals, at least until puberty [9], although the assessment of this may be complicated by systemic or topical steroid therapy.

REFERENCES

1 Bleiker TO, Shahidullah H, Dutton E et al. The prevalence and incidence of atopic dermatitis in a birth cohort: the importance of a family history. Arch Dermatol 2000; **136**: 274.
2 Balato N, Lembo G, Patruno C et al. Patch-testing in children. Contact Dermatitis 1989; **20**: 305–7.
3 Ridley CM. Lichen sclerosus et atrophicus. Semin Dermatol 1989; **8**: 54–63.
4 Holder JE, Berth-Jones J, Graham-Brown RAC. Lichen sclerosus et atrophicus presenting in childhood: a follow-up study. Br J Dermatol 1994; **131** (Suppl. 44): 50.
5 Berth-Jones J, Graham-Brown RAC. Childhood sexual abuse: a dermatological perspective. Clin Exp Dermatol 1990; **15**: 321–30.
6 Hanson RM, Glasson M, McCrossin I et al. Anogenital warts in childhood. Child Abuse Neglect 1989; **13**: 225–33.
7 Massoud AF, Hindmarsh PC, Brock CGD. Disorders of stature. In: Grossman A, ed. Clinical Endocrinology, 2nd edn. Oxford: Blackwell Science, 1998: 855–84.
8 Tanner JM, Goldstein H, Whitehouse RH. Standards for children's height at ages 2–9 years allowing for height of parents. Arch Dis Child 1970; **45**: 755–62.
9 Verbov J. Atopic and other dermatitis. In: Essential Paediatric Dermatology. Bristol: Clinical Press, 1988: 29–46.

Often severe	Moderate
Rothmund–Thomson syndrome	Turner's syndrome
Bloom's syndrome	Hypohidrotic ectodermal dysplasia
Cockayne's syndrome	Marinesco–Sjögren syndrome
Bird-headed dwarfism	Xeroderma pigmentosum
Progeria	Trichorhinophalangeal syndrome
Cornelia de Lange syndrome	Focal dermal hypoplasia
Cartilage–hair hypoplasia	Werner's syndrome
Conradi's disease	Darier's disease
Polydysplastic epidermolysis bullosa	Atopic dermatitis
Ataxia–telangiectasia	
Leprechaunism	
GAPO	
Short stature, alopecia and macular degeneration	

Table 70.1 Disorders in which short stature may occur with cutaneous changes.

GAPO, growth retardation, alopecia, pseudo-anodontia, optic atrophy.

Puberty and adolescence

Hormonal events and cutaneous changes

Puberty is the period over which the secondary sexual characteristics gradually become manifest as the reproductive system develops to full capacity, and there is rapid somatic growth [1–3]. The term adolescence embraces these events, but is also used in a wider sense to include the phase of psychological and social adjustment to the physical changes. Thus, depending on the society, adolescence may be prolonged well beyond the completion of puberty.

The onset of puberty in the male is heralded by an increase in testicular volume resulting from the appearance of a lumen in each seminiferous tubule and an increase in the size and number of the testosterone-producing Leydig cells. Testosterone is responsible for most of the secondary changes such as enlargement of the penis and larynx, growth of pubic, axillary and beard hair, and also for a rise in sebum excretion and increased axillary sweating. Slight growth of pubic hair, probably provoked by adrenal androgens, may precede the rest and be one of the earliest visible signs of impending puberty. Facial hair usually only starts to appear about 2 years later. A full account of the patterns of hair development is given in Chapter 63.

The age at which these changes occurs is highly variable but Tanner's data on white British boys give some guidance [4–6]. In 95%, the genitalia started to enlarge at between 9.5 and 13.5 years (mean 11.6 ± 0.9 years of age), and functional maturity, indicated by ability to ejaculate, was achieved between the ages of 13 and 17 (mean 14.9 ± 1.1) years. The adolescent growth spurt, when the average gain in height reached a peak of 10 cm/year, a velocity of growth similar to that at the age of 2 years, usually occurred between 12.5 and 15 (mean 14.1 ± 0.9) years, approximately 3 years after the first signs of genital enlargement.

In girls, one of the first signs of puberty is the onset of breast development (thelarche), indicated by the elevation of the breast and papilla to form a small mound known as the breast bud [5,7]. The average age in white North American girls is 9.96 ± 1.82 years and 8.87 ± 1.93 years in their African American compatriots [8], but the breasts continue to enlarge for approximately 2 more years. Breast growth is provoked by the secretion of ovarian oestrogens; the further development of the secretory alveoli during pregnancy requires the action of progesterone as well. Pubic hair also starts to develop early (see Chapter 63). The most obvious feature of puberty, namely first menstruation or menarche, occurs at an average age of 13 years, but within an age range of 10–16.5 years. The early menstrual cycles do not usually involve ovulation, so full reproductive function is generally delayed for a further year or two. The growth spurt, with a peak height gain of 8 cm/year occurs between 10.5 and 13 years of age in white British girls [7]. This is approximately 2 years earlier than in boys. It is also noteworthy that rapid somatic growth precedes the major events of sexual maturation in girls but accompanies or succeeds them in boys.

The pubertal growth spurt appears, in both sexes, to be dependent on androgenic steroids as well as on growth hormone. Boys with growth hormone deficiency respond less well to testosterone than do normal subjects, not only in relation to acceleration of growth but also for development of the secondary sexual characteristics [9].

Gonadal function in both sexes is initiated by two gonadotrophic hormones of the pituitary, namely follicle-stimulating hormone (FSH) and luteinizing hormone (LH). In the male, initiation of spermatogenesis requires both hormones, but secretion of testosterone by the Leydig cells needs only LH. It may be noted that when the earliest sign of puberty in the female is the appearance of pubic hair, this probably results from stimulation by androgens from the adrenal cortex, so-called adrenarche, and is thus dependent on an output of hypophyseal adrenocorticotrophic hormone (ACTH).

Levels of serum FSH and LH rise in both sexes between the ages of 6 and 17 years [10]. As puberty develops, LH is released in pulses, at first only at night but later also during the day [11,12]. The secretion of both gonadotrophins from the pituitary is controlled by a single releasing hormone, gonadotrophin-releasing hormone (GnRH), a decapeptide produced in the hypothalamus. This is influenced by negative feedback of the gonadotrophins, steroid hormones and a peptide called inhibin, which is produced by the gonads [13].

The important question therefore is what initiates the pulsatile release of GnRH to invoke the onset of puberty [14,15]? Animal studies show that the central component of the neuroendocrine mechanism that governs gonadal function is fully mature by birth [14]. Pulsatile GnRH release occurs during infancy, but there is then a hiatus in GnRH release between infancy and puberty [16]. The mechanisms that control this juvenile quiescence and eventual pubertal reawakening remain uncertain.

It has long been assumed that the initiation of puberty depends on the achievement of a particular body size or composition, suggesting the existence of a central growth tracking device or 'somatometer', rather than chronological age [14,17]. It is not understood how the central nervous system detects such changes in somatic development. The metabolites or hormones that are used by the brain as signals of metabolic maturity have yet to be identified. One suggestion is that developing bone produces a peptide that enters the circulation and imposes the prepubertal hiatus. This would explain the congruence of puberty with bone age rather than with chronological age. For example, it is known that in children with constitutional delay of growth and puberty or with isolated growth hormone deficiency, sexual maturity is chronologically delayed but occurs at normal skeletal age [14].

It is also unclear whether season influences the timing of puberty, as it does for the majority of species that live in changing habitats (see [18] for a review). An annual rhythm in human reproductive success exists in most societies, but it has long been controversial whether this is related to biological or sociological factors [19]. Marked seasonal effects on the timing of puberty have been noted in the female rhesus monkey [20], and, in common with most mammals in temperate latitudes, it is the changing photoperiod that is used to time puberty [18]. Studies in sheep and various species of hamster establish unequivocally that the daily pattern of melatonin secretion from the pineal gland provides an endocrine measure of day length, and mediates its effect on reproductive function. Melatonin is secreted during the hours of darkness, and provides an accurate measure of the length of night. Melatonin is not directly pro- or antigonadotrophic; it solely provides a seasonal cue. Humans show a clear daily rhythm of mela-

tonin secretion [21], so the question arises whether it has a role in triggering puberty. Tumours of the pineal gland have been associated with both precocious and delayed puberty [22,23], although there is no experimental evidence that abnormal melatonin secretion causes reproductive malfunction in such cases. The amplitude of the nocturnal rise in melatonin secretion declines over the period of childhood, and has led to a hypothesis that puberty results from a decrease in melatonin secretion [24]. This view is not supported by animal studies. In both the rhesus monkey and sheep, puberty occurs in the autumn, when the periods of melatonin secretion are actually increasing [18,20]. It may be noted that the initial increase in LH secretion in the pubertal human first occurs at night, when melatonin secretion is high, rather than during the day when melatonin secretion is basal [25]. It seems likely that, although the human has retained a melatonin secretory system, the seasonal information that it conveys, at least, has become disregarded in the course of evolution.

Social cues may also play a part in the induction of gonadal activity, as demonstrated in many mammalian species. For example, introduction of a ram can induce an increase in LH pulse frequency and ovulation in both the seasonally anoestrus and prepubertal sheep, and this appears to be effected through a pheromonal mechanism [16,26]. The demonstration that extracts of male axillary secretions can affect the menstrual cycle when applied to the female upper lip [27] suggests that similar cues may have a role in humans.

REFERENCES

1 Falkner F, Tanner JM, eds. *Human Growth*, Vols 1–3. New York: Plenum Press, 1986.
2 Sinclair D. *Human Growth After Birth*, 5th edn. Oxford: Oxford University Press, 1989.
3 Underwood LE, Van Wyk JJ. Normal and aberrant growth. In: Wilson JD, Farber DW, eds. *Williams' Textbook of Endocrinology*, 7th edn. Philadelphia: Saunders, 1985: 155–205.
4 Marshall WA, Tanner JM. Variations in the pattern of pubertal changes in boys. *Arch Dis Child* 1970; **45**: 13–23.
5 Tanner JM. *Growth at Adolescence*. Oxford: Blackwell Scientific Publications, 1962.
6 Tanner JM, Whitehouse RH. Clinical longitudinal standards for height, weight, height velocity, weight velocity and stages of puberty. *Arch Dis Child* 1976; **51**: 170–9.
7 Marshall WA, Tanner JM. Variations in pattern of pubertal changes in girls. *Arch Dis Child* 1969; **44**: 291–303.
8 Gilli D, Schenker J. The evolving story of female puberty. *Gynecol Endocrinol* 2002; **16**: 163–71.
9 Zachmann M, Aynsley-Green A, Prader A. Interrelations of the effects of growth hormone and testosterone in hypopituitarism. In: Pecile A, Müller EE, eds. *Growth Hormone and Related Peptides*. Amsterdam: Excerpta Medica, 1976: 286–96.
10 Faiman C, Winter JSD. Gonadotrophins and sex hormone patterns in puberty: clinical data. In: Grumbach MM, Grave GD, Mayer FE, eds. *Control of the Onset of Puberty*. New York: Wiley, 1974: 33–5.
11 Plant TM. Puberty in primates. In: Knobil E, Neill JD, Ewing LL *et al.*, eds. *The Physiology of Reproduction*. New York: Raven Press, 1988: 1763–88.
12 Wu FCW, Borrow SM, Nicol K *et al.* Ontogeny of pulsatile gonadotrophin secretion and pituitary responsiveness in male puberty in man: a mixed longitudinal and cross-sectional study. *J Endocrinol* 1989; **123**: 347–59.

13 O'Riordan JLH, Malan PG, Gould RP. *Essentials of Endocrinology.* Oxford: Blackwell Scientific Publications, 1988.

14 Plant TM, Fraser MO, Medhamurthy R *et al.* Somatogenic control of GnRH neuronal synchronization during development in primates: a speculation. In: Delemarre-van de Waal HA, Plant TM, van Rees GP *et al.*, eds. *Control of the Onset of Puberty*, Vol. 3. Amsterdam: Excerpta Medica, 1989: 111–21.

15 Terasawa E, Claypool LE, Gore AC *et al.* The timing of the onset of puberty in the female rhesus monkey. In: Delemarre-van de Waal HA, Plant TM, van Rees GP *et al.*, eds. *Control of the Onset of Puberty*, Vol. 3. Amsterdam: Excerpta Medica, 1989: 123–36.

16 Foster DL, Ebling FJP, Ryan KD *et al.* Mechanisms timing puberty: a comparative approach. In: Delemarre-van de Waal HA, Plant TM, van Rees GP *et al.*, eds. *Control of the Onset of Puberty*, Vol. 3. Amsterdam: Excerpta Medica, 1989: 227–45.

17 Frisch RE. Body fat, puberty and fertility. *Biol Rev* 1984; **59**: 161–88.

18 Ebling FJP, Foster DL. Pineal melatonin rhythms and the timing of puberty in mammals. *Experientia* 1989; **45**: 946–54.

19 Roenneberg T, Aschoff J. Annual rhythm of human reproduction. I. Biology, sociology or both. *J Biol Rhythm* 1990; 5: 195–216.

20 Wilson ME, Gordon TP. Season determines timing of first ovulation in outdoor-housed rhesus monkeys. *J Reprod Fertil* 1989; **85**: 583–91.

21 Arendt J. Melatonin and the human circadian system. In: Miles A, Philbrick DRS, Thompson C, eds. *Melatonin: Clinical Perspectives.* Oxford: Oxford University Press, 1988: 43–61.

22 Reichlin S. Neuroendocrinology. In: Williams RH, ed. *Textbook of Endocrinology.* Philadelphia: Saunders, 1981: 492–567.

23 Weinberger LM, Grant FC. Precocious puberty and tumors of the hypothalamus. *Arch Intern Med* 1941; **67**: 762–92.

24 Waldhauser F, Weizsenbacher G, Tatzer E *et al.* Alterations in nocturnal serum melatonin levels with growth and aging. *J Clin Endocrinol Metab* 1988; **66**: 648–52.

25 Fevre M, Segel T, Marks JM *et al.* LH and melatonin secretion patterns in pubertal boys. *J Clin Endocrinol Metab* 1979; **47**: 1383–6.

26 Ebling FJP, Foster DL. Seasonal breeding: a model for puberty? In: Delemarre-van de Waal HA, Plant TM, van Rees GP *et al.*, eds. *Control of the Onset of Puberty*, Vol. 3. Amsterdam: Excerpta Medica, 1989: 253–64.

27 Cutler WB, Preti G, Krieger A *et al.* Human axillary secretions influence women's menstrual cycles: the role of donor extract from men. *Horm Behav* 1986; **20**: 463–73.

Dermatoses of puberty and adolescence

Adolescence is a difficult period for most people. It is a time when the whole emphasis of relationships is supposed to change from the herd bond of the 'gang' to the pair bond of courtship and sexual involvement, but this does not happen all at once or completely. Most of us retain a need for the approbation of our peers throughout life, as well as a desire to develop a close one-to-one relationship. The tensions involved in this are at their most acute during adolescence and, for this reason, many skin diseases, which first presented during childhood, only begin to exert their most damaging influences after the onset of puberty. Adolescence is a bad time to have skin disease, especially on the face or on the extremities.

The physiological changes that occur in the skin during puberty and adolescence also have several effects, and may result in sufficient distress to cause the individual to seek medical advice. There are several examples of this: the increase in sebum production often results in unacceptably greasy hair, on which many hours and much money is expended; teenagers often present with secondary sexual hair that they perceive to be abnormal, largely as a result of the pressure exerted by the media; young

Table 70.2 Disorders that present in or cause particular problems during adolescence.

Acne vulgaris
Acne excoriée and neurotic excoriation
Self-mutilation and dermatitis artefacta
Seborrhoeic dermatitis
Pityriasis versicolor
Hyperhidrosis
Axillary bromhidrosis (body odour)
Hidradenitis suppurativa
Fox–Fordyce disease
Polymorphic light eruption
Epidermolysis bullosa simplex (Weber–Cockayne syndrome)
Psoriasis
Atopic dermatitis

men become anguished when male-pattern balding begins in the teenage years; members of both sexes become disturbed by the onset of 'body odour'.

It has been pointed out that the pressures of coping with a maturing skin are particularly acute for a girl who is persuaded by advertisers that she should have plenty of hair on her head, but none on her face, under her arms or on her legs. Her skin should be free from grease, spots and wrinkles and, moreover, should be odourless [1]. Puberty makes this ideal image virtually impossible to achieve. Several disorders cause special problems or make their first appearance in adolescence. The classic example is acne vulgaris but there are several others (Table 70.2).

Teenagers may present with a variety of skin disorders in which self-inflicted injury is an important component (Fig. 70.1), varying from mild excoriated acne to severe habitual mutilation. The mental state of these individuals ranges from simple mild anxiety to gross personality disorder, psychotic disturbance and instability. Extreme forms of deliberate self-harm almost invariably begin in adolescence, but most continue for many years [2].

Seborrhoeic dermatitis is generally seen only from adolescence onwards, as is pityriasis versicolor in temperate climates. An explanation for this may lie in the alterations in sebum that appear to occur at puberty [3], especially if it is accepted that yeast organisms have a role in seborrhoeic dermatitis (see Chapter 17). This alteration in sebum is also said to be responsible for the virtual disappearance of scalp ringworm after puberty.

Teenagers may seek help for a number of different axillary problems. Severe eccrine hyperhidrosis can be a very distressing complaint, but usually responds well to treatment (see Chapter 45), as does axillary odour (bromhidrosis). More difficult to deal with are abnormalities of the apocrine glands (hidradenitis and Fox–Fordyce disease).

Polymorphic light eruption often presents for the first time in adolescence, and can ruin summer holidays. So does psoriasis [4]; 25% of 5600 patients with psoriasis

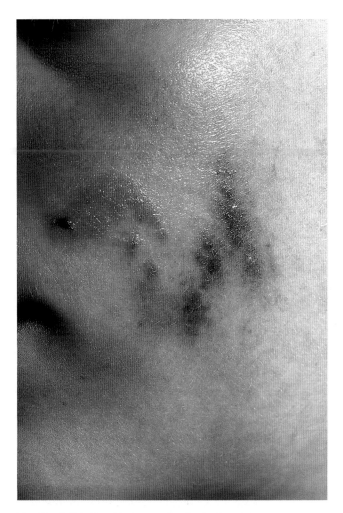

Fig. 70.1 Self-inflicted lesions on the cheek of a teenager.

dated the onset of their disease to between the ages of 10 and 20 years [5]. The impact of the appearance of psoriasis on a teenager should not be underestimated. The patient will be told that psoriasis is probably genetic, that it is likely to continue to be a lifelong problem and that there is no satisfactory cure. All this has to be assimilated during a period of increasing awareness of the importance of being attractive.

Atopic dermatitis can also be a major problem for the teenager and his or her family. It may present for the first time in adolescence, but this is rare. More commonly, children do not grow out of it as they have been led to believe, or atopic dermatitis may disappear during childhood only to reappear in adolescence. In this situation, the skin changes and pruritus are often severe, and usually have already affected the enjoyment of childhood. The adolescent is then quite abruptly faced with the prospect of the skin problem continuing for an apparently indefinite period into adult life. Many, if not all, affected teenagers become increasingly depressed and frustrated, and a sense of hopelessness can descend on the whole family.

Many patients completely lose faith in orthodox medicine and seek advice from homeopaths, herbalists, naturopaths and others. A truly sympathetic and holistic approach is therefore required if the dermatologist is to retain the confidence of his or her young patient and their relatives through this difficult period. Good communication needs to be cultivated and maintained. Professional counselling facilities can be very helpful, but are often neglected or not available.

Another troublesome aspect of atopic dermatitis in adolescence is that there is a greater tendency to develop involvement of the hands (and feet) as the years go by. This can lead to difficulties in choosing a suitable occupation (see below). Furthermore, treatment parameters usually differ in adolescents and adults from those in childhood atopic dermatitis [6]. In particular, the information and support needs differ and, in practical therapeutic terms, steroid-sparing strategies may become more important.

Some congenital and genetic diseases, such as tuberous sclerosis and neurofibromatosis, may progress during the teenage years, causing increasing physical and cosmetic disability. Others (e.g. ichthyotic disorders, pigmentary anomalies and port-wine stains), even though largely static, may exert a greater effect because of the social and psychological tensions of adolescence.

However, some disorders improve at puberty. For example, atopic dermatitis clears in many individuals, and autosomal dominant ichthyosis tends to improve.

Skin disease and career

Young people with skin disease are often not aware that they may be at a major disadvantage in pursuing some occupations.

The armed forces medically examine all recruits, and are unlikely to accept anyone with psoriasis, significant atopic dermatitis or bad acne. It is therefore preferable for acne to be eradicated before rather than after application.

Psoriasis and eczema of the hands can be troublesome for those hoping to work in catering. Although they may be accepted by colleges to study, such individuals often find it difficult to obtain subsequent employment.

Hand dermatitis among hairdressers is a far greater problem in those with active atopic dermatitis and in those who have been troubled in the past than in those who are unaffected [7]. A teenager with atopic dermatitis may work in a hair salon for months or even years suffering with hand dermatitis before eventually giving up. The same applies to nursing, where many committed individuals are rejected at the occupational health screen because of eczema. The reasons given include the exposure to irritants that the skin will inevitably have during a nurse's normal duties, and the increased risk of contracting hepatitis and acquired immune deficiency syndrome (AIDS) through broken skin.

Any teenager with a chronic skin disease, especially of the hands, should therefore be made aware of the potential difficulties that he or she may face in the choice of a future occupation. It is better that a change be made early on than after working hard to achieve a set of educational and vocational goals that are unobtainable.

REFERENCES

1 Cotterill JA. Infantile cutaneous ideas. *Br J Dermatol* 1987; **117** (Suppl. 32): 22–3.
2 Favazza AR, Conterio K. Female habitual self-mutilators. *Acta Psychiatr Scand* 1989; **79**: 283–9.
3 Stewart ME, Steele WA, Downing DT. Changes in the relative amounts of endogenous and exogenous fatty acids in sebaceous lipids during early adolescence. *J Invest Dermatol* 1989; **92**: 371–8.
4 Ingram JT. The significance and management of psoriasis. *BMJ* 1954; **ii**: 823–8.
5 Farber EM, Nall LM. The natural history of psoriasis in 5600 patients. *Dermatologica* 1974; **148**: 1–18.
6 Graham-Brown RAC. Managing adults with atopic dermatitis. *Dermatol Clin* 1996; **124**: 531–7.
7 Cronin E. Hairdresser. *Contact Dermatitis*. Edinburgh: Churchill Livingstone, 1980: 134–9.

Premature and delayed puberty and hypogonadism

Although it must be acknowledged that the measurement of the onset and progress of puberty remains somewhat controversial [1], the dermatologist will occasionally see patients with what is a clearly abnormally early or delayed puberty, or with various hypogonadal syndromes. The appearance or non-appearance of sexual hair, or the onset of acne lesions in late childhood are the usual reasons for such referrals. Premature and delayed puberty are matters for endocrinological investigations, but the dermatologist should at least be aware of the range of diagnostic possibilities.

Premature puberty

Signs of puberty before the age of 10 years are generally held to be abnormal. This may result from an early onset of complete (or true) puberty, in which the changes are triggered by early activation of the normal hypothalamo–pituitary–gonadal axis. In some instances, early signs of puberty are caused by false (or pseudo-) puberty, in which sex hormone secretion is independent of the normal control mechanisms. Partial or incomplete puberty is also recognized, and there are two forms: thelarche (isolated breast development) and pubarche (isolated development of pubic and axillary hair). The former may be unilateral and be confused with tumours. It is not clear what causes isolated breast enlargement, although tissue hypersensitivity to oestrogen has been suggested (see Chapter 67). Pubarche is often associated with adrenal androgen secretion, and this may be a priming phenomenon in the early

Table 70.3 Classification of premature puberty. (From Rayner [3].)

Complete (true)	*False (pseudopuberty)*
Constitutional	Adrenal lesions
Sporadic	Congenital adrenal hyperplasia
Familial	Tumours
Cerebral/neurogenic	Cushing's syndrome/hyperplasia
Tumours	Ovarian tumours
Development defects	Testicular tumours
CNS infections	Iatrogenic (sex hormones)
CNS trauma	
McCune–Albright syndrome	*Extrapituitary gonadotrophin-secreting tumours*
Neurofibromatosis	Teratoma
Tuberous sclerosis	Chorionepithelioma
Silver's syndrome	Hepatoblastoma
Hypothyroidism	
Pineal lesions	
Incomplete	
Premature thelarche, pubarche	

CNS, central nervous system.

phases of normal pubertal development [2]. Indeed, the very early, isolated appearance of sexual hair may presage a true early puberty, and the distinction can be a very fine one. Table 70.3 gives a clinical classification of early puberty.

Most instances of premature, complete puberty are constitutional. Although this may be sporadic, there is often a strong family history. Indeed, it seems likely that many families never present at all, accepting that it is quite normal for them. This is particularly true for girls, in whom approximately 80% of premature puberty is thought to be constitutional [3]. There is no difference in the order of events, but mental and emotional development may lag behind the physical changes. In boys, where the event is rarer, there is more often an underlying pathological condition [4].

The investigation of complete premature puberty is obviously a complex process, especially if a neurogenic origin is suspected, but the dermatologist should always look for other features of the specific syndromes listed in Table 70.3: McCune–Albright syndrome, neurofibromatosis, tuberous sclerosis and Silver's syndrome (short stature, craniofacial disproportion and clinodactyly [4]), as well as hypothyroidism.

REFERENCES

1 Coleman L, Coleman J. The measurement of puberty: a review. *J Adolesc* 2002; **25**: 535–50.
2 Ducharme JR, Forest MG, De Peretti E *et al.* Plasma adrenal and gonadal sex steroids in human pubertal development. *J Clin Endocrinol Metab* 1976; **42**: 468–76.
3 Rayner PHW. Early puberty. In: Brook CGD, ed. *Clinical Paediatric Endocrinology*. Oxford: Blackwell Scientific Publications, 1981: 224–39.
4 Silver HK. Asymmetry, short stature, and variations in sexual development: a syndrome of congenital malformations. *Am J Dis Child* 1964; **107**: 495–515.

Delayed puberty and hypogonadism

Puberty can be considered delayed if there is no sign of sexual development by the age of 15 years in boys and 14 years in girls [1]. There are a number of important causes, listed in Table 70.4. Constitutional delay accounts for at least 50% of male cases, and is much more common than in girls [1].

As with premature puberty, pubertal delay requires endocrinological investigation. However, a dermatologist can make a useful contribution if the patient presents first in the skin clinic. Examination can reveal the obesity, short stature and mental retardation of the Prader–Willi syndrome, the polydactyly of the Laurence–Moon–Biedl syndrome, or the increased height and gynaecomastia of Klinefelter's syndrome.

Table 70.4 Causes of delayed puberty. (From Chaussain [1], Kulin [2] and Santen & Kulin [3].)

Constitutional delay
Hypogonadotrophism
  Isolated gonadotrophin deficiency
    Hypogonadotrophic eunuchoidism (Kallmann's syndrome)
  Multiple hormonal deficiency states
    Idiopathic
    Tumours
    Langerhans' cell histiocytosis
    Tuberculosis
    Sarcoidosis
    Vascular disease
    Haemochromatosis
  Hyperprolactinaemia
  Specific syndromes with hypogonadotrophism
    Prader–Willi
    Laurence–Moon–Biedl
    Multiple lentigines
    Rud's
    Cerebellar ataxia
  Systemic disease
    Chronic renal failure
    Congenital heart disease
    Cystic fibrosis
    Thalassaemia major
    Diabetes mellitus
    Hypothyroidism
    Gluten intolerance
    Anorexia nervosa
  Excessive exercise
Hypergonadotrophic hypogonadism
  Klinefelter's syndrome
  Ullrich–Turner syndrome
  Dystrophia myotonica
  Trisomy 21 (Down's syndrome)
  17β-Hydroxylase deficiency
  Androgen insensitivity (testicular feminization syndrome)
  Surgical accidents (e.g. during herniorraphy)
  Testicular torsion
  Anorchia and bilateral cryptorchidism
  Irradiation and cytotoxic drugs
  Orchitis (e.g. mumps)
  Polycystic ovarian disease

Many extraneous factors can also affect the onset of puberty. Malnutrition and extreme forms of exercise, such as long-distance running and ballet training, may markedly delay onset of puberty, probably by interfering with hypothalamic triggering mechanisms [4,5].

REFERENCES

1 Chaussain J-L. Late puberty. In: Brook CGD, ed. *Clinical Paediatric Endocrinology.* Oxford: Blackwell Scientific Publications, 1981: 240–7.
2 Kulin HE. Disorders of sexual maturation: delayed adolescence and precocious puberty. In: De Groot LJ, ed. *Endocrinology,* 2nd edn. Philadelphia: Saunders, 1989: 1873–99.
3 Santen RJ, Kulin HE. *Evaluation of Delayed Puberty and Hypogonadism.* In: Santen RJ, Swerdloff RS, eds. *Male Reproductive Dysfunction.* New York: Dekker, 1986: 145–89.
4 MacConnie SE, Barkan A, Lampman RM *et al.* Decreased hypothalamic gonadotrophin releasing hormone secretion in male marathon runners. *N Engl J Med* 1986; **315**: 411–7.
5 Warren PW. Effects of undernutrition on reproductive function in the human. *Endocrinol Rev* 1983; **4**: 363–77.

The menstrual cycle

Hormonal influences [1,2]

The menstrual cycle involves changes in the genital tract, which are brought about by two hormones from the ovary. At the start of each cycle, after menstruation is completed, the repair and proliferation of the endometrium, and the synthesis of receptors for progesterone and oestradiol within its cells, are effected by the rising secretion of oestradiol. Following ovulation and the formation of the corpus luteum, the rise in progesterone causes the endometrium to double in thickness and the tubular glands to become tortuous and sacculated. The maintenance of this secretory phase is dependent on both oestradiol and progesterone, and the breakdown of the endometrium that causes menstrual bleeding is a consequence of the withdrawal of these hormones. The cyclic hormonal changes also affect the vaginal epithelium, which can be monitored through desquamated cells in vaginal smears, the consistency and pH of the cervical mucus, and several features of the skin.

Synthesis of oestrogens in the ovary first involves the production of the androgens androstenedione and testosterone, in the theca interna cells of the follicle, and then their conversion to oestrone and oestradiol in the granulosa cells. These processes are stimulated by LH from the pituitary. However, the increased production of oestradiol between the eighth and tenth days of the cycle is also dependent on FSH in the sense that this is responsible for the development of numbers of primary follicles in the early follicular phase, which increases the number of granulosa cells.

Ovulation in the middle of the cycle is associated with surges in both LH and, to a lesser extent, FSH. The surge in LH lasts for approximately 36 h, and is affected by pulsatile output of GnRH from the hypothalamus. It appears that feedback by oestradiol is responsible: in the early follicular phase, oestradiol acts to inhibit secretion of gonadotrophin but, as the follicle ripens, a threshold is exceeded which switches the feedback from negative to positive.

REFERENCES

1 O'Riordan JLH, Malan PG, Gould RP, eds. *Essentials of Endocrinology.* Oxford: Blackwell Scientific Publications, 1988.
2 Ross GT. Disorders of the ovary and female reproductive tract. In: Wilson JD, Foster DW, eds. *Textbook of Endocrinology.* Philadelphia: Saunders, 1985: 206–58.

Cutaneous changes

Many women notice changes in their skin and hair during the course of the monthly cycle. For example, 70% of Scottish women reported a few acne papules during the premenstrual phase of their cycle, and a significant number of others experienced textural variations. Some found the skin and hair greasier (35%), others drier (16%) [1], despite the fact that sebum production has not reliably been shown to alter significantly. Pre-existing skin disorders, other than acne, may also undergo premenstrual exacerbation; examples are psoriasis, rosacea, atopic dermatitis, lupus erythematosus, anogenital pruritus, recurrent aphthae and herpes simplex [2,3].

Some women experience premenstrual flushing identical in quality to that associated with the menopause. In one study of 120 women with classical features of the so-called premenstrual syndrome, 72% were observed to have such flushing episodes [4]. This phenomenon may be related in part to the general increase in cutaneous vascularity during the second half of the menstrual cycle [5], but detailed investigation of one of these women revealed that each flush (recorded using skin resistance and finger temperature) coincided with a measurable pulse of LH. Identical findings are reported in menopausal flushes (see p. 70.20), suggesting a common pathogenesis.

Other cutaneous disturbances described in the 'premenstrual syndrome', include minor non-specific abnormalities and recurrent boils. Premenstrual oedema has also been described, most commonly of the feet and ankles, but occasionally involving the hands and even the face. In rare individuals this may be very marked.

It is not at all clear what causes most of the symptoms associated with the 'premenstrual syndrome', but there have been many suggestions, including hormonal influences, abnormalities of fluid balance, nutritional changes (including essential fatty acid depletion), neurotransmitters and psychological factors. It seems most probable that the syndrome is a complex of interrelated problems, each with a different basic cause or causes [6].

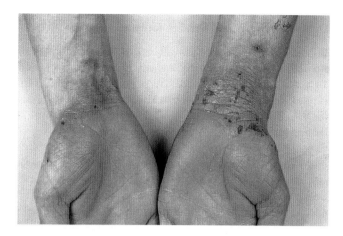

Fig. 70.2 Autoimmune progesterone dermatitis. (Courtesy of Dr J.D. Wilkinson, Amersham Hospital, Amersham, UK.)

Autoimmune progesterone dermatitis (Fig. 70.2)

There are also patients in whom the regular appearance of skin changes in the premenstrual period is associated with evidence of hypersensitivity to progesterone. This has generally been established by skin testing, deliberate challenge with progesterone or the presence of antibodies [7], and the term autoimmune progesterone dermatitis has been coined for this syndrome. The cutaneous lesions that have been described are very variable, resembling eczema, particularly the pompholyx type; urticaria; erythema multiforme [8]; or dermatitis herpetiformis [9]. Many patients develop the eruption after receiving exogenous synthetic progesterone preparations.

Treatment of autoimmune progesterone dermatitis can be difficult. Most patients are unresponsive to topical steroids and antihistamines, but some respond to oestrogen or tamoxifen therapy [7]. One resistant patient required bilateral oophorectomy [9].

REFERENCES

1 Sutherland H, Stewart I. A critical analysis of the premenstrual syndrome. *Lancet* 1965; **i**: 1180–3.
2 Anderson RH. Autoimmune progesterone dermatitis. *Cutis* 1984; **33**: 490–1.
3 Dalton K. Premenstrual tension: an overview. In: Friedmann RC, ed. *Behavior and the Menstrual Cycle.* New York: Dekker, 1982: 217–42.
4 Casper RF, Graves GR, Reid RL. Objective measurement of hot flushes associated with the premenstrual syndrome. *Fertil Steril* 1987; **47**: 341–4.
5 Edwards EA, Duntley SQ. Cutaneous vascular changes in women in reference to the menstrual cycle and ovariectomy. *Am J Obstet Gynecol* 1949; **57**: 501–9.
6 Hart RJ, Magos AL. Premenstrual tension and the premenstrual syndrome. In: Grossman A, ed. *Clinical Endocrinology*, 2nd edn. Oxford: Blackwell Science, 1998: 731–9.
7 Stephens CJM, Wojnarowska FT, Wilkinson JD. Autoimmune progesterone dermatitis responding to tamoxifen. *Br J Dermatol* 1989; **121**: 135–7.
8 Wojnarowska FT, Greaves MW, Peachey RGD *et al.* Progesterone-induced erythema multiforme. *J R Soc Med* 1985; **78**: 407–8.
9 Shelley WB, Purcel R, Spount S. Autoimmune progesterone dermatitis. *JAMA* 1964; **190**: 35–8.

Pregnancy, childbirth and the puerperium

Pregnancy, childbirth and the puerperium are associated with profound physiological endocrine upheavals. Many of the consequent cutaneous changes should be considered normal, although not every woman is happy to accept them in this light. The physiological events of pregnancy and its resolution can also modify a number of concomitant dermatoses and tumours, and there are also some pathological skin conditions that are virtually pregnancy-specific.

Endocrine background [1–3]

Pregnancy is characterized by the advent of a new and unique endocrine organ (the placenta). The endocrine changes of pregnancy start soon after the fertilized ovum becomes implanted in the endometrium, when the developing trophoblast begins to secrete chorionic gonadotrophin. This, in turn, stimulates production of oestrogen and progesterone by the corpus luteum. The increase in the concentration of these steroids suppresses the production of FSH by the pituitary and thus prevents further ovulation. At about the ninth week of pregnancy the fetoplacental unit begins to synthesize pregnenolone and progesterone. Pregnenolone crosses to the fetus and is converted to dehydroepiandrosterone by the developing fetal adrenal. This, in turn, returns to the placenta to be aromatized to oestriol. From about the 12th week there are increasing amounts of oestriol and progesterone, and the corpus luteum of pregnancy regresses.

The placenta also produces lactogen (hPL) in quantities as great as 1 g/day by late pregnancy. This hormone has some somatotrophic as well as lactogenic properties. A human chorionic thyrotrophin (hCT), structurally different from pituitary thyroid-stimulating hormone (TSH), has also been isolated.

Placental hormones are partly responsible for the physiological adaptations that occur in pregnancy including, for example, a considerable increase in blood volume. The thyroid enlarges and takes up more iodine. The pituitary also enlarges and increases its output of ACTH, prolactin and gonadotrophins. Circulating cortisol rises, caused mainly by a decrease in its rate of clearance combined with an increase in cortisol-binding globulin.

The breasts enlarge during pregnancy, most noticeably towards term. In the early phases of a first pregnancy there is a rapid growth and branching of the terminal portions of glandular tissue, together with an increase in the vascularity of the breast as a whole. Later, true acini appear for the first time, and alveolar secretion begins during the second trimester. In the last weeks there is considerable parenchymal cell enlargement and the alveoli become distended with colostrum [3].

The state of pregnancy is ended, at least in part, by an alteration in the balance of the antagonistic actions of oestrogen and progesterone. This is probably 'fine-tuned' by the fetal pituitary–adrenal axis and its effect on oestrogen production [1]. Thus, abnormalities of the fetal brain, such as anencephaly, may lead to abnormally early or late onset of parturition. The tendency of labour to be delayed in mothers bearing children with X-linked ichthyosis is caused by a reduction in the processing of hormones by the placental enzyme steroid sulphatase (see Chapter 34).

After birth, the mother's hormonal status changes yet again. Levels of prolactin rise steadily towards the end of pregnancy, and at childbirth the apparently inhibitory effect of the fetoplacental steroid hormones is suddenly lost, leaving prolactin acting unopposed. This initiates lactation [3].

REFERENCES

1 Casey ML, Macdonald PC, Simpson ER. Endocrinological changes of pregnancy. In: Wilson JD, Foster DW, eds. *Williams' Textbook of Endocrinology*, 7th edn. Philadelphia: Saunders, 1985: 422–37.
2 Buster JE, Simon JA. Placental hormones, hormonal preparation for and control of parturition, and hormonal diagnosis of pregnancy. In: De Groot LJ, ed. *Endocrinology*, 2nd edn. Philadelphia: Saunders, 1989: 2043–73.
3 Friesen HG, Cowden EA. Lactation and galactorrhoea. In: De Groot LJ, ed. *Endocrinology*, 2nd edn. Philadelphia: Saunders, 1989: 2074–86.

Physiological skin changes related to pregnancy

Pigmentation (see Chapter 39)

Most women notice a generalized increase in skin pigmentation during pregnancy, and the change is more marked in dark-haired than in fair-haired women. Areas that are already pigmented become darker, in particular the nipples, areolae, genital areas and the midline of the abdominal wall. In consequence, the 'linea alba' ('white line') may become brown. The pigmentation usually fades after delivery, but seldom to its previous level. Many women also notice an increase in the size, activity and number of melanocytic naevi.

In approximately 70% of women, especially those of dark complexion, chloasmal pigmentation also develops during the second half of pregnancy. Its intensity is not necessarily proportional to that of the general melanosis. Irregular, sharply marginated areas of pigmentation develop in a roughly symmetrical pattern either on the forehead and temples, or on the central part of the face, or both. It usually fades completely after parturition, but may persist.

Similar changes occur in other species. The pigmentary changes of pregnancy have been induced experimentally in non-pregnant guinea pigs by the injection of small doses of oestrogen and progesterone [1]. The extent to which human pigmentary changes are brought about by these steroids or by melanocyte-stimulating hormones derived from pro-opiomelanocortin (see Chapter 39) is uncertain [2–4].

Hair and nail changes

Many women maintain that hair growth on the scalp is more vigorous during pregnancy. In the latter part, the proportion of follicles in anagen rises, but a compensatory decrease after parturition associated with shedding of hairs may result in noticeable postpartum alopecia [5,6]. Spontaneous recovery is usual. Mild frontoparietal recession may also occur [7].

Minor degrees of hypertrichosis are not uncommon. Hirsutism, accompanied by acne and, in severe cases, by other evidence of virilization, occurs rarely, usually during the second half of pregnancy. It may result from an androgen-secreting tumour, luteoma, lutein cysts or polycystic ovary disease [8,9]. All cases should be thoroughly investigated. A female fetus may be masculinized. In the absence of a tumour that can be eradicated, the problem tends to recur in subsequent pregnancies. Hirsutism may regress between pregnancies, but this is not always complete.

Pregnant women often report brittleness of the nail plate, and some develop distal onycholysis, similar to that seen occasionally in thyrotoxicosis [7].

Eccrine, apocrine and sebaceous gland activity

Eccrine activity may be noticeably increased during pregnancy [7], although palmar sweating diminishes [10]. This may be responsible for the recognized increased frequency of miliaria. It is often said that apocrine gland activity is reduced during pregnancy, but the evidence is conflicting. Hurley and Shelley [11] were unable to find any increase in apocrine sweating immediately postpartum, but they pointed out that Fox–Fordyce disease usually improves in pregnancy, which suggests that apocrine activity has been reduced.

Although there is considerable individual variation, the rate of sebum excretion tends to increase during pregnancy and return to normal after delivery [12].

The rise in sebum excretion during the last trimester of pregnancy, at a time when oestrogens, which suppress sebum secretion, are being produced in large quantities, suggests that a powerful sebotrophic stimulus is released. The sebum excretion rate in women with twins or triplets is no greater than the rate in women with a single fetus, suggesting that the sebotrophic factor comes from the pituitary rather than the placenta [13]. Sebum excretion does not fall in women who are lactating [14], and suckling presumably promotes secretion of pituitary factors, such as prolactin, which either stimulate sebaceous glands directly or enhance their response to androgens.

REFERENCES

1 Snell RS, Bischitz PG. The effect of large doses of estrogen and progesterone on melanin pigmentation. *J Invest Dermatol* 1960; **35**: 73–82.
2 Dahlberg BCG. Melanocyte stimulating substances in the urine of pregnant women. *Acta Endocrinol* 1961; **60** (Suppl.): 1–51.
3 McGuinness BW. The pigment cell: molecular, biological, clinical aspects. II. Melanocyte stimulating hormone: a clinical and laboratory study. *Ann NY Acad Sci* 1963; **100**: 640–57.
4 Thody AJ, Plummer NA, Burton JL *et al.* Plasma b-melanocyte stimulating hormone levels in pregnancy. *J Obstet Gynaecol Br Comm* 1974; **81**: 875–7.
5 Lynfield YL. Effect of pregnancy on the human hair cycle. *J Invest Dermatol* 1960; **35**: 323–7.
6 Pecoraro V, Barman JM, Astore I. The normal trichogram of pregnant women. In: Montagna W, Dobson RL, eds. *Advances in Biology of Skin*, Vol. 9. *Hair Growth*. Oxford: Pergamon, 1969: 203–20.
7 Winton GB, Lewis CW. Dermatoses of pregnancy. *J Am Acad Dermatol* 1982; **6**: 977–8.
8 Fayez JA, Bunch TR, Miller GL. Virilization in pregnancy associated with polycystic ovary disease. *Obstet Gynecol* 1974; **44**: 511–21.
9 Judd HL, Benirschke K, De Vane G *et al.* Maternal virilization developing during a twin pregnancy. *N Engl J Med* 1973; **288**: 118–22.
10 MacKinnon PCB, MacKinnon IL. Palmar sweating in pregnancy. *J Obstet Gynaecol Br Emp* 1955; **62**: 298–9.
11 Hurley HL, Shelley WB. *The Human Apocrine Gland in Health and Disease.* Springfield: Thomas, 1960: 65–6.
12 Burton JL, Cunliffe WJ, Millar DG *et al.* Effect of pregnancy on sebum excretion. *BMJ* 1970; **ii**: 769–71.
13 Burton JL, Shuster S, Cartlidge M. The sebotrophic effect of pregnancy. *Acta Derm Venereol (Stockh)* 1975; **55**: 11–3.
14 Burton JL, Shuster S, Cartlidge M *et al.* Lactation, sebum excretion and melanocyte-stimulating hormone. *Nature* 1973; **243**: 349–50.

Vascular changes

The vascular changes of pregnancy do not differ qualitatively from those in hyperthyroidism or cirrhosis. All are thought to be brought about by the sustained high levels of circulating oestrogen. Vascular 'spiders' are very common in white women but said to be less so in black women [1]. They usually disappear postpartum. Palmar erythema is also common, affecting at least 70% of white women and 30% of black women [2]. In some, it takes the form of a diffuse pink mottling of the whole palm, whereas in others the changes are confined to the thenar and hypothenar eminences [3]. Palmar erythema and vascular spiders commonly occur together.

Less commonly, pregnant women develop small haemangiomas [4,5]. These usually affect the head and neck (Fig. 70.3), and occur in approximately 5% of pregnancies [4].

Varicose veins of the legs and haemorrhoids are frequent complications of pregnancy. A rarer but more serious event is the development of deep-vein thrombosis, which can lead to permanent damage to the leg veins and, occasionally, death from pulmonary embolism. Many pregnant women (possibly 50%) also develop non-pitting oedema of the face, eyelids, feet and hands [6]. The swelling is usually most pronounced in the early morning and disappears during the course of the day. There is no known treatment, but it is important to recognize and differentiate the condition from cardiac, renal or pre-eclamptic oedema.

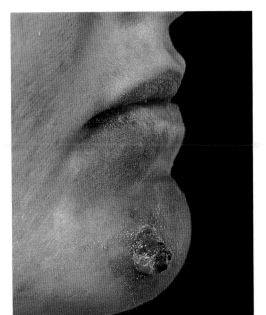

Fig. 70.3 Pyogenic granuloma in a port-wine stain during pregnancy. This woman had similar lesions in three successive pregnancies.

Gingivitis and pregnancy 'epulis'

Eighty per cent or more of pregnant women develop some gingival oedema and redness [6,7]. This can become painful and ulcerative, especially if oral hygiene is poor. In approximately 2%, the gingival changes are associated with the appearance of a small vascular lesion similar to a pyogenic granuloma, known as a pregnancy epulis or granuloma gravidarum. This may bleed profusely on contact. These phenomena, like palmar erythema and vascular spiders, are probably brought about by the general increase in vascularity associated with high oestrogen levels.

In most women, gum changes resolve after parturition. Vitamin C has been used to try to improve the symptomatology.

REFERENCES

1 Winton GB, Lewis CW. Dermatoses of pregnancy. *J Am Acad Dermatol* 1982; **6**: 977–98.
2 Cummings K, Derbes VJ. Dermatoses associated with pregnancy. *Cutis* 1967; **3**: 120–5.
3 Black MM, Mayou SC. Skin diseases in pregnancy. In: de Swiet M, ed. *Medical Disorders in Obstetric Practice*, 2nd edn. Oxford: Blackwell Scientific Publications, 1989: 808–29.
4 Hellreich PD. The skin changes of pregnancy. *Cutis* 1974; **13**: 82–6.
5 Letterman G, Schuster M. Cutaneous haemangiomas of the face in pregnancy. *Plast Reconstr Surg* 1962; **29**: 293–300.
6 Kroumpouzos G, Cohen LM. Dermatoses of pregnancy. *J Am Acad Dermatol* 2001; **45**: 1–19.
7 Hilming F. Gingivitis gravidarum: studies on clinic and on etiology with special reference to the influence of vitamin C. *Oral Surg Oral Med Oral Pathol* 1952; **5**: 734–51.

Dermatoses modified by pregnancy

Some dermatoses worsen during pregnancy, some improve, and many are unpredictable. Table 70.5 lists those dermatoses and tumours that are commonly modified by pregnancy and the puerperium. The details of most of these are discussed elsewhere in this book; however, some specific points should be noted here.

Infections and immunity in pregnancy

Cell-mediated immunity is depressed during normal pregnancy [1], which probably accounts for the increased frequency and severity of certain infections such as candidiasis. Condylomata acuminata too can be exacerbated, growing very rapidly and occasionally obstructing the birth canal. *Candida*, genital warts and herpes simplex can be transmitted to the baby during childbirth. In babies

Table 70.5 Dermatoses and tumours modified by pregnancy.

Infections
Candidiasis
Trichomoniasis
Condylomata acuminata
Pityrosporum folliculitis
Herpes simplex
Herpes varicella/zoster
Leprosy

Autoimmune disorders
Lupus erythematosus
Dermatomyositis/polymyositis
Pemphigus
Systemic sclerosis

Metabolic disorders
Porphyria cutanea tarda
Acrodermatitis enteropathica

Disorders of connective tissue
Ehlers–Danlos syndrome
Pseudoxanthoma elasticum

Tumours
Bowenoid papulosis
Langerhans' cell histiocytosis
Mycosis fungoides
Malignant melanoma
Neurofibromatosis

Miscellaneous
Atopic dermatitis
Erythema multiforme
Erythrokeratoderma variabilis
Psoriasis (and 'impetigo herpetiformis')
Acne
Hidradenitis suppurativa
Fox–Fordyce disease

of very low birth weight, candidiasis and herpes simplex can be life-threatening [2]. In view of the known oncogenic potential of some strains, there is a debate about whether mothers infected with human papillomavirus should routinely be offered caesarean section, as generally practised for active herpes simplex infection. However, there is doubt whether this practice prevents neonatal infection [3] either by herpesvirus or by genital warts [4]. Bowenoid papulosis (see Chapter 68), a condition closely linked with wart virus infection, may appear for the first time or deteriorate during pregnancy [5].

Podophyllin should never be used in the treatment of warts during pregnancy because of potential maternal and fetal toxicity; physical treatments are preferable [6].

The immune alterations of pregnancy, childbirth and the puerperium have an adverse effect on leprosy in more than one-third of patients [7]. Leprosy reactional states are more common, and the decline in immune reactivity may also lead to an increase in drug resistance [7]. Furthermore, there are specific problems with some antileprosy drugs: thalidomide cannot be used because of its teratogenicity, and clofazimine has been associated with unexplained fetal deaths [8].

Autoimmune disorders

The outcome of most pregnancies in women with systemic lupus erythematosus is undoubtedly better than was once thought, although a few develop renal damage, and disease exacerbation may be severe enough to cause death [6]. Lupus in the mother may affect the baby (neonatal lupus; see Chapter 14). Cutaneous lupus does not appear to be affected by pregnancy [9].

Most women with systemic sclerosis do not experience major problems, and some appear to improve [10]. Occasionally, however, there is severe progressive deterioration of renal function, with hypertension and preeclampsia. This may lead to fetal loss or even maternal death [11].

Dermatomyositis and polymyositis are generally unaffected by pregnancy, but some patients may deteriorate.

Metabolic disease

There is no consensus about the effects of pregnancy on porphyria cutanea tarda. Some women experience few problems, and Marks [12] suggested that endogenous oestrogen might be less harmful than exogenous compounds because of the complete absence of deterioration of the porphyria during one normal pregnancy. However, some cases do show clinical and biochemical deterioration, and on one occasion this was shown to be parallel to the physiological rise in oestrogen [13]. Acrodermatitis enteropathica is said always to deteriorate in pregnancy [14].

Disorders of connective tissue

Women with Ehlers–Danlos syndrome types I and IV often have major problems, including bleeding, wound dehiscence and uterine lacerations (see Chapter 46) [6]. They should probably be counselled to avoid pregnancy altogether. Some patients with pseudoxanthoma elasticum have suffered major gastrointestinal bleeds necessitating blood transfusion [15].

Tumours

The relationship between malignant melanoma and pregnancy (and, indeed, exogenous oestrogens) has been discussed for many years [6]. One large series suggests that melanoma developing during pregnancy carries a slightly worse prognosis, but that pregnancy following excision of a tumour does not affect prognosis [16]. Epidemiological studies from the USA have failed to show significant associations between melanoma and reproductive and other hormonal factors in women [17]. Neurofibromas may grow during pregnancy, or appear for the first time. Rupture of major blood vessels in neurofibromatosis has also been reported [18,19], and hypertension is a common complication. Pregnancy may exacerbate mycosis fungoides [20] and the eosinophilic granuloma form of Langerhans' cell histiocytosis [21].

Miscellaneous dermatoses

Atopic dermatitis often improves in pregnancy, but this is unpredictable; in some patients it is exacerbated. Breast-feeding is often a problem for those suffering from atopic dermatitis because of nipple eczema, and the puerperium may herald a deterioration in hand eczema because of exposure to irritants.

Pregnancy may trigger erythema multiforme, and vaginal stenosis has been described in severe Stevens–Johnson syndrome occurring in pregnancy [22].

Marked deterioration in erythrokeratoderma variabilis occurred during pregnancy in two related women [23].

The effects of pregnancy on psoriasis are variable, although often consistent in the same individual. A rare occurrence is the sudden eruption of acute pustular psoriasis. This used to be considered as a distinct entity called *impetigo herpetiformis*, but this term is probably best discarded.

Acne may improve, but is occasionally exacerbated during pregnancy. This can cause management problems, because a number of antiacne drugs are contraindicated in pregnancy.

Hidradenitis suppurativa and Fox–Fordyce disease often improve considerably, and it is generally presumed that this is a result of a reduction in apocrine gland activity.

REFERENCES

1 Weinberg ED. Pregnancy-associated depression of cell-mediated immunity. *Rev Infect Dis* 1984; **5**: 814–31.
2 Chapel TA, Gagliardi C, Nichols W. Congenital cutaneous candidiasis. *J Am Acad Dermatol* 1982; **6**: 926–8.
3 Prober CG, Sullender WM, Yasukawa LL *et al*. Low risk of herpes simplex virus infections in neonates exposed to the virus at the time of vaginal delivery to mothers with recurrent genital herpes simplex virus infections. *N Engl J Med* 1989; **314**: 240–4.
4 Chuang TY. Condylomata acuminata (genital warts). *J Am Acad Dermatol* 1987; **16**: 376–84.
5 Patterson JW, Kao GF, Graham JH *et al*. Bowenoid papulosis: a clinicopathologic study with ultrastructural observations. *Cancer* 1986; **57**: 823–36.
6 Winton GB. Skin diseases aggravated by pregnancy. *J Am Acad Dermatol* 1989; **20**: 1–13.
7 Duncan ME, Pearson JMH, Ridley DS *et al*. Pregnancy and leprosy: the consequences of alterations of cell-mediated and humoral immunity during pregnancy and lactation. *Lepr Rev* 1982; **55**: 129–42.
8 Farb H, West DP, Pedvis-Leftick A. Clofazimine in pregnancy complicated by leprosy. *Obstet Gynecol* 1982; **59**: 122–3.
9 Yell JA, Burge SM. The effect of hormonal changes on cutaneous disease in lupus erythematosus. *Br J Dermatol* 1993; **129**: 18–22.
10 Johnson TR, Banner EA, Winkelmann RK. Scleroderma and pregnancy. *Obstet Gynecol* 1964; **23**: 467–9.
11 Karlen JR, Cook WA. Renal scleroderma and pregnancy. *Obstet Gynecol* 1974; **44**: 349–54.
12 Marks R. Porphyria cutanea tarda. *Arch Dermatol* 1982; **118**: 452.
13 Lamon JM, Frykholm BC. Pregnancy and porphyria cutanea tarda. *Genet Clin Johns Hopkins Hosp* 1979; **145**: 235–7.
14 Bronson DM, Barsky R, Barsky S. Acrodermatitis enteropathica: recognition at long last during a recurrence in pregnancy. *J Am Acad Dermatol* 1983; **9**: 140–4.
15 Lao TT, Walters BNJ, de Swiet M. Pseudoxanthoma elasticum and pregnancy: two case reports. *Br J Obstet Gynaecol* 1984; **91**: 1049–50.
16 MacKie RM, Bufalino R, Sutherland C. The effect of pregnancy on melanoma prognosis. *Br J Dermatol* 1990; **123** (Suppl. 37): 40.
17 Holly EA, Cress RD, Ahn DK. Cutaneous melanoma in women. III. Reproductive factors and oral contraceptive use. *Am J Epidemiol* 1995; **141**: 943–50.
18 Brade DB, Bolan JC. Neurofibromatosis and spontaneous hemothorax in pregnancy: two case reports. *Obstet Gynecol* 1984; **63** (Suppl.): 35–8.
19 Tapp E, Hickling RS. Renal artery rupture in a pregnant woman with neurofibromatosis. *J Pathol* 1969; **97**: 398–402.
20 Vonderheid EC, Dellatore DL, van Scott EJ. Prolonged remission of tumor-stage mycosis fungoides by topical immunotherapy. *Arch Dermatol* 1981; **117**: 586–9.
21 Growdon WA, Cline M, Tesler A *et al*. Adverse effects of pregnancy on multifocal eosinophilic granuloma. *Obstet Gynecol* 1986; **67** (Suppl.): 2–6.
22 Graham-Brown RAC, Cochrane GW, Swinhoe JR *et al*. Vaginal stenosis due to bullous erythema multiforme (Stevens–Johnson syndrome). *Br J Obstet Gynaecol* 1981; **88**: 1156–7.
23 Gewirtzman GB, Winkler NW, Dobson RL. Erythrokeratoderma variabilis: a family study. *Arch Dermatol* 1978; **114**: 112–4.

AIDS and pregnancy

AIDS is a worldwide problem, and there have now been many pregnancies in women infected by human immunodeficiency virus (HIV). The infection has often only become apparent after birth when the children developed AIDS. Although it appears that pregnancy may subsequently accelerate the development of AIDS symptoms [1,2], there does not seem to be a tendency for HIV disease to progress during pregnancy itself [3]. If opportunistic infections, such as *Pneumocystis* pneumonia or listeriosis, develop in a pregnant woman with AIDS, the outcome is generally fatal [4,5]. This contrasts with the more usual

70% recovery rate in non-pregnant AIDS patients and suggests that the immune suppression of pregnancy may be additive to that of HIV infection. Kaposi's sarcoma has also been reported in AIDS in pregnancy [6]. The effects of maternal HIV infection on the child can be devastating [7].

REFERENCES

1 Minkoff H, Nanda D, Menez R *et al*. Pregnancies resulting in infants with acquired immunodeficiency syndrome or AIDS-related complex. *Obstet Gynecol* 1987; **69**: 285–7.
2 Minkoff H, Nanda D, Menez R *et al*. Pregnancies resulting in infants with acquired immunodeficiency syndrome or AIDS-related complex: follow-up of mothers, children, and subsequently born siblings. *Obstet Gynecol* 1987; **69**: 288–91.
3 Weisser M, Rudin C, Battegay M *et al*. Does pregnancy influence the course of HIV infection? Evidence from two large Swiss cohort studies. *J AIDS* 1998; **17**: 404–10.
4 Minkoff H, de Regt RH, Landesman S *et al*. *Pneumocystis carinii* pneumonia associated with acquired immunodeficiency syndrome in pregnancy: a report of three maternal deaths. *Obstet Gynecol* 1986; **67**: 284–7.
5 Wetli CV, Roldan ED, Fujaco RM. Listeriosis as a cause of maternal death: an obstetric complication of acquired immunodeficiency syndrome (AIDS). *Am J Obstet Gynecol* 1983; **147**: 7–9.
6 Rawlinson KF, Zubrow AB, Harris MA *et al*. Disseminated Kaposi's sarcoma in pregnancy: a manifestation of acquired immune deficiency syndrome. *Obstet Gynecol* 1984; **63** (Suppl.): 2–6.
7 Winton GB. Skin disease aggravated by pregnancy. *J Am Acad Dermatol* 1989; **20**: 1–13.

The dermatoses of pregnancy

Irritation, rashes and other skin changes are common in pregnancy [1]. The possibility that the patient has an unrelated skin condition such as scabies must not be overlooked. However, there are several skin changes that appear to be specifically related to pregnancy and the puerperium, distinct from physiological events, and not caused by exacerbation of a pre-existing condition.

Pruritus gravidarum

Itching in pregnancy is dealt with here because it is uncertain whether it is an extension of the physiological changes or a specific dermatosis [2,3].

As many as one-fifth of pregnant women experience some itching [4]. In most, this can be attributed to some identifiable skin disorder such as scabies, eczema, urticaria, a drug eruption or one of the specific pregnancy-related inflammatory dermatoses discussed below. However, there is also a small group of women who experience intense pruritus without evident primary cutaneous changes, and it is to these patients that the term pruritus gravidarum is applied.

It is generally considered that pruritus gravidarum is a mild variant of recurrent cholestasis of pregnancy, and occurs in 0.02–2.4% of pregnancies [5]. The itching begins in the second or third trimester and is often localized to the abdomen, or the palms and soles, although it may also be very widespread. The patient may be mildly icteric.

Liver function tests are occasionally abnormal, with a raised alkaline phosphatase [2].

The cause is thought to be multifactorial [6], although it is probable that the irritation itself results from abnormal hepatic excretion of bile acids induced by metabolites of both oestrogen and progesterone, both of which have been shown to affect the handling of bile acids [6,7]. The condition also occurs more commonly in mothers of patients with rare inborn cholestatic syndromes [6].

The itching usually subsides rapidly after childbirth, but may persist for some weeks into the puerperium. It may also recur with subsequent pregnancies and the use of oral contraceptive pills. Recurrent attacks increase the liability to cholelithiasis [4]. Treatment with ursodeoxycholic acid is effective in reducing itch and abnormal liver function tests [6].

Striae

Striae distensae (striae gravidarum) are a common and striking feature of most pregnancies. They are dealt with fully in Chapter 46.

Skin tags
SYN. MOLLUSCUM FIBROSUM GRAVIDARUM

Multiple tags often appear in the second half of pregnancy. These are most common on the face, the side of the neck, in the axillae and under the breasts. The histological features are those of ordinary skin tags [8]. They are usually small, but may reach 5 mm in size. They generally regress in the puerperium, and it has been suggested that they are probably a result of hormonal factors [2].

'Cracked' and sore nipples

Many women experience discomfort, irritation and fissuring of the nipples, especially early in the puerperium as they are trying to establish breastfeeding. Anatomical features, such as relatively flat nipples, contribute to the development of this problem. Mastitis and deep abscesses may occur because of penetration of the broken skin by pyogenic bacteria. The problem is, in essence, one of friction and irritation, and can be eased considerably by the judicious use of gentle cleansing and emollients.

Inflammatory dermatoses specific to pregnancy

Classification. The older literature is confusing. Dermatoses considered distinct by some authors are lumped together by others. Holmes and Black [9] have suggested a rationalization of the terminology, and have proposed a classification that seems the most logical for practical use (Table 70.6), even though alternatives are still employed. Ackerman *et al.* [10] argue that there really are only two

Table 70.6 Specific dermatoses of pregnancy. (From Shornick [12].)

Pemphigoid (herpes) gestationis
Polymorphic eruption of pregnancy
Prurigo of pregnancy
Pruritic folliculitis of pregnancy

dermatoses in this category: pruritic urticarial papules and plaques of pregnancy (PUPPP) and pemphigoid gestationis. However, some of the other dermatoses that have been reported as being pregnancy-associated are discussed here, drawing attention to those descriptions that appear to be at least clinically distinct from PUPPP or pemphigoid gestationis, and reviewing whether others are really distinct entities or not.

Pemphigoid (herpes) gestationis [11,12]

This rare and highly characteristic disorder affects approximately 1 in 150 000 pregnancies and is considered in detail in Chapter 41. The disease usually appears in the second or third trimester, and presents with an intensely itchy urticarial or vesiculobullous eruption. Immunofluorescence reveals a linear band of immunoglobulin G (IgG) at the basement-membrane zone, identical to that seen in bullous pemphigoid. Recent studies involving tissue typing have supported earlier suggestions of a genetic predisposition [13].

Polymorphic eruption of pregnancy
SYN. PRURITIC URTICARIAL PAPULES AND PLAQUES OF PREGNANCY

In addition to the above designations, these skin changes have been known as toxaemic rash of pregnancy [14], toxic erythema of pregnancy [15] and 'late onset' prurigo of pregnancy [16]. It is probable also that some patients with this condition have been recorded in the literature as prurigo gestationis (see below), erythema multiforme and pemphigoid (herpes) gestationis.

If there is agreement that all these disorders are one and the same, there is still no consensus on which name to use. In the UK, as proposed by Holmes and Black [9,11], the term polymorphic eruption of pregnancy is favoured. Elsewhere, the lengthy descriptive phrase 'pruritic urticarial papules and plaques of pregnancy' or 'PUPPP', as suggested by Lawley *et al.* [17], still finds favour, especially in the USA [18].

Incidence. Polymorphic eruption of pregnancy occurs in approximately 1 in 240 pregnancies [2]. The eruption begins in the third trimester, usually of a first pregnancy, but is occasionally delayed until a few days postpartum. It rarely recurs in subsequent pregnancies [11,17,18], but when it does it is often less severe [2].

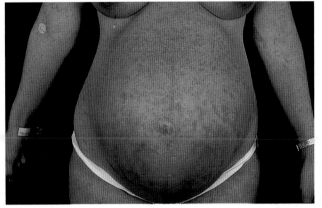

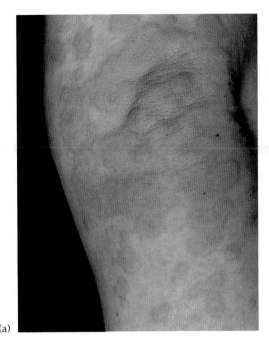

Fig. 70.4 Typical lesions of polymorphic eruption of pregnancy: (a) on the arm, and (b) on the abdomen. (Courtesy of Dr D.A. Burns, Leicester Royal Infirmary, Leicester, UK.)

Aetiology. The cause remains obscure, although the condition has been related to abnormal weight gains in the mother and the newborn, and to twin pregnancy [19]. As the disorder occurs predominantly in primigravidae in the third trimester, it has been postulated that excessive abdominal distension may act as a trigger for the skin changes. The typical distribution (see below) may lend some credence to this view. It has also been shown that serum cortisol levels are low in patients with polymorphic eruption of pregnancy, while human chorionic gonadotrophin (hCG) and oestradiol are normal [20].

Pathology [11,16,17]. The histology of this condition is non-specific, and there are many similarities with the early prebullous phase of pemphigoid gestationis. Most biopsies show epidermal and upper dermal oedema, with a perivascular infiltrate of lymphocytes and histiocytes. There may be a striking number of eosinophils (as there may be in pemphigoid gestationis). Spongiotic vesicles are also seen, and there may be patchy parakeratosis.

Immunofluorescence is uniformly negative, even by immunoelectron microscopy, and this provides the best means of distinguishing this disorder from pemphigoid gestationis, should there be any diagnostic doubt [21].

Clinical features [11,16,17]. The patient usually complains of intense itching. The skin lesions closely resemble the very early stage of pemphigoid gestationis. The eruption consists predominantly of urticated papules and plaques. Less commonly, vesicles, target lesions and polycyclic erythematous areas are seen.

The most striking feature, however, is the distribution of the lesions. They usually begin and predominate on the abdomen, often closely following the lines of the striae, where present (Fig. 70.4). The umbilicus is frequently spared. Lesions often also appear on the upper arms and thighs.

Despite the outdated term toxaemic rash of pregnancy, there is no suggestion that polymorphic eruption has any adverse effect on the outcome of the pregnancy. Indeed, the babies tend to be larger than normal [19].

Treatment. Some patients improve with topical calamine or steroids and systemic sedative antihistamines. Most women are relieved to learn that the condition is not serious, that all should be well with them and their baby, and that the rash will disappear at or soon after childbirth.

Prurigo of pregnancy [16]
SYN. EARLY ONSET PRURIGO OF PREGNANCY;
PRURIGO GESTATIONIS OF BESNIER

The main differences between this disorder and polymorphic eruption of pregnancy are that it begins earlier—usually between 25 and 30 weeks' gestation—and that there are no urticated lesions. It occurs in 1 in 300 pregnancies. Clinically, there are multiple excoriated papules over the abdomen and on the extensor surfaces of the limbs. Histology reveals acanthosis and parakeratosis, with perivascular lymphocytic infiltration around upper dermal vessels. Immunofluorescence is negative. The lesions tend to persist throughout pregnancy, and may continue well into the puerperium, although the pruritic element often settles shortly after delivery [2]. As with polymorphic eruption of pregnancy, the mother and fetus are unaffected, but prurigo of pregnancy may recur in successive pregnancies, which can cause significant distress to the pregnant woman. It has been suggested that cases labelled 'prurigo of pregnancy' may, in fact, have been eczema [20].

Only symptomatic treatment is available, and this is often rather unsatisfactory.

Pruritic folliculitis of pregnancy [22]

This disorder begins in the second or third trimester, and usually resolves within 2 weeks of delivery. The eruption consists of masses of itchy red follicular papules. It strongly resembles steroid-induced acne. Histology reveals a non-specific folliculitis. Immunofluorescence is negative. There is no adverse effect on mother or baby.

Less well-defined dermatoses

Papular dermatitis of pregnancy

Considerable controversy surrounds this entity. It was first described by Spangler *et al.* [23] in 1962, who reported a widespread papular eruption, which they estimated to occur only once in every 2400 pregnancies. In the original description, the rash consisted of widespread, 3–5 mm, intensely itchy papules with a smaller central crust. There were several laboratory abnormalities, including markedly raised urinary chorionic gonadotrophin levels and low urinary oestriol. Of most significance was the observation that there appeared to be a 30% fetal mortality with this eruption. However, there have been no other convincing reports, and a recent review of 85 patients found no evidence of increased fetal loss [24]. The confusion may have arisen because Spangler *et al.* [23] included fetal deaths in pregnancies unaffected by a rash, and spontaneous abortions, without qualifying these by gestational age [2].

It is now generally accepted that the changes reported as papular dermatitis of pregnancy are probably those of pregnancy prurigo, and that the fetal loss in Spangler *et al.*'s series was overestimated.

Autoimmune progesterone dermatitis of pregnancy

There is a single case report of a patient who developed an odd acneiform rash on the extremities and buttocks in two successive pregnancies [25]. There was an associated arthritis and a positive skin test reaction to progesterone. The author used the term autoimmune progesterone dermatitis to describe this phenomenon, thereby leading to confusion with the condition of the same name that is not pregnancy-associated (see above). However, the clinical features of the two disorders are quite distinct.

Prurigo annularis

Two reported cases [7] had annular scaly lesions that persisted for years postpartum. Whether it really had anything to do with the pregnancy must be in doubt.

REFERENCES

1 Vaughan Jones SA, Black MM. Pregnancy dermatoses. *J Am Acad Dermatol* 1999; **40**: 233–41.
2 Black MM, Mayou SC. Skin diseases in pregnancy. In: de Swiet M, ed. *Medical Disorders in Obstetric Practice*, 2nd edn. Oxford: Blackwell Scientific Publications, 1989: 808–29.
3 Winton GB, Lewis CW. Dermatoses of pregnancy. *J Am Acad Dermatol* 1982; **6**: 977–98.
4 Furhoff WR. Itching in pregnancy: a 15-year follow-up study. *Acta Med Scand* 1974; **196**: 403–10.
5 Alcalay J, Wolf JE. Pruritic urticarial papules and plaques of pregnancy: the enigma and the confusion. *J Am Acad Dermatol* 1988; **19**: 1115–6.
6 Milkiewicz P, Elias E, Williamson C *et al.* Obstetric cholestasis. *BMJ* 2002; **324**: 123–4.
7 Sasseville D, Wilkinson RD, Schnader JY. Dermatoses of pregnancy. *Int J Dermatol* 1981; **20**: 223–41.
8 Cummings K, Derbes VJ. Dermatoses associated with pregnancy. *Cutis* 1967; **3**: 120–5.
9 Holmes RC, Black MM. The specific dermatoses of pregnancy. *J Am Acad Dermatol* 1983; **8**: 405–12.
10 Ackerman AB, Cavegn BM, Robinson MJ, Abad-Casintahan MF. *Ackerman's Resolving Quandaries in Dermatology, Pathology and Dermatopathology*. Baltimore: Williams & Wilkins, 1995: 219–21.
11 Holmes RC, Black MM. The specific dermatoses of pregnancy: a reappraisal with special emphasis on a proposed simplified clinical classification. *Clin Exp Dermatol* 1982; **7**: 65–73.
12 Shornick JK. Herpes gestationis. *J Am Acad Dermatol* 1987; **17**: 539–56.
13 Shornick JK, Jenkins RD, Artlett CM *et al.* Class II MHC typing in pemphigoid gestationis. *Clin Exp Dermatol* 1995; **20**: 123–6.
14 Bourne G. Toxaemic rash of pregnancy. *Proc R Soc Med* 1962; **55**: 462–4.
15 Holmes RC, Black MM, Dann J *et al.* A comparative study of toxic erythema of pregnancy and herpes gestationis. *Br J Dermatol* 1982; **106**: 499–510.
16 Nurse DS. Prurigo of pregnancy. *Australas J Dermatol* 1968; **9**: 258–67.
17 Lawley TJ, Hertz KC, Wade TR *et al.* Pruritic urticarial papules and plaques of pregnancy. *JAMA* 1979; **241**: 1696–9.
18 Kroumpouzos G, Cohen LM. Dermatoses of pregnancy. *J Am Acad Dermatol* 2001; **45**: 1–19.
19 Cohen LM, Capeless EL, Krusinski PA *et al.* Pruritic urticarial papules and plaques of pregnancy and its relationship to maternal–fetal weight gain and twin pregnancy. *Arch Dermatol* 1989; **125**: 1534–6.
20 Vaughan Jones SA, Hern S, Nelson-Piercy C *et al.* A prospective study of 200 women with dermatoses of pregnancy correlating clinical findings with hormonal and immunopathological profiles. *Br J Dermatol* 1999; **141**: 71–81.
21 Jurecka W, Holmes RC, Black MM *et al.* An immunoelectron microscopy study of the relationship between herpes gestationis and polymorphic eruption of pregnancy. *Br J Dermatol* 1983; **108**: 147–51.
22 Zoberman E, Farmer ER. Pruritic folliculitis of pregnancy. *Arch Dermatol* 1981; **117**: 20–2.
23 Spangler AS, Reddy W, Bardiwal WA *et al.* Papular dermatitis of pregnancy. *JAMA* 1962; **181**: 577–81.
24 Vaughan Jones SA, Bhogal BS, Black MM. A prospective study of the specific dermatoses of pregnancy in 85 pregnant women including hormone profiles and effects on pregnancy outcome. *Br J Dermatol* 1996; **135** (Suppl. 47): 18.
25 Bierman SM. Autoimmune progesterone dermatitis. *Arch Dermatol* 1973; **107**: 896–901.

The menopause

Hormonal and physiological changes

Strictly speaking, the term *menopause* is used to define the fixed single point in a woman's life characterized by her last menstrual period [1–4]. This is established formally after 12 months of amenorrhoea in the middle years of life [5]. The surrounding years, or climacteric, are a time of change and readjustment to the new phase heralded by the menopause and its loss of fertility: literally, *climacteric* means a step up the ladder. It is a crucial phase for a woman, preparing her for the years to come which, in modern societies at least, may now represent as much as 30 years, or one-third of her life [6,7]. It has been estimated that by 2030, there will be 1.2 billion postmenopausal women worldwide [8].

The age of onset of menopause has been the subject of much study, and some of the data have been criticized because of flaws in their collection and interpretation [5,9]. However, menopause occurs between the ages of 45 and 55 years in 65–70% of women, and the median age in most Western populations is around 50 years. Factors that may influence menopausal age include heredity (age of mother's menopause is highly predictive), smoking, parity, socio-economic factors, exposure to toxins and nutrition [5]. The onset appears to occur a little earlier in developing countries than in Western societies [9].

True premature menopause before the age of 40 years occurs in less than 1% of women [10], but can follow surgery, irradiation, viral infections (especially mumps), accompany various enzymatic and hormonal defects, or be associated with a number of systemic disorders such as Addison's disease, rheumatoid arthritis, diabetes or myasthenia gravis [1].

During the reproductive years, oestrogen is produced mainly by ovarian follicles, but at the menopause there are major changes. There are very few follicles left, the ovaries become atrophic, and the levels of ovary-derived oestrogen fall. The endocrinology of this period of a woman's life results from the interrelationship of reduced ovarian function and resultant changes in gonadotrophins. Although there may be intermittent bursts of oestrogen in the immediate postmenopausal period because of residual follicular activity, the level of plasma oestradiol ultimately falls to less than 20 pg/L and remains there for the rest of the woman's life [9]. The ratio of oestradiol : oestrone changes, with oestrone becoming the more abundant hormone [11], and most oestrogens being derived from the direct peripheral conversion to oestrone of androstenedione, which has been produced by the adrenals. Some oestrone may arise through the alternative pathway via testosterone and oestradiol [6]. The pituitary–gonadal feedback loop is virtually absent, and levels of gonadotrophins are elevated in consequence. In addition, a number of granulosa cell-derived peptide hormones influence FSH levels [12].

These hormonal changes are reflected in a number of physiological alterations [1]. In the breast, glandular tissue decreases and fibrous tissue increases. The body of the uterus becomes smaller and its muscle is partly replaced by fibrous tissue, and the endometrium regresses and becomes atrophic. However, it still retains the capacity to respond to exogenous hormones. The vagina becomes shorter and narrower, and the vaginal epithelium atrophies. The pH of the vagina rises, and infections become more frequent. The external genitalia atrophy, with a loss of vulval subcutaneous fat and thinning of the vulval epithelium. Pubic hair diminishes.

The epithelium of the lower urinary tract also atrophies and this, together with the increased tendency to prolapse, increases the frequency of urinary tract infections. There is a loss of elasticity in the pelvic supporting ligaments, contributing to prolapse and urinary incontinence [13].

There are no structural cutaneous changes that are specifically associated with the menopause, but there are oestrogen receptors in the skin, suggesting that the skin is a target organ for oestrogen and that its withdrawal may be important [14]. It is interesting that there is a far greater concentration of oestrogen receptors in facial skin than in skin on the breasts or thigh. Some of the changes seen after the menopause, such as dryness, epidermal thinning and loss of dermal elasticity, may result, in part, from lower circulating oestrogen levels. Certainly, administration of oestrogen to castrated animals leads to thickening of the dermis and decreased breakdown of collagen. Oestrogen given to postmenopausal women also increases dermal thickness [15], and in preliminary studies has been shown to improve skin elasticity and deformability [16]. The application of topical oestrogens to the face in menopausal women has also been reported to improve various parameters, including reduction in the depth of wrinkles [17]. However, the picture is not as clear-cut with regard to the epidermis. Hormone replacement therapy (HRT) may increase the skin's water-holding capacity [18].

REFERENCES

1 Barbo DM. The physiology of the menopause. *Med Clin North Am* 1987; **71**: 11–22.
2 Hammond CB. Menopause: an American view. In: Campbell S, ed. *The Management of the Menopause and Post-Menopausal Years*. London: MTP, 1976: 405–21.
3 London DR, Shaw RW. Gynaecological endocrinology. In: O'Riordan JLH, ed. *Recent Advances in Endocrinology and Metabolism*. Edinburgh: Churchill Livingstone, 1981: 91–110.
4 Ross GT. Disorders of the ovary and female reproductive tract. In: Wilson JD, Foster DW, eds. *Williams' Textbook of Endocrinology*, 7th edn. Philadelphia: Saunders, 1981: 206–58.
5 Houmard BS, Seifer DB. Predicting the onset of menopause. In: Seifer DB, Kennard EA, eds. *Menopause: Endocrinology and Management*. NJ: Humana, 1999: 1–19.
6 Khaw KT. Epidemiology of the menopause. *Br Med Bull* 1992; **48**: 249–61.
7 Brenner S, Politi Y. Dermatologic diseases and problems of women throughout the life cycle. *Int J Dermatol* 1995; **34**: 369–79.
8 Hill K. The epidemiology of the menopause. *Maturitas* 1996; **23**: 113–27.
9 Gosden RG. *Biology of Menopause*. London: Academic Press, 1985: 1–15.
10 Coulam CB, Anderson SC, Annegan JF. Incidence of primary ovarian failure. *Obstet Gynecol* 1986; **67**: 604–6.
11 Baird DT. Synthesis and secretion of steroid hormones by the ovary *in vivo*. In: Zuckerman L, Weir JB, eds. *The Ovary*, Vol. 3, 2nd edn. New York: Academic Press, 1977: 305–57.
12 Ying S. Inhibins, activins and follistatins: gonadal proteins modulating the secretion of follicle-stimulating hormone. *Endocr Rev* 1988; **9**: 267–93.
13 Caputo R. Lower urinary tract changes of ageing women. In: Seifer DB, Kennard EA, eds. *Menopause: Endocrinology and Management*. NJ: Humana, 1999: 81–96.
14 Hasselquist M, Goldberg N, Schreter A *et al*. Isolation and characterisation of the estrogen receptors in human skin. *J Clin Endocrinol Metab* 1980; **50**: 76–82.

15 Marks R, Shahrad F. Skin changes at the time of the climacteric. *Clin Obstet Gynecol* 1977; **4**: 207–26.
16 Pierard GE, Letawae C, Dowlatti A *et al.* Effect of hormone replacement therapy for menopause on the mechanical properties of skin. *J Am Geriatr Soc* 1995; **43**: 662–5.
17 Schmidt JB, Binder M, Macheiner W *et al.* Treatment of skin ageing symptoms in perimenopausal females with estrogen compounds: a pilot study. *Maturitas* 1994; **20**: 25–30.
18 Pierard-Franchimont C, Letawe C, Goffin V *et al.* Skin water-holding capacity and transdermal estrogen therapy for menopause: a pilot study. *Maturitas* 1995; **22**: 151–4.

Skin disorders of the menopause

Atrophic vulvovaginitis

It has been known for many years that the atrophic changes in the female external genitalia described above respond, at least partially, to topical oestrogens [1].

Menopausal flushing

The most consistent and distressing complaint associated with the menopause is flushing [2]. This is usually described as a sudden feeling of intense heat in the face, neck and chest, often accompanied by discomfort and sweating. Although the intensity and duration vary, it typically lasts 3–5 min. Visible changes occur in approximately 50% of women, and generally consist of a blotchy erythema on the face, neck, upper chest and breasts. Some women also develop palpitations, throbbing in the head and neck, headaches, waves of nausea and anxiety attacks. Sleep disturbance is not uncommon [3]. It is possible to measure several physiological changes during hot flushes, including increased temperature, pulse rate and respiratory rate [4,5].

Flushes are associated with pulsatile release of LH [6], presumably because of failure of the normal feedback mechanisms. However, flushing can occur after hypophysectomy [7], and so LH itself cannot be responsible for the observed vasomotor instability. One suggested mechanism involves alteration of hypothalamic catecholamine levels, and a failure of normal central thermoregulatory centres through LH-releasing hormone neurones [2]. Flushes similar to those seen in the menopause can be induced by an enkephalin analogue and blocked by naloxone infusions [8], indicating that menopausal hot flushes may also be mediated by an opiate-dependent central mechanism [9].

The consensus is that oestrogen therapy is the most effective treatment for symptomatic hot flushes [2], although not all authorities have always agreed [5]. Alternatives that can be considered when oestrogens are contraindicated include various progestins [10], clonidine [11] and methyldopa [12]. A mixture of ergotamine, belladonna alkaloids and phenobarbital failed to stand up to double-blind trial analysis [13], but may still be worth trying if all else fails.

Keratoderma climactericum

This term has been used to describe the appearance of hard skin on the palms and soles, especially around the heels. Although originally reported as a specific association with the menopause [14], the same changes are seen in men and women at other ages, many of whom are obese. It may therefore be a non-specific effect. There has been a report of a therapeutic response to systemic retinoids [15].

Lichen sclerosus et atrophicus

This disorder is considered in detail in Chapters 56 and 68 but is mentioned here because of its frequent presentation at or around the menopause, and because of the significant symptomatology it may cause.

Complications of HRT

The increasing use of HRT, largely to prevent osteoporosis and cardiovascular disease, has revealed a number of problems associated with this treatment. There is an ongoing debate regarding the relationship between HRT and cancers of the breast and genital tract, but this is beyond the scope of this chapter. However, HRT may be responsible for a number of cutaneous problems, which should at least receive a mention here.

Oestrogen therapy may trigger or exacerbate, amongst others, chloasma (melasma); spider angiomas; darkening of naevi; the skin changes of porphyria cutanea tarda; and acanthosis nigricans [16,17]. Many clinicians also report encountering urticarial or eczematous dermatoses that appear in patients on HRT and subside on cessation of treatment. Allergic reactions have been reported to the transdermal patches frequently used as delivery systems for HRT. These may be to the adhesives or to the oestrogens themselves [18].

REFERENCES

1 Artner J, Gitsch E. Über lokalwirkungen von Östriol. *Gerburtshilfe Frauenheilk* 1959; **19**: 812–9.
2 Barbo DM. The physiology of the menopause. *Med Clin North Am* 1987; **71**: 11–22.
3 Erlick Y, Tataryn IV, Meldrum DR *et al.* Association of waking episodes with menopausal hot flushes. *JAMA* 1981; **245**: 1741–4.
4 Molnar GW. Body temperatures during menopausal hot flushes. *J Appl Physiol* 1975; **38**: 499–503.
5 Mulley G, Mitchell JRA. Menopausal flushing: does oestrogen therapy make sense? *Lancet* 1976; **i**: 1397–8.
6 Ravnikar V, Elkind-Hirsch K, Schiff I *et al.* Vasomotor flushes and the release of peripheral immunoreactive luteinizing hormone releasing hormone in postmenopausal women. *Fertil Steril* 1985; **41**: 881–7.
7 Mulley G, Mitchell JRA, Tattersall RB. Hot flushes after hypophysectomy. *BMJ* 1977; **2**: 1062.
8 Stubbs WA, Delitala G, Jones A *et al.* Hormonal and metabolic responses to an enkephalin analogue in normal man. *Lancet* 1978; **ii**: 1225–7.
9 Casper RF, Yen SSC. Neuroendocrinology of 3 menopausal flushes: an hypothesis of flush mechanism. *Clin Endocrinol* 1985; **22**: 293–312.

10 Loprinzi CL, Michalak JC, Quella SK *et al.* Megestrol acetate for the prevention of hot flashes. *N Engl J Med* 1994; **331**: 347–52.

11 Nagamani M, Kelver M, Smith E. Treatment of menopausal hot flushes with transdermal administration of clonidine. *Am J Obstet Gynecol* 1987; **156**: 561–5.

12 Nesheim BI, Saetre T. Reduction of menopausal hot flushes by methyl dopa. *Eur J Clin Pharmacol* 1981; **20**: 413–6.

13 Bergmans M, Merkins J, Corbey R, Schellekens L. Effect of Bellergal Retard on climacteric complaints: a double-blind, placebo-controlled study. *Maturitas* 1987; **9**: 227–34.

14 Haxthausen H. Keratoderma climactericum. *Br J Dermatol* 1934; **46**: 161–7.

15 Deschamps P, Leory D, Pedailles S *et al.* Keratoderma climactericum (Haxthausen's disease): clinical signs, laboratory findings and response to etretinate in 10 patients. *Dermatologica* 1986; **172**: 259–62.

16 Graham-Brown RAC. Dermatologic problems of the menopause. *Clin Dermatol* 1997; **15**: 143–5.

17 Banuchi SR, Cohen L, Lorincz AL *et al.* Acanthosis nigricans following diethylstilboestrol therapy. *Arch Dermatol* 1974; **109**: 544–6.

18 Angelini G. Topical drugs. In: Rycroft RJG, Menné T, Frosch PJ, eds. *Textbook of Contact Dermatitis*, 2nd edn. Berlin: Springer-Verlag, 1995: 493.

Old age

Introduction

Senescence in the skin is a gradual process that ultimately results in the appearances and functional differences that we associate with old age. However, by no means all of these changes are purely intrinsic. The skin is particularly vulnerable to the 'ageing' effects of a number of environmental insults, especially UV radiation, and in women there are additional hormonal changes at the menopause (see p. 70.18). These factors are superimposed on the background changes of intrinsic senescence, and care needs to be exercised in interpreting which are most important in determining any particular aspect of the appearance and function of the skin in an elderly person. However, there have been increasing efforts to disengage the roles of these intertwined and contemporaneous processes.

Biology of ageing

Ageing is the decline in the power of self-maintenance, the increase in susceptibility to disease and the growing probability of death as age advances. Ultimate senescence is as much a biological necessity as initial survival; evolutionary progress has occurred because animals are programmed for both. In the words of Macfarlane Burnet [1], 'The two basic evolutionary needs of all species of higher animal are survival to reproductive age, and death when survival offers no reproductive advantages to the species.'

Modern theories of ageing fall into two categories that, philosophically speaking, start from opposite poles. The first views ageing as an ordered process delicately programmed by the genes [2]; the second suggests that ageing is caused by the progressive retention and amplification of errors in the replication of genetic information in the somatic cells [1]. From the practical viewpoint, both types of theory emphasize the intrinsic inevitability of the process.

If the ageing of most of the bodily organs has, however reluctantly, to be accepted, the ageing of the facial skin appears to be a matter of widespread concern. The reason is that the skin plays a major part in our social and sexual interactions; the concern is not so much to do with physiological functions, which may remain adequate in old age, but about continuing effectiveness, particularly of the facial skin, in communication. To display sexuality or assert social status it is necessary to have skin and hair that look, feel and smell attractive.

The ageing of skin has so far been studied for social and commercial reasons in affluent white populations. Some of these subjects are ill adapted for the environments they now occupy or the lifestyles they endure or enjoy. It must not therefore be assumed that the data obtained will necessarily apply to skin with greater pigmentation, especially that of Mongoloid and Negroid populations.

The most obvious signs of an ageing skin are atrophy, laxity, wrinkling, sagging, dryness, yellowness, a multiplicity of pigmented and other blemishes, and sparse grey hair. Some of these stigmata clearly have genetic components, and some are mimicked by heritable disorders. The abnormal texture of the dermis in cutis laxa makes young children look old; in progeria, on the other hand, the connective tissue remains evenly dense, although the epidermis shows mottled pigmentation [3].

Intrinsic changes of ageing fall into two categories: those that appear to be engendered within the tissues themselves, and those that are the result of alterations, including hormonal, caused by senile changes in other organs. An example of the former is the greying of hair, and of the latter, the lowering of sebaceous gland activity consequent upon reduction of androgen secretion.

Into a third category must be put changes that are mainly the result of environmental factors. These may be overriding; for example, it has been stated that on exposed skin more than 90% of age-associated cosmetic problems are caused by UV radiation [4].

REFERENCES

1 Burnet M. *Intrinsic Mutagenesis: a Genetic Approach to Ageing.* Lancaster: MTP, 1974.

2 Bergsma D, Harrison DE. *Genetic Effects on Aging.* New York: Alan R Liss, 1978.

3 Lapiere CM. The ageing dermis: the main cause of the appearance of old skin. *Br J Dermatol* 1990; **122** (Suppl. 35): 5–11.

4 Leyden JJ. Clinical features of ageing skin. *Br J Dermatol* 1990; **122** (Suppl. 35): 1–3.

The ageing skin

Dermis

It cannot be doubted that wrinkling of senescent skin is almost entirely the result of changes in the dermis. The debatable questions concern the nature of these changes and the extent to which they are intrinsic or environmentally caused [1,2].

The dermis diminishes in bulk, and in absolute terms the collagen per unit area of unexposed skin decreases with age [3]. There also appears to be a steady decrease in the number and size of mast cells and fibroblasts [2]. Although it is often assumed that the lax skin of the aged results from lack of water, there is evidence that, on the contrary, water content increases between the fourth and ninth decades [4].

Gross morphological changes, especially in the collagen and elastin fibres, have been revealed by electron and light microscopy. Their relationship to molecular changes as determined by physical and chemical methods requires interpretation. Moreover, it has long been clear that such changes are largely the result of exposure to solar radiation (photoageing) [5].

Accumulating evidence indicates that intrinsically aged skin shares a number of features with photoaged (environmentally aged) skin. Commercial interests have dictated a more detailed interrogation of the mechanisms underlying photoageing. However, the same research techniques are now being applied to intrinsically aged skin. There is an age-related loss of fibroblast frequency and size, coupled with a decrease in their synthetic ability [6]. Over the age of 70 years, there is loss of collagens I and III in the papillary dermis with an associated increase in matrix metalloproteinases [7]. Reactive oxygen species and free radicals are key drivers of degeneration so characteristic of aged skin. This oxidative damage is produced in part by the action of mitogen-activated protein (MAP) kinases. In aged skin, stress-activated MAP kinase activity is elevated [8].

In the dermis of young adults, the collagen bundles are well organized. They form a rhomboid network with the individual bundles lying at angles to one another. Intertwined among the collagen bundles lie single branching elastic fibres, apparently aligned haphazardly, in planes parallel with the surface at all levels beneath the dermal–epidermal junction. The network of collagen bundles, although composed of inextensible fibres, is itself extensible as the bundles rotate relative to one another to form parallel alignments. It seems likely that the return of the network to its unstretched state is brought about by the interwoven elastic fibres [9]. Thus, in cutis laxa, an uncommon disorder in which the skin hangs in folds, the elastic fibres appear to be reduced in number and degenerate (see Chapter 46).

The various descriptions of changes in ageing based on histological staining techniques are often confusing. In general, it appears that the collagen bundles become fragmented and disorientated, and elastin fibres become progressively reduced [10]. However, in senile skin from exposed areas there may, paradoxically, be a striking increase in fibres that take up elastin stains in actinic elastosis (see Chapter 46).

Elastic fibres gradually disintegrate with age, even in protected skin, and after the age of 70 years most fibres appear abnormal [11–13]. These changes are most likely a combination of reduced synthesis and elastolysis. Similar changes can be produced in protected buttock skin within hours by incubating it with pancreatic elastase and bovine chymotrypsin [11].

Epidermis

Many differences between a senile and young epidermis have been described, but a consistent interpretation of the ageing process has proved difficult. In part, this is because the epidermis varies from site to site. Young skin from the back [14], like that from the scalp and axilla [15], has deep and complex rete ridges, whereas that of the face [15] has a fairly flat dermal–epidermal junction. It is widely agreed that in areas where the junction is corrugated in youth, it becomes flattened in the aged [15–20].

Similarly, there are differences in epidermal thickness, even in young skin. On the face or on the dorsum of the hand, for example, it is considerably greater than on the arms, legs or trunk [15]. In many areas, the whole epidermis becomes thinner with age, and the cells become less evenly aligned on the basement membrane and less regular in size, shape and staining properties [15,19–22].

The question of whether these changes result from alterations in the rate of cell replication has also engendered controversy, largely because of differing methods of study [23]. However, there is now some consensus that the cell turnover rate is halved between the third and seventh decades of life [21,24,25], notwithstanding an earlier finding that the frequency of mitoses in abdominal skin increases from childhood until the fifth decade and then levels out [26]. The evidence that the rate of epidermal repair and wound healing declines with age [27] is consonant with the view that epidermopoiesis is decreased.

The permeability of the skin also changes with age, although some of the data are contradictory [28]. According to Christophers and Kligman [16], the capacity of the isolated horny layer *in vitro* to restrict water loss does not differ between young adults and persons over 70 years of age, but the aged skin is decidedly more permeable to chemical substances. However, *in vivo*, they found that the percutaneous absorption of testosterone appeared to be reduced in old age. A possible explanation is that, although substances enter aged skin more easily than young skin, they are removed more slowly into the circulation because of changes in the dermal matrix and reduction in the vasculature [4]. The response to blistering agents, such as 50% ammonium hydroxide, is initially quicker in elderly than in young subjects, but the formation of the full blister takes longer [29].

These physiological differences must be largely related to changes in the stratum corneum, yet neither its thickness nor the number of cell layers seem to vary with age, at least on the back [16]. However, Marks [30] showed that the surface area of individual corneocytes from unexposed areas of the arms, thighs and lower abdomen increases with age, and suggested that this might reflect an increased transit time [31].

A change in the nature of the corneocytes is also indicated by the tendency of the senescent epidermal surface, especially that of the lower legs, to become dry, flaky and sometimes itchy. Apart from reduced function of the skin glands, the water-binding capacity of the stratum corneum appears to be reduced [32], coupled with an increase in renewal time if damaged [33].

Pigmentation

The most obvious senile change in white skin is irregularity of pigmentation. Yellow or brown macules, known as 'liver spots' or 'age spots', develop on the backs of the hands and exposed parts of the face in more than 50% of persons over 45 years of age. Very rarely, such *senile lentigines* develop into *lentigo maligna*, which is a precancerous condition, although it progresses very slowly [33].

The senile lentigo consists of a localized proliferation of melanocytes at the dermal–epidermal junction [34]. In general, however, the number of dopa-positive melanocytes in both exposed and unexposed skin decreases in old age, although their size increases. The reduction is in the order of 8–20% per decade compared with young adult skin [35]. Their reaction to dopa becomes variable, and some no longer donate pigment [33,36,37].

Even heavily pigmented skin darkens. A study of 578 adult natives of New Guinea revealed that pigmentation increased with age in skin exposed to the sun, but not in axillary skin, and that males darkened more than females [38].

Greying of hair

Greying usually becomes evident around the age of 50 years, by which time about half the population has approximately 50% grey or white body hairs and an even greater proportion has some depigmented scalp hair [39].

The bulbs of grey or white hairs show various abnormalities, but it is uncertain which are critical. In general, the bulbs appear to lack or be deficient in tyrosinase, the enzyme necessary for the first stages of melanin synthesis [40]. Structurally, the follicles of grey hairs still have melanocytes placed normally over the dermal papilla, but the cytoplasm may contain large vacuoles and the melanosomes may be only lightly melanized [33]. The follicles of fully white hairs may completely lack melanocytes. However, among grey or white hairs, there may be a few normal bulbs producing dark hairs.

An unexplained fact is that at all ages from their appearance on the chest in males, and probably elsewhere, grey hairs tend to be thicker and longer than pigmented ones [38].

Premature greying of hair, even before the age of 20 years, is a feature of several hereditary syndromes, and is also associated with a number of disorders induced by organ-specific antibodies. A survey of the age prevalence of normal greying of hair in men [41] showed that it fitted a simple mathematical model of ageing consonant with the view that the condition is 'autoaggressive' or 'autoimmune' in character and arises from somatic gene mutations.

Hair follicles [42]

Changes in the hair follicles vary greatly between sites. For example, it can be widely observed that hair becomes sparse on the vertex while it is still luxuriant on the occiput, and that greying usually starts at the temples.

In the scalp, the density of hair follicles steadily decreases with age, more rapidly in bald than in non-bald persons [43]. The overall capacity of the follicles to produce long hairs is progressively reduced, at least on the vertex, and especially in males. This cannot be accounted for by any diminution in the rate of growth, which remains substantially unchanged [44]. It must therefore result from a shortening of the duration of anagen. This is reflected by the gradual rise in the proportion of follicles in telogen, both in non-bald subjects [45] and in persons with pattern alopecia, where it becomes evident in advance of visible baldness [46].

Scalp hair also becomes finer, especially in persons with visible alopecia. In a group of 58 white women with diffuse alopecia, 13 of whom were clinically hypothyroid, there was a gradual reduction in mean diameter which appeared to be an exaggeration of a trend also found in normal subjects [47]. The diameters showed a wide range, with a single peak around 0.08 mm in normal persons, but two peaks at 0.04 and 0.06 mm, respectively, in patients with alopecia, suggesting that not all the follicles behave identically.

The weight of beard grown per day reaches a peak in the fourth decade, and starts to decrease slightly in the seventh decade [48]. As the density of the hairs remains constant, the decrease in weight must be accounted for by a reduction in the rate of growth, in diameter, or in both. Evidence that the linear growth of beard hair is correlated solely with levels of 5α-dihydrotestosterone (DHT) in the plasma, not with testosterone, whereas hair density is significantly correlated solely with testosterone, not with DHT [49], suggests that the age changes may result not so much from reduced production of testosterone as by lessened peripheral metabolism.

Chest hairs, which are also androgen-dependent, reach a maximum in number, breadth and length around the fifth decade, and then start to diminish markedly [39].

Axillary hair reaches a peak in mass and in rate of production towards the end of the third decade in males and females alike, and this is followed by a rapid decline, somewhat more severe in females [48,50]. Pubic hair appears to follow a similar pattern.

If most of the changes with ageing involve reductions in the amount of hair, this is not true of all sites. In the male, the eyebrows may become more bushy, and visible hairs develop around the external auditory meati. In the female, hirsutism may occur as a result of endocrine changes associated with the menopause (see p. 70.18).

Sebaceous and apocrine glands

Sebum production is at its greatest in early adulthood, and lessens in old age. A view that it remains unchanged until past the age of 70 years in men, but falls after the menopause in women, has not been entirely sustained [51,52].

Measurements of the sustainable rate of wax ester secretion after depletion of the sebum reservoir by absorption with bentonite clay suggest that sebum secretion declines steadily through each decade by approximately 23% in men and 32% in women [53]. The fatty acid composition also changes [54].

The predominant belief is that, in spite of their decreased output, the sebaceous glands increase in size because turnover of cells is slower in senility [55,56]. However, in one study in 14 women the glands appeared to become smaller and the sebocytes flatter with age [57].

The axillary apocrine glands also regress with age and produce less odour [15].

Eccrine glands

Spontaneous sweating on the fingertips declines in old age, as a result of a combination of a reduction in the number of glands [58] and of the output per gland [59]. On the forearm, the response to epinephrine has been shown to be reduced by ageing equally in men and women, suggesting an intrinsic deterioration of the glands, an interpretation supported by histological evidence. In contrast, the effect of age on the response to acetylcholine is much greater in the male than in the female, suggesting that ageing affects cholinergic sweating indirectly through the hormonal balance in the blood [59]. Such a hypothesis is borne out by the evidence that the maximum rate of cholinergic sweating is much greater in adult males than in females or in juveniles, and is thus probably androgen-dependent [60].

Nail growth

The rate of linear nail growth increases until well into the third decade. From about the age of 25 years it starts to decrease. Until the age of 70 years, nail growth is greater in men than in women, but thereafter the situation appears to be reversed [61]. Nails are more brittle in the

elderly and are characterized by beaded ridging—sometimes called 'sausage links'. Brittleness may be caused by a reduction in the nail content of lipophilic sterols and free fatty acids [62].

Nerves and sensation

Age often decreases sensory perception and increases the threshold for pain [29,63]. There is evidence for progressive disorganization or loss of some sense organs; for example, the density of Meissner corpuscles in the little finger falls from over $30/mm^2$ in young adults to approximately $12/mm^2$ by the age of 70 years [64].

Langerhans' cells and immune functions

Langerhans' cells become considerably reduced in number in elderly people, even in light-protected areas [65,66]. Recent work has confirmed the reduction in number of epidermal Langerhans' cells with age, coupled with a reduced ability to migrate from the epidermis in response to tumour necrosis factor-α [67]. T cells, similarly, are reduced in percentage and absolute number, and lose their responsiveness to specific antigens [4,68]. The number of B cells does not seem to be affected by age, but their dysfunction is reflected by increased autoantibody formation and serum levels of IgA and IgG [68–71]. Elderly skin appears to have a much reduced capacity to produce cytokines such as interleukin-2 (IL-2) [72]. However, the production of some cytokines (e.g. IL-4) increases with age [72]. The decreased intensity of delayed hypersensitivity reactions [73], the increased risk of photocarcinogenesis and the greater susceptibility to chronic skin infections are some consequences of the ageing of the immune system [24].

REFERENCES

1 Ebling FJG. Physiological background to skin ageing. *Int J Cosmet Sci* 1982; **4**: 103–10.
2 Kligman AM, Lavker RM. Cutaneous aging: the differences between intrinsic aging. *J Cutan Ageing, Cosmetol Dermatol* 1988; **1**: 5–12.
3 Shuster S, Bottoms E. Senile degeneration of skin collagen. *Clin Sci* 1963; **25**: 487–91.
4 Kligman AM. Perspectives and problems in cutaneous gerontology. *J Invest Dermatol* 1979; **73**: 39–46.
5 Knox JM, Cockerell EG, Freeman RG. Etiological factors and premature aging. *JAMA* 1962; **179**: 630–6.
6 Andrew W, Behnke R, Sato T. Changes with advancing age in the cell population of human dermis. *Gerontologica* 1964; **10**: 1–19.
7 Varani J, Fisher GJ, Kang S, Voorhees JJ. Molecular mechanisms of intrinsic skin aging and retinoid induced repair and reversal. *J Invest Dermatol Symp Proc* 1998; **3**: 57–60.
8 Chung JH, Kang S, Varani J *et al*. Decreased extracellular-signal-regulated kinase and increased stress-activated MAP kinase activities in aged human skin *in vivo*. *J Invest Dermatol* 2000; **115**: 177–82.
9 Hall DA. *The Ageing of Connective Tissue*. New York: Academic Press, 1976.
10 Robert L, Robert B, eds. *Frontiers of Matrix Biology*, Vol. 1. *Ageing of Connective Tissue, Skin*. Basel: Karger, 1973: 190.
11 Braverman IM, Fonferko E. Studies in cutaneous aging: I. The elastic fibre network. *J Invest Dermatol* 1982; **78**: 434–43.

12 Stadler R, Orfanos CE. Reifung und Alterung der elastischen Fasern: Electronenmikroskopische Studien in verschiedenen Altersperioden. *Arch Dermatol Res* 1978; **262**: 97.

13 Tsuji T, Hamada T. Age-related changes in human dermal elastic fibres. *Br J Dermatol* 1981; **105**: 57–63.

14 Eller JJ, Eller WD. Oestrogenic ointments: cutaneous effects of topical applications of natural oestrogens with report of 321 biopsies. *Arch Dermatol Syphilol* 1949; **59**: 449–64.

15 Montagna W. Morphology of the aging skin: the cutaneous appendages. In: Montagna W, ed. *Advances in Biology of Skin*, Vol. 6. *Aging*. Oxford: Pergamon, 1965: 1–16.

16 Christophers E, Kligman AM. Percutaneous absorption in aged skin. In: Montagna W, ed. *Advances in Biology of Skin*, Vol. 6. *Aging*. Oxford: Pergamon, 1965: 163–75.

17 Hill WR, Montgomery H. Regional changes and changes caused by age in the normal skin. *J Invest Dermatol* 1940; **3**: 321–45.

18 Lavker RM, Zheng P, Dong G. Morphology of aged skin. *Dermatol Clin* 1986; **4**: 379–84.

19 Montagna W, Carlisle K. Structural changes in aging human skin. *J Invest Dermatol* 1979; **73**: 47–53.

20 Montagna W, Carlisle K. Structural changes in ageing skin. *Br J Dermatol* 1990; **122** (Suppl. 35): 61–70.

21 Gilchrest BA. *Skin and Aging Processes*. Boca Raton, FL: CRC Press, 1984.

22 Lavker RM. Structural alterations in exposed and unexposed aged skin. *J Invest Dermatol* 1979; **73**: 59–66.

23 Epstein WL, Maibach HT. Cell renewal in the human epidermis. *Arch Dermatol* 1965; **92**: 462–8.

24 Cerimele D, Celleno L, Serri F. Physiological changes in ageing skin. *Br J Dermatol* 1990; **122** (Suppl. 35): 13–20.

25 Grove GL, Kligman AM. Age-associated changes in human epidermal cell renewal. *J Gerontol* 1983; **38**: 137–42.

26 Thuringer JM, Katzberg AA. The effect of age on mitosis in the human epidermis. *J Invest Dermatol* 1959; **33**: 35–9.

27 Goodson WH III, Hunt TK. Wound healing and aging. *J Invest Dermatol* 1979; **73**: 88–91.

28 Roskos KV, Guy RH, Maibach H. Percutaneous absorption in the aged. In: Gilchrest BA, ed. *Dermatologic Clinics: the Aging Skin*. Philadelphia: Saunders, 1986: 455–65.

29 Grove GL, Duncan S, Kligman AM. Effect of ageing on the blistering of human skin with ammonium hydroxide. *Br J Dermatol* 1982; **107**: 393–400.

30 Marks R. Measurement of biological ageing in human epidermis. *Br J Dermatol* 1981; **104**: 627–33.

31 Baker H, Blair CP. Cell replacement in the human stratum corneum in old age. *Br J Dermatol* 1968; **80**: 367–72.

32 Raab WP. The skin surface and stratum corneum. *Br J Dermatol* 1990; **122** (Suppl. 35): 37–41.

33 Fitzpatrick TB, Szabo G, Mitchell RE. Age changes in the human melanocyte system. In: Montagna W, ed. *Advances in Biology of Skin*, Vol. 6. *Aging*. Oxford: Pergamon, 1965: 35–50.

34 Cawley EP, Curtis AC. Lentigo senilis. *Arch Dermatol Syphilol* 1950; **62**: 635–41.

35 Quevedo WC, Szabo G, Virks J. Influence of age and UV on the populations of dopa-positive melanocytes in human skin. *J Invest Dermatol* 1969; **52**: 287–90.

36 Gilchrest BA, Blog FB, Szabo G. Effect of aging and chronic sun exposure on melanocytes in human skin. *J Invest Dermatol* 1979; **73**: 141–3.

37 Ortonne JP. Pigmentary changes in the ageing skin. *Br J Dermatol* 1990; **122** (Suppl. 35): 21–8.

38 Walsh RJ. Variation in the melanin content of the skin of New Guinea natives at different ages. *J Invest Dermatol* 1964; **42**: 261–5.

39 Hamilton JB, Terada H, Mestler GE *et al.* I. Coarse sternal hairs, a male secondary sex character that can be measured quantitatively: the influence of sex, age and genetic factors. II. Other sex-differing characters: relationship to age, to one another, and to values for coarse sternal hairs. In: Montagna W, Dobson RL, eds. *Advances in Biology of Skin*, Vol. 9. *Hair Growth*. Oxford: Pergamon, 1969: 129–51.

40 Fitzpatrick TB, Brunet P, Kukita A. The nature of hair pigment. In: Montagna W, Ellis RA, eds. *The Biology of Hair Growth*. New York: Academic Press, 1958: 255–303.

41 Burch PRJ, Murray JJ, Jackson D. The age-prevalence of arcus senilis, greying of hair, and baldness: etiological considerations. *J Gerontol* 1971; **26**: 364–72.

42 Ebling FJG. Age changes in the cutaneous appendages. *J Appl Cosmetol* 1985; **3**: 243–56.

43 Giacometti L. The anatomy of the human scalp. In: Montagna W, ed. *Advances in Biology of Skin*, Vol. 6. *Aging*. Oxford: Pergamon, 1965: 97–120.

44 Barman JM, Astore I, Pecoraro V. The normal trichogram of people over 50 years but apparently not bald. In: Montagna W, Dobson RL, eds. *Advances in Biology of Skin*, Vol. 9. *Hair Growth*. Oxford: Pergamon, 1969: 211–20.

45 Pecoraro V, Astore I, Barman JM. The pre-natal and post-natal hair cycles in man. In: Baccaredda-Boy A, Moretti G, Frey JR, eds. *Biopathology of Pattern Alopecia, Proceedings of the International Symposium, Rapallo, Italy, July 1967*. Basel: Karger, 1968: 29–38.

46 Braun-Falco O, Christophers E. Hair root pattern in male pattern alopecia. In: Baccaredda-Boy A, Moretti G, Frey JR, eds. *Biopathology of Pattern Alopecia, Proceedings of the International Symposium, Rapallo, Italy, July 1967*. Basel: Karger, 1968: 141–5.

47 Jackson D, Church RE, Ebling FJ. Hair diameter in female baldness. *Br J Dermatol* 1972; **87**: 361–7.

48 Hamilton JB. Age, sex and genetic factors in the regulation of hair growth in man: a comparison of Caucasian and Japanese populations. In: Montagna W, Ellis RA, eds. *The Biology of Hair Growth*. New York: Academic Press, 1958: 399–433.

49 Farthing MJG, Mattei AM, Edwards CRW *et al.* Relationship between plasma testosterone and dihydrotestosterone concentrations and male facial hair growth. *Br J Dermatol* 1982; **107**: 559–67.

50 Pecoraro V, Astore I, Barman JM. Growth rate and hair density of the human axilla: a comparative study of normal males and females and pregnant and post-partum females. *J Invest Dermatol* 1971; **56**: 362–5.

51 Pochi PE, Strauss JS. The effect of aging on the activity of the sebaceous gland in man. In: Montagna W, eds. *Advances in Biology of Skin*, Vol. 6. *Aging*. Oxford: Pergamon, 121–7.

52 Pochi PE, Strauss JS, Downing DT. Age-related changes in sebaceous gland activity. *J Invest Dermatol* 1979; **73**: 108–11.

53 Jacobsen E, Billings JK, Frantz RA *et al.* Age-related changes in sebaceous wax ester secretion rates in men and women. *J Invest Dermatol* 1985; **85**: 483–5.

54 Yamamoto A, Serizawa S, Ito M *et al.* Effect of aging on sebaceous gland activity and on the fatty acid composition of wax esters. *J Invest Dermatol* 1987; **89**: 507–12.

55 Kumar P, Barton SP, Marks R. Tissue measurements in senile sebaceous gland hyperplasia. *Br J Dermatol* 1988; **118**: 397–402.

56 Plewig G, Kligman AM. Proliferative activity of the sebaceous glands of the aged. *J Invest Dermatol* 1978; **70**: 314–7.

57 Ito N, Mashiko T, Sato Y. Morphological changes of sebaceous glands with ageing in human females: computer graphic analysis and ultrastructural study. *J Invest Dermatol* 1988; **90**: 570.

58 Oberste-Lehn H. Effects of aging on the papillary body of the hair follicles and on the eccrine sweat glands. In: Montagna W, ed. *Advances in Biology of Skin*, Vol. 6. *Aging*. Oxford: Pergamon, 1965: 17–34.

59 Silver AF, Montagna W, Karacan I. The effect of age on human eccrine sweating. In: Montagna W, ed. *Advances in Biology of Skin*, Vol. 6. *Aging*. Oxford: Pergamon, 1965: 129–50.

60 Rees J, Shuster S. Pubertal induction of sweat gland activity. *Clin Sci (Lond)* 1980; **60**: 689–92.

61 Orentreich N, Markofsky J, Vogelman JH. The effect of aging on the rate of linear nail growth. *J Invest Dermatol* 1979; **73**: 126–30.

62 Helmdach M, Thielitz A, Röpke E-V, Gollnick H. Age and sex variation in lipid composition of human fingernail plates. *Skin Pharmacol Appl Skin Physiol* 2000; **13**: 111–9.

63 Schludermann E, Zubeck JP. Effect of age on pain sensibility. *Percept Mot Skills* 1962; **14**: 295–301.

64 Winkelmann RK. Nerve changes in aging skin. In: Montagna, W, ed. *Advances in Biology of Skin*, Vol. 6. *Aging*. Oxford: Pergamon, 1965: 51–61.

65 Gilchrest BA, Murphy G, Soter NA. Effect of chronologic aging and ultraviolet irradiation on Langerhans' cells in human epidermis. *J Invest Dermatol* 1982; **79**: 85–8.

66 Thiers H, Maize JC, Spicer SS *et al.* The effect of aging and chronic sun exposure on human Langerhans' cell population. *J Invest Dermatol* 1984; **82**: 223–6.

67 Bhushan M, Cumberbatch M, Dearman RJ *et al.* Tumour necrosis factor-α induced migration of human Langerhans' cells: the influence of ageing. *Br J Dermatol* 2002; **146**: 32–40.

68 Makinodan T. Immunodeficiencies of ageing. In: Doria G, Eshkol A, eds. *The Immune System: Functions and Therapy of Dysfunction*. New York: Academic Press, 1980: 55–63.

69 Diaz-Jouanen E, Strickland RG, Williams RC Jr. Studies of human lymphocytes in the newborn and the aged. *Am J Med* 1975; **58**: 620–8.
70 Kay MMB, Makinodan T. Immunobiology of aging: evaluation of current status. *Clin Immunol Immunopathol* 1976; **6**: 394–413.
71 Reddy MM, Goh K. B- and T-lymphocytes in man. IV. Circulating B-, T-, and null lymphocytes in aging population. *J Gerontol* 1979; **34**: 5–8.
72 Ben-Yahuda A, Weksler ME. Host resistance and the immune system. *Clin Geriatr Med* 1992; **8**: 701–11.
73 Walford DS, Willkens RF, Decker JL. Impaired delayed hypersensitivity in an aging population: association with antinuclear reactivity and rheumatoid factor. *JAMA* 1968; **203**: 831–5.

Skin disease in old age

The demography of most nations is changing. Higher standards of housing, hygiene and nutrition, together with improvements in health care services have meant that the average lifespan has increased considerably over the last century. Added to this, many couples are now limiting their families to two or three children at most. Virtually every Western society is therefore experiencing an increase in the average age of its population. The provision of health care for elderly people is consequently becoming more and more important, and disease of the skin is no exception to this [1]. Elderly patients present in dermatology clinics and consulting rooms with a wide variety of skin problems; a few are more or less specific to old age, but most are familiar skin disorders whose clinical expression, physical and emotional consequences, and management may be altered by the age of the patient and the problems that increasing age bring with it.

The reasons an individual seeks advice for skin changes in old age may be as much influenced by personality and social conditioning as by the absolute severity of the problem. Although some societies are still said to view the outward signs of age, such as wrinkles and grey hair, as marks of distinction, it is clear that in much of the world, 'Westernization' is resulting in an increasing degree of social stigmatization associated with looking old. Furthermore, it has long been recognized that, contrary to the popular belief of the young, elderly people are often anxious to look attractive [2].

Thus, particularly in rich and highly developed societies, there is an increasing reluctance to accept the physiological consequences of old age and the effects of environmental exposure. A myth has begun to develop that these ageing changes are abnormal, and many older people with plentiful spare time and financial resources have become obsessed with the pursuit of an eternally youthful appearance (Fig. 70.5). One reason for this is that the pharmaceutical and cosmetic industries have invested heavily in the promotion of the concept that 'young is beautiful'. A great deal of money is being and will continue to be devoted to the study of compounds that may arrest or reverse the visible effects of ageing. Some are claiming success, most notably with retinoic acid for wrinkles. Such research is also increasingly gaining credence in mainstream medical circles, and dermatologists are becoming more and more involved in this area of practice.

However, most people accept (albeit increasingly reluctantly) that ageing is a natural process, and only seek medical advice when skin changes are particularly troublesome or severe, or develop earlier than might otherwise have been expected.

Skin changes of sufficient severity to warrant medical attention in elderly patients may result from the interplay of several factors:
1 Alterations in structure and function of the ageing skin
2 Cumulative effects of exposure to a variety of environmental insults, especially UV radiation
3 Cutaneous consequences of ageing or age-related disease in other organ systems
4 Changes in the environment—decreasing occupational exposure, increasing leisure exposure to potential irritants and sensitizers
5 Social circumstances, with poor nutrition, home care and mobility often contributing to the expression, perpetuation and failure to resolve of skin problems
6 Physiological problems, such as dementia, increasing rigidity of attitude and refusal to accept advice
7 Increasing physical frailty, resulting in a relative incapacity to carry out tasks correctly.

Of particular practical importance are the latter three problems, which are frequently ignored. An elderly patient may be too proud to point out that physical incapacity prevents the twice daily application of a cream, or may deliberately refuse or forget to relate relevant facts about the home situation. The onus is very much on the dermatologist to consider these factors when dealing with skin disease in the elderly patient.

Incidence of skin problems in old age

It is hard to estimate the true frequency of skin disease in the population as a whole, let alone specifically in older age groups. One problem is that the line between that which is physiological and the 'truly' pathological becomes increasingly difficult to draw with advancing years. Another is that studies of skin problems in the elderly have used different types of population and diagnostic groupings which are not directly comparable (Table 70.7). It is probably better therefore to think of skin problems rather than just skin disease in this age group.

However, it is clear that skin problems are common in elderly people. The general scale of this can be gauged from the findings of a large US study, in which dermatological examination of 20 000 non-institutionalized US citizens revealed that 40% of those aged between 65 and 74 years had some significant dermatological problem [3]. 'Significant', in this context, was defined as requiring, in the view of the examining doctor, a dermatological

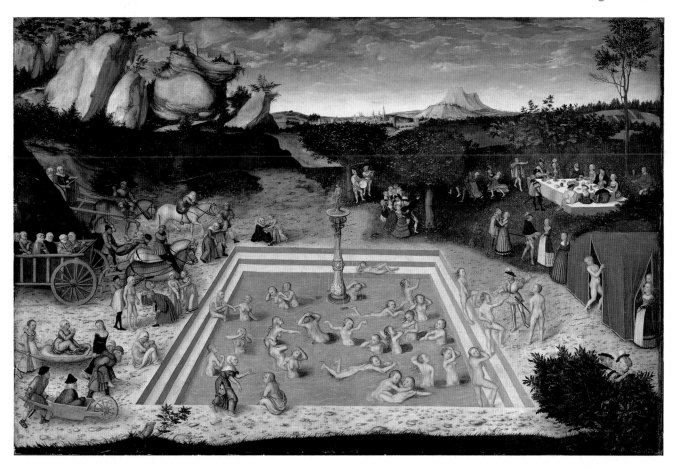

Fig. 70.5 *Der Jungbrunnen.* Lucas Cranach the Elder painted this picture of the Fountain of Youth in 1546, when he was 72 years of age. On the left, a succession of aged and decrepit women are brought to the fountain by an interesting variety of primitive transport. As they move through the basin they are transformed into lovely young maidens. The eternal desire for and, indeed, the possible advantages of rejuvenation are wonderfully expressed. (Courtesy of Staatliche Museen zu Berlin, Gemäldegalerie, Berlin, Germany.)

opinion. Smaller studies on elderly individuals selected randomly and not from skin clinics give much the same impression [4–7]. For example, of 68 volunteers aged between 50 and 91 years, living in Boston, USA, two-thirds of the entire group and 83% of those aged over 80 years complained of skin problems of some kind [4]. In a European study, 77.4% of a population of 584 elderly residents of a municipal old peoples' home in Denmark were found to have a skin problem [7].

Many of the skin problems that are found most commonly on random examination of elderly people are not those for which elderly patients necessarily seek attention from specialist or non-specialist doctors. Although eczemas, pruritus, easy bruising and dryness (under various headings) are certainly seen in skin clinics, tumours, both benign and malignant, tend to figure more prominently than inflammatory problems [8–12].

Table 70.7 Studies on the incidence of skin disease in elderly people.

Reference	No. of patients	Population studied
Droller [5]	476	Random; at home
Young [8]	330	Ambulatory outpatients from skin clinic; chosen 'at random'
Epstein [9]	687	US private practice
Tindall & Smith [6]	163	Volunteers; at home; black and white people
Verbov [12]	170	Mainly outpatients; some in-patients
Weisman *et al.* [7]	584	Residents of old peoples' homes
Beauregard & Gilchrest [4]	68	Volunteers: housing projects, geriatric home visits, medical centre employees
McFadden & Hande [10]	257	Dermatology outpatients

REFERENCES

1 Gilchrest BA. Demography of skin disease in the elderly. In: *Skin and Aging Processes*. Boca Raton, FL: CRC Press, 1984: 1.
2 Kligman AM, Graham JA. The psychology of appearance in the elderly. *Dermatol Clin* 1986; **4**: 501–7.
3 Johnson M-LT. Skin conditions and related need for medical care among persons 1–74 years, United States 1971–74. *Vital Health Statistics*. Series 11, Data from the National Health Survey; no. 212, DHEW Publication no. (PHS) 79–1660. Hyattsville, ML: US Department of Health, Education and Welfare, 1978.
4 Beauregard S, Gilchrest BA. A survey of skin problems and skin care regimens in the elderly. *Arch Dermatol* 1987; **123**: 1638–43.
5 Droller H. Dermatologic findings in a random sample of old persons. *Geriatrics* 1955; **10**: 421–4.
6 Tindall JP, Smith JG. Skin lesions of the aged and their association with internal changes. *JAMA* 1963; **186**: 1039–42.
7 Weisman K, Krakauer R, Wanscher B. Prevalence of skin disease in old age. *Acta Derm Venereol (Stockh)* 1980; **60**: 352–3.
8 Young AW. Dermatologic complaints presented by 330 geriatric patients. *Geriatrics* 1958; **13**: 428–34.
9 Epstein NN. The aging skin. I. Some problems of the aging skin with particular reference to environmental factors. In: Rees RB, ed. *Dermatoses due to Environmental and Physical Factors*. Springfield: Thomas, 1962: 28–38.
10 McFadden N, Hande K-H. A survey of elderly new patients at a dermatology outpatient clinic. *Acta Derm Venereol (Stockh)* 1987; **69**: 260–2.
11 Stern RS, Johnson M-L, DeLozier J. Utilization of physician services for dermatologic complaints. *Arch Dermatol* 1977; **113**: 1062–6.
12 Verbov J. Skin problems in the older patient. *Practitioner* 1975; **215**: 612–22.

Specific skin problems in old age

Most of the skin disorders that are particularly troublesome in the elderly patient are described elsewhere in this book. However, one or two points should be emphasized about certain specific disorders.

Wrinkles and elastosis

These changes, together with greying of the hair, are most readily associated with an aged appearance. The different clinical forms of wrinkles, and the clinical syndromes associated with elastosis, are described in Chapter 46, and the histological changes of the ageing dermis are discussed above. Plastic surgeons and dermatologists are becoming increasingly involved in their management. Chemical peels, collagen implants and facelift operations are in widespread use, and topical retinoids are employed in the treatment and prevention of wrinkling [1–3].

Pruritus

Itching in old age can be so severe that it ruins quality of life completely [4]. The itch may be localized or generalized, and may or may not be accompanied by skin changes. It is crucial to examine an itchy elderly person carefully for primary cutaneous disease. In one study, 142 of 162 elderly patients had an identifiable cause for their itching (including xerosis), leaving only 20 to whom the term senile pruritus was applicable [5]. Diagnoses that are particularly easy to miss are scabies (often caused by the inadequate examination facilities in residential homes for the elderly) and bullous pemphigoid, which often begins with a non-specific or even no rash [6]. Non-specific skin changes in anogenital itch may also conceal important diagnoses: candidiasis in undiagnosed diabetes; lichen sclerosus et atrophicus, the classical signs of which may easily be obscured by secondary excoriation and inflammation.

If a primary skin disorder has been ruled out, it is important to investigate any elderly patient with generalized itching for systemic causes: renal disease, cholestasis (especially chronic liver disease), thyroid disease, anaemia or cancer. The relationship between carcinomas and pruritus in the elderly patient is controversial, but there is no doubt that lymphomas, leukaemias and other myelodysplastic disorders may present in this way [7]. The frequency with which a systemic cause is found varies, but is high enough to justify a routine search [4], and a useful algorithm for this has been provided by Champion [8].

When all these causes have been excluded, there remains a small core of elderly patients with intractable pruritus. In some, the itching is accompanied by xeroderma, but in others the skin feels relatively normal to the touch. The management of such patients is extremely difficult, and is often totally unsatisfactory for all concerned. The topical use of emollients, soothing preparations such as menthol in calamine, and potent topical steroids may be helpful. However, many of those with the worst pruritus are quite unable to manage topical therapy by themselves, and it is necessary to resort to relatively sedative systemic drugs, such as phenothiazine-type antihistamines. These, too, have their drawbacks, not the least of which is the development of confusion and disorientation.

Senile xerosis and asteatotic eczema
SYN. ECZÉMA CRAQUELÉ

The ageing skin often feels 'dry' to the touch, although the reason for this is not clear. Water loss is not increased in aged skin [9], but the water content of the epidermis appears to be somewhat reduced [10]. It has been suggested that xerosis reflects minor abnormalities in epidermal maturation [7].

The dryness is often worse in the winter, a fact that has given rise to many of the alternative names used for these changes: winter eczema, prurigo or pruritus hiemalis. The changes are often most pronounced on the legs. In some patients, the surface texture of the skin assumes a cracked appearance resembling crazy paving. This is known as asteatotic eczema or eczéma craquelé (Fig. 70.6). Frequent washing is certainly a causative factor in susceptible individuals [11], and central heating may also play a part by reducing atmospheric humidity. Perhaps it is not surprising that this problem is commonly seen in geriatric in-patients.

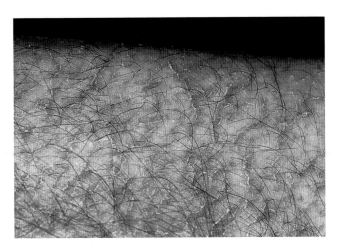

Fig. 70.6 Eczéma craquelé.

The use of emollients to reduce requirements for soaps and detergents will improve xerosis in most patients and, because high water temperature appears to increase the tendency to irritant reactions [12], so will reducing the bath temperature. Moisturizing preparations in the bath are generally held to be effective [4], but bath oils can make the bath very slippery, which has its risks in the elderly and frail patient.

Eczema

The aged may suffer from any of the clinical types of eczema. Atopic dermatitis, for example, occasionally continues into old age or even appears for the first time. However, certain patterns such as asteatotic eczema are more common and more troublesome in elderly subjects.

Seborrhoeic dermatitis may be more common in the elderly infirm and in those confined to bed [13]. In the aged patient, especially the obese, a flexural pattern is often encountered, which may mimic intertrigo and flexural psoriasis.

Some elderly patients present for the first time with a discoid or nummular eczema, and most patients with Sulzberger–Garbe disease (generally considered to be a variant of discoid eczema) are elderly.

Gravitational eczema is much more common in the elderly patient (see Chapter 17), and may be complicated by contact sensitivity.

Contact dermatitis of irritant or allergic origin is generally considered to be less common in elderly people, partly because of decreased occupational exposure [14]. This may also reflect the decline in immune reactivity that occurs with age [15] and the fact that irritant responses to some substances are reduced in intensity [16]. However, patch-test positivity remains quite common, presumably from exposure earlier in life. Allergic contact dermatitis remains a significant problem in elderly people, especially resulting from local medicaments, such as aminoglyco-

sides, lanolin, parabens, antihistamines and anaesthetics. Other sensitizers that continue to cause trouble in old age include rubber in gloves and shoes, plastics in hearing aids and spectacle frames, plants and hair dyes [14].

Marked secondary lichenification and chronic lichen simplex are also often seen in older patients.

Bullous disorders

Pemphigoid (see Chapter 41) is much more frequent in the elderly than in other age groups. Old age modifies the management of all blistering diseases because of unwanted effects of drugs, or because of physical and social circumstances. Steroids precipitate glucose intolerance more often in the elderly, and sulfapyridine or sulfamethoxypyridazine may be better first-line drugs than dapsone for dermatitis herpetiformis because of the tendency for dapsone to cause haemolysis [17]. Drug regimens should be kept simple, and written down where necessary.

Psoriasis

There is a distinct peak of onset of psoriasis in later life that is not as clearly associated with a family history as in patients whose disease begins earlier. This is reflected in different human leukocyte antigen (HLA) associations [18].

Psoriasis causes increased problems in the elderly patient. Disease of lesser extent and severity may be relatively more disabling in old age than in youth, and the systemic effects of widespread or acute pustular psoriasis are less well tolerated than in younger individuals. Flexural psoriasis is a particular problem in the elderly patient [19], but other patterns are also seen. Eruptive guttate disease, however, is rare in old age.

Treatment can be difficult. The patient may be unable to apply topical therapies, and there may be problems in travelling to and from the hospital for outpatient dithranol, or in standing for psoralen and UVA (PUVA) therapy. One solution is the use of systemic therapy, especially methotrexate. There is less reason for concern over long-term toxicity in the elderly patient, relatively small doses may keep the patient comfortable (perhaps because of diminished renal clearance) and the drug is generally well tolerated.

Leg ulcers (see Chapter 50)

Leg ulcers are a major problem. Most are caused by venous hypertension, but arterial disease becomes increasingly important with advancing years. Poor wound healing in elderly people [20], perhaps associated with other illnesses and poor nutrition, may also have a role in the perpetuation of some ulcers.

In managing chronic leg ulcers in the elderly patient it is important to take an overview of the whole situation. Strenuous efforts to heal a stable ulcer in someone who is coping independently at home may be inappropriate in some cases if long-stay in-patient treatment will be required.

Decubitus ulcers [21]

See Chapter 22.

Herpes zoster and post-herpetic neuralgia [22]

Shingles is much more common in old age, the relative incidence rising from 4 in 1000/year at age 55 years to 10 in 1000/year at age 90 years. It has been estimated that 25% of people over the age of 65 years develop shingles at some time, and that all who have had chickenpox would do so were they to live to 100 years old. Post-herpetic neuralgia is also much more common in elderly people. Approximately 50% of patients over the age of 60 years experience pain, and the incidence rises to as many as 75% of the over-70s.

Skin tumours

Most skin tumours are more common in elderly people: benign, such as seborrhoeic keratoses, senile lentigines and skin tags; dysplastic, such as actinic keratoses; and cancers, especially basal and squamous cell carcinomas. Lentigo maligna is seen predominantly in the elderly, and the highest age-specific incidence rates for invasive malignant melanoma are also in those over 60 years [23]. There is also an association between increasing age and decreasing 5-year survival in malignant melanoma [24]. It is not clear why this should be, but elderly patients seem to present with thicker lesions [24,25], and recent evidence suggests that the proportion of nodular melanomas may rise with increasing age [25]. The tendency to wait longer before presenting for treatment also extends to other tumours, and lesions such as that shown in Fig. 70.7 are essentially restricted to elderly people.

Infections with ectoparasites

Outbreaks of scabies in residential homes for the elderly are not uncommon, and are usually attributable to one individual with a heavy infection, verging on Norwegian or crusted scabies. Clothing lice (see Chapter 33) are, in the UK, almost exclusively seen in elderly vagrants.

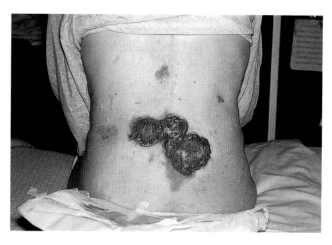

Fig. 70.7 A large neglected basal cell carcinoma on the back of an elderly lady.

2 Kligman AM, Grove GL, Hirose R *et al.* Topical tretinoin to photoaged skin. *J Am Acad Dermatol* 1986; **15**: 836–59.
3 Marks R, Lever L. Studies on the effects of topical retinoic acid on photoageing. *Br J Dermatol* 1990; **122** (Suppl. 35): 93–5.
4 Graham-Brown RAC, Monk BE. Pruritus and xerosis. In: Monk BE, Graham-Brown RAC, Sarkany I, eds. *Skin Disorders in the Elderly*. Oxford: Blackwell Scientific Publications, 1988: 133–46.
5 Young AW. The diagnosis of pruritus in the elderly. *J Am Geriat Soc* 1967; **15**: 750–8.
6 Barker DJ. Generalised pruritus as the presenting feature of bullous pemphigoid. *Br J Dermatol* 1986; **109**: 237–9.
7 Gilchrest BA. Pathologic processes associated with aging. In: *Skin and Aging Processes*. Boca Raton, FL: CRC Press, 1984: 37–56.
8 Champion RH. Generalised pruritus. *BMJ* 1984; **289**: 751–3.
9 Kligman AM. Perspectives and problems in cutaneous gerontology. *J Invest Dermatol* 1979; **73**: 39–46.
10 Potts RO, Buras EM, Chrisman DA. Changes with age in the moisture content of human skin. *J Invest Dermatol* 1984; **82**: 97–100.
11 Graham-Brown RAC. Soaps and detergents in the elderly. *Clin Dermatol* 1996; **14**: 85–7.
12 Lazar AP, Lazar P. Dry skin, water and lubrication. *Dermatol Clin* 1991; **9**: 45–51.
13 Tager A, Berlin C, Scen RJ. Seborrhoeic dermatitis in acute cardiac disease. *Br J Dermatol* 1964; **76**: 367–9.
14 Monk BE, Graham-Brown RAC. Eczema. In: Monk BE, Graham-Brown RAC, Sarkany I, eds. *Skin Disorders in the Elderly*. Oxford: Blackwell Scientific Publications, 1988: 147–57.
15 Bach J-F. Immunosenescence. *Triangle* 1986; **25**: 25–31.
16 Bettley FR, Donoghue E. The irritant effect of soap on normal skin. *Br J Dermatol* 1960; **72**: 67–76.
17 Leonard JN. Dermatitis herpetiformis, bullous pemphigoid, cicatricial pemphigoid and linear IgA disease. In: Fry L, ed. *Skin Problems in the Elderly*. Edinburgh: Churchill Livingstone, 1985: 182–201.
18 Henseler T, Christophers E. Psoriasis of early and late onset: characterization of two types of psoriasis vulgaris. *J Am Acad Dermatol* 1985; **13**: 450–6.
19 Marks R. *Skin Disease in Old Age*. London: Dunitz, 1987: 49–63.
20 Eaglstein WH. Wound healing and aging. *Dermatol Clin* 1986; **4**: 481–4.
21 Bliss MR, Silvers JR. Pressure sores. In: Monk BE, Graham-Brown RAC, Sarkany I, eds. *Skin Disorders in the Elderly*. Oxford: Blackwell Scientific Publications, 1988: 97–112.
22 Peto TEA, Juel-Jensen BE. Varicella zoster virus disease. In: Monk BE, Graham-Brown RAC, Sarkany I, eds. *Skin Disorders in the Elderly*. Oxford: Blackwell Scientific Publications, 1988: 80–96.
23 Elwood JM, Lee JAH. Recent data on the epidemiology of malignant melanoma. *Semin Oncol* 1975; **2**: 149–54.
24 Morris BT, Sober AJ. Cutaneous malignant melanoma in the older patient. *Dermatol Clin* 1986; **4**: 473–80.
25 Keefe M, White JE, Perkins P. Nodular melanomas in the over-50 age group: the next target for health education. *Br J Dermatol* 1990; **123** (Suppl. 37): 59.

REFERENCES

1 Ellis CN, Weiss JS, Hamilton TA *et al.* Sustained improvement with prolonged topical tretinoin (retinoic acid) for photoaged skin. *J Am Acad Dermatol* 1990; **23**: 629–37.

Chapter 71

General Aspects of Treatment

J.A. Cotterill & A.Y. Finlay

General principles

The general principles for the treatment of skin diseases are essentially the same as for other branches of medicine. There are, however, important aspects and details peculiar to dermatology that readily escape the non-specialist, attention to which may make so much difference to the success or otherwise of therapy. In particular, topical therapy in many situations may be in danger of being relegated to an unimportant role. Patients may decry local applications. During history taking, many patients say they have had no treatment, 'only a few ointments'. They may also be unaware of the potential harm that can be done by topical therapy, whether self-administered or iatrogenic. Careful nursing and instruction of the patient on how to use any remedy can be much more important than in other branches of medicine.

Although dermatologists have available to them many more agents of proven beneficial pharmacological activity than were available to their predecessors, they still have to persuade, console and counsel and must convince many patients that no specific treatment is available for their particular problem.

Thus, the central aspect of dermatological management is the consultation, which often demands great skill in communication techniques. Improving doctor–patient communication is not an option but a necessity [1].

The dermatological consultation

The various manoeuvres employed by patients and doctors in the consultation 'gamesmanship' have been described [2].

The individual dermatologist will, however, develop his or her own preferred technique of consultation as he or she matures in the specialty over the years. Thus, there are those dermatologists who like to see their patients completely naked so that they can be sure they are missing no other dermatological pathology. However, seeing a patient initially entirely naked may lead to a considerable loss of valuable data. The patient's dress provides psychosocial information, and the gait of the patient as he or she walks into the consulting room can give some useful information. In particular, the depressed patient often has a characteristic 'droop', whilst the anxious patient is moving in all directions at the same time, typically sitting on the edge of the chair. The depressed patient may be slow in all his or her responses to questions. An anxious person may continuously twirl a ring on a finger, and the quivering lips or the moistening of an eye in response to a question may indicate important stress-provoking factors. The language employed by the patient in describing the symptoms is also important. Whilst photosensitivity eruptions such as porphyria may produce a burning sensation in the skin, very few other skin conditions do this, and symptoms described emotively in this way may indicate that functional factors are important in pathogenesis. The patient who brings in an enormous bag of medicaments, all of which have done 'nothing at all' to help, may also indicate a psychological or psychiatric aspect to the case. A 'hollow' history and the *'belle indifference'* of the classical patient with dermatitis artefacta can be appreciated only by taking a good history. Little matchboxes and plastic bags containing detritus are very characteristic of patients with delusions of parasitosis.

What do patients want? [3–8]

Patients consult dermatologists because they want help with their skin problems. Patients require not only information and medical treatment, but also explanation, understanding and emotional support [3,4]. Whilst patients may hold elaborate, and sometimes sophisticated, theories about their own skin problems, most patients need to know the answers to three basic questions: 'Why me?', 'Why now?' and 'Why this particular illness?' [3]. Sadly patients may receive no diagnosis, few explanations, inadequate advice and leave the consultation feeling the doctor is uninterested and believes all symptoms are unimportant [5]. Above all, the patient values a doctor who listens, although not all doctors may yet have learned to hear what their patients are saying [6]. The doctor must recognize that the patient is now a key medical decision maker in reaching an optimal management choice tailored to the particular needs and views of an individual patient [7]. A paternalistic consultation style is of historical interest only, and care should be patient rather than disease centred.

Eye contact is vital if meaningful data are to be gathered from the patient [8]. Doctors with a mechanistic interrogative style who offer no eye contact usually turn off any meaningful verbal communication from the patient.

Body image, self-esteem and the leper complex

An individual's body image is largely cutaneous, so skin disease affecting any part of the body surface may produce considerable depression in body image, self-esteem, confidence and secondary depression [9]. This is particularly true where skin disease affects areas such as the scalp, hair, face, hands and genital area. The stigma of skin disease can readily produce a 'leper complex' in the individual patient, which compels the patient to withdraw from society and physical contact with other human beings [10,11]. It is vital therefore that the dermatologist provides reassurance by touching the patient at some stage during the consultation.

REFERENCES

1 Meryn S. Improving doctor–patient communication. Not an option but a necessity (Editorial). *BMJ* 1998; **316**: 1922.
2 Cotterill JA. Dermatological games. *Br J Dermatol* 1981; **105**: 311–20.
3 Armstrong D. What do patients want? Someone who will hear their questions. *BMJ* 1991; **303**: 261–2.
4 Finlay AY. Dermatology patients—what do they really need? *Clin Exp Dermatol* 2000; **25**: 444–50.
5 Price J, Leaver L. ABC of psychological medicine. Beginning treatment. *BMJ* 2002; **325**: 33–5.
6 Smith C, Armstrong D. Comparisons of criteria derived by governments for evaluating general practitioner services. *BMJ* 1989; **299**: 494–6.
7 Deyo RA. A key medical decision maker: the patient. *BMJ* 2001; **323**: 466–7.
8 Davenport S, Goldberg D, Millar T. How psychiatric disorders are missed during medical consultations. *Lancet* 1987; **i**: 439–41.
9 Hardy GE, Cotterill JA. A study of depression and obsessionality in dysmorphophobic and psoriatic patients. *Br J Psychiatry* 1982; **140**: 19–22.
10 Ginsburg IA, Link BG. Feelings of stigmatization in patients with psoriasis. *J Am Acad Dermatol* 1989; **20**: 53–63.
11 MacKenna RMB. Psychiatric factors in cutaneous disease. *Lancet* 1944; **ii**: 679–81.

Timing

A dermatosis is rarely a static event. The effect of the patient's actions and attitudes, the frequent development of anxiety or depression and the daily variations in the internal and external milieu require frequent reappraisal and adjustment of treatment. Topical corticosteroids should be reduced in strength as the disease recedes.

The timing of a return to work often involves a difficult decision; even the return of a patient from hospital to his or her environment may be misjudged. In either case, a relapse may cause the patient to lose confidence. In all dermatological therapy, Napoleon's dictum may be remembered with advantage: 'la puissance ne consiste pas à frapper fort ou à frapper souvent, mais à frapper juste'.

Failure to appreciate the natural history of disease has been responsible for much unnecessary therapy, and for a wrong assessment of therapeutic needs. For instance, in alopecia areata, specific therapy is lacking, and the average duration is unaffected by empirical measures. Infantile eczema tends to improve with time and nummular eczema 'burns itself out' in months or years. In these diseases, the patient is ill-served by measures that can only alter the immediate situation without an additional planned campaign to sustain him or her over this prolonged period. A diminishing concentration of topical corticosteroids, measures designed to distract attention from the disease and manoeuvres designed to help morale are necessary parts of the whole treatment. In diseases with a short-lived but hectic course, such as erythema multiforme exudativum, oral steroids, if given at all, should be 'tailed off' once the expected peak of the disease is past. In chronic diseases, such as psoriasis, systemic sclerosis, lichen sclerosus of the vulva, ichthyosiform erythroderma or dermatitis herpetiformis, therapy should be on the lines of a siege operation or, sometimes, as a deliberately planned retreat in which the disease is contained and held in check. Whenever possible, it is a wise precaution to hold a therapeutic reserve for periods of exceptional activity of the disease process.

Compliance

Hippocrates warned that '(the physician) should be aware . . . that patients often lie when they state they have taken their medicine'. Dermatology patients may not deliberately lie, but there may be many reasons why patients are not able to carry out a therapy regimen. It is essential that the clinician understands these potential difficulties and takes steps within the consultation to plan therapy which is practical and with which the patient agrees. The term 'concordance' or 'adherence' is now preferred over 'compliance', as the concept of compliance with treatment implies a patient passive in the treatment decision process —a situation likely to ensure inadequate or inappropriate use of therapy. Although concordance issues are of relevance to every dermatology consultation [1], there is relatively little published on the subject; there have however, been two workshops at international meetings [2,3].

Influences on adherence include the degree of motivation of patients, the extent to which their quality of life is impaired by their disease and the attitude of the patient towards their disease and their relationship with their doctor [4]. A longitudinal study [5] has shown that dissatisfaction with care and psychiatric morbidity are significantly and independently associated with poor medication adherence: the physician's interpersonal skills play a major influence in medication adherence. The strongest predictor of adherence to skin-care treatment in childhood atopic dermatitis is a good doctor–patient (mother) relationship [6]. Other factors that are likely to improve adherence with therapy include patient education about how to apply topical preparations, the use of as few different preparations as possible and the use of preparations that are cosmetically acceptable. Realistic and simple regimens with preferably once daily applications are much better than regimens with frequent applications, but a simple manoeuvre such as using a cream in the morning and an ointment at night may improve adherence [7].

The use of therapy that gives early improvement is preferable but where this is not possible the patient must understand the reality of the likelihood of speed of improvement. The patient must have the opportunity to express concerns about treatment so that unfounded fears can be allayed. For patients with psoriasis, even more important than the speed of action of a topical treatment is the opportunity to be involved in the decision taking [8]. Joint discussion and decisions between doctor and patient should be taken. Patients need information about possible side effects and how to handle them: for example if a patient is warned that there may be transient stinging, the patient may continue to use a drug instead of being alarmed and stopping it. The cost and affordability of therapy is an obvious factor in many health care settings.

When systemic drugs are used in an outpatient setting in cardiology and internal medicine clinics, there are widespread discrepancies in drug usage with 76% of patients not taking the planned medication correctly [9]. There are similar problems with patients using topical preparations [10]. The likelihood of a patient taking oral medication as planned is inversely proportional to the number of times per day that the drug should be taken [11]. Even in a controlled research setting, when a patient is asked to record the therapy used for skin disease there is poor correlation between reported treatment use and weighed ointment usage [12]: the use of electronic monitoring may be helpful in the future to monitor medication adherence [13].

There are particular cultural and age-related issues in trying to maximize the likelihood of adolescents taking medication effectively. This is of particular relevance to acne therapy [14]: the use of topical therapy that has a more rapid onset of action is likely to be an advantage in increasing usage.

When topical corticosteroids were introduced into clinical practice in the 1950s their great benefit to patients with inflammatory disease was immediately apparent. It is unlikely that the phobia surrounding their use, especially in children, would have been predicted. The phobia comes from a lack of understanding about the different potencies of corticosteroids available and a concern over side effects, the risk of which is minimal if they are used correctly. The phobia may lead to inappropriate under use and consequent poor control, especially of atopic dermatitis [15]. Surprisingly, however, the mother's anxiety about using topical steroids did not influence reported use of topical steroids in a Japanese study [6]. It is important that clinicians are aware of this issue and address it in discussions about advising their use. An approach to improving treatment compliance in occupational dermatitis has been the concept of a specialist nurse-led 'eczema school' to contribute to the education of patients and carers [16].

Only 33% of patients with psoriasis who were asked to apply an ointment twice daily actually did so [10]. Patients with psoriasis who report that they have not complied with treatment are more likely to believe that both psoriasis and their treatment interfered with their quality of life [17]. Self-reported non-adherer patients with psoriasis demonstrate more negative views towards all aspects of health care [18]. In both psoriasis [19] and in acne [20] adherence with therapy is poorer the greater the severity of the disease. It is possible that having severe skin disease leads to poor life quality, which in turn leads to a degree of depression and a sense of 'giving up'. This may result in poor concordance with therapy and in turn further deterioration in the disease. Strategies are needed to break this negative feedback loop. It is likely that treatment failure is much more often due to non-adherence than has been previously recognized.

There is a major challenge for dermatologists to identify those factors that contribute to non-adherence and to develop strategies that make it more likely that a patient will use medication appropriately and in their best interests.

REFERENCES

1 Witkowski JA. Compliance: the dermatologic patient. *Int J Dermatol* 1988; **27**: 608–11.

2 Finlay AY, de Korte J, Taieb A *et al*. The science of compliance. Workshop abstracts, European Academy of Dermatology and Venereology, Amsterdam 1999. *J Eur Acad Dermatol Venereol* 1999; **12** (Suppl. 2): S77–8.

3 Finlay AY, Draelos ZD, Hashiro M *et al*. Quality of life issues and treatment compliance in dermatology. Workshop abstracts, World Congress of Dermatology, Paris 2002. *Ann Dermatol Vénéréol* 2002; **129**: 1 S182–4.

4 Chren M-M. Rethinking compliance in dermatology. *Arch Dermatol* 2002; **138**: 393–4.

5 Renzi C, Picardi A, Abeni D *et al*. Association of dissatisfaction with care and psychiatric morbidity with poor treatment compliance. *Arch Dermatol* 2002; **138**: 337–42.

6 Ohya Y, Williams H, Steptoe A *et al*. Psychosocial factors and adherence to treatment advice in childhood atopic dermatitis. *J Invest Dermatol* 2001; **117**: 852–7.

7 Van de Kerkhof PC, Franssen M, de la Brassine M, Kuipers M. Calcipotriol cream in the morning and ointment in the evening: a novel regimen to improve compliance. *J Dermatolog Treat* 2001; **12**: 75–9.

8 Van de Kerkhof PC, de Hoop D, de Korte J, Cobelens SA, Kuipers MV. Patient compliance and disease management in the treatment of psoriasis in the Netherlands. *Dermatology* 2000; **200**: 292–8.

9 Bedell SE, Jabbour S, Goldberg R. *et al*. Discrepancies in the use of medications: their extent and predictors in an outpatient practice. *Arch Intern Med* 2000; **160**: 2129–34.

10 Van de Kerkhof PCM, Steegers-Theunissen RPM, Kuipers MV. Evaluation of topical drug treatment in psoriasis. *Dermatology* 1998; **197**: 31–6.

11 Nelson JD. Clinical compliance and patient tolerance. *Infect Dis Clin Prac* 1994; **3**: 158–60.

12 Goodwin RG, Finlay AY. Structured patient reporting of compliance is very inaccurate. *Br J Dermatol* 2002; **147** (Suppl. 62): 17.

13 Koehler AM, Maibach HI. Electronic monitoring in medication adherence measurement. Implications for Dermatology. *Am J Clin Dermatol* 2001; **2**: 7–12.

14 Finlay AY. Better quality treatments for your patients. *J Dermatolog Treat* 1998; **9** (Suppl. 2): S3–6.

15 Charman CR, Morris AD, Williams HC. Topical corticosteroids phobia in patients with atopic eczema. *Br J Dermatol* 2000; **142**: 931–6.

16 Kalimo K, Kautiainen H, Niskanen T, Niemi L. 'Eczema school' to improve compliance in an occupational dermatology clinic. *Contact Dermatitis* 1999; **41**: 315–9.

17 Richards HL, Fortune DG, O'Sullivan TM *et al*. Patients with psoriasis and their medication. *J Am Acad Dermatol* 1999; **41**: 581–3.

18 Richards HL, Mason DL, Fortune DG *et al*. Adherence to treatment; does satisfaction with healthcare provision predict compliance in psoriasis? *Br J Dermatol* 2002; **147**: 1070.

19 Zaghloul S, Gonzalez M, Judodihardjo H, Finlay AY. In psoriasis, the greater the disability, the poorer the topical treatment compliance. *Br J Dermatol* 1999; **141** (Suppl. 55): 48.

20 Zaghloul SS, Cunliffe WJ, Goodfield MJD. Compliance in acne is highly correlated to psychological well-being and self preservation. *Br J Dermatol* 2002; **147** (Suppl. 62): 43.

Side effects

Worldwide more and more people, especially the elderly, are taking not only prescription but also over-the-counter drugs, including herbal remedies. Moreover the pharmaceutical industry is constantly introducing new drugs. The individual doctor is faced with a massive task in keeping up to date with all these drugs, including side effects and cross-reactions. Whilst information technology may help this is no substitute but can complement the practice of a well-informed and competent medical practitioner. The consultation is all-important in warning the patient about possible side effects [1], but skill and care are necessary. The doctor may be guilty of negligence if major side effects are not explained, but, on the other hand, if too much emphasis is placed on side effects the doctor may invite non-compliance. Particular care must be taken

during pregnancy [2–4] and lactation [3,4]. Children pose special problems and neonates are at special risk of side effects because of immature renal and liver function [5]. Poor renal function leads to the accumulation of drug and metabolite(s) in the body increasing the risk of side effects [6,7]. In liver disease the reduction in first-pass metabolism may lead to toxic drug levels whilst reduced protein binding may lead to increased bioavailability and side effects [8].

REFERENCES

1 Price J, Leaver L. ABC of psychological medicine. Beginning treatment. *BMJ* 2002; **325**: 33–5.

2 Rubin P. Drug treatment during pregnancy. *BMJ* 1998; **196**: 135–9.

3 Reed BR. Dermatological drug use during pregnancy and lactation. *Dermatol Clin* 1997; **15**: 197–206.

4 Reed BR. Dermatologic drugs, pregnancy and lactation. A conservative guide. *Arch Dermatol* 1997; **133**: 894–8.

5 Atherton D, Gan C. Treatment in childhood. In: Wakelin SH, ed. *Handbook of Systemic Drug Treatment in Dermatology*. London: Manson, 2002: 223–32.

6 Arnoff ER, Bern JS, Brier MR. Drugs prescribing in renal failure. In: Aronoff GR *et al*., eds. *Dosing Guidelines for Adults*, 4th edn. Philadelphia, PA: American College of Physicians, 1999.

7 Tarzi R, Palmer A. Treatment in patients with renal disease. In: Wakelin SH, ed. *Handbook of Systemic Drug Treatment in Dermatology*. London: Manson, 2002: 233–241.

8 Teare J, Puleston J. Treatment in patients with liver disease. In: Wakelin SH, ed. *Handbook of Systemic Drug Treatment in Dermatology*. London: Manson, 2002: 242–9.

Therapy

General management

Explanation

Like all doctors, but perhaps more than most, dermatologists must achieve rapid rapport with their patients and be seen either to assuage the symptoms and signs of visible disease or to bring the patient—and the relatives or parents—to accept chronicity or irreversible changes. Dermatology has been called an 'applied intuitive art': if so, an easy understanding must be achieved between the artist and sitter. Allowance must be made for symptoms of anxiety—aggression, lack of faith, mistrust. If necessary, the dermatologist must gradually overcome these to become therapeutic in the clinical situation.

Patients nowadays demand and deserve a far fuller explanation of their disease than was formerly either possible or even considered desirable. No longer is it appropriate to give a learned diagnosis, a prescription and little else.

Patients may be well-informed or misinformed, but they are informed. Recourse to the Book of Proverbs or Job is not received with the understanding it used to command. It is never easy to explain autoimmune diseases or the aetiology of atopic dermatitis in easily comprehensible terms. The intelligence of the patient must be gauged; a suitable metaphor or simile is often apt. In any case, the patient's questions must be answered. In seeking clues to the causation of conditions such as contact dermatitis or chronic urticaria, one should always listen attentively to the patient's explanation. He or she may well be wrong, but occasionally the patient is right, however, unexpected the answer.

Nevertheless, his or her account of the onset and course of the disease may have become distorted by time or for medicolegal reasons, and can never be believed in cases of dermatitis artefacta. The patient's memory (or suppression of memory) of drug or topical medicaments given is usually defective, especially if self-administered.

Avoidance of aggravating factors

General advice that might be considered common sense to the dermatologist may be quite unfamiliar to some patients. Such advice includes care with environmental temperature and, at times, humidity. Advice should be given on appropriate clothing, which should not be too constricting, too hot or too harsh. Irritants and sensitizers should be avoided where possible. Many patients retain the belief that skin disease is a manifestation of dirt or germs to be expunged with vigour and exorcized with soap and water or worse. Care should indeed be taken with soap, but it is seldom necessary to proscribe bathing. It is surprising how often patients will be applying inappropriate household germicides, and in totally inappropriate concentrations. Advice to stop scratching usually causes more frustration and alienation unless something is done to help the sensation of itching.

Regimen

Rest and relaxation can play a major part in treating many dermatoses. With others there are positive benefits in remaining at work or at school. Decisions, including economic ones, are often neatly balanced, but the patient will often require positive guidance on how much activity is to be encouraged.

The arguments for and against admission to hospital clearly depend on so many variables other than the purely medical ones. The last 30 years have seen a great reduction in beds for dermatology patients in many countries. The reasons include better treatments, which remove the need for admission, improved facilities for home nursing, and better transport to outpatient facilities. The dramatic rises in cost of maintaining patients in hospital, whether at the expense of themselves or of their health services, also militate against admission.

No firm guidelines can be laid down about which particular diseases need to be treated on an inpatient basis. These will vary from culture to culture and even from town to town. No doubt many diseases might benefit from time in hospital but this may not be feasible. Sometimes, a short stay before complete remission has been achieved will allow the acute crisis to be averted, allow patients to be taught how to manage themselves, and also build up a better relationship between patient, doctors and nurses.

Recent years have seen the emergence of dermatological intensive care units for the management of such acute, life-threatening emergencies as toxic epidermal necrolysis, pemphigus and erythroderma. These have been pioneered at Creteil, France [1,2] and have pointed the way forward to improving what can be a poor prognosis.

Quite often, the need for hospitalization is avoided if the patient is given precise instructions on how to do at home almost everything that might have been done in hospital.

REFERENCES

1 Revuz J, Roujeau JC, Guillaume JC. Treatment of toxic epidermal necrolysis, Creteil's experience. *Arch Dermatol* 1987; **123**: 1156–8, 1160–5.
2 Roujeau JC, Revuz J. Intensive care in dermatology. In: Champion RH, Pye RJ, eds. *Recent Advances in Dermatology*, Vol. 8. Edinburgh: Churchill Livingstone, 1990: 85–99.

Systemic drug therapy

Drug therapy may be specific, empirical or placebo in its effect. Dermatology has suffered more than most specialties from an abundance of empirics and placebos. It has not been shown that dermatological patients respond more to placebos than others, but the presence of an obvious and visible disease and the anxiety that this engenders endow all forms of treatment with an aura of suggestibility that often confuses the judgement of the patient and physician alike. The past records of dermatological therapy give abundant evidence of the 'wish to believe'. The results of 'double-blind' trials have destroyed the edifice of this belief. Drugs should not be despised if they help the patient, but they should never be regarded as pharmacologically active without unequivocal evidence of their effectiveness. There must be no confusion in the dermatologist's mind. At his or her command there are a few specific remedies, a number of empirical ones and many placebos. The first are accepted because their action is known. The second are effective in 'double-blind' trials, although their mode of action remains unknown. The third are effective in a manner that bears no relation to the pharmacology of the drug or the pathogenesis of the disease; often, the physician endows them with his or her personality. It is important to be acquainted with the concept of the doctor as a drug and that problems may arise, as with any drug, with overdose, underdose or idiosyncratic reactions [1,2].

The placebo [2–5]

Potentially any treatment may have a dual effect related to the intrinsic property of the active drug and also to the perception that treatment is being received [3]. This latter is known as the placebo effect [4]. Distinction must be made between placebo and placebo effect [2] as any sort of therapy can act as a placebo but the response of the individual patient determines whether there is a placebo effect. Despite claims to the contrary, no consistent placebo-reactor profile has been demonstrated [2,3] but the effects of placebos can be very specific depending on patient information, i.e. patient expectations. Thus, placebos can induce opposite effects on blood pressure or heart rate depending on whether they are administered as perceived tranquillizers or stimulants and this makes a precise definition of the placebo effect difficult [3]. Moreover, variations in the placebo response to tablets of different colours—green is best for anxiety—has been demonstrated [5].

Recent evidence suggests that the placebo effect is mediated by dopaminergic reward mechanisms in the human brain and related also to the expectation of clinical benefit [3].

The placebo response in dermatology

The less effective any existing treatment, the more likely are any favourable effects to be of placebo type. Lichen planus, alopecia areata and chronic urticaria have been 'cured' in the past with many different preparations, which have not been shown to be pharmacologically effective in these diseases. But the patient has been sustained through the natural course by receiving a potion or a lotion that at least sustains the faith and the hope and, at most, is free from potential toxicity. The placebo effect is also apparent in the control of insomnia and pruritus, and extends to physical methods of treatment, notably acupuncture.

Preparations. Placebos must be harmless. Many drugs that are *not* harmless are really only being given as placebos. Lactose tablets are commonly given but even this substance is not totally harmless. Aspirin should be avoided. Carefully worded instructions may reinforce a placebo effect [3], as may an unusual size or shape of tablet.

No official placebo is included in the British National Formulary, but many manufacturers will supply inert preparations matched to their own products.

In general, physicians should be aware that the effect of a drug they are prescribing may be a placebo effect. On the other hand, it has been cogently argued that a placebo works better if the physician also believes in it!

Ethics. Most but not all physicians would agree that the administration of a placebo as a therapeutic measure is justifiable if no known effective treatment exists. In any case, it is less likely to harm the patient than a poorly tested or a powerful 'new' drug of uncertain value. In some cases, the deliberate use of a placebo initially may be

valuable in ensuring rapport with a patient who claims to be prone to all the side effects known for all drugs taken; and to assess the placebo response reactions. It also gains time for the anxious patient to accept a prolonged or incurable condition while a situation of rapport is being built up. This presupposes, of course, that no widely accepted active agent is available that is likely to be more beneficial.

In all cases, particularly in drug trials, the overriding consideration must always be the benefit to the patient. The doctor is always in a particularly authoritative position and must not abuse this authority. The patient's fully informed consent (with a witness) must always be obtained if a 'controlled' trial is embarked on. It is doubtful whether the use of 'dummy' preparations is ever justified in children, even with the parents' consent.

It is very important that none of us loses sight of the fact that we should not do harm to the patient, especially in an experimental situation. The so-called experiment where a mother aged 80 years was injected with malignant melanoma cells from her 50-year-old daughter, which led to the mother's most unpleasant death from metastatic malignant melanoma, must never be repeated [6]. It is essential that any proposed research is vetted by a well-qualified ethical committee before any projects are undertaken.

REFERENCES

1 Balint M, ed. *The Doctor, His Patient and the Illness.* London: Pitman Medical, 1975: 5.
2 Bridy H. The doctor as therapeutic agent: a placebo effect research agenda. In: Harrington A, ed. *The Placebo Effect: an Interdisciplinary Exploration.* Cambridge, MA: Harvard University Press, 1997: 77–92.
3 Fuente-Fernandez R, Schulzer M, Stoessl AJ. The placebo effect in neurological disorders. *Lancet Neurol* 2002; **1**: 85–91.
4 Beecher HK. The powerful placebo. *JAMA* 1955; **159**: 1602–6.
5 Shapirak K, McClelland HA, Griffiths NR *et al.* Study on the effects of tablet colour in the treatment of anxiety states. *BMJ* 1970; **ii**: 446–9.
6 Papworth M. *Human Guinea Pigs.* Middlesex: Penguin Books, 1967: 156–7.

Antihistamines

These are discussed in Chapter 72. In the hands of many non-dermatologists, the sight of a rash evokes a reflex desire to prescribe antihistamines. These drugs are, of course, no panacea. If they are to be prescribed, there should be some thought whether they are being used for their ability to antagonize other mediators such as acetylcholine (usually considered as a side effect), or for a central effect. Otherwise, their use must be considered as placebo, albeit usually a harmless placebo. The advent of new 'non-sedating' antihistamines, said not to cross the blood–brain barrier, makes it important not to thoughtlessly prescribe the newest antihistamine for the management of all types of pruritus (Chapters 16 & 72). Every general practitioner should have a working knowledge of short-acting, long-acting, sedative and non-sedative types of antihistamine.

Psychopharmacological agents

In recent years, there has been a marked trend, in the UK at least, away from reliance on psychopharmacological agents or willingness to take them on the part of the patient. Even the conservative dermatologist, who may feel on occasions that the short-term administration of sedatives or hypnotics would be of help in reducing itching or restoring normal sleep patterns, may encounter unexpected resistance by the patient. Unfortunately, reasonable alternatives—discussion, the encouragement of the development of relaxation or autosuggestive techniques—are time-consuming and seldom carried out by busy practitioners. Thus, anxiety may intensify until the acute 'emergency' situation, so well known to dermatologists, develops. In such cases, rest, adequate sleep and some form of sedation become imperative and may be obtained only by removal of the patient from his or her environment to hospital.

Two situations in which the rational use of psychopharmacological agents may be necessary are anxiety and depression. Many agents are available for the treatment of these conditions, and national and individual differences in prescribing are widespread. One drug often replaces another for reasons of improved efficacy. The dermatologist is best advised to choose two or three, preferably having short- or medium-term and more prolonged effects, and to use them appropriately.

Anxiety

Environmental sources of anxiety and tension have increased in modern industrialized life. Anxiety, not always recognized or acknowledged by the patient, may be an essential driving force in some individuals ('trait' anxiety) [1]; only when this increases, as a result of extra stresses or the presence of disease, may it become marked ('state' anxiety). Then, the symptoms themselves, for example the intensity of pruritus, may become part of a general stress response characterized by emotional over-arousal [2]. It is recognized that pathological anxiety is more common in patients with a chronic medical problem than in those without [3]. So detecting and treating anxiety is an integral part of dermatological management. Successful treatment has several benefits including better quality of life, less disability and less use of resources. Rather than prescribe an anxiolytic initial management should include effective communication, information giving and reassurance. Whilst behavioural therapy is one of the most effective treatments for anxiety [4] most dermatologists are not skilled in this technique. Developing an effective liaison with an interested clinical psychologist or psychiatrist, or even in a dermatological liaison clinic, is the optimal way of delivering this type of care to anxious dermatological patients.

Whilst the benzodiazepines [2–4] are the safest and most effective anxiolytics, there is concern about habituation and addiction to these drugs [5,6] so these drugs should only be used in the short term and for emergencies [3]. Their use in adequate dosage in the short term to prevent nocturnal pruritus and to give the very itchy patient a good night's sleep can be justified. However, conventional doses of sedative antihistamines such as hydroxyzine may be equally effective and not accompanied by the risk of addiction or habituation. A large number are available: the main difference lies in their different plasma half-lives [2]. They are equally effective for treating both anxiety and insomnia, although the causes of the latter should be examined before recourse to drug therapy [7]. They are widely used, especially by older females in the lower socio-economic groups [8]. Diazepam and chlordiazepoxide are the best known. Nitrazepam, used as a hypnotic, has a half-life of about 30 h and may thus accumulate on repeated use. A single dose of diazepam is frequently given to allay apprehension in young children before minor operative procedures [9,10]. When appropriate, a suitable analgesic should be given before the diazepam [11]. The intravenous use of benzodiazepines carries a risk of thrombosis or ischaemia [12,13]. This drug should be diluted with blood and given slowly [12] and resuscitation facilities should be to hand. The benzodiazepines have no antidepressive effect and may, in fact, enhance depression. The side effects are those of any drug affecting the central nervous system, including oversedation [14]. Effects of alcohol are potentiated [15].

Depressive states

Depression is common in dermatological patients and may present in many different guises. It is unusual for the patient to say 'I am depressed'. However, the condition is so common in dermatological patients that the attending dermatologist should always ask him- or herself 'is this particular patient depressed or not?' Dermatologists therefore should become adept at recognizing depression in their patients. Whilst criteria for major depression [16] (Table 71.1) are recognized, it has been claimed that simply asking two questions may be as effective in detecting depression as longer screening instruments [17] (Table 71.2).

Depression with suicidal ideation is common, both in patients with psoriasis [18] and Darier's disease [19], and any extensive skin disease, particularly if it affects important body image areas such as the face, may produce a very severe reactive depression. It is known that patients with chronic urticaria and generalized pruritus are more likely to be depressed than controls [20], and acne scarring, particularly in males, may produce severe reactive depression and even suicide [21]. Dermatological patients may become significantly depressed when they are treated

Table 71.1 Symptoms of depression.*

Depressed mood
Substantial weight loss or gain
Insomnia or hypersomnia
Feelings of guilt or worthlessness
Suicide ideation or suicide attempt
Decreased interest or pleasure*
Psychomotor agitation or retardation
Fatigue or loss of energy
Diminished ability to think or concentrate

* One of these symptoms must be present. Two or more of the above should be present within the same 21-week period.

Table 71.2 Two simple questions to detect depression [17].

1 Over the past 2 weeks have you ever felt down, depressed or hopeless?
2 Have you ever felt little interest or pleasure in doing things?

Table 71.3 Main classes of antidepressants.

Tricyclics
Selective serotonin inhibitors
Monoamine oxidase inhibitors
Norepinephrine (noradrenaline) reuptake inhibitors
Others

with corticosteroids orally or parenterally, and depressed dermatological patients are twice as likely to be admitted to hospital, and to remain as inpatients twice as long as non-depressed dermatological patients [22]. The commonest psychiatric disease present in patients with dermatological delusional disease and with body dysmorphic disorder (dermatological non-disease), in particular, is depression [23]. Depression is a well-recognized risk factor for non-compliance with medical treatment so depressed patients are three times more likely to be non-compliant than non-depressed patients [24].

Finally, dermatological patients who go to litigation are more likely to be depressed than their non-litiginous peers [25]. The treatment of depression therefore is of vital importance in dermatological practice.

The main classes of antidepressants available are shown in Table 71.3.

Rather than continuously experimenting with a wide range of available antidepressants the clinician is best advised to become familiar with one drug from each class [16]. The response to treatment may be slow and there may be little clinical benefit during the first month of therapy. Moreover, side effects are usually worse at this time, especially during the first 2 weeks of treatment [16]. Many patients with significant depression are treated with inadequate doses of antidepressants for an inadequate time. 4–6 months of treatment are necessary to avoid relapse and continuous maintenance therapy is

necessary if the patient has had two or more episodes of depression within the previous 5 years [16].

The generally lower side effect profile of selective serotonin reuptake inhibitors compared to, for example, the tricyclic group of antidepressants, and, in particular, lower cardiotoxicity, make these drugs the first-line treatment of depression [26]. It may be difficult to make a clear clinical distinction between anxiety and depression and the depression may become more apparent when a patient fails to respond to anxiolytics. Whilst tricyclic antidepressants such as amitriptyline in adequate dosage are effective in anxious, depressed patients, they also have some sedative properties and are not particularly helpful in patients with pure primary anxiety [2].

Doxepin is both a potent antidepressant and has very marked antihistamine activity. This antidepressant is useful in the itchy, depressed, elderly patient and in some patients with neurodermatitis [26].

Other drugs in use

Butyrophenone derivations such as haloperidol are also used for anxiety, depression and alcohol withdrawal symptoms. Chloral hydrate (0.3–2.0 g) should not be despised as a hypnotic, particularly in children. The unpleasant taste of paraldehyde has limited its oral use, but it is an effective and quick-acting hypnotic, especially for hypomanic states, given by intramuscular injection (5–10 mL). Beta-adrenoceptor antagonists ('β-blockers') have not found much place in dermatology, although symptoms mediated by the β-division of the sympathetic nervous system have been helped by propranolol [27]. A number of side effects have been reported [28]. Pimozide has a special place in the management of patients with delusions of parasitosis [29,30].

Topical therapy

The dictum 'primum non nocere' has a special significance in relation to the vulnerability of damaged skin, often with an impaired barrier function, to develop either sensitivity or irritant reactions to local applications that the same patient might find harmless at other times. There is a particular temptation to be overzealous in treatment when faced with a disease that fails to react to initial therapy. Visual evidence of failure is particularly hard to accept with equanimity. Full details of topical therapy are given in Chapter 75.

EMLA cream (a eutectic mixture of 5% lidocaine (lignocaine) and prilocaine) is particularly useful as a local anaesthetic cream in children to try and ensure pain-free venepuncture, and may also be used to try and minimize distress during curettage of lesions of molluscum contagiosum or in removing genital warts. Its use may ensure that the injection of keloids in children causes minimal distress, and it has a place in anaesthetizing the skin in children with port-wine stains during laser therapy. The cream is best applied under occlusion 1–4 h before the planned procedure [31]. An amethocaine-containing gel has been claimed to be more effective than the EMLA local anaesthetic in patients with port-wine stains [32].

Cosmetic camouflage

Cosmetic camouflage is very useful in the management of a wide range of dermatological problems ranging from scarring to vitiligo, and vascular anomalies such as port-wine stains. In the UK, the Red Cross offers a voluntary service and in some hospitals the occupational therapists are trained to do this work. Cosmetic camouflage has been shown to improve quality of life [33].

REFERENCES

1 Spielberger CD. Anxiety as an emotional state. In: Spielberger CD, ed. *Anxiety. Current Trends in Theory and Research*, Vol. 1. New York: Academic Press, 1972: 23–49.
2 Lader M, Peturrson H. Rational use of anxiolytic/sedative drugs. *Drugs* 1983; **25**: 514–28.
3 House A, Stark D. ABC of psychological medicine. Anxiety in medical patients. *BMJ* 2002; **325**: 207–9.
4 Westra HA, Stewart SH. Cognitive behavioural therapy and pharmacotherapy: complimentary or contradictory approach to the treatment of anxiety? *Clin Psychol Rev* 1998; **18**: 307–40.
5 Marks J, ed. *The Benzodiazepines. Use, Overuse, Misuse, Abuse*. Lancaster: MTP Press, 1978.
6 Petursson H, Lader MH. Withdrawal from long-term benzodiazepine treatment. *BMJ* 1981; **283**: 643–5.
7 Editorial. Temazepam for insomnia? *Drug Ther Bull* 1978; **16**: 21–2.
8 Lader M. Benzodiazepines—the opium of the masses? *Neuroscience* 1978; **3**: 159–65.
9 Gordon NY, Turner DJ. Oral paediatric premedication. A comparative trial of either phenobarbitone, trimeprazine or diazepam with hyoscine, prior to guillotine tonsillectomy. *Br J Anaesth* 1968; **41**: 136–42.
10 Haq IU, Dundee JW. Studies of drugs given before anaesthesia. XVI. Oral diazepam and trimeprazine for adenotonsillectomy. *Br J Anaesth* 1968; **40**: 972–8.
11 Editorial. Sedation for minor procedures. *Drug Ther Bull* 1976; **14**: 19–20.
12 Driscoll EJ, Gelfman SS, Sweet JB et al. Thrombophlebitis after intravenous use of anesthesia and sedation: its incidence and natural history. *J Oral Surg* 1979; **37**: 809–15.
13 Editorial. Coronary artery bypass. *Drug Ther Bull* 1981; **19**: 9–11.
14 Edwards JG. Adverse effects of antianxiety drugs. *Drugs* 1981; **22**: 495–514.
15 Linnoila M, Mattila MJ, Kitchell BS. Drug interactions with alcohol. *Drugs* 1979; **18**: 299–311.
16 Peveler R, Carson A, Rodin G. ABC of psychological medicine. Depression in medical patients. *BMJ* 2002; **325**: 149–53.
17 Pignome MP, Gaynes BN, Rushton JL et al. Screening for depression in adults: a summary of the evidence for the US Preventative Services Task Force. *Ann Intern Med* 2002; **136**: 765–76.
18 Gupta MA, Schork NJ, Gupta AK et al. Suicidal ideation in psoriasis. *Int J Dermatol* 1993; **32**: 188–90.
19 Denicoff KD, Lehman ZA, Rubinow DR et al. Suicidal ideation in Darier's disease. *J Am Acad Dermatol* 1990; **22**: 196–8.
20 Sheehan-Dare R, Cotterill JA. Anxiety and depression in patients with chronic urticaria and generalised pruritus. *Br J Dermatol* 1990; **123**: 769–74.
21 Cotterill JA, Cunliffe WJ. Suicide in dermatological patients. *Br J Dermatol* 1997; **137**: 246–50.
22 Pulimood S, Rajagopalan B, Rajagopalan M et al. Psychiatric morbidity among dermatology in-patients. *Natl Med J India* 1996; **9**: 208–10.
23 Hardy G, Cotterill JA. A study of depression and obsessionality in dysmorphophobic and psoriatic patients. *Br J Psychiatry* 1982; **140**: 19–22.
24 DiMatteo RM, Lepper HS, Crogham W. Depression is a risk factor for non-compliance with medical treatment. Meta analysis of the effects of anxiety and depression on patient adherence. *Arch Intern Med* 2000; **160**: 2101–7.
25 Cotterill JA. Why do patients sue? Paper presented at the Vth Congress of the European Academy of Dermatology and Venereology, October 1996.
26 Gupta MA, Gupta AK. The use of antidepressant drugs in dermatology. *J Eur Acad Dermatol Venereol* 2001; **15**: 512–8.
27 Tyrer P. Use of beta-blocking drugs in psychiatry and neurology. *Drugs* 1980; **20**: 300–8.
28 Clerens A, Guilmot-Bruneau MM, Defresne C et al. Revue: a propos des beta-bloquants en dermatologie. *Dermatologica* 1981; **163**: 5–11.
29 Koblenzer CS, ed. *Psychocutaneous Disease*. New York: Grune & Stratton, 1987: 20.
30 Driscoll MS, Rothe MJ, Grant-Kels JM, Hale MS. Delusional parasitosis. A dermatology, psychiatric and pharmacologic approach. *J Am Acad Dermatol* 1993; **29**: 1023–343.
31 Clarke S, Radford M. Topical anaesthesia for venepuncture. *Arch Dis Child* 1986; **61**: 1132–5.
32 Armstrong DKB, Handley J, Allen GE. Effect of percutaneous local anaesthesia on pain caused by pulsed dye laser treatment of port wine stains. *Br J Dermatol* 1996; **135** (Suppl. 47): 14.
33 Holme SA, Beattie PE, Flemming CJ. Cosmetic camouflage advice improves quality of life. *Br J Dermatol* 2002; **147**: 946–9.

Physical measures

Physiotherapy

The role of physiotherapists has assumed increased importance in recent years. Their duties have extended far from massage and simple forms of heat and light therapy of the past. They have become valuable members of a team devoted to a wide range of physiotherapeutic manoeuvres and to rehabilitation in the widest context.

In dermatology, the physiotherapist is probably not sufficiently invited to participate in the overall management of the patient with chronic or disabling diseases. Rehabilitation is discussed below, but techniques of relaxation are of benefit to many tense patients with irritable or vasolabile skin disease. Muscular relaxation is a key that opens the door to emotional relaxation, but it requires some experience and training to use the key effectively. Relaxation techniques [1] are a valuable adjunct to drug therapy and may even supplant it. Massage and re-education in limb movement are of great practical value in patients with constricting scars and deforming linear scleroderma, for which we have so little to offer. The influence of communal participation of physiotherapeutic activities, in which warmth, touch and encouragement combine to create an ambience conducive to relaxation and to a feeling of positive activity, should not be underestimated.

Massage [2] is valuable in the treatment of lymphoedema (Chapter 51) and rosacea.

Some physiotherapists have expertise in the management of venous leg ulceration and can participate in treatment from an early stage through the period of healing and rehabilitation.

Tap water iontophoresis is performed by many physiotherapy departments and is particularly useful in patients with hyperhidrosis of the hands, feet and axillae [3]. The need for this therapeutic approach has probably lessened following the introduction of botulinum toxin for the management of not only hyperhidrosis of the axillae and, to a lesser extent, the palms [4,5] but also dyshidrotic hand eczema [6].

Other modes of physical medicine, such as short-wave diathermy, play a small part in dermatological management.

Ultrasound has found a secure place in the treatment of soft-tissue disease and injury [7,8] and may occasionally be of adjuvant value in conditions such as scleroderma [9], panniculitis and other dermatological conditions affecting deeper tissues.

Phototherapy, often performed by physiotherapists, is discussed in Chapter 35.

Acupuncture

The empirical basis on which this technique rested for so long has been dramatically changed by the discovery of the endorphins, and that the response to acupuncture can be mediated centrally by endorphins and enkephalins [10]. It has been shown that acupuncture can reduce the effect of histamine-induced itch and flare in healthy subjects [11]. The acupuncture points described in ancient Chinese medical literature correspond to some of the so-called trigger points described in Western medicine, and are said to represent areas of low electrical resistance.

Low-dose helium neon laser light and other types of lasers directed at acupuncture points have been claimed to be effective in a wide variety of conditions, but no valid double-blind clinical trials have been carried out. Anecdotally, post-herpetic neuralgia and atopic dermatitis seem to be helped in some patients by acupuncture, but it is difficult to assess the results of treatment. However, there are few risks as long as the needles are properly sterilized [12].

Biofeedback techniques

These involve the induction of a learned response aimed at controlling or modifying vascular responses [13] or inappropriate bodily responses to various centrally mediated stimuli. They may reduce emotional intensification of erythema and have been used to control flushing, for patients with dyshidrosis whose disease flared with stress [14] and in patients with atopic dermatitis [15]. Thirty-three patients with eczema were trained to decrease or increase electrical conductivity of the skin. Those who were trained to decrease skin conductance showed clinical improvement, while the controls who were trained in the opposite direction did not. The positive response was accompanied by a significant decrease in measured conductance and anxiety [16]. Eleven of 14 patients with

chronic hyperhidrosis improved following biofeedback training. The most important aspect of the treatment was thought to be relaxation [17]. However, there is considerable individual variability in responses [1], and the main value may lie in anxiety reduction [18] and in the active involvement of the patient in self-help. It has been suggested that the techniques may be the 'ultimate placebo' [19] and their place in dermatology may remain limited by the time and patience required. Nevertheless, further developments in these methods may prove rewarding in specific dermatological situations, given a highly motivated and suitable subject.

Behaviour therapy

The use of behaviour therapy in dermatology was well summarized by Bar and Kuypers, who described four main therapeutic approaches [20].

Systemic desensitization is employed mainly in neurotic disorders where anxiety is the main clinical feature. An attempt is made to induce inhibition of anxiety following repeated exposures to weak anxiety-raising stimuli, after which progressively stronger stimuli are introduced. This type of behaviour therapy has limited application in dermatological practice.

In aversion therapy, patients with persistent behaviour disorders such as compulsive scratching or pathological hair pulling can be treated. The patient is given an unpleasant stimulus, for example a mild electric shock, whenever the unadaptive habit is demonstrated or displayed.

Operant techniques can be used to modify compulsive habits, and awards are given to reinforce good behaviour and bad behaviour is either punished or ignored. In children, a token may be given after a period of good (non-scratching) behaviour as part of a so-called token economy system.

Assertiveness training is employed in patients who are afraid of expressing their emotions and also experience extreme social fear. This technique is said to be most useful in patients with facial erythema or erythrophobia and also has a place in the treatment of patients with hyperhidrosis.

An operant technique was used successfully to modify the scratching behaviour in a patient with long-standing severe dermatitis, which had defied all traditional therapy [21]. As soon as the patient was observed scratching he was asked to fold his arms and think of something pleasant. Normal social attention was then withheld as a mild punishment. This man improved. The technique of habit reversal has an important place in the management of both adults and children with atopic eczema [22,23]. The patients were taught situation awareness so that they could recognize situations that made them itch. The patients were also instructed either to grasp an object or to keep the hands firmly on the itching area and pinch it if necessary but not scratch it. A strong correlation was demonstrated between a reduction in scratching and an improvement in skin status [22,23].

REFERENCES

1 Volow MR, Erwin CW, Cipolat AL. Biofeedback control of skin potential level. *Biofeedback Self Regul* 1979; **4**: 133–43.
2 Foldi M, Casley-Smith JR. *Lymphangiology*. Stuttgart: Schattauer, 1983: 677.
3 Abel E, Morgan K. The treatment of idiopathic hyperhidrosis by glycopyrronium bromide and tap water iontophoresis. *Br J Dermatol* 1974; **91**: 87–91.
4 Naumann M, Hofman U, Bergman NI et al. Facial hyperhidrosis: effective treatment with intracutaneous botulinum toxin. *Arch Dermatol* 1998; **134**: 301–4.
5 Shelley WB, Talamin NY, Shelley ED. Botulinum toxin therapy for palmar hyperhidrosis. *J Am Acad Dermatol* 1998; **134**: 301–4.
6 Wollina U, Karamfilov T. Adjurant botulinum toxin A in dyshidrotic hand eczema: a controlled perspective pilot study with left–right comparision. *J Eur Acad Dermatol Venereol* 2002; **16**: 40–2.
7 Dyson M, Suckling J. Stimulation of tissue repair by ultrasound. A survey of the mechanisms involved. *Physiotherapy* 1978; **64**: 105–8.
8 Dyson M, Franks C, Suckling J. Stimulation of healing of varicose ulcers by ultrasound. *Ultrasonics* 1976; **14**: 232–6.
9 Rudolph RI, Leyden JJ. Physiatrics for deforming linear scleroderma. *Arch Dermatol* 1976; **112**: 995–7.
10 Mayer DJ, Price DD, Rafil A. Antagonism of acupuncture analgesia in man by the narcotic antagonist naloxone. *Brain Res* 1977; **121**: 368–72.
11 Belgrade MJ, Solomon LM, Lichter EA. The effect of acupuncture on experimentally-induced itch. *Acta Derm Venereol Suppl (Stockh)* 1984; **64**: 129–33.
12 Vincent C. The safety of acupuncture. Acupuncture is safe in the hands of the competent practitioners. *BMJ* 2001; **323**: 467–8.
13 Friar LR, Beatty J. Migraine. Management by trained control of vasoconstriction. *J Consult Clin Psychol* 1976; **44**: 46–53.
14 Koldys KW, Meyer RP. Biofeedback training in the therapy of dyshidrosis. *Cutis* 1979; **24**: 219–21.
15 Haynes SN, Wilson CC, Jaffe PE, Britton BT. Biofeedback treatment of atopic dermatitis controlled case studies of eight cases. *Biofeedback Self Regul* 1979; **4**: 195–209.
16 Miller RM, Coger RW. Skin conductance conditioning with dyshidrosis eczema patients. *Br J Dermatol* 1986; **115**: 435–40.
17 Duller P, Doyle Gemtry W. Use of biofeedback in treating chronic hyperhydrosis. *Br J Dermatol* 1980; **103**: 143–6.
18 Green EE, Green AM, Walters ED. Biofeedback training for anxiety tension reduction. *Ann NY Acad Soc* 1974; **233**: 157–61.
19 Stroebel CF, Glueck BC. Biofeedback treatment of medicine and psychiatry: an ultimate placebo? In: Birk L, ed. *Biofeedback: Behavioural Medicine*. New York: Grave & Stratton, 1973: 19–33.
20 Bar LHJ, Kuypers BRM. Behaviour therapy in dermatological practice. *Br J Dermatol* 1973; **88**: 591–8.
21 Cataldo MF, Varni JW, Russo DC, Estes SA. Behaviour therapy techniques in treatment of exfoliative dermatitis. *Arch Dermatol* 1980; **116**: 919–22.
22 Bridgett C, Noren P, Staughton R. *Atopic Skin Disease. A Manual for Practitioners*. Petersfield, Hampshire: Wrightson Biomedical, 1996: 43–7.
23 Melin L, Frederiksen T, Noren P et al. Behavioural treatment of scratching in patients with atopic dermatitis. *Br J Dermatol* 1986; **115**: 467–74.

Hypothermia and hyperthermia

Cooling of the scalp to 25°C with ice turban packs or chemical coolants has been used to prevent or reduce hair loss during the critical period after administration of chemotherapeutic drugs [1]. Cooling of port-wine stains prior to treatment with the argon laser has also been tried to improve the efficacy of laser therapy and also to minimize scarring [2]. Some controversy still surrounds the use of skin cooling in laser dermatological surgery [3].

Resulting from the demonstration of the potential of hyperthermia as an antitumour agent [4,5], there have been occasional reports of its value in treating deep mycoses [6], leishmaniasis and myobacterial infections. Some similarity between the kinetics of tumour cells and psoriasis cells has prompted its use in the form of ultrasound in this disease [7]. Chemically generated heat in exothermic bags was used in 22 psoriatics in comparison with Goeckerman's regime [8], with apparent success and without side effects. This convenient and simple form of treatment may have a place in difficult therapeutic situations and merits further study [9].

REFERENCES

1 Guy R, Shah S, Parker H et al. Scalp cooling by thermocirculator. *Lancet* 1982; i: 937–8.
2 Gilchrest BA, Rosen S, Noe JM. Chilling port wine stains improves response to argon laser. *Plast Reconstr Surg* 1982; **69**: 278–83.
3 Nelson JS, Majoram B, Kelly KM. Active skin cooling in conjunction with laser dermatologic surgery. *Semin Cutan Med Surg* 2000; **19**: 253–66.
4 Cavaliere R, Ciocatto EC, Giovanella BC et al. Selective heat sensitivity of cancer cells. Biochemical and clinical studies. *Cancer* 1967; **20**: 1351–81.
5 Suit HD, Shwayder M. Hyperthermia: potential as an anti-tumor agent. *Cancer* 1974; **34**: 122–9.
6 Tagami H, Ohi M, Aoshima T et al. Topical heat therapy for cutaneous chromomycosis. *Arch Dermatol* 1979; **115**: 740–1.
7 Orenberg EK, Deneau DG, Farber EM. Response of chronic psoriatic plaques to localized heating induced by ultrasound. *Arch Dermatol* 1980; **116**: 893–7.
8 Urabe H, Nishitani K, Konda H. Hyperthermia in the treatment of psoriasis. *Arch Dermatol* 1981; **117**: 770–4.
9 Fesneau H, Guillot B, Mon Point S et al. Therapeutic use of hyperthermia in dermatology. *Ann Dermatol Vénéréol* 1993; **120**: 926–30.

Homeopathy [1–3]

Homeopathy is a system of therapy originated by Samuel Hahnemann in the latter part of the 18th century. Central to the theory of homeopathy is the thesis that those agents that produce symptoms of any given disease will, in a much smaller dosage, cure that disease. Others have described homeopathy as a harnessing of an energy unknown to orthodox science.

Proponents of homeopathy state that there are three essential processes in the preparation of remedies, namely dilution, succussion and trituration. By diluting the drug, the toxicity of the original product disappears and during succussion and trituration some supposed mechanical energy is imparted to the remedy, imprinting the pharmacological message of the original drug upon the molecules in the diluent. From the practical point of view there seems no doubt that many patients are happy to consult with homeopathic practitioners, and most of these consultations do no harm unless a patient is advised to stop their oral or topical steroids suddenly. There is no doubt that homeopathic practitioners spend a great deal of time with the patient and some patients undoubtedly benefit from this enhanced level of communication which they are unlikely to find in a busy National Health Service clinic.

Despite two centuries of work, there are very few controlled clinical trials that allow homeopathy to be assessed [1].

In a study of alternative medicine, utilized by patients with atopic dermatitis and psoriasis, it was found that over 50% of patients with atopic eczema and over 40% of patients with psoriasis reported previous or current use of one or more forms of alternative medicine, and homeopathy, health-food preparations and herbal remedies were used the most. The use was related to disease duration and disease severity and inefficiency of therapy prescribed by physicians as judged by the patients. The author concluded that the use of alternative medicine is commonplace and should be of concern to dermatologists [4]. This work was confirmed by a later study [5].

REFERENCES

1 Cotterill JA. Alternative medicine and dermatology. In: Champion RH, ed. *Recent Advances in Dermatology*, Vol. 7. Edinburgh: Churchill Livingstone, 1986: 257–8.
2 Burgdorf WH, Happle R. What every dermatologist should know about homeopathy. *Arch Dermatol* 1996; **132**: 955–8.
3 Pimgel S, Homeopathy. Basic aspects and principles of use in dermatology. *Hautarzt* 1992; **43**: 475–82.
4 Jenssen P. Use of alternative medicine by patients with atopic dermatitis and psoriasis. *Acta Derm Venereol (Stockh)* 1990; **70**: 421–4.
5 Ernst E. The usage of complementary therapies by dermatological patients: a systematic review. *Br J Dermatol* 2000; **142**: 857–61.

Occupational therapy and rehabilitation

A person conditioned to an active life does not take kindly to bed rest. Patients with skin diseases should be encouraged to become mobile as soon as their state allows it. Those with venous leg ulcers should not be kept in bed for long periods (although periodic elevation of the leg is important), but should have active and passive leg exercises to reduce the risk of thrombosis, foot drop and atrophy of the leg muscles. They should be encouraged to walk for increasing periods, rather than sitting, in order to re-educate their leg movements. The elderly patient with exfoliative dermatitis or pemphigus should be stimulated to pass his or her time without boredom, which passes imperceptibly in the aged into depression and despondency. In the alien milieu of a hospital ward, the elderly patient quickly deteriorates mentally and physically. Subsequent discharge or rehabilitation may then be extremely difficult. Occupational therapy should not only engage manual skill but also satisfy the emotional and intellectual needs of the patient of any age.

Patient self-help groups [1]

Increasingly, patients want to know more about their skin disease and its treatment. It is not always possible to meet all the patient's needs in an outpatient appointment, and,

moreover, there is a limit to how much a patient can take in at one outpatient visit. This is where the self-help groups are increasingly important. The concept of self-help is that patients 'own' their disease find out more about their disease for themselves and are not just passively reliant on doctors and nurses for information and help. Such groups generate information, emotional support and advice. Patients can meet others with similar skin diseases and so realize that they are not alone. Patient self-help groups usually raise funds to support their activities, which will include research grants. They also lobby Members of Parliament to ensure that the needs of skin patients are heard and met. Pressure is often put on the purchasing health authority and the provider units to improve their service and to increase the amount of money spent on dermatology. Lastly, such groups attempt to diminish the stigma of skin disease that still exists in the community. The role of the patients' self-help group in dermatology is increasingly important to patients with skin disease and their general practitioners, dermatologists and nurses alike.

REFERENCE

1 Funnell C. Importance of patients' self-help groups—a British perspective. *Retinoids Today Tomorrow* 1995; **41**: 6–8.

Quality of life impairment by skin disease

What does quality of life mean?

Being able to assess the impact of skin disease on patients is essential in order to understand and meet what dermatology patients really need [1]. There is however, considerable controversy about the definition of quality of life and whether it can be meaningfully assessed [2,3]. There have been several attempts to define quality of life and the closely associated concept of health-related quality of life (HRQoL) [4]. The need for all outcome measures used in dermatology, including quality of life measures, to be properly validated has been emphasized [5]. There is however, very little information in the literature about the absolute meaning of different overall quality of life measurement scores or the interpretation of degrees of change in scores [6]. Concepts relating to life quality in dermatology are well reviewed in a book by Rajagopalan *et al.* [7].

Why measure quality of life?

All clinical dermatologists are aware of the impact that skin disease may have on their patients. However it is only over the last two decades [8] that there have been attempts to develop methodology to measure the adverse impact of skin disease on quality of life. There are several reasons why measurement may be helpful.

Clinical therapeutic research. When new drugs are assessed, the outcome measures used are usually clinical measures such as the degree of scaling or the area of skin affected. Pharmaceutical companies and regulatory authorities are realizing that although these measures of disease activity are of course important, it is necessary to have in addition a patient-orientated outcome. There may be a 50% improvement in a psoriasis area severity index (PASI), but if the handicap experienced by the patient is only slightly improved because visible skin remains abnormal, the intervention may not have been very successful from the patient's point of view. It has been argued that a quality of life standard is better than a body-surface-area measurement for identifying patients with severe psoriasis [9]. The addition of (not the replacement by) a HRQoL measure may be essential to make a proper assessment. The introduction of several new therapies in dermatology over the last 10 years has been supported by such information [10,11].

Health service research and audit. Within many health care systems it is becoming mandatory to produce evidence of the effectiveness of care given, and to have systems in place to monitor effectiveness and assess improvement against agreed criteria. An essential part of this process has to involve having patient-orientated measures and simple but well-validated HRQoL questionnaires are well suited for this need [12–15]. The use of these measures can give additional insight into the acceptability of new methods of providing dermatology advice, such as teledermatology [16]. Sound epidemiological data are essential for the planning of health services: HRQoL data can measure the extent of problems caused by skin disorders in a community [17] and be used to compare the HRQoL of people with specific skin diseases, such as psoriasis, to the general population [18].

Research into psychological aspects of dermatology and patient behaviour. Quality of life measures can be used to gain insight into patient attitudes: stress resulting from the anticipation of other people's reactions to their psoriasis contributed more to the variance in patients' disability than any other variable [19]. It is important that the problems relating to compliance with treatment, often not recognized by dermatologists, are better understood. Quality of life indices have been used to provide patient-orientated measures in studies of compliance in psoriasis and acne.

Political/resource allocation. Patients with skin diseases are rarely given any priority for resource allocation in any health care systems. Conditions that result in death are much more likely to find political support for service development. It is the responsibility of dermatologists to argue for appropriate resource allocation and appropriate funding of dermatology services and of the education of doctors about skin problems. One way in which the arguments for this can be strengthened is by using HRQoL data that demonstrate the devastating effects of skin disease on patients' lives. If general HRQoL measures are used it is possible to quantify the effects of skin disease compared to other system disease [20,21]. It may be necessary to demonstrate to managers or politicians and defend the value of dermatology clinical services that is self-evident to clinicians, e.g. in-patient dermatology beds [22–24], patch testing [25], cosmetic camouflage advice [26] and outpatient clinical services [12]. Dermatology-specific measures can also be used to demonstrate the value from the patients' point of view of expensive or unusual therapy such as climate therapy [27].

Informing clinical decisions. Most dermatologists probably consider that they have a reasonably accurate insight into the impact of skin disease on individual patients. The assumptions made about this influence clinical decisions; for example, whether or not to start a patient on a systemic therapy which has risks of side effects. Unfortunately, dermatologists may not have as much insight as they think they have into the degree of their patients' problems [28–30]. The use of a standard HRQoL measure may therefore potentially inform a clinician more accurately about their patient and allow better judgement concerning risk/benefit of therapy change. This will only become relevant on a routine basis if the absolute meaning of HRQoL scores can be more clearly defined than at present [6].

How do quality of life measures relate to other clinical indices?

It is self evident there is likely to be a relationship between the clinical severity of skin disease and the impact that the disease has on life quality. This has been demonstrated in atopic dermatitis in children where the Children's Dermatology Life Quality Index (CDLQI) was shown to be significantly correlated with the Severity Scoring of Atopic Dermatitis (SCORAD) [31]. However there are many influences on the disability experienced and individual patients show a wide variation in their responses to similar degrees of disease [8]. Particular body site affected is an important factor with visible sites such as the face having much greater significance to a patient. The psychological attitudes of patients to their disease vary widely and these attitudes have a major influence on the degree of disability experienced. Clinical scoring systems may reflect sign changes which are not of relevance to a patient's life. For example, in psoriasis, the successful reduction of scaling and thickness may result in a large percentage reduction in PASI, but if the redness persists the quality of life improvement may be much less [32]. Quality of life measures therefore should not be used instead of clinical measures, as they are designed to assess a completely different, though interrelated, aspect of skin disease.

REFERENCES

1 Finlay AY. Dermatology patients: what do they really need? *Clin Exp Dermatol* 2000; **25**: 444–50.
2 Downie RS. The value and quality of life. *J R Coll Physicians Lond* 1999; **33**: 378–81.
3 Koller M, Lorenz W. Quality of life: a deconstruction for clinicians. *J R Soc Med* 2002; **95**: 481–8.
4 Calman KC. Quality of life in cancer patients—an hypothesis. *J Med Ethics* 1984; **10**: 124–7.
5 Chren M-M. Giving 'scale' new meaning in dermatology. *Arch Dermatol* 2000; **136**: 788–90.
6 Khilji FA, Gonzalez M, Finlay AY. Clinical meaning of change in Dermatology Life Quality Index scores. *Br J Dermatol* 2002; **147** (Suppl. 62): 50.
7 Rajagopalan R, Sherertz EF, Anderson RT. *Care Management of Skin Diseases: Life Quality and Economic Impact*. New York: Marcel Dekker, 1998.
8 Finlay AY, Kelly SE. Psoriasis—an index of disability. *Clin Exp Dermatol* 1987; **12**: 8–11.
9 Krueger GG, Feldman SR, Camisa C *et al.* Two considerations for patients with psoriasis and their clinicians: what defines mild, moderate and severe psoriasis? What constitutes a clinically significant improvement when treating psoriasis? *J Am Acad Dermatol* 2000; **43**: 281–5.
10 Drake L, Prendergast M, Maher R *et al.* The impact of tacrolimus ointment on Health-Related Quality of Life of adult and pediatric patients with atopic dermatitis. *J Am Acad Dermatol* 2001; **44**: S65–72.
11 Wall ARJ, Poyner TF, Menday AP. A comparison of treatment with dithranol and calcipotriol on the clinical severity and quality of life in patients with psoriasis. *Br J Dermatol* 1998; **139**: 1005–11.
12 Finlay AY, Coles EC, Lewis-Jones MS *et al.* Quality of life improves after seeing a dermatologist. *Br J Dermatol* 1998; **139** (Suppl. 51): 15.
13 Shum KW, Lawton S, Williams HC, Docherty G, Jones J. The British Association of Dermatologists audit of atopic eczema management in secondary care. Phase 3: audit of service outcome. *Br J Dermatol* 2000; **12**: 721–7.
14 Chinn DJ, Poyner T, Sibley G. Randomised controlled trial of a single dermatology nurse consultant in primary care on the quality of life of children with atopic eczema. *Br J Dermatol* 2002; **146**: 432–9.
15 Gradwell C, Thomas KS, English JSC, Williams HC. A randomised controlled trial of nurse follow-up clinics: do they help patients and do they free up consultants' time? *Br J Dermatol* 2002; **147**: 513–7.
16 Williams TL, May CR, Esmail A *et al.* Patient satisfaction with teledermatology is related to perceived quality of life. *Br J Dermatol* 2001; **145**: 911–7.
17 Bingefors K, Lindberg M, Isacson D. Self-reported dermatological problems and use of prescribed topical drugs correlate with decreased quality of life: an epidemiological survey. *Br J Dermatol* 2002; **147**: 285–90.
18 Wahl A, Loge JH, Wiklund I, Hanestad BR. The burden of psoriasis: a study concerning Health-Related Quality of Life among Norwegian adult patients with psoriasis compared with general population norms. *J Am Acad Dermatol* 2000; **43**: 803–8.
19 Fortune DG, Main CJ, O'Sullivan TM, Griffiths CEM. Quality of life in patients with psoriasis: the contribution of clinical variables and psoriasis-specific stress. *Br J Dermatol* 1997; **137**: 755–60.
20 Finlay AY, Khan GK, Luscombe DK, Salek MS. Validation of Sickness Impact Profile and Psoriasis Disability Index in psoriasis. *Br J Dermatol* 1990; **123**: 751–6.
21 Rapp SR, Feldman SR, Exum L *et al.* Psoriasis causes as much disability as other major medical diseases. *J Am Acad Dermatol* 1999; **41**: 401–7.
22 Kurwa H, Finlay AY. Dermatology inpatient management greatly improves life quality. *Br J Dermatol* 1995; **133**: 575–8.
23 Vensel E, Hilley T, Trent J *et al.* Sustained improvement of the quality of life of patients with psoriasis after hospitalization. *J Am Acad Dermatol* 2000; **43**: 858–60.
24 Ayyalaraju RS, Finlay AY, Dykes PJ *et al.* Hospitalization for severe skin disease improves quality of life in the United Kingdom and the United States: a comparative study. *J Am Acad Dermatol* 2003; **49**: 249–54.
25 Thompson KF, Wilkinson SM, Sommer S, Pollock B. Eczema: quality of life by body site and the effect of patch testing. *Br J Dermatol* 2002; **146**: 627–30.
26 Holme SA, Beattie PE, Fleming CJ. Cosmetic camouflage advice improves quality of life. *Br J Dermatol* 2002; **147**: 946–9.
27 Mork C, Wahl A. Improved quality of life among patients with psoriasis after supervised climate therapy at the Canary Islands. *J Am Acad Dermatol* 2002; **47**: 314–6.
28 Jemec GBE, Wulf HC. Patient–physician consensus and quality of life in dermatology. *Clin Exp Dermatol* 1996; **21**: 177–9.
29 Hermansen SE, Helland CA, Finlay AY. Patients' and doctors' assessment of skin disease handicap. *Clin Exp Dermatol* 2002; **27**: 1–3.
30 Jayaprakasam A, Darvay A, Osborne G, McGibbon D. Comparison of assessments of severity and quality of life in cutaneous disease. *Clin Exp Dermatol* 2002; **27**: 306–9.
31 Ben-Gashir MA, Seed PT, Hay RJ. Are quality of life and disease severity correlated in children with atopic eczema? *J Eur Acad Dermatol Venereol* 2002; **16**: 455–62.
32 Parry EJ, Tillman DM, Long J, MacKie RM. Audit of UVB phototherapy in the treatment of psoriasis. *Br J Dermatol* 1995; **133** (Suppl. 45): 16.

Methods of measuring quality of life in dermatology

There are several different approaches to the measurement of HRQoL. One depends on the use of fixed repeatable questionnaires that are scored. A second approach uses questionnaires that allow a variable response from the patient, taking into account the particular values of the patient. Another method is to assess the value that a patient or society places on the presence or absence of particular disease states—the utility approach. Decisions concerning which measures are appropriate to use can be confusing: general guidance is given in a review article [1]. Comparisons of assessment of quality of life in cutaneous disease [2] and in psoriasis [3] have been reviewed, and advice has been given [4] concerning understanding research about quality of life.

Some techniques are designed to be used across all disease states, some for use across a range of diseases of the same organ system and some for use in patients with specific diseases. Most published questionnaires are for use in adults, but there have been techniques described for measuring HRQoL in children with skin disease, infants with atopic dermatitis and the secondary impact of having a child with dermatitis on the family.

HRQoL measures are usually designed to assess the impact of skin disease at a particular time (e.g. 'today') or over a fixed period of time (e.g. 'over the last week'). Measures are usually designed in this way so that they can be used for example to compare data before and after intervention. However it should be noted that the long-term 'importance' or impact on a patient's life may therefore not be captured by these indices. Patients with basal cell carcinomas at the time of presentation to dermatologists generally have little or no reduction in their current quality of life [5], but of course if the disease was not treated there could be major problems in the future. It is therefore important that if HRQoL measures are used to inform priorities for resources in a health care organization, these measures should not be used in isolation.

Examples of quality of life measures

General health measures

General health measures are designed to be used across a wide range of disease states. Their use is essential if comparisons are to be drawn between the impact of skin diseases, the impact of diseases of other systems and the general population. Examples of tools available include the 36-Item Short-Form Health Survey (SF-36) [6], the Sickness Impact Profile (SIP) [7], the Nottingham Health Profile (NHP) [8] and the EuroQol and EuroQol Five Dimensions (EQ-5D) [9]. The General Health Questionnaire (GHQ) [10] is designed to detect psychiatric disorder.

Many of these general health measures have been used in dermatology. The UK SIP has been used in psoriasis [11] and atopic dermatitis [12]. The SF-36 has been used in psoriasis [13–15] and acne [16]. The twelve-question version of the GHQ (GHQ-12) has been shown to be of value in assessing psychological distress in patients with skin disease [17], and specifically in vitiligo [18]. In many investigations both a generic measure and a dermatology-specific measure have been used together [14] and the advantages of this have been emphasized in a study using the EuroQol and EG-5D in acne [16].

Dermatology-specific measures

Dermatology-specific measures are useful when comparisons need to be made between the impact of different skin diseases and where there is a need to measure change before or after intervention in any skin disease. Having a single simple measure that can be used across all skin disease is of great practical advantage, especially in a busy clinical setting.

The two dermatology-specific measures that have been most widely used are the Dermatology Life Quality Index (DLQI) [19] and Skindex [20]. Other measures that have been described include the Dermatology Quality of Life Scales [21], the Dermatology-specific Quality of Life instrument [22] and a German instrument, the Deutsches Instrument zur Erfassung der Lebensqualität bei Hauterkrankungen (DIELH) [23].

The DLQI consists of 10 questions covering a wide range of ways in which patients' lives are affected by skin disease (Fig. 71.1). They are answered by a simple tickbox method and each scored 0–3. The DLQI takes on average only 2 min to complete [24]. There are over 170 references describing the use of the DLQI in a wide range of skin conditions and in many languages worldwide [25]. Validation studies have been carried out in the UK in secondary care [19] and primary care [26], and in Spain [27,28], Germany [29], Denmark [30], the USA [31] and Norway [32]. Its use has also been described from France, The Netherlands, Belgium, Sweden, Switzerland, Russia, Yugoslavia, Canada, India, Australia, Malaysia, Hong Kong, South Africa, Tanzania, the Canary Islands and Guyana. When illustrations are added next to the text of the DLQI, the questionnaire tends to be completed more rapidly but there is an influence on the way the questionnaire is answered [24].

Skindex has been developed and thoroughly validated in three versions with 61 [20], 29 [33] or 16 [34] questions. Further validation studies have been carried out in Spain [35], Italy [36] and Japan [37]. The appropriateness of using Skindex-29 in psoriasis along with the generic SF-36 has been emphasized [3].

The aim of this questionnaire is to measure how much your skin problem has affected your life OVER THE LAST WEEK. Please tick one box for each question.

1 Over the last week, how **itchy, sore, painful** or **stinging** has your skin been?

2 Over the last week, how **embarrassed** or **self conscious** have you been because of your skin?

3 Over the last week, how much has your skin interfered with you going **shopping** or looking after your **home** or **garden**?

4 Over the last week, how much has your skin influenced the **clothes** you wear?

5 Over the last week, how much has your skin affected any **social** or **leisure** activities?

6 Over the last week, how much has your skin made it difficult for you to do any **sport**?

7 Over the last week, has your skin prevented you from **working** or **studying**?

If 'no', over the last week how much has your skin been a problem at **work** or **studying**?

8 Over the last week, how much has your skin created problems with your **partner** or any of your **close friends** or **relatives**?

9 Over the last week, how much has your skin caused any **sexual difficulties**?

10 Over the last week, how much of a problem has the **treatment** for your skin been, for example by making your home messy, or by taking up time?

Please check you have answered every question. Thank you.

© A.Y. Finlay, G.K. Khan, April 1992. This must not be copied without the permission of the authors.

Each question is answered either 'Very much' (score 3), 'A lot' (score 2), 'A little' (score 1) or 'Not at all' (score 0). Questions 3–10 also have the option 'Not relevant' (score 0). The first part of question 7 has the choices 'Yes' (score 3), 'No' or 'Not relevant'. The second part of question 7 has the choices 'A lot', 'A little' or 'Not at all'. The maximum score (indicating highest possible impairment of quality of life) is 30 and the minimum 0. Further information: www.ukdermatology.co.uk.

Fig. 71.1 The Dermatology Life Quality Index (DLQI) [19].

REFERENCES

1 Finlay AY. Quality of life measurement in dermatology: a practical guide. *Br J Dermatol* 1997; **136**: 305–14.

2 Jayaprakasam A, Darvey A, Jisborne G, McGibbon D. Comparisons of assessment of severity and quality of life in cutaneous disease. *Clin Exp Dermatol* 2002; **27**: 306–8.

3 De Korte J, Mombers FM, Sprangers MA, Bos JD. The suitability of quality of life questionnaires for psoriasis research: a systematic literature review. *Arch Dermatol* 2002; **138**: 1221–7.

4 Chren MM. Understanding research about quality of life and other health outcomes. *J Cutan Med Surg* 1999; **3**: 312–6.

5 Blackford S, Roberts DL, Salek MS, Finlay AY. Basal cell carcinomas cause little handicap. *Qual Life Res* 1996; **5**: 191–4.

6 Ware JE, Sherbourne CD. The MOS 36-Item Short-Form Health Survey (SF-36). 1. Conceptual framework and item selection. *Med Care* 1992; **30**: 437–83.

7 Bergner M, Bobbit RA, Carter WB *et al.* The Sickness Impact Profile: development and final revision of a health status measure. *Med Care* 1981; **19**: 787–805.

8 Hunt SM, McEwen J, McKenna SP. Measuring health status. A new tool for clinicians and epidemiologists. *J R Coll Gen Pract* 1985; **35**: 185–8.

9 Kind P, Gudex C, Dolan P, Williams A. Practical and methodological issues in the development of the EuroQol: the York experience. *Adv Med Sociol* 1994; **5**: 219–53.

10 Banks MH. Validation of the General Health Questionnaire in a young community sample. *Psychol Med* 1983; **13**: 349–53.

11 Finlay AY, Khan GK, Luscombe DK, Salek MS. Validation of Sickness Impact Profile and Psoriasis Disability Index in psoriasis. *Br J Dermatol* 1990; **123**: 751–6.

12 Salek MS, Finlay AY, Luscombe DK *et al.* Cyclosporin greatly improves the quality of life of adults with severe atopic dermatitis. *Br J Dermatol* 1993; **129**: 422–30.

13 Nichol MB, Margoilies JE, Lippa E *et al.* The application of multiple quality of life instruments in individuals with mild-to-moderate psoriasis. *Pharmacoeconomics* 1996; **10**: 644–53.

14 Lundberg L, Johannesson M, Silverdahl M *et al.* Health related quality of life in patients with psoriasis and atopic dermatitis measured with SF-36, DLQI and a subjective measure of disease activity. *Acta Derm Venereol* 2000; **80**: 430–4.

15 Ellis CN, Mordin MM, Adler EY. Effects of alefacept on Health-Related Quality of Life in patients with psoriasis: results from a randomised placebo controlled phase II trial. *Am J Clin Dermatol* 2003; **4**: 131–9.

16 Klassen AF, Newton JN, Mallon E. Measuring quality of life in people referred for specialist care of acne: comparing generic and disease-specific measures. *J Am Acad Dermatol* 2000; **43**: 229–33.

17 Picardi A, Abeni D, Pasquini P. Assessing psychological distress in patients with skin diseases. Reliability, validity and factor structure of the GHQ-12. *J Eur Acad Dermatol Venereol* 2001; **15**: 410–7.

18 Mattoo SK, Handa S, Kaur I *et al.* Psychiatric morbidity in vitiligo: prevalence and correlates in India. *J Eur Acad Dermatol Venereol* 2002; **16**: 573–8.

19 Finlay AY, Khan GK. Dermatology Life Quality Index (DLQI): a simple practical measure for routine clinical use. *Clin Exp Dermatol* 1994; **19**: 210–6.

20 Chren MM, Lasek RJ, Quinn LM *et al.* Skindex, a quality-of-life measure for patients with skin diseases: reliability, validity, and responsiveness. *J Invest Dermatol* 1996; **107**: 707–13.

21 Morgan M, McCreedy R, Simpson J, Hay RJ. Dermatology Quality of Life Scales—a measure of the impact of skin diseases. *Br J Dermatol* 1997; **136**: 202–6.

22 Anderson RT, Rajagopalan R. Development and validation of a quality of life instrument for cutaneous diseases. *J Am Acad Dermatol* 1997; **37**: 41–50.

23 Schäfer T, Staudt A, Ring J. German instrument for the assessment of quality of life in skin diseases (DIELH). Internal consistency, reliability, convergent and discriminant validity and responsiveness. *Hautarzt* 2001; **52**: 624–8.

24 Loo WJ, Diba V, Chawla M, Finlay AY. Dermatology Life Quality Index. Influence of an illustrated version. *Br J Dermatol* 2003; **148**: 279–84.

25 Dermatology Life Quality Index (DLQI) and Children's Dermatology Life Quality Index (CDLQI) list of references: www.ukdermatology.co.uk.

26 Harlow D, Poyner T, Finlay AY, Dykes PJ. Impaired quality of life of adults with skin disease in primary care. *Br J Dermatol* 2000; **143**: 979–82.

27 De Tiedra AG, Mercadal J, Badia X *et al.* Adaptacion transcultural al Espanol del cuestionario Dermatology Life Quality Index (DLQI): el Indice de Calidad de Vida en Dermatologia. *Actas Dermosifiliogr* 1998; **89**: 692–700.

28 Badia X, Mascaro JM, Lozano R. Measuring Health-Related Quality of Life in patients with mild to moderate eczema and psoriasis: clinical validity, reliability and sensitivity to change of the DLQI. *Br J Dermatol* 1999; **141**: 698–702.

29 Augustin M, Zschocke I, Lange S *et al.* Quality of life in skin diseases: methological and practical comparison of different quality of life questionnaires in psoriasis and atopic dermatitis. *Hautarzt* 1999; **50**: 715–22.

30 Zachariae R, Zachariae C, Ibsen H *et al.* Dermatology Life Quality Index: data from Danish inpatients and outpatients. *Acta Derm Venereol* 2000; **80**: 272–6.

31 Hahn BH, Melfi CA, Chuang TY *et al.* Use of the Dermatology Life Quality Index (DLQI) in a Midwestern US urban clinic. *J Am Acad Dermatol* 2001; **45**: 44–8.

32 Mork C, Wahl A, Moum T. The Norwegian version of the Dermatology Life Quality Index: a study of validity and reliability in psoriatics. *Acta Derm Venereol* 2002; **82**: 327–51.

33 Chren MM, Lasek RJ, Flocke SA, Zyzanski SJ. Improved discriminative and evaluative capability of a refined version of Skindex, a quality-of-life instrument for patients with skin diseases. *Arch Dermatol* 1997; **133**: 1433–40.

34 Chren MM, Lasek RJ, Sahav AP, Sands LP. Measurement properties of Skindex-16: a brief quality-of-life measure for patients with skin diseases. *J Cutan Med Surg* 2001; **5**: 105–10.

35 Jones-Caballero M, Penas PF, Garcia-Diaz A *et al.* The Spanish version of Skindex-29. *Int J Dermatol* 2000; **39**: 907–12.

36 Abeni D, Picardi A, Pasquini P *et al.* Further evidence of the validity and reliability of the Skindex-29: an Italian study on 2242 dermatological outpatients. *Dermatology* 2002; **204**: 43–9.

37 Higaki Y, Kawamoto K, Kamo T *et al.* The Japanese version of Skinned-16: a brief quality-of-life measure for patients with skin disease. *J Dermatol* 2002; **29**: 693–8.

Disease-specific measures

Because the questions in disease-specific measures reflect as closely as possible the problems encountered by patients with that disease, disease-specific measures have the potential of being the most sensitive to change. They are therefore particularly suitable for comparative purposes within a cohort of same-disease patients. In many skin diseases however, for example in the widespread inflammatory skin diseases, patients lives are broadly affected in similar ways, and so dermatology-specific measures can also be used. There is therefore no need for every skin disease to have its own disease-specific measure.

Psoriasis. A landmark study of quality of life issues in over 17 000 patients with psoriasis [1], using a study-specific questionnaire, demonstrated the major impact that psoriasis can have on patients' lives and revealed that many patients with psoriasis do not feel that their physicians are aggressive enough with their therapy.

The Psoriasis Disability Index (PDI), originally described in 1987 [2] and revised in 1995 [3] has been extensively used in international studies [4], and is available in several languages.

The stigmatizing effects of psoriasis can be recorded using a 33-item questionnaire [5]. Another technique for measuring this effect has been described [6] and used to demonstrate the high stigmatization experienced by patients with psoriasis compared to patients with other skin diseases [7]. The stress that can be caused by the impact of psoriasis on quality of life can be measured by the Psoriasis Life Stress Inventory, in its 41- [8] or 15-item versions [9].

A new construct for psoriasis which allows separate recording of signs (disease activity), psychosocial disability and history of interventions has been proposed [10]. The Salford Psoriasis Index (SPI) consists of three independent scores describing each of these aspects. This approach may be of great value in the recording and monitoring of this chronic disease.

Atopic dermatitis. The CDLQI and the DLQI have been used extensively in the monitoring of patients with atopic dermatitis. In a large managed care organization in the USA, patient-assessed severity of atopic dermatitis demonstrated a stronger correlation with the DLQI and CDLQI than did provider-assessed severity, emphasizing the importance of directly assessing the patients' attitudes [11]. The disease-specific measures for use in infants (Infant's Dermatitis Quality of Life Index, IDQOLI) and in families (Dermatitis Family Impact questionnaire, DFI) are described below. Assessment of quality of life in atopic dermatitis has been reviewed [12].

Acne. An initial attempt to produce an Acne Disability Index (ADI) [13] has been largely superseded by the more compact five-question Cardiff Acne Disability Index (CADI) [14], which was derived from it. This simple instrument has demonstrated good reliability and validity [15]. The 'Assessments of the Psychological and Social Effects of Acne' (APSEA) questionnaire [16] has 15 questions some of which relate to the overall impact and some to the recent past. A nine-item Acne Quality of Life Scale [17] has been proposed for use in acne: the questions relate specifically to the social impact of acne. The Acne-specific Quality of Life questionnaire (Acne-QoL) [18] is a 19-question tool which has been validated but not yet widely used.

Other disease-specific measures. Other disease-specific measures have been described for ulcers [19], urticaria [20], excessive axillary sweating [21], scalp dermatitis [22] and for women with androgenetic alopecia [23].

REFERENCES

1 Kreuger G, Koo J, Lebwohl M et al. The impact of psoriasis on quality of life: results of a 1998 National Psoriasis Foundation patient–membership survey. Arch Dermatol 2001; **58**: 280–4.
2 Finlay AY, Kelly SE. Psoriasis—an index of disability. Clin Exp Dermatol 1987; **12**: 8–11.
3 Finlay AY, Coles EC. The effect of severe psoriasis on the quality of life of 369 patients. Br J Dermatol 1995; **132**: 236–44.
4 Zachariae H, Zachariae R, Blomquist K et al. Quality of life and prelevance of arthritis reported by 5795 members of the Nordic Psoriasis Associations—data from the Nordic quality of life study. Acta Derm Venereol 2002; **82**: 108–13.
5 Ginsberg IH, Link BG. Feelings of stigmatisation in patients with psoriasis. J Am Acad Dermatol 1989; **20**: 53–63.
6 Schmid-Ott G, Jaeger B, Ott R, Lamprecht F. Dimensions of stigmatisation in patients with psoriasis in a 'questionnaire on experience with skin complaints'. Dermatology 1996; **193**: 304–10.
7 Vardy D, Besser A, Amir M et al. Experiences of stigmatisation play a role in mediating the impact of disease severity on quality of life in psoriasis patients. Br J Dermatol 2002; **147**: 736–42.
8 Gupta MA, Gupta AK, Kirby S et al. A psychcutaneous profile of psoriasis patients who are stress reactors. Gen Hosp Psychiatry 1989; **11**: 166–73.
9 Gupta MA, Gupta AK. The Psoriasis Life Stress Inventory. a preliminary index of psoriasis-related stress. Acta Dermatol Venereol Suppl (Stockh) 1995; **75**: 240–3.
10 Kirby B, Fortune DG, Bhushan M et al. The Salford Psoriasis Index: an holistic measure of psoriasis severity. Br J Dermatol 2000; **142**: 728–32.
11 Fivenson D, Arnold RJG, Kaniecki DJ et al. The effect of atopic dermatitis on total burden of illness and quality of life on adults and children in a large managed care organisation. J Manag Care Pharm 2002; **8**: 333–42.
12 Finlay AY. Quality of life in atopic dermatitis. J Am Acad Dermatol 2001; **45**: S64–6.
13 Motley RJ, Finlay AY. How much disability is caused by acne? Clin Exp Dermatol 1989; **14**: 194–8.
14 Motley RJ, Finlay AY. Practical use of a disability index in the routine management of acne. Clin Exp Dermatol 1992; **17**: 1–3.
15 Salek MS, Khan GK, Finlay AY. Questionnaire techniques in assessing acne handicap. Reliability and validity study. Qual Life Res 1996; **5**: 131–8.
16 Layton AM. Psychological assessment of skin disease. Interfaces Dermatol 1994; **1**: 37–9.
17 Gupta MA, Johnson AM, Gupta AK. The development of an acne Quality of Life Scale: reliability, validity, and relation to subjective acne severity in mild to moderate acne vulgaris. Acta Derm Venereol (Stockh) 1998; **78**: 451–6.
18 Martin AR, Lookingbill DP, Botek A et al. Health-Related Quality of Life among patients with facial acne—assessment of a new acne-specific questionnaire. Clin Exp Dermatol 2001; **26**: 380–5.
19 Hyland ME. Quality of life of leg ulcer patients: questionnaire and preliminary findings. J Wound Care 1994; **3**: 294–8.
20 O'Donnell BF, Lawlor F, Simpson J et al. The impact of chronic urticaria on the quality of life. Br J Dermatol 1997; **136**: 197–201.
21 Naumann MK, Hamm H, Lowe NJ. Effect of botulinum toxin type A on quality of life measures in patients with excessive axillary sweating: a randomised controlled trial. Br J Dermatol 2002; **147**: 1218–26.
22 Chen SC, Yeung J, Chren MM. Scalpdex. A quality of life instrument for scalp dermatitis. Arch Dermatol 2002; **138**: 803–7.
23 Dolte KS, Girman CJ, Hartmaier S et al. Development of a Health-Related Quality of Life questionnaire for women with androgenetic alopecia. Exp Dermatol 2000; **25**: 637–42.

Patient-specific and utility measures

HRQoL measures are, or should be, derived from information gathered from patients' experiences and not from health care professionals' concepts of what they suppose to be the impact of disease. Despite this all fixed questionnaires suffer from the disadvantage that for an individual patient, the weighting given to different aspects of life quality impairment may be different from that assigned in the questionnaire, or the specific issues may be missed. The Patient Generated Index [1] overcomes these problems by being structured in a different way: patients are asked to identify the five ways in which their life is most affected and then assign them comparative values. This technique is effective for identifying individual's specific problems as in atopic dermatitis [2] but it is difficult to incorporate in large scale before and after studies.

Utility measures are methods to assess the hypothetical value placed by people on their health. There are a variety of different approaches described. Standard gamble, time trade-off and vertical rating scales have been proposed [3] as a method to inform decisions relating to methotrexate therapy for psoriasis. A simple 'financial value' method is to ask patients how much they would be prepared to pay for a cure of their disease if such a cure existed. This has been used in acne [4], psoriasis [5] and atopic dermatitis [6].

Another approach is to ask patients to consider how much time they would be prepared to give up for the sake of a cure. These 'trade off' questions can be related to years of shortening of life, as in the Quality Adjusted Life Year (QALY), or be related to hours trade off. The hours trade off method has been described in psoriasis [5] and in atopic dermatitis [6], whereas the QALY method has been described in acne [7]. In contrast to the concept of hypothetical time that a patient would be prepared to give up, there is no correlation between the measurement of actual time spent on treatment and quality of life scores [8].

REFERENCES

1 Ruta DA, Garratt AM, Leng M et al. A new approach to the measurement of quality of life. The Patient Generated Index. Med Care 1994; 32: 1109–26.
2 Herd RM, Tidman MJ, Ruta DA, Hunter JAA. Measurement of quality of life in atopic dermatitis: correlation and validation of two different methods. Br J Dermatol 1997; 136: 502–7.
3 Zug KA, Littenberg B, Baughman RD et al. Assessing the preferences of patients with psoriasis. Arch Dermatol 1995; 131: 561–8.
4 Motley RJ, Finlay AY. How much disability is caused by acne? Clin Exp Dermatol 1989; 14: 194–8.
5 Finlay AY, Coles EC. The effect of severe psoriasis on the quality of life of 369 patients. Br J Dermatol 1995; 132: 236–44.
6 Finlay AY. Measures of the effect of adult severe atopic eczema on quality of life. J Eur Acad Dermatol Venereol 1996; 7: 149–54.
7 Simpson NB. Social and economic aspects of acne and the cost-effectiveness of isotretinoin. J Dermatolog Treat 1993; 4 (Suppl. 2): S6–9.
8 Jemec GBE, Kynemund L. Time spent on treatment in dermatology—how much time do outpatients use and is it a measure of morbidity? Acta Dermatoven APA 2001; 10: 17–9.

Children, infants and family impact

Children. The assessment of quality of life impairment in children is more difficult than in adults because of issues relating to communication, rapid change in lifestyle at different ages and differing rates of maturing. The different general measures and disease-specific measures have been reviewed [1].

The Children's Dermatology Life Quality Index (CDLQI) [2] is designed to be used by children aged 4–15 years old. It can be completed unaided by older children but parents can help younger children as necessary. An illustrated cartoon version, using the same text, has been validated [3]. Overall, children preferred the cartoon version and completed it more rapidly than the text only version. The CDLQI has been used in the assessment on children's lives of the effects of atopic dermatitis, the impact of admission for treatment, the impact of a nurse

consultant, and the effect of new topical and systemic anti-inflammatory agents. There are several different validated language translations of the CDLQI. Another measure that has been used in paediatric dermatology is the Pediatric Symptom Checklist [4], which consists of 35 questions answered by the parent. It has been used for psychosocial screening in paediatric dermatology clinics.

The lives of infants with atopic dermatitis may be severely disrupted, even though the affected children may not be able to explain their distress, or have the insight to know that what they are experiencing is abnormal. The Infant's Dermatitis Quality of Life Index (IDQOL) [5] has been proposed to encapsulate and attempt to measure the impact of atopic dermatitis on infants.

Family impact. When a patient is affected by a skin disease, those closest to the person are usually also affected. Having a child with atopic dermatitis can have a major impact on the functioning of a family. Two methods [6,7] have been proposed to measure this secondary impact. The Dermatitis Family Impact (DFI) questionnaire [6] has been used to demonstrate the relationship of dermatitis severity to family life quality [8].

REFERENCES

1 Eiser C, Morse R. Quality-of-life measures in chronic diseases in childhood. Health Technol Assess 2001; 5: 1–157.
2 Lewis-Jones MS, Finlay AY. The Children's Dermatology Life Quality Index (CDLQI). Initial validation and practical use. Br J Dermatol 1995; 132: 942–9.
3 Holme SA, Mann I, Sharpe JL et al. The Children's Dermatology Life Quality Index: validation of the cartoon version. Br J Dermatol 2003; 148: 285–90.
4 Rauch PK, Jellinek MS, Murphy JM et al. Screening for psychosocial dysfunction in pediatric dermatology practice. Clin Pediatr 1991; 30: 493–7.
5 Lewis-Jones MS, Finlay AY, Dykes PJ. The Infant's Dermatitis Quality of Life Index. Br J Dermatol 2001; 144: 104–10.
6 Lawson V, Lewis-Jones SM, Finlay AY. The family impact of childhood atopic dermatitis: the Dermatitis Family Impact Questionnaire. Br J Dermatol 1998; 138: 107–13.
7 Von Reuden U, Staab D, Kehrt R, Wahn U. Development of a questionnaire to measure Health-Related Quality of Life in parents of children with atopic dermatitis. Qual Life Res 1998; 7: 656–7.
8 Ben-Gashir MA, Seed PT, Hay RJ. Are quality of family life and disease severity related in childhood atopic dermatitis? J Eur Acad Dermatol Venereol 2002; 16: 455–62.

Declaration of interest. The author (AYF) is joint copyright holder of the following questionnaires described above: DLQI, CDLQI, PDI, IDQOL, CADI, ADI and DFI.

Some specific groups for whom problems of readjustment and rehabilitation may be important are outlined below.

Infants with atopic eczema. The main need is for dialogue with the parents and sustained contact to help relieve the inevitable tensions and emotional stresses that the condition imposes on them. Special problems arise in children where hospital admission is required. This is best dealt with in children's units. Joint management with nursing staff trained for the special requirements of sick children and expertise in basic dermatological therapy is invaluable. The parents should be encouraged to participate in the ward activity and will gain confidence in helping in the management of the problem.

The young adult atopic eczema patient. The problems here are often those of personality and environmental stresses rather than of working conditions. Apparent resolution in the protected environment of a hospital ward does not always survive exposure to the harsher emotional stresses of outside life. However, a temporary withdrawal from an adverse environment is usually helpful. It is important that the dermatologist discusses with both the patient and his or her family possible future employment. For instance, the youngster with severe hand eczema is unlikely to be able to nurse or become a hairdresser, or be able to follow a successful career in catering or engineering involving the continued exposure to coolant oils. Early counselling about future work prospects can prevent a lot of misery later on.

The older child. Children with disabling or disfiguring diseases demand special attention towards adjustment to the various epochs of their life relationships with other children, the first school, and passage through puberty. Play and companionship in the early years mark the transition from maternal social relationships. Disfigurement or disease is always a source of childish cruelty and integration into the social group requires much skilled help from nursing staff and mother figures. The transition to school and pressure of examinations call for guidance and careful management. The difficulties of a spastic, deaf or mute child are evident enough to arouse sympathy. The emotionally volatile, scratching atopic or the obviously disfigured child receives less sympathy and attention, although his or her needs are as great.

The young manual worker. There will be much anxiety about the manual worker's future working capacity. After all relevant investigations have been carried out, the work possibilities should be assessed. With the patient's consent, contact with his or her firm's medical officer and general practitioner should be routine, and the results of patch tests, etc. should be conveyed with an interpretation that is relevant to the occupation. To a worker, persistent hand eczema may mean the difference between a livelihood or disablement. Anxieties may not be readily revealed and may require patience to uncover. Re-education in working procedure, an explanation of irritant (or allergic) dermatitis and attention to the causes of persistence and relapse should be part of the normal procedure of treatment. After suffering a severe attack of dermatitis, a patient is likely to be suspicious of any agent to be handled on return to work, but he or she should be encouraged to persist at work during the first critical weeks in which

non-specific factors may temporarily exacerbate the condition. The patient should be seen at intervals for at least 3 months after return to work. The employers should be willing to grant time to attend hospital for this purpose.

Medicolegal aspects of dermatology [1]

A survey among members of the British Association of Dermatologists indicated that a significant proportion of dermatologists in the UK were concerned about the possibility of being sued, and an even greater percentage had altered their practice because of this concern [2].

The problem is not confined to the UK, with major concerns about potential litigation amongst dermatologists in the USA, Irish Republic and, more recently, in several other European countries.

There are several measures that minimize the possibility of litigation, and good and effective communication between the dermatologist and the patient is the most important. Moreover, continuing effective communication is necessary after the patient has been seen, especially if there has been dermatological surgery, so that if there are any problems these can be dealt with rapidly and effectively. There is nothing more frustrating for the patient than to find the dermatologist elusive, and resulting patient anger can initiate speedy legal retribution. It is important that not only the dermatologist but also all associated staff adopt an open and easy policy as far as communication with patients is concerned.

A second necessary line of defence against possible litigation involves making adequate and comprehensive case notes. This is particularly important as far as pigmented lesions are concerned, where it is prudent to record the variability or otherwise of the shape, the size and degree of pigmentation of the lesion. There has been a recent increase in litigation involving patients with malignant melanoma, not only over allegations about failure to make an accurate diagnosis, but also in regard to possible delay in seeing the patient after referral by the general practitioner. It is good practice for the dermatologist to see all the referral letters from the primary care physician so an informed assessment of urgency can be made. Even so, the vast numbers of anxious patients referred on account of recent change in pigmented lesions, the majority of which turn out to be absolutely benign, makes running an effective dermatological service very difficult. Particular difficulties arise when the general practitioner does not label the referral letter 'Urgent' and the patient subsequently turns out to have a malignant melanoma. In this instance, the information given by the general practitioner in the referral letter may or may not be sufficient to allocate an urgent appointment.

Dissatisfaction with scars after lesion removal is another potential area of litigation. It is good practice to explain that spread scars are the almost universal accompaniment of excision of lesions on the back and legs and the development of not only hypertrophic scarring but also keloid scarring should be emphasized, particularly in keloid-prone areas such as presternal skin and over the deltoid area. Comprehensive notes recording that a full discussion has taken place about the future cosmetic appearance of the scar, including possible diagrams of how a lesion will be excised, are both very helpful in rebutting potential litigation.

Consultant dermatologists have a responsibility to train others, and faulty technique using liquid nitrogen is a relatively common cause of litigation against general practitioners. Skin necrosis, and even peripheral neuropathy, are the commonest causes for litigation following inappropriate liquid nitrogen treatment.

Skin and subcutaneous atrophy following injections of triamcinolone in inappropriate sites, such as the arm, or too superficially, or at the same site in the buttock are also relatively common causes of cosmetic litigation as far as the general practitioner dermatologist is concerned.

It is very important that colleagues refrain from making disparaging remarks about other colleagues in front of patients. It is also important not to use emotive words, such as 'dermatitis' to, for example, an engineering worker, who may equate this diagnosis immediately with a diagnosis of industrial dermatitis, and therefore financial compensation.

One other potential pitfall for the dermatologist is the side effects from the use, not only of oral, but also of topical, steroids. Skin atrophy, striae, depression of the pituitary–adrenal axis and avascular necrosis of the femoral neck are particular examples. Avascular necrosis of the femoral neck is more common in alcoholic individuals and special care should be exercised, not only using oral steroids, but also topical steroids, in such patients [3]. It should be remembered, however, that avascular necrosis of the femoral neck has also been described in patients receiving physiological corticosteroid replacement therapy [4]. Patients on long-term oral steroid therapy should be advised about prophylaxis for osteoporosis [5].

The possibility of inducing not only cataracts but also glaucoma, especially if there is a family history of glaucoma, following the long-term use of tropical corticosteroids on the face and around the eyes in particular, should be remembered in patients, for instance, with long-standing eczema of the face [6].

Particular care needs to be exercised to avoid prescribing drugs that have previously caused an allergic reaction in a particular patient [1]. Although the resulting medical problem may not be severe, there is always a chance of a much more severe allergic reaction leading to the development of potentially fatal toxic epidermal necrolysis.

Avoidance of drug interactions is also important, particularly where potent drugs, such as methotrexate, ciclosporin, warfarin and corticosteroids are concerned. A recent study of 790 claims against general practitioners has shown that the largest proportion (25%) were related to errors in prescribing, monitoring or administering medicine [7].

Careful systems of work are vital to prevent burning of normal skin during the use of various forms of ultraviolet (UV) light, including psoralen and long-wave UV radiation (PUVA) therapy and topical dithranol (anthralin) treatment. Management changes in the British National Health Service, attempting to achieve a skill mix, have led to relatively inexperienced nurses being given the task of administering dithranol or UV therapy. Hospital managers should be told about the possible disastrous consequences of such a policy in dermatological patients, where nursing treatment expertise, built up over many years, is vital to ensure best results. Care also needs to be exercised in the topical treatment of ulcers, where the prescription of topical agents containing neomycin have led to the development of deafness [8].

Why do patients go to litigation? [9]

There are four main reasons why people sue their doctors, and the decision to take legal action is not only determined by the original 'injury' but also by insensitive handling and poor communication after the original incident. The patient seeks explanations when things go wrong and these explanations are often considered inadequate by patients who sue their doctors. The four main reasons that emerged from a recent analysis of 227 patients and relatives were, firstly, a concern with standards of care. Both patients and relatives wanted to prevent similar incidents in future. Secondly, there is a need for an explanation to know how the injury happened and why. Thirdly, there was a belief that the doctor or hospital involved should have to account and apologize for their actions. Lastly, financial compensation for pain and suffering was a significant factor. Moreover, the patients and their relatives all expressed a desire for greater honesty and assurances that lessons had been learned from their experiences [9].

Litigation and patients with psychiatric problems

Whilst patients may quite correctly seek financial compensation for errors made by their dermatologist, it is possible that some patients are more likely to go to litigation than others.

In a recent study involving nearly 100 patients, suing either their doctors or their employers and seen for medicolegal purposes, a very significant past or present history of psychiatric disturbance was found in almost 70% of the litigants. The commonest psychiatric disease present was depression, but anxiety, alcoholism and personality disorder were all represented. The medicolegal patient may also be trying to deceive both the dermatologist and the court. In this series there were two patients with artefact dermatitis and one with dermatitis simulata.

It is easy to miss a diagnosis of depression in dermatological patients, and it is thought that perhaps 50% of depressed patients in medical practice go unrecognized [10]. The depressed patient with dysmorphophobia is particularly likely to be angry, and this anger can be directed at the dermatologist or general practitioner, but, more commonly, internally, resulting ultimately in suicide [11].

Dysmorphophobic patients tend to haunt dermatologists, particularly those who are undertaking cosmetic procedures, such as laser treatment and skin resurfacing. Even though the results of treatment are good, the patient may remain dissatisfied and litigious. Before any cosmetic procedures are undertaken in a depressed patient, it is very important to make sure that communication between the patient and the doctor is optimum. Photography before and after any procedure is also important, so that there is some objective measure of the outcome. Preoperative assessment by a psychiatrist may be indicated in patients with long-standing or gross psychopathology.

Preparing a medicolegal report [1]

The data necessary to prepare a medical report on a patient seen with possible occupational dermatosis are described in Chapter 21.

Dermatologists may be asked by solicitors to prepare medicolegal reports. The commonest request is to prepare a report about alleged industrial dermatitis. Less often, a report on the dermatological consequences of an accident, either on the road, in the factory or, for instance, following a badly performed perm, may be sought. Thirdly, there may be a request to prepare a report about alleged medical negligence.

Until recently in the UK it was normal practice to appoint one expert witness to prepare a report for a claimant and a second expert witness to carry out a similar role for the defence. The present position is that normally one joint expert only is appointed by the court under Civil Proceedings Rules Part 35:3. Such a joint expert owes a duty to the court and will be expected to make a detailed declaration at the end of the expert report (Table 71.4).

It should be noted that the report has to be based on a complete and detailed enquiry of the relevant events, and a conventional medical history is not sufficient [1].

It should be remembered that the medical report may eventually go before a judge in court and it is humiliating for an expert witness to be questioned by a barrister about numerous spelling and grammatical errors. It is important that the dermatologist does not become biased on one side or the other. The expert witness has a duty to the court, and the medical report should be formulated to help the court. Solicitors may try and manipulate individual reports, asking the dermatologist to omit certain sentences

Table 71.4 Expert's declaration.

1 I understand that my overriding duty is to the court, both in preparing reports and in giving oral evidence
2 I have set out in my report what I understand from those instructing me to be the questions in respect of which my opinion as an expert is required
3 I have done my best, in preparing this report, to be accurate and complete. I have mentioned all matters which I regard as relevant to the opinions I have expressed. All of the matters on which I have expressed an opinion lie within my field of expertise
4 I have drawn to the attention of the court all matters, of which I am aware, which might adversely effect my opinion
5 Where I have no personal knowledge, I have indicated the source of factual information
6 I have not included anything in this report which has been suggested to me by anyone, including the lawyers instructing me, without forming my own independent view of the matter
7 Where, in my view, there is a range of reasonable opinion, I have indicated the extent of that range in the report
8 At the time of signing the report I consider it to be complete and accurate. I will notify those instructing me if, for any reason, I subsequently consider that the report requires any correction or qualification
9 I understand that this report will be the evidence that I will give under oath, subject to any correction or qualification I may make before swearing to its veracity
10 I have attached to this report a summary of my instructions
11 I confirm that in so far as the facts stated in my report are within my own knowledge I have made clear which they are and I believe them to be true and that the opinions I have expressed represent my true and complete professional opinion

and add others. As a generalization, this type of pressure should be resisted. Although the solicitor may wish you to amend the report for a tactical reason, the best guideline to follow is that the report should not be changed to such an extent that the writer can no longer agree with the content [12].

In a civil case involving, for instance, a claim for compensation for industrial dermatitis, the test of whether there is a causal relationship between exposure to coolant oil and the development of subsequent dermatitis depends on balance of probabilities. If, on balance of probabilities, there is more than a 50% chance that an individual's skin problem was caused, for instance, by coolant oil, that is sufficient for the claimant to establish the case. In contrast, in a criminal matter, the burden of proof has to be beyond all reasonable doubt, i.e. 99% or above certainty. In a medical negligence case, the solicitor may seek a report dealing mainly with diagnosis, causation and prognosis and seek a separate report dealing with liability and negligence.

The essence of negligence is that there has been a breach of a duty of care resulting in damage, and in medical cases this occurs in a context of diagnosis and/or treatment. There are four essential components, and all four must be present and proven before the patient can succeed in the action against the doctor [13].

1 The doctor must have had a duty of care to the plaintiff.
2 There must have been a breach of that duty.
3 The plaintiff must have suffered damage.
4 The damage must be a consequence of a breach of duty of care.

The Bolam test is often used to determine whether there has been a breach of duty of care. In this particular case the judge stated that 'a doctor is not guilty of negligence if he has acted in accordance with the practice accepted as proper by a responsible body of medical men skilled in that particular art'. This Bolam principle remains vital and central to how a doctor's professional behaviour is to be judged by other doctors, and not by lawyers, politicians or administrators. The Bolam test has been modified in the last decade so that a court in the UK can now reject medical opinion if it is not reasonable or responsible [14].

It should be noted that in exercising reasonable care, there may be an act of either commission or omission and each of these categories could lay the dermatologist open to litigation if harm has occurred. Moreover, a distinction must be made between an error of clinical judgement and negligence.

It is reassuring that the medical defence organizations in the UK still regard dermatology as a low-risk specialty, with few and relatively low-cost claims. On the other hand, plastic and reconstructive surgery involves a higher risk, as does cosmetic practice, especially when not carried out by consultant dermatologists or plastic surgeons.

It is important to remember that if something has gone wrong with patient care, a full and frank explanation with as little delay as possible will do much to diffuse the anger, upset and resentment that the patient feels and ultimately may reduce the risk that the patient will go to litigation [9]. There is a need for an explanation of how the injury has happened and why [9]. The doctor adopting this open type of approach could find him- or herself in direct conflict with the 'never admit anything' insurance type of mentality and it is important that Trust managers in the UK National Health Service, for instance, do not put pressure on their medical practitioners to adopt this approach. A prompt explanation is vital, as any delay would be seen as an attempt at cover up.

Consent [15]

Any treatment that entails the physical touching of a competent adult patient without consent constitutes the tort of battery. Consent provides a defence that makes the touching lawful. From the legal profession's point of view it is important to establish whether a competent adult patient consented to treatment or not and a requirement to obtain consent is imposed by law. In English law, once a patient has been informed in broad terms of the nature of the intended procedure and gives consent, the consent is valid, although there may be difficulties in deciding what constitutes the nature of the treatment or procedure and information in broad terms. It is very important to continue to review the information given to patients before obtaining consent. The use of information leaflets and documentation for the patient to read about treatment or surgical procedures is very helpful in this regard [16] but some doctors are still not providing enough information [14]. Medicolegally, times are changing so courts of law in the UK are putting more emphasis on the needs of patients and this can be seen as part of a wider social movement to give greater respect for individual rights.

The court appearance

Fortunately, less than 1% of cases where a medical report has been requested ever threatens to reach court, and in the majority of these cases a settlement is often reached out of court before the scheduled hearing. Should your appearance be necessary as an expert witness in court, it is important to follow several rules, but usually the expert witness drifts into this type of work without any training. Good preparation before the scheduled hearing is important and the original clinical notes, taken when preparing the medical report, can also be very useful. It is important to take the attitude that you are there to help the court, rather than to take one side or the other. Speak clearly and slowly enough to allow the judge to make notes. Do not fidget and do keep your evidence simple [17]. Take your time, when you need to, before answering the barrister's questions. When you are unclear as to what the barrister is asking, you may politely ask if the question might be rephrased. Emotionally, it may be difficult to switch from the role of a caring medical practitioner to an adversarial court system. Do not try and cross swords with an aggressive barrister, and address your comments at the judge, or jury if present. Remember, you are perfectly at liberty to ask for a short break if you have been in the witness box for some time and are getting tired.

REFERENCES

1 Sanderson KV. Dermatology. In: Jackson JP, ed. *A Practical Guide to Medicine and the Law*. London: Springer-Verlag, 1991: 96–114.
2 Cotterill JA. A survey of members of the BAD on the perceived threat of litigation. Unpublished data.
3 Cunliffe WJ, Burton JL, Holti G, Wright V. Hazards of steroid therapy in hepatic failure. *Br J Dermatol* 1975; **93**: 183–5.
4 Williams PL, Corbett M. Avascular necrosis of bone complicating corticosteroid replacement therapy. *Ann Rheum Dis* 1983; **42**: 276–9.
5 Walsh LJ, Wong CA, Pingle M, Tattersfield AE. Use of oral corticosteroids in the community and the prevention of secondary osteoporosis: a cross sectional study. *BMJ* 1996; **313**: 344–6.
6 Tani Euchi H, Ohki O, Yokozeki H *et al*. Cataract and retinal detachment in patients with severe atopic dermatitis who were withdrawn from the use of topical steroids. *J Dermatol* 1999; **26**: 658–65.
7 Green S, Goodwin H, Moss J. *Problems in General Practice. Medication, Errors: Claims For Negligence Against GP Members*. London: Medical Defence Union Risk Management Team, 1996.
8 Editorial. Deafness after topical neomycin. *BMJ* 1969; **4**: 181–2.

9 Vincent C, Young M, Phillips A. Why do people sue doctors? A study of patients and relatives taking legal action. *Lancet* 1994; **343**: 1609–13.

10 Mayou R, Hawton K. Psychiatric disorder in the general hospital. *Br J Psychiatry* 1986; **149**: 172–90.

11 Cotterill JA, Cunliffe WJ. Suicide in dermatological patients. *Br J Dermatol* 1997; **137**: 246–50.

12 Cummin J. Giving evidence. In: Leadbetter S, ed. *The Civil Perspective in Limitations of Expert Evidence.* London: Royal College of Physicians and Royal College of Pathologists, 1996: 11–8.

13 Knight B. The legal basis of medical negligence. In: Jackson JP, ed. *A Practical Guide to Medicine and the Law.* London: Springer-Verlag, 1991: 278–88.

14 Skene L, Smallwood R. Informed consent: lessons from Australia. *BMJ* 2002; **324**: 39–41.

15 Palmer RN. Consent and confidentiality. In: Jackson JP, ed. *A Practical Guide to Medicine and the Law.* London: Springer-Verlag, 1991: 19–41.

16 Shah M, Lewis FM. Cutaneous surgery. Preoperative information on what the patient expects. *J Eur Acad Dermatol Venereol* 1996; **7**: 86–7.

17 Stephens M. The criminal legal perspective. In: Leadbetter S, ed. *The Civil Perspective in Limitations of Expert Evidence.* London: Royal College of Physicians and Royal College of Pathologists, 1996: 3–10.

Chapter 72

Systemic Therapy

S.M. Breathnach, C.E.M. Griffiths, R.J.G. Chalmers & R.J. Hay

Introduction

Topical therapy is generally preferable for skin diseases, because it minimizes the risk of systemic toxicity. However, there are quite a number of drugs that are only effective when administered systemically. This chapter gives a brief survey of some of the more important systemic agents used by dermatologists. The reader is also directed to additional information on drug therapy for specific conditions dispersed amongst other chapters in these volumes.

The important subject of drug reactions and interactions is referred to in Chapter 73. The particular problems of prescribing for special groups, such as children, pregnant and lactating women and elderly people are dealt with in some detail in the *British National Formulary* [1] (and other national formularies), as are the difficulties in prescribing for patients with liver failure, renal failure and diseases affecting other organs. Where there is any doubt, the advice of a clinical pharmacologist, a pharmacist or the drug manufacturer should be sought, or information obtained from such reference works as *Martindale* [2] and Goodman and Gilman [3]. The *ABPI Data Sheet Compendium* [4] is also valuable. The dosage for children is often calculated roughly on the basis of age, but should more accurately be based on body weight or, even better, body surface area [1].

REFERENCES

1 *British National Formulary*, No 46. London: British Medical Association and the Pharmaceutical Society of Great Britain, 2003.
2 Reynolds JEF. *Martindale: The Extra Pharmacopoeia*, 30th edn. London: Pharmaceutical Trade Press, 1993.
3 Gilman AG, Goodman LS, Rall TW. *Goodman and Gilman's The Pharmacological Basis of Therapeutics*, 8th edn. New York: Pergamon, 1990.
4 Association of British Pharmaceutical Industry (ABPI). *ABPI Data Sheet Compendium*. London: Datapharm, 1996–7.

Systemic corticosteroid therapy

Corticosteroids were first introduced into dermatology by Marion Sulzberger [1]. Most of their effects are mediated by the intracellular glucocorticoid receptor via activation or repression of gene expression [2,3]. Activation requires DNA binding of the receptor, while repression is mediated by protein–protein interactions with other transcription factors. The immunosuppressive and anti-inflammatory effects are exerted mainly by an interaction of the glucocorticoid receptor with the activating protein 1 (AP-1) and nuclear factor κB (NF-κB) families of transcription factors without DNA binding. Cytokines such as tumour necrosis factor-α (TNF-α) and interleukin 1 (IL-1) activate the hypothalamus–pituitary–adrenal (HPA) axis; glucocorticoids inhibit IL-1 and TNF-α forming a cytokine–HPA axis feedback circuit. In addition, glucocorticoids induce apoptosis of inflammatory cells

72.1

of the haematopoietic system, such as monocytes, macrophages and T lymphocytes, while protecting resident tissue cells [4]. Corticosteroids, by evoking formation of a cell-membrane protein termed lipocortin, also inhibit phospholipase A_2 (PLA_2), a membrane enzyme that generates a variety of pro-inflammatory lipids from membrane phospholipids, including the prostaglandins, the leukotrienes and platelet-activating factor [5]. Other proposed mechanisms of corticosteroids include a cytostatic action, a 'stabilizing' action on lysosomal membranes, and suppression of cytokine expression. Glucocorticoid effects on bone result from inhibition of bone formation because of a decrease in the number and function of osteoblasts, and increased bone resorption resulting from osteoclastogenesis (with increased expression of RANK ligand and decreased expression of its decoy receptor, osteoprotegerin), as well as stimulated expression of collagenase 3 [6].

Indications

Systemic corticosteroid treatment, rather than topical corticosteroid therapy, is indicated in special circumstances only. These include the following.

1 Acute self-limited steroid-sensitive disorders (e.g. acute contact allergic dermatitis), where the offending allergen is evident. In these circumstances a 1-week course of oral prednisone in reducing dosage may be sufficient.

2 Acute anaphylactic reactions (e.g. following a bee or wasp sting or a drug to which the patient is sensitized). Hydrocortisone should be given intravenously in a dose of 100 mg, after prior administration of epinephrine (adrenaline) 0.5 mg intramuscularly, and chlorphenamine (chlorpheniramine) 4 mg intramuscularly (adult doses).

3 Acute autoimmune connective tissue diseases and generalized immunological vascular disorders (e.g. systemic lupus erythematosus, dermatomyositis, polyarteritis nodosa, giant cell arteritis, Wegener's granulomatosis).

4 Chronic disabling immunological bullous diseases (e.g. pemphigus vulgaris, pemphigoid).

5 Acute generalized exfoliative dermatitis (e.g. resulting from a severe drug reaction).

6 A number of miscellaneous disorders including severe lichen planus, pyoderma gangrenosum and sarcoidosis, in which there is evidence of cardiac, renal, ocular or extensive pulmonary or cutaneous involvement.

7 Although systemic steroids are often used, the value of such treatment is unproven in erythema multiforme, Stevens–Johnson syndrome, toxic epidermal necrolysis, chronic urticaria and cutaneous T-cell lymphoma.

Pharmacological considerations

Corticosteroids are anti-inflammatory, immunosuppressive, antiproliferative and vasoconstrictive.

Prednisone and prednisolone

Like cortisone and hydrocortisone, prednisone and prednisolone differ chemically only in the presence of a hydroxy group instead of a keto group at C11. The biological properties are similar, but prednisone has to be metabolically transformed in the liver to the 11β-hydroxy derivative to acquire biological potency, and hence prednisone should not be given to patients with liver disease. Both drugs possess four times the glucocorticoid potency and relatively less mineralocorticoid (salt-retaining) activity than hydrocortisone and cortisone.

Route of administration

Intramuscular

The intramuscular route, especially for triamcinolone, is popular in the USA for systemic steroid administration for short-term (less than 4 weeks) treatment. Triamcinolone does not differ significantly from prednisolone in its actions on a short-term basis, although in the long term it possesses greater mineralocorticoid activity. In the longer term, intramuscular steroids, especially in depot formulation, can cause marked HPA suppression and severe local atrophic changes, although the latter partially remit after a year or more. In the event of untoward steroid-induced complications, the drugs cannot be withdrawn promptly.

Intravenous

The intravenous route is useful in emergency treatment of acute anaphylaxis and in the pre- and postoperative cover of patients who have previously been receiving systemic steroid treatment for 4 weeks or more. A suitable regimen is 25 mg hydrocortisone preoperatively at the time of induction of anaesthesia, 100 mg during the operation and 100 mg on the first postoperative day—all doses being intravenous.

Thereafter the patient can be maintained on oral therapy as required. In fact, hypotensive crises attributable to adrenal insufficiency are extremely rare in patients withdrawn from glucocorticoid therapy and subsequently undergoing surgery without supplemental corticosteroid cover.

Pulsed steroid therapy

This is usually administered as doses of 1 g of methylprednisolone given intravenously over several hours using an intravenous line. The dose can be repeated daily for up to 5 days. It may be indicated in patients with severe bullous dermatoses, especially pemphigus vulgaris. It is a potentially hazardous procedure, and thromboembolism, cardiac arrest and steroid psychosis are occasional complications [7].

Oral steroids

Route of administration and dosage. Oral steroids may be taken in a single daily dose or using an alternate-day regimen.

Single daily dose. Short-term systemic steroid therapy is best given as a single daily dose. Prednisone and prednisolone have minimal mineralocorticoid activity and have a sufficiently prolonged action to ensure the sustained effectiveness of a single daily dose. The single dose should be given first thing in the morning. This is because the maximum rate of adrenocortical cortisol secretion occurs early in the morning and therefore less pituitary–adrenal suppression occurs at this time, while therapeutic efficacy is maintained [8].

Alternate-day dosage. Prolonged therapy may be instituted using an alternate-day regimen (twice the daily dose on alternate days with no steroid treatment on the other days) [9]. Conversion from a daily to an alternate-day regimen should be carried out gradually rather than abruptly (e.g. by progressive diminution of the dose on even-numbered days while building up the dose on odd-numbered days). In order to prevent alternate-day relapses, it may be necessary to maintain a small dose on the even-numbered day. Institution of an alternate-day systemic steroid regimen reduces but does not prevent steroid toxicity. Posterior subcapsular cataracts and osteoporosis may remain problems [10,11]. Alternate-day systemic steroid therapy is not always as effective as daily treatment when given in equivalent dosage.

Systemic steroid toxicity

A comprehensive account of the range of unwanted side effects consequent upon systemic steroid therapy is beyond the scope of this text, and is addressed in Chapter 73 [12–15]. Betamethasone and deflazacort may be used in emergencies in patients with adverse immunoglobulin E (IgE)-mediated allergic reactions to hydrocortisone and methylprednisolone [16].

The approximate physiological daily cortisol secretion by the adrenal cortex is 20 mg/day for an average adult (prednisone equivalent 5 mg/day). Short courses of prednisolone (e.g. up to 30 mg/day for less than 2 weeks), although suppressing pituitary–adrenal function, do not require tapering because recovery is rapid. However, for patients with a longer history of oral steroid treatment, gradual reduction of dosage prior to discontinuation is important, because abrupt reduction may lead to the 'steroid-withdrawal' syndrome, which resembles the

clinical features of adrenocortical insufficiency. Random plasma-cortisol determination may be within normal limits and stimulation tests of pituitary and adrenal function may also be normal [17].

One of the major problems with prolonged systemic corticosteroid therapy is osteoporosis. Patients receiving the equivalent of prednisolone 7.5 mg/day or more for over 3 months should receive prophylactic therapy to prevent bone resorption, such as calcium, bisphosphonates (alendronate, etidronate or risedronate), calcitriol or gonadal steroids (hormone replacement therapy in women, testosterone in men) [18,19].

Tests of pituitary–adrenal function

Baseline plasma-cortisol levels and study of diurnal variation of plasma cortisol are crude estimates of HPA integrity. The adrenocorticotrophic hormone (ACTH) stimulation test measures adrenal but not hypothalamo-pituitary integrity. The metyrapone test is based upon inhibition of an enzyme involved in synthesis of a cortisol precursor (2-deoxycortisol) resulting in reduction in cortisol levels and a consequent increase in ACTH. The cortisol precursors are measured in the urine and the resultant values give an indication of HPA integrity. Stress tests including insulin-induced hypoglycaemia measure the integrity of the whole HPA system, and are best carried out with the assistance of a specialized unit.

Systemic corticosteroids and pregnancy

There is little concrete evidence that systemic corticosteroids are harmful in pregnancy. Although the literature contains sporadic reports of stillbirth, spontaneous abortion and cleft palate associated with systemic corticosteroids [20], a recent review concluded that they are not teratogenic. Very little corticosteroid ingested by a mother enters her breast milk [21].

Systemic corticosteroids and cataracts

Posterior subcapsular cataracts are a recognized complication of systemic corticosteroid therapy. Screening by slit-lamp examination for patients in whom prolonged treatment with systemic corticosteroids is contemplated may help to obviate medicolegal consequences [10].

ACTH and tetracosactide

Although these agents are not corticosteroids, they provoke increased secretion of endogenous adrenal corticoids. There is little or no evidence to support the use of ACTH or tetracosactide (tetracosactrin) in place of systemic steroids. Their anti-inflammatory actions depend entirely upon increased hydrocortisone production by the adrenal cortex. They also suffer from the disadvantage that they stimulate adrenal androgen as well as hydrocortisone production, and therefore cause more salt and water retention than prednisolone [22]. Maximum response of adult adrenals is no more than 100 mg/day cortisol. ACTH and tetracosactide have to be given by injection and can cause severe anaphylactic reactions. There is no sound evidence for the often asserted view that these drugs are associated with less growth retardation in children than with oral corticosteroids. The only arguable advantage of ACTH or tetracosactide therapy is a reduced likelihood of pituitary–adrenal suppression, and this view has been challenged [22]. Certainly, overall, and dose for dose, manifestations of steroid toxicity are at least as frequent as in oral corticosteroid treatment.

REFERENCES

1 Sulzberger MB, Witten VH. The effect of topically applied compound E in selected dermatoses. *J Invest Dermatol* 1952; **19**: 101–2.
2 Schaaf MJ, Cidlowski JA. Molecular mechanisms of glucocorticoid action and resistance. *J Steroid Biochem Mol Biol* 2002; **83**: 37–48.
3 Neeck G, Renkawitz R, Eggert M. Molecular aspects of glucocorticoid hormone action in rheumatoid arthritis. *Cytokines Cell Mol Ther* 2002; **7**: 61–9.
4 Amsterdam A, Sasson R. The anti-inflammatory action of glucocorticoids is mediated by cell type specific regulation of apoptosis. *Mol Cell Endocrinol* 2002; **189**: 1–9.
5 Flower RJ. Background and discovery of lipocortins. *Agents Actions* 1986; **17**: 255–62.
6 Canalis E, Delany AM. Mechanisms of glucocorticoid action in bone. *Ann N Y Acad Sci* 2002; **966**: 73–81.
7 White KP, Driscoll MS, Rothe MJ, Grant-Kels JM. Severe adverse cadiovascular effects of pulse steroid therapy: is continuous cardiac monitoring necessary? *J Am Acad Dermatol* 1994; **30**: 768–73.
8 Nugent CA, Ward J, MacDiamid WD *et al*. Glucocorticoid toxicity: single versus divided daily doses of prednisolone. *J Chron Dis* 1965; **18**: 323–32.
9 Reichling GH, Kligman AM. Alternate-day corticosteroid therapy. *Arch Dermatol* 1961; **83**: 980–3.
10 Castrow FF. Atopic cataracts versus steroid cataracts. *J Am Acad Dermatol* 1981; **5**: 64–6.
11 MacGregor RR, Sheagren JN, Lipsett MB *et al*. Alternate-day prednisone therapy: evaluation of delayed hypersensitivity responses, control of disease and steroid side-effects. *N Engl J Med* 1969; **280**: 1427–31.
12 Gallant C, Kenny P. Oral glucocorticoids and their complications: a review. *J Am Acad Dermatol* 1986; **14**: 161–77.
13 Truhan AP, Ahmed AR. Corticosteroids: a review with emphasis on complications of prolonged systemic therapy. *Ann Allergy* 1989; **62**: 375–90.
14 Imam G, Halpern GM. Uses, adverse effects of abuse of corticosteroids. Part II. *Allergol Immunopathol (Madr)* 1995; **23**: 2–15.
15 Lester RS, Knowles SR, Shear NH. The risks of systemic corticosteroid use. *Dermatol Clin* 1998; **16**: 277–88.
16 Ventura MT, Calogiuri GF, Matino MG *et al*. Alternative glucocorticoids for use in cases of adverse reaction to systemic glucocorticoids: a study on 10 patients. *Br J Dermatol* 2003; **148**: 139–41.
17 Amatruda TT, Hollingsworth DR, D'Esopo G *et al*. A study of the mechanism of the steroid withdrawal syndrome: evidence for integrity of the hypothalamic–pituitary–adrenal system. *J Clin Endocrinol* 1960; **20**: 339–54.
18 Yosipovitch G, Hoon TS, Leok GC. Suggested rationale for prevention and treatment of glucocorticoid-induced bone loss in dermatologic patients. *Arch Dermatol* 2001; **137**: 477–81.
19 Iqbal MM, Sobhan T. Osteoporosis: a review. *Mol Med* 2002; **99**: 19–24.
20 Reinisch JM, Simon NG, Karow WG *et al*. Prenatal exposure to prednisolone in humans and animals retards uterine growth. *Science* 1978; **202**: 436–8.
21 Lockshin MD, Sammaritano LR. Corticosteroids during pregnancy. *Scand J Rheumatol Suppl* 1998; **107**: 136–8.
22 Hirschmann JV. Some principles of systemic glucocorticoid therapy. *Clin Exp Dermatol* 1986; **11**: 27–33.

Sex hormones and related compounds

Androgens

Testosterone is the most potent androgen and is currently only used for replacement therapy. Although many derivatives of testosterone have been developed with a pronounced anabolic action (the 'anabolic steroids'), they nevertheless retain significant and often troublesome virilizing activity.

Anabolic steroids

Danazol (100–600 mg/day). Danazol is a synthetic steroid derived from ethisterone. It has a high affinity for androgen receptors, and although itself a weak androgen, it has marked antiandrogenic activity. It also inhibits gonadal steroid production and reduces secretion of follicle-stimulating hormone (FSH) and luteinizing hormone (LH) by the pituitary. It increases the hepatic synthesis of a number of proteins including complement C1-esterase inhibitor and antitrypsin [1,2], and is of great value in hereditary angio-oedema because of C1-esterase inhibitor deficiency [3]. It causes enhanced production by the liver of functional C1-esterase inhibitor, but its beneficial effect is probably a result of more complex actions [4]. It can also be used to treat more severely affected patients with cholinergic urticaria who are unresponsive to antihistamines [5], probably because of its ability to enhance hepatic synthesis of antitrypsin, and can be used to inhibit ovulation in autoimmune progesterone dermatitis. Apart from its troublesome virilizing actions, it may cause hepatotoxicity; liver function tests should be carried out before and at monthly intervals during treatment.

Stanozolol (2.5–10 mg/day). Stanozolol is also a potent anabolic steroid with mild virilizing activity. It is just as effective as danazol in hereditary angio-oedema and with similar side effects, but considerably cheaper. Additionally, it has marked fibrinolytic properties, and has been advocated in the management of lipodermatosclerosis [6]. Its side effects are similar to those of danazol.

Anti-androgens [7–9]

Pregnancy must be avoided during therapy with anti-androgens because of the possible risk of abnormal development of a male fetus.

Cyproterone acetate. Cyproterone is a potent anti-androgen that competes with androgens at receptor sites and inhibits gonadotrophin secretion. In low doses (2 mg/day), usually in combination with ethinylestradiol in a reverse sequential regimen, it can be used for treatment of acne in females. It can also be used to treat hirsutism and other signs of virilization in females (at 12.5–50 mg/day in a reverse sequential regimen). Liver toxicity is an occasional problem and the drug is contraindicated in pregnancy.

Spironolactone [10]. Spironolactone blocks androgen receptors, but at low dosage it is less effective than other anti-androgens; high dosage (200 mg/day) is very effective at the cost of several adverse effects (particularly dysfunctional uterine bleeding). The concomitant use of a combined oral contraceptive may prevent these.

Flutamide. This also blocks androgen receptors, and at 250–500 mg/day for 6 months may be effective at treating hirsutism. Dry skin is very frequent, and hepatotoxicity is possible with high dosage.

Finasteride. Finasteride, a 5α-reductase type 2 inhibitor that blocks conversion of testosterone to dihydrotestosterone in the skin, is the least effective anti-androgen, but a dosage of 5 mg/day may decrease hirsutism without adverse effects. At a dosage of 1 mg/day, the drug produced clinical improvement in up to 66% of men with androgenetic alopecia treated for 2 years [11,12].

Oestrogens

Oestrogens prevent skin ageing [13], and may be useful in the management of autoimmune progesterone dermatitis [14].

Ethinylestradiol (10–35 μg/day). Ethinylestradiol (ethinyl oestradiol) is valuable replacement therapy in the treatment of postmenopausal symptoms including hot flushes, vaginitis and vaginal atrophy [15]. Plasma levels of FSH and LH, which are elevated in postmenopausal females, are useful guides to dosage. Ethinylestradiol should be avoided in patients with a history of breast cancer, liver or thromboembolic disease.

Anti-oestrogens

Tamoxifen (20 mg/day). Tamoxifen is an anti-oestrogenic drug that acts at receptor sites to block oestrogen binding. It therefore inhibits ovulation in fertile women. It may be useful in the treatment of progesterone-induced dermatitis or erythema multiforme [16]. Side effects are those associated with the menopause, together with abnormal vaginal bleeding. Bone density may be affected in the course of long-term treatment.

REFERENCES

1 Gadek JE, Fulmer JD, Gelfand JA *et al.* Danazol-induced augmentation of serum α-antitrypsin levels in individuals with marked deficiency of this antiprotease. *J Clin Invest* 1980; **66**: 82–7.

2 Gelfand JA, Sherins RJ, Alling DW, Frank MM. Treatment of hereditary angioedema with danazol: reversal of clinical and biochemical abnormalities. *N Engl J Med* 1976; **295**: 1444–8.

3 Nzeako UC, Frigas E, Tremaine WJ. Hereditary angioedema: a broad review for clinicians. *Arch Intern Med* 2001; **161**: 2417–29.

4 Warin AP, Greaves MW, Gatecliff M *et al.* Treatment of hereditary angioedema by low dose attenuated androgens: disassociation of clinical response from levels of C1-esterase inhibitor and C4. *Br J Dermatol* 1980; **103**: 405–9.

5 Wong E, Eftekhari N, Greaves MW, Milford Ward A. Beneficial effects of danazol on symptoms and laboratory changes in cholinergic urticaria. *Br J Dermatol* 1987; **116**: 553–6.

6 Burnand K, Clemenson G, Morland M *et al.* Venous lipodermatosclerosis: treatment by fibrinolytic enhancement and elastic compression. *BMJ* 1980; **280**: 7–11.

7 Thiboutot D, Chen W. Update and future of hormonal therapy in acne. *Dermatology* 2003; **206**: 57–67.

8 Azziz R. The evaluation and management of hirsutism. *Obstet Gynecol* 2003; **101**: 995–1007.

9 Falsetti L, Gambera A, Platto C, Legrenzi L. Management of hirsutism. *Am J Clin Dermatol* 2000; **1**: 89–99.

10 Farquhar C, Lee O, Toomath R, Jepson R. Spironolactone versus placebo or in combination with steroids for hirsutism and/or acne. *Cochrane Database Syst Rev* 2001; **4**: CD000194.

11 Wolff H, Kunte C. Current management of androgenetic alopecia in men. *Eur J Dermatol* 1999; **9**: 606–9.

12 Tosti A, Camacho-Martinez F, Dawber R. Management of androgenetic alopecia. *J Eur Acad Dermatol Venereol* 1999; **12**: 205–14.

13 Shah MG, Maibach HI. Estrogen and skin: an overview. *Am J Clin Dermatol* 2001; **2**: 143–50.

14 Oskay T, Kutluay L, Kaptanoglu A, Karabacak O. Autoimmune progesterone dermatitis. *Eur J Dermatol* 2002; **12**: 589–91.

15 Tzingouris VA, Aksu MF, Greenblatt RB. Estriol in the management of the menopause. *JAMA* 1978; **239**: 1638–41.

16 Wojnarowska F, Greaves MW, Peachey RDG *et al.* Progesterone-induced erythema multiforme. *J R Soc Med* 1985; **78**: 407–8.

Antihistamines

Historical note

The first effective and safe antihistamine, neoantergan, was based upon a molecule '2786 RP' discovered by Parisian investigators, Bovet and Walthert, in 1944 [1]. This antihistamine, known as anthisan or mepyramine maleate, was one of a series of diamethylamino-*N*-propyl phenothiazine compounds. Soon afterwards in the USA, diphenhydramine (Benadryl®) was launched and found to be effective by O'Leary and Faber [2] in chronic urticaria. In the UK, definition of the actions and potential role of the first-generation antihistamines was pioneered by Bain *et al.* [3,4] in urticaria.

It had long been recognized that not all of the actions of histamine, notably that of stimulation of gastric acid secretion, could be blocked by antihistamines. This puzzle was unravelled by Black *et al.* [5] who described a subset of histamine receptors designated H_2, which led to the development of the first clinically useful H_2 antihistamine, cimetidine, subsequently to be found effective in the management of chronic urticaria [6]. The later discovery of a third subset of histamine autoreceptors, H_3 [7], has as yet not generated any clinically useful applications in dermatology. However, the new class of H_1 antihistamines, in which troublesome sedative side effects of the classical

Table 72.1 Histamine receptors.

Receptors	Main action relevant to skin	Expression in skin	Antagonist
H_1	Vasodilatation Vasopermeability Itch	Yes	Chlorphenamine Terfenadine
H_2	Vasodilatation Vasopermeability	Yes	Cimetidine Ranitidine
H_3	Regulation of histamine Neurotransmitter release	?	Thioperamide*
H_{ic}	Intracellular messenger for promotion of cell growth	?	DPPE*

DPPE, *N,N*-diethyl-2-[4-(phenyl methyl) phenoxy] ethanamine HCl.
* Experimental antagonists.

antihistamines are minimalized by substitutions on the basic imidazole ring, thus preventing the drug from crossing the blood–brain barrier, has been the biggest recent milestone in the long history of antihistamines [8–12]. In 2002, 17 different oral H_1 antihistamines were available in the UK for treating allergic disorders [13].

Histamine receptors

Four classes of histamine receptor are presently recognized (Table 72.1). The discovery of H_2 receptors [5], alluded to above, was followed by demonstration of expression of H_1 and H_2 receptors in human skin. Histamine-induced vasodilatation and wealing are mediated by both classes of receptor, whereas itching is only served by H_1 receptors [14–16]. H_3 receptors are responsible for the ability of histamine in some tissues to regulate, by inhibitory feedback, its own biosynthesis and release. H_3 receptors, which also regulate transmitter release at autonomic nerve terminals, have not been convincingly shown to be represented in skin. On the other hand, the recently described intracellular (H_{ic}) histamine receptors that are responsible for the ability of histamine to promote cell and tissue growth (e.g. in embryonic tissue and wound healing) [17] are probably expressed in skin, although this has not yet been specifically demonstrated.

Other actions of antihistamines

Most H_1 antihistamines also express anticholinergic activity, resulting in the well-known side effects of the earlier 'classic' antihistamines, which include dryness of the mouth, blurring of vision and constipation. Drowsiness is also a feature of many early antihistamines. Available evidence suggests that histamine plays a part in the maintenance of the waking state, which may go some way towards explaining the sedative actions of some H_1 antihistamines. Many H_1 antagonists also prevent release of mediators from activated mast cells, although in most cases only in a higher concentration than that achieved

Table 72.2 Pharmacokinetic and pharmacodynamic activity of representative first- and second-generation antihistamines [8,23].

H_1 antagonist	T_{max} (h)	Half-life (h)	Weal suppression duration (h)
Chlorphenamine	2.8	27.9	24
Hydroxyzine	2.1	20.0	24
Diphenhydramine	1.7	9.2	12–24
Terfenadine	1.0	17	12–24
Astemizole	3.0	9.5 days	Variable
Loratadine	1.0	7.8–11.0	12–24
Cetirizine	0.9	7.4	24

T_{max}, time of maximum plasma concentration.

clinically. This response does not involve H_1 receptors [18]. Two H_1 antagonists, ketotifen and cetirizine, deserve mention as they have been claimed to be potent inhibitors of release of mast cell products [19–21]. However, no evidence of reduced urinary excretion of histamine or its metabolites was detected in patients with mastocytosis treated by the H_1 antihistamine, ketotifen [20]. Cetirizine has also been claimed to possess selective inhibitory activity against eosinophil-rich dermatoses [21,22] but the clinical relevance of this action is unclear.

H_1 antihistamines (Table 72.2 [8,23])

These are conveniently classified as first- and second-generation H_1 antihistamines. The first-generation drugs, although potent, are accompanied by troublesome atropine-like side effects, and also cause drowsiness [24], which may be useful or disadvantageous depending upon the clinical context.

First-generation H_1 antihistamines

These are exemplified by chlorphenamine (an alkylamine), diphenhydramine (an aminoalkyl ether) and hydroxyzine (a piperazine). Plasma half-lives of these drugs are variable (chlorphenamine approximately 24 h; hydroxyzine

20 h; diphenhydramine 9 h), although peak plasma concentrations are reached in approximately 2 h. Protein binding is almost total, and metabolism occurs via the hepatic microsomal cytochrome P-450 system. Thus, the half-life of certain H_1 antihistamines may be prolonged in patients receiving microsomal oxygenase inhibitors such as ketoconazole, erythromycin, doxepin or cimetidine.

The principal actions of H_1 antihistamines are on vasodilatation and increased vascular permeability, thus reducing the redness, weal and axon reflex flare reactions in acute urticaria, and suppressing the associated itching. The clinical effects of these H_1 antihistamines usually persist longer than measurable plasma levels would suggest, because of persistence of tissue levels or because of active metabolites. Once-daily administration is therefore adequate. In urticaria, first-generation H_1 antagonists reduce the size, duration and frequency of weals and greatly alleviate the itching. Although more often a nuisance, the sedative effects of first-generation H_1 antihistamines have been claimed to be highly beneficial in suppressing itching in some patients with atopic eczema [25]. Their effect is enhanced by other sedative drugs, especially alcohol. Other side effects of these antihistamines include tachycardia, with prolongation of the Q–T interval on the electrocardiogram and other arrythmias, as well as psychological disturbances.

Second-generation H_1 antihistamines [8]

These are exemplified by terfenadine, astemizole, loratadine and cetirizine, none of which produces sedation significantly greater than that caused by an otherwise identical placebo, provided recommended dosage is used. The absorption and metabolism of second-generation H_1 antihistamines resembles that of the first generation described above. The plasma half-lives of terfenadine, astemizole and cetirizine are listed in Table 72.2. These drugs in recommended regimens do not significantly cross the blood–brain barrier, thus accounting for their minimally sedating characteristics. Terfenadine is almost completely devoid of histamine H_2 or cholinergic receptor blockade and is effective in the treatment of chronic urticaria [26]. Agents including grapefruit juice and certain drugs (ketoconazole, itraconazole, erythromycin, other macrolide antibiotics, cimetidine and doxepin), which inhibit hepatic metabolism via the cytochrome P-450 system, should not be given concurrently with terfenadine, because they may promote adverse effects including cardiac arrhythmias, Q–T interval prolongation and torsades de pointes (ventricular tachycardia) [27–29]. Terfenadine is also contraindicated in patients with liver or heart disease. Terfenadine may cause rashes, which occasionally (and paradoxically) include urticaria [30,31]. The UK Committee on Safety of Medicines withdrew terfenadine from over-the-counter sale, as did the US Food and Drug Administration, because of the cardiac complications. Recently, fexofenadine, the major active metabolite of terfenadine, has been introduced as an alternative to terfenadine [32].

Astemizole also undergoes first-pass metabolism via the liver cytochrome P-450 system but its half-life together with its active metabolite dimethylastemizole is prolonged at 9.5 days [8]. It binds with greater avidity to H_1-receptor sites than any other H_1 antihistamine, evidence of histamine weal suppression being evident 4 weeks or more after discontinuation [33], but it has not been shown to be teratogenic. Like terfenadine, it must not be co-administered with macrolide antibiotics, imidazole antifungals or doxepin, because of the risk of cardiac arrhythmia [34]. Patients with a pre-existing Q–T interval prolongation are especially at risk. Other side effects of astemizole include increase in appetite and excessive weight gain [8].

Loratadine is a potent minimal-sedation antihistamine that is also substantially free of anticholinergic side effects. Loratadine is not metabolized through the liver cytochrome P-450 enzyme system to any great extent and is therefore believed free of cardiac arrhythmic complications. It inhibits evoked release of leukotrienes from human lung *in vitro* but is less active in suppressing histamine release [35]. How relevant these 'antiallergic' properties are to its therapeutic action is unclear. Desloratadine has now replaced loratadine in the UK.

Like loratadine, cetirizine, which is an active metabolite of hydroxyzine, is only minimally metabolized via the liver and therefore can be administered safely with macrolide antibiotics, imidazole antifungals and doxepin. In recommended dosage it has minimal sedative and anticholinergic actions. Cetirizine is claimed to be effective in diseases involving heavy eosinophil infiltration [21,22]. It has been proposed, on this basis, that cetirizine is especially valuable in patients with the common physical urticaria, delayed pressure urticaria [36], although adequate confirmation of this claim is lacking. Levocetirizine is also available.

H_1-antihistamine therapy in childhood

The second-generation low-sedation antihistamines are probably safer in children than the older 'classic' antihistamines; liquid formulations of astemizole, cetirizine and loratadine are available in the UK. Overdose of the first-generation antihistamines may cause severe toxicity including hyperpyrexia and convulsions in children.

H_1-antihistamine therapy in pregnancy

No antihistamines administered systemically should be deemed safe in the first trimester of pregnancy. However, of the available H_1 antihistamines, chlorphenamine [37] and tripelennamine [38] have shown little or no evidence of teratogenicity experimentally and are probably the least risky to use.

Development of tolerance during H₁-antihistamine therapy

Although tolerance of the first-generation H_1 antihistamines was reported soon after their introduction into medical practice [39], little or no information is available on the molecular basis of this phenomenon [40]. Suppression of wealing because of mast cell activation and histamine progressively dwindled in response to single doses of 75 mg hydroxyzine given daily for 3 weeks; no tolerance was demonstrated in response to chlorphenamine 16 mg/day in the same study [41]. Interestingly, this study showed that hydroxyzine, but not chlorphenamine, caused tolerance not only to itself but to several other first-generation antihistamines.

H₂ antihistamines

Cimetidine and ranitidine

The presence of H_2 receptors expressed on human skin blood vessels [14,15] prompted exploration of the value of H_2 antihistamines, co-administered with H_1 antihistamines, in the treatment of chronic urticaria. The object was to achieve an H_1-antihistamine-sparing effect, thus mitigating unwanted first-generation H_1 antihistamine side effects including drowsiness and atropine-like side effects. This strategy proved modestly successful [6,12,42–44]. However, the subsequent availability of the second-generation low-sedation antihistamines has undermined the need for an H_1-antihistamine-sparing regimen. Because ranitidine, unlike cimetidine, is not metabolized via the liver cytochrome P-450 system, it should probably be used in preference to cimetidine if H_2 antihistamine therapy is instituted.

REFERENCES

1 Bovet D, Walthert F. Structure chemique et activit? Pharmacodynamique des antihistaminiques de synthese. *Ann Pharm Fr* 1944; Suppl. 4.
2 O'Leary PA, Faber EM. Benadryl in the treatment of urticaria. *Proc Staff Meet Mayo Clin* 1945; **20**: 429–32.
3 Bain WA, Broadbent JL, Warin RP. Comparison of anthisan (mepyramine maleate) and phenergan as histamine antagonists. *Lancet* 1949; **ii**: 47–52.
4 Bain WD, Hellier FF, Warin RP. Some aspects of the action of histamine antagonists. *Lancet* 1948; **ii**: 964–6.
5 Black JW, Duncan WA, Durrant CJ et al. Definition and antagonism of histamine H₂ receptors. *Nature* 1972; **236**: 385–90.
6 Commens CA, Greaves MW. Cimetidine in chronic idiopathic urticaria: a randomized double blind study. *Br J Dermatol* 1978; **99**: 675–9.
7 Arrang JM, Garbarg M, Schwartz JC. Autoinhibition of brain histamine release mediated by a novel (H₃) class of histamine receptor. *Nature* 1983; **302**: 832–7.
8 Simons FER. Recent advances in H₁ antagonist treatment. *J Allergy Clin Immunol* 1990; **86**: 995–9.

9 Greaves MW. Antihistamines. *Dermatol Clin* 2001; **19**: 53–62.
10 Zuberbier T, Greaves MW, Juhlin et al. Management of urticaria: a consensus report. *J Investig Dermatol Symp Proc* 2001; **6**: 128–31.
11 Lee EE, Maibach HI. Treatment of urticaria: an evidence-based evaluation of antihistamines. *Am J Clin Dermatol* 2001; **2**: 27–32.
12 Black AK, Greaves MW. Antihistamines in urticaria and angioedema. *Clin Allergy Immunol* 2002; **17**: 249–86.
13 Anonymous. Oral antihistamines for allergic disorders. *Drug Ther Bull* 2002; **40**: 59–62.
14 Marks R, Greaves MW. Vascular reactions to histamine and compound 48/80 in human skin: suppression by a histamine H₂ receptor blocking agent. *Br J Clin Pharmacol* 1977; **4**: 367–9.
15 Robertson I, Greaves MW. Responses of human skin blood vessels to synthetic histamine analogues. *Br J Clin Pharmacol* 1978; **5**: 319–22.
16 Davies MG, Greaves MW. Sensory responses of human skin to synthetic histamine analogues and histamine. *Br J Clin Pharmacol* 1980; **9**: 461–5.
17 Brandes LJ, LaBella FS, Glavin GB et al. Histamine as an intracellular messenger. *Biochem Pharmacol* 1990; **40**: 1677–81.
18 Rimmer SJ, Church MK. The pharmacology and mechanism of action of histamine H₁ antagonists. *Clin Exp Allergy* 1990; **20** (Suppl. 2): 3–17.
19 Huston DP, Bressler RB, Kaliner M et al. Prevention of mast cell degranulation by ketotifen in patients with physical urticarias. *Ann Intern Med* 1986; **104**: 507–10.
20 Mallet AI, Norris P, Rendell NB et al. The effect of disodium cromoglycate and ketotifen on the excretion of histamine and N-methylimidazole acetic acid in urine of patients with mastocytosis. *Br J Clin Pharmacol* 1989; **27**: 88–91.
21 Charlesworth EN, Kagey-Sobotka A, Norman PS, Lichtenstein LM. Effect of cetirizine on mast cell mediator release and cellular traffic during the cutaneous late phase reaction. *J Allergy Clin Immunol* 1989; **83**: 905–12.
22 Leprevost C, Capron M, De Vos C et al. Inhibition of eosinophil chemotaxis by a new anti allergic compound (cetirizine). *Int Arch Allergy Appl Immunol* 1988; **87**: 9–13.
23 Simons FER, Simons KJ. The pharmacology and use of H₁ receptor-antagonist drugs. *N Engl J Med* 1994; **330**: 1663–70.
24 Monti JM. Involvement of histamine in the control of the waking state. *Life Sci* 1993; **53**: 1331–8.
25 Krause L, Shuster S. Mechanism of action of antipruritic drugs. *BMJ* 1983; **287**: 1199–200.
26 Grant JA, Bernstein DI, Buckley CE et al. Double blind comparison of terfenadine, chlorpheniramine and placebo in the treatment of chronic idiopathic urticaria. *J Allergy Clin Immunol* 1988; **81**: 574–9.
27 Thomas SHL. Drugs, QT interval abnormalities and ventricular arrhythmias. *Adverse Drug React Toxicol Rev* 1994; **13**: 77–102.
28 Woosley RL. Cardiac actions of antihistamines. *Annu Rev Pharmacol Toxicol* 1996; **36**: 233–52.
29 Thomas SHL. Drugs and the QT interval. *Adverse Drug React Bull* 1997; **182**: 691–4.
30 Stricker BHCH, Van Dijke CHP, Isaacs AJ, Lindquist M. Skin reactions to terfenadine. *BMJ* 1986; **293**: 536.
31 McClintock AD, Ching DW, Hutchinson C. Skin reactions and terfenadine. *N Z Med J* 1995; **108**: 208.
32 Kawashima M, Harada S, Tango T. Review of fexofenadine in the treatment of chronic idiopathic urticaria. *Int J Dermatol* 2002; **41**: 701–6.
33 Kailasam V, Matthews KP. Controlled clinical assessment of astemizole in the treatment of chronic idiopathic urticaria and angioedema. *J Am Acad Dermatol* 1987; **16**: 797–804.
34 Broadhurst P, Nathan AW. Cardiac arrest in a young woman with the long QT syndrome and concomitant astemizole ingestion. *Br Heart J* 1993; **70**: 469–70.
35 Temple DM, McClusky M. Loratidine, an antihistamine, blocks antigen and ionophore-induced leukotriene release from human lung *in vitro*. *Prostaglandins* 1988; **35**: 549–54.
36 Kontou-Fili K, Maniatakou G, Demaka P et al. Therapeutic effects of cetirizine in delayed pressure urticaria: clinicopathologic findings. *J Am Acad Dermatol* 1991; **24**: 1090–3.
37 Pratt WR. Allergic diseases in pregnancy and breast feeding. *Ann Allergy* 1981; **47**: 355.
38 Schatz M, Hoffman CP, Zeiger RS et al. The course and management of asthma and allergic diseases during pregnancy. In: Middleton E, Reed CE, Ellis EE et al., eds. *Allergy Principles and Practice*; Vol. 2, 4th edn. St Louis: Mosby Year Book, 1993: 1301–42.
39 Wyngaarden JB, Seevers MH. The toxic effects of antihistamine drugs. *JAMA* 1951; **145**: 277–82.

40 Monash S. Development of refractory condition of skin towards antihistaminic drugs after antihistamine therapy as determined by histamine iontopheresis. *J Invest Dermatol* 1950; **15**: 1.
41 Long WF, Taylor RJ, Wagner CJ *et al*. Skin test suppression by antihistamines and the development of subsensitivity. *J Allergy Clin Immunol* 1985; **76**: 113–17.
42 Breathnach SM, Allen R, Milford Ward A, Greaves MW. Symptomatic dermographism: natural history, clinical features, laboratory investigations and response to therapy. *Clin Exp Dermatol* 1983; **8**: 463–76.
43 Kaur S, Greaves MW, Eftekhari N. Factitious urticaria (dermographism) treatment by cimetidine and chlorpheniramine in a randomized double blind study. *Br J Dermatol* 1981; **104**: 185–90.
44 Bleehen SS, Thomas SE, Greaves MW *et al*. Cimetidine and chlorpheniramine in the treatment of chronic idiopathic urticaria: a multicentre randomized double blind study. *Br J Dermatol* 1987; **117**: 81–8.

Other antiallergic drugs

Sodium cromoglycate. Although ineffective in suppressing mast cell activation in the skin [1], it inhibits release of histamine and other mast cell-derived mediators from mast cells of lung, conjunctiva, nose and gastrointestinal tracts. It therefore has no proven role in the skin; however, it does ameliorate the diarrhoea associated with mastocytosis [2].

Leukotriene receptor antagonists. Montelukast and zafirlukast may be useful in chronic urticaria [3].

REFERENCES

1 Pearce CA, Greaves MW, Plummer VM, Yamamoto S. Effect of disodium cromoglycate on antigen-evoked histamine release from human skin. *Clin Exp Immunol* 1974; **17**: 437–40.
2 Soter NA, Austen KF, Wasserman SI. Oral disodium cromoglycate in the treatment of systemic mastocytosis. *N Engl J Med* 1979; **301**: 465–9.
3 Tedeschi A, Airaghi L, Lorini M, Asero R. Chronic urticaria: a role for newer immunomodulatory drugs? *Am J Clin Dermatol* 2003; **4**: 297–305.

Systemic non-steroidal anti-inflammatory therapy

Non-steroidal anti-inflammatory drugs (NSAIDs) are defined as substituted phenolic or benzene-ring compounds that owe their pharmacological actions mainly to inhibition of the enzyme cyclo-oxygenase (COX) (prostaglandin synthetase). This enzyme complex was shown by Vane [1] in 1971 to transform arachidonic acid into prostaglandins. However, NSAIDs undoubtedly influence other pro-inflammatory molecular pathways. NSAIDs have been advocated in a large number of common and uncommon dermatoses, including acne, psoriasis, sunburn, erythema nodosum, cryoglobulinaemia, Sweet's syndrome and systemic mastocytosis, as well as in urticarial, livedoid and nodular vasculitis [2].

Transformation of arachidonic acid and the mode of action of NSAIDs

There are two forms of COX: a constitutive enzyme (COX-

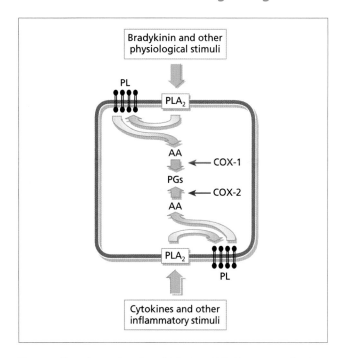

Fig. 72.1 Transformation of arachidonic acid (AA) to prostaglandins (PGs) by cyclo-oxygenases (COX) 1 and 2. PLA$_2$, phospholipase (PL) A$_2$.

1) and an induced enzyme (COX-2) (Fig. 72.1). NSAIDs act mainly by inhibition of COX-2 [3]. In contrast, inhibition of COX-1 by NSAIDs probably accounts for some of their unwanted side effects including gastric ulceration.

Arachidonic acid is also transformed via the lipoxygenase pathways (5-lipoxygenase; 12-lipoxygenase) to form a group of strongly pro-inflammatory hydroxy fatty acids of which the best known is leukotriene B$_4$ (LTB$_4$) (Fig. 72.2) [4]. Because of the proposed role of the leukotrienes and other hydroxy fatty acid products of arachidonic acid in the pathogenesis of psoriasis [5] and other inflammatory dermatoses [6], several generally unsuccessful attempts have been made to develop selective lipoxygenase-inhibiting NSAIDs for clinical dermatological use [7]. These compounds have generally proved ineffective, toxic or both.

Acetylsalicylic acid (aspirin) is the archetypal NSAID and has been shown to owe its anti-inflammatory action to inhibition of COX-2 [1]. Its role in the management of skin diseases is limited. Administration of aspirin has been shown to suppress ultraviolet erythema in humans [8]. Furthermore, Roberts *et al*. [9] have proposed that aspirin be co-administered with H$_1$ and H$_2$ antihistamines in the management of the diarrhoea of systemic mastocytosis, which is believed to be mainly caused by overproduction of prostaglandin D$_2$ by the increased population of mast cells in the involved tissues. Although originally proposed to be antipruritic, aspirin administration probably does not allay the itching of atopic eczema [10].

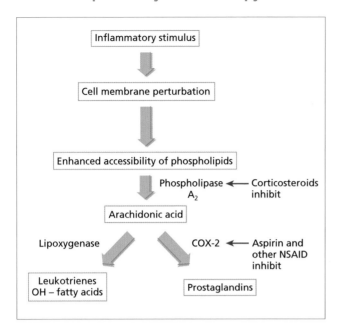

Fig. 72.2 Generation of eicosanoids from cell membrane lipids in the inflammatory response. Arachidonic acid, released from cell membrane phospholipid by the action of phospholipase A_2, is further transformed by cyclo-oxygenase 2 (COX-2) to prostaglandin, and by lipoxygenase to leukotrienes and related fatty acids. NSAID, non-steroidal anti-inflammatory drugs.

The early phase of UVB-induced erythema is caused, at least in part, by release of vasoactive prostaglandins [11]. Oral administration of indometacin (indomethacin) has been demonstrated to reduce the erythema and concurrently to suppress the increased tissue levels of COX products in UVB-irradiated skin [12]. Proposed clinical indications for oral indometacin include cutaneous vasculitis [13] and erythema nodosum [14], although these indications have not yet been confirmed by placebo-controlled double-blind trials. The value of oral indometacin in the management of psoriatic arthritis is well established; reports that oral indometacin may exacerbate the skin lesions of psoriasis have not been substantiated (see Chapter 73).

Adverse reactions to systemic NSAIDs, including urticaria and angio-oedema, are unfortunately commonplace (see Chapter 73) [15]. Reactions occur most frequently in response to piroxicam, sulindac, meclofenamate, tolmetin and phenylbutazone [16]. The best known and probably the most severe include Stevens–Johnson syndrome and toxic epidermal necrolysis. Photosensitivity is very common, especially with piroxicam, but the underlying mechanisms, which involve phototoxicity in many instances, are unknown [17].

REFERENCES

1 Vane JR. Inhibition of prostaglandin synthesis as a mechanism of action for aspirin-like drugs. *Nature New Biol* 1971; **231**: 232–5.

2 Friedman ES, LaNatra N, Stiller MJ. NSAIDs in dermatologic therapy: review and preview. *J Cutan Med Surg* 2002; **6**: 449–59.

3 Mitchell JA, Larkin S, Williams TJ. Cyclo-oxygenase-2 regulation and relevance in inflammation. *Biochem Pharmacol* 1995; **50**: 1535–42.

4 Samuelsson B, Hammarstrom S. Nomenclature for leukotrienes. *Prostaglandins* 1980; **19**: 645–8.

5 Brain S, Camp RDR, Dowd P et al. The release of leukotriene B_4-like material in biologically active amounts from the lesional skin of patients with psoriasis. *J Invest Dermatol* 1984; **83**: 70–3.

6 Barr RM, Brain S, Camp RD et al. Levels of arachidonic acid and its metabolites in human allergic and irritant contact dermatitis. *Br J Dermatol* 1984; **111**: 23–8.

7 Barr RM, Black AK, Dowd PM et al. The in vitro 5-lipoxygenase and cyclo-oxygenase inhibitor L-652, 343 does not inhibit 5-lipoxygenase in vivo in human skin. *Br J Clin Pharmacol* 1988; **25**: 23–6.

8 Miller WS, Ruderman FR, Smith JG Jr. Aspirin and ultraviolet light-induced erythema in man. *Arch Dermatol* 1967; **95**: 357–8.

9 Roberts LJ, Sweetman BJ, Lewis RA et al. Increased production of prostaglandin D_2 in patients with systemic mastocytosis. *N Engl J Med* 1980; **303**: 1400–4.

10 Daly BM, Shuster S. Effect of aspirin on pruritus. *BMJ* 1986; **293**: 907.

11 Black AK, Fincham N, Greaves MW, Hensby CN. Time course changes in levels of arachidonic acid and prostaglandin D_2, E_2 and F_2 in human skin following ultraviolet B irradiation. *Br J Pharmacol* 1980; **10**: 453–7.

12 Black AK, Greaves MW, Hensby CN et al. Effects of indomethacin on prostaglandins E_2 $F_{2\alpha}$ and arachidonic acid in human skin 24 h after UV-B and UV-C irradiation. *Br J Clin Pharmacol* 1978; **6**: 261–6.

13 Millns JL, Randle HW, Solley GO, Dicken CH. The therapeutic response of urticaria vasculitis to indomethacin. *J Am Acad Dermatol* 1980; **3**: 349–55.

14 Callen JP. Erythema nodosum. In: Provost T, Farmer ER, eds *Current Therapy in Dermatology, 1985–1986.* Toronto: Dekker, 1988: 158–60.

15 Sanchez-Borges M, Capriles-Hulett A, Caballero-Fonseca F. Cutaneous reactions to aspirin and non-steroidal anti-inflammatory drugs. *Clin Rev Allergy Immunol* 2003; **24**: 125–36.

16 Bigby M, Stern R. Cutaneous reactions to non-steroidal anti-inflammatory drugs. *J Am Acad Dermatol* 1985; **12**: 866–76.

17 Kaidbey KH, Mitchell FN. Photosensitizing potential of certain non-steroidal anti-inflammatory agents. *Arch Dermatol* 1989; **125**: 783–6.

Cytokines

Cytokines are small polypeptides, molecular mass less than 60 kDa, which act as intercellular messengers; they have a pivotal role in cutaneous inflammation. They can be either pro-inflammatory or anti-inflammatory; however, a single cytokine may have several different functions and may act on many cellular targets. DNA technology has facilitated the large-scale manufacture of recombinant human cytokines, several of which have been used to treat skin disease.

Interferons

Interferons are naturally occurring endogenous glycoproteins, which are now available for therapeutic use through recombinant DNA technology. This group of compounds exhibits antiviral, cytostatic and immunomodulatory properties and has therefore found application in both malignant and inflammatory dermatoses. Three types of interferon are available: interferon-α (IFN-α), IFN-β and IFN-γ. Unfortunately, side effects are common, including influenza-like symptoms with fever, hepatotoxicity and leukopenia; this has limited clinical usage.

Kaposi's sarcoma

Because of its antiviral, antiangiogenic and tumoristatic properties, interferon ought to be an ideal treatment for acquired immune deficiency syndrome (AIDS)-related Kaposi's sarcoma, which is probably caused by human herpesvirus 8. There have been numerous reports of remissions induced by IFN-α, invariably at the cost of troublesome side effects. In earlier studies [1], high doses did induce remissions, especially in patients without associated opportunistic infections [2]. Subsequent studies suggested that better results were obtained in the presence of sustained CD4 T-lymphocyte counts [3]. There is some evidence of synergism between IFN-α and zidovudine [4,5]. Patients who respond to treatment with IFN-α appear to have fewer opportunistic infections [6]. Co-administration of granulocyte–macrophage colony-stimulating factor (GM-CSF) with IFN-α has been shown to limit the bone marrow-suppressant side effects of the latter [7]. Both IFN-α and IFN-β inhibit neoangiogenesis—a further explanation for their effectiveness in Kaposi's sarcoma [8]. IFN-γ is ineffective in Kaposi's sarcoma.

Melanoma

There has been considerable interest in the use of IFN-α to treat metastatic melanoma. Approximately 5% of treated patients may achieve total remission. The optimal drug regimens of IFN-α are not known but up to 20% of patients may respond [9]. This response rate can be significantly increased by combination therapy with cisplatin and other antimetabolites [10]. Despite the mixed results, IFN-α is approved in the USA and Europe for high-risk melanoma patients [11]. IFN-α has been administered subsequent to melanoma lysate vaccine, leading to a response rate higher than that produced by either IFN-α or vaccine alone [12].

Cutaneous T-cell lymphoma

Cutaneous T-cell lymphoma (CTCL) is a Th2 cytokine disease in that peripheral blood mononuclear cells secrete increased amounts of IL-4 and IL-5. IFN-α, which suppresses IL-4 and IL-5 production, is effective in up to 50% of patients—particularly those with Sézary syndrome [13]. Remission rates as high as 70% have been reported when subcutaneously administered IFN-α-2a is used in combination with psoralen with UVA treatment (PUVA) or extracorporeal photopheresis [14].

Atopic dermatitis

Recombinant IFN-γ has been administered on a double-blind placebo-controlled basis to patients with atopic dermatitis with demonstrably superior effect compared with placebo control [15]. The rationale for IFN-γ treatment is based upon the findings of high-serum IgE levels and predominant Th2 cells producing IL-4 and IL-5, coupled with low production of IFN-γ by Th1 cells in atopic subjects. Administration of IFN-γ, according to this scheme, results in isotype switching away from IgE production, because of inhibition of growth of IL-4- and IL-5-producing Th2 cells [16]. Approximately one-half of the IFN-γ treated patients, but only one-quarter of the placebo-treated patients, experienced significant clinical improvement [15]. There was no reduction in serum IgE in the IFN-γ-treated group but the blood eosinophil count fell in these patients. Side effects including leukopenia were frequent in the actively treated patients. Long-term studies have demonstrated efficacy and safety for up to 2 years if IFN-γ is delivered subcutaneously at $50\,\mu g/m^2$ three times weekly. The most commonly reported side effects are influenza-like symptoms [17,18].

REFERENCES

1 Krown SE, Real FX, Cunningham RS et al. Preliminary observations on the effect of recombinant leukocyte alpha interferon in homosexual men with Kaposi's sarcoma. N Engl J Med 1983; **308**: 1071–6.
2 Groopman JE, Gottlieb MS, Goodman J et al. Recombinant α2-interferon therapy for Kaposi's sarcoma associated with the acquired immune deficiency syndrome: clinical response and prognostic parameters. Ann Intern Med 1984; **100**: 671–6.
3 Lane HC, Feinberg J, Kovaks JA et al. Antiretroviral effects of interferon-α in AIDS-associated Kaposi's sarcoma. Lancet 1988; **ii**: 1218–22.
4 Stadler R, Bratzke B, Schaart F, Orfanos CE. Long-term combined rIFN-α-2a and zidovudine therapy for HIV-associated Kaposi's sarcoma: clinical consequences and side-effects. J Invest Dermatol 1990; **95**: 170–5S.
5 Podzamczer D, Bolao F, Clotet B et al. Low-dose interferon-α combined with zidovudine in patients with AIDS-associated Kaposi's sarcoma. J Intern Med 1993; **233**: 247–53.
6 Schaart FM, Bratzke B, Rusczak Z et al. Long-term therapy of HIV-associated Kaposi's sarcoma with recombinant interferon-α-2a. Br J Dermatol 1991; **124**: 62–8.
7 Scadden DT, Bering HA, Levine JD et al. Granulocyte–monocyte colony-stimulating factor mitigates neutropenia of combined interferon-α and zidovudine treatment of acquired immunodeficiency syndrome-associated Kaposi's sarcoma. J Clin Oncol 1991; **9**: 802–8.
8 Marchisone C, Benelli R, Albini A, Santi L, Noonan DM. Inhibition of angiogenesis by type I interferons in models of Kaposi's sarcoma. Int J Biol Markers 1999; **14**: 257–62.
9 Kirkwood JM, Strawderman MH, Ernstoff MS et al. Interferon α-2b adjuvant therapy of high-risk resected cutaneous melanoma: the Eastern Cooperative Group Trial EST 1684. J Clin Oncol 1996; **14**: 7–17.
10 Legha SS. Durable complete responses in metastatic melanoma treated with interleukin-2 in combination with interferon α and chemotherapy. J Clin Oncol 1996; **14**: 7–17.
11 Kirkwood JM, Ibrahim JG, Sondak VK et al. High- and low-dose interferon α-2b in high-risk melanoma: first analysis of intergroup trial E1690/S9111/C9190. J Clin Oncol 2000; **18**: 2444–58.
12 Mitchell MS. Immunotherapy of melanoma: epidemiology and clinical manifestations. J Investig Dermatol Symp Proc 1996; **1**: 215–8.
13 Stadler R, Otte HG, Luger T et al. Prospective randomized multicenter clinical trial on the use of interferon-2a plus acitretin versus interferon-2a plus PUVA in patients with cutaneous T-cell lymphoma stages I and II. Blood 1998; **92**: 357–81.
14 Dippel E, Schrag H, Goerdt S, Orfanos CE. Extracorporeal photopheresis and interferon-α in advanced cutaneous T-cell lymphoma. Lancet 1997; **350**: 32–3.
15 Hanifin JM, Schneider LC, Leung DYM et al. Recombinant interferon-γ therapy for atopic dermatitis. J Am Acad Dermatol 1993; **28**: 189–97.

16 Gajewski TF, Fitch FW. Antiproliferative effect of IFN-γ inhibits proliferation of Th2 but not Th1 murine helper T-lymphocyte clones. *J Immunol* 1988; **140**: 4245–52.

17 Stevens SR, Hanifin JM, Hamilton T, Tofte SJ, Cooper KD. Long-term effectiveness and safety of recombinant human interferon-γ therapy for atopic dermatitis despite unchanged serum IgE levels. *Arch Dermatol* 1998; **134**: 799–804.

18 Schneider LC, Baz Z, Zarcone C, Zurakowski D. Long-term therapy with recombinant interferon-gamma (rIFN-gamma) for atopic dermatitis. *Ann Allergy Asthma Immunol* 1998; **80**: 263–8.

Interleukins

Interleukins are an expanding group of endogenous soluble mediators in use for therapy of inflammatory dermatoses, malignancy and infection.

Melanoma

IL-2 is the most widely used of the interleukins for therapy of melanoma in a variety of regimens ranging from IL-2 monotherapy to combinations with lymphokine-activated killer cells or polychemotherapy. Following a trial that demonstrated that high-dose IL-2 could induce complete remission in 6% of patients with metastatic melanoma, this approach has been approved for the indication in the USA [1]. Combining IL-2 with chemotherapy or IFN-α does not appear to improve efficacy [2].

GM-CSF as adjuvant therapy appears to prolong overall and disease-free survival in patients with stage III or IV melanoma [3].

Psoriasis

Psoriasis is a Th1-mediated disease—with a predominance of Th1 cytokines in plaques. Systemic administration of Th2 cytokines, such as IL-4, IL-10 or IL-11, is a logical cytokine-modulating approach to restore the cytokine balance in psoriasis. Recombinant human IL-4 administered five times weekly over 6 weeks in an open study produced a highly significant reduction in psoriasis severity [4]. IL-10 inhibits antigen presentation and production of pro-inflammatory cytokines such as TNF-α. Several studies [5–7] have confirmed the effectiveness of subcutaneously administered IL-10 (8 μg/kg/day or 20 μg/kg three times weekly). An open study of recombinant IL-11 (approved for treatment of chemotherapy-induced thrombocytopenia) indicated significant reduction in psoriasis severity [8].

REFERENCES

1 Rosenberg SA, Yang JC, Topalian SL *et al.* Treatment of 283 consecutive patients with metastatic melanoma or renal cell cancer using high-dose bolus interleukin-2. *JAMA* 1994; **271**: 707–13.

2 Hauschild A, Garbe C, Stolz W *et al.* Dacarbazine and interferon α with or without interleukin-2 in metastatic melanoma: a randomized phase III multicentre trial of the Dermatologic Cooperative Oncology Group (DeCOG). *Br J Cancer* 2001; **84**: 1036–42.

3 Asadullah K, Sterry W, Trefzer U. Cytokine therapy in dermatology. *Clin Exp Dermatol* 2002; **27**: 578–84.

4 Ghoreschi K, Thomas P, Breit S *et al.* Interleukin-4 therapy of psoriasis induces Th2 responses and improves human autoimmune disease. *Nat Med* 2003; **9**: 40–6.

5 Asadullah K, Sterry W, Stephanek K *et al.* IL-10 is a key cytokine in psoriasis: proof of principle by IL-10 therapy—a new therapeutic approach. *J Clin Invest* 1998; **101**: 783–94.

6 Reich K, Bruck M, Grafe A *et al.* Treatment of psoriasis with interleukin-10. *J Invest Dermatol* 1998; **6**: 1235–6.

7 Asadullah K, Döcke WD, Ebeling M *et al.* Interleukin 10 treatment of psoriasis: clinical results of a phase 2 trial. *Arch Dermatol* 1999; **135**: 187–92.

8 Trepicchio WL, Ozawa M, Walters IB *et al.* Interleukin-11 therapy selectively downregulates type I cytokine pro-inflammatory pathways in psoriasis lesions. *J Clin Invest* 1999; **104**: 1527–37.

Cytokine blocking agents

DNA technology has allowed large-scale production of neutralizing or inhibitory antibodies to pro-inflammatory cytokines. This approach to the therapy of inflammatory disease has been pioneered in the fields of rheumatoid arthritis and Crohn's disease. In dermatology, the anticytokine agents have been most extensively trialled in psoriasis with very little controlled trial evidence from other dermatoses.

TNF-α, as a key pro-inflammatory cytokine, is perhaps the most attractive target for anticytokine approaches for the treatment of inflammatory skin disease. The two agents used currently to neutralize activity of TNF-α are infliximab and etanercept.

Infliximab is a chimeric (human–mouse) monoclonal antibody against TNF-α composed of a human constant and a murine variable region of the IgG antibody [1]. Infliximab was developed initially for treatment of rheumatoid arthritis and Crohn's disease. It is now licensed, with different regimens, for treatment of both conditions. In rheumatoid arthritis the preferred regimen is combination with methotrexate, infliximab being given as 3–5 mg/kg infusions at baseline and at weeks 2 and 6 followed by regular infusions every 8 weeks, irrespective of disease activity. For Crohn's disease, a single 5 mg/kg infusion is given and repeated at 2 and 6 weeks if fistulae are present.

Following anecdotal reports [2] of effectiveness of infliximab for concurrent psoriasis in patients receiving it for Crohn's disease, a double-blind placebo-controlled trial [3] was performed in severe plaque psoriasis. Infliximab infusions of 5 or 10 mg/kg were compared with placebo delivered as monotherapy at baseline and at weeks 2 and 6. Eighty-two per cent and 91% of patients treated with 5 and 10 mg/kg infusions, respectively, achieved a highly significant reduction in clinical severity of psoriasis. Subsequent studies have borne out this remarkable and rapid response [4]. Combination with methotrexate [5] is also effective. It is probable that if licensed for psoriasis, the preferred regimen for use will be 5 mg/kg infusions according to the above loading dose, with infusions repeated at 8-week intervals. Side effects include risk of infections, reactivation of pulmonary tuberculosis [6], infusion reactions and development of antibodies against double-stranded DNA [3].

Case reports attest to the efficacy of infliximab in Behçet's disease [7], pyoderma gangrenosum [8], graft-versus-host disease [9], subcorneal pustular dermatosis [10], toxic epidermal necrolysis [11] and hidradenitis suppurativa [12].

Etanercept is a recombinant fusion protein comprising two extracellular ligand-binding proteins of the p75 TNF receptor linked to the Fc portion of human IgG [13]. The drug is administered subcutaneously twice weekly. In the USA, etanercept is approved for the treatment of rheumatoid arthritis and psoriatic arthritis; in the UK for rheumatoid arthritis only. Most trials of etanercept have been for the treatment of psoriasis—some as a secondary end point in studies on psoriatic arthritis [14]. Etanercept significantly reduces clinical severity of psoriasis in approximately 26% of patients over the course of 12 weeks [14]. Side effects include respiratory tract infections, headaches, rhinitis and, rarely, demyelination [15]. Etanercept is also reported anecdotally to show some efficacy in the treatment of scleroderma [16] and cicatricial pemphigoid [17].

There is little doubt that cytokine blockers will become commonplace in the treatment of psoriasis and perhaps other inflammatory skin diseases. Their utility will be improved by the development of oral agents that block TNF-α indirectly by approaches that include inhibition of mitogen-activated protein (MAP) kinases.

REFERENCES

1 Knight DM, Trinh H, Le J et al. Construction and initial characterization of a mouse-humoral chimeric anti-TNF antibody. *Mol Immunol* 1993; **30**: 1443–53.
2 Oh CJ, Das KM, Gottlieb AB. Treatment with anti-tumor necrosis factor-α (TNF-α) monoclonal antibody dramatically decreases the clinical activity of psoriasis lesions. *J Am Acad Dermatol* 2000; **42**: 829–30.
3 Chaudhari U, Romano P, Mulcahy LD et al. Efficacy and safety of infliximab monotherapy for plaque-type psoriasis: a randomized trial. *Lancet* 2001; **357**: 1842–7.
4 Gottlieb AB, Chaudhari U, Mulcahy LD et al. Infliximab monotherapy provides rapid and sustained benefit for plaque-type psoriasis. *J Am Acad Dermatol* 2003; **48**: 829–35.
5 Kirby B, Marsland AM, Carmichael AJ, Griffiths CEM. Successful treatment of severe recalcitrant psoriasis with combination infliximab and methotrexate. *Clin Exp Dermatol* 2001; **26**: 27–9.
6 Keane J, Gershon S, Wise RP et al. Tuberculosis associated with infliximab, a tumor necrosis factor-α neutralizing agent. *N Engl J Med* 2001; **345**: 1098–104.
7 Goossens PH, Verbug RJ, Breedveld FC. Remission of Behçet's syndrome with tumour necrosis factor-α blocking therapy. *Ann Rheum Dis* 2001; **60**: 637.
8 Tan MH, Gordon M, Lebwohl O et al. Improvement of pyoderma gangrenosum and psoriasis associated with Crohn's disease with anti-tumor necrosis factor-α monoclonal antibody. *Arch Dermatol* 2001; **137**: 930–3.
9 Kobbe G, Scheider P, Rohr U et al. Treatment of severe steroid refractory acute graft-versus-host disease with infliximab, a chimeric human–mouse anti-TNF-α antibody. *Bone Marrow Transplant* 2001; **28**: 47–9.
10 Voitglander C, Luftl M, Schuler G, Hertl M. Infliximab: a novel, highly effective treatment of recalcitrant subcorneal pustular dermatosis (Sneddon–Wilkinson disease). *Arch Dermatol* 2001; **137**: 1571–4.
11 Fischer M, Fiedler E, Marsch WC, Wohlrab J. Antitumour necrosis factor-α antibodies (infliximab) in the treatment of a patient with toxic epidermal necrolysis. *Br J Dermatol* 2002; **146**: 707–8.
12 Martinez F, Nos P, Benlloch S, Ponce J. Hidradenitis suppurativa and Crohn's disease: response to treatment with infliximab. *Inflamm Bowel Dis* 2001; **7**: 323–6.
13 Mohler LM, Torrence DS, Smith CA et al. Soluble tumor necrosis factor (TNF) receptors are effective therapeutic agents in lethal endotoxaemia and function simultaneously as both TNF carriers and TNF antagonists. *J Immunol* 1993; **151**: 1548–61.
14 Mease PJ, Goffe BS, Metz J et al. Etanercept in the treatment of psoriatic arthritis and psoriasis: a randomized trial. *Lancet* 2000; **356**: 385–90.
15 Mohan N, Edwards ET, Cupps TR et al. Demyelination occurring during anti-tumor necrosis factor-α therapy for inflammatory arthritides. *Arthritis Rheum* 2001; **44**: 2862–9.
16 Ellman MH, MacDonald PA, Kayes FA. Etanercept as treatment for diffuse scleroderma: a pilot study [Abstract]. *Arthritis Rheum* 2000; **43** (Suppl.): S392.
17 Sacher C, Rubbert A, Konig C et al. Treatment of recalcitrant cicatricial pemphigoid with tumor necrosis factor-α antagonist etanercept. *J Am Acad Dermatol* 2002; **46**: 113–5.

Receptor targeted therapies

Monoclonal antibodies can either be humanized, consisting of a human Fc fragment and a mixed human–mouse Fab (antigen binding) portion; or chimeric, in which the Fc fragment is human and the Fab portion is murine. Fusion proteins link a human or murine Fab domain to a human molecule, usually an immunoglobulin. These biotechnological approaches have been intensively trialled for the treatment of psoriasis but to date only one compound has been approved for use in treatment of skin disease. These agents are delivered parentally by intravenous, intramuscular or subcutaneous injection; overall they are well tolerated with low immunogenicity.

Monoclonal antibodies directed at the CD4 molecule on T cells have been used for the therapy of psoriasis. The first in 1991—a murine IgG1 antibody—produced significant improvement in three patients with severe psoriasis [1]. The only formal placebo-controlled trial [2] was for the use of a humanized anti-CD4 IgG4 monoclonal antibody in severe psoriasis. Patients only responded after a second course of treatment, with a reduction of 66% in clinical severity at 3 months.

Most new biological therapies under development for treatment of psoriasis are targeted at the co-stimulatory or accessory molecule ligand pairs binding T cells to antigen-presenting cells. Alefacept, a recombinant human LFA-3–IgG1 fusion protein, blocks the binding between CD2 on T cells and LFA-3 on antigen-presenting cells thereby inhibiting T-cell activation. Furthermore, this approach selectively targets the disease-causing CD45RO+ memory-effector T cells and produces apoptosis of circulating T cells. Once weekly intravenous or intramuscular administration over a 12-week cycle produces significant clinical improvement in approximately one-third of patients, some of whom achieve prolonged remission [3]. Alefacept appears safe in the short to medium term, although there are significant decreases in circulating peripheral blood T cells [4]. In 2003, alefacept became the first biological agent to be licensed for the treatment of severe psoriasis. At the time of writing this approval is limited to the USA.

Other agents targeting co-stimulatory molecules and under development for psoriasis include efalizumab, a monoclonal antibody against CD11a (LFA-1), which blocks CD11a–ICAM-1 binding and may inhibit lymphocyte binding to endothelium via the same mechanism. Efalizumab is delivered subcutaneously once weekly and produces significant clinical improvement in approximately one-quarter of patients treated over a 12-week cycle [5]. A primatized antibody to CD80 (IDEC-114) blocks binding of CD80 to CD28; intravenous administration results in modest improvement in psoriasis [6].

Cytotoxic T-lymphocyte-associated antigen 4 (CTLA4) is expressed on T cells and binds CD80 and CD86 on antigen-presenting cells. CTLA4-Ig is a chimeric protein that binds CD80 and CD86 thereby inhibiting co-stimulation. An open study of intravenous administration demonstrated efficacy in psoriasis [7].

CD25 is the high-affinity IL-2 receptor expressed on T cells. Two monoclonal antibodies against CD25—basiliximab and daclizumab—are licensed for treatment of allograft rejection. Both agents are effective in psoriasis—daclizumab as monotherapy [8] and basiliximab in combination with ciclosporin [9,10]. It appears that the anti-CD25 approach is only effective if used in patients with rapidly progressive and/or generalized pustular psoriasis rather than in stable but extensive disease. Basiliximab has also been reported effective, in a case report, in atopic dermatitis [11] but ineffective for graft-versus-host disease [12].

REFERENCES

1 Morel P, Revillard JP, Nicolas JF et al. Anti-CD4 monoclonal antibody therapy in severe psoriasis. *J Autoimmun* 1992; **5**: 465–77.
2 Gottlieb AB, Lebwohl M, Shirin S et al. Anti-CD4 monoclonal antibody treatment of moderate to severe psoriasis vulgaris: results of a pilot, multicenter, multiple-dose, placebo-controlled study. *J Am Acad Dermatol* 2000; **43**: 595–604.
3 Ellis CN, Krueger GG. Treatment of chronic plaque psoriasis by selective targeting of memory effort T lymphocytes. *N Engl J Med* 2001; **345**: 248–55.
4 Ortonne JP, Lebwohl M, Griffiths CEM. Alefacept-induced decreases in circulating blood lymphocyte counts correlate with clinical response in patients with chronic plaque psoriasis. *Eur J Dermatol* 2003; **13**: 117–23.
5 Lebwohl M, Tyring SK, Hamilton SK et al. A novel targeted T-cell modulator, efalizumab, for plaque psoriasis. *N Engl J Med* 2003; **349**: 2004–13.
6 Gottlieb A, Abdulghani A, Totoritis M et al. Results of a single-dose, dose-escalating trial of an anti-B7.1 monoclonal antibody (IDEC-114) in patients with psoriasis. *J Invest Dermatol* 2000; **114**: 840.
7 Abrams JR, Lebwohl MG, Guzzo CA et al. CTLA4Ig-mediated blockade of T-cell co-stimulation in patients with psoriasis vulgaris. *J Clin Invest* 1999; **103**: 1243–52.
8 Krueger JG, Walters IB, Miyazawa M et al. Successful *in vivo* blockade of CD25 (high-affinity interleukin 2 receptor) on T cells by administration of humanized anti-Tac antibody to patients with psoriasis. *J Am Acad Dermatol* 2000; **43**: 448–58.
9 Owen CM, Harrison PV. Successful treatment of severe psoriasis with basiliximab, an interleukin-2 receptor monoclonal antibody. *Clin Exp Dermatol* 2000; **25**: 195–7.
10 Mrowietz U, Zhu K, Christophers E. Treatment of severe psoriasis with anti-CD25 monoclonal antibodies. *Arch Dermatol* 2000; **136**: 675–6.
11 Kägi MK, Heyer G. Efficacy of basiliximab, a chimeric anti-interleukin-2 receptor monoclonal antibody, in a patient with severe chronic atopic dermatitis. *Br J Dermatol* 2001; **145**: 350–1.
12 Willenbacher W, Basara N, Blau IW et al. Treatment of steroid refractory acute and chronic graft-versus-host disease with daclizumab. *Br J Haematol* 2001; **112**: 820–3.

Essential fatty acids

Essential fatty acids are simply defined as those that cannot be synthesized by humans. The major essential fatty acids found in humans are the ω-6 fatty acids linoleic acid and its products, γ-linolenic acid and arachidonic acid, precursors of important mediators of inflammation, the eicosanoids. Arachidonic acid is synthesized from linoleic acid in the liver. Although vertebrates cannot synthesize linoleic acid *de novo*, plants can synthesize both linoleic and γ-linolenic acids, important constituents of evening primrose oil. Skin, unlike liver, is devoid of δ-5 desaturase and cannot convert γ-linolenic acid to arachidonic acid directly. Thus, arachidonic acid found in skin is not directly dietary in origin.

Linoleic acid and γ-linoleic acid in atopic dermatitis

Current interest in essential fatty acids in atopic dermatitis originates in an observation by Hansen [1] that patients with this disorder had elevated serum levels of linoleic acid but reduced levels of its δ-6-desaturase products, γ-linoleic acid and dihomo-γ-linolenic acid. A number of reports suggested that oral replacement therapy using oil from the seed of evening primrose caused clinical improvement in the skin of patients with atopic dermatitis [2]. The evidence base from controlled trials of evening primrose oil indicated that there is no good evidence to support a useful therapeutic effect in atopic dermatitis [3].

Eicosapentaenoic acid and related fatty acids

These polyunsaturated fatty acids possess a longer chain length than linoleic acid and more double bonds, and are found in large quantities in fish oils, in which eicosapentaenoic acid (EPA) and docosahexaenoic acid predominate. Attempts have been made to modify the severity of psoriasis by long-term administration of diet supplemented by fish oil [4]. Subsequent experience [5] suggests that EPA dietary supplementation, which by itself causes only marginal improvement of psoriasis, may enhance the efficacy of co-administered conventional psoriatic therapy such as phototherapy [6]. The most frequently prescribed dietary source of fish oil is Maxepa®, a concentrated fish oil product. The daily intake is 60–75 g flavoured with fruit juice and containing 180 mg EPA and 120 mg docosahexaenoic acid per gram of oil.

REFERENCES

1 Hansen AE. Serum lipid changes and therapeutic effects of various oils in infantile eczema. *Proc Soc Exp Biol Med* 1933; **31**: 160–1.
2 Lovell CR, Burton JL, Horrobin DF. Treatment of atopic eczema with evening primrose oil. *Lancet* 1981; **i**: 278.
3 Hoare C, Li Wan Po A, Williams H. Systematic review of treatments for atopic eczema. *Health Technol Assess* 2000; **4**: 1–191.
4 Ziboh VA, Cohen KA, Ellis CN *et al.* Effects of dietary supplementation of fish oil on neutrophil and epidermal fatty acids. *Arch Dermatol* 1986; **122**: 1277–82.
5 Maurice PDL, Allen BR, Barkley ASJ *et al.* The effects of dietary supplementation with fish oil in patients with psoriasis. *Br J Dermatol* 1987; **117**: 599–606.
6 Gupta AK, Ellis CN, Tellner DC, Anderson TF, Voorhees JJ. Double-blind, placebo-controlled study to evaluate the efficacy of fish oil and low-dose UVB in the treatment of psoriasis. *Br J Dermatol* 1989; **120**: 801–7.

Retinoids

This class of compounds covers both the synthetic and the natural forms of vitamin A (the term vitamin A includes the preformed vitamin A alcohol, retinol; its aldehyde, retinal; and its acid, *trans*-retinoic acid, as well as the pro-vitamin, β-carotene). Chemical manipulation of retinol has led to numerous new compounds that are less toxic than the parent molecule.

The mode of action of the retinoids has not been completely elucidated but they have profound effects on differentiation, cell growth and immune response. They are used especially in dermatology but also have a role or a potential role in cancer prevention and perhaps cancer therapy.

Effect on differentiation

It has been known for many years that vitamin A deficiency results in epithelial squamous metaplasia and that vitamin supplements reverse this effect. Retinoids have now been shown to induce differentiation in a number of cell types (e.g. mouse teratocarcinoma and human myeloid leukaemia cells), and to cause regression of bronchial metaplasia in heavy smokers [1]. Epidermis undergoes profound changes and shows hypergranulosis and hyper-plasia with decreased numbers of tonofilaments and desmosomes and widening of intercellular spaces [2]. The effect on desmosomes appears to contribute to the kerato-lytic effect of retinoids in hyperkeratotic disorders.

Effect on carcinogenesis [2,3]

In models of carcinogenesis, induction of the enzyme ornithine decarboxylase occurs during transformation [4]. The enzyme induction is inhibited by retinoids and this inhibition has been used to test the anticarcinogenic effect of new retinoids.

Tumour growth [3]

The growth of a number of human tumour cell lines (e.g.

melanoma) seems to be inhibited by retinoids but the response may be variable. Retinoids have not yet established themselves as of major importance in cancer treatment. High concentrations of retinoids cause cytotoxicity through membrane labilization, although at lower doses membrane stabilization may occur.

Receptors

There are specific retinol and retinoic acid receptors. The activity of retinoids is mediated through these in a similar manner to steroid hormones. There are at least six retinoic acid and retinoid X receptors, all of which belong to the family of steroid–thyroid–vitamin D receptors. The receptors have a more significant effect on differentiation [5] than on the inhibition of tumour growth.

Cell surface effects

Retinoids affect transformed cell surfaces and lead to loss of anchorage-independent growth, cell adhesiveness and density-dependent growth [6]. It is not clear whether these effects are exerted directly by the retinoid involvement in glycosyl transfer reactions or through changes in gene expression.

Immunostimulation

In animal models, retinoids may act as an adjuvant and stimulate antibody formation to antigens that were previously not immunogenic [7,8]. In addition, retinoids may stimulate cell-mediated cytotoxicity.

Neutrophil migration

The migration of neutrophils is reduced by retinoids, both in experimental models of inflammation [9] and in patients with acne [10]. The mode of action is unknown.

Skin flora

Retinoids do not seem to have an appreciable direct action on the skin flora.

Ageing

The effects of retinoids on the ageing process, particularly ageing skin, are complex. The emphasis is currently on topical therapy.

Isotretinoin (13-*cis*-retinoic acid)

Oral isotretinoin has been shown to be very effective in the treatment of severe recalcitrant cystic acne unresponsive to antibacterial agents and to be superior to etretinate.

Dose ranges have varied considerably from 0.1 to 2.0 mg/kg/day, but the most widely used regimen at present is 1.0 mg/kg/day as a 16-week course. This produces prolonged remission in the majority of patients (see Chapter 43). Topical isotretinoin also appears to suppress acne [11].

In a long-term study of up to 10 years (mean 9 years), post-isotretinoin, 85% clinical improvement has resulted from a 4-month course and 69% of patients were still free of acne. Twenty-three per cent required a second course, the relapse occurring within 3 years in 96% of patients [12]. The need for a second course of isotretinoin is more likely if low-dose regimens are used (0.1 and 0.5 mg/kg). The most effective dose commensurate with side effects is 1 mg/kg/day for 4 months [13]. In addition to acne, isotretinoin has been used in the treatment of Gram-negative folliculitis, rosacea and, rather less successfully, in hidradenitis suppurativa and steatocystoma multiplex.

In acne, the major therapeutic effect seems to be a profound reduction in sebaceous gland size and activity. There are reductions in bacterial flora, but it is likely that these changes are secondary to the reduction in sebum secretion. The anti-inflammatory and desquamating effects of retinoids may also have a beneficial role.

A wide range of disorders of keratinization have been found to be responsive to isotretinoin. In Europe, this group of disorders is now usually treated with acitretin.

Etretinate

This retinoid has now been superceded by acitretin, which is the hydrolysis product and active metabolite of etretinate [14]. The major disadvantage of etretinate is its binding to body fat for up to 2 years after a course has been completed, during which it is advised that female patients should not become pregnant. Etretinate is 50 times more lipophilic than acitretin [15]. The elimination half-life of etretinate is over 100 days, whereas for acitretin it is 2 days [16,17].

Acitretin

In most respects, this drug resembles the parent compound. It is less bound to fat than etretinate, and it had been hoped that the advisable time interval in which female patients should avoid pregnancy after stopping the drug might be shortened. However, it has been shown in some patients that there is reverse metabolism to etretinate (particularly in the presence of alcohol) and therefore the same restriction of 2 years is advised between the end of a course and pregnancy [18]. The efficacy of acitretin is very similar to etretinate and in general is used in slightly lower doses. Acitretin is effective in various forms of psoriasis, although in plaque psoriasis the results are often disappointing [19,20]. The efficacy can be improved by adding UVA, photochemotherapy (PUVA) or UVB phototherapy (see Chapter 35) [19].

Acitretin is effective in pustular psoriasis, both palmoplantar or generalized (von Zumbusch) [21,22], also in erythrodermic psoriasis.

In many skin conditions, reports have been confined to etretinate prior to the development of acitretin. Most clinicians would agree that the effects are similar with slightly lower doses of acitretin being required. The following disorders of keratinization are often responsive to retinoids: epidermolytic hyperkeratosis, keratoderma, X-linked ichthyosis, ichthyosis vulgaris, erythrokeratoderma variabilis, pityriasis rubra pilaris, discoid lupus erythematosus and lichen planus, Darier's disease, lamellar ichthyosis and non-bullous ichthyosiform erythroderma. Long-term treatment is required as worthwhile remissions following cessation of treatment have not been reported. Toxicity therefore may prove to be a problem in these patients.

A range of skin tumours may sometimes clear with retinoids. These include solar keratoses, keratoacanthoma, epidermodysplasia verruciformis, basal cell epithelioma and leukoplakia. However, these preparations may be of particular value in the prevention of tumours in those patients with high-risk disorders such as xeroderma pigmentosum, porokeratosis of Mibelli, familial self-healing squamous epithelioma of the skin and in those transplantation patients with extensive sunlight-damaged skin.

A number of side effects are common to all the retinoids. These appear to be dose-related and are largely cutaneous. They include cheilitis, conjunctivitis, dryness of mucous membranes and epistaxis, desquamation of hands and feet, pruritus, myalgia, arthralgia, lethargy and alopecia [23–25]. Intracranial hypertension may occur and is a reason not to combine isotretinoin with tetracyclines. Likewise, it is better to avoid supplementary therapy with vitamin A in patients on synthetic retinoids. Retinoids also appear to increase the hepatotoxicity of methotrexate. There are reports [26] of depression and suicidal intention in patients taking isotretinoin, but a causal relationship has not been demonstrated [27,28].

Patients may develop abnormal liver enzyme levels during therapy with retinoids; not all values have returned to normal on cessation of the drug [29].

Increase in very-low-density lipoprotein (VLDL) cholesterol and reduction in high-density lipoprotein (HDL) cholesterol have been reported with retinoid therapy. Many patients receiving isotretinoin have been reported with elevated serum VLDL triglyceride in the absence of a preceding hyperlipoproteinaemia. These levels have returned to normal on cessation of treatment, but all patients should be screened for hyperlipoproteinaemia prior to treatment with any retinoid.

An ossification disorder resembling idiopathic skeletal hyperostosis has been reported in patients receiving long-term retinoids. These drugs should only be given to younger children when there are good indications [30–32].

Teratogenicity

Retinoids are known to be teratogenic. Maternal ingestion of retinoids early in pregnancy can lead to fetal abnormalities [33] and the infants seem to have a characteristic appearance [34,35].

It is important that women are not pregnant prior to starting treatment. Effective contraception is mandatory during and after a course of treatment. Isotretinoin has a short half-life and therefore contraceptive measures need to be taken for only 1 month after cessation of treatment, but etretinate has a long half-life. The manufacturers recommend that conception should not occur for 2 years after cessation of acitretin therapy. It is preferable to check blood levels at that time to confirm that no drug is detectable, even though it is recognized that only a minority of patients back-metabolize acitretin to etretinate. Males can safely father children even when they are taking the drug.

Bexarotene

Synthetic third-generation oral retinoids are under development. Bexarotene is a retinoid X receptor (RXR)-selective retinoid 'rexinoid' approved for the treatment of cutaneous T-cell lymphoma [36]. A 45% response rate for monotherapy is reported in regimens of $300 \, mg/m^2/day$; the main side effects are hypertriglyceridaemia (79%) and central hypothyroidism. Combination therapy with either PUVA, interferon-α or extracorporeal photopheresis is reported to enhance the response [37].

REFERENCES

1 Gouveia J, Mathé G, Hercent T *et al.* Degree of bronchial metaplasia in heavy smokers and its regression after treatment with a retinoid. *Lancet* 1982; **i**: 710–2.
2 Elias PM, Williams ML. Retinoids, cancer, and the skin. *Arch Dermatol* 1981; **117**: 160–80.
3 Editorial. Retinoids and control of cutaneous malignancy. *Lancet* 1988; **ii**: 545–6.
4 Boutwell RK. Retinoids and inhibition of ornithine decarboxylase activity. *J Am Acad Dermatol* 1982; **6** (Suppl.): 796–800.
5 Jetten AM, Jetten MER. Possible role of retinoic acid binding protein in retinoid stimulation of embryonal carcinoma cell differentiation. *Nature* 1979; **278**: 180–2.
6 Dron LD, Blalock JE, Gifford GE. Retinoic acid and the restoration of anchorage dependent growth to transformed mammalian cells. *Exp Cell Res* 1978; **117**: 15–22.
7 Dresser DW. Adjuvancity of vitamin A. *Nature* 1968; **217**: 527–9.
8 Sporn MB, Roberts AB, Goodman DS, eds. *The Retinoids*, Vols 1 and 2. Orlando: Academic Press, 1984.
9 Dubertret L, Lebreton C, Touraine R. Inhibition of neutrophil migration by etretinate and its main metabolite. *Br J Dermatol* 1982; **107**: 681–5.
10 Norris DA, Tonnesen MG, Lee LA *et al.* 13-*cis*-retinoic acid has major anti-inflammatory activity *in vivo* [Abstract]. *Clin Res* 1983; **31**: 593.

11 Chalker DK, Lesher JL, Graham-Smith J *et al.* Efficacy of topical istotretinoin 0.05% gel in acne vulgaris: results of a multicenter, double blind investigation. *J Am Acad Dermatol* 1987; **17**: 251–4.
12 Layton AM, Knaggs H, Taylor J *et al.* Isotretinoin for acne vulgaris: 10 years later—safe and effective treatment. *Br J Dermatol* 1993; **129**: 292–6.
13 Stainforth JM, Layton AM, Taylor JP *et al.* Isotretinoin for the treatment of acne vulgaris: which factors may predict the need for more than one course? *Br J Dermatol* 1993; **129**: 297–301.
14 Paravicini U. On the metabolism and pharmacokinetics of an oral aromatic retinoid. *Ann N Y Acad Sci* 1981; **359**: 55–67.
15 Brindley C. An overview of recent clinical pharmacokinetic studies with acitretin (Ro 10-1670 etretin). *Dermatologica* 1989; **178**: 179–87.
16 Larsen FG, Jacobsen P, Larsen CG *et al.* Pharmacokinetics of etretin and etretinate during long-term treatment of psoriasis patients. *Pharmacol Toxicol* 1988; **62**: 159–65.
17 Parvicini U, Camenzind M, Gower M *et al.* Multiple dose pharmacokinetics of Ro 10-1670, the main metabolite of etretinate (Tigason). In: Saurat JH, ed. *Retinoids: New Trends in Research and Therapy*, Basel: Karger, 1985: 289–92.
18 Weigand UW, Jenson BK. Pharmacokinetics of acitretin in humans. In: Saurat JH, ed. *Retinoids: 10 Years On*. Basel: Karger, 1991: 192–203.
19 Geiger JM, Czarnetzki BM. Acitretin (R0 10-1670, etretin): overall evaluation of clinical studies. *Dermatologica* 1988; **176**: 182–90.
20 White SI, Marks JM, Shuster S. Etretinate in pustular psoriasis of palms and soles. *Br J Dermatol* 1985; **113**: 581–5.
21 Kingston T, Matt L, Lowe N. Etretin therapy for severe psoriasis. *Arch Dermatol* 1987; **123**: 55–8.
22 Wolska H, Jablonska S, Bounameaux Y. Etretinate in severe psoriasis. *J Am Acad Dermatol* 1983; **9**: 883–9.
23 Orfanos CE, Ehlert R, Gollmick K. The retinoids: a review of their clinical pharmacology and therapeutic use. *Drugs* 1987; **34**: 459.
24 Strauss JS. Retinoids and acne. *J Am Acad Dermatol* 1982; **6**: 546.
25 Ward A, Brogden RN, Heel RC *et al.* Isotretinoin: a review of its pharmacological properties and therapeutic efficacy in acne and other skin disorders. *Drugs* 1984; **28**: 6–37.
26 Ng CH, Tam MM, Hook SJ. Acne, isotretinoin treatment and acute depression. *World J Psychiatry* 2001; **2**: 159–61.
27 Jick SS, Kremers HM, Vasilakis-Scaramozza C. Isotretinoin use and risk of depression, psychotic symptoms, suicide, and attempted suicide. *Arch Dermatol* 2000; **136**: 1231–6.
28 Enders SJ, Enders JM. Isotretinoin and psychiatric illness in adolescents and young adults. *Ann Pharmacother* 2003; **37**: 1124–7.
29 Thune P, Mark NJ. A case of centrolobular toxic necrosis of the liver due to aromatic retinoid tigason (Ro 10-935). *Dermatologica* 1980; **160**: 405–8.
30 Carey BM, Parker GJS, Cunliffe WJ *et al.* Skeletal toxicity with isotretinoin therapy; a clinico-radiological evaluation. *Br J Dermatol* 1988; **119**: 609–14.
31 Pittsley RA, Yoder FW. Retinoid hyperostosis: skeletal toxicity associated with long-term administration of 13-*cis*-retinoic acid for refractory ichthyosis. *N Engl J Med* 1983; **308**: 1012–4.
32 Wilson DJ, Kay V, Charig M *et al.* Skeletal hyperostosis and extraosseous calcification in patients receiving long-term etretinate (Tigason). *Br J Dermatol* 1988; **119**: 597–607.
33 Rosa FW. Teratogenicity of isotretinoin. *Lancet* 1983; **ii**: 513.
34 Benke EP. The isotretinoin teratogen syndrome. *JAMA* 1984; **251**: 3267–9.
35 de la Cruz E, Sun S, Van Guanichyakorn K *et al.* Multiple congenital malformations associated with maternal isotretinoin therapy. *Pediatrics* 1984; **74**: 428–30.
36 Duvic M, Hymes K, Heald P *et al.* Bexarotene is effective and safe for treatment of refractory, advanced-stage cutaneous T-cell lymphoma: multinational phase II–III trial results. *J Clin Oncol* 2001; **19**: 2456–71.
37 Talpur R, Ward S, Apisarnthanarax N, Breuer-Mcham J, Duvic M. Optimizing bexarotene therapy for cutaneous T-cell lymphoma. *J Am Acad Dermatol* 2002; **47**: 672–88.

Immunosuppressive and cytotoxic drugs

These drugs, which have been primarily developed for use in oncology, must be approached with great caution when they become part of a dermatologist's armamentarium; it is essential that the treatment is not more disabling than the disease. An understanding of the clinical pharmacology of these drugs and their possible side effects is required for the proper management of patients [1]. Brief details are given below of those drugs that may be of value in dermatological practice. A more complete review can be found in Friedmann [2].

Alkylating agents

The effect of these drugs is dependent on proliferation and is expressed only when cells enter the S phase. Alkylation of DNA by these drugs leads to impaired replication.

Cyclophosphamide [3]

Dose: 1–3 mg/kg body weight daily in two or three divided doses. Cyclophosphamide is inactive *in vitro* but is metabolized to an active antimitotic agent that also has profound immunosuppressive activity. It has been successfully used together with corticosteroids in the treatment of pemphigus and pemphigoid, Wegener's granulomatosis, systemic lupus erythematosus, polymyositis, mycosis fungoides and histiocytosis X.

Chlorambucil

Dose: 0.1–0.2 mg/kg/day in one or two doses. Chlorambucil is slow acting and rather less toxic than cyclophosphamide. It has been successfully used in the treatment of mycosis fungoides, Behçet's disease, lupus erythematosus, Wegener's granulomatosis, steroid-resistant sarcoidosis and in combination with prednisone for Sézary syndrome. Benefit has been reported in lichen myxoedematosus [4], granuloma annulare [5] and as a steroid-sparing agent for patients with recalcitrant dermatomyositis [6].

Dacarbazine

Dose: 2–4.5 mg/kg/day intravenously for 10 days. This is an imidazole derivative whose mode of action is unknown. It is used particularly for the treatment of metastatic malignant melanoma (see Chapter 38).

REFERENCES

1 Calabresi P, Parks RE Jr. Antiproliferate agents and drugs used for immunosuppression. In: Gilman AG, Goodman LS, Rall TW *et al.*, eds. *Goodman and Gilman's The Pharmacological Basis of Therapeutics*, 7th edn. New York: Macmillan, 1985: 1247–306.
2 Friedmann PS. Cutaneous immunotherapy. *Clin Exp Dermatol* 2002; **27**: 545–613.
3 Razzaque Ahmed A, Honibal SM. Cyclophosphamide (cytoxan): a review on relevant pharmacology and clinical uses. *J Am Acad Dermatol* 1984; **11**: 1115–26.
4 Wieder JM, Barton KL, Baron JM *et al.* Lichen myxedematosus treated with chlorambucil. *J Dermatol Surg Oncol* 1993; **19**: 475–6.
5 Winkelmann RK, Stevens JC. Successful treatment response of granuloma annulare and carpal tunnel syndrome to chlorambucil. *Mayo Clin Proc* 1994; **69**: 1163–5.
6 Sinoway PA, Callen JP. Chlorambucil: an effective corticosteroid-sparing agent for patients with recalcitrant dermatomyositis. *Arthritis Rheum* 1993; **36**: 319–24.

Antimetabolites

Methotrexate

Methotrexate has been used for the treatment of severe psoriasis and psoriatic arthritis since the 1950s [1–6]. It is a structural analogue of folic acid and is a potent competitive inhibitor of dihydrofolate reductase, which converts dietary folic acid via dihydrofolate to tetrahydrofolate. These steps are essential in the generation of 1-carbon fragments needed for the synthesis of nucleic acids. Methotrexate is converted to methotrexate polyglutamates, which have prolonged intracellular storage. They block not only dihydrofolate reductase but also other essential enzymes involved in nucleotide synthesis including thymidylate synthase and AICAR (5-aminoimidazole-4-carboxamide ribonucleotide) transformylase [7,8]. The latter is involved in purine biosynthesis and indirectly inhibits the metabolism of intracellular adenosine, which is known to be toxic to T lymphocytes and is potently anti-inflammatory. Indirect evidence of adenosine accumulation has been shown in psoriasis patients, whose adenosine excretion was found to be double that of controls following each methotrexate dose; greater increases were seen in those showing clinical improvement than in those without [9]. Although originally hypothesized that the effects of methotrexate in psoriasis were brought about by a direct interference in epidermal cell division [10,11], it is now recognized that it significantly inhibits proliferating lymphoid cells but has little effect on epidermal cells at therapeutic doses [12]. Inhibition of epidermal proliferation, on the other hand, is probably relevant in the context of acute methotrexate toxicity.

REFERENCES

1 Zachariae H. Methotrexate. In: van de Kerkhof PCM, ed. *Textbook of Psoriasis*. Oxford: Blackwell Science, 1999: 196–232.
2 Gubner R, August S, Ginsberg V. Therapeutic suppression of tissue reactivity: effect of aminopterin in rheumatoid arthritis and psoriasis. *Am J Med Sci* 1951; **221**: 176–82.
3 Gubner R. Effect of 'aminopterin' on epithelial tissues. *Arch Dermatol* 1983; **119**: 513–24.
4 Weinstein GD. Commentary: three decades of folic acid antagonists in dermatology. *Arch Dermatol* 1983; **119**: 525–7.
5 Jones G, Crotty M, Brooks P. Interventions for treating psoriatic arthritis (Cochrane Review). In: The Cochrane Library, Issue 1, 2003. Oxford: Update Software, 2003.
6 Roenigk HH, Maibach HI. Methotrexate. In: Roenigk HH, Maibach HI, eds. *Psoriasis*, 3rd edn. New York: Marcel Dekker, 1998: 609–29.
7 Baggott JE, Morgan SL, Ha TS *et al.* Antifolates in rheumatoid arthritis: a hypothetical mechanism of action. *Clin Exp Rheumatol* 1993; **11** (Suppl. 8): S101–5.
8 Cronstein BN. The mechanism of action of methotrexate. *Rheum Dis Clin North Am* 1997; **23**: 739–55.

9 Baggott JE, Morgan SL, Sams WM, Linden J. Urinary adenosine and aminoimidazolecarboxamide excretion in methotrexate-treated patients with psoriasis. *Arch Dermatol* 1999; **135**: 813–7.

10 Bleyer WA. The clinical pharmacology of methotrexate: new applications of an old drug. *Cancer* 1978; **41**: 36–51.

11 Olsen EA. The pharmacology of methotrexate. *J Am Acad Dermatol* 1991; **25**: 306–18.

12 Jeffes EW III, McCullough JL, Pittelkow MR *et al.* Methotrexate therapy of psoriasis: differential sensitivity of proliferating lymphoid and epithelial cells to the cytotoxic and growth-inhibitory effects of methotrexate. *J Invest Dermatol* 1995; **104**: 183–8.

Therapeutic indications and efficacy

Psoriasis and psoriatic arthritis. Methotrexate is of particular value in the management of acute generalized pustular psoriasis and psoriatic erythroderma [1–3], but has been most widely employed for inducing and then maintaining control of psoriasis in patients with extensive chronic plaque disease, especially in those who also have psoriatic arthritis [4]. Published studies suggest that methotrexate can produce a reduction in disease severity of at least 50% in more than three-quarters of patients treated [5–10]. Its efficacy in a controlled trial was slightly less than that of ciclosporin [11].

Cutaneous sarcoidosis. Small open studies have demonstrated improvement in skin lesions of various morphologies [12,13]. However, methotrexate was less effective in pulmonary sarcoidosis where improvement in lung function was seen in only one-third of patients [13], and it is important to be aware that improvement in skin lesions is often slow. The side effect profile appears to be similar to that seen in psoriasis patients, although the significance of liver biopsy abnormalities may be more difficult to assess because many patients with sarcoidosis will show granulomatous infiltration in the liver [13].

Dermatomyositis. Methotrexate is increasingly advocated for cutaneous lesions. Eight of 13 patients given weekly low-dose oral methotrexate (2.5–30 mg) for skin disease inadequately controlled either by topical and systemic corticosteroids or by antimalarials, were considered to have had a good or excellent response and in all 13 it was possible to reduce or discontinue corticosteroid therapy [14]. Early introduction of methotrexate in children with juvenile dermatomyositis has been claimed to hasten recovery and allow a more rapid reduction in corticosteroid dosage [15,16].

Cutaneous lupus erythematosus (LE). Small studies suggest benefit from methotrexate for cutaneous lesions of LE [17–20]. In a larger prospective randomized controlled trial of patients with mild systemic LE only three of 18 patients receiving low-dose methotrexate (15–20 mg/ week) had residual cutaneous disease after 6 months of therapy compared to 16 of 19 patients given placebo [21]. Although there is less evidence in chronic discoid LE [22], there is thus reasonable evidence to suggest that methotrexate may enable corticosteroid dosage to be reduced in patients with systemic lupus and that it is worth considering for patients with cutaneous LE unresponsive to more standard therapies.

Systemic sclerosis and morphoea. In one randomized double-blind study of 29 patients with active systemic sclerosis allocated to weekly injections of either methotrexate 15 mg or placebo for 24 weeks, a predefined favourable response was seen in a significantly greater proportion of patients in the methotrexate group (8 of 17; 47%) than in the placebo group (1 of 12; 8%) [23]. However, a larger double-blind controlled trial of 71 patients with early diffuse systemic sclerosis randomized to the same interventions failed to demonstrate significant benefit after 12 months' treatment [24], although even this study was insufficiently powered. However, both studies showed improvement in skin scores. In a small open study, nine of 10 children with active localized morphoea responded to a combination of pulsed intravenous methylprednisolone and weekly low-dose methotrexate within a median of 3 months [25]. Methotrexate has been advocated for arresting progression of linear morphoea en coup de sabre and facial hemiatrophy in children [26]. A small uncontrolled study of methotrexate 15 mg/week for 24 weeks claimed some benefit in nine patients with widespread morphoea but these claims must be treated with caution in a disease where spontaneous improvement is not uncommon [27].

Atopic dermatitis. There are no good case series let alone randomized controlled trials of the use of methotrexate for atopic dermatitis. Recently, however, it has been claimed that, whereas the weekly regimen used in psoriasis appears not be effective, methotrexate taken as 2.5 mg on four consecutive days each week can help to control selected patients with widespread moderately severe atopic dermatitis [28]. However, there must be concerns that long-term use of such a regimen may increase the risks of liver toxicity and further data are required before this approach can be generally recommended.

Other dermatoses. Benefit from weekly low-dose methotrexate has been claimed in individual case reports or small series for polyarteritis nodosa [29], Behçet's disease [30], cutaneous small vessel vasculitis [31], antiphospholipid syndrome [32], pyoderma gangrenosum [33], pityriasis lichenoides [34–36], bullous pemphigoid [37], pemphigus [38], multicentric reticulohistiocytosis [39], scleromyxoedema [40] and Langerhans' cell histiocytosis [41].

REFERENCES

1 Ryan TJ, Baker H. Systemic corticosteroids and folic acid antagonists in the treatment of generalized pustular psoriasis: evaluation and prognosis based on the study of 104 cases. *Br J Dermatol* 1969; **81**: 134–45.

2 Ozawa A, Ohkido M, Haruki Y *et al.* Treatments of generalized pustular psoriasis: a multicenter study in Japan. *J Dermatol* 1999; **26**: 141–9.

3 Collins P, Rogers S. The efficacy of methotrexate in psoriasis: a review of 40 cases. *Clin Exp Dermatol* 1992; **17**: 257–60.

4 Jones G, Crotty M, Brooks P. Interventions for treating psoriatic arthritis (Cochrane Review). In: The Cochrane Library, Issue 1, 2003. Oxford: Update Software, 2003.

5 Griffiths CEM, Clark CM, Chalmers RJ, Li Wan Po A, Williams HC. A systematic review of treatments for severe psoriasis. *Health Technol Assess* 2000; **4**: 1–125.

6 Weinstein GD, Frost P. Methotrexate for psoriasis: a new therapeutic schedule. *Arch Dermatol* 1971; **103**: 33–8.

7 Van Scott E, Auerbach R, Weinstein GD. Parenteral methotrexate in psoriasis. *Arch Dermatol* 1964; **89**: 550–6.

8 Nyfors A, Brodthagen H. Methotrexate for psoriasis in weekly oral doses without any adjunctive therapy. *Dermatologica* 1970; **140**: 345–55.

9 Jeffes E, Weinstein GD. Methotrexate and other chemotherapeutic agents used to treat psoriasis. *Dermatol Clin* 1995; **13**: 875–90.

10 Nyfors A. Benefits and adverse drug experiences during long-term methotrexate treatment of 248 psoriatics. *Dan Med Bull* 1978; **25**: 208–11.

11 Heydendael VMR, Spuls PI, Opmeer BC *et al.* Methotrexate versus cyclosporine in moderate-to-severe chronic plaque psoriasis. *N Engl J Med* 2003; **349**: 658–65.

12 Veien NK, Brodthagen H. Cutaneous sarcoidosis treated with methotrexate. *Br J Dermatol* 1977; **97**: 213–6.

13 Lower EE, Baughman RP. Prolonged use of methotrexate for sarcoidosis. *Arch Intern Med* 1995; **155**: 846–51.

14 Kasteler JS, Callen JP. Low-dose methotrexate administered weekly is an effective corticosteroid-sparing agent for the treatment of the cutaneous manifestations of dermatomyositis. *J Am Acad Dermatol* 1997; **36**: 67–71.

15 Fischer TJ, Rachelefsky GS, Klein RB, Paulus HE, Stiehm ER. Childhood dermatomyositis and polymyositis: treatment with methotrexate and prednisone. *Am J Dis Child* 1979; **133**: 386–9.

16 Reed AM, Lopez M. Juvenile dermatomyositis: recognition and treatment. *Paediatr Drugs* 2002; **4**: 315–21.

17 Miescher PA, Reithmuller D. Diagnosis and treatment of systemic lupus erythematosus. *Semin Hematol* 1965; **2**: 1–28.

18 Rothenberg RJ, Graziano FM, Grandone JT *et al.* The use of methotrexate in steroid-resistant systemic lupus erythematosus. *Arthritis Rheum* 1988; **31**: 612–5.

19 Bottomley WW, Goodfield M. Methotrexate for the treatment of severe mucocutaneous lupus erythematosus. *Br J Dermatol* 1995; **133**: 311–4.

20 Boehm IB, Boehm GA, Bauer R. Management of cutaneous lupus erythematosus with low-dose methotrexate: indication for modulation of inflammatory mechanisms. *Rheumatol Int* 1998; **18**: 59–62.

21 Carneiro J, Sato E. Double blind, randomized, placebo controlled clinical trial of methotrexate in systemic lupus erythematosus. *J Rheumatol* 1999; **26**: 1275–9.

22 Bottomley WW, Goodfield M. Methotrexate for the treatment of discoid lupus erythematosus. *Br J Dermatol* 1995; **133**: 655–6.

23 van den Hoogen FH, Boerbooms AM, Swaak AJ *et al.* Comparison of methotrexate with placebo in the treatment of systemic sclerosis: a 24-week randomized double-blind trial, followed by a 24-week observational trial. *Br J Rheumatol* 1996; **35**: 364–72.

24 Pope JE, Bellamy N, Seibold JR *et al.* A randomized, controlled trial of methotrexate versus placebo in early diffuse scleroderma. *Arthritis Rheum* 2001; **44**: 1351–8.

25 Uziel Y, Feldman BM, Krafchik BR, Yeung RS, Laxer RM. Methotrexate and corticosteroid therapy for pediatric localized scleroderma. *J Pediatr* 2000; **136**: 91–5.

26 Atherton D. Systemic immunosuppressant therapy in childhood. *Clin Exp Dermatol* 2002; **27**: 328–37.

27 Seyger MM, van den Hoogen FH, de Boo T, de Jong EM. Low-dose methotrexate in the treatment of widespread morphoea. *J Am Acad Dermatol* 1998; **39**: 220–5.

28 Sidbury R, Hanifin JM. Systemic therapy of atopic dermatitis. *Clin Exp Dermatol* 2000; **25**: 559–66.

29 Brody M, Bohm I, Biwer E, Bauer R. Erfolgreiche Behandlung einer Panarteritis nodosa mit Methotrexat Low-dose-therapie. *Hautarzt* 1994; **45**: 476–9.

30 Jorizzo JL, White WL, Wise CM, Zanolli MD, Sherertz EF. Low-dose weekly methotrexate for unusual neutrophilic vascular reactions: cutaneous polyarteritis nodosa and Behçet's disease. *J Am Acad Dermatol* 1991; **24**: 973–8.

31 Lotti T, Ghersetich I, Comacchi C, Jorizzo JL. Cutaneous small-vessel vasculitis. *J Am Acad Dermatol* 1998; **39**: 667–87.

32 Bauer R, Brody M, Boehm I. Methotrexat-low-dose-Therapie zur Behandlung inflammatorischer and autoaggressiver Dermatosen. In: Tebbe B, Goerdt S, Orfanos CE, eds. Dermatologie—Heutiger Stand: Ergebnisse and Berichte der 38. Tagung der Deutschen Dermatologischen Gesellschaft in Berlin vom 29, April bis 3, Mai 1995. Stuttgart: Thieme, 1995: 318–20.

33 Teitel AD. Treatment of pyoderma gangrenosum with methotrexate. *Cutis* 1996; **57**: 326–8.

34 Lynch PJ, Saied NK. Methotrexate treatment of pityriasis lichenoides and lymphomatoid papulosis. *Cutis* 1979; **23**: 634–6.

35 Fink-Puches R, Soyer HP, Kerl H. Febrile ulceronecrotic pityriasis lichenoides et varioliformis acuta. *J Am Acad Dermatol* 1994; **30**: 261–3.

36 Suarez J, Lopez B, Villalba R, Perera A. Febrile ulceronecrotic Mucha–Habermann disease: a case report and review of the literature. *Dermatology* 1996; **192**: 277–9.

37 Paul MA, Jorizzo JL, Fleischer AB Jr, White WL. Low-dose methotrexate treatment in elderly patients with bullous pemphigoid. *J Am Acad Dermatol* 1994; **31**: 620–5.

38 Schaumburg-Lever G. Die Therapie des Pemphigus und Pemphigoid. *Z Hautkr* 1986; **61**: 811–2.

39 Franck N, Amor B, Ayral X *et al.* Multicentric reticulohistiocytosis and methotrexate. *J Am Acad Dermatol* 1995; **33**: 524–5.

40 McAdam LP, Pearson CM, Pitts WH, Sadoff L, Verity MA. Papular mucinosis with myopathy, arthritis, and eosinophilia: a histopathologic study. *Arthritis Rheum* 1977; **20**: 989–96.

41 Steen AE, Steen KH, Bauer R, Bieber T. Successful treatment of cutaneous Langerhans' cell histiocytosis with low-dose methotrexate. *Br J Dermatol* 2001; **145**: 137–40.

Safety precautions and side effects

Haematological or renal abnormality. Myelosuppression is the most important cause of methotrexate-associated death. Methotrexate should be avoided in patients with significant haematological abnormalities or renal impairment. Because methotrexate is eliminated largely via the kidneys, toxic levels may build up rapidly in patients with renal impairment, and even low doses of the drug may then produce acute myelosuppression [1]. This is particularly liable to occur in the elderly when concomitant drug administration or illness such as fever or diarrhoea may result in sudden deterioration of renal function; elderly patients especially should be warned to omit methotrexate doses whenever they are at risk of acute dehydration.

Drug interactions. Certain drugs may increase toxicity of methotrexate by increased antifolate effect (e.g. sulphonamides, trimethoprim, phenytoin) or by decreasing renal elimination (e.g. aspirin and NSAIDs, probenecid, ciclosporin) [2]. As life-threatening myelosuppression may result from interactions between methotrexate and such drugs, patients and all their medical attendants should be made aware of these risks.

Liver disease, alcohol and diabetes. Methotrexate should not be administered to patients with significant current or previous liver disease, especially if caused by viral hepatitis or to alcohol. Any patient suspected of alcohol abuse is unsuitable for methotrexate, although many dermatologists allow patients receiving methotrexate to continue taking small amounts of alcohol (e.g. 4–6 units of alcohol weekly). Obese diabetic patients are also at increased risk of liver damage from methotrexate [3].

Fertility. Because methotrexate is both arbortifacient and teratogenic [4–7], it is strictly contraindicated in pregnancy. Adequate contraceptive measures must be taken by women of child-bearing potential during methotrexate therapy and for at least one menstrual cycle after stopping the drug [8]. It should also be avoided during lactation. Although low-dose methotrexate has not been found to be mutagenic in sperm [9] and normal children have been born where the father was taking methotrexate at the time of conception [10], the drug may depress spermatogenesis [11]. It is customary to advise men to avoid fathering children during therapy and for at least 3 months thereafter [8].

Miscellaneous precautions. Other important contraindications to the use of low-dose methotrexate include active peptic ulceration, hepatitis virus infection, active infectious disease such as tuberculosis, immunodeficiency states and unreliability of the patient.

Management of the patient

The risks and benefits of therapy should be clearly explained to the patient both verbally and in writing. Adequate contraceptive measures must be commenced where appropriate and baseline blood tests obtained.

Methotrexate is usually given orally and is given as a single weekly dose as it is well-established that the toxicity for a given total dose is considerably increased when it is administered daily [12]. Unambiguous instructions including which day of the week the tablets are to be taken should be given to the patient and specified on the prescription. Deaths have occurred where prescribers, dispensers or patients have confused 10 mg for 2.5-mg tablets. It is thus good practice always to specify 2.5-mg tablets for inflammatory diseases. The rationale proposed for giving methotrexate in three divided doses once weekly [13] is now thought unlikely to be valid [14] and may have higher risk of hepatic fibrosis [15].

Most serious problems and the rare deaths associated with low-dose methotrexate arise because of an absolute or relative overdosage. A small test dose, usually 5 mg, should be given in order to detect those patients who may be unduly sensitive to the drug [16]. If the full blood count is stable at 7 days then subsequent doses may be gradually increased (usually in 2.5–5 mg steps) according to clinical response and any accompanying toxicity. The aim of therapy should not be to induce complete clearance of psoriasis but to achieve sufficient control that it may readily be managed with topical therapy. Most patients are adequately controlled on doses of 7.5–15 mg weekly and few patients require more than 20 mg. Even lower doses may suffice, particularly in the elderly.

Folic acid supplementation. There is little evidence that folate supplementation diminishes methotrexate efficacy

[17,18], although methotrexate toxicity is enhanced by folate depletion. Recent studies in both rheumatoid arthritis and psoriasis patients have shown that low-dose methotrexate increases circulating concentrations of homocysteine and that this rise can be reversed by folic acid administration [19,20]; elevated homocysteine levels are associated with increased risk of cardiovascular disease. Given the fact that folic acid also has protective effects on the bone marrow, it seems appropriate to recommend that all patients treated with methotrexate should receive supplemental folic acid. There is as yet insufficient information to determine the most appropriate dosage but 1–5 mg/day appears to be adequate to correct these problems without affecting clinical response to therapy [17,18].

Monitoring schedule. Initially, patients should be assessed weekly by clinical examination and laboratory measurement of full blood count, plasma urea, electrolytes and creatinine, and liver enzyme tests. Once therapy has been stabilized, assessments should be performed every 2–3 months. Results should be carefully monitored; recording of results such as haemoglobin or platelets in a table or graph makes it easier to detect abnormal trends. In any individual, the dosage of methotrexate required to maintain adequate control of psoriasis will vary from time to time and should be adjusted accordingly.

As alcohol abuse greatly increases the risks of liver damage in patients receiving methotrexate, they should be reminded regularly of the need to restrict alcohol intake. Liver damage cannot be reliably detected by standard liver enzyme tests or imaging techniques and regular liver biopsy for all patients receiving low-dose methotrexate for psoriasis is still advocated by several authorities [8,21]. However, several studies suggest that the risk of serious liver damage in carefully monitored patients receiving once weekly low-dose methotrexate is small [22–24] and that the cost and morbidity of repeated biopsy may be difficult to justify when compared with the low yield of significant liver pathology. If there are concerns about pre-existing liver damage then it may be appropriate to obtain a liver biopsy as a baseline soon after successful methotrexate therapy has been established.

It can reasonably be argued that liver biopsy need no longer be performed routinely in all patients receiving long-term methotrexate but, to provide greater reassurance that significant damage is not overlooked, several investigators have recommended the use of a serological marker of fibrosis, the aminoterminal peptide of type III procollagen (PIIINP). They have concluded that patients whose PIIINP levels are consistently normal are very unlikely to have significant liver damage [25–27]. If PIIINP assay is available it should be performed 3 monthly and liver biopsy may be restricted to the small minority in whom PIIINP levels are repeatedly elevated.

Management of problems

Inadequate response. A small minority of patients are unable to absorb methotrexate adequately but may respond satisfactorily if it is given intramuscularly or intravenously. Patients with psoriasis who relapse while receiving methotrexate may frequently be brought satisfactorily under control by a course of intensive topical therapy and/or UVB phototherapy [28]; in contrast to the combination of methotrexate and PUVA, which should be avoided, a major increased risk of skin cancer from combining UVB with methotrexate has not been demonstrated [29]. Combination of methotrexate with other systemic agents is discussed further in Chapter 35.

Nausea. This occurs in 25%, usually appears within 12 h of methotrexate ingestion, and may last up to 3 days. It is usually mild but may limit therapy [30]. Folic acid 5 mg/day has been found to be more helpful than antiemetics, taking methotrexate with the evening meal or dividing the dose, although any of these manoeuvres may help some patients. Ondansetron 8 mg orally 2 h before and, if necessary, 12 and 24 h after the weekly methotrexate dose, can be dramatically effective [31].

Liver inflammation and fibrosis. An acute rise in liver enzymes to greater than three times the upper limit of normal is usually an indication to discontinue methotrexate. If PIIINP levels are repeatedly abnormal over a 12-month period then liver biopsy should be considered. The decision to discontinue methotrexate depends not only on the results of liver biopsy but also on the ease with which an individual patient's psoriasis may be managed by other means. In general, severe fibrosis and cirrhosis are considered contraindications to further methotrexate therapy. Nevertheless, some dermatologists have continued treatment in patients with documented cirrhosis without encountering significant deterioration of liver disease [32]. In patients with hepatic inflammation or mild to moderate fibrosis without cirrhosis, continuation of methotrexate therapy is probably still safe so long as alcohol is strictly avoided and patients are closely monitored. If PIIINP remains elevated then a further liver biopsy should be considered after 12 months to 2 years of continued therapy.

Respiratory disease. Methotrexate-induced pneumonitis is rare in psoriasis. It is characterized by acute onset with fever, cough and dyspnoea. Chest X-ray shows pulmonary infiltration. It resolves rapidly with withdrawal of methotrexate and systemic corticosteroids [29]. Pulmonary fibrosis is a rare complication.

Haematological abnormalities. A rise in mean corpuscular volume (MCV) is common in patients receiving long-term methotrexate and usually indicates relative folate deficiency although it is important to exclude other causes of macrocytosis. If MCV rises above 106 fl despite folate replacement then further methotrexate therapy is probably contraindicated [33]. Falls in haemoglobin, white cell or platelet counts should prompt a reduction in dose or, if severe, withdrawal of methotrexate.

Acute toxicity and overdosage. Absolute or relative overdosage of methotrexate can result in acute toxicity, manifested clinically by myelosuppression, mucosal ulceration and, rarely, cutaneous necrolysis. Early treatment may be life-saving. The metabolic effects of methotrexate can be bypassed by administration of folinic acid. As soon as overdose is suspected, serum should be collected for measurement of methotrexate levels and folinic acid should be administered intravenously. The dose of folinic acid should be at least as high as the total dose of methotrexate thought to be responsible for the overdose and should in any event not be less than 20 mg. Subsequent doses (which may be taken orally if no more than 20 mg) should be given at 6-hourly intervals until the serum methotrexate is less than 0.01 μmol/L. The dose of folinic acid required will vary according to the serum methotrexate concentration. A dose of 20 mg suffices where the methotrexate concentration is 0.5 μmol/L or less, but at higher concentrations the dose can be calculated at 100 mg for every 1 μmol/L of measured serum methotrexate concentration [34].

REFERENCES

1 Shupack JL, Webster GF. Pancytopenia following low-dose oral methotrexate therapy for psoriasis. *JAMA* 1988; **259**: 3594–6.
2 Evans WE, Christensen ML. Drug interactions with methotrexate. *J Rheumatol* 1985; **12**: 15–20.
3 West SG. Methotrexate hepatotoxicity. *Rheum Dis Clin North Am* 1997; **23**: 883–915.
4 Kozlowski RD, Steinbrunner JV, MacKenzie AH *et al.* Outcome of first-trimester exposure to low-dose methotrexate in eight patients with rheumatic disease. *Am J Med* 1990; **88**: 589–92.
5 Milunsky A, Graef JW, Gaynor MF. Methotrexate-induced congenital malformations. *J Pediatr* 1968; **72**: 790–5.
6 Nguyen C, Duhl AJ, Escallon CS, Blakemore KJ. Multiple anomalies in a fetus exposed to low-dose methotrexate in the first trimester. *Obstet Gynecol* 2002; **99**: 599–602.
7 Powell HR, Ekert H. Methotrexate-induced congenital malformations. *Med J Aust* 1971; **2**: 1076–7.
8 Roenigk HH Jr, Auerbach R, Maibach H, Weinstein G, Lebwohl M. Methotrexate in psoriasis: consensus conference. *J Am Acad Dermatol* 1998; **38**: 478–85.
9 Estop AM. Sperm chromosome studies in patients taking low-dose methotrexate. *Am J Hum Genet* 1992; **51** (Suppl. 4): A314.
10 Perry WH. Methotrexate and teratogenesis. *Arch Dermatol* 1983; **119**: 874.
11 Sussman A, Leonard JM. Psoriasis, methotrexate, and oligospermia. *Arch Dermatol* 1980; **116**: 215–7.
12 Dahl MG, Gregory MM, Scheuer PJ. Methotrexate hepatotoxicity in psoriasis: comparison of different dose regimens. *BMJ* 1972; **1**: 654–6.
13 Weinstein GD, Frost P. Methotrexate for psoriasis: a new therapeutic schedule. *Arch Dermatol* 1971; **103**: 33–8.
14 Zanolli MD, Sherertz EF, Hedberg AE. Methotrexate: anti-inflammatory or antiproliferative? *J Am Acad Dermatol* 1990; **22**: 523–4.
15 Roenigk HH, Auerbach R, Bergfeld WF *et al.* A cooperative prospective study of the effects of psoriasis on liver biopsies. In: Farber EM, Cox AJ, eds.

Psoriasis: Proceedings of the Second International Symposium. New York: Yorke Medical, 1977: 243–8.

16 Jih DM, Werth VP. Thrombocytopenia after a single test dose of methotrexate. *J Am Acad Dermatol* 1998; **39**: 349–51.

17 Kirby B, Lyon CC, Griffiths CE, Chalmers RJ. The use of folic acid supplementation in psoriasis patients receiving methotrexate: a survey in the United Kingdom. *Clin Exp Dermatol* 2000; **25**: 265–8.

18 Ortiz Z, Shea B, Suarez Almazor M *et al.* Folic acid and folinic acid for reducing side-effects in patients receiving methotrexate for rheumatoid arthritis (Cochrane Review). In: The Cochrane Library, Issue 1, 2003. Oxford: Update Software, 2003.

19 van Ede AE, Laan RFJM, Blom HJ *et al.* Homocysteine and folate status in methotrexate-treated patients with rheumatoid arthritis. *Rheumatology* 2002; **41**: 658–65.

20 Hanrahan E, Barnes L. Elevated serum homocysteine levels in patients with psoriasis receiving long-term, low-dose methotrexate therapy. *Br J Dermatol* 2001; **145** (Suppl. 59): 43.

21 Kuijpers AL, van de Kerkhof PC. Risk–benefit assessment of methotrexate in the treatment of severe psoriasis. *Am J Clin Dermatol* 2000; **1**: 27–39.

22 Boffa MJ, Chalmers RJ, Haboubi NY, Shomaf M, Mitchell DM. Sequential liver biopsies during long-term methotrexate treatment for psoriasis: a reappraisal. *Br J Dermatol* 1995; **133**: 774–8.

23 Lanse SB, Arnold GL, Gowans JD, Kaplan MM. Low incidence of hepatotoxicity associated with long-term, low-dose oral methotrexate in treatment of refractory psoriasis, psoriatic arthritis, and rheumatoid arthritis: an acceptable risk–benefit ratio. *Dig Dis Sci* 1985; **30**: 104–9.

24 Aithal GP, Haugk B, Gumustop B, Burt AD, Record CO. Monitoring methotrexate induced hepatic fibrosis in patients with psoriasis: are serial biopsies justified? *Hepatology* 2001; **34**: 342A.

25 Boffa MJ, Smith A, Chalmers RJ *et al.* Serum type III procollagen aminopeptide for assessing liver damage in methotrexate-treated psoriatic patients. *Br J Dermatol* 1996; **135**: 538–44.

26 Zachariae H, Heickendorff L, Sogaard H. The value of amino-terminal propeptide of type III procollagen in routine screening for methotrexate-induced liver fibrosis: a 10-year follow-up. *Br J Dermatol* 2001; **144**: 100–3.

27 Kirby B, Smith A, Burrows P *et al.* The impact of the introduction of serum aminoterminal peptide of procollagen III monitoring for hepatotoxicity in psoriasis patients receiving methotrexate. *Br J Dermatol* 2001; **145** (Suppl. 59): 26.

28 Roenigk HH, Maibach HI. Methotrexate. In: Roenigk HH, Maibach HI, eds. *Psoriasis*, 3rd edn. New York: Marcel Dekker, 1998: 609–29.

29 Zachariae H. Methotrexate. In: van de Kerkhof PCM, ed. *Textbook of Psoriasis*. Oxford: Blackwell Science, 1999: 196–232.

30 Duhra P. Treatment of gastrointestinal symptoms associated with methotrexate therapy for psoriasis. *J Am Acad Dermatol* 1993; **28**: 466–9.

31 Walker SL, Kirby B, Griffiths CEM, Harrison PV, Chalmers RJG. The use of oral ondansetron for severe methotrexate-induced nausea in psoriasis. *Br J Dermatol* 2002; **147** (Suppl. 62): 38.

32 Zachariae H, Sogaard H, Heickendorff L. Methotrexate-induced liver cirrhosis: clinical, histological and serological studies—a further 10-year follow-up. *Dermatology* 1996; **192**: 343–6.

33 Dodd HJ, Kirby JD, Munro DD. Megaloblastic anaemia in psoriatic patients treated with methotrexate. *Br J Dermatol* 1985; **112**: 630–1.

34 Chalmers RJG, Boffa MJ. Current management of psoriasis: methotrexate. *J Dermatolog Treat* 1997; **8**: 41–4.

Azathioprine

Azathioprine is one of many immunosuppressive drugs used in dermatology following original use in transplant surgery. It is converted in the body to 6-mercaptopurine (6-MP), an inhibitor of purine synthesis and an immunosuppressive agent; this in turn is metabolized to purine thioanalogues by hypoxanthine guanine phosphoribosyl transferase (HGPRT). Additionally, an imidazole metabolite appears to have powerful anti-inflammatory properties. It is now known that thiopurine methyltransferase (TPMT) is a major enzyme involved in the metabolism of azathioprine. TPMT activity is determined by an allelic polymorphism for either high or low enzymic activity. Homozygotes for the low activity allele (0.5% of the population) are known to be at high risk for myelosuppression [1,2]. It is recommended that patients starting azathioprine should have blood TPMT levels measured beforehand and the dose titrated accordingly [3].

Indications

The licensed indications for azathioprine are dermatomyositis [4], systemic lupus erythematosus (also useful in severe cutaneous disease [5]) and pemphigus vulgaris [6,7]. Other dermatological conditions in which it may be useful include bullous pemphigoid [8,9], intractable atopic dermatitis [3,10], chronic actinic dermatitis [11], Behçet's disease [12], Wegener's granulomatosis [13] and other vasculitides [5], pyoderma gangrenosum [14], psoriasis [15] and perhaps pityriasis rubra pilaris in adults [16]. It appears to be inferior to methotrexate in the treatment of psoriasis but may be useful for psoriatic arthritis.

Management of the patient

The usual azathioprine regimen is 1–3 mg/kg/day. Baseline TMPT assay is recommended, with dose adjustment if necessary. Doses at the lower end of this range are generally recommended in the elderly. Azathioprine is usually used as a steroid-sparing agent, but has been used as monotherapy (e.g. in atopic dermatitis or psoriasis). It takes a few weeks to reach a steady state; dose titration may be required. Weekly blood monitoring is required initially (probably for 4 weeks), gradually extending to every 3 months.

Contraindications include low TPMT activity, pregnancy, hypersensitivity, concurrent malignancy and concurrent allopurinol therapy (because of risk of marrow toxicity). Other drugs that may interact with azathioprine include sulfsalazine, warfarin, angiotensin-converting enzyme inhibitors and any drug that suppresses bone marrow function.

Complications of treatment

Myelosuppression is a relatively common side effect of azathioprine and can develop very quickly, certainly between regular blood monitoring, and can be severe. It is more common at the start of treatment, especially in those with TPMT deficiency, but may also occur in those with normal TPMT activity.

Hypersensitivity may be manifest by rash or hepatitis, often with eosinophilia. Pancreatitis may occur [17]. Azathioprine-induced shock in dermatology patients has only been reported rarely but can be life-threatening [18].

REFERENCES

1 Snow JL, Gibson LE. The role of genetic variation in thiopurine methyl-transferase activity and the efficacy and/or side-effects of azathioprine therapy in dermatologic patients. *Arch Dermatol* 1995; **131**: 193–7.

2 Anstey A. Azathioprine in dermatology: a review in the light of advances in the understanding of methylation pharmacokinetics. *J R Soc Med* 1995; **88**: 155–60.

3 Meggitt SJ, Reynolds NJ. Azathioprine for atopic dermatitis. *Clin Exp Dermatol* 2001; **26**: 369–75.

4 Fam AG. Recent advances in the management of adult myositis. *Expert Opin Investig Drugs* 2001; **10**: 1265–77.

5 Callen JP, Spencer LV, Burruss JB et al. Azathioprine: an effective, cortico-steroid-sparing therapy for patients with recalcitrant cutaneous lupus erythematosus or with recalcitrant cutaneous leukocytoclastic vasculitis. *Arch Dermatol* 1991; **127**: 515–22.

6 Aberer W, Wolff-Schreiner EC, Stingl G, Wolff K. Azathioprine in the treatment of pemphigus vulgaris. *J Am Acad Dermatol* 1987; **16**: 527–33.

7 Harman KE, Albert S, Black MM. Guidelines for the management of pemphigus vulgaris. *Br J Dermatol* 2003; **149**: 926–37.

8 Burton JL, Harman RMM, Peachey RDG, Warin RP. A controlled trial of azathioprine in the treatment of pemphigoid. *BMJ* 1978; **2**: 1190–1.

9 Wojnarowska F, Kirtschig G, Highet AS et al. Guidelines for the management of bullous pemphigoid. *Br J Dermatol* 2003; **147**: 214–21.

10 Berth-Jones J, Takwale A, Tan E et al. Azathioprine in severe adult atopic dermatitis: a double-blind, placebo-controlled, crossover trial. *Br J Dermatol* 2002; **147**: 324–30.

11 Murphy GM, Maurice PM, Norris PG et al. Azathioprine in the treatment of chronic actinic dermatitis: a double-blind controlled trial with monitoring of exposure to ultraviolet radiation. *Br J Dermatol* 1989; **121**: 639–46.

12 Yazici H, Pazarli H, Barnes CG et al. A controlled trial of azathioprine in Behçet's syndrome. *N Engl J Med* 1990; **322**: 281–5.

13 Wisehart JM. Wegener's granulomatosis: controlled by azathioprine and corticosteroids. *Br J Dermatol* 1975; **92**: 461–7.

14 Chow RKP, Ho VC. Treatment of pyoderma gangrenosum. *J Am Acad Dermatol* 1996; **34**: 1047–60.

15 du Vivier A, Munro DD, Verbov J. Treatment of psoriasis with azathioprine. *BMJ* 1974; **1**: 49–51.

16 Hunter GA, Forbes IJ. Treatment of pityriasis rubra pilaris with azathioprine. *Br J Dermatol* 1972; **87**: 42–5.

17 Sturdevant RAL, Singleton JW, Deren JJ et al. Azathioprine-related pancreatitis in patients with Crohn's disease. *Gastroenterology* 1979; **77**: 883–6.

18 Jones JJ, Ashworth J. Azathioprine-induced shock in dermatology patients. *J Am Acad Dermatol* 1993; **29**: 795–6.

Bleomycin

This is a polypeptide antibiotic given parenterally. It has no immunosuppressive action and its toxicity is confined to the skin (pigmentation, inflammatory lesions especially on the palms and fingers) and the lungs. It is effective against squamous cell carcinoma of the skin and elsewhere, and in inducing remission in mycosis fungoides and other lymphomas. It has been used intralesionally for the treatment of intractable virus warts [1,2] but vasospasm, sometimes severe, is a potential side effect.

Hydroxyurea

Dose: 500 mg two or three times daily. Hydroxyurea blocks pyrimidine synthesis. It causes much more short-term marrow suppression than methotrexate, necessitating frequent blood counts. However, it is less effective than methotrexate and has little effect on psoriatic arthropathy. A combination of hydroxyurea with retinoids has been reported to be particularly effective [3]. Hydroxyurea is easy to administer, relatively inexpensive and has few contraindications or side effects. Leukopenia can develop and regular blood monitoring is needed. Hydroxyurea does have a place for those patients who cannot take other drugs because of systemic disorders such as hyperlipidaemia, mild renal impairment, cardiopulmonary disease and mild liver disease [4]. It may occasionally cause a dermatomyositis-like rash or leg ulceration.

Mycophenolate mofetil

Dose: 0.5–1 g twice daily. Mycophenolate mofetil (MMF) is the ester of mycophenolic acid (MPA), but provides advantages over MPA in that it has increased bioavailability. After ingestion, MMF is hydrolysed to MPA—the active acid form. MPA inhibits the enzyme inosine monophosphate dehydrogenase (IMPDH), a key enzyme in *de novo* purine synthesis. Thus, MPA blocks the production of guanosine nucleotides needed for RNA and DNA synthesis. MPA is particularly effective in blocking the type II isoform of IMPDH expressed mainly in T and B cells, thereby inhibiting T- and B-cell activation and proliferation. Monotherapy with MMF for psoriasis is not as effective as ciclosporin [5]; indeed MMF is probably best used in psoriasis as combination therapy as a ciclosporin-sparing agent [6]. Efficacy in atopic dermatitis is uncertain, with efficacy at 1 g twice daily reported with long-term remission for up to 20 weeks [7] but other studies not being able to discern benefit [8]. MMF is understandably beneficial for therapy of autoimmune bullous diseases, particularly bullous pemphigoid and pemphigus, and may be used as a steroid-sparing agent [9,10]. Beneficial use of MMF has been reported in a variety of skin diseases including pyoderma gangrenosum [11], bowel-associated dermatitis–arthritis syndrome [12], systemic lupus erythematosus [13], chronic actinic dermatitis [14] and extensive lichen planus [15].

Adverse effects include mild to moderate leukopenia and anaemia [16], immunosuppression and gastrointestinal symptoms. There is no significant toxic effect on renal or hepatic function.

Melphalan

This is used mainly in the treatment of myelomatosis and polycythaemia. Other indications include scleromyxoedema (see Chapter 57) [17].

REFERENCES

1 Cohen IS, Mosher MB, O'Keefe EJ et al. Cutaneous toxicity of bleomycin therapy. *Arch Dermatol* 1973; **107**: 553–5.

2 James MP, Collier PM, Aherne W et al. Histologic, pharmacologic, and immunocytochemical effects of injection of bleomycin into viral warts. *J Am Acad Dermatol* 1993; **28**: 933–7.

3 Wright S, Baker H, Warin AP. Treatment of psoriasis with a combination of etretinate and hydroxyurea. *J Dermatolog Treat* 1990; **1**: 211–4.

4 Wolverton SE. Hydroxyurea therapy [Review]. *J Am Acad Dermatol* 1991; **25**: 518–24.

5 Davison SC, Morris-Jones R, Powles AV, Fry L. Change of treatment from cyclosporin to mycophenolate mofetil in severe psoriasis. *Br J Dermatol* 2000; **143**: 405–7.

6 Ameen M, Smith HR, Barker JNWN. Combined mycophenolate mofetil and cyclosporin therapy for severe recalcitrant psoriasis. *Clin Exp Dermatol* 2001; **26**: 480–3.

7 Grundmann-Kollmann M, Podda M, Ochsendorf F et al. Mycophenolate mofetil is effective in the treatment of atopic dermatitis. *Arch Dermatol* 2001; **137**: 870–3.

8 Hansen ER, Buus S, Deleuran M, Andersen KE. Treatment of atopic dermatitis with mycophenolate mofetil. *Br J Dermatol* 2000; **143**: 1324–6.

9 Bohm M, Beissert S, Schwarz T, Metze D, Luger T. Bullous pemphigoid treated with mycophenolate mofetil. *Lancet* 1997; **349**: 541.

10 Enk AH, Knop J. Mycophenolate is effective in the treatment of pemphigus vulgaris. *Arch Dermatol* 1999; **135**: 54–6.

11 Hohenleutner U, Mohr VD, Michel S, Landthaler M. Mycophenolate mofetil and cyclosporin treatment for recalcitrant pyoderma gangrenosum. *Lancet* 1997; **350**: 1748.

12 Cox NH, Palmer JG. Bowel-associated dermatitis-arthritis syndrome associated with ileo-anal pouch anastamosis, and treatment with mycophenolate mofetil. *Br J Dermatol* 2003; **149**: 1296–7.

13 Goyal S, Nousari HC. Treatment of resistant discoid lupus erythematosus of the palms and soles with mycophenolate mofetil. *J Am Acad Dermatol* 2001; **45**: 142–4.

14 Pickenacker A, Luger TA, Schwarz T. Dyshidrotic eczema treated with mycophenolate mofetil. *Arch Dermatol* 1998; **134**: 378–9.

15 Frieling U, Bonsmann G, Schwarz T, Luger TA, Beissert S. Mycophenolatmofetil-eine neue therapeutische Alternative bei therapieresisten tem Lichen planus [Abstract]. *H + G Z Haut-Krankheiten* 2001; **76**: 3.

16 Lipsky JJ. Mycophenolate mofetil. *Lancet* 1996; **348**: 1357–9.

17 Nieves DS, Bondi EE, Wallmark J, Raps EC, Seykora JT. Scleromyxoedema: successful treatment of cutaneous and neurologic symptoms. *Cutis* 2000; **65**: 89–92.

Ciclosporin [1]

This drug was isolated and purified in 1972 from a soil fungus found in Norway. Its main use until recently has been as an immunosuppressant in patients following kidney, liver, heart, bone marrow or other transplants. It has increasing uses in dermatology, but its use demands careful monitoring. Ciclosporin is a cyclic polypeptide made up of 11 amino acids. The main mode of action is on helper T cells whose cell cycle is blocked in G0 or early G1 and whose production of various lymphokines, notably IL-2, is inhibited. It may also have some direct effect on DNA synthesis and on proliferation of keratinocytes [2]. Apart from its use in transplant patients, ciclosporin has been used to treat a wide range of general medical diseases in which T cells contribute—rheumatoid arthritis, systemic lupus erythematosus, polymyositis and dermatomyositis, uveitis, thyrotoxicosis, diabetes, biliary cirrhosis, various nephropathies, colitis, Crohn's disease and others. Dermatological uses [3–5] include notably psoriasis [6], pustular psoriasis [7] and psoriatic arthritis. Ciclosporin is particularly effective in widespread plaque psoriasis. Treatment at low dosage (3–5 mg/kg/day) for 1–3 months will produce substantial improvement in over 60% of patients [8]. The preferred treatment regimen for psoriasis is short-course inter-mittent therapy—using ciclosporin for no more than 3 months at a time but reinstituting therapy on relapse [9]. Using this regimen, most patients require four or fewer courses of ciclosporin (average dosage 3.4 mg/kg/day) over 2 years [10]. Most patients relapse once ciclosporin is discontinued.

The other main use of ciclosporin in skin diseases is atopic dermatitis. It is a very effective treatment [11], but relapse occurs within a few weeks of discontinuing the drug, although at 1 year later and still off the drug, the disease was only approximately 50% of the severity before ciclosporin treatment was started [12]. Ciclosporin has also been reported to benefit patients with chronic hand dermatitis [13].

Ciclosporin is also used for pemphigus and pemphigoid. There are reports of benefit of ciclosporin in dermatomyositis [14], pyoderma gangrenosum [15] and chronic idiopathic urticaria [16].

Absorption of the drug from the gut is variable, often approximately 30%, although a microemulsion formulation of ciclosporin that has better absorption has replaced the original product. Excretion is mainly via the liver but again the rate is variable. For practical purposes, assessment of blood levels of ciclosporin is unnecessary when using 'dermatological doses' in otherwise well patients, and monitoring renal function (by serum creatinine estimations) and blood pressure suffice.

Ciclosporin has little toxicity on the bone marrow or liver but does have a considerable and largely reversible toxicity on the kidney [17]. Short-term (mean 2.4 months) ciclosporin at a dosage of 5 mg/kg/day was associated with a significant but small and reversible increase in blood pressure, but only a transient mild reduction in glomerular filtration rate (GFR), which did not reach significance [18]. Renal function and biopsy findings have been studied in patients who have taken ciclosporin continuously for 5 years (average 3.3 mg/kg/day). Six of eight patients who had renal biopsies showed tubular atrophy and arteriolar hyalinosis, four had increase in interstitium and two showed increased instance of glomerular obsolescence. Renal function was assessed by GFR and serum creatinine. Both a fall in the GFR and a rise in serum creatinine correlated with the severity of the ciclosporin nephrotoxicity seen on biopsy [19]. Other side effects include nausea and vomiting, hypertension, hypertrichosis, tremor and hyperkalaemia.

Long-term toxicity may include an increased tendency for lymphomas. Although a recent epidemiological study of 1252 patients over 5 years did not demonstrate an increased incidence of lymphoma, it did reveal a sixfold increase in skin cancer, particularly in those patients who had received prior PUVA [20]. There are notable interactions with ketoconazole, erythromycin and other drugs that increase blood levels; with rifampicin and hydantoinates, which decrease blood levels; and with

NSAIDs, which seem to increase the nephrotoxicity without changing the blood levels.

New oral calcineurin inhibitors, structurally dissimilar to ciclosporin but with similar mechanisms of action, have been developed, such as pimecrolimus (a derivative of ascomycin). Oral pimecrolimus appears effective in the treatment of moderate to severe psoriasis but apparently without risk of nephrotoxicity or hypertension [21].

REFERENCES

1 Kahan BD. Cyclosporine. *N Engl J Med* 1989; **321**: 1725–38.
2 Furue M, Gaspari AH, Katz SI. Effect of cyclosporin A on epidermal cells. II. Cyclosporin A inhibits proliferation of normal and transformed keratinocytes. *J Invest Dermatol* 1988; **90**: 796–800.
3 Biren CA, Barr RJ. Dermatologic application of cyclosporine. *Arch Dermatol* 1986; **122**: 1028–32.
4 Gupta AK, Brown MD, Ellis CN *et al.* Cyclosporine in dermatology. *J Am Acad Dermatol* 1989; **21**: 1245–56.
5 Page EH, Wexler DM, Guenther LC. Cyclosporin A. *J Am Acad Dermatol* 1986; **14**: 785–91.
6 Bos JD, Mevinharde MMHM, Van Joost T *et al.* Use of cyclosporin in psoriasis. *Lancet* 1989; **ii**: 1500–2.
7 Reitamo S, Erkko P, Remitz A *et al.* Cyclosporine in the treatment of palmoplantar pustulosis. *Arch Dermatol* 1993; **129**: 1273–79.
8 Ellis CN, Fradin MS, Messana JM *et al.* Cyclosporine for plaque-type psoriasis: results of a multidose, double-blind trial. *N Engl J Med* 1991; **324**: 277–84.
9 Berth-Jones J, Henderson CA, Munro CS *et al.* Treatment of psoriasis with intermitten short course cyclsporin (Neoral): a multicentre study. *Br J Dermatol* 1997; **136**: 527–30.
10 Ho VCY, Griffiths CEM, Berth-Jones J *et al.* Intermittent short courses of cyclosporine microemulsion for the long-term management of psoriasis: a 2-year cohort study. *J Am Acad Dermatol* 2001; **44**: 643–51.
11 Van Joost TH, Heule F, Korstanje M *et al.* Cyclosporin in atopic dermatitis; a multicentre placebo-controlled study. *Br J Dermatol* 1994; **130**: 634–40.
12 Granlund H, Erkko P, Sinisalo M *et al.* Cyslosporin in atopic dermatitis: time to relapse and effect of intermittent therapy. *Br J Dermatol* 1995; **132**: 106–12.
13 Reitamo S, Granlund H. Cyclosporin A in the treatment of chronic dermatitis of the hands. *Br J Dermatol* 1994; **130**: 75–8.
14 Kavanagh GM, Ross JS, Black MM. Dermatomyositis treated with cyclosporin. *J R Soc Med* 1991; **184**: 306.
15 de Hijas C, del-Rio E, Gorospe MA *et al.* Large peristomal pyoderma gangrenosum successfully treated with cyclosporine and corticosteroids. *J Am Acad Dermatol* 1993; **29**: 1034–5.
16 Grattan CE, O'Donnell BF, Francis DM *et al.* Randomized, double-blind study of cyclosporin in chronic 'idiopathic' urticaria. *Br J Dermatol* 2000; **43**: 365–72.
17 Editorial. Cyclosporin hypertension. *Lancet* 1988; **ii**: 1234.
18 Brown AL, Wilkinson R, Thomas TH *et al.* The effect of short-term low-dose cyclosporin on renal function and blood pressure in patients with psoriasis. *Br J Dermatol* 1993; **128**: 550–5.
19 Powles AV, Cook T, Hulme B *et al.* Renal function and biopsy findings after 5 years' treatment with low-dose cyclosporin for psoriasis. *Br J Dermatol* 1993; **128**: 159–65.
20 Paul CF, Ho VC, McGeown C *et al.* Risk of malignancies in psoriasis patients treated with cyclosporine: a 5-year cohort study. *J Invest Dermatol* 2003; **120**: 211–6.
21 Rappersberger K, Komar M, Ebelin ME *et al.* Pimcrolimus identifies a common genomic anti-inflammatory profile, is clinically highly effective in psoriasis and is well-tolerated. *J Invest Dermatol* 2002; **119**: 876–9.

Fumaric acid esters (fumarates)

For more than 20 years fumarates have been used extensively in northern Europe, particularly German-speaking countries, for the treatment of moderate to severe psoriasis [1,2]. The commercially available preparation of fumarates, Fumaderm®, comprises a mixture of dimethylfumarate and the calcium, magnesium and zinc salts of monoethylfumaric acid. After ingestion, dimethylfumarate is hydrolysed to momomethylfumarate—the main active metabolite. Clinical trials [3–5] attest to the efficacy of fumarates. The drug is introduced gradually, starting at 30 mg/day, building up over several weeks to a maximum dose of 240 mg three times daily. It is estimated that, if they tolerate the drug, approximately 57% of patients will achieve a 70% reduction in severity of psoriasis. Two-thirds of treated patients develop gastrointestinal symptoms such as dyspepsia and diarrhoea; one-third of patients develop flushing. In most patients these side effects settle down over time. Lymphocyte counts fall in nearly all treated patients, sometimes by 50% [3–5]. Renal function and liver function should be monitored but impairment is unusual. The mechanism of action of fumarates appears to be an ability to promote the secretion of Th2 cytokines [6], such as IL-10, which are beneficial in psoriasis.

REFERENCES

1 Schweckendiek W. Heilung von Psoriasis. *Med Monutschr* 1959; **13**: 103–4.
2 Mrowietz U, Christophers E, Altmeyer P. The German Fumaric Acid Ester Consensus Conference: treatment of severe psoriasis with fumaric acid ester, scientific background and guidelines for therapeutic use. *Br J Dermatol* 1999; **141**: 424–9.
3 Altmeyer PJ, Matthes U, Pawlak F *et al.* Antipsoriatic effects of fumaric acid derivatives: results of a multicenter double-blind study in 100 patients. *J Am Acad Dermatol* 1994; **30**: 977–81.
4 Nugteren-Huying WM, van der Schroeff JG, Hermans J, Saarmond D. Fumaric acid therapy for psoriasis: a randomized, double-blind, placebo-controlled study. *J Am Acad Dermatol* 1990; **22**: 311–2.
5 Mrowietz U, Christophers E, Altmeyer P. Treatment of psoriasis with fumaric acid esters: results of a prospective multicentre study. German Multicentre Study. *Br J Dermatol* 1998; **138**: 456–60.
6 Ockenfels HM, Schaltewolter T, Ockenfels G, Funk R, Goos M. The antipsoriatic agent dimethylfumarate immunomodulates T-cell cytokine secretion and inhibits cytokines of the psoriatic cytokine network. *Br J Dermatol* 1998; **139**: 390–5.

PUVA [1]

Photochemotherapy with 8-methoxypsoralen followed by UVA radiation for psoriasis is considered in detail in Chapter 35. If necessary, 5-methoxypsoralen can be substituted, or 8-methoxypsoralen bath PUVA used, especially if a patient is nauseated by 8-methoxypsoralen.

PUVA is also of value in mycosis fungoides (MF) (see Chapter 54) [2]. Seventy-three patients with MF were treated with PUVA, which produced clinical and histological clearance in a very high proportion of patients with pretumour-stage MF. The response of patients with tumours was less satisfactory, such patients requiring, in addition, radiotherapy.

PUVA may be used in selected children with severe atopic dermatitis [3]. Fifty-three children (mean age 11.2 years) had twice-weekly PUVA; 39 (74%) of them achieved a clear or nearly clear skin. The mean duration of treatment to remission was 37 weeks, with mean cumulative UVA dose of 1118 J/cm. This relatively high UVA exposure is of concern. However, 22 children remained in remission 1 year after discontinuing PUVA.

PUVA has been described to be of benefit in a whole range of dermatological conditions. Some of the reports involve large numbers of patients and others only single-case reports. For an excellent review of the uses of PUVA in conditions other than psoriasis, including hand eczema, nodular prurigo, vitiligo, the various photodermatoses, granuloma annulare, lichen planus, lyphomatoid papulosis, urticaria, aquagenic pruritus, urticaria pigmentosa, idiopathic pruritus and many other conditions, refer to [4].

It is undisputed that solar UV radiation is a major aetiological factor in squamous and basal cell carcinoma and malignant melanoma in humans. Tumours have been induced in the skin of hairless albino mice by PUVA exposure using both 8-MOP and 5-MOP [5]. An early report suggested that PUVA therapy accelerated the development of skin tumours in patients with xeroderma pigmentosum [6], and it appeared to have an obvious promoter effect in a patient previously exposed to X-irradiation, arsenic and several cytotoxic drugs, who developed 25 basal or squamous cell carcinomas, the first within 21 months of onset of PUVA therapy [7].

There is now substantial literature dealing with the incidence of skin tumours in groups of PUVA-treated patients. Although certain studies have failed to show a clear relationship between PUVA and tumour development [8–10], long-term follow-up of a large US cohort has provided conclusive evidence for the carcinogenicity of PUVA [11]. In this study, an initial cohort of 1380 PUVA patients was followed up for a mean of 13.2 years. Squamous cell carcinoma (SCC) developed in one-quarter of patients exposed to high doses of PUVA, giving a relative risk of SCC of 5.9-fold by comparison with patients receiving low-dose PUVA. High-dose PUVA was regarded as a total of over 299 treatments; low-dose less than 160 [11]. Precise UVA doses were not given, but taking an average dose of 11 J/cm^2 after clearing, the high-dose group can be estimated to have had more than approximately 3200 J and the low-dose group less than 1760 J. The latter figure may therefore be taken as a cumulative dose, which should ideally not be exceeded. However, a study in Northern Ireland, where there is a high population of sun-sensitive Celtic subjects, indicated increased risk for non-melanoma skin cancer (including particularly basal cell carcinoma) with cumulative UVA doses above only 250 J/cm^2 [12]. Therefore, far more conservative UVA limits may be needed with certain populations, and safety limits may be better expressed as numbers of treatments rather than cumulative UVA doses. In the Northern Ireland study, a cumulative UVA dosage of 250 J/cm^2 equated with

approximately 100 treatments. The US study showed that fair-skinned persons had an approximately twofold higher risk of SCC than those with skin types III or IV. Overall, there was no substantial increase in the risk of basal cell carcinoma with high-dose PUVA in the US study [11]. Metastatic SCC was seen in seven patients, but two of these were elderly and had had little PUVA. Four were younger (41–57 years) and had had moderate- to high-dose PUVA, although methotrexate or ionizing radiation may have played an additional part [11].

The substantially increased risk of SCC with high-dose PUVA therapy has been supported by a large Swedish study [13]. The male genitalia appear to be particularly at risk [14–16]. In a prospective cohort study [11,16] of 892 men first exposed to PUVA in 1975–76, 24 (2.7%) had developed a total of 51 genital neoplasms. It appears that increased risk is associated with high-dose PUVA in association with UVB and coal tar. Shielding of the genitalia during PUVA therapy reduces the risk.

PUVA lentigines may exhibit cytologically atypical melanocytes [17]. There is an increased risk (incidence rate ratio 8.4) in patients who have received PUVA—the 1380 patient cohort study of patients who first received PUVA in 1975–76 calculated that high-dose PUVA (more than 250 treatments) and passage of time were contributing factors. PUVA is best avoided in those predisposed to malignant melanoma (e.g. those with numerous melanocytic naevi or atypical moles, and a family history of melanoma) [18,19].

There is no evidence of any internal carcinoma hazard, but acute leukaemia [20,21] and a preleukaemic state [22] have been reported. In addition, a patient transformed from myelodysplasia to acute fatal myeloid leukaemia after 4 months of PUVA [23].

These findings have led to a recommendation that PUVA patients should not receive more than 1000 J/cm or more than 150 treatments in a lifetime unless there are strong indications otherwise [24]. The male genitalia should be protected while receiving PUVA treatment.

REFERENCES

1 Moseley H, Ferguson J. Photochemotherapy: a reappraisal of its use in dermatology. *Drugs* 1989; **38**: 822–37.
2 Briffa DV, Warin AP, Harrington CI et al. Photochemotherapy in mycosis fungoides: a study of 73 patients. *Lancet* 1980; **ii**: 49–53.
3 Sheenan MP, Atherton DJ, Norris P et al. Oral psoralen photochemotherapy in severe childhood atopic eczema: an update. *Br J Dermatol* 1993; **129**: 431–6.
4 Honig B, Morison WL, Karp D. Photochemotherapy beyond psoriasis. *J Am Acad Dermatol* 1994; **31**: 775–90.
5 Young AR, Magnus IA, Davies AC et al. A comparison of the photo-tumorigenic potential of 8-MOP and 5-MOP in hairless albino mice exposed to solar simulated radiation. *Br J Dermatol* 1983; **108**: 507–18.
6 Reed WB. Treatment of psoriasis with oral psoralens and longwave ultraviolet light [Letter]. *Acta Derm Venereol (Stockh)* 1976; **56**: 315.
7 Baker H, Darley CR, Johnson-Smith J et al. Skin neoplasia associated with PUVA therapy. *Br J Dermatol* 1981; **105** (Suppl. 19): 65–6.
8 Roenigk HH, Caro WA. Skin cancer in the PUVA-48 cooperative study. *J Am Acad Dermatol* 1981; **4**: 319–24.

9 Ros A-M, Wennersten G, Lagerholm B. Long-term photochemotherapy for psoriasis. *Acta Derm Venereol (Stockh)* 1983; **63**: 215–21.

10 Henseler T, Christophers E, Hönigsmann H *et al.* Skin tumours in the European PUVA study. *J Am Acad Dermatol* 1987; **16**: 108–16.

11 Stern RS, Laird N. The carcinogenic risk of treatments for severe psoriasis. *Cancer* 1994; **73**: 2759–64.

12 McKenna KE, Patterson CC, Hanley J *et al.* Cutaneous neoplasia following PUVA therapy for psoriasis. *Br J Dermatol* 1996; **134**: 693–42.

13 Lindelöf B, Sigurgeirsson B, Tegner E *et al.* PUVA and cancer: a large-scale epidemiological study. *Lancet* 1991; **338**: 11–3.

14 Stern RS. Genital tumours among men with psoriasis exposed to psoralens and ultraviolet-A radiation (PUVA) and ultraviolet B radiation. *N Engl J Med* 1990; **322**: 1093–7.

15 Perkins W, Lamont D, MacKie RM. Cutaneous malignancy in males treated with photochemotherapy. *Lancet* 1990; **336**: 1248.

16 Stern RS, Bagheri S, Nichols K. PUVA follow-up study: the persistent risk of genital tumours among men treated with psoralen plus ultraviolet A (PUVA) for psoriasis. *J Am Acad Dermatol* 2002; **47**: 33–9.

17 Rhodes AR, Harrist TJ, Momtaz TK. The PUVA-induced pigmented macule: a lentiginous proliferation of large, sometimes cytologically atypical, melanocytes. *J Am Acad Dermatol* 1983; **9**: 47–58.

18 Stern RS, Nichols KT, Vakeva LH. Malignant melanoma in patients treated for psoriasis with methoxsalen (psoralen) and ultraviolet A radiation (PUVA): the PUVA follow-up study. *N Engl J Med* 1997; **336**: 1041–5.

19 Stern RS. PUVA follow-up study: the risk of melanoma in association with long-term exposure to PUVA. *J Am Acad Dermatol* 2001; **44**: 755–61.

20 Hansen NE. Development of acute myeloid leukaemia in a patient with psoriasis treated with oral 8-methoxypsoralen and longwave ultraviolet light. *Scand J Haematol* 1979; **22**: 57–60.

21 Freeman K, Warin AP. Acute myelomonocytic leukaemia developing in a patient with psoriasis treated with oral 8-methoxypsoralen and longwave ultraviolet light. *Clin Exp Dermatol* 1985; **10**: 144–6.

22 Wagner J, Manthorpe R, Philip P *et al.* Preleukaemia (haemopoietic dysplasia) developing in a patient with psoriasis treated with 8-methoxypsoralen and ultraviolet light (PUVA treatment). *Scand J Haematol* 1978; **21**: 299–304.

23 Sheehan-Dare RA, Cotterill JA, Barnard DL. Transformation of myelodysplasia to acute myeloid leukaemia during psoralen photochemotherapy (PUVA) treatment of psoriasis. *Acta Derm Venereol (Stockh)* 1989; **69**: 262–4.

24 British Photodermatology Group. British Photodermatology Group guidelines for PUVA. *Br J Dermatol* 1994; **130**: 246–55.

Photopheresis

The use of extracorporeal photoimmunochemotherapy (ECP; photopheresis) was pioneered in the early 1980s. Primarily developed for the treatment of cutaneous T-cell lymphoma (CTCL), ECP has been used to treat a variety of dermatological diseases. Derived from PUVA treatment, ECP involves the extracorporeal exposure of peripheral blood mononuclear cells (PBMC) to 8-methoxypsoralen and UVA irradiation before being returned to the patient. The machine used for this process provides the leukopheresis step prior to UVA exposure. 8-Methoxypsoralen is delivered directly to the collected buffy coat containing the PBMCs (for a detailed review of the procedure refer to Knobler and Jantschitsch [1]). Various protocols are under development for ECP but the one used most widely is photopheresis on two successive days, repeated at 2–4-week intervals. It is estimated that during one treatment session 5–10% of the circulating T-cell pool is treated. The exact mechanism of action is not fully understood but it is believed that the patient's immune system is stimulated to destroy the altered and/or damaged malignant T cells.

CTCL was the first disease for which ECP was evaluated and as a consequence most evidence of efficacy comes from treatment of this disease. Indeed, ECP is approved in the USA for palliative treatment of Sézary syndrome. The original study by Edelson *et al.* [2] demonstrated partial or complete remission in 27 out of 37 CTCL patients. Subsequent studies [3,4] confirmed this observation and it is accepted that complete remission may occur in 25% of patients with no response in a further 25%. A good therapeutic response is dictated by short disease duration, normal numbers of CD8 cells and a normal CD4 : CD8 ratio [5]. An advantage of ECP is the low side effect profile [3]. Some patients with Sézary syndrome are less responsive to ECP, and combination therapy with IFN-α, methotrexate, PUVA, bexarotene or superficial electron beam therapy may be required [6–8]. It should be noted that although the Sézary syndrome form of CTCL is responsive to ECP, some workers have questioned this high rate of response, mainly disputing the definition of Sézary syndrome—if a strict definition of clonal disease is instituted, only 16% of patients have a complete response [9]. Long-term survival is good with survival rates of 100 months from time of diagnosis [7]. Unsurprisingly, ECP has been used to treat a variety of inflammatory disease where autoreactive T cells are believed to be an important contributor to the disease process. ECP may be an important therapy for graft-versus-host disease after allogeneic bone marrow transplantation [10], and perhaps in the treatment of acute or chronic rejection of organ transplants [11]. Systemic sclerosis [12], systemic lupus erythematosus [13], atopic dermatitis [14], pemphigus vulgaris [15] and psoriatic arthritis [16] have all been reported to respond to ECP.

REFERENCES

1 Knobler R, Jantschitsch C. Extracorporeal photochemoimmunotherapy in cutaneous T-cell lymphoma. *Transf Apher Sci* 2003; **28**: 81–9.

2 Edelson RL, Berger CL, Gasparro FP *et al.* Treatment of cutaneous T-cell lymphoma by extracorporeal photochemotherapy. *N Engl J Med* 1987; **316**: 297–303.

3 Knobler RM, Girardi M. Extracorporeal photochemoimmunotherapy in cutaneous T-cell lymphomas. *Ann N Y Acad Sci* 2001; **941**: 123–38.

4 Rook A, Prystowsky MB, Cassin M, Boufal M, Lessin RS. Combined therapy for Sézary syndrome with extracorporeal photochemotherapy and low-dose interferon-α therapy. *Arch Dermatol* 1991; **127**: 1535–40.

5 Zic J, Strick GP, Greer JP *et al.* Long-term follow-up with cutaneous T-cell lymphoma treated with extracorporeal photochemotherapy. *J Am Acad Dermatol* 1996; **356**: 935–45.

6 Duvic M, Hester JP, Lemak NA. Photopheresis therapy for cutaneous T-cell lymphoma. *J Am Acad Dermatol* 1996; **35**: 573–9.

7 Gottlieb S, Wofe J, Fox FE *et al.* Treatment of cutaneous T-cell lymphoma with extracorporeal photopheresis monotherapy and in combination with recombinant interferon-α: a 10-year experience at a single institution. *J Am Acad Dermatol* 1996; **35**: 946–7.

8 Fimiani M, Rubegni P, De Aloe G, Andreasssi L. Role of extracorporeal photochemotherapy alone and in combination with interferon-α in the treatment of cutaneous T-cell lymphoma. *J Am Acad Dermatol* 1999; **41**: 502–3.

9 Russell-Jones AR. Extracorporeal photopheresis in Sézary syndrome. *Lancet* 1997; **350**: 886.

10 Owsianowski M, Gollnick H, Siegert W *et al.* Successful treatment of chronic graft-versus-host disease with extracorporeal photopheresis. *Bone Marrow Transplant* 1994; **14**: 845–8.

11 Costanzonordia MR, Hubbell EA, O'Sullivan EJ *et al.* Photopheresis versus corticosteroids in the therapy of heart transplant rejection: preliminary clinical report. *Circulation* 1992; **86**: 242–50.

12 Wollina U, Liebold K, Kautz M. Extracorporeal photopheresis for scleroderma. *J Am Acad Dermatol* 2001; **44**: 146–8.

13 Knobler RM. Extracorporeal photochemotherapy for the treatment of lupus erythematosus: preliminary observations. *Springer Semin Immunopathol* 1994; **6**: 323–5.

14 Richter HI, Billmann-Eberwein C, Grewe M *et al.* Successful monotherapy of severe and intractable atopic dermatitis by photopheresis. *J Am Acad Dermatol* 1998; **38**: 585–8.

15 Gollnick HP, Owsianowski M, Taube KM, Orfanos CE. Unresponsive severe generalized pemphigus vulgaris successfully controlled by extracorporeal photopheresis. *J Am Acad Dermatol* 1993; **28**: 122–4.

16 Vahlquist C, Larsson M, Ernerudh J *et al.* Treatment of psoriatic arthritis with extracorporeal photochemotherapy and conventional psoralen-ultraviolet A irradiation. *Arthritis Rheum* 1996; **39**: 1519–23.

Plasmapheresis

Plasmapheresis (plasma exchange) has been used for many years in patients with severe systemic lupus erythematosus in whom high-dose corticosteroids and immunosuppressants were not controlling their disease [1,2]. However, the evidence that it is effective when added to immunosuppressive treatment with prednisolone and ciclosporin in severe lupus nephritis is lacking [3]. It can also be life-saving in Goodpasture's syndrome [4]. It is used in myaesthenia gravis, Waldenström's macroglobulinaemia, cryoglobulinaemia, thrombotic thrombocytopenic purpura and Guillain–Barré syndrome. Plasmapheresis is occasionally used in acute polymyositis or dermatomyositis, but in a controlled trial involving 39 patients, it was shown to be no more effective than sham apheresis [5].

Plasmapheresis is an effective treatment for pemphigus vulgaris and bullous pemphigoid unresponsive to conventional therapy—it is particularly useful for rapid control of severe active disease and as a means of reducing the dosage of corticosteroid and other immunosuppressive therapy. Between seven and 14 therapeutic plasma exchanges are required [6]. Side effects of plasmapheresis may include hypertension.

Plasmapheresis was effective in a series of eight patients with pemphigus vulgaris, in whom the treatment was added to their glucocorticoid and immunosuppressive therapy, which had not been controlling their disease [7]. Bullous pemphigoid seems to be less successfully treated by plasmapheresis. In a study involving 100 patients, it was found that neither azathioprine nor plasmapheresis was effective as an adjuvant to corticosteroid [8]. Solar urticaria has been reported to respond to plasmapheresis when added to photochemotherapy (PUVA) that had not been effective on its own [9].

REFERENCES

1 Euler HH, Schroeder JO, Harten P *et al.* Treatment-free remission in severe systemic lupus erythematosus following synchronization of plasmapheresis with subsequent pulse cyclosphosphamide. *Arthritis Rheum* 1994; **37**: 1784–94.

2 Erickson RW, Franklin WA, Emlen W. Treatment of hemorrhagic lupus pneumonitis with plasmapheresis [Review]. *Semin Arthritis Rheum* 1994; **24**: 114–23.

3 Lewis EJ, Hunsicker LG, Lan SP *et al.* A control trial of plasmapheresis therapy in severe lupus nephritis. *N Engl J Med* 1992; **326**: 1371–9.

4 Shumak KH, Rock GA. Therapeutic plasma exchange. *N Engl J Med* 1984; **310**: 762–71.

5 Miller RW, Leitman SF, Cronin ME *et al.* Controlled trial of plasma exchange and leukapheresis in polymyositis and dermatomyositis. *N Engl J Med* 1992; **326**: 1380–4.

6 Mazzi G, Rainen A, Zanolli FA *et al.* Plasmapheresis therapy in pemphigus vulgaris and bullous pemphigoid. *Transf Apher Sci* 2003; **28**: 13–8.

7 Sondergaard K, Carstens J, Jorgensen J *et al.* The steroid-sparing effect of long-term plasmapheresis in pemphigus. *Acta Derm Venereol (Stockh)* 1995; **75**: 150–2.

8 Guillaume JC, Vaillant L, Bernard P *et al.* Controlled trial of azathioprine and plasma exchange in addition to prednisolone in the treatment of bullous pemphigoid. *Arch Dermatol* 1993; **129**: 49–53.

9 Hudson-Peacock MJ, Farr PM, Diffey BL *et al.* Combined treatment of solar urticaria with plasmapheresis and PUVA. *Br J Dermatol* 1993; **128**: 440–2.

Intravenous immunoglobulin [1]

High-dose intravenous immunoglobulin (IVIg) is produced from pooled human plasma. There are at least seven licensed IVIg preparations available, but differences between these preparations may affect outcome. IVIg has been used to treat a variety of autoimmune bullous and inflammatory dermatoses. Most reports are anecdotal with few randomized controlled trials. Treatment with IVIg is best performed in an inpatient setting but if patients are low risk, then infusions can be performed in an ambulatory setting. High doses (1–2 g/kg) are recommended, usually delivered as a 5 consecutive day cycle of 0.4 mg/kg/day, although a 3-day cycle may be used. Each infusion is given over 4–4$^{1}/_{2}$ h. Initially, cycles are repeated every 3–4 weeks until there is effective control of disease—once this has been achieved the time intervals between cycles can be gradually increased. A proposed end point is two infusions 16 weeks apart. Adverse effects are usually mild and self-limiting—common side effects include headache, chills, flushing and vomiting. More serious adverse events have included aseptic meningitis, thrombosis and anaphylaxis, particularly in IgA-deficient patients who have anti-IgA antibodies. There is a potential risk of transference of infectious agents but batches are screened for human immunodeficiency virus (HIV), syphilis and hepatitis [1].

IVIg is believed to work as an immunomodulatory agent—reducing levels of IL-1 in serum [2], it may also down-regulate expression of Fas and Fas ligand on keratinocytes, thereby preventing apoptosis [3].

Most use of IVIg in dermatology is for therapy of autoimmune mucocutaneous blistering diseases [1]. Small case series of pemphigus vulgaris [4–6] indicate that 2 g/kg IVIg produces prolonged clinical remission sustained after cessation of therapy. IVIg also has a corticosteroid-sparing effect in pemphigus vulgaris [5]. Pemphigus foliaceus is responsive to IVIg and prolonged remission has been achieved [7]. In 27 of 32 cases of bullous pemphigoid non-responsive to conventional therapy reported in the literature as having received IVIg therapy, there was significant and long-lasting clinical improvement [1]. Mucous membrane pemphigoid appears, on the basis of case reports and small uncontrolled series, to respond to IVIg to the extent that disease progression (particularly eye disease) is halted [8]. Cases of epidermolysis bullosa acquisita [9], pyoderma gangrenosum [10], dermato-myositis [11], atopic dermatitis [12] and psoriasis [13], amongst a large list of dermatoses [14], have all been treated successfully with IVIg. The use of IVIg for the treatment of toxic epidermal necrolysis is perhaps the most contentious—a rationale for its use is the ability to prevent keratinocyte apoptosis. No randomized controlled trial has been performed, but some groups [3,15] advocate it as the treatment of choice while others believe it has no benefit [16].

REFERENCES

1 Ahmed AR, Dahl MV. Consensus statement on the use of intravenous immunoglobulin therapy in the treatment of autoimminue mucocutaneous blistering disease. *Arch Dermatol* 2003; **139**: 1051–9.
2 Kumari S, Bhol KC, Rehman F, Foster CS, Ahmed AR. Interleukin-1 components in cicatricial pemphigoid: role in intravenous immunoglobulin therapy. *Cytokine* 2001; **14**: 218–24.
3 Viard I, Wehrli P, Bullani R et al. Inhibitor of toxic epidermal necrolysis by blockade of CD95 with human intravenous immunoglobulin. *Science* 1998; **282**: 490–3.
4 Ahmed AR. Intravenous immunoglobulin therapy in the treatment of patients with pemphigus vulgaris unresponsive to conventional immuno-suppressive treatment. *J Am Acad Dermatol* 2001; **45**: 679–90.
5 Sami N, Qureshi A, Ruocco E, Ahmed AR. Corticosteroid-sparing effect on intravenous immunoglobulin therapy in patients with pemphigus vulgaris. *Arch Dermatol* 2002; **138**: 1158–62.
6 Bystryn JC, Jiao D, Natow S. Treatment of pemphigus with intravenous immunoglobulin. *J Am Acad Dermatol* 2002; **47**: 358–63.
7 Sami N, Qureshi A, Ahmed AR. Steroid-sparing effect of intravenous immunoglobulin therapy in patients with pemphigus foliaceus. *Eur J Dermatol* 2002; **12**: 174–8.
8 Sami N, Bhol K, Ahmed AR. Treatment of oral pemphigoid with intra-venous immunoglobulin as monotherapy long-term follow-up: influence of treatment on autoantibody titers to human alpha 6 integrin. *Clin Exp Immunol.* 2002; **129**: 533–40.
9 Meir F, Sonnichsen K, Scaumber-Lever G, Dopfer R, Rassner G. Epidermolysis bullosa acquisita: efficacy of high-dose intravenous immunoglobulins. *J Am Acad Dermatol* 1993; **29**: 334–7.
10 Hagman JH, Carrozzo AM, Campione E, Romanelli P, Chimenti S. The use of high-dose immunoglobulin in the treatment of pyoderma gangrenosum. *J Dermatolog Treat* 2001; **12**: 19–22.
11 Oddis CV. Current approach to the treatment of polymyositis and dermato-myositis. *Curr Opin Rheumatol* 2000; **12**: 492–7.
12 Paul C, Lahfa M, Bachelez H, Chevret S, Dubertret L. A randomized controlled evaluation: blinded trial of intravenous immunoglobulin in adults with severe atopic dermatitis. *Br J Dermatol* 2002; **147**: 518–22.
13 Gurmia V, Mediwake R, Fernando M et al. Psoriasis: response to high-dose intravenous immunoglobulin in three patients. *Br J Dermatol* 2002; **147**: 554–7.
14 Jolles S, Hughes SJ, Whittaker S. Dermatological uses of high-dose intra-venous immunoglobulin. *Arch Dermatol* 1998; **134**: 80–6.
15 Trent JT, Kinsner RS, Romanelli P, Kerdel FA. Analysis of intravenous immunoglobulin for the treatment of toxic epidermal necrolysis using SCORTEN: the University of Miami experience. *Arch Dermatol* 2003; **139**: 39–43.
16 Bachot N, Revuz J, Roujeau JC. Intravenous immunoglobulin treatment for Stevens–Johnson syndrome and toxic epidermal necrolysis: a prospective non-comparative study showing no benefit on mortality or progression. *Arch Dermatol* 2003; **139**: 33–6.

Gold (sodium aurothiomalate)

Dose: 10 mg intramuscularly as a test dose, followed by 50 mg at weekly intervals. Although this regimen was devised for treatment of rheumatoid arthritis it has been successfully used in the treatment of pemphigus [1]. If there has been no improvement by the time the total dose reaches 1 g, treatment should be stopped. If improvement does occur, the frequency of the injections is reduced to every 2–3 weeks. Renal, hepatic and marrow damage must be looked for and rashes are common.

Auranofin is an oral preparation of gold, rather less effective than the parenteral preparation. Its main advantage is that its tissue half-life is much less than with injectible gold. Dose: 3–6 mg/day, increasing to 9 mg/day after 3–6 months. It has also been used in discoid lupus erythematosus.

REFERENCE

1 Penneys NS, Eaglstein WH, Frost P. Management of pemphigus with gold compounds. *Arch Dermatol* 1976; **112**: 185–7.

Chelating agents

Chelating agents are available that form complexes with a number of heavy metals. They are only occasionally of use in dermatology.

d-Penicillamine [1]

This is a degradation product of penicillin and chelates copper, mercury, zinc and lead. It is used for Wilson's disease, lead poisoning, cystinuria and rheumatoid arthritis [1,2]. Its dermatological interest lies in its ability to cause a variety of diseases, including systemic lupus erythematosus-like syndrome, pemphigus-like bullous eruptions, lichenoid and other eruptions and elastosis perforans serpiginosa (see Chapter 73). Earlier reports of possible benefit in scleroderma have not been substantiated [3–5].

Desferrioxamine

This is used in the treatment of various iron-storage diseases. In general, acute iron overload seems to respond much more satisfactorily. However, it is logical to use it in porphyria cutanea tarda as long as iron overload is present, although its value has yet to be proved (see Chapter 57).

REFERENCES

1 Editorial. d-Penicillamine in rheumatoid arthritis. *Lancet* 1975; i: 1123–5.
2 Multicentre Trial Group. Controlled trial of d-penicillamine in severe rheumatoid arthritis. *Lancet* 1973; i: 275–80.
3 Steen VD. Treatment of systemic sclerosis. *Am J Clin Dermatol* 2001; **2**: 315–25.
4 Sapadin AN, Fleischmajer R. Treatment of scleroderma. *Arch Dermatol* 2002; **138**: 99–105.
5 Furst DE, Clements PJ. d-Penicillamine is not an effective treatment in systemic sclerosis. *Scand J Rheumatol* 2001; **30**: 189–91.

Antibiotics and antibacterial agents

Antibiotics were originally substances synthesized by microorganisms that were toxic to other microorganisms at high dilution. The term is now more widely applied to any drug with therapeutic activity against living organisms, particularly bacteria. Antifungals and antivirals are drugs with activity against fungi and viruses, respectively.

Most modern antibiotics are synthetic or semi-synthetic. They are usually divided into bacteriostatic and bactericidal groups, although the distinction is not complete; erythromycin, for example, may be either bactericidal or bacteriostatic depending on the nature of the infecting organism and the drug concentration achieved.

In clinical use, antibiotics are divided into those with a narrow spectrum of activity and those broad-spectrum drugs that act against Gram-positive and Gram-negative organisms. In the laboratory, antibiotics can be further divided into five main groups:
1 Antibiotics that interfere with bacterial cell wall synthesis (e.g. the penicillins, cephalosporins and glycopeptide antimicrobials such as vancomycin and teicoplanin)
2 Antibiotics affecting bacterial cell-membrane permeability (e.g. the polymyxins)
3 Antibiotics that inhibit bacterial protein biosynthesis (e.g. the tetracyclines, aminoglycosides, macrolides, lincosamides and chloramphenicol)
4 Antibiotics that affect bacterial nucleic acid metabolism (e.g. the rifamycins and quinolones)
5 *Para*-aminobenzoic acid (PABA) antagonists (e.g. the sulphonamides).

Drug resistance

Bacterial resistance can emerge in three ways. When all sensitive bacteria have been eradicated, any remaining inherently resistant bacteria are free to multiply; this is the most common form of resistance. Less frequently, bacteria may acquire resistance, by mutation, to a drug to which they were initially sensitive. The third form, which is cause for concern, is transferable drug resistance. Here, extrachromosomal genetic information affecting the expression of resistance contained in a plasmid or a transposable section of chromosomal DNA can be transferred from one bacterium, which may be non-pathogenic, to another previously susceptible bacterium. This often takes place in the bowel or skin and may involve a variety of different organisms. Information on multiple drug resistance can be transferred with a single plasmid.

The mechanisms of drug resistance are variable and include changes in permeability of the cell membrane or antibiotic efflux, alterations in ribosomes, altered cell-wall precursors or target enzymes and the emergence of auxotrophs that have different growth substrates.

Sulphonamides

These antibacterial drugs were introduced into clinical practice in the 1930s, but the frequency of resistance combined with adverse events have limited their use. The combination of a sulphonamide (sulfamethoxazole) with trimethoprim, known as co-trimoxazole, however, is still used in dermatology although less frequently than previously. Resistance is widespread.

Sulphonamides are derivatives of *para*-amino-benzene-sulphonamide. They act by inhibiting the bacterial enzyme dihydrofolic acid synthetase, which converts PABA to dihydrofolic acid. Mammalian cells and resistant bacteria do not synthesize folic acid and are unaffected.

Sulphonamides are bacteriostatic and most are well absorbed orally. They are distributed through all body tissues, metabolized in the liver and excreted mainly by the kidneys.

Adverse effects. Although the frequency of serious adverse events is low, sulphonamides can cause a number of serious problems. Besides crystalluria, a risk if there is inadequate fluid intake, they may rarely cause blood dyscrasias such as acute haemolytic anaemia (particularly in patients with glucose-6-phosphate dehydrogenase deficiency), fever, serum sickness and a large variety of skin reactions including erythema nodosum and erythema multiforme. Potentially fatal cases of the severe form of erythema multiforme have followed the use of long-acting sulphonamides [1]. Because of the relatively high incidence of this reaction, the long-acting sulphonamides are little used.

Uses. There are now very few situations where they are drugs of first choice. They are of value in lymphogranuloma venereum, chancroid, nocardiosis and toxoplasmosis (combined with pyrimethamine). Sulfapyridine is now used only as an alternative to dapsone in dermatitis herpetiformis and allied conditions.

Sulfapyridine

Dose: 0.5–1.5 g/day as an alternative to dapsone in dermatitis herpetiformis.

Silver sulfadiazine

This has a role as a topical non-absorbable antimicrobial with a broad spectrum.

REFERENCE

1 Baker H. Drug reactions. IV. Erythema multiforme gravis and long-acting sulphonamides. *Br J Dermatol* 1968; **80**: 844–6.

Trimethoprim [1]

Trimethoprim is a synthetic antimicrobial agent in its own right. It is a potent inhibitor of bacterial dihydrofolic acid reductase, which converts dihydrofolic acid to tetrahydrofolic acid, but has many thousand times less effect on the comparable mammalian enzyme. Trimethoprim is very well absorbed orally, distributed widely through most body tissues and is excreted almost completely by the kidney. Although available as a separate drug, it has been used mainly in combination with sulfamethoxazole in the proportions 1 to 5 as co-trimoxazole. This is a logical mix as these drugs inhibit successive stages in bacterial folate metabolism and it is not surprising that their combined effect is synergistic. Both drugs used singly are bacteriostatic but co-trimoxazole appears to be bactericidal.

Co-trimoxazole tablets BP

There are two strengths containing sulfamethoxazole 400 or 800 mg and trimethoprim 80 or 160 mg, respectively. The dose is two tablets twice daily. The combination is effective against a wide range of Gram-positive and Gram-negative bacteria as well as *Nocardia* and actinomycetoma agents and is in general well tolerated. However, it is best avoided in pregnancy and in infants under 6 weeks and therefore in lactating mothers feeding young babies. Adverse reactions are similar to those seen with sulphonamides. Typical skin reactions may occur in up to 8% of patients and this has limited its use for relatively benign conditions such as acne. Impairment of red cell folate utilization may occur, particularly in the elderly, and supplements of folinic acid may be necessary [1]. Rarer side effects include renal impairment and hepatic reactions.

Co-trimoxazole may be used for urinary tract and respiratory infections but, in infections affecting the skin, is of value in chancroid, atypical mycobacterial infections [2] and mycetoma. Co-trimoxazole has potential value in the treatment of *Pneumocystis* infections, particularly in AIDS patients in whom, unfortunately, there is a high frequency of adverse reactions.

REFERENCES

1 Kuces A, Crowe SM, Grayson ML, Hoy JF. *The Use of Antibiotics*, 5th edn. Oxford: Butterworth Heinemann, 1997.

2 Barrow GI, Hewitt M. Skin infection with *Mycobacterium marinum* from a tropical fish tank. *BMJ* 1971; **ii**: 505–6.

Penicillins

The basic structure of a penicillin consists of a thiazolidine ring, a β-lactam ring and a variable side-chain. The starting point for the semi-synthetic penicillins, of which there are now many, is 6-aminopenicillamic acid. It is convenient to divide the penicillins into five main groups according to their antibacterial properties and consequent clinical usage [1]:
1 Penicillinase-sensitive penicillins (natural penicillins) (e.g. benzyl penicillin (penicillin G), and phenoxymethyl penicillin (penicillin V))
2 Penicillinase-resistant penicillins (e.g. methicillin, flucloxacillin)
3 Amino penicillins, which are broad-spectrum penicillins (vulnerable to penicillinase) (e.g. ampicillin, amoxicillin). By combining clavulanic acid, a potent β-lactamase inhibitor, with amoxicillin (Augmentin®), the spectrum of activity has been broadened to cover penicillin-resistant staphylococci
4 Carboxy penicillins (e.g. carbenicillin)
5 Other penicillins, which include extended-spectrum penicillins (e.g. piperacillin), aminopenicillins and penicillins that are stable against Gram-negative lactamases (e.g. temocillin).

Toxicity. The main problems with their use are hypersensitivity reactions, which are not uncommon. An incidence between 1 and 10% is usually accepted [2], and it appears that administration of these drugs by the oral route is associated with a lower frequency of adverse reactions than the intravenous route [3]. These reactions range from urticaria and vasculitis to anaphylaxis. Cross-reactivity in this allergy is usual. Rare side effects include interstitial nephritis, haemolytic anaemia and pancytopenia.

Penicillinase-sensitive penicillins (penicillin)

Penicillin is the drug of choice against *Streptococcus pyogenes* group A, *Treponema pallidum* and meningococcal septicaemia as well as in yaws, actinomycosis and diphtheria. Because of the emergence of resistant strains of the organism, its use in the treatment of gonorrhoea has largely been superceded. In most serious infections, penicillin is given by injection as benzyl penicillin but treatment may be continued with oral penicillin V and this drug also has a role in prophylaxis against streptococcal cellulitis in patients with lymphoedema.

Benzyl penicillin injection BP (penicillin G). Dose: 300 mg (0.5 mega-units) four times daily up to 1.8 g (3 mega-units) daily. Long-acting injectable preparations are available.

Phenoxymethyl penicillin (penicillin V). Dose: 250–500 mg orally every 6 h.

Penicillinase-resistant penicillins

For practical purposes this means cloxacillin or flucloxacillin, which are resistant to staphylococcal β-lactamase and are drugs of choice against penicillin-resistant staphylococci [4]. Flucloxacillin is somewhat less effective against other Gram-positive infections. Adequate levels are achieved by the oral route but parenteral administration is preferred in serious infections.

Flucloxacillin. Dose: 250–500 mg every 6 h and at least 30 min before food.

Amino penicillins

Ampicillin is commonly used, having a spectrum of activity against Gram-positive and Gram-negative bacteria. It is acid stable and therefore absorbed orally, but is not resistant to penicillinase. It is little used in dermatology but is important as a cause of drug rashes. These occur in about 5–10% of all patients treated but in a majority of those with infectious mononucleosis, cytomegalovirus infections or lymphatic leukaemia [2]. The typical morbilliform rash is thought to be toxic in nature and unrelated to true penicillin hypersensitivity. Amoxicillin is almost identical, is twice as well absorbed as ampicillin but is more expensive. It should probably only replace ampicillin in the patient known to be susceptible to antibiotic-induced diarrhoea [5]. Where an even broader spectrum is needed, perhaps in the treatment of heavily infected leg ulcers with surrounding cellulitis, amoxicillin with clavulanic acid (Augmentin) is worth consideration [6,7]. However, its role in dermatology is a limited one.

Ampicillin. Dose: 250 mg to 1 g every 6 h and at least 30 min before a meal.

Amoxicillin capsules. Dose: 250–500 mg every 8 h.

Amoxicillin 250 mg and clavulanic acid (Augmentin) tablets. Dose: 1–2 tablets every 8 h.

Other penicillins

Carbenicillin, piperacillin, ticarcillin and azlocillin must all be given by injection or infusion and have little place in dermatology.

Imipenem

Imipenem is a carbapenem, a bi-cyclic β-lactam compound with a broad spectrum [8]. It shows considerable activity against many Gram-positive bacteria as well as *Neisseria* spp. It is also used in *Nocardia* infections. It is seldom used in dermatology and is given intravenously.

REFERENCES

1 O'Grady F, Lambert H, Finch RG *et al. Antibiotics and Chemotherapy*, 7th edn. Edinburgh: Churchill Livingstone, 1997.
2 Beeley L. Allergy to penicillin. *BMJ* 1984; **228**: 511–2.
3 Saxon A. Immediate hypersensitivity reactions to β-lactam antibiotics. *Rev Infect Dis* 1983; **5** (Suppl. 2): 368–73.
4 Neu HC. Antistaphylococcal penicillins. *Med Clin North Am* 1982; **66**: 51–66.
5 Dyas A, Wise R. Ampicillin and alternatives. *BMJ* 1983; **286**: 583–5.
6 Anonymous. Augmentin—nice idea, but more trials please. *Drug Ther Bull* 1982; **20**: 21–4.
7 Rolinson GN, Watson A, eds. Augmentin clavulanate: potentiated amoxycillin. Proceedings of First Symposium. Amsterdam: Excerpta Medica, 1980.
8 Symposium on imipenem/cilastatin. *Am J Med* 1985; **78**: 6A.

Cephalosporins [1,2]

The cephalosporins are derivatives of 7-amino-cephalosporamic acid and are similar in structure and properties to the penicillins. They are bactericidal, acting on peptidoglycans in bacterial cell walls, and have wide spectra of activity encompassing Gram-negative organisms and staphylococci—penicillin-resistant staphylococci are generally susceptible but the degree of effectiveness varies between cephalosporins. Many are given parenterally but some orally effective ones are available (e.g. cefalexin, cefaclor). They are excreted by the kidney but unlike penicillin may cause tubular damage. Their main role is perhaps as alternative therapy in penicillin hypersensitivity, but this is not without risk as some 8–10% of all penicillin-allergic patients react to cephalosporins. Apart from this they have little dermatological use.

REFERENCES

1 Anonymous. Cephalosporins: now and tomorrow. *Drug Ther Bull* 1982; **20**: 85–8.
2 Donowitz GR, Mandell GL. β-Lactam antibiotics. *N Engl J Med* 1988; **318**: 490–500.

Quinolones [1]

The chief quinolone antibiotics are more correctly classified as fluoroquinolones or 4-quinolones. Their mode of action is via inhibition of DNA synthesis. Their spectrum of activity is broad and generally includes both Gram-positive and Gram-negative bacteria. The principal quinolone in wide use is ciprofloxacin; others include norfloxacin and ofloxacin. This can be given orally in doses of 750 mg twice daily for soft-tissue infections [2]. Ciprofloxacin is active *in vitro* against a wide range of bacteria from *Escherichia coli* to *Bacillus anthracis* and *Yersinia enterocolitica*. It is also active against staphylococci and streptococci as well as *Mycobacterium tuberculosis*, although atypical mycobacteria are generally less sensitive. In dermatology, ciprofloxacin is best reserved for severe infections such as those occurring in the immuno-compromised patient, but other indications include Gram-negative folliculitis, rhinoscleroma and cutaneous anthrax. It is an alternative treatment for chancroid and genital chlamydial infections.

REFERENCES

1 Gentry LO. Review of quinolones in treatment of infections of the skin and skin structure. *J Antimicrob Chemother* 1991; **28** (Suppl. C): 97–110.
2 Fass RJ. Treatment of skin and soft-tissue infections with oral ciprofloxacin. *J Antimicrob Chemother* 1986; **18** (Suppl.): 153–7.

Tetracyclines

These are orally effective broad-spectrum antibiotics with relatively low toxicity. The original three tetracyclines were chlortetracycline, oxytetracycline and tetracycline. Later derivatives include demethylchlortetracycline, methacycline, doxycycline and minocycline (the last three being synthetic). They act by inhibition of protein synthesis through ribosomal binding. With the exception of minocycline they all have similar spectra of activity; differing, however, in their absorption, distribution and excretion.

Both streptococci and staphylococci may be resistant to tetracyclines, although the incidence of staphylococcal resistance is less than previously and such strains are sensitive to minocycline [1]. However, as much more effective agents are available for these organisms, the tetracyclines are generally not used in these infections.

The tetracyclines are bacteriostatic against many Gram-positive and Gram-negative bacteria and are also active against rickettsiae, *Mycoplasma*, *Chlamydia*, which cause lymphogranuloma venerum, psittacosis and trachoma, as well as amoebae.

Absorption of some tetracyclines is impaired by simultaneously taking milk, aluminium, calcium or magnesium salts or iron preparations, because of chelation. However, food does not interfere with the absorption of doxycycline or minocycline. All tetracyclines are concentrated in the liver and excreted into the bile, whence they enter an enterohepatic circulation. Urinary excretion is significant and renal failure may be exacerbated by all except doxycycline [2].

Side effects [3–5]. A variety of rashes has been described (see Chapter 77), including phototoxicity, especially shown by demethylchlortetracycline [6]. Glossitis, cheilitis and persistent pruritus ani may occur. Gastrointestinal disturbances are dose dependent [7] and are much more common with doses of 2 g/day or more, which are rarely used in dermatology. Nausea and vomiting are direct irritant effects; diarrhoea may be the result of superinfection, resistant staphylococci being especially dangerous. Minocycline can cause vertigo and hyperpigmentation.

The latter is usually slate grey and can affect the skin, nails and sclerae [8]. Tetracyclines are deposited in growing teeth and bones [9] and their use should be avoided in pregnancy, during lactation and in childhood. Rarely, there may be diffuse fatty degeneration of the liver. An uncommon dermatological problem is the development of Gram-negative folliculitis after tetracycline therapy of acne [10,11].

Dermatological uses. Apart from the infections mentioned above, tetracyclines are rarely drugs of first choice. The exception, of course, is the treatment of acne vulgaris (see Chapter 42) [12,13] and rosacea (see Chapter 46).

Tetracycline, chlortetracycline, oxytetracycline

Dose: daily doses range from 500 mg (for acne) up to 3 g.

Doxycycline, minocycline

Dose: 100–200 mg/day. Doxycycline is the ordinary tetracycline of choice in patients with renal impairment. Minocycline is usually effective against staphylococci resistant to other tetracyclines and is used increasingly as a first-line treatment of acne (50 mg twice daily).

Preparations are also available as syrups, and injections for intramuscular, intravenous or intralesional use. Tetracycline resistance has been reported in *Propionibacterium acnes* and caution should be exercised over the use of repeated courses of these antibiotics. Resistance may also be passed to other bacteria [13].

REFERENCES

1 Finland M. Commentary. Twenty-fifth anniversary of the discovery of aureomycin: the place of the tetracyclines in antimicrobial chemotherapy. *Clin Pharmacol Ther* 1974; **15**: 3–8.
2 Ribush N, Morgan T. Tetracyclines and renal failure. *Med J Aust* 1972; **i**: 53–5.
3 Ad Hoc Committee Report. Systemic antibiotics for treatment of acne vulgaris. *Arch Dermatol* 1975; **111**: 1630–6.
4 Clendenning WE. Complications of tetracycline therapy. *Arch Dermatol* 1965; **91**: 628–32.
5 Kunin CM. The tetracyclines. *Pediatr Clin North Am* 1968; **15**: 43–55.
6 Falk MS. Light sensitivity due to demethylchlortetracycline: report of four cases. *JAMA* 1960; **172**: 1156–7.
7 Alestig K. Tetracyclines and chloramphenicol. In: Cohen J, Powderly WG, eds. *Infectious Diseases*. London: Mosby, 2004: 1843–7.
8 Angeloni VL, Salasche SJ, Ortiz R. Nail, skin and scleral pigmentation induced by minocycline. *Cutis* 1987; **40**: 229–33.
9 Macaulay JC, Leistyna JA. Preliminary observations on the prenatal administration of demethylchlortetracycline. *Pediatrics* 1964; **34**: 423–4.
10 Fulton JE, McGinley K, Leyden J et al. Gram-negative folliculitis in acne vulgaris. *Arch Dermatol* 1968; **98**: 349–53.
11 Leyden JL, Marples RR, Mills OH et al. Gram-negative folliculitis: complication of antibiotic therapy in acne vulgaris. *Br J Dermatol* 1973; **88**: 533–8.
12 Fry L, Ramsay CA. Tetracycline in acne vulgaris: clinical evaluation and sebum production. *Br J Dermatol* 1966; **78**: 653–60.
13 Moller JM, Leth Bak A, Stenderup A et al. Canging patterns of plasmid-mediated drug resistance during tetracycline therapy. *Antimicrob Agents Chemother* 1977; **11**: 388–94.

Macrolides

The main macrolide antibiotics are erythromycin and its derivatives azithromycin and clarithromycin. They work by binding to ribosomes and inhibiting protein synthesis.

Erythromycin [1]

Dose: 1–2 g/day in divided doses. This is the most widely used member of the macrolide group of antibiotics. It is active mainly against Gram-positive organisms such as staphylococci and streptococci. Staphylococci may rapidly develop resistance, especially in hospital, where in some studies as many as 50% of strains may be resistant; streptococci are also occasionally resistant.

Side effects include an allergic cholestatic hepatitis that occurs only with erythromycin estolate. Otherwise gastrointestinal problems such as dyspepsia and diarrhoea are not uncommon. Erythromycin is an extremely useful drug for the outpatient treatment of staphylococcal or streptococcal pyodermas, especially in the penicillin-allergic patient. It may also be used for atypical mycobacterial infections. Particular dermatological uses are for erythrasma and acne; it may safely be given in renal failure as less than 5% is excreted in the urine.

Azithromycin and clarithromycin [2]

These are newer macrolide agents with a somewhat different spectrum of activity than erythromycin and longer half-life. At present they are little used in dermatology, although they show promise as treatment for atypical mycobacterial infections, particularly those caused by the *Mycobacterium avium* complex, but *M. marinum* is also responsive [3].

REFERENCES

1 Washington JA, Wilson WR. Erythromycin: a microbial and clinical perspective after 30 years of clinical use. I. *Mayo Clin Proc* 1984; **60**: 189–203.
2 Piscitelli SC, Danziger LH, Rodvold KA. Clarithromycin and azithromycin. *Clin Pharm* 1992; **11**: 137–52.
3 Bonnet E, Debat-Zoguerch D, Petit N *et al.* Clarithromycin: a potent agent against infections due to *Mycobacterium marinum*. *Clin Infect Dis* 1994; **18**; 664–9.

Aminoglycosides

This group includes streptomycin (see below), neomycin, gentamicin, amikacin and tobramycin. They are little used in dermatological practice, their chief use being against Gram-negative infections. They inhibit protein synthesis; bacteria may rapidly become resistant, and cross-resistance occurs within the group. Normally there is almost no absorption by mouth. They are ototoxic and, to a lesser degree, nephrotoxic.

Dermatological uses. These are few. Streptomycin is still used in some countries for tuberculosis, is effective in tularaemia and some forms of actinomycetoma and can be used as an alternative to tetracyclines in granuloma venereum. The topical use of neomycin is discussed in Chapter 78.

Gentamicin [1] and amikacin [2]

Amikacin is now more widely used than gentamicin [2]. Its use is mainly restricted to the treatment of serious Gram-negative infections, especially those caused by *Pseudomonas aeruginosa* [3,4] and to *Nocardia* infections [5]. Gentamicin has a synergistic effect with carbenicillin against *Pseudomonas* and other Gram-negative organisms and is used in combination with penicillin for some forms of endocarditis. Aminoglycosides should not be used in pregnancy and should be controlled by measurements of plasma concentration.

REFERENCES

1 Second International Conference of Gentamicin. An aminoglycoside antibiotic. *J Infect Dis* 1971; **124** (Suppl.).
2 Sande MA, Mandell GL. Antimicrobial agents: the aminoglycosides. In: Gilman AG, Goodman LS, Rall TW, Murad F, eds. *Goodman and Gilman's The Pharmacological Basis of Therapeutics*, 7th edn. New York: Macmillan, 1985: 1150–69.
3 Bulger RJ, Sidell S, Kirby WMM. Laboratory and clinical studies of gentamicin: a new broad-spectrum antibiotic. *Ann Intern Med* 1963; **59**: 593–604.
4 Jao RL, Jackson GG. Gentamicin sulfate: new antibiotic against Gram-negative bacilli. *JAMA* 1964; **189**: 817–22.
5 Gombert ME, Berkowitz LB, Aulicino TM *et al.* Therapy of pulmonary nocardiosis in immunocompromised mice. *Antimicrob Agents Chemother* 1990; **34**: 1766–70.

Spectinomycin

This is an aminocyclitol antibiotic derived from a streptomycete species and is related to the aminoglycosides. Its use in dermatology is limited but it is very effective in the management of gonorrhoea as a single intramuscular injection [1].

REFERENCE

1 Holloway WJ. Spectinomycin. *Med Clin North Am* 1982; **66**: 169–84.

Lincosamides

Lincomycin and its derivative clindamycin (which ought to be used in preference to lincomycin) act against Gram-positive cocci including some penicillin-resistant staphylococci. They are highly active against *Bacteroides* infections and penetrate well into bone.

Side effects. Diarrhoea may occur in up to 20% of cases; pseudomembranous colitis may supervene and may last for weeks after the drug has been withdrawn [1,2]. There have been a number of deaths from this complication; one severe case has been reported in a patient treated for acne.

Clindamycin

This is an effective alternative drug for the treatment of acne [3]; however, in view of its known toxicity, it is now rarely used systemically for this condition. It is useful in a 1% formulation for the topical treatment of mild to moderate acne.

REFERENCES

1 Tedesco FJ, Barton RW, Alpers DH. Clindamycin associated colitis: a prospective study. *Ann Intern Med* 1974; **81**: 429–33.
2 Bartlett JG. *Clostridum difficile*: history of its role as an enteric pathogen and the current state of knowledge about the organism. *Clin Infect Dis* 1994; **18** (Suppl. 4): 265–9.
3 Christian GL, Krueger GG. Clindamycin vs placebo as adjunctive therapy in moderately severe acne. *Arch Dermatol* 1975; **111**: 997–1000.

Chloramphenicol

This would be a useful drug for a number of infections were it not for bone marrow aplasia, which occurs in 1 in 40 000 courses of treatment [1]. This has been known for 25 years, and yet a survey of 576 cases of blood dyscrasia caused by chloramphenicol concluded that in most cases there had been no indication to justify its use. Nevertheless, it remains an alternative treatment for typhoid fever and *Haemophilus influenzae* meningitis.

REFERENCE

1 Polak BCP, Wesseling H, Schut D *et al.* Blood dyscrasias attributed to chloramphenicol: a review of 576 published and unpublished cases. *Acta Med Scand* 1972; **192**: 409–14.

Rifamycins

See p. 72.37.

Polymyxins

Polymyxin B and polymyxin E (colistin) are relatively toxic drugs that are not absorbed from the gastrointestinal tract. Their use for Gram-negative infections has been largely superceded by gentamicin and ciprofloxacin. Polymyxin B is used topically.

Glycopeptide antibiotics

The two main examples of this group are vancomycin and teicoplanin. They act by inhibition of peptidoglycan polymer formation in bacterial cell walls. Vancomycin is chiefly used for the treatment of serious staphylococcal infections such as septicaemia as well as other life-threatening conditions such as pseudomembranous colitis. It has no obvious use in skin disease [1].

REFERENCE

1 Wise RI, Kory M, eds. Reassessments of vancomycin: a potentially useful antibiotic. *Rev Infect Dis* 1981; **3** (Suppl.): 199–300.

Fusidic acid [1]

This is produced by a strain of *Fusidium coccineum* and has the basic structure of a steroid, although it shows little in the way of metabolic effects. It is a very safe drug, primarily used for staphylococcal infections, although it is also active against other Gram-positive bacteria and the Gram-negative cocci. Nearly all strains of staphylococci are outstandingly sensitive to fusidic acid [2] but there have been increasing reports of resistant mutants, which can multiply rapidly. However, concomitant administration of penicillin can be used to kill any resistant mutants as they emerge. It is available for oral use, as an injection and for topical application. It is a useful drug for staphylococcal osteomyelitis in particular, and its indiscriminate prescription for minor infections should be discouraged for fear of encouraging resistant strains that are now emerging.

REFERENCE

1 Verbist L. The antimicrobial activity of fusidic acid. *J Antimicrob Chemother* 1990; **25** (Suppl. B): 1–5.
2 Drugeon HB, Caillon J, Juvin ME. *In vitro* antibacteral activity of fusidic acid alone and in combination with other antibiotics against methicillin sensitive and resistant *Staphylococcus aureus*. *J Antimicrob Chemother* 1994; **34**: 899–903.

Metronidazole [1,2]

Metronidazole is a synthetic agent active against protozoa and anaerobic bacteria. It is particularly useful in trichomoniasis, bacterial vaginosis [2], amoebiasis and giardiasis, and has proved extremely valuable against *Bacteroides* and *Helicobacter* species [3]. For the dermatologist it has a limited role in the treatment of tetracycline-failed rosacea [4]. Metronidazole is well absorbed by the oral or rectal route and it may be applied topically. It may also be given intravenously. It is available as 200 and 400 mg tablets, the usual adult oral dosage being 200 mg twice daily for rosacea, 200 mg every 8 h for *Trichomonas* infections, 400 mg every 8 h for anaerobic bacterial infections and 800 mg every 8 h for amoebiasis. The suppositories contain 500 mg, and in anaerobic infections are prescribed in the adult dosage of 1 g every 8 h at first, dropping to 1 g every 12 h. Topical formulations are available for the treatment of rosacea.

The fate and mode of excretion of metronidazole are not fully understood [5]; it is generally regarded as safe in hepatic and renal disease. There is no evidence that it is a human teratogen, and it may be given to lactating mothers, although it causes darkening of milk and may give it a bitter taste. In normal doses and for short periods it is generally a remarkably safe drug but minor gastrointestinal side effects such as nausea and an unpleasant taste in the mouth are not uncommon. Vomiting, abdominal pain and diarrhoea may follow. Darkening of urine, headache and drowsiness also occur, and leukopenia may be noted. Much less common adverse reactions are peripheral neuropathy, particularly associated with prolonged treatment, and central nervous system effects (dizziness, ataxia and fits) from high dosage. The only important interaction is with alcohol, which produces a disulfiram-like reaction in some patients.

REFERENCES

1 Phillips I, Collier J, eds. *Metronidazole*. London: Royal Society of Medicine International Congress and Symposium Series, No. 18, 1979.
2 Centers for Disease Control (CDC). Sexually transmitted diseases: treatment guidelines. *MMWR* 42 (No RR-14).
3 Rosenblatt JE, Edson RS. Metronidazole. *Mayo Clin Proc* 1983; **53**: 154–62.
4 Saihan EM, Burton JL. A double-blind trial of metronidazole versus oxytetracycline therapy for rosacea. *Br J Dermatol* 1980; **102**: 443–5.
5 Somogyi AA, Kong CE, Gurr FW *et al.* Metronidazole pharmacokinetics in patients with acute renal failure. *J Antimicrob Chemother* 1984; **13**: 183–9.

Antituberculous drugs (see Chapter 28)

The important first-line drugs for the treatment of *Mycobacterium tuberculosis* infections are isoniazid, rifampicin, ethambutol and, in some cases, streptomycin [1,2]. In the initial period of treatment, usually 60 days or until sensitivities are available, three of these drugs are used concurrently. For the continuation phase of therapy, two drugs to which the organism is sensitive are sufficient for cure without the occurrence of resistant strains (for details see Chapter 28).

Second-line drugs such as pyrazinamide, ethionamide, cycloserine, PABA or thiacetazone may be required where drug resistance or adverse reactions preclude the use of more than one of the four first-line agents.

The emergence of multidrug-resistant strains of *Mycobacterium tuberculosis* (MDR-TB) is a major potential threat [3], particularly as they may affect AIDS patients who expectorate large numbers of bacilli.

Isoniazid

This is a synthetic, orally absorbed bactericidal agent usually given in a dosage of 300 mg/day to adults (5–10 mg/kg every 24 h). It is excreted mainly by the kidney after acetylation and further metabolism. It can be used in pregnancy [4] but during lactation should be supplemented with pyridoxine because of the theoretical risk of toxic side effects (see below). In severe renal failure, the adult dosage should be reduced to 200 mg/day. Adverse reactions may be divided into toxic and allergic. Toxic reactions are more common in slow acetylators and include most commonly peripheral neuropathy but also convulsions, mental disturbances and a pellagra-like rash [5]. They are usually reversible on cessation of therapy. Pyridoxine 10 mg/day given prophylactically will reduce the incidence of these problems where high doses are used. The main allergic reactions are rashes, agranulocytosis and hepatitis, this last being apparently more common in patients with pre-existing liver disease [6].

Rifampicin

This is a synthetically modified antibiotic of the rifamycin group. It is bactericidal and very effective against *M. tuberculosis*, many atypical myobacteria and Grampositive cocci. It is also useful in leprosy. To counter the emergence of resistant strains, it is always used in combination with other antimicrobials.

Rifampicin is well absorbed orally and is available as 150 mg capsules and a 100 mg/5 mL mixture. In adults it is usual to prescribe 450–600 mg/day as a single dose before breakfast (10 mg/kg/day). Excretion is predominantly in the bile and so hepatic impairment is an indication for avoidance or at least lower dosage. In pregnancy, rifampicin is best avoided but where it has been used the incidence of abnormalities noted at birth has not been excessively high—4.3% compared with 1.8% in tuberculous controls [7]. If used in late pregnancy it may cause haemorrhagic problems in neonates. Rifampicin is generally regarded as a relatively non-toxic antituberculous drug but many different adverse reactions have been described: mild gastrointestinal disturbances and rashes —particularly flushing [8,9]. Transient impairment of liver function as revealed by elevation of transaminase levels is common but need not usually interrupt therapy. Orangered discoloration of urine, saliva and sweat may be noticed. Thrombocytopenia, however, is an uncommon side effect that must not be ignored. Three other serious adverse reactions are a flu-like illness, a syndrome of dyspnoea, wheezing and hypotension, and the occurrence of renal failure, all of which are characteristically associated with intermittent or irregular medication [10]. Drug interactions occur with warfarin (diminished anticoagulant effect), oral contraceptives (possibly) and corticosteroids (diminished steroid effect).

Other rifamycins. Rifabutin has particular activity against *M. avium–intracellulare* in addition to *M. tuberculosis*. It is used, for instance, as prophylaxis in patients with low CD4 counts. It may also be useful where there is a high risk of rifampicin resistance.

Streptomycin

This is an aminoglycoside antibiotic used mainly in the treatment of tuberculosis. It must be administered parenterally and is commonly given in a dosage of 500–1000 mg/day by intramuscular injection. Lower dosage is preferred in patients over 40 years [11]. Excretion is by the kidney so that dosage should be reduced in renal impairment. Dosage reduction is also important in the premature infant. Of the important side effects, the most common is vertigo, which is especially troublesome in elderly people. Deafness may also develop and both these eighth-nerve effects are dose related [12]. These two adverse reactions provide a strong contraindication to the use of streptomycin in pregnancy and lactation as the infant may be affected, and in patients with pre-existing vestibular or auditory impairment. Allergic reactions include skin eruptions from the trivial to exfoliative dermatitis, eosinophilia and drug fever. Contact sensitization to streptomycin is a well-recognized hazard among nurses, justifying precautions to avoid skin contamination (e.g. by wearing gloves). Because streptomycin is a neuromuscular-blocking agent, it may increase the effects of suxamethonium and other similar drugs, and should be used only with extreme caution in myasthenia gravis.

Ethambutol

This is a synthetic agent effective only against *M. tuberculosis* and some atypical mycobacteria. It is orally absorbed and is available on its own as 100 and 400 mg tablets and in combination with isoniazid in a variety of strengths. The usual initial dosage is 15 mg/kg/day in adults and 25 mg/kg/day in children, reducing later in that age group to 15 mg/kg/day. It may also be used as intermittent treatment in a dosage of 45–50 mg/kg twice weekly. Excretion is mainly via the kidney, necessitating reduction of dosage in renal impairment. Optic (retrobulbar) neuritis with diminished visual acuity and red-green colour blindness, slowly reversible on cessation of therapy, was a relatively common side effect of higher dosage regimens but should be rare with currently recommended levels [13,14]. It seems to be more effective to train patients to check their own vision regularly when on this drug than to rely on periodic ophthalmic examinations. Ethambutol may also, although rarely, cause peripheral neuropathy and renal damage, and may precipitate attacks of gout. It appears not to be a teratogen in humans and is not contraindicated during lactation.

Para-aminosalicylic acid

This drug is much less active than the above drugs, but has a role in preventing the emergence of resistant strains of *M. tuberculosis*. It is given in the high dosage of 10–20 g/day and unfortunately is associated with a high incidence of minor but unpleasant side effects [15]—gastrointestinal symptoms occur in nearly all patients. Allergic reactions with rashes and fever are common and there seems to be either cross-hypersensitivity with streptomycin or potentiation of streptomycin allergy. Although once a valued drug in triple therapy, its use is now largely restricted to poorer countries where its low cost is a major consideration.

Other antituberculous drugs [2]

A number of other antituberculous drugs are available and may be required if resistance or hypersensitivity reactions preclude the use of standard treatment. They include pyrazinamide, capreomycin, ethionamide and cycloserine. Pyrazinamide is bactericidal and low-priced [16].

REFERENCES

1 Grange J. Antimycobacterial agents. In: Finch RG, Greenwood D, Norrby SR, Whitley RJ, eds. *Antibiotics and Chemotherapy*, 8th edn. Edinburgh: Churchill Livingstone, 2003: 507–32.
2 Inderlied CB. Mycobacteria. In: Cohen J, Powderly WG, eds. *Infectious Diseases*. London: Mosby, 2004: 2285–308.
3 Frieden TR, Sterling T, Pablos-Mendez A *et al.* The emergence of drug-resistant tuberculosis in New York City. *N Engl J Med* 1993; **328**: 521–6.
4 Ludford J, Doster B, Woolpert SF. Effect of isoniazid on reproduction. *Am Rev Respir Dis* 1973; **108**: 1170–4.
5 Horne NW. Side-effects of isoniazid. *Practitioner* 1972; **208**: 263–4.
6 Girling DJ. The hepatic toxicity of antituberculosis regimens containing isoniazid, rifampicin and pyrazinamide. *Tubercle* 1978; **59**: 13–32.
7 Steen JSM, Stainton-Ellis DM. Rifampicin in pregnancy. *Lancet* 1977; **ii**: 604–5.
8 Girling DJ. Adverse reactions to rifampicin in antituberculous regimens. *J Antimicrob Chemother* 1977; **3**: 115–32.
9 Girling DJ, Hitze KL. Adverse reactions to rifampicin. *Bull WHO* 1979; **57**: 45–9.
10 Flynn CT, Rainford DJ, Hope E. Acute renal failure and rifampicin: danger of unsuspected intermittent dosage. *BMJ* 1974; **ii**: 482.
11 Line DH, Poole GW, Waterworth PM. Serum streptomycin levels and dizziness. *Tubercle* 1970; **51**: 76–81.
12 Ballantyne J. Iatrogenic deafness. *J Laryngol Otol* 1970; **84**: 967–1000.
13 Clarke GEM, Cuthbert J, Cuthbert RJ *et al.* Isoniazid plus ethambutol in the initial treatment of pulmonary tuberculosis. *Br J Dis Chest* 1972; **66**: 272–5.
14 Lees AW, Allan GW, Smith J *et al.* Toxicity for rifampicin plus isoniazid and rifampicin plus ethambutol therapy. *Tubercle* 1971; **52**: 182–90.
15 Russouw JE, Saunders SJ. Hepatic complications of antituberculous chemotherapy. *Q J Med* 1975; **44**: 1–16.
16 Heifets LB, Lindholm-Levy PJ. Is pyrazinamide bactericidal against *Mycobacterium tuberculosis*? *Am Rev Respir Dis* 1990; **141**: 250–3.

Antileprosy agents

Sulphones

The sulphones were the first effective compounds used for the treatment of leprosy. The principal agent is 4,4-diaminodiphenyl sulphone (dapsone). The sulphones are related to the sulphonamides, and probably act in the same way. *Mycobacterium leprae* is usually extremely sensitive [1] but may become resistant. The sulphones are bacteriostatic, not bactericidal.

Dapsone. This drug is orally absorbed and is available in the form of 50 and 100 mg tablets. The usual adult dosage in leprosy is 50–100 mg/day. It is excreted mainly in the urine [2]. Some degree of haemolysis is an extremely common adverse reaction [3,4]. In pregnancy and lactation there is clearly a risk of haemolysis and methaemoglobinaemia in the baby, but the presence of dapsone in breast milk may have prophylactic value against leprosy [5]. Resistance to dapsone is known to occur in approximately 20% of patients who receive the drug for the treatment of leprosy as a single agent. With the use of multiple-drug regimens, this complication is thought to be much rarer. Leprosy apart, dapsone is a well-established means of suppressing the cutaneous lesions of dermatitis herpetiformis [6] and several other diseases. Most dermatologists are more familiar with the use of the drug in this way and further details are described in Chapter 41.

Clofazimine (Lamprene®) [7,8]

This oral synthetic drug is a phenazine dye. The usual dosage is 100 mg three times a week or 100 mg/day in combination with rifampicin if sulphone resistance has occurred [9]. It has an anti-inflammatory effect that may prevent erythema nodosum from developing. For lepra reactions, 300 mg/day is recommended. Clofazimine has a very long half-life: 70 days or more. It accumulates in the tissues and is slowly excreted in urine, sweat, sebum and milk.

The main side effect is the emergence of red-brown to black discoloration of skin and conjunctivae, but urine and sputum become red too and breast milk may be discolored. Mild gastrointestinal reactions may occur and ichthyosiform rashes [10]. In general, clofazimine is a well-tolerated drug that may be prescribed in pregnancy and during lactation. In renal and hepatic impairment, biochemical tests of function are recommended from time to time but the drug may be used. Clofazimine may be valuable in treating pyoderma gangrenosum [11] and perhaps also in discoid lupus erythematosus.

Rifampicin

This drug has been discussed previously (under Antituberculosis drugs). It seems to be bactericidal for *M. leprae* in very low dosage and acts much more rapidly than dapsone, rendering the patient non-contagious in a few days or weeks [12]. It does not shorten the total duration of treatment, which should be continued with dapsone.

Thiambutosine

This is a diphenylthiourea, useful as a second-line drug when dapsone cannot be used. Resistance may develop, especially after 1 year of treatment.

REFERENCES

1 Shepard CC, Levy L, Fasal P. The sensitivity to dapsone (DDS) of *Mycobacterium leprae* from patients with and without previous treatment. *Am J Trop Med Hyg* 1969; **18**: 258–63.
2 Alexander JO'D, Young E, McFadyen T *et al.* Absorption and excretion of 35S dapsone in dermatitis herpetiformis. *Br J Dermatol* 1970; **83**: 620–31.
3 Anonymous. Adverse reactions to dapsone. *Lancet* 1981; **ii**: 184–5.
4 Cream JJ, Scott GL. Anaemia in dermatitis herpetiformis: the role of dapsone-induced haemolysis and malabsorption. *Br J Dermatol* 1970; **82**: 333–42.
5 Forrest JM. Drugs in pregnancy and lactation. *Med J Aust* 1976; **ii**: 138–41.
6 Fry L, Walkden V, Wojnarowska F *et al.* A comparison of IgA-positive and IgA-negative dapsone responsive dermatoses. *Br J Dermatol* 1980; **102**: 371–82.
7 Levy L. Pharmacological studies of clofazimine. *Am J Trop Med Hyg* 1974; **23**: 1097–109.
8 Rodriguez JN, Albalos RM, Reich CV *et al.* Effects of the administration of B663 (Lamprene®, clofazimine) on three groups of lepromatous and borderline cases of leprosy. *Int J Leprosy* 1974; **42**: 276–88.
9 Yawalker SJ, Vischer W. Lamprene (clofazimine) in leprosy. *Leprosy Rev* 1979; **50**: 135–44.
10 Michaelsson G, Molin L, Ohman S *et al.* Clofazimine: a new agent for the treatment of pyoderma gangrenosum. *Arch Dermatol* 1976; **112**: 344–9.
11 Kark EC, Davis BR, Pomeranz JR. Pyoderma gangrenosum treated with clofazimine: report of three cases. *J Am Acad Dermatol* 1981; **4**: 152–9.
12 Browne SG. The drug treatment of leprosy. *Practitioner* 1975; **215**: 493–500.

Antifungal drugs [1–3]

The drugs available for systemic use against fungal diseases are few in number. There are three main families of antifungals: the polyenes (amphotericin B); the azoles, which include the imidazoles (e.g. ketoconazole, miconazole) and the triazoles (fluconazole and itraconazole); and the allylamines. There is also a miscellaneous group of drugs such as griseofulvin, tolnaftate and flucytosine. Most antifungals work through damage to or inhibition of the fungal cell membrane. The main exceptions are the pyrimidine analogue, flucytosine, which affects RNA and DNA synthesis, and potassium iodide which probably affects phagocytic function.

Polyenes [4]

Nystatin [4]

Nystatin was the first polyene antibiotic discovered and is still valuable today as a topical anti-*Candida* agent. It is not absorbed from the gut in significant amounts.

Amphotericin B [1,4]

This is a polyene antibiotic derived from *Streptomyces nodosus*. It has a very wide range of activity against *Candida* spp. and almost all deep fungal pathogens. Resistance is rare. Absorption from the gut is negligible and so, as with nystatin, tablets and lozenges are for practical purposes topical therapy for the mouth or prophylaxis. For systemic use, amphotericin B must be given by slow intravenous infusion in 5% dextrose. This solution is unstable; it should be used promptly and other drugs should not be added, except heparin or hydrocortisone. The definitive adult dosage range is normally in the range of 0.4–1 mg/kg/day but toxicity is minimized if there is a build-up from a very low dose (1 mg) on the first day, to full dosage by days 3–5. In the seriously ill patient, a more rapid build-up to full dosage over 24–48 h is necessary.

The fate of amphotericin in the body is not fully understood [5]. Only small amounts appear in urine; much is probably bound to sterol-containing membranes. Adverse reactions are common: initially, fever, rigors, hypotension, nausea, vomiting, tinnitus and bronchospasm. Phlebitis at the site of infusion is also frequent. Hypokalaemia and hypochromic anaemia may occur and, rarely, liver function abnormalities. Nephrotoxicity is of great importance; renal clearance may be decreased and tubular damage may develop. These are particularly problems of extended treatment but are potentially reversible. If renal impairment is severe, therapy must be interrupted and should be restarted at a lower dosage.

Amphotericin B is used principally for systemic mycoses such as candidosis, aspergillosis, mucormycosis and cryptococcosis as well as the endemic respiratory infections such as histoplasmosis.

Lipid-associated amphotericins

Three formulations of lipid-associated amphotericin B have been developed: a liposomal formulation (AmBisome), a colloidal dispersion (Amphocil®) and a lipid complex (Abelcet®). They can be used at much higher dosage (usually 3 mg/day) without nephrotoxicity [6].

Flucytosine [7]

This is a synthetic cytosine analogue that is converted to 5-fluorouracil in the body. It is effective against yeasts, including *Candida* spp., *Cryptococcus neoformans* and many of the fungi involved in chromoblastomycosis. It is orally absorbed but may be given intravenously too. The tablets contain 500 mg, the usual adult dosage being 150 mg/kg/day. Lower doses are necessary in renal failure. It is important to monitor serum levels, aiming to achieve 40–60 mg/L and to avoid toxic levels—above 120 mg/L. Because resistance, both primary and secondary, is well recognized, sensitivity testing initially and at intervals is strongly recommended. It is rarely used on its own. In cryptococcal meningitis in the non-AIDS patient, flucytosine and amphotericin B are given in combination. They appear to be more effective as a combination than amphotericin B on its own and the daily dosage of the latter can be reduced to 0.4–0.6 mg/kg.

The main side effects are nausea, vomiting, diarrhoea and rashes, but thrombocytopenia and neutropenia may also occur.

Azoles

Miconazole

This is a commonly used topical imidazole, poorly absorbed by the oral route. It may be administered intravenously by slow infusion three times in 24 h, the usual adult dosage being 1.8–3 g/day. Side effects are not particularly common. They include pruritus, rashes, fever, faintness and venous thrombosis at the infusion site. Anorexia, nausea, vomiting and diarrhoea occur and anaphylaxis is a rare but genuine problem. It is seldom used now except in infections caused by *Scedosporium apiospermum* [8].

Ketoconazole [9,10]

Ketoconazole is a broad-spectrum imidazole, which is available in different topical formulations from cream to shampoo or as an oral agent. The drug is well absorbed after oral administration, although lower levels are seen in patients who are neutropenic. It is effective in chronic mucocutaneous candidosis and widespread dermatophytosis. It can also be used topically for pityriasis versicolor. It also appears to be effective in mycetoma infections caused by *Madurella mycetomatis* but not in sporotrichosis. Certain systemic mycoses such as paracoccidioidomycosis and those with soft-tissue lesions are the most sensitive [10].

Adverse events are not common but include headache, vomiting and giddiness as well as nausea. It also leads to blockade of androgen biosynthesis by interference with cytochrome P-450 at high dosage [11]. This results in symptoms such as gynaecomastia in men and menstrual irregularities in women. In addition, it causes asymptomatic changes in liver function and overt hepatitis on occasions [12]. The true frequency of the latter is estimated to be about 1 in 10 000 but it may be more common in patients receiving treatment for nail disease. It is more common also in those with a prior history of liver disease. While this is a comparatively uncommon complaint, it is sufficient to limit the use of the drug in superficial fungal disease. Also, much of its function has been assumed by the development of itraconazole and fluconazole (see below). Drug resistance is also seen rarely [13].

Itraconazole [14]

Itraconazole is a triazole antifungal drug that is avidly bound in tissue, including skin. Its serum levels are generally low after a 100–200-mg dose. It is given orally and has a broad spectrum of action against the main fungal pathogens. It is effective in dermatophytosis, candidosis and *Malassezia* infections. Originally used in a dosage of 100 mg/day, it is now often given at 200 or 400 mg. At higher doses it is possible to use shorter courses such as 400 mg/day for 1 week in tinea corporis. Because it is retained for very long periods in the nail, it is used in pulses of 400 mg/day for 1 week per month for 3–4 months [15].

In vaginal candidosis it is given as a single treatment of 600 mg/day and it produces responses in oropharyngeal candidiasis in doses of 100–200 mg/day. For recalcitrant pityriasis versicolor, a total dose of 1000 mg is necessary. Other infections responding to itraconazole include sporotrichosis, chromomycosis, paracoccidioidomycosis and histoplasmosis [14]. It has also been reported to be effective in cryptococcal meningitis, particularly as a long-term suppressive therapy of HIV-positive patients. Itraconazole is unusual amongst azoles in producing responses against aspergillosis.

Although itraconazole may occasionally cause nausea and headache, more serious adverse reactions, such as hepatic reactions and anaphylaxis, are extremely rare.

A new formulation of itraconazole in cyclodextrin, as well as an intravenous form, are also available. This oral solution is much better absorbed in AIDS patients than the conventional formulation.

Fluconazole [16]

Fluconazole is a triazole antifungal that is well absorbed after oral administration. It may also be given intravenously. Unusually for an azole, it is mainly excreted via the kidney. It is active against a range of fungal pathogens.

The principal uses of fluconazole in dermatology are in the treatment of oropharyngeal and vaginal candidosis [17]. In the latter disease, it is effective in a single dose of 150 mg; with oropharyngeal infections, treatment responses are rapid, often within 3 days of starting therapy with 50–100 mg/day [18]. For dermatophytosis, it has been found that weekly doses of 150 mg may be effective after 2–3 weeks and a similar weekly pulse has been used for onychomycosis. In systemic mycoses it is used in the management of cryptococcosis, either as primary therapy or long-term suppression, and in systemic candidosis [19].

Few adverse effects apart from nausea and dyspepsia have been attributed to fluconazole. The dosage of the drug has to be reduced in patients with renal impairment.

Certain fungi such as *Candida krusei*, *C. glabrata* and some strains of *C. albicans* may be primarily resistant to fluconazole and secondary resistance may develop in immunocompromised patients [16].

Other azoles

Two new orally active triazoles in development, voriconazole and posaconazole, have not been evaluated in superficial fungal disease. They show promise in the management of a range of systemic infections.

Allylamines

Terbinafine [20]

Terbinafine is a fungicidal allylamine antifungal, similar to naftifine. It works by the inhibition of squalene epoxidation in the synthesis of the ergosterol in the fungal cell membrane [21]. The accumulation of squalene in the cell is thought to contribute to its *in vitro* fungicidal activity. It may be given orally or topically in a dosage of 125 mg twice daily. Its chief use is in dermatophytosis, where it is highly effective even in patients with chronic infections of the hands and feet. In onychomycosis it is given in a regimen of 250 mg/day for 6 weeks for fingernails and 12 weeks for toenails [22]. It is less active when given orally in superficial candidosis and pityriasis versicolor. In dermatophytosis there is a particularly low relapse rate with this drug. Recently, it has been shown to be active in a range of other deep fungal infections, from sporotrichosis to chromoblastomycosis.

There are few side effects apart from the occasional episode of gastrointestinal discomfort. Loss of taste may occur but is reversible. Skin rashes have also been reported. Hepatic reactions are extremely rare.

Griseofulvin [23]

Griseofulvin is derived from a number of *Penicillium* species. It is a fungistatic drug whose principal activity is directed against dermatophytes. Its mode of action is via the inhibition of the formation of intracellular microtubules.

The usual human dosage is 10 mg/kg/day in tablet or, in children, solution form. Treatment duration varies between 2 and 4 weeks for tinea corporis to over 1 year for onychomycosis. The success rate even after 1 year of treatment for toenail infections is less than 30–40%.

Drug interaction with phenobarbital and coumarin anticoagulants occur. Side effects include headaches and nausea, but serious reactions are extremely rare. There are a few reports of apparent precipitation or exacerbation of systemic lupus erythematosus and porphyrias by griseofulvin.

Potassium iodide [2]

In the form of a saturated aqueous solution (100 g in 100 mL water), this is the preferred treatment for lymphocutaneous sporotrichosis and subcutaneous zygomycosis (basidiobolomycosis). It is administered orally, starting with 0.6 mL three times daily and gradually increasing until a level of four or five times the dose is attained in an adult. The mode of action is obscure. Progress must be expected to be slow and treatment should be continued until 4 weeks after apparent cure. Iodides are best avoided in pregnancy because of the risk of goitre and hypothyroidism in the infant. Adverse reactions include iododerma, salivary and lacrimal gland swelling and hypersecretion, and gastrointestinal disturbances, as well as anxiety, depression and hypothyroidism.

Cell wall antagonists

A number of new antifungals are in development that have a different site of action, the inhibition of the cell wall. Caspofungin is an echinocandin that blocks glucan synthase [24]. It is available as an intravenous drug for use in the treatment of aspergillosis or candidosis, particularly caused by resistant *Candida* species.

REFERENCES

1 Bennett JE. Chemotherapy of systemic mycoses. *N Engl J Med* 1974; **290**: 30–2.
2 Roberts DT. The current status of systemic antifungal agents. *Br J Dermatol* 1982; **106**: 597–602.
3 Speller DCE, ed. *Antifungal Chemotherapy*. Chichester: John Wiley, 1980.
4 Medoff G, Kobayashi GA. The polyenes. In: Speller DCE, ed. *Antifungal Chemotherapy*. Chichester: John Wiley, 1980: 3–33.
5 Atkinson AJ, Bennett JE. Amphotericin B pharmacokinetics in humans. *Antimicrob Agents Chemother* 1978; **13**: 271–6.
6 Hay RJ. Lipid amphotericin B combinations: 'la crème de la crème'? *J Infect* 1999; **38**: 16–20.
7 Bennett JE. Flucytosine. *Ann Intern Med* 1977; **86**: 319–22.
8 Lutwick LI, Rytel MW, Yanez JP *et al.* Deep infections of *Petriellidium boydii* treated with miconazole. *JAMA* 1979; **241**: 272–3.
9 Cox FW, Stiller RL, South DA *et al.* Oral ketoconazole for dermatophyte infections. *J Am Acad Dermatol* 1982; **6**: 455–62.
10 Jones HE. *Ketoconazole Today*. Manchester: Adis, 1987.
11 Stern RS. Ketoconazole: assessing the risks. *J Am Acad Dermatol* 1982; **6**: 544.
12 Heidberg JK, Svejgaard E. Toxic hepatitis during ketoconazole treatment. *BMJ* 1981; **283**: 825–6.
13 Ryley JF, Wilson RG, Barrett-Bee KJ. Azole resistance in *Candida albicans*. *Sabouraudia* 1984; **22**: 53–63.
14 Grant SM, Clissold SP. Itraconazole. *Drugs* 1989; **37**: 310–44.
15 Hay RJ, ed. *Itraconazole*. Manchester: Adis, 1994.
16 Powderly WB, Van't Wout JW, eds. *Fluconazole*. York: Marius, 1992.
17 Brammer KW. Treatment of vaginal candidiasis with a single oral dose of fluconazole. *Eur J Clin Microbiol Infect Dis* 1988; **7**: 364–7.
18 Dupont B, Drouhet E. Fluconazole in the management of oropharyngeal candidosis in a predominantly HIV antibody positive group of patients. *J Med Vet Mycol* 1988; **26**: 67–71.
19 Stern JJ, Hartman BJ, Sharkey P *et al.* Oral fluconazole therapy for patients with acquired immunodeficiency syndrome and cryptococcosis: experience with 22 patients. *Am J Med* 1988; **85**: 477–80.
20 Jones TC, Villars VV. Terbinafine. In: Ryley J, ed. *Chemotherapy of Fungal Diseases*. Berlin: Springer, 1990: 455–82.
21 Ryder NS, Meith H. Allylamine antifungal drugs In: Borgers M, Hay R, Rinaldi MG, eds. *Current Topics in Medical Mycology*, Vol. 4. New York: Springer, 1992: 158–88.
22 Crawford F. Young P. Godfrey C *et al.* Oral treatments for toenail onychomycosis: a systematic review. *Arch Dermatol* 2002; **138**: 811–6.
23 Davies RR. Griseofulvin. In: Speller DCE, ed. *Antifungal Chemotherapy*. Chichester: John Wiley, 1980: 149–82.
24 Abruzzo GK. Gill CJ. Flattery AM *et al.* Efficacy of the echinocandin caspofungin against disseminated aspergillosis and candidiasis in cyclophosphamide-induced immunosuppressed mice. *Antimicrob Agents Chemother* 2000; **44**: 2310–8.

Antiviral drugs

With the spread of HIV infection, considerable efforts have now been expended in searching for new antiviral drugs. Despite this there are still few effective antiviral agents [1]. Because there are fewer steps involved in the assembly of viruses, and these are inextricably associated with human metabolic and other cellular functions, the ratio between antiviral activity and host toxicity is often a narrow one. Many agents employed in the treatment of viral infections of the skin have one of three viral targets: inhibition of viral polymerase (e.g. aciclovir), inhibition of reverse transcriptase (e.g. zidovudine) or protease inhibition (e.g. indinavir). The two latter groups are mainly used for the treatment of retroviral infections.

Other approaches to treatment have involved the use of interferons, which have proved to be of limited value in most viral infections apart from some genital papillomavirus infections, and many of the available preparations are associated with dose-limiting side effects when given intravenously.

Drug resistance will occur with antivirals but often it involves a modification of the viral genome that may, in turn, affect viral pathogenetic mechanisms. This alteration in viruses may affect their capacity to cause disease except in severely immunocompromised patients such as those with AIDS.

Vidarabine (adenosine arabinoside, ARA-A)

This purine nucleoside acts by inhibiting viral DNA synthesis. It has effects mainly against the herpes group of viruses and appears to be effective in early cases of herpes simplex encephalitis and in varicella-zoster infections of immunocompromised subjects. However, its use has largely been superceded by aciclovir. At a dosage of 10 mg/kg/day intravenously it causes mainly mild gastrointestinal side effects, and rashes in 5% of subjects. CNS and haematological side effects have also been reported [2]. A 3% ointment has an established place in the topical treatment of herpes simplex keratoconjunctivitis.

Idoxuridine

This synthetic nucleoside is effective against DNA viruses, particularly the herpes group. Its use is now restricted to topical application because of severe bone marrow and hepatic toxicity when given intravenously. It has been used in 5–40% concentration in dimethyl sulfoxide (DMSO) to shorten the duration of clinical symptoms in herpes zoster infections. It can also be used in herpes keratitis but is less effective in genital herpes simplex infections [3].

Aciclovir [4–7]

This antiviral agent works by inhibition of DNA synthesis. Its mode of action involves activation by thymidine kinase and subsequent inhibition of viral polymerase. Resistance to aciclovir has been recorded sometimes, following alterations to or deficiency of thymidine kinase. This has been associated with lack of response to therapy [8,9].

Aciclovir is very active against herpesviruses. In serious infections it has been used intravenously but it is also available as 200-mg tablets, as an ophthalmic ointment and as a cream [5]. Unfortunately, it has no effect on the latent phase of either herpes simplex or zoster and is apparently ineffective in clinical practice against other viruses. The intravenous dosage for serious systemic herpes simplex infections is 5 mg/kg every 8 h by slow infusion (over 1 h). In herpes zoster, 10 mg/kg every 8 h is advised. Orally, 200 mg every 4 h (five times daily) is effective and a remarkably safe treatment for severe vulvovaginal herpes simplex [10], for example.

Studies with aciclovir have shown that it is possible to suppress recurrences of herpes simplex by intermittent administration over a long period. This has given rise to concerns over the risk of drug resistance and this approach is really only indicated in a few patients with incapacitating recurrent attacks of infection [11].

Aciclovir is less effective against herpes zoster unless given in higher dosage (e.g. 10 mg/kg intravenously 8 hourly [12]. It is therefore mainly used for treatment of varicella-zoster infection in immunocompromised patients.

The main route of excretion is renal [13]. Side effects include elevation of blood urea and creatinine, which may rarely progress to acute renal failure. In patients with established renal impairment, lower doses are indicated. Although animal and human evidence shows no teratogenic activity, aciclovir is best avoided in pregnancy. Levels are reported to be higher in human milk than in serum when given during lactation.

Newer drugs related to aciclovir

These include famciclovir, penciclovir, ganciclovir and valaciclovir [14].

Famciclovir. This is well absorbed after oral administration. It is used at a dosage of 250–500 mg up to three times daily. At these dosages it appears to be as effective as the higher dose regimen of intravenous aciclovir and is well tolerated. There is also a lower frequency of post-herpetic neuralgia after its use.

Penciclovir. This is a promising treatment for severe herpes simplex infections and, because of its pharmacokinetic properties, is given less frequently than aciclovir.

Ganciclovir [15]. This is another deoxyguanosine analogue, which can be used in the treatment or prophylaxis of cytomegalovirus (CMV) infections. It is also active against other herpesviruses. Its use is generally reserved for CMV infections in severely immunocompromised patients when it is given in a starting dosage of 5 mg/kg/12 h intravenously. It can also be used as long-term suppressive therapy to prevent relapse. However, there is a high frequency of nephrotoxicity as well as metabolic disturbances such as hypokalaemia or hypocalcaemia.

Valaciclovir. This has a similar antiviral spectrum to aciclovir. It is mainly used for the treatment of herpes zoster infections (1000 mg for 7–14 days). It is also used for shorter periods (5 days) for herpes simplex infections [16].

Zidovudine (AZT, Retrovir®) [17]

AZT has been developed for the treatment of human retrovirus infections. Its principal site of action is the inhibition of virus-RNA-dependent DNA polymerase (reverse transcriptase) [18]. AZT is given by the oral route and the normal dosage is 250–500 mg/day; variations to this regimen and drug combinations are under assessment. The use of AZT in patients with AIDS or symptomatic HIV infections has been found to result in higher levels of circulating CD4 lymphocytes and, in some studies, a decrease in mortality over the short term. Treated patients are still infectious and the therapy does not cure the infection. It is currently used to treat HIV patients with CD4 counts lower than $500/mm^3$ [19]. It has been suggested that AZT may benefit some skin complications of AIDS such as psoriasis. Administration of AZT to infected women in the second and third trimesters of pregnancy significantly reduces the risk of neonatal infection [20].

The main toxic side effects of zidovudine are neutropenia and anaemia, which occur in the majority of patients, particularly at higher doses. This is a particular problem in advanced disease. Other side effects include headache, myalgia and nausea. Progressive nail pigmentation has been described in black patients [21]. Resistance to AZT occurs regularly with long-term use.

Other antiretroviral agents

These include zalcitabine (DDC), a dideoxynucleotide analogue, and stavudine, which is a thymidine analogue. Both have been used for the treatment of patients with very low CD4 counts or where there is AZT resistance. Zalcitabine causes a painful neuropathy. Pancreatitis, rashes, ulceration and hepatitis have been described. Stavudine also causes a painful neuropathy.

Protease inhibitors

In order to circumvent the rising problem of drug resistance with antiretrovirals, a new family of drugs whose main focus of action is on the inhibition of aspartic proteases encoded by retroviruses has been developed. These cleave the Gag and Gag-Pol proteins into smaller moieties needed for maturation. The main compounds are saquinavir, indinavir, ritonavir and nelfinavir but there are others in development. Most work by mimicking the transitional state that occurs during peptide bond cleavage by aspartic proteases. Generally, they are used in combination, usually with AZT or other reverse transcriptase inhibitors and/or further protease inhibitors to prevent viral replication and increase CD4 counts. These compounds differ in structure and in the specific sites inhibited [22–24]. At present, treatment using combinations of these drugs is known as highly active antiretroviral therapy (HAART), and successful maintenance therapy can be given for HIV-infected individuals. However, it is likely that resistance will ultimately develop.

Foscarnet phosphonoformate [25]

Foscarnet is a pyrophosphate analogue that inhibits herpesvirus polymerase. It is active against most herpesviruses including CMV. It also inhibits reverse transcriptase and has activity *in vitro* against HIV, particularly in combination with AZT. It is given intravenously in severe herpes simplex and CMV infections, or topically. It is an alternative drug for severe aciclovir-resistant herpes simplex infections and for this indication the usual initial treatment is 40 mg/kg every 8 h. Adverse effects include renal tubular damage, malaise, nausea and headache. Tremor and hallucination may occur at high dosage.

REFERENCES

1 Hirsch MS, Swartz MN. Antiviral agents. *N Engl J Med* 1980; **302**: 903–7, 949–53.
2 Whitley RJ, Spruance S, Hayden F. Vidarabine therapy of mucocutaneous herpes simplex virus infection in the immunocompromised host. *J Infect Dis* 1984; **149**: 1–8.
3 Silvestri DL, Corey L, Holmes KK. Ineffectiveness of topical idoxuridine in dimethyl sulfoxide for therapy of genital herpes. *JAMA* 1982; **248**: 953–9.
4 Elion GB. The biochemistry and mechanisms of action of acyclovir. *J Antimicrob Chemother* 1983; **12** (Suppl. B): 9–17.
5 Fiddian AP, Yeo JM, Clark AE. Treatment of herpes labialis. *J Infect* 1983; **6** (Suppl. 1): 41–7.
6 King DH, Galasso G, eds. Symposium on acyclovir. *Am J Med* 1982; **73** (Suppl. 1).
7 Field HJ, Phillips I, eds. Acyclovir. Based on the Second International Acyclovir Symposium. *J Antimicrob Chemother* 1983; **12** (Suppl. B): 1–11.
8 Field HJ, Larder BA, Darby G. Isolation and characterization of acyclovir resistant strains of herpes simplex virus. *Am J Med* 1982; **73** (Suppl. 1): 369–71.
9 Dekker C, Ellis MN, Hunter G *et al.* Virus resistance in clinical practice. *J Antimicrob Chemother* 1983; **12** (Suppl. B): 137–52.
10 Bryson YJ. Current status and prospects for oral acyclovir treatment of first episode and recurrent genital herpes simplex virus. *J Antimicrob Chemother* 1983; **12** (Suppl. B): 61–9.
11 Thomas RHM, Dodd HJ, Yeo JM *et al.* Oral acyclovir in the suppression of recurrent non-genital herpes simplex virus infection. *Br J Dermatol* 1985; **113**: 731–5.
12 Huff JC, Bean B, Balfour HH *et al.* Therapy of herpes zoster with oral acyclovir. *Am J Med* 1988; **85** (Suppl. 2A): 84–9.
13 De Miranda P, Blum MR. Pharmacokinetics of acyclovir after intravenous and oral administration. *J Antimicrob Chemother* 1983; **12** (Suppl. B): 27–37.
14 Vere Hodge RA. Review antiviral portraits series. 3. Famciclovir and penciclovir. *Antiviral Chem Chemother* 1993; **4**: 67–84.
15 Laskin OL, Cederberg DM, Mills J *et al.* Ganciclovir for the treatment and suppression of serious infections caused by cytomegalovirus. *Am J Med* 1987; **83**: 201–7.
16 Beutner KR, Friedman DJ, Forszpaniak C *et al.* Valciclovir compared with aciclovir for improved therapy for herpes zoster in immunocompetent adults. *Antimicrob Agents Chemother* 1995; **39**: 546–8.
17 Hirsch MS. AIDS commentary: azidothymidine. *J Infect Dis* 1988; **157**: 427–31.
18 Yaschoan R, Broder S. Development of antiretroviral therapy for the acquired immunodeficiency syndrome and related disorders. *N Engl J Med* 1988; **316**: 557–64.
19 McLeod GX, Hammer SM. Zidovudine: five years later. *Ann Intern Med* 1992; **117**: 487–501.
20 Graham NMH, Zeger SL, Park LP *et al.* The effects on survival of early treatment of human immunodeficiency virus infection. *N Engl J Med* 1992; **326**: 1037–42.
21 Furth PA, Kazakis AM. Nail pigmentation changes associated with azidothymidine (zidovudine). *Ann Intern Med* 1988; **107**: 350.
22 Coleman RS, Cheife RT. Proteinase inhibitors: the result of rational drug design. *Pharmacotherapy* 1994; **14**: 1S.
23 Grant RM, Hecht FM, Warmerdam M *et al.* Time trends in primary HIV-1 drug resistance among recently infected persons. *JAMA* 2002; **288**: 181–8.
24 Barreiro P, Soriano V, Casas E *et al.* Different degree of immune recovery using antiretroviral regimens with protease inhibitors or non-nucleosides. *AIDS* 2002; **16**: 245–9.
25 Oleg B, Behrmetz S, Eriksson B. Clinical use of foscarnet (phosphonoformate). In: De Clerq E, ed. *Clinical Use of Antiviral Drugs.* Amsterdam: Martinus Nijhoff, 1991: 223–40.

Antiparasitic agents

Drugs that are used to treat parasitic infections which affect the skin include antibacterial agents such as metronidazole and co-trimoxazole as well as those with specific activity against parasites. This section is largely concerned with the latter group.

Drugs used to treat roundworms

The benzimidazoles. Mebendazole and albendazole are the best known of these compounds. Mebendazole (methyl 5-benzoylbenzimidazole-2 carbamate) is a synthetic drug that is active against diverse species such as *Ascaris*, *Enterobius* and *Trichuris* [1]. It is also active against the adult forms of *Trichinella spiralis* and some filariae such as *Loa loa*. It works through blocking the assembly of microtubules. It is poorly absorbed from the gastrointestinal tract. Adverse events are not common and are mainly seen at high dosage. The more common but trivial side effects are abdominal pain and diarrhoea.

Albendazole (methyl 5-N-propoxythio-2-benzimidazole carbamate) has broad-spectrum activity for parasites from *Ascaris* to *Trichuris* [2,3]. Albendazole is absorbed after oral administration but this is enhanced in the presence of a fatty meal. Once again it is well tolerated and abdominal pain and diarrhoea are the main side effects. Liver and bone marrow toxicity occur only at high dosage.

Tiabendazole is less used than previously. It is well absorbed and is active against a range of nematodes as well as some fungi. However, side effects such as nausea and vomiting are common.

Diethylcarbamazine

Diethylcarbamazine (DEC) is discussed in Chapter 32. It is a piperazine derivative used in the treatment of microfilariae [4]. It rapidly kills these microorganisms, an event that leads to considerable inflammation, which can cause damage in the eye and skin. It acts by affecting microfilarial muscle activity and affects their membranes, leading to increased host killing capacity. In onchocerciasis it can cause severe itching, oedema, erythema and hypotension—the DEC reaction. The dosage is usually built up from an initial 50-mg dose, depending on the infection.

Ivermectin

This is a macrocyclic lactone derived from avermectin B1, which is used for intestinal parasites in animals and for the management of onchocerciasis and other nematode infections [5–7]. It blocks the transmission of signals from interneurones to excitatory motor neurones. It is also effective against *Sarcoptes scabiei*. Its advantage in onchocerciasis is that it is microfilaricidal but does not lead to severe inflammatory responses. Ivermectin is well absorbed after oral administration. Side effects are not common but include fever, itching and headache. A mild DEC-like reaction may occur in some patients. Its usual dose is 150 μg/kg orally, repeated when necessary every 6–12 months.

Pentavalent antimony

The main variants used for the treatment of leishmaniasis are sodium stibogluconate and meglumine antimoniate. Neither is orally active and both have to be given parenterally (intramuscularly or intravenously) [8]. There is a slow elimination phase, which may give rise to toxicity at high dosage. Common adverse events include abdominal pain, nausea and headache [9]. Other effects are renal impairment, pancreatitis and alterations in electrocardiogram (ECG) and cardiac arrhythmias. In particular the Q–T interval may be prolonged.

REFERENCES

1 Keystone JS, Murdoch JK. Mebendazole. *Ann Intern Med* 1979; **91**: 582–6.
2 Jones SK, Reynolds NJ, Oliwiecki S *et al*. Oral albendazole for the treatment of cutaneous larva migrans. *Br J Dermatol* 1990; **122**: 99–101.
3 Pugh RNH, Teesdale CH, Burnham GM. Albendazole in children with hookworm infection. *Ann Trop Med Parasitol* 1986; **80**: 565–7.
4 Hawking F. Diethyl carbamazine and new compounds for the treatment of filariasis. *Adv Pharmacol Chemother* 1979; **16**: 129–94.
5 Grover JK, Vats V, Uppal G *et al*. Antihelmintics: a review. *Trop Gastroenterol* 2001; **22**: 180–9.
6 Collins RC, Gonzalez-Peralta C, Castro J *et al*. Ivermectin: reduction in prevalence and infection intensity of *Onchocerca volvulus* following biannual treatments in five Guatemalan communities. *Am J Trop Med Hyg* 1992; **47**: 156–69.
7 Pacque M, Greene BM, Munoz B *et al*. Ivermectin therapy: a 5-year follow-up. *J Infect Dis* 1991; **164**: 1035–6.
8 Navin TR, Arana BA, Arana FA *et al*. Placebo-controlled clinical trial of sodium stibogluconate (pentostam) versus ketoconazole for treating cutaneous leishmaniasis in Guatemala. *J Infect Dis* 1992; **165**: 528–34.
9 Ballou WR, McClain JB, Gordon DM *et al*. Safety and efficacy of high dose stibogluconate therapy for American cutaneous leishmaniasis. *Lancet* 1987; **2**: 13–6.

Drugs to improve the peripheral circulation

Raynaud's phenomenon and perniosis are the principal dermatological indications for systemic vasodilator therapy. Raynaud's phenomenon occurs in a primary, usually mild, form unassociated with systemic disease, or secondary to various underlying causes. The most common of these is connective tissue diseases; others include hyperviscosity disorders, cervical rib, drugs with a vasoconstrictor action and, rarely, occupational causes (see Chapter 23). The management of Raynaud's phenomenon has been extensively reviewed [1–4], and includes the use of calcium-channel blockers, angiotensin II receptor antagonists, prostacyclin analogues, serotonin antagonists, calcitonin gene-related peptides and newer agents such as endothelin-1 receptor antagonists and nitric oxide donors.

Calcium-channel blocking agents are of moderate benefit, and of these nifedipine is the treatment of choice [5,6]. It acts by inhibiting contraction of smooth muscle cells by reducing the cellular uptake of calcium, a process fundamental to vasospasm; it also reduces platelet aggregability. Modified release nifedipine 20–60 mg/day is usually effective. Diltiazem is also useful, but verapamil less so. Side effects include flushing, headaches and peripheral oedema. The response of primary Raynaud's phenomenon is usually more impressive than that secondary to connective tissue disease. Use of calcium-channel antagonists can occasionally precipitate erythromelalgia [7]. The angiotensin II receptor type 1 losartan has been recorded as useful in Raynaud's phenomenon [8].

Severe Raynaud's phenomenon (see Chapter 23), especially that secondary to systemic sclerosis and other connective tissue diseases, is more difficult to treat and may be poorly responsive to nifedipine. For these patients, intravenous prostacyclin or one of its stable analogues such as iloprost may be necessary [9–14]. Prostacyclin inhibits platelet adhesion and aggregation, and vascular smooth muscle proliferation, increases red cell deformability, and decreases blood viscosity. For reasons that are poorly understood, it causes sustained clinical benefit, a single low-dose infusion (0.5 ng/kg/min) often causing clinical remission for several weeks. Side effects include flushing, headaches and hypotension.

The serotonin antagonist ketanserin is not clinically beneficial [15], but fluoxetine, a selective serotonin-reuptake inhibitor, has been reported to be effective [16], as have dazoxiben, a thromboxane synthetase inhibitor

[17], and prazosin [18]. α-Adrenergic-blocking agents (e.g. thymoxamine, a non-selective α-adrenoceptor blocker) 40 mg three times daily, or prazosin, a selective α-adrenergic-blocking agent, 0.5–1.0 mg three times daily, may suffice in mild cases. The use of intravenous calcitonin gene-related peptide (CGRP) has been recommended for severe Raynaud's phenomenon [19]. CGRP, which was given in a dosage of 0.6 μg/min for 3 h/day on 5 consecutive days, causes flushing, diarrhoea, headache and hypotension.

Perniosis also responds well to calcium-channel antagonists. A double-blind cross-over placebo-controlled study of nifedipine in 10 patients [20] showed a convincing response in the nifedipine phase of the trial. Other drugs reported anecdotally to improve the peripheral circulation include oxpentifylline (pentoxifylline), fibrinolytic agents including stanozolol, and low-molecular-weight dextran infusion.

REFERENCES

1 Block JA, Sequeira W. Raynaud's phenomenon. *Lancet* 2001; **357**: 2042–8.
2 Herrick AL. Treatment of Raynaud's phenomenon: new insights and developments. *Curr Rheumatol Rep* 2003; **5**: 168–74.
3 Generini S, Del Rosso A, Pignone A, Matucci Cerinic M. Current treatment options in Raynaud's phenomenon. *Curr Treat Options Cardiovasc Med* 2003; **5**: 147–61.
4 Hummers LK, Wigley FM. Management of Raynaud's phenomenon and digital ischaemic lesions in scleroderma. *Rheum Dis Clin North Am* 2003; **29**: 293–313.
5 Thompson AE, Shea B, Welch V *et al.* Calcium-channel blockers for Raynaud's phenomenon in systemic sclerosis. *Arthritis Rheum* 2001; **44**: 1841–7.
6 Smith CD, McKendry RJR. Controlled trial of nifedipine in the treatment of Raynaud's phenomenon. *Lancet* 1982; **ii**: 1299–301.
7 Drenth JPH, Michiels JJ, Van Joost T, Vuzeuski VD. Verapamil-induced secondary erythermalgia. *Br J Dermatol* 1992; **127**: 292–4.
8 Dziadzio M, Denton CP, Smith R *et al.* Losartan therapy for Raynaud's phenomenon and scleroderma: clinical and biochemical findings in a 15-week, randomized, parallel-group, controlled trial. *Arthritis Rheum* 1999; **42**: 2646–55.
9 Fink AN, Frishman WH, Azizad M, Agarwal Y. Use of prostacyclin and its analogues in the treatment of cardiovascular disease. *Heart Dis* 1999; **1**: 29–40.
10 Pope J, Fenlon D, Thompson A *et al.* Iloprost and cisaprost for Raynaud's phenomenon in progressive systemic sclerosis. *Cochrane Database Syst Rev* 2000; CD000953.
11 Stratton R, Shiwen X, Martini G *et al.* Iloprost suppresses connective tissue growth factor production in fibroblasts and in the skin of scleroderma patients. *J Clin Invest* 2001; **108**: 241–50.
12 Scorza R, Caronni M, Mascagni B *et al.* Effects of long-term cyclic iloprost therapy in systemic sclerosis with Raynaud's phenomenon: a randomized, controlled study. *Clin Exp Rheumatol* 2001; **19**: 503–8.
13 Mittag M, Beckheinrich P, Haustein UF. Systemic sclerosis-related Raynaud's phenomenon: effects of iloprost infusion therapy on serum cytokine, growth factor and soluble adhesion molecule levels. *Acta Derm Venereol (Stockh)* 2001; **81**: 294–7.
14 Bettoni L, Geri A, Airo P *et al.* Systemic sclerosis therapy with iloprost: a prospective observational study of 30 patients treated for a median of 3 years. *Clin Rheumatol* 2002; **21**: 244–50.
15 Pope J, Fenlon D, Thompson A *et al.* Ketanserin for Raynaud's phenomenon in progressive systemic sclerosis. *Cochrane Database Syst Rev* 2000; CD000954.
16 Coleiro B, Marshall SE, Denton CP *et al.* Treatment of Raynaud's phenomenon with the selective serotonin reuptake inhibitor fluoxetine. *Rheumatology (Oxford)* 2001; **40**: 1038–43.
17 Tindell H, Tooke JE, Menys VC *et al.* Effect of dazoxiben, a thromboxane synthetase inhibitor on skin blood flow following cold challenge in patients with Raynaud's phenomenon. *Eur J Clin Invest* 1985; **15**: 20–3.
18 Pope J, Fenlon D, Thompson A *et al.* Prazosin for Raynaud's phenomenon in progressive systemic sclerosis. *Cochrane Database Syst Rev* 2000; CD000956.
19 Bunker CB, Reavley C, O'Shaungmessy DJ, Dowd PM. Calcitonin gene related peptide in treatment of severe peripheral vascular insufficiency in Raynaud's phenomenon. *Lancet* 1993; **342**: 80–3.
20 Dowd PM, Rustin MHA, Lanigan S. Nifedipine in the treatment of chilblains. *BMJ* 1986; **293**: 923–4.

Miscellaneous drugs used in special ways in dermatology

Antimalarials

A variety of drugs have been used in the treatment of malaria. However, for over 35 years it has been well known that several of these drugs may have other useful properties in the management of skin diseases [1,2]. There are several diseases where there is an undoubted beneficial effect: discoid and systemic lupus erythematosus, polymorphic light eruption and solar urticaria (see Chapters 56 and 24). They are of some value in rheumatology, where there is a resurgence of their use, as well as their more obvious application in diseases caused by some protozoa. Their use in porphyria cutanea tarda and sarcoidosis is discussed elsewhere (see Chapters 57 and 58).

The mode of action of antimalarials is complex and their usage is largely on empirical grounds. They can interfere with many biological processes. They bind to DNA, stabilize membranes, inhibit hydrolytic enzymes, interfere with prostaglandin synthesis and block chemotaxis [1,2].

The major problem with chloroquine is retinopathy and potential blindness [3,4]. There are considerable problems in defining the criteria for the diagnosis of retinopathy and the estimate that 3–5% of patients who receive the drug may develop this complication is almost certainly too high. A number of questions remain unanswered. It is generally agreed that the risk to the retina of giving chloroquine sulphate 250 mg/day for 3 months is virtually negligible, although the drug is cumulative to some extent from one year to another. It has long been thought that it is the total cumulative dose that determines the retinal toxicity. It has been suggested that it is the daily dose that counts and that 4 mg/kg/day chloroquine is likely to be safe [5].

Because of the potential retinopathy with chloroquine, hydroxychloroquine or mepacrine are the two antimalarial drugs now used. Hydroxychloroquine is more effective than mepacrine but is said to have some ocular toxicity, albeit less than with chloroquine. It is likely that in the dosage used by dermatologists (up to 400 mg/day) the risk of ocular toxicity is negligible. In many hospitals, the ophthalmologists will not agree to screen or monitor patients as they think the risk is so small, but if hydroxychloroquine is continued for more than a few months it would seem prudent to obtain ophthalmological screening, which should also be sought before starting treatment. Mepacrine lacks ocular toxicity, and is often an effective drug, especially in discoid lupus erythematosus and Hutchinson's chilblain lupus. In effective dosage (200 mg/day), it usually causes the skin to turn yellow and occasionally produces lichenoid reactions. Ocular toxicity of antimalarials as used in dermatology is well reviewed by Cox and Paterson [6].

REFERENCES

1 Isaacson D, Elgart M, Turner ML. Antimalarials in dermatology. *Int J Dermatol* 1982; **21**: 379–95.
2 Koranda FC. Antimalarials. *J Am Acad Dermatol* 1981; **4**: 650–5.
3 Olansky AJ. Antimalarials and ophthalmologic safety. *J Am Acad Dermatol* 1982; **6**: 19–23.
4 Portnoy JZ, Callen JP. Ophthalmologic aspects of chloroquine and hydroxychloroquine therapy. *Int J Dermatol* 1983; **22**: 273–8.
5 Ochsendorf FR, Runne U. Chloroquin-Retinopathie: Vermeidbar durch Beachtung der maximalen Tagesdosis. *Hautarzt* 1988; **39**: 341–2.
6 Cox NH, Paterson WD. Ocular toxicity of antimalarials in dermatology; a survey of current practice. *Br J Dermatol* 1994; **131**: 878–22.

Dapsone and sulfapyridine [1–5]

Dapsone (DDS) has been the mainstay in the treatment of leprosy for many years (see Chapter 29). It also has some action against malaria and other parasites, and has also proved a very valuable drug in the management of a wide range of mainly uncommon dermatoses. Its mode of action is not fully understood. Although many of the diseases found empirically to respond to this drug have in common the involvement of either polymorphs or immune complexes, the metabolic action of dapsone cannot be explained simply in these terms. The diseases for which dapsone is particularly effective are dermatitis herpetiformis and erythema elevatum diutinum. Other diseases also favourably but not invariably influenced include other bullous diseases (pemphigoid, mucous membrane pemphigoid, linear IgA disease, chronic bullous disease of childhood, bullous eruption of systemic lupus erythematosus, subcorneal pustular dermatosis), pyoderma gangrenosum, rheumatoid arthritis and collagen diseases, relapsing polychondritis, acne conglobata, leukocytoclastic vasculitis and granuloma faciale.

Toxicity is a considerable problem with dapsone but overall the drug has probably fewer long-term side effects than do corticosteroids or sulfapyridine. The main toxic side effect is haemolysis, which is not usually dependent on glucose-6-phosphate dehydrogenase deficiency, although that enzyme defect may compound the problem. Some haemolysis is almost invariably found on therapeutic dosage. Methaemoglobinaemia is also common and is responsible for the bluish lips commonly seen in patients on this drug. A level of 3% methaemoglobinaemia is often

unnoticed, 12% may be acceptable, but 20% is usually not. Regular blood checks of haemoglobin and reticulocytes but also including white cells and platelets should therefore be undertaken in all patients for the first few months after starting dapsone. Dapsone has several other but less common side effects, including agranulocytosis, peripheral neuropathy, drug rashes, renal damage, hypoalbuminaemia, cholestasis, psychoses and reversible male infertility. A dosage of 100 mg/day is often used as a starting dose. Many patients with dermatitis herpetiformis can be controlled on very much less. Some diseases can only be controlled by larger doses, but the incidence of side effects then rises very sharply and most dermatologists prefer not to exceed a dosage of 100–150 mg/day. It is possible to reduce dapsone-dependent methaemoglobinaemia by the concomitant administration of cimetidine (400 mg three times daily) [6].

Other drugs that share some of the useful assets of dapsone include sulfapyridine and, to a lesser extent, sulfamethoxypyridazine. Sulfapyridine is in general less effective than dapsone and, in doses that are effective, tends to cause more side effects, especially marrow suppression, although not haemolysis. The usual dose is 0.5 g twice or three times daily.

Clofazimine

This antileprotic drug has also been used especially in pyoderma gangrenosum and in lupus erythematosus and Sweet's disease.

REFERENCES

1 Stern RS. Systemic dapsone. *Arch Dermatol* 1993; **129**: 301.
2 Zhu YI, Stiller MJ. Dapsone and sulfones in dermatology: overview and update. *J Am Acad Dermatol* 2001; **45**: 420–34.
3 Paniker U, Levine N. Dapsone and sulfapyridine. *Dermatol Clin* 2001; **19**: 79–86, viii.
4 Wolf R, Matz H, Orion E, Tuzun B, Tuzun Y. Dapsone. *Dermatol Online J* 2002; **8**: 2.
5 Pfeiffer C, Wozel G. Dapsone and sulfones in dermatology: overview and update. *J Am Acad Dermatol* 2003; **48**: 308–9.
6 Coleman MD, Scott AK, Breckenridge AM *et al.* The use of cimetidine as a selective inhibitor of dapsone N-hydroxylation in man. *Br J Clin Pharmacol* 1990; **30**: 761–7.

Sulfasalazine

This drug is best known for its activity in inflammatory bowel disease and rheumatoid arthritis with their associated skin problems. The mode of action is uncertain [1,2]. It is not very well absorbed from the gut and does have side effects. Among other activities it may be a 5-lipoxygenase inhibitor. It has been found to be of some value in pustular psoriasis, arthropathic psoriasis and psoriasis vulgaris [1–5]. Its use in other conditions such as dermatitis herpetiformis, scleroderma and acne [6] has been recommended but is less well established. Sulfasalazine has been reported to be useful in metastatic cutaneous Crohn's disease [7,8]. A recent report suggested benefit in a minority of patients with alopecia areata [9].

REFERENCES

1 Farr M, Kitas GD, Waterhouse L *et al.* Treatment of psoriatic arthritis with sulfasalazine: a one year open study. *Clin Rheumatol* 1988; **7**: 372.
2 Stenson WG, Lobos E. Sulfasalazine inhibits the synthesis of chemotactic lipids by neutrophils. *J Clin Invest* 1982; **69**: 494–7.
3 Gupta AK, Ellis CN, Siegel MT *et al.* Sulfasalazine: a potential psoriasis therapy. *J Am Acad Dermatol* 1989; **20**: 797–800.
4 Gupta AK, Ellis CN, Siegel MT *et al.* Sulfasalazine improves psoriasis: a double blind analysis. *Arch Dermatol* 1990; **126**: 487–93.
5 Newman ED, Perruquet JL, Harrington TM. Sulfasalazine therapy in psoriatic arthritis: clinical and immunologic response. *J Rheumatol* 1997; **18**: 1379–82.
6 Schoch EP, McCuiston CH. Effect of salicylazosulfapyridine (azulfidine) on pustular acne and certain other dermatoses. *J Invest Dermatol* 1955; **25**: 123–6.
7 Peltz S, Vetsey JP, Ferguson A *et al.* Disseminated metastatic cutaneous Crohn's disease. *Clin Exp Dermatol* 1993; **18**: 55–9.
8 Kolansky G, Kimbrough-Green C, Dubin HV. Metastatic Crohn's disease of the face. *Arch Dermatol* 1993; **129**: 1348–9.
9 Ellis CN, Brown MF, Voorhees JJ. Sulfasalazine for alopecia areata. *J Am Acad Dermatol* 2002; **46**: 541–4.

Thalidomide

Thalidomide is an interesting drug but it is linked with the causation of severe birth defects, so that its use is very restricted, and it must never be given to pregnant women. It also has other toxic side effects, notably peripheral neuropathy [1–3]. It can be helpful in severe leprosy reactions (see Chapter 29). It may also be beneficial in some but by no means all patients with nodular prurigo [4], lupus erythematosus [5–7], actinic prurigo and other light-sensitive dermatoses, aphthosis [8], Behçet's disease, Weber–Christian disease, pyoderma gangrenosum, sarcoidosis, graft-versus-host disease, adult Langerhans' cell histiocytosis [9] and certain dermatological conditions associated with HIV infection [10]. It is a drug the use of which must always be kept under the strictest control and it must be used only by patients who are able to understand the problems. It is important to check regularly for peripheral neuropathy. Guidelines for the clinical use and dispensing of thalidomide have been drawn up [11–13].

REFERENCES

1 Aronson IK, Yu R, West DP *et al.* Thalidomide-induced peripheral neuropathy. *Arch Dermatol* 1984; **120**: 1466–70.
2 Clemmensen OJ, Olsen PZ, Andersen KE. Thalidomide neurotoxicity. *Arch Dermatol* 1984; **120**: 338–41.
3 Wulff CH, Asboe-Hansen G, Brodthagen H. Development of polyneuropathy during thalidomide therapy. *Br J Dermatol* 1985; **112**: 475–80.
4 Johnke H, Zachariae H. Thalidomide treatment of prurigo nodularis [in Danish]. *Ugeskr Laeger* 1993; **155**: 3028–30.
5 Holm AL, Bowers KE, McMeekin TO, Gaspari AA. Chronic cutaneous lupus erythematosus treated with thalidomide. *Arch Dermatol* 1993; **129**: 1548–50.

6 Knop J, Bonsmann G, Happle R *et al.* Thalidomide in the treatment of 60 cases of chronic discoid lupus erythematosus. *Br J Dermatol* 1983; **108**: 461–6.
7 Housman TS, Jorizzo JL, McCarty MA *et al.* Low-dose thalidomide therapy for refractory cutaneous lesions of lupus erythematosus. *Arch Dermatol* 2003; **139**: 50–4.
8 Bowers PW, Powell RJ. Effect of thalidomide on orogenital ulceration. *BMJ* 1983; **287**: 799–800.
9 Thomas L, Ducros B, Secchi T *et al.* Sussessful treatment of adults' Langerhans' cell histiocytosis with thalidomide. *Arch Dermatol* 1993; **129**: 1261.
10 Stirling DI. Thalidomide and its impact in dermatology. *Semin Cutan Med Surg* 1998; **17**: 231–42.
11 Judge MR, Kobza-Black A, Hawk JL. Guidelines for the clinical use and dispensing of thalidomide. *Postgrad Med J* 1995; **71**: 123.
12 Chave TA, Finlay AY, Knight AG *et al.* Thalidomide usage in Wales: the need to follow guidelines. *Br J Dermatol* 2001; **144**: 310–5.
13 Wines NY, Cooper AJ, Wines MP. Thalidomide in dermatology. *Australas J Dermatol* 2002; **43**: 229–38.

Colchicine [1–3]

Colchicine has been used in the treatment of gout for many centuries and is still a valuable remedy. It is also of use in familial Mediterranean fever. It has an antimitotic action (for which it is sometimes used topically) but its useful anti-inflammatory effects in skin diseases probably depend more on its suppression of various aspects of polymorph activity, notably chemotaxis. It may also inhibit histamine release from mast cells. Its use is somewhat restricted by its side effects, especially those on the gastrointestinal tract, but the bone marrow and kidney may also be affected. It should be avoided in pregnancy. It is not therefore a first-line drug but can prove of value in Behçet's disease [4], chronic bullous dermatosis of childhood (linear IgA disease) [5], pustular psoriasis [6], relapsing polychondritis [7], leukocytoclastic vasculitis, urticarial vasculitis [8], epidermolysis bullosa acquisita [9] and Sweet's syndrome—all diseases in which polymorphs are presumed to have a role. A common regimen is 0.5–1 mg/day orally, although larger doses are used by rheumatologists.

REFERENCES

1 Malkinson FD. Colchicine: new uses of an old, old drug. *Arch Dermatol* 1982; **118**: 453–7.
2 Aram H. Colchicine in dermatologic therapy. *Int J Dermatol* 1983; **22**: 566–9.
3 Sullivan TP, King LE Jr, Boyd AS. Colchicine in dermatology. *J Am Acad Dermatol* 1998; **39**: 993–9.
4 deBois MH, Geelhoed-Duvijvestijn PH, Westdt ML. Behçet's syndrome treated with colchicine. *Neth J Med* 1991; **38**: 175–6.
5 Zeharia A, Hodak E, Mukamel M *et al.* Successful treatment of chronic bullous dermatosis of childhood with colchicine. *J Am Acad Dermatol* 1994; **30**: 660–1.
6 Takigawa M, Miyachi Y, Uehara M *et al.* Treatment of pustulosis palmaris et plantaris with oral doses of colchicine. *Arch Dermatol* 1982; **118**: 458–602.
7 Askari AD. Colchicine for treatment of relapsing polychondritis. *J Am Acad Dermatol* 1984; **10**: 506–10.
8 Asherson RA, Buchanan N, Kenwright S *et al.* The normocomplementemic urticarial vasculitis syndrome: report of a case and response to colchicine. *Clin Exp Dermatol* 1991; **16**: 424–7.
9 Megahed M, Scharffetter-Kochanek K. Epidermolysis bullosa acquisita: successful treatment with colchicine. *Arch Dermatol Res* 1994; **286**: 35–46.

Traditional Chinese herbal medicine

The treatment involves taking a 'tea' prepared from a decoction of plant materials. Usually 10 or so plant materials are included. Trials have also been performed using a tablet form of treatment (Zemaphyte®) and showed a beneficial response in children [1] and adults [2] with atopic eczema. Even when treatment is effective and continued, the benefit often wears off after 6–12 months. Relapses occur once treatment is stopped. Of concern are the reports of hepatotoxicity [3–6] and renal toxicity [7] potentially associated with Chinese herbal remedies. While Chinese herbs cannot yet be recommended for the routine treatment of children with atopic eczema, they did help approximately half of the children who took part in the Great Ormond Street Hospital Trial [8]. Further adequate randomized controlled trials are necessary [9]. Chinese herbs have also been advocated for psoriasis [10].

REFERENCES

1 Sheehan MP, Atherton DJ. A controlled trial of traditional Chinese medical plants in widespread non-exudative atopic eczema. *Br J Dermatol* 1992; **126**: 179–84.
2 Sheehan MP, Rustin MHA, Atherton DJ *et al.* Efficacy of traditional Chinese herbal therapy in adult atopic dermatitis. *Lancet* 1992; **340**: 13–17.
3 Davies EG, Pollock I, Steele HM. Chinese herbs for eczema. *Lancet* 1990; **336**: 177.
4 Graham-Brown R. Toxicity of Chinese herbal remedies. *Lancet* 1992; **340**: 673.
5 Perharic-Walton L, Murray V. Toxicity of Chinese herbal remedies. *Lancet* 1992; **340**: 673.
6 Mostefa-Cara N, Pauwels A, Pinus E *et al.* Fatal hepatitis after herbal tea. *Lancet* 1992; **340**: 674.
7 Lord GM, Tagore R, Cook T *et al.* Nephropathy caused by Chinese herbs in the UK. *Lancet* 1999; **354**: 481–2.
8 Sheehan MP, Atherton DJ. One year follow-up of children treated with Chinese medicinal herbs for atopic eczema. *Br J Dermatol* 1994; **130**: 488–93.
9 Armstrong NC, Ernst E. The treatment of eczema with Chinese herbs: a systematic review of randomized clinical trials. *Br J Clin Pharmacol* 1999; **48**: 262–4.
10 Tse TW. Use of common Chinese herbs in the treatment of psoriasis. *Clin Exp Dermatol* 2003; **28**: 469–75.

Transdermal delivery systems

The blood is the target for penetration in transdermal delivery systems. There are two major routes for drug penetration through skin: the stratum corneum, and shunts via hair follicles and eccrine sweat gland ducts [1].

With drugs metabolized in the liver, achievement of therapeutic blood levels is enhanced by transdermal delivery because the 'first pass' effect inherent in oral administration is avoided. Thus, transdermally delivered drugs show reduced differences in 'peak' and 'trough' blood levels, and a different profile of metabolites [2]. Efficiency of transdermal delivery is greater with lipid-soluble drugs. Additional advantages include ability to use short half-life drugs, better patient compliance, reduced dosage frequency, avoidance of unpredictable intestinal absorption and gastric irritation, and fewer complications.

Recent examples of drugs marketed in a transdermal form include scopolamine, clonidine, nitroglycerine, estradiol, nicotine and prostaglandin E1 ethyl ester for the treatment of trophic acral skin lesions in systemic scleroderma [3]. Within the transdermal 'patch', the drug, which may be formulated in a liquid, solid, ointment or cream form, behaves as a reservoir. The blood levels are proportional to the active surface area of the 'patch', and drug delivery occurs over a period of 1–7 days. Skin irritation and sensitization are significant difficulties with transdermal delivery systems, which contain several sources of problems besides the drug itself, including the adhesive, vehicle penetration enhancers and polymers. More advanced transdermal delivery systems are now available that should enable continuous or pulsed delivery of new drugs including genetically engineered products [3].

REFERENCES

1 Scheuplein RJ, Blank IH. Permeability of the skin. *Physiol Rev* 1971; **51**: 702–47.
2 Powers MS. Pharmacokinetics and pharmacodynamics of transdermal dosage forms of 17b-oestradiol: comparison with conventional oral oestrogen used for hormone replacement. *Am J Obstet Gynecol* 1985; **152**: 1099–106.
3 Schlez A, Kittel M, Scheurle B *et al.* Transdermal application of prostaglandin E1 ethyl ester for the treatment of trophic acral skin lesions in a patient with systemic scleroderma. *J Eur Acad Dermatol Venereol* 2002; **16**: 526–8.

Chapter 73

Drug Reactions

S.M. Breathnach

Introduction [1–4]

A drug may be defined as a chemical substance, or combination of substances, administered for the investigation, prevention or treatment of diseases or symptoms, real or imagined. The distinction between drugs and 'other chemicals' is not always easily made, as chemicals of very diverse structure are increasingly added to foods and beverages as dyes, flavours or preservatives. Such chemicals may cause harmful side effects. Moreover, chemicals used in agriculture or in veterinary medicine may contaminate human food. In addition, with the advent of therapeutic agents that may be useful for improving the appearance, as with minoxidil for androgenetic alopecia and tretinoin for photo-aged skin, the distinction between drugs and cosmetics has become blurred [5].

An adverse drug reaction (ADR) may be defined as an undesirable clinical manifestation resulting from administration of a particular drug; this includes reactions due to overdose, predictable side effects and unanticipated adverse manifestations. Another definition is that of 'an appreciably harmful or unpleasant reaction, resulting from an intervention related to the use of a medicinal product, which predicts hazard from future administration and warrants prevention or specific treatment, or alteration of the dosage regimen, or withdrawal of the product' [6]. It has been proposed that therapeutic ineffectiveness should also be regarded as an ADR [7]. ADRs may be said to be the inevitable price we pay for the benefits of modern drug therapy [8]. They are costly both in terms of the human illness caused and in economic terms, and can undermine the doctor–patient relationship.

Sometimes, ADRs result from human error [9]. In one study, 0.9% of 530 medication errors resulted in ADRs [10]; these usually involved errors at the ordering stage, but also occurred at the administration stage [11]. In hospitals, medication errors occur at a rate of about one per patient per day; dispensing errors made by pharmacy staff range from 0.87 to 2.9% [12]. ADRs are under-reported and are an underestimated cause of morbidity and mortality; it has been estimated that ADRs represent the fourth to the sixth leading cause of death [13]. The actual frequency of fatal adverse drug events is unknown; estimates in the USA are as high as 140 000/year, although this number is heavily disputed [14]. In one study, 68% of fatal ADRs were judged to have been preventable; of these, a pharmacist could have prevented 57% [15]. Approximately 1 in 2000 of all deaths for which there were records of coroner's inquests in one district were related to drugs; of these, 20% were due to errors [16]. During 1995, 206 deaths were attributed to ADRs on death certificates in the USA, but the spontaneous post-marketing surveillance system (MedWatch) of the Food and Drug Administration (FDA) tabulated 6894 fatalities. The numbers of deaths in these datasets varied 34-fold and were up to several 100-fold less than values based on extrapolations of surveillance programmes [17]. Confusion may occur between drugs with similar spelling of their brand names [18,19]. It has been proposed that licensing authorities should exercise more control over the naming of new proprietary formulations, that non-proprietary and new proprietary names should be internationalized, and that doctors should issue printed prescriptions if possible [20].

The average extra length of stay for patients with an adverse drug event in one study in the USA was 1.9 days, and the average extra cost of hospitalization was $1939 [21]. In another study, at a university-affiliated hospital, the mean cost of an ADR or medication error varied from $95 for additional laboratory tests to $2640 for intensive care; the estimated total cost for the medication-related problems reported in 1994 was almost $1.5 million [22]. In a European study, ADRs occurred at 10.1 per 1000 patient-days, and the cost of ADRs leading to hospitalization was estimated at €11 357 per hospital bed per year [23]. Another estimate of the cost of an ADR during hospitalization or leading to hospitalization was approximately €2800 [24]. Litigation was reported for 14% of fatal ADR cases at one centre; judgements and settlements averaged $1.1 million [15]. Drug reactions, principally to corticosteroids and methotrexate, accounted for 32% of claims and 26% of dollar losses in dermatology malpractice suits in the USA from 1963 to 1973 inclusive [25]. Medication side effects, most frequently to corticosteroids, antibiotics and chemo-

therapeutic agents, represented 26% of lawsuits in a study of dermatology residency programmes in the USA between 1964 and 1988 [26]. If legal consequences are to be avoided, consistent care is needed at every stage from drug manufacture to administration [27].

It is in everyone's interests to minimize the chances of their occurrence, and to this end government regulatory bodies and the pharmaceutical industry collaborate to ensure adequate screening of new products. In addition to extensive *in vitro* and animal testing, prolonged and strictly controlled clinical trials are essential. Even so, hazards cannot be completely eliminated, for a serious reaction of low incidence may not be suspected until a very large number of patients have been treated with a new drug. Premarketing clinical trials conducted before a new drug is licensed will not identify adverse reactions occurring in less than 0.1–1% of patients, or those occurring only after prolonged administration, or with a long latency period, or only in susceptible patients, or when the drug is combined with some other factor, such as another drug [28,29].

Another problem is that only a very small fraction of all adverse reactions are ever reported to monitoring agencies, and first warning is still often given by anecdotal reports published in medical journals [30,31]. Many of these reports are subsequently validated but a substantial proportion of poorly documented reports are not [31,32]. In an analysis of 5737 articles from 80 countries between 1972 and 1979, only half the reports contained enough information for the calculation of the frequency of a particular reaction [32]. The usefulness of anecdotal case reports has again been called into question [33]. As incorrect reports may have serious legal and other consequences, a heavy responsibility rests with medical editors; a chance association or coincidental reaction should not be allowed to enter the literature. Criteria for assessment of potential drug reactions have been promulgated and include recurrence on challenge; existence of a pharmacological basis for the reactions; the occurrence of immediate acute or local reactions at the time of administration, of previously known reactions with a new route of administration, or of repeated rare reactions; and the presence of immunological abnormalities [31,34]. In the assessment of an unrecorded new reaction, the existence of similar but unpublished reports to the manufacturer or to the Committee on Safety of Medicines is of particular importance.

REFERENCES

1 Bork K. *Cutaneous Side Effects of Drugs*. Philadelphia: Saunders, 1988.
2 Breathnach SM, Hintner H. *Adverse Drug Reactions and the Skin*. Oxford: Blackwell Scientific Publications, 1992.
3 Zürcher L, Krebs A. *Cutaneous Drug Reactions*. Basel: Karger, 1992.
4 Litt JZ, Pawlak WA Jr. *Drug Eruption Reference Manual*. New York: Parthenon, 1997.
5 Lavrijsen APM, Vermeer BJ. Cosmetics and drugs. Is there a need for a third group: cosmeceutics? *Br J Dermatol* 1991; **124**: 503–4.

6 Edwards IR, Aronson JK. Adverse drug reactions: definitions, diagnosis, and management. *Lancet* 2000; **356**: 1255–9.

7 Meyboom RH, Lindquist M, Flygare AK *et al.* The value of reporting therapeutic ineffectiveness as an adverse drug reaction. *Drug Saf* 2000; **23**: 95–9.

8 Nolan L, O'Malley K. Adverse drug reactions in the elderly. *Br J Hosp Med* 1989; **41**: 446–57.

9 Wright D, Mackenzie SJ, Buchan I *et al.* Critical events in the intensive therapy unit. *Lancet* 1991; **338**: 676–8.

10 Bates DW, Boyle DL, Vander Vliet MB *et al.* Relationship between medication errors and adverse drug events. *J Gen Intern Med* 1995; **10**: 199–205.

11 Bates DW, Cullen DJ, Laird N *et al.* Incidence of adverse drug events and potential adverse drug events. Implications for prevention. ADE Prevention Study Group. *JAMA* 1995; **274**: 29–34.

12 Allan EL, Barker KN. Fundamentals of medication error research. *Am J Hosp Pharm* 1990; **47**: 555–71.

13 Brown SD Jr, Landry FJ. Recognizing, reporting, and reducing adverse drug reactions. *South Med J* 2001; **94**: 370–3.

14 Kelly WN. Can the frequency and risks of fatal adverse drug events be determined? *Pharmacotherapy* 2001; **21**: 521–7.

15 Kelly WN. Potential risks and prevention. Part 1: fatal adverse drug events. *Am J Health Syst Pharm* 2001; **58**: 1317–24.

16 Ferner RE, Whittington RM. Coroner's cases of death due to errors in prescribing or giving medicines or to adverse drug reactions: Birmingham 1986–1991. *J R Soc Med* 1994; **87**: 145–8.

17 Chyka PA. How many deaths occur annually from adverse drug reactions in the United States? *Am J Med* 2000; **109**: 122–30.

18 Fine SN, Eisdorfer RM, Miskovitz PF, Jacobson IM. Losec or Lasix? *N Engl J Med* 1990; **322**: 1674.

19 Faber J, Azzugnuni M, Di Romana S, Vanhaeverbeek M. Fatal confusion between 'Losec' and 'Lasix'. *Lancet* 1991; **337**: 1286–7.

20 Aronson JK. Confusion over similar drug names. Problems and solutions. *Drug Saf* 1995; **12**: 55–60.

21 Evans RS, Classen DC, Stevens LE *et al.* Using a hospital information system to assess the effects of adverse drug events. In: *Proceedings of the Ann Symp Comp Appl Medical Care.* 1993: 161–5.

22 Schneider PJ, Gift MG, Lee YP *et al.* Cost of medication-related problems at a university hospital. *Am J Health System Pharm* 1995; **52**: 2415–8.

23 Lagnaoui R, Moore N, Fach J *et al.* Adverse drug reactions in a department of systemic diseases-oriented internal medicine: prevalence, incidence, direct costs and avoidability. *Eur J Clin Pharmacol* 2000; **56**: 181–6.

24 Gautier S, Bachelet H, Bordet R, Caron J. The cost of adverse drug reactions. *Expert Opin Pharmacother* 2003; **4**: 319–26.

25 Altman J. Survey of malpractice claims in dermatology. *Arch Dermatol* 1975; **111**: 641–4.

26 Hollabaugh ES, Wagner RF Jr, Weedon VW, Smith EB. Patient personal injury litigation against dermatology residency programs in the United States 1964–1988. *Arch Dermatol* 1990; **126**: 618–22.

27 Day AT. Adverse drug reactions and medical negligence. *Adverse Drug React Bull* 1995; **172**: 651–4.

28 Bruinsma W. Drug monitoring in dermatology. *Int J Dermatol* 1986; **25**: 166–7.

29 Committee of Management Prescribers' Journal. Adverse drug reactions. *Prescribers J* 1991; **31**: 1–3.

30 Anonymous. Crying wolf on drug safety. *BMJ* 1982; **284**: 219–20.

31 Venning GR. Validity of anecdotal reports of suspected adverse drug reactions: the problem of false alarms. *BMJ* 1982; **284**: 249–52.

32 Venulet J, Blattner R, von Bülow J, Berneker GC. How good are articles on adverse drug reactions? *BMJ* 1982; **284**: 252–4.

33 Stern RS, Chan H-L. Usefulness of case report literature in determining drugs responsible for toxic epidermal necrolysis. *J Am Acad Dermatol* 1989; **21**: 317–22.

34 Stern RS, Wintroub BU. Adverse drug reactions: reporting and evaluating cutaneous reactions. *Adv Dermatol* 1987; **2**: 3–18.

Incidence of drug reactions [1,2]

Data collection

It is difficult to obtain reliable information on the incidence of drug reactions, despite attempts at monitoring by government and the pharmaceutical industry. One problem is the lack of standardized coding for drug reactions [3]. Moreover, the information that is available must be interpreted with considerable care, because data will be biased, depending on the method of collection [1,2]. Thus, data on medical in-patients, especially from acute care facilities, may indicate a relatively high incidence, because these patients are generally sicker and receive more intensive drug treatment. In contrast, spontaneous reporting may underestimate the true incidence [4]. National schemes for collating reported ADRs exist in many countries, and the World Health Organization's Adverse Reaction Collaborating Centre, in Uppsala, provides a very large database [2], as does the Adverse Event Reporting System of the US FDA [5,6]. The UK's 'yellow card' reporting scheme solicits ADR reports from doctors, dentists, coroners, and drug manufacturers; the wide availability of reporting forms is important in encouraging reporting [2]. The scheme has recently encouraged reporting by nursing staff, midwives and health visitors [7]. Yellow reporting cards may be obtained electronically on http://www.mca.gov.uk/yellowcard. Pharmacists also play an important role in reporting ADRs [8]. The advisability of direct reporting of ADRs by patients is becoming an increasingly important topic for discussion in the world of pharmacovigilance [9]. 'Pharmacovigilance' in France, which involves reporting to regional centres, along with most other national schemes, also relies entirely on spontaneous reporting [10,11]. Institution of an ADR reporting project in Rhode Island in the USA increased the rate of reporting of such reactions more than 17-fold over a 2-year period [12]. The quality of ADR reporting to the FDA improved following introduction of the MedWatch scheme [13]. Specialty-based systems for spontaneous reporting of ADRs (e.g. the Adverse Drug Reaction Reporting System of the American Academy of Dermatology [14] and the Gruppo Italiano Studi Epidemiologici in Dermatologia [15]) have been introduced. In the UK, in contrast, the speciality-based Cutaneous Reactions Database established at the Institute of Dermatology in 1988 was unfortunately closed in 1990 because of a meagre response [16].

Reporting of ADRs in clinical trials is neglected, compared with efficacy outcomes; of 192 randomized trials analysed, only 46% specified reasons for withdrawals due to toxicity, and only 39% of clinical adverse effects and 29% of laboratory-determined toxicity were adequately documented [17]. Inherent difficulties with spontaneous reporting are that reactions associated with newly marketed drugs, those of unusual morphology, and reactions starting soon after initiation of therapy are more likely to be notified; at best only a crude estimate of true incidence is provided [18–20]. Thus, drugs with a high potential for eliciting clinically significant ADRs are usually detected and either withdrawn from the market or placed on restricted use within the first year or two of marketing [21]. In contrast, spontaneous reports do not reliably detect ADRs widely separated in time from the original use of the drug, or that occur more commonly in populations not usually exposed to the drug [22]. They are an unreliable measure of risk, and may simply provide evidence of the relative awareness among physicians of specific toxic effects [23].

All national spontaneous reporting systems are compromised by under-reporting [2,4]; in the UK, surveys suggest that only around 10% of serious reactions are notified to the Committee on Safety of Medicines [24,25]. A survey of 44 000 patients receiving one or other of seven new drugs suggested that under-reporting by the spontaneous system may be as high as 98% when compared with information collected by the more objective 'event monitoring' system [10]. Heavy prescribing by a minority of doctors immediately following licensing may place patients at unnecessary risk, and affects safety monitoring of new drugs; the 10% of doctors who prescribed most heavily accounted for 42% of total prescribing in a survey of 28 402 general practitioners asked to supply post-marketing data on 27 new drugs dispensed in England between September 1984 and June 1991, but returned proportionately far fewer questionnaires [26]. Reasons for under-reporting include lack of time, lack of report forms and the misconception that absolute confidence in the diagnosis of an adverse reaction was important [27]; workload may affect reporting [28]. Another factor is the perceived deterrent to reporting ADRs caused by fear of involvement in litigation [29]; reporting of errors should be free of recrimination [30]. The offer of a small fee increased the rate of reporting in one hospital study almost 50-fold [31].

Pharmacoepidemiology, the epidemiological assessment of adverse drug effects, and pharmacovigilance, the process of identifying and responding to safety issues about marketed drugs, necessitate making use of information from clinical trials, spontaneous reporting systems, specialty-based reporting systems, case reports, prescription monitoring, case series, cohort studies, case–control studies, population-based registries using computerized material, and special surveillance programmes (e.g. Boston Collaborative Drug Surveillance Program in the USA) [32–34]. Crude inspection of lists of spontaneously reported drug-event combinations can be supplemented by quantitative and automated numerator-based methods such as Bayesian data mining; pharmacovigilance specialists should not be intimidated by the mathematics [35]. Computerized detection of adverse events may soon be practical on a widespread basis [36]. This is just as well, as it has been estimated that the top 20 drug companies will each need to launch four to six times the number of drugs they currently produce merely to maintain shareholder returns, with more trials, and more safety reports for evaluation [37].

REFERENCES

1 Breathnach SM, Hintner H. *Adverse Drug Reactions and the Skin*. Oxford: Blackwell Scientific Publications, 1992.
2 Rawlins MD, Breckenridge AM, Wood SM. National adverse drug reaction reporting: a silver jubilee. *Adverse Drug React Bull* 1989; **138**: 516–9.
3 Bonnetblanc JM, Roujeau JC, Benichou C. Standardized coding is needed for reports of adverse drug reactions. *BMJ* 1996; **312**: 776–7.
4 Edwards IR. The management of adverse drug reactions: from diagnosis to signal. *Therapie* 2001; **56**: 727–33.
5 Rodriguez EM, Staffa JA, Graham DJ. The role of databases in drug post-marketing surveillance. *Pharmacoepidemiol Drug Saf* 2001; **10**: 407–10.
6 Ahmad SR. Adverse drug event monitoring at the Food and Drug Administration. *J Gen Intern Med* 2003; **18**: 57–60.
7 Morrison-Griffiths S, Walley TJ, Park BK *et al*. Reporting of adverse drug reactions by nurses. *Lancet* 2003; **361**: 1347–8.
8 van Grootheest AC, van Puijenbroek EP, de Jong-van den Berg LT. Contribution of pharmacists to the reporting of adverse drug reactions. *Pharmacoepidemiol Drug Saf* 2002; **11**: 205–10.
9 van Grootheest K, de Graaf L, de Jong-van den Berg LT. Consumer adverse drug reaction reporting: a new step in pharmacovigilance? *Drug Saf* 2003; **26**: 211–7.
10 Fletcher AP. Spontaneous adverse drug reaction reporting vs event monitoring: a comparison. *J R Soc Med* 1991; **84**: 341–4.
11 Moore N, Paux G, Begaud B *et al*. Adverse drug reaction monitoring: doing it the French way. *Lancet* 1985; **ii**: 1056–8.
12 Scott HD, Thacher-Renshaw A, Rosenbaum SE *et al*. Physician reporting of adverse drug reactions. Results of the Rhode Island Adverse Drug Reaction Reporting Project. *JAMA* 1990; **263**: 1785–8.
13 Piazza-Hepp TD, Kennedy DL. Reporting of adverse events to MedWatch. *Am J Health Syst Pharm* 1995; **52**: 1436–9.
14 Stern RS, Bigby M. An expanded profile of cutaneous reactions to non-steroid anti-inflammatory drugs. Reports to a specialty-based system for spontaneous reporting of adverse reactions to drugs. *JAMA* 1984; **252**: 1433–7.
15 Gruppo Italiano Studi Epidemiologici in Dermatologia. Spontaneous monitoring of adverse reactions to drugs by Italian dermatologists: a pilot study. *Dermatologica* 1991; **182**: 12–7.
16 Kobza Black A, Greaves MM. Cutaneous reactions database closure. *Br J Dermatol* 1990; **123**: 277.
17 Ioannidis JP, Lau J. Improving safety reporting from randomised trials. *Drug Saf* 2002; **25**: 77–84.
18 Griffin JP, Weber JCP. Voluntary systems of adverse reaction reporting: Part I. *Adverse Drug React Acute Poisoning Rev* 1985; **4**: 213–30.
19 Griffin JP, Weber JCP. Voluntary systems of adverse reaction reporting: Part II. *Adverse Drug React Acute Poisoning Rev* 1986; **5**: 23–55.
20 Griffin JP, Weber JCP. Voluntary systems of adverse reaction reporting: Part III. *Adverse Drug React Acute Poisoning Rev* 1989; **8**: 203–15.
21 Ajayi FO, Sun H, Perry J. Adverse drug reactions: a review of relevant factors. *J Clin Pharmacol* 2000; **40**: 1093–101.
22 Brewer T, Colditz GA. Postmarketing surveillance and adverse drug reactions: current perspectives and future needs. *JAMA* 1999; **281**: 824–9.
23 Miwa LJ, Jones JK, Pathiyal A, Hatoum H. Value of epidemiologic studies in determining the true incidence of adverse events. The nonsteroidal anti-inflammatory drug story. *Arch Intern Med* 1997; **157**: 2129–36.
24 Rawlins MD. Spontaneous reporting of adverse drug reactions I: the data. *Br J Clin Pharmacol* 1988; **26**: 1–5.
25 Bem JL, Mann RD, Rawlins MD. Review of yellow cards 1986 and 1987. *BMJ* 1988; **296**: 1319.
26 Inman W, Pearce G. Prescriber profile and post-marketing surveillance. *Lancet* 1993; **342**: 658–61.
27 Belton KJ, Lewis SC, Payne S *et al*. Attitudinal survey of adverse drug reaction reporting by medical practitioners in the United Kingdom. *Br J Clin Pharmacol* 1995; **39**: 223–6.
28 Bateman DN, Sanders GL, Rawlins MD. Attitudes to adverse drug reaction reporting in the Northern Region. *Br J Clin Pharmacol* 1992; **34**: 421–6.
29 Kaufman MB, Stoukides CA, Campbell NA. Physicians' liability for adverse drug reactions. *South Med J* 1994; **87**: 780–4.
30 Upton DR, Cousins DH. Avoiding drug errors. Reporting of errors should be free of recrimination. *BMJ* 1995; **311**: 1367.
31 Feely J, Moriarty S, O'Connor P. Stimulating reporting of adverse drug reactions by using a fee. *BMJ* 1990; **300**: 22–3.

32 Stern RS, Wintroub BU. Adverse drug reactions: reporting and evaluating cutaneous reactions. *Adv Dermatol* 1987; **2**: 3–18.

33 Stern RS. Epidemiologic assessment of adverse drug effects. *Semin Dermatol* 1989; **8**: 136–40.

34 Rawlins MD. Pharmacovigilance: paradise lost, regained or postponed? *J R Coll Physicians Lond* 1995; **29**: 41–5.

35 Hauben M, Zhou X. Quantitative methods in pharmacovigilance: focus on signal detection. *Drug Saf* 2003; **26**: 159–86.

36 Bates DW, Evans RS, Murff H *et al*. Detecting adverse events using information technology. *J Am Med Inform Assoc* 2003; **10**: 115–28.

37 Peachey J. From pharmacovigilance to pharmacoperformance. *Drug Saf* 2002; **25**: 399–405.

General incidence of adverse drug reactions

The incidence of ADRs varies from 6% [1] to 30% [2], with at least 90 million courses of drug treatment given yearly in the USA [3]. The reported percentage of patients who develop an ADR during hospitalization varies markedly in different studies from 1.4 to 44%, although in most studies the incidence is about 10–20% [4–6], of which about one-third are allergic or pseudoallergic [6]. In one study, 0.23% of a total of 90 910 admissions had drug allergy; antimicrobials and antiepileptic drugs comprised 75% of the drug allergies reported [7]. The incidence of drug allergy in hospitalized patients was 4.2 per 1000; drug allergy developed during in-patient treatment in 2.07 per 1000 hospitalizations [7]. About 3–8% of hospital admissions are a consequence of ADRs [8–10]. A survey of 30 195 randomly selected hospital records in 51 hospitals in the state of New York found that 19% of adverse events caused by medical treatment were the result of drug complications; the most frequently implicated classes of drugs were antibiotics, antitumour agents and anticoagulants [11]. Negligence accounted for 18% of ADRs, while allergic/cutaneous complications constituted 14% of all drug-related complications.

Less information is available about the incidence among outpatients. It has been estimated that about 1 in 40 consultations in general practice is the result of ADRs [12], and eventually 41% of patients develop a reaction [13]. In one multicentre general practice study in the UK, the percentage of consultations involving an ADR increased from 0.6% for patients aged 0–20 years to 2.7% for patients aged over 50 years [14]; in another study, 2.5% of consultations were the result of iatrogenic illness [15].

Fatal reactions to drugs are more common than is generally realized. It was previously estimated that penicillin caused 300 deaths each year in the USA alone [16]. Anaphylactic reactions to penicillin were reported in 1968 to occur in about 0.015%, and fatal reactions in up to 0.002% (i.e. 1 per 50 000), of treatment courses [17]. These figures may be somewhat less today, with use of newer β-lactam antibiotics. The risk of fatal aplastic anaemia with chloramphenicol therapy was reported as at least 1 in 60 000 [18], and the risk of a fatal outcome from treatment with monoamine oxidase inhibitors may be of the same order. It has been estimated that the incidence of fatality as a result of a drug reaction among in-patients is between 0.1 and 0.3% [5,19,20]; fatality due to allergy occurs at a rate of 0.09 per 1000 cases [7].

REFERENCES

1 Deswarte RD. Drug allergy: problems and strategies. *J Allergy Clin Immunol* 1984; **74**: 209–21.

2 Jick H. Adverse drug reactions: the magnitude of the problem. *J Allergy Clin Immunol* 1984; **74**: 555–7.

3 Goldstein RA. Foreword. Symposium proceedings on drug allergy: prevention, diagnosis, treatment. *J Allergy Clin Immunol* 1984; **74**: 549–50.

4 Breathnach SM, Hintner H. *Adverse Drug Reactions and the Skin*. Oxford: Blackwell Scientific Publications, 1992.

5 Gruchalla R. Understanding drug allergies. *J Allergy Clin Immunol* 2000; **105**: S637–S644.

6 Demoly P, Bousquet J. Epidemiology of drug allergy. *Curr Opin Allergy Clin Immunol* 2001; **1**: 305–10.

7 Thong BY, Leong KP, Tang CY, Chung HH. Drug allergy in a general hospital: results of a novel prospective inpatient reporting system. *Ann Allergy Asthma Immunol* 2003; **90**: 342–7.

8 McKenney JM, Harrison WL. Drug-related hospital admissions. *Am J Hosp Pharm* 1976; **33**: 792–5.

9 Levy M, Kewitz H, Altwein W *et al*. Hospital admissions due to adverse drug reactions: a comparative study from Jerusalem and Berlin. *Eur J Clin Pharmacol* 1980; **17**: 25–31.

10 Black AJ, Somers K. Drug-related illness resulting in hospital admission. *J R Coll Physicians Lond* 1984; **18**: 40–1.

11 Leape LL, Brennan TA, Laird N *et al*. The nature of adverse events in hospitalized patients. Results of the Harvard Medical Practice Study II. *N Engl J Med* 1991; **324**: 377–84.

12 Kellaway GSM, McCrae E. Intensive monitoring of adverse drug effects in patients discharged from acute medical wards. *NZ Med J* 1973; **78**: 525–8.

13 Martys CR. Adverse reactions to drugs in general practice. *BMJ* 1979; **ii**: 1194–7.

14 Lumley LE, Walker SR, Hall CG *et al*. The under-reporting of adverse drug reactions seen in general practice. *Pharm Med* 1986; **1**: 205–12.

15 Mulroy R. Iatrogenic disease in general practice: its incidence and effects. *BMJ* 1973; **ii**: 407–10.

16 Parker CW. Allergic reactions in man. *Pharmacol Rev* 1983; **34**: 85–104.

17 Idsøe O, Guthe T, Willcox RR, De Weck AL. Nature and extent of penicillin side reactions, with particular reference to fatalities from anaphylactic shock. *Bull WHO* 1968; **38**: 159–88.

18 Witts LJ. Adverse reactions to drugs. *BMJ* 1965; **ii**: 1081–6.

19 Davies DM, ed. *Textbook of Adverse Drug Reactions*, 3rd edn. Oxford: Oxford University Press, 1985: 1–11.

20 Caranasos GJ, May FE, Stewart RB, Cluff LE. Drug-associated deaths of medical inpatients. *Arch Intern Med* 1976; **136**: 872–5.

Risk of adverse drug reactions among different patient groups

Certain patient groups are at increased risk of developing an ADR. Women are more likely than men to develop ADRs [1]. The incidence of such reactions increases with the number of drugs taken in both hospital in-patients [2–4] and outpatients [5,6]. Although data are somewhat conflicting [7], the burden of evidence suggests that the incidence of adverse reactions increases with patient age [1,8,9]. Although those over 65 years of age comprise only 12% of the population in the USA, 33% of all drugs are prescribed for this age group, and the elderly have a significantly higher incidence of ADRs, related to decreased organ reserve capacity, altered pharmacokinetics and pharmacodynamics, and polypharmacy [10]. Similarly, in the UK the elderly are dispensed twice as many prescriptions as the national average [11]. Potential adverse drug interactions are more common in elderly patients because of the higher number of concurrent medications, rather than age-based factors [12].

ADRs contribute to the need for hospitalization in 10–17% of elderly inpatients [13–15]. Inappropriate medication is a major cause of ADRs in elderly patients; 27% of elderly patients on medication admitted to a teaching hospital experienced ADRs, of which almost 50% were due to drugs with absolute contraindications and/or that were unnecessary [16]. ADRs occur in 6–17% of children admitted to specialist paediatric hospitals [17].

Patients with Sjögren's syndrome (SS) have also been reported to have a high frequency of drug allergy. In different series, drug allergy has been reported in 43% of SS patients compared with 9% of patients with systemic lupus erythematosus (SLE) without SS [18], in 62% of SS patients [19], and in 41% of rheumatoid arthritis patients with SS compared with 17% of those without SS [20]. Antibiotic allergy is increased in SLE [21].

REFERENCES

1 Davies DM, ed. *Textbook of Adverse Drug Reactions*, 3rd edn. Oxford: Oxford University Press, 1985: 1–11.
2 Vakil BJ, Kulkarni RD, Chabria NL et al. Intense surveillance of adverse drug reactions. An analysis of 338 patients. *J Clin Pharmacol* 1975; **15**: 435–41.
3 May FE, Stewart RB, Cluff LE. Drug interactions and multiple drug administration. *Clin Pharmacol Ther* 1977; **22**: 322–8.
4 Steel K, Gertman PM, Crescenzi C, Anderson J. Iatrogenic illness on a general medical service at a university hospital. *N Engl J Med* 1981; **304**: 638–42.
5 Kellaway GSM, McCrae E. Intensive monitoring of adverse drug effects in patients discharged from acute medical wards. *NZ Med J* 1973; **78**: 525–8.
6 Hutchinson TA, Flegel KM, Kramer MS et al. Frequency, severity, and risk factors for adverse reactions in adult outpatients: a prospective study. *J Chron Dis* 1986; **39**: 533–42.
7 Gurwitz JH, Avorn J. The ambiguous relation between aging and adverse drug reactions. *Ann Intern Med* 1991; **114**: 956–66.
8 Nolan L, O'Malley K. Adverse drug reactions in the elderly. *Br J Hosp Med* 1989; **41**: 446–57.
9 Sullivan JR, Shear NH. Drug eruptions and other adverse drug effects in aged skin. *Clin Geriatr Med* 2002; **18**: 21–42.
10 Sloan RW. Principles of drug therapy in geriatric patients. *Am Fam Physician* 1992; **45**: 2709–18.
11 Black D, Denham MJ, Acheson RM et al. Medication for the elderly. A report of the Royal College of Physicians. *J R Coll Physicians Lond* 1984; **18**: 7–17.
12 Heininger-Rothbucher D, Bischinger S, Ulmer H et al. Incidence and risk of potential adverse drug interactions in the emergency room. *Resuscitation* 2001; **49**: 283–8.
13 Col N, Fanale JE, Kronholm P. The role of medication noncompliance and adverse drug reactions in hospitalizations of the elderly. *Arch Intern Med* 1990; **150**: 841–5.
14 Levy M, Kewitz H, Altwein W et al. Hospital admissions due to adverse drug reactions: a comparative study from Jerusalem and Berlin. *Eur J Clin Pharmacol* 1980; **17**: 25–31.
15 Williamson J, Chopin JM. Adverse reactions to prescribed drugs in the elderly: a multicentre investigation. *Age Ageing* 1980; **9**: 73–80.
16 Lindley CM, Tully MP, Paramsothy V, Tallis RC. Inappropriate medication is a major cause of adverse drug reactions in elderly patients. *Age Ageing* 1992; **21**: 294–300.
17 Rylance G, Armstrong D. Adverse drug events in children. *Adverse Drug React Bull* 1997; **184**: 689–702.
18 Katz J, Marmary Y, Livneh A, Danon Y. Drug allergy in Sjögren's syndrome. *Lancet* 1991; **337**: 239.
19 Bloch KJ, Buchanan WW, Wohl MJ, Bunim JJ. Sjögrens's syndrome: a clinical, pathological and serological study of 62 cases. *Medicine (Baltimore)* 1965; **44**: 187–231.
20 Williams BO, Onge RAST, Young A et al. Penicillin allergy in rheumatoid arthritis with special reference to Sjögren's syndrome. *Ann Rheum Dis* 1969; **28**: 607–11.
21 Petri M, Allbritton J. Antibiotic allergy in systemic lupus erythematosus: a case–control study. *J Rheumatol* 1992; **19**: 265–9.

Acquired immune deficiency syndrome

Patients with acquired immune deficiency syndrome (AIDS) appear to be at increased risk for ADRs [1–7], up to 100-fold by some estimates [7]. The reasons are likely to be multifactorial, and include changes in drug metabolism, oxidative stress, cytokine profiles and immune hyperactivation. Human immunodeficiency virus (HIV)-positive individuals have been postulated to have a systemic glutathione deficiency, resulting in a decreased capacity to scavenge reactive hydroxylamine derivatives of sulphonamides, although this has been disputed (see pharmacogenetic mechanisms of drug reactions, p. 73.13). In the past, drugs especially implicated included sulphonamides such as co-trimoxazole (trimethoprim–sulfamethoxazole) [8–14], other sulphur congeners, for example dapsone [15], pentamidine, antituberculosis regimens containing thioacetazone (thiacetazone) [16,17] or isoniazid and rifampicin, amoxicillin–clavulanate [18,19], clindamycin, pyrimethamine [20] and thalidomide. Patients with AIDS are more likely to have particularly severe reactions, ranging from erythema multiforme to toxic epidermal necrolysis (TEN) (especially with sulphonamides, clindamycin, phenobarbital (phenobarbitone) and chlormezanone) [21,22], and to demonstrate multiple cutaneous drug reactions [3] (see Chapter 74). Drugs that are implicated in hypersensitivity have changed since the advent of highly active antiretroviral therapy, including abacavir, nonnucleoside reverse transcriptase inhibitors such as nevirapine, and protease inhibitors such as amprenavir [7]. There has been a decrease in the use of antimicrobials such as co-trimoxazole, and in Europe nevirapine has replaced sulphonamides as the leading cause of Stevens–Johnson syndrome and TEN related to AIDS [23] (see also Chapter 74).

REFERENCES

1 Coopman SA, Stern RS. Cutaneous drug reactions in human immunodeficiency virus infection. *Arch Dermatol* 1991; **127**: 714–7.
2 Bayard PJ, Berger TG, Jacobson MA. Drug hypersensitivity reactions and human immunodeficiency virus disease. *J Acquir Immune Defic Syndr* 1992; **5**: 1237–57.
3 Carr A, Tindall B, Penny R, Cooper DA. Patterns of multiple-drug hypersensitivities in HIV-infected patients. *AIDS* 1993; **7**: 1532–3.
4 Sadick NS, McNutt NS. Cutaneous hypersensitivity reactions in patients with AIDS. *Int J Dermatol* 1993; **32**: 621–7.
5 Coopman SA, Johnson RA, Platt R, Stern RS. Cutaneous disease and drug reactions in HIV infection. *N Engl J Med* 1993; **328**: 1670–4.
6 Heller HM. Adverse cutaneous drug reactions in patients with human immunodeficiency virus-1 infection. *Clin Dermatol* 2000; **18**: 485–9.

7 Pirmohamed M, Park BK. HIV and drug allergy. *Curr Opin Allergy Clin Immunol* 2001; **1**: 311–6.
8 Kletzel M, Beck S, Elser J *et al.* Trimethoprim–sulfamethoxazole oral desensitization in hemophiliacs infected with human immunodeficiency virus with a history of hypersensitivity reactions. *Am J Dis Child* 1991; **145**: 1428–9.
9 Carr A, Swanson C, Penny R, Cooper DA. Clinical and laboratory markers of hypersensitivity to trimethoprim–sulfamethoxazole in patients with *Pneumocystis carinii* pneumonia and AIDS. *J Infect Dis* 1993; **167**: 180–5.
10 Mathelier-Fusade P, Leynadier F. Intolerance aux sulfamides chez les sujets infectés par le VIH. Origine toxique et allergique. *Presse Med* 1993; **22**: 1363–5.
11 Chanock SJ, Luginbuhl LM, McIntosh K, Lipshultz SE. Life-threatening reaction to trimethoprim/sulfamethoxazole in pediatric human immunodeficiency virus infection. *Pediatrics* 1994; **93**: 519–21.
12 Roudier C, Caumes E, Rogeaux O *et al.* Adverse cutaneous reactions to trimethoprim–sulfamethoxazole in patients with the acquired immunodeficiency syndrome and *Pneumocystis carinii* pneumonia. *Arch Dermatol* 1994; **130**: 1383–6.
13 Rabaud C, Charreau I, Izard S *et al.* Adverse reactions to cotrimoxazole in HIV-infected patients: predictive factors and subsequent HIV disease progression. *Scand J Infect Dis* 2001; **33**: 759–64.
14 Eliaszewicz M, Flahault A, Roujeau JC *et al.* Prospective evaluation of risk factors of cutaneous drug reactions to sulfonamides in patients with AIDS. *J Am Acad Dermatol* 2002; **47**: 40–6.
15 Jorde UP, Horowitz HW, Wormser GP. Utility of dapsone for prophylaxis of *Pneumocystis carinii* pneumonia in trimethoprim–sulfamethoxazole-intolerant, HIV-infected individuals. *AIDS* 1993; **7**: 355–9.
16 Nunn P, Kibuga D, Gathua S *et al.* Cutaneous hypersensitivity reactions due to thiacetazone in HIV-1 seropositive patients treated for tuberculosis. *Lancet* 1991; **337**: 627–30.
17 Pozniak AL, MacLeod GA, Mahari M *et al.* The influence of HIV status on single and multiple drug reactions to antituberculous therapy in Africa. *AIDS* 1992; **6**: 809–14.
18 Battegay M, Opravil M, Würich B, Lüthy R. Rash with amoxycillin–clavulanate therapy in HIV-infected patients. *Lancet* 1989; **ii**: 1100.
19 Paparello SF, Davis CE, Malone JL. Cutaneous reactions to amoxicillin–clavulanate among Haitians. *AIDS* 1994; **8**: 276–7.
20 Piketty C, Weiss L, Picard-Dahan C *et al.* Toxidermies à la pyriméthamine chez les patients infectés par le virus de l'immunodeficience acquise. *Presse Med* 1995; **24**: 1710.
21 Porteous DM, Berger TG. Severe cutaneous drug reactions (Stevens–Johnson syndrome and toxic epidermal necrolysis) in human immunodeficiency virus infection. *Arch Dermatol* 1991; **127**: 740–1.
22 Saiag P, Caumes E, Chosidow O *et al.* Drug-induced toxic epidermal necrolysis (Lyell syndrome) in patients infected with the human immunodeficiency virus. *J Am Acad Dermatol* 1992; **26**: 567–74.
23 Fagot JP, Mockenhaupt M, Bouwes-Bavinck JN *et al.* Nevirapine and the risk of Stevens–Johnson syndrome or toxic epidermal necrolysis. *AIDS* 2001; **15**: 1843–8.

Drug reaction frequency in relation to types of medication

The incidence of reactions to a particular drug must obviously be related to the quantity prescribed [1]. Nearly one in every 10 prescriptions in the USA in 1981 contained either hydrochlorothiazide or codeine [2]. One in every five prescriptions was for a diuretic or other cardiovascular drug; analgesics and antiarthritics constituted 13%, anti-infectives 13%, and sedatives and other psychotropics 11% of prescriptions. Of the 10 drugs most frequently reported by the yellow-card system to the UK Committee on Safety of Medicines in the first 6 months of 1986, seven were non-steroidal anti-inflammatory drugs (NSAIDs) (accounting for 74% of serious adverse reactions); the remaining drugs were the angiotensin-converting enzyme (ACE) inhibitors enalapril and captopril (accounting for

19% of serious reactions) and co-trimoxazole (accounting for 7% of serious adverse reactions) [3]. In another study, anti-inflammatory agents were the drugs responsible for almost 50% of the reactions necessitating admission to a general medical ward; most of the drug-related admissions to the hospital as a whole were caused by digoxin, phenytoin, tranquillizers, antihypertensives, cardiac depressants and antineoplastic agents [4]. ADRs accounted for 8% of 1999 consecutive admissions to medical wards in yet another study [5]; the drugs most frequently involved were antirheumatics and analgesics (27%), cardiovascular drugs (23%), psychotropic drugs (14%), antidiabetics (12%), antibiotics (7%) and corticosteroids (5%). Nitrofurantoin and insulin were associated with admission rates of 617 and 182 per million daily doses, compared with 10 for diuretics and seven for benzodiazepines. ADRs were responsible for the admission of 2% of 5227 consecutive patients to the University Hospital Centre in Zagreb [6]; drugs incriminated included acetylsalicylic acid (aspirin) (38%), other NSAIDs (23%), cardiovascular agents (20%) and antimicrobials (3%).

REFERENCES

1 Committee on Safety of Medicines. CSM update: non-steroidal anti-inflammatory drugs and serious gastrointestinal reactions-2. *BMJ* 1986; **292**: 1190–1.
2 Baum C, Kennedy DL, Forbes MB, Jones JK. Drug use in the United States in 1981. *JAMA* 1984; **251**: 1293–7.
3 Mann RD. The yellow card data: the nature and scale of the adverse drug reactions problem. In: Mann RD, ed. *Adverse Drug Reactions*. Carnforth: Parthenon, 1987: 5–66.
4 Black AJ, Somers K. Drug-related illness resulting in hospital admission. *J R Coll Physicians Lond* 1984; **18**: 40–1.
5 Hallas J, Gram LF, Grodum E *et al.* Drug related admissions to medical wards: a population based survey. *Br J Clin Pharmacol* 1992; **33**: 61–8.
6 Huic M, Mucolic V, Vrhovac B *et al.* Adverse drug reactions resulting in hospital admission. *Int J Clin Pharmacol Ther* 1994; **32**: 675–82.

Incidence of drug eruptions (adverse cutaneous drug reactions)

Drug eruptions are probably the most frequent of all manifestations of drug sensitivity, at 24% of all ADRs in one study [1], although their incidence is difficult to determine. Even where the eruption is apparently the only manifestation, death can result from exfoliative dermatitis, erythema multiforme or TEN. For information on the incidence of drug-induced erythema multiforme, Stevens–Johnson syndrome and TEN, the reader is referred to Chapter 74. Epidemiological data suggest that a relatively small number of drugs are responsible most often for the most serious reactions [2]. Cutaneous reactions to common drugs such as digoxin, antacids, paracetamol (acetaminophen in the USA), glyceryl trinitrate, spironolactone, meperidine, aminophylline, propranolol, prednisone, salbutamol and diazepam are very rare.

The baseline rate of rash development, reflecting a variety of different causes, was similar for 36 marketed drugs in the UK, at around 1 per 1000 patients per month from the second to the sixth month of one study; however, the rate for rash in the first month after prescription varied substantially from 0.9 to 6.4 per 1000 patients per month, and was highest for diltiazem [3]. Most estimates of the incidence of drug eruptions are inaccurate, because many mild and transitory eruptions are not recorded and because skin disorders are sometimes falsely attributed to drugs. There have been several studies of the incidence of drug eruptions [3–13]. The reaction rate has been reported as about 2% [6,9], or 5.5 adverse skin reactions per 100 000 of the population in four Italian regions [10].

A survey [8] of adverse cutaneous drug reactions (ACDRs) among in-patients found that one-third were fixed drug reactions, one-third were exanthematous and 20% were urticaria or angio-oedema; the high frequency of fixed drug reactions in this series reflects the fact that patients under study had been admitted to hospital. Antimicrobial agents were most frequently incriminated (42%), then antipyretic/anti-inflammatory analgesics (27%), with drugs acting on the central nervous system accounting for 10% of reactions. A few drugs gave specific reactions (e.g. phenazone salicylate caused a fixed eruption, and penicillin and salicylates caused urticaria); however, most were capable of causing several types of eruption. Morbilliform exanthematous eruptions, urticaria and generalized pruritus were the commonest reactions in other large series [9,13]. The average patient had received eight different medications, which contributed considerably to the difficulties in identifying the causative drugs [9]. Antibiotics, blood products and inhaled mucolytics together caused 75% of the eruptions; amoxicillin (51 cases/1000 exposed), trimethoprim–sulfamethoxazole (33 cases/1000 exposed) and ampicillin (33 cases/1000 exposed) caused the most reactions. Reaction rates varied in the range of 1–8% for several classes of antibiotic [13]. In a study of ACDRs among children and adolescents in northern India, antibiotics were responsible for most eruptions, followed by antiepileptics; co-trimoxazole was the commonest antibacterial culprit, followed by penicillin and its semi-synthetic derivatives, and then sulphonamides, with antiepileptics being the most frequently incriminated drugs in erythema multiforme, Stevens–Johnson syndrome and TEN [11]. A more recent study from India found that the drugs most often incriminated included antimicrobials (especially sulphonamides), anticonvulsants and NSAIDs [12]. Antimicrobials, NSAIDs, analgesics and radiological contrast media were the most frequent culprits in a study from Italy [10], and the most common drug classes involved in yet another study were cardiovascular agents (36%), contrast media (20%), drugs affecting blood clotting (13%) and anti-infectives (14%) [1].

Desensitizing vaccines, muscle relaxants, intravenous anaesthetics and radiological contrast media were the most frequent causes of anaphylaxis or anaphylactoid reactions reported to the UK Committee on Safety of Medicines in 1986/1987 [14]. The chairman of the Committee accordingly advised in 1986 that desensitizing vaccines only be given where full cardiorespiratory resuscitation facilities are available. Quinidine, cimetidine, phenylbutazone, hydrochlorothiazide (especially in combination with amiloride) and furosemide (frusemide) have also been frequently implicated in drug eruptions [15,16]. In the USA and the UK, antibiotics, hypnotics and tranquillizers are the most frequent offenders; on a reaction per dose basis, penicillin, warfarin and imipramine are the three drugs most frequently incriminated [17]. The prevalence of a history of penicillin allergy in the US population has been estimated to be between 5 and 10% [18]. An international study of 1790 patients from 11 countries documented the frequency of allergic reactions to long-term benzathine benzylpenicillin (benzathine penicillin) prophylaxis for rheumatic fever at 3.2%; anaphylaxis occurred in 0.2% (1.2/10 000 injections) and the fatality rate was 0.05% (0.31/10 000 injections) [19]. Reactions to sulphonamides may affect up to 5% of those treated [20]. Rashes occurred in 7.3% of children given commonly used oral antibiotics [21]. Based on the number of patients treated, the frequency of rash with cefaclor was 12.3%, with penicillins 7.4%, with sulphonamides 8.5%, and with other cephalosporins 2.6%.

REFERENCES

1 Bordet R, Gautier S, Le Louet H *et al*. Analysis of the direct cost of adverse drug reactions in hospitalised patients. *Eur J Clin Pharmacol* 2001; **56**: 935–41.
2 Stern RS, Steinberg LA. Epidemiology of adverse cutaneous reactions to drugs. *Dermatol Clin* 1995; **13**: 681–8.
3 Kubota K, Kubota N, Pearce GL *et al*. Signalling drug-induced rash with 36 drugs recently marketed in the United Kingdom and studied by Prescription-Event Monitoring. *Int J Clin Pharmacol Ther* 1995; **33**: 219–25.
4 Kaplan AP. Drug-induced skin disease. *J Allergy Clin Immunol* 1984; **74**: 573–9.
5 Kauppinen K. Cutaneous reactions to drugs. With special reference to severe mucocutaneous bullous eruptions and sulphonamides. *Acta Derm Venereol Suppl (Stockh)* 1972; **68**: 1–89.
6 Arndt KA, Jick H. Rates of cutaneous reactions to drugs. A report from the Boston Collaborative Drug Surveillance Program. *JAMA* 1976; **235**: 918–22.
7 Kauppinen K, Stubb S. Drug eruptions: causative agents and clinical types. A series of inpatients during a 10-year period. *Acta Derm Venereol (Stockh)* 1984; **64**: 320–4.
8 Alanko K, Stubb S, Kauppinen K. Cutaneous drug reactions: clinical types and causative agents. A five year survey of in-patients (1981–1985). *Acta Derm Venereol (Stockh)* 1989; **69**: 223–6.
9 Bigby M, Jick S, Jick H, Arndt K. Drug-induced cutaneous reactions. A report from the Boston Collaborative Drug Surveillance Program on 15438 consecutive inpatients, 1975 to 1982. *JAMA* 1986; **256**: 3358–63.
10 Naldi L, Conforti A, Venegoni M *et al*. Cutaneous reactions to drugs. An analysis of spontaneous reports in four Italian regions. *Br J Clin Pharmacol* 1999; **48**: 839–46.
11 Sharma VK, Dhar S. Clinical pattern of cutaneous drug eruption among children and adolescents in north India. *Pediatr Dermatol* 1995; **12**: 178–83.
12 Sharma VK, Sethuraman G, Kumar B. Cutaneous adverse drug reactions: clinical pattern and causative agents. A 6 year series from Chandigarh, India. *J Postgrad Med* 2001; **47**: 95–9.
13 Bigby M. Rates of cutaneous reactions to drugs. *Arch Dermatol* 2001; **137**: 765–70.

14 Bem JL, Mann RD, Rawlins MD. Review of yellow cards 1986 and 1987. *BMJ* 1988; **296**: 1319.
15 Kalish RS. Drug eruptions: a review of clinical and immunological features. *Adv Dermatol* 1991; **6**: 221–37.
16 Thestrup-Pedersen K. Adverse reactions in the skin from antihypertensive drugs. *Dan Med Bull* 1987; **34**: 3–5.
17 Davies DM, ed. *Textbook of Adverse Drug Reactions*, 3rd edn. Oxford: Oxford University Press, 1985: 1–11.
18 Green CR, Rosenblum A. Report of the Penicillin Study Group: American Academy of Allergy. *J Allergy Clin Immunol* 1971; **48**: 331–43.
19 International Rheumatic Fever Study Group. Allergic reactions to long-term benzathine penicillin prophylaxis for rheumatic fever. *Lancet* 1991; **337**: 1308–10.
20 Anonymous. Hypersensitivity to sulphonamides: a clue? *Lancet* 1986; **ii**: 958–9.
21 Ibia EO, Schwartz RH, Wiedermann BL. Antibiotic rashes in children: a survey in a private practice setting. *Arch Dermatol* 2000; **136**: 849–54.

Classification and mechanisms of drug reactions [1–11]

Drug reactions may arise as a result of immunological allergy directed against the drug itself, a reactive metabolite or some contaminant of the drug or, more commonly, by non-immunological mechanisms, such as pseudoallergic reactions caused by non-immune-mediated degranulation of mast cells and basophils. Autoimmune reactions, in which the drug elicits an immune reaction to autologous structures, may also occur. Drug reactions may be predictable (type A) or unpredictable (type B) (Table 73.1). About 80% of drug reactions are predictable, usually dose related, are a function of the known pharmacological actions of the drug and occur in otherwise normal individuals. Side effects are unavoidable at the regular prescribed dose. Unpredictable reactions are dose independent, are not related to the pharmacological action of the drug, and may have a basis in pharmacogenetic variation in drug bioactivation and drug or metabolite detoxification or clearance. Intolerance refers to an expected drug reaction occurring at a lower dose, and idiosyncratic and hypersensitivity reactions are qualitatively abnormal unexpected responses. Type C reactions include those associated with prolonged therapy (e.g. analgesic nephropathy), and type D reactions consist of delayed reactions (e.g. carcinogenesis and teratogenicity). The skin has a limited repertoire of morphological reaction patterns in response to a wide variety of stimuli, and it is therefore often impossible to identify an offending drug, or the pathological mechanism involved, on the basis of clinical appearances alone. We therefore remain relatively ignorant about the mechanisms underlying many clinical drug eruptions.

Table 73.1 Classification of adverse drug reactions.

Non-immunological
Predictable
  Overdosage
  Side effects
  Cumulation
  Delayed toxicity
  Facultative effects
  Drug interactions
  Metabolic alterations
  Teratogenicity
  Non-immunological activation of effector pathways
  Exacerbation of disease
  Drug-induced chromosomal damage
Unpredictable
  Intolerance
  Idiosyncrasy

Immunological (unpredictable)
IgE-dependent drug reactions
Immune complex-dependent drug reactions
Cytotoxic drug-induced reactions
Cell-mediated reactions

Miscellaneous
Jarisch–Herxheimer reactions
Infectious mononucleosis–ampicillin reaction

REFERENCES

1 Rawlins MD, Thompson JW. Mechanisms of adverse drug reactions. In: Davies DM, ed. *Textbook of Adverse Drug Reactions*, 3rd edn. Oxford: Oxford University Press, 1985: 12–38.
2 Wintroub BU, Stern R. Cutaneous drug reactions: pathogenesis and clinical classification. *J Am Acad Dermatol* 1985; **13**: 833–45.
3 Stern RS, Wintroub BU, Arndt KA. Drug reactions. *J Am Acad Dermatol* 1986; **15**: 1282–8.
4 Breathnach SM, Hintner H. *Adverse Drug Reactions and the Skin*. Oxford: Blackwell Scientific Publications, 1992.
5 Weiss ME. Drug allergy. *Med Clin North Am* 1992; **76**: 857–82.
6 Gibaldi M. Adverse drug effect-reactive metabolites and idiosyncratic drug reactions: Part I. *Ann Pharmacother* 1992; **26**: 416–21.
7 Anderson JA. Allergic reactions to drugs and biological agents. *JAMA* 1992; **268**: 2844–57.
8 Pichler WJ. Medikamentenallergien. *Ther Umsch* 1994; **51**: 55–60.
9 Rieder MJ. Mechanisms of unpredictable adverse drug reactions. *Drug Saf* 1994; **11**: 196–212.
10 Breathnach SM. Mechanisms of drug eruptions: Part I. *Australas J Dermatol* 1995; **36**: 121–7.
11 Bonnetblanc JM, Vaillant L, Wolkenstein P. Facteurs prédisposants des réactions cutanées aux médicaments. *Ann Dermatol Vénéréol* 1995; **122**: 484–6.

Non-immunological drug reactions

Overdosage

The manifestations are a predictable exaggeration of the desired pharmacological actions of the drug, and are directly related to the total amount of drug in the body. Overdosage may be absolute, as a result of a prescribing or dispensing error or due to deliberate excess intake by the patient. It may also occur despite standard dosage due to varying individual rates of absorption, metabolism or excretion (see below). An inappropriately large dose may be given to an infant or very old person or to one with renal impairment. Drug interaction (see below) may also cause drug overdosage.

Side effects

These include unwanted or toxic effects, which are not separable from the desired pharmacological action of the drug. Examples are the drowsiness induced by antihistamines; the atropine-like anticholinergic properties of some phenothiazines, many antihistamines, and tricyclic antidepressants; and the anagen alopecia caused by cytotoxic drugs.

Cumulative toxicity

Prolonged exposure may lead to cumulative toxicity. Accumulation of drugs in the skin may lead to colour disturbance, as a result of either deposition within phagocytic cells or mucous membranes (e.g. prolonged administration of gold, silver, bismuth or mercury) or binding of the drug or a metabolite to a skin component (e.g. high-dose chlorpromazine therapy).

Delayed toxicity

Examples are the keratoses and skin tumours that appear many years after inorganic arsenic, and the delayed hepatotoxicity associated with methotrexate therapy.

Facultative effects

These include the consequences of drug-induced alterations in skin or mucous membrane flora. Antibiotics that destroy Gram-positive bacteria may allow the multiplication of resistant Gram-negative species. Broad-spectrum antibiotics, corticosteroids and immunosuppressive drugs may promote multiplication of *Candida albicans* and favour its transition from saprophytism to pathogenicity. Corticosteroids promote the spread of tinea and erythrasma. Antibiotics such as clindamycin and tetracycline may be associated with pseudomembranous enterocolitis following bowel superinfection with *Clostridium difficile*.

Drug interactions

Interactions between two or more drugs administered simultaneously may occur before entry into the body (in an intravenous drip), in the intestine, in the blood and/or at tissue receptor sites; interaction may also occur indirectly as a result of acceleration or slowing in the rate of drug metabolism or excretion. It should be remembered that the adverse consequences of drug interactions may occur not only on introduction of a drug but also on removal of a drug that causes acceleration of drug metabolism, as this may result in effective overdosage of the remaining drug. The subject of drug interactions has been extensively reviewed [1,2]. Combinations of drugs with potential adverse interactions continue to be prescribed [3].

Intestinal drug interactions. Examples include inhibition of griseofulvin absorption by phenobarbital [1], inhibition of tetracycline absorption by antacids [4] and decreased absorption of the oral contraceptive by tetracycline [5]. Whether the latter is of real significance is a matter of debate [6].

Displacement from carrier or receptor sites. Most drugs are reversibly bound to carrier proteins in plasma or extracellular fluid; bound drug acts as a reservoir, preventing excessive fluctuation in the level of the active unbound fraction. Displacement from a carrier protein augments drug activity, whereas displacement from a receptor site diminishes it. Many acidic drugs such as salicylates, coumarins, sulphonamides and phenylbutazone are bound to plasma albumin, and compete for binding sites. Thus, a sulphonamide may displace tolbutamide from albumin leading to hypoglycaemia; or aspirin, sulphonamides, clofibrate or phenylbutazone may displace warfarin from albumin, causing bleeding and ecchymoses. Similarly, sulphonamides and aspirin may increase methotrexate toxicity. Ciprofloxacin increases plasma levels of theophylline.

Enzyme stimulation or inhibition [2]. A drug may either stimulate or inhibit metabolic enzymes important to its own degradation or that of another agent, with significant clinical consequences. Thus, some drugs induce synthesis of drug-metabolizing enzymes in liver microsomes. The liver microsomal hydroxylating system (which mediates metabolism of phenytoin and debrisoquine) is based on cytochrome P-450, and appears to be a family of enzymes capable of acting on different substrates including barbiturates, fatty acids and endogenous steroids. The cytochrome P-450-dependent system also catalyses deamination (e.g. amfetamine (amphetamine)), dealkylation (e.g. morphine, azathioprine), sulphoxidation (e.g. chlorpromazine, phenylbutazone), desulphuration (thiopental (thiopentone)) and dehalogenation (e.g. halogenated anaesthetics). This lack of specificity accounts for the ability of an inducing agent to stimulate metabolism of many other drugs, and of one drug to inhibit metabolism of a structurally unrelated drug. Antibiotics, if administered over a period of time (e.g. rifampicin for tuberculosis), can be enzyme inducers. Barbiturates stimulate metabolism of griseofulvin, phenytoin and coumarin anticoagulants, and griseofulvin induces increased metabolism of coumarins. Similarly, rifampicin, phenytoin and carbamazepine increase the metabolism of ciclosporin [7]. Drugs causing enzyme inhibition include chloramphenicol, cimetidine, monoamine oxidase inhibitors, *p*-aminosalicylic acid, pethidine and morphine. Dicoumarol, chloramphenicol and phenylbutazone inhibit metabolic inactivation of tolbutamide. Allopurinol inhibits metabolism of azathioprine and mercaptopurine by xanthine oxidase. Cimetidine inhibits liver enzymes and decreases hepatic blood flow, thereby potentiating the action of some β-blockers (propranolol) and benzodiazepines, carbamazepine, warfarin, morphine, phenytoin and theophylline. Ketoconazole may potentiate oral anticoagulants [8] and erythromycin may potentiate carbamazepine [9]; both may potentiate ciclosporin. Nifedipine and ciclosporin are both metabolized by the same cytochrome P-450 enzyme, P-450cpn; ciclosporin potentiates the action of nifedipine, phenytoin and to a lesser extent valproate by decreasing P-450cpn availability by competitive inhibition [10].

Altered drug excretion. Examples include the well-known probenecid-induced reduction in the renal excretion of penicillin, and aspirin-induced reduction in renal clearance of methotrexate.

REFERENCES

1 Griffin JP, D'Arcy PF, Speirs CJ. *A Manual of Adverse Drug Interactions*, 4th edn. London: Wright (Butterworth), 1988.
2 Shapiro LE, Shear NH. Drug interactions: proteins, pumps, and P-450s. *J Am Acad Dermatol* 2002; **47**: 467–84.
3 Beers MH, Storrie MS, Lee G. Potential adverse drug interactions in the emergency room. An issue in the quality of care. *Ann Intern Med* 1990; **112**: 61–4.
4 Garty M, Hurwitz A. Effect of cimetidine and antacids on gastrointestinal absorption of tetracycline. *Clin Pharmacol Ther* 1980; **28**: 203–7.
5 Bacon JF, Shenfield GM. Pregnancy attributable to interaction between tetracycline and oral contraceptives. *BMJ* 1980; **280**: 293.
6 Fleischer AB, Resnick SD. The effect of antibiotics on the efficacy of oral contraceptives. *Arch Dermatol* 1989; **125**: 1562–4.
7 Schofield OMV, Camp RDR, Levene GM. Cyclosporin A in psoriasis: interaction with carbamazepine. *Br J Dermatol* 1990; **122**: 425–6.
8 Smith AG. Potentiation of oral anticoagulants by ketoconazole. *BMJ* 1984; **288**: 188–9.
9 Wroblewski BA, Singer WD, Whyte J. Carbamazepine–erythromycin interaction: case studies and clinical significance. *JAMA* 1986; **255**: 1165–7.
10 McFadden JP, Pontin JE, Powles AV *et al.* Cyclosporin decreases nifedipine metabolism. *BMJ* 1989; **299**: 1224.

Metabolic changes

Drugs may induce cutaneous changes by their effects on nutritional or metabolic status. Thus, drugs such as phenytoin that interfere with folate absorption or metabolism increase the risk of aphthous stomatitis, and isotretinoin may cause xanthomas by elevation of very low-density lipoproteins [1].

REFERENCE

1 Dicken CH. Eruptive xanthomas associated with isotretinoin (13-*cis*-retinoic acid). *Arch Dermatol* 1980; **116**: 951–2.

Teratogenicity and other effects on the fetus [1–6]

The advent of isotretinoin has focused the attention of dermatologists considerably on the problem of teratogenicity in general [5]. The fetus is particularly at risk from drug-induced developmental malformations during the period of organogenesis, which lasts from about the third to the tenth week of gestation. Thalidomide, retinoids and cytotoxic drugs are proven teratogens. Heavy alcohol intake (which produces fetal alcohol syndrome), smoking, anticonvulsants (especially phenytoin and trimethadione (troxidone)), warfarin and antiplatelet drugs, inhalational anaesthetics, lithium, quinine, ACE inhibitors, misoprostol, certain antimicrobials (e.g. trimethoprim, aminoglycosides, 4-quinolones and itraconazole) and cocaine are probably teratogenic. High-dose corticosteroids have been linked to cleft palate. A major correlation has been found between the incidence of glucocorticoid-induced cleft palate and the chromosome 8 segment identified by *N*-acetyltransferase in mice [7]. 6-Aminonicotinamide-induced cleft palate and phenytoin-induced cleft lip with or without cleft palate are also influenced by this genetic region but not as strongly. Sex hormones, psychotropic drugs, benzodiazepines, tetracycline, rifampicin, penicillamine and the folate antagonist pyrimethamine are possibly teratogenic and should be avoided in the first trimester of pregnancy. Chlorpheniramine appears safe to use. The potential adverse effects on the fetus and on the breastfed infant of a number of drugs not infrequently used by the dermatologist have been reviewed [4].

Drugs may also cause fetal damage later in pregnancy. Warfarin may cause haemorrhage, and phenytoin near to term produces a coagulation defect in the neonate, which is correctable by vitamin K. Antithyroid drugs and iodides may cause neonatal goitre and hypothyroidism. Fetal adrenal atrophy may follow high-dose maternal corticosteroid therapy. NSAIDs have various ill effects, although aspirin has been advocated in pregnancy for the prevention of fetal growth retardation. Tetracyclines are deposited in developing bones and cause discoloration and enamel hypoplasia of teeth [8]. Aminoglycoside antibiotics are ototoxic, and chloroquine has caused a neonatal chorioretinitis. Androgens and progestogens may virilize the fetus. Diethylstilbestrol (stilboestrol) administered from early pregnancy for several months has been associated with female and male genital tract abnormalities, and carcinoma of the vagina 20 years later in the offspring.

REFERENCES

1 Ellis C, Fidler J. Drugs in pregnancy: adverse reactions. *Br J Hosp Med* 1982; **28**: 575–84.
2 Kalter H, Warkany J. Congenital malformations: etiologic factors and their role in prevention. *N Engl J Med* 1983; **308**: 424–31, 491–7.
3 Ashton CH. Disorders of the fetus and infant. In: Davis DM, ed. *Textbook of Adverse Drug Reactions*, 3rd edn. Oxford: Oxford University Press, 1985: 77–127.
4 Stockton DL, Paller AS. Drug administration to the pregnant or lactating woman: a reference guide for dermatologists. *J Am Acad Dermatol* 1990; **23**: 87–103.
5 Mitchell AA. Teratogens and the dermatologist. New knowledge, responsibilities, and opportunities. *Arch Dermatol* 1991; **127**: 399–401.

6 Ferner RE. Teratogenic drugs: an update. *Adverse Drug React Bull* 1993; **161**: 607–10.
7 Karolyi J, Erickson RP, Liu S, Killewald L. Major effects on teratogen-induced facial clefting in mice determined by a single genetic region. *Genetics* 1990; **126**: 201–5.
8 Witkop CJ, Wolf RO. Hypoplasia and intrinsic staining of enamel following tetracycline therapy. *JAMA* 1963; **185**: 1008–11.

Effects on spermatogenesis

Most chemotherapeutic agents potentially damage sperm; conception should also be avoided after griseofulvin for 3 months. A number of drugs cause oligospermia [1], which may come to light only as a result of infertility investigations; oestrogens, androgens, cyproterone acetate, cytotoxic drugs, including methotrexate given for psoriasis [2], colchicine, most monoamine oxidase inhibitors, ketoconazole and sulfasalazine (sulphasalazine) have all been incriminated. The synthetic retinoids isotretinoin and etretinate do not seem to affect the numbers of sperm [3,4].

REFERENCES

1 Drife JO. Drugs and sperm. *BMJ* 1982; **284**: 844–5.
2 Sussman A, Leonard J. Psoriasis, methotrexate, and oligospermia. *Arch Dermatol* 1980; **116**: 215–7.
3 Schill W-B, Wagner A, Nikolowski JM, Plewig G. Aromatic retinoid and 13-*cis*-retinoic acid: spermatological investigations. In: Orfanos CE, Braun-Falco O, Farber EM *et al.*, eds. *Retinoids, Advances in Basic Research and Therapy*. Berlin: Springer, 1981: 389–95.
4 Töröck L, Kása M. Spermatological and endocrinological examinations connected with isotretinoin treatment. In: Saurat JH, ed. *Retinoids: New Trends in Research and Therapy*. Basel: Karger, 1985: 407–10.

Non-immunological activation of effector pathways (anaphylactoid reactions)

Certain drugs, such as opiates, codeine, amfetamine, polymyxin B, D-tubocurarine, atropine, hydralazine, pentamidine, quinine and radiocontrast media, may release mast cell mediators directly to produce urticaria or angio-oedema [1–7]. Some drugs, such as radiocontrast media, may activate complement by an antibody-independent method [8]. Anaphylaxis-like responses to cyclo-oxygenase inhibitors such as aspirin and other NSAIDs may lead to amplified mast cell degranulation and enhanced biosynthesis of lipoxygenase products of arachidonic acid, which cause vasodilatation and oedema [9,10]. ACE inhibitors, which cause or exacerbate angio-oedema, may potentiate bradykinin activity; they have been reported to enhance bradykinin-induced cutaneous weals in normal individuals [11,12].

REFERENCES

1 Schoenfeld MR. Acute allergic reactions to morphine, codeine, meperidine hydrochloride and opium alkaloids. *NY State J Med* 1960; **60**: 2591–3.
2 Comroe JH, Dripps RD. Histamine-like action of curare and tubocurarine injected intracutaneously and intra-arterially in man. *Anesthesiology* 1946; **7**: 260–2.
3 Greenberger PA. Contrast media reactions. *J Allergy Clin Immunol* 1984; **74**: 600–5.
4 Assem ESK, Bray K, Dawson P. The release of histamine from human basophils by radiological contrast agents. *Br J Radiol* 1983; **56**: 647–52.
5 Rice MC, Lieberman P, Siegle RL, Mason J. *In vitro* histamine release induced by radiocontrast media and various chemical analogs in reactor and control subjects. *J Allergy Clin Immunol* 1983; **72**: 180–6.
6 Watkins J. Markers and mechanisms of anaphylactoid reactions. *Monogr Allergy* 1992; **30**: 108–29.
7 Bircher AJ. Drug-induced urticaria and angioedema caused by non-IgE mediated pathomechanisms. *Eur J Dermatol* 1999; **9**: 657–63.
8 Arroyave CM, Bhatt KN, Crown NR. Activation of the alternative pathway of the complement system by radiographic contrast media. *J Immunol* 1976; **117**: 1866–9.
9 Stevenson DD, Lewis RA. Proposed mechanisms of aspirin sensitivity reactions. *J Allergy Clin Immunol* 1987; **80**: 788–90.
10 Morassut P, Yang W, Karsh J. Aspirin intolerance. *Semin Arthritis Rheum* 1989; **19**: 22–30.
11 Wood SM, Mann RD, Rawlins MD. Angio-oedema and urticaria associated with angiotensin converting enzyme inhibitors. *BMJ* 1987; **294**: 91–2.
12 Ferner RE. Effects of intradermal bradykinin after inhibition of angiotensin converting enzyme. *BMJ* 1987; **294**: 1119–20.

Exacerbation of disease

Examples of adverse drug effects on pre-existing skin conditions include lithium exacerbation of acne and psoriasis, β-blocker induction of a psoriasiform dermatitis [1] and corticosteroid withdrawal resulting in exacerbation of psoriasis; cimetidine, penicillin or sulphonamide exacerbation of lupus erythematosus (LE); and vasodilator exacerbation of rosacea. Sometimes, a drug may unmask a latent condition, as when barbiturates precipitate symptoms of porphyria.

REFERENCE

1 Abel EA, Dicicco LM, Orenberg EK *et al.* Drugs in exacerbation of psoriasis. *J Am Acad Dermatol* 1986; **15**: 1007–22.

Intolerance

The characteristic effects of the drug are produced to an exaggerated extent by an abnormally small dose. This may simply represent an extreme within normal biological variation. Alternatively, the intolerance may be contributed to by delayed metabolism or excretion due to impaired hepatic or renal function, or by genetic variation in the rate of drug metabolism (see below).

Idiosyncrasy

This describes an uncharacteristic response, not predictable from animal experiments, and not mediated by an immunological mechanism. The cause is often unknown, but genetic variation in metabolic pathways may be involved. Such genetic abnormalities include glucose-6-phosphate dehydrogenase deficiency, hereditary methaemoglobinaemia, porphyria, glucocorticoid glaucoma and malignant hyperthermia of anaesthesia, all of which are characterized by unusual pharmacological responses to various drugs.

Pharmacogenetic mechanisms and genetic influences underlying intolerance and idiosyncratic reactions [1–4]

The pharmacokinetics of drugs, including their absorption, plasma protein binding, distribution, metabolism and elimination, may be influenced by genetic factors. Oxidation, hydrolysis and acetylation are the three metabolic pathways most subject to genetic influence. Genetic factors also influence pharmacodynamics, i.e. tissue or organ responsiveness. Thus, genetic variations in all these areas may underlie both intolerance and idiosyncrasy. Variation in the regulation and expression of the human cytochrome P-450 enzyme system may play a key role in both interindividual variation in sensitivity to drug toxicity and tissue-specific damage [5]. Pharmacogenetic variability probably underlies reactions such as TEN. It has been proposed that most patients who have a severe ACDR have an abnormal metabolism of the offending drug [6].

Examples of genetically mediated intolerance include pupil size responses to phenylephrine and parasympatholytics, and the very rare dominantly inherited familial resistance to coumarin anticoagulants, the result of mutation in the receptor for vitamin K and anticoagulants. Low levels of red cell glucose-6-phosphate dehydrogenase, inherited as a sex-linked dominant trait, are common in black people, certain Levantine peoples and Filipinos, and result in a chronic deficit of reduced glutathione sulphydryl (SH) groups. Affected individuals are at risk of acute haemolysis on exposure to antimalarials, sulphonamides, dapsone, nitrofurantoin, phenacetin, aspirin and chloramphenicol, all of which may oxidize the few reduced SH groups in older red cells. Genetic variation in thiopurine methyltransferase activity may be linked to the side effects of azathioprine therapy, as homozygotes for the low-activity allele are at risk of myelosuppression, whereas homozygotes for high activity are inadequately immunosuppressed with conventional doses of azathioprine [7]. Increased susceptibility to aminoglycoside-induced deafness in two Japanese pedigrees was associated with a particular mitochondrial DNA polymorphism [8].

REFERENCES

1 Rawlins MD, Thompson JW. Mechanisms of adverse drug reactions. In: Davies DM, ed. *Textbook of Adverse Drug Reactions*, 3rd edn. Oxford: Oxford University Press, 1985: 12–38.
2 Shear NH, Bhimji S. Pharmacogenetics and cutaneous drug reactions. *Semin Dermatol* 1989; **8**: 219–26.
3 Lennard MS, Tucker GT, Woods HF. Inborn 'errors' of drug metabolism. Pharmacokinetic and clinical implications. *Clin Pharmacokinet* 1990; **19**: 257–63.
4 Knowles SR, Uetrecht J, Shear NH. Idiosyncratic drug reactions: the reactive metabolite syndromes. *Lancet* 2000; **356**: 1587–91.
5 Park BK, Pirmohamed M, Kitteringham NR. The role of cytochrome P450 enzymes in hepatic and extrahepatic human drug toxicity. *Pharmacol Ther* 1995; **68**: 385–424.
6 Chosidow O, Bourgault L, Roujeau JC. Drug rashes. What are the targets of cell-mediated cytotoxicity? *Arch Dermatol* 1994; **130**: 627–9.
7 Snow JL, Gibson LE. The role of genetic variation in thiopurine methyltransferase activity and the efficacy and/or side effects of azathioprine therapy in dermatologic patients. *Arch Dermatol* 1995; **131**: 193–7.
8 Hutchin T, Haworth I, Higashi K et al. A molecular basis for human hypersensitivity to aminoglycoside antibiotics. *Nucleic Acids Res* 1993; **21**: 4174–9.

Oxidation. Anticonvulsants, many hypnotics, tricyclic antidepressants, anticoagulants and various anti-inflammatory and anxiolytic agents are eliminated by oxidation. For many drugs, oxidation rates vary as a continuous spectrum within the population. Genetic differences in metabolism of sulphonamides may underlie idiosyncratic toxicity [1–6]. Oxidative metabolism of sulphonamides by cytochrome P-450 enzymes and *N*-acetylation yields a reactive hydroxylamine intermediate [7], which is inactivated by glutathione conjugation. The hydroxylamine metabolite is toxic to lymphocytes, and the lymphocyte toxicity is markedly increased in patients with a history of hypersensitivity or with glutathione synthetase deficiency. HIV-positive individuals have been reported in some studies to have a systemic glutathione deficiency, resulting in a decreased capacity to scavenge hydroxylamine derivatives of sulphonamides, which may partially explain the increased frequency of sulphonamide reactions [8–10]. However, other studies have not been able to confirm intracellular glutathione deficiency in peripheral blood cells of HIV-infected patients [11,12].

Phenytoin, phenobarbital and carbamazepine are oxidized by the cytochrome P-450 enzyme system into potentially reactive arene-oxide intermediates; liver microsomal epoxide hydrolase converts such reactive intermediates to non-toxic dihydrodiols [13–17]. Phenytoin hypersensitivity syndrome appears to be associated with an inherited deficiency of epoxide hydrolase, which is primarily responsible for detoxifying the toxic arene-oxide intermediate [13–16]. Activated phenytoin has been shown to be toxic to lymphocytes from patients with phenytoin reactions and, to a lesser degree, to lymphocytes from their parents [15]. However, in another study a genetic defect altering the structure and function of the microsomal epoxide hydrolase protein was thought unlikely to be responsible for predisposing patients to anticonvulsant adverse reactions [17].

Culprit drug-reactive metabolites, generated by a microsomal oxidation system, had increased toxic effects on lymphoid cells from patients with TEN (13 each with sulphonamide and anticonvulsant reactions) and on those from first-degree relatives, whereas oxygen free radical and/or aldehyde detoxification pathways were normal [18].

Impaired metabolism of phenacetin and phenformin, inherited as a result of genetic polymorphism in liver microsomal oxidation, may result in adverse reactions [19,20]. The induction of liver enzymes responsible for drug oxidation may itself be under genetic control [21]. There is a fourfold increase in toxicity to penicillamine in patients with rheumatoid arthritis with a genetically determined poor capacity to sulphoxidate the structurally related mucolytic agent, carbocysteine [22].

REFERENCES

1 Shear NH, Spielberg SP. *In vitro* evaluation of a toxic metabolite of sulfadiazide. *Can J Physiol Pharmacol* 1985; **63**: 1370–2.
2 Shear NH, Spielberg SP. An *in vitro* lymphocytotoxicity assay for studying adverse reactions to sulphonamides. *Br J Dermatol* 1985; **113**: 112–3.
3 Shear N, Spielberg S, Grant D *et al.* Differences in metabolism of sulfonamides predisposing to idiosyncratic toxicity. *Ann Intern Med* 1986; **105**: 179–84.
4 Anonymous. Hypersensitivity to sulphonamides: a clue? *Lancet* 1986; **ii**: 958–9.
5 Rieder MJ, Uetrecht J, Shear NH *et al.* Synthesis and *in vitro* toxicity of hydroxylamine metabolites of sulphonamides. *J Pharmacol Exp Ther* 1988; **244**: 724–8.
6 Rieder MJ, Uetrecht J, Shear NH *et al.* Diagnosis of sulfonamide hypersensitivity reactions by *in-vitro* 'rechallenge' with hydroxylamine metabolites. *Ann Intern Med* 1989; **110**: 286–9.
7 Meekins CV, Sullivan TJ, Gruchalla RS. Immunochemical analysis of sulfonamide drug allergy: identification of sulfamethoxazole-substituted human serum proteins. *J Allergy Clin Immunol* 1994; **94**: 1017–24.
8 Buhl R, Jaffe HA, Holroyd KJ *et al.* Systemic glutathione deficiency in symptom-free HIV-seropositive individuals. *Lancet* 1989; **334**: 1294–8.
9 van der Ven AJAM, Koopmans PP, Vree TB, van der Meer JWM. Adverse reactions to co-trimoxazole in HIV infection. *Lancet* 1991; **338**: 431–3.
10 Koopmans PP, van der Ven AJ, Vree TB, van der Meer JWM. Pathogenesis of hypersensitivity reactions to drugs in patients with HIV infection: allergic or toxic? *AIDS* 1995; **9**: 217–22.
11 Aukrust P, Svardal AM, Muller F *et al.* Increased levels of oxidized glutathione in CD4$^+$ lymphocytes associated with disturbed intracellular redox balance in human immunodeficiency type 1 infection. *Blood* 1995; **86**: 258–67.
12 Pirmohamed M, Williams D, Tingle MD *et al.* Intracellular glutathione in the peripheral blood cells of HIV-infected patients: failure to show a deficiency. *AIDS* 1996; **10**: 501–7.
13 Shear NH, Spielberg SP. Anticonvulsant hypersensitivity syndrome. *In vitro* assessment of risk. *J Clin Invest* 1988; **82**: 1826–32.
14 Spielberg SP, Gordon GB, Blake DA *et al.* Predisposition to phenytoin hepatotoxicity assessed *in vitro*. *N Engl J Med* 1981; **305**: 722–7.
15 Spielberg SP. *In vitro* assessment of pharmacogenetic susceptibility to toxic drug metabolites in humans. *Fed Proc* 1984; **43**: 2308–13.
16 Yoo JH, Kang DS, Chun WH *et al.* Anticonvulsant hypersensitivity syndrome with an epoxide hydrolase defect. *Br J Dermatol* 1999; **140**: 181–3.
17 Gaedigk A, Spielberg SP, Grant DM. Characterization of the microsomal epoxide hydrolase gene in patients with anticonvulsant adverse drug reactions. *Pharmacogenetics* 1994; **4**: 142–53.
18 Wolkenstein P, Charue D, Laurent P *et al.* Metabolic predisposition to cutaneous adverse drug reactions. Role in toxic epidermal necrolysis caused by sulfonamides and anticonvulsants. *Arch Dermatol* 1995; **131**: 544–51.
19 Shahidi NT. Acetophenetidin sensitivity. *Am J Dis Child* 1967; **113**: 81–2.
20 Eichelbaum M. Defective oxidation of drugs: pharmacokinetic and therapeutic implications. *Clin Pharmacokinet* 1982; **7**: 1–22.
21 Vessell ES, Passananti T, Greene FE, Page JG. Genetic control of drug levels and of the induction of drug-metabolizing enzymes in man: individual variability in the extent of allopurinol and nortriptyline inhibition of drug metabolism. *Ann NY Acad Sci* 1971; **179**: 752–3.
22 Dasgupta B. Adverse reactions profile: 2. Penicillamine. *Prescribers J* 1991; **31**: 72–7.

Hydrolysis. Genetic influence on drug hydrolysis is well illustrated in the case of suxamethonium, which normally results in only very brief neuromuscular blockade due to rapid hydrolysis by plasma pseudocholinesterase. Genetically determined atypical cholinesterases cannot hydrolyse the drug, leading to prolonged apnoea in affected individuals; conversely, dominantly inherited resistance to suxamethonium, mediated by a highly active cholinesterase, has been reported.

Acetylation. Isoniazid, many sulphonamides, hydralazine, dapsone, procainamide, etc. are inactivated by conversion to acetyl conjugates. Acetylation rates vary greatly, with a bimodal frequency distribution, and there is marked ethnic variation. Rapid inactivation is dominantly inherited, and is commonest among Eskimos and Japanese and least common among certain Mediterranean Jews. The LE-like syndrome due to procainamide may occur more in fast acetylators, implying that a conjugate and not the parent compound is responsible [1]. Slow acetylators, in whom higher and more persistent drug levels occur, are more liable to develop adverse reactions to isoniazid (pellagra-like syndrome and peripheral neuritis), dapsone (haemolysis) [2] and hydralazine (LE-like syndrome) [3,4]. A slow acetylation phenotype is a risk factor for hypersensitivity to trimethoprim–sulfamethoxazole in HIV-infected subjects [5,6], and for sulphonamide-induced TEN and Stevens–Johnson syndrome independent of HIV infection [7,8].

REFERENCES

1 Davies DM, Beedie MA, Rawlins MD. Antinuclear antibodies during procainamide treatment and drug acetylation. *BMJ* 1975; **iii**: 682–4.
2 Ellard GA, Gammon PT, Savin LA, Tan RSH. Dapsone acetylation in dermatitis herpetiformis. *Br J Dermatol* 1974; **90**: 441–4.
3 Perry HM JR, Sakamoto A, Tan EM. Relationship of acetylating enzyme to hydralazine toxicity. *J Lab Clin Med* 1967; **70**: 1020–1.
4 Russell GI, Bing RF, Jones JA *et al.* Hydralazine sensitivity: clinical features, autoantibody changes and HLA-DR phenotype. *Q J Med* 1987; **65**: 845–52.
5 Carr A, Gross AS, Hoskins JM *et al.* Acetylation phenotype and cutaneous hypersensitivity to trimethoprim–sulphamethoxazole in HIV-infected patients. *AIDS* 1994; **8**: 333–7.
6 Delomenie C, Grant DM, Mathelier-Fusade P *et al.* N-Acetylation genotype and risk of severe reactions to sulphonamides in AIDS patients. *Br J Clin Pharmacol* 1994; **38**: 581–2.
7 Wolkenstein P, Carriere V, Charue D *et al.* A slow acetylator genotype is a risk factor for sulphonamide-induced toxic epidermal necrolysis and Stevens–Johnson syndrome. *Pharmacogenetics* 1995; **5**: 255–8.
8 Dietrich A, Kawakubo Y, Rzany B *et al.* Low N-acetylating capacity in patients with Stevens–Johnson syndrome and toxic epidermal necrolysis. *Exp Dermatol* 1995; **4**: 313–6.

Influence of human leukocyte antigen (HLA) types. An association between HLA types and susceptibility to drug eruptions has been reported on several occasions, particularly in relation to gold (HLA-DRw3, HLA-DR5 and HLA-B8) and penicillamine toxicity [1–6]. Penicillamine toxicity is associated with HLA phenotypes as follows [1]: HLA-DR3 and HLA-B8 with renal toxicity; HLA-DR3, HLA-B7 and HLA-DR2 with haematological toxicity; HLA-A1 and HLA-DR4 with thrombocytopenia; and HLA-DRw6 with cutaneous adverse reactions. DR1/DR4 heterozygosity, or the DR5 subtypes DRB1*1102 or DRB1*1201, have been found in 61% of patients with intolerance to tiopronin given for rheumatoid arthritis [7].

A positive association with HLA-Aw33 and HLA-B17/Bw58 haplotypes, and a negative association with the HLA-A2 haplotype, has been reported in southern Chinese patients with drug eruptions after exposure to allopurinol [8]. Aspirin-sensitive asthma is associated with HLA-DQw2 [9]. HLA-linkage associations with certain bullous disorders have been reported [10,11]. Hydralazine-induced LE is commonest in female patients with the HLA-DRw4 haplotype [12,13]. Fixed drug eruptions to feprazone and trimethoprim–sulfamethoxazole are linked, respectively, to HLA-B22 and HLA-A30 B13 Cw6 [14,15]. The above findings indicate that there may be genetic predisposition to develop certain drug eruptions.

REFERENCES

1 Dasgupta B. Adverse reactions profile: 2. Penicillamine. *Prescribers J* 1991; **31**: 72–7.
2 Wooley PH, Griffin J, Payani GS *et al.* HLA-DR antigens and toxic reaction to sodium aurothiomalate and D-penicillamine in patients with rheumatoid arthritis. *N Engl J Med* 1980; **303**: 300–2.
3 Latts JR, Antel JP, Levinson DJ *et al.* Histocompatibility antigens and gold toxicity: a preliminary report. *J Clin Pharmacol* 1980; **20**: 206–9.
4 Bardin T, Dryll A, Debeyre N *et al.* HLA system and side effects of gold salts and D-penicillamine treatment of rheumatoid arthritis. *Ann Rheum Dis* 1982; **41**: 599–601.
5 Emery P, Panayi GS, Huston G *et al.* D-penicillamine induced toxicity in rheumatoid arthritis: the role of sulphoxidation status and HLA-DR3. *J Rheumatol* 1984; **11**: 626–32.
6 Rodriguez-Perez M, Gonzalez-Dominguez J, Mataran L *et al.* Association of HLA-DR5 with mucocutaneous lesions in patients with rheumatoid arthritis receiving gold sodium thiomalate. *J Rheumatol* 1994; **21**: 41–3.
7 Ju LY, Paolozzi L, Delecoeuillerie G *et al.* A possible linkage of HLA-DRB haplotypes with tiopronin intolerance in rheumatoid arthritis. *Clin Exp Rheumatol* 1994; **12**: 249–54.
8 Chan SH, Tan T. HLA and allopurinol drug eruption. *Dermatologica* 1989; **179**: 32–3.
9 Mullarkey MF, Thomas PS, Hansen JA *et al.* Association of aspirin-sensitive asthma with HLA-DQw2. *Am Rev Respir Dis* 1986; **133**: 261–3.
10 Roujeau J-C, Bracq C, Huyn NT *et al.* HLA phenotypes and bullous cutaneous reactions to drugs. *Tissue Antigens* 1986; **28**: 251–4.
11 Mobini N, Ahmed AR. Immunogenetics of drug-induced bullous diseases. *Clin Dermatol* 1993; **11**: 449–60.
12 Batchelor JR, Welsh KI, Mansilla Tinoco R *et al.* Hydralazine-induced systemic lupus erythematosus: influence of HLA-DR and sex on susceptibility. *Lancet* 1980; **i**: 1107–9.
13 Russell GI, Bing RF, Jones JA *et al.* Hydralazine sensitivity: clinical features, autoantibody changes and HLA-DR phenotype. *Q J Med* 1987; **65**: 845–52.
14 Pellicano R, Lomuto M, Ciavarella G *et al.* Fixed drug eruptions with feprazone are linked to HLA-B22. *J Am Acad Dermatol* 1997; **36**: 782–4.
15 Özkaya-Bayazit E, Akar U. Fixed drug eruption induced by trimethoprim–sulfamethoxazole: evidence for a link to HLA-A30 B13 Cw6 haplotype. *J Am Acad Dermatol* 2001; **45**: 712–7.

Drug-induced chromosomal damage [1–3]

This may be studied by examining the chromosomes of patients or animals exposed to drugs, or *in vitro* by the addition of drugs to cell cultures; substances capable of inducing chromosomal damage are termed clastogens.

Effects may be dose related, but *in vitro* results may not be representative of the *in vivo* situation. Antimitotic and antibiotic agents have been the most studied, although psychotropics, anticonvulsants, hallucinogens, immunosuppressants and oral contraceptives have also been investigated and shown to cause, in varying degree, chromosomal damage. Damage ranges from staining variations through 'gaps' in staining, chromosome breaks, gross aberrations (such as deletions, fragments, translocations and inversions) to polyploidy. Such damage may be stable and retained over a succession of cell divisions, or transient.

REFERENCES

1 Shaw MW. Human chromosome damage by chemical agents. *Annu Rev Med* 1970; **21**: 409–32.
2 Bender MA, Griggs HG, Bedford JS. Mechanisms of chromosomal aberration production. III. Chemicals and ionizing radiation. *Mutat Res* 1974; **23**: 197–212.
3 Rawlins MD, Thompson JW. Mechanisms of adverse drug reactions. In: Davies DM, ed. *Textbook of Adverse Drug Reactions*, 3rd edn. Oxford: Oxford University Press, 1985: 12–38.

Miscellaneous

Jarisch–Herxheimer reaction

This is the focal exacerbation of lesions of infective origin when potent antimicrobial therapy is initiated, and is classically observed in the treatment of early syphilis with penicillin; it may also occur 3 days after starting griseofulvin therapy, during therapy with diethylcarbamazine for onchocerciasis and tiabendazole (thiabendazole) for strongyloidiasis, and with penicillin or minocycline for erythema chronicum migrans due to *Borrelia burgdorferi* infection [1]. The reaction has been attributed to sudden release of pharmacologically and/or immunologically active substances from killed microorganisms or damaged tissues. However, there is little evidence that it is an allergic reaction [2]. Clinically there may be fever, rigors, lymphadenopathy, arthralgia, and transient macular urticarial eruptions; a vesicular eruption has also been described [3].

REFERENCES

1 Weber K. Jarisch–Herxheimer-Reaktion bei Erythema-migrans-Krankheit. *Hautarzt* 1984; **35**: 588–90.
2 Skog E, Gudjónsson H. On the allergic origin of the Jarisch–Herxheimer reaction. *Acta Derm Venereol (Stockh)* 1966; **46**: 136–43.
3 Rosen T, Rubin H, Ellner K *et al.* Vesicular Jarisch–Herxheimer reaction. *Arch Dermatol* 1989; **125**: 77–81.

Infectious mononucleosis–ampicillin reaction

Ampicillin almost always causes a severe morbilliform eruption when given to a patient with infectious mononucleosis or lymphatic leukaemia (see later). The reaction occurs much less frequently with amoxicillin. The exact mechanism is not known, although a recent report suggests that real sensitization to ampicillin and amoxicillin occurs, and is detectable *in vivo* and *in vitro* by skin tests and the lymphocyte transformation test [1].

REFERENCE

1 Renn CN, Straff W, Dorfmüller A *et al.* Amoxicillin-induced exanthema in young adults with infectious mononucleosis: demonstration of drug-specific lymphocyte reactivity. *Br J Dermatol* 2003; **147**: 1166–7.

Immunological drug reactions

Allergic hypersensitivity reactions are caused by immunological sensitization to a drug, as a result of previous exposure to that drug or to a chemically related cross-reacting substance [1–7]. It has been estimated that only about 6–10% of ADRs are immunologically mediated [8]. Although drugs frequently elicit an immune response, clinically evident hypersensitivity reactions are manifest only in a small proportion of exposed individuals. Thus, using highly sensitive passive haemagglutination assays, IgM class antibodies to the penicilloyl group (the major hapten determinant derived from penicillin) are detectable in almost 100% of normal individuals, even in the absence of a history of penicillin therapy; 40% of patients receiving more than 2 g of penicillin for more than 10 days develop IgG class antibodies [9]. Macromolecular drugs such as protein or peptide hormones, insulin or dextran are antigenic in their own right. In contrast, most drugs are small organic molecules with a molecular mass of less than 1 kDa; conjugation of free drug as a hapten with a macromolecular carrier is then required to initiate an immune response [10]. Fortunately, many drugs have only a limited capacity to form covalent bonds with tissue proteins. Clinical sensitization may also result from allergy to reactive drug metabolites as haptens, or to minor contaminants.

Clinical features distinguishing allergic from non-allergic drug reactions. Prior exposure before sensitization should have been without adverse effect. If there has been no previous exposure, there should be a latent period of several days of uneventful therapy before the reaction supervenes, during which primary sensitization occurs. Thereafter, reactions may develop within minutes (or even seconds) and certainly within 24 h. Allergic reactions do not resemble the pharmacological action of the drug, may follow exposure to doses far below the therapeutic level, and are reproducible on readministration (if judged safe).

Factors concerned in the development of hypersensitivity. The route of administration of a drug may affect its immunogenicity and the nature of any allergy. Topical drug exposure is more likely to result in sensitization than oral administration, and favours development of contact dermatitis; thus, poison ivy is a potent contact sensitizer but oral ingestion may promote tolerance. Anaphylaxis is more likely to be associated with intravenous drug administration. However, anaphylaxis may sometimes occur as quickly after oral penicillin administration [11]. Whether allergy develops may also depend on the antigenic load in terms of degree of drug exposure, and individual genetic variation in drug absorption and metabolism. Thus, as stated above, an LE-like syndrome with antinuclear antibody formation following hydralazine therapy occurs more frequently in slow acetylators of the drug [12]. Hydralazine-related SLE is 10 times more frequent in HLA-DR4-positive patients than in the population at large, and is commoner in females. Allergic drug reactions are less common in childhood and possibly in the aged; in the latter, this may be related to impaired immunological responsiveness. Immunosuppression may increase the risk by inhibiting the regulatory function of suppressor T cells [13]. Environmental factors may also affect susceptibility to drug hypersensitivity, as for example the well-recognized increase in ampicillin-induced morbilliform eruptions associated with infectious mononucleosis, and photoallergic reactions to drugs such as thiazide diuretics or phenothiazines.

Duration of hypersensitivity. The duration of allergic sensitivity is unpredictable. Although there is a general tendency for immunological responses to a drug to fall off with time, provided the patient is not re-exposed to the drug or a related substance, this can never be relied on; where necessary, safe confirmatory procedures (if available) should be carried out.

REFERENCES

1 de Weck AL. Pathophysiologic mechanisms of allergic and pseudo-allergic reactions to foods, food additives and drugs. *Ann Allergy* 1984; **53**: 583–6.
2 Wintroub BU, Stern R. Cutaneous drug reactions: pathogenesis and clinical classification. *J Am Acad Dermatol* 1985; **13**: 833–45.
3 Rawlins MD, Thompson JW. Mechanisms of adverse drug reactions. In: Davies DM, ed. *Textbook of Adverse Drug Reactions*, 3rd edn. Oxford: Oxford University Press, 1985: 12–38.
4 De Swarte RD. Drug allergy: an overview. *Clin Rev Allergy* 1986; **4**: 143–69.
5 Stern RS, Wintroub BU, Arndt KA. Drug reactions. *J Am Acad Dermatol* 1986; **15**: 1282–8.
6 Blaiss MS, de Shazo RD. Drug allergy. *Pediatr Clin North Am* 1988; **35**: 1131–47.
7 Kalish RS. Drug eruptions: a review of clinical and immunological features. *Adv Dermatol* 1991; **6**: 221–37.
8 Gruchalla RS. Drug allergy. *J Allergy Clin Immunol* 2003; **111** (2 Suppl.): S548–S559.
9 Weiss ME, Adkinson NF. Immediate hypersensitivity reactions to penicillin and related antibiotics. *Clin Allergy* 1988; **18**: 515–40.
10 Park BK, Naisbitt DJ, Gordon SF *et al.* Metabolic activation in drug allergies. *Toxicology* 2001; **158**: 11–23.
11 Simmonds J, Hodges S, Nicol F, Barnett D. Anaphylaxis after oral penicillin. *BMJ* 1978; **ii**: 1404.

12 Perry HM Jr, Sakamoto A, Tan EM. Relationship of acetylating enzyme to hydralazine toxicity. *J Lab Clin Med* 1967; **70**: 1020–1.
13 Lakin JD, Grace WR, Sell KW. IgE antipolymyxin B antibody formation in a T-cell depleted bone marrow transplant patient. *J Allergy Clin Immunol* 1975; **56**: 94–103.

Drug eruptions may occur as a result of a variety of different immunological mechanisms as described below.

IgE-dependent (type I) drug reactions: urticaria and anaphylaxis [1]

In vivo cross-linkage by polyvalent drug–protein conjugates of two or more specific IgE molecules, fixed to sensitized tissue mast cells or circulating basophil leukocytes, triggers the cell to release a variety of chemical mediators, including histamine, peptides such as eosinophil chemotactic factor of anaphylaxis, lipids such as leukotriene C_4 or prostaglandin D_2, and a variety of pro-inflammatory cytokines [2]. Interleukin-5 (IL-5) and eotaxin play a role in activating and recruiting eosinophils in drug-induced cutaneous eruptions [3]. Such cytokines in turn have effects on a variety of target tissues including skin, respiratory, gastrointestinal and/or cardiovascular systems. Eosinophil degranulation may also result in release of pro-inflammatory mediators [4]. Dilatation and increased permeability of small blood vessels with resultant oedema and hypotension, contraction of bronchiolar smooth muscle and excessive mucus secretion, and chemotaxis of inflammatory cells, including polymorphs and eosinophils, occurs. Clinically, this may produce pruritus, urticaria, bronchospasm and laryngeal oedema, and in severe cases anaphylactic shock with hypotension and possible death. Immediate reactions occur within minutes of drug administration; accelerated reactions may occur within hours or days, and are generally urticarial but may involve laryngeal oedema. Penicillins are the commonest cause of IgE-dependent drug eruptions.

REFERENCES

1 Champion RH, Greaves MW, Kobza Black A, eds. *The Urticarias*. Edinburgh: Churchill Livingstone, 1985.
2 Schwartz LB. Mast cells and their role in urticaria. *J Am Acad Dermatol* 1991; **25**: 190–204.
3 Yawalkar N, Shrikhande M, Hari Y *et al*. Evidence for a role for IL-5 and eotaxin in activating and recruiting eosinophils in drug-induced cutaneous eruptions. *J Allergy Clin Immunol* 2000; **106**: 1171–6.
4 Leiferman KM. A current perspective on the role of eosinophils in dermatologic diseases. *J Am Acad Dermatol* 1991; **24**: 1101–12.

Antibody-mediated (type II) drug reactions

Binding of antibody to cells may lead to cell damage following complement-mediated cytolysis. The classical example of immune complex formation between a drug (as hapten) bound to the surface of a cell (in this case, platelets) and IgG-class antibody, with subsequent complement fixation, was the purpura caused by apronalide (Sedormid). A further example is the thrombocytopenic purpura that may result from antibodies to quinidine–platelet conjugates [1,2]. A number of drugs, including penicillin, quinine and sulphonamides, may rarely produce a haemolytic anaemia via this mechanism. Methyldopa very occasionally induces a haemolytic anaemia mediated by autoantibodies directed against red cell antigens.

REFERENCES

1 Christie DJ, Weber RW, Mullen PC *et al*. Structural features of the quinidine and quinine molecules necessary for binding of drug-induced antibodies to human platelets. *J Lab Clin Med* 1984; **104**: 730–40.
2 Gary M, Ilfeld D, Kelton JG. Correlation of a quinidine-induced platelet-specific antibody with development of thrombocytopenia. *Am J Med* 1985; **79**: 253–5.

Immune complex-dependent (type III) drug reactions

Urticaria and anaphylaxis. Immune complexes may activate the complement cascade, with resultant formation of anaphylatoxins such as the complement protein fragments C3a and C5a, which trigger release of mediators from mast cells and basophils directly, resulting in urticaria or anaphylaxis.

Serum sickness. Serum sickness-like reactions and other immune complex-mediated conditions necessitate a drug antigen to persist in the circulation for long enough for antibody, largely of IgG or IgM class, to be synthesized and to combine with it to form circulating antibody–antigen immune complexes. They therefore develop about 6 days or more after drug administration. Serum sickness occurs when antibody combines with antigen in antigen excess, leading to slow removal of persistent complexes by the mononuclear phagocyte system. It was usually seen in the context of serum therapy with large doses of heterologous antibody, as with horse antiserum for the treatment of diphtheria. It has been reported more recently with antilymphocyte globulin therapy [1]. Clinical manifestations of serum sickness include fever, arthritis, nephritis, neuritis, oedema, and an urticarial or papular rash.

Vasculitis [2–4]. Drug-induced immune complexes play a part in the pathogenesis of cutaneous necrotizing vasculitis. Deposition of immune complexes on vascular endothelium results in activation of the complement cascade, with generation of the anaphylatoxins C3a and C5a, which have chemotactic properties. Vasoactive amines and pro-inflammatory cytokines are released from basophils and mast cells, with resultant increased vascular permeability and attraction of neutrophil polymorphonuclear cells. Immune complex interaction with platelets via their Fc receptors causes platelet aggregation and microthrombus formation. Release by neutrophils of lysosomal enzymes contributes further to local inflammation. These events lead to the histological appearance of leukocytoclastic vasculitis. Deposition of immunoglobulins and complement in and around blood vessel walls is detectable by direct immunofluorescence staining of skin biopsies. Hydralazine and the hydroxylamine metabolite of procainamide bind to complement component C4 and inhibit its function; this may impair clearance of immune complexes, and predispose to development of an LE syndrome [4].

Arthus reaction. The Arthus reaction is a localized form of immune complex vasculitis. Intradermal or subcutaneous injection of antigen such as a vaccine into a sensitized individual with circulating precipitating antibodies, usually of IgG1 class, leads to local immune complex formation and the cascade of events described above. Clinically, there is erythema and oedema, haemorrhage and occasionally necrosis at the injection site, which reaches a peak at 4–10 h, and then gradually wanes.

REFERENCES

1 Lawley TJ, Bielory L, Gascon P *et al.* A prospective clinical and immunologic analysis of patients with serum sickness. *N Engl J Med* 1984; **311**: 1407–13.
2 Mackel SE, Jordon RE. Leukocytoclastic vasculitis. A cutaneous expression of immune complex disease. *Arch Dermatol* 1983; **118**: 296–301.
3 Sams WM. Hypersensitivity angiitis. *J Invest Dermatol* 1989; **93**: 78S–81S.
4 Sim E. Drug-induced immune complex disease. *Complement Inflamm* 1989; **6**: 119–26.

Cell-mediated (type IV) reactions

The role of delayed-type cell-mediated immune reactions in contact drug hypersensitivity, as with penicillin [1], is well established, but the importance of such mechanisms involving specific effector lymphocytes in other varieties of cutaneous drug allergy is uncertain. Nevertheless, it is thought that a number of ACDRs, including some morbilliform and bullous ACDRs, fixed drug reactions, lichenoid reactions, LE-like reactions and erythema multiforme, Stevens–Johnson syndrome and TEN, involve T-lymphocyte responses to altered self. An intercurrent infectious disease (especially respiratory tract and urinary tract infections in the case of maculopapular eruptions) was documented in 58.5% of patients with ACDRs, compared with 7.5% of a control group [2]. It has been proposed that viruses may non-specifically stimulate cytotoxicity in general, which spills over to affect target cells altered by drug antigen [3]. Viruses incriminated, especially in the drug hypersensitivity syndrome, include human herpesvirus 6, Epstein–Barr virus, cytomegalovirus and hepatitis C virus [4–10].

The involvement of the skin immune system in cell-mediated drug eruptions, and graft-versus-host disease as a model for cutaneous drug eruptions, have been reviewed [11,12]. There is increasing evidence of a role for T cells and cell-mediated immunity in some drug eruptions. Sulfamethoxazole-reactive lymphocytes can be detected in peripheral blood of patients with drug-induced eruptions, at a frequency of 1/172 000, within the frequency range of urushiol-reactive T cells in patients with urushiol (poison ivy) dermatitis [13]. Patients with acute drug allergy to carbamazepine, phenytoin, sulfamethoxazole, allopurinol or paracetamol had activated drug-specific CD4+ or CD8+ T cells in the circulation [14]. In one study, predominant CD8+ T-cell activation was associated with more severe (bullous) skin lesions or liver involvement, whereas predominant activation of CD4+ cells elicited mainly maculopapular reactions [15]. Drug-specific T-cell clones from drug-induced exanthems contained heterogeneous T-cell subsets with distinct phenotypes (CD4+ > CD8+, perforin and granzyme B positive) and cell functions (strong IL-5 production, moderate interferon-γ (IFN-γ) production, and cytotoxic potential) [16,17]. Perivascular predominantly CD4+ T cells, with 30% CD8+ cells, basal keratinocyte HLA-DR and intercellular adhesion molecule (ICAM)-1 expression, and E selectin expression by endothelial cells, were seen in maculopapular or exfoliative antibiotic-induced ACDRs [18,19]. However, in other studies CD8+ T cells predominated in the epidermis in drug-induced maculopapular and bullous eruptions and patch-test reactions to β-lactam antibiotics [20,21]. β-lactam-specific peripheral and epidermal T lymphocytes from bullous exanthems were predominantly CD8+CD4−, displayed a Th1-like cytokine pattern, proliferated in an antigen- and major histocompatibility complex (MHC)-specific manner and were cytotoxic against epidermal keratinocytes in lectin-induced cytotoxicity assays. In contrast, T-cell lines from patients with penicillin-induced urticarial exanthems were predominantly CD4+CD8−, with a Th2-like cytokine pattern. Drug-specific T-cell clones and cell lines from a phenobarbital-induced eruption were heterogeneous with regard to CD4/CD8 phenotype, T-cell receptor Vβ repertoire, antigen recognition pattern and cytokine production [22]. Epicutaneous test reactions to antibiotics contained a heterogeneous population of drug-specific T cells [23]; it has been proposed that T cells producing IL-5 might contribute to eosinophilia, whereas cytotoxic CD4+ T cells might account for tissue damage [23–25]. Drug-specific T cells also contribute to the neutrophil infiltration in drug-induced acute generalized exanthematous pustulosis, by secreting the chemokine IL-8 [26–28].

Proliferation of CD8+ dermal T cells, from a sulfamethoxazole-induced bullous exanthem, to sulfamethoxazole was significantly increased in the presence of liver microsomes, suggesting that microsomal enzymes, such as the cytochrome P-450 system, generate highly reactive metabolites, which are the nominal antigens for T-cell activation

[29,30]. The expression of ICAM-1 by target keratinocytes plays an important role in the cytotoxicity of epidermal T cells in bullous drug eruptions [31]. Penicilloyl-modified MHC-associated peptides may act as T-cell epitopes; T cells may have specificity for both the backbone and the side-chain of penicillin [32]. Penicillin G may also stimulate T cells directly by binding to MHC molecules on the cell surface. Alternatively, it may bind to soluble proteins like human serum albumin, which require processing for presentation in an immunogenic form. These different modes of presentation, which elicit a variety of immunological reactivities, may explain the heterogeneity of clinical pictures seen in penicillin allergy [33]. Morbilliform drug hypersensitivity reactions in HIV-infected subjects showed spongiosis, hydropic generation of the basal layer, Civatte bodies, an epidermal lymphocytic infiltrate, and perivascular lymphocytes and macrophages [34]. Immunohistochemistry demonstrated CD8+ HLA-DR-positive T lymphocytes, marked depletion of epidermal Langerhans' cells and strong keratinocyte IL-6, tumour necrosis factor-α (TNF-α) and, to a lesser degree, IFN-γ expression.

REFERENCES

1 Stejskal VDM, Forsbeck M, Olin R. Side chain-specific lymphocyte responses in workers with occupational allergy induced by penicillins. *Int Arch Allergy Appl Immunol* 1987; **82**: 461–4.
2 Cohen AD, Friger M, Sarov B, Halevy S. Which intercurrent infections are associated with maculopapular cutaneous drug reactions? A case–control study. *Int J Dermatol* 2001; **40**: 41–4.
3 Chosidow O, Bourgault L, Roujeau JC. Drug rashes. What are the targets of cell-mediated cytotoxicity? *Arch Dermatol* 1994; **130**: 627–9.
4 Mizukawa Y, Shiohara T. Virus-induced immune dysregulation as a triggering factor for the development of drug rashes and autoimmune diseases: with emphasis on EB virus, human hepesvirus 6 and hepatitis C virus. *J Dermatol Sci* 2000; **22**: 169–80.
5 Le Cleach L, Fillet AM, Agut H, Chosidow O. Human herpesviruses 6 and 7. *Arch Dermatol* 1998; **134**: 1155–7.
6 Descamps V, Bouscarat F, Laglenne S et al. Human herpesvirus 6 infection associated with anticonvulsant hypersensitivity syndrome and reactive haemophagocytic syndrome. *Br J Dermatol* 1997; **137**: 605–8.
7 Tohyama M, Yahat Y, Yasukawa M et al. Severe hypersensitivity syndrome due to sulfasalazine associated with reactivation of human herpesvirus 6. *Arch Dermatol* 1998; **134**: 1113–7.
8 Suzuki Y, Inagi R, Aonon T et al. Human herpesvirus 6 infection as a risk factor for the development of severe drug-induced hypersensitivity syndrome. *Arch Dermatol* 1998; **134**: 1108–12.
9 Descamps V, Valance A, Edlinger C et al. Association of human herpesvirus 6 infection with drug reaction with eosinophilia and systemic symptoms. *Arch Dermatol* 2001; **137**: 301–4.
10 Aihara M, Sugita Y, Takahashi S et al. Anticonvulsant hypersensitivity syndrome associated with reactivation of cytomegalovirus. *Br J Dermatol* 2001; **144**: 1231–4.
11 Breathnach SM, Hintner H. *Adverse Drug Reactions and the Skin.* Oxford: Blackwell Scientific Publications, 1992.
12 Breathnach SM. Mechanisms of drug eruptions: Part I. *Australas J Dermatol* 1995; **36**: 121–7.
13 Kalish RS, Laporte A, Wood JA, Johnson KL. Sulfonamide-reactive lymphocytes detected at very low frequency in the peripheral blood of patients with drug-induced eruptions. *J Allergy Clin Immunol* 1994; **94**: 465–72.
14 Mauri-Hellweg D, Bettens F, Mauri D. Activation of drug-specific CD4+ and CD8+ T cells in individuals allergic to sulfonamides, phenytoin, and carbamazepine. *J Immunol* 1995; **155**: 462–72.
15 Hari Y, Frutig-Schnyder K, Hurni M et al. T cell involvement in cutaneous drug eruptions. *Clin Exp Allergy* 2001; **31**: 1398–408.
16 Yawalkar N, Egli F, Hari Y et al. Infiltration of cytotoxic T cells in drug-induced cutaneous eruptions. *Clin Exp Allergy* 2000; **30**: 847–55.
17 Yawalkar N, Pichler WJ. Pathogenesis of drug-induced exanthema. *Int Arch Allergy Immunol* 2001; **124**: 336–8.
18 Barbaud AM, Béné M-C, Schmutz J-L et al. Role of delayed cellular hypersensitivity and adhesion molecules in amoxicillin-induced morbilliform rashes. *Arch Dermatol* 1997; **133**: 481–6.
19 Barbaud AM, Béné MC, Reichert-Penetrat S et al. Immunocompetent cells and adhesion molecules in 14 cases of cutaneous drug reactions induced with antibiotics. *Arch Dermatol* 1998; **134**: 1040–1.
20 Hertl M, Geisel J, Boecker C, Merk HF. Selective generation of CD8+ T-cell clones from the peripheral blood of patients with cutaneous reactions to beta-lactam antibiotics. *Br J Dermatol* 1993; **128**: 619–26.
21 Hertl M, Bohlen H, Jugert F et al. Predominance of epidermal CD8+ T lymphocytes in bullous cutaneous reactions caused by β-lactam antibiotics. *J Invest Dermatol* 1993; **101**: 794–9.
22 Hashizume H, Takigawa M, Tokura Y. Characterization of drug-specific T cells in phenobarbital-induced eruption. *J Immunol* 2002; **168**: 5359–68.
23 Yawalkar N, Hari Y, Frutig K et al. T cells isolated from positive epicutaneous test reactions to amoxicillin and ceftriaxone are drug specific and cytotoxic. *J Invest Dermatol* 2000; **115**: 647–52.
24 Choquet-Kastylevsky G, Intrator L, Chenal C et al. Increased levels of interleukin 5 are associated with the generation of eosinophilia in drug-induced hypersensitivity syndrome. *Br J Dermatol* 1998; **139**: 1026–32.
25 Mikami C, Ochiai K, Umemiya K et al. Eosinophil activation and *in situ* interleukin-5 production by mononuclear cells in skin lesions of patients with drug hypersensitivity. *J Dermatol* 1999; **26**: 633–9.
26 Britschgi M, Steiner UC, Schmid S et al. T-cell involvement in drug-induced acute generalized exanthematous pustulosis. *J Clin Invest* 2001; **107**: 1433–41.
27 Schmid S, Kuechler PC, Britschgi M et al. Acute generalized exanthematous pustulosis: role of cytotoxic T cells in pustule formation. *Am J Pathol* 2002; **161**: 2079–86.
28 Britschgi M, Pichler WJ. Acute generalized exanthematous pustulosis, a clue to neutrophil-mediated inflammatory processes orchestrated by T cells. *Curr Opin Allergy Clin Immunol* 2002; **2**: 325–31.
29 Hertl M, Merk HF. Lymphocyte activation in cutaneous drug reactions. *J Invest Dermatol* 1995; **105** (Suppl.): S95–S98.
30 Hertl M, Jugert F, Merk HF. CD8+ dermal T cells from a sulphamethoxazole-induced bullous exanthem proliferate in response to drug-modified liver microsomes. *Br J Dermatol* 1995; **132**: 215–20.
31 Hertl M, Rönnau A, Bohlen H et al. The cytotoxicity of epidermal T lymphocytes in bullous drug reactions is strongly but not completely abrogated by inhibition of ICAM-1 on target cells (abstract). *Arch Dermatol Res* 1993; **285**: 63.
32 Weltzien HU, Padovan E. Molecular features of penicillin allergy. *J Invest Dermatol* 1998; **110**: 203–6.
33 Brander C, Mauri-Hellweg D, Bettens F et al. Heterogeneous T cell responses to beta-lactam-modified self-structures are observed in penicillin-allergic individuals. *J Immunol* 1995; **155**: 2670–8.
34 Carr A, Vasak E, Munro V et al. Immunohistological assessment of cutaneous drug hypersensitivity in patients with HIV infection. *Clin Exp Immunol* 1994; **97**: 260–5.

Erythema multiforme, Stevens–Johnson syndrome and TEN. The reader is referred to Chapter 74.

Lichenoid drug eruptions. The mechanisms underlying lichenoid drug eruptions are essentially unknown, but they may develop as a result of autoreactive cytotoxic T-cell clones directed against a drug–class II MHC antigen complex, such that keratinocytes and Langerhans' cells are viewed by the immune system as 'non-self'. Cloned murine autoreactive T cells produce a lichenoid reaction in recipient animals following injection [1]. The presence of epidermotropic T cells correlates with that of class II MHC (HLA-DR)-expressing keratinocytes and Langerhans' cells in lichenoid eruptions [2].

REFERENCES

1 Shiohara T. The lichenoid tissue reaction. An immunological perspective. *Am J Dermatopathol* 1988; **10**: 252–6.
2 Shiohara T, Moriya N, Tanaka Y *et al.* Immunopathological study of lichenoid skin diseases: correlation between HLA-DR-positive keratinocytes or Langerhans cells and epidermotropic T cells. *J Am Acad Dermatol* 1988; **18**: 67–74.

LE-like syndrome induced by drugs. Drug-induced LE, with production of antihistone antibodies, may result from interaction between the drug and nuclear material to produce a drug–nucleoprotein complex that is immunogenic. Alternatively, drugs may alter immunoregulation in such a way that autoantibody production is favoured; procainamide and hydralazine modulate lymphocyte function directly and induce autoreactivity. Thus, drugs may cause an SLE-like condition by a mechanism analogous to that in immunostimulatory graft-versus-host disease [1]. Hydralazine, isoniazid and the hydroxylamine metabolites of procainamide and practolol may also predispose to the development of an LE-like syndrome by inhibiting binding of C4 and in turn of C3 to immune complexes, thus preventing complement-mediated clearance of immune complexes by solubilization and opsonization [2].

REFERENCES

1 Gleichman E, Pals ST, Rolinck AG *et al.* Graft-versus-host reactions: clues to the etiopathogenesis of a spectrum of immunological diseases. *Immunol Today* 1984; **5**: 324–32.
2 Sim E. Drug-induced immune complex disease. *Complement Inflamm* 1989; **6**: 119–26.

Drug-induced pemphigus. Immunoprecipitation studies have shown that patients with drug-induced pemphigus foliaceus and pemphigus vulgaris often have circulating autoantibodies with the same antigenic specificity at a molecular level as autoantibodies from patients with idiopathic pemphigus [1]. Binding of an active thiol group in a drug to the pemphigus antigen complex might result in autoantibody production, or culprit drugs may result in immune dysregulation. In addition, drugs with thiol groups in their molecule, such as penicillamine, captopril and thiopronine, and piroxicam can cause acantholysis directly *in vitro* in the absence of autoantibody [2].

REFERENCES

1 Korman NJ, Eyre RW, Stanley JR. Drug-induced pemphigus: autoantibodies directed against the pemphigus antigen complexes are present in penicillamine and captopril-induced pemphigus. *J Invest Dermatol* 1991; **96**: 273–6.
2 Ruocco V, Pisani M, de Angelis E, Lombardi ML. Biochemical acantholysis provoked by thiol drugs. *Arch Dermatol* 1990; **126**: 965–6.

Fixed drug eruptions. Graft autotransplantation investigations carried out in the 1930s demonstrated cutaneous memory in involved skin in fixed drug eruption [1]. Serum factors from patients with fixed drug eruption have been reported to cause inflammation on injection into a previously involved site, but not when injected into normal skin [2], and to induce lymphocyte blast transformation [3,4]. However, cell-mediated rather than humoral immunity is thought to play the major role in the development of lesions in this condition.

Lesional skin contains increased numbers of both helper and suppressor T lymphocytes [5–8], and T suppressor/cytotoxic T cells may be seen adjacent to necrotic keratinocytes in the epidermis [6]. T cells may persist within lesional skin and contribute to immunological memory [7,9]; CD8+ suppressor/cytotoxic T cells were present in suprabasal epidermis in involved skin 3 weeks after challenge [5]. Intraepidermal CD8+ T cells phenotypically resembling effector memory T cells are greatly enriched in the resting lesions of fixed drug eruption; upon activation, they can rapidly produce large amounts of IFN-γ followed by localized epidermal injury [10].

T cells from lesional epidermis in two patients with fixed drug eruption utilized a very limited range of Vα and Vβ genes compared with peripheral blood T cells, indicating some expansion or preferential migration of T cells recognizing a restricted set of antigens [11]. Keratinocytes in lesional skin express ICAM-1 [12], which is involved in interaction between keratinocytes and lymphocytes, HLA-DR [6] and the chemotactic protein IP-10 [8], findings that suggest a role for cytokines in the evolution of the histological changes [8,13]. ICAM-1 was noted to be induced on endothelium and keratinocytes 1.5 h after drug challenge, and there was increased reactivity in lesional skin *in vitro* to TNF-α and IFN-γ, as well as to the causative drug [13]; drug-induced, TNF-α-dependent keratinocyte ICAM-1 expression in lesional skin may provide a localized initiating stimulus for epidermal T-cell activation. Early release of histamine from mast cells or basophils has been reported in fixed drug eruption, based on suction blister fluid levels [14]. Significantly higher frequencies of HLA-B22 and HLA-Cw1 antigens were found in 36 patients with fixed drug eruption, and familial cases occur, suggesting a genetic predisposition [15].

REFERENCES

1 Korkij W, Soltani K. Fixed drug eruption. A brief review. *Arch Dermatol* 1984; **120**: 520–4.
2 Wyatt E, Greaves M, Søndergaard J. Fixed drug eruption (phenolphthalein). *Arch Dermatol* 1972; **106**: 671–3.
3 Gimenez-Camarasa JM, Garcia-Calderon P, De Moragas JM. Lymphocyte transformation test in fixed drug eruption. *N Engl J Med* 1975; **292**: 819–21.
4 Suzuki S, Asai Y, Toshio H *et al.* Drug-induced lymphocyte transformation in peripheral lymphocytes from patients with drug eruption. *Dermatologica* 1978; **157**: 146–53.
5 Hindsén M, Christensen OB, Gruic V, Löfberg H. Fixed drug eruption: an immunohistochemical investigation of the acute and healing phase. *Br J Dermatol* 1987; **116**: 351–6.
6 Murphy GF, Guillén FJ, Flynn TC. Cytotoxic T lymphocytes and phenotypically abnormal epidermal dendritic cells in fixed cutaneous eruption. *Hum Pathol* 1985; **16**: 1264–71.

7 Visa K, Käyhkö K, Stubb S, Reitamo S. Immunocompetent cells of fixed drug eruption. *Acta Derm Venereol (Stockh)* 1987; **67**: 30–5.
8 Smoller BR, Luster AD, Krane JF *et al.* Fixed drug eruptions: evidence for a cytokine-mediated process. *J Cutan Pathol* 1991; **18**: 13–9.
9 Scheper RJ, Von Blomberg M, Boerrigter GH *et al.* Induction of immunological memory in the skin. Role of local T cell retention. *Clin Exp Immunol* 1983; **51**: 141–8.
10 Shiohara T, Mizukawa Y, Teraki Y. Pathophysiology of fixed drug eruption: the role of skin-resident T cells. *Curr Opin Allergy Clin Immunol* 2002; **2**: 317–23.
11 Komatsu T, Moriya N, Shiohara T. T cell receptor (TCR) repertoire and function of human epidermal T cells: restricted TCR V alpha-V beta genes are utilized by T cells residing in the lesional epidermis in fixed drug eruption. *Clin Exp Immunol* 1996; **104**: 343–50.
12 Shiohara T, Nickoloff BJ, Sagawa Y *et al.* Fixed drug eruption. Expression of epidermal keratinocyte intercellular adhesion molecule-1 (ICAM-1). *Arch Dermatol* 1989; **125**: 1371–6.
13 Teraki Y, Moriya N, Shiohara T. Drug-induced expression of intercellular adhesion molecule-1 on lesional keratinocytes in fixed drug eruption. *Am J Pathol* 1994; **145**: 550–60.
14 Alanko K, Stubb S, Salo OP, Reitamo S. Suction blister fluid histamine in fixed drug eruption. *Acta Derm Venereol (Stockh)* 1992; **72**: 89–91.
15 Pellicano R, Ciavarella G, Lomuto M, Di Giorgio G. Genetic susceptibility to fixed drug eruption: evidence for a link with HLA-B22. *J Am Acad Dermatol* 1994; **30**: 52–4.

Histopathology of drug reactions [1]

In most patterns of reaction to drugs, the histological changes are no more distinctive than are the clinical features. For example, urticaria, erythema multiforme, TEN and exfoliative dermatitis provoked by drugs cannot be differentiated from the same reactions resulting from other causes. Graft-versus-host disease-type drug eruptions in the acute phase show a predominance of epidermal CD8+ T cells, reduced epidermal OKT6-positive Langerhans' cells, and increased keratinocyte expression of HLA-DR and ICAM-1 [2]. In contrast, Langerhans' cells from lesional maculopapular drug eruptions reportedly increased in number by 66% and displayed more intense staining and more prominent dendrites in one study [3].

The histological changes in the vegetating iododermas and bromodermas, certain lichenoid eruptions and fixed drug eruptions are not pathognomonic, but are sufficiently characteristic to be of importance in differential diagnosis. The histology of a number of other drug eruptions has been reviewed [4]. Amiodarone-induced hyperpigmentation shows a lymphocytic dermatitis and yellowish-brown granules within several cell types; the drug or a metabolite composes at least a portion of the deposits. Clofazimine-induced hyperpigmentation involves accumulation of a ceroid lipofuscin within lipid-laden macrophages. The cutaneous eruption of lymphocyte recovery after chemotherapeutic agents is a maculopapular eruption with a non-specific superficial perivascular dermatitis. Chemotherapy-induced acral erythema reveals a non-specific interface dermatitis. Specific reactions occur with etoposide (starburst cells) and busulfan (busulphan) (large atypical keratinocytes), and other chemotherapeutic agents may involve sweat glands: neutrophilic eccrine hidradenitis is characterized by neutrophil infiltration and by necrosis; syringosquamous metaplasia involves squamous metaplasia of the sweat duct. Drug-induced generalized pustular toxic erythema is characterized by subcorneal pustules and occasional eosinophils. Cephalosporins may produce a syndrome clinically and histologically like pemphigus, and naproxen produces one like porphyria cutanea tarda. The photosensitive dermatitis associated with quinine and piroxicam is histologically a non-specific spongiotic dermatitis. A lichenoid giant cell dermatitis may be caused by methyldopa or chlorothiazide, and phenytoin and carbamazepine dermatitis histologically imitates mycosis fungoides.

Bromodermas and iododermas

In bromoderma, verrucous pseudoepitheliomatous hyperplasia is associated with abscesses containing neutrophils and eosinophils in the epidermis, and a dense dermal infiltrate initially consisting mainly of neutrophils and eosinophils and later containing many lymphocytes, plasma cells and histiocytes. The abundant dilated blood vessels may show endothelial proliferation. In iododermas, ulceration is more marked, but there is usually less epithelial hyperplasia. Both conditions must be differentiated from blastomycosis and coccidioidomycosis, and from pemphigus vegetans.

Fixed eruptions

In the acute stage, the epidermal changes may be indistinguishable from erythema multiforme, with loss of cell outlines and necrosis of the lower epidermis. In less acute lesions, the epidermis may show little abnormality but the dermis is oedematous and there is a conspicuous perivascular lymphocytic infiltrate. Later, there is increased melanin in the epidermis and within melanophages in the dermis.

Lichenoid eruptions

The changes may be non-specific or may resemble idiopathic lichen planus, although the cellular infiltrate tends to be more pleomorphic and less dense, and the presence of focal parakeratosis, focal interruption of the granular layer, and cytoid bodies in the cornified and granular layers suggest a drug cause [5]. Later, there may be scarring, with destruction of the sweat glands.

REFERENCES

1 Elder D, Elenitsas R, Jaworsky C, Johnson B Jr, eds. *Lever's Histopathology of the Skin*, 8th edn. Philadelphia: Lippincott, 1997.
2 Osawa J, Kitamura K, Saito S *et al.* Immunohistochemical study of graft-versus-host reaction (GVHR)-type drug eruptions. *J Dermatol* 1994; **21**: 25–30.

3 Dascalu DI, Kletter Y, Baratz M, Brenner S. Langerhans' cell distribution in drug eruption. *Acta Derm Venereol (Stockh)* 1992; **72**: 175–7.
4 Fitzpatrick JE. New histopathologic findings in drug eruptions. *Dermatol Clin* 1992; **10**: 19–36.
5 Van den Haute V, Antoine JL, Lachapelle JM. Histopathological discriminant criteria between lichenoid drug eruption and idiopathic lichen planus: retrospective study on selected samples. *Dermatologica* 1989; **179**: 10–3.

Types of clinical reaction [1–13]

The mucocutaneous reactions that may result from ADRs have been the subject of extensive reviews, to which the reader is referred for further information. The following section details a number of different drug-induced reaction patterns; see also the discussion of adverse effects of individual drugs later. It is unfortunate that although certain drugs are commonly associated with a specific reaction, most drugs are capable of causing several different types of eruption.

REFERENCES

1 Davies DM, ed. *Textbook of Adverse Drug Reactions*, 3rd edn. Oxford: Oxford University Press, 1985.
2 Stern RS, Wintroub BU. Adverse drug reactions: reporting and evaluating cutaneous reactions. *Adv Dermatol* 1987; **2**: 3–18.
3 Seymour RA, Walton JG. *Adverse Drug Reactions in Dentistry*. Oxford: Oxford University Press, 1988.
4 Bork K. *Cutaneous Side Effects of Drugs*. Philadelphia: Saunders, 1988.
5 Dukes MNG, ed. *Meyler's Side Effects of Drugs*, 11th edn. Amsterdam: Elsevier, 1988.
6 Alanko K, Stubbs S, Kauppinen K. Cutaneous drug reactions: clinical types and causative agents. A five year survey of in-patients (1981–1985). *Acta Derm Venereol (Stockh)* 1989; **69**: 223–6.
7 Shear NH, ed. Adverse reactions to drugs. *Semin Dermatol* 1989; **8**: 135–226.
8 Kalish RS. Drug eruptions: a review of clinical and immunological features. *Adv Dermatol* 1991; **6**: 221–37.
9 Pavan-Langston D, Dunkel EC. *Handbook of Ocular Drug Therapy and Ocular Side Effects of Systemic Drugs*. Boston: Little, Brown, 1991.
10 Breathnach SM, Hintner H. *Adverse Drug Reactions and the Skin*. Oxford: Blackwell Scientific Publications, 1992.
11 Zürcher L, Krebs A. *Cutaneous Drug Reactions*. Basel: Karger, 1992.
12 Bruinsma WA. *A Guide to Drug Eruptions: File of Side Effects in Dermatology*, 6th edn. Oosthuizen, The Netherlands: File of Medicines, 1996.
13 Litt JZ, Pawlak WA Jr. *Drug Eruption Reference Manual*. New York: Parthenon, 1997.

Exanthematic (maculopapular) reactions

These are the most frequent of all cutaneous reactions to drugs, and can occur after almost any drug at any time up to 3 (but usually 2) weeks after administration; they may be accompanied by fever, pruritus and eosinophilia. It is not possible to identify the offending drug by the nature of the eruption. The clinical features are variable; the lesions may be scarlatiniform, rubelliform or morbilliform, or may consist of a profuse eruption of small papules showing no close resemblance to any infective exanthem (Fig. 73.1). Less common are eruptions with large macules, polycylic and gyrate erythema, reticular eruptions and sheet-like erythema. The distribution is

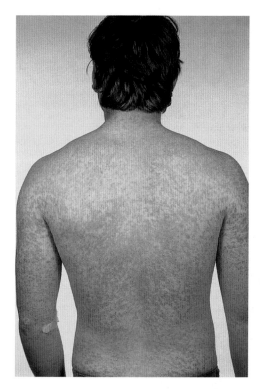

Fig. 73.1 Maculopapular erythema caused by ampicillin.

also variable but is generally symmetrical. The trunk and extremities are usually involved, and not uncommonly intertriginous areas may be favoured, but the face may be spared. Palmar and plantar lesions may occur, and sometimes the eruption is generalized. Purpuric lesions, especially on the legs, and erosive stomatitis may develop. There may be relative sparing of pressure areas. If the administration of the drug is continued, an exfoliative dermatitis may develop, although occasionally the eruption subsides despite continuation of the medication.

Morbilliform drug eruptions usually, but not always, recur on rechallenge. The main differential diagnosis is from viral rashes. In a recent series of atypical exanthems, morphology and laboratory investigations led to an aetiological diagnosis in about 70% of cases [1]. It is useful, in differentiating exanthematic drug eruptions from viral exanthems, to remember that viral rashes may start on the face and progress to involve the trunk, and are more often accompanied by conjunctivitis, lymphadenopathy and fever. Maculopapular drug eruptions usually fade with desquamation, sometimes with post-inflammatory hyperpigmentation. Commoner causes are listed in Table 73.2.

REFERENCE

1 Drago F, Rampini PR, Rampini E, Rebora A. Atypical exanthems: morphology and laboratory investigations may lead to an aetiological diagnosis in about 70% of cases. *Br J Dermatol* 2002; **147**: 255–60.

Table 73.2 Drugs causing exanthematic reactions.

Most common	Less common
Ampicillin and penicillin	Cephalosporins
Phenylbutazone and other pyrazolones	Barbiturates
Sulphonamides	Thiazides
Phenytoin	Naproxen
Carbamazepine	Isoniazid
Gold	Phenothiazines
Gentamicin	Quinidine
	Meprobamate
	Atropine

Purpura

A purpuric element to a drug eruption is not uncommon, but primarily purpuric drug-induced rashes also occur. Many drugs may interfere with platelet aggregation [1] but, with the exception of aspirin, this does not usually result in bleeding. A number of drugs have been implicated in the development of drug-induced purpura [2–4]. Several mechanisms may be involved. These include altered coagulation after anticoagulants or some cephalosporins, allergic and non-allergic thrombocytopenia, altered platelet function (as after valproic acid) or vascular causes, including steroid-induced fragility and loss of support. Cytotoxic drug therapy may result in non-allergic purpura due to bone marrow depression, with a platelet count of less than 30 000/mm^3. Bleomycin may induce thrombocytopenia by causing endothelial damage and consequent platelet aggregation [5]. A large number of drugs have been reported to cause allergic thrombocytopenia [2–4]. Heparin may cause purpura with overdosage or due to an allergic thrombocytopenia [6]. The classical example of complement-mediated destruction of platelets, following immune complex formation between a drug (as hapten) bound to the platelet surface and IgG class antibody, was the purpura caused by apronalide (Sedormid). Quinine, quinidine [7,8] and chlorothiazide may also cause allergic purpura. Tissue plasminogen activator (alteplase) has been associated with painful purpura [9]. A purpuric vasculitis-like rash followed secondary spread of a contact dermatitis to balsam of Peru [10].

Capillaritis (pigmented purpuric eruption) may be due to aspirin, carbromal or more rarely to thiamine or meprobamate [11–14], carbamazepine, phenacetin, as well as glipizide, pefloxacin, lorazepam, aspirin, paracetamol, polyvinyl pyrrolidone plasma expander, ciclosporin and griseofulvin [15,16]; it may be due to formation of antibody to a drug–capillary endothelial cell complex [12]. Chronic pigmented purpura is recorded with thiamine propyldisulphide and chlordiazepoxide [13] and aminoglutethimide [17]. NSAIDs, diuretics, meprobamate and ampicillin were the commonest drug cause of pigmented purpuric eruptions in one study [18].

REFERENCES

1 George JN, Shattil SJ. The clinical importance of acquired abnormalities of platelet function. *N Engl J Med* 1991; **324**: 27–39.
2 Miescher PA, Graf J. Drug-induced thrombocytopenia. *Clin Haematol* 1980; **9**: 505–19.
3 Moss RA. Drug-induced immune thrombocytopenia. *Am J Hematol* 1980; **9**: 439–46.
4 Bork K. *Cutaneous Side Effects of Drugs.* Philadelphia: Saunders, 1988.
5 Hilgard P, Hossfeld DK. Transient bleomycin-induced thrombocytopenia. A clinical study. *Eur J Cancer* 1978; **14**: 1261–4.
6 Babcock RB, Dumper CW, Scharfman WB. Heparin-induced thrombocytopenia. *N Engl J Med* 1976; **295**: 237–41.
7 Christie DJ, Weber RW, Mullen PC *et al.* Structural features of the quinidine and quinine molecules necessary for binding of drug-induced antibodies to human platelets. *J Lab Clin Med* 1984; **104**: 730–40.
8 Gary M, Ilfeld D, Kelton JG. Correlation of a quinidine-induced platelet-specific antibody with development of thrombocytopenia. *Am J Med* 1985; **79**: 253–5.
9 Detrana C, Hurwitz RM. Painful purpura: an adverse effect to a thrombolysin. *Arch Dermatol* 1990; **126**: 690–1.
10 Bruynzeel DP, van den Hoogenband HM, Koedijk F. Purpuric vasculitis-like eruption in a patient sensitive to balsam of Peru. *Contact Dermatitis* 1984; **11**: 207–9.
11 Peterson WC, Manick KP. Purpuric eruptions associated with use of carbromal and meprobamate. *Arch Dermatol* 1967; **95**: 40–2.
12 Carmel WJ, Dannenberg T. Nonthrombocytopenic purpura due to Miltown (2-methyl-2-*n*-propyl-1,3-propanediol dicarbamate). *N Engl J Med* 1956; **255**: 7701.
13 Nishioka K, Katayama I, Masuzawa M *et al.* Drug-induced chronic pigmented purpura. *J Dermatol* 1989; **16**: 220–2.
14 Abeck D, Gross GE, Kuwert C *et al.* Acetaminophen-induced progressive pigmentary purpura (Schamberg's disease). *J Am Acad Dermatol* 1992; **27**: 123–4.
15 Tsao H, Lerner LH. Pigmented purpuric eruption associated with injection medroxyprogesterone acetate. *J Am Acad Dermatol* 2000; **43**: 308–10.
16 Adams BB, Gadenne AS. Glipizide-induced pigmented purpuric dermatosis. *J Am Acad Dermatol* 1999; **41**: 827–9.
17 Stratakis CA, Chrousos GP. Capillaritis (purpura simplex) associated with use of aminoglutethimide in Cushing's syndrome. *Am J Hosp Pharm* 1994; **51**: 2589–91.
18 Pang BK, Su D, Ratnam KV. Drug-induced purpura simplex: clinical and histological characteristics. *Ann Acad Med Singapore* 1993; **22**: 870–2.

Annular erythema

Erythema annulare centrifugum has been reported in association with chloroquine and hydroxychloroquine [1], oestrogens, cimetidine [2], penicillin, salicylates and piroxicam, as well as with hydrochlorothiazide [3], spironolactone [4], thioacetazone [5], the phenothiazine levomepromazine [6] and etizolam [7]. Annular erythema has occurred with vitamin K [8].

REFERENCES

1 Ashurst PJ. Erythema annulare centrifugum due to hydroxychloroquine sulfate and chloroquine sulfate. *Arch Dermatol* 1967; **95**: 37–9.
2 Merrett AC, Marks R, Dudley FJ. Cimetidine-induced erythema annulare centrifugum: no cross-sensitivity with ranitidine. *BMJ* 1981; **283**: 698.
3 Goette DK, Beatrice E. Erythema annulare centrifugum caused by hydrochlorothiazide-induced interstitial nephritis. *Int J Dermatol* 1988; **27**: 129–30.
4 Carsuzaa F, Pierre C, Dubegny M. Érytheme annulaire centrifuge a l'aldactone. *Ann Dermatol Vénéréol* 1987; **114**: 375–6.
5 Ramesh V. Eruption resembling erythema annulare centrifugum. *Australas J Dermatol* 1987; **28**: 44.
6 Blazejak T, Hölzle E. Phenothiazin-induziertes Pseudolymphom. *Hautarzt* 1990; **41**: 161–3.

Table 73.3 Drugs causing pityriasis rosea-like drug reactions.

Arsenicals	Captopril
Bismuth	Griseofulvin
Gold	Isotretinoin
Barbiturates	Metronidazole
β-Blockers	Pyribenzamine
Clonidine	Methoxypromazine
	Omeprazole

Table 73.4 Drugs reported to exacerbate psoriasis.

Antimalarials
β-Blockers
Lithium salts
Non-steroidal anti-inflammatory drugs
   Ibuprofen
   Indometacin (indomethacin) (disputed)
   Meclofenamate sodium
   Pyrazolone derivatives (phenylbutazone, oxyphenbutazone)
Miscellaneous
   Captopril
   Chlortalidone (chlorthalidone)
   Cimetidine
   Clonidine
   Gemfibrozil
   Interferon
   Methlydopa
   Penicillamine
   Penicillin
   Terfenadine
   Trazodone

7 Kuroda K, Yabunami H, Hisanaga Y. Etizolam-induced superficial erythema annulare centrifugum. *Clin Exp Dermatol* 2002; **27**: 34–6.
8 Kay MH, Duvic M. Reactive annular erythema after intramuscular vitamin K. *Cutis* 1986; **37**: 445–8.

Pityriasis rosea-like reactions

The best-known drug cause of a pityriasiform rash is gold therapy [1], but several other drugs have been implicated, including metronidazole [2], captopril [3], isotretinoin [4] and omeprazole [5] (Table 73.3).

REFERENCES

1 Wile UJ, Courville CJ. Pityriasis rosea-like dermatitis following gold therapy: report of two cases. *Arch Dermatol* 1940; **42**: 1105–12.
2 Maize JC, Tomecki J. Pityriasis rosea-like drug eruption secondary to metronidazole. *Arch Dermatol* 1977; **113**: 1457–8.
3 Wilkin JK, Kirkendall WM. Pityriasis rosea-like rash from captopril. *Arch Dermatol* 1982; **118**: 186–7.
4 Helfman RJ, Brickman M, Fahey J. Isotretinoin dermatitis simulating acute pityriasis rosea. *Cutis* 1984; **33**: 297–300.
5 Buckley C. Pityriasis rosea-like eruption in a patient receiving omeprazole. *Br J Dermatol* 1996; **135**: 660–1.

Psoriasiform eruptions

See Chapter 35 and Table 73.4.

Table 73.5 Drugs causing erythroderma and exfoliative dermatitis.

Allopurinol	Hydantoins
p-Aminosalicylic acid	Isoniazid
Ampicillin	Lithium
Barbiturates	Nitrofurantoin
Captopril	Penicillamine
Carbamazepine	Penicillin
Cefoxitin	Phenylbutazone
Chloroquine	Quinidine
Chlorpromazine	Streptomycin
Cimetidine	Sulphonamides
Diltiazem	Sulphonylureas
Gold	Thioacetazone (thiacetazone)
Griseofulvin	

Exfoliative dermatitis

Exfoliative dermatitis is one of the most dangerous patterns of cutaneous reaction to drugs [1–5]. It may follow exanthematic eruptions or may develop, as in some reactions to arsenicals and the heavy metals, as erythema and exudation in the flexures, rapidly generalizing. The eruption may start several weeks after initiation of the therapy. A dermatitis in patients previously sensitized by contact may also become universal.

The main drugs implicated are listed in Table 73.5. In one large series, sulphonamides, antimalarials and penicillin were most frequently implicated [1]. In another series from India [3], the commonest associated drugs were isoniazid (20%), thioacetazone (15%), topical tar (15%) and a variety of homeopathic medicines (20%), with phenylbutazone, streptomycin and sulfadiazine (sulphadiazine) each accounting for 5% of cases. Phenytoin is a well-recognized cause [6]. Recently incriminated drugs have included captopril, cefoxitin, cimetidine and ampicillin.

REFERENCES

1 Nicolis GD, Helwig EB. Exfoliative dermatitis. A clinicopathologic study of 135 cases. *Arch Dermatol* 1973; **108**: 788–97.
2 Hasan T, Jansén DT. Erythroderma: a follow-up of fifty cases. *J Am Acad Dermatol* 1983; **8**: 836–4.
3 Sehgal VN, Srivastava G. Exfoliative dermatitis. A prospective study of 80 patients. *Dermatologica* 1986; **173**: 278–84.
4 Sage T, Faure M. Conduite à tenir devant les érythrodermies de l'adulte. *Ann Dermatol Vénéréol* 1989; **116**: 747–52.
5 Irvine C. 'Skin failure'—a real entity: discussion paper. *J R Soc Med* 1991; **84**: 412–3.
6 Danno K, Kume M, Ohta M *et al*. Erythroderma with generalized lymphadenopathy induced by phenytoin. *J Dermatol* 1989; **16**: 392–6.

Anaphylaxis and anaphylactoid reactions

This systemic reaction, which usually develops within minutes to hours (the vast majority within the first hour), is often severe and may be fatal [1–3]. Fatal drug-induced anaphylactic shock was estimated at 0.3 cases per million

Table 73.6 Drugs causing urticaria or anaphylaxis.

Animal sera	Dextrans	
Vaccines containing egg protein	Mannitol	
Desensitizing agents including pollen vaccines	Sorbitol complexes	
Antibiotics	Enzymes	
Penicillins	Trypsin	
Cephalosporins	Streptokinase	
Aminoglycosides	Chymopapain	
Tetracyclines	Steroids	
Sulphonamides	Progesterone	
Antifungal agents	Hydrocortisone	
Fluconazole	Polypeptide hormones	
Ketoconazole	Insulin	
Blood products	Corticotrophin	
Angiotensin-converting enzyme inhibitors	Vasopressin	
Radiographic contrast media	Food and drug additives	
Non-steroidal anti-inflammatory drugs (NSAIDs)	Benzoates	
Salicylates	Sulphites	
Other NSAIDs (e.g. phenylbutazone, aminopyrine,	Tartrazine dyes	
propyphenazone, metamizole, tolmetin)	Hydantoins	
Narcotic analgesics	Hydralazine	
Anaesthetic agents: local and general	Quinidine	
Muscle relaxants	Anticancer drugs	
Suxamethonium	Vitamins	
Curare	Protamine	

inhabitants per year, based on notifications to the Danish Committee on Adverse Drug Reactions and to the Central Death Register during the period 1968–90 [3]. The most frequent causes were contrast media for X-ray examinations, antibiotics and extracts of allergens. In less severe cases, there may be premonitory dizziness or faintness, skin tingling and reddening of the bulbar conjunctiva, followed by urticaria, angio-oedema, bronchospasm, abdominal pain and vasomotor collapse. It usually develops on second exposure to a drug, but may develop during the first treatment if this lasts sufficiently long for sensitization to occur. Anaphylaxis is unlikely to occur with a drug taken continuously for several months; in contrast, intermittent administration may predispose to anaphylaxis [1]. It is commoner after parenteral than oral drug administration. The β-blockers enhance anaphylactic reactions caused by other allergens, and may make resuscitation more difficult [4].

The principal drug causes are shown in Table 73.6. Antibiotics (especially penicillin) and radiocontrast media are the most common known causes of anaphylactic events [2]; the incidence of such reactions for each is about 1 in 5000 exposures [5,6], of which less than 10% are fatal [2]. The risk for recurrent anaphylactic reactions is 10–20% for penicillins [5] and 20–40% for radiocontrast media [7]. Anaphylaxis to paracetamol-containing tablets has occurred, although it was the additive polyvinyl pyrrolidone that was reponsible [8].

Anaphylactoid reactions are those that clinically resemble an immediate immune response but in which

the mechanism is undetermined. Some drugs and agents, such as mannitol and radiographic contrast media, can stimulate mediator release by an as yet unknown direct mechanism independent of IgE or complement. Anaphylactoid reactions may be produced by non-steroidal analgesics and anti-inflammatory agents (NSAIDs) [9,10], including aspirin and other salicylates, indometacin (indomethacin), phenylbutazone, propyphenazone, metamizole and tolmetin [11], as well as by radiographic contrast media, *d*-tubocurarine, benzoic acid preservatives [12], tartrazine dyes, sulphite preservatives [13] and ciprofloxacin [14]. The HLA-DRB1*11 allele showed a positive association with NSAID-induced anaphylactoid systemic reactions but not with purely cutaneous reactions [15].

REFERENCES

1 Sussman GL, Dolovich J. Prevention of anaphylaxis. *Semin Dermatol* 1989; **8**: 158–65.
2 Bochner BS, Lichtenstein LM. Anaphylaxis. *N Engl J Med* 1991; **324**: 1785–90.
3 Lenler-Petersen P, Hansen D, Andersen M *et al.* Drug-related fatal anaphylactic shock in Denmark 1968–1990. A study based on notifications to the Committee on Adverse Drug Reactions. *J Clin Epidemiol* 1995; **48**: 1185–8.
4 Toogood JH. Risk of anaphylaxis in patients receiving beta-blocker drugs. *J Allergy Clin Immunol* 1988; **81**: 1–5.
5 Weiss ME, Adkinson NF. Immediate hypersensitivity reactions to penicillin and related antibiotics. *Clin Allergy* 1988; **18**: 515–40.
6 Ansell G, Tweedie MCK, West DR *et al.* The current status of reactions to intravenous contrast media. *Invest Radiol* 1980; **15** (Suppl. 6): S32–S39.
7 Greenberger P, Patterson R, Kelly J *et al.* Administration of radiographic contrast media in high-risk patients. *Invest Radiol* 1980; **15** (Suppl. 6): S40–S43.
8 Rönnau AC, Wulferink M, Gleichmann E *et al.* Anaphylaxis to polyvinylpyrrolidone in an analgesic preparation. *Br J Dermatol* 2000; **143**: 1055–8.

9 Antépara I, Martín-Gil D, Dominguez MA, Oehling A. Adverse drug reactions produced by analgesic drugs. *Allergol Immunopathol* 1981; **9**: 545–54.

10 Stevenson DD. Diagnosis, prevention and treatment of adverse reactions to aspirin (ASA) and nonsteroidal anti-inflammatory drugs (NSAID). *J Allergy Clin Immunol* 1984; **74**: 617–22.

11 Rossi AC, Knapp DE. Tolmetin-induced anaphylactoid reactions. *N Engl J Med* 1982; **307**: 499–500.

12 Michils A, Vandermoten G, Duchateau J, Yernault J-C. Anaphylaxis with sodium benzoate. *Lancet* 1991; **337**: 1424–5.

13 Twarog FJ, Leung DYM. Anaphylaxis to a component of isoetharine (sodium bisulfite). *JAMA* 1982; **248**: 2030–1.

14 Davis H, McGoodwin E, Reed TG. Anaphylactoid reactions reported after treatment with ciprofloxin. *Ann Intern Med* 1989; **111**: 1041–3.

15 Quiralte J, Sanchez-Garcia F, Torres MJ *et al.* Association of HLA-DR11 with the anaphylactoid reaction caused by nonsteroidal anti-inflammatory drugs. *J Allergy Clin Immunol* 1999; **103**: 685–9.

Urticaria

Urticaria (see Chapter 47) is, after an exanthematous eruption, the second most common type of ACDR [1] (Fig. 73.2). Drug-induced urticaria is seen in 0.16% of medical in-patients and accounts for 9% of chronic urticaria or angio-oedema seen in dermatology outpatient departments [1]. Occurring within 24–36 h of drug ingestion, it is most commonly caused by penicillins, sulphonamides and NSAIDs. Drug-induced urticaria is seen in association with anaphylaxis, angio-oedema and serum sickness. On rechallenge, lesions may develop within minutes. Angio-oedema, involving oedema of the deep dermis or subcutaneous and submucosal areas, is more rarely seen than urticaria as an ACDR, and occurs in less than 1% of patients receiving the particular drug.

The commoner drug causes of urticaria/angio-oedema are listed in Table 73.6. The frequency of urticaria/angio-oedema or anaphylactic responses to aspirin and other NSAIDs is about 1% in an outpatient population and is familial [2]. Aspirin (salicylates) may also aggravate chronic urticaria [3,4]. In addition, an unsuspected agent, for example the yellow dye tartrazine, may really be responsible for an urticaria attributed to aspirin or another

drug. The analgesic codeine is also a cause of urticaria [5]. Penicillin is a very well-documented cause of acute urticaria, but the role of this drug in chronic urticaria is controversial [6]. Urticaria develops in about 1% of patients receiving blood transfusions [7]. There have been numerous papers on the potential role of food and drug additives [8–16], including preservatives such as benzoic acid, butylated hydroxyanisole, butylated hydroxytoluene, sulphites and rarely aspartame, as well as tartrazine dyes, in the development of chronic urticaria. However, one study suggested that common food additives are seldom if ever of significance in urticaria [9]. Urticaria may follow alcohol consumption [17], intra-articular methylprednisolone [18] and even cetirizine [19].

Certain drugs, such as opiates, codeine, amfetamine, polymyxin B, *d*-tubocurarine, atropine, hydralazine, pentamidine, quinine and radiocontrast media, may release mast cell mediators directly. Cyclo-oxygenase inhibitors, such as aspirin and indometacin, and ACE inhibitors, such as captopril and enalapril, may cause urticaria or angio-oedema by pharmacological mechanisms. ACE inhibitors may cause increased frequency, intensity and duration of bouts of idiopathic angio-oedema during long-term use [20,21].

REFERENCES

1 Shipley D, Ormerod AD. Drug-induced urticaria. Recognition and treatment. *Am J Clin Dermatol* 2001; **2**: 151–8.

2 Settipane GA, Pudupakkam RK. Aspirin intolerance. III. Subtypes, familial occurrence and cross reactivity with tartrazine. *J Allergy Clin Immunol* 1975; **56**: 215–21.

3 Settipane RA, Constantine HP, Settipane GA. Aspirin intolerance and recurrent urticaria in normal adults and children. Epidemiology and review. *Allergy* 1980; **35**: 149–54.

4 Grattan CEH. Aspirin sensitivity and urticaria. *Clin Exp Dermatol* 2003; **28**: 123–7.

5 De Groot AC, Conemans J. Allergic urticarial rash from oral codeine. *Contact Dermatitis* 1986; **14**: 209–14.

6 Boonk WJ, Van Ketel WG. The role of penicillin in the pathogenesis of chronic urticaria. *Br J Dermatol* 1982; **106**: 183–90.

7 Shulman IA. Adverse reactions to blood transfusion. *Texas Med* 1990; **85**: 35–42.

8 Simon RA. Adverse reactions to drug additives. *J Allergy Clin Immunol* 1984; **74**: 623–30.

9 Hannuksela M, Lahti A. Peroral challenge tests with food additives in urticaria and atopic dermatitis. *Int J Dermatol* 1986; **25**: 178–80.

10 Supramaniam G, Warner JO. Artificial food additives intolerance in patients with angioedema and urticaria. *Lancet* 1986; **ii**: 907–9.

11 Juhlin L. Additives and chronic urticaria. *Ann Allergy* 1987; **59**: 119–23.

12 Goodman DL, McDonnell JT, Nelson HS *et al.* Chronic urticaria exacerbated by the antioxidant food preservatives, butylated hydroxyanisole (BHA) and butylated hydroxytoluene (BHT). *J Allergy Clin Immunol* 1990; **86**: 570–5.

13 Settipane GA. Adverse reactions to sulfites in drugs and foods. *J Am Acad Dermatol* 1984; **10**: 1077–80.

14 Kulczycki A Jr. Aspartame-induced urticaria. *Ann Intern Med* 1986; **104**: 207–8.

15 Neuman I, Elian R, Nahum H *et al.* The danger of 'yellow dyes' (tartrazine) to allergic subjects. *J Allergy* 1972; **50**: 92–8.

16 Miller K. Sensitivity to tartrazine. *BMJ* 1982; **285**: 1597–8.

17 Ormerod AD, Holt PJA. Acute urticaria due to alcohol. *Br J Dermatol* 1983; **108**: 723–4.

18 Pollock B, Wilkinson SM, MacDonald Hull SP. Chronic urticaria associated with intra-articular methylprednisolone. *Br J Dermatol* 2001; **144**: 1228–30.

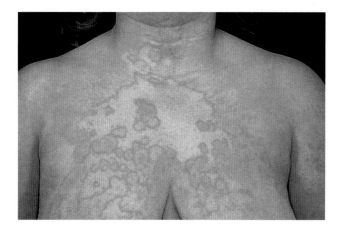

Fig. 73.2 Urticaria induced by acetylsalicylic acid. (Courtesy of St John's Institute of Dermatology, London, UK.)

19 Calista D, Schianchi S, Morri M. Urticaria induced by cetirizine. *Br J Dermatol* 2001; **144**: 196.

20 Chin HL. Severe angioedema after long-term use of an angiotensin-converting enzyme inhibitor. *Ann Intern Med* 1990; **112**: 312.

21 Kozel MMA, Mekkes JR, Bos JD. Increased frequency and severity of angio-oedema related to long-term therapy with angiotensin-converting enzyme inhibitor in two patients. *Clin Exp Dermatol* 1995; **20**: 60–1.

Serum sickness

Serum sickness, a type III immune complex-mediated reaction, may occur between 5 days and 3 weeks after initial exposure [1–5], and in its complete form combines fever, urticaria, angio-oedema, joint pain and swelling, lymphadenopathy, and occasionally nephritis or endocarditis, with eosinophilia. In minor forms of serum sickness, fever, urticaria and transitory joint tenderness may be the only manifestations.

Drugs implicated include heterologous serum [1,2], immune globulin (as treatment for Kawasaki disease) [6], aspirin, antibiotics [7,8] such as penicillin [3,7,9], amoxicillin [7], flucloxacillin [7], cefaclor [10–14], cefprozil [15], piperacillin [16], ciprofloxacin [17], cefatrizine [18], co-trimoxazole [7], troleandomycin (triacetyloleandomycin) [7], streptomycin, sulphonamides and sulfasalazine [19], thiouracils, intravenous streptokinase [20,21], *N*-acetylcysteine [22], staphylococcal protein A immunomodulation [23] and amfebutamone (bupropion) [24]. Of 32 women in an *in vitro* fertilization programme, 15% developed serum sickness 8–12 days after oocyte retrieval by echographic puncture, when a medium containing bovine serum was employed for rinsing follicles [25]. Patients had specific IgG antibodies against, and positive intradermal skin testing to, bovine serum albumin. A characteristic serpiginous, erythematous and purpuric eruption developed on the hands and feet at the borders of palmar and plantar skin in a series of patients treated with intravenous infusions of horse antithymocyte globulin for bone marrow failure [1,2]. Circulating immune complexes, low serum C4 and C3 levels, and elevated plasma C3a anaphylatoxin levels were found. Direct immunofluorescence revealed the presence of immunoreactants including IgM, C3, IgE and IgA in the walls of dermal blood vessels.

REFERENCES

1 Lawley TJ, Bielory L, Gascon P et al. A prospective clinical and immunologic analysis of patients with serum sickness. *N Engl J Med* 1984; **311**: 1407–13.

2 Bielory L, Yancey KB, Young NS et al. Cutaneous manifestations of serum sickness in patients receiving antithymocyte globulin. *J Am Acad Dermatol* 1985; **13**: 411–7.

3 Erffmeyer JE. Serum sickness. *Ann Allergy* 1986; **56**: 105–9.

4 Lin RY. Serum sickness syndrome. *Am Fam Physician* 1986; **33**: 157–62.

5 Virella G. Hypersensitivity reactions. *Immunol Ser* 1993; **58**: 329–41.

6 Comenzo RL, Malachowski ME, Meissner HC et al. Immune hemolysis, disseminated intravascular coagulation, and serum sickness after large doses of immune globulin given intravenously for Kawasaki disease. *J Pediatr* 1992; **120**: 926–8.

7 Martin J, Abbott G. Serum sickness-like illness and antimicrobials in children. *NZ Med J* 1995; **108**: 123–4.

8 Smith JM. Serum sickness-like reactions with antibiotics. *NZ Med J* 1995; **108**: 258.

9 Tatum AJ, Ditto AM, Patterson R. Severe serum sickness-like reaction to oral penicillin drugs: three case reports. *Ann Allergy Asthma Immunol* 2001; **86**: 330–4.

10 Vial T, Pont J, Pham E et al. Cefaclor-associated serum sickness-like disease: eight cases and review of the literature. *Ann Pharmacother* 1992; **26**: 910–4.

11 Parra FM, Igea JM, Martin JA et al. Serum sickness-like syndrome associated with cefaclor therapy. *Allergy* 1992; **47**: 439–40.

12 Kearns GL, Wheeler JG, Childress SH, Letzig LG. Serum sickness-like reactions to cefaclor: role of hepatic metabolism and individual susceptibility. *J Pediatr* 1994; **125**: 805–11.

13 Grammer LC. Cefaclor serum sickness. *JAMA* 1996; **275**: 1152–3.

14 Isaacs D. Serum sickness-like reaction to cefaclor. *J Paediatr Child Health* 2001; **37**: 298–9.

15 Lowery N, Kearns GL, Young RA, Wheeler JG. Serum sickness-like reactions associated with cefprozil therapy. *J Pediatr* 1994; **125**: 325–8.

16 Rye PJ, Roberts G, Staugas RE, Martin AJ. Coagulopathy with piperacillin administration in cystic fibrosis: two case reports. *J Paediatr Child Health* 1994; **30**: 278–9.

17 Guharoy SR. Serum sickness secondary to ciprofloxacin use. *Vet Hum Toxicol* 1994; **36**: 540–1.

18 Plantin P, Milochau P, Dubois D. Maladie serique medicamenteuse apres prise de cefatrizine. Premier cas reporté. *Presse Med* 1992; **21**: 1915.

19 Brooks H, Taylor HG, Nichol FE. The three week sulphasalazine syndrome. *Clin Rheumatol* 1992; **11**: 566–8.

20 Patel A, Prussick R, Buchanan WW, Sauder DN. Serum sickness-like illness and leukocytoclastic vasculitis after intravenous streptokinase. *J Am Acad Dermatol* 1991; **24**: 652–3.

21 Clesham GJ, Terry HJ, Jalihal S, Toghill PJ. Serum sickness and purpura following intravenous streptokinase. *J R Soc Med* 1992; **85**: 638–9.

22 Mohammed S, Jamal AZ, Robison LR. Serum sickness-like illness associated with N-acetylcysteine therapy. *Ann Pharmacother* 1994; **28**: 285.

23 Smith RE, Gottschall JL, Pisciotta AV. Life-threatening reaction to staphylococcal protein A immunomodulation. *J Clin Apheresis* 1992; **7**: 4–5.

24 Davis JS, Boyle MJ, Hannaford R, Watson A. Bupropion and serum sickness-like reaction. *Med J Aust* 2001; **174**: 479–80.

25 Morales C, Braso JV, Pellicer A et al. Serum sickness due to bovine serum albumin sensitization during in vitro fertilization. *J Invest Allergol Clin Immunol* 1994; **4**: 246–9.

Erythema multiforme, Stevens–Johnson syndrome and toxic epidermal necrolysis

See Chapter 74.

Drug hypersensitivity syndrome

The drug hypersensitivity syndrome [1–3], also known as *d*rug *r*ash with *e*osinophilia and *s*ystemic *s*ymptoms (DRESS) syndrome [4] or as *d*rug-*i*nduced *d*elayed *m*ulti-*o*rgan *h*ypersensitivity *s*yndrome (DIDMOHS) [2], has been reported with the anticonvulsants phenytoin, carbamazepine, phenobarbital and lamotrigine (see also anticonvulsant hypersensitivity syndrome, p. 73.45), and with trimethoprim–sulfamethoxazole, minocycline, procarbazine, allopurinol, terbinafine and dapsone. Superimposed viral infection may have a role in the aetiology [5] (see also mechanisms of drug reactions, cell-mediated immune reactions, p. 73.18). The syndrome comprises fever, facial oedema with infiltrated papules, generalized papulopustular or exanthematous rash which may extend to exfoliative dermatitis, lymphadenopathy, haematological abnormalities (hypereosinophilia in 90% of cases, atypical lymphocytes/mononucleosis in 40% of cases), and organ involvement such as hepatitis, possible nephritis, pneumonitis, myocarditis and hypothyroidism, occurring after 3–6 weeks of drug therapy. The cutaneous histological pattern shows a lymphocytic infiltrate, sometimes mimicking a cutaneous lymphoma. The mortality is of the order of 10%; the syndrome may proceed to Stevens–Johnson syndrome or TEN (see Chapter 74). Management is usually with oral corticosteroids. This syndrome should be distinguished from drug-induced pseudolymphoma syndrome, which has a more insidious beginning with nodules and infiltrated plaques appearing several weeks after starting the drug, without constitutional symptoms (see below).

REFERENCES

1 Sullivan JR, Shear NH. The drug hypersensitivity syndrome: what is the pathogenesis ? *Arch Dermatol* 2001; **137**: 357–64.
2 Sontheimer RD, Houpt KR. DIDMOHS: a proposed consensus nomenclature for the drug-induced delayed multiorgan hypersensitivity syndrome. *Arch Dermatol* 1998; **134**: 874–5.
3 Carroll MC, Yueng-Yue KA, Esterly NB, Drolet BA. Drug-induced hypersensitivity syndrome in pediatric patients. *Pediatrics* 2001; **108**: 485–92.
4 Bocquet H, Bagot M, Roujeau JC. Drug-induced pseudolymphoma and drug hypersensitivity syndrome (drug rash with eosinophilia and systemic symptoms: DRESS). *Semin Cutan Med Surg* 1996; **15**: 250–7.
5 Aihara Y, Ito S-I, Kobayashi Y *et al.* Carbamazepine-induced hypersensitivity syndrome associated with transient hypogammaglobulinaemia and reactivation of human herpesvirus 6 infection demonstrated by real-time quantitative polymerase chain reaction. *Br J Dermatol* 2003; **149**: 165–9.

Fixed eruptions [1–9]

A fixed drug eruption characteristically recurs in the same site or sites each time the drug is administered; with each exposure, however, the number of involved sites may increase. Usually, just one drug is involved, although independent lesions from more than one drug have been described [10]. Cross-sensitivity to related drugs may occur, such as between phenylbutazone and oxyphenbutazone, between tetracycline-type drugs, and between anticonvulsants [11]. There may be a refractory period after the occurrence of a fixed eruption.

Acute lesions usually develop 30 min to 8 h after drug administration as sharply marginated, round or oval itchy plaques of erythema and oedema becoming dusky violaceous or brown, and sometimes vesicular or bullous (Fig. 73.3). The eruption may initially be morbilliform, scarlatiniform or erythema multiforme-like; urticarial, nodular or eczematous lesions are less common. Lesions are sometimes solitary at first, but with repeated attacks new lesions usually appear and existing lesions may increase in size. A multifocal bullous fixed drug eruption due to mefenamic acid resembled erythema multiforme [12]. Occasionally, involvement is so extensive as to mimic TEN [13,14].

Lesions are commoner on the limbs than on the trunk; the hands and feet, genitalia and perianal areas are

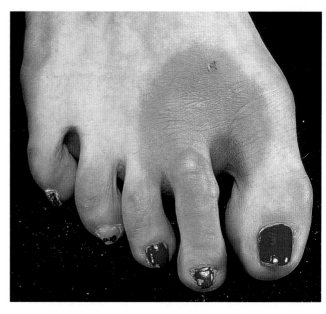

Fig. 73.3 Bullous fixed drug eruption with hyperpigmentation. (Courtesy of St John's Institute of Dermatology, London, UK.)

favoured sites. Perioral and periorbital lesions may occur. Genital [15] and oral mucous membranes [16] may be involved in association with skin lesions, or alone. In the case of isolated male genital fixed drug eruption (often affecting only the glans penis), the drugs most commonly implicated in one series were co-trimoxazole (trimethoprim–sulfamethoxazole), tetracycline and ampicillin [15]. With oral fixed drug eruption, co-trimoxazole, oxyphenbutazone and tetracycline were the most common causative drugs [16]. Pigmentation of the tongue may occur as a form of fixed drug eruption in heroin addicts [17]. As healing occurs, crusting and scaling are followed by pigmentation, which may be very persistent and occasionally extensive, especially in pigmented individuals; pigmentation may be all that is visible between attacks. Non-pigmenting fixed reactions have been reported in association with the sympathomimetic agents pseudoephedrine [18,19] and tetryzoline (tetrahydrozoline) hydrochloride, diflunisal, thiopental (thiopentone), piroxicam, the radiopaque contrast medium iothalamate, arsphenamine [20], paracetamol [21], intra-articular triamcinolone acetonide [22] and eperisone hydrochloride [23].

The number of drugs capable of producing fixed drug eruption is very large. However, most fixed drug eruptions are due to one or other of the substances listed in Table 73.7. Earlier series incriminated particularly analgesics, sulphonamides and tetracyclines. In a report from Finland, phenazones caused most eruptions, with barbiturates, sulphonamides, tetracyclines and carbamazepine causing fewer reactions [24]. A series from India reported that acetylsalicylic acid was the drug most commonly

Table 73.7 Drugs causing fixed eruptions.

Antibacterial substances	*Non-steroidal anti-inflammatory drugs*
Sulphonamides (co-trimoxazole)	Aspirin (acetylsalicylic acid)
Tetracyclines	Oxyphenbutazone
Penicillin	Phenazone (antipyrine)
Ampicillin	Metamizole
Amoxicillin	Paracetamol (acetaminophen)
Erythromycin	Ibuprofen
Trimethoprim	Various non-proprietary analgesic combinations
Nystatin	
Griseofulvin	*Phenolphthalein and related compounds*
Dapsone	
Arsenicals	*Miscellaneous*
Mercury salts	Codeine
p-Aminosalicylic acid	Hydralazine
Thioacetazone (thiacetazone)	Oleoresins
Quinine	Sympathomimetics
Metronidazole	Sympatholytics
Clioquinol	Parasympatholytics: hyoscine butylbromide
	Magnesium hydroxide
Barbiturates and other tranquillizers	Magnesium trisilicate
Barbiturate derivatives	Anthralin
Opium alkaloids	Chlorthiazone
Chloral hydrate	Chlorphenesin carbamate
Benzodiazepines: chlordiazepoxide	Food substitutes and flavours
Anticonvulsants	
Dextromethorphan	

implicated in children [25]; a more recent study found that co-trimoxazole was the usual culprit in children [26]. Co-trimoxazole has been implicated as the most frequent cause in many studies [6,8,27]. A fixed drug eruption apparently caused by co-trimoxazole was reported in a man following intercourse with his wife, who was taking the drug [28]. Trimethoprim has caused a linear fixed drug eruption [29]. A report in 1991 showed that co-trimoxazole caused the maximum incidence (36.3%), followed by tetracycline (15.9%), pyrazolones (14.2%), sulfadiazine (12.4%), dipyrine (9.3%), paracetamol (7.9%), aspirin (1.7%), thioacetazone (0.88%) and levamisole (0.88%) [27]. Co-trimoxazole was also the most common cause of fixed drug eruption (75%), followed by naproxen sodium (12.5%), dipyrone (9.5%), dimenhydrinate (1.5%) and paracetamol (1.5%) in a study in 2000 [8]. However, a survey of current causes of fixed drug eruption in the UK listed NSAIDs including aspirin, paracetamol, antibacterial agents, systemic antifungal agents, psychotropic drugs, proton pump inhibitors, calcium channel blockers, ACE inhibitors and hormonal preparations [9], reflecting the decreased use of co-trimoxazole.

A drug-specific clinical pattern in fixed drug eruptions based on a study of 113 patients has been reported [8,27]. Sulphonamides, including co-trimoxazole, induced lesions on the lips, trunk and limbs, with only minimal involvement of mucosae. Naproxen predominantly affected the lips and face. Tetracycline and co-trimoxazole caused lesions mainly on the glans penis. Pyrazolones affected mainly the lips and mucosae, with a few lesions of the

trunk and limbs. Dipyrine, aspirin and paracetamol caused lesions of the trunk and limbs, sparing the lips, genitalia and mucosae. Levamisole caused associated constitutional disturbances with extensive skin lesions, as did thioacetazone [27]. Paracetamol is a rare cause of fixed drug eruption [30–33]; other drugs implicated have included codeine [34], naproxen [35], rofecoxib [36], ciprofloxacin [37], clarithromycin [38], rifampicin [39], metronidazole [40], terbinafine [41], fluconazole [42], lamotrigine [43], dimenhydrinate [44], cetirizine [45], loratadine [46], ticlopidine [47], phenylpropanolamine hydrochloride [48], and lactulose in an injected botulinum toxin preparation [49]. Familial fixed drug eruption has occurred occasionally [50,51].

REFERENCES

1 Korkij W, Soltani K. Fixed drug eruption. A brief review. *Arch Dermatol* 1984; **120**: 520–4.
2 Kauppinen K, Stubb S. Fixed eruptions: causative drugs and challenge tests. *Br J Dermatol* 1985; **112**: 575–8.
3 Sehgal VN, Gangwani OP. Fixed drug eruption. Current concepts. *Int J Dermatol* 1987; **26**: 67–74.
4 Kanwar AJ, Bharija SC, Singh M, Belhaj MS. Ninety-eight fixed drug eruptions with provocation tests. *Dermatologica* 1988; **177**: 274–9.
5 Sehgal VN, Gangwani OP. Fixed drug eruptions. A study of epidemiological, clinical and diagnostic aspects of 89 cases from India. *J Dermatol* 1988; **15**: 50–4.
6 Mahboob A, Haroon TS. Drugs causing fixed eruptions: a study of 450 cases. *Int J Dermatol* 1998; **37**: 833–8.
7 Lee A-Y. Topical provocation in 31 cases of fixed drug eruption: change of causative drugs in 10 years. *Contact Dermatitis* 1998; **38**: 258–60.
8 Özkaya-Bayazit E, Bayazit H, Ozarmagan G. Drug related clinical pattern in fixed drug eruption. *Eur J Dermatol* 2000; **10**: 288–91.

9 Savin JA. Current causes of fixed drug eruption in the UK. *Br J Dermatol* 2001; **145**: 667–8.

10 Kivity S. Fixed drug eruption to multiple drugs: clinical and laboratory investigation. *Int J Dermatol* 1991; **30**: 149–51.

11 Chan HL, Tan KC. Fixed drug eruption to three anticonvulsant drugs: an unusual case of polysensitivity. *J Am Acad Dermatol* 1997; **36**: 259.

12 Sowden JM, Smith AG. Multifocal fixed drug eruption mimicking erythema multiforme. *Clin Exp Dermatol* 1990; **15**: 387–8.

13 Saiag P, Cordoliani F, Roujeau JC et al. Érytheme pigmenté fixe bulleux disséminé simulant un syndrome de Lyell. *Ann Dermatol Vénéréol* 1987; **114**: 1440–2.

14 Baird BJ, De Villez RL. Widespread bullous fixed drug eruption mimicking toxic epidermal necrolysis. *Int J Dermatol* 1988; **27**: 170–4.

15 Gaffoor PMA, George WM. Fixed drug eruptions occurring on the male genitals. *Cutis* 1990; **45**: 242–4.

16 Jain VK, Dixit VB, Archana. Fixed drug eruption of the oral mucous membrane. *Ann Dent* 1991; **50**: 9–11.

17 Westerhof W, Wolters EC, Brookbakker JTW et al. Pigmented lesions of the tongue in heroin addicts: fixed drug eruption. *Br J Dermatol* 1983; **109**: 605–10.

18 Vidal C, Prieto A, Perez-Carral C, Armisen M. Nonpigmenting fixed drug eruption due to pseudoephedrine. *Ann Allergy Asthma Immunol* 1998; **80**: 309–10.

19 Hindioglu U, Sahin S. Nonpigmenting solitary fixed drug eruption caused by pseudoephedrine hydrochloride. *J Am Acad Dermatol* 1998; **38**: 499–500.

20 Krivda SJ, Benson PM. Nonpigmenting fixed drug eruption. *J Am Acad Dermatol* 1994; **31**: 291–2.

21 Galindo PA, Borja J, Feo F et al. Nonpigmented fixed drug eruption caused by paracetamol. *J Invest Allergol Clin Immunol* 1999; **9**: 399–400.

22 Sener O, Caliskaner Z, Yazicioglu K et al. Nonpigmenting solitary fixed drug eruption after skin testing and intra-articular injection of triamcinolone acetonide. *Ann Allergy Asthma Immunol* 2001; **86**: 335–6.

23 Choonhakarn C. Non-pigmenting fixed drug eruption: a new case due to eperisone hydrochloride. *Br J Dermatol* 2001; **144**: 1288–9.

24 Stubb S, Alanko K, Reitamo S. Fixed drug eruptions: 77 cases from 1981 to 1985. *Br J Dermatol* 1989; **120**: 583.

25 Kanwar AJ, Bharija SC, Belhaj MS. Fixed drug eruptions in children: a series of 23 cases with provocative tests. *Dermatologica* 1986; **172**: 315–8.

26 Morelli JG, Tay YK, Rogers M et al. Fixed drug eruptions in children. *J Pediatr* 1999; **134**: 365–7.

27 Thankappan TP, Zachariah J. Drug-specific clinical pattern in fixed drug eruptions. *Int J Dermatol* 1991; **30**: 867–70.

28 Gruber F, Stasic A, Lenkovic M, Brajac I. Postcoital fixed drug eruption in a man sensitive to trimethoprim–sulphamethoxazole. *Clin Exp Dermatol* 1997; **22**: 144–5.

29 Özkaya-Bayazit E, Baykal C. Trimethoprim-induced linear fixed drug eruption. *Br J Dermatol* 1997; **137**: 1028–9.

30 Zemtsov A, Yanase DJ, Boyd AS, Shehata B. Fixed drug eruption to Tylenol: report of two cases and review of the literature. *Cutis* 1992; **50**: 281–2.

31 Hern S, Harman K, Clement M, Black MM. Bullous fixed drug eruption due to paracetamol with an unusual immunofluorescence pattern. *Br J Dermatol* 1998; **139**: 1129–31.

32 Silva A, Proenca E, Carvalho C et al. Fixed drug eruption induced by paracetamol. *Pediatr Dermatol* 2001; **18**: 163–4.

33 Hayashi H, Shimizu T, Shimizu H. Multiple fixed drug eruption caused by acetaminophen. *Clin Exp Dermatol* 2003; **28**: 455–6.

34 Gonzalo-Garijo MA, Revenga-Arranz F. Fixed drug eruption due to codeine. *Br J Dermatol* 1996; **135**: 498–9.

35 Gonzalo MA, Alvarado MI, Fernandez L et al. Fixed drug eruption due to naproxen: lack of cross-reactivity with other propionic acid derivatives. *Br J Dermatol* 2001; **144**: 1291–2.

36 Kaur C, Sarkar R, Kanwar AJ. Fixed drug eruption to rofecoxib with cross-reactivity to sulfonamides. *Dermatology* 2001; **203**: 351.

37 Dhar S, Sharma VK. Fixed drug eruption due to ciprofloxacin. *Br J Dermatol* 1996; **134**: 56–8.

38 Hamamoto Y, Ohmura A, Kinoshita E, Muto M. Fixed drug eruption due to clarithromycin. *Clin Exp Dermatol* 2001; **26**: 48–9.

39 Goel A, Balachandran C. Bullous necrotizing fixed drug eruption with hepatitis due to rifampicin. *Ind J Leprosy* 2001; **73**: 159–62.

40 Vila JB, Bernier MA, Gutierrez JV et al. Fixed drug eruption caused by metronidazole. *Contact Dermatitis* 2002; **46**: 122.

41 Munn SE, Russell Jones R. Terbinafine and fixed drug eruption. *Br J Dermatol* 1995; **133**: 815–6.

42 Ghislain PD, Ghislain E. Fixed drug eruption due to fluconazole: a third case. *J Am Acad Dermatol* 2002; **46**: 467.

43 Hsiao CJ, Lee JY, Wong TW, Sheu HM. Extensive fixed drug eruption due to lamotrigine. *Br J Dermatol* 2001; **144**: 1289–91.

44 Smola H, Kruppa A, Hunzelmann N et al. Identification of dimenhydrinate as the causative agent in fixed drug eruption using patch-testing in previously affected skin. *Br J Dermatol* 1998; **138**: 920–1.

45 Kranke B, Kern T. Multilocalized fixed drug eruption to the antihistamine cetirizine. *J Allergy Clin Immunol* 2000; **106**: 988.

46 Ruiz-Genao DP, Hernandez-Nunez A, Sanchez-Perez J, Garcia-Diez A. Fixed drug eruption due to loratadine. *Br J Dermatol* 2002; **146**: 528–9.

47 Garcia CM, Carmena R, Garcia R et al. Fixed drug eruption from ticlopidine, with positive lesional patch test. *Contact Dermatitis* 2001; **44**: 40–1.

48 Heikkilä H, Kariniemi A-L, Stubb S. Fixed drug eruption due to phenylpropanolamine hydrochloride. *Br J Dermatol* 2000; **142**: 845–7.

49 Cox NH, Duffey P, Royle J. Fixed drug eruption caused by lactulose in an injected botulinum toxin preparation. *J Am Acad Dermatol* 1999; **40**: 263–4.

50 Pellicano R, Silvestris A, Iannantuono M et al. Familial occurrence of fixed drug eruptions. *Acta Derm Venereol (Stockh)* 1992; **72**: 292–3.

51 Hatzis J, Noutsis K, Hatzidakis E et al. Fixed drug eruption in a mother and her son. *Cutis* 1992; **50**: 50–2.

Lichenoid eruptions

Lichenoid drug eruptions and lichen planus are discussed in Chapter 42. Some of the drugs that induce this pattern of reaction are listed in Table 73.8 [2]. Photodistributed lichenoid lesions may occur with a number of drugs, including thiazide diuretics (Fig. 73.4).

Photosensitivity

Drug–light reactions, which cause eruptions on exposed areas, with sparing of upper eyelids, submental and retroauricular areas, may be phototoxic or photoallergic; these cannot always be distinguished clinically, and some drugs may produce cutaneous involvement by both mechanisms [1–5]. The main drugs implicated in photosensitivity reactions are listed in Table 73.9.

REFERENCES

1 Johnson BE, Ferguson J. Drug and chemical photosensitivity. *Semin Dermatol* 1990; **9**: 39–46.

2 Elmets CA. Cutaneous phototoxicity. In: Lim HW, Soter NA, eds. *Clinical Photomedicine*. New York: Marcel Dekker, 1993: 207–26.

3 Deleo VA. Photoallergy. In: Lim HW, Soter NA, eds. *Clinical Photomedicine*. New York: Marcel Dekker, 1993: 227–39.

4 Gould JW, Mercurio MG, Elmets CA. Cutaneous photosensitivity diseases induced by exogenous agents. *J Am Acad Dermatol* 1995; **33**: 551–73.

5 González E, González S. Drug photosensitivity, idiopathic photodermatoses, and sunscreens. *J Am Acad Dermatol* 1996; **35**: 871–5.

Phototoxic reactions

Phototoxic reactions are commoner than photoallergic reactions, and can be produced in almost all individuals given a high enough dose of drug and sufficient light irradiation. They occur within 5–20 h of the first exposure, and resemble exaggerated sunburn. Erythema, oedema, blistering, weeping, desquamation and residual hyperpig-

Table 73.8 Drugs causing lichenoid eruptions.

Gold salts	Antitubercular drugs
Antimalarials	Ethambutol
Mepacrine (quinacrine, atabrine)	Isoniazid
Chloroquine	p-Aminosalicylic acid
Quinine	Streptomycin
Quinidine	Cycloserine
Pyrimethamine	Antifungal drugs: ketoconazole
Penicillamine	Chemotherapeutic agents
Diuretics	Hydroxyurea
Thiazides	5-Fluorouracil
Furosemide (frusemide)	Heavy metals
Spironolactone	Mercurials
Diazoxide	Arsenicals
Antihypertensive agents	Bismuth
β-Blockers	Miscellaneous
Angiotensin-converting enzyme inhibitors:	Tetracyclines
captopril, enalapril	Carbamazepine
Methyldopa	Phenytoin
Calcium channel blockers	Procainamide
Nifedipine	Allopurinol
Phenothiazine derivatives	Iodides and radiocontrast media
Metopromazine	Tiopronin
Levomepromazine	Pyritinol
Chlorpromazine	Cyanamide
Sulphonylurea hypoglycaemic agents	Dapsone
Chlorpropamide	Amiphenazole
Tolazamide	Levamisole
Non-steroidal anti-inflammatory drugs: phenylbutazone	Nandrolone furylpropionate
Sulfasalazine (sulphasalazine) and mesalazine	Cinnarizine
	Flunarizine

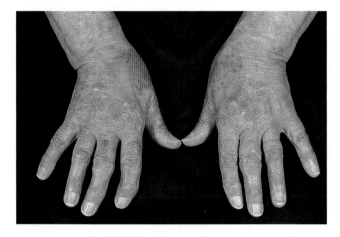

Fig. 73.4 Lichenoid photosensitivity eruption caused by thiazide diuretic. (Courtesy of A. Ive, Durham, UK.)

mentation occur on exposed areas; there may be photo-onycholysis. The following are well-recognized causes of phototoxicity:

• tetracyclines [1–4], especially demeclocycline, less frequently doxycycline, oxytetracycline and tetracycline, and rarely minocycline and methacycline;
• other antibacterials including sulphonamides and fluoroquinolones [4];
• phenothiazines, especially chlorpromazine, promethazine and less commonly thioridazine;
• furosemide [5] and nalidixic acid [4,6], both of which produce a pseudoporphyria syndrome, with blistering of the exposed areas;
• NSAIDs, including ibuprofen [7], piroxicam [8–11], carprofen and tiaprofenic acid [12];
• psoralens;
• amiodarone (which causes photosensitivity in over 50% of cases) [13];
• certain anticancer drugs [14], including dacarbazine [14,15], 5-fluorouracil, mitomycin and vinblastine;
• coal tar and its derivatives;
• fibric acid derivatives, including bezafibrate and fenofibrate [16,17];
• the non-steroid antiandrogen flutamide given for prostatic carcinoma [18,19].

REFERENCES

1 Cullen SI, Catalano PM, Helfmann RS. Tetracycline sun sensitivity. *Arch Dermatol* 1966; **93**: 77.
2 Frost P, Weinstein GP, Gomez EC. Phototoxic potential of minocycline and doxycycline. *Arch Dermatol* 1972; **105**: 681–3.
3 Layton AM, Cunliffe WJ. Phototoxic eruptions due to doxycycline: a dose-related phenomenon. *Clin Exp Dermatol* 1993; **18**: 425–7.
4 Wainwright NJ, Collins P, Ferguson J. Photosensitivity associated with antibacterial agents. *Drug Saf* 1993; **9**: 437–40.

Frequent	*Less frequent: systemic*	

Frequent	*Less frequent: systemic*
Amiodarone	Ampicillin
Phenothiazines	Antidepressants (tricyclic)
Chlorpromazine	Imipramine
Promethazine	Protriptyline
Psoralens	Antidepressants (monoamine oxidase
Sulphonamides: co-trimoxazole	inhibitors): phenelzine
Tetracyclines: demeclocycline	Antifungal agents
Thiazides	Griseofulvin
Non-steroidal anti-inflammatory drugs	Ketoconazole
Azapropazone	β-Blockers
Piroxicam	Carbamazepine
Carprofen	Cimetidine
Tiaprofenic acid	Cytotoxic agents
Benoxaprofen (withdrawn)	Dacarbazine
Nalidixic acid	Fluorouracil
Coal tar	Mitomycin
	Vinblastine
Less frequent: topical	Diazepam
Antihistamines	Furosemide (frusemide)
Local anaesthetics	Methyldopa
Benzydamine	Oral contraceptives
Hydrocortisone	Quinine
Sunscreens	Quinidine
p-Aminobenzoic acid	Sulphonylureas
Benzophenone	Chlorpropamide
Halogenated salicylanilides	Tolbutamide
	Retinoids
	Isotretinoin
	Etretinate
	Triamterene

Table 73.9 Drugs causing photosensitivity.

5 Burry JN, Lawrence JR. Phototoxic blisters from high frusemide dosage. *Br J Dermatol* 1976; **94**: 495–9.

6 Ramsay CA, Obreshkova E. Photosensitivity from nalidixic acid. *Br J Dermatol* 1974; **91**: 523–8.

7 Bergner T, Przybilla B. Photosensitisation caused by ibuprofen. *J Am Acad Dermatol* 1992; **26**: 114–6.

8 Stern RS. Phototoxic reactions to piroxicam and other nonsteroidal anti-inflammatory agents. *N Engl J Med* 1983; **309**: 186–7.

9 Serrano G, Bonillo J, Aliaga A *et al.* Piroxicam-induced photosensitivity. *In vivo* and *in vitro* studies of its photosensitizing potential. *J Am Acad Dermatol* 1984; **11**: 113–20.

10 Figueiredo A, Fontes Ribeiro CA, Conçalo S *et al.* Piroxicam-induced photosensitivity. *Contact Dermatitis* 1987; **17**: 73–9.

11 Serrano G, Fortea JM, Latasa JM. Oxicam-induced photosensitivity. Patch and photopatch testing studies with tenoxicam and piroxicam photoproducts in normal subjects and in piroxicam–droxicam photosensitive patients. *J Am Acad Dermatol* 1992; **26**: 545–8.

12 Przybilla B, Ring J, Galosi A, Dorn M. Photopatch test reactions to tiaprofenic acid. *Contact Dermatitis* 1984; **1**: 55–6.

13 Ferguson J, Addo HA, Jones S *et al.* A study of cutaneous photosensitivity induced by amiodarone. *Br J Dermatol* 1985; **113**: 537–49.

14 Kerker BJ, Hood AF. Chemotherapy-induced cutaneous reactions. *Semin Dermatol* 1989; **8**: 173–81.

15 Bonifazi E, Angelini G, Meneghini CL. Adverse photoreaction to dacarbazine (DITC). *Contact Dermatitis* 1981; **7**: 161.

16 Leenutaphong V, Manuskiatti W. Fenofibrate-induced photosensitivity. *J Am Acad Dermatol* 1996; **35**: 775–7.

17 Serrano G, Fortea JM, Latasa JM *et al.* Photosensitivity induced by fibric acid derivatives and its relation to photocontact dermatitis to ketoprofen. *J Am Acad Dermatol* 1992; **27**: 204–8.

18 Fujimoto M, Kikuchi K, Imakado S, Furue M. Photosensitive dermatitis induced by flutamide. *Br J Dermatol* 1996; **135**: 496–7.

19 Kaur C, Thami GP. Flutamide-induced photosensitivity: is it a forme fruste of lupus? *Br J Dermatol* 2003; **148**: 603–4.

Photoallergic reactions

Photoallergic reactions require a latent period during which sensitization occurs, and usually appear within 24 h of re-exposure to drug and light in a sensitized individual; unlike phototoxic reactions, they may spread beyond irradiated areas. Most systemic drugs causing photoallergy also cause phototoxicity. There may be cross-reactivity with chemically related substances.

Photoallergic reactions may occur as a result of local photocontact dermatitis to a topical photoallergen. Photocontact dermatitis is a relatively common cause of photosensitivity, accounting for 9% of cases in a multicentre study [1]. Topical photoallergens include antihistamines, chlorpromazine, local anaesthetics, benzydamine, hydrocortisone, desoximetasone (desoxymethasone) and sunscreens containing *p*-aminobenzoic acid (PABA) and its derivatives. Contact allergy and photoallergy to benzophenones in PABA-free sunscreens may be commoner than is realized [2]. Halogenated salicylanilides, previously used as a disinfectant in soaps, and related compounds also cause photocontact dermatitis.

Photoallergic reactions may also occur as a result of systemically administered drugs [3], such as phenothiazines (chlorpromazine, promethazine), sulphonamides, aromatic sulphonamides such as thiazide diuretics

[4,5] and oral hypoglycaemic agents (chlorpropamide and tolbutamide), griseofulvin [6] and quinidine [7,8]. Quinidine-induced photo-eruptions may be either eczematous or lichenoid; a persistent livedo reticularis-like eruption may be seen in severe cases of quinidine photosensitivity. Enalapril has caused a photosensitive lichenoid eruption [9]. Tricyclic antidepressants may cause allergy as well as photosensitivity [10]. NSAIDs, disinfectants, sunscreens, phenothiazines and fragrances caused photoallergic reactions most often in a 5-year survey by the German, Austrian and Swiss photopatch test group [11].

REFERENCES

1 Wennersten G, Thune P, Brodthagen H *et al*. The Scandinavian multi-center photopatch study. Preliminary results. *Contact Dermatitis* 1984; **10**: 305–9.
2 Knobler E, Almeida L, Ruxkowski AM *et al*. Photoallergy to benzophenone. *Arch Dermatol* 1989; **125**: 801–4.
3 Giudici PA, Maguire HC. Experimental photoallergy to systemic drugs. *J Invest Dermatol* 1985; **85**: 207–11.
4 Robinson HN, Morison WL, Hood AF. Thiazide diuretic therapy and chronic photosensitivity. *Arch Dermatol* 1985; **121**: 522–4.
5 Addo HA, Ferguson J, Frain-Bell W. Thiazide-induced photosensitivity: a study of 33 subjects. *Br J Dermatol* 1987; **116**: 749–60.
6 Kojima T, Hasegawa T, Ishida H *et al*. Griseofulvin-induced photodermatitis. Report of six cases. *J Dermatol* 1988; **15**: 76–82.
7 Bruce S, Wolf JE Jr. Quinidine-induced photosensitive livedo reticularis-like eruption. *J Am Acad Dermatol* 1985; **12**: 332–6.
8 Schurer NY, Holzle E, Plewig G, Lehmann P. Photosensitivity induced by quinidine sulfate: experimental reproduction of skin lesions. *Photodermatol Photoimmunol Photomed* 1992; **9**: 78–82.
9 Kanwar AJ, Dhar S, Ghosh S. Photosensitive lichenoid eruption due to enalapril. *Dermatology* 1993; **187**: 80.
10 Ljunggren B, Bojs G. A case of photosensitivity and contact allergy to systemic tricyclic drugs, with unusual features. *Contact Dermatitis* 1991; **24**: 259–65.
11 Hölzle E, Neumann N, Hausen B *et al*. Photopatch testing: the 5-year experience of the German, Austrian and Swiss photopatch test group. *J Am Acad Dermatol* 1991; **25**: 59–68.

Porphyria and pseudoporphyria

A number of drugs may precipitate porphyria cutanea tarda with resultant photosensitivity, or cause a pseudoporphyria syndrome with bulla formation. The reader is referred to Chapter 57.

Photorecall reactions

A curious photorecall-like eruption, restricted to an area of sunburn sustained 1 month previously, occurred in a patient treated with cefazolin (cephazolin) and gentamicin [1]. An ultraviolet recall-like eruption has been reported with piperacillin, tobramycin and ciprofloxacin [2]. A recurrent cutaneous reaction localized to the site of pelvic radiotherapy for adenocarcinoma of the prostate followed sun exposure in one patient [3]. Methotrexate is associated with severe reactivation of sunburn [4,5].

REFERENCES

1 Flax SH, Uhle P. Photo recall-like phenomenon following the use of cefazolin and gentamicin sulfate. *Cutis* 1990; **46**: 59–61.
2 Krishnan RS, Lewis AT, Kass JS, Hsu S. Ultraviolet recall-like phenomenon occurring after piperacillin, tobramycin, and ciprofloxacin therapy. *J Am Acad Dermatol* 2001; **44**: 1045–7.
3 Del Guidice SM, Gerstley JK. Sunlight-induced radiation recall. *Int J Dermatol* 1988; **27**: 415–6.
4 Mallory SB, Berry DH. Severe reactivation of sunburn following methotrexate use. *Pediatrics* 1986; **78**: 514–5.
5 Westwick TJ, Sherertz EF, McCarley D, Flowers FP. Delayed reactivation of sunburn by methotrexate: sparing of chronically sun-exposed skin. *Cutis* 1987; **39**: 49–51.

Photo-onycholysis

Photo-onycholysis may be caused by tetracycline, psoralens and UVA (PUVA) therapy, and the fluoroquinolone antibiotics pefloxacin and ofloxacin.

Pigmentation reactions

Hyperpigmentation (Table 73.10)

Drug-induced alteration in skin colour [1–3] may result from increased (or more rarely decreased) melanin synthesis, increased lipofuscin synthesis, cutaneous deposition of drug-related material, or most commonly as a result of post-inflammatory hyperpigmentation (e.g. fixed drug eruption). Oral contraceptives may induce chloasma [4]. Other drugs implicated in cutaneous hyperpigmentation include minocycline [5,6], antimalarials [7,8], chlorpromazine [9,10], imipramine (photodistributed) [11–13] and desimipramine [14], amiodarone [15], carotene and heavy metals. Long-term (more than 4 months) antimalarial therapy may result in brownish or blue-black pigmentation, especially on the shin, face and hard palate or subungually. Yellowish discoloration may occur with mepacrine (quinacrine) or amodiaquine. Long-term high-dose phenothiazine (especially chlorpromazine) therapy results in a blue-grey or brownish pigmentation of sun-exposed areas, the result of a phototoxic reaction, with

Table 73.10 Drugs causing pigmentation.

Oral contraceptives	Chemotherapeutic agents
Minocycline	Miscellaneous
Antimalarials	Amiodarone
Chloroquine	Carotene
Hydroxychloroquine	Clofazimine
Mepacrine	Pefloxacin
Antidepressants	Sulfasalazine (sulphasalazine)
Chlorpromazine	
Imipramine	
Heavy metals	
Gold	
Lead	
Silver	

pigment deposits in the lens and cornea [10]. The cancer chemotherapeutic agents may be associated with pigmentation as follows [16]. Skin pigmentation may be caused by bleomycin, busulfan, topical carmustine, cyclophosphamide, daunorubicin, fluorouracil, hydroxyurea, topical mechlorethamine, methotrexate, mithramycin, mitomycin and thiotepa. Busulfan and doxorubicin cause mucous membrane pigmentation. Nail pigmentation may result from bleomycin, cyclophosphamide, daunorubicin, doxorubicin and fluorouracil. Methotrexate may induce pigmentation of the hair, and cyclophosphamide of teeth. Sulfasalazine has caused reversible hyperpigmentation [17], and pefloxacin blue-black pigmentation of the legs [18].

Gold may cause blue-grey pigmentation in light-exposed areas (*chrysiasis*) [19,20] and silver may cause a similar discoloration (*argyria*) [21]. Lead poisoning can cause a blue-black line at the gingival margin and grey discoloration of the skin. Clofazimine produces red-brown discoloration of exposed skin and the conjunctivae, together with red sweat, urine and faeces [22]. Slate-grey to blue-black pigmentation may occur after long-term topical application of hydroquinone, causing ochronosis [23].

REFERENCES

1 Levantine A, Almeyda J. Drug reactions: XXII. Drug induced changes in pigmentation. *Br J Dermatol* 1973; **89**: 105–12.
2 Granstein RD, Sober AJ. Drug- and heavy metal-induced hyperpigmentation. *J Am Acad Dermatol* 1981; **5**: 1–18.
3 Ferguson J, Frain-Bell W. Pigmentary disorders and systemic drug therapy. *Clin Dermatol* 1989; **7**: 44–54.
4 Smith AG, Shuster S, Thody AJ et al. Chloasma, oral contraceptives, and plasma immunoreactive beta-melanocyte-stimulating hormone. *J Invest Dermatol* 1977; **68**: 169–70.
5 Dwyer CM, Cuddihy AM, Kerr RE et al. Skin pigmentation due to minocycline treatment of facial dermatoses. *Br J Dermatol* 1993; **129**: 158–62.
6 Pepine M, Flowers FP, Ramos-Caro FA. Extensive cutaneous hyperpigmentation caused by minocycline. *J Am Acad Dermatol* 1993; **28**: 292–5.
7 Tuffanelli D, Abraham RK, Dubois EJ. Pigmentation from antimalarial therapy. Its possible relationship to the ocular lesions. *Arch Dermatol* 1963; **88**: 419–26.
8 Leigh IM, Kennedy CTC, Ramsey JD, Henderson WJ. Mepacrine pigmentation in systemic lupus erythematosus. New data from an ultrastructural, biochemical and analytical electron microscope investigation. *Br J Dermatol* 1979; **101**: 147–53.
9 Benning TL, McCormack KM, Ingram P et al. Microprobe analysis of chlorpromazine pigmentation. *Arch Dermatol* 1988; **124**: 1541–4.
10 Wolf ME, Richer S, Berk MA, Mosnaim AD. Cutaneous and ocular changes associated with the use of chlorpromazine. *Int J Clin Pharmacol Ther Toxicol* 1993; **31**: 365–7.
11 Hashimoto K, Joselow SA, Tye MJ. Imipramine hyperpigmentation: a slate-gray discoloration caused by long-term imipramine administration. *J Am Acad Dermatol* 1991; **25**: 357–61.
12 Ming ME, Bhawan J, Stefanato CM et al. Imipramine-induced hyperpigmentation: four cases and a review of the literature. *J Am Acad Dermatol* 1999; **40**: 159–66.
13 Sicari MC, Lebwohl M, Baral J et al. Photoinduced dermal pigmentation in patients taking tricyclic antidepressants: histology, electron microscopy, and energy dispersive spectroscopy. *J Am Acad Dermatol* 1999; **40**: 290–3.
14 Steele TE, Ashby J. Desipramine-related slate-gray skin pigmentation. *J Clin Psychopharmacol* 1993; **13**: 76–7.
15 Zachary CB, Slater DN, Holt DW et al. The pathogenesis of amiodarone-induced pigmentation and photosensitivity. *Br J Dermatol* 1984; **110**: 451–6.
16 Kerber BJ, Hood AF. Chemotherapy-induced cutaneous reactions. *Semin Dermatol* 1989; **8**: 173–81.
17 Gabazza EC, Taguchi O, Yamakami T et al. Pulmonary infiltrates and skin pigmentation associated with sulfasalazine. *Am J Gastroenterol* 1992; **87**: 1654–7.
18 Le Cleach L, Chosidow O, Peytavin G et al. Blue-black pigmentation of the legs associated with pefloxacin therapy. *Arch Dermatol* 1995; **131**: 856–7.
19 Leonard PA, Moatamed F, Ward JR et al. Chrysiasis: the role of sun exposure in dermal hyperpigmentation secondary to gold therapy. *J Rheumatol* 1986; **13**: 58–64.
20 Smith RW, Leppard B, Barnett NL et al. Chrysiasis revisited: a clinical and pathological study. *Br J Dermatol* 1995; **133**: 671–8.
21 Gherardi R, Brochard P, Chamak B et al. Human generalized argyria. *Arch Pathol Lab Med* 1984; **108**: 181–2.
22 Thomsen K, Rothenborg HW. Clofazimine in the treatment of pyoderma gangrenosum. *Arch Dermatol* 1979; **115**: 851–2.
23 Williams H. Skin lightening creams containing hydroquinone. The case for a temporary ban. *BMJ* 1992; **305**: 903–4.

Hypopigmentation

Topical thiotepa has produced periorbital leukoderma [1]. Hypopigmentation has occurred as a result of occupational exposure to monobenzyl ether of hydroquinone, *p*-tertiary-butylcatechol, *p*-tertiary-butylphenol, *p*-tertiary-amylphenol, monomethyl ether of hydroquinone and hydroquinone [2]. In addition, hypopigmentation may result from phenolic detergent germicides [3], and following use of diphencyprone for alopecia areata [4,5]. Depigmentation of the skin and hair occurred after a phenobarbital-induced eruption [6]. Photoleukomelanodermatitis occurred due to afloqualone for cervical spondylosis; photopatch and oral challenge tests were positive [7]. Generalized cutaneous depigmentation followed a sulphamide-induced ADR [8].

REFERENCES

1 Harben DJ, Cooper PH, Rodman OG. Thiotepa-induced leukoderma. *Arch Dermatol* 1979; **115**: 973–4.
2 Stevenson CJ. Occupational vitiligo: clinical and epidemiological aspects. *Br J Dermatol* 1981; **105** (Suppl. 21): 51–6.
3 Kahn G. Depigmentation caused by phenolic detergent germicides. *Arch Dermatol* 1970; **102**: 177–87.
4 Hatzis J, Gourgiotou K, Tosca A et al. Vitiligo as a reaction to topical treatment with diphencyprone. *Dermatologica* 1988; **177**: 146–8.
5 Henderson CA, Ilchyshyn A. Vitiligo complicating diphencyprone sensitization therapy for alopecia universalis. *Br J Dermatol* 1995; **133**: 496–7.
6 Mion N, Fusade T, Mathelier-Fusade P et al. Depigmentation cutaneophanerienne consecutive à une toxidermie au phenobarbital. *Ann Dermatol Vénéréol* 1992; **119**: 927–9.
7 Ishikawa T, Kamide R, Niimura M. Photoleukomelanodermatitis (Kobori) induced by afloqualone. *J Dermatol* 1994; **21**: 430–3.
8 Martinez-Ruiz E, Ortega C, Calduch L et al. Generalized cutaneous depigmentation following sulfamide-induced drug eruption. *Dermatology* 2000; **201**: 252–4.

Acneiform and pustular eruptions

The term 'acneiform' is applied to eruptions that resemble acne vulgaris [1,2] (see Chapter 43). Lesions are papulopustular but comedones are usually absent. Adrenocorticotrophic hormone (ACTH), corticosteroids

[3], dexamethasone in neurosurgical patients, anabolic steroids for body-building [4], androgens (in females), oral contraceptives, iodides and bromides may produce acneiform eruptions. Isoniazid may induce acne, especially in slow inactivators of the drug [5]. Other drugs implicated in the production of acneiform rashes include dantrolene [6], danazol [7], quinidine [8], lithium [9,10] and azathioprine [11]. Acne rosacea was temporally associated with daily high-dose vitamin B supplement therapy in one patient [12], and eosinophilic pustular folliculitis (Ofuji's disease) developed in association with use of the cerebral activator indeloxazine hydrochloride [13].

REFERENCES

1 Hitch JM. Acneform eruptions induced by drugs and chemicals. *JAMA* 1967; **200**: 879–80.
2 Bedane C, Souyri N. Les acnés induites. *Ann Dermatol Vénéréol* 1990; **117**: 53–8.
3 Hurwitz RM. Steroid acne. *J Am Acad Dermatol* 1989; **21**: 1179–81.
4 Merkle T, Landthaler M, Braun-Falco O. Acne-conglobata-artige Exazerbation einer Acne vulgaris nach Einnahme von Anabolika und Vitamin-B-Komplex-haltigen Präparaten. *Hautarzt* 1990; **41**: 280–2.
5 Cohen LK, George W, Smith R. Isoniazid-induced acne and pellagra. Occurrence in slow inactivators of isoniazid. *Arch Dermatol* 1974; **109**: 377–81.
6 Pembroke AC, Saxena SR, Kataria M, Zilkha KD. Acne induced by dantrolene. *Br J Dermatol* 1981; **104**: 465–8.
7 Greenberg RD. Acne vulgaris associated with antigonadotrophic (danazol) therapy. *Cutis* 1979; **24**: 431–2.
8 Burkhart CG. Quinidine-induced acne. *Arch Dermatol* 1981; **117**: 603–4.
9 Heng MCY. Cutaneous manifestations of lithium toxicity. *Br J Dermatol* 1982; **106**: 107–9.
10 Kanzaki T. Acneiform eruption induced by lithium carbonate. *J Dermatol* 1991; **18**: 481–3.
11 Schmoeckel C, von Liebe V. Akneiformes Exanthem durch Azathioprin. *Hautarzt* 1983; **34**: 413–5.
12 Sherertz EF. Acneiform eruption due to 'megadose' vitamins B6 and B12. *Cutis* 1991; **48**: 119–20.
13 Kimura K, Ezoe K, Yokozeki H *et al.* A case of eosinophilic pustular folliculitis (Ofuji's disease) induced by patch and challenge tests with indeloxazine hydrochloride. *J Dermatol* 1996; **23**: 479–83.

Acute generalized exanthematous pustulosis (toxic pustuloderma)

Pustular reactions (toxic pustuloderma, acute generalized exanthematous pustulosis) have been reported in association with a number of drugs [1]. The main differential diagnosis of a generalized pustular drug eruption is pustular psoriasis [2]. Two histological patterns may be seen: (i) a toxic pustuloderma with spongiform intraepidermal pustules, papillary oedema and a mixed upper dermal perivascular inflammatory infiltrate; or (ii) a leukocytoclastic vasculitis with neutrophil collections both below and within the epidermis, suggesting passive neutrophil elimination via the overlying epidermis [3,4]. The presence of eosinophils in the inflammatory infiltrate is a helpful pointer to a drug cause [2]. A responsible drug was found in 87% of a series of 63 patients with acute generalized exanthematous pustulosis; antibiotics were implic-

ated as the causative agent in 80% of individuals [4]. The latter included particularly ampicillin, amoxicillin, spiramycin, erythromycin and cyclins. Hypersensitivity to mercury was also recorded as a precipitating cause. Pustulosis developed within 24 h of drug administration. It often started on the face or in flexural areas, rapidly became disseminated, with fever, and settled spontaneously with desquamation. Facial oedema, purpura, vesicles, blisters and erythema multiforme-like lesions were also seen; transient renal failure was noted in 32% of cases. Occasionally, TEN may be mimicked [5].

Acute generalized exanthematic pustulosis is usually due to penicillins or macrolides [6,7]. There have been individual reports of pustular drug reactions with ampicillin (which may be localized [8]), amoxicillin (with or without clavulanic acid) [9], propicillin [10], imipenem [11], the cephalosporins cefalexin (cephalexin) and cefradine (cephradine) [12,13], co-trimoxazole [14], doxycycline [15], chloramphenicol [16], norfloxacin [17], ofloxacin [18], teicoplanin [19], streptomycin [20], isoniazid, metronidazole [21], terbinafine [22–24], fluconazole [25], itraconazole [26], nystatin [27], salazosulfapyridine/salazopyrine [28], mesalazine [29], diltiazem [30], captopril [31] and enalapril [32], furosemide [33], hydrochlorothiazide [34], cytarabine [35], high-dose chemotherapy [36], sertraline [37], chlorpromazine [38], nitrazepam, acetylsalicylic acid [39], naproxen [40], allopurinol [41], hydroxychloroquine [42], pyrimethamine, piperazine ethionamide, the mucolytic agent eprazinone [43], dextropropoxyphene [44], icodextrin [45] and mexiletine [46]. Cases of generalized pustulation in association with the anticonvulsant hypersensitivity syndrome caused by phenytoin [47] and carbamazepine [48] have been recorded. Patch testing with the culprit drug may be positive in patients with acute generalized exanthematous pustulosis [49].

REFERENCES

1 Webster GF. Pustular drug reactions. *Clin Dermatol* 1993; **11**: 541–3.
2 Spencer JM, Silvers DN, Grossman ME. Pustular eruption after drug exposure: is it pustular psoriasis or a pustular drug eruption? *Br J Dermatol* 1994; **130**: 514–9.
3 Burrows NP, Russell Jones RR. Pustular drug eruptions: a histopathological spectrum. *Histopathology* 1993; **22**: 569–73.
4 Roujeau J-C, Bioulac-Sage P, Bourseau C *et al.* Acute generalized exanthematous pustulosis. Analysis of 63 cases. *Arch Dermatol* 1991; **127**: 1333–8.
5 Cohen AD, Cagnano E, Halevy S. Acute generalized exanthematous pustulosis mimicking toxic epidermal necrolysis. *Int J Dermatol* 2001; **40**: 458–61.
6 Manders SM, Heymann WR. Acute generalized exanthemic pustulosis. *Cutis* 1994; **54**: 194–6.
7 Trevisi P, Patrizi A, Neri I, Farina P. Toxic pustuloderma associated with azithromycin. *Clin Exp Dermatol* 1994; **19**: 280–1.
8 Jay S, Kang J, Watcher MA *et al.* Localized pustular skin eruption. Localized pustular drug eruption secondary to ampicillin. *Arch Dermatol* 1994; **130**: 787, 790.
9 Armster H, Schwarz T. Arzneimittelreaktion auf Amoxicillin unter dem Bild eines toxischen Pustuloderms. *Hautarzt* 1991; **42**: 713–6.
10 Gebhardt M, Lustig A, Bocker T, Wollina U. Acute generalized exanthematous pustulosis (AGEP): manifestation of drug allergy to propicillin. *Contact Dermatitis* 1995; **33**: 204–5.

11 Escallier F, Dalac S, Foucher JL *et al*. Pustulose exanthématique aiguë généralisée imputabilité a l'imipéneme (Tienam®). *Ann Dermatol Vénéréol* 1989; **116**: 407–9.

12 Kalb RE, Grossman ME. Pustular eruption following administration of cephradine. *Cutis* 1986; **38**: 58–60.

13 Jackson H, Vion B, Levy PM. Generalized eruptive pustular drug rash due to cephalexin. *Dermatologica* 1988; **177**: 292–4.

14 MacDonald KJS, Green CM, Kenicer KJA. Pustular dermatosis induced by co-trimoxazole. *BMJ* 1986; **293**: 1279–80.

15 Trueb RM, Burg G. Acute generalized exanthematous pustulosis due to doxycycline. *Dermatology* 1993; **186**: 75–8.

16 Lee AY, Yoo SH. Chloramphenicol induced acute generalized exanthematous pustulosis proved by patch test and systemic provocation. *Acta Derm Venereol (Stockh)* 1999; **79**: 412–3.

17 Shelley ED, Shelley WB. The subcorneal pustular eruption: an example induced by norfloxacin. *Cutis* 1988; **42**: 24–7.

18 Tsuda S, Kato K, Karashima T *et al*. Toxic pustuloderma induced by ofloxacin. *Acta Derm Venereol (Stockh)* 1993; **73**: 382–4.

19 Chu CY, Wu J, Jean SS, Sun CC. Acute generalized exanthematous pustulosis due to teicoplanin. *Dermatology* 2001; **202**: 141–2.

20 Kushimoto H, Aoki T. Toxic erythema with generalized follicular pustules caused by streptomycin. *Arch Dermatol* 1981; **117**: 444–5.

21 Watsky KL. Acute generalised exanthematous pustulosis induced by metronidazole: the role of patch testing. *Arch Dermatol* 1999; **135**: 93–4.

22 Kempinaire A, De Raeve L, Merckx M *et al*. Terbinafine-induced acute generalized exanthematous pustulosis confirmed by positive patch-test result. *J Am Acad Dermatol* 1997; **37**: 653–5.

23 Condon CA, Downs AMR, Archer CB. Terbinafine-induced acute generalized exanthematous pustulosis. *Br J Dermatol* 1998; **138**: 709–10.

24 Bennett ML, Jorizzo JL, White WL. Generalized pustular eruptions associated with oral terbinafine. *Int J Dermatol* 1999; **38**: 596–600.

25 Alsadhan A, Taher M, Krol A. Acute generalized exanthematous pustulosis induced by oral fluconazole. *J Cutan Med Surg* 2002; **6**: 122–4.

26 Heymann WR, Manders SM. Itraconazole-induced acute generalised exanthematic pustulosis. *J Am Acad Dermatol* 1996; **33**: 130–1.

27 Kuchler A, Hamm H, Weidenthaler-Barth B *et al*. Acute generalized exanthematous pustulosis following oral nystatin therapy: a report of three cases. *Br J Dermatol* 1997; **137**: 808–11.

28 Kawaguchi M, Mitsuhashi Y, Kondo S. Acute generalized exanthematous pustulosis induced by salazosulfapyridine in a patient with ulcerative colitis. *J Dermatol* 1999; **26**: 359–62.

29 Gibbon KL, Bewley AP, Thomas K. Mesalazine-induced pustular drug eruption. *J Am Acad Dermatol* 2001; **45**: S220–S221.

30 Vincente-Calleja JM, Aguirre A, Landa N *et al*. Acute generalized exanthematous pustulosis due to diltiazem: confirmation by patch testing. *Br J Dermatol* 1997; **137**: 837–9.

31 Carroll J, Thaler M, Grossman E *et al*. Generalized pustular eruption associated with converting enzyme inhibitor therapy. *Cutis* 1995; **56**: 276–8.

32 Ferguson JE, Chalmers RJ. Enalapril-induced toxic pustuloderma. *Clin Exp Dermatol* 1996; **21**: 54–5.

33 Noce R, Paredes BE, Pichler WJ, Krahenbuhl S. Acute generalized exanthematic pustulosis (AGEP) in a patient treated with furosemide. *Am J Med Sci* 2000; **320**: 331–3.

34 Petavy-Catala C, Martin L, Fontes V *et al*. Hydrochlorothiazide-induced acute generalized exanthematous pustulosis. *Acta Derm Venereol (Stockh)* 2001; **81**: 209.

35 Chiu A, Kohler S, McGuire J, Kimball AB. Cytarabine-induced acute generalised exanthematous pustulosis. *J Am Acad Dermatol* 2002; **45**: 633–5.

36 Valks R, Fraga J, Munoz E *et al*. Acute generalized exanthematous pustulosis in patients receiving high-dose chemotherapy. *Arch Dermatol* 1999; **135**: 1418–20.

37 Thedenat B, Loche F, Albes B *et al*. Acute generalized exanthematous pustulosis with photodistribution pattern induced by sertraline. *Dermatology* 2001; **203**: 87–8.

38 Burrows NP, Ratnavel RC, Norris PG. Pustular eruptions after chlorpromazine. *BMJ* 1994; **309**: 97.

39 Ballmer-Weber BK, Widmer M, Burg G. Acetylsalicylsaure-induzierte generalisierte Pustulose. *Schweiz Med Wochenschr* 1993; **123**: 542–6.

40 Grattan CEH. Generalized pustular drug rash due to naproxen. *Dermatologica* 1989; **179**: 57–8.

41 Boffa MJ, Chalmers RJ. Allopurinol-induced toxic pustuloderma. *Br J Dermatol* 1994; **131**: 447.

42 Lotem M, Ingber A, Segal R, Sandbank M. Generalized pustular drug rash induced by hydroxychloroquine. *Acta Derm Venereol (Stockh)* 1990; **70**: 250–1.

43 Faber M, Maucher OM, Stengel R, Goerttler E. Epraxinonenexanthem mit subkornealer Pustelbildung. *Hautarzt* 1984; **35**: 200–3.

44 Machet L, Martin L, Machet MC *et al*. Acute generalized exanthematous pustulosis induced by dextropropoxyphene and confirmed by patch testing. *Acta Derm Venereol (Stockh)* 2000; **80**: 224–5.

45 Al-Hoqail IA, Crawford RI. Acute generalized exanthematous pustulosis induced by icodextrin. *Br J Dermatol* 2001; **145**: 1026–7.

46 Sasaki K, Yamamoto T, Kishi M *et al*. Acute exanthematous pustular drug eruption induced by mexiletine. *Eur J Dermatol* 2001; **11**: 469–71.

47 Kleier RS, Breneman DL, Boiko S. Generalized pustulation as a manifestation of the anticonvulsant hypersensitivity syndrome. *Arch Dermatol* 1991; **127**: 1361–4.

48 Commens CA, Fischer GO. Toxic pustuloderma following carbamazepine therapy. *Arch Dermatol* 1988; **124**: 178–9.

49 Moreau A, Dompmartin A, Castel B *et al*. Drug-induced acute generalized exanthematous pustulosis with positive patch tests. *Int J Dermatol* 1995; **34**: 263–6.

Eczematous eruptions

Allergic contact dermatitis is discussed in Chapter 20. This section concerns the entity termed 'systemic contact-type dermatitis medicamentosa' [1–5] (Table 73.11). A patient initially sensitized to a drug by way of allergic contact dermatitis may develop an eczematous reaction when the same, or a chemically related, substance is subsequently administered systemically. The eruption tends to be symmetrical, and may involve first, or most severely, the site(s) of the original dermatitis, before becoming generalized. Patients with a contact allergy to ethylenediamine may develop urticaria or systemic eczema following injection of aminophylline preparations containing ethylenediamine as a solubilizer for theophylline [6,7]. Patients with contact allergy to parabens may develop systemic eczema on medication with a drug containing parabens as a preservative [8]. Similarly, sensitized patients may develop eczema following oral ingestion of neomycin or hydroxyquinolines [9]. Diabetic patients sensitized by topical preparations containing *p*-amino compounds, such as *p*-phenylenediamine hair dyes, PABA sunscreens and certain local anaesthetic agents (e.g. benzocaine), may develop a systemic contact dermatitis with the hypoglycaemic agents tolbutamide or chlorpropamide. Sulphonylureas may also induce eczematous eruptions in sulphanilamide-sensitive patients as a result of cross-reactivity. Phenothiazines can produce allergic contact dermatitis, photoallergic reactions and eczematous contact-type dermatitis, and may cross-react with certain antihistamines. Tetraethylthiuram disulphide (disulfiram, Antabuse) for the management of alcoholism can cause eczematous reactions in patients sensitized to thiurams via rubber gloves. 'Systemic contact-type dermatitis' reactions have also been described with [4] acetylsalicylic acid, codeine [10], phenobarbital, pseudoephedrine hydrochloride and norephedrine hydrochloride [11], ephedrine [12], erythromycin [13], isoniazid [14], dimethylsulfoxide, hydroxyquinone, nystatin, subcutaneous hydromorphone

Table 73.11 Systemic drugs that can reactivate allergic contact eczema to chemically related topical medicaments. (From Fisher [1].)

Systemic drug	Topical medicament
Ethylenediamine antihistamines Aminophylline Piperazine	Aminophylline suppositories and ethylenediamine hydrochloride
Organic and inorganic mercury compounds	Ammoniated mercury
Tincture of benzoin inhalation	Balsam of Peru
Procaine Acetohexamide p-Aminosalicylic acid Azo dyes in foods and drugs Chlorothiazide Chlorpropamide Tolbutamide	Benzocaine (p-amino compound) and glyceryl p-aminobenzoic acid sunscreens
Chloral hydrate	Chlorobutanol
Iodochlorhydroxyquinoline	Halogenated hydroxyquinoline creams (Vioform)
Iodides, iodinated organic compounds, radiographic contrast media	Iodine
Streptomycin, kanamycin, paromycin, gentamicin	Neomycin sulphate
Glyceryl trinitrate tablets	Glyceryl trinitrate ointment
Disulfiram (Antabuse)	Thiuram (rubber chemical)

given for cancer pain [15], amlexanox [16], enoxolone [17], vitamin B_1, vitamin C, parabens, butylated hydroxyanisole, hydroxytoluene and tea-tree oil [18]. Allergic eczematous reactions to endogenous or exogenous systemic corticosteroids, including hydrocortisone and methylprednisolone, have been documented in patients who are patch-test positive to topical corticosteroids [19,20].

The term 'baboon syndrome' denotes a characteristic pattern of systemic allergic contact dermatitis [21–23], in which there is diffuse erythema of the buttocks, upper inner thighs and axillae, provoked by penicillin [24], ampicillin, amoxicillin [25], nickel, heparin, mercury (including that found in a homeopathic medicine [26]), terbinafine [27] and hydroxyurea [28]. Patch tests are commonly positive and usually vesicular, although histology of the eruption itself may show leukocytoclastic vasculitis; oral challenge with the suspected antigen may be required to substantiate the diagnosis. Disulfiram therapy of a nickel-sensitive alcoholic patient may induce this syndrome, as the drug leads to an initial acute increase in blood nickel concentration [21]. Cases have been described from Japan under the name 'mercury exanthem' following inhalation of mercury vapour from crushed thermometers in patients with a history of mercury allergy.

The term 'endogenic contact eczema' [29] refers to the occurrence of an eczematous contact drug reaction following primary sensitization by oral therapy, as in the case of a patient with a drug-related exanthem who later develops localized dermatitis due to topical therapy. Thus, ecze-

matous eruptions may develop following therapy with penicillin [30], methyldopa, allopurinol, indometacin, sulphonamides, gold, quinine, chloramphenicol, clonidine or bleomycin [31]. The alkylating agent mitomycin C administered intravesically for carcinoma of the bladder has been associated with an eczematous eruption, particularly on the face, palms and soles in some patients; these may have positive patch tests to the drug [32,33].

Some of the more important causes of eczematous drug reactions are listed in Table 73.11. Sensitivity to the suspected drug may be confirmed by subsequent patch testing, when the skin reaction has settled.

REFERENCES

1 Fisher AA. *Contact Dermatitis*. Philadelphia: Lea & Febiger, 1986.
2 Rycroft RJG, Menné T, Frosch PJ, Benezra CM, eds. *Textbook of Contact Dermatitis*. Berlin: Springer, 1992.
3 Cronin E. Contact dermatitis XVII. Reactions to contact allergens given orally or systemically. *Br J Dermatol* 1972; **86**: 104–7.
4 Menné T, Veien NK, Maibach HI. Systemic contact-type dermatitis due to drugs. *Semin Dermatol* 1989; **8**: 144–8.
5 Aquilina C, Sayag J. Eczéma par réactogenes internes. *Ann Dermatol Vénéréol* 1989; **116**: 753–65.
6 Berman BA, Ross RN. Ethylenediamine: systemic eczematous contact-type dermatitis. *Cutis* 1983; **31**: 594–8.
7 Hardy C, Schofield O, George CF. Allergy to aminophylline. *BMJ* 1983; **286**: 2051–2.
8 Aeling JL, Nuss DD. Systemic eczematous 'contact-type' dermatitis medicamentosa caused by parabens. *Arch Dermatol* 1974; **110**: 640.
9 Ekelund E-G, Möller H. Oral provocation in eczematous contact allergy to neomycin and hydroxy-quinolines. *Acta Derm Venereol (Stockh)* 1969; **49**: 422–6.

10 Estrada JL, Puebla MJ, de Urbina JJ *et al.* Generalized eczema due to codeine. *Contact Dermatitis* 2001; **44**: 185.

11 Tomb RR, Lepoittevin JP, Espinassouze F *et al.* Systemic contact dermatitis from pseudoephedrine. *Contact Dermatitis* 1991; **24**: 86–8.

12 Villas Martinez F, Badas AJ, Garmendia Goitia JF, Aguirre I. Generalized dermatitis due to oral ephedrine. *Contact Dermatitis* 1993; **29**: 215–6.

13 Fernandez Redondo V, Casas L, Taboada M, Toribio J. Systemic contact dermatitis from erythromycin. *Contact Dermatitis* 1994; **30**: 311.

14 Meseguer J, Sastre A, Malek T, Salvador MD. Systemic contact dermatitis from isoniazid. *Contact Dermatitis* 1993; **28**: 110–1.

15 de Cuyper C, Goeteyn M. Systemic contact dermatitis from subcutaneous hydromorphone. *Contact Dermatitis* 1992; **27**: 220–3.

16 Hayakawa R, Ogino Y, Aris K, Matsunaga K. Systemic contact dermatitis due to amlexanox. *Contact Dermatitis* 1992; **27**: 122–3.

17 Villas Martinez F, Joral Badas A, Garmendia Goitia JF, Aguirre I. Sensitization to oral enoxolone. *Contact Dermatitis* 1994; **30**: 124.

18 de Groot AC, Weyland JW. Systemic contact dermatitis from tea tree oil. *Contact Dermatitis* 1992; **27**: 279–80.

19 Lauerma AI, Reitamo S, Maibach HI. Systemic hydrocortisone/cortisol induces allergic skin reactions in presensitized subjects. *J Am Acad Dermatol* 1991; **24**: 182–5.

20 Murata Y, Kumano K, Ueda T *et al.* Systemic contact dermatitis caused by systemic corticosteroid use. *Arch Dermatol* 1997; **133**: 1053–4.

21 Andersen KE, Hjorth N, Menné T. The baboon syndrome: systemically-induced allergic contact dermatitis. *Contact Dermatitis* 1984; **10**: 97–100.

22 Herfs H, Schirren CG, Przybilla B, Plewig G. Das 'Baboon-Syndrom'. Eine besondere Manifestation einer hamatogenen Kontaktreaktion. *Hautarzt* 1993; **44**: 466–9.

23 Duve S, Worret W, Hofmann H. The baboon syndrome: a manifestation of haematogenous contact-type dermatitis. *Acta Derm Venereol (Stockh)* 1994; **74**: 480–1.

24 Panhans-Gross A, Gall H, Peter RU. Baboon syndrome after oral penicillin. *Contact Dermatitis* 1999; **41**: 352–3.

25 Kick G, Przybilla B. Delayed prick test reaction identifies amoxicillin as elicitor of baboon syndrome. *Contact Dermatitis* 2000; **43**: 366–7.

26 Audicana M, Bernedo N, Gonzalez I *et al.* An unusual case of baboon syndrome due to mercury present in a homeopathic medicine. *Contact Dermatitis* 2001; **45**: 185.

27 Weiss JM, Mockenhaupt M, Schopf E, Simon JC. Reproducible drug exanthema to terbinafine with characteristic distribution of baboon syndrome. *Hautarzt* 2001; **52**: 1104–6.

28 Chowdhury MM, Patel GK, Inaloz HS, Holt PJ. Hydroxyurea-induced skin disease mimicking the baboon syndrome. *Clin Exp Dermatol* 1999; **24**: 336–7.

29 Pirilä V. Endogenic contact eczema. *Allerg Asthma* 1970; **16**: 15–9.

30 Girard JP. Recurrent angioneurotic oedema and contact dermatitis due to penicillin. *Contact Dermatitis* 1978; **4**: 309.

31 Lincke-Plewig H. Bleomycin-Exantheme. *Hautarzt* 1980; **31**: 616–8.

32 Colver GB, Inglis JA, McVittie E *et al.* Dermatitis due to intravesical mitomycin C: a delayed-type hypersensitivity reaction? *Br J Dermatol* 1990; **122**: 217–24.

33 De Groot AC, Conemans JMH. Systemic allergic contact dermatitis from intravesical instillation of the antitumor antibiotic mitomycin C. *Contact Dermatitis* 1991; **24**: 201–9.

Bullous eruptions

Bullous drug eruptions encompass many different clinical reactions and pathomechanisms [1,2]. Isolated blisters, often located preferentially on the extremities, may be caused by a wide variety of chemically distinct drugs. Fixed drug eruptions and drug-induced vasculitis may have a bullous component; these are reviewed elsewhere in this chapter. Erythema multiforme, Stevens–Johnson syndrome and drug-induced TEN are discussed in Chapter 74. The specific drug-induced entities of porphyria and pseudoporphyria, bullous pemphigoid, pemphigus and linear IgA disease are discussed here.

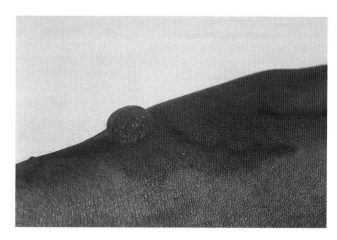

Fig. 73.5 Bullous eruption in barbiturate overdose. (Courtesy of Charing Cross Hospital, London, UK.)

Bullous eruption in drug overdosage

Bullae, often at pressure areas, may be seen in patients comatose after overdosage with barbiturates (Fig. 73.5), methadone, meprobamate, imipramine, nitrazepam or glutethimide [1–5].

REFERENCES

1 Bork K. *Cutaneous Side Effects of Drugs.* Philadelphia: Saunders, 1988.

2 Breathnach SM, Hintner H. *Adverse Drug Reactions and the Skin.* Oxford: Blackwell Scientific Publications, 1992.

3 Brehmer-Andersson E, Pedersen NB. Sweat gland necrosis and bullous skin changes in acute drug intoxication. *Acta Derm Venereol (Stockh)* 1969; **49**: 157–62.

4 Mandy S, Ackerman AB. Characteristic traumatic skin lesions in drug-induced coma. *JAMA* 1970; **213**: 253–6.

5 Herschtal D, Robinson MJ. Blisters of the skin in coma induced by amitriptyline and chlorazepate dipotassium. Report of a case with underlying sweat gland necrosis. *Arch Dermatol* 1979; **115**: 499.

Drug-induced porphyria

Porphyria is discussed in Chapter 57. Drugs reported to exacerbate the acute hepatic porphyrias are listed in Table 73.12; these either cause excess destruction of haem or inhibit haem synthesis [1–3].

Pseudoporphyria

Pseudoporphyria, in which porphyria-like blistering of exposed areas on the extremities occurs in the absence of abnormal porphyrin metabolism, may be caused by high-dose furosemide [4], naproxen [5,6] and other NSAIDs [7–9], combined carisoprodol and aspirin [10], nalidixic acid [11], tetracyclines [12] and sulphonylureas. Phototoxic mechanisms have been implicated in some cases. A similar syndrome has been reported in a patient taking very large doses of pyridoxine (vitamin B_6) [13].

Table 73.12 Drugs that are unsafe to use in patients with acute intermittent porphyria, porphyria cutanea tarda or variegate porphyria.

Aminoglutethimide	Meprobamate
Barbiturates	Novobiocin
Carbamazepine	Oestrogens
Carbromal	Primidone
Chlorpropamide	Progestogens
Danazol	Pyrazolone derivatives
Diclofenac	Rifampicin
Diphenylhydantoin (phenytoin)	Sulphonamides
Ergot preparations	Tolbutamide
Glutethimide	Trimethadione
Griseofulvin	Valproic acid

REFERENCES

1 Targovnick SE, Targovnik JH. Cutaneous drug reactions in porphyrias. *Clin Dermatol* 1986; **4**: 111–7.
2 Köstler E, Seebacher C, Riedel H, Kemmer C. Therapeutische und pathogenetische Aspekte der Porphyria cutanea tarda. *Hautarzt* 1986; **37**: 210–6.
3 Ayala F, Santoianni P. Drug-induced cutaneous porphyria. *Clin Dermatol* 1993; **11**: 535–9.
4 Burry JN, Lawrence JR. Phototoxic blisters from high frusemide dosage. *Br J Dermatol* 1976; **94**: 495–9.
5 Judd LE, Henderson DW, Hill DC. Naproxen-induced pseudoporphyria: a clinical and ultrastructural study. *Arch Dermatol* 1986; **122**: 451–4.
6 Lang BA, Finlayson LA. Naproxen-induced pseudoporphyria in patients with juvenile rheumatoid arthritis. *J Pediatr* 1994; **124**: 639–42.
7 Stern RS. Phototoxic reactions to piroxicam and other nonsteroidal anti-inflammatory agents. *N Engl J Med* 1983; **309**: 186–7.
8 Taylor BJ, Duffill MB. Pseudoporphyria from nonsteroidal anti-inflammatory drugs. *NZ Med J* 1987; **100**: 322–3.
9 Meggitt SJ, Farr PM. Pseudoporphyria and propionic acid non-steroidal anti-inflammatory drugs. *Br J Dermatol* 1999; **141**: 591–2.
10 Hazen PG. Pseudoporphyria in a patient receiving carisoprodol/aspirin therapy. *J Am Acad Dermatol* 1994; **31**: 500.
11 Keane JT, Pearson RW, Malkinson FD. Nalidixic acid-induced photosensitivity in mice: a model for pseudoporphyria. *J Invest Dermatol* 1984; **82**: 210–3.
12 Hawk JLM. Skin changes resembling hepatic cutaneous porphyria induced by oxytetracycline photosensitization. *Clin Exp Dermatol* 1980; **5**: 321–5.
13 Baer R, Stilman RA. Cutaneous skin changes probably due to pyridoxine abuse. *J Am Acad Dermatol* 1984; **10**: 527–8.

Drug-induced bullous pemphigoid

Idiopathic bullous pemphigoid is discussed in Chapter 41. In drug-induced bullous pemphigoid, patients tend to be younger; tissue-bound and circulating anti-basement-membrane zone IgG antibodies may be absent, or additional antibodies such as intercellular or antiepidermal cytoplasmic antibodies may be detected. Some cases of drug-induced bullous pemphigoid are short-lived, whereas others become chronic. Drug-induced bullous or cicatricial pemphigoid have been reported with a number of medications [1–5], especially furosemide [6,7] but also bumetanide [8], spironolactone [9,10], penicillamine [11,12], the penicillamine analogue tiobutarit [13], penicillin [14] and its derivatives [15], ciprofloxacin [16], sulfasalazine, salicylazosulfapyridine, phenacetin [17], enalapril [18], fluoxetine [19], novoscabin, topical fluorouracil, and PUVA therapy [20]. In the case of enalapril-induced bullous pemphigoid, the IgG antibody was directed against the 230-kDa bullous pemphigoid antigen [18]. Cicatricial pemphigoid has been described in association with penicillamine [12] and clonidine [21]. An association with vaccination for influenza and with tetanus toxoid and induction of bullous pemphigoid has been noted rarely [22–25].

REFERENCES

1 Ahmed AR, Newcomer VD. Drug-induced bullous pemphigoid. *Clin Dermatol* 1987; **5**: 8–10.
2 Ruocco V, Sacerdoti G. Pemphigus and bullous pemphigoid due to drugs. *Int J Dermatol* 1991; **30**: 307–12.
3 Fellner MJ. Drug-induced bullous pemphigoid. *Clin Dermatol* 1993; **11**: 515–20.
4 Van Joost T, Van't Veen AJ. Drug-induced cicatricial pemphigoid and acquired epidermolysis bullosa. *Clin Dermatol* 1993; **11**: 521–7.
5 Vassileva S. Drug-induced pemphigoid: bullous and cicatricial. *Clin Dermatol* 1998; **16**: 379–87.
6 Fellner MJ, Katz JM. Occurrence of bullous pemphigoid after furosemide therapy. *Arch Dermatol* 1976; **112**: 75–7.
7 Castel T, Gratacos R, Castro J et al. Bullous pemphigoid induced by furosemide. *Clin Exp Dermatol* 1981; **6**: 635–8.
8 Boulinguez S, Bernard P, Bedane C et al. Bullous pemphigoid induced by bumetanide. *Br J Dermatol* 1998; **138**: 548–9.
9 Bastuji-Garan S, Joly P, Picard-Dahan C et al. Drugs associated with bullous pemphigoid. *Arch Dermatol* 1996; **132**: 272–6.
10 Grange F, Koessler A, Scrivener Y et al. Pemphigoide bulleuse induite par la spironolactone. *Ann Dermatol Venereol* 1996; **123**: S110–S111.
11 Rasmussen HB, Jepsen LV, Brandrup F. Penicillamine-induced bullous pemphigoid with pemphigus-like antibodies. *J Cutan Pathol* 1989; **16**: 154–7.
12 Bialy-Golan A, Brenner S. Penicillamine-induced bullous dermatoses. *J Am Acad Dermatol* 1996; **35**: 732–42.
13 Yamaguchi R, Oryu F, Hidano A. A case of bullous pemphigoid induced by tiobutarit (D-penicillamine analogue). *J Dermatol* 1989; **16**: 308–11.
14 Alcalay J, David M, Ingber A et al. Bullous pemphigoid mimicking bullous erythema multiforme: an untoward side effect of penicillins. *J Am Acad Dermatol* 1988; **18**: 345–9.
15 Hodak E, Ben-Shetrit A, Ingber A, Sandbank M. Bullous pemphigoid: an adverse effect of ampicillin. *Clin Exp Dermatol* 1990; **15**: 50–2.
16 Kimyai-Asadi A, Usman A, Nousari HC. Ciprofloxacin-induced bullous pemphigoid. *J Am Acad Dermatol* 2000; **42**: 847.
17 Kashihara M, Danno K, Miyachi Y et al. Bullous pemphigoid-like lesions induced by phenacetin: report of a case and an immunopathologic study. *Arch Dermatol* 1984; **120**: 1196–9.
18 Pazderka Smith E, Taylor TB, Meyer LJ, Zone JJ. Antigen identification in drug-induced bullous pemphigoid. *J Am Acad Dermatol* 1993; **29**: 879–82.
19 Rault S, Grosieux-Dauger C, Verraes S et al. Bullous pemphigoid induced by fluoxetine. *Br J Dermatol* 1998; **139**: 1092–6.
20 Abel EA, Bennett A. Bullous pemphigoid. Occurrence in psoriasis treated with psoralens plus long-wave ultraviolet radiation. *Arch Dermatol* 1979; **115**: 988–9.
21 Van Joost T, Faber WR, Manuel HR. Drug-induced anogenital cicatricial pemphigoid. *Br J Dermatol* 1980; **102**: 715–8.
22 Bodokh I, Lacour JP, Bourdet JF et al. Réactivation de pemphigoïde bulleuse apres vaccination antigrippale. *Thérapie* 1994; **49**: 154.
23 Venning VA, Wojnarowska F. Induced bullous pemphigoid. *Br J Dermatol* 1995; **132**: 831–2.
24 Fournier B, Descamps V, Bouscarat F et al. Bullous pemphigoid induced by vaccination. *Br J Dermatol* 1996; **135**: 153–4.
25 Downs AMR, Lear JT, Bower CPR, Kennedy CTC. Does influenza vaccination induce bullous pemphigoid? A report of four cases. *Br J Dermatol* 1998; **138**: 363.

Table 73.13 Drugs implicated in the development of pemphigus.

Thiol drugs
Penicillamine
Captopril, ramipril
Gold sodium thiomalate
Pyritinol
Thiamazole (methimazole)
Tiopronin (mercaptopropionylglycine)

Non-thiol drugs
Antibiotics
Penicillin and derivatives
Rifampicin
Cefalexin (cephalexin)
Cefadroxil
Ceftazidine

Pyrazolone derivatives
Aminophenazone
Aminopyrine
Azapropazone
Oxyphenbutazone
Phenylbutazone

Miscellaneous
Glibenclamide
Hydantoin
Levodopa
Lysine acetylsalicylate
Nifedipine
Phenobarbital (phenobarbitone)
Piroxicam
Progesterone
Propranolol
Interferon-β and interleukin-2
Heroin

Drug-induced pemphigus

The variants of idiopathic pemphigus are discussed in Chapter 41. A number of drugs have been implicated in drug-induced pemphigus (Table 73.13) [1,2], usually of foliaceus type, although the erythematosus, herpetiformis and urticaria-like forms also occur; drug-induced pemphigus vulgaris is rare. Most patients with drug-induced pemphigus have tissue-bound and/or low-titre circulating autoantibodies with the same antigenic specificity at a molecular level as autoantibodies from patients with the corresponding subtype of idiopathic pemphigus [3,4]; however, in the case of penicillamine-induced pemphigus, 10% do not have tissue-bound, and more than 30% do not have circulating, autoantibodies. About 80% of cases are caused by drugs associated with a thiol group in the molecule, especially penicillamine [5–11], but also the structurally related ACE inhibitors captopril [3,12–14] and ramipril [15], gold sodium thiomalate, drugs with disulphide bonds such as pyritinol [16], *S*-thiopyridoxine, tiopronin (mercaptopropionylglycine; which is chemically related to penicillamine and used as an alternative therapy in penicillamine intolerance) [4,17,18], and bucillamine

[19], as well as those with a sulphur-containing ring that may undergo metabolic change to the thiol form, such as piroxicam [20]. Penicillin [21,22], and its derivatives ampicillin [22], procaine penicillin and amoxicillin, may also cause pemphigus. Other drugs that cause pemphigus may contain an active amide group [23].

Rifampicin [24], cefalexin [25], cefadroxil, ceftazidime [26], pyrazolone derivatives [27] including dipyrone [28], propranolol, propranolol–meprobamate [29], optalidon, pentachlorophenol, phenobarbital [30], nifedipine [31], phosphamide, hydantoin, combinations of indometacin and aspirin [32], glibenclamide [33], as well as heroin [34], have all been established as rare causes of a pemphigus-like reaction. Fatal pemphigus vulgaris has been recorded after IFN-β and IL-2 therapy for lymphoma [35]. Fludarabine has been implicated in the development of paraneoplastic pemphigus [36,37].

REFERENCES

1 Brenner S, Wolf R, Ruocco V. Drug-induced pemphigus. I. A survey. *Clin Dermatol* 1993; **11**: 501–5.
2 Ruocco V, De Angelis E, Lombardi ML. Drug-induced pemphigus. II. Pathomechanisms and experimental investigations. *Clin Dermatol* 1993; **11**: 507–13.
3 Korman NJ, Eyre RW, Stanley JR. Drug-induced pemphigus: autoantibodies directed against the pemphigus antigen complexes are present in penicillamine and captopril-induced pemphigus. *J Invest Dermatol* 1991; **96**: 273–6.
4 Verdier-Sevrain S, Joly P, Thomine E *et al.* Thioproine-induced herpetiform pemphigus: report of a case studied by immunoelectron microscopy and immunoblot analysis. *Br J Dermatol* 1994; **130**: 238–40.
5 Goldberg I, Kashman Y, Brenner S. The induction of pemphigus by phenol drugs. *Int J Dermatol* 1999; **38**: 888–92.
6 Kishimoto K, Iwatsuki K, Akiba H *et al.* Subcorneal pustular dermatosis-type IgA pemphigus induced by thiol drugs. *Eur J Dermatol* 2001; **11**: 41–4.
7 Zillikens D, Zentner A, Burger M *et al.* Pemphigus foliaceus durch Penicillamin. *Hautarzt* 1993; **44**: 167–71.
8 Jones E, Sobkowski WW, Murray SJ, Walsh NMG. Concurrent pemphigus and myasthenia gravis as manifestations of penicillamine toxicity. *J Am Acad Dermatol* 1993; **28**: 655–6.
9 Bialy-Golan A, Brenner S. Penicillamine-induced bullous dermatoses. *J Am Acad Dermatol* 1996; **35**: 732–42.
10 Peñas PF, Buezo GF, Carvajal I *et al.* D-Penicillamine-induced pemphigus foliaceus with autoantibodies to desmoglein-1 in a patient with mixed connective tissue disease. *J Am Acad Dermatol* 1997; **37**: 121–3.
11 Toth GG, Jonkman MF. Successful treatment of recalcitrant penicillamine-induced pemphigus foliaceus by low-dose intravenous immunoglobulins. *Br J Dermatol* 1999; **141**: 583–5.
12 Clement M. Captopril-induced eruptions. *Arch Dermatol* 1981; **117**: 525–6.
13 Katz RA, Hood AF, Anhalt GJ. Pemphigus-like eruption from captopril. *Arch Dermatol* 1987; **123**: 20–1.
14 Kaplan RP, Potter TS, Fox JN. Drug-induced pemphigus related to angiotensin-converting enzyme inhibitors. *J Am Acad Dermatol* 1992; **26**: 364–6.
15 Vignes S, Paul C, Flageul B, Dubertret L. Ramipril-induced superficial pemphigus. *Br J Dermatol* 1996; **135**: 657–8.
16 Civatte J, Duterque M, Blanchet P *et al.* Deux cas de pemphigus superficiel induit par le pyritinol. *Ann Dermatol Vénéréol* 1978; **105**: 573–7.
17 Alinovi A, Benoldi D, Manganelli P. Pemphigus erythematosus induced by thiopronin. *Acta Derm Venereol (Stockh)* 1982; **62**: 452–4.
18 Lucky PA, Skovby F, Thier SO. Pemphigus foliaceus and proteinuria induced by α-mercaptopropionylglycine. *J Am Acad Dermatol* 1983; **8**: 667–72.
19 Ogata K, Nakajima H, Ikeda M *et al.* Drug-induced pemphigus foliaceus with features of pemphigus vulgaris. *Br J Dermatol* 2001; **144**: 421–2.

20 Martin RL, McSweeny GW, Schneider J. Fatal pemphigus vulgaris in a patient taking piroxicam. *N Engl J Med* 1983; **309**: 795–6.

21 Duhra PL, Foulds IS. Penicillin-induced pemphigus vulgaris. *Br J Dermatol* 1988; **118**: 307.

22 Fellner MJ, Mark AS. Penicillin- and ampicillin-induced pemphigus vulgaris. *Int J Dermatol* 1980; **19**: 392–3.

23 Wolf R, Brenner S. An active amide group in the molecule of drugs that induce pemphigus: a casual or causal relationship? *Dermatology* 1994; **189**: 1–4.

24 Lee CW, Lim JH, Kang HJ. Pemphigus foliaceus induced by rifampicin. *Br J Dermatol* 1984; **111**: 619–22.

25 Wolf R, Dechner E, Ophir J, Brenner S. Cephalexin. A nonthiol drug that may induce pemphigus vulgaris. *Int J Dermatol* 1991; **30**: 213–5.

26 Pellicano R, Iannantuono M, Lomuto M. Pemphigus erythematosus induced by ceftazidime. *Int J Dermatol* 1993; **32**: 675–6.

27 Chorzelski TP, Jablonska S, Blaszczyk M. Autoantibodies in pemphigus. *Acta Derm Venereol (Stockh)* 1966; **46**: 26.

28 Brenner S, Bialy-Golan A, Crost N. Dipyrone in the induction of pemphigus. *J Am Acad Dermatol* 1997; **36**: 488–90.

29 Goddard W, Lambert D, Gavanou J, Chapius JL. Pemphigus acquit après traitement par l'association propranolol–méprobamate. *Ann Dermatol Vénéréol* 1980; **107**: 1213–6.

30 Dourmishev AL, Rahman MA. Phenobarbital-induced pemphigus vulgaris. *Dermatologica* 1986; **173**: 256–8.

31 Kim SC, Won JH, Ahn SK. Pemphigus foliaceus induced by nifedipine. *Acta Derm Venereol (Stockh)* 1993; **73**: 210–1.

32 Demento FJ, Grover RW. Acantholytic herpetiform dermatitis. *Arch Dermatol* 1973; **107**: 883–7.

33 Paterson AJ, Lamey PJ, Lewis MA *et al.* Pemphigus vulgaris precipitated by glibenclamide therapy. *J Oral Pathol Med* 1993; **22**: 92–5.

34 Fellner MJ, Winiger J. Pemphigus erythematosus and heroin addiction. *Int J Dermatol* 1978; **17**: 308–11.

35 Ramseur WL, Richards F, Duggan DB. A case of fatal pemphigus vulgaris in association with beta interferon and interleukin-2 therapy. *Cancer* 1989; **63**: 2005–7.

36 Anhalt GJ. Paraneoplastic pemphigus: the role of tumours and drugs. *Br J Dermatol* 2001; **144**: 1102–4.

37 Gooptu C, Littlewood TJ, Frith P *et al.* Paraneoplastic pemphigus: an association with fludarabine? *Br J Dermatol* 2001; **144**: 1255–61.

Linear IgA disease

Idiopathic linear IgA disease is discussed in Chapter 41. The drugs implicated as a cause of this condition have been reviewed [1–3], and include vancomycin especially [1–9], but also amiodarone, ampicillin, atorvastatin [10], captopril [11], carbamazepine [12], cefamandole (cephamandole), diclofenac, furosemide [13], glibenclamide, IFN-γ, iodine, lithium, penicillin [14,15], phenytoin [16] and somatostatin, as well as tea-tree oil [17]. Most patients lack circulating antibodies to the basement membrane; resolution of the rash follows discontinuation of medication.

REFERENCES

1 Collier PM, Wojnarowska F. Drug-induced linear immunoglobulin A disease. *Clin Dermatol* 1993; **11**: 529–33.

2 Kuechle ML, Stegemeir E, Maynard B *et al.* Drug-induced linear IgA bullous dermatosis: report of six cases and review of the literature. *J Am Acad Dermatol* 1994; **30**: 187–92.

3 Geissmann C, Beylot-Barry M, Doutre MS, Beylot C. Drug-induced linear IgA bullous dermatosis. *J Am Acad Dermatol* 1995; **32**: 296.

4 Carpenter S, Berg D, Sidhu-Malik N *et al.* Vancomycin-associated linear IgA dermatosis. A report of three cases. *J Am Acad Dermatol* 1992; **26**: 45–8.

5 Piketty C, Meeus F, Nochy D *et al.* Linear IgA dermatosis related to vancomycin. *Br J Dermatol* 1994; **130**: 130–1.

6 Whitworth JM, Thomas I, Peltz S *et al.* Vancomycin-induced linear IgA bullous dermatosis (LABD). *J Am Acad Dermatol* 1996; **34**: 890–1.

7 Palmer RA, Ogg G, Allen J *et al.* Vancomycin-induced linear IgA disease with autoantibodies to BP180 and LAD285. *Br J Dermatol* 2001; **145**: 816–20.

8 Ahkami R, Thomas I. Linear IgA bullous dermatosis associated with vancomycin and disseminated varicella-zoster infection. *Cutis* 2001; **67**: 423–6.

9 Dellavalle RP, Burch HM, Tyal S *et al.* Vancomycin-associated linear IgA bullous dermatosis mimicking toxic epidermal necrolysis. *J Am Acad Dermatol* 2003; **48**: S56–S57.

10 Konig C, Eickert A, Scharfetter-Kochanek K *et al.* Linear IgA bullous dermatosis induced by atorvastatin. *J Am Acad Dermatol* 2001; **44**: 689–92.

11 Friedman IS, Rudikoff D, Phelps RG, Sapadin AN. Captopril-triggered linear IgA bullous dermatosis. *Int J Dermatol* 1998; **37**: 608–12.

12 Cohen LM, Ugent RB. Linear IgA bullous dermatosis occurring after carbamazepine. *J Am Acad Dermatol* 2002; **46**: S32–S33.

13 Cerottini J-P, Ricci C, Guggisberg D, Panizzon RG. Drug-induced linear IgA bullous dermatosis probably induced by furosemide. *J Am Acad Dermatol* 1999; **41**: 103–5.

14 Combemale P, Gavaud C, Cozzani E *et al.* Dermatose a IgA lineaire (DIAL) induite par penicilline G. *Ann Dermatol Vénéréol* 1993; **120**: 847–8.

15 Wakelin S, Allen J, Zhou S, Wojnorowska F. Drug-induced linear IgA disease with antibodies to collagen VII. *Br J Dermatol* 1998; **138**: 310–4.

16 Acostamadiedo JM, Perniciaro C, Rogers RS III. Phenytoin-induced linear IgA bullous disease. *J Am Acad Dermatol* 1998; **38**: 352–6.

17 Perett CM, Evans AV, Russell-Jones R. Tea tree oil dermatitis associated with linear IgA disease. *Clin Exp Dermatol* 2003; **28**: 167–70.

Drug-induced epidermolysis bullosa acquisita

This entity has been linked to antibiotics, including vancomycin [1].

REFERENCE

1 Delbaldo C, Chen M, Friedli A *et al.* Drug-induced epidermolysis bullosa acquisita with antibodies to type VII collagen. *J Am Acad Dermatol* 2002; **46**: S161–S164.

Vasculitis

Drug-induced cutaneous necrotizing vasculitis [1–3] may also involve internal organs, including the heart, liver and kidneys, with fatal results. The patterns of polyarteritis nodosa, Henoch–Schönlein vasculitis and hypocomplementaemic vasculitis are not seen commonly with drugs. Drugs that have been implicated are listed in Table 73.14. These include ampicillin, sulphonamides, furosemide [4], thiazide diuretics, phenylbutazone and other NSAIDs, quinidine, amiodarone [5], hydralazine [6], enalapril [7], propylthiouracil [8,9], mefloquine [10], cimetidine [11], coumadin [12,13], anticonvulsants including phenytoin and in isolated cases carbamazepine and trimethadione [14,15], zidovudine (azidothymidine) [16], indinavir [17], fluoxetine [18], didanosine [19], piperazine [20], centrally acting appetite suppressants [21], hyposensitization therapy [22,23], bacille Calmette–Guérin (BCG) vaccination (which may cause a papulonecrotic type of vasculitis) [24], radiographic contrast media [25], food and drug additives including dye excipients such as tartrazine (FD&C yellow no. 5), ponceau, sodium benzoate, 4-hydroxybenzoic acid [26,27], vitamin B_6 [28] and the use of a nicotine patch [29].

Table 73.14 Drugs recorded as inducing vasculitis.

Additives	Levamisole
Allopurinol	Maprotiline
Aminosalicylic acid	Mefloquine
Amiodarone	Methotrexate
Amfetamine (amphetamine)	Penicillin
Ampicillin	Phenacetin
Aspirin	Phenothiazines
Arsenic	Phenylbutazone
Captopril	Phenytoin
Carbamazepine	Piperazine
Cimetidine	Procainamide
Coumadin	Propylthiouracil
Didanosine	Quinidine
Enalapril	Radiocontrast media
Erythromycin	Streptomycin
Etacrynic acid (ethacrynic acid)	Sulphonamides
Fluoroquinolone antibiotics	Trazodone
Fluoxetine	Tetracycline
Furosemide (frusemide)	Thiazides
Griseofulvin	Trimethadione
Guanethidine	Vaccines
Hydralazine	Zidovudine
Iodides	

Leukocytoclastic vasculitis and necrotizing angiitis have also been documented in drug abusers [30–32].

REFERENCES

1 Mullick FG, McAllister HA Jr, Wagner BM, Fenoglio JJ Jr. Drug-related vasculitis. Clinicopathologic correlations in 30 patients. *Hum Pathol* 1979; **10**: 313–25.
2 Mackel SE, Jordon RE. Leukocytoclastic vasculitis. A cutaneous expression of immune complex disease. *Arch Dermatol* 1983; **118**: 296–301.
3 Sanchez NP, Van Hale HM, Su WPD. Clinical and histopathologic spectrum of necrotizing vasculitis. Report of findings in 101 cases. *Arch Dermatol* 1985; **121**: 220–4.
4 Hendricks WM, Ader RS. Furosemide-induced cutaneous necrotizing vasculitis. *Arch Dermatol* 1977; **113**: 375–6.
5 Staubli M, Zimmerman A, Bircher J. Amiodarone-induced vasculitis and polyserositis. *Postgrad Med J* 1985; **61**: 245–7.
6 Peacock A, Weatherall D. Hydralazine-induced necrotizing vasculitis. *BMJ* 1981; **282**: 1121–2.
7 Carrington PR, Sanusi ID, Zahradka S, Winder PR. Enalapril-associated erythema and vasculitis. *Cutis* 1993; **51**: 121–3.
8 Vasily DB, Tyler WB. Propylthiouracil-induced cutaneous vasculitis. Case presentation and review of literature. *JAMA* 1980; **243**: 458–61.
9 Gammeltoft M, Kristensen JK. Propylthio-uracil-induced cutaneous vasculitis. *Acta Derm Venereol (Stockh)* 1982; **62**: 171–3.
10 Scerri L, Pace JL. Mefloquine-associated cutaneous vasculitis. *Int J Dermatol* 1993; **32**: 517–8.
11 Mitchell GG, Magnusson AR, Weiler JM. Cimetidine-induced cutaneous vasculitis. *Am J Med* 1983; **75**: 875–6.
12 Tanay A, Yust I, Brenner S *et al.* Dermal vasculitis due to coumadin hypersensitivity. *Dermatologica* 1982; **165**: 178–85.
13 Tamir A, Wolf R, Brenner S. Leukocytoclastic vasculitis: another coumarin-induced hemorrhagic reaction. *Acta Derm Venereol (Stockh)* 1994; **74**: 138–9.
14 Drory VE, Korczyn AD. Hypersensitivity vasculitis and systemic lupus erythematosus induced by anticonvulsants. *Clin Neuropharmacol* 1993; **16**: 19–29.
15 Kaneko K, Igarashi J, Suzuki Y *et al.* Carbamazepine-induced thrombocytopenia and leucopenia complicated by Henoch–Schonlein purpura symptoms. *Eur J Pediatr* 1993; **152**: 769–70.
16 Torres RA, Lin RY, Lee M, Barr MR. Zidovudine-induced leukocytoclastic vasculitis. *Arch Intern Med* 1992; **152**: 850–1.
17 Rachline A, Lariven S, Descamps V *et al.* Leucocytoclastic vasculitis and indinavir. *Br J Dermatol* 2000; **143**: 1112–3.
18 Roger D, Rolle F, Mausset J *et al.* Urticarial vasculitis induced by fluoxetine. *Dermatology* 1995; **191**: 164.
19 Herranz P, Fernandez-Diaz ML, de Lucas R *et al.* Cutaneous vasculitis associated with didanosine. *Lancet* 1994; **344**: 680.
20 Balzan M, Cacciottolo JM. Hypersensitivity vasculitis associated with piperazine therapy. *Br J Dermatol* 1994; **131**: 133–4.
21 Papadavid E, Yu RC, Tay A, Chu AC. Urticarial vasculitis induced by centrally acting appetite suppressants. *Br J Dermatol* 1996; **134**: 990–1.
22 Phanuphak P, Kohler PF. Onset of polyarteritis nodosa during allergic hyposensitisation treatment. *Am J Med* 1980; **68**: 479–85.
23 Merk H, Kober ML. Vasculitis nach spezifischer Hyposensibilisierung. *Z Hautkr* 1982; **57**: 1682–5.
24 Lübbe D. Vasculitis allergica vom papulonekrotischen Typ nach BCG-Impfung. *Dermatol Monatsschr* 1982; **168**: 186–92.
25 Kerdel FA, Fraker DL, Haynes HA. Necrotizing vasculitis from radiographic contrast media. *J Am Acad Dermatol* 1984; **10**: 25–9.
26 Michäelsson G, Petterson L, Juhlin L. Purpura caused by food and drug additives. *Arch Dermatol* 1974; **109**: 49–52.
27 Lowry MD, Hudson CF, Callen FP. Leukocytoclastic vasculitis caused by drug additives. *J Am Acad Dermatol* 1994; **30**: 854–5.
28 Ruzicka T, Ring J, Braun-Falco O. Vasculitis allergica durch vitamin B$_6$. *Hautarzt* 1984; **35**: 197–9.
29 Van der Klauw MM, Van Hillo B, Van den Berg WH *et al.* Vasculitis attributed to the nicotine patch (Nicotinell). *Br J Dermatol* 1996; **34**: 361–4.
30 Citron BP, Halpen M, McCarron M *et al.* Necrotizing angiitis associated with drug abuse. *N Engl J Med* 1970; **283**: 1003–11.
31 Lignelli GJ, Bucheit WA. Angiitis in drug abusers. *N Engl J Med* 1971; **284**: 112–3.
32 Gendelman H, Linzer M, Barland P *et al.* Leukocytoclastic vasculitis in an intravenous heroin abuser. *NY State J Med* 1983; **83**: 984–6.

Lupus erythematosus-like syndrome

A reaction resembling idiopathic LE has been reported in association with a large variety of drugs [1–9], although only about 5% of cases of SLE are drug induced. Cutaneous manifestations are in general rare: 18% and 26%, respectively, of patients with procainamide- and hydralazine-induced LE had skin changes in one series [6]. Photosensitivity may be prominent; some patients develop discoid LE lesions; urticarial or erythema multiforme-like lesions may also be seen. Constitutional symptoms may be present, and there may be evidence of Raynaud's disease, arthritis or polyserositis. Renal involvement is rare, as is central nervous system involvement. The condition usually, but not always, resolves after discontinuation of the drug. Abnormal laboratory findings include the presence of LE cells, and of antinuclear antibodies directed against ribonucleoprotein, single-stranded DNA and especially histones [10,11]. Antibodies against native double-stranded DNA are rarely found in drug-induced LE, and complement levels are normal; deposition of immunoreactants in uninvolved skin is rare. Patients with drug-induced LE may have the lupus anticoagulant [12,13].

A partial list of drugs reported to induce an SLE-like syndrome or exacerbate idiopathic LE is given in Table 73.15. Drugs most commonly implicated in inducing LE include especially hydralazine [14,15] and procainamide [16,17], and less commonly β-blockers, methyldopa [18,19], isoniazid, most anticonvulsants in clinical use

Table 73.15 Drugs inducing lupus erythematosus-like syndromes.

Angiotensin-converting enzyme inhibitors (captopril)	Lithium
	Methyldopa
Anticonvulsants	Methysergide
Carbamazepine	Nitrofurantoin
Hydantoins	Oral contraceptives
Primidone	Penicillin
Trimethadione	Penicillamine
Valproate	Phenothiazines
Allopurinol	(chlorpromazine)
Aminoglutethimide	Phenylbutazone
p-Aminosalicylic acid	Procainamide
β-Blockers	Quinidine
Calcium channel blockers	Streptomycin
Clonidine	Sulfasalazine
Co-trimoxazole	(sulphasalazine)
Ethosuximide	Sulphonamides
Gold salts	Terbinafine
Griseofulvin	Tetracycline
Hydralazine	Thiazide diuretics
Ibuprofen	Thionamide
Isoniazid	Thiouracils

including phenytoin, carbamazepine, ethosuximide, trimethadione, primidone and valproate (but not phenobarbital or benzodiazepines) [20], and quinidine [21,22]. LE following penicillamine therapy [23,24], 2-mercaptopropionylglycine [25], rifampicin [26], etanercept [27] and the tetracycline derivative COL-3 used in antiangiogenesis [28] has also been documented. Minocycline may induce an autoimmune syndrome of which LE may form part [29–31].

Subacute LE with positive Ro/SSA antibodies has been reported in association with a number of drugs [9], including phenytoin [32], thiazide diuretics such as hydrochlorothiazide [33–36], ACE inhibitors [37,38], calcium channel blockers [39], terbinafine [40–42], griseofulvin [43], piroxicam, oxprenolol, interferons and statins. The oral contraceptive induced LE lesions on the palms and feet of a patient [44]. In addition, a number of drugs may exacerbate pre-existing SLE, such as griseofulvin, β-blockers, sulphonamides [45], testosterone and oestrogens.

REFERENCES

1 Reidenberg MM. The chemical induction of systemic lupus erythematosus and lupus-like illnesses. *Arthritis Rheum* 1981; **24**: 1004–9.
2 Harmon CE, Portnova JP. Drug-induced lupus: clinical and serological studies. *Clin Rheum Dis* 1982; **8**: 121–35.
3 Stratton MA. Drug-induced systemic lupus erythematosus. *Clin Pharm* 1985; **4**: 657–63.
4 Totoritis MC, Rubin RL. Drug-induced lupus. Genetic, clinical, and laboratory features. *Postgrad Med* 1985; **78**: 149–52.
5 Moureaux P. Les formes cutanées du lupus. *Allerg Immunol* 1995; **27**: 196–9.
6 Dubois EL. Serologic abnormalities in spontaneous and drug-induced systemic lupus erythematosus. *J Rheumatol* 1975; **2**: 204–14.
7 Callen JP. Drug-induced cutaneous lupus erythematosus, a distinct syndrome that is frequently unrecognised. *J Am Acad Dermatol* 2001; **45**: 315–6.
8 Callen JP. How frequently are drugs associated with the development or exacerbation of subacute cutaneous lupus ? *Arch Dermatol* 2003; **139**: 89–90.
9 Srivastava M, Rencic A, Diglio G *et al*. Drug-induced, Ro/SSA-positive cutaneous lupus erythematosus. *Arch Dermatol* 2003; **139**: 45–9.
10 Hobbs RN, Clayton AL, Bernstein RM. Antibodies to the five histones and poly(adenosine diphosphateribose) in drug-induced lupus: implications for pathogenesis. *Ann Rheum Dis* 1987; **46**: 408–16.
11 Totoritis MC, Tan EM, McNally EM *et al*. Association of antibody to histone complex H2A-H2B with symptomatic procainamide-induced lupus. *N Engl J Med* 1988; **318**: 1431–6.
12 Bell WR, Boss GR, Wolfson JS. Circulating anticoagulant in the procainamide-induced lupus syndrome. *Arch Intern Med* 1977; **137**: 1471–3.
13 Canoso RT, Sise HS. Chlorpromazine-induced lupus anticoagulant and associated immunologic abnormalities. *Am J Hematol* 1982; **13**: 121–9.
14 Mansilla Tinoco R, Harland SJ, Ryan PJ *et al*. Hydralazine, antinuclear antibodies, and the lupus syndrome. *BMJ* 1982; **284**: 936–9.
15 Russell GI, Bing RF, Jones JA *et al*. Hydralazine sensitivity: clinical features, autoantibody changes and HLA-DR phenotype. *Q J Med* 1987; **65**: 845–52.
16 Dubois EL. Procainamide induction of a systemic lupus erythematosus-like syndrome. Presentation of six cases, review of the literature, and analysis and follow up of reported cases. *Medicine (Baltimore)* 1969; **48**: 217–28.
17 Blomgren SE, Condemi JJ, Vaughan JH. Procainamide-induced lupus erythematosus. Clinical and laboratory observations. *Am J Med* 1972; **52**: 338–48.
18 Harrington TM, Davis DE. Systemic lupus-like syndrome induced by methyldopa therapy. *Chest* 1981; **79**: 696–7.
19 Dupont A, Six R. Lupus-like syndrome induced by methyldopa. *BMJ* 1982; **285**: 693–4.
20 Drory VE, Korczyn AD. Hypersensitivity vasculitis and systemic lupus erythematosus induced by anticonvulsants. *Clin Neuropharmacol* 1993; **16**: 19–29.
21 McCormack GD, Barth WF. Quinidine induced lupus syndrome. *Semin Arthritis Rheum* 1985; **15**: 73–9.
22 Cohen MG, Kevat S, Prowse MV *et al*. Two distinct quinidine-induced rheumatic syndromes. *Ann Intern Med* 1988; **108**: 369–71.
23 Chalmers A, Thompson D, Stein HE *et al*. Systemic lupus erythematosus during penicillamine therapy for rheumatoid arthritis. *Ann Intern Med* 1982; **97**: 659–63.
24 Condon C, Phelan M, Lyons JF. Penicillamine-induced type II bullous systemic lupus erythematosus. *Br J Dermatol* 1997; **136**: 474–5.
25 Katayama I, Nishioka K. Lupus like syndrome induced by 2-mercaptopropionylglycine. *J Dermatol* 1986; **13**: 151–3.
26 Patel GK, Anstey AV. Rifampicin-induced lupus erythematosus. *Clin Exp Dermatol* 2001; **26**: 260–2.
27 Shakoor N, Michalska M, Harris CA, Block JA. Drug-induced systemic lupus erythematosus associated with etanercept therapy. *Lancet* 2002; **359**: 45–9.
28 Ghate JV, Turner ML, Rudek MA *et al*. Drug-induced lupus associated with COL-3. Report of 3 cases. *Arch Dermatol* 2001; **137**: 471–4.
29 Crosson J, Stillman MT. Minocycline-related lupus erythematosus with associated liver disease. *J Am Acad Dermatol* 1997; **36**: 867–8.
30 Elkayam O, Yaron M, Caspi D. Minocycline-induced autoimmune syndromes: an overview. *Semin Arthritis Rheum* 1999; **28**: 392–7.
31 Dunphy J, Oliver M, Rands AL *et al*. Antineutrophil cytoplasmic antibodies and HLA class II alleles in minocycline-induced lupus-like syndrome. *Br J Dermatol* 2000; **142**: 461–7.
32 Ross S, Dywer C, Ormerod AD *et al*. Subacute cutaneous lupus erythematosus associated with phenytoin. *Clin Exp Dermatol* 2002; **27**: 474–6.
33 Darken M, McBurney EI. Subacute cutaneous lupus erythematosus-like drug eruption due to combination diuretic hydrochlorothiazide and triamterene. *J Am Acad Dermatol* 1988; **18**: 38–42.
34 Wollenberg A, Meurer M. Thiazid-Diuretika-induzierter subakut-kutaner Lupus erythematodes. *Hautarzt* 1991; **42**: 709–12.
35 Goodrich AL, Kohn SR. Hydrochlorothiazide-induced lupus erythematosus: a new variant? *J Am Acad Dermatol* 1993; **28**: 1001–2.
36 Brown CW Jr, Deng JS. Thiazide diuretics induce cutaneous lupus-like adverse reaction. *J Toxicol Clin Toxicol* 1995; **33**: 729–33.
37 Callen JP, Fernandez-Diaz MC, Herranz P *et al*. Subacute cutaneous lupus erythematosus associated with cilazapril. *J Am Acad Dermatol* 1997; **37**: 781.
38 Patri P, Nigro A, Rebora A. Lupus erythematosus-like eruption from captopril. *Acta Derm Venereol (Stockh)* 1985; **65**: 447–8.
39 Crowson AN, Magro CM. Subacute cutaneous lupus erythematosus arising in the setting of calcium channel blocker therapy. *Hum Pathol* 1997; **28**: 67–73.
40 Brooke R, Coulson IH, Al-Dawoud A. Terbinafine-induced subacute cutaneous lupus erythematosus. *Br J Dermatol* 1998; **139**: 1132–3.

41 Bonsmann G, Schiller M, Luger TA. Terbinafine-induced subacute cutaneous lupus erythematosus. *J Am Acad Dermatol* 2001; **44**: 925–31.

42 Callen JP, Hughes AP, Kulp-Shorten CL. Terbinafine-exacerbated/induced subacute cutaneous lupus erythematosus: a report of 5 patients. *Arch Dermatol* 2001; **137**: 1196–8.

43 Miyagawa S, Okuchi T, Shiomo Y *et al.* Subacute cutaneous lupus erythematosus lesions precipitated by griseofulvin. *J Am Acad Dermatol* 1989; **21**: 343–6.

44 Furukawa F, Tachibana T, Imamura S, Tamura T. Oral contraceptive-induced lupus erythematosus in a Japanese woman. *J Dermatol* 1991; **18**: 56–8.

45 Petri M, Allbritton J. Antibiotic allergy in systemic lupus erythematosus: a case–control study. *J Rheumatol* 1992; **19**: 265–9.

Dermatomyositis reactions

Dermatomyositis has been reported to be precipitated by a variety of drugs, including penicillamine [1–3], NSAIDs (niflumic acid and diclofenac) [4], carbamazepine [5] and vaccination, as with BCG [6]. Acral skin lesions simulating chronic dermatomyositis have been reported during long-term hydroxyurea therapy [7]. Allergy to benzalkonium chloride has caused a dermatomyositis-like reaction [8].

REFERENCES

1 Simpson NB, Golding JR. Dermatomyositis induced by penicillamine. *Acta Derm Venereol (Stockh)* 1979; **59**: 543–4.

2 Wojnorowska F. Dermatomyositis induced by penicillamine. *J R Soc Med* 1980; **73**: 884–6.

3 Carroll GC, Will RK, Peter JB *et al.* Penicillamine induced polymyositis and dermatomyositis. *J Rheumatol* 1987; **14**: 995–1001.

4 Grob JJ, Collet AM, Bonerandi JJ. Dermatomyositis-like syndrome induced by nonsteroidal anti-inflammatory agents. *Dermatologica* 1989; **178**: 58–9.

5 Simpson JR. 'Collagen disease' due to carbamazepine (Tegretol). *BMJ* 1966; **ii**: 1434.

6 Kass E, Staume S, Mellbye OJ *et al.* Dermatomyositis associated with BCG vaccination. *Scand J Rheumatol* 1979; **8**: 187–91.

7 Richard M, Truchetet F, Friedel J *et al.* Skin lesions simulating chronic dermatomyositis during long-term hydroxyurea therapy. *J Am Acad Dermatol* 1989; **21**: 797–9.

8 Cox NH. Allergy to benzalkonium chloride simulating dermatomyositis. *Contact Dermatitis* 1994; **31**: 50.

Scleroderma-like reactions

Penicillamine [1,2], bleomycin [3,4], bromocriptine [5], vitamin K (phytomenadione) [6,7], sodium valproate [8] and 5-hydroxytryptophan combined with carbidopa [9,10] (see also the eosinophilia–myalgia syndrome below) have all been implicated in either localized or generalized morphoea-like, or systemic sclerosis-like, reactions. Eosinophilic fasciitis has been associated with tryptophan ingestion in some cases [11], as well as with phenytoin [12].

REFERENCES

1 Bernstein RM, Hall MA, Gostelow BE. Morphea-like reaction to D-penicillamine therapy. *Ann Rheum Dis* 1981; **40**: 42–4.

2 Miyagawa S, Yoshioka A, Hatoko M *et al.* Systemic sclerosis-like lesions during long-term penicillamine therapy for Wilson's disease. *Br J Dermatol* 1987; **116**: 95–100.

3 Finch WR, Rodnan GP, Buckingham RB *et al.* Bleomycin-induced scleroderma. *J Rheumatol* 1980; **7**: 651–9.

4 Snauwaert J, Degreef H. Bleomycin-induced Raynaud's phenomenon and acral sclerosis. *Dermatologica* 1984; **169**: 172–4.

5 Leshin B, Piette WW, Caplin RM. Morphea after bromocriptine therapy. *Int J Dermatol* 1989; **28**: 177–9.

6 Brunskill NJ, Berth-Jones J, Graham-Brown RAC. Pseudosclerodermatous reaction to phytomenadione injection (Texier's syndrome). *Clin Exp Dermatol* 1988; **13**: 276–8.

7 Pujol RM, Puig L, Moreno A *et al.* Pseudoscleroderma secondary to phytonadione (vitamin K1) injections. *Cutis* 1989; **43**: 365–8.

8 Goihman-Yahr M, Leal G, Essenfeld-Yahr E. Generalized morphea: a side effect of valproate sodium? *Arch Dermatol* 1980; **116**: 621.

9 Chamson A, Périer C, Frey J. Syndrome sclérodermiforme et poïkilodermique observé au cours d'un traitement par carbidopa et 5-hydroxytryptophanne. Culture de fibroblastes avec analyse biochimique du métabolisme du collagene. *Ann Dermatol Vénéréol* 1986; **113**: 71.

10 Joly P, Lampert A, Thomine E, Lauret P. Development of pseudo-bullous morphea and scleroderma-like illness during therapy with L-5-hydroxytryptophan and carbidopa. *J Am Acad Dermatol* 1991; **25**: 332–3.

11 Gordon ML, Lebwohl MG, Phelps RG *et al.* Eosinophilic fasciitis associated with tryptophan ingestion. A manifestation of eosinophilia–myalgia syndrome. *Arch Dermatol* 1991; **127**: 217–20.

12 Buchanan RR, Gordon DA, Muckle TJ *et al.* The eosinophilic fasciitis syndrome after phenytoin (Dilantin) therapy. *J Rheumatol* 1980; **7**: 733–6.

Chemical and industrial causes of scleroderma-like reactions [1]

Scleroderma-like changes formed part of the clinical spectrum of the Spanish toxic oil syndrome, which resulted from contamination of rapeseed cooking oil with acetanilide [2]. Scleroderma-like changes have been induced by industrial exposure to vinyl chloride [3], epoxy resins [1,4], organic solvents [5] including perchlorethylene [6], trichlorethylene and trichlorethane [7], and in coalminers due to silica exposure [8,9].

REFERENCES

1 Ishikawa O, Warita S, Tamura A, Miyachi Y. Occupational scleroderma. A 17-year follow-up study. *Br J Dermatol* 1995; **133**: 786–9.

2 Rush PJ, Bell MJ, Fam AG. Toxic oil syndrome (Spanish oil disease) and chemically induced scleroderma-like conditions. *J Rheumatol* 1984; **11**: 262–4.

3 Harris DK, Adams WGF. Acroosteolysis occurring in men engaged in the polymerisation of vinyl chloride. *BMJ* 1967; **3**: 712–24.

4 Yamakage A, Ishikawa H, Saito Y, Hattori A. Occupational scleroderma-like disorders occurring in men engaged in the polymerization of epoxy resins. *Dermatologica* 1980; **161**: 33–44.

5 Yamakage A, Ishikawa H. Generalized morphea-like scleroderma occurring in people exposed to organic solvents. *Dermatologica* 1982; **165**: 186–93.

6 Sparrow GP. A connective tissue disease similar to vinyl chloride disease in a patient exposed to perchlorethylene. *Clin Exp Dermatol* 1977; **2**: 17–22.

7 Flindt-Hansen H, Isager H. Scleroderma after occupational exposure to trichlorethylene and trichlorethane. *Acta Derm Venereol (Stockh)* 1987; **67**: 263–4.

8 Rodnan GP, Benedek TG, Medsger TA Jr, Cammarata RJ. The association of progressive systemic sclerosis (scleroderma) with coalminers' pneumoconiosis and other forms of silicosis. *Ann Intern Med* 1967; **66**: 323–4.

9 Rustin MHA, Bull HA, Ziegler V *et al.* Silica-associated systemic sclerosis is clinically, serologically and immunologically indistinguishable from idiopathic systemic sclerosis. *Br J Dermatol* 1990; **123**: 725–34.

Eosinophilia–myalgia syndrome

Ingestion of tryptophan, taken as a mild antidepressant, a 'natural hypnotic', or by athletes to increase pain tolerance, was associated with eosinophilia–myalgia syndrome [1–4], characterized by eosinophilia, myalgia, arthralgia, limb swelling, fever, weakness and fatigue, respiratory complaints, pulmonary hypertension, arrhythmias, ascending polyneuropathy and a variety of cutaneous manifestations. The latter included diffuse morbilliform erythema, urticaria, angio-oedema, dermatographism, livedo reticularis, alopecia and papular mucinosis. Some patients developed chronic muscle weakness, with diffuse scleroderma-like or fasciitis-like skin changes. The eosinophilia–myalgia syndrome is now thought to have been caused by a contaminant of L-tryptophan following a change in the manufacturing process between October 1988 and June 1989 [5,6].

REFERENCES

1 Kaufman LD, Seidman RJ, Phillips ME, Gruber BL. Cutaneous manifestations of the L-tryptophan-associated eosinophilia–myalgia syndrome: a spectrum of sclerodermatous skin disease. *J Am Acad Dermatol* 1990; **23**: 1063–9.
2 Reinauer S, Plewig G. Das Eosinophilie-Myalgie Syndrom. *Hautarzt* 1991; **42**: 137–9.
3 Gordon ML, Lebwohl MG, Phelps RG *et al.* Eosinophilic fasciitis associated with tryptophan ingestion. A manifestation of eosinophilia–myalgia syndrome. *Arch Dermatol* 1991; **127**: 217–20.
4 Connolly SM, Quimby SR, Griffing WL, Winkelmann RK. Scleroderma and L-tryptophan: a possible explanation of the eosinophilia–myalgia syndrome. *J Am Acad Dermatol* 1991; **23**: 451–7.
5 Slutsker L, Hoesly FC, Miller LM *et al.* Eosinophilia–myalgia syndrome associated with exposure to tryptophan from a single manufacturer. *JAMA* 1990; **264**: 213–7.
6 Mayeno AN, Lin F, Foote CS *et al.* Characterization of 'peak E', a novel amino acid associated with eosinophilia–myalgia syndrome. *Science* 1990; **250**: 1707–8.

Erythema nodosum [1]

Sulphonamides, other antibiotics [2], a variety of analgesics, antipyretics and anti-infectious agents, as well as the contraceptive pill [2–5], oestrogen replacement therapy [6], treatment of haematological disorders with granulocyte colony-stimulating factor [7], all-*trans*-retinoic acid [8] and *Echinacea* herbal therapy [9] have all been implicated in the aetiology of erythema nodosum. Erythema nodosum leprosum was induced by prolonged treatment with recombinant IFN-γ (in 60% of patients within 7 months) [10] and by co-trimoxazole [11].

REFERENCES

1 Bork K. *Cutaneous Side Effects of Drugs.* Philadelphia: Saunders, 1988.
2 Puavilai S, Sakuntabhai A, Sriprachaya-Anunt S *et al.* Etiology of erythema nodosum. *J Med Assoc Thailand* 1995; **78**: 72–5.
3 Posternal F, Orusco MMM, Laugier P. Eythème noueux et contraceptifs oraux. *Bull Dermatol* 1974; **81**: 642–5.
4 Bombardieri S, Di Munno O, Di Punzio C, Pasero G. Erythema nodosum associated with pregnancy and oral contraceptives. *BMJ* 1977; **i**: 1509–10.
5 Muller-Ladner U, Kaufmann R, Adler G, Scherbaum WA. Rezidivierendes Erythema nodosum nach Einnahme eines niedrig dosierten oralen Antikonzeptivums. *Med Klin* 1994; **89**: 100–2.
6 Yang SG, Han KH, Cho KH, Lee AY. Development of erythema nodosum in the course of oestrogen replacement therapy. *Br J Dermatol* 1997; **137**: 319–20.
7 Nomiyama J, Shinohara K, Inoue H. Erythema nodosum caused by the administration of granulocyte colony-stimulating factor in a patient with refractory anemia. *Am J Hematol* 1994; **47**: 333.
8 Hakimian D, Tallman MS, Zugerman C, Caro WA. Erythema nodosum associated with all-*trans*-retinoic acid in the treatment of acute promyelocytic leukemia. *Leukemia* 1993; **7**: 758–9.
9 Soon SL, Crawford RI. Recurrent erythema nodosum associated with *Echinacea* herbal therapy. *J Am Acad Dermatol* 2001; **44**: 298–9.
10 Sampaio EP, Moreira AL, Sarno EN *et al.* Prolonged treatment with recombinant interferon-gamma induces erythema nodosum leprosum in lepromatous leprosy patients. *J Exp Med* 1992; **175**: 1729–37.
11 Nishioka SA, Goulart IM, Burgarelli MK *et al.* Necrotizing erythema nodosum leprosum triggered by cotrimoxazole? *Int J Lepr Other Mycobact Dis* 1994; **62**: 296–7.

Pseudolymphomatous syndrome: anticonvulsant hypersensitivity syndrome

This syndrome should be differentiated from the drug hypersensitivity syndrome, which has a more acute onset (see above). A number of drugs may produce a reaction pattern that simulates a lymphoma [1–6]. Skin involvement may consist of erythematous plaques, multiple infiltrative papules or solitary nodules; there may be facial oedema. Pseudolymphomatous syndrome develops between 2 weeks and 5 years after starting drug therapy, but usually within 7 weeks. Histopathologically, there is epidermotropism of atypical lymphocytes, often with Pautrier's microabscess-like structures; pseudolymphomatous syndrome differs from mycosis fungoides in that there may be moderate to marked spongiosis, necrotic keratinocytes, epidermal eosinophils, papillary dermal oedema and extravasated erythrocytes, and a mixed dermal inflammatory infiltrate including neutrophils. Misdiagnosis of pseudolymphomatous syndrome as malignant lymphoma may lead to patients being treated unnecessarily with chemotherapy.

Phenytoin especially, but also phenobarbital and carbamazepine, mephenytoin, trimethadione and sodium valproate have been implicated [7–12]. Cutaneous lesions in patients with reactions to phenytoin or carbamazepine may show histological features of mycosis fungoides; cutaneous lesions resembling those of mycosis fungoides in the absence of fever have been reported with phenytoin and carbamazepine. Phenobarbital has produced a hypersensitivity syndrome resembling Langerhans' cell histiocytosis [13].

Other drugs have been associated with mycosis fungoides-like drug eruptions, including allopurinol, antidepressants (e.g. fluoxetine [14,15] and amitriptyline [15]), phenothiazines [16], thioridazine, benzodiazepines, antihistamines [4], β-blockers (e.g. atenolol [17]), ACE inhibitors [18], calcium channel blockers, salazosulfapyridine [19], lipid-lowering agents, mexiletine, ciclosporin [20], penicillamine, amiloride hydrochloride with hydrochlorothiazide, bromocriptine [21] and gemcitabine [22]. A generalized cutaneous B-cell pseudolymphoma was induced by neuroleptics [23]. Cutaneous T-cell lymphoma and Sézary syndrome have been reported in association with silicone breast implants [24,25].

Pseudolymphomatous syndrome usually responds to drug withdrawal, although not for many months in some cases [5]. Occasionally, a true lymphoma may develop.

REFERENCES

1 Kardaun SH, Scheffer E, Vermeer BJ. Drug-induced pseudolymphomatous skin reactions. *Br J Dermatol* 1988; **118**: 545–52.
2 Sigal M, Pulik M. Pseudolymphomes medicamenteux a expression cutanée predominante. *Ann Dermatol Vénéréol* 1993; **120**: 175–80.
3 Handfield-Jones SE, Jenkins RE, Whittaker SJ *et al.* The anticonvulsant hypersensitivity syndrome. *Br J Dermatol* 1993; **129**: 175–7.
4 Magro CM, Crowson AN. Drugs with antihistaminic properties as a cause of atypical cutaneous lymphoid hyperplasia. *J Am Acad Dermatol* 1995; **32**: 419–28.
5 Magro CM, Crowson AN. Drug-induced immune dysregulation as a cause of atypical cutaneous lymphoid infiltrates: a hypothesis. *Hum Pathol* 1996; **27**: 125–32.
6 Choi TS, Doh KS, Kim SH *et al.* Clinicopathological and genotypic aspects of anticonvulsant-induced pseudolymphoma syndrome. *Br J Dermatol* 2003; **148**: 730–6.
7 Wolf R, Kahane E, Sandbank M. Mycosis fungoides-like lesions associated with phenytoin therapy. *Arch Dermatol* 1985; **121**: 1181–2.
8 Rijlaarsdam U, Scheffer E, Meijer CJLM *et al.* Mycosis fungoides-like lesions associated with phenytoin and carbamazepine therapy. *J Am Acad Dermatol* 1991; **24**: 216–20.
9 Shuttleworth D, Graham-Brown RAC, Williams AJ *et al.* Pseudo-lymphoma associated with carbamazepine. *Clin Exp Dermatol* 1984; **9**: 421–3.
10 Welykyj S, Gradini R, Nakao J, Massa M. Carbamazepine-induced eruption histologically mimicking mycosis fungoides. *J Cutan Pathol* 1990; **17**: 111–6.
11 Nathan DL, Belsito DV. Carbamazepine-induced pseudolymphoma with CD-30 positive cells. *J Am Acad Dermatol* 1998; **38**: 806–9.
12 Cogrel O, Beylot-Barry M, Vergier B *et al.* Sodium valproate-induced cutaneous pseudolymphoma followed by recurrence with carbamazepine. *Br J Dermatol* 2001; **144**: 1235–8.
13 Nagata T, Kawamura N, Motoyama T *et al.* A case of hypersensitivity syndrome resembling Langerhans cell histiocytosis during phenobarbital prophylaxis for convulsion. *Jpn J Clin Oncol* 1992; **22**: 421–7.
14 Gordon KB, Guitart J, Kuzel T *et al.* Pseudomycosis fungoides in a patient taking clonazepam and fluoxetine. *J Am Acad Dermatol* 1996; **34**: 304–6.
15 Crowson AN, Magro CM. Antidepressant therapy. A possible cause of atypical cutaneous lymphoid hyperplasia. *Arch Dermatol* 1995; **131**: 925–9.
16 Blazejak T, Hölzle E. Phenothiazin-induziertes Pseudolymphom. *Hautarzt* 1990; **41**: 161–3.
17 Henderson CA, Shamy HK. Atenolol-induced pseudolymphoma. *Clin Exp Dermatol* 1990; **15**: 119–20.
18 Furness PN, Goodfield MJ, MacLennan KA *et al.* Severe cutaneous reactions to captopril and enalapril: histological study and comparison with early mycosis fungoides. *J Clin Pathol* 1986; **39**: 902–7.
19 Gallais V, Grange F, De Bandt M *et al.* Toxidermie a la salazosulfapyridine. Erythrodermie pustuleuse et syndrome pseudolymphomateux: 2 observations. *Ann Dermatol Vénéréol* 1994; **121**: 11–4.
20 Harman KE, Morris SD, Higgins EM. Persistent anticonvulsant hypersensitivity syndrome responding to ciclosporin. *Clin Exp Dermatol* 2003; **28**: 364–5.
21 Wiesli P, Joos L, Galeazzi RL, Dummer R. Cutaneous pseudolymphoma associated with bromocriptine therapy. *Clin Endocrinol* 2000; **53**: 656–7.
22 Marucci G, Sgarbanti E, Maestri A *et al.* Gemcitabine-associated CD8+ CD30+ pseudolymphoma. *Br J Dermatol* 2001; **145**: 650–2.
23 Luelmo Aguilar J, Mieras Barcelo C, Martin-Urda MT *et al.* Generalized cutaneous B-cell pseudolymphoma induced by neuroleptics. *Arch Dermatol* 1992; **128**: 121–3.
24 Duvic M, Moore D, Menter A, Vonderheid EC. Cutaneous T-cell lymphoma in association with silicone breast implants. *J Am Acad Dermatol* 1995; **32**: 939–42.
25 Sena E, Ledo A. Sézary syndrome in association with silicone breast implant. *J Am Acad Dermatol* 1995; **33**: 1060–1.

Acanthosis nigricans-like and ichthyosiform eruptions

See Chapter 34.

Erythromelalgia [1]

Drugs implicated include iodide contrast media, vaccines (influenza and hepatitis), nifedipine, felodipine, nicardipine, bromocriptine, norephedrine, pergolide and ticlopidine.

REFERENCE

1 Cohen JS. Erythromelalgia: new theories and new therapies. *J Am Acad Dermatol* 2000; **43**: 841–7.

Hair changes (see also Chapter 63)

Drug-induced alopecia

A considerable number of drugs have been reported to cause hair loss [1–5]; the most important causes are listed in Table 73.16. Cytotoxic drugs may cause alopecia by either anagen or telogen effluvium. Chemotherapeutic agents implicated in the production of alopecia include amsacrine, bleomycin, cyclophosphamide, cytarabine, dactinomycin, daunorubicin, doxorubicin, etoposide, fluorouracil, methotrexate and the nitrosoureas [2]. Telogen alopecia has been caused by anticoagulants (heparins and coumarins), antithyroid drugs (carbimazole and thiouracils), levodopa, propranolol, albendazole and oral contraceptives. Retinoids cause alopecia by disrupting

Table 73.16 Drugs causing alopecia.

Anticoagulants	Retinoids
Coumarins	Acitretin
Dextran	Etretinate
Heparin	Isotretinoin
Heparinoids	Miscellaneous
Anticonvulsants	Albendazole
Carbamazepine	Allopurinol
Valproic acid	Amfetamine (amphetamine)
Cytotoxic agents	Antithyroid drugs
Drugs acting on the central	Bromocriptine
nervous system	Captopril
Amitriptyline	Cholestyramine
Doxepin	Cimetidine
Haloperidol	Dixyrazine
Lithium	Gentamicin
Hypocholesterolaemic agents	Gold
Clofibrate	Ibuprofen
Nicotinic acid	Levodopa
Triparanol	Metoprolol
Antithyroid drugs	Oral contraceptives
Carbimazole	Propranolol
Thiouracils	Trimethadione

Table 73.17 Drugs causing hypertrichosis.

Androgens	Penicillamine
Corticosteroids	Phenytoin
Ciclosporin	Psoralens
Diazoxide	Streptomycin
Minoxidil	

keratinization. Hydantoins may cause scalp alopecia and hypertrichosis elsewhere, and clofibrate may cause alopecia by interfering with keratinization. Temporary hair loss has been described after 5-aminosalicylic acid enemas [6] and bromocriptine [7], and danazol has induced generalized alopecia [8]. Certain β-blockers have caused increased hair loss [9–11] as have dixyrazine [12] and ibuprofen [13].

Drug-induced hirsutism and hypertrichosis

The hirsutism induced in women by corticosteroids, androgens and certain progestogens is well recognized. Other drugs that may cause hypertrichosis are listed in Table 73.17 [3,4]. Up to 50% of children treated with diazoxide, and up to 40% of patients on ciclosporin, develop hypertrichosis. Zidovudine has caused excessive growth of eyelashes [14].

REFERENCES

1 Brodin MB. Drug-related alopecia. *Dermatol Clin* 1987; **5**: 571–9.
2 Kerber BJ, Hood AF. Chemotherapy-induced cutaneous reactions. *Semin Dermatol* 1989; **8**: 173–81.
3 Rook A, Dawber R. *Diseases of the Hair and Scalp*, 2nd edn. Oxford: Blackwell Scientific Publications, 1990.
4 Merk HF. Drugs affecting hair growth. In: Orfanos CE, Happle R, eds. *Hair and Hair Diseases*. Berlin: Springer, 1990: 601–9.
5 Pillans PI, Woods DJ. Drug-associated alopecia. *Int J Dermatol* 1995; **34**: 149–58.
6 Kutty PK, Raman KRK, Hawken K, Barrowman JA. Hair loss and 5-aminosalicylic acid enemas. *Ann Intern Med* 1982; **97**: 785–6.
7 Blum I, Leiba S. Increased hair loss as a side effect of bromocriptine treatment. *N Engl J Med* 1980; **303**: 1418.
8 Duff P, Mayer AR. Generalized alopecia: an unusual complication of danazol therapy. *Am J Obstet Gynecol* 1981; **141**: 349–50.
9 England JR, England JD. Alopecia and propranolol therapy. *Aust Fam Physician* 1982; **11**: 225–6.
10 Graeber CW, Lapkin RA. Metoprolol and alopecia. *Cutis* 1981; **28**: 633–4.
11 Fraunfelder FT, Meyer SM, Menacker SJ. Alopecia possibly secondary to topical ophthalmic β-blockers. *JAMA* 1990; **263**: 1493–4.
12 Poulsen J. Hair loss, depigmentation of hair, ichthyosis, and blepharoconjunctivitis produced by dixyrazine. *Acta Derm Venereol (Stockh)* 1981; **61**: 85–8.
13 Meyer HC. Alopecia associated with ibuprofen. *JAMA* 1979; **242**: 142.
14 Klutman NE, Hinthorn DR. Excessive growth of eyelashes in a patient with AIDS being treated with zidovudine. *N Engl J Med* 1991; **324**: 1896.

Drug-induced hair discoloration (see Chapter 63)

Drug-induced change in hair colour, usually occurring 3–12 months after the onset of treatment, is a rare but well-recognized phenomenon [1,2]. Darkening of hair has occurred during treatment with verapamil [3], tamoxifen [4], carbidopa [5] and PABA. Etretinate has caused darkening as well as lightening, curling and kinking of hair [6]. Greying of hair has been reported with chloroquine and mephenesin [7]. Chloroquine depigmentation is reversible and occurs only in red- or blonde-haired individuals; both IFN-α [8] and chloroquine are capable of arresting phaeomelanin synthesis.

REFERENCES

1 Rook A. Some chemical influences on hair growth and pigmentation. *Br J Dermatol* 1965; **77**: 115–29.
2 Bublin JG, Thompson DF. Drug-induced hair colour changes. *Clin Pharmacol Ther* 1992; **17**: 297–302.
3 Read GM. Verapamil and hair colour change. *Lancet* 1991; **338**: 1520.
4 Hampson JP, Donnelly A, Lewisones MS, Pye JK. Tamoxifen induced hair colour change. *Br J Dermatol* 1995; **132**: 483–4.
5 Reynolds NJ, Crossley J, Ferguson I, Peachey RDG. Darkening of white hair in Parkinson's disease. *Clin Exp Dermatol* 1989; **14**: 317–8.
6 Vesper JL, Fenske A. Hair darkening and new growth associated with etretinate therapy. *J Am Acad Dermatol* 1996; **34**: 860.
7 Spillane JD. Brunette to blonde. Depigmentation of hair during treatment with oral mephenesin. *BMJ* 1963; **i**: 997–8.
8 Fleming CJ, MacKie RM. Alpha interferon-induced hair discolouration. *Br J Dermatol* 1996; **135**: 337–8.

Nail changes

Drug-induced nail abnormalities have been the subject of several reviews [1–7] (see Chapter 62). Heavy metals may induce the following changes: arsenic causes transverse, broad, white lines (Mee's lines); silver causes blue discoloration of the lunulae; gold results in thin and brittle nails with longitudinal streaking, yellow-brown discoloration and onycholysis; and lead produces partial leukonychia. Penicillamine therapy is associated with the yellow nail syndrome and nail dystrophy. Cytotoxic agents may produce transverse or longitudinal pigmentation, splinter haemorrhages, Beau's lines, leukonychia, Mee's lines, onycholysis, shortening of lunulae, pallor, atrophy, nail shedding and slow growth; acute paronychia has occurred with methotrexate. The β-blockers may induce a psoriasiform nail dystrophy, with onycholysis and subungual hyperkeratosis. Thiazide diuretics may result in onycholysis. Discoloration or pigmentation occurs with antimalarials (blue-brown discoloration), lithium (golden discoloration), phenolphthalein (dark-blue discoloration), phenothiazines (blue-black or purple pigmentation), phenytoin (pigmentation), psoralens and tetracyclines (yellow pigmentation). Oral contraceptives may induce photo-onycholysis and onycholysis, and are associated with an increased growth rate and reduced splitting and fragility. In contrast, heparin reduces nail growth and causes transverse banding and subungual haematomas. Retinoids cause thinning and increased fragility, onychoschizia, onycholysis, temporary nail shedding, onychomadesis, ingrowing nails, periungual granulation tissue and paronychia.

Table 73.18 Drugs causing onycholysis.

Antibiotics	*Miscellaneous*
Cefaloridine (cephaloridine)	Acridine
Cloxacillin	Captopril
Chloramphenicol	Norethindrone and mestranol
Chlortetracycline	Practolol (discontinued)
Demethylchlortetracycline	Psoralens
Doxycycline	Phenothiazines
Fluoroquinolones	Retinoids
Minocycline	Sulpha-related drugs
Tetracycline hydrochloride	Thiazides
Chemotherapeutic agents	*Photo-onycholysis*
Adriamycin	Oral contraceptives
Bleomycin	Psoralens
5-Fluorouracil	Fluoroquinolones
Mitoxantrone	Tetracyclines

Onycholysis

Drugs causing onycholysis [6,7] and photo-onycholysis are listed in Table 73.18.

REFERENCES

1 Daniel CR III, Scher RK. Nail changes secondary to systemic drugs or ingestants. *J Am Acad Dermatol* 1984; **10**: 250–8.
2 Fenton DA. Nail changes due to drugs. In: Samman PD, Fenton DA, eds. *The Nails in Disease*, 4th edn. London: Heinemann, 1986: 121–5.
3 Fenton DA, Wilkinson JD. The nail in systemic diseases and drug-induced changes. In: Baran R, Dawber RPR, eds. *Diseases of the Nails and Their Management*. Oxford: Blackwell Scientific Publications, 1984: 205–65.
4 Daniel CR III, Scher RK. Nail changes secondary to systemic drugs or ingestants. In: Scher RK, Daniel CR III, eds. *Nails: Therapy, Diagnosis, Surgery*. Philadelphia: Saunders, 1990: 192–201.
5 Zaias N. *The Nail in Health and Disease*, 2nd edn. East Norwalk, CT: Appleton Lange, 1990.
6 Baran R, Juhlin L. Drug-induced photo-onycholysis. Three subtypes identified in a study of 15 cases. *J Am Acad Dermatol* 1987; **17**: 1012–6.
7 Daniel CR. Onycholysis: an overview. *Semin Dermatol* 1991; **10**: 34–40.

Oral conditions (see also Chapter 66)

ADRs affecting the mouth have been extensively reviewed [1–4]. Disturbance of taste has been reported with a wide variety of drugs [5,6], including captopril, griseofulvin, metronidazole and protease inhibitor antiretrovirals. Orofacial effects of antiretroviral therapies have been reviewed [6]. These include mouth ulcers due to bone marrow suppression, erythema multiforme (e.g. with didanosine), lichenoid reactions with zidovudine, xerostomia (seen in up to one-third of patients taking didanosine), oral and perioral paraesthesiae (especially with ritonavir), and cheilitis with indinavir.

Xerostomia

Dryness of the mouth (xerostomia) may result from anticholinergic side effects of drugs. Xerostomia has been recorded in association with antidepressants, tranquil-

Table 73.19 Drugs associated with xerostomia.

Antidepressants (tricyclic)	Minor tranquillizers
Amitriptyline	Diazepam
Doxepin	Chordiazepoxide
Imipramine	Hydroxyzine
Antidepressants (monoamine	Antiparkinsonian drugs
oxidase inhibitors)	Antihypertensives (ganglion
Isocarboxazid	blockers)
Phenelzine	Gastrointestinal antispasmodics
Psychotropic agents	Atropine
Chlorpromazine	Propantheline bromide
Thioridazine	Phenobarbital (phenobarbitone)
Haloperidol	
Prochlorperazine	

lizers, antiparkinsonian drugs, antihypertensives and gastrointestinal antispasmodics (Table 73.19). Parotitis with salivary sialadenitis has been reported in up to 15% of patients taking phenylbutazone, and may be associated with fever and a rash [7]. A similar syndrome may occur with repeated administration of iodinated contrast media [8] and with nitrofurantoin [9].

REFERENCES

1 Zelickson BD, Rogers RS III. Drug reactions involving the mouth. *Clin Dermatol* 1986; **4**: 98–109.
2 Korstanje MJ. Drug-induced mouth disorders. *Clin Exp Dermatol* 1995; **20**: 10–8.
3 Parks ET. Lesions associated with drug reactions. *Dermatol Clin* 1996; **14**: 327–37.
4 Porter SR, Scully C. Adverse drug reactions in the mouth. *Clin Dermatol* 2000; **18**: 525–32.
5 Griffin JP. Drug-induced disorders of taste. *Adverse Drug React Toxicol Rev* 1992; **11**: 229–39.
6 Scully C, Diz Dios P. Orofacial effects of antiretroviral therapies. *Oral Dis* 2001; **7**: 205–10.
7 Speed BR, Spelman DW. Sialadenitis and systemic reactions associated with phenylbutazone. *Aust NZ J Med* 1982; **12**: 261–4.
8 Chohen JC, Roxe DM, Said R *et al.* Iodide mumps after repeated exposure to iodinated contrast media. *Lancet* 1980; **i**: 762–3.
9 Meyboom RH, van Gent A, Zinkstok DJ. Nitrofurantoin-induced parotitis. *BMJ* 1982; **285**: 1049.

Stomatitis

Type I immediate hypersensitivity and type IV delayed hypersensitivity reactions may be involved in allergic stomatitis [1]. The allergic stomatitides may present with clinical appearances that mimic classic oral vesiculobullous and ulcerative lesions. Stomatitis may form a part of drug-induced lichenoid reactions, fixed drug reactions or erythema multiforme, but may also arise separately from these conditions as a side effect of a number of drugs (Table 73.20). Chemotherapeutic agents causing stomatitis or buccal ulceration include [2] actinomycin D, adriamycin, amsacrine, bleomycin, busulfan, chlorambucil, cyclophosphamide, dactinomycin, daunorubicin, doxorubicin, fluorouracil, IL-2, mercaptopurine, methotrexate, mithramycin, mitomycin, nitrosoureas, procar-

Table 73.20 Drugs causing stomatitis or buccal ulceration.

Chemotherapeutic agents	Antihypertensive agents
Antirheumatic drugs	Captopril
Gold	Hydralazine
Naproxen	Methyldopa (rare)
Indometacin (indomethacin)	Miscellaneous
Penicillamine	Chlorpromazine
Zomepirac	Valproic acid
Antidepressants	
Amitriptyline	
Doxepin	
Imipramine	

bazine and vincristine. Penicillamine may induce stomatitis or ulceration as part of drug-induced pemphigus [3] or a lichenoid drug eruption. Gold therapy is another well-recognized cause of stomatitis [4–6]. Allergic reactions to dental materials and therapy may cause stomatitis. Positive patch tests to mercuric chloride were seen in 42%, and to copper sulphate in 16%, of patients with oral mucosal lesions associated with amalgam restorations, compared with 9% of controls, in one series [7]. It has been postulated that mercury released from dental amalgams can cause hypersensitivity/toxic reactions resulting in lichen planus lesions, and may play a major role in the pathogenesis of gingivitis, periodontitis and periodontal disease [8]. Mercuric chloride caused statistically significant increased IFN-γ release, but not proliferation, in lymphocyte cultures from patients with hypersensitivity to amalgam restorations [9]. β-Blockers have been implicated in aphthous ulcers [10].

REFERENCES

1 Jainkittivong A, Langlais RP. Allergic stomatitis. *Semin Dermatol* 1994; **13**: 91–101.
2 Kerker BJ, Hood AF. Chemotherapy-induced cutaneous reactions. *Semin Dermatol* 1989; **8**: 173–81.
3 Hay KD, Muller HK, Rade PC. D-Penicillamine-induced mucocutaneous lesions with features of pemphigus. *Oral Surg* 1978; **45**: 385–95.
4 Glenert U. Drug stomatitis due to gold therapy. *Oral Surg* 1984; **58**: 52–6.
5 Gall H. Allergien auf zahnärztliche Werkstoffe und Dentalpharmaka. *Hautarzt* 1983; **34**: 326–31.
6 Wiesenfeld D, Ferguson MM, Forsyth A *et al.* Allergy to dental gold. *Oral Surg* 1984; **57**: 158–60.
7 Nordlind K, Liden S. Patch test reactions to metal salts in patients with oral mucosal lesions associated with amalgam restorations. *Contact Dermatitis* 1992; **27**: 157–60.
8 Swartzendruber DE. The possible relationship between mercury from dental amalgam and diseases. I. Effects within the oral cavity. *Med Hypotheses* 1993; **41**: 31–4.
9 Nordlind K, Liden S. In vitro lymphocyte reactivity to heavy metal salts in the diagnosis of oral mucosal hypersensitivity to amalgam restorations. *Br J Dermatol* 1993; **128**: 38–41.
10 Boulinguez S, Reix S, Bedane C *et al.* Role of drug exposure in aphthous ulcers: a case–control study. *Br J Dermatol* 2000; **143**: 1261–5.

Hyperpigmentation

Hyperpigmentation of the buccal mucosa may occur with chemotherapeutic agents [1]. Oestrogen is associated with gingival hypermelanosis [2]. Amalgam tattoos with localized hyperpigmentation of the buccal mucosa result from implantation of amalgam in soft tissues, especially of the gingival or alveolar mucosa [3].

Reactions caused by antibacterial, antifungal and immunosuppressive therapy

Systemic antibiotics or immunosuppressive medication [4], and corticosteroids administered by aerosol [5], may lead to the development of candidiasis of the buccal mucosa. Black hairy tongue may be associated with broad-spectrum antibiotic therapy and with griseofulvin treatment.

Gingival hyperplasia

Gingival hyperplasia may be caused by phenytoin [6], nifedipine [7], diltiazem [8], felodipine, verapamil and ciclosporin [9].

REFERENCES

1 Krutchik AN, Buzdar AU. Pigmentation of the tongue and mucous membranes associated with cancer chemotherapy. *South Med J* 1979; **72**: 1615–6.
2 Hertz RS, Beckstead PC, Brown WJ. Epithelial melanosis of the gingiva possibly resulting from the use of oral contraceptives. *J Am Dent Assoc* 1980; **100**: 713–4.
3 Buchner A, Hansen LS. Amalgam pigmentation (amalgam tattoo) of the oral mucosa: a clinicopathologic study of 268 cases. *Oral Surg* 1980; **49**: 139–47.
4 Torack RM. Fungus infections associated with antibiotic and steroid therapy. *Am J Med* 1957; **22**: 872–82.
5 Chervinsky P, Petraco AJ. Incidence of oral candidiasis during therapy with triamcinolone acetonide aerosol. *Ann Allergy* 1979; **43**: 80–3.
6 Hassell TM, Page RC, Narayanan AS, Cooper CG. Diphenylhydantoin (Dilantin) gingival hyperplasia: drug induced abnormality of connective tissue. *Proc Natl Acad Sci USA* 1976; **73**: 2909–12.
7 Benini PL, Crosti C, Sala F *et al.* Gingival hyperplasia by nifedipine. Report of a case. *Acta Derm Venereol (Stockh)* 1985; **65**: 362–5.
8 Giustiniani S, Robustelli della Cuna F, Marieni M. Hyperplastic gingivitis during diltiazem therapy. *Int J Cardiol* 1987; **15**: 247–9.
9 Frosch PJ, Ruder H, Stiefel A *et al.* Gingivahyperplasie und Seropapeln unter Cyclosporinbehandlung. *Hautarzt* 1988; **39**: 611–6.

Important or widely prescribed drugs

Antibacterial agents

β-Lactam antibiotics

Inaccurate histories of allergy to antibiotics are frequently documented in medical records by hospital doctors [1]. Reactions to β-lactam antibiotics may be immediate, accelerated or delayed [2–5]. Non-immediate reactions to penicillins are a reproducible phenomenon, suggesting that a specific mechanism is responsible [6]. In one study, 39% of 74 subjects with a cutaneous reaction to a penicillin derivative had a non-immediate reaction, in 93% to an aminopenicillin (10.3% ampicillin, 82.7% amoxicillin).

There was a positive delayed direct challenge and a delayed skin-test response in 65% of cases, and a lympho-monocytic infiltrate on skin biopsy [6]. Cross-reactivity exists between several members of this group of antibiotics, but restricted sensitivity to a single penicillin derivative also occurs [7]. As a group, penicillins had a higher frequency of allergic reactions than cephalosporins in a study of patients with cystic fibrosis treated with parenteral β-lactam antibiotics [8]. Serum sickness reactions occur [9]. (See also acute generalized exanthematous pustulosis, p. 73.35.)

REFERENCES

1 Absy M, Glatt AE. Antibiotic allergy: inaccurate history taking in a teaching hospital. *South Med J* 1994; **87**: 805–7.
2 Vega JM, Blanca M, Garcia JJ *et al.* Immediate allergic reactions to amoxicillin. *Allergy* 1994; **49**: 317–22.
3 Warrington RJ, Silviu-Dan F, Magro C. Accelerated cell-mediated immune reactions in penicillin allergy. *J Allergy Clin Immunol* 1993; **92**: 626–8.
4 Ortiz-Frutos FJ, Quintana I, Soto T *et al.* Delayed hypersensitivity to penicillin. *Allergy* 1996; **51**: 134–5.
5 Lopez Serrano C, Villas F, Cabanas R, Contreras J. Delayed hypersensitivity to beta-lactams. *J Invest Allergol Clin Immunol* 1994; **4**: 315–9.
6 Terrados S, Blanca M, Garcia J *et al.* Nonimmediate reactions to betalactams: prevalence and role of the different penicillins. *Allergy* 1995; **50**: 563–7.
7 Blanca M, Vega JM, Garcia J *et al.* New aspects of allergic reactions to betalactams: crossreactions and unique specificities. *Clin Exp Allergy* 1994; **24**: 407–15.
8 Pleasants RA, Walker TR, Samuelson WM. Allergic reactions to parenteral beta-lactam antibiotics in patients with cystic fibrosis. *Chest* 1994; **106**: 1124–8.
9 Tatum AJ, Ditto AM, Patterson R. Severe serum sickness-like reaction to oral penicillin drugs: three case reports. *Ann Allergy Asthma Immunol* 2001; **86**: 330–4.

Penicillin

Toxic reactions to penicillin are extremely rare and usually only follow massive doses, but can occur with normal doses in patients with renal impairment; encephalopathy with epilepsy may result from binding of the β-lactam ring to γ-aminobutyric acid receptors [1]. In contrast, immunological reactions are common [2–4]; allergy to penicillin has been reported in up to 10% of patients treated [5]. All forms of penicillin, including the semisynthetic penicillins, are potentially cross-allergenic; in general, allergic reactions to semi-synthetic compounds are commoner than to natural penicillins. All four types of immunological reaction may occur: urticaria and anaphylactic shock (type I), haemolytic anaemia or agranulocytosis (type II), allergic vasculitis or serum sickness-like reaction (type III) and allergic contact dermatitis [6] (type IV). Immediate reactions occur within 1 h, and take the form of urticaria, laryngeal oedema, bronchospasm and/or anaphylactic shock. So-called accelerated reactions with the same clinical features develop 1–72 h later. Reactions occurring more than 72 h after exposure are termed late reactions; these include maculopapular rashes with scarlatiniform and morbilliform exanthems, urticaria,

serum sickness, erythema multiforme, haemolytic anaemia, thrombocytopenia and neutropenia. Fever is the commonest reaction.

The antigenic structures responsible for penicillin allergy include a 'major determinant', the penicilloyl group formed by spontaneous hydrolysis of penicillin (penicilloyl polylysine is used for skin testing), and additional antigenic compounds to which benzylpenicillin is metabolized, termed 'minor determinants' [3]. Most immediate-type anaphylactic hypersensitivity reactions are mediated by IgE antibodies to minor antigenic determinants, whereas accelerated reactions are usually the result of IgE antibodies directed against the major antigenic determinant [3,7]. For information on skin testing for penicillin, see the diagnosis section at the end of the chapter (p. 73.174).

Anaphylactic reactions to penicillin reportedly occur in about 0.015% of treatment courses; fatal reactions occur in 0.0015–0.002% (i.e. 1 in 50 000 to 1 in 100 000) of treatment courses [8]. Young and middle-aged adults aged 20–49 years are at most risk [9]. Atopy does not augment the risk of a reaction to β-lactam antibiotics, but may increase the risk of any reaction being severe [3]. Anaphylaxis is commoner after parenteral administration, and is very rare, but has been recorded, after oral ingestion [9]. Maculopapular reactions occur in about 2% of treatment courses [3]; where there is a history of a prior penicillin reaction, the risk of a subsequent reaction increases to about 10% [10]. A fair proportion (33% in one study) of children may lose their skin-test reactivity within a year [11]. In practice, when penicillin is given to children said to be allergic to penicillin, very few experience an adverse reaction [7]. In adults, the rate of disappearance of penicillin-specific IgE is highly variable, from 10 days to indefinite persistence [3]. For a group of penicillin-allergic patients, the time lapsed since a previous reaction is inversely related to the risk of a further IgE-mediated reaction [10]. In one study, 80–90% of patients were skin-test positive 2 months after an acute allergic reaction, but less than 20% were skin-test positive 10 years later [12]. Nevertheless, patients with a prior history of an IgE-dependent reaction remain at risk of recurrence, even though IgE antibodies become undetectable by skin testing [13]. Most serious and fatal allergic reactions to β-lactam antibiotics occur in individuals who have never had a prior allergic reaction; a negative history should therefore not induce a false sense of security [3]. Continuous prophylactic treatment is associated with a very low incidence of reactions [14].

Activation of allergy in a sensitized individual may require only minute amounts of the drug, as from contaminated syringes, dental root-canal fillings, viral vaccines, contaminated milk or meat products, and contamination of transfused blood [15]. Urticaria and wheezing occurred in the penicillin-sensitive spouse of a man receiving parenteral mezlocillin, and was postulated to have arisen as a result of seminal fluid transmission of penicillin [16]. Hypersensitivity reactions have occurred after intrauterine placement, in penicillin-sensitive patients, of spermatozoa or embryos exposed to penicillin *in vitro* [17].

Penicillin has been reported to cause erythema multiforme [18], vesicular and bullous eruptions, exfoliative dermatitis [19], vascular purpura or fixed eruptions, postinflammatory elastolysis (cutis laxa), which was generalized and eventually fatal in one case [20], and a very few cases of pemphigus vulgaris [21,22], pemphigoid [23] and pustular psoriasis [24]. It has been proposed that penicillin may have a role in chronic 'idiopathic' urticaria [25].

Cloxacillin and flucloxacillin

Cloxacillins cross-react with penicillins, but unlike ampicillin do not produce distinctive eruptions. Flucloxacillin rarely elicits primary penicillin hypersensitivity. In one case report, parenteral cloxacillin was tolerated but oral administration caused progressive generalized erythema with pruritus, facial angio-oedema and tachycardia [27]. Flucloxacillin has been implicated as a cause of cholestatic jaundice; this complication is rare, and the risk is greater in elderly patients and those receiving therapy for more than 2 weeks [27].

REFERENCES

1 Barrons RW, Murray KM, Richey RM. Populations at risk for penicillin-induced seizures. *Ann Pharmacother* 1992; **26**: 26–9.
2 Erffmeyer JE. Penicillin allergy. *Clin Rev Allergy* 1986; **4**: 171–88.
3 Weiss ME, Adkinson NF. Immediate hypersensitivity reactions to penicillin and related antibiotics. *Clin Allergy* 1988; **18**: 515–40.
4 Weber EA, Knight A. Testing for allergy to antibiotics. *Semin Dermatol* 1989; **8**: 204–12.
5 Van Arsdael PP. The risk of penicillin reactions. *Ann Intern Med* 1968; **69**: 1071.
6 Stejskal VDM, Forsbeck M, Olin R. Side chain-specific lymphocyte responses in workers with occupational allergy induced by penicillins. *Int Arch Allergy Appl Immunol* 1987; **82**: 461–4.
7 Anonymous. Penicillin allergy in childhood. *Lancet* 1989; **i**: 420.
8 Idsøe O, Guthe T, Willcox RR, de Weck AL. Nature and extent of penicillin side reactions, with particular reference to fatalities from anaphylactic shock. *Bull WHO* 1968; **38**: 159–88.
9 Simmonds J, Hodges S, Nicol F, Barnett D. Anaphylaxis after oral penicillin. *BMJ* 1978; **ii**: 1404.
10 Sogn DD. Penicillin allergy. *J Allergy Clin Immunol* 1984; **74**: 589–93.
11 Chandra RK, Joglekar SA, Tomas E. Penicillin allergy: anti-penicillin IgE antibodies and immediate hypersensitivity skin reactions employing major and minor determinants of penicillin. *Arch Dis Child* 1980; **55**: 857–60.
12 Sullivan TJ, Wedner JH, Shatz GS et al. Skin testing to detect penicillin allergy. *J Allergy Clin Immunol* 1981; **68**: 171–80.
13 Adkinson NF Jr. Risk factors for drug allergy. *J Allergy Clin Immunol* 1984; **74**: 567–72.
14 Wood HF, Simpson R, Feinstein AR et al. Rheumatic fever in children and adolescents. A long-term epidemiologic study of subsequent prophylaxis, streptococcal infections, and clinical sequelae. I. Description of the investigative techniques and the population studied. *Ann Intern Med* 1964; **60** (Suppl. 5): 6–17.
15 Michel J, Sharon R. Non-haemolytic adverse reaction after transfusion of a blood unit containing penicillin. *BMJ* 1980; **i**: 152–3.
16 Burks JH, Fliegalman R, Sokalski SJ. An unforeseen complication of home parenteral antibiotic therapy. *Arch Intern Med* 1989; **149**: 1603–4.
17 Smith YR, Hurd WW, Menge AC et al. Allergic reactions to penicillin during in vitro fertilization and intrauterine insemination. *Fertil Steril* 1992; **58**: 847–9.
18 Staretz LR, Deboom GW. Multiple oral and skin lesions occurring after treatment with penicillin. *J Am Dent Assoc* 1990; **121**: 436–7.
19 Levine BB. Skin rashes with penicillin therapy: current management. *N Engl J Med* 1972; **286**: 42–3.
20 Kerl H, Burg G, Hashimoto K. Fatal, penicillin-induced, generalized, post-inflammatory elastolysis (cutis laxa). *Am J Dermatopathol* 1983; **5**: 267–76.
21 Duhra PL, Foulds IS. Penicillin-induced pemphigus vulgaris. *Br J Dermatol* 1988; **118**: 307.
22 Fellner MJ, Mark AS. Penicillin- and ampicillin-induced pemphigus vulgaris. *Int J Dermatol* 1980; **19**: 392–3.
23 Alcalay J, David M, Ingber A et al. Bullous pemphigoid mimicking bullous erythema multiforme: an untoward side effect of penicillins. *J Am Acad Dermatol* 1988; **18**: 345–9.
24 Katz M, Seidenbaum M, Weinrauch L. Penicillin-induced generalized pustular psoriasis. *J Am Acad Dermatol* 1988; **17**: 918–20.
25 Boonk WJ, Van Ketel WG. The role of penicillin in the pathogenesis of chronic urticaria. *Br J Dermatol* 1982; **106**: 183–90.
26 Torres MJ, Blanca M, Fernandez J et al. Selective allergic reaction to oral cloxacillin. *Clin Exp Allergy* 1996; **26**: 108–11.
27 Fairley CK, McNeil JJ, Desmond P et al. Risk factors for development of flucloxacillin-associated jaundice. *BMJ* 1993; **306**: 233–5.

Ampicillin

A morbilliform rash, with onset on the extremities and becoming generalized, occurs in 5–10% of patients treated with ampicillin, and usually develops 7–12 days after onset of therapy. This time interval suggests an allergic mechanism, although the rash disappears spontaneously even if ampicillin is continued, and may not develop on re-exposure [1]. Skin tests are generally negative. An urticarial reaction, present in about 1.5% of patients, indicates the presence of type I IgE-mediated general penicillin allergy [2,3]. Administration of ampicillin when a patient has infectious mononucleosis leads to florid morbilliform and sometimes purpuric eruptions in up to 100% of patients [4–6]. Cutaneous reactions to ampicillin are increased in cytomegalovirus infection [7], chronic lymphatic leukaemia [8], renal insufficiency or when allopurinol is administered concomitantly [9]. Ampicillin has been reported to cause a fixed drug eruption [10], erythema multiforme and Stevens–Johnson syndrome [11,12], TEN [13], Henoch–Schönlein purpura [14], serum sickness [15] and pemphigus vulgaris [16] in individual cases. Administration of ampicillin to a patient with a history of psoriasis resulted in erythroderma on two separate occasions [17]. A recurrent, localized, pustular skin eruption developed on the cheeks with ampicillin in one case [18].

Delayed intradermal skin tests and patch tests, indicating delayed hypersensitivity, were positive in about half of 60 subjects with maculopapular reactions to the aminopenicillins ampicillin and amoxicillin [19]; in another study, hypersensitivity to an antigenic determinant in the side-chain structure was suggested, as intradermal and patch tests were positive to ampicillin but there was good tolerance to benzylpenicillin [20]. Re-exposure of patients to ampicillins and other penicillins is contraindicated after urticarial reactions; anaphylactic reactions to ampicillin have been recorded. The risk is far less after morbilliform rashes but is not negligible.

REFERENCES

1 Adcock BB, Rodman DP. Ampicillin-specific rashes. *Arch Fam Med* 1996; **5**: 301–4.
2 Bass JW, Crowley DM, Steele RW *et al.* Adverse effects of orally administered ampicillin. *J Pediatr* 1973; **83**: 106–8.
3 Anonymous. Ampicillin rashes. *BMJ* 1975; **ii**: 708–9.
4 Weiss ME, Adkinson NF. Immediate hypersensitivity reactions to penicillin and related antibiotics. *Clin Allergy* 1988; **18**: 515–40.
5 Pullen H, Wright N, Murdoch JMcC. Hypersensitivity reactions to anti-bacterial drugs in infectious mononucleosis. *Lancet* 1967; **ii**: 1176–8.
6 Renn CN, Straff W, Dorfmüller A *et al.* Amoxicillin-induced exanthema in young adults with infectious mononucleosis: demonstration of drug-specific lymphocyte reactivity. *Br J Dermatol* 2003; **147**: 1166–7.
7 Klemola E. Hypersensitivity reactions to ampicillin in cytomegalovirus mononucleosis. *Scand J Infect Dis* 1970; **2**: 29.
8 Cameron SJ, Richmond J. Ampicillin hypersensitivity in lymphatic leuk-aemia. *Scott Med J* 1972; **16**: 425–7.
9 Jick H, Slone D, Shapiro S *et al.* Excess of ampicillin rashes associated with allopurinol or hyperuricemia. A report from the Boston Collaborative Drug Surveillance Program, Boston University Medical Center. *N Engl J Med* 1972; **286**: 505–7.
10 Arndt KA, Parrish J. Ampicillin rashes. *Arch Dermatol* 1973; **107**: 74.
11 Gupta HL, Dheman R. Ampicillin-induced Stevens–Johnson syndrome. *J Indian Med Assoc* 1979; **72**: 188–9.
12 Garty BZ, Offer I, Livni E, Danon YL. Erythema multiforme and hypersens-itivity myocarditis caused by ampicillin. *Ann Pharmacother* 1994; **28**: 730–1.
13 Tagami H, Tatsuta K, Iwatski K, Yamada M. Delayed hypersensitivity in ampicillin-induced toxic epidermal necrolysis. *Arch Dermatol* 1983; **119**: 910–3.
14 Beeching NJ, Gruer LD, Findlay CD, Geddes AM. A case of Henoch–Schönlein purpura syndrome following oral ampicillin. *J Antimicrob Chemother* 1982; **10**: 479–82.
15 Caldwell JR, Cliff LE. Adverse reactions to antimicrobial agents. *JAMA* 1974; **230**: 77–80.
16 Fellner MJ, Mark AS. Penicillin- and ampicillin-induced pemphigus vul-garis. *Int J Dermatol* 1980; **19**: 392–3.
17 Saito S, Ikezawa Z. Psoriasiform intradermal test reaction to ABPC in a patient with psoriasis and ABPC allergy. *J Dermatol* 1990; **17**: 677–83.
18 Lim JT, Ng SK. An unusual drug eruption to ampicillin. *Cutis* 1995; **56**: 163–4.
19 Romano A, Di Fonso M, Papa G *et al.* Evaluation of adverse cutaneous reactions to aminopenicillins with emphasis on those manifested by macu-lopapular rashes. *Allergy* 1995; **50**: 113–8.
20 Lopez Serrano C, Villas F, Cabanas R, Contreras J. Delayed hypersensitivity to beta-lactams. *J Invest Allergol Clin Immunol* 1994; **4**: 315–9.

Amoxicillin

Cutaneous eruptions including urticaria or morbilliform or maculopapular rashes occur in 1–2% of treatment courses with amoxicillin [1–3]. Immediate allergy (ana-phylaxis or urticaria/angio-oedema) to amoxicillin has occurred in patients with good tolerance of benzylpeni-cillin, aztreonam and ceftazidime [4,5]. However, amoxi-cillin has been reported to cross-react with penicillin on first exposure [6]. Amoxicillin caused an unusual intertriginous eruption in two patients [7]. Serum sick-ness has been reported with amoxicillin in children [8]. Amoxicillin has caused a fixed eruption [9], and a curious, recurrent, localized, pustular eruption [10]. This drug has also been implicated in the development of an acute gen-eralized exanthematous pustulosis [11]. There may be an increased frequency of rash with amoxicillin and clavu-lanate therapy in HIV-positive patients [12]. Amoxicillin, like clavulanic acid and flucloxacillin, may cause a cho-lestatic hepatitis [13]. This occurs at a frequency of 1 in 6000 adults when the drug is combined with clavulanic acid (co-amoxiclav) [14]. Amoxicillin has also been implicated in the baboon syndrome [15], palmar exfoliative exan-them [16] and localized peri-buccal pustulosis [17].

Methicillin

Methicillin caused reappearance of a recently faded ampi-cillin rash in a patient with glandular fever [18].

REFERENCES

1 Wise PJ, Neu HC. Experience with amoxicillin: an overall summary of clin-ical trials in the United States. *J Infect Dis* 1974; **129** (Suppl.): S266–S267.
2 Levine LR. Quantitative comparison of adverse reactions to cefaclor versus amoxicillin in a surveillance study. *Pediatr Infect Dis* 1985; **4**: 358–61.
3 Bigby M, Jick S, Jick H, Arndt K. Drug-induced cutaneous reactions. A report from the Boston Collaborative Drug Surveillance Program on 15438 consecutive inpatients, 1975 to 1982. *JAMA* 1986; **256**: 3358–63.
4 Vega JM, Blanca M, Garcia JJ *et al.* Immediate allergic reactions to amoxi-cillin. *Allergy* 1994; **49**: 317–22.
5 Martin JA, Igea JM, Fraj J *et al.* Allergy to amoxicillin in patients who toler-ated benzylpenicillin, aztreonam, and ceftazidime. *Clin Infect Dis* 1992; **14**: 592–3.
6 Fellner MJ. Amoxicillin cross reacts with penicillin on first exposure. *Int J Dermatol* 1993; **32**: 308–9.
7 Wolf R, Brenner S, Krakowski A. Intertriginous drug eruption. *Acta Derm Venereol (Stockh)* 1992; **72**: 441–2.
8 Chopra R, Roberts J, Warrington RJ. Severe delayed-onset hypersensitivity reactions to amoxicillin in children. *Can Med Assoc J* 1989; **140**: 921–3.
9 Chowdhury FH. Fixed genital drug eruption. *Pract Med* 1982; **226**: 1450.
10 Shuttleworth D. A localized, recurrent pustular eruption following amoxy-cillin administration. *Clin Exp Dermatol* 1989; **14**: 367–8.
11 Roujeau J-C, Bioulac-Sage P, Bourseau C *et al.* Acute generalized exanthe-matous pustulosis. Analysis of 63 cases. *Arch Dermatol* 1991; **127**: 1333–8.
12 Battegay M, Opravil M, Wütrich B, Lüthy R. Rash with amoxycillin–clavulanate therapy in HIV-infected patients. *Lancet* 1989; **ii**: 1100.
13 Anonymous. Drug-induced cholestatic hepatitis from common antibiotics. *Med J Aust* 1992; **157**: 531.
14 Anonymous. Revised indications for co-amoxiclav (Augmentin). *Curr Probl Pharmacovig* 1997; **23**: 8.
15 Kick G, Przybilla B. Delayed prick test reaction identifies amoxicillin as elicitor of baboon syndrome. *Contact Dermatitis* 2000; **43**: 366–7.
16 Gastaminza G, Audicana MT, Fernandez E *et al.* Palmar exfoliative exan-thema to amoxicillin. *Allergy* 2000; **55**: 510–1.
17 Novalbos A, Bombin C, Figueredo E *et al.* Localized pustulosis induced by betalactams. *J Invest Allergol Clin Immunol* 2000; **10**: 178–9.
18 Fields DA. Methicillin rash in infectious mononucleosis. *West J Med* 1981; **133**: 521.

Cephalosporins [1]

In general, cephalosporins are fairly well tolerated [1–3], adverse reactions ranging from 1 to 10% [1]; parenteral administration may cause minor adverse reactions, including thrombophlebitis and pain. The most common adverse effects are allergic reactions, occurring in 1–3% of patients [2]; haematological toxicity occurs in less than 1% of patients. Anaphylaxis is rare (less than 0.02%) [1]. Other reactions include localized gastrointestinal disturbances, hepatotoxicity, nephrotoxicity and mild central nervous system effects. Cephalosporin reactions are minimally, if at all, increased in patients with histories of penicillin allergy [1]. Post-marketing studies of second- and third-generation cephalosporins showed no increase in allergic reactions in patients with a history of penicillin allergy. Cephalosporin antibiotics are safe in penicillin-allergic patients and penicillin skin tests do not identify potential reactors [1]. Isolated independent hypersensitivity to individual cephalosporins, such as cefazolin [4,5], cefonicid [6] and cefuroxime [7], with good tolerance to other β-lactam antibiotics, has been described.

Hypersensitivity reactions include various exanthems and contact urticaria [8]; cases of anaphylaxis to cefaclor [9] and of fatal anaphylactic shock related to cefalotin (cephalothin) [10] have been reported. Vulvovaginitis and pruritus ani are not uncommon. Delayed reactions have been reported with cefonicid [6] and cefuroxime [11]. Serum sickness reactions occur [12–15], especially with cefaclor; the latter drug may also cause urticaria and erythema multiforme [15]. Exfoliative dermatitis has been attributed to cefoxitin [16]. Disulfiram-like reactions to alcohol have been described with newer members of this group. Pustular reactions have been documented with cefradine, cefalexin and cefazolin [17–19]. Ceftazidime has been implicated in the development of erythema multiforme [20]. Cephalosporins [21] including cefalexin [22] have been reported to cause TEN, and cefalexin has precipitated pemphigus vulgaris [23]. Cefazolin has caused an unusual fixed drug eruption [24]. A curious photo-recall-like phenomenon followed the use of cefazolin and gentamicin sulphate, in that the eruption was restricted to an area of sunburn sustained 1 month previously [25]. Cefotaxime has caused a photodistributed phototoxic telangiectasia [26].

REFERENCES

1 Anne S, Reisman RE. Risk of administering cephalosporin antibiotics to patients with histories of penicillin allergy. *Ann Allergy Asthma Immunol* 1995; **74**: 167–70.
2 Thompson JW, Jacobs RF. Adverse effects of newer cephalosporins. An update. *Drug Saf* 1993; **9**: 132–42.
3 Matsuno K, Kunihiro E, Yamatoya O et al. Surveillance of adverse reactions due to ciprofloxacin in Japan. *Drugs* 1995; **49** (Suppl. 2): 495–6.
4 Igea JM, Fraj J, Davila I et al. Allergy to cefazolin: study of in vivo cross reactivity with other betalactams. *Ann Allergy* 1992; **68**: 515–9.
5 Warrington RJ, McPhillips S. Independent anaphylaxis to cefazolin without allergy to other beta-lactam antibiotics. *J Allergy Clin Immunol* 1996; **98**: 460–2.
6 Martin JA, Alonso MD, Lazaro M et al. Delayed allergic reaction to cefonicid. *Ann Allergy* 1994; **72**: 341–2.
7 Marcos Bravo C, Luna Ortiz I, Gonzalez Vazquez R. Hypersensitivity to cefuroxime with good tolerance to other betalactams. *Allergy* 1995; **50**: 359–61.
8 Tuft L. Contact urticaria from cephalosporins. *Arch Dermatol* 1975; **111**: 1609.
9 Nishioka K, Katayama I, Kobayashi Y, Takijiri C. Anaphylaxis due to cefaclor hypersensitivity. *J Dermatol* 1986; **13**: 226–7.
10 Spruell FG, Minette LJ, Sturner WQ. Two surgical deaths associated with cephalothin. *JAMA* 1974; **229**: 440–1.
11 Romano A, Pietrantonio F, Di Fonso M, Venuti A. Delayed hypersensitivity to cefuroxime. *Contact Dermatitis* 1992; **27**: 270–1.
12 Kearns GL, Wheeler JG, Childress SH, Letzig LG. Serum sickness-like reactions to cefaclor: role of hepatic metabolism and individual susceptibility. *J Pediatr* 1994; **125**: 805–11.
13 Grammer LC. Cefaclor serum sickness. *JAMA* 1996; **275**: 1152–3.
14 Isaacs D. Serum sickness-like reaction to cefaclor. *J Paediatr Child Health* 2001; **37**: 298–9.
15 Joubert GI, Hadad K, Matsui D et al. Selection of treatment of cefaclor-associated urticarial, serum sickness-like reactions and erythema multiforme by emergency pediatricians: lack of a uniform standard of care. *Can J Clin Pharmacol* 1999; **6**: 197–201.
16 Kannangara DW, Smith B, Cohen K. Exfoliative dermatitis during cefoxitin therapy. *Arch Intern Med* 1982; **142**: 1031–2.
17 Kalb R, Grossman ME. Pustular eruption following administration of cephradine. *Cutis* 1986; **38**: 58–60.
18 Jackson H, Vion B, Levy PM. Generalized eruptive pustular drug rash due to cephalexin. *Dermatologica* 1988; **177**: 292–4.
19 Fayol J, Bernard P, Bonnetblanc JM. Pustular eruption following the administration cefazolin: a second case report. *J Am Acad Dermatol* 1988; **19**: 571.
20 Pierce TH, Vig SJ, Ingram PM. Ceftazidime in the treatment of lower respiratory tract infection. *J Antimicrob Chemother* 1983; **12** (Suppl. A): 21–5.
21 Nichter LS, Harman DM, Bryant CA et al. Cephalosporin-induced toxic epidermal necrolysis. *J Burn Care Rehabil* 1983; **4**: 358–60.
22 Hogan DJ, Rooney ME. Toxic epidermal necrolysis due to cephalexin. *J Am Acad Dermatol* 1987; **17**: 852.
23 Wolf R, Dechner E, Ophir J, Brenner S. Cephalexin. A non-thiol drug that may induce pemphigus vulgaris. *Int J Dermatol* 1991; **30**: 213–5.
24 Sigal-Nahum M, Konqui A, Gauliet A, Sigal S. Linear fixed drug eruption. *Br J Dermatol* 1988; **118**: 849–51.
25 Flax SH, Uhle P. Photo recall-like phenomenon following the use of cefazolin and gentamicin sulfate. *Cutis* 1990; **46**: 59–61.
26 Borgia F, Vaccaro M, Guarneri F, Cannavo SP. Photodistributed telangiectasia following use of cefotaxime. *Br J Dermatol* 2000; **143**: 674–8.

Monobactams

Monobactams (e.g. aztreonam) show weak and rare cross-reactivity with IgE antibodies to penicillin [1–3], although immediate hypersensitivity on first exposure to aztreonam in penicillin-allergic patients has been recorded [4,5]. In general, aztreonam is well tolerated in high-risk patients allergic to other β-lactam antibiotics, but there is a 20% sensitization rate following exposure [6]. However, aztreonam and the monobactams can be safely given to penicillin-allergic patients [7]. Generalized urticaria to aztreonam but good tolerance of the other β-lactams has been recorded [8].

Carbapenems

Cross-reactivity and allergic reactions to imipenem occur in patients known to be allergic to penicillin [9]. Carbapenems should be avoided in patients with penicillin allergy [7]. Imipenem combined with cilastatin, a non-antibiotic enzyme inhibitor that prevents breakdown of imipenem to nephrotoxic metabolites, may cause phlebitis or pain at the site of infusion [10]. Imipenem has been associated with a pustular eruption [11], and imipenem–cilastatin with palmoplantar pruritus during infusion in a child with AIDS [12].

REFERENCES

1 Adkinson NF, Saxon A, Spence MR, Swabb EA. Cross-allergenicity and immunogenicity of aztreonam. *Rev Infect Dis* 1985; **7** (Suppl. 4): S613–S621.

2 Saxon A, Hassner A, Swabb EA et al. Lack of cross-reactivity between aztreonam, a monobactam antibiotic, and penicillin-allergic subjects. *J Infect Dis* 1984; **149**: 16.

3 Adkinson NF Jr. Beta-lactam crossreactivity. *Clin Exp Allergy* 1998; **28** (Suppl. 4): 37–40.

4 Hantson P, de Coninck B, Horn JL, Mahieu P. Immediate hypersensitivity to aztreonam and imipenem. *BMJ* 1991; **302**: 294–5.

5 Alvarez JS, Del Castillo JAS, Garcia IS, Ortiz MJA. Immediate hypersensitivity to aztreonam. *Lancet* 1990; **335**: 1094.

6 Moss RB. Sensitization to aztreonam and cross-reactivity with other beta-lactam antibiotics in high-risk patients with cystic fibrosis. *J Allergy Clin Immunol* 1991; **87**: 78–88.

7 Kishiyama JL, Adelman DC. The cross-reactivity and immunology of beta-lactam antibiotics. *Drug Saf* 1994; **10**: 318–27.

8 de la Fuente Prieto R, Armentia Medina A, Sanchez Palla P et al. Urticaria caused by sensitization to aztreonam. *Allergy* 1993; **48**: 634–6.

9 Saxon A, Adelman DC, Patel A et al. Imipenem cross-reactivity with penicillin in humans. *J Allergy Clin Immunol* 1988; **82**: 213–7.

10 Anonymous. Imipenem + cilastatin: a new type of antibiotic. *Drug Ther Bull* 1991; **29**: 43–4.

11 Escallier F, Dalac S, Foucher JL et al. Pustulose exanthématique aiguë généralisée: imputabilité a l'imipéneme (Tienam®). *Ann Dermatol Vénéréol* 1989; **116**: 407–9.

12 Machado ARL, Silva CLO, Galvão NAM. Unusual reaction to imipenem–cilastatin in a child with the acquired immunodeficiency syndrome. *J Allergy Clin Immunol* 1991; **87**: 754.

Tetracyclines

Many of the side effects are common to all drugs within the group, and cross-sensitivity occurs [1]. Nausea, vomiting and diarrhoea are well-recognized dose-related effects. Oral or vaginal candidiasis may occur as a result of overgrowth of commensals. Resumption of therapy does not necessarily lead to recurrence of the vaginitis [2].

Photosensitivity

All tetracyclines, but especially demethylchlortetracycline, may cause phototosensitive eruptions [1,3–6], which clinically resemble exaggerated sunburn, sometimes with blistering. Phototoxicity is thought to be involved, in that high serum levels predispose to its occurrence. Reactions to both UVA and UVB have been reported. High concentrations of tetracycline are found in sun-damaged skin [3]. Symptoms may persist for months [1]. Photo-onycholysis may develop in fingernails and (if exposed) toenails; the thumb (normally less exposed) may be spared [7,8]. Tetracycline therapy is best avoided if there is a prospect of considerable sun exposure. Porphyria cutanea tarda-like changes may develop after chronic sun exposure [6,9]. A photosensitive lichenoid rash has been attributed to demethylchlortetracycline [10].

REFERENCES

1 Wright AL, Colver GB. Tetracyclines: how safe are they? *Clin Exp Dermatol* 1988; **13**: 57–61.

2 Hall JH, Lupton ES. Tetracycline therapy for acne: incidence of vaginitis. *Cutis* 1977; **20**: 97–8.

3 Blank H, Cullen SI, Catalano PM. Photosensitivity studies with demethylchlortetracycline and doxycycline. *Arch Dermatol* 1968; **97**: 1–2.

4 Frost P, Weinstein GP, Gomez EC. Phototoxic potential of minocycline and doxycycline. *Arch Dermatol* 1972; **105**: 681–3.

5 Kaidbey KH, Kligman AM. Identification of systemic phototoxic drugs by human intradermal assay. *J Invest Dermatol* 1978; **70**: 272–4.

6 Hawk JLM. Skin changes resembling hepatic cutaneous porphyria induced by oxytetracycline photosensitization. *Clin Exp Dermatol* 1980; **5**: 321–5.

7 Baker H. Photo-onycholysis caused by tetracyclines. *BMJ* 1977; **ii**: 519–20.

8 Kestel JL Jr. Photo-onycholysis from minocycline. Side effects of minocycline therapy. *Cutis* 1981; **28**: 53–4.

9 Epstein JH, Tuffanelli DL, Seibert JS, Epstein WL. Porphyria-like cutaneous changes induced by tetracycline hydrochloride photosensitization. *Arch Dermatol* 1976; **112**: 661–6.

10 Jones HE, Lewis CW, Reisner JE. Photosensitive lichenoid eruption associated with demeclocycline. *Arch Dermatol* 1972; **106**: 58–63.

Pigmentation

Methacycline is a rare cause [1]. Long-term minocycline therapy for acne may result in pigmentation. Although this is generally held to be a rare event, it may occur in about 1.4% of patients [2–5]. The average time for the development of pigmentary changes was 5 months, and onset of this complication did not seem to be related to cumulative dosage of the drug [3]. Facial hyperpigmentation was reported in two sisters on long-term minocycline therapy, who were also being treated with Dianette (cyproterone acetate and ethinylestradiol); it was suggested that pigmentation occurred either as a result of a genetic alteration in the metabolic handling of the drug or because of accentuation by the concomitant therapy [6]. Other drugs, including amitriptyline [2], phenothiazines and 13-*cis*-retinoic acid, have been implicated in the accentuation of minocycline-related hyperpigmentation.

Three types of pigmentation are described with minocycline and may occur in combination or isolation [3]. A focal type with well-demarcated blue-black macules is seen in areas of previous inflammation or scarring, especially in relation to acne scars. Minocycline has been associated with post-inflammatory hyperpigmentation in women who have undergone sclerotherapy [7]. Macular or more diffuse hyperpigmentation may appear distant from acne sites, especially on the extensor surface of the lower legs and forearms and on sun-exposed areas. These two types resolve on cessation of therapy, with a mean time to resolution of 12 months [3]. A more persistent diffuse brown-grey change may develop, especially in sun-exposed areas [5]. Minocycline pigmentation may respond well to laser therapy [8–11].

The oral cavity and lips may be involved [12,13]. Conjunctival pigmentation may occur with tetracyclines [14,15] and scleral pigmentation with minocycline [16,17]. Minocycline can cause nail pigmentation and longitudinal melanonychia [5,18,19], and tetracycline may produce yellow discoloration of the nail [20]. Cutaneous osteomas presenting as blue skin nodules that fluoresce yellow under UV light may rarely develop in patients being treated with tetracycline [21] or minocycline [22] for acne.

Black galactorrhoea occurred in a patient taking both minocycline and phenothiazines [23].

Pigmentation may also involve bones, teeth, thyroid, aorta and endocardium [19,24]. Histological and electron microscopic studies have demonstrated increased melanin, haemosiderin and either minocycline or a metabolite in the skin [25–27]; pigment may be seen in dermal histiocytes and eccrine myoepithelial cells [26]. Minocycline is metabolized to form a brown-black degradation product [28].

REFERENCES

1 Möller H, Rausing A. Methacycline pigmentation: a five-year follow-up. *Acta Derm Venereol (Stockh)* 1980; **60**: 495–501.
2 Basler RSW, Goetz CS. Synergism of minocycline and amitriptyline in cutaneous hyperpigmentation. *J Am Acad Dermatol* 1985; **12**: 577.
3 Layton AM, Cunliffe WJ. Minocycline induced pigmentation in the treatment of acne: a review and personal observations. *J Dermatol Treat* 1989; **1**: 9–12.
4 Dwyer CM, Cuddihy AM, Kerr RE et al. Skin pigmentation due to minocycline treatment of facial dermatoses. *Br J Dermatol* 1993; **129**: 158–62.
5 Pepine M, Flower FP, Ramos-Caro FA. Extensive cutaneous hyperpigmentation caused by minocycline. *J Am Acad Dermatol* 1993; **28**: 292–5.
6 Eedy DJ, Burrows D. Minocycline-induced pigmentation occurring in two sisters. *Clin Exp Dermatol* 1991; **16**: 55–7.
7 Leffell DJ. Minocycline hydrochloride hyperpigmentation complicating treatment of venous ectasia of the extremities. *J Am Acad Dermatol* 1991; **24**: 501–2.
8 Collins P, Cotterill JA. Minocycline-induced pigmentation resolves after treatment with the Q-switched ruby laser. *Br J Dermatol* 1996; **135**: 317–9.
9 Wilde JL, English JC III, Finley EM. Minocycline-induced hyperpigmentation. Treatment with the neodymium:Yag laser. *Arch Dermatol* 1997; **133**: 1344–6.
10 Wood B, Munro CS, Bilsland D. Treatment of minocycline-induced pigmentation with the neodymium-Yag laser. *Br J Dermatol* 1998; **139**: 562.
11 Green D, Friedman KJ. Treatment of minocycline-induced cutaneous pigmentation with the Q-switched Alexandrite laser and a review of the literature. *J Am Acad Dermatol* 2001; **44**: 342–7.
12 Siller GM, Tod MA, Savage NW. Minocycline-induced oral pigmentation. *J Am Acad Dermatol* 1994; **30**: 350–4.
13 Chu PSL, Yen TS, Berger TG. Minocycline hyperpigmentation localized to the lips: an unusual fixed drug reaction? *J Am Acad Dermatol* 1994; **30**: 802–3.
14 Brothers DM, Hidayat AA. Conjunctival pigmentation associated with tetracycline medication. *Ophthalmology* 1981; **88**: 1212–5.
15 Messmer E, Font RL, Sheldon G, Murphy D. Pigmented conjunctival cysts following tetracycline/minocycline therapy. Histochemical and electron microscopic observations. *Ophthalmology* 1983; **90**: 1462–8.
16 Angeloni VL, Salasche SJ, Ortiz R. Nail, skin, and scleral pigmentation induced by minocycline. *Cutis* 1988; **42**: 229–33.
17 Sabroe RA, Archer CB, Harlow D et al. Minocycline-induced discolouration of the sclerae. *Br J Dermatol* 1996; **135**: 314–6.
18 Mallon E, Dawber RPR. Longitudinal melanonychia induced by minocycline. *Br J Dermatol* 1995; **130**: 794–5.
19 Wolfe ID, Reichmister J. Minocycline hyperpigmentation: skin, tooth, nail, and bone involvement. *Cutis* 1984; **33**: 475–8.
20 Hendricks AA. Yellow lunulae with fluorescence after tetracycline therapy. *Arch Dermatol* 1980; **116**: 438–40.
21 Walter JF, Macknet KD. Pigmentation of osteoma cutis caused by tetracycline. *Arch Dermatol* 1979; **115**: 1087–8.
22 Moritz DL, Elewski B. Pigmented postacne osteoma cutis in a patient treated with minocycline: report and review of the literature. *J Am Acad Dermatol* 1991; **24**: 851–3.
23 Basler RSW, Lynch PJ. Black galactorrhea as a complication of minocycline and phenothiazine therapy. *Arch Dermatol* 1985; **121**: 417–8.
24 Butler JM, Marks R, Sutherland R. Cutaneous and cardiac valvular pigmentation with minocycline. *Clin Exp Dermatol* 1985; **10**: 432–7.
25 Sato S, Murphy GF, Bernard JD et al. Ultrastructural and x-ray microanalytical observations on minocycline-related hyperpigmentation of the skin. *J Invest Dermatol* 1981; **77**: 264–71.
26 Argenyi ZB, Finelli L, Bergfeld WF et al. Minocycline-related cutaneous hyperpigmentation as demonstrated by light microscopy, electron microscopy and x-ray energy spectroscopy. *J Cutan Pathol* 1987; **14**: 176–80.
27 Okada N, Moriya K, Nishida K et al. Skin pigmentation associated with minocycline therapy. *Br J Dermatol* 1989; **121**: 247–54.
28 Nelis HJCF, DeLeenheer AP. Metabolism of minocycline in humans. *Drug Metab Dispos* 1982; **10**: 142–6.

Other cutaneous side effects

Allergic reactions are far less common than with penicillin. Morbilliform, urticarial, erythema multiforme-like and bullous eruptions [1,2], exfoliative dermatitis and erythema nodosum [3] have been reported, as well as a recurrent follicular acneiform eruption in one patient [4]. Minocycline has caused eosinophilic cellulitis and pustular folliculitis with eosinophilia [5]. Gram-negative folliculitis of the face is uncommon but well recognized; *Proteus* may be responsible, and the condition responds to ampicillin [6]. Tetracyclines are a well-known cause of fixed drug eruptions [7–9], and minocycline [10] and doxycycline [11] have caused Stevens–Johnson syndrome. TEN has been recorded [12]. It has been suggested that tetracyclines may exacerbate psoriasis [13,14]. An eruption resembling Sweet's syndrome has occurred with minocycline, tetracycline and doxycycline [15–17]. Pruritus at the site of active acne has been recorded within 2–6 weeks of starting oral tetracyclines (oxytetracycline, doxycycline or minocycline) [18].

REFERENCES

1 Shelley WB, Heaton CL. Minocycline sensitivity. *JAMA* 1973; **224**: 125–6.
2 Fawcett IW, Pepys J. Allergy to a tetracycline preparation: a case report. *Clin Allergy* 1976; **6**: 301–4.
3 Bridges AJ, Graziano FM, Calhoun W, Reizner GT. Hyperpigmentation, neutrophilic alveolitis, and erythema nodosum resulting from minocycline. *J Am Acad Dermatol* 1990; **22**: 959–62.
4 Bean SF. Acneiform eruption from tetracycline. *Br J Dermatol* 1971; **85**: 585–6.
5 Kaufmann D, Pichler W, Beer JH. Severe episode of high fever with rash, lymphadenopathy, neutropenia, and eosinophilia after minocycline therapy for acne. *Arch Intern Med* 1994; **154**: 1983–4.
6 Leyden JJ, Marples RR, Mills OH Jr, Kligman AM. Gram-negative folliculitis: a complication of antibiotic therapy in acne vulgaris. *Br J Dermatol* 1973; **88**: 533–8.
7 Jolly HW, Sherman IJ Jr, Carpenter CL et al. Fixed drug eruptions to tetracyclines. *Arch Dermatol* 1978; **114**: 1484–5.
8 Fiumara NJ, Yaqub M. Pigmented penile lesions (fixed drug eruptions) associated with tetracycline therapy for sexually transmitted diseases. *Sex Transm Dis* 1980; **8**: 23–5.
9 Chan HL, Wong SN, Lo FL. Tetracycline-induced fixed drug eruptions: influence of dose and structure of tetracyclines. *J Am Acad Dermatol* 1985; **13**: 302–3.
10 Shoji A, Someda Y, Hamada T. Stevens–Johnson syndrome due to minocycline therapy. *Arch Dermatol* 1987; **123**: 18–20.
11 Curley RK, Verbov JL. Stevens–Johnson syndrome due to tetracyclines: a case report (doxycycline) and review of the literature. *Clin Exp Dermatol* 1987; **12**: 124–5.
12 Tatnall FM, Dodd HJ, Sarkany I. Elevated serum amylase in a case of toxic epidermal necrolysis. *Br J Dermatol* 1985; **113**: 629–30.

13 Tsankov M, Botev-Zlatkov M, Lazarova AZ *et al.* Psoriasis and drugs: influence of tetracyclines on the course of psoriasis. *J Am Acad Dermatol* 1988; **19**: 629–32.

14 Bergner T, Przybilla B. Psoriasis and tetracyclines. *J Am Acad Dermatol* 1990; **23**: 770.

15 Mensing H, Kowalzick L. Acute febrile neutrophilic dermatosis (Sweet's syndrome) caused by minocycline. *Dermatologica* 1991; **182**: 43–6.

16 Thibault MJ, Billick RC, Srolovitz H. Minocycline-induced Sweet's syndrome. *J Am Acad Dermatol* 1992; **27**: 801–4.

17 Khan Durani B, Jappe U. Drug-induced Sweet's syndrome in acne caused by different tetracyclines: case report and review of the literature. *Br J Dermatol* 2002; **147**: 558–62.

18 Yee KC, Cunliffe WJ. Itching in acne: an unusual complication of therapy. *Dermatology* 1994; **189**: 117–9.

Gastrointestinal absorption and drug interactions

Absorption of tetracyclines is reduced when taken with meals, especially those containing calcium or iron such as milk, or with drugs such as iron or antacids [1]. The decrease in serum levels following a test meal has been reported as follows: oxytetracycline 50% [1], minocycline 13% [1] and doxycycline 20% [2]. Oxytetracycline may have a hypoglycaemic effect in insulin-dependent diabetics [3]. Tetracyclines can potentiate the action of warfarin by depressing prothrombin activity, and elevate serum levels of lithium given simultaneously [4].

REFERENCES

1 Leyden JJ. Absorption of minocycline HCl and tetracycline hydrochloride. Effect of food, milk and iron. *J Am Acad Dermatol* 1985; **12**: 308–12.

2 Welling PG, Koch PA, Lau CC, Craig WA. Bioavailability of tetracycline and doxycycline in fasted and nonfasted subjects. *Antimicrob Agents Chemother* 1977; **11**: 462–9.

3 Miller JB. Hypoglycaemic effect of oxytetracycline. *BMJ* 1966; **2**: 1007.

4 McGennis AJ. Lithium carbonate and tetracycline interaction. *BMJ* 1978; **i**: 1183.

Systemic side effects of tetracyclines

Long-term use of tetracycline for acne may rarely result in benign intracranial hypertension [1,2]. As retinoids may potentiate this effect, it is safest not to use them in combination with tetracycline therapy for acne. Oesophageal ulceration has been described in a number of patients [3]. With the exception of doxycycline and minocycline, tetracyclines may exacerbate renal failure. Combination therapy with tetracyclines and nephrotoxic drugs such as gentamicin or diuretics should be avoided [4]. Deteriorated tetracyclines have caused nephropathy accompanied by an exanthematic eruption. Patients should be warned not to use outdated or poorly stored tetracycline, because degraded tetracycline can cause a Fanconi-type syndrome comprising renal tubular acidosis and proteinuria [5,6] and lactic acidosis [7]. Dose-related vestibular disturbance has been reported with minocycline [8]. Reversible pulmonary infiltration with eosinophilic or neutrophilic alveolitis has been rarely described in association with tetracycline [9] and especially minocycline [10–12] ther-apy. There have been isolated case reports linking tetracycline with SLE [13].

Minocycline has been reported to cause other serious, albeit rare, adverse events. Serum sickness-like reactions occur at about 15 days [14,15]. A hypersensitivity syndrome may develop at about 23–35 days, with a severe self-limiting eruption, sometimes exfoliative dermatitis, associated with eosinophilia and acute hepatic failure, occasionally fatal [16–20]. A drug-induced autoimmune syndrome with hepatitis or vasculitis and some features of SLE occurs rarely with minocycline, on average 1–2 years after the start of therapy, and is commoner in women [20–25]. Hepatitis, sometimes with the histological features of chronic active hepatitis, may be associated with polyarthralgia and positive antinuclear antibodies but negative or only weakly positive anti-DNA antibodies, and is only rarely fatal; patients usually recover within 3 months of drug cessation. Perinuclear antineutrophilic cytoplasmic antibody (p-ANCA) may be a marker for development of minocycline-induced autoimmunity [26–28]; in one study, all such patients were p-ANCA positive and had the haplotype HLA-DR4 or HLA-DR2, and all had the HLA-DQB1 allele, suggesting genetic susceptibility [28]. Systemic reactions to minocycline are certainly more frequent than those to oxytetracycline or doxycycline [29], and it has therefore been suggested that the use of minocycline in acne should be restricted to patients unresponsive to other tetracyclines [30].

REFERENCES

1 Walters BNJ, Gubbay SS. Tetracycline and benign intracranial hypertension: report of five cases. *BMJ* 1979; **282**: 19–20.

2 Pearson MG, Littlewood SM, Bowden AN. Tetracycline and benign intracranial hypertension. *BMJ* 1981; **282**: 568–9.

3 Channer KS, Hollanders D. Tetracycline-induced oesophageal ulceration. *BMJ* 1981; **282**: 1359–60.

4 Wright AL, Colver GB. Tetracyclines: how safe are they? *Clin Exp Dermatol* 1988; **13**: 57–61.

5 Moser RH. Bibliographies on diseases: medical progress. Reactions to tetracyclines. *Clin Pharmacol Ther* 1966; **7**: 117–31.

6 Frimpter GW, Timpanelli AE, Eisenmenger WJ *et al.* Reversible 'Fanconi syndrome' caused by degraded tetracycline. *JAMA* 1963; **184**: 111–3.

7 Montoliu J, Carrera M, Darnell A *et al.* Lactic acidosis and Fanconi's syndrome due to degraded tetracycline. *BMJ* 1981; **281**: 1576–7.

8 Allen JC. Minocycline. *Ann Intern Med* 1976; **85**: 482–7.

9 Ho D, Tashkin DP, Bein ME, Sharma O. Pulmonary infiltrates with eosinophilia associated with tetracycline. *Chest* 1979; **76**: 33–5.

10 Bando T, Fujimura M, Noda Y *et al.* Minocycline-induced pneumonitis with bilateral hilar lymphadenopathy and pleural effusion. *J Intern Med* 1994; **33**: 177–9.

11 Sitbon O, Bidel N, Dussopt C *et al.* Minocycline and pulmonary eosinophilia. A report on eight patients. *Arch Intern Med* 1994; **154**: 1633–40.

12 Dykhuizen RS, Zaidi AM, Godden DJ *et al.* Minocycline and pulmonary eosinophilia. *BMJ* 1995; **310**: 1520–1.

13 Domz CA, Minamara DH, Hozapfel HF. Tetracycline provocation in lupus erythematosus. *Ann Intern Med* 1959; **50**: 1217.

14 Landau M, Shachar E, Brenner S. Minocycline-induced serum sickness-like reaction. *J Eur Acad Dermatol Venereol* 2000; **14**: 67–8.

15 Malakar S, Dhar S, Shah Malakar R. Is serum sickness an uncommon adverse effect of minocycline treatment? *Arch Dermatol* 2001; **137**: 100–1.

16 Davies MG, Kersey PJW. Acute hepatitis and exfoliative dermatitis associated with minocycline. *BMJ* 1989; **298**: 1523–4.

17 Kaufmann D, Pichler W, Beer JH. Severe episode of high fever with rash, lymphadenopathy, neutropenia, and eosinophilia after minocycline therapy for acne. *Arch Intern Med* 1994; **154**: 1983–4.

18 Knowles SR, Shapiro L, Shear NH. Serious adverse reactions induced by minocycline. Report of 13 patients and review of the literature. *Arch Dermatol* 1996; **132**: 934–9.

19 MacNeil M, Haase DA, Tremaine R, Marrie TJ. Fever, lymphadenopathy, eosinophilia, lymphocytosis, hepatitis, and dermatitis: a severe adverse reaction to minocycline. *J Am Acad Dermatol* 1997; **36**: 347–50.

20 Lawrenson RA, Seaman HE, Sundstrom A *et al.* Liver damage associated with minocycline use in acne: a systematic review of the published literature and pharmacovigilance data. *Drug Saf* 2000; **23**: 333–49.

21 Elkayam O, Yaron M, Caspi D. Minocycline-induced autoimmune syndromes: an overview. *Semin Arthritis Rheum* 1999; **28**: 392–7.

22 Byrne PAC, Williams BD, Pritchard MH. Minocycline-related lupus. *Br J Rheumatol* 1994; **33**: 674–6.

23 Gordon PM, White MI, Herriot R *et al.* Minocyline-associated lupus erythematosus. *Br J Dermatol* 1995; **132**: 120–1.

24 Gough A, Chapman S, Wagstaff K *et al.* Minocycline-induced autoimmune hepatitis and systemic lupus erythematosus-like syndrome. *BMJ* 1996; **312**: 169–72.

25 Crosson J, Stillman MT. Minocycline-related lupus erythematosus with associated liver disease. *J Am Acad Dermatol* 1997; **36**: 867–8.

26 Shapiro LE, Uetrecht J, Shear NH. Minocycline, perinuclear antineutrophilic cytoplasmic antibody, and pigment: the biochemical basis. *J Am Acad Dermatol* 2001; **45**: 787–9.

27 Schaffer JV, Davidson DM, McNiff JM, Bolognia JL. Perinuclear antineutrophilic cytoplasmic antibody-positive cutaneous polyarteritis nodosa associated with minocycline therapy for acne vulgaris. *J Am Acad Dermatol* 2001; **44**: 198–206.

28 Dunphy J, Oliver M, Rands AL *et al.* Antineutrophil cytoplasmic antibodies and HLA class II alleles in minocycline-induced lupus-like syndrome. *Br J Dermatol* 2000; **142**: 461–7.

29 Shapiro LE, Knowles SR, Shear NH. Comparative safety of tetracycline, minocycline, and doxycycline. *Arch Dermatol* 1997; **133**: 1224–30.

30 Ferner RE, Moss C. Minocycline for acne. First line antibacterial treatment of acne should be with tetracycline or oxytetracycline. *BMJ* 1996; **312**: 138.

Effects on the fetus and on teeth

There is little evidence that tetracycline is teratogenic [1]. There is an isolated case report of congenital abnormalities in a child whose mother took clomocycline for acne [2]. Yellow discoloration of the teeth due to tetracycline exposure during mineralization of the deciduous or permanent teeth is well known [3–5]. A yellow-brown fluorescent discoloration is formed as a result of a complex with calcium orthophosphate. Tetracyclines should not be given to pregnant women or children under the age of 12 years. Tetracyclines are excreted in breast milk, but chelation with calcium decreases their absorption so that tooth discoloration is probably prevented [1].

Tetracycline may be deposited up to late adolescence in calcifying teeth such as the molars, but as these are not normally visible this is not a problem [5]. Minocycline may rarely stain the teeth of adults [6–8].

REFERENCES

1 Wright AL, Colver GB. Tetracyclines: how safe are they? *Clin Exp Dermatol* 1988; **13**: 57–61.

2 Corcoran R, Castles JM. Tetracycline for acne vulgaris and possible teratogenesis. *BMJ* 1977; **ii**: 807–8.

3 Conchie JM, Munroe JD, Anderson DO. The incidence of staining of permanent teeth by the tetracyclines. *Can Med Assoc J* 1970; **103**: 351–6.

4 Moffitt JM, Cooley RO, Olsen NH, Hefferren JJ. Prediction of tetracycline-induced tooth discolouration. *J Am Dent Assoc* 1974; **88**: 547–52.

5 Grossman ER. Tetracycline and staining of the teeth. *JAMA* 1986; **225**: 2442.

6 Poliak SC, DiGiovanna JJ, Gross EG *et al.* Minocycline-associated tooth discoloration in young adults. *JAMA* 1985; **254**: 2930–2.

7 Rosen T, Hoffmann TJ. Minocycline-induced discoloration of the permanent teeth. *J Am Acad Dermatol* 1989; **21**: 569.

8 Berger RS, Mandel EN, Hayes TJ, Grimwood RR. Minocycline staining of the oral cavity. *J Am Acad Dermatol* 1989; **21**: 1300–1.

Tetracyclines and the contraceptive pill

Tetracyclines have been reported to interfere with the action of the contraceptive pill [1,2], and it is standard practice to inform female patients of this and to suggest use of an additional or alternative method of contraception while on medication. However, there is controversy as to whether there is really a significant risk of interaction [3–6]. It has been argued that there is a baseline pill failure rate of at least 1% per year, and that antibiotics commonly used in dermatology do not increase the risk of pregnancy [6].

REFERENCES

1 Bacon JF, Shenfield GM. Pregnancy attributable to interaction between tetracycline and oral contraceptives. *BMJ* 1980; **280**: 293.

2 Hughes BR, Cunliffe WJ. Interactions between the oral contraceptive pill and antibiotics. *Br J Dermatol* 1990; **122**: 717–8.

3 Fleischer AB Jr, Resnick SD. The effect of antibiotics on the efficacy of oral contraceptives. *Arch Dermatol* 1989; **125**: 1562–4.

4 Orme ML'E, Back DJ. Interactions between oral contraceptive steroids and broad-spectrum antibiotics. *Clin Exp Dermatol* 1986; **11**: 327–31.

5 De Groot AC, Eshuis H, Stricker BHC. Oral contraceptives and antibiotics in acne. *Br J Dermatol* 1991; **124**: 212.

6 Helms SE, Bredle DL, Zajic J *et al.* Oral contraceptive failure rates and oral antibiotics. *J Am Acad Dermatol* 1997; **36**: 705–10.

Sulphonamides and trimethoprim

Reactions occur in 1–5% of those exposed [1–5]. They are commoner in patients with AIDS [6–8], and slow acetylators are at greater risk [9]. Type I reactions (urticaria and anaphylaxis) are rare but recorded. Phototoxic and photoallergic eruptions occur [10,11]. Morbilliform and rubelliform rashes are seen, and erythema multiforme, Stevens–Johnson syndrome and TEN [12–17], erythema nodosum [1], generalized exfoliative dermatitis [1,18,19] and fixed eruptions [20] are all well known. In addition, an LE-like syndrome and allergic vasculitis [21] are documented. Agranulocytosis or haemolytic anaemia is occasionally precipitated.

REFERENCES

1 Koch-Weser J, Sidel VW, Dexter M *et al.* Adverse reactions to sulfisoxazole, sulfamethoxazole, and nitrofurantoin. Manifestations and specific reaction rates during 2,118 courses of therapy. *Arch Intern Med* 1971; **128**: 399–404.

2 Kauppinen K, Stubb S. Drug eruptions: causative agents and clinical types. A series of inpatients during a 10-year period. *Acta Derm Venereol (Stockh)* 1984; **64**: 320–4.

3 Bigby M, Jick S, Jick H, Arndt K. Drug-induced cutaneous reactions. A report from the Boston Collaborative Drug Surveillance Program on 15438 consecutive inpatients, 1975 to 1982. *JAMA* 1986; **256**: 3358–63.

4 Anonymous. Hypersensitivity to sulphonamides: a clue? *Lancet* 1986; **ii**: 958–9.

5 Rieder MJ, Uetrecht J, Shear NH *et al*. Diagnosis of sulfonamide hypersensitivity reactions by in-vitro 'rechallenge' with hydroxylamine metabolites. *Ann Intern Med* 1989; **110**: 286–9.

6 De Raeve L, Song M, Van Maldergem L. Adverse cutaneous drug reactions in AIDS. *Br J Dermatol* 1988; **119**: 521–3.

7 van der Ven AJAM, Koopmans PP, Vree TB, van der Meer JWM. Adverse reactions to co-trimoxazole in HIV infection. *Lancet* 1991; **338**: 431–3.

8 Roudier C, Caumes E, Rogeaux O *et al*. Adverse cutaneous reactions to trimethoprim–sulfamethoxazole in patients with the acquired immunodeficiency syndrome and *Pneumocystis carinii* pneumonia. *Arch Dermatol* 1994; **130**: 1383–6.

9 Carr A, Gross AS, Hoskins JM *et al*. Acetylation phenotype and cutaneous hypersensitivity to trimethoprim–sulphamethoxazole in HIV-infected patients. *AIDS* 1994; **8**: 333–7.

10 Epstein JH. Photoallergy. A review. *Arch Dermatol* 1972; **106**: 741–8.

11 Hawk JLM. Photosensitizing agents used in the United Kingdom. *Clin Exp Dermatol* 1984; **9**: 300–2.

12 Kauppinen K. Cutaneous reactions to drugs. With special reference to severe mucocutaneous bullous eruptions and sulphonamides. *Acta Derm Venereol Suppl (Stockh)* 1972; **68**: 1–89.

13 Jick H, Derby LE. A large population-based follow-up study of trimethoprim–sulfamethoxazole, trimethoprim, and cephalexin for uncommon serious drug toxicity. *Pharmacotherapeutica* 1995; **15**: 428–32.

14 Carrol OM, Bryan PA, Robinson RJ. Stevens–Johnson syndrome associated with long-acting sulfonamides. *JAMA* 1966; **195**: 691–3.

15 Aberer W, Stingl G, Wolff K. Stevens–Johnson-Syndrom und toxische epidermale Nekrolyse nach Sulfonamideinahme. *Hautarzt* 1982; **33**: 484–90.

16 Chan H-L, Stern RS, Arndt KA *et al*. The incidence of erythema multiforme, Stevens–Johnson syndrome, and toxic epidermal necrolysis. A population-based study with particular reference to reactions caused by drugs among outpatients. *Arch Dermatol* 1990; **126**: 43–7.

17 Schöpf E, Stühmer A, Rzany B *et al*. Toxic epidermal necrolysis and Stevens–Johnson syndrome. An epidemiologic study from West Germany. *Arch Dermatol* 1991; **127**: 839–42.

18 Nicolis GD, Helwig EB. Exfoliative dermatitis. A clinicopathologic study of 135 cases. *Arch Dermatol* 1973; **108**: 788–97.

19 Sehgal VN, Srivastava G. Exfoliative dermatitis. A prospective study of 80 patients. *Dermatologica* 1986; **173**: 278–84.

20 Sehgal VN, Gangwani OP. Fixed drug eruption. Current concepts. *Int J Dermatol* 1987; **26**: 67–74.

21 Lehr D. Sulfonamide vasculitis. *J Clin Pharmacol* 1972; **2**: 181–9.

Sulfasalazine

Rashes occur in 1–5% of patients, and may be widespread as part of a hypersensitivity syndrome with hepatitis and encephalopathy [1–5], but desensitization is possible [6]. Blood disorders attributable to sulfasalazine occur at a rate of 3 per 1000 users [7]. An autoimmune syndrome has been described [8]. Photosensitivity [9] and a fixed eruption [10] have been documented. TEN, erythroid hypoplasia and agranulocytosis have been reported [11]. Bronchiolitis obliterans and alveolitis are well-recognized complications, and acute hypersensitivity pneumonia is recorded. LE, including cerebral LE, may be induced [12]. Reversible oligospermia may occur [13], and reversible hair loss has been attributed to use of this drug in enemas [14]. Many of the above adverse effects are attributable to the carrier molecule, sulfapyridine, which delivers 5-aminosalicylic acid, the component of sulfasalazine active in ulcerative colitis, to its site of action in the colon;

patients who are slow acetylators may be especially prone to side effects [15]. Urticaria, and possibly the renal toxicity, are due to the 5-aminosalicylic acid component [16].

Mesalazine (5-aminosalicylic acid)

Fever, erythematous skin eruption and lung involvement [17], and fever, diarrhoea, exfoliative dermatitis, marked atypical lymphocytosis and severe hepatotoxicity [18] have been described in patients with a previous history of sulfasalazine hypersensitivity. Additional cutaneous hypersensitivity reactions including vasculitis [19], a Kawasaki-like syndrome [20] and an LE-like syndrome [21] have been documented. This drug may cause renal damage, and is associated with blood dyscrasia [22] including fatal bone marrow suppression and thrombocytopenia [23]. A pustular reaction is recorded [24].

Olsalazine

This drug, which consists of a dimer of two molecules of 5-aminosalicylic acid linked by an azo bond, dispenses with the unwanted effects of sulfapyridine. Nonetheless, up to one in five patients experience diarrhoea, rash, nausea and abdominal pain severe enough to stop treatment with the drug [16].

Sulfamethoxypyridazine

Obliterative bronchiolitis and alveolitis have been documented in a patient with linear IgA disease of adults [25].

REFERENCES

1 Leroux JL, Ghezail M, Chertok P, Blotman F. Hypersensitivity reaction to sulfasalazine: skin rash, fever, hepatitis and activated lymphocytes. *Clin Exp Rheumatol* 1992; **10**: 427.

2 Gran JT, Myklebust G. Toxicity of sulphasalazine in rheumatoid arthritis. Possible protective effect of rheumatoid factors and corticosteroids. *Scand J Rheumatol* 1993; **22**: 229–32.

3 Gabay C, De Bandt M, Palazzo E. Sulphasalazine-related life-threatening side effects: is N-acetylcysteine of therapeutic value? *Clin Exp Rheumatol* 1993; **11**: 417–20.

4 Schoonjans R, Mast A, Van Den Abeele G *et al*. Sulfasalazine-associated encephalopathy in a patient with Crohn's disease. *Am J Gastroenterol* 1993; **88**: 1416–20.

5 Rubin R. Sulfasalazine-induced fulminant hepatic failure and necrotizing pancreatitis. *Am J Gastroenterol* 1994; **89**: 789–91.

6 Koski JM. Desensitization to sulphasalazine in patients with arthritis. *Clin Exp Rheumatol* 1993; **11**: 169–70.

7 Jick H, Myers MW, Dean AD. The risk of sulfasalazine- and mesalazine-associated blood disorders. *Pharmacotherapeutica* 1995; **15**: 176–81.

8 Vyse T, So AK. Sulphasalazine-induced autoimmune syndrome. *Br J Rheumatol* 1992; **31**: 115–6.

9 Watkinson G. Sulfasalazine: a review of 40 years' experience. *Drugs* 1986; **32**: 1–11.

10 Kanwar AJ, Singh M, Yunus M, Belhaj MS. Fixed eruption to sulphasalazine. *Dermatologica* 1987; **174**: 104.

11 Maddocks JL, Slater DN. Toxic epidermal necrolysis, agranulocytosis and erythroid hypoplasia associated with sulphasalazine. *J R Soc Med* 1980; **73**: 587–8.

12 Rafferty P, Young AC, Haeny MR. Sulphasalazine-induced cerebral lupus erythematosus. *Postgrad Med J* 1982; **58**: 98–9.

13 Drife JO. Drugs and sperm. *BMJ* 1982; **284**: 844–5.

14 Kutty PK, Raman KRK, Hawken K, Barrowman JA. Hair loss and 5-aminosalicylic acid enemas. *Ann Intern Med* 1982; **97**: 785–6.

15 Das KM, Eastwood MA, McManus JPA, Sircus W. Adverse reactions during salicylazosulfapyridine therapy and the relation with drug metabolism and acetylator phenotype. *N Engl J Med* 1973; **289**: 491–5.

16 Anonymous. Olsalazine: a further choice in ulcerative colitis. *Drug Ther Bull* 1990; **28**: 57–8.

17 Hautekeete ML, Bourgeois N, Potvin P et al. Hypersensitivity with hepatotoxicity to mesalazine after hypersensitivity to sulfasalazine. *Gastroenterology* 1992; **103**: 1925–7.

18 Aparicio J, Carnicer F, Girona E, Gomez A. Cutaneous hypersensitivity reaction to mesalazine. *Am J Gastroenterol* 1996; **91**: 620–1.

19 Lim AG, Hine KR. Fever, vasculitic rash, arthritis, pericarditis, and pericardial effusion after mesalazine. *BMJ* 1994; **308**: 113.

20 Waanders H, Thompson J. Kawasaki-like syndrome after treatment with mesalazine. *Am J Gastroenterol* 1991; **86**: 219–21.

21 Dent MT, Ganatpathy S, Holdworth CD, Channer KC. Mesalazine-induced lupus-like syndrome. *BMJ* 1992; **305**: 159.

22 Anonymous. Blood dyscrasias and mesalazine. *Curr Probl Pharmacovig* 1995; **21**: 5.

23 Daneshmend TK. Mesalazine-associated thrombocytopenia. *Lancet* 1991; **337**: 1297–8.

24 Gibbon KL, Bewley AP, Thomas K. Mesalazine-induced pustular drug eruption. *J Am Acad Dermatol* 2002; **46**: S220–S221.

25 Godfrey KM, Wojnarowska F, Friedland JS. Obliterative bronchiolitis and alveolitis associated with sulphamethoxypyridazine (Lederkyn) therapy for linear IgA disease of adults. *Br J Dermatol* 1990; **123**: 125–31.

Sulfadoxine

This sulphonamide is used in malaria prophylaxis in combination with pyrimethamine. The risk of reactions seems to be very low, but drug fever, TEN and photodermatitis have been recorded [1]. Stevens–Johnson syndrome may occur with Fansidar (pyrimethamine and sulfadoxine) for malaria prophylaxis [1–4] or with sulfadoxine alone [5]. TEN has occurred with Fansidar in an AIDS patient [6].

REFERENCES

1 Koch-Weser J, Hodel C, Leimer R, Styk S. Adverse reactions to pyrimethamine/sulfadoxine. *Lancet* 1982; **ii**: 1459.

2 Hornstein OP, Ruprecht KW. Fansidar-induced Stevens–Johnson syndrome. *N Engl J Med* 1982; **307**: 1529–30.

3 Miller KD, Lobel HO, Satriale RF et al. Severe cutaneous reactions among American travelers using pyrimethamine–sulfadoxine (Fansidar) for malaria prophylaxis. *Am J Trop Med Hyg* 1986; **35**: 451–8.

4 Ortel B, Sivayathorn A, Hönigsmann H. An unusual combination of phototoxicity and Stevens–Johnson syndrome due to antimalarial therapy. *Dermatologica* 1989; **178**: 39–42.

5 Hernborg A. Stevens–Johnson syndrome after mass prophylaxis with sulfadoxine for cholera in Mozambique. *Lancet* 1985; **i**: 1072–3.

6 Raviglione MC, Dinan WA, Pablos-Mendez A et al. Fatal toxic epidermal necrolysis during prophylaxis with pyrimethamine and sulfadoxine in a human immunodeficiency virus-infected person. *Arch Intern Med* 1988; **148**: 2863–5.

Trimethoprim–sulfamethoxazole (co-trimoxazole)

The general incidence and patterns of reactions to this mixture of sulfamethoxazole and trimethoprim are about the same as for sulphonamides in general; cutaneous reactions are seen in 3.3% of patients [1–3]. Severe cutaneous reactions of all types occur in about 1 per 100 000 users of the drug [2,3]. In view of these severe reactions, the drug is now indicated primarily for *Pneumocystis carinii* pneumonia, and for acute exacerbations of chronic bronchitis and urinary tract infections, and otitis media in children, only where there is good reason to prefer this combination [4]. There is a greatly increased incidence of reactions in patients with AIDS [5–13]. In one study, 18 of 38 patients with AIDS and *P. carinii* pneumonia treated with trimethoprim–sulfamethoxazole developed cutaneous reactions within a median of 11 days. It is sometimes possible to continue treatment through a hypersensitivity reaction, as reported for 67% of cases in the above study [14]. Adjuvant corticosteroids reduce the incidence of adverse cutaneous reactions to co-trimoxazole in patients with AIDS who are treated for hypoxaemic *P. carinii* pneumonia, but the incidence of mucocutaneous herpes simplex virus infection is higher [15]. If it is deemed essential to continue the drug, desensitization can be attempted [16,17].

Fixed eruptions occur [18–22], and may be due to the sulphonamide or trimethoprim components; a widespread fixed eruption mimicking TEN has been documented in one case [23]. Pustular reactions [24] and Sweet's syndrome [25] have been documented. Severe reactions have included erythema multiforme or Stevens–Johnson syndrome [26,27] that has been fatal [27], TEN in AIDS patients [5,11,12], cutaneous vasculitis [28] and fatal agranulocytosis [29]. One patient developed a rapidly progressive subepidermal bullous eruption within hours of intravenous trimethoprim–sulfamethoxazole [30].

REFERENCES

1 Jick J. Adverse reactions to trimethoprim–sulphamethoxazole in hospitalized patients. *Rev Infect Dis* 1982; **4**: 426–8.

2 Lawson DH, Paice BJ. Adverse reactions to trimethoprim–sulfamethoxazole. *Rev Infect Dis* 1982; **4**: 429–33.

3 Huisman MV, Buller HR, TenCate JW. Co-trimoxasole toxicity. *Lancet* 1984; **ii**: 1152.

4 Anonymous. Revised indications for co-trimoxazole (Septrin, Bactrim, various generic preparations). *Curr Probl Pharmacovig* 1995; **21**: 5.

5 Coopman SA, Johnson RA, Platt R, Stern RS. Cutaneous disease and drug reactions in HIV infection. *N Engl J Med* 1993; **328**: 1670–4.

6 Mitsuyasu R, Groopman J, Volberding P. Cutaneous reaction to trimethoprim–sulfamethoxazole in patients with AIDS and Kaposi's sarcoma. *N Engl J Med* 1983; **308**: 1535–6.

7 Gordin FM, Simon GL, Wofsy CB et al. Adverse reactions to trimethoprim sulfamethoxazole in patients with the acquired immune deficiency syndrome. *Ann Intern Med* 1984; **100**: 495–9.

8 Cohn DL, Penley KA, Judson FN et al. The acquired immunodeficiency syndrome and a trimethoprim–sulfamethoxazole-adverse reaction. *Ann Intern Med* 1984; **100**: 311.

9 Kovacs JA, Hiemenz JW, Macher AM et al. *Pneumocystis carinii* pneumonia: a comparison between patients with the acquired immunodeficiency syndrome and patients with other immunodeficiencies. *Ann Intern Med* 1984; **100**: 663–71.

10 De Raeve L, Song M, Van Maldergem L. Adverse cutaneous drug reactions in AIDS. *Br J Dermatol* 1988; **119**: 521–3.

11 Arnold P, Guglielmo J, Hollander H. Severe hypersensitivity reaction upon rechallenge with trimethoprim–sulfamethoxazole in a patient with AIDS. *Drug Intell Clin Pharmacol* 1988; **22**: 43–4.

12 Coopman SA, Stern RS. Cutaneous drug reactions in human immuno-deficiency virus infection. *Arch Dermatol* 1991; **127**: 714–7.
13 Chanock SJ, Luginbuhl LM, McIntosh K, Lipshultz SE. Life-threatening reaction to trimethoprim/sulfamethoxazole in pediatric human immuno-deficiency virus infection. *Pediatrics* 1994; **93**: 519–21.
14 Roudier C, Caumes E, Rogeaux O et al. Adverse cutaneous reactions to trimethoprim–sulfamethoxazole in patients with the acquired immuno-deficiency syndrome and *Pneumocystis carinii* pneumonia. *Arch Dermatol* 1994; **130**: 1383–6.
15 Caumes E, Roudier C, Rogeaux O et al. Effect of corticosteroids on the incid-ence of adverse cutaneous reactions to trimethoprim–sulfamethoxazole during treatment of AIDS-associated *Pneumocystis carinii* pneumonia. *Clin Infect Dis* 1994; **18**: 319–23.
16 Kletzel M, Beck S, Elser J et al. Trimethoprim–sulfamethoxazole oral desens-itization in hemophiliacs infected with human immunodeficiency virus with a history of hypersensitivity reactions. *Am J Dis Child* 1991; **145**: 1428–9.
17 Carr A, Penny R, Cooper DA. Efficacy and safety of rechallenge with low-dose trimethoprim–sulphamethoxazole in previously hypersensitive HIV-infected patients. *AIDS* 1993; **7**: 65–71.
18 Talbot MD. Fixed genital drug reaction. *Practitioner* 1980; **224**: 823–4.
19 Varsano I, Amir Y. Fixed drug eruption due to co-trimoxazole. *Dermato-logica* 1989; **178**: 232.
20 Van Voorhees A, Stenn KS. Histological phases of Bactrim-induced fixed drug eruption. The report of one case. *Am J Dermatopathol* 1987; **9**: 528–32.
21 Bharija SC, Belhaj MS. Fixed drug eruption due to cotrimoxazole. *Australas J Dermatol* 1989; **30**: 43–4.
22 Lim JT, Chan HL. Fixed drug eruptions due to co-trimoxazole. *Ann Acad Med Singapore* 1992; **21**: 408–10.
23 Baird BJ, De Villez RL. Widespread bullous fixed drug eruption mimicking toxic epidermal necrolysis. *Int J Dermatol* 1988; **27**: 170–4.
24 MacDonald KJS, Green CM, Kenicer KJA. Pustular dermatosis induced by co-trimoxazole. *BMJ* 1986; **293**: 1279–80.
25 Walker DC, Cohen PR. Trimethoprim–sulfamethoxazole-associated acute febrile neutrophilic dermatosis: case report and review of drug-induced Sweet's syndrome. *J Am Acad Dermatol* 1996; **34**: 918–23.
26 Azinge NO, Garrick GA. Stevens–Johnson syndrome (erythema multi-forme) following ingestion of trimethoprim–sulfamethoxazole on two sep-arate occasions in the same person. A case report. *J Allergy Clin Immunol* 1978; **62**: 125–6.
27 Beck MH, Portnoy B. Severe erythema multiforme complicated by fatal gastro-intestinal involvement following co-trimoxasole therapy. *Clin Exp Dermatol* 1979; **4**: 201–4.
28 Wåhlin A, Rosman N. Skin manifestations with vasculitis due to co-trimoxazole. *Lancet* 1976; **ii**: 1415.
29 Lawson DH, Henry DA, Jick H. Fatal agranulocytosis attributed to co-trimoxazole therapy. *BMJ* 1976; **ii**: 316.
30 Roholt NS, Lapiere JC, Traczyk T et al. A nonscarring sublamina densa bullous drug eruption. *J Am Acad Dermatol* 1995; **32**: 367–71.

Trimethoprim

Used alone, this substance causes less reactions than sulphonamides; fixed eruption has been proven [1–3] and was linear in one case [4]. Two patients experienced life-threatening immediate reactions and one patient devel-oped generalized urticaria following oral trimethoprim–sulfamethoxazole; prick tests and oral challenge tests were positive with trimethoprim but not sulfamethox-azole [5].

REFERENCES

1 Kanwar AJ, Bharija SC, Singh M, Belhaj MS. Fixed drug eruption to trimetho-prim. *Dermatologica* 1986; **172**: 230–1.
2 Hughes BR, Holt PJA, Marks R. Trimethoprim associated fixed drug erup-tion. *Br J Dermatol* 1987; **116**: 241–2.
3 Lim JT, Chan HL. Fixed drug eruptions due to co-trimoxazole. *Ann Acad Med Singapore* 1992; **21**: 408–10.
4 Özkaya-Bayazit E, Baykal C. Trimethoprim-induced linear fixed drug erup-tion. *Br J Dermatol* 1997; **137**: 1028–9.
5 Alonso MD, Marcos C, Davila I et al. Hypersensitivity to trimethoprim. *Allergy* 1992; **47**: 340–2.

Aminoglycosides

Gentamicin, tobramycin, streptomycin and kanamycin cross-react and are all potentially ototoxic and nephro-toxic. Exanthematic eruptions are common with strepto-mycin, developing in 5% or more of patients. Continued treatment may lead to generalized exfoliative dermatitis with these drugs [1] in a minority, but in a proportion of patients the rash subsides and treatment can be con-tinued. Fever and eosinophilia may be associated with the reactions. Urticaria [2], maculopapular rashes, fever and eosinophilia are well recognized with this group of drugs. Skin necrosis following subcutaneous injection of aminoglycoside antibiotics (gentamicin, sisomicin and netilmicin) has been reported in elderly females with a history of thrombosis being treated with heparin anti-coagulant therapy [3–5]. The reaction has also occurred following intramuscular sisomicin in a patient with defect-ive fibrinolysis and abnormal neutrophil function [6]. A toxic erythema with generalized follicular pustulosis has been documented with streptomycin [7]. Deafness has rarely followed topical therapy with neomycin, including administration of aerosol preparations in the treatment of extensive burns. An anaphylactic reaction due to strepto-mycin occurred during *in vitro* fertilization immediately after embryo transfer [8].

REFERENCES

1 Karp S, Bakris G, Cooney A et al. Exfoliative dermatitis secondary to tobramycin sulfate. *Cutis* 1991; **47**: 331–2.
2 Schretlen-Doherty JS, Troutman WG. Tobramycin-induced hypersensitivity reaction. *Ann Pharmacother* 1995; **29**: 704–6.
3 Taillandier J, Manigaud G, Fixy P, Dumont D. Nécroses cutanées induites par la gentamicine sous-cutanée. *Presse Med* 1984; **13**: 1574–5.
4 Duterque M, Hubert Asso AM, Corrard A. Lésions nécrotiques par injections sous cutanées de gentamicine et de sisomicine. *Ann Dermatol Vénéréol* 1985; **112**: 707–8.
5 Bernard P, Paris M, Cantanzano G, Bonnetblanc JM. Vascularite cutanée localisée induite par la Nétilmicine. *Presse Med* 1987; **16**: 915–6.
6 Grob JJ, Mege JL, Follano J et al. Skin necrosis after injection of aminogly-cosides. Arthus reaction, local toxicity, thrombotic process or pathergy? *Dermatologica* 1990; **181**: 258–62.
7 Kushimoto H, Aoki T. Toxic erythema with generalized follicular pustules caused by streptomycin. *Arch Dermatol* 1981; **117**: 444–5.
8 Abeck D, Kuwert C, Segnini-Torres M et al. Streptomycin-induced anaphy-lactic reaction during in vitro fertilization (IVF). *Allergy* 1994; **49**: 388–9.

Macrolide antibiotics

Macrolides account for 10–15% of the worldwide oral antibiotic market, with severe adverse reactions being rare [1]. Gastrointestinal reactions occur in 15–20% of patients on erythromycins and in 5% or fewer patients treated with some recently developed macrolide derivatives that seldom or never induce endogenous release of motilin, such as roxithromycin, clarithromycin, dirithromycin, azithromycin and rikamycin. Except for troleandomycin and some erythromycins administered at high dose and for long periods of time, the hepatotoxic potential of macrolides is low. Transient deafness and allergic reactions to macrolide antibacterials are highly unusual and are more common with the erythromycins than with the recently developed 14-, 15- and 16-membered macrolides.

Azithromycin

This drug has caused toxic pustuloderma [2].

Clarithromycin

Fixed drug eruption is recorded [3].

Erythromycin

This is one of the most innocuous antibiotics in current use. Cholestasis caused by the estolate ester is the only potentially serious side effect. Hypersensitivity skin reactions are rare but when they occur skin tests may be positive [4,5]. Erythema multiforme, Stevens–Johnson syndrome, toxic pustuloderma [6], systemic contact dermatitis [7] and vasculitis have all been recorded.

Spiramycin

Rashes, usually transient erythema, may occur in up to 1% of cases. Spiramycin, given for toxoplasmosis in pregnancy, was associated in one case with an erythematous maculopapular pruritic eruption with eosinophilia and raised γ-glutamyl transpeptidase [8]. The drug has caused an allergic vasculitis [9].

REFERENCES

1 Periti P, Mazzei T, Mini E, Novelli A. Adverse effects of macrolide antibacterials. *Drug Saf* 1993; **9**: 346–64.
2 Trevisi P, Patrizi A, Neri I, Farina P. Toxic pustuloderma associated with azithromycin. *Clin Exp Dermatol* 1994; **19**: 280–1.
3 Rosina P, Chieregato C, Schena D. Fixed drug eruption from clarithromycin. *Contact Dermatitis* 1998; **38**: 105.
4 Van Ketel WG. Immediate and delayed-type allergy to erythromycin. *Contact Dermatitis* 1976; **2**: 363–4.
5 Shirin H, Schapiro JM, Arber N *et al*. Erythromycin base-induced rash and liver function disturbances. *Ann Pharmacother* 1992; **26**: 1522–3.
6 Roujeau J-C, Bioulac-Sage P, Bourseau C *et al*. Acute generalized exanthematous pustulosis. Analysis of 63 cases. *Arch Dermatol* 1991; **127**: 1333–8.
7 Fernandez Redondo V, Casas L, Taboada M, Toribio J. Systemic contact dermatitis from erythromycin. *Contact Dermatitis* 1994; **30**: 311.
8 Ostlere LS, Langtry JAA, Staughton RCD. Allergy to spiramycin during prophlyactic treatment of fetal toxoplasmosis. *BMJ* 1991; **302**: 970.
9 Galland MC, Rodor F, Jouglard J. Spiramycin allergic vasculitis: first report. *Therapie* 1987; **42**: 227–9.

Clindamycin and lincomycin

These antibiotics have become particularly associated with a potentially lethal pseudomembranous colitis due to superinfection with *Clostridium difficile* [1–3]. Vancomycin or metronidazole is the treatment of choice for this complication. Hypersensitivity skin reactions are rare with lincomycin but common with clindamycin, occurring in up to 10% of patients [4]. Erythema multiforme and anaphylaxis are very rare [5].

REFERENCES

1 Dantzig PI. The safety of long-term clindamycin therapy for acne. *Arch Dermatol* 1976; **112**: 53–4.
2 Tan SG, Cunliffe WJ. The unwanted effects of clindamycin in acne. *Br J Dermatol* 1976; **94**: 313–5.
3 Anonymous. Antibiotic-associated colitis: a progress report. *BMJ* 1978; i: 669–71.
4 Lammintausta K, Tokola R, Kalimo K. Cutaneous adverse reactions to clindamycin: results of skin tests and oral exposure. *Br J Dermatol* 2002; **146**: 643–8.
5 Lochmann O, Kohout P, Vymola F. Anaphylactic shock following the administration of clindamycin. *J Hyg Epidemiol Microbiol Immunol* 1977; **21**: 441–7.

Miscellaneous antibiotics

Chloramphenicol

Although contact dermatitis from topical application is common, hypersensitivity skin reactions to oral therapy are rare. Macular, papular and urticarial eruptions are reported [1], as is acute generalized exanthematous pustulosis [2]. Pruritus may be prominent. Erythema multiforme and TEN [3] occur rarely. There is a risk of aplastic anaemia [4] and death has exceptionally followed the use of eye drops [5].

REFERENCES

1 Unsdek HE, Curtiss WP, Neill EJ. Skin eruption due to chloramphenicol (Chloromycetin®). *Arch Dermatol Syphilol* 1951; **64**: 217.
2 Lee AY, Yoo SH. Chloramphenicol induced acute generalized exanthematous pustulosis proved by patch test and systemic provocation. *Acta Derm Venereol (Stockh)* 1999; **79**: 412–3.
3 Mathe P, Aubert L, Labouche F *et al*. Syndrome de Lyell. Etiologie médicamenteuse: rôle probable de chloramphénicol. *J Méd Bordeaux* 1965; **42**: 1367–76.
4 Hargraves MM, Mills SD, Heck FJ. Aplastic anemia associated with the administration of chloramphenicol. *JAMA* 1952; **149**: 1293–300.
5 Fraunfelder FT, Bagby GC. Ocular chloramphenicol and aplastic anemia. *N Engl J Med* 1983; **308**: 1536.

Fusidic acid

Topical use can lead to contact dermatitis but hypersensitivity reactions to oral or parenteral use are very rare; jaundice has accompanied intravenous use. Acanthosis nigricans-like lesions have been reported after local application [1].

REFERENCE

1 Teknetzis A, Lefaki I, Joannides D, Minas A. Acanthosis nigricans-like lesions after local application of fusidic acid. *J Am Acad Dermatol* 1993; **28**: 501–2.

Metronidazole and tinidazole

Metronidazole. Pruritus, fixed eruptions and generalized erythema [1–4] are rare. A pityriasis rosea-like eruption has been described [5]. A reversible peripheral neuropathy may complicate prolonged therapy.

Tinidazole. A fixed eruption with cross-reactivity with metronidazole has been reported [6,7].

REFERENCES

1 Naik RPC, Singh G. Fixed drug eruption due to metronidazole. *Dermatologica* 1977; **155**: 59–60.
2 Shelley WB, Shelley ED. Fixed drug eruption due to metronidazole. *Cutis* 1987; **39**: 393–4.
3 Gastaminza G, Anda M, Audicana MT *et al*. Fixed-drug eruption due to metronidazole with positive topical provocation. *Contact Dermatitis* 2001; **44**: 36.
4 Knowles S, Choudhury T, Shear NH. Metronidazole hypersensitivity. *Ann Pharmacother* 1994; **28**: 325–6.
5 Maize JC, Tomecki KJ. Pityriasis rosea-like drug eruption secondary to metronidazole. *Arch Dermatol* 1977; **113**: 1457–8.
6 Kanwar AJ, Sharma R, Rajagopalan M, Kaur S. Fixed drug eruption due to tinidazole with cross-reactivity with metronidazole. *Dermatologica* 1990; **181**: 277.
7 Mishra D, Mobashir M, Zaheer MS. Fixed drug eruption and cross-reactivity between tinidazole and metronidazole. *Int J Dermatol* 1990; **29**: 740.

Nitrofurantoin

Pruritus, morbilliform rashes and urticaria may be seen occasionally. Erythema multiforme, erythema nodosum [1], exfoliative dermatitis and an LE-like syndrome [2] are documented. Acute or chronic pulmonary reactions may accompany these skin manifestations, and may lead to pulmonary fibrosis [3]. Polyneuritis is a dose-dependent toxic reaction. Hepatitis, cholestatic jaundice and marrow suppression may occur rarely. Abnormal immunoelectrophoretic patterns may be induced [4].

REFERENCES

1 Chisholm JC, Hepner M. Nitrofurantoin induced erythema nodosum. *J Natl Med Assoc* 1981; **73**: 59–61.
2 Selross O, Edgren J. Lupus-like syndrome associated with pulmonary reaction to nitrofurantoin. *Acta Med Scand* 1975; **197**: 125–9.
3 Rantala H, Kirvelä O, Anttolainen I. Nitrofurantoin lung in a child. *Lancet* 1979; **ii**: 799–80.
4 Teppo AM, Haltia K, Wager O. Immunoelectrophoretic 'tailing' of albumin line due to albumin–IgG antibody complexes: a side effect of nitrofurantoin treatment? *Scand J Immunol* 1976; **5**: 249–61.

Quinolones

These compounds are related to nalidixic acid; central nervous system toxicity, upper gastrointestinal tract reactions and phototoxicity have been recorded [1–7]. Cross-reactivity occurs [8]. Gastrointestinal side effects occur in up to 6% of patients. Hypersensitivity reactions involving the skin have been reported in 0.5–2% of patients, and in up to 2.4% of patients receiving cinoxacin; they most frequently manifest themselves as rash or pruritus. Fever, urticaria, angio-oedema and anaphylactoid reactions are rare. Anaphylactic or anaphylactoid reactions have been documented with cinoxacin [9], ciprofloxacin (1.2 per 100 000 prescriptions) [10,11] and pipemidic acid [12]. Fixed drug eruption due to pipemidic acid is recorded [13]. Norfloxacin [14] and ofloxacin [15] have caused a pustular eruption. Ciprofloxacin [16,17], pefloxacin, fleroxacin [18] and enoxacin [19] have been associated with photosensitivity. Pefloxacin and ofloxacin have caused photo-onycholysis [20], and sparfloxacin has been implicated in photosensitivity and a lichenoid tissue reaction [21]. Hypersensitivity leukocytoclastic vasculitis has been reported with both ofloxacin and ciprofloxacin [22,23] and serum sickness with ciprofloxacin [24]. Intravenous administration of ciprofloxacin through small veins on the dorsa of the hands may be associated with local reactions at the site of infusion [25]. Stevens–Johnson syndrome or TEN has been described with quinolones [26] including ciprofloxacin [27]. Ciprofloxacin has caused bullous pemphigoid [28].

Nalidixic acid. Cutaneous reactions are common, occurring in up to 5% of patients; various hypersensitivity reactions are seen, including exfoliative dermatitis. Phototoxicity is now well recognized [29–33]. A bullous photodermatitis may occur, usually on the hands or feet; chronic scarring and increased skin fragility may mimic porphyria cutanea tarda. Long-wave UV light is responsible [32]. An LE-like syndrome has been reported [34], as well as transient alopecia.

REFERENCES

1 Christ W, Lehnert T, Ulbrich B. Specific toxicologic aspects of the quinolones. *Rev Infect Dis* 1988; **10** (Suppl. 1): S141–S146.
2 Wolfson JS, Hooper DC. Fluoroquinolone antimicrobial agents. *Clin Microbiol Rev* 1989; **2**: 378–424.
3 Hooper DC, Wolfson JS. Fluoroquinolone antimicrobial agents. *N Engl J Med* 1991; **324**: 384–94.
4 Sisca TS, Heel RC, Romankiewicz JA. Cinoxacin: a review of its pharmacological properties and therapeutic efficacy in the treatment of urinary tract infections. *Drugs* 1983; **25**: 544–69.
5 Campoli-Richards DM, Monck JP, Price A *et al*. Ciprofloxacin. A review of its antibacterial activity, pharmacokinetic properties and therapeutic use. *Drugs* 1988; **35**: 373–447.
6 Norrby SR, Lietman PS. Safety and tolerability of fluoroquinolones. *Drugs* 1993; **45** (Suppl. 3): 59–64.
7 Matsuno K, Kunihiro E, Yamatoya O *et al*. Surveillance of adverse reactions due to ciprofloxacin in Japan. *Drugs* 1995; **49** (Suppl. 2): 495–6.
8 Davila I, Diez ML, Quirce S *et al*. Cross-reactivity between quinolones. Report of three cases. *Allergy* 1993; **48**: 388–90.
9 Stricker BHC, Slagboom G, Demaeseneer R *et al*. Anaphylactic reactions to cinoxacin. *BMJ* 1988; **297**: 1434–5.

10 Davis H, McGoodwin E, Reed TG. Anaphylactoid reactions reported after treatment with ciprofloxacin. *Ann Intern Med* 1989; **111**: 1041–3.
11 Deamer RL, Prichard JG, Loman GJ. Hypersensitivity and anaphylactoid reactions to ciprofloxacin. *Ann Pharmacother* 1992; **26**: 1081–4.
12 Gerber D. Anaphylaxis caused by pipemidic acid. *S Afr Med J* 1985; **67**: 999.
13 Miyagawa S, Yamashina Y, Hirota S, Shirai T. Fixed drug eruption due to pipemidic acid. *J Dermatol* 1991; **18**: 59–60.
14 Shelley ED, Shelley WB. The subcorneal pustular drug eruption: an example induced by norfloxacin. *Cutis* 1988; **42**: 24–7.
15 Tsuda S, Kato K, Karashima T *et al*. Toxic pustuloderma induced by ofloxacin. *Ann Dermatol Vénéréol* 1993; **73**: 382–4.
16 Nederost ST, Dijkstra JWE, Handel DW. Drug-induced photosensitivity reaction. *Arch Dermatol* 1989; **125**: 433–4.
17 Ferguson J, Johnson BE. Ciprofloxacin-induced photosensitivity: in vitro and in vivo studies. *Br J Dermatol* 1990; **123**: 9–20.
18 Bowie WR, Willetts V, Jewesson PJ. Adverse reactions in a dose-ranging study with a new long-acting fluoroquinolone, fleroxacin. *Antimicrob Agents Chemother* 1989; **33**: 1778–82.
19 Izu R, Gardeazabal J, Gonzalez M *et al*. Enoxacin-induced photosensitivity: study of two cases. *Photodermatol Photoimmunol Photomed* 1992; **9**: 86–8.
20 Baran R, Brun P. Photo-onycholysis induced by the fluoroquinolones pefloxacine and ofloxacine. Report on 2 cases. *Dermatologica* 1986; **173**: 185–8.
21 Hamanaka H, Mizutani H, Shimizu M. Sparfloxacin-induced photosensitivity and the occurrence of a lichenoid tissue reaction after prolonged exposure. *J Am Acad Dermatol* 1998; **38**: 945–9.
22 Huminer C, Cohen JD, Majafla R, Dux S. Hypersensitivity vasculitis due to ofloxacin. *BMJ* 1989; **299**: 303.
23 Choc U, Rothschield BM, Laitman L. Ciprofloxacin-induced vasculitis. *N Engl J Med* 1989; **320**: 257–8.
24 Guharoy SR. Serum sickness secondary to ciprofloxacin use. *Vet Hum Toxicol* 1994; **36**: 540–1.
25 Thorsteinsson SB, Bergan T, Johannesson G *et al*. Tolerance of ciprofloxacin at injection site, systemic safety and effect on electroencephalogram. *Chemotherapy* 1987; **33**: 448–51.
26 Roujeau JC, Kelly JP, Naldi L *et al*. Medication use and the risk of Stevens–Johnson syndrome or toxic epidermal necrolysis. *N Engl J Med* 1995; **333**: 1600–7.
27 Tham TCK, Allen G, Hayes D *et al*. Possible association between toxic epidermal necrolysis and ciprofloxacin. *Lancet* 1991; **338**: 522.
28 Kimyai-Asadi A, Usman A, Nousari HC. Ciprofloxacin-induced bullous pemphigoid. *J Am Acad Dermatol* 2000; **42**: 847.
29 Baes H. Photosensitivity caused by nalidixic acid. *Dermatologica* 1968; **136**: 61–4.
30 Birkett DA, Garretts M, Stevenson CJ. Phototoxic bullous eruptions due to nalidixic acid. *Br J Dermatol* 1969; **81**: 342–4.
31 Ramsay CA, Obreshkova E. Photosensitivity from nalidixic acid. *Br J Dermatol* 1974; **91**: 523–8.
32 Rosén K, Swanbeck G. Phototoxic reactions from some common drugs provoked by a high-intensity UVA lamp. *Acta Derm Venereol (Stockh)* 1982; **62**: 246–8.
33 Nederost ST, Dijkstra JWE, Handel DW. Drug-induced photosensitivity reaction. *Arch Dermatol* 1989; **125**: 433–4.
34 Rubinstein A. LE-like disease caused by nalidixic acid. *N Engl J Med* 1979; **301**: 1288.

Synergistins

An eczema-like drug eruption is recorded after oral antibiotic synergistins, pristinamycin and virginiamycin, following contact sensitization with topical virginiamycin [1].

REFERENCE

1 Michel M, Dompmartin A, Szczurko C *et al*. Eczematous-like drug eruption induced by synergistins. *Contact Dermatitis* 1996; **34**: 86–7.

Vancomycin

Allergic skin reactions are not uncommon, occurring in up to 5% of patients. Rapid intravenous infusion of vancomycin can cause a histamine-induced anaphylactoid reaction characterized by flushing, a maculopapular eruption of the neck, face, trunk and extremities (so-called 'red man syndrome'), prolonged hypotension and, in rare cases, cardiac arrest [1–3]. Desensitization has been successfully achieved in patients with vancomycin hypersensitivity [4–6]. TEN has occurred [7]. Vancomycin has been reported to have induced linear IgA bullous dermatosis [8–12], which may mimic TEN [13].

REFERENCES

1 Pau AK, Khakoo R. Red-neck syndrome with slow infusion of vancomycin. *N Engl J Med* 1985; **313**: 756–7.
2 Valero R, Gomar C, Fita G *et al*. Adverse reactions to vancomycin prophylaxis in cardiac surgery. *J Cardiothor Vasc Anesth* 1991; **5**: 574–6.
3 Killian AD, Sahai JV, Memish ZA. Red man syndrome after oral vancomycin. *Ann Intern Med* 1991; **115**: 410–31.
4 Lin RY. Desensitization in the management of vancomycin hypersensitivity. *Arch Intern Med* 1990; **150**: 2197–8.
5 Anne S, Middleton E Jr, Reisman RE. Vancomycin anaphylaxis and successful desensitization. *Ann Allergy* 1994; **73**: 402–4.
6 Wong JT, Ripple RE, MacLean JA *et al*. Vancomycin hypersensitivity: synergism with narcotics and 'desensitization' by a rapid continuous intravenous protocol. *J Allergy Clin Immunol* 1994; **94**: 189–94.
7 Vidal C, Gonzalez Quintela A, Fuente R. Toxic epidermal necrolysis due to vancomycin. *Ann Allergy* 1992; **68**: 345–7.
8 Baden LA, Apovian C, Imber MJ, Dover JS. Vancomycin-induced linear IgA bullous dermatosis. *Arch Dermatol* 1988; **124**: 1186–8.
9 Carpenter S, Berg D, Sidhu-Malik N *et al*. Vancomycin-associated linear IgA dermatosis. A report of three cases. *J Am Acad Dermatol* 1992; **26**: 45–8.
10 Piketty C, Meeus F, Nochy D *et al*. Linear IgA dermatosis related to vancomycin. *Br J Dermatol* 1994; **130**: 130–1.
11 Whitworth JM, Thomas I, Peltz S *et al*. Vancomycin-induced linear IgA bullous dermatosis (LABD). *J Am Acad Dermatol* 1996; **34**: 890–1.
12 Palmer RA, Ogg G, Allen J *et al*. Vancomycin-induced linear IgA disease with autoantibodies to BP180 and LAD285. *Br J Dermatol* 2001; **145**: 816–20.
13 Dellavalle RP, Burch HM, Tyal S *et al*. Vancomycin-associated linear IgA bullous dermatosis mimicking toxic epidermal necrolysis. *J Am Acad Dermatol* 2003; **48**: S56–S57.

Topical antibiotics

The side effects of topical antibiotics have been reviewed [1]. Allergic contact dermatitis is rare with topical clindamycin, erythromycin and tetracycline, polymyxin B, gentamicin and mupirocin, but is more frequent with neomycin.

Bacitracin

Anaphylaxis due to bacitracin allergy has followed topical application of this antibiotic [2–5]. The patients had had multiple prior exposures and previous local reactions of pruritus, urticaria or possible allergic contact dermatitis. Two patients with anaphylactic reactions to Polyfax ointment, containing polymyxin B and bacitracin, have been reported; one had previously documented positive patch tests to Polyfax, and the other had clinical intolerance to the preparation [5]. Another patient developed anaphylaxis to a similar proprietary mixture (Polysporin) [6]. Intracutaneous injection of bacitracin in sensitive individuals induces histamine release with large weal-and-flare reactions [7].

Chloramphenicol

Urticaria and angio-oedema have been described with topical use [8]. Fatal aplastic anaemia has followed the use of eye drops containing this antibiotic [9].

Sulphonamides

Erythema multiforme and Stevens–Johnson syndrome have been reported from topical preparations [10,11].

REFERENCES

1 Hirschmann JV. Topical antibiotics in dermatology. *Arch Dermatol* 1988; **124**: 1691–700.
2 Roupe G, Strannegård Ö. Anaphylactic shock elicited by topical administration of bacitracin. *Arch Dermatol* 1969; **100**: 450–2.
3 Shechter JF, Wilkinson RD, Del Carpio J. Anaphylaxis following the use of bacitracin ointment: report of a case and review of the literature. *Arch Dermatol* 1984; **120**: 909–11.
4 Katz BE, Fisher AA. Bacitracin: a unique topical antibiotic sensitiser. *J Am Acad Dermatol* 1987; **17**: 1016–24.
5 Eedy DJ, McMillan JC, Bingham EA. Anaphylactic reactions to topical antibiotic combinations. *Postgrad Med J* 1990; **66**: 858–9.
6 Knowles SR, Shear NH. Anaphylaxis from bacitracin and polymyxin B (Polysporin) ointment. *Int J Dermatol* 1995; **34**: 572–3.
7 Bjorkner B, Moller H. Bacitracin: a cutaneous allergen and histamine releaser. *Acta Derm Venereol (Stockh)* 1973; **53**: 487–91.
8 Schewach-Millet M, Shapiro D. Urticaria and angioedema due to topically applied chloramphenicol ointment. *Arch Dermatol* 1985; **121**: 587.
9 Fraunfelder FT, Bagby GC. Ocular chloramphenicol and aplastic anemia. *N Engl J Med* 1983; **308**: 1536.
10 Genvert GI, Cohen EJ, Donnenfeld ED, Blecher MH. Erythema multiforme after use of topical sulfacetamide. *Am J Ophthalmol* 1985; **99**: 465–8.
11 Gottschalk HR, Stone OJ. Stevens–Johnson syndrome from ophthalmic sulphonamide. *Arch Dermatol* 1976; **112**: 513–4.

Antituberculous drugs

Severe cutaneous reactions (such as Stevens–Johnson syndrome and TEN) and multiple drug reactions to antituberculous drugs (including thioacetazone, streptomycin and isoniazid) occur more often in HIV-positive patients [1–5]. The World Health Organization has advised against the use of thioacetazone in tuberculosis patients with known, or suspected, HIV infection in view of the severe cutaneous hypersensitivity [3–5]. The following drugs are reported to cause contact dermatitis: isoniazid, rifampicin, ethambutol, *p*-aminosalicylic acid, streptomycin and kanamycin [6]. The incidence of other reactions to individual drugs is difficult to assess because several drugs are usually used in combination.

Cycloserine

A lichenoid drug eruption with positive patch tests and resolution 4 months after withdrawal has been reported [7].

Ethambutol

Hypersensitivity reactions are very rare. Side effects are largely confined to visual disturbances, with loss of acuity, colour blindness and restricted visual fields; these are usually reversible if the drug is stopped promptly. Patients should have ophthalmic assessments prior to and during therapy. Lichenoid reactions occur and may be restricted to light-exposed sites [8,9].

Ethionamide

Eczema chiefly affecting the forehead, acneiform eruptions, butterfly eruptions on the face, stomatitis, alopecia and purpura have been reported.

Isoniazid

Allergic skin reactions occur in fewer than 1% of patients. An acneiform eruption, usually occurring in slow inactivators of the drug, is well recognized [10,11]. Urticaria, purpura and an LE-like syndrome [12,13] have been reported, as have photosensitive lichenoid eruptions [14]. Rarely, a pellagra-like syndrome has been induced in malnourished patients, due to metabolic antagonism of nicotinic acid with resultant pyridoxine deficiency [10,15]. Exfoliative dermatitis [16] and Stevens–Johnson syndrome [2] have been reported.

Pyrazinamide

Hepatitis, arthralgia, flushing, photosensitivity, lichenoid photodermatitis, maculopapular rashes, urticaria and pellagra are recorded [17].

Rifampicin

Cutaneous hypersensitivity reactions are very uncommon. There have been isolated reports of LE [18], erythema nodosum leprosum-like eruption in borderline lepromatous leprosy [19], exacerbation of bullous erythema multiforme, TEN [20] and pemphigus [21,22]; existing pemphigus may also be exacerbated [23]. Altered liver function, usually transient, and thrombocytopenic purpura may occur. Rifampicin has precipitated porphyria cutanea tarda [24]. It induces liver enzymes and may thus reduce the effectiveness of a number of drugs, including oral contraceptives.

Streptomycin

See aminoglycosides section on p. 73.60.

Thioacetazone

Severe cutaneous hypersensitivity reactions have been reported, including maculopapular rashes (which progress to mucosal involvement with constitutional symptoms), Stevens–Johnson syndrome and TEN, especially in HIV-seropositive patients [2,3,5,25,26]. Cutaneous hypersensitivity reactions have been reported in 20% of HIV-seropositive patients compared with 1% of HIV-seronegative patients who receive the drug as part of treatment for tuberculosis [26]. Figurate erythematous eruptions resembling erythema annulare centrifugum may occur [27].

REFERENCES

1 Pozniak AL, MacLeod GA, Mahari M *et al.* The influence of HIV status on single and multiple drug reactions to antituberculous therapy in Africa. *AIDS* 1992; **6**: 809–14.
2 Dukes CS, Sugarman J, Cegielski JP, Lallinger GJ, Mwakyusa DH. Severe cutaneous hypersensitivity reactions during treatment of tuberculosis in patients with HIV infection in Tanzania. *Trop Geogr Med* 1992; **44**: 308–11.
3 Chintu C, Luo C, Bhat G *et al.* Cutaneous hypersensitivity reactions due to thiacetazone in the treatment of tuberculosis in Zambian children infected with HIV-I. *Arch Dis Child* 1993; **68**: 665–8.
4 Nunn P, Porter J, Winstanley P. Thiacetazone: avoid like poison or use with care? *Trans R Soc Trop Med Hyg* 1993; **87**: 578–82.
5 Kelly P, Buve A, Foster SD *et al.* Cutaneous reactions to thiacetazone in Zambia: implications for tuberculosis treatment strategies. *Trans R Soc Trop Med Hyg* 1994; **88**: 113–5.
6 Holdiness MR. Contact dermatitis to antituberculous drugs. *Contact Dermatitis* 1986; **15**: 282–8.
7 Shim JH, Kim TY, Kim HO, Kim CW. Cycloserine-induced lichenoid drug eruption. *Dermatology* 1995; **191**: 142–4.
8 Frentz G, Wadskov S, Kssis V. Ethambutol-induced lichenoid eruption. *Acta Derm Venereol (Stockh)* 1981; **61**: 89–91.
9 Grossman ME, Warren K, Mady A, Satra KH. Lichenoid eruption associated with ethambutol. *J Am Acad Dermatol* 1995; **33**: 675–6.
10 Cohen LK, George W, Smith R. Isoniazid-induced acne and pellagra. Occurrence in slow acetylators of isoniazid. *Arch Dermatol* 1974; **109**: 377–81.
11 Oliwiecki S, Burton JL. Severe acne due to isoniazid. *Clin Exp Dermatol* 1988; **13**: 283–4.
12 Grunwald M, David M, Feuerman EJ. Appearance of lupus erythematosus in a patient with lichen planus treated by isoniazid. *Dermatologica* 1982; **165**: 172–7.
13 Sim E, Gill EW, Sim RB. Drugs that induce systemic lupus erythematosus inhibit complement C4. *Lancet* 1984; **ii**: 422–4.
14 Lee AY, Jung SY. Two patients with isoniazid-induced photosensitive lichenoid eruptions confirmed by photopatch test. *Photodermatol Photoimmunol Photomed* 1998; **14**: 77–8.
15 Schmutz JL, Cuny JF, Trechot P *et al.* Les érythèmes pellagroïdes médicamenteux. Une observation d'érythème pellagroïde secondaire a l'isoniazide. *Ann Dermatol Vénéréol* 1987; **114**: 569–76.
16 Rosin MA, King LE Jr. Isoniazid-induced exfoliative dermatitis. *South Med J* 1982; **75**: 81.
17 Choonhakarn C, Janma J. Pyrazinamide-induced lichenoid photodermatitis. *J Am Acad Dermatol* 1999; **40**: 645–6.
18 Patel GK, Anstey AV. Rifampicin-induced lupus erythematosus. *Clin Exp Dermatol* 2001; **26**: 260–2.
19 Karthikeyan K, Thappa DM, Kadhiravan T. Rifampicin-induced erythema nodosum leprosum-like eruption in borderline lepromatous leprosy. *Ind J Leprosy* 2001; **73**: 167–9.
20 Okano M, Kitano Y, Igarashi T. Toxic epidermal necrolysis due to rifampicin. *J Am Acad Dermatol* 1987; **17**: 303–4.
21 Gange RW, Rhodes EL, Edwards CO, Powell MEA. Pemphigus induced by rifampicin. *Br J Dermatol* 1976; **95**: 445–8.
22 Lee CW, Lim JH, Kang HJ. Pemphigus foliaceus induced by rifampicin. *Br J Dermatol* 1984; **111**: 619–22.
23 Miyagawa S, Yamanashi Y, Okuchi T *et al.* Exacerbation of pemphigus by rifampicin. *Br J Dermatol* 1986; **114**: 729–32.
24 Millar JW. Rifampicin-induced porphyria cutanea tarda. *Br J Dis Chest* 1980; **74**: 405–8.
25 Fegan D, Glennon J. Cutaneous sensitivity to thiacetazone. *Lancet* 1991; **337**: 1036.
26 Nunn P, Kibuga D, Gathua S *et al.* Cutaneous hypersensitivity reactions due to thiacetazone in HIV-1 seropositive patients treated for tuberculosis. *Lancet* 1991; **337**: 627–30.
27 Ramesh V. Eruption resembling erythema annulare centrifugum. *Australas J Dermatol* 1987; **28**: 44.

Antileprotic drugs

Clofazimine

This drug regularly causes a reversible, dose-dependent, brown-orange pigmentation of the skin [1–3]. Biopsy specimens from two lepromatous leprosy patients on long-term clofazimine therapy revealed ceroid-lipofuscin pigment as well as clofazimine inside macrophage phagolysosomes [3]. Reddish-blue pigmentation occurred in scarred areas of LE in one patient [4]. Xeroderma, pruritus, phototoxicity, acne and non-specific rashes are described [2]. Gastrointestinal symptoms may occur early due to direct irritation of the gut and are quickly reversible; ulcerative enteritis may occur after 9–14 months of treatment. After prolonged high-dose therapy, persistent diarrhoea, abdominal pain and weight loss, associated with deposition of crystalline clofazimine in the small intestinal submucosa and mesenteric lymph nodes, may occur [5,6]. Splenic infarction has been associated with this syndrome [7,8].

REFERENCES

1 Thomsen K, Rothenborg HW. Clofazimine in the treatment of pyoderma gangrenosum. *Arch Dermatol* 1979; **115**: 851–2.
2 Yawalker SJ, Vischer W. Lamprene (clofazimine) in leprosy. Basic information. *Lepr Rev* 1979; **50**: 135–44.
3 Job CK, Yoder L, Jacobson RR, Hastings RC. Skin pigmentation from clofazimine therapy in leprosy patients: a reappraisal. *J Am Acad Dermatol* 1990; **23**: 236–41.
4 Kossard S, Doherty E, McColl I, Ryman W. Autofluorescence of clofazimine in discoid lupus erythematosus. *J Am Acad Dermatol* 1987; **17**: 867–71.
5 Harvey RF, Harman RRM, Black C *et al.* Abdominal pain and malabsorption due to tissue deposition of clofazimine (Lamprene) crystals. *Br J Dermatol* 1977; **97** (Suppl. 15): 19.
6 Venencie PY, Cortez A, Orieux G *et al.* Clofazimine enteropathy. *J Am Acad Dermatol* 1986; **15**: 290–1.
7 Jopling WAH. Complications of treatment with clofazimine (Lamprene: B.663). *Lepr Rev* 1976; **47**: 1–3.
8 McDougal AC, Horsfall WR, Hede JE, Chaplin AJ. Splenic infarction and tissue accumulation of crystals associated with the use of clofazimine (Lamprene: B.663) in the treatment of pyoderma gangrenosum. *Br J Dermatol* 1980; **102**: 227–30.

Dapsone

Reactions have been reviewed [1]. Fixed eruptions occur in 3% of West Africans being treated for leprosy. Erythema multiforme [2] and exfoliative dermatitis [3] have been described during leprosy treatment. Another uncommon side effect is a hypersensitivity reaction (dapsone or sulphone syndrome) within the first month or so, with fever, a widespread erythematous eruption studded with pustules, exfoliative dermatitis, hepatitis, lymphadenopathy and anaemia [4–10]. In Vanuatu, 24% of 37 patients treated over 4 years with daily dapsone 100 mg, clofazimine, and monthly rifampicin and clofazimine for leprosy developed the dapsone syndrome, with a fatality rate of 11% [11]. The increase in reactions may have related to a high starting dose of dapsone, possibly enhanced by the combination with clofazimine and rifampicin and by a genetic susceptibility of the Melanesian population.

Red cell life is always shortened, but clinical haemolytic anaemia is uncommon; patients with low red cell glucose-6-phosphate dehydrogenase levels [12] and those who are slow acetylators [13] are at a special risk of developing this complication. Methaemoglobinaemia and Heinz body formation are seen [14]. Agranulocytosis is rare but well recognized and may occur in the first weeks of therapy [15–17]. For patients receiving the drug for dermatitis herpetiformis, this side effect occurred at a median dosage of 100 mg/day and a median duration of therapy of 7 weeks [16]. The total risk was one case per 3000 patient-years of exposure to the drug; however, agranulocytosis was estimated to occur in 1 in 240 to 1 in 425 new patients receiving dapsone for dermatitis herpetiformis [16]. Agranulocytosis occurred in approximately 1 in 10 000 to 1 in 20 000 US soldiers receiving dapsone for malarial prophylaxis [18]. Elderly patients do not tolerate dapsone well, and sulfapyridine or sulfamethoxypyridazine (the latter obtainable on a named-patient basis from Lederle Laboratories) is to be preferred for IgA-related diseases. A fatal haematological reaction developed in a Burmese boy during induction of treatment for lepromatous leprosy [19].

Severe but usually reversible hypoalbuminaemia due to failure of albumin production [20,21] or an atypical nephrotic syndrome may occur. Rarely, dapsone causes a peripheral neuropathy, usually purely motor or mixed sensorimotor and usually recovering within a year [22–25], and optic atrophy [25]. Permanent retinal damage has followed overdosage [26]. Headaches [27], and occasionally a psychosis [28], may be precipitated.

REFERENCES

1 Zhu YI, Stiller MJ. Dapsone and sulfones in dermatology. Overview and update. *J Am Acad Dermatol* 2001; **45**: 420–34.

2 Dutta RK. Erythema multiforme bullosum due to dapsone. *Lepr India* 1980; **52**: 306–9.
3 Browne SG. Antileprosy drugs. *BMJ* 1971; **iv**: 558–9.
4 Tomecki KJ, Catalano CJ. Dapsone hypersensitivity: the sulfone syndrome revisited. *Arch Dermatol* 1981; **117**: 38–9.
5 Mohle-Boetani J, Akula SK, Holodniy M *et al*. The sulfone syndrome in a patient receiving dapsone prophylaxis for *Pneumocystis carinii* pneumonia. *West J Med* 1992; **156**: 303–6.
6 Barnard GF, Scharf MJ, Dagher RK. Sulfone syndrome in a patient receiving steroids for pemphigus. *Am J Gastroenterol* 1994; **89**: 2057–9.
7 Saito S, Ikezawa Z, Miyamoto H, Kim S. A case of the 'dapsone syndrome'. *Clin Exp Dermatol* 1994; **19**: 152–6.
8 Chalasani P, Baffoe-Bonnie H, Jurado RL. Dapsone therapy causing sulfone syndrome and lethal hepatic failure in an HIV-infected patient. *South Med J* 1994; **87**: 145–6.
9 Bocquet H, Bourgault-Villada I, Delfau-Larue MH *et al*. Syndrome d'hypersensibilité à la dapsone. Clone T circulant transitoire. *Ann Dermatol Vénéréol* 1995; **122**: 514–6.
10 Prussick R, Shear NH. Dapsone hypersensitivity syndrome. *J Am Acad Dermatol* 1996; **35**: 346–9.
11 Reeve PA, Ala J, Hall JJ. Dapsone syndrome in Vanuatu: a high incidence during multidrug treatment (MDT) of leprosy. *J Trop Med Hyg* 1992; **95**: 266–70.
12 Beutler E. Glucose-6-phosphate dehydrogenase deficiency. *Lancet* 1991; **324**: 169–74.
13 Ellard GA, Gammon PT, Savin LA, Tan RSH. Dapsone acetylation in dermatitis herpetiformis. *Br J Dermatol* 1974; **90**: 441–4.
14 Wagner A, Marosi C, Binder M *et al*. Fatal poisoning due to dapsone in a patient with grossly elevated methaemoglobin levels. *Br J Dermatol* 1995; **133**: 816–7.
15 Potter MN, Yates P, Slade R, Kennedy CTC. Agranulocytosis caused by dapsone therapy for granuloma annulare. *J Am Acad Dermatol* 1989; **20**: 87–8.
16 Hörnstein P, Keisu M, Wiholm B-E. The incidence of agranulocytosis during treatment of dermatitis herpetiformis with dapsone as reported in Sweden, 1972 through 1988. *Arch Dermatol* 1990; **126**: 919–22.
17 Cockburn EM, Wood SM, Waller PC, Bleehen SS. Dapsone-induced agranulocytosis: spontaneous reporting data. *Br J Dermatol* 1993; **128**: 702–3.
18 Ognibene AJ. Agranulocytosis due to dapsone. *Ann Intern Med* 1970; **75**: 521–4.
19 Frey HM, Gershon AA, Borkowsky W, Bullock WE. Fatal reaction to dapsone during treatment of leprosy. *Ann Intern Med* 1981; **94**: 777–9.
20 Kingham JG, Swain P, Swarbrick ET *et al*. Dapsone and severe hypoalbuminaemia: a report of two cases. *Lancet* 1979; **ii**: 662–4.
21 Cowan RE, Wright JT. Dapsone and severe hypoalbuminaemia in dermatitis herpetiformis. *Br J Dermatol* 1981; **104**: 201–4.
22 Waldinger TP, Siegle RJ, Weber W *et al*. Dapsone-induced peripheral neuropathy. Case report and review. *Arch Dermatol* 1984; **120**: 356–9.
23 Ahrens EM, Meckler RJ, Callen JP. Dapsone-induced peripheral neuropathy. *Int J Dermatol* 1986; **25**: 314–6.
24 Rhodes LE, Coleman MD, Lewis-Jones MS. Dapsone-induced motor peripheral neuropathy in pemphigus foliaceus. *Clin Exp Dermatol* 1995; **20**: 155–6.
25 Homeida M, Babikr A, Daneshmend TK. Dapsone-induced optic atrophy and motor neuropathy. *BMJ* 1980; **281**: 1180.
26 Kenner DJ, Holt K, Agnello R, Chester GH. Permanent retinal damage following massive dapsone overdose. *Br J Ophthalmol* 1980; **64**: 741–4.
27 Guillet G, Krausz I, Guillet MH, Carlhant D. Survenue de céphalées en cours de traitement par dapsone. *Ann Dermatol Vénéréol* 1992; **119**: 46.
28 Fine J-D, Katz SI, Donahue MJ, Hendricks AA. Psychiatric reaction to dapsone and sulfapyridine. *J Am Acad Dermatol* 1983; **9**: 274–5.

Thalidomide

Teratogenicity (phocomelia), gastric intolerance, drowsiness, neuropsychiatric upset and a sensory peripheral neuropathy developing after several months have been reported [1]. Minor to moderate skin eruptions occur in up to 46% of patients taking thalidomide, including morbilliform, seborrhoeic, maculopapular and non-specific rashes; severe skin reactions such as exfoliative erythroderma, erythema multiforme and TEN are rare [2]. A dermatitis associated with eosinophilia develops in a few cases of erythema nodosum leprosum treated with thalidomide over several years [3]. Hypersensitivity reactions characterized by fever, tachycardia and an extensive erythematous macular eruption developed on rechallenge in a number of patients with HIV infection treated with thalidomide for severe aphthous oropharyngeal ulceration [4]. In addition, brittle fingernails, exfoliative erythroderma [5], toxic pustuloderma [6], face or limb oedema, pruritus, red palms and xerostomia have been described [7].

REFERENCES

1 Revuz J. Actualité du thalidomide. *Ann Dermatol Vénéréol* 1990; **117**: 313–21.
2 Hall VC, El-Azhary RA, Bouwhuis S, Rajkumar SV. Dermatologic side effects of thalidomide in patients with multiple myeloma. *J Am Acad Dermatol* 2003; **48**: 548–52.
3 Waters MFR. An internally controlled double blind trial of thalidomide in severe erythema nodosum leprosum. *Lepr Rev* 1971; **42**: 26–42.
4 Williams I, Weller IVD, Malin A *et al.* Thalidomide hypersensitivity in AIDS. *Lancet* 1991; **337**: 436–7.
5 Bielsa I, Teixido J, Ribera M, Ferrandiz C. Erythroderma due to thalidomide: report of two cases. *Dermatology* 1994; **189**: 179–81.
6 Darvay A, Basarab T, Russell-Jones R. Thalidomide-induced toxic pustuloderma. *Clin Exp Dermatol* 1997; **22**: 297–9.
7 Tseng S, Pak G, Washenik K *et al.* Rediscovering thalidomide: a review of its mechanism of action, side effects, and potential uses. *J Am Acad Dermatol* 1996; **35**: 969–79.

Antifungal drugs

Dermatological aspects of antifungal drugs have been reviewed [1–3]. Rashes occur as follows.
• Itraconazole: in 1.1% of cases, with pruritus in 0.7%; the drug is teratogenic.
• Fluconazole: in 1.8% of cases; exfoliative dermatitis is recorded.
• Terbinafine: in 2.7% of cases, including erythema, urticaria, eczema, pruritus, and isolated Stevens–Johnson syndrome and TEN [3].
Relevant interactions between itraconazole, fluconazole and terbinafine have been discussed [4].

REFERENCES

1 Lesher JL, Smith JG Jr. Antifungal agents in dermatology. *J Am Acad Dermatol* 1987; **17**: 383–94.
2 Gupta AK, Sauder DN, Shear NH. Antifungal agents: an overview. Part I. *J Am Acad Dermatol* 1994; **30**: 677–98.
3 Gupta AK, Sauder DN, Shear NH. Antifungal agents: an overview. Part II. *J Am Acad Dermatol* 1994; **30**: 911–33.
4 Gupta AK, Katz HI, Shear NH. Drug interactions with itraconazole, fluconazole, and terbinafine and their management. *J Am Acad Dermatol* 1999; **41**: 237–49.

Amphotericin

Skin reactions are rare. The 'grey syndrome', characterized by ashen colour, acral cyanosis and prostration, may occur as an immediate reaction to infusion. Allergic reactions occur to liposomal amphotericin [1,2].

Fluconazole

Angio-oedema has occurred [3], as has fixed drug eruption [4]. An anaphylactic reaction developed in a patient who had previously received ketoconazole and metronidazole, suggesting cross-sensitization [5], and Stevens–Johnson syndrome has been reported in a patient with AIDS [6]. Thrombocytopenia is described [7].

Itraconazole

Serum sickness [8] and acute generalized exanthematous pustulosis [9] are recorded.

Flucytosine

Transitory macular and urticarial rashes have been seen. A toxic erythema occurred in a patient [10]. Anaphylaxis has been reported in a patient with AIDS [11]. Bone marrow depression can occur.

REFERENCES

1 Tollemar J, Ringden O, Andersson S *et al.* Randomized double-blind study of liposomal amphotericin B (AmBisome) prophylaxis of invasive fungal infections in bone marrow transplant recipients. *Bone Marrow Transplant* 1993; **12**: 577–82.
2 Ringden O, Andstrom E, Remberger M *et al.* Allergic reactions and other rare side-effects of liposomal amphotericin. *Lancet* 1994; **344**: 1156–7.
3 Abbott M, Hughes DL, Patel R, Kinghorn GR. Angio-oedema after fluconazole. *Lancet* 1991; **338**: 633.
4 Heikkila H, Timonen K, Stubb S. Fixed drug eruption due to fluconazole. *J Am Acad Dermatol* 2000; **42**: 883–4.
5 Neuhaus G, Pavic N, Pletscher M. Anaphylactic reaction after oral fluconazole. *BMJ* 1991; **302**: 1341.
6 Gussenhoven MJE, Haak A, Peereboom-Wynia JDR, van't Wout JW. Stevens–Johnson syndrome after fluconazole. *Lancet* 1991; **338**: 120.
7 Mercurio MG, Elewski BE. Thrombocytopenia caused by fluconazole therapy. *J Am Acad Dermatol* 1996; **32**: 525–6.
8 Park H, Knowles S, Shear NH. Serum sickness-like reaction to itraconazole. *Ann Pharmacother* 1998; **32**: 1249.
9 Park YM, Kim JW, Kim CW. Acute generalised exanthematous pustulosis induced by itraconazole. *J Am Acad Dermatol* 1997; **36**: 794–7.
10 Thyss A, Viens P, Ticchioni M *et al.* Toxicodermie au cours d'un traitement par 5 fluorocytosine. *Ann Dermatol Vénéréol* 1987; **114**: 1131–2.
11 Kotani S, Hirose S, Niiya K *et al.* Anaphylaxis to flucytosine in a patient with AIDS. *JAMA* 1988; **260**: 3275–6.

Griseofulvin

Reactions to griseofulvin are uncommon and usually mild; headaches and gastrointestinal disturbances are the most frequent. Morbilliform, erythematous or, rarely, haemorrhagic eruptions are occasionally seen [1,2]. Photodermatitis [3,4] with sensitivity to wavelengths above 320 nm is by no means rare; clinically, the features are mainly eczematous, although pellagra-like changes may be seen [4]. The reaction is thought to be photoallergic and photopatch tests are positive in some cases; there may be photo cross-reactivity with penicillin [4]. Histology may be non-specific; direct immunofluorescence showed immunoglobulin and complement at the dermal–epidermal junction and around papillary blood vessels in one series [4]. Urticaria and a fixed drug eruption [5,6], cold urticaria [7], severe angio-oedema [8], erythema multiforme [9,10], serum sickness [11], exfoliative dermatitis [12] and TEN [13,14] are recorded. Exacerbation of LE has been reported [15–19], with fatality in one case [18]. Patients with anti-SSA/Ro and SSB/La antibodies may be at increased risk of developing a drug eruption [19,20]. Temporary granulocytopenia has been reported, and proteinuria may occur. Hepatitis and a morbilliform eruption are recorded [21]. Griseofulvin may interfere with the action of anticoagulants and the contraceptive pill [22], and should be avoided in pregnancy as potentially teratogenic; men should avoid conception for 6 months after taking the drug.

Ketoconazole

Pruritus and gastrointestinal upset are the most frequent side effects [1]. Urticaria and angio-oedema are recorded [2]. Severe anaphylaxis has been observed in two patients, one of whom had previously reacted to topical miconazole [3]. Other adverse reactions include exfoliative erythroderma [4]. The drug may block testosterone synthesis, causing dose-dependent lowering of serum testosterone and resultant oligospermia, impotence, decreased libido and gynaecomastia in some men [5–7]. It also blocks the cortisol response to ACTH, and may lead to adrenal insufficiency [7–9]. Hypothyroidism has been documented [10]. The most serious side effect is idiosyncratic hepatitis, which occurs in about 1 in 10 000 patients, and which may lead to fulminant and potentially fatal hepatic necrosis [11–17]. Trichoptilosis has resulted from misuse of ketoconazole 2% shampoo [18].

REFERENCES

1 Faergemann J, Maibach H. Griseofulvin and ketoconazole in dermatology. *Semin Dermatol* 1983; **2**: 262–9.
2 Von Pöhler H, Michalski H. Allergisches Exanthem nach Griseofulvin. *Dermatol Monatsschr* 1972; **58**: 383–90.
3 Jarratt M. Drug photosensitization. *Int J Dermatol* 1976; **15**: 317–23.
4 Kojima T, Hasegawa T, Ishida H *et al.* Griseofulvin-induced photodermatitis. Report of six cases. *J Dermatol* 1988; **15**: 76–82.
5 Feinstein A, Sofer E, Trau H, Schewach-Millet M. Urticaria and fixed drug eruption in a patient treated with griseofulvin. *J Am Acad Dermatol* 1984; **10**: 915–7.
6 Savage J. Fixed drug eruption to griseofulvin. *Br J Dermatol* 1977; **97**: 107–8.
7 Chang T. Cold urticaria and photosensitivity due to griseofulvin. *JAMA* 1965; **193**: 848–50.
8 Goldblatt S. Severe reaction to griseofulvin: sensitivity investigation. *Arch Dermatol* 1961; **83**: 936–7.
9 Rustin NHA, Bunker CB, Dowd P, Robinson TWE. Erythema multiforme due to griseofulvin. *Br J Dermatol* 1989; **120**: 455–8.
10 Thami GP, Kaur S, Kanwar AJ. Erythema multiforme due to griseofulvin with positive re-exposure test. *Dermatology* 2001; **203**: 84–5.
11 Prazak G, Ferguson JS, Comer JE, McNeil BS. Treatment of tinea pedis with griseofulvin. *Arch Dermatol* 1960; **81**: 821–6.
12 Reaves LE III. Exfoliative dermatitis occurring in a patient treated with griseofulvin. *J Am Geriatr Soc* 1964; **12**: 889–92.
13 Taylor B, Duffill M. Toxic epidermal necrolysis from griseofulvin. *J Am Acad Dermatol* 1988; **19**: 565–7.
14 Mion G, Verdon G, Le Gulluche Y *et al.* Fatal toxic epidermal necrolysis after griseofulvin. *Lancet* 1989; **ii**: 1331.
15 Alexander S. Lupus erythematosus in two patients after griseofulvin treatment of *Trichophyton rubrum* infection. *Br J Dermatol* 1962; **74**: 72–4.
16 Anderson WA, Torre D. Griseofulvin and lupus erythematosus. *J Med Soc NJ* 1966; **63**: 161–2.
17 Watsky MS, Linfield YL. Lupus erythematosus exacerbated by griseofulvin. *Cutis* 1976; **17**: 361–3.
18 Madhok R, Zoma A, Capell H. Fatal exacerbation of systemic lupus erythematosus after treatment with griseofulvin. *BMJ* 1985; **291**: 249–50.
19 Miyagawa S, Okuchi T, Shiomi Y, Sakamoto K. Subacute cutaneous lupus erythematosus lesions precipitated by griseofulvin. *J Am Acad Dermatol* 1989; **21**: 343–6.
20 Miyagawa S, Sakamoto K. Adverse reactions to griseofulvin in patients with circulating anti-SSA/Ro and SSB/La autoantibodies. *Am J Med* 1989; **87**: 100–2.
21 Gaudin JL, Bancel B, Vial T, Bel A. Hepatite aigue cytolytique et eruption morbiliforme imputables à la prise de griseofulvin. *Gastroenterol Clin Biol* 1993; **17**: 145–6.
22 Coté J. Interaction of griseofulvin and oral contraceptives. *J Am Acad Dermatol* 1990; **22**: 124–5.

REFERENCES

1 Faergemann J, Maibach H. Griseofulvin and ketoconazole in dermatology. *Semin Dermatol* 1983; **2**: 262–9.
2 Gonzalez-Delgado P, Florido-Lopez F, Saenz de San Pedro B *et al.* Hypersensitivity to ketoconazole. *Ann Allergy* 1994; **73**: 326–8.
3 Van Dijke CPH, Veerman FR, Haverkamp HC. Anaphylactic reactions to ketoconazole. *BMJ* 1983; **287**: 1673.
4 Rand R, Sober AJ, Olmstead PM. Ketoconazole therapy and exfoliative erythroderma. *Arch Dermatol* 1983; **119**: 97–8.
5 Graybill JR, Drutz DJ. Ketoconazole: a major innovation for treatment of fungal disease. *Ann Intern Med* 1980; **93**: 921–3.
6 Moncada B, Baranda L. Ketoconazole and gynecomastia. *J Am Acad Dermatol* 1982; **7**: 557–8.
7 Pont A, Graybill JR, Craven PC *et al.* High-dose ketoconazole therapy and adrenal and testicular function in humans. *Arch Intern Med* 1984; **144**: 2150–3.
8 Pont A, Williams P, Loose D *et al.* Ketoconazole blocks adrenal steroid synthesis. *Ann Intern Med* 1982; **97**: 370–2.
9 Sonino N. The use of ketoconazole as an inhibitor of steroid production. *N Engl J Med* 1987; **317**: 812–8.
10 Kitching NH. Hypothyroidism after treatment with ketoconazole. *BMJ* 1986; **293**: 993–4.
11 Horsburgh CR Jr, Kirkpatrick CJ, Teutsch CB. Ketoconazole and the liver. *Lancet* 1982; **i**: 860.
12 Stern RS. Ketoconazole: assessing its risks. *J Am Acad Dermatol* 1982; **6**: 544.
13 Rollman O, Lööf L. Hepatic toxicity of ketoconazole. *Br J Dermatol* 1983; **108**: 376–8.
14 Duarte PA, Chow CC, Simmons F, Ruskin J. Fatal hepatitis associated with ketoconazole therapy. *Arch Intern Med* 1984; **144**: 1069–70.
15 Lewis J, Zimmerman HJ, Benson GD, Ishak KG. Hepatic injury associated with ketoconazole therapy: analysis of 33 cases. *Gastroenterology* 1984; **86**: 503–13.
16 Lake-Bakaar G, Scheuer PJ, Sherlock S. Hepatic reactions associated with ketoconazole in the United Kingdom. *BMJ* 1987; **294**: 419–22.
17 Knight TE, Shikuma CY, Knight J. Ketoconazole-induced fulminant hepatitis necessitating liver transplantation. *J Am Acad Dermatol* 1991; **25**: 398–400.
18 Aljabre SH. Trichoptilosis caused by misuse of ketoconazole 2% shampoo. *Int J Dermatol* 1993; **32**: 150–1.

Nystatin

A fixed drug eruption has been reported [1], as has Stevens–Johnson syndrome in an isolated case [2].

REFERENCES

1 Pareek SS. Nystatin-induced fixed eruption. *Br J Dermatol* 1980; **103**: 679–80.
2 Garty B-Z. Stevens–Johnson syndrome associated with nystatin treatment. *Arch Dermatol* 1991; **127**: 741–2.

Terbinafine

This drug is well tolerated with relatively few side effects [1]. Idiosyncratic hepatitis has been reported [2], with serious hepatobiliary dysfunction occurring in 1 in 54 000 [3]. Neutropenia, pancytopenia and thrombocytopenia are recorded [4–8]. Cutaneous adverse effects occur in 3% of patients [3,9]; these include severe urticaria, pityriasiform rashes, erythroderma, erythema multiforme [10,11] and TEN [12], serum sickness-like reactions, acute generalized exanthematous pustulosis [13–17], LE-like rashes [18–20], induction or exacerbation of psoriasis which may be pustular [21–24], baboon syndrome [25], fixed drug eruption [26] and alopecia [27].

REFERENCES

1 Villars V, Jones TC. Present status of the efficacy and tolerability of terbinafine (Lamisil) used systemically in the treatment of dermatomycoses of skin and nails. *J Dermatol Treat* 1990; **1** (Suppl. 2): 33–8.
2 Lowe G, Green C, Jennings P. Hepatitis associated with terbinafine treatment. *BMJ* 1993; **306**: 248.
3 Gupta AK, Kopstein JB, Shear NH. Hypersensitivity reaction to terbinafine. *J Am Acad Dermatol* 1997; **36**: 1018–9.
4 Kovacs MJ, Alshammari S, Guenther L, Bourcier M. Neutropenia and pancytopenia associated with oral terbinafine. *J Am Acad Dermatol* 1994; **31**: 806.
5 Gupta AK, Soori G, Del Rosso JQ et al. Severe neutropenia associated with oral terbinafine therapy. *J Am Acad Dermatol* 1998; **38**: 765–7.
6 Ornstein DL, Ely P. Reversible agranulocytosis associated with oral terbinafine for onychomycosis. *J Am Acad Dermatol* 1998; **39**: 1023–4.
7 Shapiro M, Li L-J, Miller J. Terbinafine-induced neutropenia. *Br J Dermatol* 1999; **140**: 1196–7.
8 Tsai H-H, Lee W-R, Hu C-H. Isolated thrombocytopenia associated with oral terbinafine. *Br J Dermatol* 2002; **147**: 627–8.
9 Gupta AK, Lynde CW, Lauzon GJ et al. Cutaneous adverse effects associated with terbinafine therapy: 10 case reports and a review of the literature. *Br J Dermatol* 1998; **138**: 529–32.
10 McGregor JM, Rustin MHA. Terbinafine and erythema multiforme. *Br J Dermatol* 1994; **131**: 587–8.
11 Todd P, Halpern S, Munro DD. Oral terbinafine and erythema multiforme. *Clin Exp Dermatol* 1995; **20**: 247–8.
12 White SI, Bowen-Jones D. Toxic epidermal necrolysis induced by terbinafine in a patient on long-term anti-epileptics. *Br J Dermatol* 1996; **134**: 188–9.
13 Kempinaire A, De Raeve L, Merckx M et al. Terbinafine-induced acute generalized exanthematous pustulosis confirmed by positive patch-test result. *J Am Acad Dermatol* 1997; **37**: 653–5.
14 Condon CA, Downs AMR, Archer CB. Terbinafine-induced acute generalized exanthematous pustulosis. *Br J Dermatol* 1998; **138**: 709–10.
15 Bennett ML, Jorizzo JL, White WL. Generalized pustular eruptions associated with oral terbinafine. *Int J Dermatol* 1999; **38**: 596–600.
16 Hall AP, Tate B. Acute generalized exanthematous pustulosis associated with oral terbinafine. *Australas J Dermatol* 2000; **41**: 42–5.
17 Lombardo M, Cerati M, Pazzaglia A. Acute generalized exanthematous pustulosis induced by terbinafine. *J Am Acad Dermatol* 2003; **49**: 158–9.
18 Brooke R, Coulson IH, Al-Dawoud A. Terbinafine-induced subacute cutaneous lupus erythematosus. *Br J Dermatol* 1998; **139**: 1132–3.
19 Holmes S, Kemmett D. Exacerbation of systemic lupus erythematosus induced by terbinafine. *Br J Dermatol* 1998; **139**: 1133.
20 Murphy M, Barnes L. Terbinafine-induced lupus erythematosus. *Br J Dermatol* 1998; **138**: 708–9.
21 Wach F, Stolz W, Hein R, Landthaler M. Severe erythema anulare centrifugum-like psoriatic drug eruption induced by terbinafine. *Arch Dermatol* 1995; **131**: 960–1.
22 Gupta AK, Sibbald RG, Knowles SR et al. Terbinafine therapy may be associated with the development of psoriasis de novo or its exacerbation: four case reports and a review of drug-induced psoriasis. *J Am Acad Dermatol* 1997; **36**: 858–62.
23 Papa CA, Miller OF. Pustular psoriasiform eruption with leukocytosis associated with terbinafine. *J Am Acad Dermatol* 1998; **39**: 115–7.
24 Wilson NJE, Evans S. Severe pustular psoriasis provoked by oral terbinafine. *Br J Dermatol* 1998; **139**: 168.
25 Weiss JM, Mockenhaupt M, Schopf E, Simon JC. Reproducible drug exanthema to terbinafine with characteristic distribution of baboon syndrome. *Hautarzt* 2001; **52**: 1104–6.
26 Munn SE, Russell Jones R. Terbinafine and fixed drug eruption. *Br J Dermatol* 1995; **133**: 815–6.
27 Richert B, Uhoda I, de la Brassinne M. Hair loss after terbinafine treatment. *Br J Dermatol* 2001; **145**: 842.

Antiviral agents

Aciclovir (acyclovir)

In general, there are very few side effects [1]. Vesicular reactions, palm and sole dermatitis, peripheral oedema, erythema nodosum, exanthems, hyperhidrosis, acne, lichenoid eruption, pruritus, urticaria, vasculitis, alopecia and fixed drug eruption are recorded [2–4]. Intravenous use may cause inflammation and phlebitis. A nephropathy may develop with intravenous use, especially in patients with renal failure, due to renal precipitation of the drug; the dose should be reduced in patients with impaired renal function. An encephalopathy may occur. Peripheral oedema has been reported very rarely [5,6].

REFERENCES

1 Arndt KA. Adverse reactions to acyclovir: topical, oral, and intravenous. *J Am Acad Dermatol* 1988; **18**: 188–90.
2 Buck ML, Vittone SB, Zaglul HF. Vesicular eruptions following acyclovir administration. *Ann Pharmacother* 1993; **27**: 1458–9.
3 Carrasco L, Pastor MA, Izquierdo MJ et al. Drug eruption secondary to acyclovir with recall phenomenon in a dermatome previously affected by herpes zoster. *Clin Exp Dermatol* 2002; **27**: 132–4.
4 Montoro J, Basomba A. Fixed drug eruption due to acyclovir. *Contact Dermatitis* 1997; **36**: 225.
5 Hisler BM, Daneshvar SA, Aronson PJ, Hashimoto K. Peripheral edema and oral acyclovir. *J Am Acad Dermatol* 1988; **18**: 1142–3.
6 Medina S, Torrelo A, España A, Ledo A. Edema and oral acyclovir. *Int J Dermatol* 1991; **30**: 305–6.

Idoxuridine

This drug is used only topically for herpes simplex and herpes zoster, in view of its toxicity on systemic administration. Severe alopecia and loss of nails followed parenteral use [1].

REFERENCE

1 Nolan DC, Carruthers MM, Lerner AM. Herpesvirus hominis encephalitis in Michigan: report of thirteen cases, including six treated with idoxuridine. *N Engl J Med* 1970; **282**: 10–3.

Foscarnet

This drug is used for cytomegalovirus retinitis in AIDS, and for mucocutaneous herpes simplex virus unresponsive to aciclovir in immunocompromised patients. A generalized cutaneous rash has been reported with use of this drug in AIDS [1]. Genital ulceration, both of the penis [2,3] and vulva [4], is documented. In one study [2], 15% of 60 patients treated with intravenous foscarnet developed penile ulceration [2]. Eosinophilic folliculitis has been reported [5].

REFERENCES

1 Green ST, Nathwani D, Goldberg DJ et al. Generalised cutaneous rash associated with foscarnet usage in AIDS. J Infect 1990; 21: 227–8.
2 Katlama C, Dohin E, Caumes E et al. Foscarnet induction therapy for cytomegalovirus retinitis in AIDS: comparison of twice-daily and three-times-daily regimens. J Acquir Immune Defic Syndr 1992; 5 (Suppl. 1): S18–S24.
3 Evans LM, Grossman ME. Foscarnet-induced penile ulcer. J Am Acad Dermatol 1992; 27: 124–6.
4 Caumes E, Gatineau M, Bricaire F et al. Foscarnet-induced vulvar erosion. J Am Acad Dermatol 1993; 28: 799.
5 Roos TC, Albrecht H. Foscarnet-associated eosinophilic folliculitis in a patient with AIDS. J Am Acad Dermatol 2001; 44: 546–7.

Ribavirin (tribavirin)

This synthetic guanosine analogue used in the treatment of relapsing chronic hepatitis C infection has been implicated in the development of Grover's disease [1].

REFERENCE

1 Antunes I, Azevedo F, Mesquita-Guimaraes J et al. Grover's disease secondary to ribavirin. Br J Dermatol 2000; 142: 1257–8.

Antiretroviral drugs

Cutaneous side effects of antiretroviral agents have been reviewed [1–4]. There are three categories of agent: nucleoside reverse transcriptase inhibitors, non-nucleoside reverse transcriptase inhibitors and protease inhibitors. Nucleoside reverse transcriptase inhibitors have resulted in alterations of the nails, nail and mucocutaneous pigmentation, hair changes, vasculitis and morbilliform eruptions. Drug hypersensitivity is associated with the non-nucleoside reverse transcriptase inhibitors nevirapine, delavirdine and efavirenz, as well as the nucleoside reverse transcriptase inhibitor abacavir and the protease inhibitor amprenavir [2]. Protease inhibitors have been associated with lipodystrophy syndrome, hypersensitivity reactions, urticaria, morbilliform eruptions and a large number of drug interactions.

REFERENCES

1 Carr A, Cooper DA. Adverse effects of antiretroviral therapy. Lancet 2000; 356: 1423–30.

2 Ward HA, Russo GG, Shrum J. Cutaneous manifestations of antiretroviral therapy. J Am Acad Dermatol 2002; 46: 284–93.
3 Rotunda A, Hirsch RJ, Scheinfeld N, Weinberg JM. Severe cutaneous reactions associated with the use of human immunodeficiency virus medications. Acta Derm Venereol (Stockh) 2003; 83: 1–9.
4 Phillips EJ, Knowles SR, Shear N. Cutaneous manifestations of antiviral therapy. J Am Acad Dermatol 2003; 48: 985–6.

Nucleoside reverse transcriptase inhibitors

Abacavir. This drug is associated with a hypersensitivity syndrome in 4% of cases [1]. Stevens–Johnson syndrome is recorded [2].

Zidovudine. This drug may cause gastrointestinal upset and marrow suppression (with serious anaemia in 32% and leukopenia in 37%), myalgia, headache and insomnia [3–6]. Such side effects have been reported in healthcare workers treated with zidovudine for attempted prophylaxis of HIV infection following accidental needlestick injury [7,8]. Zidovudine-related thrombocytopenia resulted in ecchymoses around Kaposi's sarcoma lesions in a patient with AIDS, simulating rapid intracutaneous spread of neoplasm [9]. Vaginal tumours have been documented in rodents. Diffuse pigmentation, as well as isolated hyperpigmented spots on the palms, soles and fingers, and pigmentation of the fingernails and toenails (usually starting at 4–8 weeks into therapy but up to 1 year) and buccal mucosa have been described [10–15]. Postural hypotension has been recorded [16]. Hypertrichosis of the eyelids has occurred [17]. A possible link with neutrophilic eccrine hidradenitis has been postulated in HIV-infected patients [18]. Hypersensitivity reactions from rash to anaphylaxis have been documented [19,20]. Other reported cutaneous reactions include acne, pruritus, urticaria and leukocytoclastic vasculitis [21].

Lamivudine. Paronychia is recorded [22].

Dideoxycytidine. A maculopapular reaction with oral ulceration developed in 70% of patients treated with this anti-AIDS agent, but resolved spontaneously in those who continued on therapy [23].

REFERENCES

1 Phillips EJ, Knowles SR, Shear N. Cutaneous manifestations of antiviral therapy. J Am Acad Dermatol 2003; 48: 985–6.
2 Bossi P, Roujeau JC, Bricaire F, Caumes E. Stevens–Johnson syndrome associated with abacavir therapy. Clin Infect Dis 2002; 35: 902.
3 Gill PS, Rarick M, Brynes RK et al. Azidothymidine associated with bone marrow failure in AIDS. Ann Intern Med 1987; 107: 502–5.
4 Richman DD, Fiscal MA, Grieco MH et al. The toxicity of azidothymidine (AZT) in the treatment of patients with AIDS or AIDS-related complex: a double blind, placebo-controlled trial. N Engl J Med 1987; 317: 192–7.
5 Gelmon K, Montaner JS, Fanning M et al. Nature, time course and dose dependence of zidovudine-related side-effects: results from the Multicenter Canadian Azidothymidine Trial. AIDS 1989; 3: 555–61.
6 Moore RD, Creagh-Kirk T, Keruly J et al. Long-term safety and efficacy of zidovudine in patients with advanced human immunodeficiency virus infection. Arch Intern Med 1991; 151: 981–6.

7 Centers for Disease Control. Public health service statement on management of occupational exposure to human immunodeficiency virus, including considerations regarding zidovudine post-exposure use. *MMWR* 1990; **39**: 1–14.
8 Jeffries DJ. Zidovudine after occupational exposure to HIV. Hospitals should be able to give it within an hour. *BMJ* 1991; **302**: 1349–51.
9 Barnett JH, Gilson E. Zidovudine-related thrombocytopenia simulating rapid growth of Kaposi's sarcoma. *Arch Dermatol* 1991; **127**: 1068–9.
10 Azon-Masoliver A, Mallolas J, Gatell J, Castel T. Zidovudine-induced nail pigmentation. *Arch Dermatol* 1988; **124**: 1570–1.
11 Fisher CA, McPoland PR. Azidothymidine-induced nail pigmentation. *Cutis* 1989; **43**: 552–4.
12 Bendick C, Rasokat H, Steigleder GK. Azidothymidine-induced hyperpigmentation of skin and nails. *Arch Dermatol* 1989; **125**: 1285–6.
13 Greenberg RG, Berger TG. Nail and mucocutaneous hyperpigmentation with azidothymidine therapy. *J Am Acad Dermatol* 1990; **22**: 327–30.
14 Grau-Massanes M, Millan F, Febrer MI *et al.* Pigmented nail bands and mucocutaneous pigmentation in HIV-positive patients treated with zidovudine. *J Am Acad Dermatol* 1990; **22**: 687–8.
15 Tadini G, D'Orso M, Cusini M *et al.* Oral mucosa pigmentation: a new side effect of azidothymidine therapy in patients with acquired immunodeficiency syndrome. *Arch Dermatol* 1991; **127**: 267–8.
16 Loke RHT, Murray-Lyon IM, Carter GD. Postural hypotension related to zidovudine in a patient infected with HIV. *BMJ* 1990; **300**: 163–4.
17 Klutman NE, Hinthorn DR. Excessive growth of eyelashes in a patient with AIDS being treated with zidovudine. *N Engl J Med* 1991; **324**: 1896.
18 Smith KJ, Skelton HG III, James WD *et al.* Neutrophilic eccrine hidradenitis in HIV-infected patients. *J Am Acad Dermatol* 1990; **23**: 945–7.
19 Carr A, Penny R, Cooper DA. Allergy and desensitization to zidovudine in patients with acquired immunodeficiency syndrome (AIDS). *J Allergy Clin Immunol* 1993; **91**: 683–5.
20 Wassef M, Keiser P. Hypersensitivity of zidovudine: report of a case of anaphylaxis and review of the literature. *Clin Infect Dis* 1995; **20**: 1387–9.
21 Torres RA, Lin RY, Lee M, Barr MR. Zidovudine-induced leukocytoclastic vasculitis. *Arch Intern Med* 1992; **152**: 850–1.
22 Tosti A, Piraccini BM, D'Antuono A *et al.* Paronychia associated with antiretroviral therapy. *Br J Dermatol* 1999; **140**: 1165–8.
23 McNeely MC, Yarchoan R, Broder S, Lawley TJ. Dermatologic complications associated with administration of 2′,3′-dideoxycytidine in patients with human immunodeficiency virus infection. *J Am Acad Dermatol* 1989; **21**: 1213–7.

Non-nucleoside reverse transcriptase inhibitors

Delavirdine. Various rashes occur in 18–50% of cases.

Efavirenz. Mild rashes are recorded within the first 2 weeks of therapy [1].

Nevirapine. Severe rashes have been observed in 3% of patients taking nevirapine in clinical trials, 85% of whom were men [2,3]. A hypersensitivity syndrome is well recorded [4,5]. The drug is the leading cause of Stevens–Johnson syndrome and TEN related to AIDS in Europe [6–9].

REFERENCES

1 Phillips EJ, Knowles SR, Shear N. Cutaneous manifestations of antiviral therapy. *J Am Acad Dermatol* 2003; **48**: 985–6.
2 Bersoff-Matcha SJ, Miller WC, Aberg JA *et al.* Sex differences in nevirapine rash. *Clin Infect Dis* 2001; **32**: 124–9.
3 Anonymous. From the Centers for Disease Control and Prevention. Serious adverse events attributed to nevirapine regimens for postexposure prophylaxis after HIV exposures: worldwide, 1997–2000. *JAMA* 2001; **285**: 402–3.
4 Claudio GA, Martin AF, de Dios Perrino S, Velasco AA. DRESS syndrome associated with nevirapine therapy. *Arch Intern Med* 2001; **161**: 2501–2.

5 Lanzafame M, Rovere P, De Checchi G *et al.* Hypersensitivity syndrome (DRESS) and meningoencephalitis associated with nevirapine therapy. *Scand J Infect Dis* 2001; **33**: 475–6.
6 Wetterwald E, Le Cleach L, Michel C *et al.* Nevirapine-induced overlap Stevens–Johnson syndrome/toxic epidermal necrolysis. *Br J Dermatol* 1999; **140**: 980–2.
7 Metry DW, Lahart CJ, Farmer KL, Hebert AA. Stevens–Johnson syndrome caused by the antiretroviral drug nevirapine. *J Am Acad Dermatol* 2001; **44** (2 Suppl.): 354–7.
8 Fagot JP, Mockenhaupt M, Bouwes-Bavinck JN *et al.* Nevirapine and the risk of Stevens–Johnson syndrome or toxic epidermal necrolysis. *AIDS* 2001; **15**: 1843–8.
9 Dodi F, Alessandrini A, Camera M *et al.* Stevens–Johnson syndrome in HIV patients treated with nevirapine: two case reports. *AIDS* 2002; **16**: 1197–8.

Protease inhibitors

Saquinivir causes rashes, and indinavir causes taste disturbance and dry skin [1]. Indinavir has been associated with the development of cheilitis in 40% of cases, diffuse cutaneous dryness and pruritus in 12%, asteatotic dermatitis on the trunk, arms and thighs, and scalp hair loss in 12% [2]. Multiple pyogenic granulomas were observed in the toenails in 6% and softening of the nail plate in 5% of subjects. Multiple subcutaneous lipomas are associated with protease inhibitors [3]. Paronychia is a recognized complication [4,5]. Angiolipomas shortly after initiation of therapy [6] and leukocytoclastic vasculitis [7] have been documented with indinavir. A peripheral lipodystrophy syndrome has been linked to therapy with protease inhibitors [8–12] and was noted in 14% of patients on indinavir [2]. It comprises peripheral lipoatrophy, relative central adiposity, sometimes with a 'buffalo hump', insulin resistance and serum lipid abnormalities. The mix of features is variable in individual patients.

REFERENCES

1 Anonymous. Safety issues with anti-HIV drugs. *Curr Probl Pharmacovig* 1997; **23**: 5.
2 Calista D, Boschini A. Cutaneous side effects induced by indinavir. *Eur J Dermatol* 2000; **10**: 292–6.
3 Bornhovd E, Sakrauski AK, Bruhl H *et al.* Multiple circumscribed subcutaneous lipomas associated with use of human immunodeficiency virus protease inhibitors? *Br J Dermatol* 2000; **143**: 1113–4.
4 Tosti A, Piraccini BM, D'Antuono A *et al.* Paronychia associated with antiretroviral therapy. *Br J Dermatol* 1999; **140**: 1165–8.
5 Daudén E, Pascual-López M, Martínez-Garcia C, García-Díez A. Paronychia and excess granulation tissue of the toes and finger in a patient treated with indinavir. *Br J Dermatol* 2000; **142**: 1063–4.
6 Dank JP, Colven R. Protease inhibitor-associated angiolipomatosis. *J Am Acad Dermatol* 2000; **42**: 129–31.
7 Rachline A, Lariven S, Descamps V *et al.* Leucocytoclastic vasculitis and indinavir. *Br J Dermatol* 2000; **143**: 1112–3.
8 Ward HA, Russo GG, Shrum J. Cutaneous manifestations of antiretroviral therapy. *J Am Acad Dermatol* 2002; **46**: 284–93.
9 Williamson K, Reboli AC, Manders SM. Protease-inhibitor-induced lipodystrophy. *J Am Acad Dermatol* 1999; **40**: 635–6.
10 Panse I, Vasseur E, Raffin-Sanson ML *et al.* Lipodystrophy associated with protease inhibitors. *Br J Dermatol* 2000; **142**: 496–500.
11 Pujol RM, Domingo P, Guiu X-M *et al.* HIV-1 protease inhibitor-associated partial lipodystrophy: clinicopathologic review of 14 cases. *J Am Acad Dermatol* 2000; **42**: 193–8.
12 Mallon PW, Cooper DA, Carr A. HIV-associated lipodystrophy. *HIV Med* 2001; **2**: 166–73.

Antimalarials [1–4]

Pruritus, lichenoid eruptions, exfoliative dermatitis, pigment changes, bleaching of hair, alopecia, photosensitivity with exacerbation of psoriasis and porphyria cutanea tarda, retinopathy and corneal opacities have all been reported.

REFERENCES

1 Ribrioux A. Antipaludéens de synthese et peau. *Ann Dermatol Vénéréol* 1990; **117**: 975–90.
2 Ochsendorf FR, Runne U. Chloroquin und Hydroxychloroquin: Nebenwirkungsprofil wichtiger Therapeutika. *Hautarzt* 1991; **42**: 140–6.
3 Ziering CL, Rabinowitz LG, Esterly NB. Antimalarials for children. Indications, toxicities, and guidelines. *J Am Acad Dermatol* 1993; **28**: 764–70.
4 Sowunmi A, Falade AG, Adedeji AA, Falade CO. Comparative clinical characteristics and responses to oral 4-aminoquinoline therapy of malarious children who did and did not develop 4-aminoquinoline-induced pruritus. *Ann Trop Med Parasitol* 2001; **95**: 645–53.

Chloroquine and hydroxychloroquine

Adverse cutaneous reactions to hydroxychloroquine are commoner in patients with dermatomyositis than in those with cutaneous LE [1]. Pruritus is common in Africans on acute or prolonged treatment, but rare in Europeans [2–5]. Pigmentary changes develop in about 25% of patients receiving any of the antimalarials for more than 4 months [6–9]; chloroquine binds to melanin [9]. Blackish-purple patches on the shins are often seen, and brown-grey pigmentation may appear in light-exposed skin [8]. The nail beds may be pigmented diffusely or in transverse bands, and the hard palate is diffusely pigmented. In contrast, red-blonde (but not dark) hair may be bleached [10]. Chloroquine has been associated with vitiligo-like depigmentation [11].

Photosensitivity may be seen [12]; in addition, certain types of porphyria may be provoked [13]. Effects on psoriasis are unpredictable, but precipitation of severe psoriasis has long been recognized [14–19], including erythroderma [19]. However, 88% of a series of 50 psoriatics who were treated with standard doses of chloroquine noted no change in their psoriasis [20]. Lichenoid eruptions are uncommon, and erythema annulare centrifugum is rare [21]. TEN with oral involvement has been documented. A pustular eruption with hydroxychloroquine has been reported [22]. Toxic psychosis has been described with hydroxychloroquine [23]. All antimalarials are potentially teratogenic.

Chloroquine and hydroxychloroquine may cause serious ophthalmic side effects [24,25]. Corneal deposits occur in 95% of patients on long-term therapy, but of these 95% are asymptomatic [26]. A potentially irreversible retinopathy leading to blindness may develop in 0.5–2% of cases [27,28]. The retinal changes may progress after the drug is stopped. Use of less than 250 mg (or 4 mg/kg)

daily of chloroquine, with pretreatment and 6-monthly ophthalmological assessment using an Amsler grid, is recommended. Malaria prophylaxis with two tablets weekly is said not to carry an appreciable risk. Ocular toxicity with hydroxychloroquine is rare below 6.5 mg/kg; guidelines for screening include baseline renal and liver function tests, assessment of near visual acuity and yearly visual acuity [29].

REFERENCES

1 Pelle MT, Callen JP. Adverse cutaneous reactions to hydroxychloroquine are more common in patients with dermatomyositis than in patients with cutaneous lupus erythematosus. *Arch Dermatol* 2002; **138**: 1231–3.
2 Spencer HC, Poulter NR, Lury JD, Poulter CJ. Chloroquine-associated pruritus in a European. *BMJ* 1982; **285**: 1703–4.
3 Salako LA. Toxicity and side-effects of antimalarials in Africa: a critical review. *Bull WHO* 1984; **62** (Suppl.): 63–8.
4 Mnyika KS, Kihamia CM. Chloroquine-induced pruritus: its impact on chloroquine utilization in malaria control in Dar es Salaam. *J Trop Med Hyg* 1991; **94**: 27–31.
5 Ezeamuzie IC, Igbigbi PS, Ambakederemo AW *et al.* Halofantrine-induced pruritus amongst subjects who itch to chloroquine. *J Trop Med Hyg* 1991; **94**: 184–8.
6 Dall JLC, Keane JA. Disturbances of pigmentation with chloroquine. *BMJ* 1959; **i**: 1387–9.
7 Tuffanelli D, Abraham RK, Dubois EJ. Pigmentation from antimalarial therapy: its possible relationship to the ocular lesions. *Arch Dermatol* 1963; **88**: 419–26.
8 Levy H. Chloroquine-induced pigmentation. Case reports. *S Afr Med J* 1982; **2**: 735–7.
9 Sams WM, Epstein JH. The affinity of melanin for chloroquine. *J Invest Dermatol* 1965; **45**: 482–8.
10 Dupré A, Ortonne J-P, Viraben R, Arfeux F. Chloroquine-induced hypopigmentation of hair and freckles. Association with congenital renal failure. *Arch Dermatol* 1985; **121**: 1164–6.
11 Martín-García RF, Camacho N del R, Sánchez JL. Chloroquine-induced, vitiligo-like depigmentation. *J Am Acad Dermatol* 2003; **48**: 981–3.
12 Van Weelden H, Boling HH, Baart de la Faille H, Van Der Leun JC. Photosensitivity caused by chloroquine. *Arch Dermatol* 1982; **118**: 290.
13 Davis MJ, Vander Ploeg DE. Acute porphyria and coproporphyrinuria following chloroquine therapy: a report of two cases. *Arch Dermatol* 1957; **75**: 796–800.
14 O'Quinn SE, Kennedy CB, Naylor LZ. Psoriasis, ultraviolet light and chloroquine. *Arch Dermatol* 1964; **90**: 211–6.
15 Baker H. The influence of chloroquine and related drugs on psoriasis and keratoderma blenorrhagicum. *Br J Dermatol* 1966; **78**: 161–6.
16 Abel EA, Dicicco LM, Orenberg EK *et al.* Drugs in exacerbation of psoriasis. *J Am Acad Dermatol* 1986; **15**: 1007–22.
17 Nicolas J-F, Mauduit G, Haond J *et al.* Psoriasis grave induit par la chloroquine (nivaquine). *Ann Dermatol Vénéréol* 1988; **115**: 289–93.
18 Luzar MJ. Hydroxychloroquine in psoriatic arthropathy: exacerbation of psoriatic skin lesions. *J Rheumatol* 1982; **9**: 462–4.
19 Slagel GA, James WD. Plaquenil-induced erythroderma. *J Am Acad Dermatol* 1985; **12**: 857–62.
20 Katugampola G, Katugampola S. Chloroquine and psoriasis. *Int J Dermatol* 1990; **29**: 153–4.
21 Ashurst PJ. Erythema annulare centrifugum. Due to hydroxychloroquine sulfate and chloroquine sulfate. *Arch Dermatol* 1967; **95**: 37–9.
22 Lotem M, Ingber A, Segal R, Sandbank M. Generalized pustular drug rash induced by hydroxychloroquine. *Acta Derm Venereol (Stockh)* 1990; **70**: 250–1.
23 Ward WQ, Walter-Ryan WG, Shehi GM. Toxic psychosis: a complication of antimalarial therapy. *J Am Acad Dermatol* 1985; **12**: 863–5.
24 Olansky AJ. Antimalarials and ophthalmologic safety. *J Am Acad Dermatol* 1982; **6**: 19–23.
25 Portnoy JZ, Callen JP. Ophthalmologic aspects of chloroquine and hydroxychloroquine safety. *Int J Dermatol* 1983; **22**: 273–8.
26 Easterbrook M. Ocular side effects and safety of antimalarial agents. *Am J Med* 1988; **85**: 23–9.

27 Marks JS. Chloroquine retinopathy: is there a safe daily dose? *Ann Rheum Dis* 1982; **41**: 52–8.
28 Easterbrook M. Dose relationships in patients with early chloroquine retinopathy. *J Rheumatol* 1987; **14**: 472–5.
29 Jones SK. Ocular toxicity and hydroxychloroquine: guidelines for screening. *Br J Dermatol* 1999; **140**: 3–7.

Mefloquine

Dizziness, nausea, erythema and neurological disturbance are documented. Pruritus occurs in 4–10% and maculopapular rash in up to 30% of cases; urticaria, facial lesions, cutaneous vasculitis, Stevens–Johnson syndrome and TEN [1,2], and exfoliative dermatitis [3] have been recorded.

REFERENCES

1 Van Den Enden E, Van Gompel A, Colebunders R, Van Den Ende J. Mefloquine-induced Stevens–Johnson syndrome. *Lancet* 1991; **337**: 683.
2 Smith HR, Croft AM, Black MM. Dermatological adverse effects with the antimalarial drug mefloquine: a review of 74 published case reports. *Clin Exp Dermatol* 1999; **24**: 249–54.
3 Martin GJ, Malone JL, Ross EV. Exfoliative dermatitis during malarial prophylaxis with mefloquine. *Clin Infect Dis* 1993; **16**: 341–2.

Mepacrine (atabrine, quinacrine)

This drug constantly causes yellow staining of the skin, which may involve the conjunctiva and may mimic jaundice [1]. Lichenoid eruptions are well known. Large numbers of military personnel given mepacrine for malaria prophylaxis in the Second World War developed a tropical lichenoid dermatitis, which was quickly followed by anhidrosis, cutaneous atrophy, alopecia, nail changes, altered pigmentation and keratoderma [2,3]. A few patients developed localized bluish-black hyperpigmentation confined to the palate, face, pretibial area and nail beds after prolonged administration of more than a year. Years later, lichenoid nodules, scaly red plaques, atrophic lesions on the soles, erosions and leukoplakia of the tongue, and fungating warty growths appeared [3,4]. Progression to squamous cell carcinoma, especially on the palm, has occurred. Ocular toxicity is much less than with chloroquine.

REFERENCES

1 Leigh JM, Kennedy CTC, Ramsey JD, Henderson WJ. Mepacrine pigmentation in systemic lupus erythematosus. *Br J Dermatol* 1979; **101**: 147–53.
2 Bauer F. Late sequelae of atabrine dermatitis: a new premalignant entity. *Aust J Dermatol* 1978; **19**: 9–12.
3 Bauer F. Quinacrine hydrochloride drug eruption (tropical lichenoid dermatitis). Its early and late sequelae and its malignant potential. A review. *J Am Acad Dermatol* 1981; **4**: 239–48.
4 Callaway JL. Late sequelae of quinacrine dermatitis, a new premalignant entity. *J Am Acad Dermatol* 1979; **1**: 456.

Pyrimethamine

This folate antagonist can cause agranulocytosis even in very low dosage, especially when combined with dapsone [1]. A lichenoid eruption has been reported [2], as has photosensitivity. The reported rate for all serious reactions to pyrimethamine–sulfadoxine (Fansidar) in one study was 1 in 2100 prescriptions and for cutaneous reactions including Stevens–Johnson syndrome 1 in 4900, with a fatality rate of 1 in 11 100 [3]. In another study [4], severe cutaneous adverse reactions to Fansidar, including erythema multiforme, Stevens–Johnson syndrome and TEN, were estimated at 1.1 (0.9–1.3) per million. Similar rates for severe reactions to pyrimethamine–dapsone (Maloprim) were 1 in 9100 prescriptions and for blood dyscrasias 1 in 20 000, with a fatality rate of 1 in 75 000. For developing countries with mainly single-dose use, the risk was estimated at 0.1 per million, compared with mainly prophylactic use in Europe and North America at a risk of 10 and 36 per million respectively. Prophylactic use thus had a 40 times higher risk than single-dose therapeutic use [4]. Reactions to pyrimethamine are more common in patients with HIV infection [5]. Epidermal necrolysis, angiooedema, bullous disorders and serious hepatic disorders also occurred. Because few serious reactions have been recorded with chloroquine and proguanil, it has been recommended that use of compound antimalarials should be restricted [3].

REFERENCES

1 Friman G, Nyström-Rosander C, Jonsell G *et al.* Agranulocytosis associated with malaria prophylaxis with Maloprim. *BMJ* 1983; **286**: 1244–5.
2 Cutler TP. Lichen planus caused by pyrimethamine. *Clin Exp Dermatol* 1980; **5**: 253–6.
3 Phillips-Howard PA, West LJ. Serious adverse drug reactions to pyrimethamine–sulphadoxine, pyrimethamine–dapsone and to amodiaquine in Britain. *J R Soc Med* 1990; **83**: 82–5.
4 Sturchler D, Mittelholzer ML, Kerr L. How frequent are notified severe cutaneous adverse reactions to Fansidar? *Drug Saf* 1993; **8**: 160–8.
5 Piketty C, Weiss L, Picard-Dahan C *et al.* Toxidermies a la pyrimethamine chez les patients infectés par le virus de l'immunodeficience acquise. *Presse Med* 1995; **24**: 1710.

Quinine

Purpura due to quinine may or may not be thrombocytopenic [1,2]. Erythematous, urticarial, photoallergic [3–5], bullous and fixed eruptions are recorded. Lichenoid eruptions are rare. If contact allergic sensitivity is already present, eczematous reactions may occur, as in 'systemic contact-type eczema' [6]. Splinter haemorrhages, and a maculopapular and a photosensitive papulonecrotic eruption, due to a lymphocytic vasculitis, have been recorded in one case [7].

REFERENCES

1 Belkin GA. Cocktail purpura. An unusual case of quinine sensitivity. *Ann Intern Med* 1967; **66**: 583–6.
2 Helmly RB, Bergin JJ, Shulman NR. Quinine-induced purpura: observation on antibody titers. *Arch Intern Med* 1967; **20**: 59–62.

3 Ljunggren B, Sjövall P. Systemic quinine photosensitivity. *Arch Dermatol* 1986; **122**: 909–11.
4 Ferguson J, Addo HA, Johnson BE *et al*. Quinine induced photosensitivity: clinical and experimental studies. *Br J Dermatol* 1987; **117**: 631–40.
5 Diffey BL, Farr PM, Adams SJ. The action spectrum in quinine photosensitivity. *Br J Dermatol* 1988; **118**: 679–85.
6 Calnan CD, Caron GA. Quinine sensitivity. *BMJ* 1961; **ii**: 1750–2.
7 Harland CC, Millard LG. Another quirk of quinine. *BMJ* 1991; **302**: 295.

Anthelmintics

Amocarzine (CGP 6140)

This macrofilaricidal and microfilaricidal drug used for the therapy of onchocerciasis may be associated with dizziness and pruritus with or without a rash [1].

Benzimidazole compounds

These are used for the therapy of both intestinal helminthiasis and hydatid disease; fever, gastrointestinal upset, reversible neutropenia and transient abnormalities in liver function are reported. Telogen effluvium has been documented with both albendazole [2,3] and mebendazole.

Ivermectin

Fever, rash, pruritus, local swelling and tender regional lymphadenopathy are documented [4]. The incidence of moderate adverse reactions including pruritus, localized rash and fever was 4% in a study of patients with onchocerciasis from Ecuador [5], and increased itching and/or rash occurred in 8% of cases in another study [6]. Patients with reactive onchodermatitis (sowda) may have severe pruritus and limb swelling with ivermectin [7]. A 3-year, placebo-controlled, double-blind trial involving 7148 patients given ivermectin annually for onchocerciasis by mass distribution identified musculosketetal pains, oedema of the face or extremities, itching and papular rash as adverse reactions; bullous skin lesions that did not recur developed in five persons [8].

Levamisole

Prolonged use at high dosage as an immunostimulant is associated with type I reactions, with itching, pruritus and urticaria. Lichenoid [9] and non-specific [10] rashes, leukocytoclastic vasculitis with a reticular livedo pattern due to circulating immune complexes [11] and cutaneous necrotizing vasculitis [12] have been reported. A distinctive purpuric eruption of the ears is recorded [13].

Niridazole

Urticaria and a pellagra-like dermatitis have been described.

Piperazine

Occupational dermatitis has been caused [14]. Previous contact sensitization induced by ethylenediamine has led to severe cross-reactions on subsequent oral administration of piperazine, including generalized exfoliative dermatitis [15].

Tetrachlorethylene

This drug has caused TEN.

Tiabendazole

An unusual body odour is well known after the administration of this drug. Skin reactions, consisting of urticaria or maculopapular rashes, are infrequent and usually mild and transient. Erythema multiforme [16] and TEN [17] have been reported.

REFERENCES

1 Poltera AA, Zea-Flores G, Guderian R *et al*. Onchocercacidal effects of amocarzine (CGP 6140) in Latin America. *Lancet* 1991; **337**: 583–4.
2 Karawifa MA, Yasawi MI, Mohamed AE. Hair loss as a complication of albendazole therapy. *Saudi Med J* 1988; **9**: 530.
3 Garcia-Muret MP, Sitjas D, Tuneu L, de Moragas JM. Telogen effluvium associated with albendazole therapy. *Int J Dermatol* 1990; **29**: 669–70.
4 Bryan RT, Stokes SL, Spencer HC. Expatriates treated with ivermectin. *Lancet* 1991; **337**: 304.
5 Guderian RH, Beck BJ, Proano S Jr, Mackenzie CD. Onchocerciasis in Ecuador, 1980–86: epidemiological evaluation of the disease in the Esmerldas province. *Eur J Epidemiol* 1989; **5**: 294–302.
6 Whitworth JAG, Maude GH, Luty AJF. Expatriates treated with ivermectin. *Lancet* 1991; **337**: 625–6.
7 Guderian RH, Anselmi M, Sempertegui R, Cooper PJ. Adverse reactions to ivermectin in reactive onchodermatitis. *Lancet* 1991; **337**: 188.
8 Burnham GM. Adverse reactions to ivermectin treatment for onchocerciasis. Results of a placebo-controlled, double-blind trial in Malawi. *Trans R Soc Trop Med Hyg* 1993; **87**: 313–7.
9 Kirby JD, Black MM, McGibbon D. Levamisole-induced lichenoid eruptions. *J R Soc Med* 1980; **73**: 208–11.
10 Parkinson DR, Cano PO, Jerry LM *et al*. Complications of cancer immunotherapy with levamisole. *Lancet* 1977; **ii**: 1129–32.
11 Macfarlane DG, Bacon PA. Levamisole-induced vasculitis due to circulating immune complexes. *BMJ* 1978; **i**: 407–8.
12 Scheinberg MA, Bezera JBG, Almeida LA, Silveira LA. Cutaneous necrotising vasculitis induced by levamisole. *BMJ* 1978; **i**: 408.
13 Rongioletti F, Ghio L, Ginevri F *et al*. Purpura of the ears: a distinctive vasculopathy with circulating autoantibodies complicating long-term treatment with levamisole in children. *Br J Dermatol* 1999; **140**: 948–51.
14 Calnan CD. Occupational piperazine dermatitis. *Contact Dermatitis* 1975; **1**: 126.
15 Burry JN. Ethylenediamine sensitivity with a systemic reaction to piperazine treatment. *Contact Dermatitis* 1978; **4**: 380.
16 Humphreys F, Cox NH. Thiabendazole-induced erythema multiforme with lesions around melanocytic naevi. *Br J Dermatol* 1988; **118**: 855–6.
17 Robinson HM, Samorodin CS. Thiabendazole-induced toxic epidermal necrolysis. *Arch Dermatol* 1976; **112**: 1757–60.

Drugs for *Pneumocystis*

Pentamidine

This drug is increasingly being used in the treatment and

prophylaxis of *Pneumocystis carinii* pneumonia in patients with AIDS. Urticaria, including contact urticaria [1], or maculopapular eruption proceeding to erythroderma have been reported with nebulized therapy [2,3]. TEN may occur with systemic therapy [4,5].

REFERENCES

1 Belsito DV. Contact urticaria from pentamidine isethionate. *Contact Dermatitis* 1993; **29**: 158–9.
2 Leen CLS, Mandal BK. Rash due to nebulised pentamidine. *Lancet* 1988; **ii**: 1250–1.
3 Berger TG, Tappero JW, Leoung GS, Jacobson MA. Aerosolized pentamidine and cutaneous eruptions. *Ann Intern Med* 1989; **110**: 1035–6.
4 Wang JJ, Freeman AI, Gaeta JF, Sinks LF. Unusual complications of pentamidine in the treatment of *Pneumocystis carinii* pneumonia. *J Pediatr* 1970; **77**: 311–4.
5 Walzer PD, Perl DP, Krogstadt DJ *et al*. *Pneumocystis carinii* pneumonia in the United States: epidemiologic, diagnostic and clinical features. *Ann Intern Med* 1974; **80**: 83–93.

Non-steroidal anti-inflammatory drugs

Acetylsalicylic acid and related compounds

Aspirin

Reactions to aspirin [1–4] occur in 0.3% of normal subjects [2,4]. These are usually sporadic, but occasionally more than one family member may be affected, and an HLA linkage has been reported [5]. Urticaria or angio-oedema is the commonest reaction [1]. Two types of specific IgE antibody were found in sera from aspirin-sensitive patients with salicyloyl and *O*-methylsalicyloyl discs using radioallergosorbent tests, favouring an IgE-dependent mechanism [6]. Chronic idiopathic urticaria is often aggravated by aspirin [7,8]; this exacerbation probably has a non-allergic basis. It has been estimated that patients with chronic urticaria or angio-oedema have a risk of up to 30% of developing a flare in the condition following administration of aspirin or an NSAID [3]. The reaction is dose dependent and is greater when the urticaria is in an active phase. Aspirin may render the skin of such patients more reactive to histamine [5]. The syndrome of nasal polyposis, bronchial asthma and aspirin intolerance is well known [4,9]; up to 40% of patients with nasal polyps, and 4% of patients with asthma, may develop broncho-constriction on exposure to aspirin, but only 2% develop urticaria [4]. Anaphylactoid responses may occur [3]; these may involve abnormalities of platelet function [10]. Cross-sensitivity between aspirin and tartrazine is now thought to be rare [3]. Oral desensitization is feasible if essential, and may be maintained by daily aspirin intake [3].

Other reported reactions include purpura, scarlatiniform erythema, erythema multiforme, fixed eruption and a lichenoid eruption (which recurred on challenge) [11], but all are rare [1]. Neonatal petechiae may result from aspirin therapy of the mother [12]. Aspirin has been reported to provoke generalized pustular psoriasis [13]. Oral ulceration may follow prolonged chewing of aspirin [14], and at the site of an insoluble aspirin tablet placed at the side of an aching tooth.

Nephropathy, marrow depression and gastric haemorrhage are well-recognized hazards. The elderly are at increased risk of developing such complications [15]. The drug may interfere with renal clearance, for example of methotrexate. Aspirin is safe to administer to patients with glucose-6-phosphate dehydrogenase deficiency [16].

REFERENCES

1 Baker H, Moore-Robinson M. Drug reactions. IX. Cutaneous responses to aspirin and its derivatives. *Br J Dermatol* 1970; **82**: 319–21.
2 Settipane RA, Constantine HP, Settipane GA. Aspirin intolerance and recurrent urticaria in normal adults and children. *Epidemiol Rev Allergy* 1980; **35**: 149–54.
3 Stevenson DD. Diagnosis, prevention and treatment of adverse reactions to aspirin and nonsteroidal anti-inflammatory drugs. *J Allergy Clin Immunol* 1984; **74**: 617–22.
4 Morassut P, Yang W, Karsh J. Aspirin intolerance. *Semin Arthritis Rheum* 1989; **19**: 22–30.
5 Mullarkey MF, Thomas PS, Hansen JA *et al*. Association of aspirin-sensitive asthma with HLA-DQw2. *Am Rev Respir Dis* 1986; **133**: 261–3.
6 Daxun Z, Becker WM, Schulz KH, Schlaak M. Sensitivity to aspirin: a new serological diagnostic method. *J Invest Allergol Clin Immunol* 1993; **3**: 72–8.
7 Champion RH, Roberts SOB, Carpenter RG, Roger JH. Urticaria and angio-oedema. A review of 554 patients. *Br J Dermatol* 1969; **81**: 588–97.
8 Doeglas HMG. Reactions to aspirin and food additives in patients with chronic urticaria, including the physical urticarias. *Br J Dermatol* 1975; **93**: 135–44.
9 Samter M, Beers RF. Intolerance to aspirin. Clinical studies and consideration of its pathogenesis. *Ann Intern Med* 1968; **68**: 975–83.
10 Wüthrich B. Azetylsalizylsäure-Pseudoallergie. eine Anomalie der Thrombozyten-Funktion? *Hautarzt* 1988; **39**: 631–4.
11 Bharija SC, Belhaj MS. Acetylsalicylic acid may induce a lichenoid eruption. *Dermatologica* 1988; **177**: 19.
12 Stuart MJ, Gross SJ, Elrad H, Graeber JE. Effects of acetylsalicylic-acid ingestion on maternal and neonatal hemostasis. *N Engl J Med* 1982; **307**: 909–12.
13 Shelley WB. Birch pollen and aspirin psoriasis. *JAMA* 1964; **189**: 985–8.
14 Claman HN. Mouth ulcers associated with prolonged chewing of gum containing aspirin. *JAMA* 1967; **202**: 651–2.
15 Karsh J. Adverse reactions and interactions with aspirin. Considerations in the treatment of the elderly patient. *Drug Saf* 1990; **5**: 317–27.
16 Beutler E. Glucose-6-phosphate dehydrogenase deficiency. *Lancet* 1991; **324**: 169–74.

Diflunisal

Various cutaneous reactions have been reported in up to 5% of patients, including pruritus, urticaria, exanthems, Stevens–Johnson syndrome, erythroderma [1] and a lichenoid photoreactive rash [2]. A non-pigmenting fixed drug eruption has been documented [3].

REFERENCES

1 Chan L, Winearls C, Oliver D *et al*. Acute interstitial nephritis and erythroderma associated with diflunisal. *BMJ* 1980; **280**: 84–5.
2 Street ML, Winkelmann RK. Lichenoid photoreactive epidermal necrosis with diflunisal. *J Am Acad Dermatol* 1989; **20**: 850–1.
3 Roetzheim RG, Herold AH, Van Durme DJ. Nonpigmenting fixed drug eruption caused by diflunisal. *J Am Acad Dermatol* 1991; **24**: 1021–2.

Paracetamol (acetaminophen)

This drug is a major metabolite of phenacetin, and has largely replaced it. Allergic reactions are very rare, considering that it has been estimated that more than 1.4 billion tablets are sold per annum in the UK [1,2]. Urticaria [3], anaphylaxis, a widespread maculopapular eruption, a fixed eruption [2,4–8] that may be non-pigmenting [8], exfoliative dermatitis [9], delayed hypersensitivity reactions [10], linear IgA bullous dermatosis [11] and figurate purpura [12] have been seen.

REFERENCES

1 Stricker BHC, Meyboom RHB, Lindquist M. Acute hypersensitivity reactions to paracetamol. *BMJ* 1985; **291**: 938–9.
2 Thomas RH, Munro DD. Fixed drug eruption due to paracetamol. *Br J Dermatol* 1986; **115**: 357–9.
3 Cole FOA. Urticaria from paracetamol. *Clin Exp Dermatol* 1985; **10**: 404.
4 Guin JD, Haynie LS, Jackson D, Baker GF. Wandering fixed drug eruption: a mucocutaneous reaction to acetaminophen. *J Am Acad Dermatol* 1987; **3**: 399–402.
5 Guin JD, Baker GF. Chronic fixed drug eruption caused by acetaminophen. *Cutis* 1988; **41**: 106–8.
6 Valsecchi R. Fixed drug eruption to paracetamol. *Dermatologica* 1989; **179**: 51–8.
7 Duhra P, Porter DI. Paracetamol-induced fixed drug eruption with positive immunofluorescence findings. *Clin Exp Dermatol* 1990; **15**: 293–5.
8 Galindo PA, Borja J, Feo F *et al.* Nonpigmented fixed drug eruption caused by paracetamol. *J Invest Allergol Clin Immunol* 1999; **9**: 399–400.
9 Girdhar A, Bagga AK, Girdhar BF. Exfoliative dermatitis due to paracetamol. *Indian J Dermatol Venereol Lepr* 1984; **50**: 162–3.
10 Ibanez MD, Alonso E, Munoz MC *et al.* Delayed hypersensitivity reaction to paracetamol (acetaminophen). *Allergy* 1996; **51**: 121–3.
11 Avci O, Ökmen M, Cetiner S. Acetaminophen-induced linear IgA bullous dermatosis. *J Am Acad Dermatol* 2003; **48**: 299–301.
12 Kwon SJ, Lee CW. Figurate purpuric eruptions on the trunk: acetaminophen-induced rashes. *J Dermatol* 1998; **25**: 756–8.

Phenacetin

Capillaritis, vasculitis and a bullous pemphigoid-like eruption [1] have been documented.

Salicylamide

Use of teething jellies containing this substance has resulted in severe urticaria in infants [2].

REFERENCES

1 Kashihara M, Danno K, Miyachi Y *et al.* Bullous pemphigoid-like lesions induced by phenacetin. Report of a case and an immunopathologic study. *Arch Dermatol* 1984; **120**: 1196–9.
2 Bentley-Phillips B. Infantile urticaria caused by salicylamide teething powder. *Br J Dermatol* 1968; **80**: 341.

Other NSAIDs

Dermatological aspects of the NSAIDs have been extensively reviewed [1–13]. All these drugs inhibit the enzyme cyclo-oxygenase, and decrease the production of prostaglandins and thromboxanes [6]. NSAIDs represent about 5% of all prescriptions in the UK [5] and USA [2]; nearly one in seven Americans were treated with an NSAID in 1984, and in 1986 100 million prescriptions for these drugs were written in the USA [14]. NSAIDs accounted for 25% of all suspected ADRs reported to the UK Committee on Safety of Medicines in 1986 [5,15]. Reactions to NSAIDs occur in about 1 in 50 000 administrations; NSAIDs should be avoided in patients known to be intolerant of aspirin [6]. In a large series, allergic or pseudoallergic reactions were observed in 0.2% of patients exposed to minor analgesics (including aspirin and pyrazolones, mainly metamizole, propyphenazone) and in 0.8% of patients exposed to NSAIDs (including the pyrazolone oxyphenbutazone); most reactions were cutaneous, mainly maculopapular exanthems, urticaria and angio-oedema [10]. Piroxicam, meclofenamate sodium, sulindac and zomepirac sodium had the highest reaction rates relative to the number of new prescriptions in the USA [1,2]. In contrast, naproxen, fenoprofen, ibuprofen and indometacin all had low rates of reaction; ibuprofen is available as a non-prescription drug in the USA and the UK. In another study of 2747 patients with rheumatoid arthritis, toxicity index scores computed from symptoms, laboratory abnormalities and hospitalizations attributed to NSAID therapy indicated that indometacin, tolmetin sodium and meclofenamate sodium were the most toxic, and buffered aspirin, salsalate and ibuprofen the least toxic [16].

Cutaneous adverse reactions to NSAIDs were, in order of frequency in one study [11], urticaria/angio-oedema, fixed eruptions, exanthems, erythema multiforme and Stevens–Johnson syndrome. Drug exanthems and urticaria occur in 0.2–9% of patients treated with NSAIDs [2,6]. Drug exanthems develop in 1% of patients on phenylbutazone and 0.3% of patients on indometacin [6]; they are most frequently associated with diflunisal, sulindac, meclofenamate sodium, piroxicam and phenylbutazone. All the NSAIDs, but particularly aspirin and tolmetin, may cause urticaria and anaphylactoid reactions, especially in a patient with a history of aspirin-induced urticaria. Pyrazolone NSAIDs, feprazone, nimesulide, piroxicam and flurbiprofen cause fixed drug eruptions. Although all NSAIDs may precipitate exfoliative erythroderma, this is commonest with phenylbutazone [6]. All the NSAIDs, but particularly phenylbutazone, piroxicam, fenbufen and sulindac, may cause Stevens–Johnson syndrome or TEN [6]. Oral lichenoid lesions have also been recorded with NSAIDs [17]. Psoriasis has been reported anecdotally to be exacerbated by indometacin and meclofenamate sodium, but there is no definitive evidence that NSAIDs consistently exacerbate psoriasis [5]. Contact dermatitis induced by topical NSAIDs is rare but increasing; ketoprofen and bufexamac are major contact allergens [13].

Children on NSAIDs were 2.4 times as likely to have shallow facial scars, as described in drug-induced pseudoporphyria, in one study; this relative risk was increased to 6 with naproxen [18].

Most of the NSAIDs causing photosensitivity are phenylpropionic acid derivatives: carprofen, ketoprofen, tiaprofenic acid, naproxen and nabumetone [19–24]. NSAIDs that cause photosensitivity absorb UV radiation at wavelengths longer than 310 nm, resulting in the generation of singlet oxygen molecules, which damage cell membranes [12]. The cutaneous photosensitivity appears to be elicited by a phototoxic mechanism [19–21,24]. The phototoxic reactions with NSAIDs are immediate, consisting of itching, burning, erythema and at higher fluences wealing; this contrasts with the delayed reactions associated with psoralens and tetracyclines, which produce abnormal delayed erythema or exaggerated sunburn. Propionic acid derivatives may also precipitate photourticaria by mast cell degranulation [23]. Piroxicam, an enolic acid derivative structurally unrelated to phenylpropionic acid, is the most frequently cited non-phenylpropionic acid NSAID to cause photosensitivity [20,21,25]; phototoxicity to the parent drug has not been elicited in volunteers or experimental animals, although a phototoxic metabolite has been identified *in vitro*. Indometacin, sulindac [26], meclofenamate sodium and phenylbutazone have all been associated with photosensitivity [2]. NSAIDs may cause pseudoporphyria changes [27].

Apart from the cutaneous complications, NSAIDs may cause a variety of adverse effects [14,28–30], including gastrointestinal bleeding, intestinal perforations and acute deterioration in renal function with interstitial nephritis [28]; the elderly and patients with impaired renal function or receiving concomitant diuretic therapy are most at risk. NSAIDs may inhibit platelet aggregation and increase bleeding times [29]. Aplastic anaemia is a recognized complication, and has occurred in the same individual with two different NSAIDs (sulindac and fenbufen) [31]. Hepatic syndromes [30], pneumonitis (naproxen, ibuprofen, fenoprofen and sulindac can elicit pulmonary infiltrates with eosinophilia [32]) and neurological problems, such as headache, aseptic meningitis and dizziness, are recorded [14]. Niflumic acid and diclofenac both precipitated a dermatomyositis-like syndrome in a patient [33]. The potential for adverse interactions between NSAIDs and other drugs is considerable [14].

REFERENCES

1 Stern RS, Bigby M. An expanded profile of cutaneous reactions to nonsteroid anti-inflammatory drugs. Reports to a specialty-based system for spontaneous reporting of adverse reactions to drugs. *JAMA* 1984; **252**: 1433–7.

2 Bigby M, Stern R. Cutaneous reactions to non-steroidal anti-inflammatory drugs. A review. *J Am Acad Dermatol* 1985; **12**: 866–76.

3 O'Brien WM, Bagby GF. Rare reactions to nonsteroidal anti-inflammatory drugs. *J Rheumatol* 1985; **12**: 13–20.

4 Roujeau JC. Clinical aspects of skin reactions to NSAIDs. *Scand J Rheumatol* 1987; **65** (Suppl.): 131–4.

5 Greaves MW. Pharmacology and significance of nonsteroidal anti-inflammatory drugs in the treatment of skin diseases. *J Am Acad Dermatol* 1987; **16**: 751–64.

6 Bigby M. Nonsteroidal anti-inflammatory drug reactions. *Semin Dermatol* 1989; **8**: 182–6.

7 Arnaud A. Allergy and intolerance to nonsteroidal anti-inflammatory agents. *Clin Rev Allergy Immunol* 1995; **13**: 245–51.

8 Van Arsdel PP Jr. Pseudoallergic reactions to nonsteroidal anti-inflammatory drugs. *JAMA* 1991; **266**: 3343–4.

9 Bottoni A, Criscuolo D. Cutaneous adverse reactions following the administration of nonsteroidal antiinflammatory drugs and antibiotics: an Italian survey. *Int J Clin Pharmacol Ther Toxicol* 1992; **30**: 257–9.

10 Oberholzer B, Hoigne R, Hartmann K et al. Die Haufigkeit von unerwunschten Arzneimittelwirkungen nach Symptomen und Syndrome. Aus den Erfahrungen des CHDM und der SANZ. Als Beispiel: die allergischen und pseudoallergischen Reaktionen unter leichten Analgetika und NSAIDs. *Ther Umsch* 1993; **50**: 13–9.

11 Anonymous. Cutaneous reactions to analgesic-antipyretics and nonsteroidal anti-inflammatory drugs. Analysis of reports to the spontaneous reporting system of the Gruppo Italiano Studi Epidemiologici in Dermatologia. *Dermatology* 1993; **186**: 164–9.

12 Figueras A, Capella D, Castel JM, Laorte JR. Spontaneous reporting of adverse drug reactions to non-steroidal anti-inflammatory drugs. A report from the Spanish System of Pharmacovigilance, including an early analysis of topical and enteric-coated formulations. *Eur J Clin Pharmacol* 1994; **47**: 297–303.

13 Gebhardt M, Wollina U. Kutane Nebenwirkungen nichtsteroidaler Antiphlogistika (NSAID). *Z Rheumatol* 1995; **54**: 405–12.

14 Brooks PM, Day RO. Nonsteroidal antiinflammatory drugs: differences and similarities. *N Engl J Med* 1991; **324**: 1716–25.

15 Committee on Safety of Medicines. Nonsteroidal anti-inflammatory drugs and serious gastrointestinal adverse reaction: 1. *BMJ* 1986; **292**: 614.

16 Fries JF, Williams CA, Bloch DA. The relative toxicity of nonsteroidal anti-inflammatory drugs. *Arthritis Rheum* 1991; **34**: 1353–60.

17 Hamburger J, Potts AJC. Non-steroidal anti-inflammatory drugs and oral lichenoid reactions. *BMJ* 1983; **287**: 1258.

18 Wallace CA, Farrow D, Sherry DD. Increased risk of facial scars in children taking nonsteroidal antiinflammatory drugs. *J Pediatr* 1994; **125**: 819–22.

19 Ljunggren B. Propionic acid-derived nonsteroidal anti-inflammatory drugs are phototoxic in vitro. *Photodermatology* 1985; **2**: 3–9.

20 Stern RS. Phototoxic reactions to piroxicam and other nonsteroidal anti-inflammatory agents. *N Engl J Med* 1983; **309**: 186–7.

21 Diffey BL, Daymond TJ, Fairgreaves H. Phototoxic reactions to piroxicam, naproxen and tiaprofenic acid. *Br J Rheumatol* 1983; **22**: 239–42.

22 Przybilla B, Ring J, Schwab U et al. Photosensibilisierende Eigenschaften nichtsteroidaler Antirheumatika im Photopatch-Test. *Hautarzt* 1987; **38**: 18–25.

23 Kaidbey KH, Mitchell FN. Photosensitizing potential of certain nonsteroidal anti-inflammatory agents. *Arch Dermatol* 1989; **125**: 783–6.

24 Kochevar IE. Phototoxicity of nonsteroidal inflammatory drugs. Coincidence or specific mechanism? *Arch Dermatol* 1989; **125**: 824–6.

25 Serrano G, Bonillo J, Aliaga A et al. Piroxicam-induced photosensitivity and contact sensitivity to thiosalicylic acid. *J Am Acad Dermatol* 1990; **23**: 479–83.

26 Jeanmougin M, Manciet J-R, Duterque M et al. Photosensibilisation au sulindac. *Ann Dermatol Vénéréol* 1987; **114**: 1400–1.

27 Taylor BJ, Duffill MB. Pseudoporphyria from nonsteroidal anti-inflammatory drugs. *NZ Med J* 1987; **100**: 322–3.

28 Clive DM, Stoff JS. Renal syndromes associated with nonsteroidal anti-inflammatory drugs. *N Engl J Med* 1984; **310**: 563–72.

29 Ekenny GN. Potential renal, haematological and allergic adverse effects associated with nonsteroidal anti-inflammatory drugs. *Drugs* 1992; **44** (Suppl. 5): 31–7.

30 Carson JL, Willett LR. Toxicity of nonsteroidal anti-inflammatory drugs. An overview of the epidemiological evidence. *Drugs* 1993; **46** (Suppl. 1): 243–8.

31 Andrews R, Russell N. Aplastic anaemia associated with a non-steroidal anti-inflammatory drug: relapse after exposure to another such drug. *BMJ* 1990; **301**: 38.

32 Goodwin SD, Glenny RW. Nonsteroidal anti-inflammatory drug-associated pulmonary infiltrates with eosinophilia. Review of the literature and Food and Drug Administration Adverse Drug Reaction reports. *Arch Intern Med* 1992; **152**: 1521–4.

33 Grob JJ, Collet AM, Bonerandi JJ. Dermatomyositis-like syndrome induced by nonsteroidal anti-inflammatory agents. *Dermatologica* 1989; **178**: 58–9.

Propionic acid derivatives

Carprofen. This drug causes photosensitivity [1].

Fenbufen. Morbilliform and erythematous rashes, erythema multiforme [2], Stevens–Johnson syndrome and allergic vasculitis have been recorded rarely. Fenbufen has caused exfoliative dermatitis, haemolytic anaemia and hepatitis [3], and was the drug implicated most commonly in adverse reactions reported to the UK Committee on Safety of Medicines in 1986 and 1987. A florid erythematous rash with pulmonary eosinophilia has been described in four cases [4].

Fenoprofen. This drug has caused pruritus, urticaria, vesicobullous eruption, thrombocytopenic purpura and TEN [5].

Ibuprofen. Pruritus is the only common cutaneous reaction. When used in rheumatoid arthritis, rashes are rare, although patients with SLE are liable to develop a generalized rash with fever and abdominal symptoms [6]. Angiooedema/urticaria [7,8], anaphylaxis [9], fixed eruptions [8], a linear eruption [10], vesicobullous rashes, erythema multiforme, vasculitis [11] and alopecia [12] occur. Psoriasis has been reported to be exacerbated [13]. This drug is available over the counter in the UK.

Ketoprofen. Topical application has caused photoallergic contact dermatitis [14] and systemic ketoprofen has caused pseudoporphyria.

Naproxen. The incidence of side effects is low given the widespread and long-term use of naproxen. Rashes occur in about 5% of patients; pruritus is the commonest symptom. Naproxen is associated with a photosensitivity dermatitis [15] and pseudoporphyria [16–20]; most photo-urticarial reactions are evoked by the UVA band. Urticaria/angio-oedema, anaphylaxis [21], purpura and thrombocytopenia [22], hyperhidrosis, acneiform problems in women [23], vasculitis [24,25], vesicobullous and fixed drug eruptions [26], erythema multiforme, a pustular reaction [27] and lichen planus-like reaction [28] have all been reported, as has recurrent allergic sialadenitis [29].

Tiaprofenic acid. This drug may cause photosensitivity [30].

REFERENCES

1 Merot Y, Harms M, Saurat JH. Photosensibilisation au carprofén (imadyl), un nouvel anti-inflammatoire non stéroidien. *Dermatologica* 1983; **166**: 301–7.
2 Peacock A, Ledingham J. Fenbufen-induced erythema multiforme. *BMJ* 1981; **283**: 582.
3 Muthiah MM. Severe hypersensitivity reaction to fenbufen. *BMJ* 1988; **297**: 1614.
4 Burton GH. Rash and pulmonary eosinophilia associated with fenbufen. *BMJ* 1990; **300**: 82–3.
5 Stotts JS, Fang ML, Dannaker CJ, Steinman HK. Fenoprofen-induced toxic epidermal necrolysis. *J Am Acad Dermatol* 1988; **18**: 755–7.
6 Shoenfeld Y, Livni E, Shaklai M, Pinkhas J. Sensitization to ibuprofen in SLE. *JAMA* 1980; **244**: 547–8.
7 Shelley ED, Shelley WB. Ibuprofen urticaria. *J Am Acad Dermatol* 1987; **17**: 1057–8.
8 Diaz Jara M, Perez Montero A, Gracia Bara MT *et al*. Allergic reactions due to ibuprofen in children. *Pediatr Dermatol* 2001; **18**: 66–7.
9 Takahama H, Kubota Y, Mizoguchi M. A case of anaphylaxis due to ibuprofen. *J Dermatol* 2000; **27**: 337–40.
10 Alfonso R, Belinchon I. Linear drug eruption. *Eur J Dermatol* 2001; **11**: 122–3.
11 Davidson KA, Ringpfeil F, Lee JB. Ibuprofen-induced bullous leukocytoclastic vasculitis. *Cutis* 2001; **67**: 303–7.
12 Meyer HC. Alopecia associated with ibuprofen. *JAMA* 1979; **242**: 142.
13 Ben-Chetrit E, Rubinow A. Exacerbation of psoriasis by ibuprofen. *Cutis* 1986; **38**: 45.
14 Alomar A. Ketoprofen photodermatitis. *Contact Dermatitis* 1985; **12**: 112–3.
15 Shelley WB, Elpern DJ, Shelley ED. Naproxen photosensitization demonstrated by challenge. *Cutis* 1986; **38**: 169–70.
16 Farr PM, Diffey BL. Pseudoporphyria due to naproxen. *Lancet* 1985; **i**: 1166–7.
17 Judd LE, Henderson DW, Hill DC. Naproxen-induced pseudoporphyria: a clinical and ultrastructural study. *Arch Dermatol* 1986; **122**: 451–4.
18 Mayou S, Black MM. Pseudoporphyria due to naproxen. *Br J Dermatol* 1986; **114**: 519–20.
19 Burns DA. Naproxen pseudoporphyria in a patient with vitiligo. *Clin Exp Dermatol* 1987; **12**: 296–7.
20 Levy ML, Barron KS, Eichenfield A, Honig PJ. Naproxen-induced pseudoporphyria: a distinctive photodermatitis. *J Pediatr* 1990; **117**: 660–4.
21 Cistero A, Urias S, Guindo J *et al*. Coronary artery spasm and acute myocardial infarction in naproxen-associated anaphylactic reaction. *Allergy* 1992; **47**: 576–8.
22 Hunt PJ, Gibbons SS. Naproxen induced thrombocytopenia: a case report. *NZ Med J* 1995; **108**: 483–4.
23 Hamman CO. Severe primary dysmenorrhea treated with naproxen. A prospective, double-blind crossover investigation. *Prostaglandins* 1980; **19**: 651–7.
24 Grennan DM, Jolly J, Holloway LJ, Palmer DG. Vasculitis in a patient receiving naproxen. *NZ Med J* 1979; **89**: 48–9.
25 Singhal PC, Faulkner M, Venkatesham J, Molho L. Hypersensitivity angiitis associated with naproxen. *Ann Allergy* 1989; **63**: 107–9.
26 Habbema L, Bruynzeel DP. Fixed drug eruption due to naproxen. *Dermatologica* 1987; **174**: 184–5.
27 Grattan CEH. Generalized pustular drug rash due to naproxen. *Dermatologica* 1989; **179**: 57–8.
28 Heymann WR, Lerman JS, Luftschein S. Naproxen-induced lichen planus. *J Am Acad Dermatol* 1984; **10**: 299–301.
29 Knulst AC, Stengs CJ, Baart de la Faille H *et al*. Salivary gland swelling following naproxen therapy. *Br J Dermatol* 1995; **133**: 647–9.
30 Neumann RA, Knobler RM, Lindemayr H. Tiaprofenic acid-induced photosensitivity. *Contact Dermatitis* 1989; **20**: 270–3.

Phenylacetic acids

Diclofenac. A variety of cutaneous adverse effects [1,2], including pruritus, urticaria, various exanthems, papulovesicular eruptions [3], delayed allergy [4], vasculitis [5], a bullous eruption associated with linear basement membrane deposition of IgA [6] and fatal erythema multiforme [1] have been recorded.

REFERENCES

1 Ciucci AG. A review of spontaneously reported adverse drug reactions with diclofenac sodium (Voltarol). *Rheum Rehabil* 1979; Suppl. 2: 116–21.

2 O'Brien WM. Adverse reactions to nonsteroidal antiinflammatory drugs. Diclofenac compared with other nonsteroidal antiinflammatory drugs. *Am J Med* 1986; **80**: 70–80.

3 Seigneuric C, Nougué J, Plantavid M. Érythème polymorphe avec atteinte muqueuse: responsabilité du diclofénac? *Ann Dermatol Vénéréol* 1982; **109**: 287.

4 Schiavino D, Papa G, Nucera E *et al.* Delayed allergy to diclofenac. *Contact Dermatitis* 1992; **26**: 357–8.

5 Bonafé J-L, Mazières B, Bouteiller G. Trisymptôme de Gougerot induit par les anti-inflammatoires. Rôle du diclofénac? *Ann Dermatol Vénéréol* 1982; **109**: 283–4.

6 Gabrielson TØ, Staerfelt F, Thune PO. Drug induced bullous dermatosis with linear IgA deposits along the basement membrane. *Acta Derm Venereol (Stockh)* 1981; **61**: 439–41.

Oxicams

Piroxicam. This drug may cause adverse cutaneous reactions in 2–3% of patients [1,2]. More than two-thirds of affected patients have photosensitivity; lesions may be vesicobullous or eczematous, and occur within 3 days of starting therapy in 50% of cases [3–10]. Photosensitivity may result from phototoxic metabolites [7]. Photocontact dermatitis developed in three patients after the application of a gel containing 0.5% piroxicam. Patch tests were positive to thiomersal and thiosalicylic acid and photopatch tests with piroxicam were positive. Patch tests in patients with systemic photosensitivity to piroxicam were also positive for thiomersal and thiosalicylic acid. Contact allergic sensitivity to the latter is a marker for patients with a high risk of developing photosensitivity reactions to piroxicam [10,11].

Other eruptions include urticaria, maculopapular [12] or lichenoid rashes, alopecia, erythema multiforme [13] and vasculitis [14]. Piroxicam was well tolerated in patients with an urticarial reaction to a single NSAID, but provoked urticaria in 27% of patients with allergy to at least two different NSAIDs, indicating that mechanisms other than interference with prostaglandin synthesis and release of inflammatory mediators participate in allergic reactions to NSAIDs [15]. Classical fixed drug eruption [16,17] and a non-pigmenting fixed drug reaction [18], with cross-sensitivity among piroxicam, tenoxicam and droxicam in one case [19], have also been reported. Contact sensitivity to piroxicam is recorded [20]. Piroxicam was thought to have triggered subacute LE in a patient with Sjögren's syndrome and seronegative arthritis [21]. Isolated case reports of linear IgA bullous dermatosis [22], fatal pemphigus vulgaris [23] and fatal TEN [24] have appeared. The drug has caused peripheral neuropathy and erythroderma [25]. Blood dyscrasias have been reported.

REFERENCES

1 Pitts N. Efficacy and safety of piroxicam. *Am J Med* 1982; **72** (Suppl. 2A): 77–87.

2 Gerber D. Adverse reactions of piroxicam. *Drug Intell Clin Pharmacol* 1987; **21**: 707–10.

3 Stern RS. Phototoxic reactions to piroxicam and other nonsteroidal antiinflammatory agents. *N Engl J Med* 1983; **309**: 186–7.

4 Diffey BL, Daymond TJ, Fairgreaves H. Phototoxic reactions to piroxicam, naproxen and tiaprofenic acid. *Br J Rheumatol* 1983; **22**: 239–42.

5 Serrano G, Bonillo J, Aliaga A *et al.* Piroxicam-induced photosensitivity. *J Am Acad Dermatol* 1984; **11**: 113–20.

6 McKerrow KJ, Greig DE. Piroxicam-induced photosensitive dermatitis. *J Am Acad Dermatol* 1986; **15**: 1237–41.

7 Kochevar IE, Morison WL, Lamm JL *et al.* Possible mechanism of piroxicam-induced photosensitivity. *Arch Dermatol* 1986; **122**: 1283–7.

8 Kaidbey KH, Mitchell FN. Photosensitizing potential of certain nonsteroidal anti-inflammatory agents. *Arch Dermatol* 1989; **125**: 783–6.

9 Kochevar IE. Phototoxicity of nonsteroidal inflammatory drugs. Coincidence or specific mechanism? *Arch Dermatol* 1989; **125**: 824–6.

10 Serrano G, Bonillo J, Aliaga AET *et al.* Piroxicam-induced photosensitivity and contact sensitivity to thiosalicylic acid. *J Am Acad Dermatol* 1990; **23**: 479–83.

11 Trujillo MJ, de Barrio M, Rodriguez A *et al.* Piroxicam-induced photodermatitis. Cross-reactivity among oxicams. A case report. *Allergol Immunopathol* 2001; **29**: 133–6.

12 Faure M, Goujon C, Perrot H *et al.* Accidents cutanés provoqués par le piroxicam. A propos de trois observations. *Ann Dermatol Vénéréol* 1982; **109**: 255–8.

13 Bertail M-A, Cavelier B, Civatte J. Réaction au piroxicam (Feldène®). A type d'ectoderme érosive pluri-orificielle. *Ann Dermatol Vénéréol* 1982; **109**: 261–2.

14 Goebel KN, Mueller-Brodman W. Reversible overt nephropathy with Henoch–Schönlein purpura due to piroxicam. *BMJ* 1982; **284**: 311–2.

15 Carmona MJ, Blanca M, Garcia A *et al.* Intolerance to piroxicam in patients with adverse reactions to nonsteroidal antiinflammatory drugs. *J Allergy Clin Immunol* 1992; **90**: 873–9.

16 Stubb S, Reitamo S. Fixed drug eruption caused by piroxicam. *J Am Acad Dermatol* 1990; **22**: 1111–2.

17 de la Hoz B, Soria C, Fraj J *et al.* Fixed drug eruption due to piroxicam. *Int J Dermatol* 1990; **29**: 672–3.

18 Valsecchi R, Cainelli T. Nonpigmenting fixed drug reaction to piroxicam. *J Am Acad Dermatol* 1989; **21**: 1300.

19 Ordoqui E, De Barrio M, Rodriguez VM *et al.* Cross-sensitivity among oxicams in piroxicam-caused fixed drug eruption: two case reports. *Allergy* 1995; **50**: 741–4.

20 Valsecchi R, Pansera B, di Landro A, Cainelli T. Contact sensitivity to piroxicam. *Contact Dermatitis* 1993; **29**: 167.

21 Roura M, Lopez-Gil F, Umbert P. Systemic lupus erythematosus exacerbated by piroxicam. *Dermatologica* 1991; **182**: 56–8.

22 Camilleri M, Pace JL. Linear IgA bullous dermatosis induced by piroxicam. *J Eur Acad Dermatol Venereol* 1998; **10**: 70–2.

23 Martin RL, McSweeny GW, Schneider J. Fatal pemphigus vulgaris in a patient taking piroxicam. *N Engl J Med* 1983; **309**: 795–6.

24 Roujeau JC, Revuz I, Touraine R *et al.* Syndrome de Lyell au cours d'un traitement par un nouvel antiinflammatoire. *Nouv Presse Med* 1981; **10**: 3407–8.

25 Sangla I, Blin O, Jouglard J *et al.* Neuropathic axonale et toxidermie iatrogene par le piroxicam. Manifestations d'hypersensibilite? *Rev Neurol* 1993; **149**: 217–8.

Anthranilic acids

Meclofenamate sodium. Rashes occur in up to 9% of patients. More than two-thirds of reactions have been exanthematous, with prominent pruritus; vasculitic, purpuric or petechial reactions are also noted, as well as occasional urticaria, fixed drug eruption, erythema multiforme [1], exfoliative erythroderma and a vesicobullous reaction. It has been reported to exacerbate psoriasis [2]. Selective adverse reactions to glafenine and meclofenamate occurred in a patient tolerating aspirin and other cyclo-oxygenase inhibitors [3].

Mefenamic acid. Urticaria, a morbilliform eruption, fixed drug eruption [4,5], pseudoporphyria [6] and generalized exfoliative dermatitis are documented. Acute renal failure, severe thrombocytopenia and jaundice developed after a small dose of mefenamic acid in one patient with drug-dependent antibodies reacting against platelets [7].

REFERENCES

1 Harrington T, Davis D. Erythema multiforme induced by meclofenamate sodium. *J Rheumatol* 1983; **10**: 169–70.
2 Meyerhoff JO. Exacerbation of psoriasis with meclofenamate. *N Engl J Med* 1983; **309**: 496.
3 Fernandez-Rivas M, de la Hoz B, Cuevas M *et al*. Hypersensitivity reactions to anthranilic acid derivatives. *Ann Allergy* 1993; **71**: 515–8.
4 Wilson DL, Otter A. Fixed drug eruption associated with mefenamic acid. *BMJ* 1986; **293**: 1243.
5 Watson A, Watt G. Fixed drug eruption to mefenamic acid. *Australas J Dermatol* 1986; **27**: 6–7.
6 O'Hagan AH, Irvine AD, Allen GE, Walsh M. Pseudoporphyria induced by mefenamic acid. *Br J Dermatol* 1998; **139**: 1131–2.
7 Schwartz D, Gremmel F, Kurz R *et al*. Case report: acute renal failure, thrombocytopenia and nonhemolytic icterus probably caused by mefenamic acid (Parkemed)-dependent antibodies. *Beitr Infusionsther* 1992; **30**: 413–5.

Heterocyclic acetic acids

Indometacin (indomethacin). Allergic reactions are very uncommon, but pruritus, urticaria, purpura and morbilliform eruptions are documented. Stomatitis [1] and thrombocytopenia occur rarely, as well as a generalized exfoliative dermatitis and TEN [2]. Vasculitis has been documented [3]. There have been rare reports of exacerbation of psoriasis [4,5]; however, indometacin in a standard dose of 75 mg/day had no significant harmful effect on psoriasis in a series of patients treated with the Ingram regimen of coal-tar bath, suberythemal UVB phototherapy and dithranol in Lassar's paste [6]. Exacerbation of dermatitis herpetiformis has been recorded [7].

REFERENCES

1 Guggenheimer J, Ismail YH. Oral ulcerations associated with indomethacin therapy: report of three cases. *J Am Dent Assoc* 1975; **90**: 632–4.
2 O'Sullivan M, Hanly JG, Molloy M. A case of toxic epidermal necrolysis secondary to indomethacin. *Br J Rheumatol* 1983; **22**: 47–9.
3 Marsh FP, Almeyda JR, Levy IS. Non-thrombocytopenic purpura and acute glomerulonephritis after indomethacin therapy. *Ann Rheum Dis* 1971; **30**: 501–5.
4 Katayama H, Kawada A. Exacerbation of psoriasis induced by indomethacin. *J Dermatol* 1981; **8**: 323–7.
5 Powles AV, Griffiths CEM, Seifert MH, Fry L. Exacerbation of psoriasis by indomethacin. *Br J Dermatol* 1987; **117**: 799–800.
6 Sheehan-Dare RA, Goodfield MJD, Rowell NR. The effect of oral indomethacin on psoriasis treated with the Ingram regime. *Br J Dermatol* 1991; **125**: 253–5.
7 Griffiths CEM, Leonard JN, Fry L. Dermatitis herpetiformis exacerbated by indomethacin. *Br J Dermatol* 1985; **112**: 443–5.

Sulindac. Rashes occur in up to 9% of patients. The drug has caused anaphylaxis [1] and anaphylactoid reactions [2], photosensitivity [3], facial and oral erythema, a pernio-like reaction [4] and fixed drug eruption [5]. Stevens–Johnson syndrome [6–8], TEN [6,9], serum sickness and exfoliative erythroderma are documented. Blood dyscrasias, toxic hepatitis, pancreatitis, and aseptic meningitis in patients with SLE are recorded.

Tolmetin. Anaphylactoid reactions are well recognized [10]. TEN has been recorded.

REFERENCES

1 Smith F, Lindberg P. Life-threatening hypersensitivity to sulindac. *JAMA* 1980; **244**: 269–70.
2 Hyson CP, Kazakoff MA. A severe multisystem reaction to sulindac. *Arch Intern Med* 1991; **151**: 387–8.
3 Jeanmougin M, Manciet J-R, Duterque M *et al*. Photosensibilisation au sulindac. *Ann Dermatol Vénéréol* 1987; **114**: 1400–1.
4 Reinertsen J. Unusual pernio-like reaction to sulindac. *Arthritis Rheum* 1981; **24**: 1215.
5 Aram HA. Fixed drug eruption due to sulindac. *Int J Dermatol* 1984; **23**: 421.
6 Levitt L, Pearson RW. Sulindac-induced Stevens–Johnson toxic epidermal necrolysis syndrome. *JAMA* 1980; **243**: 1262–3.
7 Husain Z, Runge LA, Jabbs JM, Hyla JA. Sulindac-induced Stevens–Johnson syndrome: report of 3 cases. *J Rheumatol* 1981; **8**: 176–9.
8 Maguire FW. Stevens–Johnson syndrome due to sulindac: a case report and review of the literature. *Del Med J* 1981; **53**: 193–7.
9 Chevrant Breton J, Pibouin M, Allain H *et al*. Toxic epidermal necrolysis induced by sulindac. *Thérapie* 1985; **40**: 67–9.
10 Rossi A, Knapp D. Tolmetin-induced anaphylactoid reactions. *N Engl J Med* 1982; **307**: 499–500.

Pyrazolones

Amidopyrine (aminophenazone). This is the most dangerous of all analgesics and has caused hundreds of deaths due to blood dyscrasias. It has been withdrawn from western Europe and North America but is still available in certain parts of the world. TEN, exfoliative dermatitis and erythema multiforme are all well known.

Azapropazone. Photosensitivity is recognized [1]. A multifocal bullous fixed drug eruption resembling erythema multiforme has been reported [2]. A bullous eruption on the face and extremities, with histological features suggestive of pemphigoid but negative immunofluorescence, has been reported [3]. The drug is contraindicated in patients receiving warfarin, as the latter medication is potentiated [4].

REFERENCES

1 Olsson S, Biriell C, Boman G. Photosensitivity during treatment with azapropazone. *BMJ* 1985; **291**: 939.
2 Sowden JM, Smith AG. Multifocal fixed drug eruption mimicking erythema multiforme. *Clin Exp Dermatol* 1990; **15**: 387–8.
3 Barker DJ, Cotterill JA. Skin eruptions due to azapropazone. *Lancet* 1977; **i**: 90.
4 Win N, Mitchell DC. Azapropazone and warfarin. *BMJ* 1991; **302**: 969–70.

Phenylbutazone and oxyphenbutazone. Reactions have been frequent and often fatal [1,2]. Therefore, in the UK oxyphenbutazone has been withdrawn and phenylbutazone is restricted to hospital use for ankylosing spondylitis.

Pruritus, morbilliform eruptions, urticaria and buccal ulceration are most common; erythema multiforme, fixed eruptions (especially with oxyphenbutazone), generalized exfoliative dermatitis and TEN [3] are all well-documented hazards. Drug exanthems or erythroderma may occur in up to 4% of patients treated with phenylbutazone. Occasional reports of exacerbation of psoriasis have occurred [4]. Rarer reactions have included generalized lymphadenopathy, a Sjögren-like syndrome, non-thrombocytopenic purpura, allergic vasculitis [5] and polyarteritis nodosa. Provocation of temporal arteritis has been reported. A haemorrhagic bullous eruption of the hands was observed in three patients [6]. Cutaneous necrosis has been seen after intramuscular injection. Phenylbutazone causes fluid retention, gastrointestinal bleeding and bone marrow depression [2]; the hazards of the latter are greatly increased if the dose exceeds 200 mg/day.

REFERENCES

1 Van Joost T, Asghar SS, Cormane RH. Skin reactions caused by phenylbutazone. Immunologic studies. *Arch Dermatol* 1974; **110**: 929–33.
2 Inman WHW. Study of fatal bone marrow depression with special reference to phenylbutazone and oxyphenbutazone. *BMJ* 1977; **i**: 1500–5.
3 Montgomery PR. Toxic epidermal necrolysis due to phenylbutazone. *Br J Dermatol* 1970; **83**: 220.
4 Reshad H, Hargreaves GK, Vickers CFH. Generalized pustular psoriasis precipitated by phenylbutazone and oxyphenbutazone. *Br J Dermatol* 1983; **109**: 111–3.
5 Von Paschoud J-M. Vasculitis allergica cutis durch phenylbutazon. *Dermatologica* 1966; **133**: 76–86.
6 Millard LG. A haemorrhagic bullous eruption of the hands caused by phenylbutazone: a report of 3 cases. *Acta Derm Venereol (Stockh)* 1977; **57**: 83–6.

Cyclo-oxygenase-2 inhibitors

Celecoxib. Fixed drug eruption and Sweet's syndrome are documented [1,2].

REFERENCES

1 Bandyopadhyay D. Celecoxib-induced fixed drug eruption. *Clin Exp Dermatol* 2003; **28**: 452.
2 Fye KH, Crowley E, Berger TG *et al.* Celecoxib-induced Sweet's syndrome. *J Am Acad Dermatol* 2001; **45**: 300–2.

Miscellaneous anti-inflammatory agents

Benzydamine

Photoallergy has been described to both topical and systemic administration of this drug [1].

REFERENCE

1 Frosch PJ, Weickel R. Photokontakallergie durch Benzydamin (Tantum). *Hautarzt* 1989; **40**: 771–3.

Allopurinol

Dermatological complications occur in up to 10% of cases [1–7]. Acute sensitivity reactions are well known, including scarlatiniform erythema, morbilliform rashes, urticaria or generalized exfoliative dermatitis, which may be associated with fever, eosinophilia, hepatic abnormalities and a nephropathy. Vasculitis (perhaps triggered by oxypurinol, the principal metabolite of allopurinol, which has a long half-life and accumulates in renal failure [5]), erythema multiforme [7], Stevens–Johnson syndrome and TEN [5,8,9] have been reported. Cell-mediated immunity directed towards allopurinol and more importantly to its oxypurinol metabolite is thought to be involved in the pathogenesis of allopurinol-induced hypersensitivity [10]. Hypersensitivity reactions occur on average within 2–6 weeks of starting the drug, although the interval may be much longer. Eruptions are commoner in the setting of impaired renal function [11] and with concomitant thiazide therapy [12], and may first appear up to 3 weeks after the drug has been discontinued [13]. The mortality is about 20% [5]. Other allopurinol-induced cutaneous changes include alopecia and ichthyosis [14]. Allopurinol potentiates the risk of a reaction to ampicillin [15] and increases blood ciclosporin levels [16]. Desensitization may be successful in cases with minor rashes induced by allopurinol [17–19].

REFERENCES

1 Lupton GP. The allopurinol hypersensitivity syndrome. *J Am Acad Dermatol* 1979; **1**: 365–74.
2 McInnes GT, Lawson DH, Jick H. Acute adverse reactions attributed to allopurinol in hospitalised patients. *Ann Rheum Dis* 1981; **40**: 245–9.
3 Singer JZ, Wallace SL. The allopurinol hypersensitivity syndrome. Unnecessary morbidity and mortality. *Arthritis Rheum* 1986; **29**: 82–7.
4 Foucault V, Pibouin M, Lehry D *et al.* Accidents médicamenteux sévères et allopurinol *Ann Dermatol Vénéréol* 1988; **115**: 1169–72.
5 Arellano F, Sacristan JA. Allopurinol hypersensitivity syndrome: a review. *Ann Pharmacother* 1993; **27**: 337–43.
6 Elasy T, Kaminsky D, Tracy M, Mehler PS. Allopurinol hypersensitivity syndrome revisited. *West J Med* 1995; **162**: 360–1.
7 Kumar A, Edward N, White MI *et al.* Allopurinol, erythema multiforme, and renal insufficiency. *BMJ* 1996; **312**: 173–4.
8 Bennett TO, Sugar J, Sahgal S. Ocular manifestations of toxic epidermal necrolysis associated with allopurinol use. *Arch Ophthalmol* 1977; **95**: 1362–4.
9 Dan M, Jedwab M, Peled M *et al.* Allopurinol-induced toxic epidermal necrolysis. *Int J Dermatol* 1984; **23**: 142–4.
10 Braden GL, Warzynski MJ, Golightly M, Ballow M. Cell-mediated immunity in allopurinol-induced hypersensitivity. *Clin Immunol Immunopathol* 1994; **70**: 145–51.
11 Handke KR, Noone RM, Stone WJ. Severe allopurinol toxicity. Description and guidelines for prevention in patients with renal insufficiency. *Am J Med* 1984; **76**: 47–56.
12 Handke KR. Evaluation of a thiazide allopurinol drug interaction. *Am J Med Sci* 1986; **292**: 213–6.
13 Bigby M, Jick S, Jick H, Arndt K. Drug-induced cutaneous reactions. A report from the Boston Collaborative Drug Surveillance Program on 15438 consecutive inpatients, 1975 to 1982. *JAMA* 1986; **256**: 3358–63.
14 Auerbach R, Orentreich N. Alopecia and ichthyosis secondary to allopurinol. *Arch Dermatol* 1968; **98**: 104.
15 Jick H, Slone D, Shapiro S *et al.* Excess of ampicillin rashes associated with allopurinol or hyperuricemia. A report from the Boston Collaborative Drug

Surveillance Program, Boston University Medical Center. *N Engl J Med* 1972; **286**: 505–7.

16 Gorrie M, Beaman M, Nicholls A, Backwell A. Allopurinol interaction with cyclosporin. *BMJ* 1994; **308**: 113.

17 Fam AG, Lewtas J, Stein J, Paton TW. Desensitization to allopurinol in patients with gout and cutaneous reactions. *Am J Med* 1992; **93**: 299–302.

18 Kelso JM, Keating RM. Successful desensitization for treatment of a fixed drug eruption to allopurinol. *J Allergy Clin Immunol* 1996; **97**: 1171–2.

19 Walz-LeBlanc BA, Reynolds WJ, MacFadden DK. Allopurinol sensitivity in a patient with chronic tophaceous gout: success of intravenous desensitization after failure of oral desensitization. *Arthritis Rheum* 1991; **34**: 1329–31.

Drugs acting on the central nervous system

The adverse effects of psychotropic medication have been reviewed [1–4]; the prevalence of skin reactions to psychotropic medications is about 5% [2].

REFERENCES

1 Gupta MA, Gupta AK, Haberman HF. Psychotropic drugs in dermatology. A review and guidelines for use. *J Am Acad Dermatol* 1986; **14**: 633–45.

2 Srebrnik A, Hes JP, Brenner S. Adverse cutaneous reactions to psychotropic drugs. *Acta Derm Venereol Suppl (Stockh)* 1991; **158**: 1–12.

3 Kimyai-Asadi A, Harris JC, Nousari HC. Critical overview: adverse cutaneous reactions to psychotropic medications. *J Clin Psychiatry* 1999; **60**: 714–25.

4 Warnock JK, Morris DW. Adverse cutaneous reactions to mood stabilizers. *Am J Clin Dermatol* 2003; **4**: 21–30.

Antidepressants

Tricyclics and related compounds

Antidepressants are associated with a range of idiosyncratic reactions affecting the liver, skin, haematological and central nervous systems; reactions are mediated by chemically reactive metabolites formed by the cytochrome P-450 enzyme system either directly or indirectly via an immune mechanism. Individual susceptibility is determined by genetic and environmental factors, which result in inadequate detoxification of the chemically reactive metabolite [1]. Sedative, cardiovascular, anticholinergic and gastrointestinal side effects are well known [2,3]. Agranulocytosis may occur occasionally. Cutaneous reactions are rare [2] but include maculopapular rashes, photosensitivity (protriptyline and imipramine), urticaria, pruritus, hyperhidrosis, vasculitis or acne (maprotiline), and TEN (amoxapine).

Amineptine. Severe acne [4,5] and rosacea [6] have been reported.

Amitriptyline. A bullous reaction in a patient with overdosage of amitriptyline and clorazepate dipotassium has been reported [7]. Alopecia is documented.

Clomipramine. A photoallergic eruption has been documented [8].

Imipramine. This drug has caused urticarial or exanthematic eruptions occasionally [9] and agranulocytosis has occurred. Oedema of the feet is seen in older people. Glossitis and stomatitis are rare, as are transient erythema of the face, photosensitivity and exfoliative dermatitis. Slate-grey pigmentation of exposed skin may develop; golden-yellow granules, which ultrastructurally are electron-dense inclusion bodies in phagocytes, fibroblasts and dendrocytes, are seen in the papillary dermis [10–12]. Q-switched alexandrite and ruby lasers may be helpful in treating the pigmentation [13]. Cutaneous vasculitis is well documented. Atypical cutaneous lymphoid hyperplasia has been documented [14].

Maprotiline. Acne [15] and vasculitis [16] are recorded.

Mianserin. Erythema multiforme has recently been reported [17], as has a severe allergic reaction [18].

Trazodone. This drug has caused leukonychia [19], erythema multiforme [20] and vasculitis [21], and has been implicated in causing a psoriasiform eruption. Skin swelling is recorded [22].

REFERENCES

1 Pirmohamed M, Kitteringham NR, Park BK. Idiosyncratic reactions to antidepressants: a review of the possible mechanisms and predisposing factors. *Pharmacol Ther* 1992; **53**: 105–25.

2 Gupta MA, Gupta AK, Haberman HF. Psychotropic drugs in dermatology. A review and guidelines for use. *J Am Acad Dermatol* 1986; **14**: 633–45.

3 Gupta MA, Gupta AK, Ellis CN. Antidepressant drugs in dermatology. An update. *Arch Dermatol* 1987; **123**: 647–52.

4 Thioly-Bensoussan D, Edelson Y, Cardinne A, Grupper C. Acné monstrueuse iatrogène provoquée par le Survector®: première observation mondiale à propos de deux cas. *Nouv Dermatol* 1987; **6**: 535–7.

5 De Galvez Aranda MV, Sanchez PS, Alonso Corral MJ *et al.* Acneiform eruption caused by amineptine. A case report and review of the literature. *J Eur Acad Dermatol Venereol* 2001; **15**: 337–9.

6 Jeanmougin M, Civatte J, Cavelier-Balloy B. Toxiderme rosaceiforme a l'amineptine (Survector). *Ann Dermatol Vénéréol* 1988; **115**: 1185–6.

7 Herschtal D, Robinson MJ. Blisters of the skin in coma induced by amitriptyline and clorazepate dipotassium. Report of a case with underlying sweat gland necrosis. *Arch Dermatol* 1979; **115**: 499.

8 Ljunggren B, Bojs G. A case of photosensitivity and contact allergy to systemic tricyclic drugs, with unusual features. *Contact Dermatitis* 1991; **24**: 259–65.

9 Almeyda J. Drug reactions XIII. Cutaneous reactions to imipramine and chlordiazepoxide. *Br J Dermatol* 1971; **84**: 298–9.

10 Hashimoto K, Joselow SA, Tye MJ. Imipramine hyperpigmentation: a slate-gray discoloration caused by long-term imipramine administration. *J Am Acad Dermatol* 1991; **25**: 357–61.

11 Ming ME, Bhawan J, Stefanato CM *et al.* Imipramine-induced hyperpigmentation: four cases and a review of the literature. *J Am Acad Dermatol* 1999; **40**: 159–66.

12 Sicari MC, Lebwohl M, Baral J *et al.* Photoinduced dermal pigmentation in patients taking tricyclic antidepressants: histology, electron microscopy, and energy dispersive spectroscopy. *J Am Acad Dermatol* 1999; **40**: 290–3.

13 Atkin DH, Fitzpatrick RE. Laser treatment of imipramin-induced hyperpigmentation. *J Am Acad Dermatol* 2000; **43**: 77–80.

14 Crowson AN, Magro CM. Antidepressant therapy. A possible cause of atypical cutaneous lymphoid hyperplasia. *Arch Dermatol* 1995; **131**: 925–9.

15 Ponte CD. Maprotiline-induced acne. *Am J Psychiatry* 1982; **139**: 141.

16 Oakley AM, Hodge L. Cutaneous vasculitis from maprotiline. *Aust NZ J Med* 1985; **15**: 256–7.

17 Quraishy E. Erythema multiforme during treatment with mianserin. *Br J Dermatol* 1981; **104**: 481.

18 Bazin N, Beaufils B, Feline A. A severe allergic reaction to mianserin. *Am J Psychiatry* 1991; **148**: 1088–9.

19 Longstreth GF, Hershman J. Trazodone-induced hepatotoxicity and leukonychia. *J Am Acad Dermatol* 1985; **13**: 149–50.

20 Ford HE, Jenike MA. Erythema multiforme associated with trazodone therapy. *J Clin Psychiatry* 1985; **46**: 294–5.

21 Mann SC, Walker MM, Messenger GG *et al.* Leukocytoclastic vasculitis secondary to trazodone treatment. *J Am Acad Dermatol* 1984; **10**: 669–70.

22 Fisher S, Bryant SG, Kent TA. Postmarketing surveillance by patient self-monitoring: trazodone versus fluoxetine. *J Clin Psychopharmacol* 1993; **13**: 235–42.

Monoamine oxidase inhibitors

Iproniazid. Vasculitis and peripheral neuritis are documented.

Phenelzine. Hypersensitivity skin reactions are rare.

Selective serotonin reuptake inhibitors

Fluoxetine

This drug has caused urticaria [1], urticarial vasculitis [2] and hypersensitivity [3], and serum sickness [4]; familial cases are documented [5]. Atypical cutaneous lymphoid hyperplasia [6], including pseudomycosis fungoides [6–8], is recorded.

Paroxetine

Cutaneous vasculitis has been reported [9].

Miscellaneous selective serotonin reuptake inhibitors

The 5-HT$_3$ receptor antagonists granisetron, ondansetron and tropisetron are antiemetic medications used during chemotherapy. Effects include headache and gastrointestinal symptoms, and rarely hypersensitivity reactions [10]. There were no cross-over reactions to citalopram or paroxetine among patients hypersensitive to zimeldine [11].

REFERENCES

1 Leznoff A, Binkley KE, Joffee RT *et al.* Adverse cutaneous reactions associated with fluoxetine strategy for reintroduction of this drug in selected patients. *J Clin Psychopharmacol* 1992; **12**: 355–7.

2 Roger D, Rolle F, Mausset J *et al.* Urticarial vasculitis induced by fluoxetine. *Dermatology* 1995; **191**: 164.

3 Beer K, Albertini J, Medenica M, Busbey S. Fluoxetine-induced hypersensitivity. *Arch Dermatol* 1994; **130**: 803–4.

4 Shapiro LE, Knowles SR, Shear NH. Fluoxetine-induced serum sickness-like reaction. *Ann Pharmacother* 1997; **31**: 927.

5 Olfson M, Wilner MT. A family case history of fluoxetine-induced skin reactions. *J Nerv Ment Dis* 1991; **179**: 504–5.

6 Crowson AN, Magro CM. Antidepressant therapy. A possible cause of atypical cutaneous lymphoid hyperplasia. *Arch Dermatol* 1995; **131**: 925–9.

7 Gordon KB, Guitart J, Kuzel T *et al.* Pseudomycosis fungoides in a patient taking clonazepam and fluoxetine. *J Am Acad Dermatol* 1996; **34**: 304–6.

8 Vermeer MH, Willemze R. Is mycosis fungoides exacerbated by fluoxetine? *J Am Acad Dermatol* 1996; **35**: 635–6.

9 Margolese HC, Chouinard G, Beauclair L, Rubino M. Cutaneous vasculitis induced by paroxetine. *Am J Psychiatry* 2001; **158**: 497.

10 Kataja V, de Bruijn KM. Hypersensitivity reactions associated with 5-hydroxytryptamine(3)-receptor antagonists: a class effect? *Lancet* 1996; **347**: 584–5.

11 Bengtsson BO, Lundmark J, Walinder J. No crossover reactions to citalopram or paroxetine among patients hypersensitive to zimeldine. *Br J Psychiatry* 1991; **158**: 853–5.

Lithium

Skin reactions [1–5] are relatively uncommon. Pustular and psoriasiform lesions induced by this drug have received particular attention [6]. The pustular propensities of lithium have been attributed to lysosomal enzyme release and increased neutrophil chemotaxis [2]. Tetracycline should be avoided in treating these pustular eruptions as it may precipitate serious lithium toxicity. The acneiform 'erysipelas' eruption consists of monomorphic pustules on an erythematous base, tends to affect mainly the arms and legs, is not associated with comedones or cystic lesions, and may be very persistent. Various patterns of folliculitis may occur. Lithium can aggravate pre-existing psoriasis, making it more difficult to control [6–10], and may precipitate a palmoplantar pustular reaction [11] or even generalized pustular psoriasis [12]. Psychiatrists should avoid the use of lithium in psoriatics if possible. Darier's disease may also be exacerbated or initiated [13,14].

Additional reactions described include morbilliform rashes, erythema multiforme [15], a dermatitis herpetiformis-like rash [16], linear IgA bullous dermatosis [17] and a generalized exfoliative eruption [18]. An LE-like syndrome [19] with increased prevalence of antinuclear antibodies [20], toenail dystrophy [21] and hair loss [22,23] have been reported. Keratoderma has been documented [24], as has hidradenitis suppurativa [25]. None of these effects is related to excessive blood levels of lithium or other evidence of toxicity.

REFERENCES

1 Callaway CL, Hendrie HC, Luby ED. Cutaneous conditions observed in patients during treatment with lithium. *Am J Psychiatry* 1968; **124**: 1124–5.

2 Heng MCY. Cutaneous manifestations of lithium toxicity. *Br J Dermatol* 1982; **106**: 107–9.

3 Deandrea D, Walker N, Mehlmauer M, White K. Dermatological reactions to lithium: a review. *J Clin Psychopharmacol* 1982; **2**: 199–204.

4 Sarantidis D, Waters B. A review and controlled study of cutaneous conditions associated with lithium carbonate. *Br J Psychiatry* 1983; **143**: 42–50.

5 Albrecht G. Unerwünschte Wirkungen von Lithium an der Haut. *Hautarzt* 1985; **36**: 77–82.

6 Chan HH, Wing Y, Su R *et al.* A control study of the cutaneous side effects of chronic lithium therapy. *J Affective Disord* 2000; **57**: 107–13.

7 Lazarus GS, Gilgor RS. Psoriasis, polymorphonuclear leukocytes, and lithium carbonate. An important clue. *Arch Dermatol* 1979; **115**: 1183–4.

8 Skoven I, Thormann J. Lithium compound treatment and psoriasis. *Arch Dermatol* 1979; **115**: 1185–7.

9 Abel EA, Dicicco LM, Orenberg EK *et al*. Drugs in exacerbation of psoriasis. *J Am Acad Dermatol* 1986; **15**: 1007–22.
10 Sasaki T, Saito S, Aihara M *et al*. Exacerbation of psoriasis during lithium treatment. *J Dermatol* 1989; **16**: 59–63.
11 White SW. Palmoplantar pustular psoriasis provoked by lithium therapy. *J Am Acad Dermatol* 1982; **7**: 660–2.
12 Lowe NJ, Ridgway HB. Generalized pustular psoriasis precipitated by lithium. *Arch Dermatol* 1978; **114**: 1788–9.
13 Milton GP, Peck GL, Fu J-J *et al*. Exacerbation of Darier's disease by lithium carbonate. *J Am Acad Dermatol* 1990; **23**: 926–8.
14 Rubin MB. Lithium-induced Darier's disease. *J Am Acad Dermatol* 1996; **32**: 674–5.
15 Balldin J, Berggren U, Heijer A, Mobacken H. Erythema multiforme caused by lithium. *J Am Acad Dermatol* 1991; **24**: 1015–6.
16 Meinhold JM, West DP, Gurwich E *et al*. Cutaneous reaction to lithium carbonate: a case report. *J Clin Psychiatry* 1980; **41**: 395–6.
17 McWhirter JD, Hashimoto K, Fayne S *et al*. Linear IgA bullous dermatosis related to lithium carbonate. *Arch Dermatol* 1987; **123**: 1120–2.
18 Kuhnley EJ, Granoff AL. Exfoliative dermatitis during lithium treatment. *Am J Psychiatry* 1979; **136**: 1340–1.
19 Shukla VR, Borison RL. Lithium and lupus-like syndrome. *JAMA* 1982; **248**: 921–2.
20 Presley AP, Kahn A, Williamson N. Antinuclear antibodies in patients on lithium carbonate. *BMJ* 1976; **ii**: 280–1.
21 Hooper JF. Lithium carbonate and toenails. *Am J Psychiatry* 1981; **138**: 1519.
22 Dawber R, Mortimer P. Hair loss during lithium treatment. *Br J Dermatol* 1982; **107**: 124–5.
23 Orwin A. Hair loss following lithium therapy. *Br J Dermatol* 1983; **108**: 503–4.
24 Labelle A, Lapierre YD. Keratodermia: side effects of lithium. *J Clin Psychopharmacol* 1991; **11**: 149–50.
25 Gupta AK, Knowles SR, Gupta MA *et al*. Lithium therapy associated with hidradenitis suppurativa: case report and a review of the dermatologic side effects of lithium. *J Am Acad Dermatol* 1995; **32**: 382–6.

Hypnotics, sedatives and anxiolytics

Barbiturates

A toxic bullous eruption may appear at pressure points in comatose patients after overdosage [1–4]. In one series, 8% of patients admitted with drug-induced coma had such bullae [3] (see Fig. 73.5). The bullae are few, large and may lead to ulceration [2]. Necrotic lesions are seen in 4% of patients recovering from, and in 40% of fatalities related to, barbiturate-induced coma [4]. Allergic reactions are very uncommon and may be scarlatiniform or morbilliform. Exfoliative dermatitis has proved fatal [5], as has erythema multiforme. Urticaria and serum sickness are very rare, as is purpuric capillaritis. Fixed eruptions are well known [6] and particularly occur on the glans penis. TEN, LE-like syndrome, purpura and photosensitivity are recorded [7]. Phenobarbital is one cause of the anticonvulsant hypersensitivity syndrome (see p. 73.45) [8,9]. In one case, a syndrome resembling Langerhans' cell histiocytosis was produced [10]. Hypopigmentation may follow a severe reaction [11]. Exfoliative dermatitis is recorded [12].

REFERENCES

1 Beveridge GW, Lawson AAH. Occurrence of bullous lesions in acute barbiturate intoxication. *BMJ* 1965; **i**: 835–7.
2 Gröschel D, Gerstein AR, Rosenbaum JM. Skin lesions as a diagnostic aid in barbiturate poisoning. *N Engl J Med* 1970; **283**: 409–10.
3 Pinkus NB. Skin eruptions in drug-induced coma. *Med J Aust* 1971; **2**: 886–8.
4 Almeyda J, Levantine A. Drug reactions XVII. Cutaneous reactions to barbiturates, chloralhydrate and its derivatives. *Br J Dermatol* 1972; **86**: 313–6.
5 Sneddon IB, Leishman AWD. Severe and fatal phenobarbitone eruptions. *BMJ* 1952; **i**: 1276–8.
6 Korkij W, Soltani K. Fixed drug eruption. A brief review. *Arch Dermatol* 1984; **120**: 520–4.
7 Gupta MA, Gupta AK, Haberman HF. Psychotropic drugs in dermatology. A review and guidelines for use. *J Am Acad Dermatol* 1986; **14**: 633–45.
8 Vittorio CC, Muglia JJ. Anticonvulsant hypersensitivity syndrome. *Arch Intern Med* 1995; **155**: 2285–90.
9 De Vriese AS, Philippe J, Van Renterghem DM *et al*. Carbamazepine hypersensitivity syndrome: report of 4 cases and review of the literature. *Medicine (Baltimore)* 1995; **74**: 144–51.
10 Nagata T, Kawamura N, Motoyama T *et al*. A case of hypersensitivity syndrome resembling Langerhans cell histiocytosis during phenobarbital prophylaxis for convulsion. *Jpn J Clin Oncol* 1992; **22**: 421–7.
11 Mion N, Fusade T, Mathelier-Fusade P *et al*. Depigmentation cutaneophanerienne consecutive a une toxidermie au phenobarbital. *Ann Dermatol Vénéréol* 1992; **119**: 927–9.
12 Sawaishi Y, Komatsu K, Takeda O *et al*. A case of tubulo-interstitial nephritis with exfoliative dermatitis and hepatitis due to phenobarbital hypersensitivity. *Eur J Pediatr* 1992; **151**: 69–72.

Benzodiazepines

Allergic reactions are very rare [1].

Alprazolam. Photosensitivity has been recorded with this newer benzodiazepine [2].

Chlordiazepoxide. Morbilliform erythema, urticaria [3], fixed eruption [4], photoallergic eczema [5] and exacerbation of porphyria have been recorded. Erythema multiforme and chronic pigmented purpuric eruption occur rarely [6].

Clobazam. A generalized erythematous pruritic eruption [7] and TEN confined to light-exposed areas [8] have been reported. There has been a report of coma-induced bullae and sweat gland necrosis associated with the drug [9].

Diazepam and nitrazepam. Bullae similar to those seen after barbiturates may occur in comatose patients after overdosage [10,11]. Thrombophlebitis may follow intravenous injection of diazepam [12]. Hyperpigmentation in previously dermabraded scars has been attributed to diazepam [13]. Vasculitis is documented [14]. An eruption comprising oedema, moon face and generalized erythema, with erosions of cheeks, axillae and the genitocrural area was attributed to nitrazepam; a provocation test was positive [15].

Lormetazepam. A fixed drug eruption has been reported [16].

Temazepam. An extensive fixed drug eruption has been reported [17]. Extravasation following attempted femoral vein injection of a suspension of the contents of capsules in tap water, by an addict, resulted in extensive necrosis of genital and pubic skin [18].

REFERENCES

1 Edwards JG. Adverse effects of antianxiety drugs. *Drugs* 1981; **22**: 495–514.
2 Kanwar AJ, Gupta R, Das Mehta S, Kaur S. Photosensitivity to alprazolam. *Dermatologica* 1990; **181**: 75.
3 Almeyda J. Drug reactions XIII. Cutaneous reactions to imipramine and chlordiazepoxide. *Br J Dermatol* 1971; **84**: 298–9.
4 Blair HM III. Fixed drug eruption from chlordiazepoxide: report of a case. *Arch Dermatol* 1974; **109**: 914.
5 Luton EF, Finchum RN. Photosensitivity reaction to chlordiazepoxide. *Arch Dermatol* 1965; **91**: 362–3.
6 Nishioka K, Katayama I, Masuzawa M *et al.* Drug-induced chronic pigmented purpura. *J Dermatol* 1989; **16**: 220–2.
7 Machet L, Vaillant L, Dardaine V, Lorette G. Patch testing with clobazam: relapse of generalised drug eruption. *Contact Dermatitis* 1992; **26**: 347–8.
8 Redondo P, Vicente J, España A *et al.* Photo-induced toxic epidermal necrolysis caused by clobazam. *Br J Dermatol* 1996; **135**: 999–1002.
9 Setterfield JF, Robinson R, MacDonald D, Calonje E. Coma-induced bullae and sweat gland necrosis following clobazam. *Clin Exp Dermatol* 2000; **25**: 215–8.
10 Ridley CM. Bullous lesions in nitrazepam-overdosage. *BMJ* 1971; **iii**: 28.
11 Varma AJ, Fisher BK, Sarin MK. Diazepam-induced coma with bullae and eccrine sweat gland necrosis. *Arch Intern Med* 1977; **137**: 1207–10.
12 Langdon DE, Harlan JR, Bailey RL. Thrombophlebitis with diazepam used intravenously. *JAMA* 1973; **223**: 184–5.
13 Fereira JA. The role of diazepam in skin hyperpigmentation. *Aesthetic Plast Surg* 1980; **4**: 343–8.
14 Olcina GM, Simonart T. Severe vasculitis after therapy with diazepam. *Am J Psychiatry* 1999; **156**: 972–3.
15 Shoji A, Kitajima J, Hamada T. Drug eruption caused by nitrazepam in a patient with severe pustular psoriasis successfully treated with methotrexate and etretinate. *J Dermatol* 1987; **14**: 274–8.
16 Jafferany M, Haroon TS. Fixed drug eruption with lormetazepam (Noctamid). *Dermatologica* 1988; **177**: 386.
17 Archer CB, English JSC. Extensive fixed drug eruption induced by temazepam. *Clin Exp Dermatol* 1988; **13**: 336–8.
18 Meshikhes AN, Duthie JS. Untitled report. *BMJ* 1991; **303**: 478.

Miscellaneous hypnotics, sedatives and anxiolytics

Carbromal

This drug, now rarely used, commonly produced a characteristic capillaritis with punctate purpura and haemosiderin giving a golden-brown discoloration of the skin, especially on the legs [1].

Chloral hydrate

Hypersensitivity reactions are very rare. Chloral is now virtually given only in tablet form as dichloralphenazone, in which the phenazone may cause a fixed eruption [2].

Ethchlorvynol

Overdose has caused bullous lesions [3].

Glutethimide

Dermographism with subsequent erythema, and vesicles that lasted several days, were reported in one comatose patient [4] and bullae in another patient [5] following overdosage. Fixed eruptions are recorded [6].

Meprobamate

Anorexia, drowsiness, dizziness, flushing and gastro-intestinal symptoms may occur, especially with high doses. Fixed eruptions may occur [7]. The most characteristic cutaneous reaction, preceded by itching, malaise and fever, is an erythema starting in the limb flexures that rapidly gives way to a fierce non-thrombocytopenic purpura [8]. A widespread toxic erythema was associated with an anaphylactoid reaction in a patient in whom patch testing proved useful in diagnosis [9].

REFERENCES

1 Peterson WC Jr, Manick KP. Purpuric eruptions associated with use of carbromal and meprobamate. *Arch Dermatol* 1967; **95**: 40–2.
2 McCulloch H, Zeligman I. Fixed drug eruption and epididymitis due to antipyrine. *Arch Dermatol Syphilol* 1951; **64**: 198–9.
3 Brodin MD, Redmon WJ. Bullous eruptions due to ethchlorvynol. *J Cutan Pathol* 1980; **7**: 326–9.
4 Leavell UW Jr, Coyer JR, Taylor RJ. Dermographism and erythematous lines in glutethimide overdose. *Arch Dermatol* 1972; **106**: 724–5.
5 Burdon JGW, Cade JF. 'Barbiturate burns' caused by glutethimide. *Med J Aust* 1979; **1**: 101–2.
6 Fisher M, Lerman JS. Fixed eruption due to glutethimide. *Arch Dermatol* 1971; **104**: 87–9.
7 Gore HC Jr. Fixed drug eruption cross reaction of meprobamate and carisoprodol. *Arch Dermatol* 1965; **91**: 627.
8 Levan NE. Meprobamate reaction. *Arch Dermatol* 1957; **75**: 437–8.
9 Felix RH, Comaish JS. The value of patch and other skin tests in drug eruptions. *Lancet* 1974; **i**: 1017–9.

Antipsychotics

The most important clinical side effects include those on the central nervous and cardiovascular systems and the ocular effects [1,2]. Drugs with high potency, such as haloperidol and pimozide, tend to have fewer cardiovascular and anticholinergic effects and are less sedating, but have more neurological effects. Long-term use of antipsychotic agents results in tardive dyskinesia.

Phenothiazines

The side effects of this group of drugs have been reviewed [1–4].

Chlorpromazine. This drug is still widely used, although many related compounds are now available. Pigmentation of the skin in light-exposed areas after chronic use may be a problem, especially in women and black people [5–11]. Rarely, a purplish or slate-grey pigmentation develops [6]. There may be brown discoloration of cornea and lens [5], and bulbar conjunctiva [7]. Chlorpromazine has an affinity for melanin *in vitro* [8]. Electron microscopy shows many melanosome complexes within lysosomes of dermal macrophages, and electron-dense 'chlorpromazine bodies' in macrophages, endothelial cells and Schwann cells [9,10]; energy-dispersive X-ray microanalysis has revealed the abundant presence of sulphur in these granules, which is a constituent of the chlorpromazine molecule [10]. Similar pigmentary deposits are found in internal organs [11] and in blood neutrophils and monocytes.

Chlorpromazine has caused lichenoid eruptions [12], exfoliative dermatitis, erythema multiforme, an LE-like illness [13] with positive antinuclear factor [14] and the lupus anticoagulant [15], and Henoch–Schönlein vasculitis [16]. Phototoxicity is well known [17–19] and phenothiazine-derived antihistamines may cause photosensitivity in atopics and subsequent development of actinic reticuloid [19]. Photocontact urticaria has been documented [20]. A pustular reaction is recorded [21]. Cholestatic jaundice is an important hazard.

Fluspirilene. Subcutaneous nodules may develop at injection sites after long-term high doses of this depot preparation [22].

Thioridazine. Vasculitis is documented [23].

Thiothixene. A sensitivity reaction has been recorded [24].

Trifluoperazine. A fixed eruption has been recorded [25].

Loxapine. Dermatitis, pruritus and seborrhoea have been recorded, and photosensitivity eruptions may occur occasionally [26].

Levomepromazin. An erythema annulare centrifugum-like pseudolymphomatous eruption has been reported [27].

REFERENCES

1 Simpson GM, Pi EH, Sramek JJ Jr. Adverse effects of antipsychotic agents. *Drugs* 1981; **21**: 138–51.
2 Gupta MA, Gupta AK, Haberman HF. Psychotropic drugs in dermatology. A review and guidelines for use. *J Am Acad Dermatol* 1986; **14**: 633–45.
3 Hägermark Ö, Wennersten G, Almeyda J. Drug reactions XIV. Cutaneous side effects of phenothiazines. *Br J Dermatol* 1971; **84**: 605–7.
4 Bond WS, Yee GC. Ocular and cutaneous effects of chronic phenothiazine therapy. *Am J Hosp Pharm* 1980; **37**: 74–8.
5 Greiner AC, Berry K. Skin pigmentation and corneal and lens opacities with prolonged chlorpromazine therapy. *Can Med Assoc J* 1964; **90**: 663–5.
6 Hays GB, Lyle CB Jr, Wheeler CE Jr. Slate-grey color in patients receiving chlorpromazine. *Arch Dermatol* 1964; **90**: 471–6.
7 Satanove A. Pigmentation due to phenothiazines in high and prolonged dosage. *JAMA* 1965; **191**: 263–8.
8 Blois MS Jr. On chlorpromazine binding in vivo. *J Invest Dermatol* 1965; **45**: 475–81.
9 Hashimoto K, Wiener W, Albert J, Nelson RG. An electron microscopic study of chlorpromazine pigmentation. *J Invest Dermatol* 1966; **47**: 296–306.
10 Benning TL, McCormack KM, Ingram P *et al.* Microprobe analysis of chlorpromazine pigmentation. *Arch Dermatol* 1988; **124**: 1541–4.
11 Greiner AC, Nicolson GA. Pigment deposition in viscera associated with prolonged chlorpromazine therapy. *Can Med Assoc J* 1964; **90**: 627–35.
12 Matsuo I, Ozawa A, Niizuma K, Ohkido M. Lichenoid dermatitis due to chlorpromazine phototoxicity. *Dermatologica* 1979; **159**: 46–9.
13 Pavlidakey GP, Hashimoto K, Heller GL, Daneshvar S. Chlorpromazine-induced lupuslike disease: case report and review of the literature. *J Am Acad Dermatol* 1985; **13**: 109–15.
14 Zarrabi MH, Zucker S, Miller F *et al.* Immunologic and coagulation disorders in chlorpromazine-treated patients. *Ann Intern Med* 1979; **91**: 194–9.
15 Canoso RT, Sise HS. Chlorpromazine-induced lupus anticoagulant and associated immunologic abnormalities. *Am J Hematol* 1982; **13**: 121–9.
16 Aram H. Henoch–Schönlein purpura induced by chlorpromazine. *J Am Acad Dermatol* 1987; **17**: 139–40.
17 Johnson BE. Cellular mechanisms of chlorpromazine photosensitivity. *Proc R Soc Med* 1974; **67**: 871–3.
18 Ljunggren B. Phenothiazine phototoxicity: toxic chlorpromazine photoproducts. *J Invest Dermatol* 1977; **69**: 383–6.
19 Amblard P, Beani J-C, Reymond J-L. Photo-allergie rémanente aux phénothiazines chez l'atopique. *Ann Dermatol Vénéréol* 1982; **109**: 225–8.
20 Lovell CR, Cronin E, Rhodes EL. Photocontact urticaria from chlorpromazine. *Contact Dermatitis* 1986; **14**: 290–1.
21 Burrows NP, Ratnavel RC, Norris PG. Pustular eruptions after chlorpromazine. *BMJ* 1994; **309**: 97.
22 UK Committee on Safety of Medicines. *Curr Probl* 1981: 7.
23 Greenfield JR, McGrath M, Kossard S *et al.* ANCA-positive vasculitis induced by thioridazine: confirmed by rechallenge. *Br J Dermatol* 2003; **147**: 1265–7.
24 Matsuoka LY. Thiothixene drug sensitivity. *J Am Acad Dermatol* 1982; **7**: 405–6.
25 Kanwar AJ, Singh M, El-Sheriff AK, Belhaj MS. Fixed eruption due to trifluoperazine hydrochloride. *Br J Dermatol* 1987; **117**: 798–9.
26 Anonymous. Cloxapine and loxapine for schizophrenia. *Drug Ther Bull* 1991; **29**: 41–2.
27 Blazejak T, Hölzle E. Phenothiazin-induziertes Pseudolymphom. *Hautarzt* 1990; **41**: 161–3.

Miscellaneous antipsychotic agents

Clozapine. An acute severe adverse reaction resembling SLE is recorded [1].

Haloperidol. This drug causes reactions at injection sites [2,3].

Olanzapine. A pustular reaction is documented [4].

REFERENCES

1 Reinke M, Wiesert KN. High incidence of haloperidol decanoate injection site reactions (letter). *J Clin Psychiatry* 1992; **53**: 415–6.
2 Maharaj K, Guttmacher LB, Moeller R. Haloperidol decanoate: injection site reactions. *J Clin Psychiatry* 1995; **56**: 172–3.
3 Wickert WA, Campbell NR, Martin L. Acute severe adverse clozapine reaction resembling systemic lupus erythematosus. *Postgrad Med J* 1994; **70**: 940–1.
4 Adams BB, Mutasim DF. Pustular eruption induced by olanzapine, a novel antipsychotic agent. *J Am Acad Dermatol* 1999; **41**: 851–3.

Anticonvulsants

Allergic rashes to antiepileptic drugs are usually mild, taking the form of urticarial or morbilliform eruptions; the rare occurrence of a severe reaction indicates that the drug should be ceased, and this can be done abruptly with minimal risk of status epilepticus [1,2]. There may be cross-reactivity in terms of clinical reactions to the aromatic anticonvulsants (phenytoin, phenobarbital, carbamazepine, primidone and clonazepam), which may all cause the so-called drug hypersensitivity syndrome (see

p. 73.27), with fever, mucocutaneous eruptions, lymphadenopathy and hepatitis, 1 week to 3 months into therapy; there may be multiorgan involvement with renal and pulmonary lesions [3–10]. The reaction may develop into TEN. Arene oxide metabolites may be involved in the pathogenesis of these eruptions [3]. Sodium valproate may usually be substituted safely. The drug hypersensitivity syndrome reportedly occurs at a rate of 1 in 1000 to 1 in 10 000 exposures; siblings of patients may be at increased risk of developing this syndrome [9]. Generalized pustulation may be a manifestation of anticonvulsant hypersensitivity [11]. A severe form of hypersensitivity vasculitis, with extensive visceral involvement and poor prognosis, is seen very rarely with phenytoin and in isolated cases with carbamazepine and trimethadione [12]. Drug-induced SLE is much more frequent, and has been described with most anticonvulsants in clinical use (phenytoin, carbamazepine, ethosuximide, trimethadione, primidone and valproate) [12]. Of the newer anticonvulsant drugs, vigabatrin is usually well tolerated, but lamotrigine is associated with rashes [13,14]. Anticonvulsants may be associated with pseudolymphoma (see p. 73.45).

REFERENCES

1 Hebert AA, Ralston JP. Cutaneous reactions to anticonvulsant medications. *J Clin Psychiatry* 2001; **62** (Suppl. 14): 22–6.
2 Pelekanos J, Camfield P, Camfield C, Gordon K. Allergic rash due to antiepileptic drugs: clinical features and management. *Epilepsia* 1991; **32**: 554–9.
3 Shear N, Spielberg S. Anticonvulsant hypersensitivity syndrome. In vitro assessment of risk. *J Clin Invest* 1989; **82**: 1826–32.
4 Chang DK, Shear NH. Cutaneous reactions to anticonvulsants. *Semin Neurol* 1992; **12**: 329–37.
5 Handfield-Jones SE, Jenkins RE, Whittaker SJ *et al.* The anticonvulsant hypersensitivity syndrome. *Br J Dermatol* 1993; **129**: 175–7.
6 Gall H, Merk H, Scherb W, Sterry W. Anticonvulsiva-Hyper-sensitivitats-Syndrom auf Carbamazepin. *Hautarzt* 1994; **45**: 494–8.
7 Richens A, Davidson DL, Cartlidge NE, Easter DJ. A multicentre comparative trial of sodium valproate and carbamazepine in adult onset epilepsy. Adult EPITEG Collaborative Group. *J Neurol Neurosurg Psychiatry* 1994; **57**: 682–7.
8 Alldredge BK, Knutsen AP, Ferriero D. Antiepileptic drug hypersensitivity syndrome: in vitro and clinical observations. *Pediatr Neurol* 1994; **10**: 169–71.
9 Vittorio CC, Muglia JJ. Anticonvulsant hypersensitivity syndrome. *Arch Intern Med* 1995; **155**: 2285–90.
10 Licata AL, Louis ED. Anticonvulsant hypersensitivity syndrome. *Compr Ther* 1996; **22**: 152–5.
11 Kleier RS, Breneman DL, Boiko S. Generalized pustulation as a manifestation of the anticonvulsant hypersensitivity syndrome. *Arch Dermatol* 1991; **127**: 1361–4.
12 Drory VE, Korczyn AD. Hypersensitivity vasculitis and systemic lupus erythematosus induced by anticonvulsants. *Clin Neuropharmacol* 1993; **16**: 19–29.
13 Schmidt D, Kramer G. The new anticonvulsant drugs. Implications for avoidance of adverse effects. *Drug Saf* 1994; **11**: 422–31.
14 Brodie MJ. Lamotrigine versus other antiepileptic drugs: a star rating system is born. *Epilepsia* 1994; **35** (Suppl. 5): S41–S46.

Carbamazepine [1]

Eruptions occur in 3% [2–5] to 12% [6–8] of patients and include diffuse erythema, miliary exanthem, maculopapular or speckled morbilliform reddish rash, urticaria, purpuric petechiae or a mucocutaneous syndrome, any of which may occur from day 8 to 60. The drug hypersensitivity syndrome [9–11], erythroderma and exfoliative dermatitis, erythema multiforme and TEN [3,4,12] are well recognized. Eczema and photosensitivity [13], an LE-like syndrome and dermatomyositis [14], as well as a pustular [15–17] and a lichenoid [3,18] reaction, are very rare. Lesions with clinical and histological features suggestive of mycosis fungoides (pseudolymphoma) have been reported [18–21]. Patch testing has been advocated for the diagnosis of carbamazepine eruptions [9,10,22,23], but has resulted in reinduction of exfoliative dermatitis [24]. A psoriasiform eruption has been reported [25], as has thrombocytopenia and leukopenia complicated by Henoch–Schönlein purpura [26]. Cross-reactivity may occur with oxcarbazepine [27,28]. Other adverse effects include nausea, vomiting, ataxia, vertigo and drowsiness. Abnormal liver function [29] and bone marrow suppression with occasional deaths due to aplastic anaemia have been recorded [3]. Development of a rash may act as an early warning of marrow toxicity. Carbamazepine therapy during pregnancy carries a 1% risk of development of spina bifida in the offspring [30].

Oral steroid therapy enabled 16 of 20 patients successfully to continue on carbamazepine after development of a rash shortly after introduction of the drug [31]. Desensitization has been achieved by induction of tolerance in patients in whom there was no suitable alternative therapy [32,33].

REFERENCES

1 Pasmans SG, Bruijnzeel-Koomen CA, van Reijsen FC. Skin reactions to carbamazepine. *Allergy* 1999; **54**: 649–50.
2 Harman PRM. Carbamazepine (Tegretol) drug eruptions. *Br J Dermatol* 1967; **79**: 500–1.
3 Roberts DL, Marks R. Skin reactions to carbamazepine. *Arch Dermatol* 1981; **117**: 273–5.
4 Breathnach SM, McGibbon DH, Ive FA *et al.* Carbamazepine ('Tegretol') and toxic epidermal necrolysis: report of three cases with histopathological observations. *Clin Exp Dermatol* 1982; **7**: 585–91.
5 Chadwick D, Shan M, Foy P *et al.* Serum anticonvulsant concentrations and the risk of drug-induced skin eruptions. *J Neurol Neurosurg Psychiatry* 1984; **47**: 642–4.
6 Richens A, Davidson DL, Cartlidge NE, Easter DJ. A multicentre comparative trial of sodium valproate and carbamazepine in adult onset epilepsy. Adult EPITEG Collaborative Group. *J Neurol Neurosurg Psychiatry* 1994; **57**: 682–7.
7 Kramlinger KG, Phillips KA, Post RM. Rash complicating carbamazepine treatment. *J Clin Psychopharmacol* 1994; **14**: 408–13.
8 Konishi T, Naganuma Y, Hongo K *et al.* Carbamazepine-induced skin rash in children with epilepsy. *Eur J Pediatr* 1993; **152**: 605–8.
9 Scerri L, Shall L, Zaki I. Carbamazepine-induced anticonvulsant hypersensitivity syndrome: pathogenic and diagnostic considerations. *Clin Exp Dermatol* 1993; **18**: 540–2.
10 De Vriese AS, Philippe J, Van Renterghem DM *et al.* Carbamazepine hypersensitivity syndrome: report of 4 cases and review of the literature. *Medicine (Baltimore)* 1995; **74**: 144–51.
11 Okuyama R, Ichinohasama R, Tagami H. Carbamazepine induced erythroderma with systemic lymphadenopathy. *J Dermatol* 1996; **23**: 489–94.
12 Reed MD, Bertino JA, Blumer JL. Carbamazepine-associated exfoliative dermatitis. *Clin Pharmacol* 1982; **1**: 78–9.

13 Terui T, Tagami H. Eczematous drug eruption from carbamazepine: co-existence of contact and photocontact sensitivity. *Contact Dermatitis* 1989; **20**: 260–4.

14 Simpson JR. 'Collagen disease' due to carbamazepine (Tegretol). *BMJ* 1966; ii: 1434.

15 Staughton RCD, Harper JI, Rowland Payne CME *et al.* Toxic pustuloderma: a new entity? *J R Soc Med* 1984; **77**: 6–8.

16 Commens CA, Fischer GO. Toxic pustuloderma following carbamazepine therapy. *Arch Dermatol* 1988; **124**: 178–9.

17 Mizoguchi S, Setoyama M, Higashi Y *et al.* Eosinophilic pustular folliculitis induced by carbamazepine. *J Am Acad Dermatol* 1998; **38**: 641–3.

18 Atkin SL, McKenzie TMM, Stevenson CJ. Carbamazepine-induced lichenoid eruption. *Clin Exp Dermatol* 1990; **15**: 382–3.

19 Welykyj S, Gradini R, Nakao J, Massa M. Carbamazepine-induced eruption histologically mimicking mycosis fungoides. *J Cutan Pathol* 1990; **17**: 111–6.

20 Rijlaarsdam U, Scheffer E, Meijer CJLM *et al.* Mycosis fungoides-like lesions associated with phenytoin and carbamazepine therapy. *J Am Acad Dermatol* 1991; **24**: 216–20.

21 Nathan DL, Belsito DV. Carbamazepine-induced pseudolymphoma with CD-30 positive cells. *J Am Acad Dermatol* 1998; **38**: 806–9.

22 Houwerzijl J, De Gast GC, Nater JP *et al.* Lymphocyte-stimulation tests and patch tests in carbamazepine hypersensitivity. *Clin Exp Immunol* 1977; **29**: 272–7.

23 Silva R, Machado A, Brandao M, Gonçalo S. Patch test diagnosis in carbamazepine erythroderma. *Contact Dermatitis* 1986; **15**: 254–5.

24 Vaillant L, Camenen I, Lorette G. Patch testing with carbamazepine: reinduction of an exfoliative dermatitis. *Arch Dermatol* 1989; **125**: 299.

25 Brenner S, Wolf R, Landau M, Politi Y. Psoriasiform eruption induced by anticonvulsants. *Isr J Med Sci* 1994; **30**: 283–6.

26 Kaneko K, Igarashi J, Suzuki Y *et al.* Carbamazepine-induced thrombocytopenia and leucopenia complicated by Henoch–Schönlein purpura symptoms. *Eur J Pediatr* 1993; **152**: 769–70.

27 Beran RG. Cross-reactive skin eruption with both carbamazepine and oxcarbazepine. *Epilepsia* 1993; **34**: 163–5.

28 Dam M. Practical aspects of oxcarbazepine treatment. *Epilepsia* 1994; **35** (Suppl. 3): S23–S25.

29 Ramsey ID. Carbamazepine-induced jaundice. *BMJ* 1967; **4**: 155.

30 Rosa FW. Spina bifida in infants of women treated with carbamazepine during pregnancy. *N Engl J Med* 1991; **324**: 674–7.

31 Murphy JM, Mashman J, Miller JD, Bell JB. Suppression of carbamazepine-induced rash with prednisone. *Neurology* 1991; **41**: 144–5.

32 Eames P. Adverse reaction to carbamazepine managed by desensitization. *Lancet* 1989; i: 509–10.

33 Boyle N, Lawlor BA. Desensitization to carbamazepine-induced skin rash. *Am J Psychiatry* 1996; **153**: 1234.

Diphenylhydantoin (phenytoin, Dilantin)

Cutaneous manifestations related to phenytoin have been reviewed [1–7]. The various diverse presentations share certain histopathological findings: adhesion of the infiltrated cells to the basal layer of the epidermis, cell infiltration into the epidermis, vacuolation of the basal cells, and dyskeratotic cells in the epidermis and epidermal necrosis, with CD8+ T cells predominant in the epidermis [5].

About 5% of children develop a mild transient maculopapular rash within 3 weeks of starting treatment. This is more likely to occur if high loading doses are given initially [3,4]. In other series, between 8.5% [8] and 19% [9] of patients receiving phenytoin developed exanthematic rashes [10]. A phenytoin-induced hypersensitivity state, with generalized lymphadenopathy, hepatosplenomegaly, fever, arthralgia and eosinophilia, occurs in about 1% of patients, and may be accompanied by hepatitis, nephritis and haematological abnormalities [7,11–13]. Skin

involvement may lead to a suspicion of lymphoma, the phenytoin-induced pseudolymphoma syndrome [14–19]. Cutaneous lesions may be restricted to a few erythematous plaques [18], or cutaneous nodules [15], or consist of a generalized erythematous maculopapular rash [14], generalized exfoliative dermatitis [16,20] or TEN [21,22]. Generalized pustulation has been recorded as a manifestation of the anticonvulsant drug hypersensitivity syndrome [23]. Universal depigmentation has resulted from TEN [24]. Cutaneous histopathology in the pseudolymphoma syndrome is often indistinguishable from that of mycosis fungoides, with infiltrating cells having cerebriform nuclei and forming Pautrier microabscesses [17,19]. The rash resolves after cessation of the drug; systemic corticosteroids may aid resolution [25]. However, there is a threefold risk of true lymphoma on long-term therapy [26–28], and T-cell lymphoma has been reported in an adult [29].

Long-term treatment causes fibroblast proliferation, and may result in dose-dependent gingival hyperplasia [30,31] or coarsening of the features [32]; hypertrophic retro-auricular folds were reported in an isolated case [33]. Hypertrichosis may be seen. Other reactions have included fixed eruptions [34], including a widespread fixed drug eruption mimicking TEN [35], erythema multiforme [1,3], TEN with cholestasis [36], cutaneous vasculitis [37], an LE-like syndrome [38,39] and eosinophilic fasciitis [40]. Linear IgA bullous dermatosis has been provoked [41]. Localized reactions to intravenous phenytoin have included delayed bluish discoloration, erythema and oedema, sometimes with bullae, distal to the site of injection; immediate burning pain and swelling, and a delayed erythematous eruption with superficial sloughing, partial epidermal necrosis and frequent multinucleate keratinocytes on histology have also been reported [42,43].

Treatment during pregnancy may lead to a characteristic 'fetal hydantoin syndrome', with general underdevelopment and hypoplasia of phalanges and nails [44]; neonatal acne may be associated [45]. However, recent controlled observations suggest that acne is neither caused nor worsened by hydantoins [46], despite reports to the contrary [47].

REFERENCES

1 Silverman AK, Fairley J, Wong RC. Cutaneous and immunologic reactions to phenytoin. *J Am Acad Dermatol* 1988; **18**: 721–41.

2 Levantine A, Almeyda J. Drug reactions XX. Cutaneous reactions to anticonvulsants. *Br J Dermatol* 1972; **87**: 646–9.

3 Pollack MA, Burk PG, Nathanson G. Mucocutaneous eruptions due to anti epileptic drug therapy in children. *Ann Neurol* 1979; **5**: 262–7.

4 Wilson JT, Höjer B, Tomson G *et al.* High incidence of a concentration-dependent skin reaction in children treated with phenytoin. *BMJ* 1978; i: 1583–6.

5 Tone T, Nishioka K, Kameyama K *et al.* Common histopathological processes of phenytoin drug eruption. *J Dermatol* 1992; **19**: 27–34.

6 Potter T, DiGregorio F, Stiff M, Hashimoto K. Dilantin hypersensitivity syndrome imitating staphylococcal toxic shock. *Arch Dermatol* 1994; **130**: 856–8.
7 Conger LA Jr, Grabski WJ. Dilantin hypersensitivity reaction. *Cutis* 1996; **57**: 223–6.
8 Leppik IE, Lapora A, Loewenson R. Seasonal incidence of phenytoin allergy unrelated to plasma levels. *Arch Neurol* 1985; **42**: 120–2.
9 Rapp RP, Norton JA, Young B, Tibbs PA. Cutaneous reactions in head-injured patients receiving phenytoin for seizure prophylaxis. *Neurosurgery* 1983; **13**: 272–5.
10 Robinson HM, Stone JH. Exanthem due to diphenylhydantoin therapy. *Arch Dermatol* 1970; **101**: 462–5.
11 Stanley J, Fallon-Pellici V. Phenytoin hypersensitivity reaction. *Arch Dermatol* 1978; **114**: 1350–3.
12 Brown M, Schubert T. Phenytoin hypersensitivity hepatitis and mononucleosis syndrome. *J Clin Gastroenterol* 1986; **8**: 469–77.
13 Shear N, Spielberg S. Anticonvulsant hypersensitivity syndrome. In vitro assessment of risk. *J Clin Invest* 1989; **82**: 1826–32.
14 Charlesworth EN. Phenytoin-induced pseudolymphoma syndrome. An immunologic study. *Arch Dermatol* 1977; **113**: 477–80.
15 Adams JD. Localized cutaneous pseudolymphoma associated with phenytoin therapy: a case report. *Australas J Dermatol* 1981; **22**: 28–9.
16 Rosenthal CJ, Noguera CA, Coppola A, Kapelner SN. Pseudolymphoma with mycosis fungoides manifestations, hyperresponsiveness to diphenylhydantoin, and lymphocyte disregulation. *Cancer* 1982; **49**: 2305–14.
17 Kardaun SH, Scheffer E, Vermeer BJ. Drug-induced pseudolymphomatous skin reactions. *Br J Dermatol* 1988; **118**: 545–52.
18 Wolf R, Kahane E, Sandbank M. Mycosis fungoides-like lesions associated with phenytoin therapy. *Arch Dermatol* 1985; **121**: 1181–2.
19 Rijlaarsdam U, Scheffer E, Meijer CJLM et al. Mycosis fungoides-like lesions associated with phenytoin and carbamazepine therapy. *J Am Acad Dermatol* 1991; **24**: 216–20.
20 Danno K, Kume M, Ohta M et al. Erythroderma with generalized lymphadenopathy induced by phenytoin. *J Dermatol* 1989; **16**: 392–6.
21 Sherertz EF, Jegasothy BV, Lazarus GS. Phenytoin hypersensitivity reaction presenting with toxic epidermal necrolysis and severe hepatitis: report of a patient treated with corticosteroid 'pulse therapy'. *J Am Acad Dermatol* 1985; **12**: 178–81.
22 Schmidt D, Kluge W. Fatal toxic epidermal necrolysis following reexposure to phenytoin. A case report. *Epilepsia* 1983; **24**: 440–3.
23 Kleier RS, Breneman DL, Boiko S. Generalized pustulation as a manifestation of the anticonvulsant hypersensitivity syndrome. *Arch Dermatol* 1991; **127**: 1361–4.
24 Smith DA, Burgdorf WHC. Universal cutaneous depigmentation following phenytoin-induced toxic epidermal necrolysis. *J Am Acad Dermatol* 1984; **10**: 106–9.
25 Chopra S, Levell NJ, Cowley G, Gilkes JJ. Systemic corticosteroids in the phenytoin hypersensitivity syndrome. *Br J Dermatol* 1996; **134**: 1109–12.
26 Tashima CK, De Los Santos R. Lymphoma and anticonvulsant therapy. *JAMA* 1974; **228**: 287–8.
27 Bichel J. Hydantoin derivatives and malignancies of the haemopoietic system. *Acta Med Scand* 1975; **198**: 327–8.
28 Li FP, Willard DR, Goodman R et al. Malignant lymphoma after diphenylhydantoin (Dilantin) therapy. *Cancer* 1975; **36**: 1359–62.
29 Isobe T, Horimatsu T, Fujita T et al. Adult T cell lymphoma following diphenylhydantoin therapy. *Acta Haematol Jpn* 1980; **43**: 711–4.
30 Angelopoulos AP, Goaz PW. Incidence of diphenylhydantoin gingival hyperplasia. *Oral Surg* 1972; **34**: 898–906.
31 Hassell TM, Page RC, Narayanan AS, Cooper CG. Diphenylhydantoin (Dilantin) gingival hyperplasia: drug induced abnormality of connective tissue. *Proc Natl Acad Sci USA* 1976; **73**: 2909–12.
32 Lefebvre EB, Haining RG, Labbé RF. Coarse facies, calvarial thickening and hyperphosphatasia associated with long-term anticonvulsant therapy. *N Engl J Med* 1972; **286**: 1301–2.
33 Trunnell TN, Waisman M. Hypertrophic retroauricular folds attributable to diphenylhydantoin. *Cutis* 1982; **30**: 207–9.
34 Sweet RD. Fixed skin eruption due to phenytoin sodium. *Lancet* 1950; **i**: 68.
35 Baird BJ, De Villez RL. Widespread bullous fixed drug eruption mimicking toxic epidermal necrolysis. *Int J Dermatol* 1988; **27**: 170–4.
36 Spechler SJ, Sperber H, Doos WG, Koff RS. Cholestasis and toxic epidermal necrolysis associated with phenytoin sodium ingestion: the role of bile duct injury. *Ann Intern Med* 1981; **95**: 455–6.
37 Yermakov VM, Hitti IF, Sutton AL. Necrotizing vasculitis associated with diphenylhydantoin: two fatal cases. *Hum Pathol* 1983; **14**: 182–4.
38 Gleichman H. Systemic lupus erythematosus triggered by diphenylhydantoin. *Arthritis Rheum* 1982; **25**: 1387–8.
39 Ross S, Dywer C, Ormerod AD et al. Subacute cutaneous lupus erythematosus associated with phenytoin. *Clin Exp Dermatol* 2002; **27**: 474–6.
40 Buchanan RR, Gordon DA, Muckle TJ et al. The eosinophilic fasciitis syndrome after phenytoin (Dilantin) therapy. *J Rheumatol* 1980; **7**: 733–6.
41 Acostamadiedo JM, Perniciaro C, Rogers RS III. Phenytoin-induced linear IgA bullous disease. *J Am Acad Dermatol* 1998; **38**: 352–6.
42 Hunt SJ. Cutaneous necrosis and multinucleate epidermal cells associated with intravenous phenytoin. *Am J Dermatopathol* 1995; **17**: 399–402.
43 Kilarski DJ, Buchanan C, Von Behren L. Soft tissue damage associated with intravenous phenytoin. *N Engl J Med* 1984; **311**: 1186–7.
44 Nagy R. Fetal hydantoin syndrome. *Arch Dermatol* 1981; **117**: 593–5.
45 Stankler L, Campbell AGM. Neonatal acne vulgaris: a possible feature of the fetal hydantoin syndrome. *Br J Dermatol* 1980; **103**: 453–5.
46 Greenwood R, Fenwick PBC, Cunliffe WJ. Acne and anticonvulsants. *BMJ* 1983; **287**: 1669–70.
47 Jenkins RB, Ratner AC. Diphenylhydantoin and acne. *N Engl J Med* 1972; **287**: 148.

Lamotrigine

Dosage-related allergic rashes occur in about 5–10% of patients, usually in the first 8 weeks, leading to a withdrawal rate of 2% of patient exposures [1–4]. In one study, six of eight patients with a prior lamotrigine-related rash had no recurrence on rechallenge, and two other patients had only mild rashes [5]. Rashes leading to hospitalization, including hypersensitivity syndrome [6], Stevens–Johnson syndrome and TEN [7], occurred in 1 in 100 to 1 in 300 individuals in clinical trials, and appeared to be increased with over-rapid titration when starting therapy and with concurrent valproate medication [3,8].

REFERENCES

1 Richens A. Safety of lamotrigine. *Epilepsia* 1994; **35** (Suppl. 5): S37–S40.
2 Calabrese JR, Sullivan JR, Bowden CL et al. Rash in multicenter trials of lamotrigine in mood disorders: clinical relevance and management. *J Clin Psychiatry* 2002; **63**: 1012–9.
3 Guberman AH, Besag FM, Brodie MJ et al. Lamotrigine-associated rash: risk/benefit considerations in adults and children. *Epilepsia* 1999; **40**: 985–91.
4 Messenheimer JA. Lamotrigine. *Epilepsia* 1995; **36** (Suppl. 2): S87–S94.
5 Tavernor SJ, Wong IC, Newton R, Brown SW. Rechallenge with lamotrigine after initial rash. *Seizure* 1995; **4**: 67–71.
6 Jones D, Chhiap V, Resor S et al. Phenytoin-like hypersensitivity associated with lamotrigine. *J Am Acad Dermatol* 1997; **36**: 1016–8.
7 Sterker M, Berrouschot J, Schneider D. Fatal course of toxic epidermal necrolysis under treatment with lamotrigine. *Int J Clin Pharmacol Ther* 1995; **33**: 595–7.
8 Anonymous. Lamotrigine (Lamictal): increased risk of serious skin reactions in children. *Curr Probl Pharmacovig* 1997; **23**: 8.

Sodium valproate

Occasional transient rashes and stomatitis are documented. Temporary hair loss may be followed by increasing curliness of the regrowing hair [1]. Alteration in hair colour has been noted [2]. One case of generalized morphoea [3] and two cases of cutaneous leukocytoclastic vasculitis recurring on challenge [4] have been reported. An extrapyramidal syndrome may be induced [5], and the drug may be teratogenic [6].

REFERENCES

1 Jeavons PM, Clark JE, Harding GFA. Valproate and curly hair. *Lancet* 1977; i: 359.
2 Herranz JL, Arteaga R, Armijo JA. Change in hair colour induced by valproic acid. *Dev Med Child Neurol* 1981; **23**: 386–7.
3 Goihman-Yahr M, Leal H, Essenfeld-Yahr E. Generalized morphea: a side effect of valproate sodium? *Arch Dermatol* 1980; **116**: 621.
4 Kamper AM, Valentijn RM, Stricker BHC, Purcell PM. Cutaneous vasculitis induced by sodium valproate. *Lancet* 1991; **337**: 497–8.
5 Lautin A, Stanley M, Angrist B, Gershon S. Extrapyramidal syndrome with sodium valproate. *BMJ* 1979; ii: 1035–6.
6 Gomez MR. Possible teratogenicity of valproic acid. *J Pediatr* 1981; **98**: 508–9.

Trimethadione

Serious hypersensitivity reactions may occur, including erythema multiforme, urticaria and generalized exfoliative dermatitis.

Vigabatrin

An allergic vasculitis developed in one patient 6 months after commencement of this drug [1].

REFERENCE

1 Dieterle L, Becker EW, Berg PA *et al*. Allergische Vaskulitis durch Vigabatrin. *Nervenarzt* 1994; **65**: 122–4.

Opioid analgesics and amfetamine (amphetamine)

Cutaneous side effects common to drug abuse, most frequently cocaine, heroin and pentazocine, following parenteral injection include [1,2] infections, abscesses, septic phlebitis, subcutaneous and deep dermal cellulitis, necrosis, tetanus, widespread urticaria, cutaneous manifestations of primary and secondary syphilis, HIV infection and endocarditis. Starch and talc granulomas, lymphangitis and lymphadenitis in draining lymph nodes, pigmentary abnormalities including hyperpigmentation over the injected veins, accidental 'soot' tattoos (caused by needles sterilized over an open flame), scarring, ulceration, necrotizing angiitis and leukocytoclastic vasculitis may supervene. Skin popping refers to injection of drugs beneath the skin without concern for vascular access; this may result in ulcers being delayed for a number of years [3].

REFERENCES

1 Rosen VJ. Cutaneous manifestations of drug abuse by parenteral injections. *Am J Dermatopathol* 1985; **7**: 79–83.
2 Smith DJ, Busito MJ, Velanovich V *et al*. Drug injection injuries of the upper extremity. *Ann Plastic Surg* 1989; **22**: 19–24.
3 Pardes JB, Falanga V, Kerdel FA. Delayed cutaneous ulcerations arising at sites of prior parenteral drug abuse. *J Am Acad Dermatol* 1993; **29**: 1052–4.

Buprenorphine

An addict accidentally injected a suspension of crushed tablets into the superficial pudendal artery instead of the femoral vein, and developed pain, oedema and mottling of the penis [1].

REFERENCE

1 Naylor AR, Gordon M, Jenkins AMcL. Untitled report. *BMJ* 1991; **303**: 478.

Codeine

This drug has been associated with pruritus, urticaria (usually due to non-immunological release of histamine) [1,2], angio-oedema, macular and maculopapular eruptions, scarlatiniform rashes [1,3,4], fixed eruption, bullous eruption, generalized eczema [5], erythema multiforme and erythema nodosum.

REFERENCES

1 Hunskaar S, Dragsund S. Scarlatiniform rash and urticaria due to codeine. *Ann Allergy* 1985; **54**: 240–1.
2 De Groot AC, Conemans J. Allergic urticarial rash from oral codeine. *Contact Dermatitis* 1986; **14**: 209–14.
3 Voohost R, Sparreboom S. Four cases of recurrent pseudo-scarlet fever caused by phenanthrene alkaloids with a 6-hydroxy group (codeine and morphine). *Ann Allergy* 1980; **44**: 116–20.
4 Mohrenschlager M, Glockner A, Jessberger B *et al*. Codeine caused pruritic scarlatiniform exanthemata: patch test negative but positive to oral provocation test. *Br J Dermatol* 2000; **143**: 663–4.
5 Estrada JL, Puebla MJ, de Urbina JJ *et al*. Generalized eczema due to codeine. *Contact Dermatitis* 2001; **44**: 185.

Heroin

Use of the dorsal vein of the penis for administration of the drug has produced ulceration [1]. Systemic infections, such as candidiasis, may supervene [2]. Leukocytoclastic vasculitis and necrotizing angiitis have been reported in drug abusers [3–5]. Pigmentation of the tongue may occur as a form of fixed drug eruption in heroin addicts [6]. A possible association with development of pemphigus erythematosus has been suggested [7].

REFERENCES

1 White WB, Barrett S. Penile ulcer in heroin abuse: a case report. *Cutis* 1982; **29**: 62–3.
2 Bielsa I, Miro JM, Herrero C *et al*. Systemic candidiasis in heroin abusers. *Int J Dermatol* 1987; **26**: 314–9.
3 Citron BP, Halpern M, McCarron M *et al*. Necrotizing angiitis associated with drug abuse. *N Engl J Med* 1970; **283**: 1003–11.
4 Lignelli GJ, Bucheit WA. Angiitis in drug abusers. *N Engl J Med* 1971; **284**: 112–3.
5 Gendelman H, Linzer M, Barland P *et al*. Leukocytoclastic vasculitis in an intravenous heroin abuser. *NY State J Med* 1983; **83**: 984–6.
6 Westerhof W, Wolters EC, Brookbakker JTW *et al*. Pigmented lesions of the tongue in heroin addicts: fixed drug eruption. *Br J Dermatol* 1983; **109**: 605–10.
7 Fellner MJ, Winiger J. Pemphigus erythematosus and heroin addiction. *Int J Dermatol* 1978; **17**: 308–11.

Morphine

Morphine is a potent histamine releaser and may cause pruritus and urticaria [1]. Profuse sweating is a common effect. Morphine provokes facial flushing blocked by naloxone [2]. Local skin irritation during subcutaneous morphine infusion is recorded [3].

REFERENCES

1 McLelland J. The mechanism of morphine-induced urticaria. *Arch Dermatol* 1986; **122**: 138–9.
2 Cohen RA, Coffman JD. Naloxone reversal of morphine-induced peripheral vasodilatation. *Clin Pharmacol Ther* 1980; **28**: 541–4.
3 Shvartzman P, Bonneh D. Local skin irritation in the course of subcutaneous morphine infusion: a challenge. *J Palliat Care* 1994; **10**: 44–5.

Pentazocine

Woody induration of the skin and subcutaneous tissues at injection sites, perhaps with central ulceration and peripheral pigmentation, and a granulomatous histology, is well recognized [1–8]. Pigmentation, ulceration and a chronic panniculitis have supervened after many years of use. Phlebitis, cellulitis, fibrous myopathy [9] and limb contractures can complicate these changes. Generalized eruptions are rare [10]. There is an isolated report of TEN [11].

REFERENCES

1 Parks DL, Perry HO, Muller SA. Cutaneous complications of pentazocine injections. *Arch Dermatol* 1971; **104**: 231–5.
2 Schlicher JE, Zuehlke RL, Lynch PJ. Local changes at the site of pentazocine injection. *Arch Dermatol* 1971; **104**: 90–1.
3 Swanson DW, Weddige RL, Morse RM. Hospitalised pentazocine abusers. *Mayo Clin Proc* 1973; **48**: 85–93.
4 Schiff BL, Kern AB. Unusual cutaneous manifestations of pentazocine addiction. *JAMA* 1977; **238**: 1542–3.
5 Padilla RS, Becker LE, Hoffman H, Long G. Cutaneous and venous complications of pentazocine abuse. *Arch Dermatol* 1979; **115**: 975–7.
6 Palestine RF, Millns JL, Spigel GT *et al.* Skin manifestations of pentazocine abuse. *J Am Acad Dermatol* 1980; **2**: 47–55.
7 Mann RJ, Gostelow BE, Meacock DJ, Kennedy CTC. Pentazocine ulcers. *J R Soc Med* 1982; **75**: 903–5.
8 Jain A, Bhattacharya SN, Singal A, Baruah MC, Bhatia A. Pentazocine induced widespread cutaneous and myo-fibrosis. *J Dermatol* 1999; **26**: 368–70.
9 Johnson KR, Hsueh WA, Glusman SM, Arnett FC. Fibrous myopathy: a rheumatic complication of drug abuse. *Arthritis Rheum* 1976; **19**: 923–6.
10 Pedragosa R, Vidal J, Fuentes R, Huguet P. Tricotropism by pentazocine. *Arch Dermatol* 1987; **123**: 297–8.
11 Hunter JAA, Davison AM. Toxic epidermal necrolysis associated with pentazocine therapy and severe reversible renal failure. *Br J Dermatol* 1973; **88**: 287–90.

Methylamfetamine

A link with necrotizing angiitis has been recorded when this drug is used alone or with heroin or D-lysergic acid diethylamide [1].

REFERENCE

1 Citron BP, Halpern M, McCarron M *et al.* Necrotizing angiitis associated with drug abuse. *N Engl J Med* 1970; **283**: 1003–11.

Antiparkinsonian drugs

Amantadine

Reversible livedo reticularis has occurred in a high percentage of patients receiving amantadine, a tricyclic amine used in the treatment of Parkinson's disease [1,2].

Apomorphine

Panniculitis, ranging from mild pruritic erythema to painful nodules, has been observed [3].

Bromocriptine

Transient livedo reticularis [4], erythromelalgia [5], acrocyanosis with Raynaud's phenomenon [6,7], morphoea [8] and swelling of the legs with a sclerodermatous histology [9] have been reported rarely, as have alopecia [10], pseudolymphoma [11] and psychosis.

Carbidopa

Scleroderma-like reactions have occurred when this drug has been given in conjunction with tryptophan [12,13].

Levodopa

There have been several isolated reports of the occurrence of malignant melanoma [14–16], in certain instances involving multiple primaries, but the association may be by chance alone.

REFERENCES

1 Shealy CN, Weeth JB, Mercier D. Livedo reticularis in patients with parkinsonism receiving amantadine. *JAMA* 1970; **212**: 1522–3.
2 Vollum DI, Parkes JD, Doyle D. Livedo reticularis during amantadine treatment. *BMJ* 1971; **ii**: 627–8.
3 Acland KM, Churchyard A, Fletcher CL *et al.* Panniculitis in association with apomorphine infusion. *Br J Dermatol* 1998; **138**: 480–2.
4 Calne DB, Plotkin C, Neophytides A *et al.* Long-term treatment of Parkinsonism with bromocriptine. *Lancet* 1978; **i**: 735–7.
5 Eisler T, Hall RP, Kalavar KAR, Calne DB. Erythromelalgia-like eruption in Parkinsonian patients treated with bromocriptine. *Neurology* 1981; **37**: 1368–70.
6 Duvoisin RC. Digital vasospasm with bromocriptine. *Lancet* 1976; **ii**: 204.
7 Pearce I, Pearce JMS. Bromocriptine in Parkinsonism. *BMJ* 1978; **i**: 1402–4.
8 Leshin B, Piette WW, Caplin RM. Morphea after bromocriptine therapy. *Int J Dermatol* 1989; **28**: 177–9.
9 Dupont E, Olivarius B, Strong MJ. Bromocriptine-induced collagenosis-like symptomatology in Parkinson's disease. *Lancet* 1982; **i**: 850–1.
10 Blum I, Leiba S. Increased hair loss as a side effect of bromocriptine treatment. *N Engl J Med* 1980; **303**: 1418.
11 Wiesli P, Joos L, Galeazzi RL, Dummer R. Cutaneous pseudolymphoma associated with bromocriptine therapy. *Clin Endocrinol* 2000; **53**: 656–7.

12 Sternberg EM, Van Woert MH, Young SN *et al.* Development of a scler-oderma-like illness during therapy with L-5-hydroxytryptophan and car-bidopa. *N Engl J Med* 1980; **303**: 782–7.
13 Chamson A, Périer C, Frey J. Syndrome sclérodermiforme et poïkiloder-mique observé au cours d'un traitement par carbidopa et 5-hydroxytrypto-phane. Culture de fibroblastes avec analyse biochimique du métabolisme du collagène. *Ann Dermatol Vénéréol* 1986; **113**: 71.
14 Sober AJ, Wick MM. Levodopa therapy and malignant melanoma. *JAMA* 1978; **240**: 554–5.
15 Bernstein JE, Medenica M, Soltani K *et al.* Levodopa administration and multiple primary cutaneous melanomas. *Arch Dermatol* 1980; **116**: 1041–4.
16 Rosin MA, Braun M III. Malignant melanoma and levodopa. *Cutis* 1984; **33**: 572–4.

Antivertigo drugs and cerebrovascular dilators

Cinnarizine

This drug [1], and its derivative flunarizine [2], have been implicated in the precipitation of lichenoid eruptions. In the case of cinnarizine, clinical and immunofluores-cence features of lichen planus were combined with the presence of a circulating anti-basement-membrane zone IgG antibody [2]. Other side effects include drowsiness, depression and parkinsonism.

REFERENCES

1 Miyagawa W, Ohi H, Muramatsu T *et al.* Lichen planus pemphigoides-like lesions induced by cinnarizine. *Br J Dermatol* 1985; **112**: 607–13.
2 Suys E, De Coninck A, De Pauw I, Roseeuw D. Lichen planus induced by flunarizine. *Dermatologica* 1990; **181**: 71–2.

Miscellaneous nervous system drugs

Drugs for alcoholism

Cyanamide. This inhibitor of alcohol dehydrogenase, used in the treatment of alcoholism in some countries, has been implicated in the development of a lichen planus-like eruption with oesophageal involvement [1,2], as well as exfoliative dermatitis [2].

Disulfiram. This drug causes vasomotor flushing, morbil-liform rash and urticaria, as well as eczema in patients sensitized to rubber; it cross-reacts with rubber [3–5]. A toxic pustular eruption is recorded [6].

REFERENCES

1 Torrelo A, Soria C, Rocamora A *et al.* Lichen planus-like eruption with esophageal involvement as a result of cyanamide. *J Am Acad Dermatol* 1990; **23**: 1168–9.
2 Kawana S. Drug eruption induced by cyanamide (carbimide): a clinical and histopathologic study of 7 patients. *Dermatology* 1997; **195**: 30–4.
3 Webb PK, Gibbs SC, Mathias CT *et al.* Disulfiram hypersensitivity and rub-ber contact dermatitis. *JAMA* 1979; **241**: 2061.
4 Fischer AA. Dermatologic aspects of disulfiram use. *Cutis* 1982; **30**: 461–524.
5 Minet A, Frankart M, Eggers S *et al.* Réactions allergiques aux implants de disulfirame. *Ann Dermatol Vénéréol* 1989; **116**: 543–5.
6 Larbre B, Larbre JP, Nicolas JF *et al.* Toxicodermie pustuleuse aus disul-firame. A propos d'un cas. *Ann Dermatol Vénéréol* 1990; **117**: 721–2.

Drugs to aid smoking cessation

Amfebutamone. This antidepressant drug, structurally re-lated to the phenylethylamines (amfetamines) and used in aiding smoking cessation, has been implicated in causing liver dysfunction, pruritus and urticaria [1], serum sick-ness [2,3], and generalized pustular and erythrodermic psoriasis [4].

REFERENCES

1 Fays S, Tréchot P, Schmutz JL *et al.* Bupropion and generalised acute urticaria: eight cases. *Br J Dermatol* 2003; **148**: 177–8.
2 McCollom RA, Elbe DH, Ritchie AH. Bupropion-induced serum sickness-like reaction. *Ann Pharmacother* 2000; **34**: 471–3.
3 Davis JS, Boyle MJ, Hannaford R, Watson A. Bupropion and serum sickness-like reaction. *Med J Aust* 2001; **174**: 479–80.
4 Cox NH, Gordon PM, Dodd H. Generalized pustular and erythrodermic psoriasis associated with bupropion treatment. *Br J Dermatol* 2002; **146**: 1061–3.

Appetite suppressants and stimulants

Centrally acting appetite suppressants may induce urtic-arial vasculitis [1]. Megestrol, a synthetic orally active progesterone derivative used to stimulate appetite and weight gain in cachectic patients, caused a generalized morbilliform rash in a man; skin testing with progesterone acetate was positive [2]. Sibutramine, a centrally acting drug used in weight management, caused an erythema multiforme-like reaction [3].

Pyritinol

This drug, given for cerebral concussion, caused an unusual erythema multiforme-like eruption and severe headache after 10 days' treatment [4].

REFERENCES

1 Papadavid E, Yu RC, Tay A, Chu AC. Urticarial vasculitis induced by cent-rally acting appetite suppressants. *Br J Dermatol* 1996; **134**: 990–1.
2 Fisher DA. Drug-induced progesterone dermatitis. *J Am Acad Dermatol* 1996; **34**: 863–4.
3 Goh BK, Ng PPL, Giam YC. Severe bullous drug eruption due to sibutramine (Reductil©). *Br J Dermatol* 2003; **149**: 215–6.
4 Nachbar F, Korting HC, Vogl T. Erythema multiforme-like eruption in asso-ciation with severe headache following pyritinol. *Dermatology* 1993; **187**: 42–6.

Drugs acting on the cardiovascular system

Adverse cutaneous reactions due to cardiovascular and antiarrhythmic drug therapy have been reviewed [1,2].

REFERENCES

1 Reiner DM, Frishman WH, Luftschein S, Grossman M. Adverse cutaneous reactions from cardiovascular drug therapy. *NY State J Med* 1992; **92**: 137–47.
2 Sun DK, Reiner D, Frishman W *et al.* Adverse dermatologic reactions from antiarrhythmic drug therapy. *J Clin Pharmacol* 1994; **34**: 953–66.

Cardiac antiarrhythmic drugs

Amiodarone

This iodinated antiarrhythmic drug causes photosensitivity in around 40% of patients [1–13]. Symptoms develop within 2 h of sun exposure as a burning sensation followed by erythema; the action spectrum is UVA, extending to a degree into visible light wavebands above 400 nm [4]. Light sensitivity may persist for up to 4 months after the drug is stopped [1,2]. Blue or grey pigmentation of the face and other sun-exposed areas, resembling that in argyria, is a much less common late effect, occurring in 2–5% of cases; areas not exposed to the sun may also be involved [3,6–12]. It is induced by a phototoxic reaction involving both UVB and UVA [3,6], and is related to both duration and dosage of the drug [11]. However, although cutaneous side effects are more likely with increasing duration of treatment and cumulative dosage, neither the serum amiodarone level nor the serum metabolite level have any predictive power [13]. Amiodarone-pigmented skin contains the drug and its metabolites in higher concentrations than non-pigmented skin [3]. Iodine-rich amiodarone and its metabolites have been detected bound to lipofuscin within secondary lysosomes in perivascular dermal macrophages [7–10]. Electron-dense granules and myelin-like bodies are also found in peripheral blood leukocytes [12]. The cutaneous pigmentation slowly fades after discontinuation of therapy, but may persist for months to years [8].

Iododerma has occurred with long-term therapy. Vasculitis [14] and linear IgA disease [15] have been recorded. A fatal case of TEN has been reported [16]. The most severe adverse effect seen with amiodarone is pulmonary fibrosis, which occurs in 5–10% of exposed patients and which has a 10% mortality rate. Other problems have been cardiac dysrhythmias, thyroid dysfunction, peripheral neuropathy and reversible corneal deposits [17].

REFERENCES

1 Marcus FI, Fontaine GH, Frank R, Grosgogeat Y. Clinical pharmacology and therapeutic applications of the antiarrhythmic agent amiodarone. *Am Heart J* 1981; **101**: 480–93.
2 Chalmers RJ, Muston HL, Srinivas V, Bennett DH. High incidence of amiodarone-induced photosensitivity in North-west England. *BMJ* 1982; **285**: 341.
3 Zachary CB, Slater DN, Holt DW *et al.* The pathogenesis of amiodarone-induced pigmentation and photosensitivity. *Br J Dermatol* 1984; **110**: 451–6.
4 Ferguson J, Addo HA, Jones S *et al.* A study of cutaneous photosensitivity induced by amiodarone. *Br J Dermatol* 1985; **113**: 537–49.
5 Roupe G, Larkö O, Olsson SB *et al.* Amiodarone photoreactions. *Acta Derm Venereol (Stockh)* 1987; **67**: 76–9.
6 Waitzer S, Butany J, From L *et al.* Cutaneous ultrastructural changes and photosensitivity associated with amiodarone therapy. *J Am Acad Dermatol* 1987; **16**: 779–87.
7 McGovern B, Garan H, Kelly E, Ruskin JN. Adverse reactions during treatment with amiodarone hydrochloride. *BMJ* 1983; **287**: 175–9.
8 Miller RAW, McDonald ATJ. Dermal lipofuscinosis associated with amiodarone therapy. Report of a case. *Arch Dermatol* 1984; **120**: 646–9.
9 Holt DW, Adams PC, Campbell RWF *et al.* Amiodarone and its desethyl-metabolite: tissue distribution and ultrastructural changes in amiodarone treated patients. *Br J Clin Pharmacol* 1984; **17**: 195–6.
10 Török L, Szekeres L, Lakatos A, Szücs M. Amiodaronebedingte Hyperpigmentierung. *Hautarzt* 1986; **37**: 507–10.
11 Heger JJ, Prystowsky EN, Zipes DP. Relationships between amiodarone dosage, drug concentrations, and adverse side effects. *Am Heart J* 1983; **106**: 931–5.
12 Rappersberger K, Konrad K, Wieser E *et al.* Morphological changes in peripheral blood cells and skin in amiodarone-treated patients. *Br J Dermatol* 1986; **114**: 189–96.
13 Shukla R, Jowett NI, Thompson DR, Pohl JE. Side effects with amiodarone therapy. *Postgrad Med J* 1994; **70**: 492–8.
14 Staubli M, Zimmerman A, Bircher J. Amiodarone-induced vasculitis and polyserositis. *Postgrad Med J* 1985; **61**: 245–7.
15 Primka EJ III, Liranzo MO, Bergfeld W *et al.* Amiodarone-induced linear IgA disease. *J Am Acad Dermatol* 1996; **31**: 809–11.
16 Bencini PL, Crosti C, Sala F *et al.* Toxic epidermal necrolysis and amiodarone. *Arch Dermatol* 1985; **121**: 838.
17 Morgan DJR. Adverse reactions profile: 3. Amiodarone. *Drug Ther Bull* 1991; **31**: 104–11.

Digoxin

Allergic reactions are very rare [1], but exanthematic erythema, urticaria, bullous eruptions and thrombocytopenic purpura are documented. In one patient, a psoriasiform rash occurred, confirmed by later re-exposure [2].

REFERENCES

1 Martin SJ, Shah D. Cutaneous hypersensitivity reaction to digoxin. *JAMA* 1994; **271**: 1905.
2 David M, Livni E, Stern E *et al.* Psoriasiform eruption induced by digoxin: confirmed by reexposure. *J Am Acad Dermatol* 1981; **5**: 702–3.

Procainamide

This drug is well known for precipitating an LE-like syndrome [1–6], perhaps partly as a result of binding of the hydroxylamine metabolite of procainamide to complement component C4, with resultant impaired complement-mediated clearance of immune complexes [5,6]. A lichenoid eruption followed the occurrence of drug-induced LE in one case [7]. Urticarial vasculitis has been reported [8].

REFERENCES

1 Dubois EL. Procainamide induction of a systemic lupus erythematosus-like syndrome. Presentation of six cases, review of the literature, and analysis and follow-up of reported cases. *Medicine (Baltimore)* 1969; **48**: 217–8.
2 Blomgren SE, Condemi JJ, Vaughan JH. Procainamide-induced lupus erythematosus. Clinical and laboratory observations. *Am J Med* 1972; **52**: 338–48.
3 Whittle TS Jr, Ainsworth SK. Procainamide-induced systemic lupus erythematosus. Renal involvement with deposition of immune complexes. *Arch Pathol Lab Med* 1976; **100**: 469–74.
4 Tan EM, Rubin RL. Autoallergic reactions induced by procainamide. *J Allergy Clin Immunol* 1984; **74**: 631–4.
5 Sim E, Stanley L, Gill EW, Jones A. Metabolites of procainamide and practolol inhibit complement components C3 and C4. *Biochem J* 1988; **251**: 323–6.

6 Sim E. Drug-induced immune complex disease. *Complement Inflamm* 1989; **6**: 119–26.
7 Sherertz EF. Lichen planus following procainamide-induced lupus erythematosus. *Cutis* 1988; **42**: 51–3.
8 Knox JP, Welykyj SE, Gradini R, Massa MC. Procainamide-induced urticarial vasculitis. *Cutis* 1988; **42**: 469–72.

Quinidine

An eczematous photosensitivity is well described [1–5]; fever is common. Thrombocytopenic purpura may be induced, resulting from antibodies to drug–platelet conjugates [6,7]. Urticarial, scarlatiniform and morbilliform eruptions occur; the latter may proceed to generalized exfoliative dermatitis if the drug is continued. Fixed and lichenoid eruptions [8–14], often induced by light, are recorded, as well as an acneiform rash [15]. Livedo reticularis has been documented; the mechanism is unknown, although recent exposure to sunlight was a feature common to all cases [16–18]. Drug-induced LE [19–21] and Henoch–Schönlein vasculitis [22,23] have been seen. Psoriasis may be exacerbated [24,25]. Localized blue-grey pigmentation of the shins, hard palate, nails, nose, ears and forearms has been recorded [26].

REFERENCES

1 Berger TG, Sesody SJ. Quinidine-induced lichenoid photodermatitis. *Cutis* 1982; **29**: 595–8.
2 Marx JL, Eisenstat BA, Gladstein AH. Quinidine photosensitivity. *Arch Dermatol* 1983; **119**: 39–43.
3 Armstrong RB, Leach EE, Whitman G *et al.* Quinidine photosensitivity. *Arch Dermatol* 1985; **121**: 525–8.
4 Jeanmougin M, Sigal M, Djian B *et al.* Photo-allergie à la quinidine. *Ann Dermatol Vénéréol* 1986; **113**: 985–7.
5 Schürer NY, Lehmann P, Plewig G. Chinidininduzierte Photoallergie. Eine klinische und experimentelle Studie. *Hautarzt* 1991; **42**: 158–61.
6 Christie DJ, Weber RW, Mullen PC *et al.* Structural features of the quinidine and quinine molecules necessary for binding of drug-induced antibodies to human platelets. *J Lab Clin Med* 1984; **104**: 730–40.
7 Gary M, Ilfeld D, Kelton JG. Correlation of a quinidine-induced platelet-specific antibody with development of thrombocytopenia. *Am J Med* 1985; **79**: 253–5.
8 Anderson TE. Lichen planus following quinidine therapy. *Br J Dermatol* 1967; **79**: 500.
9 Pegum JS. Lichenoid quinidine eruption. *Br J Dermatol* 1968; **80**: 343.
10 Maltz BL, Becker LE. Quinidine-induced lichen planus. *Int J Dermatol* 1980; **19**: 96–7.
11 Bonnetblanc J-M, Bernard P, Catanzano G, Souyri N. Eruptions lichénoides photinduites aux quinidiniques. *Ann Dermatol Vénéréol* 1987; **114**: 957–61.
12 Wolf R, Dorfman B, Krakowski A. Quinidine induced lichenoid and eczematous photodermatitis. *Dermatologica* 1987; **174**: 285–9.
13 De Larrard G, Jeanmougin M, Moulonguet I *et al.* Toxidermie lichénoïde alopéciante à la quinidine. *Ann Dermatol Vénéréol* 1988; **115**: 1172–4.
14 Jeanmougin M, Elkara-Marrak H, Pons A *et al.* Éruption lichénoïde photoinduite a l'hydroxyquinidine. *Ann Dermatol Vénéréol* 1987; **114**: 1397–9.
15 Burckhart CG. Quinidine-induced acne. *Arch Dermatol* 1987; **117**: 603–4.
16 Marion DF, Terrien CM. Photosensitive livedo reticularis. *Arch Dermatol* 1973; **108**: 100–1.
17 De Groot WP, Wuite J. Livedo racemosa-like photosensitivity reaction during quinidine durettes medication. *Dermatologica* 1974; **148**: 371–6.
18 Bruce S, Wolf JE Jr. Quinidine-induced photosensitive livedo reticularis-like eruption. *J Am Acad Dermatol* 1985; **12**: 332–6.
19 Lavie CJ, Biundo J, Quinet RJ, Waxman J. Systemic lupus erythematosus (SLE) induced by quinidine. *Arch Intern Med* 1985; **145**: 446–8.
20 McCormack GD, Barth WF. Quinidine induced lupus syndrome. *Semin Arthritis Rheum* 1985; **15**: 73–9.
21 Cohen MG, Kevat S, Prowse MV *et al.* Two distinct quinidine-induced rheumatic syndromes. *Ann Intern Med* 1988; **108**: 369–71.
22 Aviram A. Henoch–Schönlein syndrome associated with quinidine. *JAMA* 1980; **243**: 432–4.
23 Zax RH, Hodge SJ, Callen JP. Cutaneous leukocytoclastic vasculitis. Serial histopathologic evaluation demonstrates the dynamic nature of the infiltrate. *Arch Dermatol* 1990; **126**: 69–72.
24 Baker H. The influence of chloroquine and related drugs on psoriasis and keratoderma blenorrhagicum. *Br J Dermatol* 1966; **78**: 161–6.
25 Brenner S, Cabili S, Wolf R. Widespread erythematous scaly plaques in an adult. Psoriasiform eruption induced by quinidine. *Arch Dermatol* 1993; **129**: 1331–2, 1334–5.
26 Mahler R, Sissons W, Watters K. Pigmentation induced by quinidine therapy. *Arch Dermatol* 1986; **122**: 1062–4.

β-Adrenoceptor-blocking agents

This group of drugs shares certain potential side effects in common [1,2]. Peripheral ischaemia may be aggravated, and cold extremities and Raynaud's phenomenon [3] may present as new symptoms. Peripheral gangrene and peripheral skin necrosis have been reported [4,5]. An LE-like syndrome [6,7], and eczematous or lichenoid eruptions [1,2] may be induced rarely. Psoriasis vulgaris is occasionally aggravated or precipitated by a number of β-blockers including atenolol, oxprenolol and propranolol [8–14]. Cross-sensitivity is not usual [15], but cross-reactivity between atenolol, oxprenolol and propranolol has been reported [16]. Peyronie's disease (induratio penis plastica) has been attributed to labetalol, metoprolol and propranolol [17,18]. Aphthous ulcers have been linked to β-blockers [19], and vasculitis occurred with sotalol [20]. β-Blockers may enhance anaphylactic reactions caused by other allergens, and may make resuscitation more difficult [21–23]. Vitiligo may be exacerbated [24]. Topical ophthalmic β-blockers, especially timolol, have been implicated in pruritus [25], alopecia [26], chronic erythroderma [27] and LE [28].

REFERENCES

1 Felix RH, Ive FA, Dahl MGC. Skin reactions to beta-blockers. *BMJ* 1975; **i**: 626.
2 Hödl S. Nebenwirkungen der Betarezeptorenblocker an der Haut. Übersicht und eigene Beobachtungen. *Hautarzt* 1985; **36**: 549–57.
3 Marshall AJ, Roberts CJC, Barritt DW. Raynaud's phenomenon as a side effect of beta-blockers in hypertension. *BMJ* 1976; **i**: 1498–9.
4 Gokal R, Dornan TL, Ledingham JGG. Peripheral skin necrosis complicating beta-blockade. *BMJ* 1979; **i**: 721–2.
5 Hoffbrand BI. Peripheral skin necrosis complicating beta-blockade. *BMJ* 1979; **i**: 1082.
6 Hughes GRV. Hypotensive agents, beta-blockers, and drug-induced lupus. *BMJ* 1982; **284**: 1358–9.
7 McGuinness M, Frye RA, Deng J-S. Atenolol-induced lupus erythematosus. *J Am Acad Dermatol* 1997; **37**: 298–9.
8 Arntzen N, Kavli G, Volden G. Psoriasis provoked by β-blocking agents. *Acta Derm Venereol (Stockh)* 1984; **64**: 346–8.
9 Abel EA, Dicicco LM, Orenberg EK *et al.* Drugs in exacerbation of psoriasis. *J Am Acad Dermatol* 1986; **15**: 1007–22.
10 Heng MCY, Heng MK. Beta-adrenoceptor antagonist-induced psoriasiform eruption. Clinical and pathogenetic aspects. *Int J Dermatol* 1988; **27**: 619–27.

11 Gold MH, Holy AK, Roenigk HH Jr. Beta-blocking drugs and psoriasis. A review of cutaneous side effects and retrospective analysis of their effects on psoriasis. *J Am Acad Dermatol* 1988; **19**: 837–41.
12 Halevy S, Livni E. Psoriasis and psoriasiform eruptions associated with propranolol: the role of an immunologic mechanism. *Arch Dermatol Res* 1990; **283**: 472–3.
13 Steinkraus V, Steinfath M, Mensing H. Beta-adrenergic blocking drugs and psoriasis. *J Am Acad Dermatol* 1992; **27**: 266–7.
14 Halevy S, Livni E. Beta-adrenergic blocking drugs and psoriasis: the role of an immunologic mechanism. *J Am Acad Dermatol* 1993; **29**: 504–5.
15 Furhoff A-K, Norlander M, Peterson C. Cross-sensitivity between practolol and other beta-blockers? *BMJ* 1976; **i**: 831.
16 Van Joost T, Smitt JHS. Skin reactions to propranolol and cross sensitivity to β-adrenoreceptor blocking agents. *Arch Dermatol* 1981; **117**: 600–1.
17 Yudkin JS. Peyronie's disease in association with metoprolol. *Lancet* 1977; **ii**: 1355.
18 Jones HA, Castleden WM. Peyronie's disease. *Med J Aust* 1981; **ii**: 514–5.
19 Boulinguez S, Reix S, Bedane C et al. Role of drug exposure in aphthous ulcers: a case–control study. *Br J Dermatol* 2000; **143**: 1261–5.
20 Rustmann WC, Carpenter MT, Harmon C, Botti CF. Leukocytoclastic vasculitis associated with sotalol therapy. *J Am Acad Dermatol* 1998; **38**: 111–2.
21 Hannaway PJ, Hopper GDK. Severe anaphylaxis and drug-induced beta-blockade. *N Engl J Med* 1983; **308**: 1536.
22 Toogood JH. Risk of anaphylaxis in patients receiving beta-blocker drugs. *J Allergy Clin Immunol* 1988; **81**: 1–5.
23 Hepner MJ, Ownby DR, Anderson JA et al. Risk of systemic reactions in patients taking beta-blocker drugs receiving allergen immunotherapy injections. *J Allergy Clin Immunol* 1990; **86**: 407–11.
24 Schallreuter KU. Beta-adrenergic blocking drugs may exacerbate vitiligo. *Br J Dermatol* 1995; **132**: 168–9.
25 Lazarov A, Amicha B. Skin reactions due to eye drops: report of two cases. *Cutis* 1996; **58**: 363–4.
26 Fraunfelder FT, Meyer SM, Menacker SJ. Alopecia possibly secondary to topical ophthalmic β-blockers. *JAMA* 1990; **263**: 1493–4.
27 Shelley WB, Shelley ED. Chronic erythroderma induced by β-blocker (timolol maleate). *J Am Acad Dermatol* 1997; **37**: 799–800.
28 Zamber RW, Starkebaum G, Rubin RL et al. Drug induced systemic lupus erythematosus due to ophthalmic timolol. *J Rheumatol* 1992; **19**: 977–9.

Acebutolol

Rashes with mixed lichenoid and LE-like features have been reported [1]. The LE syndrome may have pleuropulmonary features [2].

Atenolol

Conjunctivitis and a periocular dermatitis [3], as well as a psoriasiform rash [4], pseudolymphomatous reaction [5] and vasculitis [6], are recorded.

Cetamolol

A psoriasiform eruption has been documented [7].

Labetalol

Mixed eruptions with psoriasiform and pityriasis rubra pilaris-like changes [8], a bullous lichenoid eruption [9] and an SLE-like syndrome [10] are documented.

Metoprolol

Various psoriasiform or eczematous rashes may follow long-term therapy [11,12]. Conjunctivitis and periocular dermatitis have occurred [3]. Peyronie's disease appears to be a rare but confirmed side effect and may be reversible. Telogen effluvium has been noted [13].

Oxprenolol

This drug, like practolol, has caused an oculocutaneous syndrome [14]. An eruption combining well-defined, eroded or scaly red rings with a lichenoid histology [15,16] is recognized. Acute psoriasis with arthropathy has been described [17]. Peripheral skin necrosis associated with Raynaud's phenomenon, an LE syndrome, various patterns of dermatitis [3] and generalized pigmentation [18] are all documented.

Practolol

This drug has been withdrawn, but is discussed in view of its important side-effect profile. It caused an oculocutaneous syndrome comprising dry eyes and scarring, fibrosis and metaplasia of the conjunctiva; a psoriasiform, lichenoid or mixed eruption with a characteristic histology; pleural and pericardial reactions; fibrinous peritonitis; and serous otitis media [19,20]. Subsequent treatment with another β-blocker did not elicit cross-sensitivity reactivation of the syndrome [21]. Ocular cicatricial pemphigoid was seen [22], and exacerbation of psoriasis was recorded [23].

Pindolol

Psoriasiform [24] and lichenoid rashes with pemphigus-like antibodies demonstrated by immunofluorescence have been seen, as well as an SLE syndrome [25].

Propranolol

This is probably the most widely used β-blocker, and many adverse cutaneous reactions have been reported [26–29]. Rashes may be lichenoid [30], psoriasiform [29] or generalized and exfoliative. Other miscellaneous reported reactions include alopecia [31], erythema multiforme [32] and a cheilostomatitis with ulceration of the lips. Peyronie's disease has developed. Generalized pustular psoriasis [33] and pemphigus [34] have occurred.

REFERENCES

1 Taylor AEM, Hindson C, Wacks H. A drug eruption due to acebutolol with combined lichenoid and lupus erythematosus features. *Clin Exp Dermatol* 1982; **7**: 219–21.
2 Record NB. Acebutolol-induced pleuropulmonary lupus syndrome. *Ann Intern Med* 1981; **95**: 326–7.
3 Van Joost T, Middelkamp Hup H, Ros FE. Dermatitis as a side-effect of long-term topical treatment with certain beta-blocking agents. *Br J Dermatol* 1979; **101**: 171–6.
4 Gawkrodger DJ, Beveridge GW. Psoriasiform reaction to atenolol. *Clin Exp Dermatol* 1984; **9**: 92–4.

5 Henderson CA, Shamy HK. Atenolol-induced pseudolymphoma. *Clin Exp Dermatol* 1990; **15**: 119–20.

6 Wolf R, Ophir J, Elman M, Krakowski A. Atenolol-induced cutaneous vasculitis. *Cutis* 1989; **43**: 231–3.

7 White WB, Schulman P, McCabe EJ. Psoriasiform cutaneous eruptions induced by cetamolol hydrochloride. *Arch Dermatol* 1986; **122**: 857–8.

8 Finlay AY, Waddington E, Savage RL *et al.* Cutaneous reactions to labetalol. *BMJ* 1978; i: 987.

9 Gange RW, Wilson Jones E. Bullous lichen planus caused by labetalol. *BMJ* 1978; i: 816–7.

10 Brown RC, Cooke M, Losowsky MS. SLE syndrome, probably induced by labetalol. *Postgrad Med J* 1981; **57**: 189–90.

11 Neumann HAM, van Joost T, Westerhof W. Dermatitis as a side-effect of long-term metoprolol. *Lancet* 1979; ii: 745.

12 Neumann HAM, van Joost T. Adverse reactions of the skin to metoprolol and other beta-adrenergic-blocking agents. *Dermatologica* 1981; **162**: 330–5.

13 Graeber CW, Lapkin RA. Metoprolol and alopecia. *Cutis* 1981; **28**: 633–4.

14 Holt PJA, Waddington E. Oculocutaneous reaction to oxprenolol. *BMJ* 1975; ii: 539–40.

15 Levene GM, Gange RW. Eruption during treatment with oxprenolol. *BMJ* 1978; i: 784.

16 Gange RW, Levene GM. A distinctive eruption in patients receiving oxprenolol. *Clin Exp Dermatol* 1979; **4**: 87–97.

17 MacFarlane DG, Settas L. Acute psoriatic arthropathy precipitated by oxprenolol. *Ann Rheum Dis* 1984; **43**: 102–4.

18 Harrower ADB, Strong JA. Hyperpigmentation associated with oxprenolol administration. *BMJ* 1977; ii: 296.

19 Felix RH, Ive FA, Dahl MGC. Cutaneous and ocular reactions to practolol. *BMJ* 1974; iv: 321–4.

20 Wright P. Untoward effects associated with practolol administration: oculomucocutaneous syndrome. *BMJ* 1975; i: 595–8.

21 Furhoff A-K, Norlander M, Peterson C. Cross-sensitivity between practolol and other beta-blockers? *BMJ* 1976; i: 831.

22 Van Joost T, Crone RA, Overdijk AD. Ocular cicatricial pemphigoid associated with practolol therapy. *Br J Dermatol* 1976; **94**: 447–50.

23 Søndergaard J, Wadskov S, Ærenlund-Jensen H, Mikkelsen HI. Aggravation of psoriasis and occurrence of psoriasiform cutaneous eruptions induced by practolol (Eraldin®). *Acta Derm Venereol (Stockh)* 1976; **56**: 239–43.

24 Bonerandi J-J, Follana J, Privat Y. Apparition d'un psoriasis au cours d'un traitement par bêta-bloquants (Pindolol). *Ann Dermatol Syphiligr* 1976; **103**: 604–6.

25 Bensaid J, Aldigier J-C, Gualde N. Systemic lupus erythematosus syndrome induced by pindolol. *BMJ* 1979; i: 1603–4.

26 Ærenlund-Jensen H, Mikkelsen HI, Wadskov S, Søndergaard J. Cutaneous reactions to propranolol (Inderal®). *Acta Med Scand* 1976; **199**: 363–7.

27 Cochran REI, Thomson J, McQueen A, Beevers DG. Skin reactions associated with propranolol. *Arch Dermatol* 1976; **112**: 1173–4.

28 Scribner MD. Propranolol therapy. *Arch Dermatol* 1977; **113**: 1303.

29 Faure M, Hermier C, Perrot H. Accidents cutanés provoqués par le propranolol. *Ann Dermatol Vénéréol* 1979; **106**: 161–5.

30 Hawk JLM. Lichenoid drug eruption induced by propranolol. *Clin Exp Dermatol* 1980; **5**: 93–6.

31 Hilder RJ. Propranolol and alopecia. *Cutis* 1979; **24**: 63–4.

32 Pimstone B, Joffe B, Pimstone N *et al.* Clinical response to long-term propranolol therapy in hyperthyroidism. *S Afr Med J* 1969; **43**: 1203–5.

33 Hu C-H, Miller AC, Peppercorn R, Farber EM. Generalized pustular psoriasis provoked by propranolol. *Arch Dermatol* 1985; **121**: 1326–7.

34 Godard W, Lambert D, Gavanou J, Chapuis J-L. Pemphigus induit après traitement par l'association propranolol–méprobamate. *Ann Dermatol Vénéréol* 1980; **107**: 1213–6.

Antihypertensive drugs and vasodilators

The dermatological side effects of antihypertensive agents have been reviewed [1].

REFERENCE

1 Thestrup-Pedersen K. Adverse reactions in the skin from antihypertensive drugs. *Dan Med Bull* 1987; **34**: 3–5.

ACE inhibitors

In addition to dermatological problems, these drugs may be nephrotoxic, cause cough and electrolyte disturbances, and are teratogenic [1,2]. The overall incidence of adverse effects from ACE inhibitors is estimated at 28%, of which about 50% occur in the skin. Cutaneous reactions comprise life-threatening angio-oedema, pruritus, bullous eruptions, urticaria, other generalized rashes, photosensitivity and hair loss [3]. Angio-oedema has been reported with captopril, enalapril maleate and lisinopril [4–11]. The cumulative incidence of angio-oedema, almost always on the head and neck, has been estimated at 0.1–0.7% of cases treated; it usually occurs in the first week of treatment [5,9], although onset more than 6 weeks after starting treatment occurs in 20% of patients [6]. In addition, increased frequency, intensity and duration of bouts of angio-oedema have been recorded during long-term use of ACE inhibitors [7–9]. There may be cross-reactivity between drugs; angio-oedema has developed after substituting lisinopril for captopril [10]. Fatal angio-oedema occurred in a patient on captopril for 2 years [11]. Anaphylactoid reactions have been reported during haemodialysis with AN69 membranes in patients receiving ACE inhibitors; the role of bacterial contamination of dialysate is controversial [12–14]. Anaphylactoid reactions have also occurred with LDL apheresis with dextran sulphate [15].

ACE inhibitors have been implicated in both the exacerbation and induction of psoriasis [16–19]. ACE inhibitors most commonly produce a dose-related pruritic maculopapular eruption on the upper trunk and arms, especially with captopril (2.4–7%) and less with enalapril (1.5%), which is often transitory and rarely requires discontinuation of the drug. Urticaria, a pemphigoid-like reaction, a pityriasis rosea-like reaction, a lichenoid eruption, erythroderma, alopecia and Stevens–Johnson syndrome have been reported [20]. Captopril and enalapril may produce eruptions with histological similarities to mycosis fungoides [21]. An interstitial granulomatous drug reaction characterized by violaceous plaques with a predilection for skinfold areas and by histology resembling the diffuse interstitial phase of granuloma annulare without complete collagen necrobiosis has been documented with ACE inhibitors [22].

REFERENCES

1 Ferner RE. Adverse effects of angiotensin-converting-enzyme inhibitors. *Adverse Drug React Bull* 1990; **141**: 528–31.

2 Parish RC, Miller LJ. Adverse effects of angiotensin converting enzyme inhibitors: an update. *Drug Saf* 1992; **7**: 14–31.

3 Steckelings UM, Artuc M, Wollschlager T *et al.* Angiotensin-converting enzyme inhibitors as inducers of adverse cutaneous reactions. *Acta Derm Venereol (Stockh)* 2001; **81**: 321–5.

4 Orfan N, Patterson R, Dykewicz MS. Severe angioedema related to ACE

inhibitors in patients with a history of idiopathic angioedema. *JAMA* 1990; **264**: 1287–9.

5 Slater EE, Merill DD, Guess HA *et al*. Clinical profile of angioedema associated with angiotensin converting-enzyme inhibition. *JAMA* 1988; **260**: 967–70.

6 Hedner T, Samuelsson O, Lindholm L *et al*. Angio-oedema in relation to treatment with angiotensin converting enzyme inhibitors. *BMJ* 1992; **304**: 941–6.

7 Chin HL. Severe angioedema after long-term use of an angiotensin-converting enzyme inhibitor. *Ann Intern Med* 1990; **112**: 312.

8 Kozel MMA, Mekkes JR, Bos JD. Increased frequency and severity of angio-oedema related to long-term therapy with angiotensin-converting enzyme inhibitor in two patients. *Clin Exp Dermatol* 1995; **20**: 60–1.

9 Sabroe RA, Kobza Black A. Angiotensin-converting enzyme (ACE) inhibitors and angio-oedema. *Br J Dermatol* 1997; **136**: 153–8.

10 McElligott S, Perlroth M, Raish L. Angioedema after substituting lisinopril for captopril. *Ann Intern Med* 1992; **116**: 426–7.

11 Jason DR. Fatal angioedema associated with captopril. *J Forensic Sci* 1992; **37**: 1418–21.

12 Verresen L, Waer M, Vanrenterghem Y, Michielsen P. Angiotensin-converting-enzyme inhibitors and anaphylactoid reactions to high-flux membrane dialysis. *Lancet* 1990; **336**: 1360–2.

13 Tielemans C, Madhoun P, Lenears M *et al*. Anaphylactoid reactions during hemodialysis on AN69 membranes in patients receiving ACE inhibitors. *Kidney Int* 1990; **38**: 982–4.

14 Verresen L, Waer M, Vanrenterghem Y, Michielsen P. Anaphylactoid reactions, haemodialysis, and ACE inhibitors. *Lancet* 1991; **337**: 1294.

15 Keller C, Grutzmacher P, Bahr F *et al*. LDL-apheresis with dextran sulphate and anaphylactoid reactions to ACE inhibitors. *Lancet* 1993; **341**: 60–1.

16 Wolf R, Tamir A, Brenner S. Psoriasis related to angiotensin-converting enzyme inhibitors. *Dermatologica* 1990; **181**: 51–3.

17 Coulter DM, Pillans PI. Angiotensin-converting enzyme inhibitors and psoriasis. *NZ Med J* 1993; **106**: 392–3.

18 Tamir A, Wolf R, Brenner S. Exacerbation and induction of psoriasis by angiotensin-converting enzyme inhibitors. *J Am Acad Dermatol* 1994; **30**: 1045.

19 Ikai K. Exacerbation and induction of psoriasis by angiotensin-converting enzyme inhibitors. *J Am Acad Dermatol* 1996; **32**: 819.

20 Vollenweider Roten S, Mainetti C, Donath R, Saurat J-H. Enalapril-induced lichen planus-like eruption. *J Am Acad Dermatol* 1995; **32**: 293–5.

21 Furness PN, Goodfield MJ, MacLennan KA *et al*. Severe cutaneous reactions to captopril and enalapril: histological study and comparison with early mycosis fungoides. *J Clin Pathol* 1986; **39**: 902–7.

22 Perrin C, Lacour JP, Castanet J, Michiels JF. Interstitial granulomatous drug reaction with a histological pattern of interstitial granulomatous dermatitis. *Am J Dermatopathol* 2001; **23**: 295–8.

Captopril. Dermatological complications occur in 4% [1] to 12% [2] of patients treated with captopril, and less commonly with other ACE inhibitors; side effects are more likely with renal impairment. Loss of sense of taste, or a metallic taste (augesia), ulceration of the tongue and apthtous stomatitis [3] are reported. Early changes within the first months [4–6] include pruritus, urticaria [7] and angio-oedema, which occurs in about 1 in 1000 patients and may occasionally be fatal [8], and pityriasis rosea-like [9] and morbilliform rashes. These are dose dependent and have a good prognosis. Late changes [4–6] consist of pemphigus-like [10–12] and lichenoid [13–17] eruptions. SLE-like eruptions have been recorded [18,19]. Antinuclear antibodies may develop [20,21]. Oral changes may be due to a leukocytoclastic vasculitis [22], and a serum sickness-like syndrome has been induced [23]. Psoriasis has been reported to be exacerbated or triggered [24,25].

Severe reactions [26,27] have included exfoliative dermatitis [28–30], and marrow depression with neutropenia or agranulocytosis [31]. Lymphadenopathy may be induced [32]. Alopecia [33] and an acquired IgA deficiency [34] have been reported. The merits of skin testing in the prediction of captopril reactions have been discussed [35]. It has been postulated that some toxic effects are related to the presence of a sulphydryl group, as enalapril (another ACE inhibitor lacking this group) has been safely substituted in certain cases of captopril hypersensitivity [36].

Cilazapril. Cilazapril had more neurological (mainly headache) but fewer skin reactions than the other ACE inhibitors, lisinopril, enalapril and captopril [37].

Enalapril. Enalapril produces rashes in approximately 1.4% of patients, requiring discontinuation in about 0.4% [38]. Toxic pustuloderma is recorded [38]. A single report of pemphigus foliaceus has appeared; part of the structure of this drug is identical to that of captopril, although it does not contain a sulphydryl group [39]. Bullous eruptions [40] and lichenoid eruptions [41] occur.

Lisinopril [42]. Vasculitis has been recorded [43], as has pallor, flushing and oedema [44].

REFERENCES

1 Williams GH. Converting-enzyme inhibitors in the treatment of hypertension. *N Engl J Med* 1988; **319**: 1517–25.

2 Wilkin JK, Hammond JJ, Kirkendall WM. The captopril-induced eruption. A possible mechanism: cutaneous kinin potentiation. *Arch Dermatol* 1980; **116**: 902–5.

3 Seedat YK. Aphthous ulcers of mouth from captopril. *Lancet* 1979; **ii**: 1297–8.

4 Clement M. Captopril-induced eruptions. *Arch Dermatol* 1981; **117**: 525–6.

5 Luderer JR, Lookingbill DP, Schneck DW *et al*. Captopril-induced skin eruptions. *J Clin Pharmacol* 1982; **22**: 151–9.

6 Daniel F, Foix C, Barbet M *et al*. Captopril-induced eruptions: occurrence over a three-year period. *Ann Dermatol Vénéréol* 1983; **110**: 441–6.

7 Wood SM, Mann RD, Rawlins MD. Angio-oedema and urticaria associated with angiotensin converting enzyme inhibitors. *BMJ* 1987; **294**: 91–2.

8 Slater EE, Merrill DD, Guess HA *et al*. Clinical profile of angioedema associated with angiotensin converting-enzyme inhibition. *JAMA* 1988; **260**: 967–70.

9 Wilkin JK, Kirkendall WM. Pityriasis rosea-like rash from captopril. *Arch Dermatol* 1982; **118**: 186–7.

10 Parfrey PS, Clement M, Vandenburg MJ, Wright P. Captopril-induced pemphigus. *BMJ* 1980; **281**: 194.

11 Katz RA, Hood AF, Anhalt GJ. Pemphigus-like eruption from captopril. *Arch Dermatol* 1987; **123**: 20–1.

12 Korman NJ, Eyre RW, Stanley JR. Drug-induced pemphigus: autoantibodies directed against the pemphigus antigen complexes are present in penicillamine and captopril-induced pemphigus. *J Invest Dermatol* 1991; **96**: 273–6.

13 Reinhardt LA, Wilkin JK, Kirkendall WM. Lichenoid eruption produced by captopril. *Cutis* 1983; **31**: 98–9.

14 Bravard P, Barbet M, Eich D *et al*. Éruption lichénoïde au captopril. *Ann Dermatol Vénéréol* 1983; **110**: 433–8.

15 Flageul B, Foldes C, Wallach D *et al*. Captopril-induced lichen planus pemphigoides with pemphigus-like features. A case report. *Dermatologica* 1986; **173**: 248–55.

16 Bretin N, Dreno B, Bureau B, Litoux P. Immunohistological study of captopril-induced late cutaneous reactions. *Dermatologica* 1988; **177**: 11–5.

17 Rotstein E, Rotstein H. Drug eruptions with lichenoid histology produced by captopril. *Australas J Dermatol* 1989; **30**: 9–14.

18 Patri P, Nigro A, Rebora A. Lupus erythematosus-like eruption from captopril. *Acta Derm Venereol (Stockh)* 1985; **65**: 447–8.

19 Sieber C, Grimm E, Follath F. Captopril and systemic lupus erythematosus syndrome. *BMJ* 1990; **301**: 669.
20 Reidenberg MM, Case DB, Drayer DE *et al*. Development of antinuclear antibodies in patients treated with high doses of captopril. *Arthritis Rheum* 1984; **27**: 579–81.
21 Kallenberg CGM. Autoantibodies during captopril treatment. *Arthritis Rheum* 1985; **28**: 597–8.
22 Viraben R, Adoue D, Dupre A, Touron P. Erosions and ulcers of the mouth. *Arch Dermatol* 1982; **118**: 959.
23 Hoorntje SJ, Weening JJ, Kallenberg GGM *et al*. Serum-sickness-like syndrome with membranous glomerulopathy in a patient on captopril. *Lancet* 1979; ii: 1297.
24 Hauschild TT, Bauer R, Kreysel HW. Erstmanifestation einer eruptiv-exanthematischen Psoriasis vulgaris unter Captoprilmedikation. *Hautarzt* 1986; **37**: 274–7.
25 Wolf R, Dorfman B, Krakowski A. Psoriasiform eruption induced by captopril and chlorthalidone. *Cutis* 1987; **40**: 162–4.
26 Goodfield MJ, Millard LG. Severe cutaneous reactions to captopril. *BMJ* 1985; **290**: 1111.
27 Furness PN, Goodfield MJ, MacLennan KA *et al*. Severe cutaneous reactions to captopril and enalapril: histological study and comparison with early mycosis fungoides. *J Clin Pathol* 1986; **39**: 902–7.
28 Solinger AM. Exfoliative dermatitis from captopril. *Cutis* 1982; **29**: 473–4.
29 O'Neill PG, Rajan N, Charlat ML, Bolli R. Captopril-related exfoliative dermatitis. *Texas Med* 1989; **85**: 40–1.
30 Daniel F, Foix C, Barbet M *et al*. Toxidermies au captopril: incidences au cours d'un traitement de 1321 mois/patients. *Ann Dermatol Vénéréol* 1983; **110**: 441–6.
31 Edwards CRW, Drury P, Penketh A, Damluji SA. Successful reintroduction of captopril following neutropenia. *Lancet* 1981; i: 723.
32 Åberg H, Mörlin C, Frithz G. Captopril-associated lymphadenopathy. *BMJ* 1981; **283**: 1297–8.
33 Motel PJ. Captopril and alopecia: a case report and review of known cutaneous reactions in captopril use. *J Am Acad Dermatol* 1990; **23**: 124–5.
34 Hammarström L, Smith CIE, Berg U. Captopril-induced IgA deficiency. *Lancet* 1991; **337**: 436.
35 Smit AJ, van der Laan S, De Monchy J *et al*. Cutaneous reactions to captopril. Predictive values of skin tests. *Clin Allergy* 1984; **14**: 413–9.
36 Gavras I, Gavras H. Captopril and enalapril. *Ann Intern Med* 1983; **98**: 556–7.
37 Coulter DM. Short term safety assessment of cilazapril. *NZ Med J* 1993; **106**: 497–9.
38 Ferguson JE, Chalmers RJ. Enalapril-induced toxic pustuloderma. *Clin Exp Dermatol* 1996; **21**: 54–5.
39 Shelto RM. Pemphigus foliaceus associated with enalapril. *J Am Acad Dermatol* 1991; **24**: 503–4.
40 Mullins PD, Choudhury SL. Enalapril and bullous eruptions. *BMJ* 1994; **309**: 1411.
41 Vollenweider Roten S, Mainetti C, Donath R, Saurat J-H. Enalapril-induced lichen planus-like eruption. *J Am Acad Dermatol* 1995; **32**: 293–5.
42 Horiuchi Y, Matsuda M. Eruptions induced by the ACE inhibitor, lisinopril. *J Dermatol* 1999; **26**: 128–30.
43 Barlow RJ, Schulz EJ. Lisinopril-induced vasculitis. *Clin Exp Dermatol* 1988; **13**: 117–20.
44 Fallowfield JM, Blenkinsopp J, Raza A *et al*. Post-marketing surveillance of lisinopril in general practice in the UK. *Br J Clin Pract* 1993; **47**: 296–304.

Angiotensin II receptor antagonists

Sartans, angiotensin II receptor antagonists, have been implicated in the induction of psoriasis [1] and of Henoch–Schönlein purpura [2].

REFERENCES

1 Marquart-Elbaz C, Grosshans E, Alt M, Lipsker D. Sartans, angiotensin II receptor antagonists, can induce psoriasis. *Br J Dermatol* 2002; **147**: 617–8.
2 Brouard M, Piguet V, Chavaz P, Borradori L. Schönlein–Henoch purpura associated with losartan treatment and presence of antineutrophil cytoplasmic antibodies of x specificity. *Br J Dermatol* 2001; **145**: 362–3.

Calcium channel blockers

Cutaneous reactions are rare and have been reported in six per million prescriptions of nifedipine, 17 per million prescriptions of verapamil, and six per million prescriptions of diltiazem [1,2]. In one study, reactions to the dihydropyridine drugs (including nicardipine, nifedipine and nisoldipine), verapamil and diltiazem occurred after an average of 95 days (range 7 days to 10 years) [3]. Pruritus, maculopapular rashes, and urticaria/angio-oedema, alopecia and a hypersensitivity syndrome have been described with all these drugs, as have Stevens–Johnson syndrome and erythema multiforme; TEN has occurred with diltiazem. There is a suggestion that the more severe reactions are commoner with diltiazem. Peripheral oedema as a side effect is common to the dihydropyridine calcium antagonists, including nifedipine, nicardipine, isradipine and amlodipine; it occurs in 7–30% of patients depending on the specific drug, but is usually mild [4]. Psoriasiform eruptions are described [3], as are photosensitivity and erythromelalgia. Amlodipine has caused pruritus [5], a lichenoid eruption [6] and photosensitivity presenting as telangiectasia [7]. Felodipine has also been associated with photodistributed telangiectasia [8].

REFERENCES

1 Stern R, Khalsa JH. Cutaneous adverse reactions associated with calcium channel blockers. *Arch Intern Med* 1989; **149**: 829–32.
2 Sadick NS, Katz AS, Schreiber TL. Angioedema from calcium channel blockers. *J Am Acad Dermatol* 1989; **21**: 132–3.
3 Kitamura K, Kanasashi M, Suga C *et al*. Cutaneous reactions induced by calcium channel blockers: high frequency of psoriasiform eruptions. *J Dermatol* 1993; **20**: 279–86.
4 Maclean D, MacConnachie AM. Selected side-effects: 1. Peripheral oedema with dihydropyridine calcium antagonists. *Prescribers J* 1991; **31**: 4–6.
5 Orme S, da Costa D. Generalised pruritus associated with amlodipine. *BMJ* 1997; **315**: 463.
6 Swale VJ, McGregor JM. Amlodipine-associated lichen planus. *Br J Dermatol* 2001; **144**: 920–1.
7 Grabczynska SA, Cowley N. Amlodipine induced-photosensitivity presenting as telangiectasia. *Br J Dermatol* 2000; **142**: 1255–6.
8 Silvestre JF, Albares P, Carnero L, Botella R. Photodistributed felodipine-induced facial telangiectasia. *J Am Acad Dermatol* 2001; **45**: 323–4.

Diltiazem. Cutaneous reactions to diltiazem have been reviewed [1–3]. They include pruritic macular exanthem, toxic erythema with fever and occasionally facial angio-oedema [4–6], generalized cutaneous reactions [7], erythema multiforme [8], subcorneal pustular dermatosis, a generalized pustular dermatitis [9,10], a lichenoid photo-distributed eruption with pigmentary incontinence [11], a photosensitive erythroderma [12], psoriasiform eruptions [2], exfoliative dermatitis in a patient with psoriasis [13], a subacute cutaneous LE-like syndrome [14], vasculitis [15] and vasculitic leg ulcers [16], recurrent nail dystrophy, hyperplastic gingivitis [17], and proptosis and periorbital oedema [18]. Generalized lymphadenopathy has occurred [19]. Patch tests may be positive in diltiazem reactions

[5,6,10]. Dermatological cross-sensitivity between diltiazem and amlodipine is reported [20].

REFERENCES

1 Wittal RA, Fischer GO, Georgouras KE, Baird PJ. Skin reactions to diltiazem. *Australas J Dermatol* 1992; **33**: 11–8.
2 Kitamura K, Kanasashi M, Suga C *et al.* Cutaneous reactions induced by calcium channel blocker: high frequency of psoriasiform eruptions. *J Dermatol* 1993; **20**: 279–86.
3 Knowles S, Gupta AK, Shear NH. The spectrum of cutaneous reactions associated with diltiazem: three cases and a review of the literature. *J Am Acad Dermatol* 1998; **38**: 201–6.
4 Wakeel RA, Gavin MP, Keefe M. Severe toxic erythema caused by diltiazem. *BMJ* 1988; **296**: 1071.
5 Hammentgen R, Lutz G, Köhler U, Nitsch J. Makulopapulöses Exanthem bei Diltiazem-Therapie. *Dtsch Med Wochenschr* 1988; **113**: 1283–5.
6 Romano A, Pietrantonio F, Garcovich A *et al.* Delayed hypersensitivity to diltiazem in two patients. *Ann Allergy* 1992; **69**: 31–2.
7 Sousa-Basto A, Azenha A, Duarte ML, Pardal-Oliveira F. Generalized cutaneous reaction to diltiazem. *Contact Dermatitis* 1993; **29**: 44–5.
8 Berbis P, Alfonso MJ, Levy JL, Privat Y. Diltiazem associated erythema multiforme. *Dermatologica* 1990; **179**: 90.
9 Lambert DG, Dalac S, Beer F *et al.* Acute generalized exanthematous pustular dermatitis induced by diltiazem. *Br J Dermatol* 1988; **118**: 308–9.
10 January V, Machet L, Gironet N *et al.* Acute generalized exanthematous pustulosis induced by diltiazem: value of patch testing. *Dermatology* 1998; **197**: 274–5.
11 Scherschun L, Lee MW, Lim HW. Diltiazem-associated photodistributed hyperpigmentation: a review of 4 cases. *Arch Dermatol* 2001; **137**: 179–82.
12 Hashimoto M, Tanaka S, Horio T. Photosensibility due to diltiazem hydrochloride. *Acta Dermatol* 1979; **74**: 181–4.
13 Larvijsen APM, Van Dijke C, Vermeer B-J. Diltiazem-associated exfoliative dermatitis in a patient with psoriasis. *Acta Derm Venereol (Stockh)* 1986; **66**: 536–8.
14 Crowson AN, Magro CM. Diltiazem and subacute cutaneous lupus erythematosus-like lesions. *N Engl J Med* 1995; **333**: 1429.
15 Sheehan-Dare RA, Goodfield MJ. Severe cutaneous vasculitis induced by diltiazem. *Br J Dermatol* 1988; **119**: 134.
16 Carmichael AJ, Paul CJ. Vasculitic leg ulcers associated with diltiazem. *BMJ* 1988; **297**: 562.
17 Giustiniani S, Robustelli della Cuna F, Marieni M. Hyperplastic gingivitis during diltiazem therapy. *Int J Cardiol* 1987; **15**: 247–9.
18 Friedland S, Kaplan S, Lahav M, Shapiro A. Proptosis and periorbital edema due to diltiazem treatment. *Arch Ophthalmol* 1993; **111**: 1027–8.
19 Scolnick B, Brinberg D. Diltiazem and generalized lymphadenopathy. *Ann Intern Med* 1985; **102**: 558.
20 Baker BA, Cacchione JG. Dermatologic cross-sensitivity between diltiazem and amlodipine. *Ann Pharmacother* 1994; **28**: 118–9.

Nicardipine. Erythromelalgia is recorded [1].

Nicorandil. Oral ulceration is documented [2,3].

Nifedipine. Headache, tachycardia and flushing are common side effects. Gingival hyperplasia is well recognized [4]. Burning sensations, erythema, painful oedema and erythromelalgia have been described [5–8]. There have been isolated reports of a truncal morbilliform rash [9], fixed drug eruption [10], a generalized bullous eruption, vasculitis [11], purpura, photosensitivity [12] in one case confirmed by rechallenge [13], gynaecomastia [14], erysipelas-like lesions on the shins with erythematous plaques on the trunk [15], exfoliative dermatitis [16,17] and pemphigoid nodularis [18].

Verapamil. Erythema multiforme has been reported [19], as have gingival hyperplasia, gynaecomastia [20], alopecia, maculopapular eruptions, ecchymosis, vasculitis, urticaria and hyperkeratosis.

REFERENCES

1 Levesque H, Moore N, Wolfe LM, Courtoid H. Erythromelalgia induced by nicardipine (inverse Raynaud's phenomenon?). *BMJ* 1989; **298**: 1252–3.
2 Cribier B, Marquart-Elbaz C, Lipsker D *et al.* Chronic buccal ulceration induced by nicorandil. *Br J Dermatol* 1998; **138**: 372–3.
3 Desruelles R, Bahadoran P, Lacour J-P *et al.* Giant oral aphthous ulcers induced by nicorandil. *Br J Dermatol* 1998; **138**: 712–3.
4 Benini PL, Crosti C, Sala F *et al.* Gingival hyperplasia by nifedipine. Report of a case. *Acta Derm Venereol (Stockh)* 1985; **65**: 362–5.
5 Bridgman JF. Erythematous edema of the legs due to nifedipine. *BMJ* 1978; i: 578.
6 Fisher JR, Padnick MB, Olstein S. Nifedipine and erythromelalgia. *Ann Intern Med* 1983; **98**: 671–2.
7 Brodmerkel GJ Jr. Nifedipine and erythromelalgia. *Ann Intern Med* 1983; **99**: 415.
8 Alcalay J, David M, Sandbank M. Cutaneous reactions to nifedipine. *Dermatologica* 1987; **175**: 191–3.
9 Parish LC, Witkowski JA. Truncal morbilliform eruption due to nifedipine. *Cutis* 1992; **49**: 113–4.
10 Alcalay J, David M. Generalized fixed drug eruptions associated with nifedipine. *BMJ* 1986; **292**: 450.
11 Brenner S, Brau S. Vasculitis following nifedipine. *Harefuah* 1985; **108**: 139–40.
12 Thomas SE, Wood ML. Photosensitivity reactions associated with nifedipine. *BMJ* 1986; **292**: 992.
13 Zenarola P, Gatti S, Lomuto M. Photodermatitis due to nifedipine: report of 2 cases. *Dermatologica* 1991; **182**: 196–8.
14 Clyne CAC. Unilateral gynaecomastia and nifedipine. *BMJ* 1986; **292**: 380.
15 Leibovici V, Zlotogorski A, Heyman A *et al.* Polymorphous drug eruption due to nifedipine. *Cutis* 1988; **41**: 367.
16 Reynolds NJ, Jones SK, Crossley J, Harman RRM. Exfoliative dermatitis due to nifedipine. *Br J Dermatol* 1989; **121**: 401–4.
17 Mohammed KN. Nifedipine-induced exfoliative dermatitis and pedal edema. *Ann Pharmacother* 1994; **28**: 967.
18 Ameen M, Harman KE, Black MM. Pemphigoid nodularis associated with nifedipine. *Br J Dermatol* 2000; **142**: 575–7.
19 Kürkçüoglu N, Alaybeyi F. Erythema multiforme after verapamil treatment. *J Am Acad Dermatol* 1991; **24**: 511–2.
20 Rodriguez LaG, Jick H. Risk of gynaecomastia associated with cimetidine, omeprazole, and other antiulcer drugs. *BMJ* 1994; **308**: 503–6.

Centrally acting antihypertensive drugs

Clonidine. Hypersensitivity rashes occur in up to 5% of patients. A pityriasis rosea-like and LE-like syndrome, exacerbation of psoriasis [1] and an isolated instance of anogenital cicatricial pemphigoid [2] have been documented. Transdermally administered clonidine has caused allergic contact dermatitis, but also erythema, scaling, vesiculation, excoriation, induration and dyspigmentation [3].

REFERENCES

1 Wilkin JK. Exacerbation of psoriasis during clonidine therapy. *Arch Dermatol* 1981; **117**: 4.
2 Van Joost T, Faber WR, Manuel HR. Drug-induced anogenital cicatricial pemphigoid. *Br J Dermatol* 1980; **102**: 715–8.
3 Prisant LM. Transdermal clonidine skin reactions. *J Clin Hypertens* 2002; **4**: 136–8.

Methyldopa. An eczematous eruption of discoid or seborrhoeic pattern is characteristic, is more likely to occur in previously eczematous subjects and persists until the drug is stopped [1]. Eczema of the palms and soles has also been described and may become widespread. The reaction is probably allergic as it may be dose related. Purpuric, erythematous and lichenoid rashes occur, sometimes in association with fever and other allergic symptoms [2,3]. Lichenoid eruptions may be ulcerated [4,5] and persistent ulceration of the tongue has been described. Fixed eruptions are very rare. An LE-like syndrome is documented [6,7] and an autoimmune haemolytic anaemia is well known [5]. Psoriasis may be precipitated. An extensive erythematous skin eruption, fever, lymphadenopathy and eosinophilia due to methyldopa, recurrent on re-exposure, has been recorded [8].

REFERENCES

1 Church R. Eczema provoked by methyldopa. *Br J Dermatol* 1974; **91**: 373–8.
2 Stevenson CJ. Lichenoid eruptions due to methyldopa. *Br J Dermatol* 1971; **85**: 600.
3 Burry JN, Kirk J. Lichenoid drug reaction from methyldopa. *Br J Dermatol* 1974; **91**: 475–6.
4 Burry JN. Ulcerative lichenoid eruption from methyldopa. *Arch Dermatol* 1976; **112**: 880.
5 Furhoff A-K. Adverse reactions with methyldopa: a decade's reports. *Acta Med Scand* 1978; **203**: 425–8.
6 Harrington TM, Davis DE. Systemic lupus-like syndrome induced by methyldopa therapy. *Chest* 1981; **79**: 696–7.
7 Dupont A, Six R. Lupus-like syndrome induced by methyldopa. *BMJ* 1982; **285**: 693–4.
8 Wolf R, Tamir A, Werbin N, Brenner S. Methyldopa hypersensitivity syndrome. *Ann Allergy* 1993; **71**: 166–8.

Adrenergic neurone-blocking agents

Guanethidine. Hypersensitivity eruptions are very rare but polyarteritis nodosa has been attributed to this drug [1].

REFERENCE

1 Dewar HA, Peaston MJT. Three cases resembling polyarteritis nodosa arising during treatment with guanethidine. *BMJ* 1964; **ii**: 609–11.

Vasodilator antihypertensive drugs

Diazoxide. Transient flushing is common. During long-term treatment, up to half the patients develop hypertrichosis without other signs of virilization [1]. A clinical picture resembling hypertrichosis lanuginosa may develop [2,3]. Oedema occurs in at least 10% of patients; photosensitivity is very uncommon but well recognized. Lichenoid [3,4] and other rashes occur rarely.

REFERENCES

1 Burton JL, Schutt WH, Caldwell JW. Hypertrichosis due to diazoxide. *Br J Dermatol* 1975; **93**: 707–11.

2 Koblenzer PJ, Baker J. Hypertrichosis lanuginosa associated with diazoxide therapy in prepubertal children: a clinicopathologic study. *Ann NY Acad Sci* 1968; **150**: 373–82.
3 Menter MA. Hypertrichosis lanuginosa and a lichenoid eruption due to diazoxide therapy. *Proc R Soc Med* 1973; **66**: 326–7.
4 Okun R, Russell RP, Wilson WR. Use of diazoxide with trichlormethiazide for hypertension. *Arch Intern Med* 1963; **112**: 882–6.

Hydralazine. The LE-like syndrome due to this drug is well known [1–7]. Hydralazine binds to complement component C4 and inhibits its function; this may impair clearance of immune complexes, and predispose to development of an LE syndrome [6,7].

Orogenital ulceration may be part of the picture [8], and the syndrome has presented as a leg ulcer [9]. Cutaneous vasculitis may be severe and necrotizing [10,11]. An association between hydralazine-induced LE syndrome and the development of Sweet's syndrome has been noted rarely [12]. Fixed drug eruption has been reported [13]. Characteristic lung changes are attributed to the drug [14].

REFERENCES

1 Alarcon-Segovia D, Wakin KG, Worthington JW *et al.* Clinical and experimental studies on the hydralazine syndrome and its relationship to systemic lupus erythematosus. *Medicine (Baltimore)* 1967; **46**: 1–33.
2 Batchelor JR, Welsh KI, Mansilla Tinoco R *et al.* Hydralazine-induced systemic lupus erythematosus: influence of HLA-DR and sex upon susceptibility. *Lancet* 1980; **i**: 1107–9.
3 Dubroff LM, Reid R Jr, Papalian M. Molecular models for hydralazine-related systemic lupus erythematosus. *Arthritis Rheum* 1981; **24**: 1082–5.
4 Perry HM Jr. Possible mechanisms of the hydralazine-related lupus-like syndrome. *Arthritis Rheum* 1981; **24**: 1093–105.
5 Mansilla Tinoco R, Harland SJ, Ryan P *et al.* Hydralazine, antinuclear antibodies, and the lupus syndrome. *BMJ* 1982; **284**: 936–9.
6 Sim E, Law S-KA. Hydralazine binds covalently to complement component C4. Different reactivity of C4A and C4B gene products. *FEBS Lett* 1985; **184**: 323–7.
7 Sim E. Drug-induced immune complex disease. *Complement Inflamm* 1989; **6**: 119–26.
8 Neville E, Graham PY, Brewis RA. Orogenital ulcers, SLE and hydralazine. *Postgrad Med J* 1981; **57**: 378–9.
9 Kissin MW, Williamson RCN. Hydrallazine-induced SLE-like syndrome presenting as a leg ulcer. *BMJ* 1979; **ii**: 1330.
10 Bernstein RM, Egerton-Vernon J, Webster J. Hydrallazine-induced cutaneous vasculitis. *BMJ* 1980; **280**: 156–7.
11 Peacock A, Weatherall D. Hydralazine-induced necrotising vasculitis. *BMJ* 1981; **282**: 1121–2.
12 Servitje O, Ribera M, Juanola X, Rodriguez-Moreno J. Acute neutrophilic dermatosis associated with hydralazine-induced lupus. *Arch Dermatol* 1988; **123**: 1435–6.
13 Sehgal VN, Gangwani OP. Hydralazine-induced fixed drug eruption. *Int J Dermatol* 1986; **25**: 394.
14 Bass BH. Hydralazine lung. *Thorax* 1981; **36**: 695–6.

Minoxidil. This arterial vasodilator causes hypertrichosis, especially of the arms and face, which may be unacceptable to women [1,2]; the hair disappears slowly after the drug is withdrawn. Fluid retention may require diuretic therapy to control it. Thrombocytopenia [3], bullous eruptions [4], erythema multiforme or Stevens–Johnson syndrome [5] and pseudoacromegaly [6] have been described.

REFERENCES

1 Burton JL, Marshall A. Hypertrichosis due to minoxidil. *Br J Dermatol* 1979; **101**: 593–5.
2 Ryckmanns F. Hypertrichose durch Minoxidil. *Hautarzt* 1980; **31**: 205–6.
3 Peitzmann SJ, Martin C. Thrombocytopenia and minoxidil. *Ann Intern Med* 1980; **92**: 874.
4 Rosenthal T, Teicher A, Swartz J, Boichis H. Minoxidil-induced bullous eruption. *Arch Intern Med* 1978; **138**: 1856–7.
5 DiSantis DJ, Flanagan J. Minoxidil-induced Stevens–Johnson syndrome. *Arch Intern Med* 1981; **141**: 1515.
6 Nguyen KH, Marks JG Jr. Pseudoacromegaly induced by the long-term use of minoxidil. *J Am Acad Dermatol* 2003; **48**: 962–5.

Nitrate vasodilators

Glyceryl and pentaerythritol tetranitrate. Reactions to nitrate vasodilators are rare, but erythroderma with cross-reactivity to glyceryl trinitrate has been caused by this drug [1].

REFERENCE

1 Ryan FP. Erythroderma due to peritrate and glyceryl trinitrate. *Br J Dermatol* 1972; **87**: 498–500.

Diuretics

Carbonic anhydrase inhibitor

Acetazolamide. This drug has caused hirsutism in a child [1]. Hypersensitivity reactions are rare.

REFERENCE

1 Weiss IS. Hirsutism after chronic administration of acetazolamide. *Am J Ophthalmol* 1974; **78**: 327–8.

Loop diuretics

Bumetanide. Occasional hypersensitivity rashes occur. Pseudoporphyria has been reported wih this sulphonamide-derived drug [1].

Etacrynic acid (ethacrynic acid). A Henoch–Schönlein type of vasculitis has been documented.

Furosemide (frusemide). Reactions are rare: only two patients of 3830 receiving this medication in one study developed cutaneous complications [2]. Phototoxic blistering has followed very high dosage (2.0 g/day) in chronic renal failure [3] but erythema multiforme [4,5], bullous pemphigoid [6,7], other bullous haemorrhagic eruptions [8] and an acquired blistering disorder with skin fragility [9] have apparently been precipitated by conventional dosage. The skin changes may mimic those of porphyria. Several cases of generalized exfoliative dermatitis have been documented. Anaphylaxis [10], a necrotizing vasculitis [11] and an eruption resembling Sweet's syndrome [12] have been reported. Cross-reactivity between furosemide, hydrochlorothiazide and sulphonamides is recorded, but the use of one of these drugs in a patient known to have allergy to another involves only low risk [13].

REFERENCES

1 Leitao EA, Person JR. Bumetanide-induced pseudoporphyria. *J Am Acad Dermatol* 1990; **23**: 129–30.
2 Bigby M, Jick S, Jick H, Arndt K. Drug-induced cutaneous reactions. A report from the Boston Collaborative Drug Surveillance Program on 15438 consecutive inpatients, 1975 to 1982. *JAMA* 1986; **256**: 3358–63.
3 Burry JN, Lawrence JR. Phototoxic blisters from high frusemide dosage. *Br J Dermatol* 1976; **94**: 493–9.
4 Gibson TP, Blue P. Erythema multiforme and furosemide therapy. *JAMA* 1970; **212**: 1709.
5 Zugerman C, La Voo EJ. Erythema multiforme caused by oral furosemide. *Arch Dermatol* 1980; **116**: 518–9.
6 Fellner MI, Katz JM. Occurrence of bullous pemphigoid after furosemide therapy. *Arch Dermatol* 1976; **112**: 75–7.
7 Castel T, Gratacos R, Castro J *et al.* Bullous pemphigoid induced by frusemide. *Clin Exp Dermatol* 1981; **6**: 635–8.
8 Ebringer A, Adam WR, Parkin JD. Bullous haemorrhagic eruption associated with frusemide. *Med J Aust* 1969; **1**: 768–71.
9 Kennedy AC, Lyell A. Acquired epidermolysis bullosa due to high dose frusemide. *BMJ* 1976; **i**: 1509–10.
10 Hansbrough JR, Wedner HJ, Chaplin DD. Anaphylaxis to intravenous furosemide. *J Allergy Clin Immunol* 1987; **80**: 538–41.
11 Hendricks WM, Ader RS. Furosemide-induced cutaneous necrotizing vasculitis. *Arch Dermatol* 1977; **113**: 375.
12 Cobb MW. Furosemide-induced eruption simulating Sweet's syndrome. *J Am Acad Dermatol* 1989; **21**: 339–43.
13 Sullivan TJ. Cross-reactions among furosemide, hydrochlorothiazide, and sulfonamides. *JAMA* 1991; **265**: 120–1.

Potassium-sparing diuretics

Spironolactone. This drug, which is also used for the treatment of acne vulgaris and hirsutism [1], may cause gynaecomastia [2–4], gastrointestinal upset, hyperkalaemia and rarely agranulocytosis [1]. Spironolactone has an anti-androgenic effect [4] and may result in loss of libido and impotence or menstrual irregularities. A maculopapular eruption [5], LE-like syndrome [6], annular LE [7], erythema annulare centrifugum [8] and a lichenoid eruption [9] have been seen.

REFERENCES

1 Shaw JC. Spironolactone in dermatologic therapy. *J Am Acad Dermatol* 1991; **24**: 236–43.
2 Clarke E. Spironolactone therapy and gynecomastia. *JAMA* 1965; **193**: 157–8.
3 Loriaux DL, Meuard R, Taylor A *et al.* Spironolactone and endocrine dysfunction. *Ann Intern Med* 1976; **85**: 630–6.
4 Rose LI, Underwood RH, Newmark SR *et al.* Pathophysiology of spironolactone-induced gynecomastia. *Ann Intern Med* 1977; **87**: 398–403.
5 Gupta AK, Knowles SR, Shear NH. Spironolactone-associated cutaneous effects: a case report and a review of the literature. *Dermatology* 1994; **189**: 402–5.
6 Uddin MS, Lynfield YL, Grosberg SJ, Stiefler R. Cutaneous reaction to spironolactone resembling lupus erythematosus. *Cutis* 1979; **24**: 198–200.
7 Leroy D, Dompmartin A, Le Jean S *et al.* Toxidermie a l'aldactone® à type d'érytheme annulaire centrifuge lupique. *Ann Dermatol Vénéréol* 1987; **114**: 1237–40.

8 Carsuzaa F, Pierre C, Dubegny M. Erytheme annulaire centrifuge à l'aldactone. *Ann Dermatol Vénéréol* 1987; **114**: 375–6.
9 Downham TF III Spironolactone-induced lichen planus. *JAMA* 1978; **240**: 1138.

Thiazides and related diuretics

Photosensitivity is uncommon, occurring in 1 in 1000 to 1 in 100 000 prescriptions [1–7]. Hydrochlorothiazide causes considerably more reactions than bendroflumethiazide (bendrofluazide). The mechanism is unknown, and both phototoxic [1,4,7] and photoallergic [2,3] mechanisms have been proposed. The commonest reaction is lichenoid [8], but petechial and erythematous eruptions may occur in exposed skin. Xerostomia has been reported, as has a vasculitis [9]. An eruption resembling subacute cutaneous LE has been described in patients taking a combination of hydrochlorothiazide and triamterene [10,11] and with hydrochlorothiazide alone [12]. Other side effects include hypokalaemia, short-term elevation of LDL cholesterol, impotence, a diabetogenic effect and exacerbation of gout [13].

Chlortalidone (chlorthalidone). Pseudoporphyria has been documented with this thiazide-related diuretic [14]. Psoriasis has been triggered in a patient also receiving captopril [15].

REFERENCES

1 Diffey BL, Langtry J. Phototoxic potential of thiazide diuretics in normal subjects. *Arch Dermatol* 1989; **125**: 1355–8.
2 Harber LC, Lashinsky AM, Baer RL. Photosensitivity to chlorothiazide and hydrochlorothiazide. *N Engl J Med* 1959; **261**: 1378–81.
3 Torinuki W. Photosensitivity due to hydrochlorothiazide. *J Dermatol* 1980; **7**: 293–6.
4 Rosén K, Swanbeck G. Phototoxic reactions from some common drugs provoked by a high-intensity UVA lamp. *Acta Derm Venereol (Stockh)* 1982; **62**: 246–8.
5 Hawk JLM. Photosensitizing agents used in the United Kingdom. *Clin Exp Dermatol* 1984; **9**: 300–2.
6 Robinson HN, Morison WL, Hood AF. Thiazide diuretic therapy and chronic photosensitivity. *Arch Dermatol* 1985; **121**: 522–4.
7 Addo HA, Ferguson J, Frain-Bell W. Thiazide-induced photosensitivity: a study of 33 subjects. *Br J Dermatol* 1987; **116**: 749–60.
8 Johnston GA. Thiazide-induced lichenoid photosensitivity. *Clin Exp Dermatol* 2002; **27**: 670–2.
9 Björnberg A, Gisslén H. Thiazides: a cause of necrotising vasculitis? *Lancet* 1965; **ii**: 982–3.
10 Berbis P, Vernay-Vaisse C, Privat Y. Lupus cutané subaigu observé au cours d'un traitement par diurétiques thiazidiques. *Ann Dermatol Vénéréol* 1986; **113**: 1245–8.
11 Darken M, McBurney EI. Subacute cutaneous lupus erythematosus-like drug eruption due to combination diuretic hydrochlorothiazide and triamterene. *J Am Acad Dermatol* 1988; **18**: 38–42.
12 Reed BR, Huff JC, Jones SK *et al.* Subacute cutaneous lupus erythematosus associated with hydrochlorothiazide therapy. *Ann Intern Med* 1985; **103**: 49–51.
13 Orme M. Thiazides in the 1990s. The risk : benefit ratio still favours the drug. *BMJ* 1990; **300**: 1168–9.
14 Baker EJ, Reed KD, Dixon SL. Chlorthalidone-induced pseudoporphyria: clinical and microscopic findings of a case. *J Am Acad Dermatol* 1989; **21**: 1026–9.
15 Wolf R, Dorfman B, Krakowski A. Psoriasiform eruption induced by captopril and chlorthalidone. *Cutis* 1987; **40**: 162–4.

Miscellaneous cardiovascular drugs

Dobutamine

Two patients with local dermal hypersensitivity at the site of dobutamine hydrochloride injection, consisting of erythema, pruritus and phlebitis with or without bullae, have been described [1]. Dermal cellulitis has also been reported [2].

Dopamine

This positive inotropic agent has caused local skin necrosis, due to extravasation at the site of an intravenous cannula [3], and acral gangrene secondary to distal vasoconstriction [4,5]. Localized piloerection and vasoconstriction proximal to the site of infusion have been documented [6]. Allergic reactions may occur [7].

REFERENCES

1 Wu CC, Chen WJ, Cheng J. Local dermal hypersensitivity from dobutamine hydrochloride (Dobutrex solution) injection. *Chest* 1991; **99**: 1547–8.
2 Cernek PK. Dermal cellulitis: a hypersensitivity reaction from dobutamine hydrochloride. *Ann Pharmacother* 1994; **28**: 964.
3 Green SI, Smith JW. Dopamine gangrene. *N Engl J Med* 1976; **294**: 114.
4 Boltax RS, Dineen JP, Scarpa FJ. Gangrene resulting from infiltrated dopamine solution. *N Engl J Med* 1977; **296**: 823.
5 Park JY, Kanzler M, Swetter SM. Dopamine-associated symmetric peripheral gangrene. *Arch Dermatol* 1997; **133**: 247–8.
6 Ross M. Dopamine-induced localized cutaneous vasoconstriction and piloerection. *Arch Dermatol* 1991; **127**: 586–7.
7 Merola B, Sarnacchiaro F, Colao A *et al.* Allergy to ergot-derived dopamine agonists. *Lancet* 1992; **339**: 620.

Vasopressin

This drug, when used intravenously for control of bleeding oesophageal varices or as a local vasoconstrictor agent, has caused cutaneous necrosis at sites of extravasation, and occasionally at distant sites, with a bullous eruption [1]. Mottling, cyanosis, ecchymoses, bullae, ulcers and gangrene are often preceded by coolness and paraesthesiae [2].

REFERENCES

1 Korenberg RJ, Landau-Price D, Penneys NS. Vasopressin-induced bullous disease and cutaneous necrosis. *J Am Acad Dermatol* 1986; **15**: 393–8.
2 Maceyko RF, Vidimos AT, Steck WD. Vasopressin-associated cutaneous infarcts, alopecia, and neuropathy. *J Am Acad Dermatol* 1994; **31**: 111–3.

Rutosides (Paroven)

This mixture of oxerutins, used for relief of symptoms of oedema related to chronic venous insufficiency and for reduction of lymphoedema, has been associated with transient urticaria [1].

REFERENCE

1 Anonymous. Paroven: not much effect in trials. *Drug Ther Bull* 1992; **30**: 7–8.

Drugs acting on the respiratory system

β-Agonists

Albuterol

Patchy erythema of the hands developed in a pregnant patient following infusion [1].

Salbutamol

LE-like acral erythema developed after infusion in three pregnant patients with premature labour [2].

Salmeterol

An urticarial reaction that recurred on challenge was attributed to this drug administered from a metered dose inhaler [3].

REFERENCES

1 Morin Leport LRM, Loisel JC, Feuilly C. Hand erythema due to infusion of sympathomimetics. *Br J Dermatol* 1990; **122**: 116–7.
2 Reygagne P, Lacour JP, Ortonne J-P. Palmar and plantar erythema due to infusion of sympathomimetics in pregnant women. *Br J Dermatol* 1991; **124**: 210.
3 Hatton MQF, Allen MB, Mellor EJ, Cooke NJ. Salmeterol rash. *Lancet* 1991; **337**: 1169–70.

Aminophylline

This drug is a mixture of theophylline and ethylenediamine. Urticaria, generalized erythema and exfoliative dermatitis have followed systemic administration, probably as a result of reactions to the ethylenediamine component rather than to theophylline itself [1]. Cross-reactions may occur with ethylenediamine in antihistamines and topical preparations [1,2]. Patch tests may or may not be positive [3].

REFERENCES

1 Gibb W, Thompson PJ. Allergy to aminophylline. *BMJ* 1983; **287**: 501.
2 Elias JA, Levinson AI. Hypersensitivity reactions to ethylenediamine in aminophylline. *Am Rev Respir Dis* 1981; **123**: 550–2.
3 Kradjan WA, Lakshminarayan S. Allergy to aminophylline: lack of predictability by skin testing. *Am J Hosp Pharm* 1981; **38**: 1031–3.

Miscellaneous respiratory system drugs

Sodium cromoglicate (sodium cromoglycate)

Hypersensitivity reactions are rare, but urticaria, angio-oedema and anaphylactic shock are recorded [1].

REFERENCE

1 Scheffer AL, Rocklin RE, Goetzl EJ. Immunologic components of hypersensitivity reactions to cromolyn sodium. *N Engl J Med* 1975; **293**: 1220–4.

Pseudoephedrine

This drug is present in nasal decongestants and has caused a fixed drug eruption [1–3], recurrent pseudoscarlatina [4,5], allergic reactions [6], systemic contact dermatitis [7] and a reaction simulating recurrent toxic shock syndrome [8].

REFERENCES

1 Shelley WB, Shelley ED. Nonpigmenting fixed drug reaction pattern: examples caused by sensitivity to pseudoephedrine hydrochloride and tetra-hydrozoline. *J Am Acad Dermatol* 1987; **17**: 403–7.
2 Hauken M. Fixed drug eruption and pseudoephedrine. *Ann Intern Med* 1994; **120**: 442.
3 Quan MB, Chow WC. Nonpigmenting fixed drug eruption after pseudoephedrine. *Int J Dermatol* 1996; **35**: 367–70.
4 Taylor BJ, Duffill MB. Recurrent pseudo-scarlatina and allergy to pseudoephedrine hydrochloride. *Br J Dermatol* 1988; **118**: 827–9.
5 Rochina A, Burches E, Morales C et al. Adverse reaction to pseudoephedrine. *J Invest Allergol Clin Immunol* 1995; **5**: 235–6.
6 Heydon J, Pillans P. Allergic reaction to pseudoephedrine. *NZ Med J* 1995; **108**: 112–3.
7 Tomb RR, Lepoittevin JP, Espinassouze F et al. Systemic contact dermatitis from pseudoephedrine. *Contact Dermatitis* 1991; **24**: 86–8.
8 Cavanah DK, Ballas ZK. Pseudoephedrine reaction presenting as recurrent toxic shock syndrome. *Ann Intern Med* 1993; **119**: 302–3.

Drugs acting on the renal system

Icodextrin

This new osmotic agent used in peritoneal dialysis has caused a variety of allergic reactions [1,2], a psoriasiform eruption limited to the palms and soles [3], and acute generalized exanthematous pustulosis [4].

REFERENCES

1 Goldsmith D, Jayawardene S, Sabharawal N, Cooney K. Allergic reactions to the polymeric glucose-based peritoneal dialysis fluid icodextrin in patients with renal failure. *Lancet* 2000; **355**: 897.
2 Divino Fiho JC. Allergic reactions to icodextrin in patients with renal failure. *Lancet* 2000; **355**: 1364–5.
3 Valance A, Lebrun-Vignes B, Descamps V. Icodextrin cutaneous hypersensitivity: report of 3 psoriasiform cases. *Arch Dermatol* 2001; **137**: 309–10.
4 Al-Hoqail IA, Crawford RI. Acute generalized exanthematous pustulosis induced by icodextrin. *Br J Dermatol* 2001; **145**: 1026–7.

Drugs acting on the skeletal system

Alendronate

This drug for osteoporosis has caused urticaria [1] and a gyrate erythema [2].

REFERENCES

1 Kontoleon P, Ilias I, Stavropoulos PG, Papapetrou PD. Urticaria after administration of alendronate. *Acta Derm Venereol (Stockh)* 2000; **80**: 398.
2 High WA, Cohen JB, Wetherington W, Cockerell CJ. Superficial gyrate erythema as a cutaneous reaction to alendronate for osteoporosis. *J Am Acad Dermatol* 2003; **48**: 945–6.

Drugs for erectile dysfunction

Sildenafil (Viagra)

A lichenoid reaction is reported [1].

REFERENCE

1 Goldman BD. Lichenoid drug reaction due to sildenafil. *Cutis* 2000; **65**: 282–3.

Metals and metal antagonists

Metals

Arsenic

Features of acute [1] and chronic [2] arsenic poisoning have been reviewed. Bullous eruptions, photosensitivity, exfoliative dermatitis, erythroderma with pustulation, and alopecia may be acute manifestations of arsenic toxicity. Occupational exposure may occur, especially in agriculture. Inorganic arsenic is sometimes present in Chinese proprietary medicines [2]. Fowler's solution (containing 1% potassium arsenite) and sodium arsenate were used in the past for psoriasis; as little as 0.19 g has been carcinogenic and the interval between exposure and tumour induction may be as long as 47 years [3]. Subjects with an abnormally high retention of ingested arsenic may be at particular risk [4]. The cutaneous manifestations of arsenic exposure, including macular pigmentation, palmoplantar punctate keratoses and intraepidermal (Bowen's disease), basal cell or squamous carcinomas of the skin, are well known [2–11]. Keratoses and tumours may be present without pigmentation. In one series of patients, there was a dose-related development of palmar and plantar keratoses in 40%, and carcinomas of the skin in 8%, of patients who received arsenic in the form of Fowler's solution for 6–26 years; the minimum latent period before development of keratoses was 2.5 years, and the average was 6 years [5]. In another series, Bowen's disease occurred within 10 years and invasive carcinomas within 20 years [9]. The lag times for development of keratoses, Bowen's disease and squamous cell cancer were, respectively, 28, 39 and 41 years in another series [2]. Arsenic contamination of well water in Taiwan resulted in numerous affected individuals with arsenical keratoses and cutaneous carcinomas [7]. Carcinomas may arise in the arsenical keratoses [7]. Groundwater contamination leads to an endemic problem [12,13]. Cutaneous electron microscopic changes are said to be characteristic [10]. The diagnostic significance of the skin arsenic content is disputed. A 42-year-old man who took arsenic for 35 years for psoriasis developed melanoderma, keratoses, muscular dystrophies, hyperlipidaemia, testicular atrophy, gynaecomastia, skin tumours and an obliterating angiitis of leg vessels, which led to amputation [6]. The role of arsenic in causing internal malignancy is the subject of controversy [9,14,15].

REFERENCES

1 Bartolomé B, Córdoba S, Nieto S *et al.* Acute arsenic poisoning: clinical and histopathological features. *Br J Dermatol* 1999; **141**: 1106–9.
2 Wong SS, Tan KC, Goh CL. Cutaneous manifestations of chronic arsenicism: review of seventeen cases. *J Am Acad Dermatol* 1998; **38**: 179–85.
3 Evans S. Arsenic and cancer. *Br J Dermatol* 1977; **97** (Suppl. 15): 13–4.
4 Bettley FR, O'Shea JA. The absorption of arsenic and its relation to carcinoma. *Br J Dermatol* 1975; **92**: 563–8.
5 Fierz U. Katamnestische Untersuchungen über die Nebenwirkungen der Therapie mit anorganischem Arsen bei Hautkrankheiten. *Dermatologica* 1965; **131**: 41–58.
6 Meyhofer W, Knoth W. Über die Auswirkung einer langjährigen antipsoriatischen Arsentherapie auf mehrere Organe unter besonderer Berücksichtigung andrologischer Befunde. *Hautarzt* 1966; **117**: 309–13.
7 Yeh S. Skin cancer in chronic arsenicism. *Hum Pathol* 1973; **4**: 469–85.
8 Weiss J, Jänner M. Multiple Basaliome und Menigiom nach mehrjähriger Arsentherapie. *Hautarzt* 1980; **31**: 654–6.
9 Miki Y, Kawatsu T, Matsuda K *et al.* Cutaneous and pulmonary cancers associated with Bowen's disease. *J Am Acad Dermatol* 1982; **6**: 26–31.
10 Ohyama K, Sonoda K, Kuwahara H. Electron microscopic observations of arsenical keratoses and Bowen's disease associated with chronic arsenicism. *Dermatologica* 1982; **64**: 161–6.
11 Ratnam KV, Espy MJ, Muller SA *et al.* Clinicopathologic study of arsenic-induced skin lesions: no definite association with human papillomavirus. *J Am Acad Dermatol* 1992; **27**: 120–2.
12 Woollons A, Russell-Jones R. Chronic endemic hydroarsenicism. *Br J Dermatol* 1998; **139**: 1092–6.
13 Kurokawa M, Ogata K, Idemori M *et al.* Investigation of skin manifestations of arsenicism due to intake of arsenic-contaminated groundwater in residents of Samta, Jessore, Bangladesh. *Arch Dermatol* 2001; **137**: 102–3.
14 Reymann F, Møller R, Nielsen A. Relationship between arsenic intake and internal malignant neoplasms. *Arch Dermatol* 1978; **114**: 378–81.
15 Callen JP, Headington J. Bowen's and non-Bowen's squamous intraepidermal neoplasia of the skin. Relationship to internal malignancy. *Arch Dermatol* 1980; **116**: 422–6.

Gold

The use of gold in rheumatoid arthritis is associated with a 23–30% incidence of reactions [1–3]; most of these are minor, but about 15% may be severe or even fatal [4]. Possession of the HLA-DR3 and HLA-B8 phenotypes reportedly predisposes to thrombocytopenia, leukopenia and nephrotoxicity, HLA-DR4 is linked to leukopenia, and

HLA-B7 is associated with cutaneous adverse reactions [2]. In another study, HLA-DR5 was significantly associated with mucocutaneous lesions, whereas HLA-B8 and HLA-DR3 antigens were associated with proteinuria in rheumatoid arthritis patients after gold therapy; HLA-DR7 was negatively associated with reactions and may confer protection, and HLA-B27 was associated with chrysiasis due to gold therapy [5]. A further study showed that gold dermatitis in patients with rheumatoid arthritis was associated with HLA-B35 and disease duration [6]. Antibodies to the Ro 52-kDa antigen are associated with skin eruptions in rheumatoid arthritis patients treated with gold [7].

Rashes and mouth ulcers are common [1,2,8–13], representing about 50% of all complications with parenteral gold and 35% of those with oral gold. Localized or generalized pruritus is an important warning sign of potential toxicity. Gold reactions may simulate exanthematic eruptions [14], erythema annulare centrifugum [15], seborrhoeic dermatitis or lichen planus [16,17]; a mixture of these patterns, sometimes with discoid eczematoid lesions, is characteristic. Lichen planus is often of the hypertrophic variety especially on the scalp, and severe and irreversible alopecia may follow [18]. There may be striking and persistent post-inflammatory hyperpigmentation. Permanent nail dystrophy has followed onycholysis [19]. Yellow nails have been described [20].

In one study, eczematous or lichenoid rashes persisted up to 11 months after cessation of therapy [21]. Histology was characterized by a sparse dermal perivascular infiltrate, predominantly of CD4$^+$ HLA-DR-positive helper T lymphocytes, an increase in the number of dermal Langerhans' cells and epidermal macrophage-like cells, and Langerhans' cell apposition to mononuclear cells. A patient with a lichenoid and seborrhoeic dermatitis-like rash on gold sodium thiomalate therapy had a positive intradermal test to gold thiomalate; patch tests were positive to thiomalate (the thiol carrier of gold thiomalate) but negative to gold itself [22]. Interestingly, the same patient subsequently developed a seborrhoeic dermatitis-like eruption, but not a lichenoid eruption, while on auranofin; this time, patch tests were positive to both auranofin and gold. A previous contact dermatitis from gold jewellery may be reactivated [23].

Other reactions documented include erythema nodosum [24], severe hypersensitivity reactions [25], vasculitis [26], polyarteritis, an SLE-like syndrome, generalized exfoliative dermatitis and TEN. Psoriasis was reported to be exacerbated in a patient with arthritis treated with gold [27].

Prolonged administration of gold may cause a distinct grey, blue or purple pigmentation of exposed skin (chrysiasis), which is a dose-dependent reaction that occurs above a threshold of 20 mg/kg; gold granules are seen within dermal endothelial cells and macrophages [28–32]. Even in the absence of pigmentation, gold can be detected histochemically in the skin up to 20 years after therapy.

Localized argyria with chrysiasis has been caused by implanted acupuncture needles [33]. An unusual late cutaneous reaction involved the appearance of widespread keloid-like angiofibromatoid lesions [34].

A benign vasodilatory 'nitritoid' reaction, consisting of flushing, light-headedness and transient hypotension, may occur immediately after the first injection of gold [2,35]. It occurs in roughly 5% of patients taking gold sodium thiomalate. Non-vasomotor effects, including arthralgia, myalgia and constitutional symptoms within the first 24 h, are recognized. Mucous membrane symptoms include loss of taste, metallic taste, stomatitis, glossitis and diarrhoea. Punctate stomatitis may occur with or without skin lesions. Gold is also deposited in the cornea and may cause a keratitis with ulceration. A polyneuropathy is recorded. In general, auranofin is less toxic than intramuscular gold [2]. Eosinophilia is common and may sometimes herald another complication; serum IgE may be raised [36]. Other immunological reactions are rare, although pulmonary fibrosis is recorded [37]. Blood dyscrasias, especially thrombocytopenic purpura, and occasionally fatal neutropenia or aplastic anaemia occur in a small proportion of cases and usually present within the first 6 months of therapy. Jaundice occurs in about 3% of cases, and may result from idiosyncratic intrahepatic cholestasis [38]. Proteinuria and renal damage are well known.

REFERENCES

1 Thomas I. Gold therapy and its indications in dermatology. A review. *J Am Acad Dermatol* 1987; **16**: 845–54.
2 Pullar T. Adverse reactions profile: 1. Gold. *Prescribers J* 1991; **31**: 22–6.
3 Lemmel EM. Comparison of pyritinol and auranofin in the treatment of rheumatoid arthritis. The European Multicentre Study Group. *Br J Rheumatol* 1993; **32**: 375–82.
4 Girdwood RH. Death after taking medicaments. *BMJ* 1974; **i**: 501–4.
5 Rodriguez-Perez M, Gonzalez-Dominguez J, Mataran L *et al.* Association of HLA-DR5 with mucocutaneous lesions in patients with rheumatoid arthritis receiving gold sodium thiomalate. *J Rheumatol* 1994; **21**: 41–3.
6 van Gestel A, Koopman R, Wijnands M *et al.* Mucocutaneous reactions to gold: a prospective study of 74 patients with rheumatoid arthritis. *J Rheumatol* 1994; **21**: 1814–9.
7 Tishler M, Nyman J, Wahren M, Yaron M. Anti-Ro (SSA) antibodies in rheumatoid arthritis patients with gold-induced side effects. *Rheumatol Int* 1997; **17**: 133–5.
8 Almeyda J, Baker H. Drug reactions XII. Cutaneous reactions to antirheumatic drugs. *Br J Dermatol* 1970; **83**: 707–11.
9 Penneys NS, Ackerman AB, Gottlieb NL. Gold dermatitis: a clinical and histopathological study. *Arch Dermatol* 1974; **109**: 372–6.
10 Penneys NS. Gold therapy: dermatologic uses and toxicities. *J Am Acad Dermatol* 1979; **1**: 315–20.
11 Webster CG, Burnett JW. Gold dermatitis. *Cutis* 1994; **54**: 25–8.
12 Lizeaux-Parmeix V, Bedane C, Lavignac C *et al.* Reactions cutanées aux sels d'or. *Ann Dermatol Vénéréol* 1994; **121**: 793–7.
13 Laeijendecker R, van Joost T. Oral manifestations of gold allergy. *J Am Acad Dermatol* 1994; **30**: 205–9.
14 Möller H, Björkner B, Bruze M. Clinical reactions to systemic provocation with gold sodium thiomalate in patients with contact allergy to gold. *Br J Dermatol* 1996; **135**: 423–7.
15 Tsuji T, Nishimura M, Kimura S. Erythema annulare centrifugum associated with gold sodium thiomalate therapy. *J Am Acad Dermatol* 1992; **27**: 284–7.
16 Lasarowa AZ, Tsankov NK, Stoimenov AP. Lichenoide Eruptionen nach Goldtherapie. Bericht uber zwei Falle. *Hautarzt* 1992; **43**: 514–6.

17 Russell MA, King LE Jr, Boyd AS. Lichen planus after consumption of a gold-containing liquor. *N Engl J Med* 1996; **334**: 603.

18 Burrows NP, Grant JW, Crisp AJ, Roberts SO. Scarring alopecia following gold therapy. *Acta Derm Venereol (Stockh)* 1994; **74**: 486.

19 Voigt K, Holzegel K. Bleibende nagelveränderungen nach Goldtherapie. *Hautarzt* 1977; **28**: 421–3.

20 Roest MAB, Ratnavel R. Yellow nails associated with gold therapy for rheumatoid arthritis. *Br J Dermatol* 2001; **145**: 855–6.

21 Ranki A, Niemi K-M, Kanerva L. Clinical, immunohistochemical, and electron-microscopic findings in gold dermatitis. *Am J Dermatopathol* 1989; **11**: 22–8.

22 Ikezawa Z, Kitamura K, Nakajima H. Gold sodium thiomalate (GTM) induces hypersensitivity to thiomalate, the thiol carrier of GTM. *J Dermatol* 1990; **17**: 550–4.

23 Rennie T. Local gold toxicity. *BMJ* 1976; **ii**: 1294.

24 Stone RL, Claflin A, Penneys NS. Erythema nodosum following gold sodium thiomalate therapy. *Arch Dermatol* 1973; **107**: 603–4.

25 Walzer RA, Feinstein R, Shapiro L, Einbinder J. Severe hypersensitivity reaction to gold. Positive lymphocyte transformation test. *Arch Dermatol* 1972; **106**: 231–4.

26 Roenigk HR, Handel D. Gold vasculitis. *Arch Dermatol* 1974; **109**: 253–5.

27 Smith DL, Wernick R. Exacerbation of psoriasis by chrysotherapy. *Arch Dermatol* 1991; **127**: 268–70.

28 Beckett VL, Doyle JA, Hadley GA et al. Chrysiasis resulting from gold therapy in rheumatoid arthritis: identification of gold by X-ray microanalysis. *Mayo Clin Proc* 1982; **57**: 773–5.

29 Pelachyk IM, Bergfeld WF, McMahon JT. Chrysiasis following gold therapy for rheumatoid arthritis. *J Cutan Pathol* 1984; **11**: 491–4.

30 Smith RW, Leppard B, Barnett NL et al. Chrysiasis revisited: a clinical and pathological study. *Br J Dermatol* 1995; **133**: 671–8.

31 Fleming CJ, Salisbury ELC, Kirwan P et al. Chrysiasis after low-dose gold and UV light exposure. *J Am Acad Dermatol* 1996; **34**: 349–51.

32 Keen CE, Brady K, Kirkham N, Levison DA. Gold in the dermis following chrysotherapy: histopathology and microanalysis. *Histopathology* 1993; **23**: 355–60.

33 Suzuki H, Baba S, Uchigasaki S, Murase M. Localized argyria with chrysiasis caused by implanted acupuncture needles. Distribution and chemical forms of silver and gold in cutaneous tissue by electron microscopy and X-ray microanalysis. *J Am Acad Dermatol* 1993; **29**: 833–7.

34 Herbst WM, Hornstein OP, Grießmeyer G. Ungewöhnliche kutane Angiofibromatose nach Goldtherapie einer primär chronischen Polyarthritis. *Hautarzt* 1989; **40**: 568–72.

35 Arthur AB, Klinkhoff A, Teufel A. Nitritoid reactions: case reports, review, and recommendations for management. *J Rheumatol* 2001; **28**: 2209–12.

36 Davis P, Ezeoke A, Munro J et al. Immunological studies on the mechanism of gold hypersensitivity reactions. *BMJ* 1973; **iii**: 676–8.

37 Morley TF, Komansky HJ, Adelizzi RA et al. Pulmonary gold toxicity. *Eur J Respir Dis* 1984; **65**: 627–32.

38 Favreau M, Tannebaum H, Lough J. Hepatic toxicity associated with gold therapy. *Ann Intern Med* 1977; **87**: 717–9.

Iron

Iron-induced brownish discoloration has been noted at the site of local injection (local siderosis) [1].

REFERENCE

1 Bork K. Lokalisierte kutane Siderose nach intramuskulären Eiseninjektion. *Hautarzt* 1984; **35**: 598–9.

Mercury

Skin manifestations of mercury exposure have been reviewed [1,2]. Mercury-containing teething powders have long been banned, but occasional occupational or environmental exposure can occur. Mercury amalgam in dental fillings has caused buccal pigmentation. Stomatitis may occur as a toxic reaction. Allergic reactions may be scarlatiniform or morbilliform, and can progress to generalized exfoliative dermatitis. Eczema is recorded [3]. Pink disease or acrodynia, a distinctive pattern of reaction to chronic exposure to mercury in young infants and children, is now very rare [4]. Painful extremities, pinkish acral discoloration, peeling of the palms and soles, gingivitis and various systemic complications may occur. Acrodynia developed in a child following inhalation of mercury-containing vapours from phenyl-mercuric acetate contained in latex paint [5]. A mercury-containing drug given for 3 weeks to a patient with long-standing pustular psoriasis of the palms was associated with development of generalized pustular psoriasis [6]. (See also exogenous ochronosis from topical mercury-containing preparations, p. 73.168.) Cutaneous granulomas are recorded [1], and a nodular reaction occurred after intake of a duck soup that contained metallic mercury for a neck abscess 18 years previously [7].

REFERENCES

1 Boyd AS, Seger D, Vannucci S et al. Mercury exposure and cutaneous disease. *J Am Acad Dermatol* 2000; **43**: 81–90.

2 Chan MHM, Cheung RCK, Chan IHS, Lam CWK. An unusual case of mercury intoxication. *Br J Dermatol* 2001; **144**: 192–4.

3 Adachi A, Horikawa T, Takashima T, Ichihashi M. Mercury-induced nummular eczema. *J Am Acad Dermatol* 2000; **43**: 383–5.

4 Dinehart SM, Dillard R, Raimer SS et al. Cutaneous manifestations of acrodynia (pink disease). *Arch Dermatol* 1988; **124**: 107–9.

5 Anonymous. From the MMWR. Mercury exposure from interior latex paint: Michigan. *Arch Dermatol* 1990; **126**: 577.

6 Wehner-Caroli J, Scherwitz C, Schweinsberg F, Fierlbeck G. Exazerbation einer Psoriasis pustulosa bei Quecksilber-Intoxikation. *Hautarzt* 1994; **45**: 708–10.

7 June JB, Min PK, Kim DW et al. Cutaneous nodular reaction to oral mercury. *J Am Acad Dermatol* 1997; **37**: 131–3.

Silver

Ingestion of silver or topical application of silver preparations to the oral mucosa or upper respiratory tract can produce slate-blue discoloration, especially of exposed skin, including oral and conjunctival mucosae [1–8]. Argyria localized to the left hand occurred in an antique restorer due to polishing silver [9]. Topical application may also cause systemic argyria, in which visceral organs are also discoloured [10]. Localized argyria can result when the backs of earrings become embedded [11]. In some patients, the nail beds of the fingers but not the toes may show bluish discoloration [12]. Silver granules are found free within the dermis; melanin may be increased in the epidermis or within melanophages [13–15].

REFERENCES

1 Pariser RJ. Generalized argyria. Clinicopathologic features and histochemical studies. *Arch Dermatol* 1978; **114**: 373–7.

2 Reynold J-L, Stoebner P, Amblard P. Argyrie cutanée. Étude en microscopie electronique et en microanalyse X de 4 cas. *Ann Dermatol Vénéréol* 1980; **107**: 251–5.

3 Johansson EA, Kanerva L, Niemi K-M *et al.* Generalized argyria with low ceruloplasmin and copper levels in the serum. A case report with clinical and microscopical findings and a trial of penicillamine treatment. *Clin Exp Dermatol* 1982; **7**: 169–76.

4 Pezzarossa E, Alinovi A, Ferrari C. Generalized argyria. *J Cutan Pathol* 1983; **10**: 361–3.

5 Gherardi R, Brochard P, Chamak B *et al.* Human generalized argyria. *Arch Pathol Lab Med* 1984; **108**: 181–2.

6 Jurecka W. Generalisierte Argyrose. *Hautarzt* 1986; **37**: 628–31.

7 Mittag H, Knecht J, Arnold R *et al.* Zur Frage der Argyrie. Ein klinische, analytisch-chemische und mikromorphologische Untersuchung. *Hautarzt* 1987; **38**: 670–7.

8 Tanner LS, Gross DJ. Generalized argyria. *Cutis* 1990; **45**: 237–9.

9 Kapur N, Landon G, YuRC. Localized argryia in an antique restorer. *Br J Dermatol* 2001; **144**: 191–2.

10 Marshall IP, Schneider RP. Systemic argyria secondary to topical silver nitrate. *Arch Dermatol* 1977; **113**: 1077–9.

11 van den Nieuwenhijsen IJ, Calame JJ, Bruynzeel DP. Localized argyria caused by silver earrings. *Dermatologica* 1988; **177**: 189–91.

12 Plewig G, Lincke H, Wolff HH. Silver-blue nails. *Acta Derm Venereol (Stockh)* 1977; **57**: 413–9.

13 Hönigsmann H, Konrad K, Wolff K. Argyrose (Histologie und Ultrastruktur). *Hautarzt* 1973; **24**: 24–30.

14 Shelley WB, Shelley ED, Burmeister V. Argyria: the intradermal 'photograph', a manifestation of passive photosensitivity. *J Am Acad Dermatol* 1987; **16**: 211–7.

15 Sato S, Sueki H, Nishijima A. Two unusual cases of argyria: the application of an improved tissue processing method for X-ray microanalysis of selenium and sulphur in silver-laden granules. *Br J Dermatol* 1999; **140**: 158–63.

Metal antagonists

Deferoxamine (desferrioxamine)

Itching, erythema and urticaria are occasionally seen [1]. An indurated erythema with oedema lasting 2 weeks has been reported following infusion of this drug [2].

REFERENCES

1 Bousquet J, Navarra M, Robert G *et al.* Rapid desensitisation for desferrioxamine anaphylactoid reactions. *Lancet* 1983; **ii**: 859–60.

2 Venencie P-Y, Rain B, Blanc A, Tertian G. Toxidermie a la déféroxamine (Desféral). *Ann Derm Vénéréol* 1988; **115**: 1174.

Penicillamine

There is a fourfold increase in toxicity with this drug in patients with rheumatoid arthritis who have a genetically determined poor capacity to sulphoxidate the structurally related mucolytic agent carbocysteine [1,2]. In addition, penicillamine toxicity is independently associated with HLA phenotype [1–3]. HLA-DR3 and HLA-B8 are associated with renal toxicity, HLA-DR3, HLA-B7 and HLA-DR2 with haematological toxicity, and HLA-A1 and HLA-DR4 with thrombocytopenia. Cutaneous adverse reactions are linked to HLA-DRw6. Anti-Ro(SSA)-positive patients with rheumatoid arthritis more often developed rashes and acute febrile reactions [4].

The cutaneous side effects of this chelating agent comprise three distinct types: (i) acute hypersensitivity reactions occurring early during treatment, (ii) late reactions including disturbances of autoimmune mechanisms leading to pemphigus foliaceus or erythematosus and cicatricial pemphigoid, and (iii) lathyrogenic effects on connective tissue [2,5–9]. Hypersensitivity reactions are common and consist of urticarial or morbilliform rashes appearing within the first few weeks; the eruption clears on drug withdrawal and does not always recur on re-exposure. It is possible to desensitize patients to penicillamine [10].

Autoimmune syndromes caused by penicillamine are well documented. The development of pemphigus during the treatment of both Wilson's disease and rheumatoid arthritis with penicillamine was first noted in the French literature [11,12]. Since then, there have been numerous case reports [13–25]; about 7% of patients receiving penicillamine for more than 6 months develop drug-induced pemphigus [13]. The reader is referred to the section on drug-induced pemphigus (p. 73.40). Findings with direct immunofluorescence mimic the idiopathic disorder, with epidermal intercellular deposition of immunoreactants [16]. Most patients develop pemphigus foliaceus, although there have been isolated reports of pemphigus vulgaris [14] and of pemphigus erythematosus with both epidermal intercellular and subepidermal deposition of IgG [15,17]. In some patients, clinical appearances may resemble dermatitis herpetiformis [21,22]. Oral lesions may be indistinguishable from those seen in idiopathic pemphigus, with cheilosis, glossitis and stomatitis [23]. Painful erosive vulvovaginitis may lead to scarring. Penicillamine-induced pemphigus usually subsides rapidly after cessation of the drug; occasionally it may be more persistent [13] and fatalities have occurred [24,25]. A curious bullous dermatosis without the features of pemphigus has been described recently [26]. Other autoimmune manifestations include a bullous pemphigoid-like reaction [27], cicatricial pemphigoid [28,29], both discoid and systemic LE [30–33], dermatomyositis [34–37], and both morphoea and systemic sclerosis [38,39]. Pre-existing lichen planus [40] may be exacerbated, and lichenoid eruptions develop *de novo* [41,42]. Alopecia, facial dryness and scaling, nail changes and hypertrichosis are recorded. The yellow nail syndrome has been reported frequently in association with penicillamine [43].

Prolonged high-dose therapy for more than a year, as for Wilson's disease, has effects on collagen and elastin [44,45], resulting from inhibition of the condensation of soluble tropocollagen to insoluble collagen. There is anisodiametricity of connective tissue fibres, resulting in the 'lumpy-bumpy' elastic fibre [46–48]. The skin becomes wrinkled and thin, aged looking and abnormally fragile; asymptomatic, violaceous, friable, haemorrhagic macules, papules and plaques develop on pressure sites, and minor trauma causes ecchymoses [49]. There may be light-blue anetoderma-like lesions [50], and small white papules at

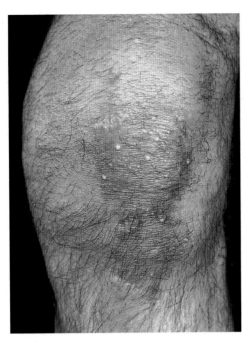

Fig. 73.6 Penicillamine dermopathy with milia. (Courtesy of St John's Institute of Dermatology, London, UK.)

venepuncture sites. Lymphangiectasis may develop [49]. Blisters may occur, with a picture resembling epidermolysis bullosa with scarring and milia formation (Fig. 73.6) [51]. Cutis laxa and elastosis perforans serpiginosa [52–58], which may be verruciform [52,53], are described. Lesions resembling pseudoxanthoma elasticum have been documented rarely [59–62].

Penicillamine may induce impaired taste sensation in up to 25% of patients, but other gastrointestinal effects are usually minor. Important non-dermatological complications [2,8] include marrow suppression; various renal problems, such as reversible proteinuria, in up to 30% of patients on therapy for more than 6 months; established nephrotic syndrome; and Goodpasture's syndrome. Thrombocytopenia occurs in up to 3% of patients, and may be either of gradual or precipitous onset. Immunological abnormalities include acquired IgA deficiency [63] and development of myasthenia gravis [64]. The bones may be involved in the connective tissue disorder. A chronic bronchoalveolitis is recognized [65]. Breast enlargement and breast gigantism [66] are documented.

REFERENCES

1 Emery P, Panayi GS, Huston G *et al*. D-Penicillamine-induced toxicity in rheumatoid arthritis: the role of sulphoxidation status and HLA-DR3. *J Rheumatol* 1984; **11**: 626–32.

2 Dasgupta B. Adverse reactions profile: 2. Penicillamine. *Prescribers J* 1991; **31**: 72–7.

3 Wooley PH, Griffin J, Panayi GS *et al*. HLA-DR antigens and toxic reaction to sodium aurothiomalate and D-penicillamine in patients with rheumatoid arthritis. *N Engl J Med* 1980; **303**: 300–2.

4 Vlachoyiannopoulos PG, Zerva LV, Skopouli FN *et al*. D-Penicillamine toxicity in Greek patients with rheumatoid arthritis: anti-Ro(SSA) antibodies and cryoglobulinemia are predictive factors. *J Rheumatol* 1991; **18**: 44–9.

5 Katz R. Penicillamine-induced skin lesions. Occurrence in a patient with hepatolenticular degeneration (Wilson's disease). *Arch Dermatol* 1967; **95**: 196–8.

6 Greer KE, Askew FC, Richardson DR. Skin lesions induced by penicillamine. *Arch Dermatol* 1976; **112**: 1267–9.

7 Sternlieb I, Fisher M, Scheinberg IH. Penicillamine-induced skin lesions. *J Rheumatol* 1981; **8** (Suppl. 7): 149–54.

8 Levy RS, Fisher M, Alter JN. Penicillamine: review and cutaneous manifestations. *J Am Acad Dermatol* 1983; **8**: 548–58.

9 Bialy-Golan A, Brenner S. Penicillamine-induced bullous dermatoses. *J Am Acad Dermatol* 1996; **35**: 732–42.

10 Chan CY, Baker AL. Penicillamine hypersensitivity: successful desensitization of a patient with severe hepatic Wilson's disease. *Am J Gastroenterol* 1994; **89**: 442–3.

11 Degos R, Touraine R, Belaïch S *et al*. Pemphigus chez un malade traité par pénicillamine pour maladie de Wilson. *Bull Soc Fr Dermatol Syphiligr* 1969; **76**: 751–3.

12 Benveniste M, Crouzet J, Homberg JC *et al*. Pemphigus induit par la D-pénicillamine dans la polyarthrite rhumatoïde. *Nouv Presse Med* 1975; **4**: 3125–8.

13 Marsden RA, Ryan TJ, Vanhegan RI *et al*. Pemphigus foliaceus induced by penicillamine. *BMJ* 1976; **ii**: 1423–4.

14 From E, Frederiksen P. Pemphigus vulgaris following D-penicillamine. *Dermatologica* 1976; **152**: 358–62.

15 Thorvaldsen J. Two cases of penicillamine-induced pemphigus erythematosus. *Dermatologica* 1979; **159**: 167–70.

16 Santa Cruz DJ, Prioleau PG, Marcus MD, Uitto J. Pemphigus-like lesions induced by D-penicillamine. Analysis of clinical, histopathological, and immunofluorescence features in 34 cases. *Am J Dermatopathol* 1981; **3**: 85–92.

17 Yung CW, Hambrick GW Jr. D-Penicillamine-induced pemphigus syndrome. *J Am Acad Dermatol* 1982; **6**: 317–24.

18 Bahmer FA, Bambauer R, Stenger D. Penicillamine-induced pemphigus foliaceus-like dermatosis. A case with unusual features, successfully treated by plasmapheresis. *Arch Dermatol* 1985; **121**: 665–8.

19 Kind P, Goerz G, Gleichmann E, Plewig G. Penicillamininduzierter Pemphigus. *Hautarzt* 1987; **38**: 548–52.

20 Civatte J. Durch Medikamente induzierte Pemphigus-Erkrankungen. *Dermatol Monatsschr* 1989; **175**: 1–7.

21 Marsden RA, Dawber RPR, Millard PR, Mowat AG. Herpetiform pemphigus induced by penicillamine. *Br J Dermatol* 1977; **97**: 451–2.

22 Weltfriend S, Ingber A, David M, Sandbank M. Pemphigus herpetiformis nach D-Penicillamin bei einem Patienten mit HLA B8. *Hautarzt* 1988; **39**: 587–8.

23 Eisenberg E, Ballow M, Wolfe SH *et al*. Pemphigus-like mucosal lesions: a side effect of penicillamine therapy. *Oral Surg* 1981; **51**: 409–14.

24 Sparrow GP. Penicillamine pemphigus and the nephrotic syndrome occurring simultaneously. *Br J Dermatol* 1978; **98**: 103–5.

25 Matkaluk RM, Bailin PL. Penicillamine-induced pemphigus foliaceus. A fatal outcome. *Arch Dermatol* 1981; **117**: 156–7.

26 Fulton RA, Thomson J. Penicillamine-induced bullous dermatosis. *Br J Dermatol* 1982; **107** (Suppl. 22): 95–6.

27 Brown MD, Dubin HV. Penicillamine-induced bullous pemphigoid-like eruption. *Arch Dermatol* 1987; **123**: 1119–20.

28 Pegum JS, Pembroke AC. Benign mucous membrane pemphigoid associated with penicillamine treatment. *BMJ* 1977; **i**: 1473.

29 Shuttleworth D, Graham-Brown RAC, Hutchinson PE, Jolliffe DS. Cicatricial pemphigoid in D-penicillamine treated patients with rheumatoid arthritis: a report of three cases. *Clin Exp Dermatol* 1985; **10**: 392–7.

30 Burns DA, Sarkany I. Penicillamine induced discoid lupus erythematosus. *Clin Exp Dermatol* 1979; **4**: 389–92.

31 Walshe JM. Penicillamine and the SLE syndrome. *J Rheumatol* 1981; **8** (Suppl. 7): 155–60.

32 Chalmers A, Thompson D, Stein HE *et al*. Systemic lupus erythematosus during penicillamine therapy for rheumatoid arthritis. *Ann Intern Med* 1982; **97**: 659–63.

33 Tsankov NK, Lazarov AZ, Vasileva S, Obreshkova EV. Lupus erythematosus-like eruption due to D-penicillamine in progressive systemic sclerosis. *Int J Dermatol* 1990; **29**: 571–4.

34 Simpson NB, Golding JR. Dermatomyositis induced by penicillamine. *Acta Derm Venereol (Stockh)* 1979; **59**: 543–4.

35 Wojnarowska F. Dermatomyositis induced by penicillamine. *J R Soc Med* 1980; **73**: 884–6.

36 Carroll GC, Will RK, Peter JB *et al*. Penicillamine induced polymyositis and dermatomyositis. *J Rheumatol* 1987; **14**: 995–1001.

37 Wilson CL, Bradlow A, Wojnarowska F. Cutaneous problems with drug therapy in rheumatoid arthritis. *Int J Dermatol* 1991; **30**: 148–9.

38 Bernstein RM, Hall MA, Gostelow BE. Morphea-like reaction to D-penicillamine therapy. *Ann Rheum Dis* 1981; **40**: 42–4.

39 Miyagawa S, Yoshioka A, Hatoko M *et al*. Systemic sclerosis-like lesions during long-term penicillamine therapy for Wilson's disease. *Br J Dermatol* 1987; **116**: 95–100.

40 Powell FC, Rogers RS III, Dickson ER. Lichen planus, primary biliary cirrhosis and penicillamine. *Br J Dermatol* 1982; **107**: 616.

41 Seehafer JR, Rogers RS III, Fleming R, Dickson ER. Lichen planus-like lesions caused by penicillamine in primary biliary cirrhosis. *Arch Dermatol* 1981; **117**: 140–2.

42 Van Hecke E, Kint A, Temmerman L. A lichenoid eruption induced by penicillamine. *Arch Dermatol* 1981; **117**: 676–7.

43 Ilchyshyn A, Vickers CFH. Yellow nail syndrome associated with penicillamine therapy. *Acta Derm Venereol (Stockh)* 1983; **63**: 554–5.

44 Poon E, Mason GH, Oh C. Clinical and histological spectrum of elastotic changes induced by penicillamine. *Australas J Dermatol* 2002; **43**: 147–50.

45 Iozumi K, Nakagawa H, Tamaki K. Penicillamine-induced degenerative dermatoses: report of a case and brief review of such dermatoses. *J Dermatol* 1997; **24**: 458–65.

46 Bardach H, Gebhart W, Niebauer G. 'Lumpy-bumpy' elastic fibers in the skin and lungs of a patient with a penicillamine-induced elastosis perforans serpiginosa. *J Cutan Pathol* 1979; **6**: 243–52.

47 Gebhart W, Bardach H. The 'lumpy-bumpy' elastic fiber. A marker for long-term administration of penicillamine. *Am J Dermatopathol* 1981; **3**: 33–9.

48 Hashimoto K, McEvoy B, Belcher R. Ultrastructure of penicillamine-induced skin lesions. *J Am Acad Dermatol* 1981; **4**: 300–15.

49 Goldstein JB, McNutt S, Hambrick GW. Penicillamine dermatopathy with lymphangiectases. A clinical, immunohistologic, and ultrastructural study. *Arch Dermatol* 1989; **125**: 92–7.

50 Davis W. Wilson's disease and penicillamine-induced anetoderma. *Arch Dermatol* 1977; **113**: 976.

51 Beer WE, Cooke KB. Epidermolysis bullosa induced by penicillamine. *Br J Dermatol* 1967; **79**: 123–5.

52 Guilane J, Benhamou JP, Molas G. Élastome perforant verruciforme chez un malade traité par pénicillamine pour maladie de Wilson. *Bull Soc Fr Derm Syph* 1972; **79**: 450–3.

53 Sfar Z, Lakhua M, Kamoun MR *et al*. Deux cas d'élastomes verruciforme après administration prolongée de D-pénicillamine. *Ann Dermatol Vénéréol* 1982; **109**: 813–4.

54 Reymond JL, Stoebner P, Zambelli P *et al*. Penicillamine induced elastosis perforans serpiginosa: an ultrastructural study of two cases. *J Cutan Pathol* 1982; **9**: 352–7.

55 Price RG, Prentice RSA. Penicillamine-induced elastosis perforans serpiginosa. Tip of the iceberg? *Am J Dermatopathol* 1986; **8**: 314–20.

56 Sahn EE, Maize JC, Garen PD *et al*. D-Penicillamine-induced elastosis perforans serpiginosa in a child with juvenile rheumatoid arthritis. Report of a case and review of the literature. *J Am Acad Dermatol* 1989; **20**: 979–88.

57 Wilhelm K, Wolff HH. Penicillamin-induzierte Elastosis perforans serpiginosa. *Hautarzt* 1994; **45**: 45–7.

58 Hill VA, Seymour CA, Mortimer PS. Penicillamine-induced elastosis perforans serpiginosa and cutis laxa in Wilson's diseases. *Br J Dermatol* 2000; **142**: 560–1.

59 Meyrick-Thomas RH, Light N, Stephens AD *et al*. Pseudoxanthoma elasticum-like skin changes induced by penicillamine. *J R Soc Med* 1984; **77**: 794–8.

60 Meyrick-Thomas RH, Kirby JDT. Elastosis perforans serpiginosa and pseudoxanthoma elasticum-like skin change due to D-penicillamine. *Clin Exp Dermatol* 1985; **10**: 386–91.

61 Light N, Meyrick Thomas RH, Stephens A *et al*. Collagen and elastin changes in D-penicillamine-induced pseudoxanthoma elasticum. *Br J Dermatol* 1986; **114**: 381–8.

62 Burge S, Ryan T. Penicillamine-induced pseudo-pseudoxanthoma elasticum in a patient with rheumatoid arthritis. *Clin Exp Dermatol* 1988; **13**: 255–8.

63 Hjalmarson O, Hanson L-Å. IgA deficiency during D-penicillamine treatment. *BMJ* 1977; **i**: 549.

64 Garlepp MJ, Dawkins RL, Christiansen FT. HLA antigens and acetylcholine receptor antibodies in penicillamine induced myasthenia gravis. *BMJ* 1983; **286**: 338–40.

65 Murphy KC, Atkins CJ, Offer RC *et al*. Obliterative bronchiolitis in two rheumatoid arthritis patients treated with penicillamine. *Arthritis Rheum* 1981; **24**: 557–60.

66 Passas C, Weinstein A. Breast gigantism with penicillamine therapy. *Arthritis Rheum* 1978; **21**: 167–8.

Tiopronin (N-(2-mercaptopropionyl) glycine)

This drug, used in Japan for the treatment of liver disease, mercury intoxication, cataracts and allergic dermatoses, dissociates disulphide bonds, like penicillamine. Morbilliform, urticarial and lichenoid eruptions, bullous in one case, have occurred [1].

REFERENCE

1 Hsiao L, Yoshinaga A, Ono T. Drug-induced bullous lichen planus in a patient with diabetes mellitus and liver disease. *J Am Acad Dermatol* 1986; **15**: 103–5.

Anticoagulants, fibrinolytic agents and antiplatelet drugs

Oral anticoagulants

Adverse reactions to oral anticoagulant drugs have been reviewed [1–3].

REFERENCES

1 Baker H, Levene GM. Drug reactions V. Cutaneous reactions to anticoagulants. *Br J Dermatol* 1969; **81**: 236–8.

2 Hirsh J. Oral anticoagulant drugs. *N Engl J Med* 1991; **324**: 1865–75.

3 Gallerani M, Manfredini R, Moratelli S. Non-haemorrhagic adverse reactions of oral anticoagulant therapy. *Int J Cardiol* 1995; **49**: 1–7.

Coumarins

There may be cross-sensitivity across the group comprising acenocoumarol (nicoumalone), phenprocoumon and warfarin [1].

Phenprocoumon. A patient on long-term anticoagulation developed repeated episodes of skin and subcutaneous fat necrosis related to episodes of excessive anticoagulation with acquired functional deficiency of protein C, thought to be due to hepatic dysfunction resulting from congestive cardiac failure [2].

Warfarin. Haemorrhage is the commonest adverse reaction. Maculopapular rashes occur [1], and may be seen after a single dose of warfarin [3]. Rarely, an oral loading dose may lead to one or more areas of painful erythema and ecchymosis, which rapidly progress to central blistering and massive cutaneous and subcutaneous necrosis

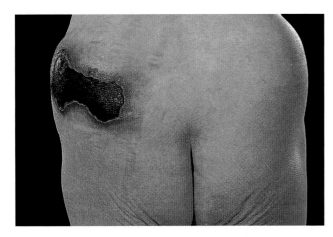

Fig. 73.7 Warfarin necrosis. (Courtesy of A. Ive, Durham, UK.)

(Fig. 73.7) [4–12]; if extensive, the condition may be fatal [3]. The lesions usually start after 2–14 days of treatment (usually 3–5 days), tend to be symmetrical, and occur over fatty areas, for example the breasts, buttocks, thighs, calves and abdomen. Most patients have been women, but lesions of the penis may occur [6]. Warfarin necrosis has been associated with the heterozygous state for deficiency of protein C, a vitamin K-dependent serine protease [8–10]. Activated protein C is a potent anticoagulant that selectively inactivates co-factors Va and VIIIa and inhibits platelet coagulant activity by inactivation of platelet factor Va. Continued coumarin therapy does not aggravate the condition, but resumption of therapy with loading doses may lead to new lesions [7]. The condition is preventable by vitamin K_1 injections. Other side effects are rare, and include urticaria [13], dermatitis, gastrointestinal upset, purple erythema of the dependent parts (purple toe syndrome) [14–16], acral purpura [17] and alopecia [18].

Oral anticoagulants and quinidine act synergistically to depress vitamin K-sensitive hepatic clotting synthesis [19]. Their combined use can precipitate serious hypoprothrombinaemic haemorrhage. Azapropazone displaces warfarin from protein-binding sites and also alters renal clearance of R and S isomers of warfarin; this may lead to effective warfarin overdosage [20]. Itraconazole may potentiate the action of warfarin [21].

REFERENCES

1 Kruis-de Vries MH, Stricker BHC, Coenraads PJ, Nater JP. Maculopapular rash due to coumarin derivatives. *Dermatologica* 1989; **178**: 109–11.
2 Teepe RGC, Broekmans AW, Vermeer BJ *et al*. Recurrent coumarin-induced skin necrosis in a patient with an acquired functional protein C deficiency. *Arch Dermatol* 1986; **122**: 1408–12.
3 Antony SJ, Krick SK, Mehta PM. Unusual cutaneous adverse reaction to warfarin therapy. *South Med J* 1993; **86**: 1413–4.
4 Lacy JP, Goodin RR. Warfarin-induced necrosis of skin. *Ann Intern Med* 1975; **82**: 381–2.
5 Schleicher SM, Fricker MP. Coumarin necrosis. *Arch Dermatol* 1980; **116**: 444–5.
6 Weinberg AC, Lieskovsky G, McGehee WG, Skinner DG. Warfarin necrosis of the skin and subcutaneous tissue of the male external genitalia. *J Urol* 1983; **130**: 352–4.
7 Slutzki S, Bogokowsky H, Gilboa Y, Halpern Z. Coumadin-induced skin necrosis. *Int J Dermatol* 1984; **23**: 117–9.
8 Kazmier FJ. Thromboembolism, coumarin necrosis, and protein C. *Mayo Clin Proc* 1985; **60**: 673–4.
9 Gladson CL, Groncy P, Griffin JH. Coumarin necrosis, neonatal purpura fulminans, and protein C deficiency. *Arch Dermatol* 1988; **123**: 1701a–1706a.
10 Auletta MJ, Headington JT. Purpura fulminans. A cutaneous manifestation of severe protein C deficiency. *Arch Dermatol* 1988; **124**: 1387–91.
11 Sharafuddin MJ, Sanaknaki BA, Kibbi AG. Erythematous, hemorrhagic, and necrotic plaques in an elderly man. Coumarin-induced skin necrosis. *Arch Dermatol* 1992; **128**: 105, 108.
12 Comp PC. Coumarin-induced skin necrosis. Incidence, mechanisms, management and avoidance. *Drug Saf* 1993; **8**: 128–35.
13 Sheps ES, Gifford RW. Urticaria after administration of warfarin sodium. *Am J Cardiol* 1959; **3**: 118–20.
14 Feder W, Auerbach R. 'Purple toes': an uncommon sequela of oral coumarin drug therapy. *Ann Intern Med* 1961; **55**: 911–7.
15 Akle CA, Joiner CL. Purple toe syndrome. *J R Soc Med* 1981; **74**: 219.
16 Lebsack CS, Weibert RT. Purple toes syndrome. *Postgrad Med* 1982; **71**: 81–4.
17 Stone MS, Rosen T. Acral purpura: an unusual sign of coumarin necrosis. *J Am Acad Dermatol* 1986; **14**: 797–802.
18 Umlas J, Harken DE. Warfarin-induced alopecia. *Cutis* 1988; **42**: 63–4.
19 Koch-Weser J. Quinidine-induced hypoprothrombinemic hemorrhage in patients on chronic warfarin therapy. *Ann Intern Med* 1968; **68**: 511–7.
20 Win N, Mitchell DC. Azapropazone and warfarin. *BMJ* 1991; **302**: 969–70.
21 Yeh J, Soo SC, Summerton C, Richardson C. Potentiation of action of warfarin by itraconazole. *BMJ* 1990; **301**: 669.

Indandiones

Hypersensitivity reactions occur in up to 0.3% of patients within 3 months of onset of treatment with phenindione. Scarlatiniform, eczematous, erythema multiforme-like or generalized exfoliative eruptions are seen [1,2]. Alopecia and stomatitis may accompany the rash. Brownish-yellow or orange discoloration of the palmar or finger skin on handling the tablets develops after contact with soap alkali [3]. Cutaneous necrosis occurs rarely.

REFERENCES

1 Hollman A, Wong HO. Phenindione sensitivity. *BMJ* 1964; **ii**: 730–2.
2 Copeman PWM. Phenindione toxicity. *BMJ* 1965; **ii**: 305.
3 Silverton NH. Skin pigmentation by phenindione. *BMJ* 1966; **i**: 675.

Heparin: parenteral anticoagulant

The most frequent side effect is haemorrhage [1,2]. Other common side effects include osteoporosis and (temporary) telogen effluvium 6–16 weeks after administration. Hypoaldosteronism may occur. Hypersensitivity reactions including urticaria and anaphylactic shock are well documented but very uncommon [3]. Rapid desensitization was achieved in a patient with heparin urticarial hypersensitivity who required cardiac surgery [4]. Hypereosinophilia is recorded [5]. Vasospastic reactions, including pain, cyanosis and severe itching or burning plantar sensations, are described.

Erythematous infiltrated plaques developing 3–21 days after commencement of heparin therapy [6–14] may closely mimic contact dermatitis both clinically and histologically, and patch tests may be positive [8,9]. Delayed-type hypersensitivity reactions in patients receiving heparin may occur with both unfractionated and low-molecular-weight heparins. Delayed-type hypersensitivity to heparins is characterized by considerable cross-reactivity between low-molecular-weight heparins, unfractionated heparins and danaparoid [13]. Unfractionated heparins may be tolerated even if low-molecular-weight heparins are not. Subcutaneous provocation testing with a panel of heparins, danaparoid and desirudin (hirudin) is recommended for determining acceptable treatment options for patients allergic to specific heparins. Low-molecular-weight heparin analogues may be satisfactorily substituted in some patients with this reaction [6,15], but are not always tolerated [7,16,17]; a panel of different low-molecular-weight heparin preparations should be checked by subcutaneous provocation tests before reinstitution of heparin therapy. Chlorocresol may be responsible for some reactions attributed to heparin [7,18], including anaphylactoid reactions.

Skin necrosis occurring 6–8 days after onset of subcutaneous heparin is rare, but may occur at injection sites and occasionally at distal sites elsewhere [19–27]. Diabetic women on high-dose antibiotics are predisposed to this complication. A scleroderma-like evolution has been recorded [22]. Clinically, the skin necrosis resembles that of coumarin necrosis [25]. It may occur with use of low-molecular-weight heparin [23,26].

Heparin may cause an allergic thrombocytopenia [28–35]. Thrombocytopenia is usually asymptomatic, but may be associated with arterial or venous thrombosis in about 0.4% of cases [29,33,34]; thromboembolism may occasionally be lethal [30]. Thrombocytopenia usually begins 3–15 days after initiation of therapy, but may occur within hours in previously exposed patients, and is thought to be caused by an IgG–heparin immune complex involving both the Fab and Fc portions of the IgG molecule [29]. Heparin-induced antiendothelial cell antibodies, which recognize heparin-like glycans on the cell surface of platelets and endothelial cells, may lead to platelet aggregation and endothelial cell expression of procoagulant tissue factor, with resultant thrombocytopenia and thrombosis [21]. Thrombocytopenia may occur with both unfractionated and low-molecular-weight heparins [20]. Clinical cross-reactivity between heparin and the polysulphated chondroitin-like substance Arteparon, used in the treatment of degenerative joint disease, has been described [32].

REFERENCES

1 Tuneu A, Moreno A, de Moragas JM. Cutaneous reactions secondary to heparin injections. *J Am Acad Dermatol* 1985; **12**: 1072–7.
2 Hirsh J. Heparin. *N Engl J Med* 1991; **324**: 1565–74.
3 Curry N, Bandana EJ, Pirofsky B. Heparin sensitivity: report of a case. *Arch Intern Med* 1973; **132**: 744–5.
4 Patriarca G, Rossi M, Schiavino D *et al*. Rush desensitization in heparin hypersensitivity: a case report. *Allergy* 1994; **49**: 292–4.
5 Bircher AJ, Itin PH, Buchner SA. Skin lesions, hypereosinophilia, and subcutaneous heparin. *Lancet* 1994; **343**: 861.
6 Zimmermann R, Harenberg J, Weber E *et al*. Behandlung bei heparininduzierter kutaner Reaktion mit einem niedermolekularen Heparin-Analog. *Dtsch Med Wochenschr* 1984; **109**: 1326–8.
7 Klein GF, Kofler H, Wol H, Fritsch PO. Eczema-like, erythematous, infiltrated plaques: a common side-effect of subcutaneous heparin therapy. *J Am Acad Dermatol* 1989; **21**: 703–7.
8 Guillet G, Delaire P, Plantin P, Guillet MH. Eczema as a complication of heparin therapy. *J Am Acad Dermatol* 1989; **21**: 1130.
9 Bircher AJ, Flückiger R, Buchner SA. Eczematous infiltrated plaques to subcutaneous heparin: a type IV allergic reaction. *Br J Dermatol* 1990; **123**: 507–14.
10 Koch P, Hindi S, Landwehr D. Delayed allergic skin reactions due to subcutaneous heparin-calcium, enoxaparin-sodium, pentosan polysulfate and acute skin lesions from systemic sodium-heparin. *Contact Dermatitis* 1996; **34**: 156–8.
11 Koch P, Münßinger T, Rupp-John C, Uhl K. Delayed-type hypersensitivity skin reactions caused by subcutaneous unfractionated and low-molecular-weight heparins: tolerance of a new recombinant hirudin. *J Am Acad Dermatol* 2000; **42**: 612–9.
12 Szolar-Platzer C, Aberer W, Kranke B. Delayed-type skin reaction to the heparin-alternative danaparoid. *J Am Acad Dermatol* 2000; **43**: 920–2.
13 Grassegger A, Fritsch P, Reider N. Delayed-type hypersensitivity and cross-reactivity to heparins and danaparoid: a prospective study. *Dermatol Surg* 2001; **27**: 47–52.
14 Wutschert R, Piletta P, Bounameaux H. Adverse skin reactions to low molecular weight heparins: frequency, management and prevention. *Drug Saf* 1999; **20**: 515–25.
15 Koch P, Bahmer FA, Schafer H. Tolerance of intravenous low-molecular-weight heparin after eczematous reaction to subcutaneous heparin. *Contact Dermatitis* 1991; **25**: 205–6.
16 Bosch A, Las Heras G, Martin E, Oller G. Skin reaction with low molecular weight heparins. *Br J Haematol* 1993; **85**: 637.
17 Phillips JK, Majumdar G, Hunt BJ, Savidge GF. Heparin-induced skin reaction due to two different preparations of low molecular weight heparin (LMWH). *Br J Haematol* 1993; **84**: 349–50.
18 Ainley EJ, Mackie IG, MacArthur D. Adverse reaction to chlorocresol-preserved heparin. *Lancet* 1977; **i**: 705.
19 Shelley WB, Säyen JJ. Heparin necrosis: an anticoagulant-induced cutaneous infarct. *J Am Acad Dermatol* 1982; **7**: 674–7.
20 Levine LE, Bernstein JE, Soltani K *et al*. Heparin-induced skin necrosis unrelated to injection sites: a sign of potentially lethal complications. *Arch Dermatol* 1983; **119**: 400–3.
21 Mathieu A, Avril MF, Schlumberger M *et al*. Un cas de nécrose cutanée induite par l'héparine. *Ann Dermatol Vénéréol* 1984; **111**: 733–4.
22 Barthelemy H, Hermier C, Perrot H. Nécrose cutanée avec évolution sclérodermiforme après l'injection souscutanée d'heparinate de calcium. *Ann Dermatol Vénéréol* 1985; **112**: 245–7.
23 Cordoliani F, Saiag P, Guillaume J-C *et al*. Nécrose cutanés étendues induites par la fraxiparine. *Ann Dermatol Vénéréol* 1987; **114**: 1366–8.
24 Rongioletti F, Pisani S, Ciaccio M, Rebora A. Skin necrosis due to intravenous heparin. *Dermatologica* 1989; **178**: 47–50.
25 Gold JA, Watters AK, O'Brien E. Coumadin versus heparin necrosis. *J Am Acad Dermatol* 1987; **16**: 148–50.
26 Ojeda E, Perez MC, Mataix R *et al*. Skin necrosis with a low molecular weight heparin. *Br J Haematol* 1992; **82**: 620.
27 Yates P, Jones S. Heparin skin necrosis: an important indicator of potentially fatal heparin hypersensitivity. *Clin Exp Dermatol* 1993; **18**: 138–41.
28 Cine DB, Tomaski A, Tannenbaum S. Immune endothelial cell injury in heparin-associated thrombocytopenia. *N Engl J Med* 1987; **316**: 581–9.
29 Warkentin TE, Kelton JG. Heparin-induced thrombocytopenia. *Annu Rev Med* 1989; **40**: 31–44.
30 Jaffray B, Welch GH, Cooke TG. Fatal venous thrombosis after heparin therapy. *Lancet* 1991; **337**: 561.
31 Eichinger S, Kyrle PA, Brenner B *et al*. Thrombocytopenia associated with low-molecular-weight heparin. *Lancet* 1991; **337**: 1425–6.
32 Greinacher A, Michels I, Schafer M *et al*. Heparin-associated thrombocytopenia in a patient treated with polysulphated chondroitin sulphate:

evidence for immunological crossreactivity between heparin and polysulphated glycosaminoglycan. *Br J Haematol* 1992; **81**: 252–4.

33 Gross AS, Thompson FL, Arzubiaga MC *et al.* Heparin-associated thrombocytopenia and thrombosis (HATT) presenting with livedo reticularis. *Int J Dermatol* 1993; **32**: 276–9.
34 O'Bryan-Tear G. Heparin induced thrombosis. Datasheet warns of risk. *BMJ* 1993; **307**: 561.
35 Ouellette D, Menkis AH. Heparin-induced thrombocytopenia. *Ann Thorac Surg* 1993; **55**: 809.

Protamine: heparin antagonist

This low-molecular-weight protein, derived from salmon sperm and/or testes, is used for neutralization of heparin anticoagulation after cardiac surgery. Adverse reactions have been reviewed [1]. Idiosyncratic responses or those related to complement generation of anaphylatoxins are recorded [2]. IgE-dependent anaphylaxis [3], as well as delayed reactions causing skin nodules [4–6], which may be granulomatous [6], may occur in diabetics treated with protamine-containing insulin.

REFERENCES

1 Cormack JG, Levy JH. Adverse reactions to protamine. *Coron Artery Dis* 1993; **4**: 420–5.
2 Sussman GL, Dolovich J. Prevention of anaphylaxis. *Semin Dermatol* 1989; **8**: 158–65.
3 Kim R. Anaphylaxis to protamine masquerading as an insulin allergy. *Del Med J* 1993; **65**: 17–23.
4 Sarche MB, Paolillo M, Chacon RS *et al.* Protamine as a cause of generalized allergic reactions to NPH insulin. *Lancet* 1982; **i**: 1243.
5 Kollner A, Senff H, Engelmann L *et al.* Protaminallergie vom Spattyp und Insulinallergie vom Soforttyp. *Dtsch Med Wochenschr* 1991; **116**: 1234–8.
6 Hulshof MM, Faber WR, Kniestedt WF *et al.* Granulomatous hypersensitivity to protamine as a complication of insulin therapy. *Br J Dermatol* 1992; **127**: 286–8.

Fibrinolytic drugs

Haemorrhage is the most common untoward effect from use of thrombolysins [1]. Allergic complications are rare, particularly with alteplase or urokinase. These agents should be used electively in all patients previously exposed to streptokinase or anistreplase [2].

Alteplase (tissue-type plasminogen activator)

Painful purpura occurring within hours of administration has been recorded [3].

Aminocaproic acid

A maculopapular eruption occurring 12–72 h after administration of ε-aminocaproic acid, with positive patch tests to the drug, has been described [4]. A transient, non-inflammatory, subepidermal, bullous eruption on the legs, with fibrin thrombi in papillary dermal vessels, has also been recorded [5].

Anistreplase (anisoylated plasminogen streptokinase activator complex)

Anistreplase given for acute myocardial infarction was associated with leukocytoclastic vasculitis [6]. Maculopapular rashes and urticaria are described; patients with maculopapular rashes had significantly higher rises in serum IgM, IgG, IgA and IgE antistreptokinase level [7].

REFERENCES

1 Chesebro JH, Knatterud G, Roberts R *et al.* Thrombolysis in myocardial infarction (TIMI) trial, phase I: a comparison between intravenous tissue plasminogen activator and intravenous streptokinase. *Circulation* 1987; **76**: 142–54.
2 de Bono DP. Complications of thrombolysis and their clinical management. *Z Kardiol* 1993; **82** (Suppl. 2): 147–51.
3 DeTrana C, Hurwitz RM. Painful purpura: an adverse effect to a thrombolysin. *Arch Dermatol* 1990; **126**: 690–1.
4 Gonzalez Gutierrez ML, Esteban Lopez MI, Ruiz Ruiz MD. Positivity of patch tests in cutaneous reaction to aminocaproic acid: two case reports. *Allergy* 1995; **50**: 745–6.
5 Brooke CP, Spiers EM, Omura EF. Noninflammatory bullae associated with epsilon-aminocaproic acid infusion. *J Am Acad Dermatol* 1992; **27**: 880–2.
6 Burrows N, Russell Jones R. Vasculitis occurring after intravenous anistreplase. *J Am Acad Dermatol* 1992; **26**: 508.
7 Dykewicz MS, McMorrow NK, Davison R *et al.* Drug eruptions and isotypic antibody responses to streptokinase after infusions of anisoylated plasminogen–streptokinase complex (APSAC, anistreplase). *J Allergy Clin Immunol* 1995; **95**: 1020–8.

Streptokinase

Allergic reactions have been reported in up to 6% of patients [1–3], ranging from minor rashes to angio-oedema or anaphylaxis (which may be fatal [4–6]), bleeding, strokes and a syndrome resembling adult respiratory distress syndrome [3]. Patients who develop reactions to streptokinase cannot be predicted on the basis of antistreptokinase IgG antibody titres at presentation; minor reactions to streptokinase would not appear to be antibody mediated [7]. However, streptokinase-related thrombolytic agents should be avoided in reinfarction thrombolysis therapy in patients with raised antistreptokinase antibody titres, as hypersensitivity reactions including serum sickness may occur [8–10]. This drug has been reported in association with a hypersensitivity vasculitis [11,12], serum sickness with leukocytoclastic vasculitis [13,14] and a lymphocytic angiitis [15]. Skin necrosis is recorded [16].

Urokinase

Haemorrhagic bullae occurred as a complication of urokinase therapy for haemodialysis catheter thrombosis [17].

REFERENCES

1 Dykewicz MS, McGratt KG, Davison R *et al.* Identification of patients at risk for anaphylaxis due to streptokinase. *Arch Intern Med* 1986; **146**: 305–7.

2 ISIS-2 (Second International Study of Infarct Survival) Collaborative Group. Randomized trial of intravenous streptokinase, oral aspirin, both, or neither among 17187 cases of suspected acute myocardial infarction: ISIS-2. *Lancet* 1988; **ii**: 349–60.

3 Siebert WJ, Ayres RW, Bulling MT *et al.* Streptokinase morbidity: more common than previously recognised. *Aust NZ J Med* 1992; **22**: 129–33.

4 Allpress SM, Cluroe AD, Vuletic JC, Kolemeyer TD. Death after streptokinase. *NZ Med J* 1993; **106**: 295.

5 Hohage H, Schulte B, Pfeiff B, Pullmann H. Anaphylaktische Reaktion unter Streptokinase-Therapie. *Wien Klin Wochenschr* 1993; **105**: 176–8.

6 Cooper JP, Quarry DP, Beale DJ, Chappell AG. Life-threatening, localized angio-oedema associated with streptokinase. *Postgrad Med J* 1994; **70**: 592–3.

7 Lynch M, Pentecost BL, Littler WA, Stockley RA. Why do patients develop reactions to streptokinase? *Clin Exp Immunol* 1993; **94**: 279–85.

8 Lee HS, Yule S, McKenzie A *et al.* Hypersensitivity reactions to streptokinase in patients with high pretreatment antistreptokinase antibody and neutralisation titres. *Eur Heart J* 1993; **14**: 1640–3.

9 Cross DB. Should streptokinase be readministered? Insights from recent studies of antistreptokinase antibodies. *Med J Aust* 1994; **161**: 100–1.

10 Jennings K. Antibodies to streptokinase. *BMJ* 1996; **312**: 393–4.

11 Ong ACM, Handler CE, Walker JM. Hypersensitivity vasculitis complicating intravenous streptokinase therapy in acute myocardial infarction. *Int J Cardiol* 1988; **21**: 71–3.

12 Thompson RF, Stratton MA, Heffron WA. Hypersensitivity vasculitis associated with streptokinase. *Clin Pharmacol* 1985; **4**: 383–8.

13 Patel IA, Prussick R, Buchanan WW, Sauder DN. Serum sickness-like illness and leukocytoclastic vasculitis after intravenous streptokinase. *J Am Acad Dermatol* 1991; **24**: 652–3.

14 Totto WG, Romano T, Benian GM *et al.* Serum sickness following streptokinase therapy. *Am J Rheumatol* 1982; **138**: 143–4.

15 Sorber WA, Herbst V. Lymphocytic angiitis following streptokinase therapy. *Cutis* 1988; **42**: 57–8.

16 Penswick J, Wright AL. Skin necrosis induced by streptokinase. *BMJ* 1994; **309**: 378.

17 Ejaz AA, Aijaz M, Nawab ZM *et al.* Hemorrhagic bullae as a complication of urokinase therapy for hemodialysis catheter thrombosis. *Am J Nephrol* 1995; **15**: 178–9.

Antiplatelet drugs

Clopidogrel

This drug, a novel thienopyridine derivative chemically related to ticlopidine and used in patients at risk of thromboembolic disorders, has caused a photosensitive lichenoid eruption [1].

Ticlopidine

This antiplatelet drug, indicated for coronary artery disease, cerebrovascular disease, peripheral vascular disease and diabetic retinopathy, is also a thienopyridine derivative [2,3]. Gastrointestinal symptoms, thrombocytopenia with minor bleeding including bruising, neutropenia, rashes in 10–15% of patients, and hepatic dysfunction in 4% of cases have been reported. Thrombotic thrombocytopenic purpura has also been documented [4]. Cutaneous reactions, including urticaria, pruritus, maculopapular and fixed drug eruptions, erythromelalgia and erythema multiforme, are recorded in up to 11.8% of patients [5]. Acute generalized exanthematous pustulosis has been documented [6].

REFERENCES

1 Dogra S, Kanwar AJ. Clopidrogel bisulphate-induced photosensitive lichenoid eruption: first report. *Br J Dermatol* 2003; **148**: 593–611.

2 McTavish D, Faulds D, Goa KL. Ticlopidine. An updated review of its pharmacology and therapeutic use in platelet-dependent disorders. *Drugs* 1990; **40**: 238–59.

3 Anonymous. Ticlopidine. *Lancet* 1991; **337**: 459–60.

4 Page Y, Tardy B, Zeni F *et al.* Thrombotic thrombocytopenic purpura related to ticlopidine. *Lancet* 1991; **337**: 774–6.

4 Yosipovitch G, Rechavia E, Feinmesser M, David M. Adverse cutaneous reactions to ticlopidine in patients with coronary stents. *J Am Acad Dermatol* 1999; **41**: 473–6.

5 Cannavò SP, Borgia F, Guarneri F, Vaccaro M. Acute generalized exanthematous pustulosis following use of ticlopidine. *Br J Dermatol* 2000; **142**: 577–8.

Vitamins including retinoids

Vitamin A

Generalized peeling may be a delayed manifestation of acute intoxication [1]. Chronic intoxication produces the following epithelial problems: pruritus, erythema, hyperkeratosis, dryness of mouth, nose and eyes, epistaxis, fissuring, dryness and scaling of the lips, peeling of the palms and soles, and alopecia. A yellow-orange skin discoloration, photosensitivity and nail changes have also been observed [2–5]. Headache, pseudotumour cerebri, anaemia, hepatomegaly and skeletal pain may be present. Cortical hyperostoses and periosteal reaction of tubular bone [6], and more rarely premature epiphyseal closure and change in the contour of long bones [7], are seen.

REFERENCES

1 Nater P, Doeglas HMG. Halibut liver poisoning in 11 fishermen. *Acta Derm Venereol (Stockh)* 1970; **50**: 109–13.

2 Oliver TK. Chronic vitamin A intoxication. Report of a case in an older child and a review of the literature. *Am J Dis Child* 1959; **95**: 57–67.

3 Muenter MD, Perry HO, Ludwig J. Chronic vitamin A intoxication in adults. Hepatic, neurologic and dermatologic complications. *Am J Med* 1971; **50**: 129–36.

4 Teo ST, Newth J, Pascoe BJ. Chronic vitamin A intoxication. *Med J Aust* 1973; **2**: 324–6.

5 Bobb R, Kieraldo JH. Cirrhosis due to hypervitaminosis A. *West J Med* 1978; **128**: 244–6.

6 Frame B, Jackson CE, Reynolds WA, Umphrey JE. Hypercalcemia and skeletal effects in chronic hypervitaminosis A. *Ann Intern Med* 1974; **80**: 44–8.

7 Ruby LK, Mital MA. Skeletal deformities following chronic hypervitaminosis A. *J Bone Joint Surg* 1974; **56**: 1283–7.

Retinoids

The cutaneous and systemic side effects of these synthetic vitamin A-related compounds resemble those of hypervitaminosis A, and have been extensively reviewed [1–12].

REFERENCES

1 Orfanos CE, Braun-Falco O, Farber EM *et al.*, eds. *Retinoids. Advances in Basic Research and Therapy.* Berlin: Springer, 1981.

2 Foged E, Jacobsen F. Side-effects due to Ro 10-3959 (Tigason). *Dermatologica* 1982; **164**: 395–403.

3 Windhorst DB, Nigra T. General clinical toxicology of oral retinoids. *J Am Acad Dermatol* 1982; **4**: 675–82.

4 Cunliffe WJ, Miller AJ, eds. *Retinoid Therapy. A Review of Clinical and Laboratory Research*. Lancaster: MTP Press, 1984.

5 Saurat JH, ed. *Retinoids: New Trends in Research and Therapy*. Basel: Karger, 1985.

6 Yob EH, Pochi PE. Side effects and long-term toxicity of synthetic retinoids. *Arch Dermatol* 1987; **123**: 1375–8.

7 Bigby M, Stern RS. Adverse reactions to isotretinoin. A report from the Adverse Drug Reaction Reporting System. *J Am Acad Dermatol* 1988; **18**: 543–52.

8 Saurat J-H. Side effects of systemic retinoids and their clinical management. *J Am Acad Dermatol* 1992; **27**: S23–S28.

9 Vahlquist A. Long-term safety of retinoid therapy. *J Am Acad Dermatol* 1992; **27**: S29–S33.

10 Gollnick HPM. Oral retinoids: efficacy and toxicity in psoriasis. *Br J Dermatol* 1996; **135** (Suppl. 49): 6–17.

11 Mørk N-J, Kolbenstvedt A, Austad J. Skeletal side-effects of 5 years' acitretin treatment. *Br J Dermatol* 1996; **134**: 1156–7.

12 Hermann G, Jungblut RM, Goerz G. Skeletal changes after long-term therapy with synthetic retinoids. *Br J Dermatol* 1997; **136**: 469–70.

Acitretin

The side effects of this principal metabolite of etretinate are similar to those of the parent compound [1–6], comprising cheilitis, alopecia, conjunctivitis, peeling of the palms and soles, xerosis, myalgia and pancreatitis; elevated levels of serum triglyceride, cholesterol and liver transaminase are seen. There has been no biopsy-proven hepatotoxicity [7]. Alopecia is particularly frequent [4], and scaling of the palms and soles appears more prominent than with etretinate [5]. There is a higher occurrence of vulvovaginal candidiasis during acitretin exposure [8]. Multiple milia have occurred [9]. Skeletal effects may be significant, but are not an absolute contraindication to therapy [10]. Acitretin does not seem to cause osteoporosis [11].

Persistent levels of etretinate have been detected in plasma following a change to acitretin therapy. Detectable plasma etretinate was present in 45% of current acitretin users and 18% of those who had stopped acitretin, whereas detectable subcutaneous tissue etretinate was present in 83% of current acitretin users and 86% of those who had discontinued the drug [12]. Inability to detect plasma etretinate is therefore a poor predictor of the absence of etretinate in fat. Acitretin and/or etretinate were detectable in fat and in some cases plasma from women who had ceased acitretin therapy for up to 29 months [12]. It has been proposed that subcutaneous tissue levels of acitretin and etretinate should be monitored when plasma measurements are negative, and that the recommended contraception period of 2 years after cessation of acitretin therapy should be reconsidered to avoid the risk of teratogenicity [13]. It has been suggested that acitretin is only converted to etretinate following alcohol intake [14].

REFERENCES

1 Geiger J-M, Czarnetzki BM. Acitretin (Ro 10-1670, Etretin): overall evaluation of clinical studies. *Dermatologica* 1988; **176**: 182–90.

2 Gupta AK, Goldfarb MT, Ellis CN, Voorhees JJ. Side-effect profile of acitretin therapy in psoriasis. *J Am Acad Dermatol* 1989; **21**: 1088–93.

3 Ruzicka T, Sommerburg C, Braun-Falco O *et al.* Efficiency of acitretin in combination with UV-B in the treatment of severe psoriasis. *Arch Dermatol* 1990; **126**: 482–6.

4 Murray HE, Anhalt AW, Lessard R *et al.* A 12-month treatment of severe psoriasis with acitretin: results of a Canadian open multicenter study. *J Am Acad Dermatol* 1991; **24**: 598–602.

5 Blanchet-Bardon C, Nazzaro V, Rognin C *et al.* Acitretin in the treatment of severe disorders of keratinization. Results of an open study. *J Am Acad Dermatol* 1991; **24**: 982–6.

6 Katz HI, Waalen J, Leach EE. Acitretin in psoriasis: an overview of adverse effects. *J Am Acad Dermatol* 1999; **41**: S7–S12.

7 Roenigk HH Jr, Callen JP, Guzzo CA *et al.* Effects of acitretin on the liver. *J Am Acad Dermatol* 1999; **41**: 584–8.

8 Sturkenboom MC, Middelbeek A, de Jong van den Berg LT *et al.* Vulvovaginal candidiasis associated with acitretin. *J Clin Epidemiol* 1995; **48**: 991–7.

9 Chang A, Kuligowski ME, van de Kerkhof PC. Multiple milia during treatment with acitretin for mycosis fungoides. *Acta Derm Venereol (Stockh)* 1993; **73**: 235.

10 Mørk N-J, Kolbenstvedt A, Austad J. Skeletal side-effects of 5 years' acitretin treatment. *Br J Dermatol* 1996; **134**: 1156–7.

11 McMullen EA, McCarron P, Irvine D *et al.* Association between long-term acitretin therapy and osteoporosis: no evidence of increased risk. *Clin Exp Dermatol* 2003; **28**: 307–9.

12 Lambert WE, De Leenheer AP, De Bersaques JP, Kint A. Persistent etretinate levels in plasma after changing the therapy to acitretin. *Arch Dermatol Res* 1990; **282**: 343–4.

13 Sturkenboom MC, de Jong van den Berg LT, van Voorst Vader PC *et al.* Inability to detect plasma etretinate and acitretin is a poor predictor of the absence of these teratogens in tissue after stopping acitretin treatment. *Br J Clin Pharmacol* 1994; **38**: 229–35.

14 Grønhøy Larsen F, Steinkjer B, Jakobsen P *et al.* Acitretin is converted to etretinate only during concomitant alcohol intake. *Br J Dermatol* 2000; **143**: 1164–9.

Etretinate

This drug has been largely superseded by acitretin. The dermatological side effects are dose dependent, and resemble those associated with isotretinoin therapy [1–3]. With dosage over 0.5 mg/kg, cheilitis with dryness, scaling and fissuring of the lips is almost universal. There may be pruritus, a dry mouth, dry nose, epistaxis, meatitis, desquamation including the face, hands and feet, and reduced tolerance of sunlight [4] and therapeutic products such as tar or dithranol. Pseudoporphyria has been reported in a renal transplant recipient treated with etretinate to suppress cutaneous neoplasia [5]. A 'retinoid dermatitis' resembling asteatotic eczema may develop in up to 50% of patients [6]. Increased stickiness of the palms and soles, possibly due to increased quantities of carcinoembryonic antigen and other glycoproteins in eccrine sweat [7,8], has been reported. Mucosal erosions, conjunctivitis, paronychia, alopecia [9] and curling, kinking or darkening of hair [10] are all well documented. Intertriginous erosions have also been described [11]. Oedema [12], excess granulation tissue [13] and multiple pyogenic granulomas [14] develop rarely. Erythroderma has been reported [15].

Prolonged therapy may lead to skin fragility [16,17]; blistering, erosions and scarring have been reported in one patient [18]. Softening of the nails is seen [19], and chronic paronychia, onycholysis, onychomadesis, nail shedding, onychoschizia and fragility may occur [20,21]. Parakeratotic digitate keratoses appearing after treatment of disseminated superficial actinic porokeratosis may arise as a result of etretinate-resistant regions in the ring of the cornoid lamella [22]. There has been a single case of generalization of palmoplantar pustulosis following cessation of etretinate therapy [23].

Systemic side effects of etretinate include benign intracranial hypertension [24]. Minor disturbances in tests of liver function are not uncommon, and may not always be reversible; liver changes range from non-specific reactive hepatitis to acute hepatitis, chronic active hepatitis and severe fibrosis or cirrhosis [25–28]. Fatal liver necrosis occurred in a patient with ichthyosiform erythroderma [29], but other factors may have been relevant. However, several studies involving liver biopsies have indicated good tolerance of etretinate without significant hepatotoxic side effects [30–32]; in one study, patients were followed for 3 years [32]. Etretinate, like isotretinoin, can cause increase in triglycerides and cholesterol [33–36] but to a lesser extent [36]. There have been isolated reports of possible etretinate-related thrombocytopenia [37]. Retinal toxicity has been postulated [38], although a recent report has not confirmed this [39]. Erectile dysfunction has been documented occasionally [40].

Skeletal abnormalities, such as periosteal thickening, vertebral hyperostosis, disc degeneration, osteoporosis and calcification of spinal ligaments, occur in a significant number of adults receiving long-term therapy for disorders of keratinization, but the severity of the changes is minor [41,42]. Radiological evidence of thinning of long bones may be seen in children [43], and premature epiphyseal closure has been recorded [44].

Etretinate, like isotretinoin, is grossly teratogenic, and because of its deposition in body fat stores is excreted only very slowly, especially in the obese [45]. Detectable serum levels have been found in some patients more than 2 years after discontinuation of therapy. It is therefore recommended that female patients of child-bearing years should be advised to prevent pregnancy not only during the course of treatment but also for at least 2 years after stopping therapy; if pregnancy is contemplated after this period of time, an estimation of circulating levels of retinoid metabolites should be obtained.

REFERENCES

1 Foged E, Jacobsen F. Side-effects due to Ro 10-3959 (Tigason). *Dermatologica* 1982; **164**: 395–403.
2 Ellis CN, Voorhees JJ. Etretinate therapy. *J Am Acad Dermatol* 1987; **16**: 267–91.
3 Halioua B, Saurat J-H. Risk : benefit ratio in the treatment of psoriasis with systemic retinoids. *Br J Dermatol* 1990; **122** (Suppl. 36): 135–50.
4 Collins MRL, James WD, Rodman OG. Etretinate photosensitivity. *J Am Acad Dermatol* 1986; **14**: 274.
5 McDonagh AJG, Harrington CI. Pseudoporphyria complicating etretinate therapy. *Clin Exp Dermatol* 1989; **14**: 437–8.
6 Taieb A, Maleville J. Retinoid dermatitis mimicking 'eczéma craquelé'. *Acta Derm Venereol (Stockh)* 1985; **65**: 570.
7 Pennys NS, Hernandez D. A sticky problem with etretinate. *N Engl J Med* 1991; **325**: 521.
8 Higgins EM, Pembroke AC. Sticky palms: an unusual side-effect of etretinate therapy. *Clin Exp Dermatol* 1993; **18**: 389–90.
9 Berth-Jones J, Shuttleworth D, Hutchinson PE. A study of etretinate alopecia. *Br J Dermatol* 1990; **122**: 751–5.
10 Vesper JL, Fenske A. Hair darkening and new growth associated with etretinate therapy. *J Am Acad Dermatol* 1996; **34**: 860.
11 Shelley ED, Shelley WB. Inframammary, intertriginous, and decubital erosion due to etretinate. *Cutis* 1991; **47**: 111–3.
12 Allan S, Christmas T. Severe edema associated with etretinate. *J Am Acad Dermatol* 1988; **19**: 140.
13 Hodak E, David M, Feuerman EJ. Excess granulation tissue during etretinate therapy. *J Am Acad Dermatol* 1984; **11**: 1166–7.
14 Williamson DM, Greenwood R. Multiple pyogenic granulomata occurring during etretinate therapy. *Br J Dermatol* 1983; **109**: 615–7.
15 Levin J, Almeyda J. Erythroderma due to etretinate. *Br J Dermatol* 1985; **112**: 373.
16 Williams ML, Elias PM. Nature of skin fragility in patients receiving retinoids for systemic effect. *Arch Dermatol* 1981; **117**: 611–9.
17 Neild VS, Moss RF, Marsden RA et al. Retinoid-induced skin fragility in a patient with hepatic disease. *Clin Exp Dermatol* 1985; **10**: 459–65.
18 Ramsay B, Bloxham C, Eldred A et al. Blistering, erosions and scarring in a patient on etretinate. *Br J Dermatol* 1989; **121**: 397–400.
19 Lindskov R. Soft nails after treatment with aromatic retinoids. *Arch Dermatol* 1982; **118**: 535–6.
20 Baran R. Action thérapeutique et complications du rétinoïde aromatique sur l'appareil unguéal. *Ann Dermatol Vénéréol* 1982; **109**: 367–71.
21 Baran R. Etretinate and the nails (study of 130 cases): possible mechanisms of some side-effects. *Clin Exp Dermatol* 1986; **11**: 148–52.
22 Carmichael AJ, Tan CY. Digitate keratoses: a complication of etretinate used in the treatment of disseminated superficial actinic porokeratosis. *Clin Exp Dermatol* 1990; **15**: 370–1.
23 Miyagawa S, Muramatsu T, Shirai T. Generalization of palmoplantar pustulosis after withdrawal of etretinate. *J Am Acad Dermatol* 1991; **24**: 305–6.
24 Viraben R, Mathieu C. Benign intracranial hypertension during etretinate therapy for mycosis fungoides. *J Am Acad Dermatol* 1985; **13**: 515–7.
25 Schmidt H, Foged E. Some hepatotoxic side effects observed in patients treated with aromatic retinoid (Ro 10-9359). In: Orfanos CE, Braun-Falco O, Farber EM et al., eds. *Retinoids. Advances in Basic Research and Therapy.* Berlin: Springer, 1981: 359–62.
26 Van Voorst Vader P, Houthoff H, Eggink H, Gips C. Etretinate (Tigason) hepatitis in two patients. *Dermatologica* 1984; **168**: 41–6.
27 Kano Y, Fukuda M, Shiohara T, Nagashima M. Cholestatic hepatitis occurring shortly after etretinate therapy. *J Am Acad Dermatol* 1994; **31**: 133–4.
28 Sanchez MR, Ross B, Rotterdam H et al. Retinoid hepatitis. *J Am Acad Dermatol* 1993; **28**: 853–8.
29 Thune P, Mørk NJ. A case of centrolobular necrosis of the liver due to aromatic retinoid: Tigason (Ro-10-9359). *Dermatologica* 1980; **160**: 405–8.
30 Foged E, Bjerring P, Kragballe K et al. Histologic changes in the liver during etretinate treatment. *J Am Acad Dermatol* 1984; **11**: 580–3.
31 Zachariae H, Foged E, Bjerring P et al. Liver biopsy during etretinate (Tigason®) treatment. In: Saurat JH, ed. *Retinoids: New Trends in Research and Therapy.* Basel: Karger, 1985: 494–7.
32 Roenigk HH Jr. Retinoids: effect on the liver. In: Saurat JH, ed. *Retinoids: New Trends in Research and Therapy.* Basel: Karger, 1985: 476–88.
33 Ellis CN, Swanson NA, Grekin RC et al. Etretinate therapy causes increases in lipid levels in patients with psoriasis. *Arch Dermatol* 1982; **118**: 559–62.
34 Michaëlsson G, Bergquist A, Vahlquist A, Vessby B. The influence of Tigason (R 10-9359) on the serum lipoproteins in man. *Br J Dermatol* 1981; **105**: 201–5.
35 Vahlquist C, Michaëlsson G, Vahlquist A, Vessby B. A sequential comparison of etretinate (Tigason) and isotretinoin (Roaccutane) with special regard to their effects on serum lipoproteins. *Br J Dermatol* 1985; **112**: 69–76.

36 Marsden J. Hyperlipidaemia due to isotretinoin and etretinate: possible mechanisms and consequences. *Br J Dermatol* 1986; **114**: 401–7.

37 Naldi L, Rozzoni M, Finazzi G *et al.* Etretinate therapy and thrombocytopenia. *Br J Dermatol* 1991; **124**: 395.

38 Weber U, Melink B, Goerz G, Michaelis L. Abnormal retinal function associated with long-term etretinate? *Lancet* 1988; **i**: 235–6.

39 Pitts JF, MacKie RM, Dutton GN *et al.* Etretinate and visual function: a 1-year follow-up study. *Br J Dermatol* 1991; **125**: 53–5.

40 Reynolds OD. Erectile dysfunction in etretinate treatment. *Arch Dermatol* 1991; **127**: 425–6.

41 DiGiovanna JJ, Gerber LH, Helfgott RK *et al.* Extraspinal tendon and ligament calcification associated with long-term therapy with etretinate. *N Engl J Med* 1986; **315**: 1177–82.

42 Halkier-Sørensen L, Andresen J. A retrospective study of bone changes in adults treated with etretinate. *J Am Acad Dermatol* 1989; **20**: 83–7.

43 Halkier-Sørensen L, Laurberg G, Andresen J. Bone changes in children on long-term treatment with etretinate. *J Am Acad Dermatol* 1987; **16**: 999–1006.

44 Prendiville J, Bingham EA, Burrows D. Premature epiphyseal closure: a complication of etretinate therapy in children. *J Am Acad Dermatol* 1986; **15**: 1259–62.

45 DiGiovanna JJ, Zech LA, Ruddel ME *et al.* Etretinate: persistent serum levels after long-term therapy. *Arch Dermatol* 1989; **125**: 246–51.

Isotretinoin (13-cis-retinoic acid)

Dermatological complications have been reviewed [1,2]; erythema and scaling of the face, generalized xerosis, skin fragility, pruritus, epistaxis, dry nose and dry mouth may be seen in up to 80% of cystic acne patients. A dose-related cheilitis occurs in over 90% and conjunctivitis in about 40% of patients. Transient exacerbation of acne may occur, especially in the early stages of therapy. Exuberant granulation tissue, or pyogenic granulomas at the site of healing acne lesions, has been reported frequently [3–7].

Rashes, including erythema, and thinning of the hair (in rare cases persistent) occur in fewer than 10% of patients. Both isotretinoin and etretinate may cause curliness or kinking of hair [8]. Nasolabial follicular sebaceous casts have been reported [9]. The following have occurred in approximately 5% of cases: peeling of the palms and soles, skin infections and possible increased susceptibility to sunburn. Phototesting confirmed photosensitivity in some patients in one study [10] but not another [11]. A photoaggravated allergic reaction has been documented in which the patient had positive patch tests to isotretinoin [12]. Reversible melasma is recorded [13], as is facial cellulitis [14]. Scarring, which may be keloidal, may occur after dermabrasion or laser therapy within a year of isotretinoin therapy; such procedures are best postponed during this period [15–17].

REFERENCES

1 Yob EH, Pochi PE. Side effects and long-term toxicity of synthetic retinoids. *Arch Dermatol* 1987; **123**: 1375–8.

2 Bigby M, Stern RS. Adverse reactions to isotretinoin. A report from the Adverse Drug Reaction Reporting System. *J Am Acad Dermatol* 1988; **18**: 543–52.

3 Campbell JP, Grekin RC, Ellis CN *et al.* Retinoid therapy is associated with excess granulation tissue responses. *J Am Acad Dermatol* 1983; **9**: 708–13.

4 Exner JH, Dahod S, Pochi PE. Pyogenic granuloma-like acne lesions during isotretinoin therapy. *Arch Dermatol* 1983; **119**: 808–11.

5 Valentic JP, Barr RJ, Weinstein GD. Inflammatory neovascular nodules associated with oral isotretinoin treatment of severe acne. *Arch Dermatol* 1983; **119**: 871–2.

6 Stary A. Acne conglobata: Ungewöhnlicher Verlauf unter 13-*cis*-Retinsäuretherapie. *Hautarzt* 1986; **37**: 28–30.

7 Blanc D, Zultak M, Wendling P, Lonchampt F. Eruptive pyogenic granulomas and acne fulminans in two siblings treated with isotretinoin. A possible common pathogenesis. *Dermatologica* 1988; **177**: 16–8.

8 Bunker CB, Maurice PDL, Dowd PM. Isotretinoin and curly hair. *Clin Exp Dermatol* 1990; **15**: 143–5.

9 Plewig G. Nasolabial follicular sebaceous casts: a novel complication of isotretinoin therapy. *Br J Dermatol* 2001; **144**: 919.

10 Ferguson J, Johnson BE. Photosensitivity due to retinoids: clinical and laboratory studies. *Br J Dermatol* 1986; **115**: 275–83.

11 Wong RC, Gilber M, Woo TY *et al.* Photosensitivity and isotretinoin therapy. *J Am Acad Dermatol* 1986; **15**: 1095–6.

12 Auffret N, Bruley C, Brunetiere RA *et al.* Photoaggravated allergic reaction to isotretinoin. *J Am Acad Dermatol* 1990; **23**: 321–2.

13 Burke H, Carmichael AJ. Reversible melasma associated with isotretinoin. *Br J Dermatol* 1996; **135**: 862.

14 Boffa MJ, Dave VK. Facial cellulitis during oral isotretinoin treatment for acne. *J Am Acad Dermatol* 1994; **31**: 800–2.

15 Rubenstein R, Roenigk HH Jr, Stegman SJ *et al.* Atypical keloids after dermabrasion of patients taking isotretinoin. *J Am Acad Dermatol* 1986; **15**: 280–5.

16 Zachariae H. Delayed wound healing and keloid formation following argon laser treatment or dermabrasion during isotretinoin treatment. *Br J Dermatol* 1988; **118**: 703–6.

17 Katz BE, MacFarlane DF. Atypical facial scarring after isotretinoin therapy in a patient with previous dermabrasion. *J Am Acad Dermatol* 1994; **30**: 852–3.

Systemic side effects. These include headache, which is not uncommon; anorexia, nausea and vomiting are much more common than with etretinate, as are lethargy, irritability and fatigue [1]. Isotretinoin therapy has been associated with benign intracranial hypertension [2]; in some cases, there was concomitant use of tetracyclines, so this combination should be avoided. A variety of central nervous system reactions have been reported, but may bear no relationship to therapy. The issue of whether isotretinoin may be associated with initiation or exacerbation of depression is a particular matter of controversy [3,4]. Anecdotal reports suggested this possibility; resolution usually, but not always [5], occurs within a few weeks of cessation of therapy. Psychiatric symptoms occurred in seven of 700 patients in one study, with recurrence of depression following rechallenge in some cases [6]. Of 5 million individuals exposed to isotretinoin in the USA between 1982 and 2000, 37 patients committed suicide, 100 were hospitalized for treatment of depression and 284 were managed as outpatients [7]. This incidence of suicide is less than that predicted for a group of comparable age and sex distribution. A large study comparing 7195 patients treated with isotretinoin with 13 700 patients treated with antibiotics, drawn from Canadian and UK databases, concluded that there was no increase in depression or suicide in the isotretinoin-treated group [8]. However, the study has been criticized as flawed with regard to the UK data, because it was provided by general practitioners who were not responsible for prescribing the drug, and there may have been selection bias in the ascertainment of mental disorders. A recent study of 2821 patients found no evidence to support an association between use of isotretinoin and onset of depression [9]. The field is complicated by the fact that there may be a confounding effect of acne on the development of psychological or psychiatric effects [10,11]. In addition, there is an increased frequency of pretreatment anxiety in patients and their families [7]. Conversely, isotretinoin therapy may lead to an improvement in mental state [10,11].

Patients treated for disorders of keratinization have developed corneal opacities, which improved when the drug was withdrawn [12]. Blepharoconjunctivitis, dry eyes with decreased tolerance of contact lenses and blurred vision due to myopia may occur [13]. Decreased night vision has been documented rarely, as have cataracts and other visual disturbances [13–17]; decreased night vision after isotretinoin therapy may be more permanent than generally suspected [17], and many asymptomatic patients have abnormal electroretinograms [14]. Loss of sense of taste is recorded [18].

Transient chest pain is uncommon. Non-specific urogenital findings and non-specific gastrointestinal symptoms have occurred in approximately 5% of cases. Isotretinoin therapy has been associated with onset of inflammatory bowel disease [19] and with impairment of pulmonary function in patients with systemic sclerosis [20,21].

Approximately 16% of patients develop musculoskeletal symptoms, including arthralgia, of mild to moderate degree; cases of acute knee aseptic arthritis have been documented [22]. High-dose prolonged therapy in a child for epidermolytic hyperkeratosis was associated with premature closure of epiphyses [23]. A high prevalence of skeletal hyperostosis has been noted in patients on prolonged (1 year or more), relatively high-dose (2 mg/kg daily) isotretinoin therapy for disorders of keratinization [24–28]. The syndrome of *diffuse idiopathic skeletal hyperostosis* (DISH) includes ossification of ligaments and accretion of bone onto vertebral bodies, especially of the cervical spine. Mild osteoporosis has also been seen. X-ray changes have been minimal in prospective studies of patients with cystic acne treated with a single course of isotretinoin at recommended doses [29–31]. Nasal bone osteophytosis has been described with short-term therapy for acne [32].

Mild to moderate elevation of liver enzymes occurs in about 15% of cases; in some patients these return to normal despite continued administration of the drug. A single case of fatty liver developing in a patient (with low to normal levels of α_1-antitrypsin) on low-dose isotretinoin has been reported [33]. Elevated sedimentation rates occur in about 40% of patients. Between 10 and 20% of patients show decreased red blood cell parameters and white blood cell counts, elevated platelet counts and pyuria. Thrombocytopenia may occur [34].

Isotretinoin induces reversible changes in serum lipids in a significant number of treated subjects [35–40]. A dose-related increase in triglycerides occurs in about 25% of individuals according to the Roche data sheet; five of 135 cystic acne patients, and 32 of 298 patients treated for all diagnoses, showed triglyceride levels above 500 mg/ dL. In another study, 17% of patients taking isotretinoin for 20 weeks exhibited hypertriglyceridaemia, but in 15% this was of only mild to moderate degree [38]. About 15% showed a mild to moderate decrease in serum highdensity lipoprotein levels, and 7% experienced minimal elevations of serum cholesterol during therapy; some patients had increases in LDL cholesterol [38]. Lipid abnormalities peaked within 4 weeks in men, but not until 12 weeks in women. If sustained over a long period, these alterations in lipoproteins might be risk factors for coronary artery disease. Patients with an increased tendency to develop hypertriglyceridaemia include those with diabetes mellitus, obesity, increased alcohol intake or a familial history. Some patients have been able to reverse triglyceride elevation by reduction in weight, restriction of dietary fat and alcohol, and reduction in dose while continuing the drug. An obese male patient with Darier's disease developed elevated triglycerides and subsequent eruptive xanthomas [41].

Major human fetal abnormalities related to isotretinoin therapy during pregnancy have been documented [42–45]. The most frequently reported abnormalities involve the central nervous system (microcephaly or hydrocephalus and cerebellar malformation) and cardiovascular system (anomalies of the great vessels). Microtia or absence of external ears, microphthalmia, facial dysmorphia and thymus gland abnormalities have also been reported. There is an increased risk of spontaneous abortion. Women of child-bearing potential should sign a consent form and be instructed that they should not be pregnant when isotretinoin therapy is started (preferably on the second or third day of the next normal menstrual period) and should use effective contraception during, and for 1 month after stopping, therapy. Isotretinoin has a much shorter halflife than etretinate, so that pregnancy is permissible 1 month after stopping therapy. Analysis of data voluntarily reported to Hoffmann La Roche Inc. in the USA enabled prospective study of 88 patients who had completed or discontinued isotretinoin therapy prior to becoming pregnant; 90% of all pregnancies occurred within 2 months after cessation of therapy, and 64% within 1 month [46]. There were no significant increases in the rates of spontaneous abortion or of congenital malformations among the live births. There appears to be no adverse effect of isotretinoin on male reproductive function [47,48].

REFERENCES

1 Windhorst DB, Nigra T. General clinical toxicology of oral retinoids. *J Am Acad Dermatol* 1982; **4**: 675–82.

2 Anonymous. Adverse effects with isotretinoin. *J Am Acad Dermatol* 1984; **10**: 519–20.

3 Ellis CN, Krach KJ. Uses and complications of isotretinoin therapy. *J Am Acad Dermatol* 2001; **45** (Suppl.): S150–S157.

4 O'Connell KA, Wilkin JK, Pitts M. Isotretinoin (Accutane) and serious psychiatric adverse events. *J Am Acad Dermatol* 2003; **48**: 306–8.

5 Gatti S, Serri F. Acute depression from isotretinoin. *J Am Acad Dermatol* 1991; **25**: 132.

6 Scheinman PL, Peck GL, Rubinow DR *et al.* Acute depression from isotretinoin. *J Am Acad Dermatol* 1990; **23**: 1112–4.

7 Wysowski DK, Pitts M, Beitz J. An analysis of reports of depression and suicide in patients treated with isotretinoin. *J Am Acad Dermatol* 2001; **45**: 515–9.

8 Jick SS, Kremers HM, Vasilakis-Scaramozza C. Isotretinoin use and risk of depression, psychotic symptoms, suicide and attempted suicide. *Arch Dermatol* 2000; **136**: 1231–6.

9 Hersom K, Neary MP, Levaux HP *et al.* Isotretinoin and antidepressant pharmacotherapy: a prescription sequence symmetry analysis. *J Am Acad Dermatol* 2003; **49**: 424–32.

10 Rubinow DR, Peck GL, Sqillace KM Gantt GG. Reduced anxiety and depression in cystic acne patients after successful treatment with oral isotretinoin. *J Am Acad Dermatol* 1987; **17**: 25–32.

11 Kellett SC, Gawkrodger DJ. The psychological and emotional impact of acne and the effect of treatment with isotretinoin. *Br J Dermatol* 1999; **140**: 273–82.

12 Cunningham WJ. Use of isotretinoin in the ichthyoses. In: Cunliffe WJ, Miller AJ, eds. *Retinoid Therapy. A Review of Clinical and Laboratory Research*. Lancaster: MTP Press, 1984: 321–5.

13 Fraunfelder FT, La Braico JM, Meyer SM. Adverse ocular reactions possibly associated with isotretinoin. *Am J Ophthalmol* 1985; **100**: 534–7.

14 Brown RD, Grattan CEH. Visual toxicity of synthetic retinoids. *Br J Ophthalmol* 1989; **73**: 286–8.

15 Gold JA, Shupack JL, Nemec MA. Ocular side effects of the retinoids. *Int J Dermatol* 1989; **28**: 218–25.

16 Denman ST, Welebar RG, Hanifin JM *et al.* Abnormal night vision and altered dark adaptometry in patients treated with isotretinoin for acne. *J Am Acad Dermatol* 1986; **14**: 692–3.

17 Maclean H, Wright M, Choie D, Tidman MJ. Abnormal night vision with isotretinoin therapy for acne. *Clin Exp Dermatol* 1995; **20**: 86.

18 Halpern SM, Todd PM, Kirby JD. Loss of taste associated with isotretinoin. *Br J Dermatol* 1996; **134**: 378.

19 Gold MH, Roenigk HH. The retinoids and inflammatory bowel disease. *Arch Dermatol* 1988; **124**: 325–6.

20 Bunker CB, Sheron N, Maurice PDL *et al.* Isotretinoin and eosinophilic pleural effusion. *Lancet* 1989; **i**: 435–6.

21 Bunker CB, Maurice PDL, Little S *et al.* Isotretinoin and lung function in systemic sclerosis. *Clin Exp Dermatol* 1991; **16**: 11–3.

22 Matsuoka LY, Wortsman J, Pepper JJ. Acute arthritis during isotretinoin treatment for acne. *Arch Intern Med* 1984; **144**: 1870–1.

23 Milstone LM, McGuire J, Ablow RC. Premature epiphyseal closure in a child receiving oral 13-cis-retinoic acid. *J Am Acad Dermatol* 1982; **7**: 663–6.

24 Pittsley R, Yoder K. Retinoid hyperostosis. Skeletal toxicity associated with long-term administration of 13 *cis*-retinoic acid for refractory ichthyosis. *N Engl J Med* 1983; **308**: 1012–4.

25 Ellis CN, Madison KC, Pennes DR *et al.* Isotretinoin is associated with early skeletal radiographic changes. *J Am Acad Dermatol* 1984; **10**: 1024–9.

26 Gerber L, Helfgott R, Gross E *et al.* Vertebral abnormalities associated with synthetic retinoid use. *J Am Acad Dermatol* 1984; **10**: 817–23.

27 Pennes D, Ellis C, Madison K *et al.* Early skeletal hyperostosis secondary to 13-cis-retinoic acid. *Am J Roentgenol* 1984; **142**: 979–83.

28 McGuire J, Milstone L, Lawson J. Isotretinoin administration alters juvenile and adult bone. In: Saurat JH, ed. *Retinoids: New Trends in Research and Therapy*. Basel: Karger, 1985: 419–39.

29 Ellis CN, Pennes DR, Madison KC *et al.* Skeletal radiographic changes during retinoid therapy. In: Saurat JH, ed. *Retinoids: New Trends in Research and Therapy*. Basel: Karger, 1985: 440–4.

30 Kilcoyne RF, Cope R, Cunningham W *et al.* Minimal spinal hyperostosis with low-dose isotretinoin therapy. *Invest Radiol* 1986; **21**: 41–4.

31 Carey BM, Parkin GJS, Cunliffe WJ, Pritlove J. Skeletal toxicity with isotretinoin therapy: a clinico-radiological evaluation. *Br J Dermatol* 1988; **119**: 609–14.

32 Novick NL, Lawson W, Schwartz IS. Bilateral nasal bone osteophytosis associated with short-term oral isotretinoin therapy for cystic acne vulgaris. *Am J Med* 1984; **77**: 736–9.

33 Taylor AEM, Mitchison H. Fatty liver following isotretinoin. *Br J Dermatol* 1991; **124**: 505–6.

34 Johnson TM, Rainin R. Isotretinoin-induced thrombocytopenia. *J Am Acad Dermatol* 1987; **17**: 838–9.

35 Nigra TP, Katz RA, Jorgensen H. Elevation of serum triglyceride levels from oral 13-cis-retinoic acid. In: Orfanos CE, Braun-Falco O, Farber EM *et al.*, eds. *Retinoids. Advances in Basic Research and Therapy*. Berlin: Springer, 1981: 363–9.

36 Lyons F, Laker MF, Marsden JR *et al.* Effect of oral 13-cis-retinoic acid on serum lipids. *Br J Dermatol* 1982; **107**: 591–5.

37 Zech LA, Gross EG, Peck GL, Brewer HB. Changes in plasma cholesterol and triglyceride levels after treatment with oral isotretinoin. A prospective study. *Arch Dermatol* 1983; **119**: 987–93.

38 Bershad S, Rubinstein A, Paterniti JR Jr. *et al.* Changes in plasma lipids and lipoproteins during isotretinoin therapy for acne. *N Engl J Med* 1985; **313**: 981–5.

39 Gollnick H, Schwartzkopff W, Pröschle W *et al.* Retinoids and blood lipids: an update and review. In: Saurat JH, ed. *Retinoids: New Trends in Research and Therapy*. Basel: Karger, 1985: 445–60.

40 Marsden J. Hyperlipidaemia due to isotretinoin and etretinate: possible mechanisms and consequences. *Br J Dermatol* 1986; **114**: 401–7.

41 Dicken CH, Connolly SM. Eruptive xanthomas associated with isotretinoin (13-cis-retinoic acid). *Arch Dermatol* 1980; **16**: 951–2.

42 Hill RM. Isotretinoin teratogenicity. *Lancet* 1984; **i**: 1465.

43 Stern RS, Rosa F, Baum C. Isotretinoin and pregnancy. *J Am Acad Dermatol* 1984; **10**: 851–4.

44 Chen DT. Human pregnancy experience with the retinoids. In: Saurat JH, ed. *Retinoids: New Trends in Research and Therapy*. Basel: Karger, 1985: 398–406.

45 Rosa FW, Wilk AL, Kelsey FO. Teratogen update: vitamin A cogeners, the outcome of pregnancies in patients who had taken isotretinoin. *Teratology* 1986; **33**: 355–64.

46 Dai WS, Hsu M-A, Itri L. Safety of pregnancy after discontinuation of isotretinoin. *Arch Dermatol* 1989; **125**: 362–5.

47 Schill W-B, Wagner A, Nikolowski J, Plewig G. Aromatic retinoid and 13-cis-retinoic acid: spermatological investigations. In: Orfanos CE, Braun-Falco O, Farber EM *et al.*, eds. *Retinoids. Advances in Basic Research and Therapy*. Berlin: Springer, 1981: 389–95.

48 Töröck L, Kása M. Spermatological and endocrinological examinations connected with isotretinoin treatment. In: Saurat JH, ed. *Retinoids: New Trends in Research and Therapy*. Basel: Karger, 1985: 407–10.

Tazarotene

Pyogenic granuloma-like lesions have been associated with the use of this topical retinoid in the treatment of psoriasis [1,2].

Tretinoin

Oral tretinoin administered as differentiation therapy of acute promyelocytic leukaemia was associated with mild rashes, the nature of which was unspecified [3]. An acute neutrophilic dermatosis with a myeloblastic infiltrate occurred in a leukaemic patient receiving all-*trans*-retinoic acid therapy [4].

REFERENCES

1 Dawkins MA, Clark AR, Feldman SR. Pyogenic granuloma-like lesion associated with topical tazarotene therapy. *J Am Acad Dermatol* 2000; **43**: 154–5.

2 Pierson JC, Owens NM. Pyogenic granuloma-like lesions associated with topical retinoid therapy. *J Am Acad Dermatol* 2001; **45**: 967–8.

3 Warrell RP, Frankel SR, Miller WH *et al.* Differentiation therapy of acute promyelocytic leukemia with tretinoin (all-*trans*-retinoic acid). *N Engl J Med* 1991; **324**: 1385–93.

4 Piette WW, Trapp JF, O'Donnell MJ et al. Acute neutrophilic dermatosis with myeloblastic infiltrate in a leukemia patient receiving all-*trans*-retinoic acid therapy. *J Am Acad Dermatol* 1994; **30**: 293–7.

Vitamin B

Vitamin B₁

Anaphylaxis following intravenous administration has occurred [1].

Vitamin B₆ (pyridoxine)

Vasculitis is recorded [2], as is a pseudoporphyria syndrome with megadosage [3]. A photosensitive eruption [4] and rosacea fulminans are documented [5].

Nicotinic acid

Flushing is common; other transient rashes, urticaria, pruritus, scaling, hyperpigmentation and an acanthosis nigricans-like eruption [6,7] are all documented. Persistent rashes and hair loss have rarely occurred.

REFERENCES

1 Kolz R, Lonsdorf G, Burg G. Unverträglichkeitsreaktionen nach parenteraler Gabe von Vitamin B₁. *Hautarzt* 1980; **31**: 657–9.
2 Ruzicka T, Ring J, Braun-Falco O. Vasculitis allergica durch Vitamin B₆. *Hautarzt* 1984; **35**: 197–9.
3 Baer R, Stilman MA. Cutaneous skin changes probably due to pyridoxine abuse. *J Am Acad Dermatol* 1984; **10**: 527–8.
4 Murata Y, Kumano K, Ueda T et al. Photosensitive dermatitis caused by pyridoxine hydrochloride. *J Am Acad Dermatol* 1998; **39**: 314–7.
5 Jansen T, Romiti R, Kreuter A, Altmeyer P. Rosacea fulminans triggered by high-dose vitamins B6 and B12. *J Eur Acad Dermatol Venereol* 2001; **15**: 484–5.
6 Tromovitch TA, Jacobs PH, Kern S. Acanthosis nigricans-like lesions from nicotinic acid. *Arch Dermatol* 1964; **89**: 222–3.
7 Elgart ML. Acanthosis nigricans and nicotinic acid. *J Am Acad Dermatol* 1981; **5**: 709–10.

Vitamin C (ascorbic acid)

Patients with cutaneous and respiratory allergy have been described.

Vitamin E (α-tocopherol)

White hair developed at injection sites in infants given intramuscular vitamin E for epidermolysis bullosa, probably due to quinones formed during vitamin E degradation [1].

REFERENCE

1 Sehgal VN. Vitamin E: a melanotoxic agent. A preliminary report. *Dermatologica* 1972; **145**: 56–9.

Vitamin K

Skin reactions with vitamin K have been reviewed [1–11]. Three distinct types of cutaneous reaction are seen: (i) localized eczematous at the injection site (onset 4–16 days, dose range 10–410 mg); (ii) localized morphoea-form (average onset 8.5 months, range 5 weeks to 1.5 years, dose range 30–2080 mg); and (iii) very rarely, a diffuse maculopapular eruption [10,11]. The pruritic, erythematous, macular lesions or plaques may last for up to 6 months, whereas the prognosis for resolution of the morphoea-form changes is very poor. Patch and intradermal skin tests may be positive, suggesting an immunological basis. Most, but not all [3,6,8], cases have occurred in patients with liver disease. In addition, a proportion of these reactions progress to produce scleroderma-like changes [9,12–16]. An annular erythema has been documented [17].

REFERENCES

1 Barnes HM, Sarkany I. Adverse skin reactions from vitamin K₁. *Br J Dermatol* 1976; **95**: 653–6.
2 Bullen AW, Miller JP, Cunliffe WJ, Losowsky MS. Skin reactions caused by vitamin K in patients with liver disease. *Br J Dermatol* 1978; **98**: 561–5.
3 Sanders MN, Winkelmann RK. Cutaneous reactions to vitamin K. *J Am Acad Dermatol* 1988; **19**: 699–704.
4 Mosser C, Janin-Mercier A, Souteyrand P. Les réactions cutanées apres administration parentérale de vitamine K. *Ann Dermatol Vénéréol* 1987; **114**: 243–51.
5 Finkelstein H, Champion MC, Adam JE. Cutaneous hypersensitivity to vitamin K₁ injection. *J Am Acad Dermatol* 1987; **16**: 540–5.
6 Joyce JP, Hood AF, Weiss MM. Persistent cutaneous reaction to intramuscular vitamin K injection. *Arch Dermatol* 1988; **124**: 27–8.
7 Tuppal R, Tremaine R. Cutaneous eruption from vitamin K₁ injection. *J Am Acad Dermatol* 1992; **27**: 105–6.
8 Lee MM, Gellis S, Dover JS. Eczematous plaques in a patient with liver failure. Fat-soluble vitamin K hypersensitivity. *Arch Dermatol* 1992; **128**: 257, 260.
9 Lemlich G, Green M, Phelps R et al. Cutaneous reactions to vitamin K₁ injections. *J Am Acad Dermatol* 1993; **28**: 345–7.
10 Wong DA, Freeman S. Cutaneous allergic reaction to intramuscular vitamin K1. *Australas J Dermatol* 1999; **40**: 147–52.
11 Wilkins K, DeKoven J, Assaad D. Cutaneous reactions associated with vitamin K1. *J Cutan Med Surg* 2000; **4**: 164–8.
12 Texier L, Gendre PH, Gauthier O et al. Hypodermites sclérodermiformes lombo-fessières induites par des injections médicamenteuses intramusculaires associées a la vitamine K₁. *Ann Dermatol Syphiligr* 1972; **99**: 363–71.
13 Janin-Mercier A, Mosser C, Souteyrand P, Bourges M. Subcutaneous sclerosis with fasciitis and eosinophilia after phytonadione injections. *Arch Dermatol* 1985; **121**: 1421–3.
14 Brunskill NJ, Berth-Jones J, Graham-Brown RAC. Pseudosclerodermatous reaction to phytomenadione injection (Texier's syndrome). *Clin Exp Dermatol* 1988; **13**: 276–8.
15 Pujol RM, Puig L, Moreno A et al. Pseudoscleroderma secondary to phytonadione (vitamin K1) injections. *Cutis* 1989; **43**: 365–8.
16 Guidetti MS, Vincenzi C, Papi M, Tosti A. Sclerodermatous skin reaction after vitamin K1 injections. *Contact Dermatitis* 1994; **31**: 45–6.
17 Kay MH, Duvic M. Reactive annular erythema after intramuscular vitamin K. *Cutis* 1986; **37**: 445–8.

Hormones and related compounds

ACTH and systemic corticosteroids

The side effects of these agents have been reviewed [1–13].

Well-known side effects include acne, cutaneous thinning and atrophy, telangiectasia, striae distensae, purpura and ecchymoses, hypertrichosis, impaired wound healing, pigmentary changes, cushingoid (moon) facies, truncal adiposity [14] and buffalo hump of the upper back. Acne occurred in one of 51 patients treated with intravenous corticosteroids in one study [15]. Other systemic side effects include fluid and electrolyte abnormalities, weight gain, oedema, hypertension, cardiac failure, peptic ulcer disease, pancreatitis, diabetes, muscular weakness, myopathy, tendon rupture, glaucoma, posterior subcapsular cataracts, mental changes including psychosis, osteoporosis, vertebral collapse, necrosis of the femoral head, growth suppression in children, opportunistic infection, masking of infection or reactivation of a dormant infection (e.g. tuberculosis), polycythaemia and suppression of the hypothalamic–pituitary axis. Pulse steroid therapy with systemic methylprednisolone has resulted in sudden death due to anaphylaxis, arrhythmia or ischaemic heart disease, but not particularly in dermatological patients [16].

Adrenocorticotrophic hormone

Allergic reactions to ACTH are recorded but are uncommon. Urticaria and dizziness, nausea and weakness are the most frequent, but severe anaphylactic shock has occurred. Synthetic ACTH is usually tolerated by patients sensitive to animal ACTH [17]. Depot preparations containing tetracosactide (tetracosactrin) adsorbed on a zinc phosphate complex have produced reactions [18] and may induce melanoderma [19].

REFERENCES

1 Lucky AW. Principles of the use of glucocorticosteroids in the growing child. *Pediatr Dermatol* 1984; **1**: 226–35.
2 Fritz KA, Weston WL. Systemic glucocorticosteroid therapy of skin disease in children. *Pediatr Dermatol* 1984; **1**: 236–45.
3 Davis GF. Adverse effects of corticosteroids. II. Systemic. *Clin Dermatol* 1986; **4**: 161–9.
4 Gallant C, Kenny P. Oral glucocorticoids and their complications. A review. *J Am Acad Dermatol* 1986; **14**: 161–77.
5 Seale PS, Compton MR. Side-effects of corticosteroid agents. *Med J Aust* 1986; **144**: 139–42.
6 Chosidow O, Étienne SD, Herson S, Puech AJ. Pharmacologie des corticoïdes. Notions classiques et nouvelles. *Ann Dermatol Vénéréol* 1989; **116**: 147–66.
7 Fine R. Glucocorticoids (1989). *Int J Dermatol* 1990; **29**: 377–9.
8 Kyle V, Hazleman BL. Treatment of polymyalgia rheumatica and giant cell arteritis. II. Relation between steroid dose and steroid associated side effects. *Ann Rheum Dis* 1989; **48**: 662–6.
9 Truhan AP, Ahmed AR. Corticosteroids: a review with emphasis on complications of prolonged systemic therapy. *Ann Allergy* 1989; **62**: 375–90.
10 Weiss MM. Corticosteroids in rheumatoid arthritis. *Semin Arthritis Rheum* 1989; **19**: 9–21.
11 Rasanen L, Hasan T. Allergy to systemic and intralesional corticosteroids. *Br J Dermatol* 1993; **128**: 407–11.
12 Dooms-Goossens A. Sensitisation to corticosteroids. Consequences for anti-inflammatory therapy. *Drug Saf* 1995; **13**: 123–9.
13 Imam AP, Halpern GM. Uses, adverse effects of abuse of corticosteroids. Part II. *Allergol Immunopathol* 1995; **23**: 2–15.
14 Horber HH, Xurcher RM, Herren H *et al.* Altered body fat distribution in patients with glucocorticoid treatment and in patients on long-term dialysis. *Am J Clin Nutr* 1986; **43**: 758–69.
15 Fung MA, Berger TG. A prospective study of acute-onset steroid acne associated with administration of intravenous corticosteroids. *Dermatology* 2000; **200**: 43–4.
16 White KP, Driscoll MS, Rothe MJ, Grant-Kels JM. Severe adverse cardiovascular effects of pulse steroid therapy: is continuous cardiac monitoring necessary? *J Am Acad Dermatol* 1994; **30**: 768–73.
17 Patriarca G. Allergy to tetracosactrin-depot. *Lancet* 1971; **i**: 138.
18 Clee MD, Ferguson J, Browning MCK *et al.* Glucocorticoid hypersensitivity in an asthmatic patient: presentation and treatment. *Thorax* 1985; **40**: 477–8.
19 Khan SA. Melanoderma caused by depot tetracosactrin. *Trans St John's Hosp Dermatol Soc* 1970; **56**: 168–71.

Systemic corticosteroids

In addition to those listed above, the cutaneous side effects of systemic corticosteroids include allergic and immediate reactions [1,2]. In one study, seven of 25 patients with cutaneous delayed-type hypersensitivity to hydrocortisone had an immediate reaction following intradermal injection of hydrocortisone sodium succinate, and had significantly increased levels of IgG antibodies to hydrocortisone. These patients are at risk of developing type III and possibly type I reactions following systemic hydrocortisone [3].

Protein binding of hydrocortisone or a degradation product may be important in the development of corticosteroid allergy [4]. Urticarial reactions have followed the intra-arterial injection of prednisone, prednisolone, hydrocortisone [5] or methylprednisolone [6], but are rare. Anaphylaxis occurred after intradermal injection of triamcinolone for alopecia areata [7]. Anaphylactoid reactions have been reported to topical and parenteral hydrocortisone, but may represent pseudoallergic reactions rather than IgE-mediated immediate hypersensitivity [8,9].

Generalized skin reactions, including urticaria and maculopapular eruptions, developed in patients after therapy with oral triamcinolone acetonide [10], prednisone [11], or dexamethasone and betamethasone [12]; the patients were subsequently shown to be patch-test positive to these corticosteroids. In another study, five patients reacted with diffuse erythema principally on the trunk or on the face, appearing within a few hours to 24 h and fading in 1–3 days, on treatment with systemic or intralesional hydrocortisone, methylprednisolone, prednisolone or betamethasone [2]. On patch testing, one patient reacted to prednisolone and methylprednisolone and two patients were positive to pivalone. Patients sensitive to hydrocortisone or methylprednisolone reacted to these corticosteroids in intradermal tests. A combination of intradermal and patch tests is recommended when allergy to systemic or intralesional corticosteroids is suspected [2].

Other cases of generalized delayed systemic corticosteroid reactions, including eczematous or exanthematous eruptions and erythroderma, with or without bullae or purpura, often with positive patch or intradermal testing, have been recorded [13–18]. Systemic administration of hydrocortisone, and provocation of endogenous cortisol secretion by injection of the ACTH analogue tetracosactide, provoked dose-dependent allergic skin reactions at sites of previous allergic reactions to topical steroids in two patients with proven topical corticosteroid sensitivity (i.e. systemic allergic contact-type dermatitis); in one case, this was at a positive patch-test site to hydrocortisone 17-butyrate [19]. Thus, it has been postulated that high stress levels, which cause increased secretion of endogenous adrenocortical hormones, could be implicated in exacerbations of eczema in corticosteroid-sensitive patients, and a persistent autoimmune skin reaction to cortisol might occur following topical sensitization to topical hydrocortisone [19]. The fact that, in steroid-sensitive patients, systemic provocation testing with hydrocortisone results in a reaction confined to the skin may be partly explained by the observation *in vitro* that only enriched Langerhans' cells, and not peripheral blood mononuclear antigen-presenting cells, are capable of presenting corticosteroid to T cells of corticosteroid-sensitive subjects [20].

Perioral dermatitis has been recorded in renal transplant recipients on corticosteroids and immunosuppressive therapy [21]. Panniculitis following short-term high-dose steroid therapy in children manifests as subcutaneous nodules on the cheeks, arms and trunk [22]. Reversible panniculitis occurred in a child treated with steroids for hepatic encephalopathy [23]. Juxta-articular adiposis dolorosa developed in a patient treated with high doses of prednisone for the L-tryptophan-induced eosinophilia myalgia syndrome [24]. Acanthosis nigricans may occur with corticosteroid therapy [25]. Immunosuppression with corticosteroids has been associated with the development of Kaposi's sarcoma during the treatment of temporal arteritis [26].

Inhaled corticosteroids have been associated with purpura and dermal thinning [27] as well as acne [28,29], perioral dermatitis and tongue hypertrophy [30], allergic reactions [31], an eczematous dermatitis [32] and adrenal suppression [29]. Nasal corticosteroids may cause nasal congestion, pruritus, burning and perforation of the septum, urticaria and eczema of the face [33]. Intralesional corticosteroid injection may also lead to allergic reactions [34], including a disseminated morbilliform and persistent urticarial dermatitis following intra-articular triamcinolone acetonide [35], erythroderma following intradermal budesonide [36] and erythema multiforme after intradural injection of prednisolone acetate [37]. Facial flushing and/or generalized erythema has followed epidural steroid injection [38]. Anaphylactic shock has been recorded after intra-articular injections of corticosteroids containing carboxymethylcellulose, benzylic acid, polysorbate 80 and merthiolate; skin tests to carboxymethylcellulose were positive [39].

REFERENCES

1 Preuss L. Allergic reactions to systemic glucocorticoids: a review. *Ann Allergy* 1985; **55**: 772–5.
2 Rasanen L, Hasan T. Allergy to systemic and intralesional corticosteroids. *Br J Dermatol* 1993; **128**: 407–11.
3 Wilkinson SM, Mattey DL, Beck MH. IgG antibodies and early intradermal reactions to hydrocortisone in patients with cutaneous delayed-type hypersensitivity to hydrocortisone. *Br J Dermatol* 1994; **131**: 495–8.
4 Wilkinson SM, English JS, Mattey DL. *In vitro* evidence of delayed-type hypersensitivity to hydrocortisone. *Contact Dermatitis* 1993; **29**: 241–5.
5 Ashford RF, Bailey A. Angioneurotic oedema and urticaria following hydrocortisone: a further case. *Postgrad Med J* 1980; **56**: 437.
6 Pollock B, Wilkinson SM, MacDonald Hull SP. Chronic urticaria associated with intra-articular methylprednisolone. *Br J Dermatol* 2001; **144**: 1228–30.
7 Downs AMR, Lear JT, Kennedy CTC. Anaphylaxis to intradermal triamcinolone acetonide. *Arch Dermatol* 1998; **134**: 1163–4.
8 King RA. A severe anaphylactoid reaction to hydrocortisone. *Lancet* 1960; **ii**: 1093–4.
9 Peller JS, Bardana EL Jr. Anaphylactoid reaction to corticosteroid: case report and review of the literature. *Ann Allergy* 1985; **54**: 302–5.
10 Brambilla L, Boneschi V, Chiappino G et al. Allergic reactions to topical desoxymethasone and oral triamcinolone. *Contact Dermatitis* 1989; **21**: 272–3.
11 De Corres LF, Bernaola G, Urrutia I et al. Allergic dermatitis from systemic treatment with corticosteroids. *Contact Dermatitis* 1990; **22**: 104–5.
12 Maucher O, Faber M, Knipper H et al. Kortikoidallergie. *Hautarzt* 1987; **38**: 577–82.
13 Whitmore SE. Delayed systemic allergic reactions to corticosteroids. *Contact Dermatitis* 1995; **32**: 193–8.
14 Torres V, Tavares-Bello R, Melo H, Soares AP. Systemic contact dermatitis from hydrocortisone. *Contact Dermatitis* 1993; **29**: 106.
15 Vidal C, Tome S, Fernandex-Redondo V, Tato F. Systemic allergic reaction to corticosteroids. *Contact Dermatitis* 1994; **31**: 273–4.
16 Whitmore SE. Dexamethasone injection-induced generalised dermatitis. *Br J Dermatol* 1994; **131**: 296–7.
17 Fernandez de Corres L, Urrutia I, Audicana M et al. Erythroderma after intravenous injection of methylprednisolone. *Contact Dermatitis* 1991; **25**: 68–70.
18 Yawalkar N, Hari Y, Helbling A et al. Elevated serum levels of interleukins 5, 6, and 10 in a patient with drug-induced exanthem caused by systemic corticosteroids. *J Am Acad Dermatol* 1998; **39**: 790–3.
19 Lauerma AI, Reitamo S, Maibach HI. Systemic hydrocortisone/cortisol induces allergic skin reactions in presensitized subjects. *J Am Acad Dermatol* 1991; **24**: 182–5.
20 Lauerma AI, Räsänen L, Reunala T, Reitamo S. Langerhans cells but not monocytes are capable of antigen presentation *in vitro* in corticosteroid contact hypersensitivity. *Br J Dermatol* 1991; **123**: 699–705.
21 Adams SJ, Davison AM, Cunliffe WJ, Giles GR. Perioral dermatitis in renal transplant recipients maintained on corticosteroids and immunosuppressive therapy. *Br J Dermatol* 1982; **106**: 589–92.
22 Roenigk HH, Haserick JR, Arundell FD. Poststeroid panniculitis. *Arch Dermatol* 1964; **90**: 387–91.
23 Saxena AK, Nigam PK. Panniculitis following steroid therapy. *Cutis* 1988; **42**: 341–2.
24 Greenbaum SS, Varga J. Corticosteroid-induced juxta-articular adiposis dolorosa. *Arch Dermatol* 1991; **127**: 231–3.
25 Brown J, Winkelmann RK. Acanthosis nigricans: a study of 90 cases. *Medicine (Baltimore)* 1968; **47**: 33–51.
26 Leung F, Fam AG, Osoba D. Kaposi's sarcoma complicating corticosteroid therapy for temporal arteritis. *Am J Med* 1981; **71**: 320–2.
27 Capewell S, Reynolds S, Shuttleworth D et al. Purpura and dermal thinning associated with high-dose inhaled corticosteroids. *BMJ* 1990; **300**: 1548–51.
28 Monk B, Cunliffe WJ, Layton AM, Rhodes DJ. Acne induced by inhaled corticosteroids. *Clin Exp Dermatol* 1993; **18**: 148–50.
29 Bong JL, Connell JM, Lever R. Intranasal betamethasone induced acne and adrenal suppression. *Br J Dermatol* 2000; **142**: 579–80.
30 Dubus JC, Marguet C, Deschildre A et al. Local side-effects of inhaled corticosteroids in asthmatic children: influence of drug, dose, age, and device. *Allergy* 2001; **56**: 944–8.
31 Lauerma AH, Kiistala R, Makinen-Kiljunen S et al. Allergic skin reaction after inhalation of budesonide. *Clin Exp Allergy* 1993; **23**: 232–3.

32 Holmes P, Cowen P. Spongiotic (eczematous-type) dermatitis after inhaled budesonide. *Aust NZ J Med* 1992; **22**: 511.

33 Isaksson M. Skin reactions to inhaled corticosteroids. *Drug Saf* 2001; **24**: 369–73.

34 Saff DM, Taylor JS, Vidimos AT. Allergic reaction to intralesional triamcinolone acetonide: a case report. *Arch Dermatol* 1995; **131**: 742–3.

35 Ijsselmuiden OE, Knegt-Junk KJ, van Wijk RG, van Joost T. Cutaneous adverse reactions after intra-articular injection of triamcinolone acetonide. *Acta Derm Venereol (Stockh)* 1995; **75**: 57–8.

36 Wilkinson SM, Smith AG, English JS. Erythroderma following the intradermal injection of the corticosteroid budesonide. *Contact Dermatitis* 1992; **27**: 121–2.

37 Lavabre C, Chevalier X, Larget-Piet B. Erythema multiforme after intradural injection of prednisolone acetate. *Br J Rheumatol* 1992; **31**: 717–8.

38 DeSio JM, Kahn CH, Warfield CA. Facial flushing and/or generalized erythema after epidural steroid injection. *Anesth Analg* 1995; **80**: 617–9.

39 Beaudouin E, Kanny G, Gueant JL, Moneret-Vautrin DA. Anaphylaxie à la carboxymethylcellulose: à propos de deux cas de chocs à des corticoides injectables. *Allerg Immunol* 1992; **24**: 333–5.

Topical corticosteroids

The dermatological complications of topical corticosteroids have been reviewed [1–4]. Concerns have been expressed about the illegal availability of potent topical steroids in the UK, and their consequent unregulated use [5]. Many of the adverse reactions are related to the potency of the preparation; thus, in general, fluorinated steroids are associated with more significant side effects. Topical steroids cause decreased epidermal kinetic activity [6], decreased synthesis of dermal collagen types I and III and ground substance, and thinning of the dermis and epidermis [7–11]. Initial vasoconstriction of the superficial small vessels is followed by rebound vasodilatation, which becomes permanent in later stages. There are resultant striae, easy bruising, purpura, hypertrichosis and telangiectasia; stellate pseudoscars or ulcerated areas may be seen. Reversible hypopigmentation may develop. Local injection of a potent steroid may result in atrophy with telangiectasia, and localized lipoatrophy may occur. Perilymphatic atrophy is recorded following intradermal steroid injection. Long-term daily use of a potent steroid, especially under plastic occlusion as for fingertip eczema, may result in acroatrophy of terminal phalanges of the fingers [12,13].

Topical steroids may exacerbate acne, or lead to acne rosacea, with papules, pustules and telangiectasia, or perioral dermatitis, characterized by erythema, papules and pustules at the perioral area [14–16]. They decrease the number and antigen-presenting capacity of epidermal Langerhans' cells [17], and mask or potentiate skin infections, including fungal (tinea incognito) and bacterial infections and verruca vulgaris. Their withdrawal may provoke conversion of plaque- to pustular-type psoriasis [18]. Topical steroid therapy around the eye has been associated with development of glaucoma.

Topical corticosteroids may induce allergic contact dermatitis [19–25]. The prevalence of positive patch tests to corticosteroids in contact dermatitis clinics ranges from 2 to 5% [19,20]. The allergen may be the steroid itself, or a preservative or stabilizer such as ethylenediamine. There may be cross-reactivity between different steroids [21–23]. Cross-reactivity is more likely between steroids with similar substitutions at C-6 and C-9 positions. Intradermal tests may be a more sensitive means of detecting corticosteroid hypersensitivity than patch testing [24].

Systemic side effects of topical corticosteroids occur particularly from the use of large amounts of high-potency topical corticosteroids, especially under plastic occlusion [26,27]. Oedema due to sodium retention occurs more frequently with halogenated corticosteroids [27]. Hypothalamic–pituitary axis suppression may occur [28,29]; a single application of 25 g of 0.05% clobetasol propionate ointment suppressed plasma cortisol for 96 h [30]. Cushing's syndrome [31,32] may result, and growth retardation in children is a hazard [33]. Glycosuria and hyperglycaemia may rarely occur [34].

REFERENCES

1 Miller JA, Munro DD. Topical corticosteroids: clinical pharmacology and therapeutic use. *Drugs* 1980; **19**: 119–34.

2 Behrendt H, Korting HC. Klinische Prüfung von erwünschten und unerwünschten Wirkungen topisch applizierbarer Glukokortikosteroide am Menschen. *Hautarzt* 1990; **41**: 2–8.

3 Coskey RJ. Adverse effects of corticosteroids. I. Topical and intralesional. *Clin Dermatol* 1986; **4**: 155–60.

4 Kligman AM. Adverse effects of topical corticosteroids. In: Christophers E, Schöpf E, Kligman AM, Stoughton RB, eds. *Topical Corticosteroid Therapy: a Novel Approach to Safer Drugs*. New York: Raven Press, 1988: 181–7.

5 Keane FM, Munn SE, Taylor NF, du Vivier AW. Unregulated use of clobetasol propionate. *Br J Dermatol* 2001; **144**: 1095–6.

6 Marshall RC, Du Vivier RA. The effects on epidermal DNA synthesis of the butyrate esters of clobetasone and clobetasol, and the propionate ester of clobetasol. *Br J Dermatol* 1978; **98**: 355–9.

7 Smith JG, Wehr RF, Chalker DK. Corticosteroid-induced cutaneous atrophy and telangiectasia. *Arch Dermatol* 1976; **112**: 1115–7.

8 Winter GD, Burton JL. Experimentally induced steroid atrophy in the domestic pig and man. *Br J Dermatol* 1976; **94**: 107–9.

9 Lehmann P, Zheng P, Lacker RM, Kligman AM. Corticosteroid atrophy in human skin: a study by light, scanning and transmission electron microscopy. *J Invest Dermatol* 1983; **81**: 169–76.

10 Oikarinen A, Haapasaari KM, Sutinen M, Tasanen K. The molecular basis of glucocorticoid-induced skin atrophy: topical glucocorticoid apparently decreases both collagen synthesis and the corresponding collagen mRNA level in human skin *in vivo*. *Br J Dermatol* 1998; **139**: 1106–10.

11 Oishi Y, Fu ZW, Ohnuki Y *et al*. Molecular basis of the alteration in skin collagen metabolism in response to *in vivo* dexamethasone treatment: effects on the synthesis of collagen type I and III, collagenase, and tissue inhibitors of metalloproteinases. *Br J Dermatol* 2002; **147**: 859–68.

12 Requena L, Zamora E, Martin L. Acroatrophy secondary to long-standing applications of topical steroids. *Arch Dermatol* 1990; **126**: 1013–4.

13 Wolf R, Tur E, Brenner S. Corticosteroid-induced 'disappearing digit'. *J Am Acad Dermatol* 1990; **23**: 755–6.

14 Sneddon I. Perioral dermatitis. *Br J Dermatol* 1972; **87**: 430–2.

15 Cotterill JA. Perioral dermatitis. *Br J Dermatol* 1979; **101**: 259–62.

16 Edwards EK Jr, Edwards ED Sr. Perioral dermatitis secondary to the use of a corticosteroid ointment as moustache wax. *Int J Dermatol* 1987; **26**: 649.

17 Ashworth J, Booker J, Breathnach SM. Effect of topical corticosteroid therapy on Langerhans cell function in human skin. *Br J Dermatol* 1988; **118**: 457–69.

18 Boxley JD, Dawber RPR, Summerly R. Generalised pustular psoriasis on withdrawal of clobetasol propionate ointment. *BMJ* 1975; **2**: 225–6.

19 Wilkinson SM. Hypersensitivity to topical corticosteroids. *Clin Exp Dermatol* 1994; **19**: 1–11.

20 Bircher AJ, Thurlimann W, Hunziker T *et al*. Contact hypersensitivity to corticosteroids in routine patch test patients. A multi-centre study of the Swiss Contact Dermatitis Research Group. *Dermatology* 1995; **191**: 109–14.

21 Lepoittevin JP, Drieghe J, Dooms-Goossens A. Studies in patients with corticosteroid contact allergy. Understanding cross-reactivity among different steroids. *Arch Dermatol* 1995; **131**: 31–7.
22 Wilkinson SM, Hollis S, Beck MH. Cross-reaction patterns in patients with allergic contact dermatitis from hydrocortisone. *Br J Dermatol* 1995; **132**: 766–71.
23 Wilkinson M, Hollis S, Beck M. Reactions to other corticosteroids in patients with positive patch test reactions to budesonide. *J Am Acad Dermatol* 1995; **33**: 963–8.
24 Wilkinson SM, Heagerty AHM, English JSC. A prospective study into the value of patch and intradermal tests in identifying topical corticosteroid allergy. *Br J Dermatol* 1992; **127**: 22–5.
25 Sommer S, Wilkinson SM, English JSC *et al.* Type-IV hypersensitivity to betamethasone valerate and clobetasol propionate: results of a multicentre study. *Br J Dermatol* 2002; **147**: 266–9.
26 Vickers CFH, Fritsch WC. A hazard of plastic film therapy. *Arch Dermatol* 1963; **87**: 633–5.
27 Fitzpatrick TB, Griswold MC, Hicks JH. Sodium retention and edema from percutaneous absorption of fluorcortisone acetate. *JAMA* 1955; **158**: 1149–52.
28 Carruthers JA, August PJ, Staughton RCD. Observations on the systemic effect of topical clobetasol propionate (Dermovate). *BMJ* 1975; **4**: 203–4.
29 Weston WL, Fennessey PV, Morelli J *et al.* Comparison of hypothalamus–pituitary–adrenal axis suppression from superpotent topical steroids by standard endocrine function testing and gas chromatographic mass spectrometry. *J Invest Dermatol* 1988; **90**: 532–5.
30 Hehir M, du Vivier A, Eilon L *et al.* Investigation of the pharmacokinetics of clobetasol propionate and clobetasone butyrate after a single application of ointment. *Clin Exp Dermatol* 1983; **8**: 143–51.
31 May P, Stein ES, Ryler RJ *et al.* Cushing syndrome from percutaneous absorption of triamcinolone cream. *Arch Intern Med* 1976; **136**: 612–3.
32 Himathongkam T, Dasanabhairochana P, Pitchayayothin N, Sriphrapradang A. Florid Cushing's syndrome and hirsutism induced by desoximetasone. *JAMA* 1978; **239**: 430–1.
33 Bode HH. Dwarfism following long-term topical corticosteroid therapy. *JAMA* 1980; **244**: 813–4.
34 Gomez EC, Frost P. Induction of glycosuria and hyperglycemia by topical corticosteroid therapy. *Arch Dermatol* 1976; **112**: 1559–62.

Sex hormones

Gonadotrophins

These drugs may cause allergic reactions [1]. Menotrophin (Pergonal) has been associated with localized keratosis follicularis (Darier's disease) [2]. Intracutaneous administration of two human menopausal gonadotrophin preparations (Organon and Pergonal) caused local induration and erythema [3].

REFERENCES

1 Dore PC, Rice C, Killick S. Human gonadotrophin preparations may cause allergic reaction. *BMJ* 1994; **308**: 1509.
2 Telang GH, Atillasoy E, Stierstorfer M. Localized keratosis follicularis associated with menotropin treatment and pregnancy. *J Am Acad Dermatol* 1994; **30**: 271–2.
3 Odink J, Zuiderwijk PB, Schoen ED, Gan RA. A prospective, double-blind, split-subject study on local skin reactions after administration of human menopausal gonadotrophin preparations to healthy female volunteers. *Hum Reprod* 1995; **10**: 1045–7.

Gonadorelin analogues

Buserelin. A pigmented roseola-like eruption has been documented [1].

Leuprorelin. This drug, given for precocious puberty, has caused anaphylaxis [2], rashes [3] and local reactions [4].

REFERENCES

1 Kono T, Ishii M, Taniguchi S. Intranasal buserelin acetate-induced pigmented roseola-like eruption. *Br J Dermatol* 2000; **143**: 658–9.
2 Taylor JD. Anaphylactic reaction to LHRH analogue, leuprorelin. *Med J Aust* 1994; **161**: 455.
3 Carel JC, Lahlou N, Guazzarotti L *et al.* Treatment of central precocious puberty with depot leuprorelin. French Leuprorelin Trial Group. *Eur J Endocrinol* 1995; **132**: 699–704.
4 Manasco PK, Pescovitz OH, Blizzard RM. Local reactions to depot leuprolide therapy for central precocious puberty. *J Pediatr* 1993; **123**: 334–5.

Oestrogens and related compounds

Oestrogens. Spider naevi and melanocytic naevi may develop under oestrogen therapy, as may chloasma. Severe premenstrual exacerbation of papulovesicular eruptions, urticaria, eczema or generalized pruritus occurred in seven women; several had a positive delayed tuberculin-type skin test to oestrogen [1]. Patients with generalized chronic urticaria had an urticarial reaction to intradermal oestrogens. Elimination of oral oestrogen therapy or anti-oestrogen therapy with tamoxifen proved effective. In another patient, a premenstrual urticarial reaction was exacerbated by oestrogen; oophorectomy cured the eruption [2]. A bullous autoimmune oestrogen dermatitis has been delineated [3].

Diethylstilbestrol therapy of pregnant women has been associated with female and male genital tract abnormalities in the offspring. Diethylstilbestrol is a transplacental carcinogen and has caused adenocarcinoma of the vagina 20 years later in young women whose mothers took the drug in the first 18 weeks of pregnancy [4–6]. Acanthosis nigricans has resulted from use of diethylstilbestrol [7]. Hyperkeratosis of the nipples developed in a man treated for adenocarcinoma of the prostate with diethylstilbestrol [8]. Porphyria cutanea tarda may also be precipitated [9,10].

REFERENCES

1 Shelley WB, Shelley ED, Talanin NY, Santoso-Pham J. Estrogen dermatitis. *J Am Acad Dermatol* 1995; **32**: 25–31.
2 Mayou SC, Charles-Holmes R, Kenney A *et al.* A premenstrual urticarial eruption treated with bilateral oophorectomy and hysterectomy. *Clin Exp Dermatol* 1988; **13**: 114–6.
3 Mutasim DF, Baumbach JL. Bullous autoimmune estrogen dermatitis. *J Am Acad Dermatol* 2003; **49**: 130–1.
4 Monaghan JM, Sirisena LAW. Stilboestrol and vaginal clear-cell adenocarcinoma syndrome. *BMJ* 1978; **i**: 1588–90.
5 Wingfield M. The daughters of stilboestrol. Grown up now but still at risk. *BMJ* 1991; **302**: 1414–5.
6 Anonymous. Diethylstilboestrol: effects of exposure *in utero. Drug Ther Bull* 1991; **29**: 49–50.
7 Banuchi SR, Cohen L, Lorincz AL, Morgan J. Acanthosis nigricans following diethylstilbestrol therapy. *Arch Dermatol* 1974; **109**: 544–6.
8 Mold DE, Jegasothy BV. Estrogen-induced hyperkeratosis of the nipple. *Cutis* 1980; **26**: 95–6.

9 Becker FT. Porphyria cutanea tarda induced by estrogens. *Arch Dermatol* 1965; **92**: 252–6.
10 Roenigk HH, Gottlob ME. Estrogen-induced porphyria cutanea tarda. *Arch Dermatol* 1970; **102**: 260–6.

Oral contraceptives. Cutaneous complications of oral contraceptives have been reviewed [1–4]. These drugs combine an oestrogen with a progestogen. Candidiasis is common; the sexual partner may suffer penile irritation after coitus without physical signs or frank candidal balanoposthitis. Genital warts may increase. Facial hyperpigmentation (chloasma) is well recognized [5,6], as are hirsutism and acne. Gingival epithelial melanosis has been recorded [7]. Alopecia related to contraceptive therapy may be of either androgenic or postpartum telogen pattern following withdrawal of the drug. Erythema nodosum is a well-recognized but rare complication [8,9].

The relapse of herpes gestationis is well documented [10]. Rare lichenoid, eczematous and fixed eruptions have been described, as have a lymphocytic cutaneous vasculitis and an eruption resembling Sweet's syndrome [11]. Oral contraceptives have been implicated in both the provocation [12] and induction of remission of pityriasis lichenoides. An SLE-like reaction has also been reported [13]. An oral contraceptive-induced LE-like eruption, with erythematous lesions on the palms and feet in association with a weakly positive antinuclear factor and C1q deposition at the dermal–epidermal junction on direct immunofluorescence, developed in a patient. It resolved on cessation of medication [14].

The jaundice rarely induced by these drugs resembles cholestatic jaundice of pregnancy. The hepatotoxic effects may result in provocation of variegate porphyria, porphyria cutanea tarda [15,16] and hereditary coproporphyria [17]; onycholysis may occur [16]. Photosensitivity unrelated to porphyrin disturbances has also been reported [18,19]. Benign hepatomas may also be a hazard [20].

Other hormonal contraceptives. Keloid formation has followed levonorgestrel implantion [21]. Vaginal erythematous areas were associated with use of a levonorgestrel-releasing contraceptive ring in 48 of 139 subjects [22]. Rosacea has been associated with a progesterone-releasing intrauterine contraceptive device [23].

Hormone replacement therapy. Melasma of the arms is recorded [24–26].

REFERENCES

1 Baker H. Drug reactions VIII. Adverse cutaneous reaction to oral contraceptives. *Br J Dermatol* 1969; **81**: 946–9.
2 Jelinek JE. Cutaneous complications of oral contraceptives. *Arch Dermatol* 1970; **101**: 181–6.
3 Coskey RJ. Eruptions due to oral contraceptives. *Arch Dermatol* 1977; **113**: 333–4.
4 Girard M. Évaluation des risques cutanés de la pilule. *Ann Dermatol Vénéréol* 1990; **117**: 436–40.

5 Resnik S. Melasma induced by oral contraceptive drugs. *JAMA* 1967; **199**: 601.
6 Smith AG, Shuster S, Thody AJ et al. Chloasma, oral contraceptives, and plasma immunoreactive beta melanocyte-stimulating hormone. *J Invest Dermatol* 1977; **68**: 169–70.
7 Hertz RS, Beckstead PC, Brown WJ. Epithelial melanosis of the gingiva possibly resulting from the use of oral contraceptives. *J Am Dent Assoc* 1980; **100**: 713–4.
8 Posternal F, Orusco MMM, Laugier P. Eythème noueux et contraceptifs oraux. *Bull Dermatol* 1974; **81**: 642–5.
9 Bombardieri S, Di Munno O, Di Punzio C, Pasero G. Erythema nodosum associated with pregnancy and oral contraceptives. *BMJ* 1977; **i**: 1509–10.
10 Morgan JK. Herpes gestationis influenced by an oral contraceptive. *Br J Dermatol* 1968; **80**: 456–8.
11 Tefany FJ, Georgouras K. A neutrophilic reaction of Sweet's syndrome type associated with the oral contraceptive. *Australas J Dermatol* 1991; **32**: 55–9.
12 Hollander A, Grotts IA. Mucha–Habermann disease following estrogen–progesterone therapy. *Arch Dermatol* 1973; **107**: 465.
13 Garrovich M, Agudelo C, Pisko E. Oral contraceptives and systemic lupus erythematosus. *Arthritis Rheum* 1980; **23**: 1396–8.
14 Furukawa F, Tachibana T, Imamura S, Tamura T. Oral contraceptive-induced lupus erythematosus in a Japanese woman. *J Dermatol* 1991; **18**: 56–8.
15 Degos R, Touraine R, Kalis B et al. Porphyrie cutanée tardive après prise prolongé de contraceptifs oraux. *Ann Dermatol Syphiligr* 1969; **96**: 5–14.
16 Byrne JPH, Boss JM, Dawber RPR. Contraceptive pill-induced porphyria cutanea tarda presenting with onycholysis of the finger nails. *Postgrad Med J* 1976; **52**: 535–8.
17 Roberts DT, Brodie MJ, Moore MR et al. Hereditary coproporphyria presenting with photosensitivity induced by the contraceptive pill. *Br J Dermatol* 1977; **96**: 549–54.
18 Erickson LR, Peterka ES. Sunlight sensitivity from oral contraceptives. *JAMA* 1968; **203**: 980–1.
19 Cooper SM, George S. Photosensitivity reaction associated with use of the combined oral contraceptive. *Br J Dermatol* 2001; **144**: 641–2.
20 Baum JK, Holtz F, Bookstein JJ, Klein EW. Possible association between benign hepatomas and oral contraceptives. *Lancet* 1973; **ii**: 926–8.
21 Nuovo J, Sweha A. Keloid formation from levonorgestrel implant (Norplant System) insertion. *J Am Board Family Pract* 1994; **7**: 152–4.
22 Bounds W, Szarewski A, Lowe D, Guillebaud J. Preliminary report of unexpected local reactions to a progestogen-releasing contraceptive vaginal ring. *Eur J Obstet Gynecol Reprod Biol* 1993; **48**: 123–5.
23 Choudry K, Humphreys F, Menage J. Rosacea in association with the progesterone-releasing intrauterine contraceptive device. *Clin Exp Dermatol* 2001; **26**: 102.
24 Johnston GA, Sviland L, McLelland J. Melasma of the arms associated with hormone replacement therapy. *Br J Dermatol* 1998; **139**: 932.
25 Varma S, Roberts DL. Melasma of the arms associated with hormone replacement therapy. *Br J Dermatol* 1999; **141**: 592.
26 O'Brien TJ, Dyall-Smith D, Hall AP. Melasma of the arms associated with hormone replacement therapy. *Br J Dermatol* 1999; **141**: 592–3.

Anti-oestrogens

Clomifene (clomiphene). Hot flushes [1] and recurrent petechiae and palpable purpura of the legs with neutrophilic infiltration in a woman treated for infertility with multiple courses of clomifene [2] have been reported.

REFERENCES

1 Derman SG, Adashi EY. Adverse effects of fertility drugs. *Drug Saf* 1994; **11**: 408–21.
2 Coots NV, McCoy CE, Gehlbach DL, Becker LE. A neutrophilic drug reaction to Clomid. *Cutis* 1996; **57**: 91–3.

Tamoxifen. This oestrogen receptor antagonist used in the therapy of breast cancer in women has caused hirsutism, hair loss, dry skin and a variety of rashes [1].

REFERENCE

1 Descamps V, Bouscarat F, Boui M *et al.* Delayed appearance of maculopapular eruptions induced by tamoxifen. *Ann Dermatol Vénéreol* 1999; **126**: 716–7.

Progesterone and progestogens

Autoimmune progesterone dermatitis. A number of eruptions, including urticaria, eczema, pompholyx, erythema annulare centrifugum and erythema multiforme, have been reported to recur cyclically in the second (luteal) phase of the menstrual cycle, with the period immediately before menstruation peaking in severity [1–8]. Oral and perineal lesions may occur. It has been proposed that they result from sensitization to endogenous progesterone. There is frequently, but not always, a history of prior exposure to synthetic progesterones [1,3]. Confirmation is with a positive intradermal test with progesterone, preferably in an aqueous or aqueous alcohol solution, and/or existence of circulating antibody to progesterone, and by suppression of symptoms with agents that inhibit ovulation and result in decreased serum progesterone [7]. Two patients with recurrent premenstrual erythema multiforme and autoreactivity to 17α-hydroxyprogesterone have been described [5,6]; in one case, the eruption spread in pregnancy, cleared after abortion and was associated with a high-affinity binding factor to 17α-hydroxyprogesterone in the serum [6]. In another case with recurrent erythema multiforme, cured by oophorectomy, progesterone sensitivity was confirmed by challenge with medroxyprogesterone acetate [9].

Medroxyprogesterone acetate. A pigmented purpura [10] and skin necrosis following intramuscular Depo-Provera [11] are recorded.

Megestrol. A generalized morbilliform rash developed in a cachectic man treated with this synthetic orally active progesterone derivative to stimulate appetite and weight gain; skin testing with progesterone acetate was positive [12].

REFERENCES

1 Hart R. Autoimmune progesterone dermatitis. *Arch Dermatol* 1977; **113**: 426–30.
2 Wojnarowska F, Greaves MW, Peachey RDG *et al.* Progesterone-induced erythema multiforme. *J R Soc Med* 1985; **78**: 407–8.
3 Stephens CJM, Black MM. Perimenstrual eruptions: autoimmune progesterone dermatitis. *Semin Dermatol* 1989; **8**: 26–9.
4 Yee KC, Cunliffe WJ. Progesterone-induced urticaria: response to buserelin. *Br J Dermatol* 1994; **130**: 121–3.
5 Cheesman KL, Gaynor LV, Chatterton RT Jr *et al.* Identification of a 17α-hydroxyprogesterone-binding immunoglobulin in the serum of a woman with periodic rashes. *J Clin Endocrinol Metab* 1982; **55**: 597–9.
6 Pinta JS, Sobrinho L, da Silva MB *et al.* Erythema multiforme associated with autoreactivity to 17α-hydroxyprogesterone. *Dermatologica* 1990; **180**: 146–50.
7 Herzberg AJ, Strohmeyer CR, Cirillo-Hyland VA. Autoimmune progesterone dermatitis. *J Am Acad Dermatol* 1995; **32**: 333–8.
8 Halevy S, Cohen AD, Lunenfeld E, Grossman N. Autoimmune progesterone dermatitis manifested as erythema annulare centrifugum: confirmation of progesterone sensitivity by in vitro interferon-γ release. *J Am Acad Dermatol* 2002; **47**: 311–3.
9 Ródenas JM, Herranz MT, Tercedor J. Autoimmune progesterone dermatitis: treatment with oophorectomy. *Br J Dermatol* 1998; **139**: 508–11.
10 Tsao H, Lerner LH. Pigmented purpuric eruption associated with injection medroxyprogesterone acetate. *J Am Acad Dermatol* 2000; **43**: 308–10.
11 Clark SM, Lanigan SW. Acute necrotic skin reaction to intramuscular Depo-Provera®. *Br J Dermatol* 2000; **143**: 1356–7.
12 Fisher DA. Drug-induced progesterone dermatitis. *J Am Acad Dermatol* 1996; **34**: 863–4.

Androgens

Anabolic steroids. Exacerbation of acne vulgaris with development of acne conglobata has been reported [1]. Both the size of sebaceous glands and the rate of sebum secretion are increased [2,3]. A lichenoid eruption was reported in a patient with aplastic anaemia treated with nandrolone furylpropionate (Cemelon) [4].

Danazol. This 17-ethinyltestosterone derivative, which is an inhibitor of pituitary gonadotrophin, is a very weak androgen. Of 530 recipients of danazol, 29% reported at least one adverse event within 45 days after receiving the drug, but there were no known long-term sequelae [5]. Acne, hirsutism, seborrhoea, rash and generalized alopecia are documented [6–8]. Exacerbation of LE-like eruptions has been reported in patients receiving this drug for non-C1-esterase inhibitor-dependent angio-oedema [9] or for hereditary angio-oedema [10].

Gestrinone. This derivative of 19-nortestosterone, like danazol, may cause weight gain, hirsutism, acne, voice change or irregular menstrual bleeding [11].

Testosterone. Severe acne or acne fulminans has followed therapy with testosterone, with [2,12] or without [13] anabolic steroids.

Yohimbine. Yohimbine is an indole alkaloid obtained from the yohimbe tree in West Africa and is used in the treatment of male impotence. A case of generalized erythrodermic skin eruption, progressive renal failure and LE-like syndrome is recorded [14].

REFERENCES

1 Merkle T, Landthaler M, Braun-Falco O. Acne-conglobata-artige Exazerbation einer Acne vulgaris nach Einnahme von Anabolika und Vitamin-B-Komplex-haltigen Präparaten. *Hautarzt* 1990; **41**: 280–2.
2 Király CL, Collan Y, Alén M. Effect of testosterone and anabolic steroids on the size of sebaceous glands in power athletes. *Am J Dermatopathol* 1987; **9**: 515–9.
3 Király CL, Alén M, Rahkila P, Horsmanheimo M. Effect of androgenic and anabolic steroids on the sebaceous gland in power athletes. *Acta Derm Venereol (Stockh)* 1987; **67**: 36–40.
4 Aihara M, Kitamura K, Ikezawa Z. Lichenoid drug eruption due to nandrolone furylpropionate (Cemelon). *J Dermatol* 1989; **16**: 330–4.

5 Jick SS, Myers MW. A study of danazol's safety. *Pharmacotherapy* 1995; **15**: 40–1.
6 Spooner JB. Classification of side-effects to danazol therapy. *J Int Med Res* 1977; **5** (Suppl. 3): 15–7.
7 Greenberg RD. Acne vulgaris associated with antigonadotrophic (Danazol) therapy. *Cutis* 1979; **24**: 431–2.
8 Duff P, Mayer AR. Generalized alopecia: an unusual complication of danazol therapy. *Am J Obstet Gynecol* 1981; **141**: 349–50.
9 Fretwell MD, Altman LC. Exacerbation of a lupus-erythematosus-like syndrome during treatment of non-C1-esterase-inhibitor dependent angioedema with danazol. *J Allergy Clin Immunol* 1982; **69**: 306–10.
10 Sassolas B, Guillet G. Lupus, hereditary angioneurotic oedema and the risks of danazol treatment. *Br J Dermatol* 1991; **125**: 190–1.
11 Anonymous. Gestrinone (Dimetriose): another option in endometriosis. *Drug Ther Bull* 1991; **29**: 45.
12 Heydenreich G. Testosterone and anabolic steroids and acne fulminans. *Arch Dermatol* 1989; **125**: 571–2.
13 Traupe H, von Mühlendahl KE, Brämswig J, Happle R. Acne of the fulminans type following testosterone therapy in three excessively tall boys. *Arch Dermatol* 1988; **124**: 414–7.
14 Sandler B, Aronson P. Yohimbine-induced cutaneous drug eruption, progressive renal failure, and lupus-like syndrome. *Urology* 1993; **41**: 343–5.

Antiandrogens

Cyproterone acetate. Fixed drug eruption is recorded [1].

REFERENCE

1 Galindo PA, Borja J, Feo F *et al*. Fixed drug eruption caused by cyproterone acetate. *Allergy* 1998; **53**: 813.

Insulin

Adverse reactions to insulin [1–5] used to be relatively common, with bovine insulin having the most potential for production of allergic reactions, followed by porcine and human insulin. Insulin allergy and other local cutaneous reactions are rarely seen with highly purified and biosynthetic preparations [3,4], although local symptoms still occur in approximately 5% of patients [3]. Lipoatrophy, which was reported in 10–55% of patients treated with non-purified bovine/porcine insulin preparations, has almost disappeared since the advent of exclusive human insulin treatment. Allergic symptoms to human insulin are found in less than 1% of *de novo*-treated patients, but still occur when human insulin is used in the insulin-allergic patient [3]. Anaphylaxis may occur with recombinant human insulin [6]. Local allergic reactions are often of immediate hypersensitivity type; they are more common in the first few months, and usually subside with continued therapy. Generalized pruritus and urticaria occur rarely. Typically, more severe anaphylactoid reactions follow reintroduction of insulin in patients who have previously received long-term therapy. Delayed reactions may also occur, and take the form of pruritic erythema and induration, sometimes with papulation, within 24 h of injection [7]. Biphasic responses may be seen in the same individual, with initial immediate urticaria and a delayed reaction after 4–6 h. Allergy may develop to the insulin itself (i.e. bovine or porcine pro-

tein), to preservatives such as parabens and zinc [8,9] or to protamine (Surfen) present in depot preparations [10–13]. Sterile furunculoid lesions at injection sites, which heal with scars and which have a granulomatous histology, may result. Lipoatrophy at injection sites, or more rarely distally, occurred especially with longer-acting preparations; affected patients had lesional immunoglobulin deposits and circulating anti-insulin antibodies [14]. Exceptionally, hypertrophic lipodystrophy [15], or hyperkeratotic verrucous plaques at the site of repeated injections [16], may develop.

REFERENCES

1 Grammer L. Insulin allergy. *Clin Rev Allergy* 1986; **4**: 189–200.
2 De Shazo RD, Mather P, Grant W *et al*. Evaluation of patients with local reactions to insulin with skin tests and *in vitro* techniques. *Diabetes Care* 1987; **10**: 330–6.
3 Schernthaner G. Immunogenicity and allergenic potential of animal and human insulins. *Diabetes Care* 1993; **16** (Suppl. 3): 155–65.
4 Patrick AW, Williams G. Adverse effects of exogenous insulin. Clinical features, management and prevention. *Drug Saf* 1993; **8**: 427–44.
5 Barbaud A, Got I, Trechot P *et al*. Allergies cutanées et insulinotherapie. Aspects recents, conduite a tenir. *Ann Dermatol Vénéréol* 1996; **123**: 214–8.
6 Fineberg SE, Galloway JA, Fineberg NS *et al*. Immunogenicity of recombinant human insulin. *Diabetologica* 1983; **25**: 465–9.
7 White WN, DeMartino SA, Yoshida T. Severe delayed inflammatory reactions from injected insulin. *Am J Med* 1983; **74**: 909–13.
8 Feinglos MN, Jegasothy BV. 'Insulin' allergy due to zinc. *Lancet* 1979; **i**: 122–4.
9 Jordaan HF, Sandler M. Zinc-induced granuloma: a unique complication of insulin therapy. *Clin Exp Dermatol* 1989; **14**: 227–9.
10 Kim R. Anaphylaxis to protamine masquerading as an insulin allergy. *Del Med J* 1993; **65**: 17–23.
11 Kollner A, Senff H, Engelmann L *et al*. Protaminallergie vom Spattyp und Insulinallergie vom Soforttyp. *Dtsch Med Wochenschr* 1991; **116**: 1234–8.
12 Hulshof MM, Faber WR, Kniestedt WF *et al*. Granulomatous hypersensitivity to protamine as a complication of insulin therapy. *Br J Dermatol* 1992; **127**: 286–8.
13 Lee AY, Chey WY, Choi J, Jeon JS. Insulin-induced drug eruptions and reliability of skin tests. *Acta Derm Venereol (Stockh)* 2002; **82**: 114–7.
14 Reeves WG, Allen BR, Tattersal RB. Insulin-induced lipoatrophy: evidence for an immune pathogenesis. *BMJ* 1980; **280**: 1500–3.
15 Johnson DA, Parlette HL. Insulin-induced hypertrophic lipodystrophy. *Cutis* 1983; **32**: 273–4.
16 Fleming MG, Simon SI. Cutaneous insulin reaction resembling acanthosis nigricans. *Arch Dermatol* 1986; **122**: 1054–6.

Thyroxine

Chronic urticaria and angio-oedema was reported in a patient, associated with exogenous thyrotoxicosis, related to thyroid replacement therapy [1].

REFERENCE

1 Pandya AG, Beaudoing DL. Chronic urticaria associated with exogenous thyroid use. *Arch Dermatol* 1990; **126**: 1238–9.

Antithyroid drugs

Thiouracils

Hypersensitivity reactions include drug fever, pruritus,

urticaria, angio-oedema, exanthems, acneiform rashes, depigmentation of hair and LE-like syndromes. Propylthiouracil has caused allergic vasculitis [1–3], and methylthiouracil has resulted in erythema multiforme. Thiouracils may cause excessive hair loss. These drugs may cause marrow failure [4].

REFERENCES

1 Vasily DB, Tyler WB. Propylthiouracil-induced cutaneous vasculitis. *JAMA* 1980; **243**: 458–60.
2 Gammeltoft M, Kristensen JK. Propylthiouracil-induced cutaneous vasculitis. *Acta Derm Venereol (Stockh)* 1982; **62**: 171–3.
3 Otsuka S, Kinebuchi A, Tabata H *et al.* Myeloperoxidase-antineutrophil cytoplasmic antibody-associated vasculitis following propylthiouracil therapy. *Br J Dermatol* 2000; **142**: 828–30.
4 International Agranulocytosis and Aplastic Anemia Study. Risk of agranulocytosis and aplastic anemia in relation to use of antithyroid drugs. *BMJ* 1988; **287**: 262–5.

Chemotherapeutic (cytotoxic) agents

General side effects

There have been a number of excellent reviews of the dermatological complications of these compounds [1–10], including histopathological reactions [11,12]. Bone marrow depression, with aplastic anaemia, agranulocytosis or thrombocytopenia, and gastrointestinal intolerance may occur with any of these drugs. Mucocutaneous surfaces are especially vulnerable to the toxic effects of this group of drugs on rapidly dividing cells. Common side effects therefore include alopecia (see p. 73.46) and stomatitis [13]. Cytotoxic drugs may cause alopecia by either anagen or telogen effluvium. Severe alopecia of anagen type within 2 weeks of administration of the drug is frequently seen with cyclophosphamide, doxorubicin and the nitrosoureas; it is usually reversible with cessation of therapy. Other chemotherapeutic agents implicated in the production of alopecia include amsacrine, bleomycin, cyclophosphamide, cytarabine, dactinomycin, daunorubicin, etoposide, fluorouracil and methotrexate. Stomatitis occurs most frequently with acridinyl anisidide, dactinomycin, daunorubicin, doxorubicin, fluorouracil and methotrexate; it may respond to reduced dosage. Similarly, a number of drugs may cause pigmentation of the buccal mucosa [14] or of the nails [15–17]. Onycholysis may be induced [18].

Hypersensitivity or allergic reactions such as urticaria and angio-oedema [19,20] occur with all cancer chemotherapeutic agents except altretamine, the nitrosoureas and dactinomycin. With L-asparaginase and mitomycin (administered intravesically) they occur in about 10% of patients, and are relatively frequent with cisplatin; they are very rare with methotrexate. Type I reactions are commonest, but all four types of reactions are represented.

Many of these agents have distinctive cutaneous side effects, ranging from localized or diffuse hyperpigmentation to less usual ones, including radiation enhancement and recall phenomena, photosensitivity and hypersensitivity reactions, and phlebitis or chemical cellulitis. Confluent erythematous and hyperpigmented patches, with focal basal layer vacuolar degeneration, occurred within flexural areas during the first month after autologous peripheral stem cell transplantation [21]. Photosensitivity reactions occur with dacarbazine, fluorouracil, mitomycin and vinblastine. Radiation recall effects involve reactivation of an inflammatory response in areas irradiated months or years previously. Clinically, these range from erythema to vesiculation, with erosions and subsequent hyperpigmentation. They have most often been reported in association with dactinomycin and doxorubicin therapy [22] but also with edatrexate [23] and gemcitabine [24]; melphalan, etoposide, vinblastine, bleomycin, fluorouracil, hydroxyurea and methotrexate may also cause radiation enhancement. UV recall is recorded with mitomycin and the combination of etoposide and cyclophosphamide [25]. Rare complications such as diffuse sclerosis of the hands and feet, Raynaud's phenomenon [26], sterile folliculitis and flushing reactions may also occur. Multiple drug regimens may pose special problems in trying to elucidate the cause of a specific reaction, such as white-banded nails [27] or multiple Beau's lines [28]. A pityriasis lichenoides-like eruption occurred during therapy for myelogenous leukaemia with vincristine and mercaptopurine, antibiotics and aciclovir [29]. Fingertip necrosis occurred during chemotherapy with bleomycin, vincristine and methotrexate for HIV-related Kaposi's sarcoma [30].

Most cytotoxic drugs are teratogenic and are contraindicated during pregnancy, especially during the first trimester. Alkylating drugs usually cause sterility in males, and may shorten reproductive life in women.

REFERENCES

1 Weiss RB. Hypersensitivity reactions to cancer chemotherapy. *Semin Oncol* 1982; **9**: 5–13.
2 Bronner AK, Hood AF. Cutaneous complications of chemotherapeutic agents. *J Am Acad Dermatol* 1983; **9**: 645–63.
3 McDonald CJ. Cytotoxic agents for use in dermatology. I. *J Am Acad Dermatol* 1985; **12**: 753–5.
4 McDonald CJ. Use of cytotoxic drugs in dermatologic diseases. II. *J Am Acad Dermatol* 1985; **12**: 965–75.
5 Hood AF. Cutaneous side effects of cancer chemotherapy. *Med Clin North Am* 1986; **70**: 187–209.
6 Delaunay M. Effets cutanés indésirables de la chimiothérapie antitumorale. *Ann Dermatol Vénéréol* 1989; **116**: 347–61.
7 Kerker BJ, Hood AF. Chemotherapy-induced cutaneous reactions. *Semin Dermatol* 1989; **8**: 173–81.
8 Rapini RP. Cytotoxic drugs in the treatment of skin disease. *Int J Dermatol* 1991; **30**: 313–22.
9 Mansouri S, Dubertret L, Bastuji-Garin S *et al.* Role of drugs in cutaneous eruptions after chemotherapy for acute myelogenous leukemia. *Arch Dermatol* 1998; **134**: 881–2.
10 Susser WS, Whitaker-Worth DL, Grant-Kels JM. Mucocutaneous reactions to chemotherapy. *J Am Acad Dermatol* 1999; **40**: 367–98.
11 Fitzpatrick JE, Hood AF. Histopathologic reactions to chemotherapeutic agents. *Adv Dermatol* 1988; **3**: 161–84.

12 Fitzpatrick JE. The cutaneous histopathology of chemotherapeutic reactions. *J Cutan Pathol* 1993; **20**: 1–14.

13 Bottomley WK, Perlin E, Ross GR. Antineoplastic agents and their oral manifestations. *Oral Surg* 1977; **44**: 527–34.

14 Krutchik AN, Buzdar AU. Pigmentation of the tongue and mucous membranes associated with cancer chemotherapy. *South Med J* 1979; **72**: 1615–6.

15 Sulis E, Floris C. Nail pigmentation following cancer chemotherapy: a new genetic entity? *Eur J Cancer* 1980; **16**: 1517–9.

16 Daniel CR III, Scher RK. Nail changes secondary to systemic drugs or ingestants. *J Am Acad Dermatol* 1984; **10**: 250–8.

17 Daniel CR III, Scher PK. Nail changes secondary to systemic drugs or ingestants. In: Scher RK, Daniel CR III, eds. *Nails: Therapy, Diagnosis, Surgery.* Philadelphia: Saunders, 1990: 192–201.

18 Makris A, Mortimer P, Powles TJ. Chemotherapy-induced onycholysis. *Eur J Cancer* 1996; **32A**: 374–5.

19 Weiss RB. Hypersensitivity reactions. *Semin Oncol* 1992; **19**: 458–77.

20 O'Brien ME, Souberbielle BE. Allergic reactions to cytotoxic drugs: an update. *Ann Oncol* 1992; **3**: 605–10.

21 Brazzelli V, Ardigo M, Chiesa MG et al. Flexural erythematous eruption following autologous peripheral blood stem cell transplantation: a study of four cases. *Br J Dermatol* 2001; **145**: 490–5.

22 Solberg LA Jr, Wick MR, Bruckman JE. Doxorubicin-enhanced skin reaction after whole-body electron beam irradiation for leukemia cutis. *Mayo Clin Proc* 1980; **55**: 711–5.

23 Perez EA, Campbell DL, Ryu JK. Radiation recall dermatitis induced by edatrexate in a patient with breast cancer. *Cancer Invest* 1995; **13**: 604–7.

24 Jeter MD, Janne PA, Brooks S et al. Gemcitabine-induced radiation recall. *Int J Radiat Oncol Biol Phys* 2002; **53**: 394–400.

25 Williams BJ, Roth DJ, Callen JP. Ultraviolet recall associated with etoposide and cyclophosphamide therapy. *Clin Exp Dermatol* 1993; **18**: 452–3.

26 Vogelzang NJ, Bosl GJ, Johnson D et al. Raynaud's phenomenon: a common toxicity after combination chemotherapy for testicular cancer. *Ann Intern Med* 1981; **95**: 288–92.

27 James WD, Odom RB. Chemotherapy-induced transverse white lines in the fingernails. *Arch Dermatol* 1983; **119**: 334–5.

28 Singh M, Kaur S. Chemotherapy-induced multiple Beau's lines. *Int J Dermatol* 1986; **25**: 590–1.

29 Isoda M. Pityriasis lichenoides-like eruption occurring during therapy for myelogenous leukemia. *J Dermatol* 1989; **16**: 73–5.

30 Pechère M, Zulian GB, Vogel J-J et al. Fingertip necrosis during chemotherapy with bleomycin, vincristine and methotrexate for HIV-related Kaposi's sarcoma. *Br J Dermatol* 1996; **134**: 378–9.

Extravasation

Extravasation, leading to skin necrosis with ulceration, occurs with several agents [1–5]. Phlebitis and chemical cellulitis have been recorded with most antimitotic agents. Residual drug should be aspirated and the limb elevated; plastic surgical advice should be sought as soon as possible. High dermal concentrations of doxorubicin have been documented as late as 28 days after accidental extravasation [6]. Histological examination of doxorubicin-related extravasation lesions demonstrated exaggerated interface-type dermatitis with thrombosis of venous tributaries [7].

REFERENCES

1 Ignoffo RJ, Friedman MA. Therapy of local toxicities caused by extravasation of cancer chemotherapeutic drugs. *Cancer Treat Rev* 1980; **7**: 17–27.

2 Harwood KV, Aisner J. Treatment of chemotherapy extravasation: current status. *Cancer Treat Rep* 1984; **68**: 939–45.

3 Banerjee A, Brotherston TM, Lamberty BGH et al. Cancer chemotherapy agent-induced perivenous extravasation injury. *J Postgrad Med* 1987; **63**: 5–9.

4 Rudolph R, Larson DL. Etiology and treatment of chemotherapeutic agent extravasation injuries: a review. *J Clin Oncol* 1987; **5**: 1116–26.

5 Dufresne RG Jr. Skin necrosis from intravenously infused materials. *Cutis* 1989; **39**: 197–8.

6 Sonneveld P, Wassenaar HA, Nooter K. Long persistence of doxorubicin in human skin after extravasation. *Cancer Treat Rep* 1984; **68**: 895–6.

7 Bhawan J, Petry J, Rybak ME. Histologic changes induced in skin by extravasation of doxorubicin (adriamycin). *J Cutan Pathol* 1989; **16**: 158–63.

Acral erythema

Several cytotoxic drugs (especially cytosine arabinoside, fluorouracil, docetaxel and doxorubicin, and rarely cyclophosphamide, hydroxyurea, mercaptopurine, methotrexate and mitotane) can cause dose-dependent acral erythema, often preceded by paraesthesiae, either alone or in combination [1–17]. Bulla formation, desquamation and subsequent re-epithelialization may occur. Reactions may occur sooner (from 24 h to 3 weeks) and more severely with bolus or short-term chemotherapy than with low-dose continuous infusion, and are usually reproducible on challenge. Intravenous ciclosporin, given in bone marrow transplant patients, reportedly worsens the pain of acral erythema [12]. The condition should be distinguished from graft-versus-host disease in patients who receive chemotherapy followed by bone marrow transplantation, and from chemotherapy-induced Raynaud's phenomenon. This may not be easy, as histological changes may suggest graft-versus-host disease [18].

REFERENCES

1 Doyle LA, Berg C, Bottino G, Chabner E. Erythema and desquamation after high-dose methotrexate. *Ann Intern Med* 1983; **98**: 611–2.

2 Feldman LD, Jaffer A. Fluorouracil-associated palmar-plantar erythrodysesthesia syndrome. *JAMA* 1985; **254**: 3479.

3 Crider MK, Jansen J, Norins AL, McHale MS. Chemotherapy-induced acral erythema in patients receiving bone marrow transplantation. *Arch Dermatol* 1986; **122**: 1023–7.

4 Cox GJ, Robertson DB. Toxic erythema of palms and soles associated with high-dose mercaptopurine chemotherapy. *Arch Dermatol* 1986; **122**: 1413–4.

5 Guillaume J-C, Carp E, Rougier P et al. Effets secondaires cutanéo-muqueux des perfusions continues de 5-fluorouracile: 12 observations. *Ann Dermatol Vénéréol* 1988; **115**: 1167–9.

6 Horwitz LJ, Dreizen S. Acral erythemas induced by chemotherapy and graft-versus-host disease in adults with hematogenous malignancies. *Cutis* 1990; **46**: 397–404.

7 Baack BR, Burgdorf WHC. Chemotherapy-induced acral erythema. *J Am Acad Dermatol* 1991; **24**: 457–61.

8 Reynaert H, De Coninck A, Neven AM et al. Chemotherapy-induced acral erythema and acute graft-versus-host disease after allogeneic bone marrow transplantation. *Bone Marrow Transplant* 1992; **10**: 185–7.

9 Cohen PR. Acral erythema: a clinical review. *Cutis* 1993; **51**: 175–9.

10 Pirisi M, Soardo G. Images in clinical medicine. Chemotherapy-induced acral erythema. *N Engl J Med* 1994; **330**: 1279.

11 Komamura H, Higashiyama M, Hashimoto K et al. Three cases of chemotherapy-induced acral erythema. *J Dermatol* 1995; **22**: 116–21.

12 Kampmann KK, Graves T, Rogers SD. Acral erythema secondary to high-dose cytosine arabinoside with pain worsened by cyclosporin infusions. *Cancer* 1989; **63**: 2482–5.

13 Revenga Arranz F, Fernandez-Duran DA, Grande C et al. Acute and painful erythema of the hands and feet. Acral erythema induced by chemotherapy. *Arch Dermatol* 1997; **133**: 499–500, 502–3.

14 Nagore E, Insa A, Sanmartin O. Antineoplastic therapy-induced palmar plantar erythrodysesthesia ('hand–foot') syndrome. Incidence, recognition and management. *Am J Clin Dermatol* 2000; **1**: 225–34.

15 Tsuruta D, Mochida K, Hamada T *et al.* Chemotherapy-induced acral erythema: report of a case and immunohistochemical findings. *Clin Exp Dermatol* 2000; **25**: 386–8.
16 Soker M, Akdeniz S, Devecioglu C, Haspolat K. Chemotherapy-induced bullous acral erythema in a subject with B-cell lymphoma. *J Eur Acad Dermatol Venereol* 2001; **15**: 490–1.
17 de Bono JS, Stephenson J Jr, Baker SD *et al.* Troxacitabine, an L-stereoisomeric nucleoside analog, on a five-times-daily schedule: a phase I and pharmacokinetic study in patients with advanced solid malignancies. *J Clin Oncol* 2002; **20**: 96–109.
18 Beard JS, Smith KJ, Skelton HG. Combination chemotherapy with 5-fluorouracil, folinic acid, and α-interferon producing histologic features of graft-versus-host disease. *J Am Acad Dermatol* 1993; **29**: 325–30.

Neutrophilic eccrine hidradenitis

Neutrophilic eccrine hidradenitis may represent a reaction pattern to a variety of chemotherapeutic agents [1–8], but particularly cytarabine and bleomycin. It has been induced by granulocyte–macrophage colony stimulating factor [9]. Clinically, erythematous papules or plaques or nodules are most frequent, although hyperpigmented plaques, pustules, purpura and urticaria have been described. Lesions resolve spontaneously over several days. The histology is characterized by infiltration of eccrine coils with neutrophils and necrosis of the secretory epithelium. The condition has also been described in a patient receiving haemodialysis without chemotherapy [10] and in a patient without a malignancy who was taking paracetamol [11].

REFERENCES

1 Fitzpatrick JE, Bennion SD, Reed OM *et al.* Neutrophilic eccrine hidradenitis associated with induction chemotherapy. *J Cutan Pathol* 1987; **14**: 272–8.
2 Scallan PJ, Kettler AH, Levy ML *et al.* Neutrophilic eccrine hidradenitis. *Cancer* 1988; **62**: 2532–6.
3 Fernández Cogolludo E, Ambrojo Antunez P, Aguilar Martínez A *et al.* Neutrophil eccrine hidradenitis: a report of two additional cases. *Clin Exp Dermatol* 1989; **14**: 341–6.
4 Burg G, Bieber T, Langecker P. Lokalisierte neutrophile ekkrien Hidradenitis unter Mitoxantron: eine typische Zytostatikanebenwirkung. *Hautarzt* 1988; **39**: 233–6.
5 Allegue F, Soria C, Rocamora A *et al.* Neutrophilic eccrine hidradenitis in two neutropenic patients. *J Am Acad Dermatol* 1990; **23**: 1110–3.
6 Margolis DJ, Gross PR. Neutrophilic eccrine hidradenitis: a case report and review of the literature. *Cutis* 1991; **48**: 198–200.
7 Thorisdottir K, Tomecki KJ, Bergfeld WF *et al.* Neutrophilic eccrine hidradenitis. *J Am Acad Dermatol* 1993; **28**: 775–7.
8 Kanzki H, Takashi O, Makino E *et al.* Neutrophilic eccrine hidradenitis: report of two cases. *J Dermatol* 1995; **22**: 137–42.
9 Bachmeyer C, Chaibi P, Aractingi S. Neutrophilic eccrine hidradenitis induced by granulocyte-stimulating factor. *Br J Dermatol* 1998; **139**: 354–5.
10 Moreno A, Barnadas MA, Ravella A, Moragas JM. Infectious eccrine hidradenitis in a patient undergoing hemodialysis. *Arch Dermatol* 1985; **121**: 1106–7.
11 Kuttner BJ, Kurban RS. Neutrophilic eccrine hidradenitis in the absence of an underlying malignancy. *Cutis* 1988; **41**: 403–5.

Syringosquamous metaplasia

A related but distinct entity termed 'syringosquamous metaplasia', which may be confused with well-differentiated squamous cell carcinoma histologically, has been described in patients receiving chemotherapy for leukaemia and other cancers [1–3]. Clinically, this may appear as an erythematous, blanching, papular crusted eruption, or as erythematous oedematous plaques or confluent erythematous macular areas, in the axillae or groins, with painful erythema and oedema on the palms and soles [4].

REFERENCES

1 Bhawan J, Malhotra R. Syringosquamous metaplasia. A distinctive eruption in patients receiving chemotherapy. *Am J Dermatopathol* 1990; **12**: 1–6.
2 Hurt MA, Halvorson RD, Petr FC Jr *et al.* Eccrine squamous syringometaplasia. A cutaneous sweat gland reaction in the histologic spectrum of 'chemotherapy-associated eccrine hidradenitis' and 'neutrophilic eccrine hidradenitis'. *Arch Dermatol* 1990; **126**: 73–7.
3 Valks R, Buezo GF, Dauden E *et al.* Eccrine squamous syringometaplasia in intertriginous areas. *Br J Dermatol* 1996; **134**: 984–6.
4 Valks R, Fraga J, Porras-Luque J *et al.* Chemotherapy-induced eccrine squamous syringometaplasia. A distinctive eruption in patients receiving hematopoietic progenitor cells. *Arch Dermatol* 1997; **133**: 873–8.

Side effects related to immunosuppression

The cutaneous manifestations of immunosuppression have been reviewed [1–4]. Immunosuppressive therapy, such as azathioprine and prednisone for renal transplant patients, may encourage skin infections of various types, for example warts, herpes simplex and herpes zoster [5], pityriasis versicolor and fungal infections [6]. Development of disseminated superficial actinic porokeratosis [7–9], porokeratosis of Mibelli [10–13] and increased numbers of benign [14,15] or eruptive dysplastic [16] melanocytic naevi may be promoted. Eruptive keratoacanthomas occurred in a patient with SLE on prednisolone and cyclophosphamide [17].

REFERENCES

1 Cohen EB, Komorowski RA, Clowry LJ. Cutaneous complications in renal transplant recipients. *Am J Clin Pathol* 1987; **88**: 32–7.
2 Abel EA. Cutaneous manifestations of immunosuppression in organ transplant recipients. *J Am Acad Dermatol* 1989; **21**: 167–79.
3 Boitard C, Nach J-F. Long-term complications of conventional immunosuppressive treatment. *Adv Nephrol* 1989; **18**: 335–54.
4 Paller AS, Mallory SB. Acquired forms of immunosuppression. *J Am Acad Dermatol* 1991; **24**: 482–8.
5 Spencer ES, Anderson HK. Viral infections in renal allograft recipients treated with long-term immunosuppression. *BMJ* 1979; **2**: 829–30.
6 Shelley WB. Induction of tinea cruris by topical nitrogen mustard and systemic chemotherapy. *Acta Derm Venereol (Stockh)* 1981; **61**: 164–5.
7 Bencini PL, Crosti C, Sala F. Porokeratosis: immunosuppression and exposure to sunlight. *Br J Dermatol* 1987; **116**: 113–6.
8 Neumann RA, Knobler RM, Metze D, Jurecka W. Disseminated superficial porokeratosis and immunosuppression. *Br J Dermatol* 1988; **119**: 375–80.
9 Lederman JS, Sober AJ, Lederman GS. Immunosuppression: a cause of porokeratosis? *J Am Acad Dermatol* 1985; **13**: 75–9.
10 Grattan CEH, Christopher AP. Porokeratosis and immunosuppression. *J R Soc Med* 1987; **80**: 597–8.
11 Tatnall FM, Sarkany I. Porokeratosis of Mibelli in an immunosuppressed patient. *J R Soc Med* 1987; **80**: 180–1.
12 Wilkinson SM, Cartwright PH, English JSC. Porokeratosis of Mibelli and immunosuppression. *Clin Exp Dermatol* 1991; **16**: 61–2.

13 Herranz P, Pizarro A, De Lucas R *et al.* High incidence of porokeratosis in renal transplant recipients. *Br J Dermatol* 1997; **136**: 176–9.
14 McGregor JM, Barker JNWN, MacDonald DM. The development of excess numbers of melanocytic naevi in an immunosuppressed identical twin. *Clin Exp Dermatol* 1991; **16**: 131–2.
15 Hughes BR, Cunliffe WJ, Bailey CC. Excess benign melanocytic naevi after chemotherapy for malignancy in childhood. *BMJ* 1989; **299**: 88–91.
16 Barker JNWN, MacDonald DM. Eruptive dysplastic naevi following renal transplantation. *Clin Exp Dermatol* 1988; **13**: 123–5.
17 Dessoukey MW, Omar MF, Abdel-Dayem H. Eruptive keratoacanthomas associated with immunosuppressive therapy in a patient with systemic lupus erythematosus. *J Am Acad Dermatol* 1997; **37**: 478–80.

Internal malignancy

The frequency of internal cancers common in the general population is not increased in transplant patients. However, that of a variety of otherwise uncommon malignancies is increased [1–3], including non-Hodgkin's lymphoma (mostly B-cell, with 14% of T-cell, and less than 1% of null-cell, origin), which accounts for 21% of cancers in transplant recipients; Kaposi's sarcoma; other sarcomas; carcinoma of the vulva and perineum; carcinoma of the kidney; and hepatobiliary tumours. Non-Hodgkin's lymphoma appears commoner and develops earlier where potent immunosuppressive agents such as ciclosporin and/or the monoclonal antibody OKT3 have been used; however, although cancer develops in 6% of all transplant recipients, only 1% of patients die from this complication [3]. Leukaemia may develop following chemotherapy [4], and bladder cancer has been associated with cyclophosphamide therapy [5].

Skin cancers

Actinic keratoses, squamous cell and basal cell cancer of the lip and skin [6–12], and malignant melanoma [13] have been reported to be more common, especially in immunosuppressed renal transplant patients. The majority of these patients have received azathioprine and corticosteroids. Interestingly, the immunosuppressed renal transplant recipients have been reported to be at high risk for skin cancer unless they express the HLA class I allele A11 [14]. Furthermore, patients with long-standing renal grafts mismatched for HLA-B have a significantly higher incidence of squamous cell cancers than other mismatches, and patients who are homozygous for HLA-DR are at increased risk for actinic keratoses and skin cancer [15]. These findings imply that MHC gene products participate in the pathogenesis of skin cancer in immunosuppressed patients, probably via influences on T-cell recognition of neoantigens [16]. There was no difference from control levels in the number of CD1$^+$ HLA-DR$^+$ antigen-presenting Langerhans' cells in the epidermis of immunosuppressed renal transplant recipients treated with either azathioprine/prednisone or ciclosporin/prednisone [17].

REFERENCES

1 Penn I. Depressed immunity and the development of cancer. *Clin Exp Immunol* 1981; **146**: 459–74.
2 Penn I. Tumors of the immunocompromised patient. *Annu Rev Med* 1988; **39**: 63–73.
3 Penn I. Cancers complicating organ transplantation. *N Engl J Med* 1990; **323**: 1767–9.
4 Williams CJ. Leukaemia and cancer chemotherapy. The risk is acceptably small but may be reducible further. *BMJ* 1990; **301**: 73–4.
5 Elliot RW, Essenhigh DM, Morley AR. Cyclophosphamide treatment of systemic lupus erythematosus: risk of bladder cancer exceeds benefit. *Blood* 1970; **35**: 543–8.
6 Walder BK, Robertson MR, Jeremy D. Skin cancer and immunosuppression. *Lancet* 1971; **ii**: 1282–3.
7 Lowney ED. Antimitotic drugs and aggressive squamous cell tumors. *Arch Dermatol* 1972; **105**: 924.
8 Kinlen LJ, Sheil AGR, Peto J, Doll R. Collaborative United Kingdom–Australasian study of cancer in patients treated with immunosuppressive drugs. *BMJ* 1979; **ii**: 1461–6.
9 Boyle J, Briggs JD, MacKie RM *et al.* Cancer, warts and sunshine in renal transplant patients. *Lancet* 1984; **i**: 702–5.
10 McLelland J, Rees A, Williams G *et al.* The incidence of immunosuppression-related skin disease in long-term transplant patients. *Transplantation* 1988; **46**: 871–4.
11 Gupta AK, Cardella CJ, Haberman HF. Cutaneous malignant neoplasms in patients with renal transplants. *Arch Dermatol* 1986; **122**: 1288–93.
12 Hintner H, Fritsch P. Skin neoplasia in the immunodeficient host. *Curr Probl Dermatol* 1989; **18**: 210–7.
13 Greene MH, Young TI. Malignant melanoma in renal transplant recipients. *Lancet* 1981; **i**: 1196–9.
14 Bouwes Bavinck JN, Koottee AMM, van der Woude FJ *et al.* HLA-A11-associated resistance to skin cancer in renal-transplant recipients. *N Engl J Med* 1990; **323**: 1350.
15 Bouwes Bavinck JM, Vermeer BJ, vans der Woude FJ *et al.* Relation between skin cancer and HLA antigens in renal-transplant recipients. *N Engl J Med* 1991; **325**: 843–8.
16 Streilein JW. Immunogenetic factors in skin cancer. *N Engl J Med* 1991; **325**: 884–7.
17 Scheibner KG, Murray A, Sheil R *et al.* T6+ and HLA-DR+ cell numbers in epidermis of immunosuppressed renal transplant recipients. *J Cutan Pathol* 1987; **14**: 202–6.

Alkylating agents

These drugs interfere with cell replication by damaging DNA. Gametogenesis is often severely affected, and their use is associated with a marked increase in non-lymphocytic leukaemia, especially when used in conjunction with radiotherapy.

Alkyl sulphonates

Busulfan. Reactions are rare, but have included urticaria, bullous erythema multiforme [1], Addisonian-like pigmentation [2,3] due to increased epidermal and dermal melanin, and drug-induced porphyria cutanea tarda [4]. Vasculitis has been reported. Keratinocyte nuclear abnormalities with abundant pale cytoplasm have been described [5]. Progressive pulmonary fibrosis may occur.

REFERENCES

1 Dosik H, Hurewitz DJ, Rosner F, Schwartz JM. Bullous eruptions and elevated leukocyte alkaline phosphatase in the course of busulphan-treated chronic granulocytic leukaemia. *Blood* 1970; **35**: 543–8.

2 Harrold BP. Syndrome resembling Addison's disease following prolonged treatment with busulphan. *BMJ* 1966; **1**: 463–4.
3 Burns WA, McFarland W, Matthews MJ. Toxic manifestations of busulfan therapy. *Med Ann DC* 1971; **40**: 567–9.
4 Kyle RA, Dameshek W. Porphyria cutanea tarda associated with chronic granulocytic leukemia treated with busulfan. *Blood* 1964; **23**: 776–85.
5 Hymes SR, Simonton SC, Farmer ER *et al.* Cutaneous busulfan effect in patients receiving bone marrow transplanation. *J Cutan Pathol* 1985; **12**: 125–9.

Nitrogen mustard derivatives

Chlorambucil. Morbilliform rashes occur; urticarial plaques and periorbital oedema have been described rarely [1–4]. A delayed allergic reaction on the third cycle of chemotherapy, with generalized erythroderma with exfoliation and oedema of the face and arms, as well as immune haemolytic anaemia and TEN, have been described [5]. Alopecia is uncommon. Sterility with azoospermia and amenorrhoea is documented.

REFERENCES

1 Knisely RE, Settipane GA, Albala MM. Unusual reaction to chlorambucil in a patient with chronic lymphocytic leukemia. *Arch Dermatol* 1971; **104**: 77–9.
2 Millard LG, Rajah SM. Cutaneous reaction to chlorambucil. *Arch Dermatol* 1977; **113**: 1298.
3 Peterman A, Braunstein B. Cutaneous reaction to chlorambucil therapy. *Arch Dermatol* 1986; **122**: 1358–60.
4 Zervas J, Karkantaris C, Kapiri E *et al.* Allergic reaction to chlorambucil in chronic lymphocytic leukaemia: case report. *Leuk Res* 1992; **16**: 329–30.
5 Torricelli R, Kurer SB, Kroner T, Wuthrich B. Allergie vom Spattyp auf Chlorambucil (Leukeran). Fallbeschreibung und Literaturubersicht. *Schweiz Med Wochenschr* 1995; **125**: 1870–3.

Cyclophosphamide and mesna. Alopecia is common and occurs in 5–30% of cases [1]. Pigmentation, which may be widespread or localized to the palms, soles or nails, is well documented and usually reversible [2,3]. Nail dystrophy may be seen. Allergic exanthems are rare, but anaphylactic and urticarial reactions less so [4–7]. Type I hypersensitivity with a markedly delayed onset (from 8 to 16 h up to 10 days), associated with immediate skin-test results to cyclophosphamide metabolites but not the parent drug, has been documented [7]. There may be cross-sensitivity to other alkylating agents, especially mechlorethamine and chlorambucil [8]. Sterility may supervene.

Haemorrhagic cystitis, the result of toxicity of the metabolite acrolein, is a complication in up to 40% of cases if cyclophosphamide is used alone. Introduction of the thiol compound mesna (2-mercaptoethane sulphonate) has virtually eliminated this complication. There have been recent reports of urticaria, angio-oedema, allergic maculopapular pruritic rashes, generalized fixed drug eruption, and occasional more severe reactions with flushing, widespread erythema and ulceration or blistering of mucous membranes related to mesna; patch tests may be positive [9–13].

REFERENCES

1 Ahmed AR, Hombal SM. Cyclophosphamide (Cytoxan). *J Am Acad Dermatol* 1984; **11**: 1115–26.
2 Harrison BM, Wood CBS. Cyclophosphamide and pigmentation. *BMJ* 1972; **1**: 352.
3 Shah PC, Rao KRP, Patel AR. Cyclophosphamide induced nail pigmentation. *Br J Dermatol* 1978; **98**: 675–80.
4 Murti L, Horsman LR. Acute hypersensitivity reaction to cyclophosphamide. *J Pediatr* 1979; **94**: 844–5.
5 Lakin JD, Cahill RA. Generalized urticaria to cyclophosphamide: type I hypersensitivity to an immunosuppressive agent. *J Allergy Clin Immunol* 1976; **58**: 160–71.
6 Knysak DJ, McLean JA, Solomon WR *et al.* Immediate hypersensitivity reaction to cyclophosphamide. *Arthritis Rheum* 1994; **37**: 1101–4.
7 Popescu NA, Sheehan MG, Kouides PA *et al.* Allergic reactions to cyclophosphamide: delayed clinical expression associated with positive immediate skin tests to drug metabolites in five patients. *J Allergy Clin Immunol* 1996; **97**: 26–33.
8 Kritharides L, Lawrie K, Varigos GA. Cyclophosphamide hypersensitivity and cross-reactivity with chlorambucil. *Cancer Treat Rep* 1987; **71**: 1323–4.
9 Pratt CB, Sandlund JT, Meyer WH, Cain AM. Mesna-induced urticaria. *Drug Intell Clin Pharm* 1988; **22**: 914.
10 Seidel A, Andrassy K, Ritz E *et al.* Allergic reactions to mesna. *Lancet* 1991; **338**: 381.
11 Gross WL, Mohr J, Christophers E. Allergic reactions to mesna. *Lancet* 1991; **338**: 381.
12 D'Cruz D, Haga H-J, Hughes GRV. Allergic reactions to mesna. *Lancet* 1991; **338**: 705–6.
13 Zonzits E, Aberer W, Tappeiner G. Drug eruptions from mesna. After cyclophosphamide treatment of patients with systemic lupus erythematosus and dermatomyositis. *Arch Dermatol* 1992; **128**: 80–2.

Lomustine. Flushing has been reported.

Mechlorethamine. Angio-oedema and pruritus have been recorded [1]; however, in view of the large number of patients receiving this drug as part of the MOPP (mechlorethamine, Oncovin (vincristine), procarbazine, prednisone) regimen for lymphoma, these side effects must be exceedingly rare. Topical mechlorethamine [2] used to treat psoriasis or mycosis fungoides may cause hyperpigmentation of involved and uninvolved skin [3], contact sensitization [4,5] and rarely immediate-type hypersensitivity with urticaria or anaphylactoid reactions [6].

REFERENCES

1 Wilson KS, Alexander S. Hypersensitivity to mechlorethamine. *Ann Intern Med* 1981; **94**: 823.
2 Price NM, Deneau DG, Hoppe RT. The treatment of mycosis fungoides with ointment-based mechlorethamine. *Arch Dermatol* 1982; **118**: 234–7.
3 Flaxman BA, Sosis AC, Van Scott EJ. Changes in melanosome distribution in Caucasoid skin following topical application of nitrogen mustard. *J Invest Dermatol* 1973; **60**: 321–6.
4 Van Scott EJ, Winters PL. Responses of mycosis fungoides to intensive external treatment with nitrogen mustard. *Arch Dermatol* 1970; **102**: 507–14.
5 Ramsay DL, Halperin PS, Zeleniuch-Jacquotte A. Topical mechlorethamine therapy for early stage mycosis fungoides. *J Am Acad Dermatol* 1988; **19**: 684–91.
6 Daughters D, Zackheim H, Maibach H. Urticaria and anaphylactoid reactions after topical application of mechlorethamine. *Arch Dermatol* 1973; **107**: 429–30.

Melphalan. Trivial morbilliform rashes are relatively common [1]. Severe anaphylactic reactions may occur after intravenous use, especially in patients with IgA κ myeloma

[2]. Urticaria or angio-oedema after oral use is very rare [3]. Vasculitis has been documented, and melanonychia striata has been recorded [4]. Scleroderma has supervened after isolated limb perfusion [5]. Radiation recall is uncommon [6]. Sterility with azoospermia and amenorrhoea are recorded.

REFERENCES

1 Costa GG, Engle RL Jr, Schilling A *et al.* Melphalan and prednisone: an effective combination for the treatment of multiple myeloma. *Am J Med* 1973; **54**: 589–99.
2 Cornwell GG, Pajak TF, McIntyre OR. Hypersensitivity reactions to i.v. melphalan during the treatment of multiple myeloma: cancer and leukemia group B experience. *Cancer Treat Rep* 1979; **63**: 399–403.
3 Lawrence BV, Harvey HA, Lipton A. Anaphylaxis due to oral melphalan. *Cancer Treat Rep* 1980; **64**: 731–2.
4 Malacarne P, Zavagli G. Melphalan-induced melanonychia striata. *Arch Dermatol Res* 1977; **258**: 81–3.
5 Landau M, Brenner S, Gat A *et al.* Reticulate scleroderma after isolated limb perfusion with melphalan. *J Am Acad Dermatol* 1998; **39**: 1011–2.
6 Kellie SJ, Plowman PN, Malpas JS. Radiation recall and radio-sensitization with alkylating agents. *Lancet* 1987; **i**: 1149–50.

Ethylenemine derivatives

Thiotepa (triethylenethiophosphoramide)

Intravesical installation caused pruritus, urticaria or angio-oedema in five of 164 patients with bladder carcinoma [1]. Intravenous administration resulted in patterned hyperpigmentation confined to skin occluded by adhesive bandages or electrocardiograph pads, probably due to secretion of the drug in sweat [2]. In contrast, topical thiotepa has produced periorbital leukoderma [3].

REFERENCES

1 Veenema RJ, Dean AL, Uson AC *et al.* Thiotepa bladder installations: therapy and prophylaxis for superficial bladder tumors. *J Urol* 1969; **101**: 711–5.
2 Horn TD, Beveridge RA, Egorine MJ *et al.* Observations and proposed mechanism of N,N',N''-triethylenethiophosphoramide (thiotepa)-induced hyperpigmentation. *Arch Dermatol* 1989; **125**: 524–7.
3 Harben DJ, Cooper PH, Rodman OG. Thiotepa-induced leukoderma. *Arch Dermatol* 1979; **115**: 973–4.

Nitrosoureas

Carmustine

Topical carmustine (BCNU) used for the treatment of cutaneous T-cell lymphoma may result in erythema, skin tenderness and telangiectasia. Contact sensitization may develop [1]. Mild bone marrow suppression has been recorded.

REFERENCE

1 Zackheim HS, Epstein EH Jr, Crain WR. Topical carmustine (BCNU) for cutaneous T cell lymphoma: a 15-year experience in 143 patients. *J Am Acad Dermatol* 1990; **22**: 802–10.

Dacarbazine (DTIC)

Photosensitivity [1,2] and a fixed eruption-like rash [3] have been reported. A patient with malignant melanoma treated with DTIC developed sudden hepatic vein thrombosis (Budd–Chiari syndrome) following intravenous administration [4]. Increasing blood eosinophilia appears to be a sign of the imminent development of this complication. Chemical cellulitis occurs following extravasation.

REFERENCES

1 Bolling R, Meyer-Hamme S, Schauder S. Lichtsensibilisierung unter DTIC-Therapie beim metastasierenden malignen Melanom. *Hautarzt* 1980; **31**: 602–5.
2 Yung CW, Winston EM, Lorincz AL. Dacarbazine-induced photosensitivity reaction. *J Am Acad Dermatol* 1981; **4**: 451–3.
3 Koehn GG, Balizet LR. Unusual local cutaneous reaction to dacarbazine. *Arch Dermatol* 1982; **118**: 1018–9.
4 Swensson-Beck H, Trettel WH. Budd–Chiari-Syndrom bei DTIC-Therapie. *Hautarzt* 1981; **33**: 30–1.

Procarbazine

Type I reactions are rare; recurrent angio-oedema, urticaria and arthralgia with decreased serum complement have been reported [1,2]. Hypersensitivity to procarbazine in patients treated with mechlorethamine, vincristine and procarbazine (MOP) for high-grade glioma manifested as a maculopapular rash, fever, reversible abnormal liver function and interstitial pneumonitis [3].

REFERENCES

1 Glovsky MM, Braunwald J, Opelz G, Alenty A. Hypersensitivity to procarbazine associated with angio-edema, urticaria and low serum complement activity. *J Allergy Clin Immunol* 1976; **57**: 134–40.
2 Andersen E, Videbaeck A. Procarbazine-induced skin reactions in Hodgkin's disease and other malignant lymphomas. *Scand J Haematol* 1980; **24**: 149–51.
3 Coyle T, Bushunow P, Winfield J *et al.* Hypersensitivity reactions to procarbazine with mechlorethamine, vincristine, and procarbazine chemotherapy in the treatment of glioma. *Cancer* 1992; **69**: 2532–40.

Cytotoxic antibiotics

Bleomycin

The principal problem of systemic therapy is progressive pulmonary fibrosis. Alopecia, glossitis and buccal ulceration occur, and drug fever is common, usually 1–4 h after injection. Distinctive, localized, erythematous, tender macules, nodules or infiltrated plaques on the hands, elbows, knees and buttocks have been documented [1–3]. Their causation is uncertain, and the rash may resolve despite continued therapy [4]. Raynaud's phenomenon with or without ischaemic ulcerations, and systemic sclerosis-like changes in men, have been described [5–7]. Capillary microscopy has been advocated for the invest-

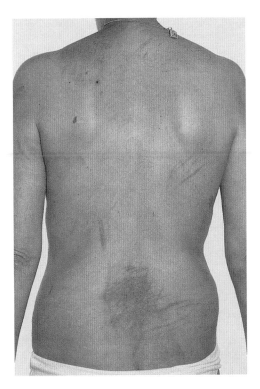

Fig. 73.8 Flagellate pigmentation caused by bleomycin. (Courtesy of Dr A. Ilchyshyn, Coventry and Warwickshire Hospital, Coventry, UK.)

igation of bleomycin acral vascular toxicity [8]. In normal human skin, intradermal bleomycin induced a localized time- and dose-dependent inflammatory reaction and persistent post-inflammatory hyperpigmentation; histology showed neutrophilic eccrine hidradenitis, with keratinocyte necrosis, HLA-DR and ICAM-1 expression, and endothelial cell ICAM-1 up-regulation and E-selectin induction [9]. Intralesional bleomycin therapy for warts induced keratinocyte apoptosis and complete epidermal necrosis with diffuse neutrophil accumulation and microabscess formation at the granular layer [10]. Clinically, intralesional therapy may cause persistent Raynaud's phenomenon [11,12] and loss of nails [13].

Cutaneous erythema or hyperpigmentation, which may be diffuse [14], patchy or linear, and prominent over pressure areas, especially the elbows or in striae distensae [15], is seen in approximately 30% of patients [16]. 'Flagellate' streaked erythema or pigmentation [17–24] on the trunk and proximal extremities is common (Fig. 73.8); it recurs in previously involved sites, and develops in new sites, within 24 h of rechallenge [21]. It has been proposed that trauma from scratching induces localized vasodilatation, with increased concentration of cutaneous bleomycin; hyperpigmentation has been documented in a patient treated with bleomycin where a heating pad had been applied [25]. There may be darkening of the nail cuticle and palmar creases.

REFERENCES

1 Lincke-Plewig H. Bleomycin-Exanthem. *Hautarzt* 1980; **31**: 616–8.
2 Cohen IS, Mosher MB, O'Keefe EJ. Cutaneous toxicity of bleomycin therapy. *Arch Dermatol* 1973; **107**: 553–5.
3 Haerslev T, Avnstorp C, Joergensen M. Sudden onset of adverse effects due to low-dosage bleomycin indicates an idiosyncratic reaction. *Cutis* 1993; **52**: 45–6.
4 Bennett JP, Burns CP. Absence of progression of recurrent bleomycin skin toxicity without postponement or attenuation of therapy. *Am J Med* 1988; **85**: 585–6.
5 Finch WR, Rodnan GP, Buckingham RB *et al.* Bleomycin-induced scleroderma. *J Rheumatol* 1980; **7**: 651–9.
6 Bork K, Korting GW. Symptomatische Sklerodermie durch Bleomyzin. *Hautarzt* 1983; **34**: 10–2.
7 Snauwaert J, Degreef H. Bleomycin-induced Raynaud's phenomenon and acral sclerosis. *Dermatologica* 1984; **169**: 172–4.
8 Bellmunt J, Navarro M, Morales S *et al.* Capillary microscopy is a potentially useful method for detecting bleomycin vascular toxicity. *Cancer* 1990; **65**: 303–9.
9 Templeton SF, Solomon AR, Swerlick RA. Intradermal bleomycin injections into normal human skin. A histopathologic and immunopathologic study. *Arch Dermatol* 1994; **130**: 577–83.
10 James MP, Collier PM, Aherne W *et al.* Histologic, pharmacologic, and immunocytochemical effects of injection of bleomycin into viral warts. *J Am Acad Dermatol* 1993; **28**: 933–7.
11 Epstein E, O'Keefe EJ, Hayes M, Bovenmyer DA. Persisting Raynaud's phenomenon following intralesional bleomycin treatment of finger warts. *J Am Acad Dermatol* 1985; **13**: 468–71.
12 Epstein E. Intralesional bleomycin and Raynaud's phenomenon. *J Am Acad Dermatol* 1991; **24**: 785–6.
13 Gonzalez FU, Gil MCC, Martinez AA *et al.* Cutaneous toxicity of intralesional bleomycin in the treatment of periungual warts. *Arch Dermatol* 1986; **122**: 974–5.
14 Wright AL, Bleehen SS, Champion AE. Reticulate pigmentation due to bleomycin: light- and electron-microscopic studies. *Dermatologica* 1990; **181**: 255–7.
15 Tsuji T, Sawabe M. Hyperpigmentation in striae distensae after bleomycin treatment. *J Am Acad Dermatol* 1993; **28**: 503–5.
16 Ohnuma T, Selawry OS, Holland JF *et al.* Clinical study with bleomycin: tolerance to twice weekly dosage. *Cancer* 1972; **30**: 914–22.
17 Cortina P, Garrido JA, Tomas JF *et al.* 'Flagellate' erythema from bleomycin, with histopathological findings suggestive of inflammatory oncotaxis. *Dermatologica* 1990; **180**: 106–9.
18 Fernandez-Obregon AC, Hogan KP, Bibro MK. Flagellate pigmentation from intrapleural bleomycin. A light and electron microscopic study. *J Am Acad Dermatol* 1985; **13**: 464–8.
19 Polla BS, Saurat JG, Merot Y, Slosman D. Flagellate pigmentation from bleomycin. *J Am Acad Dermatol* 1986; **14**: 690.
20 Rademaker M, Meyrick Thomas RH, Lowe DG, Munro DD. Linear streaking due to bleomycin. *Clin Exp Dermatol* 1987; **12**: 457–9.
21 Mowad CM, Nguyen TV, Elenitsas R, Leyden JJ. Bleomycin-induced flagellate dermatitis: a clinical and histopathological review. *Br J Dermatol* 1994; **131**: 700–2.
22 Nigro MG, Hsu S. Bleomycin-induced flagellate pigmentation. *Cutis* 2001; **68**: 285–6.
23 von Hilsheimer GE, Norton SA. Delayed bleomycin-induced hyperpigmentation and pressure on the skin. *J Am Acad Dermatol* 2002; **46**: 642–3.
24 Abess A, Keel DM, Graham BS. Flagellate hyperpigmentation following intralesional bleomycin treatment of verruca plantaris. *Arch Dermatol* 2003; **139**: 337–9.
25 Kukla LJ, McGuire WP. Heat-induced recall of bleomycin skin changes. *Cancer* 1982; **50**: 2283–4.

Dactinomycin (actinomycin D)

A papulopustular acneiform sterile folliculitis, spreading from the face to the trunk and buttocks, and which may mimic septic cutaneous emboli, is common [1]. Dactinomycin-related lesions with the histology of an interface dermatitis with syringometaplasia developed in the axillae, groins and central line exit site of two children [2]. Radiation recall occurs [3]. Persistent serpentine supravenous hyperpigmentation was recorded in combination dactinomycin and vincristine therapy [4].

REFERENCES

1 Epstein EH, Lutzner MA. Folliculitis induced by actinomycin D. *N Engl J Med* 1969; **281**: 1094–6.
2 Kanwar VS, Gajjar A, Ribeiro RC *et al.* Unusual cutaneous toxicity following treatment with dactinomycin: a report of two cases. *Med Pediatr Oncol* 1995; **24**: 329–33.
3 Coppes MJ, Jorgenson K, Arlette JP. Cutaneous toxicity following the administration of dactinomycin. *Med Pediatr Oncol* 1997; **29**: 226–7.
4 Marcoux D, Anex R, Russo P. Persistent serpentine supravenous hyperpigmented eruption as an adverse reaction to chemotherapy combining actinomycin and vincristine. *J Am Acad Dermatol* 2000; **43**: 540–6.

Daunorubicin

Angio-oedema with generalized urticaria [1], and hyperpigmentation of the oral mucosa, skin and nails [2–4] have been described.

REFERENCES

1 Freeman AI. Clinical note. Allergic reaction to daunomycin (NSC-82151). *Cancer Chemother Rep* 1970; **54**: 475–6.
2 Kelly TM, Fishman LM, Lessner HE. Hyperpigmentation with daunorubicin therapy. *Arch Dermatol* 1984; **120**: 262–3.
3 Anderson LL, Thomas ED, Berger TG *et al.* Cutaneous pigmentation after daunorubicin chemotherapy. *J Am Acad Dermatol* 1992; **26**: 255–6.
4 Kroumpouzos G, Travers R, Allan A. Generalised hyperpigmentation with daunorubicin chemotherapy. *J Am Acad Dermatol* 2002; **46**: S1–S3.

Doxorubicin (Adriamycin)

Short-lived localized erythema or urticaria with pruritus along the vein proximal to the injection site may occur in up to 3% of patients [1]. Angio-oedema, generalized urticaria with or without anaphylaxis and chronic urticaria have been reported rarely [2]. Cutaneous and nail pigmentation are well recognized [3,4]. Erythema and desquamation of palmar and plantar skin, with or without onycholysis, occurs frequently in patients receiving doxorubicin [5–7]. Liposomal doxorubicin is associated with a dose-limiting hand–foot syndrome and stomatitis [8,9] and with psoriasiform pustular reactions [10]. Allergic cross-reaction occurs with daunorubicin. Toxic epidermal injury after intra-arterial injection [11], phlebitis and chemical cellulitis with extensive tissue necrosis and ulceration following extravasation [12] are well documented.

REFERENCES

1 Vogelzang NJ. 'Adriamycin flare': a skin reaction resembling extravasation. *Cancer Treat Rep* 1979; **63**: 2067–9.
2 Hatfield AK, Harder L, Abderhalden RT. Chronic urticarial reactions caused by doxorubicin-containing regimens. *Cancer Chemother Rep* 1981; **65**: 353–4.

3 Giacobetti R, Esterly NB, Morgan ER. Nail hyperpigmentation secondary to therapy with doxorubicin. *Am J Dis Child* 1981; **135**: 317–8.
4 Curran CF. Doxorubicin-associated hyperpigmentation. *NZ Med J* 1990; **103**: 517.
5 Vogelzang NJ, Ratain MJ. Cancer chemotherapy and skin changes. *Ann Intern Med* 1985; **103**: 303–4.
6 Jones AP, Crawford SM. Anthracycline-induced toxicity affecting palmar and plantar skin. *Br J Cancer* 1989; **59**: 814.
7 Curran CF. Onycholysis in doxorubicin-treated patients. *Arch Dermatol* 1990; **126**: 1244.
8 Uziely B, Jeffers S, Isacson R *et al.* Liposomal doxorubicin: antitumor activity and unique toxicities during two complementary phase I studies. *J Clin Oncol* 1995; **13**: 1777–85.
9 Gordon KB, Tajuddin A, Guitart J *et al.* Hand–foot syndrome associated with liposome-encapsulated doxorubicin therapy. *Cancer* 1995; **75**: 2169–73.
10 Kreuter A, Gambichler T, Schlottmann R *et al.* Psoriasiform pustular eruptions from pegylated-liposomal doxorubicin in AIDS-related Kaposi's sarcoma. *Acta Derm Venereol (Stockh)* 2001; **81**: 224.
11 Von Eyben FE, Bruze M, Eksborg S *et al.* Toxic epidermal injury following intraarterial adriamycin treatment. *Cancer* 1981; **48**: 1535–8.
12 Reilly JJ, Neifeld JP, Rosenberg SA. Clinical course and management of accidental adriamycin extravasation. *Cancer* 1977; **40**: 2053–6.

Mitomycin

Urticaria and dermatitis [1–3], particularly on the face, palms and soles, or genitals and sometimes more generalized, have been reported after intravesical therapy. Sunlight-induced recall of ulceration following extravasation has been recorded [4].

REFERENCES

1 Colver GB, Inglis JA, McVittie E *et al.* Dermatitis due to intravesical mitomycin C: a delayed-type hypersensitivity reaction? *Br J Dermatol* 1990; **122**: 217–24.
2 De Groot AC, Conemans JMH. Systemic allergic contact dermatitis from intravesical instillation of the antitumor antibiotic mitomycin C. *Contact Dermatitis* 1991; **24**: 201–9.
3 Arregui MA, Aguirre A, Gil N *et al.* Dermatitis due to mitomycin C bladder instillations: study of 2 cases. *Contact Dermatitis* 1991; **24**: 368–70.
4 Fuller B, Lind M, Bonomi P. Mitomycin C extravasation exacerbated by sunlight. *Ann Intern Med* 1981; **94**: 542.

Antimetabolites

Aminoglutethimide

This inhibitor of adrenal steroid synthesis has been reported to induce SLE [1].

REFERENCE

1 McCraken M, Benson EA, Hickling P. Systemic lupus erythematosus induced by aminoglutethimide. *BMJ* 1980; **281**: 1254.

Azathioprine

The dermatological aspects of this derivative of the antimetabolite mercaptopurine have been reviewed [1–3]. Bone marrow suppression is the main problem; blood counts should be performed weekly for the first month, then monthly thereafter. Homozygotes for the low-activity allele for thiopurine methyltransferase are at risk of myelosuppression [4–7]. It is therefore recommended that thiopurine methyltransferase levels should be measured before commencing patients on azathioprine [6]. Gastro-intestinal upset is common and may necessitate discontinuation of therapy. Hypersensitivity reactions [8–10], including fever [11], maculopapular rashes, urticaria, vasculitis, erythema multiforme or erythema nodosum, cholestatic jaundice, hepatitis, liver necrosis, interstitial pneumonitis, polyneuropathy, pancreatitis, shock [12] with hypotension, nephritis and oliguria are well recognized.

An acneiform exanthem has been described, confirmed on challenge [13]. An eruption comprising tiny superficial blisters and peeling in the flexures is described [14]. Multiple large resistant warts are common on the hands of renal transplant recipients maintained on long-term azathioprine and prednisolone therapy; herpes simplex and herpes zoster infection may occur [15], and Norwegian scabies may be promoted [16]. Disseminated superficial actinic porokeratosis [17] and porokeratosis of Mibelli [18] have been documented. Keratoacanthomas and squamous cell carcinomas may develop [19]. Long-term therapy may predispose to the development of malignancy, especially non-Hodgkin's lymphoma [20]. Azathioprine crosses the placenta, although there is little evidence that azathioprine is teratogenic in humans, and detailed analysis of successful pregnancies notified to the European Dialysis and Transplant Association did not suggest an excessive rate of congenital abnormality [21]. However, depressed fetal haemopoiesis and resultant neonatal thrombocytopenia and leukopenia have been documented [22]. Pregnancy may be best avoided in patients receiving this drug [23]. Allopurinol may potentiate the effect of azathioprine by inhibiting its metabolism; the dose of azathioprine should therefore be reduced to one-quarter of the regular dose.

REFERENCES

1 Speerstra F, Boerbooms AM, van de Putte LB *et al*. Side effects of azathioprine treatment in rheumatoid arthritis: analysis of ten years of experience. *Ann Rheum Dis* 1982; **41**: 37–9.
2 Gendler E. Azathioprine for use in dermatology. *J Dermatol Surg Oncol* 1984; **10**: 462–4.
3 Younger IR, Harris DWS, Colver GB. Azathioprine in dermatology. *J Am Acad Dermatol* 1991; **25**: 281–6.
4 Snow JL, Gibson LE. The role of genetic variation in thiopurine methyltransferase activity and the efficacy and/or side effects of azathioprine therapy in dermatologic patients. *Arch Dermatol* 1995; **131**: 193–7.
5 Snow JL, Gibson LE. A pharmacogenetic basis for the safe and effective use of azathioprine and other thiopurine drugs in dermatologic patients. *J Am Acad Dermatol* 1995; **32**: 114–6.
6 Jackson AP, Hall AG, McLelland J. Thiopurine methyltransferase levels should be measured before commencing patients on azathioprine. *Br J Dermatol* 1997; **136**: 133–4.
7 Tavadia SMB, Mydlarski PR, Reis MD *et al*. Screening for azathioprine toxicity: a pharmacoeconomic analysis based on a target case. *J Am Acad Dermatol* 2000; **42**: 628–32.

8 Stetter M, Schmidl M, Krapf R. Azathioprine hypersensitivity mimicking Goodpasture's syndrome. *Am J Kidney Dis* 1994; **23**: 874–7.
9 Knowles SR, Gupta AK, Shear NH, Sauder D. Azathioprine hypersensitivity-like reactions: a case report and a review of the literature. *Clin Exp Dermatol* 1995; **20**: 353–6.
10 Parnham AP, Dittmer I, Mathieson PW *et al*. Acute allergic reactions associated with azathioprine. *Lancet* 1996; **348**: 542–3.
11 Smak Gregoor PJ, van Saase JL, Weimar W, Kramer P. Fever and rigors as sole symptoms of azathioprine hypersensitivity. *Neth J Med* 1995; **47**: 288–90.
12 Jones JJ, Ashworth J. Azathioprine-induced shock in dermatology patients. *J Am Acad Dermatol* 1993; **29**: 795–6.
13 Schmoeckel C, von Liebe V. Akneiformes Exanthem durch Azathioprin. *Hautarzt* 1983; **34**: 413–5.
14 Hermanns-Le T, Pierard GE. Azathioprine-induced skin peeling syndrome. *Dermatology* 1997; **194**: 175–6.
15 Spencer ES, Anderson HK. Viral infections in renal allograft recipients treated with long-term immunosuppression. *BMJ* 1979; **2**: 829–30.
16 Paterson WD, Allen BR, Beveridge GW. Norwegian scabies during immunosuppressive therapy. *BMJ* 1983; **4**: 211–2.
17 Neumann RA, Knobler RM, Metze D *et al*. Disseminated superficial porokeratosis and immunosuppression. *Br J Dermatol* 1988; **119**: 375–80.
18 Tatnell FM, Sarkany I. Porokeratosis of Mibelli in an immunosuppressed patient. *J R Soc Med* 1987; **80**: 180–1.
19 McLelland J, Rees A, Williams G *et al*. The incidence of immunosuppression-related skin disease in long-term transplant patients. *Transplantation* 1988; **46**: 871–4.
20 Phillips LT, Salisbury J, Leigh I, Baker H. Non-Hodgkin's lymphoma associated with long-term azathioprine therapy. *Clin Exp Dermatol* 1987; **12**: 444–5.
21 Registration Committee of the European Dialysis and Transplant Association. Successful pregnancies in women treated by dialysis and kidney transplantation. *Br J Obstet Gynaecol* 1980; **87**: 839–45.
22 Davison JM, Dellagrammatikas H, Parkin JM. Maternal azathioprine therapy and depressed haemopoiesis in the babies of renal allograft patients. *Br J Obstet Gynaecol* 1985; **92**: 233–9.
23 Gebhart DOE. Azathioprine teratogenicity: review of the literature and case report. *Obstet Gynecol* 1983; **61**: 270.

Cytarabine (cytosine arabinoside)

This drug interferes with pyrimidine synthesis. A self-limited palmoplantar erythema, occasionally with bullae, may occur [1–4]. Neutrophilic eccrine hidradenitis has been reported [5]. A syndrome with fever, malaise, arthralgia, conjunctivitis and diffuse erythematous maculopapular rash is documented [6]. The overall incidence of cutaneous reactions, including morbilliform eruptions, acral erythema, swelling and generalized urticaria, was almost 53% in one series [7].

REFERENCES

1 Walker IR, Wilson WEB, Sauder DN *et al*. Cytarabine-induced palmar-plantar erythema. *Arch Dermatol* 1985; **121**: 1240–1.
2 Shall L, Lucas GS, Whittaker JA, Holt PJA. Painful red hands: a side-effect of leukaemia therapy. *Br J Dermatol* 1988; **119**: 249–53.
3 Brown J, Burck K, Black D, Collins C. Treatment of cytarabine acral erythema with corticosteroids. *J Am Acad Dermatol* 1991; **24**: 1023–5.
4 Richards C, Wujcik D. Cutaneous toxicity associated with high-dose cytosine arabinoside. *Oncol Nurs Forum* 1992; **19**: 1191–5.
5 Flynn TC, Harrist TJ, Murphy GF *et al*. Neutrophilic eccrine hidradenitis: a distinctive type of neutrophilic dermatosis associated with cytarabine therapy and acute leukemia. *J Am Acad Dermatol* 1984; **11**: 584–90.
6 Shah SS, Rybak ME, Griffin TW. The cytarabine syndrome in an adult. *Cancer Treat Rep* 1983; **67**: 405–6.
7 Cetkovska P, Pizinger K, Cetkovsky P. High-dose cytosine arabinoside-induced cutaneous reactions. *J Eur Acad Dermatol Venereol* 2002; **16**: 481–5.

Fluorouracil

Anaphylaxis is rare; alopecia and recall phenomena [1] may be seen. Erythema followed by hyperpigmentation of sun-exposed areas occurs in up to 5% of patients [2]. Photosensitivity is recorded; pellagra may be caused by direct inhibition of the transformation of tryptophan into nicotinamide. Rarely, hyperpigmented streaks (serpentine supravenous hyperpigmentation) develop over arm veins used for injection [2–5]. Continuous infusion may be followed by the development of erythema, oedema and desquamation of the hands [6–10]. Pyridoxine may decrease the intensity and pain of fluorouracil-induced acral erythema [8]. Oral administration resulted in painful erythema multiforme-like erosions and blisters on the soles and arms in one case [9]. Systemic fluorouracil may result in marked inflammation of metastatic skin lesions [11] and of solar keratoses [12]. Topical application may lead to hyperpigmentation with or without a preceding irritant or allergic contact dermatitis [13].

Capecitabine

Capecitabine is a fluoropyrimidine carbamate that is metabolized to fluorouracil, and has been recorded as causing hand–foot syndrome in 50% of patients, and rarely leopard-like vitiligo, onycholysis and periungual pyogenic granulomas [14].

Gemcitabine

This drug has caused radiation recall [15].

REFERENCES

1 Prussick R, Thibault A, Turner ML. Recall of cutaneous toxicity from fluorouracil. *Arch Dermatol* 1993; **129**: 644–5.
2 Hrushesky WJ. Unusual pigmentary changes associated with 5-fluorouracil therapy. *Cutis* 1980; **26**: 181–2.
3 Hrushesky WJ. Serpentine supravenous 5-fluorouracil (NSC-19893) hyperpigmentation. *Cancer Treat Rep* 1976; **60**: 639.
4 Vukelja SJ, Bonner MW, McCollough M *et al.* Unusual serpentine hyperpigmentation associated with 5-fluorouracil. Case report and review of cutaneous manifestations associated with systemic 5-fluorouracil. *J Am Acad Dermatol* 1991; **25**: 905–8.
5 Pujol RM, Rocamora V, Lopez-Pousa A *et al.* Persistent supravenous erythematous eruption: a rare local complication of intravenous 5-fluorouracil therapy. *J Am Acad Dermatol* 1998; **39**: 839–42.
6 Feldman LD, Jaffer A. Fluorouracil-associated palmar–plantar erythrodysesthesia syndrome. *JAMA* 1985; **254**: 3479.
7 Guillaume J-C, Carp E, Rougier P *et al.* Effects secondaires cutanéomuqueux des perfusions continues de 5-fluorouracile: 12 observations. *Ann Dermatol Vénéréol* 1988; **115**: 1167–9.
8 Vukelja SJ, Lombardo RA, James WD *et al.* Pyridoxine for the palmar–plantar erythrodysesthesia syndrome. *Ann Intern Med* 1989; **111**: 688–9.
9 Ueki H, Namba M. Arzneimittelexanthem durch ein neues 5-Fluorouurazil-derivat. *Hautarzt* 1980; **31**: 207–8.
10 Chiara S, Nobile MT, Barzacchi C *et al.* Hand–foot syndrome induced by high-dose, short-term, continuous 5-fluorouracil infusion. *Eur J Cancer* 1997; **33**: 967–9.
11 Schlang HA. Inflammation of malignant skin involvement with fluorouracil. *JAMA* 1977; **238**: 1722.
12 Bataille V, Cunningham D, Mansi J, Mortimer P. Inflammation of solar keratoses following systemic 5-fluorouracil. *Br J Dermatol* 1996; **135**: 478–80.
13 Goette DK, Odom RB. Allergic contact dermatitis to topical fluorouracil. *Arch Dermatol* 1977; **113**: 1058–61.
14 Piguet V, Borradori L. Pyogenic granuloma-like lesions during capecitabine therapy. *Br J Dermatol* 2002; **147**: 1270–2.
15 Jeter MD, Janne PA, Brooks S *et al.* Gemcitabine-induced radiation recall. *Int J Radiat Oncol Biol Phys* 2002; **53**: 394–400.

Methotrexate

Dermatological aspects. These have been reviewed [1–3]. Methotrexate is a folic acid analogue and antagonist that inactivates dihydrofolate reductase. There is marked individual variation in absorption from the gastrointestinal tract, and hence in expression of toxic effects. Alopecia occurs in 6% of patients receiving low-dose therapy for psoriasis and in 8% of patients on high-dose regimens for malignancy, and is usually the result of telogen effluvium. Intermittent high dosage has resulted in horizontal pigmented banding of hair (the 'flag sign' of chemotherapy) [4]. Urticaria develops in about 4% of patients on low-dose oral or parenteral therapy for psoriasis [5]. Exacerbation of urticarial vasculitis has been documented [6]. Photosensitivity occurs in up to 5% of cases. Methotrexate use has been associated with severe reactivation of sunburn [7,8]; in one case, there was sparing of chronically sun-exposed skin [8]. Chronic viral wart and molluscum infections may result from immunosuppression. Cutaneous toxicity with local epidermal necrosis may occasionally occur [9,10]. A macular erythema occurring in 15% of patients, and biopsy-proven capillaritis, have been reported with high-dose therapy [3]. An eruption of erythematous indurated papules on the proximal parts of the limbs has been documented in patients with collagen vascular disease [11]. Anaphylactic reactions [12] and pain, burning, erythema and desquamation of the palms and soles [13–15] are seen with high-dose intravenous methotrexate, but are extremely rare. Vasculitis has been very rarely documented with both intermediate dosage therapy for leukaemia [16] and high-dose therapy [17]. TEN is recorded [18,19], and occurred after a single injection of 25 mg for pustular psoriasis [19].

REFERENCES

1 Plantin P, Saraux A, Guillet G. Méthotrexate en dermatologie: aspects actuels. *Ann Dermatol Vénéréol* 1989; **116**: 109–15.
2 Zachariae H. Methotrexate side-effects. *Br J Dermatol* 1990; **122** (Suppl. 36): 127–33.
3 Olsen EA. The pharmacology of methotrexate. *J Am Acad Dermatol* 1991; **25**: 306–18.
4 Wheeland RG, Burgdorf WH, Humphrey GB. The flag sign of chemotherapy. *Cancer* 1983; **51**: 1356–8.
5 Weinstein GD, Frost P. Methotrexate for psoriasis. A new therapeutic schedule. *Arch Dermatol* 1971; **103**: 33–8.
6 Borcea A, Greaves MW. Methotrexate-induced exacerbation of urticarial vasculitis: an unusual adverse reaction. *Br J Dermatol* 2000; **143**: 203–4.
7 Mallory SB, Berry DH. Severe reactivation of sunburn following methotrexate use. *Pediatrics* 1986; **78**: 514–5.

8 Westwick TJ, Sherertz EF, McCarley D, Flowers FP. Delayed reactivation of sunburn by methotrexate: sparing of chronically sun-exposed skin. *Cutis* 1987; **39**: 49–51.

9 Harrison PV. Methotrexate-induced epidermal necrosis. *Br J Dermatol* 1987; **116**: 867–9.

10 Kaplan DL, Olsen EA. Erosion of psoriatic plaques after chronic methotrexate administration. *Int J Dermatol* 1988; **27**: 59–62.

11 Goerttler E, Kutzner H, Peter HH, Requena L. Methotrexate-induced papular eruption in patients with rheumatic diseases: a distinctive adverse cutaneous reaction produced by methotrexate in patients with collagen vascular diseases. *J Am Acad Dermatol* 1999; **40**: 702–7.

12 Klimo P, Ibrahim E. Anaphylactic reaction to methotrexate used in high doses as an adjuvant treatment of osteogenic sarcoma. *Cancer Treat Rep* 1981; **65**: 725.

13 Doyle LA, Berg C, Bottino G *et al.* Erythema and desquamation after high-dose methotrexate. *Ann Intern Med* 1983; **98**: 611–2.

14 Martins da Cunha AC, Rappersberger K, Gadner H. Toxic skin reaction restricted to palms and soles after high-dose methotrexate. *Pediatr Hematol Oncol* 1991; **8**: 277–80.

15 Aractingi S, Briant E, Marolleau J *et al.* Décollements cutanés induits par le methotrexate. *Presse Med* 1992; **21**: 1668–70.

16 Fondevila CG, Milone GA, Pavlovsky S. Cutaneous vasculitis after intermediate dose of methotrexate (IDMTX). *Br J Haematol* 1989; **72**: 591–2.

17 Navarro M, Pedragosa R, Lafuerza A *et al.* Leukocytoclastic vasculitis after high-dose methotrexate. *Ann Intern Med* 1986; **105**: 471–2.

18 Collins P, Rogers S. The efficacy of methotrexate in psoriasis: a review of 40 cases. *Clin Exp Dermatol* 1992; **17**: 257–60.

19 Primka EJ III, Camisa C. Methotrexate-induced toxic epidermal necrolysis in a patient with psoriasis. *J Am Acad Dermatol* 1997; **36**: 815–8.

Systemic complications. Because folic acid is an essential co-factor for DNA synthesis and cell division, bone marrow suppression may occur even on low-dose therapy [1–4]. Thrombocytopenia may develop after a single test dose [5]. Severe bone marrow suppression [6] with the dosage used in the therapy of psoriasis is fortunately not common. Stomatitis may be a warning sign of overdosage. The risk of myelosuppression is much greater in the presence of renal impairment. Gastrointestinal upset is common. Abnormalities of taste sensation occur rarely [7].

The main hazard is hepatotoxicity with long-term use [8]. The risk of developing severe hepatotoxicity is related to the daily dose, the dose frequency and the cumulative dose [9]. Alcohol consumption, underlying liver disease and obesity, especially in the presence of diabetes, are aggravating factors. Recommendations have included obtaining baseline haematological, renal and hepatic function tests and a liver biopsy before or within 4 months of starting therapy, and repeating after every 1.5 g [10]. Liver function tests may be unreliable indicators of fibrosis or cirrhosis. These guidelines appear prudent but have never been rigorously tested, and are variously applied in clinical practice [10,11]. There seems to be a discrepancy between the degree of hepatotoxicity in rheumatoid arthritis and that in psoriasis, and many rheumatologists do not routinely carry out liver biopsy [11]. The requirement for liver biopsies in psoriasis patients on long-term, low-dose, once-weekly oral methotrexate has been questioned [12]. Radionuclide liver scans are thought to be of little value in the detection of methotrexate-induced liver disease, but liver ultrasound may be of some assistance [13]. Abnormal liver biopsy may improve after cessation

of therapy [14]. Assay of serum levels of the amino-propeptide of type III procollagen is being used in some centres to screen for patients in whom liver biopsy is mandatory [15–17].

Acute renal failure may follow high-dose methotrexate therapy, although renal damage is rare in patients treated for psoriasis. Pulmonary complications, such as pneumonitis or fibrosis, are rare [18,19]. There do not appear to be adverse effects on humoral or cellular immunity from low weekly doses as given for rheumatoid arthritis or psoriasis [20].

Methotrexate is a known teratogen, and may cause oligospermia [21,22]. It is recommended that patients avoid pregnancy or impregnation during, and for 12 weeks after cessation of, methotrexate therapy [23].

Care must be taken with regard to potential drug interactions with methotrexate [24,25]. Drugs that also interfere with folate metabolism, such as trimethoprim–sulfamethoxazole [26–28], may cause pancytopenia; both trimethoprim and sulfamethoxazole bind to dihydrofolate reductase. Drugs that displace methotrexate from plasma protein-binding sites, such as salicylates, sulphonamides and diphenylhydantoin, as well as drugs that impair the renal clearance of methotrexate, such as NSAIDs and sulphonamides, may also cause pancytopenia. A toxic reaction occurred in a patient treated with penicillin and furosemide [29].

REFERENCES

1 MacKinnon SK, Starkebaum G, Wilkens RF. Pancytopenia associated with low-dose pulse methotrexate in the treatment of rheumatoid arthritis. *Semin Arthritis Rheum* 1985; **15**: 119–26.

2 Shupack JL, Webster GF. Pancytopenia following low-dose oral methotrexate therapy for psoriasis. *JAMA* 1988; **259**: 3594–6.

3 Abel EA, Farber EM. Pancytopenia following low-dose methotrexate therapy. *JAMA* 1988; **259**: 3612.

4 Copur S, Dahut W, Chu E, Allegra CJ. Bone marrow aplasia and severe skin rash after a single low dose of methotrexate. *Anticancer Drugs* 1995; **6**: 154–7.

5 Jih DM, Werth VP. Thrombocytopenia after a single test dose of methotrexate. *J Am Acad Dermatol* 1998; **39**: 349–51.

6 Takami M, Kuniyoshi Y, Oomukai T *et al.* Severe complications after high-dose methotrexate treatment. *Acta Oncol* 1995; **34**: 611–2.

7 Duhra P, Foulds IS. Methotrexate-induced impairment of taste acuity. *Clin Exp Dermatol* 1988; **13**: 126–7.

8 Zachariae H, Kragballe K, Søgaard H. Methotrexate induced liver cirrhosis: studies including serial liver biopsies during continued treatment. *Br J Dermatol* 1980; **102**: 407–12.

9 Lewis JH, Schiff E. ACG Committee on FDA-Related Matters. Methotrexate-induced chronic liver injury: guidelines for detection and prevention. *Am J Gastroenterol* 1988; **88**: 1337–45.

10 Roenigk HH Jr, Auerbach R, Maibach HI, Weinstein GD. Methotrexate in psoriasis: revised guidelines. *J Am Acad Dermatol* 1988; **19**: 145–56.

11 Petrazzuoli M, Rothe MJ, Grin-Jorgensen C *et al.* Monitoring patients taking methotrexate for hepatotoxicity. Does the standard of care match published guidelines? *J Am Acad Dermatol* 1994; **31**: 969–77.

12 Boffa MJ, Chalmers RJG, Haboubi NY *et al.* Sequential liver biopsies during long-term methotrexate treatment for psoriasis: a reappraisal. *Br J Dermatol* 1995; **133**: 774–8.

13 Coulson IH, McKenzie J, Neild VS *et al.* A comparison of liver ultrasound with liver biopsy histology in psoriatics receiving long-term methotrexate therapy. *Br J Dermatol* 1987; **116**: 491–5.

14 Newman M, Auerbach R, Feiner H *et al.* The role of liver biopsies in psoriatic patients receiving long-term methotrexate treatment. Improvement in liver abnormalities after cessation of therapy. *Arch Dermatol* 1989; **125**: 1218–24.

15 Zachariae H, Søgaard H, Heickendorff L. Serum aminoterminal propeptide of type III procollagen. *Acta Derm Venereol (Stockh)* 1989; **69**: 241–4.

16 Boffa MJ, Smith A, Chalmer RJG *et al.* Serum type III procollagen aminopeptide for assessing liver damage in methotrexate-treated psoriatic patients. *Br J Dermatol* 1996; **135**: 538–44.

17 Zachariae H, Heickendorff L, Søgaard H. The value of amino-terminal propeptide of type III procollagen in routine screening for methotrexate-induced liver fibrosis: a 10 year follow up. *Br J Dermatol* 2001; **144**: 100–3.

18 Phillips TJ, Jones DH, Baker H. Pulmonary complications following methotrexate therapy. *J Am Acad Dermatol* 1987; **16**: 373–5.

19 Carson CW, Cannon GW, Egger MJ *et al.* Pulmonary disease during the treatment of rheumatoid arthritis with low dose pulse methotrexate. *Semin Arthritis Rheum* 1987; **16**: 186–95.

20 Andersen PA, West SG, O'Dell JR *et al.* Weekly pulse methotrexate in rheumatoid arthritis: clinical and immunologic effects in a randomized, double-blind study. *Ann Intern Med* 1985; **103**: 489–96.

21 Sussman A, Leonard JM. Psoriasis, methotrexate, and oligospermia. *Arch Dermatol* 1980; **116**: 215–7.

22 Shamberger RC, Rosenberg SA, Seipp CA *et al.* Effects of high-dose methotrexate and vincristine on ovarian and testicular functions in patients undergoing postoperative adjuvant treatment of osteosarcoma. *Cancer Treat Rep* 1981; **65**: 739–46.

23 Morris LF, Harrod MJ, Menter MA, Silverman AK. Methotrexate and reproduction in men: case report and recommendations. *J Am Acad Dermatol* 1993; **29**: 913–6.

24 Evans WE, Christensen ML. Drug interactions with methotrexate. *J Rheumatol* 1985; **12** (Suppl. 12): 15–20.

25 Liddle BJ, Marsden JR. Drug interactions with methotrexate. *Br J Dermatol* 1989; **120**: 582–3.

26 Thomas DR, Dover JS, Camp RDR. Pancytopenia induced by the interaction between methotrexate and trimethoprim–sulfamethoxazole. *J Am Acad Dermatol* 1987; **17**: 1055–6.

27 Ferrazzini G, Klein J, Sulh H *et al.* Interaction between trimethoprim–sulfamethoxazole and methotrexate in children with leukemia. *J Pediatr* 1990; **117**: 823–6.

28 Groenendal H, Rampen FHJ. Methotrexate and trimethoprim–sulphamethoxazole: a potentially hazardous combination. *Clin Exp Dermatol* 1990; **15**: 358–60.

29 Nierenberg DW, Mamelok RD. Toxic reaction to methotrexate in a patient receiving penicillin and furosemide. *Arch Dermatol* 1983; **119**: 449–50.

Vinca alkaloids and etoposide

These drugs cause metaphase arrest by interfering with microtubule assembly.

Etoposide (VP-16)

This semi-synthetic podophyllotoxin derivative causes bone marrow suppression, alopecia and gastrointestinal symptoms. It has caused Stevens–Johnson syndrome and radiation recall. Four cases of a diffuse, erythematous, maculopapular rash occurring 5–9 days after initiation of therapy, with spontaneous resolution within 3 weeks, have been reported [1]. On histology, scattered, markedly enlarged individual keratinocytes with a 'starburst' nuclear chromatin pattern were seen. Hypersensitivity reactions are generally held to be rare [2–4], but 51% of patients with newly diagnosed Hodgkin's disease had one or more acute hypersensitivity reactions to etoposide administration, including flushing, respiratory problems, changes in blood pressure and abdominal pain [5].

Vincristine

Peripheral neuropathy is well recognized with long-term therapy [6].

Vinblastine

Photosensitivity is common [7]. Acute alopecia and radiation recall are documented. Erythema multiforme-like reactions are described following intravenous injection [8].

REFERENCES

1 Yokel BK, Friedman KJ, Farmer ER, Hood AF. Cutaneous pathology following etoposide therapy. *J Cutan Pathol* 1987; **14**: 326–30.

2 Kasperek C, Black CD. Two cases of suspected immunologic-based hypersensitivity reactions to etoposide therapy. *Ann Pharmacother* 1992; **26**: 1227–30.

3 de Souza P, Friedlander M, Wilde C *et al.* Hypersensitivity reactions to etoposide. A report of three cases and review of the literature. *Am J Clin Oncol* 1994; **17**: 387–9.

4 Hoetelmans RM, Schornagel JH, ten Bokkel Huinink WW, Beijnen JH. Hypersensitivity reactions to etoposide. *Ann Pharmacother* 1996; **30**: 367–71.

5 Hudson MM, Weinstein HJ, Donaldson SS *et al.* Acute hypersensitivity reactions to etoposide in a VEPA regimen for Hodgkin's disease. *J Clin Oncol* 1993; **11**: 1080–4.

6 Watkins SM, Griffin JP. High incidence of vincristine-induced neuropathy in lymphomas. *BMJ* 1978; **i**: 610–2.

7 Breza TS, Halprin KM, Taylor JR. Photosensitivity reaction to vinblastine. *Arch Dermatol* 1975; **111**: 1168–70.

8 Arias D, Requena L, Hasson A *et al.* Localized epidermal necrolysis (erythema multiforme-like reactions) following intravenous injection of vinblastine. *J Cutan Pathol* 1991; **18**: 344–6.

Enzymes

L-Asparaginase (crisantaspase)

Dose-dependent IgE-mediated hypersensitivity reactions, including urticaria and anaphylaxis, are frequent, especially when the drug is used alone [1]. Allergic reactions to intramuscular L-asparaginase include local painful erythema, and urticaria or a general exanthem; continuous infusion is better tolerated [2].

REFERENCES

1 Ertel IJ, Nesbit ME, Hammond D *et al.* Effective dose of L-asparaginase for induction of remission in previously treated children with acute lymphocytic leukemia: a report from Children's Cancer Study Group. *Cancer Res* 1979; **39**: 3893–6.

2 Rodriguez T, Baumgarten E, Fengler R *et al.* Langzeitinfusion von L-Asparaginase: eine Alternative zur intramuskularen Injektion? *Klin Padiatr* 1995; **207**: 207–10.

Miscellaneous chemotherapeutic agents

Acridinyl anisidide (AMSA)

Skin reactions are rare but widespread erythema has been reported [1].

REFERENCE

1 Rosenfelt FP, Rosenbloom BE, Weinstein IM. Allergic reaction following administration of AMSA. *Cancer Treat Rep* 1982; **66**: 549–5.

Bromodeoxyuridine

A distinctive eruption comprising linear supravenous papules and erythroderma has been described with bromodeoxyuridine given in combination with radiotherapy for central nervous system tumours [1]. Ipsilateral facial dermatitis with epilation of eyebrows and eyelashes, ocular irritation, bilateral nail dystrophy, oral ulceration, exanthem or erythema multiforme have also been described [2].

REFERENCES

1 Fine J-D, Breathnach SM. Distinctive eruption characterized by linear supravenous papules and erythroderma following broxuridine (bromodeoxyuridine) therapy and radiotherapy. *Arch Dermatol* 1986; **122**: 199–200.
2 McCuaig CM, Ellis CN, Greenberg HS *et al.* Mucocutaneous complications of intra-arterial 5-bromodeoxyuridine and radiation. *J Am Acad Dermatol* 1989; **21**: 1235–40.

Carboplatin

Hypersensitivity reactions occur in 1–30% of patients [1–5]; acute allergic reactions include urticaria, bronchospasm, hypotension, facial erythema and facial swelling. Desensitization can be successful [5]. A pruritic maculopapular rash occurred in 10 of 40 patients treated with carboplatin, etoposide and ifosfamide plus mesna followed by autologous stem cell reinfusion; the rash was distributed at the extremities or was confluent on the trunk and face, with facial oedema and painful swelling of hands and feet, and resolved spontaneously with hyperpigmentation in all patients [6].

REFERENCES

1 Hendrick AM, Simmons D, Cantwell BM. Allergic reactions to carboplatin. *Ann Oncol* 1992; **3**: 239–40.
2 Tonkin KS, Rubin P, Levin L. Carboplatin hypersensitivity: case reports and review of the literature. *Eur J Cancer* 1993; **29A**: 1356–7.
3 Weidmann B, Mulleneisen N, Bojko P, Niederle N. Hypersensitivity reactions to carboplatin. Report of two patients, review of the literature, and discussion of diagnostic procedures and management. *Cancer* 1994; **73**: 2218–22.
4 Chang SM, Fryberger S, Crouse V *et al.* Carboplatin hypersensitivity in children. A report of five patients with brain tumors. *Cancer* 1995; **75**: 1171–5.
5 Broome CB, Schiff RI, Friedman HS. Successful desensitization to carboplatin in patients with systemic hypersensitivity reactions. *Med Pediatr Oncol* 1996; **26**: 105–10.
6 Beyer J, Grabbe J, Lenz K *et al.* Cutaneous toxicity of high-dose carboplatin, etoposide and ifosfamide followed by autologous stem cell reinfusion. *Bone Marrow Transplant* 1992; **10**: 491–4.

Cisplatin

Periungual hyperpigmentation [1] and acral erythema [2] or digital necrosis [3] have been documented. Severe hypersensitivity reactions, including flushing, erythema, maculopapular eruptions, urticaria and anaphylaxis, occur in about 5% of cases when this drug is used as a single agent, and in up to 20% when given with other chemotherapeutic agents [4,5]. Cross-reactivity with carboplatin may occur [5]. Atopic subjects are especially at risk. Local reactions follow extravasation [6]. Severe allergic exfoliative dermatitis with ischaemia and necrosis of the hands developed in a patient who had received multiple doses of cisplatin [7].

REFERENCES

1 Kim KJ, Chang SE, Choi JH *et al.* Periungal hyperpigmentation induced by cisplatin. *Clin Exp Dermatol* 2002; **27**: 118–9.
2 Vakalis D, Ioannides D, Lazaridou E *et al.* Acral erythema induced by chemotherapy with cisplatin. *Br J Dermatol* 1998; **139**: 750–1.
3 Marie I, Levesque H, Plissonier D *et al.* Digital necrosis related to cisplatin in systemic sclerosis. *Br J Dermatol* 2000; **142**: 833–4.
4 Vogl SE, Zaravinos T, Kaplan BH. Toxicity of cis-diaminedichloro-platinum II given in a two-hour outpatient regimen of diuresis and hydration. *Cancer* 1980; **45**: 11–5.
5 Shlebak AA, Clark PI, Green JA. Hypersensitivity and cross-reactivity to cisplatin and analogues. *Cancer Chemother Pharmacol* 1995; **35**: 349–51.
6 Fields S, Koeller J, Topper RL *et al.* Local soft tissue toxicity following cisplatin extravasation. *J Natl Cancer Inst* 1990; **82**: 1649–50.
7 Lee TC, Hook CC, Long HJ. Severe exfoliative dermatitis associated with hand ischemia during cisplatin therapy. *Mayo Clin Proc* 1994; **69**: 80–2.

Colchicine

Alopecia is recorded [1].

REFERENCE

1 Haarms M. Haarausfall und Haarveränderungen nach Kolchizintherapie. *Hautarzt* 1980; **31**: 161–3.

Flutamide

A photosensitive dermatitis [1,2] and pseudoporphyria [3] have been reported with this non-steroid antiandrogen used in the treatment of prostatic carcinoma.

REFERENCES

1 Fujimoto M, Kikuchi K, Imakado S, Furue M. Photosensitive dermatitis induced by flutamide. *Br J Dermatol* 1996; **135**: 496–7.
2 Yokote R, Tokura Y, Igarashi N *et al.* Photosensitive drug eruption induced by flutamide. *Eur J Dermatol* 1998; **8**: 427–9.
3 Borroni G, Brazzelli V, Baldini F *et al.* Flutamide-induced pseudoporphyria. *Br J Dermatol* 1998; **138**: 711–2.

Hydroxycarbamide (hydroxyurea)

Dermatological aspects of this drug have been reviewed [1–6]. Impaired renal function has been reported in some, but not all, studies [3]. A modest fall in haemoglobin and development of macrocytosis is almost constant.

Stomatitis occurs especially with high-dose therapy and has been accompanied by soreness, violet erythema, and oedema of the palms and soles with subsequent intense universal hyperpigmentation [7], but alopecia is rare. Morbilliform erythema occurs, and hyperpigmentation, generalized or localized to pressure areas, was recorded in up to 5% of cases [2]. A more recent survey reported mucocutaneous adverse reactions after a mean duration of 6.4 weeks of treatment in up to 65% of patients, with pigmentation of nails, skin or mucosa seen in 58.6% [6]. Other less common findings were xerosis, diffuse alopecia, oedema of the legs, oral ulcers and actinic psoriasis; scleral pigmentation and acquired ichthyosis were also noted. Nail pigmentation changes [8], such as multiple pigmented nail bands [9], or onycholysis with nail dystrophy occurs. Fixed drug eruption has been reported [3], as has baboon syndrome [10]. Dermatomyositis-like acral erythema, scaling, and atrophy especially on the dorsum of the hands, with lesser involvement of the feet [1,4,11–14], and palmar and plantar keratoderma have been rarely described with long-term therapy for chronic myeloid leukaemia. Photosensitivity is documented, and LE [15] and vasculitis have been reported. An ulcerative lichen planus-like dermatitis has been recorded [16]. Lichenoid eruptions similar to graft-versus-host disease are documented [17,18]. Several reports have recorded an association with leg ulcers [12,13,19–23]. Accelerated development of skin malignancies occurs, and eruptive squamous and basal cell cancers on light-exposed areas may be seen [24]. Radiation recall occurs [25].

REFERENCES

1 Kennedy BJ, Smith LR, Goltz RW. Skin changes secondary to hydroxyurea therapy. *Arch Dermatol* 1975; **111**: 183–7.
2 Layton AM, Sheehan-Dare RA, Goodfield MJD, Cotterill JA. Hydroxyurea in the management of therapy resistant psoriasis. *Br J Dermatol* 1989; **121**: 647–53.
3 Boyd AS, Neldner KH. Hydroxyurea therapy. *J Am Acad Dermatol* 1991; **25**: 518–24.
4 Kelly RI, Bull RH, Marsden A. Cutaneous manifestations of long-term hydroxyurea therapy. *Australas J Dermatol* 1994; **35**: 61–4.
5 Chaine B, Neonato M-G, Girot R, Aractingi S. Cutaneous adverse reactions to hydroxyurea in patients with sickle cell disease. *Arch Dermatol* 2001; **137**: 467–70.
6 Kumar B, Saraswat A, Kaur I. Mucocutaneous adverse effects of hydroxyurea: a prospective study of 30 psoriasis patients. *Clin Exp Dermatol* 2002; **27**: 8–13.
7 Brincker H, Christensen BE. Acute mucocutaneous toxicity following high-dose hydroxyurea. *Cancer Chemother Pharmacol* 1993; **32**: 496–7.
8 Aste N, Gumo G, Contu F et al. Nail pigmentation caused by hydroxyurea: report of 9 cases. *J Am Acad Dermatol* 2002; **47**: 146–7.
9 Vomvouras S, Pakula AS, Shaw JM. Multiple pigmented nail bands during hydroxyurea therapy: an uncommon finding. *J Am Acad Dermatol* 1991; **24**: 1016–7.
10 Chowdhury MM, Patel GK, Inaloz HS, Holt PJ. Hydroxyurea-induced skin disease mimicking the baboon syndrome. *Clin Exp Dermatol* 1999; **24**: 336–7.
11 Richard M, Truchetet F, Friedel J et al. Skin lesions simulating chronic dermatomyositis during long-term hydroxyurea therapy. *J Am Acad Dermatol* 1989; **21**: 797–9.
12 Suehiro M, Kishimoto S, Wakabayashi T et al. Hydroxyurea dermopathy with a dermatomyositis-like eruption and a large leg ulcer. *Br J Dermatol* 1998; **139**: 748–9.
13 Varma S, Lanigan SW. Dermatomyositis-like eruption and leg ulceration caused by hydroxyurea in a patient with psoriasis. *Clin Exp Dermatol* 1999; **24**: 164–6.
14 Dacey MJ, Callen JP. Hydroxyurea-induced dermatomyositis-like eruption. *J Am Acad Dermatol* 2003; **48**: 439–41.
15 Layton AM, Cotterill JA, Tomlinson IW. Hydroxyurea-induced lupus erythematosus. *Br J Dermatol* 1994; **130**: 687–8.
16 Renfro L, Kamino H, Raphael B et al. Ulcerative lichen planus-like dermatitis associated with hydroxyurea. *J Am Acad Dermatol* 1991; **24**: 143–5.
17 Daoud MS, Gibson LE, Pittelkow MR. Hydroxyurea dermopathy: a unique lichenoid eruption complicating long-term therapy with hydroxyurea. *J Am Acad Dermatol* 1997; **36**: 178–82.
18 Eming SA, Peters T, Hartmann K et al. Lichenoid chronic graft-versus-host disease-like acrodermatitis induced by hydroxyurea. *J Am Acad Dermatol* 2001; **45**: 321–3.
19 Weinlich G, Schuler G, Greil R et al. Leg ulcers associated with long-term hydroxyurea therapy. *J Am Acad Dermatol* 1998; **39**: 372–4.
20 Kido M, Tago O, Fujiwara H et al. Leg ulcer associated with hydroxyurea treatment in a patient with chronic myelogenous leukaemia: successful treatment with prostaglandin E$_1$ and pentoxifylline. *Br J Dermatol* 1998; **139**: 1124–6.
21 Sirieix ME, Debure C, Baudot N et al. Leg ulcers and hydroxyurea: forty-one cases. *Arch Dermatol* 1999; **135**: 818–20.
22 Weinlich G, Fritsch P. Leg ulcers in patients treated with hydroxyurea for myeloproliferative disorders: what is the trigger? *Br J Dermatol* 1999; **141**: 171–2.
23 Aragane Y, Ikamoto T, Yajima A et al. Hydroxyurea-induced foot ulcer successfully treated with a topical basic fibroblast growth factor product. *Br J Dermatol* 2003; **148**: 599–600.
24 Papi M, Didona B, DePita O et al. Multiple skin tumors on light-exposed areas during long-term treatment with hydroxyurea. *J Am Acad Dermatol* 1993; **28**: 485–6.
25 Sears ME. Erythema in areas of previous irradiation in patients treated with hydroxyurea (NSC-32065). *Cancer Chemother Rep* 1964; **40**: 31–2.

Imatinib

This protein tyrosine kinase inhibitor, used in the therapy of chronic myeloid leukaemia, has caused oedema, pruritus, and exanthematous, psoriasiform and exfoliative dermatoses [1].

REFERENCE

1 Valeyrie L, Bastuji-Garin S, Revuz J et al. Adverse cutaneous reactions to imatinib (ST1571) in Philadelphia chromosome-positive leukemias: a prospective study of 54 patients. *J Am Acad Dermatol* 2003; **48**: 201–6.

Suramin

Suramin sodium, a polysulphonated naphthylurea used in the treatment of metastatic prostatic and other cancers, has caused generalized, erythematous, maculopapular eruptions within the first 24 h of therapy (which were self-limited despite continued drug infusion), keratoacanthoma and disseminated superficial actinic porokeratosis [1–3]. Distinctive findings include scaling erythematous papules (suramin keratoses) and a predilection for previously sun-exposed areas (UV recall). Severe cutaneous reactions occur in 10% of cases [3]. Histopathological findings have included hyperkeratosis, parakeratosis, spongiosis, acanthosis, exocytosis, apoptosis, a perivascular lymphohistiocytic infiltrate, upper dermal oedema and increased dermal mucin [3]. Erythema multiforme [4] and TEN [5,6] are recorded.

REFERENCES

1 O'Donnell BP, Dawson NA, Weiss RB et al. Suramin-induced skin reactions. Arch Dermatol 1992; **128**: 75–9.
2 Wichterich K, Tebbe B, Handke A et al. Kutane Arzneimittelreaktion durch Suramin bei 4 Patienten mit metastasierendem Prostata-Karzinom. Hautarzt 1994; **45**: 84–7.
3 Lowitt MH, Eisenberger M, Sina B, Kao GF. Cutaneous eruptions from suramin. A clinical and histopathologic study of 60 patients. Arch Dermatol 1995; **131**: 1147–53.
4 Katz SK, Medenica MM, Kobayashi K et al. Erythema multiforme induced by suramin. J Am Acad Dermatol 1995; **32**: 292–3.
5 May E, Allolio B. Fatal toxic epidermal necrolysis during suramin therapy. Eur J Cancer 1991; **28A**: 1294.
6 Falkson G, Rapoport BL. Lethal toxic epidermal necrolysis during suramin therapy. Eur J Cancer 1992; **27**: 1338.

Taxanes

Docetaxel. Docetaxel, a semi-synthetic analogue of paclitaxel from the needles of the European yew *Taxus baccata* and used in the treatment of advanced and/or metastatic cancer, caused neutropenia, skin reactions (81%) and nail changes (41%), neurosensory toxicity (59%), fluid retention with oedema and hypersensitivity reactions (16–55%) [1–3]. The commonest skin reaction is characterized by discrete erythematous to violaceous patches or oedematous plaques similar to acral erythema [4]. Nail changes recorded [5,6] include horizontal banding [7], dyschromia [8] and subungual abscess [9]. Squamous syringometaplasia [10] and supravenous discoloration of the skin are documented [11].

REFERENCES

1 ten Bokkel Huinink WW, Prove AM, Piccard M et al. A phase II trial with docetaxel (Taxotene) in second line treatment with chemotherapy for advanced breast cancer. A study of the EORTC Early Clinical Trials Group. Ann Oncol 1994; **5**: 527–32.
2 Pazdur R, Lassere Y, Soh LT et al. Phase II trial of docetaxel (Taxotere) in metastatic colorectal carcinoma. Ann Oncol 1994; **5**: 468–70.
3 Mertens WC, Eisenhauer EA, Jolivet J et al. Docetaxel in advanced renal carcinoma. A phase II trial of the National Cancer Institute of Canada Clinical Trials Group. Ann Oncol 1994; **5**: 185–7.
4 Zimmerman GC, Keeling JH, Burris HA et al. Acute cutaneous reactions to docetaxel, a new chemotherapeutic agent. Arch Dermatol 1995; **131**: 202–6.
5 Valero V, Holmes FA, Walters RS et al. Phase II trial of docetaxel: a new, highly effective antineoplastic agent in the management of patients with anthracycline-resistant metastatic breast cancer. J Clin Oncol 1995; **13**: 2886–94.
6 Pavithran K, Doval DC. Nail changes due to docetaxel. Br J Dermatol 2002; **146**: 709–10.
7 Llombart-Cussac A, Pivot X. Docetaxel chemotherapy induces transverse superficial loss of the nail plate. Arch Dermatol 1997; **133**: 1466–7.
8 Jacob CI, Frunza Patten S. Nail bed dyschromia secondary to docetaxel therapy. Arch Dermatol 1998; **134**: 1167–8.
9 Vanhooteghem O, Richert B, Vindevoghel A et al. Subungual abscess: a new ungual side-effect related to docetaxel therapy. Br J Dermatol 2000; **143**: 462–4.
10 Karam A, Metges JP, Labat JP et al. Squamous syringometaplasia associated with docetaxel. Br J Dermatol 2002; **146**: 524–5.
11 Schrijvers D, van den Brande J, Vermorken JB. Supravenous discoloration of the skin due to docetaxel treatment. Br J Dermatol 2000; **142**: 1069–70.

Paclitaxel. Paclitaxel, a diterpenoid taxane derivative found in the bark and needles of the western yew *Taxus brevifolia*, interrupts mitosis by promoting and stabilizing microtubule formation, and shows substantial activity against advanced refractory cancer. Neutropenia is the major dose-limiting toxic effect; other adverse effects include severe hypersensitivity reactions including anaphylaxis, cardiac toxicity, neurotoxicity, arthralgia or myalgia, mucositis, nausea and vomiting, and alopecia [1–6]. Local necrosis has followed accidental subcutaneous extravasation of paclitaxel [7], and administration via a central vein has produced a recall reaction at a site of prior extravasation [8]. Bullous fixed drug eruption is recorded [9], as is a scleroderma-like reaction [10,11]. Desensitization is possible [12].

REFERENCES

1 Onetto N, Canetta R, Winograd B et al. Overview of Taxol safety. Monogr Natl Cancer Inst 1993; **15**: 131–9.
2 Schiller JH, Storer B, Tutsch K et al. A phase I trial of 3-hour infusions of paclitaxel (Taxol) with or without granulocyte colony-stimulating factor. Semin Oncol 1994; **21** (Suppl. 8): 9–14.
3 Gelmon K. The taxoids: paclitaxel and docetaxel. Lancet 1994; **344**: 1267–72.
4 van Herpen CM, van Hoesel QG, Punt CJ. Paclitaxel-induced severe hypersensitivity reaction occurring as a late toxicity. Ann Oncol 1995; **6**: 852.
5 Berghmans T, Klastersky J. Paclitaxel-induced cutaneous toxicity. Support Care Cancer 1995; **3**: 203–4.
6 Payne JY, Holmes F, Cohen P et al. Paclitaxel: severe mucocutaneous toxicity in a patient with hyperbilirubinemia. South Med J 1996; **89**: 542–5.
7 Raymond E, Cartier S, Canuel C et al. Extravasation de paclitaxel (Taxol). Rev Med Int 1995; **16**: 141–2.
8 Meehan JL, Sporn JR. Case report of Taxol administration via central vein producing a recall reaction at a site of prior Taxol extravasation. J Natl Cancer Inst 1994; **86**: 1250–1.
9 Young PC, Montemarano AD, Lee N et al. Hypersensitivity to paclitaxel manifested as a bullous fixed drug eruption. J Am Acad Dermatol 1996; **34**: 313–4.
10 Läuchli S, Trüeb RM, Fehr M, Hafner J. Scleroderma-like drug reaction to paclitaxel (Taxol®). Br J Dermatol 2002; **147**: 619–21.
11 Kupfer I, Balguerie X, Courville P et al. Scleroderma-like cutaneous lesions induced by paclitaxel: a case study. J Am Acad Dermatol 2003; **48**: 279–81.
12 Essayan DM, Kagey-Sobotka A, Colarusso PJ et al. Successful parenteral desensitization to paclitaxel. J Allergy Clin Immunol 1996; **97**: 42–6.

Triazinate

Acanthosis nigricans-like hyperpigmentation has been recorded [1].

REFERENCE

1 Greenspan AH, Shupack JL, Foo S-H. Acanthosis nigricans-like hyperpigmentation secondary to triazinate therapy. Arch Dermatol 1985; **121**: 232–5.

Topical nitrogen mustard

Urticaria, anaphylactoid reactions and a local bullous reaction have been recorded [1,2]. Contact dermatitis is well recognized.

REFERENCES

1 Daughters D, Zackheim H, Maibach H. Urticaria and anaphylactoid reactions after topical application of mechlorethamine. *Arch Dermatol* 1973; **107**: 429–30.
2 Goday JJ, Aguirre A, Raton JA *et al.* Local bullous reaction to topical mechlorethamine (mustine). *Contact Dermatitis* 1990; **22**: 306–7.

Drugs affecting the immune response

Ciclosporin

Ciclosporin is a ligand for the immunophilin, cyclophilin A, and is thought to block early events in T-cell gene activation by interfering with the intracellular translocation of a substance known as nuclear factor of activated T cells [1,2]. It selectively inhibits antigen-induced activation of, and IL-2 production by, CD4$^+$ helper T lymphocytes, thereby blocking T-cell proliferation [3,4]. It inhibits transcription of genes encoding for IL-2 and IFN-γ [5], and blocks expression of IL-2 receptors. Ciclosporin also inhibits Langerhans' cell antigen-presenting function [6–8] and suppresses ICAM-1 expression by papillary endothelium in inflamed skin, thus reducing T-cell recruitment [9]. Much of the information on side effects was derived from patients who underwent organ transplants, and in diseases such as rheumatoid arthritis [10]. The drug is now used by dermatologists [11–18] especially in the management of difficult psoriasis [13–16], refractory atopic eczema [17] and a number of other conditions [16].

Dermatological complications. Hypertrichosis develops in a high proportion of patients; it affects especially the face and eyebrows, the upper back along the spinal column and the lateral upper arms [18–23]. The hypertrichosis is reversible, and children and adolescents seem to be at greater risk of developing this complication [23]. Other cutaneous complications include gingival hyperplasia [21,24], angio-oedema [25] and hyperplastic pseudofolliculitis barbae [26]. Acne keloidalis is recorded [27]. Anaphylaxis may occur in response to intravenous ciclosporin [11], probably due to the solvent. A mild capillary leak syndrome has resulted in purpuric lesions in the flexures and at pressure points [28], and cutaneous vasculitis is recorded [29].

There have been isolated reports of the development of benign lymphocytic infiltrates in patients with psoriasis or alopecia areata [30,31], of pseudolymphoma after therapy of actinic reticuloid [32] and of an aggressive T-cell lymphoma after ciclosporin therapy for Sézary syndrome [33]. Squamous cell skin cancer may develop [34,35] and could potentially be predisposed to by previous PUVA [36]. A study showed no difference in the incidence of cutaneous malignancy in renal allograft recipients treated with either ciclosporin or azathioprine [34]. Kaposi's sarcoma may occur; a renal transplant patient treated with ciclosporin and methylprednisolone developed a Kaposi's sarcoma, which completely regressed on reducing the dosage of both drugs [37]. There have been isolated reports of development of malignant melanoma in ciclosporin-treated patients, but the incidence of this complication does not seem to be increased above the risk in the general population [38,39].

Systemic side effects. Headache and rarely seizures [40], gastrointestinal and musculoskeletal symptoms are well recognized. There is an increased risk of nephrotoxicity [41,42], which appears to be caused by arteriolar vasoconstriction due to local thromboxane A_2 release [43], and consequent hypertension [44]. Impaired renal function may develop after short- as well as long-term treatment for psoriasis [45]. Both renal dysfunction and hypertension are reversible, and lymphoma development unlikely, in patients on short-term low-dose (less than 5 mg/kg) therapy. Adverse effects on renal function and systolic blood pressure appear greater in psoriasis patients receiving higher doses [15]. Some degree of renal impairment is inevitable with longer term therapy [46]. Rarely, a serious capillary leak syndrome occurs, with marked fluid retention and periorbital oedema, and may be fatal; there may be associated gastrointestinal bleeding, pneumonitis, uraemia and urinary sodium loss followed by hypertension and convulsions [21].

Hepatotoxicity is a complication [47] and hypercholesterolaemia is recorded [48]. Ciclosporin may be associated with myopathy without rhabdomyolysis or with rhabdomyolysis; the latter occurs in the setting of concomitant lovastatin or colchicine therapy [49]. Lymphoma and other cancers have developed on high dosage as used for organ grafting [19,50]. Transplant patients treated with ciclosporin have not been shown to have a higher incidence of neoplasms than those receiving other immunosuppressive agents.

Successful pregnancies have occurred in patients receiving ciclosporin for psoriasis [51,52]. There is no evidence of a teratogenic effect in humans, based on the experience of 107 transplant recipients [53].

Interactions of ciclosporin and other drugs have been reviewed [54]. Ciclosporin blood levels may be increased by concomitant therapy with erythromycin or ketoconazole, as a result of inhibition of the hepatic microsomal cytochrome P-450 enzyme system [55], as well as with danazol, oral contraceptives and calcium channel antagonists. Decreased blood levels may be caused by drugs that induce hepatic enzymes, including phenytoin, phenobar-

bital and tuberculostatic therapy with rifampicin and isoniazid. Aminoglycoside antibiotics, melphalan, amphotericin and trimethoprim (alone or in combination with
sulfamethoxazole) interact with ciclosporin by altering
renal function. Patients should avoid grapefruit juice
taken within 1 h of oral ciclosporin as it contains a psoralen that inhibits the CYP 3A subfamily of cytochrome
P-450 and reduces metabolism of ciclosporin [56].

REFERENCES

1 Gallagher RB, Cambier JC. Signal transmission pathways and lymphocyte function. *Immunol Today* 1990; **11**: 187–9.
2 Anonymous. Unmasking immunosuppression. *Lancet* 1991; **338**: 789.
3 Ryffel B. Pharmacology of cyclosporine. 6. Cellular activation: regulation of intracellular events by cyclosporine. *Pharmacol Rev* 1989; **41**: 407–22.
4 Borel JF. Pharmacology of cyclosporin (Sandimmune). 4. Pharmacological properties *in vivo. Pharmacol Rev* 1989; **41**: 259–371.
5 Granelli-Piperno A. Lymphokine gene expression *in vivo* is inhibited by cyclosporin A. *J Exp Med* 1990; **171**: 533–44.
6 Furue M, Katz SI. The effects of cyclosporin on epidermal cells. I. Cyclosporin inhibits accessory cell functions of epidermal Langerhans cells *in vitro. J Immunol* 1988; **140**: 4139–43.
7 Demidem A, Taylor JR, Grammer SF, Streilein JW. Comparison of effects of transforming growth factor-beta and cyclosporin A on antigen-presenting cells of blood and epidermis. *J Invest Dermatol* 1991; **96**: 401–7.
8 Dupuy P, Bagot M, Michel L *et al.* Cyclosporin A inhibits the antigen-presenting functions of freshly isolated human Langerhans cells *in vitro. J Invest Dermatol* 1991; **96**: 408–13.
9 Petzelbauer P, Stingl G, Wolff K, Volc-Platzer B. Cyclosporin A suppresses ICAM-1 expression by papillary endothelium in healing psoriatic plaques. *J Invest Dermatol* 1991; **96**: 362–9.
10 Dougados M, Awada H, Amor B. Cyclosporin in rheumatoid arthritis: a double blind placebo controlled study in 52 patients. *Ann Rheum Dis* 1988; **47**: 127–33.
11 Gupta AK, Brown MD, Ellis CN *et al.* Cyclosporine in dermatology. *J Am Acad Dermatol* 1989; **21**: 1245–56.
12 Fradin MS, Ellis CN, Voorhees JJ. Management of patients and side effects during cyclosporine therapy for cutaneous disorders. *J Am Acad Dermatol* 1990; **23**: 1265–74.
13 De Rie MA, Meinardi MMHM, Bos JD. Analysis of side-effects of medium- and low-dose cyclosporin maintenance therapy in psoriasis. *Br J Dermatol* 1990; **123**: 347–53.
14 Mihatsch MJ, Wolff K, eds. Risk/benefit ratio of cyclosporin A (Sandimmun®) in psoriasis. *Br J Dermatol* 1990; **122** (Suppl. 36): 1–115.
15 Ellis CN, Fradin MS, Messana JM *et al.* Cyclosporine for plaque-type psoriasis. Results of a multidose, double-blind trial. *N Engl J Med* 1991; **324**: 277–84.
16 Ellis CN, ed. Cyclosporine in dermatology. Proceedings of a symposium. *J Am Acad Dermatol* 1991; **23**: 1231–4.
17 Sowden JM, Berth-Jones J, Ross JS *et al.* Double-blind, controlled, crossover study of cyclosporin in adults with severe refractory atopic dermatitis. *Lancet* 1991; **338**: 137–40.
18 Fradin MS, Ellis CN, Voorhees JJ. Management of patients and side effects during cyclosporine therapy for cutaneous disorders. *J Am Acad Dermatol* 1990; **23**: 1265–75.
19 European Multicentre Trial. Cyclosporin A as sole immunosuppressive agent in recipients of kidney allografts from cadaver donors. Preliminary results. *Lancet* 1982; **ii**: 57–60.
20 Mortimer PS, Thompson JF, Dawber RP *et al.* Hypertrichosis and multiple cutaneous squamous cell carcinomas in association with cyclosporin A therapy. *J R Soc Med* 1983; **76**: 786–7.
21 Harper JI, Kendra JR, Desai S *et al.* Dermatological aspects of the use of cyclosporin A for prophylaxis of graft-versus-host disease. *Br J Dermatol* 1984; **110**: 469–74.
22 Bencini PL, Montagnino G, Sala F *et al.* Cutaneous lesions in 67 cyclosporin-treated renal transplant recipients. *Dermatologica* 1986; **172**: 24–30.
23 Wysocki GP, Daley TD. Hypertrichosis in patients receiving cyclosporine therapy. *Clin Exp Dermatol* 1987; **12**: 191–6.
24 Bennett JA, Christian JM. Cyclosporin-induced gingival hyperplasia: case report and literature review. *J Am Dent Assoc* 1985; **3**: 272–3.
25 Isenberg DA, Snaith ML, Al-Khader AA *et al.* Cyclosporin relieves arthralgia, causes angioedema. *N Engl J Med* 1980; **303**: 754.
26 Lear J, Bourke JF, Burns DA. Hyperplastic pseudofolliculitis barbae associated with cyclosporin. *Br J Dermatol* 1997; **136**: 132–3.
27 Azurdia RM, Graham RM, Weismann K *et al.* Acne keloidalis in Caucasian patients on cyclosporin following organ transplantation. *Br J Dermatol* 2000; **143**: 465–7.
28 Ramon D, Bettloch E, Jimenez A *et al.* Remission of Sézary's syndrome with cyclosporin A. Mild capillary leak syndrome as an unusual side effect. *Acta Derm Venereol (Stockh)* 1986; **66**: 80–2.
29 Gupta MN, Sturrock RD, Gupta G. Cutaneous leucocytoclastic vasculitis caused by cyclosporin A. *Ann Rheum Dis* 2000; **59**: 319.
30 Brown MD, Ellis CN, Billings J *et al.* Rapid occurrence of nodular cutaneous T-lymphocyte infiltrates with cyclosporine therapy. *Arch Dermatol* 1988; **124**: 1097–100.
31 Gupta AK, Cooper KD, Ellis CN *et al.* Lymphocytic infiltrates of the skin in association with cyclosporine therapy. *J Am Acad Dermatol* 1990; **23**: 1137–41.
32 Thestrup-Pedersen K, Zachariae C, Kaltoft K *et al.* Development of cutaneous pseudolymphoma following ciclosporin therapy of actinic reticuloid. *Dermatologica* 1988; **177**: 376–81.
33 Catterall MD, Addis BJ, Smith JL, Coode PE. Sézary syndrome: transformation to a high grade T-cell lymphoma after treatment with cyclosporin A. *Clin Exp Dermatol* 1983; **8**: 159–69.
34 Bunney MH, Benton EC, Barr BB *et al.* The prevalence of skin disorders in renal allograft recipients receiving cyclosporin A compared with those receiving azathioprine. *Nephrol Dial Transplant* 1990; **5**: 379–82.
35 Paul C, Ho VC, McGeown C *et al.* Risk of malignancies in psoriasis patients treated with cyclosporine: a 5 year cohort study. *J Invest Dermatol* 2003; **120**: 211–6.
36 Stern RS. Risk assessment of PUVA and cyclosporine. Lessons from the past: challenges for the future. *Arch Dermatol* 1989; **125**: 545–7.
37 Pilgrim M. Spontane Manifestation und Regression eines Kaposi-Sarkoms unter Cyclosporin A. *Hautarzt* 1988; **39**: 368–70.
38 Mérot Y, Miescher PA, Balsiger F *et al.* Cutaneous malignant melanomas occurring under cyclosporin A therapy: a report of two cases. *Br J Dermatol* 1990; **123**: 237–9.
39 Arellano F, Krupp PF. Cutaneous malignant melanoma occurring after cyclosporin A therapy. *Br J Dermatol* 1991; **124**: 611.
40 Humphreys TR, Leyden JJ. Acute reversible central nervous system toxicity associated with low-dose oral cyclosporin therapy. *J Am Acad Dermatol* 1993; **29**: 490–2.
41 Myers BD, Ross J, Newton L *et al.* Cyclosporine-associated chronic nephropathy. *N Engl J Med* 1984; **311**: 699–705.
42 Myers BD, Sibley R, Newton L *et al.* The long-term course of cyclosporine-associated chronic nephropathy. *Kidney Int* 1988; **33**: 590–600.
43 Coffman TM, Carr DR, Yarger WE, Klotman PE. Evidence that renal prostaglandin and thromboxane production is stimulated in chronic cyclosporine nephrotoxicity. *Transplantation* 1987; **43**: 282–5.
44 Porter GAM, Bennett WM, Sheps SG. Cyclosporine-associated hypertension. *Arch Intern Med* 1990; **150**: 280–3.
45 Powles AV, Carmichael D, Julme B *et al.* Renal function after long-term low-dose cyclosporin for psoriasis. *Br J Dermatol* 1990; **122**: 665–9.
46 Markham T, Watson A, Rogers S. Adverse effects with long-term cyclosporin for severe psoriasis. *Clin Exp Dermatol* 2002; **27**: 111–4.
47 Lorber MI, Van Buren CT, Flechner SM *et al.* Hepatobiliary and pancreatic complications of cyclosporine therapy in 466 renal transplant recipients. *Transplantation* 1987; **43**: 35–40.
48 Ballantyne CM, Podet EJ, Patsch WP *et al.* Effects of cyclosporine therapy on plasma lipoprotein levels. *JAMA* 1989; **262**: 53–6.
49 Arellano F, Krupp P. Muscular disorders associated with cyclosporin. *Lancet* 1991; **337**: 915.
50 Penn I, First MR. Development and incidence of cancer following cyclosporin therapy. *Transplant Proc* 1986; **18** (Suppl. 1): 210–3.
51 Wright S, Glover M, Baker H. Psoriasis, cyclosporine, and pregnancy. *Arch Dermatol* 1991; **127**: 426.
52 Imal N, Tatanabe R, Fujiwara H *et al.* Successful treatment of impetigo herpetiformis with oral cyclosporine during pregnancy. *Arch Dermatol* 2002; **138**: 128–9.
53 Cockburn I, Krupp P, Monka C. Present experience of Sandimmune in pregnancy. *Transplant Proc* 1989; **21**: 3730–2.

54 Yee GC, McGuire TR. Pharmacokinetic drug interactions with cyclosporin (Part I). *Clin Pharmacokinet* 1990; **19**: 319–32.

55 Abel EA. Isotretinoin treatment of severe cystic acne in a heart transplant patient receiving cyclosporine: consideration of drug interactions. *J Am Acad Dermatol* 1991; **24**: 511.

56 Anonymous. Drug interactions with grapefruit. *Curr Probl Pharmacovig* 1997; **23**: 2.

Sirolimus

This macrolide immunosuppressant, which impairs lymphocyte activation by IL-2, IL-4 and IL-12, has caused a capillary leak syndrome [1].

REFERENCE

1 Kaplan MJ, Ellis CN, Bata-Csorgo Z *et al.* Systemic toxicity following administration of sirolimus (formerly rapamycin) for psoriasis. Association of capillary leak syndrome with apoptosis of lesional lymphocyte. *Arch Dermatol* 1999; **135**: 553–7.

PUVA therapy

See Chapter 35.

Immunotherapy

Sera

Animal immune sera can produce any type of early or late hypersensitivity reactions, from urticaria, asthma or fatal anaphylaxis to serum sickness. Clinical manifestations of serum sickness include fever, arthritis, nephritis, neuritis, myocarditis, uveitis, oedema and an urticarial or papular rash. A characteristic serpiginous, erythematous and purpuric eruption developed on the hands and feet, at the borders of palmar and plantar skin, in patients treated with equine antithymocyte globulin [1,2]. Low serum C4 and C3 levels, elevated plasma C3a anaphylatoxin levels, and circulating immune complexes were found. Immunoreactants, including IgM, C3, IgE and IgA, were deposited in the walls of dermal blood vessels on direct immunofluorescence [1,2]. Patients with autoimmune disease may have a particular liability to react to antilymphocyte globulin.

Intravenous immunoglobulin

Angio-oedema-like hypersensitivity eruptions and eczematous, purpuric, petechial/purpuric, lichenoid and vasculitic reactions are recorded [3].

REFERENCES

1 Lawley TJ, Bielory L, Gascon P *et al.* A prospective clinical and immunologic analysis of patients with serum sickness. *N Engl J Med* 1984; **311**: 1407–13.

2 Bielory L, Yancey KB, Young NS *et al.* Cutaneous manifestations of serum sickness in patients receiving antithymocyte globulin. *J Am Acad Dermatol* 1985; **13**: 411–7.

3 Smith KJ, Dutka AL, Skelton HG. Lichenoid/interface cutaneous eruptions to IVIg with the primary infusion may be related to the re-regulation of anti-idiotype network. *J Cutan Med Surg* 1998; **3**: 96–101.

Vaccines

Overall the incidence of significant side effects is very low. Egg, gelatin, antibiotics and preservatives in vaccines may cause reactions [1]. Needle gauge and length may affect the incidence of local reactions [2]. In Canada during 1990, from more than 12 million doses of vaccines there were 2832 reports of adverse events associated with immunizing agents received by the Childhood Immunization Division of the Laboratory Centre for Disease Control [3]. Only 39 of 43 618 Alaskan natives who received 101 360 doses of hepatitis B plasma-derived vaccine developed side effects, including myalgia/arthralgia lasting longer than 3 days, rashes (eight patients) and dizziness [4]. Influenza vaccination in the elderly is, however, reported to cause no more systemic side effects than placebo [5]. In contrast, another study found local reactions in 17.5% of patients, including swelling, itching and pain [6]. Leukocytoclastic vasculitis has been reported with influenza vaccination [7]. Measles and measles–mumps–rubella vaccine, hepatitis B vaccine, and diphtheria and tetanus toxoids have been statistically associated with anaphylaxis [8], and measles–mumps–rubella vaccine with thrombocytopenia and purpura [8,9] and Gianotti–Crosti syndrome [10]. A variety of reactions have been documented following hepatitis B vaccination [11], including urticaria/angio-oedema [12], erythema multiforme [13], erythema nodosum [14], polyarteritis nodosa and pityriasis rosea [15], and lichenoid eruptions [16,17].

Local reactions include erythema, swelling and tenderness, which may result from an Arthus reaction [18–20]. Keloid scarring may develop. Local inflammatory reactions, fever, lymphadenopathy, urticaria and lichenoid rashes have been observed following vaccination in patients sensitive to the preservative merthiolate; patch testing and intradermal testing may be positive [21,22]. Inflammatory nodular reactions may occur as a result of aluminium sensitization, as with hepatitis B, diphtheria and tetanus vaccination [23,24]; patch testing to aluminium may be positive [23]. Itching, eczema and circumscribed hypertrichosis developed over nodules following immunization with vaccines adsorbed on aluminium hydroxide in three children [24]. Transient subcutaneous nodule formation at the injection site, and increased regional adenopathy, have been rarely noted in patients with HIV infection treated with gpl60 vaccination [25].

Urticaria, angio-oedema or anaphylaxis may occur in patients allergic to egg protein who are vaccinated with live measles vaccine. However, in a series of children with egg allergy and a positive skin-prick test to egg white, 0.98% developed a mild reaction not requiring therapy following immunization with a full dose of vaccine [26]. Of 98 patients with a history of previous inoculations with human diploid cell rabies vaccine, 3% developed generalized urticaria or wheezing within 1 day, and a further 3% developed urticaria 6–14 days, after booster vaccination [27]. Urticaria and systemic symptoms including malaise and fever, or Stevens–Johnson syndrome may follow tetanus toxoid vaccination [28,29]. Vaccination may result in development of an autoimmune state; dermatomyositis has been provoked. Fatalities have rarely occurred following vaccination as a result of anaphylaxis [30,31]. Vaccination against Japanese encephalitis caused serious adverse reactions, including urticaria, angio-oedema, hypotension and collapse [32]. An association with vaccination for influenza and with tetanus toxoid and induction of bullous pemphigoid has been noted rarely [33–35].

REFERENCES

1 Georgitis JW, Fasano MB. Allergenic components of vaccines and avoidance of vaccination-related adverse events. *Curr Allergy Rep* 2001; **1**: 11–7.
2 Watson M. Needle length and incidence of local reactions to immunization. Needle gauge is more important than needle length. *BMJ* 2001; **322**: 492.
3 Duclos P, Pless R, Koch J, Hardy M. Adverse events temporally associated with immunizing agents. *Can Fam Physician* 1993; **39**: 1907–13.
4 McMahon BJ, Helminiak C, Wainwright RB *et al.* Frequency of adverse reactions to hepatitis B vaccine in 43,618 persons. *Am J Med* 1992; **92**: 254–6.
5 Margolis KL, Nichol KL, Poland GA, Pluhar RE. Frequency of adverse reactions to influenza vaccine in the elderly. A randomized, placebo-controlled trial. *JAMA* 1990; **264**: 1139–41.
6 Govaert TME, Dinant GJ, Aretz K *et al.* Adverse reactions to influenza vaccine in elderly people: randomised double blind placebo controlled trial. *BMJ* 1993; **307**: 988–90.
7 Tavadia S, Drummond A, Evans CD, Wainwright NJ. Leucocytoclastic vasculitis and influenza vaccination. *Clin Exp Dermatol* 2003; **28**: 154–6.
8 Stratton KR, Howe CJ, Johnson RB Jr. Adverse events associated with childhood vaccines other than pertussis and rubella. Summary of a report from the Institute of Medicine. *JAMA* 1994; **271**: 1602–5.
9 Farrington P, Pugh S, Colville A *et al.* A new method for active surveillance of adverse events from diphtheria/tetanus/pertussis and measles/mumps/rubella vaccines. *Lancet* 1995; **345**: 567–9.
10 Velangi SS, Tidman MJ. Gianotti–Crosti syndrome after measles, mumps and rubella vaccination. *Br J Dermatol* 1998; **139**: 1122–3.
11 Drago F, Rebora A. Cutaneous immunologic reactions to hepatitis B virus vaccine. *Ann Intern Med* 2002; **136**: 780.
12 Barbaud A, Trechot P, Reichert-Pénétrat S *et al.* Allergic mechanisms and urticaria/angioedema after hepatitis B immunization. *Br J Dermatol* 1998; **139**: 925–6.
13 Loche F, Schwarze HP, Thedenat B *et al.* Erythema multiforme associated with hepatitis B immunization. *Clin Exp Dermatol* 2002; **25**: 167–8.
14 Rogerson S, Nye F. Hepatitis B vaccine associated with erythema nodosum and polyarthritis. *BMJ* 1990; **301**: 345.
15 De Heyser F, Naeyaert JM, Hindryckz P *et al.* Immune-mediated pathology following hepatitis B vaccination. Two cases of polyarteritis nodosa and one case of pityriasis-rosea-like drug eruption. *Clin Exp Rheumatol* 2000; **18**: 81–5.
16 Saywell CA, Wittal RA, Kossard S. Lichenoid reaction to hepatitis B vaccination. *Australas J Dermatol* 1997; **38**: 152–4.
17 Ferrando MF, Doutre MS, Beylot-Barry M *et al.* Lichen planus following hepatitis B vaccination. *Br J Dermatol* 1998; **139**: 350.
18 Jacobs RL, Lowe RS, Lanier BQ. Adverse reactions to tetanus toxoid. *JAMA* 1982; **247**: 40–2.
19 Sutter RW. Adverse reactions to tetanus toxoid. *JAMA* 1994; **271**: 1629.
20 Marrinan LM, Andrews G, Alsop-Shields L, Dugdale AE. Side effects of rubella immunisation in teenage girls. *Med J Aust* 1990; **153**: 631–2.
21 Noel I, Galloway A, Ive FA. Hypersensitivity to thiomersal in hepatitis B vaccine. *Lancet* 1991; **338**: 705.
22 Rueff F. Nebenwirkungen durch Thiomersal und Huhnereiweiss bei Impfungen. *Hautarzt* 1994; **45**: 879–81.
23 Cosnes A, Flechet M-L, Revuz J. Inflammatory nodular reactions after hepatitis B vaccination due to aluminium sensitization. *Contact Dermatitis* 1990; **23**: 65–7.
24 Pembroke AC, Marten RH. Unusual cutaneous reactions following diphtheria and tetanus immunization. *Clin Exp Dermatol* 1979; **4**: 345–8.
25 Redfield RR, Birx DL, Ketter N *et al.* A phase I evaluation of the safety and immunogenicity of vaccination with recombinant gp160 in patients with early human immunodeficiency virus infection. *N Engl J Med* 1991; **324**: 1677–84.
26 Aickin R, Hill D, Kemp A. Measles immunisation in children with allergy to egg. *BMJ* 1994; **309**: 223–5.
27 Fishbein DB, Yenne KM, Dreesen DW *et al.* Risk factors for systemic hypersensitivity reactions after booster vaccinations with human diploid cell rabies vaccine: a nationwide prospective study. *Vaccine* 1993; **11**: 1390–4.
28 Kuhlwein A, Bleyl A. Tetanusantitoxintiter und Reaktionen nach Tetanusimpfungen. *Hautarzt* 1985; **36**: 462–4.
29 Weisse ME, Bass JW. Tetanus toxoid allergy. *JAMA* 1990; **264**: 2448.
30 Boston Collaborative Drug Surveillance Program. Drug-induced anaphylaxis. A cooperative study. *JAMA* 1973; **224**: 613–5.
31 Lockey RF, Benedict LM, Turkeltaub PC, Bukantz SC. Fatalities from immunotherapy (IT) and skin testing (ST). *J Allergy Clin Immunol* 1987; **79**: 660–77.
32 Ruff TA, Eisen D, Fuller A, Kass R. Adverse reactions to Japanese encephalitis vaccine. *Lancet* 1991; **338**: 881–2.
33 Bodokh I, Lacour JP, Bourdet JF *et al.* Réactivation de pemphigoïde bulleuse apres vaccination antigrippale. *Thérapie* 1994; **49**: 154.
34 Venning VA, Wojnarowska F. Induced bullous pemphigoid. *Br J Dermatol* 1995; **132**: 831–2.
35 Fournier B, Descamps V, Bouscarat F *et al.* Bullous pemphigoid induced by vaccination. *Br J Dermatol* 1996; **135**: 153–4.

Hyposensitization immunotherapy

Hyposensitization immunotherapy is a standard treatment for recalcitrant hay fever and bee or wasp stings in many countries in the world, including the USA, Scandinavia and the continent of Europe [1]. However, in the UK, allergen-injection immunotherapy for IgE-mediated diseases has been largely discontinued, following the recommendations of the Committee on Safety of Medicines in 1986 [2], because of concern about deaths related to bronchospasm and anaphylaxis. The Committee recommended that immunotherapy be given only where full facilities for cardiopulmonary resuscitation are available and that patients be kept under medical observation for at least 2 h. The necessity for the latter recommendation has been questioned, as serious reactions occur within minutes [1]. The British Society for Allergy and Clinical Immunology Working Party concluded that specific allergen immunotherapy for summer hay fever uncontrolled by conventional medication and for wasp and bee venom hypersensitivity has an acceptable risk/benefit ratio, provided that treatment is given by experienced practitioners in a clinic where full resuscitative facilities are immediately available; a symptom-free observation period of 60 min after injection is sufficient [3,4]. Patients with asthma should be excluded, however, in view of an increased frequency of reactions [4,5]. Fatalities from allergen immunotherapy are extremely rare [6]. In one series, β-blocker drugs did not increase the frequency of systemic reactions in patients receiving allergen immunotherapy, but patients developed more severe systemic reactions that were more refractory to therapy [7].

In contrast, local urticarial reactions are common [1]. Desensitization injections for hay fever have resulted in occasional tender nodules lasting for several months or years [8,9]; these are thought to develop as a result of allergy to aluminium, as it is present in the lesions and patch tests may be positive [9,10]. Inflammatory nodules at injection sites, first developing several years later, have also been described [11]. Injections of mixtures of grass pollens, cereal pollens and dust-mite allergens have resulted in multiple cutaneous B-cell pseudolymphomas [12]. Polyarteritis nodosa [13], vasculitis [14,15] and serum sickness [16,17] have been described following hyposensitization therapy for allergy to pollen, house-dust mite and wasp venom. Cold urticaria developed during the course of hyposensitization to wasp venom [18].

REFERENCES

1 Varney VA, Gaga M, Frew AJ et al. Usefulness of immunotherapy in patients with severe summer hay fever uncontrolled by antiallergic drugs. *BMJ* 1991; **302**: 265–9.
2 Anonymous. CSM update. Desensitising vaccines. *BMJ* 1986; **293**: 948.
3 Anonymous. Position paper on allergen immunotherapy. Report a BSACI working party, January–October 1992. *Clin Exp Allergy* 1993; **23** (Suppl. 3): 1–44.
4 British Society for Allergy and Clinical Immunology Working Party. Injection immunotherapy. *BMJ* 1993; **307**: 919–23.
5 Bousquet J, Michel FB. Safety considerations in assessing the role of immunotherapy in allergic disorders. *Drug Saf* 1994; **10**: 5–17.
6 Lockey RF, Benedict LM, Turkeltaub PC, Bukantz SC. Fatalities from immunotherapy and skin testing. *J Allergy Clin Immunol* 1987; **79**: 660–77.
7 Hepner MJ, Ownby DR, Anderson JA et al. Risk of systemic reactions in patients taking beta-blocker drugs receiving allergen immunotherapy injections. *J Allergy Clin Immunol* 1990; **86**: 407–11.
8 Osterballe O. Side effects during immunotherapy with purified grass pollen extracts. *Allergy* 1982; **37**: 553–62.
9 Frost L, Johansen S, Pedersen S et al. Persistent subcutaneous nodules in children hyposensitised with aluminium-containing allergen extracts. *Allergy* 1985; **40**: 368–72.
10 Nagore E, Martinez-Escribano JA, Tato A et al. Subcutaneous nodules following treatment with aluminium-containing allergen extracts. *Eur J Dermatol* 2001; **11**: 138–40.
11 Jones SK, Lovell CR, Peachey RDG. Delayed onset of inflammatory nodules following hay fever desensitization injections. *Clin Exp Dermatol* 1988; **13**: 376–8.
12 Goerdt S, Spieker T, Wölffer L-U et al. Multiple cutaneous B-cell pseudolymphomas after allergen injections. *J Am Acad Dermatol* 1996; **35**: 1072–4.
13 Phanuphak P, Kohler PF. Onset of polyarteritis nodosa during allergic hyposensitization treatment. *Am J Med* 1980; **68**: 479–85.
14 Merk H, Kober ML. Vasculitis nach spezifischer Hyposensibilisierung. *Z Hautkr* 1982; **57**: 1682–5.
15 Berbis P, Carena MC, Auffranc JC, Privat Y. Vascularite nécrosante cutanéo-systémique survenue en cours de désensibilisation. *Ann Dermatol Vénéréol* 1986; **113**: 805–9.
16 Umetsu DT, Hahn JS, Perez-Atayde AR, Geha RS. Serum sickness triggered by anaphylaxis: a complication of immunotherapy. *J Allergy Clin Immunol* 1985; **76**: 713–6.
17 De Bandt M, Atassi-Dumont M, Kahn MF, Herman D. Serum sickness after wasp venom immunotherapy: clinical and biological study. *J Rheumatol* 1997; **24**: 1195–7.
18 Anfosso-Capra F, Philip-Joet F, Reynaud-Gaubert M, Arnaud A. Occurrence of cold urticaria during venom desensitization. *Dermatologica* 1990; **181**: 276–7.

BCG vaccination

Vaccination with BCG causes a benign self-limiting lesion consisting of a small papule, pustule or ulcer, which heals to leave a small scar within weeks. Axillary lymphadenitis and abscesses occurred after vaccination of rural Haitian children [1], and disseminated BCG infection in children born to HIV-1-infected women [2]. Occasionally, local abscess formation may follow vaccination of strongly tuberculin-positive individuals, administration of too much vaccine, or injection of vaccine too deeply [3–5]. BCG abscesses may also rarely arise following needle-stick injury in health-care professionals [6]. In Austria, where the Ministry of Health's recommendation is for all neonates to be vaccinated, the normal complication rate is 0.3–0.6%, with suppurative lymphadenitis, generalized lymphadenopathy and osteitis [7]. Following a change to a more virulent vaccine strain, this rate temporarily increased substantially, with 5% of 659 children vaccinated at the University Hospital, Innsbruck requiring surgical excision of suppurating lymph nodes [7]. Anaphylactoid reactions to BCG vaccine, probably as a result of immune complex reactions mediated by antibodies to dextran in the vaccine, have been reported [8]. A papulonecrotic type of vasculitis has been documented [9]. Dermatomyositis may occasionally be a complication [10].

BCG immunotherapy for malignant melanoma [11] has been associated with local ulceration [11,12], local recurrent erysipelas, keloid formation, influenza-like symptoms, lymphadenopathy, urticaria and angio-oedema, granulomatous hepatitis, arthritis [13] and reactivation of pulmonary tuberculosis. Widespread miliary granulomas were present in a patient with fatal disseminated infection following intralesional immunotherapy of cutaneous malignant melanoma [14].

REFERENCES

1 Bonnlander H, Rossignol AM. Complications of BCG vaccinations in rural Haiti. *Am J Public Health* 1993; **83**: 583–5.
2 O'Brien KL, Andrae JR, Marie AL et al. Bacillus Calmette–Guérin complications in children born to HIV-1-infected women with a review of literature. *Pediatrics* 1995; **95**: 414–7.
3 Lotte A, Wasz-Hockert O, Poisson N et al. BCG complications. *Adv Tuberculosis Res* 1984; **21**: 107–93, 194–245.
4 de Souza GRM, Sant'anna CC, Lapa e Silva JR et al. Intradermal BCG complications: analysis of 51 cases. *Tubercle* 1983; **64**: 23–7.
5 Puliyel JM, Hughes A, Chiswick ML, Mughal MZ. Adverse local reactions from accidental BCG overdose in infants. *BMJ* 1996; **313**: 528–9.
6 Warren JP, Nairn DS, Robertson MH. Cold abscess after accidental BCG inoculation. *Lancet* 1984; **ii**: 289.
7 Hengster P, Fille M, Menardi G. Suppurative lymphadenitis in newborn babies after change of BCG vaccine. *Lancet* 1991; **337**: 1168–9.
8 Rudin C, Amacher A, Berglund A. Anaphylactoid reactions to BCG vaccination. *Lancet* 1991; **337**: 377.
9 Lübbe D. Vasculitis allergica vom papulonekrotischen Typ nach BCG-Impfung. *Dermatol Monatsschr* 1982; **168**: 186–92.
10 Kass E, Staume S, Mellbye OJ et al. Dermatomyositis associated with BCG vaccination. *Scand J Rheumatol* 1979; **8**: 187–91.

11 Schult C. Nebenwirkungen der BCG-Immuntherapie bei 511 Patienten mit malignen Melanom. *Hautarzt* 1984; **35**: 78–83.
12 Korting HC, Strasser S, Konz B. Multiple BCG-Ulzera nach subkutaner Impfstoffapplikation im Rahmen der Immunochemotherapie des malignen Melanoms. *Hautarzt* 1988; **39**: 170–3.
13 Torisu M, Miyahara T, Shinohara A *et al.* A new side effect of BCG immunotherapy: BCG-induced arthritis in man. *Cancer Immunol Immunother* 1978; **5**: 77–83.
14 de la Monte SM, Hutchins GM. Fatal disseminated bacillus Calmette–Guérin infection and arrested growth of cutaneous malignant melanoma following intralesional immunotherapy. *Am J Dermatopathol* 1986; **8**: 331–5.

Cytokines

Cytokines are being increasingly used in the management of neoplastic and haematological disorders and AIDS, and in addition are starting to be used for the therapy of specific dermatological disorders; side effects have been reviewed [1]. Reactions range from minor injection-site reactions, pruritus and flushing to life-threatening autoimmune disorders, severe erythroderma or bullous skin reactions [2].

REFERENCES

1 Luger TA, Schwarz T. Therapeutic use of cytokines in dermatology. *J Am Acad Dermatol* 1991; **24**: 915–26.
2 Asnis LA, Gaspari AA. Cutaneous reactions to recombinant cytokine therapy. *J Am Acad Dermatol* 1995; **33**: 393–410.

Colony-stimulating factors

Recombinant haematopoietic colony-stimulating factors used in the treatment of haematological disorders are usually well tolerated, but may induce itching and erythema or lichenoid reactions [1] at the site of injection, thrombophlebitis with intravenous infusion, facial flushing and a transient maculopapular eruption, fever, chills, myalgias, arthralgia and bone pain, transient leukopenia, decreased appetite, nausea and mild elevation of transaminase levels [2]. Neutrophilic dermatoses have been recorded in children [3]. Two types of recombinant human granulocyte colony-stimulating factor are in use for neutropenia: one is a glycosylated natural product from mammalian cells, and the other a non-glycosylated form from *Escherichia coli*. A drug eruption may occur with either type without detectable antibodies; intradermal tests may be useful and there may not be cross-reactivity [4]. Both local reactions at the site of injection and diffuse maculopapular eruptions may be seen [4–7]. Local pustular reactions [8] or subcorneal pustular dermatosis [9] are documented. Intravenous recombinant granulocyte–macrophage colony-stimulating factor (GM-CSF) therapy for leukaemia resulted in a widespread confluent maculopapular eruption in three patients, associated with a dermal lymphocyte, macrophage and granulocyte infiltration, exocytosis, and keratinocyte ICAM-1 expression [10]. Of 23 patients with advanced malignancy

treated with GM-CSF, nine had a cutaneous eruption characterized by local erythema and pruritus at the injection site, recall erythema at previous injection sites or a generalized maculopapular rash [11]. Other studies have reported widespread rashes [12,13], in one series manifested as annular erythematous papules and plaques on the extremities, becoming generalized and clearing with fine desquamation [13]. Recurrent exacerbation of acne [14], widespread folliculitis [15], toxic folliculitis [16] and a Sweet's syndrome-like rash [17–19] have been recorded. A capillary leak syndrome with pleural and pericardial effusions, ascites and large-vessel thrombosis has been noted only with high-dose GM-CSF therapy [20]. Necrotizing vasculitis developed at GM-CSF injection sites in one patient with white cell aplasia, but not in over 150 other neutropenic patients who received the drug [21]. However, vasculitis was reported in a large series [22]. Thrombotic and necrotizing panniculitis has been documented [23]. Psoriasis [24], and arthritis in Felty's syndrome with rheumatoid arthritis [25], have been reported to deteriorate.

REFERENCES

1 Viallard AM, Lavenue A, Balme B *et al.* Lichenoid cutaneous drug reaction at injection sites of granulocyte colony-stimulating factor (Filgrastim). *Dermatology* 1999; **198**: 301–3.
2 Wakefield PE, James WD, Samlaska CP, Meltzer MS. Colony-stimulating factors. *J Am Acad Dermatol* 1990; **23**: 903–12.
3 Prendiville J, Thiessen P, Mallory SB. Neutrophilic dermatoses in two children with idiopathic neutropenia: association with granulocyte colony-stimulating factor (G-CSF) therapy. *Pediatr Dermatol* 2001; **18**: 417–21.
4 Sasaki O, Yokoyama A, Uemura S *et al.* Drug eruption caused by recombinant human G-CSF. *Intern Med* 1994; **33**: 641–3.
5 Schiro JA, Kupper TS. Cutaneous eruptions during GM-CSF infusion. Clues for cytokine biology. *Arch Dermatol* 1991; **127**: 110–2.
6 Samlaska CP, Noyes DK. Localized cutaneous reactions to granulocyte colony-stimulating factor. *Arch Dermatol* 1993; **129**: 645–6.
7 Scott GA. Report of three cases of cutaneous reactions to granulocyte–macrophage colony-stimulating factor and a review of the literature. *Am J Dermatopathol* 1995; **17**: 107–14.
8 Passweg J, Buser U, Tichelli A *et al.* Pustular eruption at the site of subcutaneous injection of recombinant human granulocyte–macrophage colony-stimulating factor. *Ann Hematol* 1991; **63**: 326–7.
9 Lautenschlager S, Itin PH, Hirsbrunner P, Büchner SA. Subcorneal pustular dermatosis at the injection site of recombinant human granulocyte–macrophage colony-stimulating fator in a patient with IgA myeloma. *J Am Acad Dermatol* 1994; **30**: 783–9.
10 Horn TD, Burke PJ, Karp JE, Hood AF. Intravenous administration of recombinant human granulocyte–macrophage colony-stimulating factor causes a cutaneous eruption. *Arch Dermatol* 1991; **127**: 49–52.
11 Lieschke GJ, Maher D, Cebon J *et al.* Effects of bacterially synthesized recombinant human granulocyte–macrophage colony-stimulating factor in patients with advanced malignancy. *Ann Intern Med* 1989; **110**: 357–64.
12 Yamashita N, Natsuaki M, Morita H *et al.* Cutaneous eruptions induced by granulocyte colony-stimulating factor in two cases of acute myelogenous leukemia. *J Dermatol* 1993; **20**: 473–7.
13 Glass LF, Fotopoulos T, Messina JL. A generalized cutaneous reaction induced by granulocyte colony-stimulating factor. *J Am Acad Dermatol* 1996; **34**: 455–9.
14 Lee PK, Dover JS. Recurrent exacerbation of acne by granulocyte colony-stimulating factor administration. *J Am Acad Dermatol* 1996; **34**: 855–6.
15 Ostlere LS, Harris D, Prentice HG, Rustin MH. Widespread folliculitis induced by human granulocyte-colony-stimulating factor therapy. *Br J Dermatol* 1992; **127**: 193–4.

16 Paul C, Giachetti S, Pinquier L *et al*. Cutaneous effects of granuloycte colony-stimulating factor in healthy volunteers. *Arch Dermatol* 1998; **134**: 111–2.

17 Karp DL. The Sweet syndrome or G-CSF reaction? *Ann Intern Med* 1992; **117**: 875–6.

18 Richard MA, Grob JJ, Laurans R *et al*. Sweet's syndrome induced by granulocyte colony-stimulating factor in a woman with congenital neutropenia. *J Am Acad Dermatol* 1996; **35**: 629–31.

19 Prevost-Blank PL, Shwayder AT. Sweet's syndrome secondary to granulocyte colony-stimulating factor. *J Am Acad Dermatol* 1996; **35**: 995–7.

20 Antman KS, Griffin JD, Elias A *et al*. Effect of recombinant human granulocyte–macrophage colony-stimulating factor on chemotherapy-induced myelosuppression. *N Engl J Med* 1988; **319**: 593–8.

21 Farmer KL, Kurzrock R, Duvic M. Necrotizing vasculitis at granulocyte–macrophage-colony-stimulating factor injection sites. *Arch Dermatol* 1990; **126**: 1243–4.

22 Jain KK. Cutaneous vasculitis associated with granulocyte colony-stimulating factor. *J Am Acad Dermatol* 1994; **31**: 213–5.

23 Dereure O, Bessis D, Lavabre-Bertrand T *et al*. Thrombotic and necrotizing panniculitis associated with recombinant human granulocyte colony-stimulating factor treatment. *Br J Dermatol* 2000; **142**: 834–6.

24 Kelly RI, Marsden RA. Granulocyte–macrophage colony-stimulating factor and psoriasis. *J Am Acad Dermatol* 1994; **30**: 144.

25 McMullin MF, Finch MB. Felty's syndrome treated with rhG-CSF associated with flare of arthritis and skin rash. *Clin Rheumatol* 1995; **14**: 204–8.

Interferon

Cutaneous reactions to recombinant IFN [1–12] given to patients with chronic hepatitis C, cancer or AIDS are frequent (5–10%) but usually of moderate degree. No adverse cutaneous side effects resulted from intralesional injection of IFN-γ in 10 patients treated for keloid scarring [13]. Most patients experience influenza-like symptoms following systemic therapy; reversible leukopenia and thrombocytopenia are recorded with higher dosage. Local reactions consist of erythema, eczema, epilation, or induration at injection sites or urticaria. More serious reactions include vesiculobullous reactions, vasculitis, necrosis, ulceration, alopecia and exacerbation of psoriasis. Skin ulceration or necrosis may be a serious problem with both IFN-α and IFN-β [7–12]. Raynaud's phenomenon and digital necrosis induced by IFN-α is recorded [14].

Of 63 patients treated with IFN-γ for prophylaxis of infection in chronic granulomatous disease, one had a severe cutaneous reaction (unspecified), and rashes or injection-site erythema or tenderness occurred in 17% and 14% of cases respectively [1]. Diffuse inflammatory lesions have occurred with IFN-α and ribavirin therapy for hepatitis C [15]. Transient, localized or disseminated oedematous, erythematous and/or papular changes, vesicles or petechiae were seen in six patients during intravenous IFN-α for chronic active hepatitis C, 5–14 days after starting therapy [2]. Eruptions disappeared in 10–14 days despite continuation of IFN-α; histology revealed upper dermal perivascular CD4+ lymphoid infiltration and oedema, with endothelial cell but not keratinocyte ICAM-1 and E-selectin expression, suggesting a non-allergic mechanism.

Capillaritis is recorded with IFN-α [16], as is lichen planus [3,17]. Reactivation of oral herpes simplex and enhanced radiation toxicity have been recorded. IFN-α-2a for the treatment of cutaneous T-cell lymphoma has induced temporary alopecia [18]. In contrast, IFN-α therapy has caused increased eyelash and eyebrow growth [19], as well as straight hair [20]. Severe urticaria has been documented with IFN-α-1a [21] and mucinoses with IFN-α-1b [22]. Both IFN-α and IFN-α-1b have been associated with granulomatous or sarcoidal reactions [23–25]. IFN-α has caused hypertriglyceridaemia [26] and IFN-β has been related to squamous cell cancer following ulceration [27].

IFN-α used in the treatment of disseminated carcinoma [28,29] or intralesionally for viral warts [30], and IFN-β therapy for multiple sclerosis [11,31], have been reported to exacerbate or trigger onset of psoriasis; psoriatic arthritis has also been triggered by IFN-α [32] and IFN-γ [33], and Reiter's syndrome by IFN-α [34]. Psoriasis appeared at the site of subcutaneous injection of recombinant IFN-γ in patients with psoriatic arthritis [35], and at the site of intralesional injection in a patient receiving recombinant IFN-β for a basal cell carcinoma [36]. Exacerbation of underlying autoimmune disease is documented with IFN-α [37]. Neutralizing antibodies to recombinant IFN-α may be produced [38]. Systemic sclerosis has been associated with IFN-α [39]. Systemic LE has been recorded following IFN therapy of myelogenous leukaemia [40], and pemphigus vulgaris after IFN-β and IL-2 therapy for lymphoma [41].

REFERENCES

1 International Chronic Granulomatous Disease Cooperative Study Group. A controlled trial of interferon gamma to prevent infection in chronic granulomatous disease. *N Engl J Med* 1991; **324**: 509–16.

2 Toyofuku K, Imayama S, Yasumoto S *et al*. Clinical and immunohistochemical studies of skin eruptions: relationship to administration of interferon-alpha. *J Dermatol* 1994; **21**: 732–7.

3 Papini M, Bruni PL. Cutaneous reactions to recombinant cytokine therapy. *J Am Acad Dermatol* 1996; **35**: 1021.

4 Elgart GW, Sheremata W, Ahn YS. Cutaneous reactions to recombinant human interferon beta-1b: the clinical and histologic spectrum. *J Am Acad Dermatol* 1997; **37**: 553–8.

5 Paquet P, Pierard-Franchimont C, Arrese JE, Pierard GE. Cutaneous side effects of interferons. *Rev Med Liege* 2001; **56**: 699–702.

6 Manjon-Haces JA, Vazquez-Lopez F, Gomez-Diez S *et al*. Adverse cutaneous reactions to interferon alfa-2b plus ribavirin therapy in patients with chronic hepatitis C virus. *Acta Derm Venereol (Stockh)* 2001; **81**: 223.

7 Charron A, Bessis D, Dereure O *et al*. Local cutaneous side effects of interferons. *Presse Med* 2001; **30**: 1555–60.

8 Garcia-F-Villalta M, Dauden E, Sanchez J *et al*. Local reactions associated with subcutaneous injections of both beta-interferon 1a and 1b. *Acta Derm Venereol (Stockh)* 2001; **81**: 152.

9 Weinberg JM. Cutaneous necrosis associated with recombinant interferon injection. *J Am Acad Dermatol* 1998; **39**: 807.

10 Sheremata WA, Taylor JR, Elgart GW. Severe necrotizing cutaneous lesions complicating treatment with interferon beta-1b. *N Engl J Med* 1995; **332**: 1584.

11 Webster GF, Knobler RL, Lublin FD *et al*. Cutaneous ulcerations and pustular psoriasis flare caused by recombinant interferon beta injections in patients with multiple sclerosis. *J Am Acad Dermatol* 1996; **34**: 365–7.

12 Levesque H, Cailleux N, Moore N *et al*. Autoimmune phenomena associated with cutaneous aseptic necrosis during interferon-alpha treatment for chronic myelogenous leukaemia. *Br J Rheumatol* 1995; **34**: 582–3.

13 Granstein RD, Rook A, Flotte RJ et al. A controlled trial of intralesional recombinant interferon-γ in the treatment of keloidal scarring. Arch Dermatol 1990; **126**: 1295–302.

14 Bachmeyer C, Farge D, Gluckman E et al. Raynaud's phenomenon and digital necrosis induced by interferon-alpha. Br J Dermatol 1996; **135**: 481–3.

15 Dereure O, Faison-Peyron N, Larrey D et al. Diffuse inflammatory lesions in patients treated with interferon alfa and ribavirin for hepatitis C: a series of 20 patients. Br J Dermatol 2003; **147**: 1142–6.

16 Gupta G, Holmes SC, Spence E, Mills PR. Capillaritis associated with interferon-alfa treatment of chronic hepatitis C infection. J Am Acad Dermatol 2000; **43**: 937–8.

17 Schlesinger TE, Camisa C, Gay D, Bergfeld WF. Oral erosive lichen planus with epidermolytic hyperkeratosis during interferon alfa-2b therapy for chronic hepatitis C virus infection. J Am Acad Dermatol 1997; **36**: 1023–5.

18 Olsen EA, Rosen ST, Vollmer RT et al. Inteferon alfa-2a in the treatment of cutaneous T cell lymphoma. J Am Acad Dermatol 1989; **20**: 395–407.

19 Foon KA, Dougher G. Increased growth of eyelashes in a patient given leukocyte A interferon. N Engl J Med 1984; **311**: 1259.

20 Bessis D, Luong MS, Blanc P et al. Straight hair associated with inteferon-alfa plus ribavirin in hepatitis C infection. Br J Dermatol 2002; **147**: 392–3.

21 Mazzeo L, Ricciardi L, Fazio MC et al. Severe urticaria due to recombinant intereferon beta-1a. Br J Dermatol 2003; **148**: 172–3.

22 Benito-Leon J, Borbujo J, Cortes L. Cutaneous mucinoses complicating interferon beta-1b therapy. Eur Neurol 2002; **47**: 123–4.

23 Sanders S, Busam K, Tahan SR et al. Granulomatous and suppurative dermatitis at inteferon alfa injection sites: report of 2 cases. J Am Acad Dermatol 2002; **46**: 611–6.

24 Cogrel O, Doutre MS, Marliere V et al. Cutaneous sarcoidosis during interferon alfa and ribavirin treatment of hepatitis C virus infection: two cases. Br J Dermatol 2002; **146**: 320–4.

25 Mehta CL, Tyler RJ, Cripps DJ. Granulomatous dermatitis with focal sarcoidal features associated with recombinant interferon β-1b injections. J Am Acad Dermatol 1998; **39**: 1024–8.

26 Junghans V, Rünger TM. Hypertriglyceridaemia following adjuvant inteferon-α treatment in two patients with malignant melanoma. Br J Dermatol 1999; **140**: 183–4.

27 Fruland JE, Sandermann S, Snow SN et al. Skin necrosis with subsequent formation of squamous cell carcinoma after subcutaneous interferon beta injection. J Am Acad Dermatol 1997; **37**: 488–9.

28 Quesada JR, Gutterman JU. Psoriasis and alpha-interferon. Lancet 1986; i: 1466–8.

29 Hartmann F, von Wussow P, Deicher H. Psoriasis: exacerbation bei therapie mit alpha-Interferon. Dtsch Med Wochenschr 1989; **114**: 96–8.

30 Shiohara T, Kobayashi M, Abe K, Nagashima M. Psoriasis occurring predominantly on warts. Possible involvement of interferon alpha. Arch Dermatol 1988; **124**: 1816–21.

31 Kowalzick L. Psoriasis flare caused by recombinant interferon beta injections. J Am Acad Dermatol 1997; **36**: 501.

32 Jucgla A, Marcoval J, Curco N, Servitje O. Psoriasis with articular involvement induced by interferon alfa. Arch Dermatol 1991; **127**: 910–1.

33 O'Connell PG, Gerber LH, Digiovanna JJ, Peck GL. Arthritis in patients with psoriasis treated with gamma-interferon. J Rheumatol 1992; **19**: 80–2.

34 Cleveland MG, Mallory SB. Incomplete Reiter's syndrome induced by systemic interferon alpha treatment. J Am Acad Dermatol 1993; **29**: 788–9.

35 Fierlbeck G, Rassner G, Müller C. Psoriasis induced at the injection site of recombinant interferon gamma. Arch Dermatol 1990; **126**: 351–5.

36 Kowalzick L, Weyer U. Psoriasis induced at the injection site of recombinant interferons. Arch Dermatol 1990; **126**: 1515–6.

37 Conlon KC, Urba WJ, Smith JW II et al. Exacerbation of symptoms of autoimmune disease in patients receiving alpha-interferon therapy. Cancer 1990; **65**: 2237–42.

38 Steis RG, Smith JW, Urba WJ. Resistance to recombinant interferon alfa-2a in hairy-cell leukemia associated with neutralizing anti-interferon antibodies. N Engl J Med 1988; **318**: 1409–13.

39 Beretta L, Caronni M, Vanoli M, Scorza R. Systemic sclerosis after interferon-alfa therapy for myeloproliferative disorders. Br J Dermatol 2002; **147**: 385–6.

40 Shilling PJ, Kurzrock R, Kantarijian H et al. Development of systemic lupus erythematosus after interferon therapy for chronic myelogenous leukemia. Cancer 1991; **68**: 1536–7.

41 Ramseur WL, Richards F, Duggan DB. A case of fatal pemphigus vulgaris in association with beta interferon and interleukin-2 therapy. Cancer 1989; **63**: 2005–7.

Interleukins

IL-1. Mucositis and an erythematous eruption with erosions in intertriginous areas and under occlusive tape have been documented [1].

IL-2. Immunotherapy with IL-2, either alone or in conjunction with lymphokine-activated killer cells, is used in the treatment of metastatic cancer; mild influenza-like symptoms are common. Cutaneous complications [2–8] include mucositis, macular erythema (principally restricted to the head, neck and upper chest), burning and pruritus (which resolves with mild desquamation), erythroderma and petechiae. Transient urticaria, necrotic lesions and blisters may be seen [8]. Type I hypersensitivity reactions, ranging from pruritus, erythema and oedema to hypotension, within hours of chemotherapy in patients previously treated with high-dose IL-2 have occurred [9]. A generalized capillary leak syndrome, with non-pitting oedema and diffuse pulmonary infiltrate on chest X-ray, is recorded [6] and is also documented with denileukin difitox, formed from the fusion of human IL-2 with diphtheria toxin [10]. Exacerbation of psoriasis (including erythroderma) has been described [2–6]. IL-2 treatment predisposes to acute hypersensitivity reactions to iodine-containing contrast media [6]. Glossitis, telogen effluvium, punctate superficial ulcers and erosions in scars may be seen. Erythema nodosum has been documented [11]. Local inflammatory painful nodules with a central multi-loculated vesicle have occurred at the site of subcutaneous injections of IL-2 and IFN-α [12]. Linear IgA bullous dermatosis has been associated with IL-2 therapy [13]. TEN is a rare complication [14]. It is of interest that lymphocytes activated by IL-2 can non-specifically destroy keratinocytes *in vitro* [15].

Other side effects include hypothyroidism (antithyroid antibodies are present in 50% of patients), neurological and psychiatric disturbances, musculoskeletal disorders, impaired renal function, cardiovascular injuries, cholestasis, pancreatitis, anaemia, thrombocytopenia, lymphocytopenia and eosinophilia [6].

IL-3. Erythema and purpura at the site of injection, and urticaria [16] may be induced.

IL-4. Transient acantholytic dermatosis is recorded [17].

IL-6. Coalescent, erythematous, scaling macules and papules occurred [18].

REFERENCES

1 Prussick R, Horn TD, Wilson WH, Turner MC. A characteristic eruption associated with ifosfamide, carboplatin, and etoposide chemotherapy after pretreatment with recombinant interleukin-1α. J Am Acad Dermatol 1996; **35**: 705–9.

2 Rosenberg SA, Lotze MT, Muul LM *et al.* Clinical experience with the treatment of 157 patients with advanced cancer using lymphokine-activated killer cells and interleukin-2 or high dose interleukin 2 alone. *N Engl J Med* 1987; **316**: 889–97.

3 Gaspari A, Lotze MT, Rosenberg SA *et al.* Dermatologic changes associated with interleukin-2 administration. *JAMA* 1987; **258**: 1624–9.

4 Rosenberg SA. Immunotherapy of cancer using interleukin 2: current status and future prospects. *Immunol Today* 1988; **9**: 58–62.

5 Lee RE, Gaspari AA, Lotze MT *et al.* Interleukin 2 and psoriasis. *Arch Dermatol* 1988; **124**: 1811–5.

6 Vial T, Descotes J. Clinical toxicity of interleukin-2. *Drug Saf* 1992; **7**: 417–33.

7 Larbre B, Nicolas JF, Sarret Y *et al.* Immunotherapie par interleukine 2 et manifestations cutanées. *Ann Dermatol Vénéréol* 1993; **120**: 528–33.

8 Wolkenstein P, Chosidow O, Wechster J *et al.* Cutaneous side effects associated with interleukin 2 administration for metastatic melanoma. *J Am Acad Dermatol* 1993; **28**: 66–70.

9 Heywood GR, Rosenberg SA, Weber JS. Hypersensitivity reactions to chemotherapy agents in patients receiving chemoimmunotherapy with high-dose interleukin 2. *J Natl Cancer Inst* 1995; **87**: 915–22.

10 Railan D, Fivenson DP, Wittenberg G. Capillary leak syndrome in a patient treated with interleukin 2 fusion toxin for cutaneous T-cell lymphoma. *J Am Acad Dermatol* 2000; **43**: 323–4.

11 Weinstein A, Bujak D, Mittelman A *et al.* Erythema nodosum in a patient with renal cell carcinoma treated with interleukin 2 and lymphokine-activated killer cells. *JAMA* 1987; **258**: 3120–1.

12 Klapholz L, Ackerstein A, Goldenhersh MA *et al.* Local cutaneous reaction induced by subcutaneous interleukin-2 and interferon alpha-2a immunotherapy following ABMT. *Bone Marrow Transplant* 1993; **11**: 443–6.

13 Tranvan A, Pezen DS, Medenica M *et al.* Interleukin-2 associated linear IgA bullous dermatosis. *J Am Acad Dermatol* 1996; **35**: 865–7.

14 Wiener JS, Tucker JA Jr, Walther PJ. Interleukin-2-induced dermatotoxicity resembling toxic epidermal necrolysis. *South Med J* 1992; **82**: 656–9.

15 Kalish RS. Non-specifically activated human peripheral blood mononuclear cells are cytotoxic for human keratinocytes in vitro. *J Immunol* 1989; **142**: 74–80.

16 Bridges AG, Helm TN, Bergfeld WF *et al.* Interleukin-3-induced urticaria-like eruption. *J Am Acad Dermatol* 1996; **34**: 1076–8.

17 Mahler SJ, De Villez RL, Pulitzer DR. Transient acantholytic dermatosis induced by recombinant human interleukin 4. *J Am Acad Dermatol* 1993; **29**: 206–9.

18 Fleming TE, Mirando WS, Soohoo LF *et al.* An inflammatory eruption associated with recombinant human IL-6. *Br J Dermatol* 1994; **130**: 534–6.

Stem cell factor

Human recombinant stem cell factor, a cytokine that acts on haematopoietic progenitor cells and which is used for human anaemic disorders and for speeding haematological recovery after chemotherapy, causes reversible hyperpigmentation at sites of injection; there are increases in melanocyte numbers, dendrite extension and melanin [1].

REFERENCE

1 Grichnik JM, Crawford J, Jimenez F *et al.* Human recombinant stem-cell factor induces melanocytic hyperplasia in susceptible patients. *J Am Acad Dermatol* 1995; **33**: 577–83.

Tumour necrosis factor

Subcutaneous or intramuscular administration of TNF for advanced malignancy is limited by local pain, erythema and swelling or frank ulceration, and intravenous infusion may cause hypotension [1].

REFERENCE

1 Wakefield PE, James WD, Samlaska CP, Meltzer MS. Tumor necrosis factor. *J Am Acad Dermatol* 1991; **24**: 675–85.

Inhibitors of tumour necrosis factor

Etanercept. This fusion protein, comprising the extracellular ligand-binding domain of the 75-kDa receptor for TNF-α and the constant domain of human IgG1, has been associated with injection-site reactions [1–3], follicular hyperkeratosis at distant sites and necrotic and purpuric reactions [3], urticaria [4], autoimmune rashes [5], leukocytoclastic vasculitis [6] and onset of cutaneous squamous cell cancer [7].

Infliximab. Various dermatological complications are recorded, including an atopic dermatitis-like rash [8], eczematid-like purpura [9], erythema multiforme and lichenoid reactions [10], and necrotizing fasciitis and sepsis [11].

REFERENCES

1 Werth VP, Levinson AI. Etancercept-induced injection site reactions: mechanistic insights from clinical findings and immunohistochemistry. *Arch Dermatol* 2001; **137**: 953–5.

2 Zeltser R, Valle L, Tanck C *et al.* Clinical, histological, and immunophenotypic characteristics of injection site reactions associated with etancercept. *Arch Dermatol* 2001; **137**: 893–9.

3 Misery L, Perrot JL, Gentil-Perret A *et al.* Dermatological complications of etancercept therapy for rheumatoid arthritis. *Br J Dermatol* 2002; **146**: 334–5.

4 Skytta E, Pohjankoski H, Savolainen A. Etanercept and urticaria in patients with juvenile idiopathic arthritis. *Clin Exp Rheumatol* 2001; **18**: 533–4.

5 Brion PH, Mittal-Henkle A, Kalunian KC. Autoimmune skin rashes associated with etanercept for rheumatoid arthritis. *Ann Intern Med* 1999; **131**: 634.

6 Galaria NA, Werth VP, Schumacher HR. Leukocytoclastic vasculitis due to etanercept. *J Rheumatol* 2000; **27**: 2041–4.

7 Smith KJ, Skelton HG. Rapid onset of cutaneous squamous cell carcinoma in patients with rheumatoid arthritis after starting tumor necrosis factor α receptor IgG1-Fc fusion complex therapy. *J Am Acad Dermatol* 2002; **45**: 953–6.

8 Wright RC. Atopic dermatitis-like eruption precipitated by infliximab. *J Am Acad Dermatol* 2003; **49**: 160–1.

9 Wang LC, Medenica MM, Shea CR, Busbey S. Infliximab-induced eczematid-like purpura of Doucas and Kapetenakis. *J Am Acad Dermatol* 2003; **49**: 157–8.

10 Vegara G, Sivestre JF, Betlloch I *et al.* Cutaneous drug eruption to infliximab: report of 4 cases with an interface dermatitis pattern. *Arch Dermatol* 2002; **138**: 1258–9.

11 Chan AT, Cleeve V, Daymond TJ. Necrotising fasciitis in a patient receiving infliximab for rheumatoid arthritis. *Postgrad Med J* 2002; **78**: 47–8.

Monoclonal antibodies

Basiliximab. This IL-2 receptor monoclonal antibody has caused myalgia [1].

Cetuximab. Paronychia and aphthous ulcers [2,3], follicular papulopustules [4], and a facial acneiform follicular eruption [3] are recorded with this chimeric antiepidermal growth factor receptor antibody.

OKT3. Orthoclone OKT3, a murine monoclonal antibody directed against the CD3 subset of T lymphocytes, has been used as an immunosuppressive agent in renal transplant recipients, and has been anecdotally associated with anaphylaxis [5].

Rituximab. This murine–human chimeric antibody (IDEC-C2B8) has caused vasculitis and serum sickness [6,7].

REFERENCES

1 Bell HK, Parslew RAG. Use of basiliximab as a cyclosporin-sparing agent in palmopustular psoriasis with myalgia as an adverse effect. *Br J Dermatol* 2002; **147**: 606–7.
2 Boucher KW, Davidson K, Mirakhur B *et al.* Paronychia induced by cetuximab, an antiepidermal growth factor receptor antibody. *J Am Acad Dermatol* 2002; **45**: 632–3.
3 Busam KJ, Capodieci P, Motzer R *et al.* Cutaneous side-effects in cancer patients treated with the antiepidermal growth factor receptor antibody C225. *Br J Dermatol* 2001; **144**: 1169–76.
4 Kimyai-Asadi A, Jih MH. Follicular toxic effects of chimeric anti-epidermal growth factor receptor antibody cetuximab used to treat human solid tumors. *Arch Dermatol* 2002; **138**: 129–31.
5 Werier J, Cheung AHS, Matas AJ. Anaphylactic hypersensitivity reaction after repeat OKT3 treatment. *Lancet* 1991; **337**: 1351.
6 Dereure O, Navarro R, Rossi JF, Guilhou JJ. Rituximab-induced vasculitis. *Dermatology* 2001; **203**: 83–4.
7 D'Arcy CA, Mannik M. Serum sickness secondary to treatment with the murine–human chimeric antibody IDEC-C2B8 (rituximab). *Arthritis Rheum* 2001; **44**: 1717–8.

Miscellaneous drugs affecting the immune response

Diphencyprone

Diphencyprone [1] used for alopecia areata has resulted in urticaria [2,3] and erythema multiforme [4], and has been linked to the development of vitiligo [5–7]. Severe contact dermatitis reactions may be induced.

REFERENCES

1 Shah M, Lewis FM, Messenger AG. Hazards in the use of diphencyprone. *Br J Dermatol* 1996; **134**: 1153.
2 van der Steen PHM, van Baar HMJ, Perret CM, Happle R. Treatment of alopecia areata with diphenylcyclopropenone. *J Am Acad Dermatol* 1991; **24**: 253–7.
3 Alam M, Gross EA, Savin RC. Severe urticarial reaction to diphenylcyclopropenone therapy for alopecia areata. *J Am Acad Dermatol* 1999; **40**: 110–2.
4 Perret CM, Steijlen PM, Zaun H, Happle R. Erythema multiforme-like eruptions: a rare side effect of topical immunotherapy with diphenylcyclopropenone. *Dermatologica* 1990; **180**: 5–7.
5 Hatzis J, Gourgiotou K, Tosca A *et al.* Vitiligo as a reaction to topical treatment with diphencyprone. *Dermatologica* 1988; **177**: 146–8.
6 Duhra P, Foulds IS. Persistent vitiligo induced by diphencyprone. *Br J Dermatol* 1990; **123**: 415–6.
7 Henderson CA, Ilchyshyn A. Vitiligo complicating diphencyprone sensitization therapy for alopecia universalis. *Br J Dermatol* 1995; **133**: 496–7.

Erythropoietin

This drug has caused a generalized eczematous reaction [1].

REFERENCE

1 Hardwick N, King CM. Generalized eczematous reaction to erythropoietin. *Contact Dermatitis* 1993; **28**: 123.

Roquinimex

The incidence of graft-versus-host reactions is enhanced in patients treated with the cytokine inducer carboxamide–quinoline immunotherapeutic agent roquinimex (Linomide), used for post-transplantation immunotherapy in autologous bone marrow transplantation for acute and chronic myelogenous leukaemia [1,2]. Cutaneous graft-versus-host reactions were associated with eccrine sweat gland necrosis.

REFERENCES

1 Gaspari AA, Cheng SF, DiPersio JF, Rowe JM. Roquinimex-induced graft-versus-host reaction after autologous bone marrow transplantation. *J Am Acad Dermatol* 1995; **33**: 711–7.
2 Ohsuga Y, Rowe JM, Liesveld J *et al.* Dermatologic changes associated with roquinimex immunotherapy after autologous bone marrow transplant. *J Am Acad Dermatol* 2000; **43**: 437–41.

Antihistamines

H_1 antihistamines

All traditional H_1 antagonists cause side effects [1–4], especially sedation, most marked with the aminoalkylether and phenothiazine groups. Dizziness, poor coordination, blurred vision and diplopia, as well as nervousness, insomnia and tremor may occur. In addition, atropine-like anticholinergic effects including dryness of mucous membranes, urinary retention, palpitations, agitation, increased intraocular pressure and gastrointestinal upset are seen. Phenothiazine-derived drugs may cause photosensitivity or cholestatic jaundice. The effects of nervous system depressants, such as alcohol, hypnotics, sedatives, analgesics and anxiolytics, may be potentiated. Decreased efficacy of drugs metabolized by the liver microsomal enzyme system, including oral anticoagulants, phenytoin and griseofulvin, may occur as a result of liver-enzyme induction by antihistamines. The newer antihistamines (e.g. terfenadine, astemizole, loratadine, cetirizine) are much less likely to cause sedation [1–4].

Terfenadine and astemizole rarely cause QT interval prolongation and torsade de pointes. Arrhythmias occur when metabolism of terfenadine is impaired, as with inhibition of the cytochrome P-450 isoform CYP 3A4 by ketoconazole, itraconazole and related imidazole antifungals, erythromycin, clarithromycin and related macrolide antibiotics, grapefruit juice, or liver disease [5–7]. Patients on terfenadine or astemizole should be instructed accordingly. The UK Committee on Safety of Medicines withdrew terfenadine from over-the-counter sale, as did the US FDA. However, no increased risk of life-threatening ventricular arrhythmic events or cardiac arrest with terfenadine compared with over-the-counter antihistamines, ibuprofen or clemastine was found in one study [8].

True hypersensitivity reactions are rare. Fixed eruptions have been caused by thonzylamine and cyclizine [9], cetirizine [10], hydroxyzine [11] and loratadine [12]. Skin eruptions have been documented with terfenadine [13,14], including possible exacerbation of psoriasis [15]; alopecia has been reported rarely [16]. Cetirizine has been linked to maculopapular eruptions and precipitation of urticaria [17–20]. Lichenoid and subacute LE-like dermatoses are recorded with antihistamine therapy [21]. Hydroxyzine caused a systemic contact dermatitis in one case [22]. A pityriasis lichenoides et varioliformis acuta-like drug exanthem was reportedly caused by astemizole, with a positive challenge test [23]. Antihistamines are associated with atypical lymphoid hyperplasia, presenting as solitary or multiple nodules and plaques, or multiple papules, in some patients [24].

REFERENCES

1 Woodward JK. Pharmacology and toxicology of nonclassical antihistamines. *Cutis* 1988; **42**: 5–9.
2 Lichtenstein LM, Simons FER, eds. Advancements in antiallergic therapy: beyond conventional antihistamines. *J Allergy Clin Immunol* 1990; **86** (Suppl.): 995–1046.
3 Kennard CD, Ellis CN. Pharmacologic therapy for urticaria. *J Am Acad Dermatol* 1991; **25**: 176–89.
4 Soter NA. Treatment of urticaria and angioedema: low-sedating H1-type antihistamines. *J Am Acad Dermatol* 1991; **24**: 1084–7.
5 Thomas SHL. Drugs, QT interval abnormalities and ventricular arrhythmias. *Adverse Drug React Acute Toxicol Rev* 1994; **13**: 77–102.
6 Woosley RL. Cardiac actions of antihistamines. *Annu Rev Pharmacol Toxicol* 1996; **36**: 233–52.
7 Thomas SHL. Drugs and the QT interval. *Adverse Drug React Bull* 1997; **182**: 691–4.
8 Pratt CM, Hertz RP, Ellis BE *et al.* Risk of developing life-threatening ventricular arrhythmia associated with terfenadine in comparison with over-the-counter antihistamines, ibuprofen and clemastine. *Am J Cardiol* 1994; **73**: 346–52.
9 Griffiths WAD, Peachey RDG. Fixed drug eruption due to cyclizine. *Br J Dermatol* 1970; **82**: 616–7.
10 Inamadar AC, Palit A, Athanikar SB *et al.* Multiple fixed drug eruptions due to cetirizine. *Br J Dermatol* 2002; **147**: 1025–6.
11 Cohen HA, Barzilai A, Matalon A, Harel L, Gross S. Fixed drug eruption of the penis due to hydroxyzine hydrochloride. *Ann Pharmacother* 1997; **31**: 327–9.
12 Ruiz-Genao DP, Hernández-Núñez A, Sánchez-Pérez J, García-Díez A. Fixed drug eruption due to loratadine. *Br J Dermatol* 2002; **146**: 528–9.
13 Stricker BHCH, Van Dijke CHP, Isaacs AJ, Lindquist M. Skin reactions to terfenadine. *BMJ* 1986; **293**: 536.
14 McClintock AD, Ching DW, Hutchinson C. Skin reactions and terfenadine. *NZ Med J* 1995; **108**: 208.
15 Harrison PV, Stones RN. Severe exacerbation of psoriasis due to terfenadine. *Clin Exp Dermatol* 1988; **13**: 275.
16 Jones S, Morley W. Terfenadine causing hair loss (unreviewed report). *BMJ* 1985; **291**: 940.
17 Stingeni L, Caraffini S, Agostinelli D *et al.* Maculopapular and urticarial eruption from cetirizine. *Contact Dermatitis* 1997; **37**: 249–50.
18 Karamfilov T, Wilmer A, Hipler UC, Wollina U. Cetirizine-induced urticarial reaction. *Br J Dermatol* 1999; **140**: 979–80.
19 Calista D, Schianchi S, Morri M. Urticaria induced by cetirizine. *Br J Dermatol* 2001; **144**: 196.
20 Schröter S, Damveld B, Marsch WC. Urticarial intolerance reaction to cetirizine. *Clin Exp Dermatol* 2002; **27**: 185–7.
21 Crowson AN, Magro CM. Lichenoid and subacute cutaneous lupus erythematosus-like dermatitis associated with antihistamine therapy. *J Cutan Pathol* 1999; **26**: 95–9.
22 Menne T. Systemic contact dermatitis to hydroxyzine. *Am J Contact Dermatitis* 1997; **8**: 2–5.
23 Stosiek N, Peters KP, von den Driesch P. Pityriasis-lichenoides-et-varioliformis-acuta-ähnliches Arzneiexanthem durch Astemizol. *Hautarzt* 1993; **44**: 235–7.
24 Magro CM, Crowson AN. Drugs with antihistaminic properties as a cause of atypical cutaneous lymphoid hyperplasia. *J Am Acad Dermatol* 1995; **32**: 419–28.

H₂ antihistamines

Severe adverse reactions are rare with cimetidine, ranitidine, nizatidine and famotidine [1]. Gastrointestinal upset, headache, drowsiness, fatigue or muscular pain occur in fewer than 3% of patients. Confusion, dizziness, somnolence, gynaecomastia or galactorrhoea with increased prolactin levels (cimetidine and ranitidine only), impotence and loss of libido (with cimetidine), bone marrow depression, hepatitis, abnormal renal function or nephritis, arthralgia, myalgia, cardiac abnormalities, and minor or severe skin reactions occur in fewer than 1% of patients.

Cimetidine. Mucocutaneous reactions are rare in relation to the enormous worldwide use of this drug. Reported reactions include a seborrhoeic dermatitis-like rash [2] and asteatotic dermatitis [3], erythema annulare centrifugum [4], erythrosis [5], giant urticaria [6], transitory alopecia [7], erythema multiforme [8] and exfoliative dermatitis [9]. Other effects have included thrombocytopenia [10] and leukocytoclastic vasculitis [11]. Exacerbation of cutaneous LE [12] and SLE with granulocytopenia [13] are documented. Cimetidine binds to androgen receptors, thereby blocking the binding of dihydrotestosterone, and gynaecomastia and hypogonadism are now well-known side effects [14]. The drug augments cell-mediated immunity *in vitro* by blockade of H₂ receptors on T lymphocytes [15].

REFERENCES

1 Feldman M, Burton ME. Histamine₂-receptor antagonists. Standard therapy for acid-peptic diseases. *N Engl J Med* 1990; **323**: 1672–80.
2 Kanwar A, Majid A, Garg MP, Singh G. Seborrheic dermatitis-like eruption caused by cimetidine. *Arch Dermatol* 1981; **117**: 65–6.
3 Greist MC, Epinette WW. Cimetidine-induced xerosis and asteatotic dermatitis. *Arch Dermatol* 1982; **118**: 253–4.
4 Merrett AC, Marks R, Dudley FJ. Cimetidine-induced erythema annulare centrifugum: no cross-sensitivity with ranitidine. *BMJ* 1981; **283**: 698.
5 Angelini G, Bovo P, Vaona B, Cavallini G. Cimetidine and erythrosis-like lesions. *BMJ* 1979; **i**: 1147–8.
6 Hadfield WA Jr. Cimetidine and giant urticaria. *Ann Intern Med* 1979; **91**: 128–9.
7 Vircburger MI, Prelevic GM, Brkic S *et al.* Transitory alopecia and hypergonadotrophic hypogonadism during cimetidine treatment. *Lancet* 1981; **i**: 1160–1.
8 Ahmed AH, McLarly DG, Sharma SK, Masawe AEJ. Stevens–Johnson syndrome during treatment with cimetidine. *Lancet* 1979; **ii**: 433.

9 Yantis PL, Bridges ME, Pittman FE. Cimetidine-induced exfoliative dermatitis. *Dig Dis Sci* 1980; **25**: 73–4.
10 Rate R, Bonnell M, Chervenak C, Pavinich G. Cimetidine and hematologic effects. *Ann Intern Med* 1979; **91**: 795.
11 Dernbach WK, Taylor G. Leukocytoclastic vasculitis from cimetidine. *JAMA* 1981; **246**: 331.
12 Davidson BL, Gilliam JN, Lipsky PE. Cimetidine-associated exacerbation of cutaneous lupus erythematosus. *Arch Intern Med* 1982; **142**: 166–7.
13 Littlejohn GO, Urowitz MB. Cimetidine, lupus erythematosus, and granulocytopenia. *Ann Intern Med* 1979; **91**: 317–8.
14 Jensen RT, Collen MJ, Pandol SJ *et al*. Cimetidine-induced impotence and breast changes in patients with gastric hypersecretory states. *N Engl J Med* 1983; **308**: 883–7.
15 Mavligit GM. Immunologic effects of cimetidine: potential uses. *Pharmacotherapy* 1987; **7** (Suppl. 2): S120–S124.

Famotidine. This drug has been associated with the development of symptomatic dermographism [1], pruritic exanthem [2–4], contact eczema [4], leukocytoclastic vasculitis [5] and TEN.

REFERENCES

1 McCarley Warner D, Ramos-Caro FA, Flowers FP. Famotidine (Pepcid)-induced symptomatic dermatographism. *J Am Acad Dermatol* 1994; **31**: 677–8.
2 Reynolds JC. Famotidine in the management of duodenal ulcer: an analysis of multicenter findings worldwide. *Clin Ther* 1988; **10**: 436–49.
3 Dragosics B, Weiss W, Okulski G. Zur Therapie peptischer Ulzera mit Famotidin. Erfahrungsbericht einer offenen klinischen Studie. *Wien Med Wochenschr* 1992; **142**: 408–13.
4 Monteseirin J, Conde J. Contact eczema from famotidine. *Contact Dermatitis* 1990; **22**: 290.
5 Andreo JA, Vivancos F, Lopez VM *et al*. Vasculitis leucocitoclastica y famotidina. *Med Clin (Barc)* 1990; **95**: 234–5.

Ranitidine. Urticaria [1] and anaphylaxis [2] are recorded, as are allergic dermatitis and allergic contact dermatitis [3,4]. Immune complex-mediated rashes [5], lichenoid eruptions [6] and photosensitivity with UVA sensitivity on monochromator light testing [7] have been documented, as has cholestatic hepatitis [8]. This drug has a less marked effect on androgen receptors than cimetidine, but gynaecomastia has occurred [9].

REFERENCES

1 Picardo M, Santucci B. Urticaria from ranitidine. *Contact Dermatitis* 1983; **9**: 327.
2 Lazaro M, Compaired JA, De La Hoz B *et al*. Anaphylactic reaction to ranitidine. *Allergy* 1993; **48**: 385–7.
3 Juste S, Blanco J, Garces M, Rodriguez G. Allergic dermatitis due to oral ranitidine. *Contact Dermatitis* 1992; **27**: 339–40.
4 Alomar A, Puig L, Vilaltella I. Allergic contact dermatitis due to ranitidine. *Contact Dermatitis* 1987; **17**: 54–5.
5 Haboub N. Rash mediated by immune complexes associated with ranitidine treatment. *BMJ* 1988; **296**: 897.
6 Horiuchi Y, Katagiri T. Lichenoid eruptions due to the H2-receptor antagonists roxatidine and ranitidine. *J Dermatol* 1996; **23**: 510–2.
7 Todd P, Norris P, Hawk JLM, du Vivier AWP. Ranitidine-induced photosensitivity. *Clin Exp Dermatol* 1995; **20**: 146–8.
8 Devuyst O, Lefebvre C, Geubel A, Coche E. Acute cholestatic hepatitis with rash and hypereosinophilia associated with ranitidine treatment. *Acta Clin Belg* 1993; **48**: 109–14.
9 Tosti S, Cagnoli M. Painful gynaecomastia with ranitidine. *Lancet* 1982; **ii**: 160.

Leukotriene receptor antagonists

Montelukast. This drug for asthma, occasionally used in urticaria, has been associated with cutaneous lesions of Churg–Strauss syndrome [1].

REFERENCE

1 Gal AA, Morris RJ, Pine JR, Spraker MK. Cutaneous lesions of Churg–Strauss syndrome associated with montelukast therapy. *Br J Dermatol* 2002; **147**: 618–9.

Injections, infusions and procedures

Radiographic contrast media and radiopharmaceuticals

Radiographic contrast media

Reactions to radiographic contrast media were previously reported to occur in about 4–8% of cases; severe reactions occurred in 1 in 1000 administrations, and occasionally fatal anaphylactoid reactions developed (1 in 3000 for intravenous cholangiograms and between 1 in 10 000 and 1 in 100 000 for intravenous urography) [1–3]. Although IgE-mediated mechanisms may be involved [4], the vast majority of contrast reactions are not due to iodine allergy but rather to non-immunological release of mast cell mediators or to direct complement activation [5,6]. The risk of severe reactions is increased in atopics, asthmatics, those taking β-blockers, and with higher doses of contrast media; up to 40% of patients with a previous reaction may develop a recurrence [7,8].

Newer low-osmolality radiocontrast media are associated with fewer reactions [8–14], for example administration of iohexol in 50 660 patients undergoing excretory urography resulted in a frequency of adverse reactions of any type of 2.1% [9]. In another series, there was a 7.0% incidence of mild adverse reactions to low-osmolar iodine contrast medium in 4550 radiological procedures including computed tomography (CT), intravenous urography, arteriography, venography and myelography [12]. There were only two cases of severe anaphylactoid reactions during 783 consecutive cases undergoing voiding cystourethrography or retrograde pyelography [14]. The incidence of contrast media complications in the catheterization laboratory is 0.23%, with one death per 55 000 [15].

Low-osmolality radiocontrast media (e.g. iohexol or iopamidol) should be the contrast media of choice for patients with a prior immediate generalized reaction to conventional contrast media; in addition, patients should receive H$_1$ antihistamines and corticosteroid prophylaxis therapy [8,13,15]. However, although in one study the relative risk for all adverse drug reactions was three to six times higher for ionic vs. non-ionic contrast media [16], in another study mortality was not lower with the newer low-osmolar media than with the older high-osmolar media [17]. In this latter large study, the overall mortality was 13 per million intravenous injections of radiocontrast media, rising to 35 per million in those over 65 years of age [17]. A further study in the USA found that in a clinical trial comparing the safety of low- vs. high-osmolality radiologic contrast media in patients who underwent either cardiac angiography or contrast-enhanced body CT, 19% of 1004 patients had at least one adverse reaction [18]. The mean cost per patient of treating adverse reactions was $459 (range $0–39 057).

In addition to immediate reactions, widespread erythema and oedema at 6 h, reaching a maximum at 9–12 h, followed intravenous injection of a CT contrast medium (iotrolan) [19]. Fixed drug eruptions have been recorded with iopamidol and iomeprol [20,21]. Mild to moderate delayed allergy-like reactions to contrast media of the maculopapular exanthematous and urticarial/angio-oedematous types have been reported in 0.5–2% of recipients [22]. Isolated cases of reticulate purpura [23], bullous lichen planus [24], iododerma [25], vasculitis [26] and erythrodermic psoriasis [27] have been documented. There has been a single case report of fatal TEN following second exposure to diatrizoate solution for excretory pyelography [28].

REFERENCES

1 Lieberman P, Siegle RL, Treadwell G. Radiocontrast reactions. *Clin Rev Allergy* 1986; **4**: 229–45.
2 Grammer LC, Patterson R. Adverse reactions to radiographic contrast material. *Clin Dermatol* 1986; **4**: 149–54.
3 Katayama H, Tanaka T. Clinical survey of adverse reactions to contrast media. *Invest Radiol* 1988; **23** (Suppl.): S88–S89.
4 Kanny G, Maria Y, Mentre B, Moneret-Vautrin DA. Case report: recurrent anaphylactic shock to radiographic contrast media. Evidence supporting an exceptional IgE-mediated reaction. *Allerg Immunol* 1993; **25**: 425–30.
5 Arroyave CM, Bhatt KN, Crown NR. Activation of the alternative pathway of the complement system by radiocontrast media. *J Immunol* 1976; **117**: 1866–9.
6 Rice MC, Lieberman P, Siegle RL, Mason J. In vitro histamine release induced by radiocontrast media and various chemical analogs in reactor and control subjects. *J Allergy Clin Immunol* 1983; **72**: 180–6.
7 Enright T, Chua-Lim A, Duda E, Lim DT. The role of a documented allergic profile as a risk factor for radiographic contrast media reaction. *Ann Allergy* 1989; **62**: 302–5.
8 Porri F, Vervloet D. Les reactions aux produits de contraste iodes. *Allerg Immunol* 1994; **26**: 374–6.
9 Schrott KM, Behrends B, Clauss W *et al*. Iohexol in excretory urography: results of the drug monitoring programs. *Fortschr Med* 1986; **104**: 153–6.
10 Greenberger PA, Patterson R. The prevention of immediate generalized reactions to contrast media in high-risk patients. *J Allergy Clin Immunol* 1991; **87**: 867–71.
11 Gertz EW, Wisneski JA, Miller R *et al*. Adverse reactions of low osmolality contrast media during cardiac angiography: a prospective randomized multicenter study. *J Am Coll Cardiol* 1992; **19**: 899–906.
12 Kuwatsuru R, Katayama H, Tomita T *et al*. Adverse reactions to low osmolar iodine contrast media (second report) (in Japanese). *Nippon Acta Radiologica* 1992; **52**: 1233–46.
13 Porri F, Pradal M, Fontaine JL *et al*. Reactions aux produits de contraste iodes. *Presse Med* 1993; **22**: 543–9.
14 Weese DL, Greenberg HM, Zimmern PE. Contrast media reactions during voiding cystourethrography or retrograde pyelography. *Urology* 1993; **41**: 81–4.
15 Goss JE, Chambers CE, Heupler FA Jr. Systemic anaphylactoid reactions to iodinated contrast media during cardiac catheterization procedures: guidelines for prevention, diagnosis, and treatment. Laboratory Performance Standards Committee of the Society for Cardiac Angiography and Interventions. *Cathet Cardiovasc Diagn* 1995; **34**: 99–105.
16 Andrew E, Haider T. Incidence of roentgen contrast medium reactions after intravenous injection in pre-registration trials and post-marketing surveillances. *Acta Radiol* 1993; **34**: 210–3.
17 Cashman JD, McCredie J, Henry DA. Intravenous contrast media: use and associated mortality. *Med J Aust* 1991; **155**: 618–23.
18 Powe NR, Moore RD, Steinberg EP. Adverse reactions to contrast media: factors that determine the cost of treatment. *Am J Roentgenol* 1993; **161**: 1089–95.
19 Kanzaki T, Sakagami H. Late phase allergic reaction to a CT contrast medium (iotrolan). *J Dermatol* 1991; **18**: 528–31.
20 Yamauchi R, Morita A, Tsuji T. Fixed drug eruption caused by iopamidol, a contrast medium. *J Dermatol* 1997; **24**: 243–5.
21 Watanabe H, Sueki H, Nakada T *et al*. Multiple fixed drug eruption caused by iomeprol (Iomeron), a nonionic contrast medium. *Dermatology* 1999; **198**: 291–4.
22 Christiansen C, Pichler WJ, Skotland T. Delayed allergy-like reactions to X-ray contrast media: mechanistic considerations. *Eur Radiol* 2000; **10**: 1965–75.
23 Rinker MH, Sanguea OP, Davis LS. Reticulated purpura occurring with contrast medium after hysterosalpingography. *Br J Dermatol* 1998; **138**: 919–20.
24 Grunwald MH, Halevy S, Livni E, Feuerman EJ. Bullous lichen planus after intravenous pyelography. *J Am Acad Dermatol* 1985; **13**: 512–3.
25 Chang MW, Miner JE, Moiin A, Hashimoto K. Iododerma after computed tomographic scan with intravenous radiopaque contrast media. *J Am Acad Dermatol* 1997; **36**: 1014–6.
26 Kerdel FA, Fraker DL, Haynes HA. Necrotizing vasculitis from radiographic contrast media. *J Am Acad Dermatol* 1984; **10**: 25–9.
27 Evans AV, Parker JC, Russell-Jones R. Erythrodermic psoriasis precipitated by radiologic contrast media. *J Am Acad Dermatol* 2002; **46**: 960–1.
28 Kaftori JK, Abraham Z, Gilhar A. Toxic epidermal necrolysis after excretory pyelography. Immunologic-mediated contrast medium reaction? *Int J Dermatol* 1988; **27**: 346–7.

Radiopharmaceuticals

The reported incidence of reactions to agents used in nuclear medicine is low; these usually take the form of immediate urticaria or angio-oedema [1–3]. Urticarial or anaphylactic reactions to technetium (^{99m}Tc) sulphur colloid and ^{99m}Tc human albumin microspheres together accounted for 50% of reported reactions [2]. The bone-scanning agent ^{99m}Tc methylene diphosphonate produces a delayed-onset erythematous pruritic eruption within 4–24 h [4].

REFERENCES

1 Rhodes BA, Cordova MA. Adverse reactions to radio-pharmaceuticals: incidence in 1978, and associated symptoms. *J Nucl Med* 1980; **2**: 1107.
2 Cordova MA, Hladik WB III, Rhodes BA. Validation and characterization of adverse reactions to radiopharmaceuticals. *Noninvasive Med Imaging* 1984; **1**: 17–24.
3 Keeling D, Sampson CB. Adverse reactions to radiopharmaceuticals: incidence, reporting, symptoms, treatment. *Nuklearmedizin* 1986; **23** (Suppl.): 478–82.
4 Collins MRL, James WD, Rodman OG. Adverse cutaneous reaction to technetium Tc 99m methylene diphosphonate. *Arch Dermatol* 1988; **124**: 180–1.

Halides

Bromides

Bromides have a long half-life and are excreted slowly by the kidney; bromism may develop in patients with impaired renal function, and eruptions may not develop until as much as 2 months after the drug has been discontinued. Acneiform and vegetating lesions occur more often, and bullae less frequently, than with iodism [1,2]. Vegetating bromoderma presents as single or multiple papillomatous nodules or plaques, studded with small pustules, on the face or limbs. Bromoderma tuberosum has been caused by anticonvulsive treatment with potassium bromide [3]. Bromism is also characterized by weakness, restlessness, headache, ataxia and personality changes [2].

Iodides

Serious and even fatal reactions of anaphylactic type have been caused by radiograpic contrast media containing organic iodine [4]. Iodism, nasal congestion and conjunctivitis, often accompanied by an exanthematic eruption, may be associated with a wide variety of systemic symptoms [5,6]. Prolonged administration of small doses of iodide, as in many cough mixtures, may provoke eruptions with or without mucosal or systemic symptoms. Lesions may first develop some days after the drug is discontinued. The following may occur: urticaria, an acneiform rash, papulopustular lesions, nodules, anthracoid or carbuncular lesions, or clear or haemorrhagic bullae on the face, forearms, neck and flexures or on the buccal mucosa [6]. If the iodine is continued, the bullae may be replaced by vegetating masses, which simulate pemphigus vegetans or a granulomatous infection [7]. Iododerma has developed after administration of oral [8] and intravenous [9,10] radiographic contrast media, and during thyroid protection treatment [11]. Iododerma seems more frequent in patients with renal failure, and may be accompanied by leukocytoclastic vasculitis [2]. The eruption recurs within days of readministration in a sensitized individual [12]. Cell-mediated [5] and 'hyperinflammatory' [13] mechanisms have been postulated. Vegetating iododerma may be an idiosyncratic response that is commoner in patients with polyarteritis nodosa or paraproteinaemia [14]. Fixed eruptions occur rarely [15]. Generalized pustular psoriasis has been reportedly provoked by potassium iodide [16].

Histology of bromoderma and iododerma

In bromoderma, verrucous pseudoepitheliomatous hyperplasia is associated with abscesses containing neutrophils and eosinophils in the epidermis, and with a dense dermal infiltrate initially consisting mainly of neutrophils and eosinophils and later containing many lymphocytes, plasma cells and histiocytes. The abundant dilated blood vessels may show endothelial proliferation. In iododermas, ulceration is more marked, but there is usually less epithelial hyperplasia. Both conditions must be differentiated from blastomycosis and coccidioidomycosis, and from pemphigus vegetans [17].

REFERENCES

1 Blasik LG, Spencer SK. Fluoroderma. *Arch Dermatol* 1979; **115**: 1334–5.
2 Carney MWP. Five cases of bromism. *Lancet* 1971; **ii**: 523–4.
3 Pfeifle J, Grieben U, Bork K. Bromoderma tuberosum durch antikonvulsive Behandlung mit Kaliumbromid. *Hautarzt* 1992; **43**: 792–4.
4 Vaillant L, Pengloan J, Blanchier D *et al.* Iododerma and acute respiratory distress with leucocytoclastic vasculitis following the intravenous injection of contrast medium. *Clin Exp Dermatol* 1990; **15**: 232–3.
5 Kincaid MC, Green WR, Hoover RE, Farmer ER. Iododerma of the conjunctiva and skin. *Ophthalmology* 1981; **88**: 1216–20.
6 O'Brien TJ. Iodic eruptions. *Australas J Dermatol* 1987; **28**: 119–22.
7 Rosenberg FR, Einbinder J, Walzer RA, Nelson CT. Vegetating iododerma. An immunologic mechanism. *Arch Dermatol* 1972; **105**: 900–5.
8 Boudoulas O, Siegle RJ, Grinwood RE. Iododerma occurring after orally administered iopanoic acid. *Arch Dermatol* 1987; **123**: 387–8.
9 Heydenreich G, Larsen PO. Iododerma after high dose urography in an oliguric patient. *Br J Dermatol* 1977; **97**: 567–9.
10 Lauret P, Godin M, Bravard P. Vegetating iodides after an intravenous pyelogram. *Dermatologica* 1985; **71**: 463–8.
11 Wilkin JK, Strobel D. Iododerma during thyroid protection treatment. *Cutis* 1985; **36**: 335–7.
12 Jones LE, Pariser H, Murray PF. Recurrent iododerma. *Arch Dermatol* 1958; **28**: 353–8.
13 Stone OJ. Proliferative iododerma: a possible mechanism. *Int J Dermatol* 1985; **24**: 565–6.
14 Soria C, Allegue F, España A *et al.* Vegetating iododerma with underlying systemic diseases: report of three cases. *J Am Acad Dermatol* 1990; **22**: 418–22.
15 Baker H. Fixed drug eruption due to iodide and antipyrine. *Br J Dermatol* 1962; **74**: 310–6.
16 Shelley WB. Generalized pustular psoriasis induced by potassium iodide. *JAMA* 1967; **201**: 1009–14.
17 Elder D, Elenitsas R, Jaworsky C, Johnson B Jr, eds. *Lever's Histopathology of the Skin*, 8th edn. Philadelphia: Lippincott, 1997.

Agents used in general anaesthesia

Neuromuscular blocking agents, skeletal muscle relaxants and general anaesthetics

The incidence of life-threatening anaphylactic or anaphylactoid reactions during anaesthesia has been variously reported to occur in 1 in 1000 to 1 in 20 000, and minor reactions probably occur in more than 1% of cases; neuromuscular blocking agents are the triggering agents in 50–69% of these reactions, with latex being less frequently incriminated (about 12%) [1–10]. The mortality rate in anaphylactic reactions to drugs used in general anaesthesia is between 4 and 6% [8]. Reactions were most likely with suxamethonium and gallamine, then D-tubocurarine and alcuronium, and least likely with pancuronium and vecuronium [3,6,9]; in another study, succinylcholine and rocuronium were most frequently incriminated [10]. Mucocutaneous manifestations including erythema, urticaria and angio-oedema are reported in up to 80% of reactions, but may only be recognized after the acute phase has passed. Reactions are more frequent in women and in atopic patients. Proposed mechanisms for anaphylactic reactions include type I (IgE antibody-mediated) hypersensitivity [9,11–13], with antibodies persisting for up to 29 years [12], and direct histamine release. Only one reaction in three is likely to be IgE-mediated (type I) anaphylaxis, but non-immune reactions are no less hazardous than type I reactions [9]. Cross-reactivity is widespread with most of the drugs but is least with pancuronium. It has been suggested that pancuronium should be used where muscle relaxation during anaesthesia is essential but sensitivity to another relaxant exists [3], although others have questioned the safety of this procedure [7]. IgE-dependent sensitivity to thiopental may result in anaphylactic reactions [5].

REFERENCES

1 Fisher MMcD. Intradermal testing in the diagnosis of acute anaphylaxis during anaesthesia: results of five years experience. *Anaesth Intensive Care* 1979; **7**: 58–61.
2 Fisher MMcD. The diagnosis of acute anaphylactoid reactions to neuromuscular blocking agents: a commonly undiagnosed condition. *Anaesth Intensive Care* 1981; **9**: 235–41.
3 Galletly DC, Treuren BC. Anaphylactoid reactions during anaesthesia. Seven years' experience of intradermal testing. *Anaesthesia* 1985; **40**: 329–33.
4 Leynadier F, Sansarricq M, Didier JM, Dry J. Prick tests in the diagnosis of anaphylaxis to general anaesthesia. *Br J Anaesth* 1987; **59**: 683–9.
5 Cheema AL, Sussman GL, Jancelewicz Z et al. Update: pentothal-induced anaphylaxis. *J Allergy Clin Immunol* 1988; **81**: 220.
6 Fisher MM, Baldo BA. The incidence and clinical features of anaphylactic reactions during anesthesia in Australia. *Ann Fr Anesth Reanim* 1993; **12**: 97–104.
7 Moneret-Vautrin DA, Laxenaire MC. Anaphylaxis to muscle relaxants: predictive tests. *Anaesthesia* 1990; **45**: 246–7.
8 Moscicki RA, Sockin SM, Corsello BF et al. Anaphylaxis during induction of general anesthesia: subsequent evaluation and management. *J Allergy Clin Immunol* 1990; **86**: 325–32.
9 Watkins J. Adverse reaction to neuromuscular blockers: frequency, investigation, and epidemiology. *Acta Anaesthesiol Scand Suppl* 1994; **102**: 6–10.
10 Laxenaire MC, Mertes PM, Groupe d'Etudes des Reactions Anaphylactoides Peranesthesiques. Anaphylaxis during anaesthesia. Results of a two-year survey in France. *Br J Anaesth* 2001; **87**: 549–58.
11 Baldo BA, Fisher MM. Mechanisms in IgE-dependent anaphylaxis to anesthetic drugs. *Ann Fr Anesth Reanim* 1993; **12**: 131–40.
12 Fisher MM, Baldo BA. Persistence of allergy to anaesthetic drugs. *Anaesth Intensive Care* 1992; **20**: 143–6.
13 Assem ES. Anaphylactoid reactions to neuromuscular blockers: major role of IgE antibodies and possible contribution of IgE-independent mechanisms. *Monogr Allergy* 1992; **30**: 24–53.

Local anaesthetic agents

Local anaesthetics may cause both immediate anaphylactic reactions and contact dermatitis [1–10]. True allergic reactions caused by local anaesthetics are extremely rare [9,11]; more often, the allergic response is caused by a metabolite, preservative or unrelated substance. Acute anaphylactic reactions are uncommon, but are probably less likely to occur when amide linkage agents are used [4,5]. Necrosis of the fingertip has followed local injection

for nail extraction [12]. Dizziness and confusion due to systemic absorption followed repeated application of topical lidocaine (lignocaine) [13]. Severe lidocaine intoxication with progressive neurological and psychiatric abnormalities and cardiorespiratory arrest occurred following topical application to painful ulcerated areas in a patient with cutaneous T-cell lymphoma [14].

Tetracaine (amethocaine). Tetracaine in the form of a self-adhesive patch caused slight or moderate erythema at the site of application in 26% of patients, and slight oedema in 5% [15].

EMLA cream (proprietary name). A eutectic mixture of prilocaine and lidocaine in a cream base (EMLA cream) has been associated with methaemoglobinaemia [16–18]; two metabolites of prilocaine, namely 4-hydroxy-2-methylaniline and 2-methylaniline (*o*-toluidine), have been incriminated. A 3-month-old infant became cyanosed after application of 5 g, but concomitant sulphonamide therapy may have made a contribution [16]. Small but significant increases in methaemoglobin levels have been reported in children aged 1–6 years following routine administration of 5 g before surgery, and these may persist for at least 24 h [17], so it is recommended that the minimum effective dose be used in children requiring daily application. Blanching following application of EMLA cream is common [19]. Hyperpigmentation is recorded [20]. Contact dermatitis can arise to both lidocaine and prilocaine [21–23].

Bupivacaine. A delayed hypersensitivity rash may occur after injection of arthroscopy portals with bupivacaine [24].

REFERENCES

1 Schatz M. Skin testing and incremental challenge in the evaluation of adverse reactions of local anesthetics. *J Allergy Clin Immunol* 1984; **74**: 606–16.
2 Fisher MMcD, Graham R. Adverse responses to local anaesthetics. *Anaesth Intensive Care* 1984; **12**: 325–7.
3 Ruzicka T, Gerstmeier M, Przybilla B, Ring J. Allergy to local anesthetics: comparison of patch test with prick and intradermal test results. *J Am Acad Dermatol* 1987; **16**: 1202–8.
4 Christie JL. Fatal consequences of local anesthesia: report of five cases and a review of the literature. *J Forensic Sci* 1975; **21**: 671–9.
5 Kennedy KS, Cave RH. Anaphylactic reaction to lidocaine. *Arch Otolaryngol Head Neck Surg* 1986; **112**: 671–3.
6 Glinert RJ, Zachary CB. Local anesthetic allergy. Its recognition and avoidance. *J Dermatol Surg Oncol* 1991; **17**: 491–6.
7 Grognard C. Complications des anesthesiques locaux. *Ann Dermatol Vénéréol* 1993; **120**: 172–4.
8 Skidmore RA, Patterson JD, Tomsick RS. Local anesthetics. *Dermatol Surg* 1996; **22**: 511–22.
9 Gall H, Kaufmann R, Kalveram CM. Adverse reactions to local anesthetics: analysis of 197 cases. *J Allergy Clin Immunol* 1996; **97**: 933–7.
10 Kajimoto Y, Rosenberg ME, Kytta J et al. Anaphylactoid skin reactions after intravenous regional anaesthesia using 0.5% prilocaine with or without preservative: a double-blind study. *Acta Anaesthesiol Scand* 1995; **39**: 782–4.
11 Jackson D, Chen AH, Bennett CR. Identifying true lidocaine allergy. *J Am Dent Assoc* 1994; **125**: 1362–6.

12 Roser-Maass E. Nekrosen an Fingerendgliedern nach Lokalanästhesie bei Nagelextraktion. *Hautarzt* 1981; **32**: 39–41.

13 Goodwin DP, McMeekin TO. A case of lidocaine absorption from topical administration of 40% lidocaine cream. *J Am Acad Dermatol* 1999; **41**: 280–1.

14 Lie RL, Vermeer BJ, Edelbroek PM. Severe lidocaine intoxication by cutaneous absorption. *J Am Acad Dermatol* 1990; **23**: 1026–8.

15 Doyle E, Freeman J, Im NT, Morton NS. An evaluation of a new self-adhesive patch preparation of amethocaine for topical anaesthesia prior to venous cannulation in children. *Anaesthesia* 1993; **48**: 1050–2.

16 Jakobson B, Nilsson A. Methaemoglobinaemia associated with a prilocaine-lidocaine cream and trimethoprim–sulphamethoxazole. A case report. *Acta Anaesthesiol Scand* 1985; **29**: 453–5.

17 Frayling IM, Addison GM, Chattergee K, Meakin G. Methaemoglobinaemia in children treated with prilocaine–lignocaine cream. *BMJ* 1990; **301**: 153–4.

18 Nilsson A, Engberg G, Henneberg S *et al.* Inverse relationship between age-dependent erythrocyte activity of methaemoglobin reductase and prilocaine-induced methaemoglobinaemia during infancy. *Br J Anaesth* 1990; **64**: 72–6.

19 Villada G, Zetlaoui J, Revuz J. Local blanching after epicutaneous application of EMLA cream. *Dermatologica* 1990; **181**: 38–40.

20 Godwin Y, Brotherston M. Hyperpigmentation following the use of EMLA cream. *Br J Plast Surg* 2001; **54**: 82–3.

21 Duggan M, Burns D, Henry M, Mitchell T. Reaction to topical lignocaine in a patient with contact dermatitis. *Contact Dermatitis* 1993; **28**: 190–1.

22 van den Hove J, Decroix J, Tennstedt D, Lachapelle JM. Allergic contact dermatitis from prilocaine, one of the local anaesthetics in EMLA cream. *Contact Dermatitis* 1994; **30**: 239.

23 Thakur BK, Murali MR. EMLA cream-induced allergic contact dermatitis: a role for prilocaine as an immunogen. *J Allergy Clin Immunol* 1995; **95**: 776–8.

24 Magsamen BF. Delayed hypersensitivity rash to the knee after injection of arthroscopy portals with bupivacaine (Marcain). *Arthroscopy* 1995; **11**: 512–3.

Infusions and injections

Intravenous infusion

Pain, oedema, induration and thrombophlebitis are well-recognized complications [1–4]. Localized bullous eruptions following infusion of commonly used non-vesicant fluids, such as saline, have been described [5]. Extravasation was reported to occur in 11% of 16 380 administrations to children monitored over a 6-month period [6]. Skin necrosis following intravenous infusion of chemotherapeutic agents occurs in up to 6% of patients [1,3,5–9].

REFERENCES

1 Barton A. Adverse reactions to intravenous catheters and other devices. *Lancet* 1993; **342**: 683.

2 Dufresne RG. Skin necrosis from intravenously infused materials. *Cutis* 1987; **39**: 197–8.

3 MacCara E. Extravasation: a hazard of intravenous therapy. *Drug Intell Clin Pharm* 1987; **17**: 713–7.

4 Rudolph R, Larson DL. Etiology and treatment of chemotherapeutic agent extravasation injuries. A review. *J Clin Oncol* 1987; **5**: 1116–26.

5 Robijns BJL, de Wit WM, Bosma NJ, van Vloten WA. Localized bullous eruptions caused by extravasation of commonly used intravenous infusion fluids. *Dermatologica* 1991; **182**: 39–42.

6 Brown AS, Hoelzer DJ, Piercy SA. Skin necrosis from extravasation of intravenous fluids in children. *Plast Reconstr Surg* 1979; **64**: 145–50.

7 Ignoffo RJ, Friedman MA. Therapy of local toxicities caused by extravasation of cancer chemotherapeutic drugs. *Cancer Treat Rev* 1980; **7**: 17–27.

8 Harwood KV, Aisner J. Treatment of chemotherapeutic extravasation: current status. *Cancer Treat Rep* 1984; **68**: 939–45.

9 Banerjee A, Brotherston TM, Lamberty BGH *et al.* Cancer chemotherapy agent-induced perivenous extravasation injury. *J Postgrad Med* 1987; **63**: 5–9.

Blood transfusion

Urticaria occurs in about 1% of transfusions [1], and may be the result of allergy to soluble proteins in donor plasma. Post-transfusion purpura may rarely occur as a result of profound thrombocytopenia about 1 week after transfusion, and is associated with antiplatelet alloantibodies. Other potential side effects include transmission of infectious diseases, including syphilis, hepatitis B and HIV-related syndromes (AIDS).

Graft-versus-host disease may develop following transfusion of unirradiated blood in immunosuppressed patients [2–8], including those with malignancies [2], and infants with severe congenital immunodeficiency [3]. Isolated reports of fatal transfusion-associated graft-versus-host disease in presumed immunocompetent hosts receiving fresh unirradiated blood have been reported [9–11]. This paradoxical situation may be partly explained by situations in which recipients heterozygous for a given MHC haplotype receive a transfusion from a donor homozygous for this haplotype, as the recipient would not react to the donor haplotype but the donor lymphocytes would react to the non-identical recipient haplotype [8]. Thus, some recipients of non-irradiated blood from their offspring may be at risk of developing graft-versus-host disease. An acute fatal illness, characterized by fever, diffuse erythematous rash and progressive leukopenia, has been described in Japanese patients 10 days after surgical operation and has been termed 'postoperative erythroderma' [12]. Histologically, scattered single cell epidermal cell eosinophilic necrosis, satellite cell necrosis, basal cell liquefaction degeneration and a scanty dermal infiltrate may be seen; the reaction is compatible with an acute graft-versus-host reaction following blood transfusion [12].

REFERENCES

1 Shulman IA. Adverse reactions to blood transfusion. *Texas Med* 1990; **85**: 35–42.

2 Decoste SD, Boudreaux C, Dover JS. Transfusion-associated graft-vs-host disease in patients with malignancies. Report of two cases and review of the literature. *Arch Dermatol* 1990; **126**: 1324–9.

3 Hathaway WE, Githens JH, Blackburn WR *et al.* Aplastic anemia, histiocytosis and erythrodermia in immunologically deficient children. *N Engl J Med* 1965; **273**: 953–8.

4 Brubaker DB. Human posttransfusion graft-versus-host disease. *Vox Sang* 1983; **45**: 401–20.

5 Leitman SF, Holland PV. Irradiation of blood products: indications and guidelines. *Transfusion* 1985; **25**: 292–300.

6 Anderson KC, Weinstein HJ. Transfusion-associated graft-versus-host disease. *N Engl J Med* 1990; **323**: 315–21.

7 Ray TL. Blood transfusions and graft-vs-host disease. *Arch Dermatol* 1990; **126**: 1347–50.

8 Ferrara JLM, Deeg HJ. Graft-versus-host disease. *N Engl J Med* 1991; **324**: 667–74.

9 Arsura EL, Bertelle A, Minkowitz S *et al.* Transfusion-associated graft-vs-host disease in a presumed immunocompetent patient. *Arch Intern Med* 1988; **148**: 1941–4.

10 Capond SM, DePond WD, Tyan DB *et al.* Transfusion-associated

graft-versus-host disease in an immunocompetent patient. *Ann Intern Med* 1991; **114**: 1025–6.
11 Juji T, Takahashi K, Shibata Y *et al.* Post-transfusion graft-versus-host disease in immunocompetent patients after cardiac surgery in Japan. *N Engl J Med* 1989; **321**: 56.
12 Hidano A, Yamashita N, Mizuguchi M, Toyoda H. Clinical, histological, and immunohistological studies of postoperative erythroderma. *J Dermatol* 1989; **16**: 20–30.

Hydroxyethyl starch

Hydroxyethyl starch (hetastarch) is used as a plasma expander for hypovolaemia, to prime cardiopulmonary bypass machines, as a sedimenting agent to increase the yield of granulocytes during leukapheresis, and to improve microcirculation as in the treatment of sudden deafness. It has been implicated in the development of lichen planus [1], and severe generalized pruritus in up to 32% of recipients, beginning 2 weeks after exposure and taking up to 2 years to settle [2–6].

REFERENCES

1 Bode U, Deisseroth AB. Donor toxicity in granulocyte collections: association of lichen planus with the use of hydroxyethyl starch leukapheresis. *Transfusion* 1981; **21**: 83–5.
2 Parker NE, Porter JB, Williams HJM, Leftley N. Pruritus after administration of hetastarch. *BMJ* 1982; **284**: 385–6.
3 Gall H, Kaufmann R, von Ehr M *et al.* Persistierender Pruritus nach Hydroxyathylstarke-Infusionen. Retrospektive Langzeitstudie an 266 Fallen. *Hautarzt* 1993; **44**: 713–6.
4 Cox NH, Popple AW. Persistent erythema and pruritus, with a confluent histiocytic skin infiltrate, following the use of a hydroxyethylstarch plasma expander. *Br J Dermatol* 1996; **134**: 353–7.
5 Speight EL, MacSween RM, Stevens A. Persistent itching due to etherified starch plasma expander. *BMJ* 1997; **314**: 1466–7.
6 Murphy M, Carmichael AJ, Lawler PG *et al.* The incidence of hydroxyethyl starch-associated pruritus. *Br J Dermatol* 2001; **144**: 973–6.

Fluorescein

A psoriasiform eruption followed parenteral administration for fluorescein angiography [1].

REFERENCE

1 Mayama M, Hirayama K, Nakano H *et al.* Psoriasiform drug eruption induced by fluorescein sodium used for fluorescein angiography. *Br J Dermatol* 1999; **140**: 982–4.

Renal dialysis

Dermatological complications of renal dialysis have been reviewed [1,2]. These include marked premature ageing, hyperpigmentation, xeroderma, decreased sebaceous and sweat gland secretion, Raynaud's syndrome, generalized pruritus and carpal tunnel syndrome due to amyloid β deposition [1]. Extravasation, phlebitis and bacterial infection of the cannula, with resulting septicaemia, may occur and are related to the site of insertion of the cannula into the arteriovenous fistula. A bullous dermatosis of haemodialysis has been described [2,3]. This resembles porphyria clinically and histologically, and porphyrins may be elevated [3], although cases with pseudoporphyria in which there are no abnormalities of porphyrin metabolism have also been documented [2]. Two-thirds of patients with dialysis-associated anaphylaxis have IgE antibodies to ethylene oxide/human serum albumin [4]. Allergic contact dermatitis due to rubber chemicals in the haemodialysis equipment may be seen around the arteriovenous shunt [5]. Porokeratosis localized to the access region for haemodialysis has also been reported [6].

REFERENCES

1 Altmeyer P, Kachel H-G, Jünger M *et al.* Hautveränderungen bei Langzeitdialysepatienten. *Hautarzt* 1982; **33**: 303–9.
2 Gupta AK, Gupta MA, Cardella CJ, Haberman HF. Cutaneous complications of chronic renal failure and dialysis. *Int J Dermatol* 1986; **25**: 498–504.
3 Poh-Fitzpatrick MB, Bellet N, DeLeo VA *et al.* Porphyria cutanea tarda in two patients treated with hemodialysis for chronic renal failure. *N Engl J Med* 1978; **299**: 292–4.
4 Grammer LC, Roberts M, Wiggins CA *et al.* A comparison of cutaneous testing and ELISA testing for assessing reactivity to ethylene oxide–human serum albumin in hemodialysis patients with anaphylactic reactions. *J Allergy Clin Immunol* 1991; **87**: 674–6.
5 Kruis-De Vries M, Coenraads P, Nater J. Allergic contact dermatitis due to rubber chemicals in haemodialysis equipment. *Contact Dermatitis* 1987; **17**: 303–5.
6 Nakazawa A, Matsuo I, Ohkido M. Porokeratosis localized to the access region for hemodialysis. *J Am Acad Dermatol* 1991; **25**: 338–40.

Necrosis from intramuscular injections

Severe painful local necrosis at the site of an injected medicament (embolia cutis medicamentosa, also known as Nicolau's syndrome) may follow intramuscular therapeutic injections and was originally described with bismuth. It occurs particularly with preparations containing corticosteroids, local anaesthetics, antirheumatic drugs and antihistamines; more rarely, chlorpromazine, penicillin, phenobarbital and sulphonamides have been implicated [1,2]. The condition has also followed sclerotherapy [3]. Clinically, stellate erythema and infiltration are followed by central deep necrosis that heals with scarring.

REFERENCES

1 Bork K. *Cutaneous Side Effects of Drugs.* Philadelphia: Saunders, 1988.
2 Faucher L, Marcoux D. What syndrome is this? Nicolau syndrome. *Pediatr Dermatol* 1995; **12**: 187–90.
3 Geukens J, Rabe E, Bieber T. Embolia cutis medicamentosa of the foot after sclerotherapy. *Eur J Dermatol* 1999; **9**: 132–3.

Polidocanol

The sclerosing solution polidocanol is said to cause allergic reactions in up to 0.06% of cases; systemic allergic reactions may be more common than previously recognized [1].

REFERENCE

1 Feied CF, Jackson JJ, Bren TS *et al.* Allergic reactions to polidocanol for vein sclerosis. Two case reports. *J Dermatol Surg Oncol* 1994; **20**: 466–8.

Drugs affecting metabolism or gastrointestinal function

Hypoglycaemic drugs

Dermatological aspects of the oral hypoglycaemic drugs have been reviewed [1–4].

Biguanides

Rashes are much less frequent with metformin and phenformin than with sulphonylureas. Transient erythemas, pruritus and urticaria have been noted.

Sulphonylureas

Chlorpropamide and tolbutamide are most often prescribed, and both can give rise to toxic or allergic reactions. Angio-oedema with glibornuride, urticaria with glibenclamide and a bullous dermatitis with carbutamide have been described [5]; there was no cross-reactivity between first- and second-generation sulphonylureas.

Chlorpropamide. Eruptions occur in 2–3% of patients on chlorpropamide [2]. These include maculopapular rashes, photosensitivity [6], erythema annulare, Stevens–Johnson syndrome [7], erythema nodosum [1], lichenoid eruptions [8,9], purpura and exfoliative dermatitis [10]. Porphyria has been provoked [11]. A disulfiram-like effect, with flushing of the face, headache and palpitations after taking alcohol, occurs in up to 30% of patients [12,13]. The fact that the flush is blocked by naloxone suggests that opioids may be involved in the response.

Glibenclamide. Bullae and cholestasis have occurred together [14].

Glipizide. Pigmented purpuric eruption is documented [15].

REFERENCES

1 Beurey J, Jeandidier P, Bermont A. Les complications dermatologiques des traitements antidiabétiques. *Ann Dermatol Syphiligr* 1966; **93**: 13–42.
2 Almeyda J, Baker H. Drug reactions. X. Adverse cutaneous reactions to hypoglycaemic agents. *Br J Dermatol* 1970; **82**: 634–6.
3 Harris EL. Adverse reactions to oral antidiabetic agents. *BMJ* 1971; **3**: 29–30.
4 Perez MI, Kohn SR. Cutaneous manifestations of diabetes mellitus. *J Am Acad Dermatol* 1994; **30**: 519–31.
5 Chichmanian RM, Papasseudi G, Hieronimus S *et al.* Allergies aux sulfonylurees hypoglycemiantes. Les reactions croisées existent-elles? *Thérapie* 1991; **46**: 163–7.
6 Hitselberger JF, Fosnaugh RP. Photosensitivity due to chlorpropamide. *JAMA* 1962; **180**: 62–3.
7 Yaffee HS. Stevens–Johnson syndrome caused by chlorpropamide: report of a case. *Arch Dermatol* 1960; **82**: 636–7.
8 Dinsdale RCW, Ormerod TP, Walker AE. Lichenoid eruption due to chlorpropamide. *BMJ* 1968; **i**: 100.
9 Barnett JH, Barnett SM. Lichenoid drug reactions to chlorpropamide and tolazamide. *Cutis* 1984; **34**: 542–4.
10 Rothfeld EL, Goldman J, Goldberg HH, Einhorn S. Severe chlorpropamide toxicity. *JAMA* 1960; **172**: 54–6.
11 Zarowitz H, Newhouse S. Coproporphyrinuria with a cutaneous reaction induced by chlorpropamide. *NY State J Med* 1965; **65**: 2385–7.
12 Stakosch CR, Jefferys DB, Keen H. Blockade of chlorpropamide alcohol flush by aspirin. *Lancet* 1980; **i**: 394–6.
13 Medback S, Wass JAH, Clement-Jones V *et al.* Chlorpropamide alcohol flush and circulating met-enkephalin: a positive link. *BMJ* 1981; **283**: 937–9.
14 Wongpaitoon V, Mills PR, Russell RI, Patrick RS. Intra-hepatic cholestasis and cutaneous bullae associated with glibenclamide therapy. *Postgrad Med J* 1981; **57**: 244–6.
15 Adams BB, Gadenne AS. Glipizide-induced pigmented purpuric dermatosis. *J Am Acad Dermatol* 1999; **41**: 827–9.

Lipid-lowering drugs

Acipimox

This nicotinic acid analogue causes less prostaglandin-mediated flushing and itching than nicotinic acid [1].

Clofibrate

Erythema multiforme and a variety of other erythematous rashes have been described [2].

Gemfibrozil

This lipid-lowering drug, which mainly lowers triglycerides, has been associated with exacerbation of psoriasis [3,4].

Statins

The lipid-lowering drugs lovastatin, simvastatin and pravastatin can cause eczema [4,5]; these drugs block an early step in cholesterol biosynthesis by inhibiting the activity of 3-hydroxy-3-methylglutaryl coenzyme A (HMG-CoA) reductase. Simvastatin has caused a lichenoid eruption with skin and mucosal involvement [6,7], and chronic actinic dermatitis [8]. Pravastatin has also been associated with a lichenoid rash [9]. Atorvastatin has caused linear IgA bullous dermatosis [10] and TEN [11].

Triparanol and diazacholesterol

These drugs inhibit a late step in cholesterol biosynthesis (Δ^{24} sterol reductase) and can induce ichthyosis or palmoplantar hyperkeratosis [4].

REFERENCES

1 Anonymous. Acipimox: a nicotinic acid analogue for hyperlipidaemia. *Drug Ther Bull* 1991; **29**: 57–9.
2 Murata Y, Tani M, Amano M. Erythema multiforme due to clofibrate. *J Am Acad Dermatol* 1988; **18**: 381–2.
3 Fisher DA, Elias PM, LeBoit PL. Exacerbation of psoriasis by the hypolipidemic agent, gemfibrozil. *Arch Dermatol* 1988; **124**: 854–5.

4 Proksch E. Lipidsenker-induzierte Nebenwirkungen an der Haut. *Hautarzt* 1995; **46**: 76–80.
5 Krasovec M, Elsner P, Burg G. Generalized eczematous skin rash possibly due to HMG-CoA reductase inhibitors. *Dermatology* 1993; **186**: 248–52.
6 Feldmann R, Mainetti C, Saurat JH. Skin lesions due to treatment with simvastatin (Zocor). *Dermatology* 1993; **186**: 272.
7 Roger D, Rolle F, Labrousse F *et al*. Simvastatin-induced lichenoid drug eruption. *Clin Exp Dermatol* 1994; **19**: 88–9.
8 Granados MT, de la Torre C, Cruces MJ, Pineiro G. Chronic actinic dermatitis due to simvastatin. *Contact Dermatitis* 1998; **38**: 294–5.
9 Keough GC, Richardson TT, Grabski WJ. Pravastatin-induced lichenoid drug eruption. *Cutis* 1998; **61**: 98–100.
10 Konig C, Eickert A, Scharfetter-Kochanek K *et al*. Linear IgA bullous dermatosis induced by atorvastatin. *J Am Acad Dermatol* 2001; **44**: 689–92.
11 Pfeiffer CM, Kazenoff S, Rothberg HD. Toxic epidermal necrolysis from atorvastatin. *JAMA* 1998; **279**: 1613–4.

Drugs for gastrointestinal ulceration

Omeprazole

This proton pump inhibitor, a substituted benzimidazole, has gained widespread use in the treatment of gastric and duodenal ulceration and reflux oesophagitis. Adverse events with the drug are rare and involve mainly the gastrointestinal and central nervous systems, with diarrhoea, headache and dizziness, and confusion in the elderly, moderate elevation of aminotransferases and possible leukopenia [1–3]. The prevalence of cutaneous reactions to omeprazole is approximately 0.5–1.5% [1–4]. A variety of eruptions are recorded, including angio-oedema and urticaria [4,5], anaphylaxis [6], maculopapular rashes, lichen planus [7,8], pityriasiform eruption [9], erythema multiforme and erythroderma [10], exfoliative dermatitis [11], bullous eruption [12] and photosensitivity. Gynaecomastia is recorded [13].

Tripotassium dicitratobismuthate (De-Nol)

The Netherlands Centre for Monitoring of Adverse Reactions to Drugs has received several reports of skin reactions, on average 2 days after starting treatment, including maculopapular exanthema, angio-oedema and erythema [14].

Bismuth subsalicylate (PeptoBismol)

Black granules at follicular orifices have been reported [15]. Blue linear pigmentation of the soft palate, oral mucosa and vagina, ulcerative stomatitis, generalized pigmentation, dermatitis and erythroderma are recorded.

REFERENCES

1 McTavish D, Buckley MM, Heel RC. Omeprazole: an update review of its pharmacology and therapeutic use in acid related disorders. *Drugs* 1991; **42**: 138–70.
2 Castot A, Bidault I, Dahan R, Efthymiou ML. Bilan des effects inattendus et toxiques de l'omeprazole (Mopral) rapportés aux centres regionaux de pharmacovigilance, au cours des 22 premiers mois de commercialisation. *Thérapie* 1993; **48**: 469–74.

3 Yeomans ND. Omeprazole: short- and long-term safety. *Adverse Drug React Acute Toxicol Rev* 1994; **13**: 145–56.
4 Bowlby HA, Dickens GR. Angioedema and urticaria associated with omeprazole confirmed by drug rechallenge. *Pharmacotherapy* 1994; **14**: 119–22.
5 Haeney MR. Angio-oedema and urticaria associated with omeprazole. *BMJ* 1992; **305**: 870.
6 Ottervanger JP, Phaff RA, Vermeulen EG, Stricker BH. Anaphylaxis to omeprazole. *J Allergy Clin Immunol* 1996; **97**: 1413–4.
7 Sharma BK, Walt RP, Pounder RE *et al*. Optimal dose of oral omeprazole for maximal 24 hour decrease of intragastric acidity. *Gut* 1984; **25**: 957–64.
8 Bong JL, Lucke TW, Douglas WS. Lichenoid drug eruption with proton pump inhibitors. *BMJ* 2000; **320**: 283.
9 Buckley C. Pityriasis rosea-like eruption in a patient receiving omeprazole. *Br J Dermatol* 1996; **135**: 660–1.
10 Cockayne SE, Glet RJ, Gawkrodger DJ, McDonagh AJ. Severe erythrodermic reactions to the proton pump inhibitors omeprazole and lansoprazole. *Br J Dermatol* 1999; **141**: 173–5.
11 Epelde Gonzalo FD, Boada Montagut L, Thomas Vecina S. Exfoliative dermatitis related to omeprazole. *Ann Pharmacother* 1995; **29**: 82–3.
12 Stenier C, Fiasse R, Bourland J *et al*. Bullous skin reaction induced by omeprazole. *Br J Dermatol* 1995; **133**: 343–4.
13 Lindquist M, Edwards IR. Endocrine effects of omeprazole. *BMJ* 1992; **305**: 451–2.
14 Ottervanger JP, Stricker BH. Huidafwijkingen door bismutoxide (De-Nol). *Ned Tijdschr Geneeskd* 1994; **138**: 152–3.
15 Ruiz-Maldonado R, Contreras-Ruiz J, Sierra-Santoyo A *et al*. Black granules on the skin after bismuth subsalicylate ingestion. *J Am Acad Dermatol* 1997; **37**: 489–90.

Laxatives

Side effects of laxatives have been reviewed [1].

Dantron (danthron)

A highly characteristic irritant erythema of the buttocks and thighs has been observed in patients who are partially incontinent. The erythema results from skin soiling by faecal matter containing an anthralin (dithranol)-like breakdown product [2].

Phenolphthalein

Fixed eruptions are well known [3–5]. Bullous erythema multiforme and an LE-like reaction are documented.

REFERENCES

1 Ruoff H-J. Unerwünschte Wirkungen und Wechselwirkungen von Abführmitteln. *Med Klin* 1980; **75**: 214–8.
2 Barth JH, Reshad H, Darley CR, Gibson JRA. A cutaneous complication of Dorbanex therapy. *Clin Exp Dermatol* 1984; **9**: 95–6.
3 Shelley WB, Schlappner OL, Heiss HB. Demonstration of intercellular immunofluorescence and epidermal hysteresis in bullous fixed drug eruption due to phenolphthalein. *Br J Dermatol* 1972; **6**: 118–25.
4 Wyatt E, Greaves M, Sondergaard J. Fixed drug eruption (phenolphthalein). Evidence for a blood-borne mediator. *Arch Dermatol* 1972; **106**: 671–3.
5 Zanolli MD, McAlvany J, Krowchuk DP. Phenolphthalein-induced fixed drug eruption: a cutaneous complication of laxative use in a child. *Pediatrics* 1993; **91**: 1199–201.

Miscellaneous drugs

Food and drug additives

Dermatological complications of food and drug additives

have been reviewed [1–14]. These substances have been implicated in the causation of urticaria [4–7], anaphylaxis, purpura and vasculitis [8–12]. However, one study suggested that common food additives are seldom if ever of significance in urticaria [11]. In another study, only 0.63% of food additive provocation tests resulted in exacerbation in 1110 patients with urticaria; tests were again not positive on re-provocation [13]. The prevalence of adverse reactions to food additives is estimated to be 0.03–0.23% [15]. The necessity for double-blind, placebo-controlled testing to substantiate alleged food additive allergy has been emphasized [16]. Information about excipients ('inert ingredients') has been reported in a study that examined the sweeteners, flavourings, dyes and preservatives present in chewable and liquid preparations of 102 over-the-counter and prescription brands of antidiarrhoeal, cough and cold, antihistamine/decongestant, analgesic/antipyretic and liquid theophylline medications [17]. An average preparation contained two sweeteners, primarily saccharin and sucrose, followed by sorbitol, glucose, fructose and others. The type of flavouring was not specified in 36 of the 102 preparations; cherry was the most common flavouring, followed by vanilla and lemon. Twenty-one different dyes and colouring agents were used; red dye no. 40 was the most common, followed by yellow no. 6. Sodium benzoate and methylparabens were the commonest of eight preservatives used. Mandatory labelling of excipients in all pharmaceutical preparations is the only way that physicians and patients can be fully informed [17]. It is important to appreciate that peanut oil, to which patients may be strongly allergic, is found in certain medications [18]. Caffeine in coffee and cola beverages caused urticaria in a 10-year-old child, confirmed by prick test and oral challenge test with caffeine [19].

REFERENCES

1 Levantine AJ, Almeyda J. Cutaneous reactions to food and drug additives. *Br J Dermatol* 1977; **91**: 359–62.
2 Simon RA. Adverse reactions to drug additives. *J Allergy Clin Immunol* 1984; **74**: 623–30.
3 Ruzicka T. Diagnostik von Nahrungsmittelallergien. *Hautarzt* 1987; **38**: 10–5.
4 Juhlin LG, Michäelsson G, Zetterström O. Urticaria and asthma induced by food-and-drug additives in patients with aspirin hypersensitivity. *J Allergy* 1972; **50**: 92–8.
5 Doeglas HMG. Reactions to aspirin and food additives in patients with chronic urticaria, including the physical urticarias. *Br J Dermatol* 1975; **93**: 135–44.
6 Supramaniam G, Warner JO. Artificial food additive intolerance in patients with angio-oedema and urticaria. *Lancet* 1986; **ii**: 907–9.
7 Juhlin L. Additives and chronic urticaria. *Ann Allergy* 1987; **59**: 119–23.
8 Michäelsson G, Petterson L, Juhlin L. Purpura caused by food and drug additives. *Arch Dermatol* 1974; **109**: 49–52.
9 Kubba R, Champion RI. Anaphylactoid purpura caused by tartrazine and benzoates. *Br J Dermatol* 1975; **93** (Suppl. 2): 61–2.
10 Eisenmann A, Ring J, von der Helm D *et al.* Vasculitis allergica durch Nahrungsmittelallergie. *Hautarzt* 1988; **39**: 319–21.
11 Veien NK, Krogdahl A. Cutaneous vasculitis induced by food additives. *Acta Derm Venereol (Stockh)* 1991; **71**: 73–4.
12 Lowry MD, Hudson CF, Callen FP. Leukocytoclastic vasculitis caused by drug additives. *J Am Acad Dermatol* 1994; **30**: 854–5.
13 Hernandez Garcia J, Garcia Selles J, Negro Alvarez JM *et al.* Incidencias de reacciones adversas con aditivos. Nuestra experiencia de 10 anos. *Allergol Immunopathol* 1994; **22**: 233–42.
14 Barbaud A. Place of excipients in drug-related allergy. *Clin Rev Allergy Immunol* 1995; **13**: 253–63.
15 Wuthrich B. Adverse reactions to food additives. *Ann Allergy* 1993; **71**: 379–84.
16 Goodman DL, McDonnell JT, Nelson HS *et al.* Chronic urticaria exacerbated by the antioxidant food preservatives, butylated hydroxyanisole (BHA) and butylated hydroxytoluene (BHT). *J Allergy Clin Immunol* 1990; **86**: 570–5.
17 Kumar A, Rawlings RD, Beaman DC. The mystery ingredients: sweeteners, flavorings, dyes, and preservatives in analgesic/antipyretic, antihistamine/decongestant, cough and cold, antidiarrheal, and liquid theophylline preparations. *Pediatrics* 1993; **91**: 927–33.
18 Weeks R. Peanut oil in medications. *Lancet* 1996; **348**: 759–60.
19 Caballero T, Garcia-Ara C, Pascual C *et al.* Urticaria induced by caffeine. *J Invest Allergol Clin Immunol* 1993; **3**: 160–2.

Colouring agents

Colourings in food and medications (including some antihistamines), such as tartrazine, sunset yellow and other azo dyes, have been reported to cause adverse reactions [1,2], including urticaria [3,4] or vasculitis [5,6].

REFERENCES

1 Vandelle C, Belegaud D, Bidault I, Castol A. Allergie aux colorants des medicaments. Confrontation des cas publiés et de l'experience du Centre Regional de Pharmacovigilance. *Thérapie* 1993; **48**: 484–5.
2 Gracey-Whitman L, Ell S. Artificial colourings and adverse reactions. *BMJ* 1995; **311**: 1204.
3 Neuman I, Elian R, Nahum H *et al.* The danger of 'yellow dyes' (tartrazine) to allergic subjects. *J Allergy* 1972; **50**: 92–8.
4 Miller K. Sensitivity to tartrazine. *BMJ* 1982; **285**: 1597–8.
5 Lowry MD, Hudson CF, Callen FP. Leukocytoclastic vasculitis caused by drug additives. *J Am Acad Dermatol* 1994; **30**: 854–5.
6 Wuthrich B. Adverse reactions to food additives. *Ann Allergy* 1993; **71**: 379–84.

Flavouring agents

Aspartame. Aspartame, a synthetic dipeptide composed of aspartic acid and the methyl ester of phenylalanine and used under the trade name of NutraSweet (G.D. Searle & Co., Skokie, Illinois, USA) as a low-calorie artificial sweetener, has been associated with relatively few adverse side effects despite its widespread use [1]. Cutaneous side effects reported include urticaria, angio-oedema and other nondescript 'rashes' [2], granulomatous septal panniculitis [3] and lobular panniculitis [4]. However, in a recent study of patients with a history of aspartame sensitivity, it was not possible to identify any subject with a clearly reproducible adverse reaction [5]. Similarly, a multicentre, placebo-controlled, challenge study showed that aspartame and its conversion products are no more likely than placebo to cause urticaria and/or angio-oedema reactions in subjects with a history consistent with hypersensitivity to aspartame [6].

Cyclamates. Cyclamates, used as sweeteners in soft drinks, have caused photosensitivity [7].

Quinine. Quinine in tonic water and other bitter drinks may cause fixed eruptions [8].

REFERENCES

1 US Food and Drug Administration. Food additives permitted for direct addition to food for human consumption: aspartame. *Federal Register* 1983; **48**: 31376–82.
2 Kulczycki A Jr. Aspartame-induced urticaria. *Ann Intern Med* 1986; **104**: 207–8.
3 Novick NL. Aspartame-induced granulomatous panniculitis. *Ann Intern Med* 1985; **102**: 206–7.
4 McCauliffe DP, Poitras K. Aspartame-induced lobular panniculitis. *J Am Acad Dermatol* 1991; **24**: 298–300.
5 Garriga MM, Berkebile C, Metcalfe DD. A combined single-blind, double-blind, placebo-controlled study to determine the reproducibility of hypersensitivity reactions to aspartame. *J Allergy Clin Immunol* 1991; **87**: 821–7.
6 Geha R, Buckley CE, Greenberger P *et al.* Aspartame is no more likely than placebo to cause urticaria/angioedema: results of a multicenter, randomized, double-blind, placebo-controlled, crossover study. *J Allergy Clin Immunol* 1993; **92**: 513–20.
7 Lambert SI. A new photosensitizer. The artificial sweetener cyclamate. *JAMA* 1967; **201**: 747–50.
8 Commens C. Fixed drug eruption. *Aust J Dermatol* 1983; **24**: 1–8.

Preservatives

The antioxidant food preservatives butylated hydroxyanisole (BHA) and butylated hydroxytoluene (BHT) have been reported to exacerbate chronic urticaria [1]. Sodium benzoate has been associated with urticaria, angio-oedema, asthma and rarely anaphylaxis [2]. Parabens used as preservatives may also cause urticaria [3].

Sulphiting agents are commonly used in parenteral emergency drugs, including epinephrine (adrenaline), dexamethasone, dobutamine, dopamine, norepinephrine (noradrenaline), phenylephrine, procainamide and physostigmine [4]. Published anaphylactic or asthmatic reactions have been associated with sulphited local anaesthetics, gentamicin, metoclopramide, doxycycline and vitamin B complex. The reactions have a rapid onset and do not always coincide with a positive oral challenge, although patients with a history of positive oral challenge to 5–10 mg of sulphite may be at increased risk of developing a reaction to parenteral sulphites. Sulphites added as antioxidant preservatives may provoke urticaria, asthma, anaphylaxis and shock [4–10], as well as urticarial vasculitis [11]. Intolerance due to metabisulphite as an antioxidant in a dental anaesthetic has led to angio-oedema; patch tests were positive [12]. Basophil activation induced by sulphites may be IgE dependent [13]. It has been claimed that there is a high specificity of patch testing in the diagnosis of patients with sulphite sensitivity [14].

REFERENCES

1 Goodman DL, McDonnell JT, Nelson HS *et al.* Chronic urticaria exacerbated by the antioxidant food preservatives, butylated hydroxyanisole (BHA) and butylated hydroxytoluene (BHT). *J Allergy Clin Immunol* 1990; **86**: 570–5.
2 Michils A, Vandermoten G, Duchateau J, Yernault J-C. Anaphylaxis with sodium benzoate. *Lancet* 1991; **337**: 1424–5.
3 Nagel JE, Fuscaldo JT, Fireman P. Paraben allergy. *JAMA* 1977; **237**: 1594–5.
4 Smolinske SC. Review of parenteral sulfite reactions. *J Toxicol Clin Toxicol* 1992; **30**: 597–606.
5 Habenicht HA, Preuss L, Lovell RG. Sensitivity to ingested metabisulfites: cause of bronchospasm and urticaria. *Immunol Allergy Pract* 1983; **5**: 243–5.
6 Settipane GA. Adverse reactions to sulfites in drugs and foods. *J Am Acad Dermatol* 1984; **10**: 1077–80.
7 Belchi-Hernandez J, Florido-Lopez JF, Estrada-Rodriguez JL *et al.* Sulfite-induced urticaria. *Ann Allergy* 1993; **71**: 230–2.
8 Twarog FJ, Leung DYM. Anaphylaxis to a component of isoetharine (sodium bisulfite). *JAMA* 1982; **248**: 2030–1.
9 Przybilla B, Ring J. Sulfit-Überempfindlichkeit. *Hautarzt* 1987; **38**: 445–8.
10 Hassoun S, Bonneau JC, Drouet M, Sabbah A. Enquete sur pathologies induites par les sulfites en allergologie. *Allerg Immunol* 1994; **26**: 184, 187–8.
11 Wuthrich B. Adverse reactions to food additives. *Ann Allergy* 1993; **71**: 379–84.
12 Dooms-Goosens A, Gidi de Alan A, Degreef H, Kochuyt A. Local anaesthetic intolerance due to metabisulfite. *Contact Dermatitis* 1989; **20**: 124–6.
13 Sainte-Laudy J, Vallon C, Guerin JC. Mise en evidence des IgE specifiques du groupe des sulfites chez les intolerants à ces conservateurs. *Allerg Immunol* 1994; **26**: 132–4, 137–8.
14 Gay G, Sabbah A, Drouet M. Valeur diagnostique de l'epidermotest aux sulfites. *Allerg Immunol* 1994; **26**: 139–40.

Miscellaneous food additives

Agricultural or veterinary chemicals may leave residues in animals and plants used as human food, for example penicillin in milk or meat, with resultant urticaria [1,2]. The exposure of a rural Turkish population to flour contaminated with hexachlorobenzene induced an outbreak of cutaneous porphyria [3]. Contaminated rapeseed cooking oil containing acetanilide resulted in the Spanish 'toxic oil syndrome'; the central feature of the illness was a toxic pneumonitis, but fixed rashes and scleroderma-like changes in survivors were seen [4–6]. Outbreaks of atypical erythema multiforme and other exanthems in the Netherlands were attributed to an additive in margarine [7,8]. The high arsenic content of a rural water supply in Taiwan caused arsenicism [9]. Chemicals added to tobacco, for example menthol in cigarettes, have caused urticaria [10]. *N*-Nitroso compounds, which are known to be carcinogenic in animals, occur in food products and certain alcoholic drinks, but there is no direct proof as yet of a causal role in human disease [11].

REFERENCES

1 Boonk WJ, Van Ketel WG. The role of penicillin in the pathogenesis of chronic urticaria. *Br J Dermatol* 1982; **106**: 183–90.
2 Kanny G, Puygrenier J, Beaudoin E, Moneret-Vautrin DA. Choc anaphylactique alimentaire: implication des residus de penicilline. *Allerg Immunol* 1994; **26**: 181–3.
3 Peters HA, Gocmen A, Cripps DJ *et al.* Epidemiology of hexachlorobenzene-induced porphyria in Turkey. *Arch Neurol* 1982; **39**: 744–9.
4 Martinez-Tello FJ, Navas-Palacios JJ, Ricoy JR *et al.* Pathology of a new toxic syndrome caused by ingestion of adulterated oil in Spain. *Virchows Arch A* 1982; **397**: 261–85.
5 Anonymous. Toxic oil syndrome. *Lancet* 1983; i: 1257–8.
6 Rush PJ, Bell MJ, Fam AG. Toxic oil syndrome (Spanish oil disease) and chemically induced scleroderma-like conditions. *J Rheumatol* 1984; **11**: 262–4.

7 Sternberg TH, Bierman SM. Unique syndromes involving the skin induced by drugs, food additives, and environmental contaminants. *Arch Dermatol* 1963; **88**: 779–88.

8 Mali JW, Malten KE. The epidemic of polymorphic toxic erythema in the Netherlands in 1960. The so-called margarine disease. *Acta Derm Venereol (Stockh)* 1966; **46**: 123–35.

9 Yeh S. Skin cancer in chronic arsenicism. *Hum Pathol* 1973; **4**: 469–85.

10 McGowan EM. Menthol urticaria. *Arch Dermatol* 1966; **94**: 62–3.

11 Tannenbaum SR. N-nitroso compounds: a perspective on human exposure. *Lancet* 1983; i: 628–30.

Herbal remedies, homeopathy and naturopathy (alternative therapy)

Adverse cutaneous effects of herbal drugs have been reviewed [1–4]. Virtually all herbal remedies may cause allergic reactions, and several cause photosensitization. Some herbal medicines, particularly Ayurvedic remedies, contain arsenic or mercury that may produce typical skin lesions. Other popular remedies that can cause dermatological side effects include St John's wort, kava, aloe vera, eucalyptus, camphor, henna and yohimbine. In addition, some herbal treatments used specifically for dermatological conditions, for example Chinese oral herbal remedies for atopic eczema, have been reported to cause systemic adverse effects. There is concern that some agents, notably Chinese herbal creams, have been shown repeatedly to be adulterated with corticosteroids [5,6].

REFERENCES

1 Monk B. Severe cutaneous reactions to alternative remedies. *BMJ* 1986; **293**: 665–6.

2 Ernst E. Adverse effects of herbal drugs in dermatology. *Br J Dermatol* 2000; **143**: 923–9.

3 Ernst E. The usage of complementary therapies by dermatological patients: a systematic review. *Br J Dermatol* 2000; **143**: 857–61.

4 Bedi MK, Shenefelt PD. Herbal therapy in dermatology. *Arch Dermatol* 2002; **138**: 232–42.

5 But PPH. Herbal poisoning caused by adulterants or erroneous substitutes. *J Trop Med Hyg* 1994; **97**: 371–4.

6 Bircher AJ, Hauri U, Niederer M *et al.* Stealth triamcinolone acetonide in a phytocosmetic cream. *Br J Dermatol* 2002; **146**: 531–2.

Chinese herbal medicine

Adverse effects of Chinese herbal medicines, including life-threatening 'dazao'-induced angio-oedema and liquorice-induced hypokalaemic periodic paralysis, accounted for 0.2% of medical admissions to a hospital in Hong Kong over an 8-month period [1]. Herbal poisoning in Hong Kong, Taipei and Kuala Lumpur has occurred as a result of addition of adulterants (*Podophyllum emodi*) or erroneous substitutes (*Datura metel*) [2]. A fatality due to total liver necrosis associated with ingestion of Chinese herbal medicines is believed to have occurred because the patient prepared a decoction from a herbal mixture containing *Eurysolen gracilis* Prain (Labiatae), a herb not used in Chinese medicine [3]. A multisystem illness developed in a patient after ingestion of Chinese herbal medicines

containing the potentially toxic compounds benzaldehyde, cinnamoyl alcohol and ephedrine [4]. Some Chinese patent medicines contain mercurial ingredients, cinnabar (red mercuric sulphide) and calomel (mercurous chloride) [5]. Alopecia and sensory polyneuropathy from thallium in a Chinese herbal medication has been reported [6]. Cutaneous aspects of thallium poisoning include palmar and plantar scaling, acneiform lesions on the face and diffuse alopecia, accompanied by acute nervous system and gastrointestinal symptoms [7]. Chinese herbal medicine may contain camouflaged prescription anti-inflammatory drugs, corticosteroids and lead [8], and some practitioners of Chinese medicine supply 'herbal creams' that actually contain potent topical steroid ointments [9,10]. Fixed drug eruption has been documented with use of a Chinese traditional herbal medicine containing mainly pseudo-ephedrine and ephedrine [11].

There are major concerns about hepatotoxicity [12–16] and nephrotoxicity [17–23] with Chinese herbal medicine. In one case, hepatotoxicity was associated with ingestion of the Chinese herbal product jin bu huan anodyne tablets (*Lycopodium serratum*) [14]. A rapidly progressive fibrosing interstitial nephritis developed in young women who followed the same slimming regimen containing two Chinese herbs (*Stephania tetrandra* and *Magnolia officinalis*) [17–19]. The known carcinogen, aristolochic acid, has been suspected in some cases of nephropathy [19,20]. Urothelial malignancy has supervened [22]. Acquired Fanconi's syndrome was induced by a mixture of Chinese crude drugs [23].

The need for correct identification of herbs in herbal poisoning [24], and for monitoring of the safety of herbal medicines [25], has been emphasized. Greater awareness of their toxicity is required [26,27]. Special licensing of herbal remedies exists in Germany, France and Australia and has been advocated in the UK [28].

Analgesic and anti-inflammatory Chinese medicinal materials, especially those containing fragrance, may cause contact sensitization and can cause systemic contact dermatitis [29,30]. Erythema multiforme [30], exanthem [31] and erythroderma [32] are described. Fever with oedematous erythema was caused by a decoction of the crude drug Boi of Kampo (Sino-Japanese traditional) medicine for the alleviation of arthralgia; oral ingestion tests incriminated the constituent sinomenine [33].

A 'tea' prepared from a decoction of herbs has been reported to be of benefit in eczema [34,35]. The decoction contains paenol (2'-hydroxy-4'-methoxyacetophenone), which is known to have platelet antiaggregatory, analgesic and antipyretic properties [36]. Hepatotoxicity was described in a 9-year-old girl who consumed a Chinese herbal tea for 6 months [37] and was reported in a further patient [38]. Reversible abnormal liver function tests have been reported in two children receiving Chinese herbal therapy (Zemaphyte) [39]. Toxicology screening in a group of adults on Zemaphyte for 1 year revealed no abnormalities in haematological or biochemical parameters; transient nausea and abdominal distension, with a mild laxative effect, was noted in about one-third of patients [40]. Dilated cardiomyopathy followed therapy of atopic eczema with Chinese herbal medicine [41].

REFERENCES

1 Chan TY, Chan AY, Critchley JA. Hospital admissions due to adverse reactions to Chinese herbal medicines. *J Trop Med Hyg* 1992; **95**: 296–8.
2 But PP. Herbal poisoning caused by adulterants or erroneous substitutes. *J Trop Med Hyg* 1994; **947**: 371–4.
3 Perharic-Walton L, Murray V. Toxicity of Chinese herbal remedies. *Lancet* 1992; **340**: 674.
4 Gorey JD, Wahlqvist ML, Boyce NW. Adverse reaction to a Chinese herbal remedy. *Med J Aust* 1992; **157**: 484–6.
5 Kang-Yum E, Oransky SH. Chinese patent medicine as a potential source of mercury poisoning. *Vet Hum Toxicol* 1992; **34**: 235–8.
6 Schaumburg HH, Berger A. Alopecia and sensory polyneuropathy from thallium in a Chinese herbal medication. *JAMA* 1992; **268**: 3430–1.
7 Tromme I, Van Neste D, Dobbelaere F *et al.* Skin signs in the diagnosis of thallium poisoning. *Br J Dermatol* 1998; **138**: 321–5.
8 Goldman JA, Myerson G. Chinese herbal medicine: camouflaged prescription anti-inflammatory drugs, corticosteroids, and lead. *Arthritis Rheum* 1991; **34**: 1207.
9 Allen BR, Parkinson R. Chinese herbs for eczema. *Lancet* 1990; **336**: 177.
10 O'Driscoll J, Burden AD, Kingston TP. Potent topical steroid obtained from a Chinese herbalist. *Br J Dermatol* 1992; **127**: 543–4.
11 Matsumoto K, Mikoshiba H, Saida T. Nonpigmenting solitary fixed drug eruption caused by a Chinese traditional herbal medicine, ma huang (*Ephedra hebra*), mainly containing pseudoephedrine and ephedrine. *J Am Acad Dermatol* 2003; **48**: 628–30.
12 Mostefa-Kara N, Pauwels A, Pinus E *et al.* Fatal hepatitis after herbal tea. *Lancet* 1992; **340**: 674.
13 Graham-Brown R. Toxicity of Chinese herbal remedies. *Lancet* 1992; **340**: 673.
14 Woolf GM, Petrovic LM, Rojter SE *et al.* Acute hepatitis associated with the Chinese herbal product jin bu huan. *Ann Intern Med* 1994; **121**: 729–35.
15 Pillans PI. Toxicity of herbal products. *NZ Med J* 1995; **108**: 469–71.
16 Larrey D, Pageaux GP. Hepatotoxicity of herbal remedies and mushrooms. *Semin Liver Dis* 1995; **15**: 183–8.
17 Vanherweghem JL, Depierreux M, Tielemans C *et al.* Rapidly progressive interstitial renal fibrosis in young women: association with slimming regimen including Chinese herbs. *Lancet* 1993; **341**: 387–91.
18 Depierreux M, Van Damme B, Vanden Houte K, Vanherweghem JL. Pathologic aspects of a newly described nephropathy related to the prolonged use of Chinese herbs. *Am J Kidney Dis* 1994; **24**: 172–80.
19 Cosyns JP, Jadoul M, Squifflet JP *et al.* Chinese herbs nephropathy: a clue to Balkan endemic nephropathy? *Kidney Int* 1994; **45**: 1680–8.
20 Vanhaelen M, Vanhaelen-Fastre R, But P, Vanherweghem JL. Identification of aristolochic acid in Chinese herbs. *Lancet* 1994; **343**: 174.
21 Diamond JR, Pallone TL. Acute interstitial nephritis following use of tung shueh pills. *Am J Kidney Dis* 1994; **24**: 219–21.
22 Cosyns JP, Jadoul M, Squifflet JP *et al.* Urothelial malignancy in nephropathy due to Chinese herbs. *Lancet* 1994; **344**: 188.
23 Izumotani T, Ishimura E, Tsumura K *et al.* An adult case of Fanconi syndrome due to a mixture of Chinese crude drugs. *Nephron* 1993; **65**: 137–40.
24 But PP. Need for correct identification of herbs in herbal poisoning. *Lancet* 1993; **341**: 637.
25 Mills SY. Monitoring the safety of herbal remedies. European pilot studies are under way. *BMJ* 1995; **311**: 1570.
26 Atherton DJ. Towards the safer use of traditional remedies. Greater awareness of toxicity is needed. *BMJ* 1994; **308**: 673–4.
27 Harper J. Traditional Chinese medicine for eczema. Seemingly effective, but caution must prevail. *BMJ* 1994; **308**: 489–90.
28 De Smet PAGM. Should herbal medicine-like products be licensed as medicines? Special licensing seems the best way forward. *BMJ* 1995; **310**: 1023–4.
29 Li LF. A clinical and patch test study of contact dermatitis from traditional Chinese medicinal materials. *Contact Dermatitis* 1995; **33**: 392–5.
30 Mateo MP, Velasco M, Miquel FJ, de la Cuadra J. Erythema-multiforme-like eruption following allergic contact dermatitis from sesquiterpene lactones in herbal medicine. *Contact Dermatitis* 1995; **33**: 449–50.
31 Li LF, Zhao J, Li SY. Exanthematous drug eruption due to Chinese herbal medicines sanjieling capsule and huoxuexiaoyan pill. *Contact Dermatitis* 1994; **30**: 252–3.
32 Catlin DH, Sekera M, Adelman DC. Erythroderma associated with ingestion of an herbal product. *West J Med* 1993; **159**: 491–3.
33 Okuda T, Umezawa Y, Ichikawa M *et al.* A case of drug eruption caused by the crude drug Boi (*Sinomenium* stem/Sinomeni caulis et Rhizoma). *J Dermatol* 1995; **22**: 795–800.
34 Atherton D, Sheehan M, Rustin MHA *et al.* Chinese herbs for eczema. *Lancet* 1990; **336**: 1254.
35 Sheehan MP, Atherton DJ, Luo HD. Controlled trial of traditional Chinese medicinal plants in widespread non-exudative atopic eczema (abstract). *Br J Dermatol* 1991; **125** (Suppl. 38): 17.
36 Galloway JH, Marsh ID, Bittner SB *et al.* Chinese herbs for eczema, the active compound? *Lancet* 1991; **337**: 566.
37 Davies EG, Pollock I, Steel HM. Chinese herbs for eczema. *Lancet* 1990; **336**: 177.
38 Carlsson C. Herbs and hepatitis. *Lancet* 1990; **336**: 1068.
39 Sheehan MP, Atherton DJ. One year follow-up of children with atopic eczema treated with traditional Chinese medicinal plants. *Br J Dermatol* 1992; **127** (Suppl. 40): 13.
40 Sheehan MP, Stevens H, Ostlere LS *et al.* Follow-up of adult patients with atopic eczema treated with Chinese herbal therapy for 1 year. *Clin Exp Dermatol* 1995; **20**: 136–40.
41 Ferguson JE, Chalmers RJG, Rowlands DJ. Reversible dilated cardiomyopathy following treatment of atopic eczema with Chinese herbal medicine. *Br J Dermatol* 1997; **136**: 592–3.

Kava dermopathy

The kava plant, a member of the black-pepper family, is used ceremonially by many traditional societies of the southern Pacific in the form of an intoxicant beverage prepared from roots to induce relaxation and sociability and promote sleep. Herbal drugs containing kava have been used for insomnia, nervousness and depression. A reversible ichthyosiform kava dermopathy resulted from excessive use of kava [1,2]. Systemic contact-type dermatitis occurred after oral administration of kava extract [2].

REFERENCES

1 Norton SA, Ruze P. Kava dermopathy. *J Am Acad Dermatol* 1994; **31**: 89–97.
2 Suss R, Lehmann P. Hamatogenes Kontaktekzem durch pflanzliche Medikamente am Beispiel des Kavawurzel-extraktes. *Hautarzt* 1996; **47**: 459–61.

Homeopathic drugs

Cases of erythroderma, confluent urticaria and anaphylaxis have been reported following homeopathic medication [1]. Treatment of a diaper dermatitis and mild respiratory and enteral infections with the homeopathic mercurial medicine Mercurius 6a (cinnabar dilute 1 × 10(6)) was followed by dissemination of the dermatitis, irritability and albuminuria [2]. Baboon syndrome was associated with use of a homeopathic medicine containing mercury [3].

REFERENCES

1 Aberer W, Strohal R. Homeopathic preparations: severe adverse effects, unproven benefits. *Dermatologica* 1991; **182**: 253.
2 Montoya-Cabrera MA, Rubio-Rodriguez S, Velazquez-Gonzalez E, Avila Montoya S. Intoxicacion mercurial causada por un medicamento homeopatico. *Gaceta Med Mex* 1991; **127**: 267–70.
3 Audicana M, Bernedo N, Gonzalez I *et al*. An unusual case of baboon syndrome due to mercury present in a homeopathic medicine. *Contact Dermatitis* 2001; **45**: 185.

Naturopathy

Bizarre and unpredictable cutaneous reactions may follow topical application or ingestion of naturally occurring substances. A curious gyrate erythematous eruption was seen in a patient following local application of onion rings as a home remedy for arthralgia [1]. Substantial amounts of psoralen may be absorbed from vegetables; a patient who consumed a large quantity of celery root (*Apium graveolens*) 1 h before a visit to a suntan parlour developed a severe generalized phototoxic reaction [2]. A bullous phototoxic reaction developed after exposure to aerosolized bergamot aromatherapy oil in a sauna and subsequent UVA radiation in a tanning salon [3]. Phyto-photodermatitis followed application of *Citrus hystrix* as a mosquito repellent [4]. Phototoxicity has been reported from herbal remedies for vitiligo incorporating powdered seeds of *Psoralea corylifolia*, which contains psoralen, isopsoralen and psoralidin [5].

Contact sensitization has been caused by alternative topical medicaments containing plant extracts [6–9], including tea-tree oil [7,8], which has also caused systemic contact dermatitis [7]; allergic airborne contact dermatitis has been caused by benzaldehyde, eucalyptus oil, laurel oil, pomerance flower oil, lavender oil, rosewood oil and jasmine oil used for aromatherapy [9]. Application of henna as a decoration may cause allergic contact eczema [10]. A diffuse morbilliform eruption occurred with a *Gingko biloba* supplement [11], recurrent erythema nodosum with *Echinacea* therapy [12], erythroderma with intake of St John's wort (*Hypericum perforatum*) [13], and tea-tree oil dermatitis has been associated with linear IgA disease [14].

REFERENCES

1 Breathnach SM, Hintner H. *Adverse Drug Reactions and the Skin*. Oxford: Blackwell Scientific Publications, 1992.
2 Ljunggren B. Severe phototoxic burn following celery ingestion. *Arch Dermatol* 1990; **126**: 1334–6.
3 Kaddu S, Kerl H, Wolf P. Accidental bullous phototoxic reactions to bergamot aromatherapy oil. *J Am Acad Dermatol* 2001; **45**: 458–61.
4 Koh D, Ong C-N. Phytophotodermatitis due to the application of *Citrus hystrix* as a folk remedy. *Br J Dermatol* 1999; **140**: 737–8.
5 Maurice PDL, Cream JJ. The dangers of herbalism. *BMJ* 1989; **299**: 1204.
6 Bruynzeel DP, van Ketel WG, Young E *et al*. Contact sensitization by alternative topical medicaments containing plant extracts. The Dutch Contact Dermatoses Group. *Contact Dermatitis* 1992; **27**: 278–9.
7 de Groot AC, Weyland JW. Systemic contact dermatitis from tea tree oil. *Contact Dermatitis* 1992; **27**: 279–80.
8 Knight TE, Hausen BM. *Melaleuca* oil (tea tree oil) dermatitis. *J Am Acad Dermatol* 1994; **30**: 423–7.
9 Schaller M, Korting HC. Allergic airborne contact dermatitis from essential oils used in aromatherapy. *Clin Exp Dermatol* 1995; **20**: 143–5.
10 Lestringant GG, Bener A, Frossard PM. Cutaneous reactions to henna and associated additives. *Br J Dermatol* 1999; **141**: 598–600.
11 Chiu AE, Lane AT, Kimball AB. Diffuse morbilliform eruption after consumption of *Ginkgo biloba* supplement. *J Am Acad Dermatol* 2002; **46**: 145–6.
12 Soon SL, Crawford RI. Recurrent erythema nodosum associated with *Echinacea* herbal therapy. *J Am Acad Dermatol* 2001; **44**: 298–9.
13 Holme SA, Roberts DL. Erythroderma associated with St John's wort. *Br J Dermatol* 2000; **143**: 1127–8.
14 Perett CM, Evans AV, Russell-Jones R. Tea tree oil dermatitis associated with linear IgA disease. *Clin Exp Dermatol* 2003; **28**: 167–70.

Miscellaneous

Canthaxanthin, a synthetic non-provitamin A carotenoid deposited in epidermis and subcutaneous fat, caused fatal aplastic anaemia when ingested to promote tanning [1].

REFERENCE

1 Bluhm R, Branch R, Johnston P, Stein R. Aplastic anemia associated with canthaxanthin ingested for 'tanning' purposes. *JAMA* 1990; **264**: 1141–2.

Industrial and other exposure to chemicals

For a discussion of sclerodermatous reactions to environmental agents, see p. 73.44. A form of fluoride toxicity occurred due to industrial poisoning in the Italian town of Chizzolo, resulting in pinkish brown, round or oval macules seen in hundreds of the local population [1]. Similar small outbreaks have occurred in North America [2]. Exfoliative dermatitis has been recorded with trichloroethylene [3]. Occupational exposure to trichloroethylene has also caused Stevens–Johnson syndrome [4].

Patients exposed to dioxin after an industrial accident at Seveso, Italy developed early irritative lesions, comprising erythema and oedema of exposed areas, vesicobullous and necrotic lesions of the palms and fingertips, and papulonodular lesions; later lesions were those of chloracne [5]. Contamination of rice-bran cooking oil with polychlorinated biphenyls in Taiwan resulted in chloracne, and congenital abnormalities in offspring [6].

Pruritus, urticaria, and discoid and diffuse eczema may occur following the use of brominated disinfectant compounds such as 1-bromo-3-chlor-5,5-dimethylhydantoin (Di-halo, Aquabrome) in public swimming pools [7]. Accidental occupational exposure to high concentrations of methyl bromide during a fumigation procedure resulted in erythema with multiple vesicles and large bullae, with predilection for moist flexures and pressure areas [8]. Idiopathic thrombocytopenic purpura has been associated with industrial exposure to wood preservatives [9], turpentine [10], and to insecticides such as chlordane and heptachlor [11]. Reversible alopecia occurred with occupational exposure to borax-containing solutions [12].

REFERENCES

1 Waldbott GC, Cecilioni VA. 'Chizzolo' maculae. *Cutis* 1970; **6**: 331–4.
2 Tabuenca JM. Toxic–allergic syndrome caused by ingestion of rapeseed oil denatured with aniline. *Lancet* 1981; **ii**: 567–8.
3 Nakayama H, Kobayashi M, Takahashi M *et al.* Generalized eruption with severe liver dysfunction associated with occupational exposure to trichloroethylene. *Contact Dermatitis* 1988; **19**: 48–51.
4 Phoon WH, Chan MOY, Rahan VS *et al.* Stevens–Johnson syndrome associated with occupational exposure to trichloroethylene. *Contact Dermatitis* 1984; **10**: 270–6.
5 Caputo R, Monti M, Ermacora E *et al.* Cutaneous manifestations of tetrachlorodibenzo-*p*-dioxin in children and adolescents. *J Am Acad Dermatol* 1988; **19**: 812–9.
6 Gladen BC, Taylor JS, Wu Y-C *et al.* Dermatological findings in children exposed transplacentally to heat-degraded polychlorinated biphenyls in Taiwan. *Br J Dermatol* 1990; **122**: 799–808.
7 Rycroft RJG, Penny PT. Dermatoses associated with brominated swimming pools. *BMJ* 1983; **28**: 462.
8 Hezemans-Boer M, Toonstra J, Meulenbelt J *et al.* Skin lesions due to exposure to methyl bromide. *Arch Dermatol* 1988; **124**: 917–21.
9 Hay A, Singer CRJ. Wood preservatives, solvents, and thrombocytopenic purpura. *Lancet* 1991; **338**: 766.
10 Wahlberg P, Nyman D. Turpentine and thrombocytopenic purpura. *Lancet* 1969; **ii**: 215–6.
11 Epstein SS, Ozonoff D. Leukemias and blood dyscrasias following exposure to chloradone and heptachlor. *Carcinogen Mutagen Teratogen* 1987; **7**: 527–40.
12 Beckett WS, Oskvig R, Gaynor ME, Goldgeier MH. Association of reversible alopecia with occupational topical exposure to common borax-containing solutions. *J Am Acad Dermatol* 2001; **44**: 599–602.

Local and systemic effects of topical applications

Many topical therapeutic agents may cause serious or even dangerous systemic side effects if absorbed in sufficient quantity; such absorption may be facilitated through diseased skin, and with use of newer vehicles or occlusive polythene dressings. The risk of serious systemic effects is greatest in infancy and in the old and frail. The quantity absorbed in relation to body weight is greatest in infancy, when the surface area is relatively greater; moreover, neonatal skin is more permeable. Most dangerous or fatal reactions have occurred because either the physician was unaware of the potential hazard or the patient continued self-treatment without medical supervision.

Topical therapy

Anthralin (dithranol)

Topical anthralin, used in the therapy of stable plaque psoriasis, is well known for causing erythema, irritation and a sensation of burning in normal skin; it stains the skin and clothing [1]. Application of 10% triethanolamine following short-contact anthralin treatment has been reported to inhibit anthralin-induced inflammation without preventing the therapeutic effect [2]. Allergic contact dermatitis to anthralin is very rare. The natural and syn-

thetic anthranols have toxic effects on liver, intestines and the central nervous system, but systemic toxicity in humans under therapeutic conditions has not been established [3].

REFERENCES

1 Paramsothy Y, Lawrence CM. Time course and intensity of anthralin inflammation on involved and uninvolved psoriatic skin. *Br J Dermatol* 1987; **116**: 517–9.
2 Ramsay B, Lawrence CM, Bruce JM, Shuster S. The effect of triethanolamine application on anthralin-induced inflammation and therapeutic effect in psoriasis. *J Am Acad Dermatol* 1990; **23**: 73–6.
3 Ippen H. Basic questions on toxicology and pharmacology of anthralin. *Br J Dermatol* 1981; **105** (Suppl. 20): 72–6.

Boric acid

Poisoning has usually occurred in infants treated for napkin eruptions. Almost all cases have been caused by the use of boric ointments or lotions. However, use of borated talc proved fatal in one infant [1]. Wet boric dressings caused the death of an adult woman [2].

REFERENCES

1 Brooke C, Boggs T. Boric-acid poisoning: report of a case and review of the literature. *Am J Dis Child* 1951; **82**: 465–72.
2 Jordan JW, Crissey JT. Boric acid poisoning: report of fatal adult case from cutaneous use. A critical evaluation of this drug in dermatologic practice. *Arch Dermatol* 1957; **75**: 720–8.

Calcipotriol

This vitamin D_3 analogue has been reported to cause transient local irritation, and facial or perioral dermatitis [1]. Contact allergy is recorded [2]. Topical application of calcipotriol for 5 weeks to a mean of 16% of the body surface of psoriatic patients did not result in detectable systemic alteration of calcium metabolism [3]. The manufacturer's data sheet (Leo Laboratories) states that increased serum calcium may occur with application in daily doses of 50–100 g of the 50 µg/g ointment. Severe symptomatic hypercalcaemia developed after application of about 200 g of the ointment over 1 week to exfoliative psoriasis covering 40% of the body surface [4]. It is recommended that treatment be confined to stable mild to moderate psoriasis, and that the recommended dose of 100 g/week should not be exceeded. Hyperpigmentation occurred at the site of topical calcipotriol application in two patients receiving photochemotherapy [5].

REFERENCES

1 Kragballe K, Gjertsen BT, De Hoop D *et al.* Double-blind, right/left comparison of calcipotriol and betamethasone valerate in treatment of psoriasis vulgaris. *Lancet* 1991; **337**: 193–6.
2 de Groot AC. Contact allergy to calcipotriol. *Contact Dermatitis* 1994; **30**: 242–3.

3 Saurat J-H, Gumowski Sunek D, Rizzoli R. Topical calcipotriol and hypercalcaemia. *Lancet* 1991; **337**: 1287.
4 Dwyer C, Chapman RS. Calcipotriol and hypercalcaemia. *Lancet* 1991; **338**: 764–5.
5 Gläser R, Röwert J, Mrowietz U. Hyperpigmentation due to topical calcipotriol and photochemotherapy in two psoriatic patients. *Br J Dermatol* 1998; **139**: 148–51.

Coal tar

Coal tar vapour inhalation precipitated severe symptomatic bronchoconstriction in an atopic asthmatic subject following application of coal-tar bandages for treatment of eczema, confirmed by challenge [1].

REFERENCE

1 Ibbotson SH, Stenton SC, Simpson NB. Acute severe bronchoconstriction precipitated by coal tar bandages. *Clin Exp Dermatol* 1995; **20**: 58–9.

Chlorhexidine gluconate (Hibitane)

Urticaria, dyspnoea and anaphylactic shock have occurred following topical application as a disinfectant [1,2], as have contact urticaria, photosensitive dermatitis [3] and deafness.

REFERENCES

1 Okano M, Nomura M, Hata S *et al.* Anaphylactic symptoms due to chlorhexidine gluconate. *Arch Dermatol* 1989; **125**: 50–2.
2 Snellman E, Rantanen T. Severe anaphylaxis after a chlorhexidine bath. *J Am Acad Dermatol* 1999; **40**: 771–2.
3 Wahlberg JE, Wennersten G. Hypersensitivity and photosensitivity to chlorhexidine. *Dermatologica* 1971; **143**: 376–9.

Dequalinium chloride

Necrotic lesions have occurred following its use in the treatment of balanitis [1].

REFERENCE

1 Coles RB, Simpson WT, Wilkinson DS. Dequalinium: a possible complication of its use in balanitis. *Lancet* 1964; **ii**: 531.

Dimethylsulfoxide

Topical application can cause erythema, pruritus and urticaria, but systemic reactions are very rare; a generalized contact dermatitis-like reaction followed intravesical instillation in a sensitized individual [1].

REFERENCE

1 Nishimura M, Takano Y, Toshitani Y. Systemic contact dermatitis medicamentosa occurring after intravesical dimethyl sulfoxide treatment for interstitial cystitis. *Arch Dermatol* 1988; **124**: 182–3.

Doxepin

Doxepin cream causes allergic contact dermatitis and systemic contact dermatitis [1,2].

REFERENCES

1 Taylor JS, Praditsuwan P, Handel D, Kuffner G. Allergic contact dermatitis from doxepin cream. One-year patch test clinic experience. *Arch Dermatol* 1996; **132**: 515–8.
2 Shelley W, Shelley ED, Talanin NY. Self-potentiating allergic contact dermatitis caused by doxepin hydrochloride cream. *J Am Acad Dermatol* 1996; **34**: 143–4.

Formaldehyde

Industrial exposure is recognized to be a health hazard, and a threshold limit of 2 ppm is allowed in the UK and the USA [1]. Irritant or allergic dermatitis is common in exposed workers [2]. Systemic symptoms including breathlessness, headache and drowsiness have been attributed to prolonged exposure to very low levels in the home [3].

REFERENCES

1 Anonymous. The health hazards of formaldehyde. *Lancet* 1981; **i**: 926–7.
2 Glass WI. An outbreak of formaldehyde dermatitis. *NZ Med J* 1961; **60**: 423.
3 Harris JC, Rumack BH, Aldrich FD. Toxicology of urea formaldehyde and polyurethane foam insulation. *JAMA* 1981; **245**: 243–6.

Lindane (g-benzene hexachloride)

Lindane therapy for scabies has potential toxicity, which includes neurotoxicity with convulsions, especially in children [1–7]. Most reports have occurred with overexposure or misuse, although side effects have followed single applications, particularly when the epidermal barrier has been compromised. Whether this constitutes a significant problem in normal individuals is doubtful [6]. Nevertheless, it has been suggested that permethrin may be a safer and less toxic alternative [8].

REFERENCES

1 Lee B, Groth P. Scabies: transcutaneous poisoning during treatment. *Arch Dermatol* 1979; **115**: 124–5.
2 Pramanik AK, Hansen RC. Transcutaneous gamma benzene hexachloride absorption and toxicity in infants and children. *Arch Dermatol* 1979; **115**: 124–5.
3 Matsuoka LY. Convulsions following application of gamma benzene hexachloride. *J Am Acad Dermatol* 1981; **5**: 98–9.
4 Rasmussen JE. The problem of lindane. *J Am Acad Dermatol* 1981; **5**: 507–16.
5 Davies JE, Dehdia HV, Morgade C *et al.* Lindane poisonings. *Arch Dermatol* 1983; **119**: 142–4.
6 Rasmussen J. Lindane: a prudent approach. *Arch Dermatol* 1987; **123**: 1008–10.
7 Friedman SJ. Lindane neurotoxic reaction in nonbullous ichthyosiform erythroderma. *Arch Dermatol* 1987; **123**: 1056–8.
8 Schultz MW, Gomez M, Hansen RC *et al.* Comparative study of 5% permethrin cream and 1% lindane lotion for the treatment of scabies. *Arch Dermatol* 1990; **126**: 167–70.

Hexachlorophene (hexachlorophane)

This substance has potential neurotoxicity. Exposure of babies to a talc containing 6.3% hexachlorophene due to a manufacturing error resulted in deaths, with ulceration, skin lesions and a characteristic demyelinating encephalopathy [1]. A 3% emulsion has produced milder neurological changes but a 0.33% concentration in talc is apparently safe. Encephalopathy has occurred in burns patients [2].

REFERENCES

1 Martin-Bouyer G, Lebreton R, Toga M *et al.* Outbreak of accidental hexachlorophene poisoning in France. *Lancet* 1982; **i**: 91–5.
2 Larson DL. Studies show hexachlorophene causes burn syndrome. *J Am Hosp Assoc* 1968; **42**: 63–4.

Hydroquinone

Depigmenting creams containing 6–8% hydroquinone, used especially by black South African women, have caused rebound hyperpigmentation and coarsening of the skin, with ochronotic changes in the dermis, colloid degeneration and colloid milium [1–6]. Collagen degeneration may be seen histologically [2]. Similar changes have been seen in black women in the USA [3] and in a Mexican American woman [4]. Interestingly, ochronosis does not develop in areas of vitiligo [7]. The Q-switched ruby laser may be helpful in treating exogenous ochronosis [8]. The nails may be pigmented [9].

REFERENCES

1 Findlay GH, Morrison JGL, Simson IW. Exogenous ochronosis and pigmented colloid milium from hydroquinone bleaching creams. *Br J Dermatol* 1975; **93**: 613–22.
2 Phillips JI, Isaacson C, Carman H. Ochronosis in Black South Africans who used skin lighteners. *Am J Dermatopathol* 1986; **8**: 14–21.
3 Lawrence N, Bligard CA, Reed R, Perret WJ. Exogenous ochronosis in the United States. *J Am Acad Dermatol* 1988; **18**: 1207–11.
4 Howard KL, Furner BB. Exogenous ochronosis in a Mexican-American woman. *Cutis* 1990; **45**: 180–2.
5 Camarasa JG, Serra-Baldrich E. Exogenous ochronosis with allergic contact dermatitis from hydroquinone. *Contact Dermatitis* 1994; **31**: 57–8.
6 Snider RL, Thiers BH. Exogenous ochronosis. *J Am Acad Dermatol* 1993; **28**: 662–4.
7 Hull PR, Procter PR. The melanocyte: an essential link in hydroquinone-induced ochronosis. *J Am Acad Dermatol* 1990; **22**: 529–31.
8 Kramer KE, Lopez A, Stefanato CM, Phillips TJ. Exogenous ochronosis. *J Am Acad Dermatol* 2000; **42**: 869–71.
9 Garcia RL, White JW, Willis WF. Hydroquinone nail pigmentation. *Arch Dermatol* 1978; **114**: 1402–3.

Iodine

Povidone-iodine scrub for acne (Betadine) induced hyperthyroidism [1].

REFERENCE

1 Smit E, Whiting DA, Feld S. Iodine-induced hyperthyroidism caused by acne treatment. *J Am Acad Dermatol* 1994; **31**: 115–7.

Latanoprost

Topical latanoprost for glaucoma may induce eyelash hypertrichosis [1].

REFERENCE

1 Demitsu T, Manabe M, Harima N *et al.* Hypertrichosis induced by latanoprost. *J Am Acad Dermatol* 2001; **44**: 721–3.

Lead lotions

The continued use of wet dressings of lead subacetate in the treatment of exfoliative dermatitis caused lead poisoning, with punctate basophilia and an elevated urinary lead level [1].

REFERENCE

1 Kennedy CC, Lynas HA. Lead poisoning by cutaneous absorption from lead dressings. *Lancet* 1949; **i**: 650–2.

Mercury

Poisoning is now fortunately rare, but was seen from continued application of large amounts of a topical application, as for psoriasis [1,2]. Idiosyncratic poisoning after much smaller doses is also recognized [3]. Intoxication has followed the use of a mercury dusting powder [4] and poisoning of a suckling infant has followed the use of perchloride of mercury lotion for cracked nipples [5]. Fever, a generalized morbilliform rash and oedema of the extremities have been the usual clinical features. Exfoliative dermatitis and encephalopathy have developed; permanent damage to the renal tubules is manifest as persistent albuminuria or frank nephrotic syndrome [6]. Rarely, gross symptoms, such as loose teeth [7], swollen bleeding gums and weight loss, may be observed.

Application of a mercury-containing cream to the face over many years can produce slate-grey pigmentation, especially on the eyelids, nasolabial folds and neck folds (exogenous ochronosis) [8–10]; mercury granules lie free in the dermis or within macrophages [11]. Mercury is a moderate sensitizer and leads to contact sensitivity.

REFERENCES

1 Inman PM, Gordon B, Trinder P. Mercury absorption and psoriasis. *BMJ* 1956; **ii**: 1202–6.
2 Young E. Ammoniated mercury poisoning. *Br J Dermatol* 1960; **72**: 449–55.
3 Williams BH, Beach WC. Idiosyncrasy to ammoniated mercury: treatment with 2,3-dimercapto-propanol (BAL). *JAMA* 1950; **142**: 1286–8.
4 MacGregor ME, Rayner PHW. Pink disease and primary renal tubular acidosis: a common cause. *Lancet* 1964; **ii**: 1083–5.
5 Hunt GM. Mercury poisoning in infancy. *BMJ* 1966; **i**: 1482.
6 Silverberg DS, McCall JT, Hunt JC. Nephrotic syndrome with use of ammoniated mercury. *Arch Intern Med* 1967; **20**: 581–6.
7 Bourgeois M, Dooms-Goossens A, Knockaert D *et al.* Mercury intoxication

after topical application of a metallic mercury ointment. *Dermatologica* 1986; **172**: 48–51.
8 Lamar LM, Bliss BO. Localized pigmentation of the skin due to topical mercury. *Arch Dermatol* 1966; **93**: 450–3.
9 Prigent F, Cohen J, Civatte J. Pigmentation des paupieres probablement secondaire l'application prolongée d'une pomade ophtalmologique contenant du mercure. *Ann Dermatol Vénéréol* 1986; **113**: 357–8.
10 Aberer W. Topical mercury should be banned: dangerous, outmoded but still popular. *J Am Acad Dermatol* 1991; **24**: 150–1.
11 Burge KM, Winkelmann RK. Mercury pigmentation. An electron microscopic study. *Arch Dermatol* 1970; **102**: 51–61.

Methyl salicylate (oil of wintergreen)

Topical application of methyl salicylate and menthol as a rubifacient, with use of a heating pad, resulted in local skin necrosis and interstitial nephritis [1].

REFERENCE

1 Heng MCY. Local necrosis and interstitial nephritis due to topical methyl salicylate and menthol. *Cutis* 1987; **39**: 442–4.

Mexiletine

Mexiletine hydrochloride induced contact uriticaria in a patient receiving iontophoresis [1]. A generalized drug eruption followed topical provocation on previously involved skin [2].

REFERENCES

1 Yamazaki S, Katayama I, Kurumaji Y *et al*. Contact urticaria induced by mexiletine hydrochloride in a patient receiving iontophoresis. *Br J Dermatol* 1994; **130**: 538–40.
2 Kikuchi K, Tsunoda T, Tagami H. Generalized drug eruption due to mexiletine hydrochloride: topical provocation on previously involved skin. *Contact Dermatitis* 1991; **25**: 70–2.

Minoxidil

Topical minoxidil, as used for androgenetic alopecia, is associated with cutaneous problems in up to 10% of patients, with allergic contact dermatitis occurring in 4% of individuals [1]. The contact allergen is often propylene glycol [2]. Diffuse hypertrichosis occurred during treatment with 5% topical minoxidil in female patients [3]. Acute non-allergic eruptions of the scalp resulted from combined use of minoxidil and retinoic acid [4].

REFERENCES

1 Wilson C, Walkden V, Powell S *et al*. Contact dermatitis in reaction to 2% topical minoxidil solution. *J Am Acad Dermatol* 1991; **24**: 661–2.
2 Friedman ES, Friedman PM, Cohen DE, Washenik K. Allergic contact dermatitis to topical minoxidil solution: etiology and treatment. *J Am Acad Dermatol* 2002; **46**: 309–12.
2 Peluso AM, Misciali C, Vincenzi C, Tosti A. Diffuse hypertrichosis during treatment with 5% topical minoxidil. *Br J Dermatol* 1997; **136**: 118–20.
4 Fisher AA. Unusual acute, nonallergic eruptions of the scalp from combined use of minoxidil and retinoic acid. *Cutis* 1993; **51**: 17–8.

Non-steroidal anti-inflammatory drugs

Allergic and photoallergic contact dermatitis and phototoxicity have resulted from topical NSAIDs [1–3]. An erythema multiforme-like reaction followed acute contact dermatitis from two different bufexamac-containing topical preparations [4].

REFERENCES

1 Ophaswongse S, Maibach H. Topical nonsteroidal antiinflammatory drugs: allergic and photoallergic contact dermatitis and phototoxicity. *Contact Dermatitis* 1993; **29**: 57–64.
2 Oh VM. Ketoprofen gel and delayed hypersensitivity dermatitis. *BMJ* 1994; **309**: 512.
3 Valsecchi R, Pansera B, Leghissa P, Reseghetti A. Allergic contact dermatitis of the eyelids and conjunctivitis from diclofenac. *Contact Dermatitis* 1996; **34**: 150–1.
4 Koch P, Bahmer FA. Erythema-multiforme-like, urticarial papular and plaque eruptions from bufexamac. report of 4 cases. *Contact Dermatitis* 1994; **31**: 97–101.

Phenol

Severe systemic reactions, such as abdominal pain, dizziness, haemoglobinuria, cyanosis and sometimes fatal coma, have followed the application of phenol to extensive wounds. Accidental application of pure phenol to a small area of skin in an infant has proved fatal. The prolonged use of phenol as a dressing for a large ulcer may give rise to exogenous ochronosis, with darkening of the cornea and of the skin of face and hands.

Podophyllin

Excessive application may lead to severe local irritation or ulceration [1]. There have been occasional reports of confusional states, coma, peripheral neuropathy, vomiting and even death following the application of this resin to large areas of genital warts, especially in pregnancy [2,3]. However, careful review of the reports suggests that in the majority the effects could not be attributed with certainty to podophyllin [2]. Animal experiments suggest teratogenicity; although teratogenicity is controversial in humans, the drug is best avoided in pregnancy.

REFERENCES

1 Higgins SP, Stedman YF, Chandiok P. Severe genital ulceration in two females following self-treatment with podophyllin solutions. *Genitourin Med* 1994; **70**: 146–7.
2 Bargman H. Is podophyllin a safe drug to use and can it be used in pregnancy? *Arch Dermatol* 1988; **124**: 1718–20.
3 Sundharam JA, Bargman H. Is podophyllin safe for use in pregnancy? *Arch Dermatol* 1989; **125**: 1000–1.

Resorcinol

Acute resorcinol poisoning is very rare but an ointment

containing 12.5% resorcinol applied to the napkin area produced dusky cyanosis, a maculopapular eruption, haemolytic anaemia and haemoglobinuria in an infant [1]. The continued application to large leg ulcers of ointments containing resorcinol has caused myxoedema and widespread blue-grey pigmentation mimicking ochronosis [2]. Application for warts caused generalized urticaria with angio-oedema, pompholyx of palms and soles, or papulovesicular eczema with pompholyx [3].

REFERENCES

1 Cunningham AA. Resorcin poisoning. *Arch Dis Child* 1956; **31**: 173–6.
2 Thomas AE, Gisburn MA. Exogenous ochronosis and myxoedema from resorcinol. *Br J Dermatol* 1961; **73**: 378–81.
3 Barbaud A, Modiano P, Cocciale M *et al.* The topical application of resorcinol can provoke a systemic allergic reaction. *Br J Dermatol* 1996; **135**: 1014–5.

Salicylic acid and salicylates

The frequent application of salicylic acid ointments to extensive lesions will produce symptoms of salicylism even in adults [1–7]. Most cases of poisoning have occurred in children with psoriasis or ichthyosis [1,2]; fatal cases have been recorded [4]. Drowsiness and delusions are followed by acidosis, coma and death from respiratory failure.

REFERENCES

1 Young CJ. Salicylate intoxication from cutaneous absorption of salicylate acid: review of the literature and report of a case. *South Med J* 1952; **45**: 1075–7.
2 Cawley EP, Peterson NT, Wheeler CE. Salicylic acid poisoning in dermatological therapy. *JAMA* 1953; **151**: 372–4.
3 Von Weiss JF, Lever WF. Percutaneous salicylic acid intoxication in psoriasis. *Arch Dermatol* 1964; **90**: 614–9.
4 Lindsey LP. Two cases of fatal salicylate poisoning after topical application of an anti-fungal solution. *Med J Aust* 1969; **1**: 353–4.
5 Davies MG, Vella Briffa D, Greaves MW. Systemic toxicity from topically applied salicylic acid. *BMJ* 1979; i: 661.
6 Anderson JAR, Ead RD. Percutaneous salicylate poisoning. *Clin Exp Dermatol* 1979; **4**: 349–51.
7 Pec J, Strmenova M, Palencarova E *et al.* Salicylate intoxication after use of topical salicylic acid ointment by a patient with psoriasis. *Cutis* 1992; **50**: 307–9.

Silver sulfadiazine

Topical application has caused hyperpigmentation [1], contact sensitivity [2] and dermatitis [3].

REFERENCES

1 Dupuis LL, Shear NH, Zucker RM. Hyperpigmentation due to topical application of silver sulfadiazine cream. *J Am Acad Dermatol* 1985; **12**: 1112–4.
2 Fraser-Moodie A. Sensitivity to silver in a patient treated with silver sulphadiazine (Flamazine). *Burns* 1992; **18**: 74–5.
3 McKenna SR, Latenser BA, Jones LM *et al.* Serious silver sulphadiazine and mafenide acetate dermatitis. *Burns* 1995; **21**: 310–2.

Tretinoin

Topical tretinoin, used for the management of photo-aged skin, may cause erythema, peeling, burning and itching of the skin within days [1,2]. Pink discoloration without other signs may also develop, as may inflammation in solar keratoses.

REFERENCES

1 Weiss JS, Ellis CN, Headington JT *et al.* Topical tretinoin improves photo-aged skin: a double-blind, vehicle-controlled study. *JAMA* 1988; **259**: 527–32.
2 Weinstein GD, Nigra TP, Pochi PE *et al.* Topical tretinoin for treatment of photodamaged skin. *Arch Dermatol* 1991; **127**: 659–65.

Vitamin E

Vitamin E in deodorants has caused contact dermatitis [1].

REFERENCE

1 Minkin W, Cohen HJ, Frank SB. Contact dermatitis from deodorants. *Arch Dermatol* 1973; **107**: 774–5.

Warfarin

An epidemic of haemorrhagic disease with fatalities occurred due to warfarin-contaminated talcs [1]. Poisoning has also been attributed to preparation of rodent baits [2].

REFERENCES

1 Martin-Bouyer G, Linh PD, Tuan LC *et al.* Epidemic of haemorrhagic disease in Vietnamese infants caused by warfarin-contaminated talcs. *Lancet* 1983; i: 230–2.
2 Fristedt B, Sterner N. Warfarin intoxication from percutaneous absorption. *Arch Environ Health* 1965; **11**: 205–8.

Transdermal drug-delivery systems

Transdermal delivery systems are available for clonidine, estradiol (oestradiol), glyceryl trinitrate, scopolamine and nicotine, and systems for other drugs are being developed. Erythema, irritancy, scaling, vesiculation, excoriation, induration, pigmentary changes and contact sensitization are not uncommon; the occlusive element may lead to miliaria rubra [1–13]. Systemic reactions may occur. Allergic skin reactions occur in up to 50% of patients with clonidine, but with glyceryl trinitrate, scopolamine, estradiol and testosterone they are much less frequent [2]. Reactivation of an area of contact dermatitis may develop via oral medication rarely [2]. Transdermal compared with oral metoprolol had comparable efficacy, and systemic side effects were comparable; 69% of patients had local side effects at the patch site (erythema, papular exanthem, pruritus, localized urticarial exanthem) [4]. Allergic contact dermatitis is recorded with nicotine

[8–11], glyceryl trinitrate and estradiol [12]. Use of transdermal oestrogen patches resulted in systemic sensitization to ethanol [14]. Transdermal fentanyl patches have been associated with a diffuse rash [15].

REFERENCES

1 Hogan DJ, Maibach HI. Adverse dermatologic reactions to transdermal drug delivery systems. *J Am Acad Dermatol* 1990; **22**: 811–4.
2 Holdiness MR. A review of contact dermatitis associated with transdermal therapeutic systems. *Contact Dermatitis* 1989; **20**: 3–9.
3 Berti JJ, Lipsky JJ. Transcutaneous drug delivery: a practical review. *Mayo Clin Proc* 1995; **70**: 581–6.
4 Jeck T, Edmonds D, Mengden T et al. Betablocking drugs in essential hypertension: transdermal bupranolol compared with oral metoprolol. *Int J Clin Pharmacol Res* 1992; **12**: 139–48.
5 Kolloch RE, Mehlburger L, Schumacher H, Gobel BO. Efficacy and safety of two different galenic formulations of a transdermal clonidine system in the treatment of hypertension. *Clin Auton Res* 1993; **3**: 373–8.
6 Antihypertensive Patch Italian Study (APIS) Investigators. One year efficacy and tolerability of clonidine administered by the transdermal route in patients with mild to moderate essential hypertension: a multicentre open label study. *Clin Auton Res* 1993; **3**: 379–83.
7 Breidthardt J, Schumacher H, Mehlburger L. Long-term (5 year) experience with transdermal clonidine in the treatment of mild to moderate hypertension. *Clin Auton Res* 1993; **3**: 385–90.
8 Bircher AJ, Howard H, Rufli T. Adverse skin reactions to nicotine in a transdermal therapeutic system. *Contact Dermatitis* 1991; **25**: 230–6.
9 Farm G. Contact allergy to nicotine from a nicotine patch. *Contact Dermatitis* 1993; **29**: 214–5.
10 Dwyer CM, Forsyth A. Allergic contact dermatitis from methacrylates in a nicotine transdermal patch. *Contact Dermatitis* 1994; **30**: 309–10.
11 Sudan BJ. Nicotine skin patch treatment and adverse reactions: skin irritation, skin sensitization, and nicotine as a hapten. *J Clin Psychopharmacol* 1995; **15**: 145–6.
12 Torres V, Lopes JC, Leite L. Allergic contact dermatitis from nitroglycerin and estradiol transdermal therapeutic systems. *Contact Dermatitis* 1992; **26**: 53–4.
13 Prisant LM. Transdermal clonidine skin reactions. *J Clin Hypertens* 2002; **4**: 136–8.
14 Grebe SK, Adams JD, Feek CM. Systemic sensitization to ethanol by transdermal estrogen patches. *Arch Dermatol* 1993; **129**: 379–80.
15 Stoukides CA, Stegman M. Diffuse rash associated with transdermal fentanyl. *Clin Pharm* 1992; **11**: 222.

Management of drug reactions

Diagnosis

Drug reactions, apart from fixed drug eruption, have non-specific clinical features, and it is often impossible to identify the offending chemical with certainty, especially when a patient with a suspected reaction is receiving many drugs simultaneously. Drug reactions may be mistaken for naturally occurring conditions and may therefore be overlooked. By the same token, it may on occasion be very difficult to state that a given eruption is drug induced. Experience with the type of reaction most commonly caused by particular drugs may enable the range of suspects to be narrowed, but familiar drugs may occasionally produce unfamiliar reactions and new drugs may mimic the reactions of the familiar. The assessment of a potential adverse drug reaction always necessitates taking a careful history, and may involve a trial of drug elimination, skin tests, *in vitro* tests and challenge by re-exposure [1].

A drug reaction may first become evident after the offending medication has been stopped, and depot injections may have delayed effects. Interpretation of elimination tests should be tempered by the knowledge that drug reactions may take weeks to settle. *In vivo* and *in vitro* tests are only applicable to truly allergic reactions. Skin tests, including prick and intradermal testing and patch testing, are for the most part unreliable, even when apparently appropriate antigens are used; they may be hazardous [2–4]. *In vitro* tests are not widely available and are essentially research tools.

All too frequently therefore the diagnosis is no more than an assessment of probability. The fact that major disagreements occurred between clinical pharmacologists asked to assess the likelihood of adverse drug reaction in two series confirms that identification of a responsible drug is often a subjective judgement [5,6]. An algorithm has been reported that provides detailed criteria for ranking the probability of whether a given drug is responsible for a reaction, based on (i) previous experience, (ii) the alternative aetiological candidates, (iii) timing of events, (iv) drug level and (v) the results of drug withdrawal and rechallenge [7,8]. A number of other algorithms have been developed to assist in the diagnosis of which, if any, drug is the cause of a given eruption [9–12]. The difficulties inherent in the diagnosis of drug reactions have been reviewed [1,13,14].

REFERENCES

1 Nigen S, Knowles SR, Shear NH. Drug eruptions: approaching the diagnosis of drug-induced skin diseases. *J Drugs Dermatol* 2003; **2**: 278–99.
2 Bruynzeel D, van Ketel W. Skin tests in the diagnosis of maculopapular drug eruptions. *Semin Dermatol* 1987; **6**: 119–24.
3 Vaillant L, Camenen I, Lorette G. Patch testing with carbamazepine: reinduction of an exfoliative dermatitis. *Arch Dermatol* 1989; **125**: 299.
4 Machet L, Vaillant L, Dardaine V, Lorette G. Patch testing with clobazam: relapse of generalized drug eruption. *Contact Dermatitis* 1992; **26**: 347–8.
5 Karch FE, Smith CL, Kerzner B et al. Adverse drug reactions: a matter of opinion. *Clin Pharmacol Ther* 1976; **19**: 489–92.
6 Koch-Weser J, Sellers EM, Zacest R. The ambiguity of adverse drug reactions. *Eur J Clin Pharmacol* 1977; **11**: 75–8.
7 Kramer MS, Leventhal JM, Hutchinson TA, Feinstein AR. An algorithm for the operational assessment of adverse drug reactions. I. Background, description, and instructions for use. *JAMA* 1979; **242**: 623–32.
8 Leventhal JM, Hutchinson TA, Kramer MS, Feinstein AR. An algorithm for the operational assessment of adverse drug reactions. III. Results of tests among clinicians. *JAMA* 1979; **242**: 1991–4.
9 Naranjo CA, Busto U, Sellers EM et al. A method for estimating the probability of adverse drug reactions. *Clin Pharmacol Ther* 1981; **27**: 239–45.
10 Louick C, Lacouture P, Mitchell A et al. A study of adverse reaction algorithms in a drug surveillance program. *Clin Pharmacol Ther* 1985; **38**: 183–7.
11 Pere J, Begaud B, Harramburu F, Albin H. Computerized comparison of six adverse drug reaction assessment procedures. *Clin Pharmacol Ther* 1986; **40**: 451–61.
12 Ghajar BM, Lanctôt KL, Shear NH, Naranjo CA. Bayesian differential diagnosis of a cutaneous reaction associated with the administration of sulfonamides. *Semin Dermatol* 1989; **8**: 213–8.
13 Ring J. Diagnostik von Arzneimittel-bedingten Unverträglichkeitsreaktionz. *Hautarzt* 1987; **38**: S16–S22.
14 Shear NH. Diagnosing cutaneous adverse reactions to drugs. *Arch Dermatol* 1990; **126**: 94–7.

Drug history

Patients should be specifically questioned about laxatives, oral contraceptives, vaccines, homeopathic medicines, etc. as these may not be volunteered as medications. They should be asked when they last took a tablet for any reason. The history should include information on when each drug was first taken relative to the onset of the reaction, whether the same or a related drug has been administered previously, and whether there is a prior history of drug sensitivity or contact dermatitis. Allergic drug reactions do not usually develop for at least 4 days, more commonly 7–10 days, after initial drug administration in a previously unsensitized individual. However, this time relationship cannot be relied on to differentiate between allergic and non-allergic reactions, as a previous sensitizing exposure may not have produced a clinically evident reaction.

Drug elimination

Resolution of a reaction on withdrawal of a drug is supportive incriminatory evidence but not diagnostic. Failure of a rash to subside on drug withdrawal does not necessarily exonerate it, as traces of the drug may persist for long periods and some reactions, once initiated, continue for many days without re-exposure to the drug. The unwitting substitution of a drug that is chemically closely related may perpetuate a reaction, as when an antihistamine of phenothiazine structure is prescribed to alleviate the symptoms of a reaction caused by another phenothiazine. Elimination diets have been advocated for diagnosis of food additive intolerance leading to urticaria [1,2].

REFERENCES

1 Rudzki E, Czubalski K, Grzywa Z. Detection of urticaria with food additives intolerance by means of diet. *Dermatologica* 1980; **161**: 57–62.
2 Metcalfe DD, Sampson HA, eds. Workshop on experimental methodology for clinical studies of adverse reactions to foods and food additives. *J Allergy Clin Immunol* 1990; **86** (Suppl.): 421–42.

Skin testing

Skin testing has been reviewed [1–7]. Drug skin tests are of three types: patch tests for delayed cellular hypersensitivity, prick tests for immediate hypersensitivity, and intradermal tests for both immediate or delayed hypersensitivity [5]. The quick patch test (application under a Finn chamber for 30 min) can be used in patients with severe hypersensitivity [8]. Prick tests and intradermal tests performed with sequential dilutions may be useful in the identification of patients who present with immediate IgE-related hypersensitivity reactions, and are sensitive to one of a number of drugs, including penicillin and other β-lactam antibiotics, agents used in general anaesthesia, tetanus toxoid, streptokinase, chymopapain, heterologous sera or insulin, and may thus aid in the prevention of anaphylaxis [1]. Vasculitis related to circulating immune complexes cannot be reproduced by skin tests. Delayed cellular hypersensitivity is involved in inducing maculopapular rashes, baboon syndrome, localized or generalized eczema or acute generalized exanthematous pustulosis. In such reactions, drug patch tests or delayed positive reactions on intradermal tests occur in more than 50% of patients [5]. Significantly higher numbers of positive patch tests are seen in maculopapular than in urticarial reactions [4]. Diluted drug patch tests can be positive in the drug hypersensitivity syndrome (drug rash with eosinophilia and systemic symptoms). Drug skin tests are not of great value in investigating Stevens–Johnson syndrome or TEN; relevant positive patch tests were seen in only 9% of 22 patients with Stevens–Johnson syndrome/TEN compared with 50% of 14 patients with acute generalized exanthematous pustulosis [9].

The results of skin-test reactions, including intradermal testing and patch testing, were evaluated in 242 patients with delayed-type (non-immediate) drug eruptions [6]. Intradermal testing was positive in 89.7% of patients, and patch tests were positive in 31.5% of cases; overall, 62% of patients had either a positive intradermal or patch test. Intradermal testing was more frequently positive in maculopapular rashes, erythema multiforme and erythrodermic rashes than in eczematous reactions, whereas positive patch tests were comparatively frequent in erythroderma, eczematous reactions and anticonvulsant-induced reactions. It was concluded that a combination of patch testing and intradermal testing is useful in the demonstration of causative agents in delayed-type drug eruptions [6]. Unfortunately, the usefulness of this approach is limited, because the significant antigenic determinants are unknown for most drugs [1]. Moreover, intradermal testing is not always safe. False-negative skin testing may occur because of poor absorption through the skin, because a metabolite rather than the substance administered in the test is the sensitizing antigen, or because testing is performed either too soon after a reaction, in a refractory period, or too late, so that the patient no longer demonstrates skin-test reactivity.

Drug skin tests should be performed 6 weeks to 6 months after complete resolution of the reaction [3]. For patch tests, the commercial form of the drug should be tested diluted at 30% in petrolatum and/or water; the pure drug should be tested diluted at 10%. Lower concentrations are used in severe drug reactions. Sodium lauryl sulphate in the commercial form of some drugs can induce irritation when they are patch tested as such, and positive patch tests to drugs can be related to an excipient rather than the drug itself [4]. It is useful to carry out the test on the site most affected in the initial reaction [10].

Re-elicitation of an exfoliative dermatitis has followed patch testing [9].

Drug prick tests are performed on the volar forearm skin with the commercialized form of the drug, but with sequential dilutions in cases of urticaria. Intradermal tests are performed with sequential dilutions (10^{-4}, 10^{-3}, 10^{-2}, 10^{-1}) of 0.04 mL of a pure sterile or injectable form of the drug. Prick tests and intradermal tests should be read at 20 min and at day 1, and patch tests at day 2 and day 4; these tests also need to be read at 1 week.

The success of skin testing varies with the drug tested, with a high percentage of positive results on patch testing with β-lactam antibiotics, pristinamycin, carbamazepine and tetrazepam, or with β-lactam antibiotics and heparins on delayed readings of intradermal tests. The results of drug skin tests also depend on the clinical features of the adverse drug reaction. Appropriate controls are necessary to avoid false-positive results.

REFERENCES

1 Sussman GL, Dolovich J. Prevention of anaphylaxis. *Semin Dermatol* 1989; **8**: 158–65.
2 Deleo VA. Skin testing in systemic cutaneous drug reactions. *Lancet* 1998; **352**: 1488–90.
3 Barbaud A, Goncalo M, Bruynzeel D, Bircher A. Guidelines for performing skin tests with drugs in the investigation of cutaneous adverse drug reactions. *Contact Dermatitis* 2001; **45**: 321–8.
4 Barbaud A, Trechot P, Reichert-Penetrat S *et al.* Relevance of skin tests with drugs in investigating cutaneous adverse drug reactions. *Contact Dermatitis* 2001; **45**: 265–8.
5 Barbaud A. The use of skin testing in the investigation of toxidermia: from pathophysiology to the results of skin testing. *Therapie* 2002; **57**: 258–62.
6 Osawa J, Naito S, Aihara M *et al.* Evaluation of skin test reactions in patients with non-immediate type drug eruptions. *J Dermatol* 1990; **17**: 235–9.
7 Bruynzeel DP, Maibach HI. Patch testing in systemic drug eruptions. *Clin Dermatol* 1997; **15**: 479–84.
8 Oi M, Satoh T, Yokozeki H, Nishioka K. Detection of immediate-type reaction to the epitope of β-lactam antibiotics by the quick patch test. *Br J Dermatol* 2003; **148**: 182–3.
9 Wolkenstein P, Chosidow O, Fléchet ML *et al.* Patch testing in severe cutaneous adverse drug reactions including Stevens–Johnson syndrome and toxic epidermal necrolysis. *Contact Dermatitis* 1996; **35**: 234–6.
10 Barbaud A, Trechot P, Reichert-Penetrat S *et al.* The usefulness of patch testing on the previously most severely affected site in a cutaneous adverse drug reaction to tetrazepam. *Contact Dermatitis* 2001; **44**: 259–60.

Patch testing

Patch testing in drug eruptions may be helpful in identifying the drug responsible, especially in systemic contact-type dermatitis medicamentosa, photosensitivity (photopatch testing) or fixed drug reactions [1–7]. Positive patch tests have been found overall in about 15% of patients with drug eruptions [1,2] and 25% of patients with penicillin allergy [1–3]. Patch testing in a previously involved site, but not in normal skin, yielded a positive response in a proportion of cases of fixed drug eruption, especially with phenazone (pyrazolone) derivatives (e.g. phenylbutazone), but also with a sulphonamide, doxycycline, trimethoprim, chlormezanone, a barbiturate and

carbamazepine [5]. In a series of 30 patients [6], positive reactions were always seen with phenazone salicylate (16 patients) and carbamazepine (three patients), and in one case with chlormezanone. Both positive and negative reactions were seen with trimethoprim (three and two, respectively), doxycycline (two and one) and sulfadiazine (one and one). The vehicle used as a diluent for the drug may be important in determining whether a reaction is seen; use of dimethylsulfoxide as the vehicle may increase the number of positive patch tests [5,8,9]. Topical provocation of fixed drug eruption has also been reported with sulfamethoxazole [10], dimenhydrinate [11] and metronidazole [12]. However, other reports in the literature do not suggest that patch testing is helpful in fixed drug eruption [13].

Patch testing has supported a diagnosis of allergy, in the absence of topical sensitization, to diazepam, meprobamate and practolol [14], anticonvulsants including hydantoin derivatives and carbamazepine [15–17] (but only in patients with exfoliative dermatitis and maculopapular exanthem and not with fixed drug eruption, erythema multiforme or urticaria [16]), tartrazine dyes [18], chloramphenicol [19], diclofenac-induced maculopapular eruption [20], and in TEN induced by ampicillin [21]. Antibiotics (especially penicillin, ampicillin and other β-lactam antibiotics [22,23] and aminoglycosides), NSAIDs (pyrazolone derivatives and occasionally aspirin), neuroleptics (phenothiazines, barbiturates, meprobamate, benzodiazepines), β-blockers, gold salts, carbimazole, amantadine, corticosteroids, mitomycin, heparin and amide anaesthetics have all been associated with positive patch tests in allergic subjects. Positive patch tests to the following drugs have been found in patients with acute generalized exanthematous pustulosis: diltiazem [24,25], metronidazole [26], nystatin [27] and terbinafine [28].

However, care must be exercised, because anaphylactoid responses may occur even in response to the small amounts of drug absorbed from a patch test. Moreover, patch testing has produced exfoliative dermatitis in a patient sensitized to carbamazepine [29] and relapse of a generalized drug eruption in the case of clobazam [30]. A patch test with a solution of the drug will sometimes induce a generalized petechial reaction in patients with purpura caused by drug sensitivity, for example in carbromal or apronalide (Sedormid) purpura.

REFERENCES

1 Bruynzeel DP, van Ketel WG. Skin tests in the diagnosis of maculo-papular drug eruptions. *Semin Dermatol* 1987; **6**: 119–24.
2 Bruynzeel DP, van Ketel WG. Patch testing in drug eruptions. *Semin Dermatol* 1989; **8**: 196–203.
3 Bruynzeel DP, von Blomberg-van der Flier M, Scheper RJ *et al.* Allergy for penicillin and the relevance of epicutaneous tests. *Dermatologica* 1985; **171**: 429–34.
4 Calkin JM, Maibach HI. Delayed hypersensitivity drug reactions diagnosed by patch testing. *Contact Dermatitis* 1993; **29**: 223–33.

5 Alanko K, Stubb S, Reitamo S. Topical provocation of fixed drug eruption. *Br J Dermatol* 1987; **116**: 561–7.

6 Alanko K. Topical provocation of fixed drug eruption. A study of 30 patients. *Contact Dermatitis* 1994; **31**: 25–7.

7 Lee A-Y. Topical provocation in 31 cases of fixed drug eruption: change of causative drugs in 10 years. *Contact Dermatitis* 1998; **38**: 258–60.

8 Özkaya-Bayazit E, Güngör H. Trimethoprim-induced fixed drug eruption: positive topical provocation on previously involved and uninvolved skin. *Contact Dermatitis* 1997; **39**: 87–8.

9 Özkaya-Bayazit H, Ozarmagan G. Topical provocation in 27 cases of cotrimoxazole-induced fixed drug eruption. *Contact Dermatitis* 1999; **41**: 185–9.

10 Oleaga JM, Aguirre A, Gonzalez M, Diaz-Perez JL. Topical provocation of fixed drug eruption due to sulphamethoxazole. *Contact Dermatitis* 1993; **29**: 155.

11 Smola H, Kruppa A, Hunzelmann N *et al.* Identification of dimenhydrinate as the causative agent in fixed drug eruption using patch-testing in previously affected skin. *Br J Dermatol* 1998; **138**: 920–1.

12 Short KA, Salisbury JR, Fuller LC. Fixed drug eruption following metronidazole therapy and the use of topical provocation testing in diagnosis. *Clin Exp Dermatol* 2002; **27**: 464–6.

13 Sehgal VN, Gangwani OP. Fixed drug eruption. Current concepts. *Int J Dermatol* 1987; **26**: 67–74.

14 Felix RE, Comaish JS. The value of patch and other skin tests in drug eruptions. *Lancet* 1984; **i**: 1017–9.

15 Houwerzijl J, de Gast GC, Nater JP. Patch test in drug eruptions. *Contact Dermatitis* 1982; **8**: 155–8.

16 Alanko K. Patch testing in cutaneous reactions caused by carbamazepine. *Contact Dermatitis* 1993; **29**: 254–7.

17 Jones M, Fernandez-Herrera J, Dorado JM *et al.* Epicutaneous test in carbamazepine cutaneous reactions. *Dermatology* 1994; **188**: 18–20.

18 Roeleveld CG, Van Ketel WG. Positive patch tests to the azo dye tartrazine. *Contact Dermatitis* 1976; **2**: 180.

19 Rudzki E, Grzywa Z, Maciejowska E. Drug reaction with positive patch tests to chloramphenicol. *Contact Dermatitis* 1976; **2**: 181.

20 Romano A, Pietrantonio F, Di Fonso M *et al.* Positivity of patch tests in cutaneous reaction to diclofenac. Two case reports. *Allergy* 1994; **49**: 57–9.

21 Tagami H, Tatsuda K, Iwatski K, Yamada M. Delayed hypersensitivity in ampicillin-induced toxic epidermal necrolysis. *Arch Dermatol* 1983; **119**: 910–3.

22 Galindo Bonilla PA, Garcia Rodriguez R, Feo Brito F *et al.* Patch testing for allergy to beta-lactam antibiotics. *Contact Dermatitis* 1994; **31**: 319–20.

23 Romano A, Di Fonso M, Pietrantonio F *et al.* Repeated patch testing in delayed hypersensitivity to beta-lactam antibiotics. *Contact Dermatitis* 1993; **28**: 190.

24 Vincente-Calleja JM, Aguirre A, Landa N *et al.* Acute generalized exanthematous pustulosis due to diltiazem: confirmation by patch testing. *Br J Dermatol* 1997; **137**: 837–9.

25 January V, Machet L, Gironet N *et al.* Acute generalized exanthematous pustulosis induced by diltiazem: value of patch testing. *Dermatology* 1998; **197**: 274–5.

26 Watsky KL. Acute generalised exanthematous pustulosis induced by metronidazole: the role of patch testing. *Arch Dermatol* 1999; **135**: 93–4.

27 Kuchler A, Hamm H, Weidenthaler-Barth B *et al.* Acute generalized exanthematous pustulosis following oral nystatin therapy: a report of three cases. *Br J Dermatol* 1997; **137**: 808–11.

28 Kempinaire A, De Raeve L, Merckx M *et al.* Terbinafine-induced acute generalized exanthematous pustulosis confirmed by positive patch-test result. *J Am Acad Dermatol* 1997; **37**: 653–5.

29 Vaillant L, Camenen I, Lorette G. Patch testing with carbamazepine: reinduction of an exfoliative dermatitis. *Arch Dermatol* 1989; **125**: 299.

30 Machet L, Vaillant L, Dardaine V, Lorette G. Patch testing with clobazam: relapse of generalized drug eruption. *Contact Dermatitis* 1992; **26**: 347–8.

Penicillin

It is clearly important to exclude from treatment with penicillin those patients truly at risk of developing hypotensive episodes or fatal anaphylaxis. The role of skin testing in this situation has been reviewed [1–12]. Skin tests should be carried out using major-determinant antigens (benzylpenicilloyl polylysine, PPL) and minor-determinant mixture (benzylpenicillin, benzylpenicilloate and benzylpenilloate) antigens [13]. Procedures have been published, and the reader is referred to the original articles for details about methodology [13–15]. Epicutaneous testing should precede intradermal testing, and positive (histamine or opiate) and negative (diluent) controls should be included. False-negative results may be found after a systemic allergic reaction, as a result of a refractory period or temporary desensitization, so that skin testing should be postponed for at least 4–6 weeks [13].

There is a high incidence of wrongly diagnosed penicillin allergy on the basis of history, and a considerable proportion of patients who have had proven allergic reactions to penicillins eventually stop producing the IgE antibody responsible. In a large study, only 1% of 566 patients with a history of penicillin allergy, and negative skin tests to major determinant (PPL) and minor-determinant mixture and its components (potassium benzylpenicillin, benzylpenicilloate and benzylpenicilloyl-*N*-propylamine), had possibly IgE-mediated reactions [4]. In another study [7], 7.1% of 776 individuals with a previous history of penicillin allergy and 1.7% of 4287 subjects negative by history had positive skin tests to major determinant (PPL) and/or a minor-determinant mixture. Positive skin tests were seen in 17% and 12% of patients with a history of anaphylaxis or urticaria, respectively, but in only 4% with a history of an exanthem. Mild adverse reactions to skin tests occurred in 1% of patients positive by history and 9% of those with positive skin tests. In patients with negative skin tests who received benzylpenicillin or ampicillin, mild acute allergic reactions occurred in 0.5% of subjects negative by history and 2.9% of subjects positive by history. Thus, routine penicillin skin testing can facilitate the safe use of penicillin in 90% of individuals with a previous history of allergy [7]. Positive skin tests, an average of 5 years later, to major and minor determinants of benzylpenicillin and/or minor-determinant mixtures of ampicillin, amoxicillin or cloxacillin were found in 19% of 112 patients with a history of urticaria and angio-oedema or exanthem to penicillins and other semi-synthetic penicillins (most frequently ampicillin and amoxicillin) [8]. Skin-test reactivity was limited in about half to the semi-synthetic penicillin reagents derived from ampicillin, amoxicillin or cloxacillin. The existence of isolated skin-test positivity to reagents specific for ampicillin or amoxicillin, with good tolerance of major and minor penicillin determinants, has been confirmed in other reports [9,16,17], emphasizing the necessity for using reagents specific for the side-chains of these aminopenicillin drugs to exclude possible immediate hypersensitivity in patients who reacted to these antibiotics clinically [8–11,16,17]. Thus 7% of 288 patients with a history of penicillin allergy reacted only to skin testing with amoxicillin and not to benzylpenicillin or phenoxymethylpenicillin diagnostic reagent determinants [16]; these would have been missed if the latter agents had been used alone.

Patients treated with penicillin after a negative skin test to PPL and to minor-determinant mixture develop IgE-mediated reactions only very rarely, and these are almost always mild and self-limited [1,4,7]. Thus, when adequately performed, negative skin tests indicate that the risk of a life-threatening reaction is almost negligible, and that any β-lactam antibiotic may be safely given. In contrast, the risk of an acute allergic reaction, including respiratory obstruction or hypotension, with a positive history and positive skin test is 50–70%; the risk in a patient with a negative history but a positive skin test is about 10% [1,13,18].

Intradermal skin testing is generally safe, with few reactions, and although skin testing may rarely cause sensitization [19], it does not usually do so [13]. However, there is a risk, albeit very small, of fatality from skin testing [20]. A more major problem with skin testing is that use of the major determinant (PPL) alone misses about 10–25% of all positive subjects, and that even addition of benzylpenicillin G as the sole minor-determinant antigen misses 5–10% of positive subjects [21,22]. This is significant because patients with reactivity to minor antigenic determinants are thought to be at a higher risk for anaphylaxis [13,23]. In addition, as detailed above, reagents for detecting sensitivity to aminopenicillins (ampicillin and amoxicillin) should be used [15]. Comprehensive skin testing is therefore only practicable in specialized centres. Skin tests can give both false-positive and false-negative reactions [18]. Thus, it has been argued that a positive or negative result in an individual patient cannot be used to entirely reliably predict outcome [24].

Further difficulties are that skin tests have no predictive value in non-IgE-mediated reactions such as serum sickness, haemolytic anaemia, drug fever, interstitial nephritis, contact dermatitis, maculopapular exanthems or exfoliative dermatitis. Accelerated or late IgE-mediated reactions may occur despite a negative pretreatment skin test [1,13]. Positive intradermal skin-test reactions occurred in only 87% of patients with a history of delayed-type rashes induced by penicillins and cephalosporins and who had positive oral provocation tests [25]. Oral challenge was positive in 18 of 33 patients with positive delayed skin testing and patch testing to ampicillin or amoxicillin, but also in 16 of 27 patients with negative allergy tests [26]. Skin testing is contraindicated where there is a history of exfoliative dermatitis, Stevens–Johnson syndrome or TEN.

There is clearly individual variation in the approach to the diagnosis and management of β-lactam allergy [12], based on a survey of 3500 physician members and fellows of the American Academy of Allergy and Immunology and of allergy training programme directors in the USA.

PPL and fresh penicillin G were used for skin testing by more than 86% of both respondent groups, whereas minor-determinant mixtures were used by only 40%. Epicutaneous followed by intradermal injection was the skin-test technique used by 86% of these allergists.

REFERENCES

1 Weiss ME, Adkinson NF. Immediate hypersensitivity reactions to penicillin and related antibiotics. *Clin Allergy* 1988; **18**: 515–40.
2 Torricelli R, Wuthrich B. Diagnostisches Vorgehen bei Verdacht auf Soforttypallergie auf Penicilline. *Hautarzt* 1996; **47**: 392–3.
3 Shepherd G, Mendelson L. The role of skin testing for penicillin allergy. *Arch Intern Med* 1992; **152**: 2505.
4 Sogn DD, Evans R III, Shepherd GM et al. Results of the National Institute of Allergy and Infectious Diseases Collaborative Clinical Trial to test the predictive value of skin testing with major and minor penicillin derivatives in hospitalized adults. *Arch Intern Med* 1992; **152**: 1025–32.
5 Lin RY. A perspective on penicillin allergy. *Arch Intern Med* 1992; **152**: 930–7.
6 Weiss ME. Evaluation and treatment of patients with prior reactions to beta-lactam antibiotics. *Curr Clin Top Infect Dis* 1993; **3**: 131–45.
7 Gadde J, Spence M, Wheeler B, Adkinson NF Jr. Clinical experience with penicillin skin testing in a large inner-city STD clinic. *JAMA* 1993; **270**: 2456–63.
8 Silviu-Dan F, McPhillips S, Warrington RJ. The frequency of skin test reactions to side-chain penicillin determinants. *J Allergy Clin Immunol* 1993; **91**: 694–701.
9 Audicana M, Bernaola G, Urrutia I et al. Allergic reactions to betalactams: studies in a group of patients allergic to penicillin and evaluation of cross-reactivity with cephalosporin. *Allergy* 1994; **49**: 108–13.
10 Blanca M. The contribution of the side chain of penicillins in the induction of allergic reactions. *J Allergy Clin Immunol* 1994; **94**: 562–3.
11 Warrington RJ. The contribution of the side chain of penicillins in the induction of allergic reactions. *J Allergy Clin Immunol* 1995; **95**: 640.
12 Wickern GM, Nish WA, Bitner AS, Freeman TM. Allergy to beta-lactams: a survey of current practices. *J Allergy Clin Immunol* 1994; **94**: 725–31.
13 Weber EA, Knight A. Testing for allergy to antibiotics. *Semin Dermatol* 1989; **8**: 204–12.
14 Adkinson NF Jr. Tests for immunoglobulin drug reactions. In: Rose NF, Friedman H, eds. *Manual of Clinical Immunology*. Washington, DC: American Society for Microbiology, 1986: 692–7.
15 Lisi P, Lapomarda V, Stingeni L et al. Skin tests in the diagnosis of eruptions caused by betalactams. *Contact Dermatitis* 1997; **37**: 151–4.
16 Blanca M, Vega JM, Garcia J et al. Allergy to penicillin with good tolerance to other penicillins: study of the incidence in subjects allergic to betalactams. *Clin Exp Allergy* 1990; **20**: 475–81.
17 Vega JM, Blanca M, Garcia JJ et al. Immediate allergic reactions to amoxicillin. *Allergy* 1994; **49**: 317–22.
18 Green GR, Rosenblum AH, Sweet LC. Evaluation of penicillin hypersensitivity: value of clinical history and skin testing with penicilloyl-polylysine and penicillin G. A cooperative prospective study of the penicillin Study Group of the American Academy of Allergy. *J Allergy Clin Immunol* 1977; **60**: 339–45.
19 Nugent JS, Quinn JM, McGrath CM et al. Determination of the incidence of sensitization after penicillin skin testing. *Ann Allergy Asthma Immunol* 2003; **90**: 398–403.
20 Dogliotti M. An instance of fatal reaction to the penicillin scratch test. *Dermatologica* 1968; **136**: 489–96.
21 Gorevic PD, Levine BB. Desensitization of anaphylactic hypersensitivity specific for the penicilloate minor determinant of penicillin and carbenicillin. *J Allergy Clin Immunol* 1981; **68**: 267–72.
22 Sogn DD. Penicillin allergy. *J Allergy Clin Immunol* 1984; **74**: 589–93.
23 Adkinson NF Jr. Risk factors for drug allergy. *J Allergy Clin Immunol* 1984; **74**: 567–72.
24 Ewan P. Allergy to penicillin. *BMJ* 1991; **302**: 1462.
25 Aihara M, Ikezawa Z. Evaluation of the skin test reactions in patients with delayed type rash induced by penicillins and cephalosporins. *J Dermatol* 1987; **14**: 440–8.
26 Romano A, Di Fonso M, Papa G et al. Evaluation of adverse cutaneous reactions to aminopenicillins with emphasis on those manifested by maculopapular rashes. *Allergy* 1995; **50**: 113–8.

Agents used in general anaesthesia

Intradermal [1–4] or prick [5,6] testing may be helpful in identifying the causative drug [7], and is essential in confirming lack of sensitivity to pancuronium before use in cases of documented sensitivity to other relaxants [3]. In one series of patients with a history of anaphylaxis during induction of general anaesthesia, skin testing was performed by the prick and intracutaneous methods with dilutions of thiobarbiturates, muscle relaxants or β-lactam antibiotics [8]. No patient experienced a recurrence of anaphylaxis during subsequent general anaesthesia when agents producing positive skin tests were avoided, provided a premedication regimen of prednisone and diphenhydramine was given [8].

REFERENCES

1 Fisher MMcD. Intradermal testing in the diagnosis of acute anaphylaxis during anaesthesia: results of five years experience. *Anaesth Intensive Care* 1979; **7**: 58–61.
2 Fisher MMcD. The diagnosis of acute anaphylactoid reactions to neuromuscular blocking agents: a commonly undiagnosed condition. *Anaesth Intensive Care* 1981; **9**: 235–41.
3 Galletly DC, Treuren BC. Anaphylactoid reactions during anaesthesia. Seven years' experience of intradermal testing. *Anaesthesia* 1985; **40**: 329–33.
4 Soetens FM, Smolders FJ, Meeuwis HC *et al.* Intradermal skin testing in the investigation of suspected anaphylactic reactions during anaesthesia: a retrospective survey. *Acta Anaesthesiol Belg* 2003; **54**: 59–63.
5 Leynadier F, Sansarricq M, Didier JM, Dry J. Prick tests in the diagnosis of anaphylaxis to general anaesthetics. *Br J Anaesth* 1987; **59**: 683–9.
6 Moneret-Vautrin DA, Laxenaire MC. Anaphylaxis to muscle relaxants: predictive tests. *Anaesthesia* 1990; **45**: 246–7.
7 Moneret-Vautrin DA, Laxenaire MC. Skin tests in diagnosis of allergy to muscle relaxants and other anesthetic drugs. *Monogr Allergy* 1992; **30**: 145–55.
8 Moscicki RA, Sockin SM, Corsello BF *et al.* Anaphylaxis during induction of general anesthesia: subsequent evaluation and management. *J Allergy Clin Immunol* 1990; **86**: 325–32.

Local anaesthetics

Avoidance of local anaesthetics on the basis of a vague or equivocal history of a prior adverse reaction may result in substantial increased pain and risk. True allergic reactions probably constitute no more than 1% of all adverse reactions to these drugs, some but not the majority of which are due to preservatives, especially parabens. Skin testing and/or incremental challenge beginning with diluted drug is a safe and effective method for identifying a drug that a patient with a history of an adverse reaction can tolerate [1–7]. Patients with positive patch tests to local anaesthetics and a negative history of anaphylactoid reactions rarely have positive intradermal skin tests. The risk of anaphylactic reactions with amide local anaesthetics (except butanilicaine) is therefore low in such patients [3]. Conversely, patients with anaphylactic reactions to local anaesthetics are usually patch-test negative [3]. Skin testing may produce systemic adverse reactions, especially with undiluted drug. False-positive reactions occur, but false-negative reactions have not been reported, and most skin-tested patients who tolerate a local anaesthetic are skin-test negative to the drug. The choice of a drug for use in skin testing and incremental challenge may be facilitated by current concepts of non-cross-reacting groups of local anaesthetics. Thus, benzoic acid esters, both those with and without *p*-aminobenzoyl groups, do not cross-react with amide local anaesthetic agents.

REFERENCES

1 Schatz M. Skin testing and incremental challenge in the evaluation of adverse reactions of local anesthetics. *J Allergy Clin Immunol* 1984; **74**: 606–16.
2 Fisher MMcD, Graham R. Adverse responses to local anaesthetics. *Anaesth Intensive Care* 1984; **12**: 325–7.
3 Ruzicka T, Gerstmeier M, Przybilla B, Ring J. Allergy to local anesthetics: comparison of patch test with prick and intradermal test results. *J Am Acad Dermatol* 1987; **16**: 1202–8.
4 Glinert RJ, Zachary CB. Local anesthetic allergy. Its recognition and avoidance. *J Dermatol Surg Oncol* 1991; **17**: 491–6.
5 Hodgson TA, Shirlaw PJ, Challacombe SJ. Skin testing after anaphylactoid reactions to dental local anesthetics. A comparison with controls. *Oral Surg Oral Med Oral Pathol* 1993; **75**: 706–11.
6 Wasserfallen JB, Frei PC. Long-term evaluation of usefulness of skin and incremental challenge tests in patients with history of adverse reaction to local anesthetics. *Allergy* 1995; **50**: 162–5.
7 Gall H, Kaufmann R, Kalveram CM. Adverse reactions to local anesthetics: analysis of 197 cases. *J Allergy Clin Immunol* 1996; **97**: 933–7.

Analgesics and NSAIDs

Prick tests were positive in only 13% of 117 patients with a history suggestive of anaphylactoid reactions to a variety of mild analgesics including NSAIDs [1].

REFERENCE

1 Przybilla B, Ring J, Harle R, Galosi A. Hauttestung mit Schmerz-mittelinhaltsstoffen bei Patienten mit anaphylaktoiden Unverträgli-chkeitsreaktionen auf 'leichte' Analgetika. *Hautarzt* 1985; **36**: 682–7.

Heparin

Provocation testing may be a useful diagnostic measure [1–6]. Low-molecular-weight heparin analogues may be satisfactorily substituted in some patients with this reaction, but are not always tolerated [2]. Subcutaneous testing of a panel of heparins, danaparoid and desirudin (hirudin) is recommended for determining acceptable treatment options for patients allergic to specific heparins [3,6]. In type I reactions, or in the presence of skin necrosis with or without heparin-induced thrombocytopenia, a low-molecular-weight heparin should be replaced by danaparoid sodium or hirudin. In the presence of a negative subcutaneous provocation test, the compound can be used with little risk. If all types of low-molecular-weight heparin and danaparoid sodium show positive skin tests, oral anticoagulants should be used, and intravenous injections of any kind of heparin should be avoided because of the potential for anaphylactic shock.

REFERENCES

1 Zimmermann R, Harenberg J, Weber E *et al.* Behandlung bei heparin-induzierter kutaner Reaktion mit einem niedermolekularen Heparin-Analog. *Dtsch Med Wochenschr* 1984; **109**: 1326–8.
2 Klein GF, Kofler H, Wol H, Fritsch PO. Eczema-like, erythematous, infiltrated plaques: a common side effect of subcutaneous heparin therapy. *J Am Acad Dermatol* 1989; **21**: 703–7.
3 Wutschert R, Piletta P, Bounameaux H. Adverse skin reactions to low molecular weight heparins: frequency, management and prevention. *Drug Saf* 1999; **20**: 515–25.
4 Koch P, Münßinger T, Rupp-John C, Uhl K. Delayed-type hypersensitivity skin reactions caused by subcutaneous unfractionated and low-molecular-weight heparins: tolerance of a new recombinant hirudin. *J Am Acad Dermatol* 2000; **42**: 612–9.
5 Szolar-Platzer C, Aberer W, Kranke B. Delayed-type skin reaction to the heparin-alternative danaparoid. *J Am Acad Dermatol* 2000; **43**: 920–2.
6 Grassegger A, Fritsch P, Reider N. Delayed-type hypersensitivity and cross-reactivity to heparins and danaparoid: a prospective study. *Dermatol Surg* 2001; **27**: 47–52.

Skin testing in urticaria

Skin tests have been advocated as useful in the investigation of chronic urticaria [1,2]. Patch testing with a series of penicillins was positive in 6.9% of patients in one study [1], and there were positive intracutaneous tests to cilligen and/or penicillin G in 21.5% of patients. Avoidance of dietary dairy produce, which potentially might have contained penicillin, alleviated the urticaria in 50% of the penicillin-allergic patients. The reported prevalence of positive intracutaneous tests to penicillin was much higher in this study than in other reported series in the literature.

REFERENCES

1 Boonk WJ, van Ketel WG. Skin testing in chronic urticaria. *Dermatologica* 1981; **163**: 151–9.
2 Antony SJ, Fisher RH. Association of penicillin allergy with idiopathic anaphylaxis. *J Fam Pract* 1993; **37**: 499–502.

In vitro tests

Tests for IgE antibody

The detection of drug-specific circulating antibodies does not prove an allergy. It is important to record when a blood test is taken in relation to the evolution of a drug reaction, as the antibody response to a drug has a finite duration. For example, antipenicillin IgE antibodies begin to disappear within 10–30 days. Radioallergosorbent tests (RASTs) for drug-specific IgE class antibody are available for penicillin, insulin and ACTH. RAST detects specific IgE antibody to the penicilloyl determinant, and is positive in 60–90% of patients with a positive skin test to PPL [1,2]; however, there is no *in vitro* test for minor-determinant antigens, and therefore in practice this test is of very limited use [2,3]. Investigation of cross-reactivity of antibodies to penicillin in 123 patients with a history of penicillin allergy, using enzyme-linked immunosorbent assay, detected IgE antibodies specific to amoxicillin, ampicillin or flucloxacillin, respectively, in three patients [4]. These antibodies did not cross-react with other penicillin antigens, and would have been missed had testing involved only use of benzylpenicillin. Thus, allergy to semi-synthetic penicillins can occur without allergy to benzylpenicillin, negative tests specific for benzylpenicillin or phenoxymethylpenicillin cannot be generalized to other penicillins, and exclusive reliance on benzylpenicilloyl RAST to detect allergy to semi-synthetic penicillins could lead to serious adverse consequences [5]. IgE antibodies specific for 1-phenyl-2,3-dimethyl-3-pyrazoline-5-one were found in 17 of 19 serum samples from individuals sensitive to pyrazoline drugs with 4-amino-antipyrine discs by RAST [6].

REFERENCES

1 Wide L, Juhlin L. Detection of penicillin allergy of the immediate type by radioimmunoassay of reagins (IgE) to penicilloyl conjugates. *Clin Allergy* 1971; **1**: 171–7.
2 Weiss ME, Adkinson NF. Immediate hypersensitivity reactions to penicillin and related antibiotics. *Clin Allergy* 1988; **18**: 515–40.
3 Ewan P. Allergy to penicillin. *BMJ* 1991; **302**: 1462.
4 Christie G, Coleman J, Newby S *et al.* A survey of the prevalence of penicillin specific IgG, IgM and IgE antibodies detected by ELISA and defined by hapten inhibition in patients with suspected penicillin allergy and in healthy volunteers. *Br J Clin Pharmacol* 1988; **25**: 381–6.
5 Walley T, Coleman J. Allergy to penicillin. *BMJ* 1991; **302**: 1462–3.
6 Zhu D, Becker WM, Schulz KH *et al.* Detection of IgE antibodies specific for 1-phenyl-2,3-dimethyl-3-pyrazoline-5-one by RAST: a serological diagnostic method for sensitivity to pyrazoline drugs. *Asian Pac J Allergy Immunol* 1992; **10**: 95–101.

Miscellaneous *in vitro* tests

The histamine-release test [1], basophil degranulation test [2–4] and passive haemagglutination test [5] are of strictly limited use. A positive basophil degranulation assay, which involves binding of drug to specific IgE on the basophil surface, has been reported with penicillin, erythromycin, sulphonamides and aspirin, but false-negative results are common [3,4]. The leukocyte and macrophage migration inhibition tests [6–9], platelet-activating factor release from white blood cells after antigenic challenge as tested by platelet aggregation [10], and the lymphocyte toxicity assay [11–14] are the subject of investigation but are essentially research tools.

A number of drugs have been reported to induce lymphocyte proliferation, as determined by incorporation of ^{3}H-thymidine, in patients with drug eruptions, including penicillin, carbamazepine, phenytoin, furosemide, sulfamethoxazole and hydrochlorothiazide [15–20]. However, in general only low levels of stimulation are observed, perhaps because the antigen responsible for the reaction is a drug metabolite rather than the parent compound, and the significance of the test is difficult to interpret. Addition of human liver microsomes containing cytochrome P-450 enzymes to the reaction medium of the lymphocyte transformation test, in order to aid generation of potentially reactive drug metabolites, may increase the sensitivity of *in vitro* detection of T-cell reactivity [21,22].

REFERENCES

1 Perelmutter L, Eisen AH. Studies on histamine release from leukocytes of penicillin-sensitive individuals. *Int Arch Allergy* 1970; **38**: 104–12.
2 Shelley WB. Indirect basophil degranulation test for allergy to penicillin and other drugs. *JAMA* 1963; **184**: 171–8.
3 Sastre Dominguez J, Sastre Castillo A. Human basophil degranulation test in drug allergy. *Allergol Immunopath* 1986; **14**: 221–8.
4 Harrabi S, Loiseau P, Dehenry J. A technic for human basophil degranulation. *Allerg Immunol* 1987; **19**: 287–9.
5 Thiel JA, Mitchell S, Parker CW. The specificity of hemagglutination reactions in human and experimental penicillin hypersensitivity. *J Allergy* 1964; **35**: 399–424.
6 David JR, al-Askari S, Lawrence HS, Thomas L. Delayed hypersensitivity in vitro. I. The specificity of inhibition of cell migration by antigens. *J Immunol* 1964; **93**: 264–73.
7 Halevy S, Grunwald MH, Sandbank M *et al*. Macrophage migration inhibition factor (MIF) in drug eruption. *Arch Dermatol* 1990; **126**: 48–51.
8 Lazarov A, Livni E, Halevy S. Generalised pustular drug eruptions: confirmation by in vitro tests. *J Eur Acad Dermatol Venereol* 1998; **10**: 36–41.
9 Kivity S. Fixed drug eruption to multiple drugs: clinical and laboratory investigation. *Int J Dermatol* 1991; **30**: 149–51.
10 Dunoyer-Geindre S, Ludi F *et al*. PAF acether release on antigenic challenge. A method for the investigation of drug allergic reactions. *Allergy* 1992; **47**: 50–4.
11 Shear N, Spielberg S, Grant D *et al*. Differences in metabolism of sulfonamides predisposing to idiosyncratic toxicity. *Ann Intern Med* 1986; **105**: 179–84.
12 Shear N, Spielberg S. Anticonvulsant hypersensitivity syndrome. In vitro assessment of risk. *J Clin Invest* 1989; **82**: 1826–32.
13 Rieder MJ, Uetrecht J, Shear NH *et al*. Diagnosis of sulfonamide hypersensitivity reactions by in-vitro 'rechallenge' with hydroxylamine metabolites. *Ann Intern Med* 1989; **110**: 286–9.
14 Shear NH. Diagnosing cutaneous adverse reactions to drugs. *Arch Dermatol* 1990; **126**: 94–7.
15 Rocklin RE, David JR. Detection in vitro of cellular hypersensitivity to drugs. *J Allergy Clin Immunol* 1971; **48**: 276–82.
16 Gimenez-Camarasa JM, Garcia-Calderon P, de Moragas JM. Lymphocyte transformation test in fixed drug eruption. *N Engl J Med* 1975; **292**: 819–21.
17 Dobozy A, Hunyadi J, Kenderessy AS, Simon N. Lymphocyte transformation test in detection of drug hypersensitivity. *Clin Exp Dermatol* 1981; **6**: 367–72.
18 Sarkany I. Role of lymphocyte transformation in drug allergy. *Int J Dermatol* 1981; **8**: 544–5.
19 Roujeau JC, Albengres E, Moritz S *et al*. Lymphocyte transformation test in drug-induced toxic epidermal necrolysis. *Int Arch Allergy Appl Immunol* 1985; **78**: 22–4.
20 Zakrzewska JM, Ivanyi L. In vitro lymphocyte proliferation by carbamazepine, carbamazepine-10,11-epoxide, and oxcarbazepine in the diagnosis of drug-induced hypersensitivity. *J Allergy Clin Immunol* 1988; **82**: 1826–32.
21 Merk HF, Baron J, Kawadubo Y *et al*. Metabolites and allergic drug reactions. *Clin Exp Allergy* 1998; **28** (Suppl. 4): 21–4.
22 Sachs B, Erdmann S, Al-Masaoudi T, Merk HF. In vitro drug allergy detection system incorporating human liver microsomes in chlorazepate-induced skin rash: drug-specific proliferation associated with interleukin-5 secretion. *Br J Dermatol* 2001; **144**: 316–20.

Challenge tests

A drug suspected of causing a drug eruption may be reliably incriminated by the reaction in response to a test dose administered after recovery. However, fatal reactions have occurred to test doses, for example penicillin and quinine,

and provocation tests should only be performed in exceptional circumstances [1–6]. A history of Stevens–Johnson syndrome or TEN constitutes an absolute contraindication to drug challenge, and test dosing in reactions of anaphylactic type, blood dyscrasia or SLE-like reaction is seldom advisable. Challenge tests are open to misinterpretation [6], because a very small challenge dose may fail to elicit a reaction that a therapeutic dose would provoke, because of false positives, and because false negatives may occur as a result of a refractory period following a reaction [7].

Test dosing in patients with drug reactions such as fixed drug eruption, which are not potentially fatal, may be helpful [5]. Topical challenge in the form of patch testing in a previously involved site may yield a positive response in a high proportion of such cases [8]. Oral provocation tests using tartrazine, and other food additives such as sodium benzoate, have been advocated for the investigation of chronic urticaria or food intolerance [9–12]. Protocols for the analysis of adverse reactions to foods and food additives have been published [13].

REFERENCES

1 Kauppinen K. Cutaneous reactions to drugs. With special reference to severe mucocutaneous bullous eruptions and sulphonamides. *Acta Derm Venereol Suppl (Stockh)* 1972; **68**: 1–89.
2 Kauppinen K. Rational performance of drug challenge in cutaneous hypersensitivity. *Semin Dermatol* 1983; **2**: 117–230.
3 Kauppinen K, Stubb S. Drug eruptions. Causative agents and clinical types. *Acta Derm Venereol (Stockh)* 1984; **64**: 320–4.
4 Girard M. Conclusiveness of rechallenge in the interpretation of adverse drug reactions. *Br J Clin Pharmacol* 1987; **23**: 73–9.
5 Kauppinen K, Alanko K. Oral provocation: uses. *Semin Dermatol* 1989; **8**: 187–91.
6 Girard M. Oral provocation: limitations. *Semin Dermatol* 1989; **8**: 192–5.
7 Stevenson DD, Simon RA, Mathison DA. Aspirin-sensitive asthma: tolerance to aspirin after positive oral aspirin challenges. *J Allergy Clin Immunol* 1980; **66**: 82–8.
8 Alanko K, Stubb S, Reitamo S. Topical provocation of fixed drug eruption. *Br J Dermatol* 1987; **116**: 561–7.
9 Warin RP, Smith RJ. Challenge test battery in chronic urticaria. *Br J Dermatol* 1976; **94**: 401–6.
10 Supramaniam G, Warner JO. Artificial food additive intolerance in patients with angio-oedema and urticaria. *Lancet* 1986; **ii**: 907–9.
11 Wilson N, Scott A. A double blind assessment of additive intolerance in children using a 12 day challenge period at home. *Clin Exp Allergy* 1989; **19**: 267–72.
12 Michils A, Vandermoten G, Duchateau J, Yemault J-C. Anaphylaxis with sodium benzoate. *Lancet* 1991; **337**: 1424–5.
13 Metcalfe DD, Sampson HA, eds. Workshop on experimental methodology for clinical studies of adverse reactions to foods and food additives. *J Allergy Clin Immunol* 1990; **86** (Suppl.): 421–42.

Treatment

Clearly, prevention is better than cure [1,2]. Drugs implicated in a previous reaction should be avoided; the patient should be asked about allergies, and hypersensitivity records in the notes and on prescription charts should be checked. In the case of suspected penicillin allergy, an alternative antibiotic, preferably with a non-β-lactam structure such as erythromycin, should be substituted;

use of griseofulvin should be avoided as it has a 5–10% cross-reactivity based on non-structural mechanisms [2]. However, lack of a positive history does not eliminate the possibility of an allergic reaction, as in the case of penicillin hypersensitivity [3]. Where it is essential to readminister one of a group of drugs to a patient with a previous history of an adverse reaction to a related medication, as with radiographic contrast media and agents used in general anaesthesia, then if possible preliminary skin testing should be carried out to enable identification of safe alternative therapy. In addition, the procedure should be covered by premedication with oral corticosteroids and antihistamines, with or without epinephrine, in order to obtund the onset of an anaphylactic reaction. In the situation where there is no acceptable alternative for an essential drug, then rapid desensitization therapy should be considered.

The approach to treatment of an established presumed drug eruption obviously depends on the severity of the reaction. For many minor conditions, withdrawal of the suspected drug, and symptomatic therapy with emollients, mild to moderately potent topical corticosteroids and systemic antihistamines where indicated, is all that is necessary. When a patient is receiving multiple drugs, it is wise to withdraw all but the essential medications, and to consider substituting alternative non-cross-reacting drugs for the remainder. Because of the wide variety of patterns of drug reaction, it is only possible to summarize the therapy of individual reactions here. The reader is referred to the discussion of the more serious conditions in this book and elsewhere [1–7].

Table 73.21 Management of anaphlyaxis.

Stop drug administration
Give 0.5–1 mL epinephrine (adrenaline) 1 in 1000 i.m. immediately
Check airway and give oxygen
Antihistamines
    Chlorpheniramine maleate 10–20 mg i.v. *or*
    Hydroxyzine 25–50 mg i.m. and four times daily orally *or*
    H_1 and H_2 antagonists *or*
    Cimetidine 300 mg i.v. 6 hourly
Corticosteroids
    Hydrocortisone 250 mg i.v. and 100 mg 6 hourly
    Prednisolone 40 mg/day for 3 days
Give i.v. 0.9% NaCl or 5% glucose
Monitor blood pressure and pulse
For bronchospasm
    Aminophylline 250 mg i.v. over 5 min and 250 mg in 500 mL 0.9% NaCl over 6 h *or*
    Nebulized terbutaline, salbutamol or metaproterenol

infection, high-output cardiac failure, stress ulceration and gastrointestinal haemorrhage, malabsorption and venous thrombosis. The management [1,2] includes maintenance of body temperature and fluid and electrolyte balance, treatment of cardiac failure by use of digitalization and diuretics (avoiding vasodilator drugs), and administration of intravenous albumin for hypoalbuminaemia. If the patient does not respond rapidly to potent topical corticosteroids, prednisolone 40–60 mg/day should be given. This approach also applies to the anticonvulsant hypersensitivity syndrome; oral corticosteroid therapy has been helpful [3,4].

REFERENCES

1 Sheffer AL, Pennoyer MD. Management of adverse drug reactions. *J Allergy Clin Immunol* 1984; **74**: 580–8.
2 Fellner MJ, Ledesma GN. Current comments on cutaneous allergy. Management of antibiotic allergies. *Int J Dermatol* 1991; **30**: 184–5.
3 Weber EA, Knight A. Testing for allergy to antibiotics. *Semin Dermatol* 1989; **8**: 204–12.
4 Braun-Falco O, Plewig G, Wolff HH, Winkelmann RK. *Dermatology.* Berlin: Springer, 1991.
5 Breathnach SM, Hintner H. *Adverse Drug Reactions and the Skin.* Oxford: Blackwell Scientific Publications, 1992.
6 Breathnach SM. Management of drug eruptions. Part II. Diagnosis and treatment. *Australas J Dermatol* 1995; **36**: 187–91.
7 Drake LA, Dinehart SM, Farmer ER *et al.* Guidelines of care for cutaneous adverse drug reactions. American Academy of Dermatology. *J Am Acad Dermatol* 1996; **35**: 458–61.

Anaphylaxis

The management of severe acute urticaria and anaphylaxis is detailed in Table 73.21.

Exfoliative dermatitis/erythroderma

The complications of this potentially serious drug-induced condition include hypothermia, fluid and electrolyte loss,

REFERENCES

1 Marks J. Erythroderma and its management. *Clin Exp Dermatol* 1982; **7**: 415–22.
2 Roujeau JC, Revuz J. Intensive care in dermatology. In: Champion RH, Pye RJ, eds. *Recent Advances in Dermatology*, Vol. 8. Edinburgh: Churchill Livingstone, 1990: 85–99.
3 Murphy JM, Mashman J, Miller JD, Bell JB. Suppression of carbamazepine-induced rash with prednisone. *Neurology* 1991; **41**: 144–5.
4 Chopra S, Levell NJ, Cowley G, Gilkes JJ. Systemic corticosteroids in the phenytoin hypersensitivity syndrome. *Br J Dermatol* 1996; **134**: 1109–12.

Toxic epidermal necrolysis

See Chapter 74.

Desensitization

It is possible to induce a state of antigen-specific mast cell unresponsiveness, in patients with type I IgE-mediated reactions, if a drug is essential for a patient's well-being and no alternative is available. Desensitization markedly diminishes the risk of anaphylactic reactions but not of non-IgE-mediated reactions; it should only be carried out in an intensive care setting. Mechanisms proposed to explain the development of tolerance following desensitization procedures include mediator depletion, tachyphylaxis, production of blocking antibodies, or change in the level of specific IgE antibodies.

Desensitization is most frequently carried out for patients with penicillin allergy, with increasing doses of penicillin being administered over 3–5 h [1–3]. The drug is usually given orally; increasing doses are given, starting with a very weak concentration (e.g. one millionth of the therapeutic dose) and working up to a full dose. There have been no severe allergic reactions recorded in patients who completed oral desensitization to penicillin; about 35% experience minor cutaneous reactions including pruritus or urticaria. Although the protection is usually short-lived, tolerance can be maintained by long-term administration of low doses of oral penicillin. Patients with sensitivity to vancomycin [4], 5-aminosalicylic acid [5] and allopurinol [6] have been successfully desensitized.

Patients with HIV infection with previous cutaneous reactions to sulphonamides [7–11] or antituberculous medication [12] have also been desensitized. A 10-day oral desensitization regimen was described for trimethoprim–sulfamethoxazole in 28 HIV-infected patients [8]; 82% were successfully desensitized, and four of the 28 patients had relatively severe rashes (three maculopapular, one erythroderma) during the desensitization phase. Four patients subsequently had rashes 12–33 weeks after desensitization [8].

REFERENCES

1 Wendel GD, Stark BJ, Jamison RB et al. Penicillin allergy and desensitization in serious infections during pregnancy. *N Engl J Med* 1985; **312**: 1229–32.
2 Stark BJ, Earl HS, Gross GN et al. Acute and chronic desensitization of pencillin-allergic patients using oral penicillin. *J Allergy Clin Immunol* 1987; **79**: 523–32.
3 Weiss ME, Adkinson NF. Immediate hypersensitivity reactions to penicillin and related antibiotics. *Clin Allergy* 1988; **18**: 515–40.
4 Wong JT, Ripple RE, MacLean JA et al. Vancomycin hypersensitivity: synergism with narcotics and 'desensitization' by a rapid continuous intravenous protocol. *J Allergy Clin Immunol* 1994; **94**: 189–94.
5 Stelzle RC, Squire EN. Oral desensitization to 5-aminosalicylic acid medications. *Ann Allergy Asthma Immunol* 1999; **83**: 23–4.
6 Fam AG, Dunne SM, Iazzetta J, Paton TW. Efficacy and safety of desensitization to allopurinol following cutaneous reactions. *Arthritis Rheum* 2001; **44**: 231–8.
7 Torgovnick J. Desensitization to sulfonamides in patients with HIV infection. *Am J Med* 1990; **88**: 548–9.
8 Absar N, Daneshvar H, Beall G. Desensitization to trimethoprim/sulfamethoxazole in HIV-infected patients. *J Allergy Clin Immunol* 1994; **93**: 1001–5.
9 Belchi-Hernandez J, Espinosa-Parra FJ. Management of adverse reactions to prophylactic trimethoprim–sulfamethoxazole in patients with human immuno-deficiency virus infection. *Ann Allergy Asthma Immunol* 1996; **76**: 355–8.
10 Douglas R, Spelman D, Czarny D, O'Hehir RE. Successful desensitization of two patients who previously developed Stevens–Johnson syndrome while receiving trimethoprim-sulfamethoxazole. *Clin Infect Dis* 1997; **25**: 1480.
11 Caumes E, Guermonprez G, Lecomte C et al. Efficacy and safety of desensitization with sulfamethoxazole and trimethoprim in 48 previously hypersensitive patients infected with human immunodeficiency virus. *Arch Dermatol* 1997; **133**: 465–9.
12 Kura MM, Hira SK. Reintroducing antituberculosis therapy after Stevens–Johnson syndrome in human immunodeficiency virus-infected patients with tuberculosis: role of desensitization. *Int J Dermatol* 2001; **40**: 481–4.

Chapter 74

Erythema Multiforme, Stevens–Johnson Syndrome and Toxic Epidermal Necrolysis

S.M. Breathnach

Definition and terminology

Clinically, erythema multiforme involves macular, papular or urticarial lesions, as well as the classical iris or 'target lesions', distributed preferentially on the distal extremities. Lesions may involve the palms or trunk, as well as the oral and genital mucous membranes with erosions. Stevens–Johnson syndrome (SJS), first described in 1922, comprises extensive erythema multiforme of the trunk and mucous membranes, accompanied by fever, malaise, myalgia and arthralgia [1,2]. Toxic epidermal necrolysis (TEN; Lyell's syndrome), first described in 1956 [3], is characterized by extensive sheet-like skin erosions with widespread purpuric macules or flat atypical target lesions, accompanied by severe involvement of conjunctival, corneal, irideal, buccal, labial and genital mucous membranes [4,5]. Historically, the three presentations were considered to form a spectrum from mild to fulminatingly severe cases. More recently, there has been a re-evaluation of this concept and a tendency to consider erythema multiforme minor and major as part of one spectrum, often related to (especially herpesvirus) infections and perhaps on occasion to drug reactions, but to separate off SJS and TEN, both of which are more closely linked to drug sensitivities, and which may be regarded as severe variants of a single disease [6–10].

Erythema multiforme major occurs in younger males, frequently recurs, has less fever and milder mucosal lesions, and lacks association with collagen vascular diseases, human immunodeficiency virus (HIV) infection or cancer; herpes simplex is associated with SJS in up to 10% of cases [10]. SJS, with occasional skin blisters and erosions covering less than 10% of the body's surface area, is differentiated from TEN, in which typically sheet-like erosions involve more than 30% of the body surface. However, there are a number of cases (10–20% in adults, and a higher percentage in children) that even experienced clinicians and histopathologists are unable to classify, as they seem to have features of both groups.

There may be significant differences between countries in the clinical classification of severe cutaneous reactions, indicating the need for precise definitions [11]. Thus, the term 'acute disseminated epidermal necrosis (ADEN)' has been proposed [12], with ADEN type 1 corresponding to SJS, type 2 to transitional SJS/TEN with epidermal detachment between 10 and 29% and type 3 to full-blown TEN, while it has even been advocated by Lyell that the term 'exanthematic necrolysis' should replace TEN [13].

REFERENCES

1 Stevens AH, Johnson FC. A new eruptive fever associated with stomatitis and ophthalmia: report of two cases in children. *Am J Dis Child* 1922; **24**: 526–7.
2 Côté B, Wechsler J, Bastuji-Garin S *et al*. Clinicopathologic correlation in erythema multiforme and Stevens–Johnson syndrome. *Arch Dermatol* 1995; **131**: 1268–72.
3 Lyell A. Toxic epidermal necrolysis: an eruption resembling scalding of the skin. *Br J Dermatol* 1956; **68**: 355–61.
4 Revuz JE, Roujeau JC. Advances in toxic epidermal necrolysis. *Semin Cutan Med Surg* 1996; **15**: 258–66.
5 Wolkenstein P, Revuz J. Toxic epidermal necrolysis. *Dermatol Clin* 2000; **18**: 485–95, ix.
6 Bastuji-Garin S, Rzany B, Stern RS *et al*. A clinical classification of cases of toxic epidermal necrolysis, Stevens–Johnson syndrome, and erythema multiforme. *Arch Dermatol* 1993; **129**: 92–6.
7 Roujeau JC. The spectrum of Stevens–Johnson syndrome and toxic epidermal necrolysis: a clinical classification. *J Invest Dermatol* 1994; **102**: 28S–30S.

8 Assier H, Bastuji-Garin S, Revuz J, Roujeau JC. Erythema multiforme with mucous membrane involvement and Stevens–Johnson syndrome are clinically different disorders with distinct causes. *Arch Dermatol* 1995; **131**: 539–43.

9 Roujeau JC. Stevens–Johnson syndrome and toxic epidermal necrolysis are severity variants of the same disease which differs from erythema multiforme. *J Dermatol* 1997; **24**: 726–9.

10 Auquier-Dunant A, Mockenhaupt M, Naldi L *et al*. Correlations between clinical patterns and causes of erythema multiforme majus, Stevens–Johnson syndrome, and toxic epidermal necrolysis: results of an international prospective study. *Arch Dermatol* 2002; **138**: 1019–24.

11 Stern RS, Albengres E, Carlson J *et al*. An international comparison of case definition of severe adverse cutaneous reactions to medicines. *Drug Saf* 1993; **8**: 69–77.

12 Ruiz-Maldonado R. Acute disseminated epidermal necrosis types 1, 2, and 3: study of 60 cases. *J Am Acad Dermatol* 1985; **13**: 623–35.

13 Lyell A. Requiem for toxic epidermal necrolysis. *Br J Dermatol* 1990; **122**: 837–8.

Erythema multiforme

Aetiology

Immunology

The clinical picture would seem to be a reaction pattern to many different triggering factors; it appears to have an immunological basis. Human leukocyte antigen (HLA) studies have shown an association with HLA-B62 (B15), HLA-B35 and HLA-DR53 in recurrent cases [1–3]. Immune complexes have been demonstrated, both in the skin and circulation [4,5], autoantibodies against epithelial cells have been demonstrated [6], and autoantibodies against desmosomal plaque proteins desmoplakin I and II, with suprabasal acantholysis, were found in seven of 10 patients with erythema multiforme major [7]. However, these findings are probably simply epiphenomena. The histology suggests delayed hypersensitivity; CD4$^+$ lymphocytes have been found in the dermis and CD8$^+$ cells in the epidermis. Herpesvirus-infected peripheral blood mononuclear cells induced up-regulation of CD54 and major histocompatibility complex class I molecules in adjacent non-infected human dermal microvascular endothelial cells *in vitro*, and consequent increased endothelial binding of peripheral blood mononuclear cells [8]. Herpes simplex virus (HSV) DNA can be identified in lesions of herpes-induced erythema multiforme [9,10]. It has been proposed that peripheral blood mononuclear cells (macrophages or Langerhans' cells) pick up HSV DNA and transport fragments to distant skin sites, leading to recruitment of HSV-specific CD4$^+$ Th1 cells that produce interferon-γ (IFN-γ) [11]. This initiates an inflammatory cascade that includes expression of IFN-γ induced genes, increased sequestration of circulating leukocytes, monocytes and natural killer (NK) cells, and recruitment of autoreactive T cells. By extrapolation, drug hapten-specific T cells could be involved in the pathogenesis of drug-induced erythema multiforme. Peripheral blood mononuclear cells obtained from a patient with carba-mazepine-induced erythema multiforme at the time of disease showed increased binding to intercellular adhesion molecule-1$^+$ (ICAM-1$^+$) heterologous keratinocytes, and to autologous keratinocytes *in vitro*, which could be inhibited completely by antibodies to lymphocyte function-associated antigen-1 (LFA-1), the ligand for ICAM-1 [12]. Perforin-positive cells may mediate apoptotic cell death in erythema multiforme and SJS [13]. MCP-1, RANTES, macrophage IFN-γ inducible gene (Mig), and IFN-γ inducible protein 10 (IP 10) were expressed by basal keratinocytes above and mononuclear cells within inflammatory foci. These cytokines contribute to the cell-specific and spatially restricted recruitment of mononuclear cells in the acute inflammation of erythema multiforme [14].

REFERENCES

1 Duvic M, Reisner EG, Dawson DV *et al*. HLA-B15 associates with erythema multiforme. *J Am Acad Dermatol* 1983; **8**: 493–6.

2 Kämpgen E, Burg G, Wank R. Association of herpes simplex virus-induced erythema multiforme with the human leucocyte antigen Dqw3. *Arch Dermatol* 1988; **124**: 1372–5.

3 Schofield JK, Tatnall FM, Brown J *et al*. Recurrent erythema multiforme: tissue typing in a large series of patients. *Br J Dermatol* 1994; **131**: 532–5.

4 Bushkell LL, Mackel SE, Jordan RE. Erythema multiforme: direct immunofluorescence studies and detection of circulating immune complexes. *J Invest Dermatol* 1980; **74**: 372–4.

5 Kazmierowski JA, Wuepper KD. Erythema multiforme: clinical spectrum and immunopathogenesis. *Springer Semin Immunopathol* 1981; **4**: 45–53.

6 Matsuoka LY, Wortsmann J, Stanley JR. Epidermal autoantibodies in erythema multiforme. *J Am Acad Dermatol* 1989; **21**: 677–80.

7 Foedinger D, Sterickzy B, Elbe A *et al*. Autoantibodies against desmoplakin I and II define a subset of patients with erythema multiforme major. *J Invest Dermatol* 1996; **106**: 1012–6.

8 Larcher C, Gasser A, Hattmannstorfer R *et al*. Interaction of HSV-1 infected peripheral blood mononuclear cells with cultured dermal microvascular endothelial cells: a potential model for the pathogenesis of HSV-1 induced erythema multiforme. *J Invest Dermatol* 2001; **116**: 150–6.

9 Brice S, Krzemien D, Weston W *et al*. Detection of herpes simplex virus DNA in cutaneous lesions of erythema multiforme. *J Invest Dermatol* 1989; **93**: 183–7.

10 Aslanzadeh J, Helm KF, Espy MJ *et al*. Detection of HSV-specific DNA in biopsy of patients with erythema multiforme by polymerase chain reaction. *Br J Dermatol* 1992; **126**: 19–23.

11 Aurelian L, Ono F, Burnett J. Herpes simplex virus (HSV)-associated erythema multiforme (HAEM): a viral disease with an autoimmune component. *Dermatol Online J* 2003; **9**: 1.

12 Bruynzeel L, Van der Raaij EMH, Boorsma DM *et al*. Increased adherence to keratinocytes of peripheral blood mononuclear leucocytes of a patient with drug-induced erythema multiforme. *Br J Dermatol* 1992; **129**: 45–9.

13 Inachi S, Mizutani H, Shimizu M. Epidermal apoptotic cell death in erythema multiforme and Stevens–Johnson syndrome: contribution of perforin-positive cell infiltration. *Arch Dermatol* 1997; **133**: 845–9.

14 Spandau U, Brocker EB, Kampgen E, Gillitzer R. CC and CXC chemokines are differentially expressed in erythema multiforme *in vivo*. *Arch Dermatol* 2002; **138**: 1027–33.

Triggering factors

Potential triggering factors are listed in Table 74.1 [1–21]. In up to 50% of cases, there is no known provoking factor. The most common association is with a preceding

Table 74.1 Some causes of erythema multiforme.

Virus infections [1]
  Herpes simplex [2,3]
  'Primary atypical pneumonia', *Mycoplasma* infections [4,5]
  Acquired immune deficiency syndrome
  Adenovirus [6]
  Cytomegalovirus [7]
  Hepatitis B
  Infectious mononucleosis [8,9]
  Lymphogranuloma inguinale
  Milker's nodes
  Mumps
  Orf
  Poliomyelitis
  Psittacosis
  Variola
  Vaccinia
  Varicella [10]
Bacterial infections
  A wide range has been recorded
  Rickettsiae [11]
Fungal infections [12]
  Histoplasmosis [13,14]
  Vaccination [15]
  Drug reactions
  Contact reactions
  Carcinoma, lymphoma, leukaemia
  Lupus erythematosus (Rowell's syndrome) [16,17]
  Polyarteritis nodosa
  Pregnancy, premenstrual, 'autoimmune progesterone dermatitis' [18]
  Sarcoidosis [19]
  Wegener's granulomatosis
  X-ray therapy [20,21]
Unknown

herpes simplex infection (facial or genital) [2,3], or with a *Mycoplasma* infection [4,5]; other viral or bacterial infections have also been incriminated.

REFERENCES

1 Anderson JA, Bolin V, Sutow WW *et al*. Virus as possible aetiologic agent of erythema multiforme exudativum, bullous type. *Arch Dermatol Syphilol* 1949; **59**: 251–62.
2 Editorial. Recurrent erythema multiforme and herpes simplex virus. *Lancet* 1989; **ii**: 1311–2.
3 Schofield JK, Tatnall FM, Leigh IM. Recurrent erythema multiforme: clinical features and treatment in a large series of patients. *Br J Dermatol* 1992; **128**: 542–5.
4 Gordon AM, Lyell A. Mycoplasmas and their association with skin disease. *Br J Dermatol* 1970; **82**: 414–7.
5 Sontheimer RD, Garibaldi RA, Kruegger GG. Stevens–Johnson syndrome associated with *Mycoplasma pneumoniae* infections. *Arch Dermatol* 1978; **114**: 241–4.
6 Strom J. Febrile mucocutaneous syndromes (ectodermosis erosiva pleuriorificialis, Stevens–Johnson syndrome, etc.) in adenovirus infections. *Acta Derm Venereol (Stockh)* 1967; **47**: 281.
7 Seishima M, Oyama Z, Yamamura M. Erythema multiforme associated with cytomegalovirus infection in non-immunosuppressed patients. *Dermatology* 2001; **203**: 299–302.
8 Williamson DM. Erythema multiforme in infectious mononucleosis. *Br J Dermatol* 1974; **91**: 345–6.
9 Hughes T, Burrows NP. Infectious mononucleosis presenting as erythema multiforme. *Clin Exp Dermatol* 1993; **18**: 373–4.
10 Prais D, Grisuru-Soen G, Barzilai A, Amir J. Varicella zoster virus infection associated with erythema multiforme in children. *Infection* 2001; **29**: 37–9.
11 Lang MH, Wehrenberg O. Erythema exsudativum multiforme bei Rickettsiose. *Hautarzt* 1987; **38**: 432–4.
12 Salim A, Young E. Erythema multiforme associated with *Trichophyton mentagrophytes* infection. *J Eur Acad Dermatol Venereol* 2002; **16**: 645–6.
13 Leznoff A, Frank H, Telner P *et al*. Histoplasmosis in Montreal during the fall of 1963, with observations on erythema multiforme. *Can Med Assoc J* 1963; **91**: 1154–60.
14 Sellers TF, Price WN, Newberry WM. An epidemic of erythema multiforme and erythema nodosum caused by histoplasmosis. *Ann Intern Med* 1965; **62**: 1244–62.
15 Loche F, Schwarze HP, Thedenat B, Carriere M, Bazex J. Erythema multiforme associated with hepatitis B immunization. *Clin Exp Dermatol* 2000; **25**: 167–8.
16 Rowell NR, Beck JS, Anderson JR. Lupus erythematosus and erythema multiforme-like lesions. *Arch Dermatol* 1963; **88**: 176–80.
17 Roustan G, Salas C, Barbadillo C *et al*. Lupus erythematosus with an erythema multiforme-like eruption. *Eur J Dermatol* 2000; **10**: 459–62.
18 Warin AP. Case 2: diagnosis—erythema multiforme as a presentation of autoimmune progesterone dermatitis. *Clin Exp Dermatol* 2001; **26**: 107–8.
19 Carswell WA. A case of sarcoidosis presenting with erythema multiforme. *Am Rev Respir Dis* 1972; **106**: 462–4.
20 Davis J, Pack GT. Erythema multiforme following deep X-ray therapy. *Arch Dermatol Syphilol* 1952; **66**: 41–8.
21 Nawalkjha PL, Mathur NK, Malhotra YK *et al*. Severe erythema multiforme (Stevens–Johnson syndrome) following telecobalt therapy. *Br J Radiol* 1972; **45**: 768–9.

Drug induced

Erythema multiforme has been regarded as a well-recognized pattern of adverse cutaneous drug reaction [1–7], although in a prospective study of cases of erythema multiforme only 10% were drug related [2]. In another study, antecedent medication use, especially cephalosporins, was recorded in 59% of erythema multiforme patients and 68% of SJS patients [4]. Often drugs are blamed on inadequate evidence; confirmation of drug sensitivity necessitates re-exposure to the drug, which may carry an unacceptable risk.

Drugs implicated (Table 74.2), often on anecdotal evidence, include sulphonamides and co-trimoxazole, barbiturates, pyrazolone derivatives (phenylbutazone), phenolphthalein, rifampicin, penicillins, hydantoin derivatives, carbamazepine, phenothiazines, chlorpropamide, thiazide diuretics and sulphones. Recent reports have incriminated phenazone, minoxidil, fenbufen, mianserin, sulindac, methaqualone, ceftazidime [8], trazodone [9], progesterone [10], lithium [11], ampicillin [12], amoxicillin [13], vancomycin [14], ofloxacin [15], danazol [16], intradural prednisolone acetate [17], indapamide and sertraline [18], allopurinol [13,19], suramin [20], terbinafine [21,22], fenoterol [23], antiretroviral agents including didanosine [24], griseofulvin [25], celecoxib and rofecoxib [26,27], sulfaguanidine [28], porfirin sodium as part of photodynamic therapy [29], the H_2-blocker roxatidine [30], granulocyte macrophage stimulating factor [31], thalidomide [32] and amfebutamone [33]. Erythema multiforme may follow vaccination [34,35].

Antibiotics
Sulphonamides
  Co-trimoxazole
  Sulfadoxine–pyrimethamine
Sulphones
Penicillins and ampicillin
Cephalosporins
  Ceftazidime
Quinolones
Rifampicin
Tetracyclines
Erythromycin
Thiacetazone

Antifungal or antiyeast preparations
Terbinafine
Griseofulvin
Nystatin

Antiretroviral drugs
Abacavir
Nevirapine

Non-steroidal anti-inflammatory drugs
Salicylates
Fenbufen
Ibuprofen
Sulindac
Paracetamol (acetaminophen)
Pyrazolone derivatives
  Antipyrine
  Phenylbutazone
  Phenazone

Metals
Arsenic
Bromides
Mercury
Gold
Iodides

Anticonvulsants
Barbiturates
Carbamazepine
Hydantoin derivatives
Lamotrigine
Trimethadione

Antihypertensives
Frusemide (furosemide)
Hydralazine
Minoxidil
Thiazide diuretics

Drugs acting on the central nervous system
Danazol
Lithium
Mianserin
Phenothiazines
Trazodone

Miscellaneous
Allopurinol
Chlorpropamide
Codeine
Cyclophosphamide
Methaqualone
Nitrogen mustard
Pentazocine
Phenolphthalein
Progesterone
Topical agents (see text)
Vaccination

Table 74.2 Drugs reported as causing erythema multiforme or Stevens–Johnson syndrome.

REFERENCES

1 Kauppinen K. Cutaneous reactions to drugs: with special reference to severe mucocutaneous bullous eruptions and sulphonamides. *Acta Derm Venereol (Stockh)* 1972; **52** (Suppl. 68): 1–89.

2 Huff JC, Weston WL, Tonnesen MG. Erythema multiforme. a critical review of characteristics, diagnostic criteria, and causes. *J Am Acad Dermatol* 1983; **8**: 763–75.

3 Stewart MG, Duncan NO III, Franklin DJ *et al.* Head and neck manifestations of erythema multiforme in children. *Otolaryngol Head Neck Surg* 1994; **111**: 236–42.

4 Gebel K, Hornstein OP. Drug-induced oral erythema multiforme: results of a long-term retrospective study. *Dermatologica* 1984; **168**: 35–40.

5 Nethercott JR, Choi BC. Erythema multiforme (Stevens–Johnson syndrome): chart review of 123 hospitalized patients. *Dermatologica* 1985; **171**: 383–96.

6 Fabbri P, Panconesi E. Erythema multiforme ('minus' and 'maius') and drug intake. *Clin Dermatol* 1993; **11**: 479–89.

7 Rzany B, Hering O, Mockenhaupt M *et al.* Histopathological and epidemiological characteristics of patients with erythema exudativum multiforme major, Stevens–Johnson syndrome and toxic epidermal necrolysis. *Br J Dermatol* 1996; **135**: 6–11.

8 Pierce TH, Vig SJ, Ingram PM. Ceftazidime in the treatment of lower respiratory tract infection. *J Antimicrob Chemother* 1983; **12** (Suppl. A): 21–5.

9 Ford HE, Jenike MA. Erythema multiforme associated with trazadone therapy. *J Clin Psychiatry* 1985; **46**: 294–5.

10 Wojnarowska F, Greaves MW, Peachey RDG *et al.* Progesterone-induced erythema multiforme. *J R Soc Med* 1985; **78**: 407–8.

11 Balldin J, Berggren U, Heijer A, Mobacken H. Erythema multiforme caused by lithium. *J Am Acad Dermatol* 1991; **24**: 1015–6.

12 Garty BZ, Offer I, Livni E, Danon YL. Erythema multiforme and hypersensitivity myocarditis caused by ampicillin. *Ann Pharmacother* 1994; **28**: 730–1.

13 Perez A, Cabrerizo S, de Barrio M *et al.* Erythema-multiforme-like eruption from amoxycillin and allopurinol. *Contact Dermatitis* 2001; **44**: 113–4.

14 Padial MA, Barranco P, Lopez-Serrano C. Erythema multiforme to vancomycin. *Allergy* 2000; **55**: 1201.

15 Nettis E, Giordano D, Pierluigi T *et al.* Erythema multiforme-like rash in a patient sensitive to ofloxacin. *Acta Derm Venereol (Stockh)* 2002; **82**: 395–6.

16 Reynolds NJ, Sansom JE. Erythema multiforme during danazol therapy. *Clin Exp Dermatol* 1992; **17**: 140.

17 Lavabre C, Chevalier X, Larget-Piet B. Erythema multiforme after intradural injection of prednisolone acetate. *Br J Rheumatol* 1992; **31**: 717–8.

18 Gales BJ, Gales MA. Erythema multiforme and angioedema with indapamide and sertraline (Letter). *Am J Hosp Pharm* 1994; **51**: 118–9.

19 Kumar A, Edward N, White MI *et al.* Allopurinol, erythema multiforme, and renal insufficiency. *BMJ* 1996; **312**: 173–4.

20 Katz SK, Medenica MM, Kobayashi K *et al.* Erythema multiforme induced by suramin. *J Am Acad Dermatol* 1995; **32**: 292–3.

21 Todd P, Halpern S, Munro DD. Oral terbinafine and erythema multiforme. *Clin Exp Dermatol* 1995; **20**: 247–8.

22 Gupta AK, Kopstein JB, Shear NH. Hypersensitivity reaction to terbinafine. *J Am Acad Dermatol* 1997; **36**: 1018–9.

23 Sachs B, Renn C, al Masaoudi T, Merk HF. Fenoterol-induced erythema exudativum multiforme-like exanthem: demonstration of drug-specific lymphocyte reactivity *in vivo* and *in vitro*. *Acta Derm Venereol* 2001; **81**: 368–9.

24 Scully C, Diz Dios P. Orofacial effects of antiretroviral therapies. *Oral Dis* 2001; **7**: 205–10.

25 Thami GP, Kaur S, Kanwar AJ. Erythema multiforme due to griseofulvin with positive re-exposure test. *Dermatology* 2001; **203**: 84–5.

26 Ernst EJ, Egge JA. Celecoxib-induced erythema multiforme with glyburide cross-reactivity. *Pharmacotherapy* 2002; **22**: 637–40.

27 Sarkar R, Kaur C, Kanwar AJ. Erythema multiforme due to rofecoxib. *Dermatology* 2002; **204**: 304–5.

28 de Frutos C, de Barrio M, Tornero P *et al*. Erythema multiforme from sulfaguanidine. *Contact Dermatitis* 2002; **46**: 186–7.

29 Wolfsen HC, Ng CS. Cutaneous consequences of photodynamic therapy. *Cutis* 2002; **69**: 140–2.

30 Horiuchi Y. Erythema multiforme caused by the H_2-blocker, roxatidine. *J Dermatol* 2000; **27**: 352–3.

31 Mori T, Sato N, Watanabe R, Okamoto S, Ikeda Y. Erythema exsudativum multiforme induced by granulocyte colony-stimulating factor in an allogeneic peripheral blood stem cell donor. *Bone Marrow Transplant* 2000; **26**: 239–40.

32 Hall VC, El-Azhary RA, Bouwhuis S, Rajkumar SV. Dermatologic side effects of thalidomide in patients with multiple myeloma. *J Am Acad Dermatol* 2003; **48**: 548–52.

33 Lineberry TW, Peters GE Jr, Bostwick JM. Bupropion-induced erythema multiforme. *Mayo Clin Proc* 2001; **76**: 664–6.

34 Frey SE, Couch RB, Tacket CO *et al*. Clinical responses to undiluted and diluted smallpox vaccine. *N Engl J Med* 2002; **346**: 1265–74.

35 Karakaya G, Sahin S, Fuat Kalyoncu A. Erythema multiforme: as a complication of allergen-specific immunotherapy. *Allergol Immunopathol (Madr)* 2001; **29**: 276–8.

Topical agents and erythema multiforme-like reactions

Topical sensitivities reportedly also provoke erythema multiforme. The substances involved are usually potent sensitizers such as *Primula obconica* [1], poison ivy, a variety of weeds [2], diphenyl cyclopropenone and bromofluorene [3–5]. A large number of topical medications can induce erythema multiforme-like eruptions, including balsam of Peru, chloramphenicol, econazole, ethylenediamine, furazolidone, mafenide acetate cream used to treat burns, the muscle relaxant mephenesin, neomycin, nifuroxime, promethazine, scopolamine, sulphonamides, ophthalmic anticholinergic preparations (scopolamine hydrobromide and tropicamide drops), vitamin E, the antimycotic agent pyrrolnitrin, as well as proflavine, budesonide [6], topical nitrogen mustard [7], sesquiterpene lactones in herbal medicine [8], bufexamac [9] and phenylbutazone [10], nitroglycerin patch [11], tea tree oil [12] and a paint-on henna tattoo [13].

Erythema multiforme has also been associated with use of rubber gloves [14] and with blister beetle dermatitis [15]. In addition, contact with a number of environmental substances may induce erythema multiforme-like reactions [16], including nickel, formaldehyde, trichloroethylene, phenyl sulphone derivative, the insecticide methyl parathion, nitrogen mustard, epoxy compounds, trinitrotoluene, cutting oil [17] and bisphenol A [18].

REFERENCES

1 Lengrand F, Tellart AS, Segard M *et al*. Erythema multiforme-like eruption: an unusual presentation of primula contact allergy. *Contact Dermatitis* 2001; **44**: 35.

2 Jovanovic M, Mimica-Dukic N, Poljacki M, Boza P. Erythema multiforme due to contact with weeds: a recurrence after patch testing. *Contact Dermatitis* 2003; **48**: 17–25.

3 Agrup G, Cronin E. Contact dermatitis X. *Br J Dermatol* 1970; **82**: 428–33.

4 Fisher AA. Erythema multiforme-like eruptions due to topical medications. II. *Cutis* 1986; **37**: 158–61.

5 Perret CM, Steijlen PM, Zaun H, Happle R. Erythema multiforme-like lesions: a rare side effect of topical immunotherapy with diphenylcyclopropenone. *Dermatologica* 1990; **180**: 5–7.

6 Stingeni L, Caraffini S, Assalve D *et al*. Erythema multiforme-like contact dermatitis from budesonide. *Contact Dermatitis* 1996; **34**: 154–5.

7 Newman JM, Rindler JM, Bergfeld WF. Stevens–Johnson syndrome associated with topical nitrogen mustard therapy. *J Am Acad Dermatol* 1997; **36**: 112–4.

8 Mateo MP, Velasco M, Miquel FJ, de la Cuadra J. Erythema multiforme-like eruption following allergic contact dermatitis from sesquiterpene lactones in herbal medicine. *Contact Dermatitis* 1995; **33**: 449–50.

9 Koch P, Bahmer FA. Erythema multiforme-like, urticarial papular and plaque eruptions from bufexamac: report of four cases. *Contact Dermatitis* 1994; **31**: 97–101.

10 Kerre S, Busschots A, Dooms-Goossens A. Erythema multiforme-like contact dermatitis due to phenylbutazone. *Contact Dermatitis* 1995; **33**: 213–4.

11 Silvestre JF, Betlloch I, Guijarro J *et al*. Erythema multiforme-like eruption on the application site of a nitroglycerin patch, followed by widespread erythema multiforme. *Contact Dermatitis* 2001; **45**: 299–300.

12 Khanna M, Qasem K, Sasseville D. Allergic contact dermatitis to tea tree oil with erythema multiforme-like id reaction. *Am J Contact Dermat* 2000; **11**: 238–42.

13 Jappe U, Hausen BM, Petzoldt D. Erythema-multiforme-like eruption and depigmentation following allergic contact dermatitis from a paint-on henna tattoo, due to para-phenylenediamine contact hypersensitivity. *Contact Dermatitis* 2001; **45**: 249–50.

14 Lu CY, Sun CC. Localized erythema-multiforme-like contact dermatitis from rubber gloves. *Contact Dermatitis* 2001; **45**: 311–2.

15 Inanir I. Erythema multiforme associated with blister beetle dermatitis. *Contact Dermatitis* 2002; **46**: 175.

16 Fisher AA. Erythema multiforme-like eruptions due to topical miscellaneous compounds. III. *Cutis* 1986; **37**: 262–4.

17 Hata M, Tokura Y, Takigawa M. Erythema multiforme-like eruption associated with contact dermatitis to cutting oil. *Eur J Dermatol* 2001; **11**: 247–8.

18 Akita H, Washimi Y, Akamatsu H *et al*. Erythema multiforme-like occupational contact dermatitis due to bisphenol A. *Contact Dermatitis* 2001; **45**: 305.

Pathology [1–4]

The most important changes are in the upper dermis and lower epidermis. Some cases have prominent dermal inflammatory changes, with a lymphohistiocytic infiltrate rich in T lymphocytes around blood vessels, oedema and vasodilatation, but little epidermal change. There may also be vacuolar degeneration of the lower epidermis or individually necrotic epidermal cells (Fig. 74.1). Such changes occur especially in classical erythema multiforme with target lesions. In more severe bullous cases, there is more dramatic necrosis of the whole epidermis. Electron microscopy demonstrates the damaged basement membrane in the floor of the bulla, with a few ragged islands of epidermal cells showing some evidence of regeneration. The histology of the oral lesions is similar to that in the

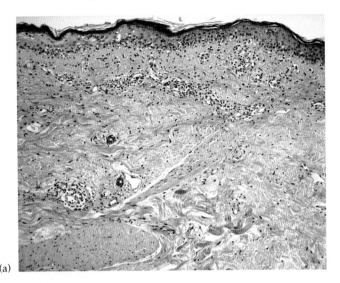

(a)

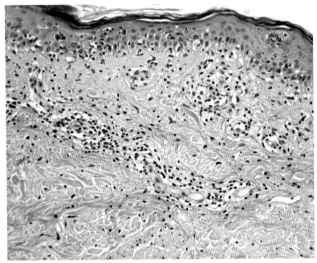

(b)

Fig. 74.1 (a,b) Histopathology of erythema multiforme. Note upper dermal perivascular lymphocytic infiltration, epidermal vaculoar degeneration and scattered individual necrotic keratinocytes (H&E). (Courtesy of Dr E. Calonje, St John's Institute of Dermatology, London, UK.)

skin, and there may be very marked degenerative changes in the epithelium [5].

REFERENCES

1 Ackerman AB. Dermal and epidermal types of erythema multiforme. *Arch Dermatol* 1975; **111**: 795.
2 Bedi TR, Pinkus H. Histopathological spectrum of erythema multiforme. *Br J Dermatol* 1976; **95**: 243–50.
3 Rzany B, Hering O, Mockenhaupt M *et al*. Histopathological and epidemiological characteristics of patients with erythema exudativum multiforme major, Stevens–Johnson syndrome and toxic epidermal necrolysis. *Br J Dermatol* 1996; **135**: 6–11.
4 Paquet P, Pierard GE. Erythema multiforme and toxic epidermal necrolysis: a comparative study. *Am J Dermatopathol* 1997; **19**: 127–32.
5 Lozada-Nur F, Gorsky M, Silverman S. Oral erythema multiforme: clinical observation and treatment of 95 patients. *Oral Surg Oral Med Oral Pathol* 1989; **67**: 36–40.

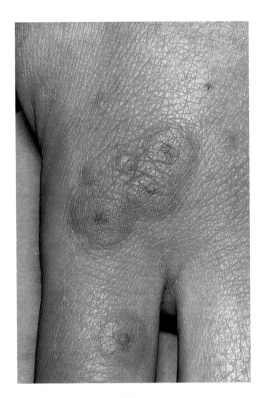

Fig. 74.2 Erythema multiforme. Typical target lesions over knuckles.

Clinical features [1–4]

Erythema multiforme can occur at any age, including neonates [5,6] or young children [7]. In general, the course is that of an eruption developing over a few days and resolving in 2–3 weeks. Repeated attacks associated with recurrent herpes simplex are frequent.

Erythema multiforme minor; papular or simplex form. This accounts for approximately 80% of cases. Clinically, macular, papular or urticarial lesions, as well as the classical iris or 'target lesions' (Fig. 74.2), are distributed preferentially on the distal extremities. Lesions may involve the palms or trunk, as well as the oral (Fig. 74.3) and genital mucous membranes. The lesions are dull red, flat or slightly raised maculopapules, which may remain small or may increase in size to reach a diameter of 1–3 cm in 48 h. Typical cases show at least some target (or iris) lesions. Target lesions are less than 3 cm in diameter, rounded and have three zones: a central area of dusky erythema or purpura, a middle paler zone of oedema and an outer ring of erythema with a well-defined edge. Atypical target lesions have only two of the zones. The lesions appear in successive crops for a few days and fade in 1–2 weeks, sometimes leaving dusky discoloration. There may be a few lesions, or they may be very profuse.

Classically, the backs of the hands, palms, wrists, feet and extensor aspects of the elbows and knees are affected;

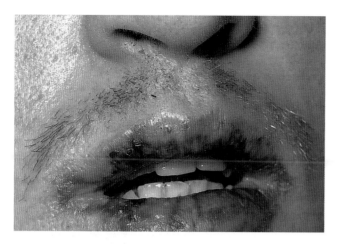

Fig. 74.3 Erythema multiforme. Mucosal lesions.

less commonly the face. Often the hands are selectively involved. Thus, the typical distribution is acral. The Koebner phenomenon is not uncommon, and accounts for some bizarre distributions. There may be occasional erythematous lesions, erosions or bullae on the mucous membranes. Photoaggravation of erythema multiforme is well recognized [8].

Localized vesiculobullous form. This form is intermediate in severity. The skin lesions present as erythematous macules or plaques, often with a central bulla and a marginal ring of vesicles (herpes iris of Bateman). Mucous membranes are quite often involved. In this type, the skin lesions tend to occur in the classical acral distribution, but may be few in number.

Erythema multiforme major. This is a severe illness associated with more extensive target lesions and mucous membrane involvement. The onset is usually sudden, although there may be a prodromal systemic illness of 1–13 days before the eruption appears.

Atypical cases. Because the diagnosis of erythema multiforme depends on the clinical and pathological appearance, criteria for the diagnosis of atypical cases are difficult to apply. However, there are cases where the clinical picture is atypical but the histology nevertheless shows the characteristic changes. Erythema multiforme-like lesions have been reported in the setting of acute generalized exanthematous pustulosis [9]. Lesions many centimetres across may remain stationary or slowly enlarge over several weeks or months (persistent erythema multiforme) [10,11]. On rare occasions, cases with otherwise typical morphology and histology may develop lesions almost continuously rather than episodically [10]. Erythema multiforme along Blaschko's lines has been reported [12],

as has disseminated granuloma annulare following erythema multiforme minor [13].

Rowell's syndrome. This syndrome comprises lupus erythematosus associated with erythema multiforme-like lesions, and immunological findings of speckled antinuclear antibodies, anti-La antibodies and a positive test for rheumatoid factor [14–19]. However, the existence of the syndrome as a defined entity has been questioned [19].

Differential diagnosis

Drug eruptions and lupus erythematosus must be excluded, along with pemphigoid and toxic erythemas of unknown cause. The distinction between atypical erythema multiforme and urticarial vasculitis can be difficult. Kawasaki disease (see Chapter 27) may resemble erythema multiforme, but the characteristic red lips, strawberry tongue, red and swollen palms and soles, and the lymphadenopathy should permit a clinical diagnosis. Differential diagnosis of mouth lesions is considered in Chapter 66.

Treatment [7,20]

Symptomatic treatment only is necessary in the papular and localized bullous forms. Ocular involvement requires the early help of an ophthalmologist. In the more severe cases, good nursing is of paramount importance; such cases may require the sort of attention used for TEN (see below), in a dermatological intensive care unit or burns unit. The value of systemic corticosteroids is still debated [7,20–22], but relief of systemic symptoms such as fever is achieved. For more severe cases, prednisolone at an initial dosage of 30–60 mg/day, decreasing over a period of 1–4 weeks, may be given.

Antiviral therapy with agents such as aciclovir for erythema multiforme following overt herpes simplex infections tends to be disappointing once the eruption has appeared; this is so for recurrent cases, even when given at the very first sign of recurrent herpes. However, long-term prophylactic use may be quite helpful [23–25]. A dosage of 200 mg three times daily may be appropriate, but smaller or larger doses may be needed. Relapses tend to occur when the drug is omitted. It is of interest that some patients who suffer from recurrent erythema multiforme without overt herpes infection are helped by prophylactic aciclovir, implying that recurrent herpes infection may nevertheless be responsible. Aciclovir prevented recurrent polyarthritis associated with erythema multiforme [26].

Thalidomide has been used in a few cases to prevent relapses of recurrent erythema multiforme [27]. Other drugs used have included dapsone [11,28], azathioprine [11] and mycophenolate mofetil [29].

REFERENCES

1 Huff JC, Weston WL. Recurrent erythema multiforme. *Medicine* 1989; **68**: 133–40.
2 Huff JC, Weston WL, Tonnesen MG. Erythema multiforme: a critical review of characteristics, diagnostic criteria and causes. *J Am Acad Dermatol* 1983; **8**: 763–75.
3 Bastuji-Garin S, Rzany B, Stern RS *et al.* A clinical classification of cases of toxic epidermal necrolysis, Stevens–Johnson syndrome, and erythema multiforme. *Arch Dermatol* 1993; **129**: 92–6.
4 Auquier-Dunant A, Mockenhaupt M, Naldi L *et al.* Correlations between clinical patterns and causes of erythema multiforme majus, Stevens–Johnson syndrome, and toxic epidermal necrolysis: results of an international prospective study. *Arch Dermatol* 2002; **138**: 1019–24.
5 Johnston GA, Ghura HS, Carter E, Graham-Brown RA. Neonatal erythema multiforme major. *Clin Exp Dermatol* 2002; **27**: 661–4.
6 Torrelo A, Moreno M, De Prada I *et al.* Erythema multiforme in a neonate. *J Am Acad Dermatol* 2003; **48** (Suppl. 5): 78–9.
7 Rasmussen JE. Erythema multiforme in children. *Br J Dermatol* 1976; **95**: 181–6.
8 Murphy GM. Diseases associated with photosensitivity. *J Photochem Photobiol B* 2001; **64**: 93–8.
9 Lin JH, Sheu HM, Lee JY. Acute generalized exanthematous pustulosis with erythema multiforme-like lesions. *Eur J Dermatol* 2002; **12**: 475–8.
10 Drago F, Parodi A, Rebora A. Persistent erythema multiforme: report of new cases and review of the literature. *J Am Acad Dermatol* 1995; **33**: 366–9.
11 Pavlovic MD, Karadaglic DM, Kandolf LO, Mijuskovic ZP. Persistent erythema multiforme: a report of three cases. *J Eur Acad Dermatol Venereol* 2001; **15**: 54–8.
12 Micalizzi C, Farris A. Erythema multiforme along Blaschko's lines. *J Eur Acad Dermatol Venereol* 2000; **14**: 203–4.
13 Abraham Z, Feuerman EJ, Schafer I, Feinmesser M. Disseminated granuloma annulare following erythema multiforme minor. *Australas J Dermatol* 2000; **41**: 238–41.
14 Rowell NR, Beck JS, Anderson JR. Lupus erythematosus and erythema multiforme-like lesions. *Arch Dermatol* 1963; **88**: 176–80.
15 Fitzgerald EA, Purcell SM, Kantor GR, Goldman HM. Rowell's syndrome: report of a case. *J Am Acad Dermatol* 1996; **35**: 801–3.
16 Marzano AV, Berti E, Gasparini G, Caputo R. Lupus erythematosus with antiphospholipid syndrome and erythema multiforme-like lesions. *Br J Dermatol* 1999; **141**: 720–4.
17 Roustan G, Salas C, Barbadillo C *et al.* Lupus erythematosus with an erythema multiforme-like eruption. *Eur J Dermatol* 2000; **10**: 459–62.
18 Zeitouni NC, Funaro D, Cloutier RA, Gagne E, Claveau J. Redefining Rowell's syndrome. *Br J Dermatol* 2000; **142**: 343–6.
19 Shteyngarts AR, Warner MR, Camisa C. Lupus erythematosus associated with erythema multiforme: does Rowell's syndrome exist? *J Am Acad Dermatol* 1999; **40**: 773–7.
20 Rasmussen JE. Erythema multiforme: a practical approach to recent advances. *Pediatr Dermatol* 2002; **19**: 82–4.
21 Renfro L, Grant-Kels JM, Feder HH *et al.* Are systemic steroids indicated in the treatment of erythema multiforme? *Pediatr Dermatol* 1989; **6**: 43–50.
22 Martinez AE, Atherton DJ. High-dose systemic corticosteroids can arrest recurrences of severe mucocutaneous erythema multiforme. *Pediatr Dermatol* 2000; **17**: 87–90.
23 Huff JC. Therapy and prevention of erythema multiforme with acyclovir. *Semin Dermatol* 1988; **7**: 212–7.
24 Lemak MA, Duvic M, Bean SF. Oral acyclovir for the prevention of herpes-associated erythema multiforme. *J Am Acad Dermatol* 1986; **15**: 50–4.
25 Tatnall FM, Schofield JK, Leigh I. A double-blind placebo controlled trial of continuous acyclovir therapy in recurrent erythema multiforme. *Br J Dermatol* 1995; **132**: 267–70.
26 Molnar I, Matulis M. Arthritis associated with recurrent erythema multiforme responding to oral acyclovir. *Clin Rheumatol* 2002; **21**: 415–7.
27 Moisson YF, Janier M, Civatte J. Thalidomide for recurrent erythema multiforme. *Br J Dermatol* 1992; **126**: 92–3.
28 Mahendran R, Grant JW, Norris PG. Dapsone-responsive persistent erythema multiforme. *Dermatology* 2000; **200**: 281–2.
29 Davis MD, Rogers RS III, Pittelkow MR. Recurrent erythema multiforme/ Stevens–Johnson syndrome: response to mycophenolate mofetil. *Arch Dermatol* 2002; **138**: 1547–50.

Stevens–Johnson syndrome and toxic epidermal necrolysis

Incidence of reactions

The incidence of TEN has been estimated at 1.2 cases per million per year in France based on nationwide surveillance between 1981 and 1985 inclusive [1]. Another study, based on the data of the Group Health Cooperative of Puget Sound, Seattle, Washington (which covers about 260 000 individuals), investigated hospitalized patients from 1972 to 1986 inclusive. The incidence of erythema multiforme, SJS and TEN was estimated at 1.8 cases per million person-years for patients aged between 20 and 64 years; the incidence for patients aged less than 20 years, and 65 years or more, increased to 7 and 9 cases per million person-years, respectively [2]. The incidence of TEN was estimated at 0.5 per million per year. Reaction rates per 100 000 exposed individuals were as follows: phenobarbital 20, nitrofurantoin 7, co-trimoxazole and ampicillin 3 and amoxicillin 2. An Italian study estimated the incidence of TEN at about 1.2 cases per million per year [3]. A study based on computerized Medicaid billing data for 1980–84 from the states of Michigan, Minnesota and Florida reported an incidence of SJS of 7.1, 2.6 and 6.8 per million per year, respectively; penicillins, especially aminopenicillins, were most frequently implicated [4]. In West Germany, the overall annual risk of TEN and of SJS was estimated over the years 1981–85 as 0.93 and 1.1 per million, respectively; drugs most frequently implicated were antibiotics (sulphonamides and beta-lactam agents), and analgesics and non-steroidal anti-inflammatory agents (NSAIDs) [5]. In this study, it was possible to attribute the cause of the TEN to a drug in 88% of cases. Another study estimated the incidence for West Germany and Berlin for SJS and TEN as up to 1.89 per million inhabitants per year [6]. An ongoing international case–control study of TEN and SJS in relation to the use of drugs is being carried out, based on data collection in France, Italy, Germany and Portugal [7]. The incidence of SJS/TEN with long-acting sulphonamides, sulphones, antibiotics, anticonvulsants, NSAIDs or allopurinol is fortunately rare, occurring only once per 10 000–100 000 courses of drug given [8,9]. The incidence of TEN (cases/million/year) has been reported to be 2.7 times higher, and the fatality twice as high (51% compared with 25%), in the elderly compared with younger adults; the same drugs (NSAIDs, antibacterials and anticonvulsants) are incriminated in both groups [10].

Patients with AIDS have a dramatically increased incidence of TEN [11]; 14 of 80 consecutive cases of TEN patients were HIV infected, and 15 cases of AIDS-associated TEN occurred in the Paris area over a study period, compared with the expected 0.04 cases [12]. Sulphonamides (sulfadiazine, co-trimoxazole, sulfadoxine), clindamycin, phenobarbital and chlormezanone were implicated [12], as were sulfadiazine and pyrimethamine/clindamycin [13]. Patients with AIDS are more likely to demonstrate multiple cutaneous drug reactions [14].

REFERENCES

1 Roujeau J-C, Guillaume J-C, Fabre J-D *et al*. Toxic epidermal necrolysis (Lyell syndrome): incidence and drug aetiology in France, 1981–85. *Arch Dermatol* 1990; **126**: 37–42.

2 Chan H-L, Stern RS, Arndt KA *et al*. The incidence of erythema multiforme, Stevens–Johnson syndrome, and toxic epidermal necrolysis: a population based study with particular reference to reactions caused by drugs among outpatients. *Arch Dermatol* 1990; **126**: 43–7.

3 Naldi L, Locati F, Marchesi L, Cainelli T. Incidence of toxic epidermal necrolysis in Italy. *Arch Dermatol* 1990; **126**: 1103–4.

4 Strom BL, Carson JL, Halpern AC *et al*. A population based study of Stevens–Johnson syndrome: incidence and antecedent drug exposures. *Arch Dermatol* 1991; **127**: 831–8.

5 Schöpf E, Stühmer A, Rzany B *et al*. Toxic epidermal necrolysis and Stevens–Johnson syndrome: an epidemiologic study from West Germany. *Arch Dermatol* 1991; **127**: 839–42.

6 Rzany B, Mockenhaupt M, Baur S *et al*. Epidemiology of erythema exudativum multiforme majus, Stevens–Johnson syndrome, and toxic epidermal necrolysis in Germany (1990–92): structure and results of a population based registry. *J Clin Epidemiol* 1996; **49**: 769–73.

7 Kaufman DW. Epidemiologic approaches to the study of toxic epidermal necrolysis. *J Invest Dermatol* 1994; **102**: 31S–33S.

8 Leenutaphong V, Sivayathorn A, Suthipinittharm P, Sunthopalin P. Stevens–Johnson syndrome and toxic epidermal necrolysis in Thailand. *Int J Dermatol* 1993; **32**: 428–31.

9 Roujeau JC, Kelly JP, Naldi L *et al*. Medication use and the risk of Stevens–Johnson syndrome or toxic epidermal necrolysis. *N Engl J Med* 1995; **333**: 1600–7.

10 Bastuji-Garin S, Zahedi M, Guillaume JC, Roujeau JC. Toxic epidermal necrolysis (Lyell syndrome) in 77 elderly patients. *Age Ageing* 1993; **22**: 450–6.

11 Porteous DM, Berger TG. Severe cutaneous drug reactions (Stevens–Johnson syndrome and toxic epidermal necrolysis) in human immunodeficiency virus infection. *Arch Dermatol* 1991; **127**: 740–1.

12 Saiag P, Caumes E, Chosidow O *et al*. Drug-induced toxic epidermal necrolysis (Lyell syndrome) in patients infected with the human immunodeficiency virus. *J Am Acad Dermatol* 1992; **26**: 567–74.

13 Caumes E, Bocquet H, Guermonprez G *et al*. Adverse cutaneous reactions to pyrimethamine/sulfadiazine and pyrimethamine/clindamycin in patients with AIDS and toxoplasmic encephalitis. *Clin Infect Dis* 1995; **21**: 656–8.

14 Carr A, Tindall B, Penny R, Cooper DA. Patterns of multiple-drug hypersensitivities in HIV-infected patients. *AIDS* 1993; **7**: 1532–3.

Aetiology

Immunology

SJS and TEN, like erythema multiforme, would seem to have an immunological pathogenesis. In general, CD4$^+$ T cells predominate in the upper dermis, while epidermal CD8$^+$ T cells and macrophages are variable and Langerhans' cells virtually disappear. Keratinocytes express HLA-DR and ICAM-1, and there is endothelial cell ICAM-1, vascular cell adhesion molecule 1 (VCAM-1) and E-selectin expression [1–7]. CD3$^+$ activated T cells expressing the skin-homing receptor (cutaneous leukocyte antigen, CLA) in both skin and peripheral blood parallel the severity of the disease, and tumour necrosis factor-α (TNF-α), IFN-γ and interleukin-2 (IL-2) are overexpressed in peripheral blood mononuclear cells, suggest-

ing an important role for T cells in TEN [7]. Soluble TNF-α (sTNF-α), sTNF-R1 and sTNF-R2 levels were significantly higher in TEN blisters than in burns [8]. sTNF-R1 and sTNF-R2 were significantly more abundant in TEN blisters than serum, indicating that TNF-α processing was mainly a local event in TEN skin [8]. Significantly higher levels of sIL-2R and lower levels of IL-1α were present in blister fluid, but not serum, of patients with TEN compared with patients with burns [9]. Cytokines released by activated mononuclear cells and keratinocytes may contribute to local cell death in TEN. Prominent involvement of the monocyte–macrophage lineage, including factor XIIIa$^+$ HLA-DR$^+$ dendrocytes and CD68$^+$ Mac387$^+$ macrophages before, during and especially after epidermal necrosis has been reported [6], with dense labelling of the epidermis for TNF-α. Factor-XIIIa$^+$ dendrocytes appear activated in the skin, and depleted from lymph nodes [10].

Keratinocytes from TEN patients have been reported to undergo extensive apoptosis [11]. Activated lymphocytes might induce apoptosis via an interaction between *Fas* antigen (CD95), expressed by keratinocytes after exposure to IFN-γ, and its ligand *Fas*-ligand (FasL), expressed on the surface of and secreted by lymphocytes [12]. Sera from TEN and SJS patients contained high concentrations of soluble FasL (sFasL), and induced abundant keratinocyte apoptosis *in vitro*, compared with sera from patients with an erythema multiforme-type drug eruption [13]. Moreover, peripheral blood mononuclear cells from TEN and SJS patients secreted high levels of sFasL on stimulation with the causal drug [13].

Alternatively, it has been proposed that keratinocyte necrosis may be mediated by cytotoxic lymphocytes via the perforin granzyme route. The key role of drug-specific T lymphocytes in the mechanisms of most drug reactions has been confirmed by *in vitro* studies of many clones of T lymphocytes [14]. CD3$^+$, CD8$^+$, CD28$^-$, KIR/KAR$^+$ (killer inhibitory receptor), CLA-positive cells demonstrating cytotoxic T lymphocyte (CTL)- and NK-like cytotoxicity predominated in blister fluid obtained early in one study [15]. In a case of co-trimoxazole-induced TEN, blister fluid lymphocytes were predominantly CD8$^+$, DR$^+$, CLA$^+$, CD56$^+$ perforin-positive T lymphocytes, cytotoxic only in the presence of the drug towards autologous Epstein–Barr virus (EBV) transformed lymphocytes and allogeneic cells sharing HLA-Cw4 [16]. Cytotoxicity occurred in the presence of either co-trimoxazole, sulfamethoxazole, or the nitroso metabolite of sulfamethoxazole, but not with the hydroxylamine metabolite of sulfamethoxazole. In a patient with carbamazepine-induced TEN, lymphocytes were more susceptible to cytotoxic killing by liver microsome-induced carbamazepine intermediates than by the parent drug [17].

Inducible nitric acid synthase is demonstrable in skin in TEN/SJS, which might indicate that nitric oxide mediates apoptosis and necrosis [18]. The matrix metalloproteinase MMP2 has a significant role in epidermal detachment, inflammation and re-epithelialization. Increased levels of the activated forms of MMP2 were higher in TEN blister fluid compared with bullous pemphigoid, second-degree burns or suction blisters, indicating a potential role for MMP2 in the inflammatory reaction and repair process in TEN skin [19].

The reason why some individuals develop such marked immune reactions against medications is unknown. A widely accepted hypothesis is that patients suffering from severe drug reactions are exposed to increased amounts of reactive (oxidative) metabolites because of decreased production of normal soluble non-toxic metabolites, and/or a lowered ability to detoxify reactive metabolites [20]. Alteration in detoxification enzymes could be explained on a genetic basis (e.g. slow acetylation genotype) or on a functional basis (e.g. enzyme dysfunction in AIDS or other diseases). This 'reactive metabolites' hypothesis for drug eruptions still lacks definitive proof.

REFERENCES

1 Merot Y, Gravallese E, Guillén FJ, Murphy GF. Lymphocyte subsets and Langerhans' cells in toxic epidermal necrolysis: report of a case. *Arch Dermatol* 1986; **122**: 455–8.
2 Villada G, Roujeau J-C, Cordonnier C et al. Toxic epidermal necrolysis after bone marrow transplantation: study of nine cases. *J Am Acad Dermatol* 1990; **23**: 870–5.
3 Miyauchi H, Hosokawa H, Akaeda T et al. T-cell subsets in drug-induced toxic epidermal necrolysis: possible pathogenic mechanism induced by CD8+ T cells. *Arch Dermatol* 1991; **127**: 851–5.
4 Villada G, Roujeau JC, Clerici T et al. Immunopathology of toxic epidermal necrolysis: keratinocytes, HLA-DR expression, Langerhans' cells, and mononuclear cells: an immunopathologic study of five cases. *Arch Dermatol* 1992; **128**: 50–3.
5 Correia O, Delgado L, Ramos JP et al. Cutaneous T-cell recruitment in toxic epidermal necrolysis: further evidence of CD8+ lymphocyte involvement. *Arch Dermatol* 1993; **129**: 466–8.
6 Paquet P, Nikkels A, Arrese JE et al. Macrophages and tumor necrosis factor-α in toxic epidermal necrolysis. *Arch Dermatol* 1994; **130**: 605–8.
7 Leyva L, Torres MJ, Posadas S et al. Anticonvulsant-induced toxic epidermal necrolysis: monitoring the immunologic response. *J Allergy Clin Immunol* 2000; **105**: 157–65.
8 Paquet P, Pierard GE. Soluble fractions of tumor necrosis factor-α, interleukin-6 and of their receptors in toxic epidermal necrolysis: a comparison with second-degree burns. *Int J Mol Med* 1998; **1**: 459–62.
9 Correia O, Delgado L, Roujeau JC et al. Soluble interleukin-2 receptor and interleukin-1α in toxic epidermal necrolysis: a comparative analysis of serum and blister fluid samples. *Arch Dermatol* 2002; **138**: 29–32.
10 Paquet P, Quatresooz P, Pierard GE. Factor-XIIIa+ dendrocytes in drug-induced toxic epidermal necrolysis (Lyell's syndrome): paradoxical activation in skin and rarefaction in lymph nodes. *Dermatology* 2003; **206**: 374–8.
11 Paul C, Wolkenstein P, Adle H et al. Apoptosis as a mechanism of keratinocyte death in toxic epidermal necrolysis. *Br J Dermatol* 1996; **134**: 710–4.
12 Sayama K, Yonehara S, Watanabe Y, Miki Y. Expression of *Fas* antigen on keratinocytes *in vivo* and induction of apoptosis in cultured keratinocytes. *J Invest Dermatol* 1994; **103**: 330–4.
13 Abe R, Shimizu T, Shibaki A et al. Toxic epidermal necrolysis and Stevens–Johnson syndrome are induced by soluble *fas* ligand. *Am J Pathol* 2003; **162**: 1515–20.
14 Schnyder B, Burkhart C, Schnyder-Frutig K et al. Recognition of sulfamethoxazole and its reactive metabolites by drug-specific CD4+ T cells from allergic individuals. *J Immunol* 2000; **164**: 6647–54.
15 Le Cleach L, Delaire S, Boumsell L et al. Blister fluid T lymphocytes during toxic epidermal necrolysis are functional cytotoxic cells which express human natural killer (NK) inhibitory receptors. *Clin Exp Immunol* 2000; **119**: 225–30.
16 Nassif A, Bensussan A, Dorothee G et al. Drug specific cytotoxic T-cells in the skin lesions of a patient with toxic epidermal necrolysis. *J Invest Dermatol* 2002; **118**: 728–33.
17 Friedmann PS, Strickland I, Pirmohamed M, Park BK. Investigation of mechanisms in toxic epidermal necrolysis induced by carbamazepine. *Arch Dermatol* 1994; **130**: 598–604.
18 Lerner LH, Qureshi AA, Reddy BV, Lerner EA. Nitric acid synthase in toxic epidermal necrolysis and Stevens–Johnson syndrome. *J Invest Dermatol* 2000; **114**: 196–9.
19 Paquet P, Nusgens BV, Pierard GE, Lapiere CM. Gelatinases in drug-induced toxic epidermal necrolysis. *Eur J Clin Invest* 1998; **28**: 528–32.
20 Shear NH, Spielberg SP, Grant DM, Tang BK, Kalow W. Differences in metabolism of sulfonamides predisposing to idiosyncratic toxicity. *Ann Intern Med* 1986; **105**: 179–84.

Drugs implicated in Stevens–Johnson syndrome

Drugs potentially causing SJS are listed in Table 74.2 [1–8]. A retrospective study from Malaysia reported that the most common causes of SJS were sulphonamides, tetracycline and the penicillin derivatives [8]. In the USA, NSAIDs were reported to be an important cause [9]. Severe SJS-like reactions have been described resulting from sulphonamides with or without trimethoprim [10–12] and following malaria prophylaxis with Fansidar (pyrimethamine and sulfadoxine) [13,14]. Patients with AIDS are at an increased risk of developing severe SJS reactions to co-trimoxazole and thiacetazone [15–17]. The culprit drugs in a study from Thailand included the following: antibiotics (penicillin, sulphonamides, tetracycline, erythromycin); anticonvulsants (phenytoin, carbamazepine, barbiturates); antitubercular drugs (thiacetazone); analgesics (acetylsalicylic acid, fenbufen); sulphonylurea; and allopurinol. The total mortality rate was 14%: 5% for SJS and 40% for TEN [7]. Data from surveillance networks in France, Germany, Italy and Portugal on 245 people hospitalized because of SJS or TEN [18] indicated that for drugs usually used for short periods, relative risks were increased as follows: co-trimoxazole and other sulphonamide antibiotics 172, chlormezanone 62, aminopenicillins 6.7, quinolones 10 and cephalosporins 14, and for paracetamol (acetaminophen) 0.6 in France but 9.3 in the other countries. For drugs used for months or years, the increased risk was largely in the first 2 months, and was as follows: carbamazepine 90, phenobarbital 45, phenytoin 53, valproic acid 25, oxicam NSAIDs 72, allopurinol 52 and corticosteroids 54. For many drugs, including thiazide diuretics and oral hypoglycaemic agents, there was no significant increase in risk. The excess risk did not exceed five cases per million users per week for any of the drugs. Acetylsalicylic acid and other salicylates are not associated with a measurable increase in the risk of SJS or TEN [19].

Other drugs implicated in SJS include the antiretroviral drugs nevirapine [20–23] and abacavir [24], lamotrigine

[25], terbinafine [26], nystatin [27], ciprofloxacin [28], the antimalarials mefloquine [29] and hydroxychloroquine [30], cyclophosphamide [31], methotrexate [32], rituximab [33], the specific tyrosine kinase inhibitor STI571 used in leukaemia therapy [34], propylthiouracil [35], ranitidine [36], mebendazole and metronidazole [37], bezafibrate [38], diltiazem, nifedipine and verapamil [39], sertraline [40], fluoxetine and fluvoxamine [41] and tetrazepam [42]. SJS has followed vaccination [43], ingestion of a health drink (Eberu) containing ophiopogonis tuber [44] and use of cocaine [45].

REFERENCES

1 Bianchine JR, Macaraeg PVJ, Lasagna L et al. Drugs as aetiologic factors in the Stevens–Johnson syndrome. Am J Med 1968; **44**: 390–405.
2 Kauppinen K. Cutaneous reactions to drugs: with special reference to severe mucocutaneous bullous eruptions and sulphonamides. Acta Derm Venereol (Stockh) 1972; **52** (Suppl. 68): 1–89.
3 Böttiger LE, Strandberg I, Westerholm B. Drug-induced febrile mucocutaneous syndrome: with a survey of the literature. Acta Med Scand 1975; **198**: 229–33.
4 Ruiz-Maldonado R. Acute disseminated epidermal necrosis types 1, 2, and 3: study of 60 cases. J Am Acad Dermatol 1985; **13**: 623–35.
5 Nethercott JR, Choi BC. Erythema multiforme (Stevens–Johnson syndrome): chart review of 123 hospitalized patients. Dermatologica 1985; **171**: 383–96.
6 Ting HC, Adam BA. Stevens–Johnson syndrome: a review of 34 cases. Int J Dermatol 1985; **24**: 587–91.
7 Leenutaphong V, Sivayathorn A, Suthipinittharm P, Sunthonpalin P. Stevens–Johnson syndrome and toxic epidermal necrolysis in Thailand. Int J Dermatol 1993; **32**: 428–31.
8 Gebel K, Hornstein OP. Drug-induced oral erythema multiforme: results of a long-term retrospective study. Dermatologica 1984; **168**: 35–40.
9 Stern R, Bigby M. An expanded profile of cutaneous reactions to non-steroidal anti-inflammatory drugs. JAMA 1984; **252**: 1433–7.
10 Carrol OM, Bryan PA, Robinson RJ. Stevens–Johnson syndrome associated with long-acting sulfonamides. JAMA 1966; **195**: 691–3.
11 Azinge NO, Garrick GA. Stevens–Johnson syndrome (erythema multiforme) following ingestion of trimethoprim–sulfamethoxazole on two separate occasions in the same person: a case report. J Allergy Clin Immunol 1978; **62**: 125–6.
12 Aberer W, Stingl G, Wolff K. Stevens–Johnson-Syndrom und toxische epidermale Nekrolyse nach Sulfonamideinahme. Hautarzt 1982; **33**: 484–90.
13 Hornstein OP, Ruprecht KW. Fansidar-induced Stevens–Johnson syndrome. N Engl J Med 1982; **307**: 1529–30.
14 Miller KD, Lobel HO, Satriale RF et al. Severe cutaneous reactions among American travelers using pyrimethamine–sulfadoxine (Fansidar) for malaria prophylaxis. Am J Trop Med Hyg 1986; **35**: 451–8.
15 De Raeve L, Song M, Van Maldergem L. Adverse cutaneous drug reactions in AIDS. Br J Dermatol 1988; **119**: 521–3.
16 Porteous DM, Berger TG. Severe cutaneous drug reactions (Stevens–Johnson syndrome and toxic epidermal necrolysis) in human immunodeficiency virus infection. Arch Dermatol 1991; **127**: 740–1.
17 van der Ven AJAM, Koopmans PP, Vree TB, van der Meer JWM. Adverse reactions to co-trimoxazole in HIV infection. Lancet 1991; **338**: 431–3.
18 Roujeau JC, Kelly JP, Naldi L et al. Medication use and the risk of Stevens–Johnson syndrome or toxic epidermal necrolysis. N Engl J Med 1995; **333**: 1600–7.
19 Kaufman DW, Kelly JP. Acetylsalicylic acid and other salicylates in relation to Stevens–Johnson syndrome and toxic epidermal necrolysis. Br J Clin Pharmacol 2001; **51**: 174–6.
20 Wetterwald E, Le Cleach L, Michel C et al. Nevirapine-induced overlap Stevens–Johnson syndrome/toxic epidermal necrolysis. Br J Dermatol 1999; **140**: 980–2.
21 Metry DW, Lahart CJ, Farmer KL, Hebert AA. Stevens–Johnson syndrome caused by the antiretroviral drug nevirapine. J Am Acad Dermatol 2001; **44** (2 Suppl.): 354–7.
22 Fagot JP, Mockenhaupt M, Bouwes-Bavinck JN et al. Nevirapine and the risk of Stevens–Johnson syndrome or toxic epidermal necrolysis. AIDS 2001; **15**: 1843–8.
23 Dodi F, Alessandrini A, Camera M et al. Stevens–Johnson syndrome in HIV patients treated with nevirapine: two case reports. AIDS 2002; **16**: 1197–8.
24 Bossi P, Roujeau JC, Bricaire F, Caumes E. Stevens–Johnson syndrome associated with abacavir therapy. Clin Infect Dis 2002; **35**: 902.
25 Guberman AH, Besag FM, Brodie MJ et al. Lamotrigine-associated rash: risk–benefit considerations in adults and children. Epilepsia 1999; **40**: 985–91.
26 Rzany B, Mockenhaupt M, Gehring W, Schöpf E. Stevens–Johnson syndrome after terbinafine therapy. J Am Acad Dermatol 1994; **30**: 509.
27 Garty B-Z. Stevens–Johnson syndrome associated with nystatin treatment. Arch Dermatol 1991; **127**: 741–2.
28 Bhatia RS. Stevens Johnson syndrome following a single dose of ciprofloxacin. J Assoc Physicians India 1994; **42**: 344.
29 Smith HR, Croft AM, Black MM. Dermatological adverse effects with the antimalarial drug mefloquine: a review of 74 published case reports. Clin Exp Dermatol 1999; **24**: 249–54.
30 Leckie MJ, Rees RG. Stevens–Johnson syndrome in association with hydroxychloroquine treatment for rheumatoid arthritis. Rheumatology (Oxford) 2002; **41**: 473–4.
31 Assier-Bonnet HJ, Aractingi S, Cadranel J et al. Stevens–Johnson syndrome induced by cyclophosphamide: report of two cases. Br J Dermatol 1996; **135**: 864–5.
32 Hani N, Casper C, Groth W et al. Stevens–Johnson syndrome-like exanthema secondary to methotrexate histologically simulating acute graft-versus-host disease. Eur J Dermatol 2000; **10**: 548–50.
33 Lowndes S, Darby A, Mead G, Lister A. Stevens–Johnson syndrome after treatment with rituximab. Ann Oncol 2002; **13**: 1948–50.
34 Hsiao LT, Chung HM, Lin JT et al. Stevens–Johnson syndrome after treatment with STI571: a case report. Br J Haematol 2002; **117**: 620–2.
35 Dysseleer A, Buysschaert M, Fonck C et al. Acute interstitial nephritis and fatal Stevens–Johnson syndrome after propylthiouracil therapy. Thyroid 2000; **10**: 713–6.
36 Lin CC, Wu JC, Huang DF et al. Ranitidine-related Stevens–Johnson syndrome in patients with severe liver diseases: a report of two cases. J Gastroenterol Hepatol 2001; **16**: 481–3.
37 Chen KT, Twu SJ, Chang HJ, Lin RS. Outbreak of Stevens–Johnson syndrome/toxic epidermal necrolysis associated with mebendazole and metronidazole use among Filipino laborers in Taiwan. Am J Public Health 2003; **93**: 489–92.
38 Sawamura D, Umeki K. Stevens–Johnson syndrome associated with bezafibrate. Acta Derm Venereol (Stockh) 2000; **80**: 457.
39 Knowles S, Gupta AK, Shear NH. The spectrum of cutaneous reactions associated with diltiazem: three cases and a review of the literature. J Am Acad Dermatol 1998; **38**: 201–6.
40 January V, Toledano C, Machet L et al. Stevens–Johnson syndrome after sertraline. Acta Derm Venereol (Stockh) 1999; **79**: 401.
41 Richard MA, Fiszenson F, Jreissati M et al. Cutaneous adverse effects during selective serotonin reuptake inhibitors therapy: two cases. Ann Dermatol Vénéréol 2001; **128**: 759–61.
42 Sanchez I, Garcia-Abujeta JL, Fernandez L et al. Stevens–Johnson syndrome from tetrazepam. Allergol Immunopathol (Madr) 1998; **26**: 55–7.
43 Ball R, Ball LK, Wise RP et al. Stevens–Johnson syndrome and toxic epidermal necrolysis after vaccination: reports to the vaccine adverse event reporting system. Pediatr Infect Dis J 2001; **20**: 219–23.
44 Mochitomi Y, Inoue A, Kawabata H et al. Stevens–Johnson syndrome caused by a health drink (Eberu) containing ophiopogonis tuber. J Dermatol 1998; **25**: 662–5.
45 Hofbauer GF, Burg G, Nestle FO. Cocaine-related Stevens–Johnson syndrome. Dermatology 2000; **201**: 258–60.

Drugs and other factors implicated in toxic epidermal necrolysis

There is a degree of overlap between SJS and TEN; SJS may evolve into TEN, and several drugs can produce both entities (Tables 74.2 & 74.3) [1–17]. A large number of

Table 74.3 Drugs causing toxic epidermal necrolysis.

Antibiotics	*Anticonvulsants*
Sulphonamides	Barbiturates
Co-trimoxazole*	Phenobarbital*
Sulfadoxine	Carbamazepine*
Sulfadiazine	Lamotrigine*
Sulfasalazine	Phenytoin*
Penicillins	Valproic acid†
Amoxicillin†	
Ampicillin†	*Antifungal agents*
Cephalosporins†	Terbinafine
Ethambutol	Griseofulvin
Fluoroquinalones†	
Isoniazid	*Antiretroviral drugs*
Streptomycin	Abacavir
Tetracycline	Nevirapine*
Thiacetazone*	
	Gastrointestinal drugs
Non-steroidal anti-inflammatory drugs	Famotidine
Phenylbutazone*	Omeprazole
Oxyphenabutazone	Ranitidine
Oxicam-derivatives	
Meloxicam*	*Miscellaneous*
Piroxicam*	Allopurinol*
Tenoxicam*	Chlorpromazine
Isoxicam	Dapsone
Diclofenac†	Gold
Fenbufen	Nitrofurantoin
Salicylates	Pentamidine
Naproxen	Tolbutamide
Pyrazolon derivatives	Vaccination

* Definite high risk.
† Probable low-risk association.

different drugs have been implicated anecdotally, but the most common triggers (Table 74.3) include antiepileptic drugs (phenytoin, barbiturates, carbamazepine and lamotrigine [18–20]), sulphonamides and trimethoprim [21], ampicillin and other β-lactam antibiotics [22], allopurinol [23], NSAIDs (especially pyrazolon derivatives, e.g. phenylbutazone, and oxicam derivatives) [23] and pentamidine. A high proportion of adult cases of SJS or TEN related to anticonvulsants occur in patients receiving radiotherapy for brain tumour. It is suspected that cancer and/or radiotherapy increases the risk.

In France, a survey showed two main classes of drug were most often responsible: antibacterial agents (especially sulphonamides); NSAIDs including oxyphenabutazone, and fenbufen; and phenytoin [24]. The incidence of erythema multiforme, SJS and TEN in a US series with the following drugs were reported as follows: phenobarbital 20, nitrofurantoin 7, co-trimoxazole and ampicillin each 3, and amoxicillin 2, per 100 000 exposed patients [7]. Review of the English language literature from 1966 to 1987 suggested that allopurinol, NSAIDs, phenytoin and the sulphonamide antibiotics were most frequently responsible [25]. A study from the USA reported that penicillins, especially aminopenicillins, were most frequently

implicated [9]. In West Germany, drugs most frequently implicated were antibiotics (sulphonamides and β-lactam agents) and analgesics and NSAIDs [10]. In India, by contrast, one-third of cases were the result of drugs used for the treatment of tuberculosis, especially thiacetazone and isoniazid [26]. The absolute incidence of phenytoin-induced TEN is very low, with nine cases reported in the USA over a decade, compared with 2 million Americans who took phenytoin [11]. Similarly, 4 in 232 390 patients on co-trimoxazole developed erythema multiforme or SJS, while only 1 in 196 397 prescribed cephalexin developed TEN [21]. The risk of SJS/TEN is highest in the first 8 weeks of therapy with phenytoin, phenobarbital, carbamazepine and lamotrigine; the risk with valproic acid is less [27]. Terbinafine [26–28] and antiretrovirals including nevirapine [29] have also been associated with TEN. In Europe, nevirapine has replaced sulphonamides as the leading cause of SJS and TEN related to AIDS [30]. By contrast, the following medications are not associated with a moderate or high risk of causing TEN: contraceptive pills, benzodiazepines, thiazide diuretics, sulphonylurea antidiabetics, angiotensin-converting enzyme inhibitors, β-blockers, acetyl salicylic acid and fibrate cholesterol-lowering agents [17].

More than 100 different medications have been reported as having caused TEN, but case reports are of limited significance because publications are biased toward 'original' and new associations. Nonetheless, other antibiotics, antifungals and antiprotozoal drugs incriminated include ciprofloxacin [31,32], vancomycin [33,34], ofloxacin [35], thiacetazone [36], fluconazole [37], griseofulvin [38,39], Fansidar [40] and foscarnet [41], as well as the antimalarials mefloquine [42] and hydroxychloroquine [43]. Miscellaneous causes include fluoxetine and fluvoxamine [44,45], tetrazepam [46], diltiazem, nifedipine and verapamil [47], thalidomide [48], methotrexate [49,50], cytosine arabinoside [51], IL-2 [52], etretinate [53], omeprazole [54], ranitidine [55], famotidine [56] and cimetidine [57], atorvastatin [58], valdecoxib and celecoxib [59,60]. Even acetaminophen (paracetamol) has rarely been recorded as causing TEN [61].

Immunization with diphtheria–pertussis–tetanus (DPT), measles, poliomyelitis, smallpox and influenza vaccines has been recorded as a cause of TEN [11,62,63]. Single cases of TEN have followed use of the radiological contrast media diatrizoate solution for excretory pyelography [64] and iopamidol for cardiac catherization [65], use of a terconazole vaginal suppository [66] and contact with a toxic fumigant, acrylonitrile [67]. TEN has been described in association with graft-versus-host reactions [68,69] and with lupus erythematosus [70]. It is not yet clear whether SJS and TEN are always drug-induced or may have other causes. A few well-documented cases have been attributed to *Mycoplasma pneumoniae* or *Klebsiella pneumoniae* infections.

REFERENCES

1 Heng MCY. Drug-induced toxic epidermal necrolysis. *Br J Dermatol* 1985; **113**: 597–60.

2 Fabrizio PJ, McCloshey WW, Jeffrey LP. Drugs causing toxic epidermal necrolysis. *Drug Intell Clin Pharmacol* 1985; **19**: 733–5.

3 Guillaume J-C, Roujeau J-C, Penso D *et al.* The culprit drugs in 87 cases of toxic epidermal necrolysis (Lyell's syndrome). *Arch Dermatol* 1987; **123**: 1166–70.

4 Ruiz-Maldonado R. Acute disseminated epidermal necrosis types 1, 2 and 3: study of 60 cases. *J Am Acad Dermatol* 1985; **13**: 623–35.

5 Roujeau J-C, Chosidow O, Saiag P, Guillaume J-C. Toxic epidermal necrolysis (Lyell syndrome). *J Am Acad Dermatol* 1990; **23**: 1039–58.

6 Roujeau J-C, Guillaume J-C, Fabre J-D *et al.* Toxic epidermal necrolysis (Lyell syndrome): incidence and drug aetiology in France, 1981–85. *Arch Dermatol* 1990; **126**: 37–42.

7 Chan H-L, Stern RS, Arndt KA *et al.* The incidence of erythema multiforme, Stevens–Johnson syndrome, and toxic epidermal necrolysis: a population based study with particular reference to reactions caused by drugs among outpatients. *Arch Dermatol* 1990; **126**: 43–7.

8 Naldi L, Locati F, Marchesi L, Cainelli T. Incidence of toxic epidermal necrolysis in Italy. *Arch Dermatol* 1990; **126**: 1103–4.

9 Strom BL, Carson JL, Halpern AC *et al.* A population based study of Stevens–Johnson syndrome: incidence and antecedent drug exposures. *Arch Dermatol* 1991; **127**: 831–8.

10 Schöpf E, Stühmer A, Rzany B *et al.* Toxic epidermal necrolysis and Stevens–Johnson syndrome: an epidemiologic study from West Germany. *Arch Dermatol* 1991; **127**: 839–42.

11 Avakian R, Flowers FP, Araujo OE, Ramos-Caro FA. Toxic epidermal necrolysis: a review. *J Am Acad Dermatol* 1991; **25**: 69–79.

12 Parsons JM. Toxic epidermal necrolysis. *Int J Dermatol* 1992; **31**: 749–68.

13 Paquet P. Les medicaments responsables de necrolyse epidermique toxique (syndrome de Lyell). *Thérapie* 1993; **48**: 133–9.

14 Lyell A. Drug-induced toxic epidermal necrolysis. I. An overview. *Clin Dermatol* 1993; **11**: 491–2.

15 Roujeau JC. Drug-induced toxic epidermal necrolysis. II. Current aspects. *Clin Dermatol* 1993; **11**: 493–500.

16 Leenutaphong V, Sivayathorn A, Suthipinittharm P, Sunthopalin P. Stevens–Johnson syndrome and toxic epidermal necrolysis in Thailand. *Int J Dermatol* 1993; **32**: 428–31.

17 Roujeau JC, Kelly JP, Naldi L *et al.* Medication use and the risk of Stevens–Johnson syndrome or toxic epidermal necrolysis. *N Engl J Med* 1995; **333**: 1600–7.

18 Creamer JD, Whittaker SJ, Kerr-Muir M, Smith NP. Phenytoin-induced toxic epidermal necrolysis: a case report. *Clin Exp Dermatol* 1996; **21**: 116–20.

19 Sterker M, Berrouschot J, Schneider D. Fatal course of toxic epidermal necrolysis under treatment with lamotrigine. *Int J Clin Pharmacol Ther* 1995; **33**: 595–7.

20 Bhushan M, Brooke R, Hewitt-Symonds M, Craven NM, August PJ. Prolonged toxic epidermal necrolysis due to lamotrigine. *Clin Exp Dermatol* 2000; **25**: 349–51.

21 Jick H, Derby LE. A large population based follow-up study of trimethoprim-sulfamethoxazole, trimethoprim, and cephalexin for uncommon serious drug toxicity. *Pharmacotherapy* 1995; **15**: 428–32.

22 Romano A, Di Fonso M, Pocobelli D *et al.* Two cases of toxic epidermal necrolysis caused by delayed hypersensitivity to beta-lactam antibiotics. *J Invest Allergol Clin Immunol* 1993; **3**: 53–5.

23 Stratigos JD, Bartsokas SK, Capetanakis J. Further experiences of toxic epidermal necrolysis incriminating allopurinol, pyrazolone, and derivatives. *Br J Dermatol* 1972; **86**: 564–7.

24 Roujeau J-C, Guillaume J-C, Fabre J-D *et al.* Toxic epidermal necrolysis (Lyell syndrome): incidence and drug aetiology in France, 1981–85. *Arch Dermatol* 1990; **126**: 37–42.

25 Stern RS, Chan H-L. Usefulness of case report literature in determining drugs responsible for toxic epidermal necrolysis. *J Am Acad Dermatol* 1989; **21**: 317–22.

26 Nanda A, Kaur S. Drug-induced toxic epidermal necrolysis in developing countries. *Arch Dermatol* 1990; **126**: 125.

25 Rzany B, Correia O, Kelly JP *et al.* Risk of Stevens–Johnson syndrome and toxic epidermal necrolysis during first weeks of antiepileptic therapy: a case–control study. Study Group of the International Case Control Study on Severe Cutaneous Adverse Reactions. *Lancet* 1999; **353**: 2190–4.

26 Carstens J, Wendelboe P, Sogaard H, Thestrup-Pedersen K. Toxic epidermal necrolysis and erythema multiforme following therapy with terbinafine. *Acta Derm Venereol (Stockh)* 1994; **74**: 391–2.

27 White SI, Bowen-Jones D. Toxic epidermal necrolysis induced by terbinafine in a patient on long-term antiepileptics. *Br J Dermatol* 1996; **134**: 188–9.

28 Gupta AK, Kopstein JB, Shear NH. Hypersensitivity reaction to terbinafine. *J Am Acad Dermatol* 1997; **36**: 1018–9.

29 Wetterwald E, Le Cleach L, Michel C *et al.* Nevirapine-induced overlap Stevens–Johnson syndrome/toxic epidermal necrolysis. *Br J Dermatol* 1999; **140**: 980–2.

30 Fagot JP, Mockenhaupt M, Bouwes-Bavinck JN *et al.* Nevirapine and the risk of Stevens–Johnson syndrome or toxic epidermal necrolysis. *AIDS* 2001; **15**: 1843–8.

31 Tham TCK, Allen G, Hayes D *et al.* Possible association between toxic epidermal necrolysis and ciprofloxacin. *Lancet* 1991; **338**: 522.

32 Moshfeghi M, Mandler HD. Ciprofloxacin-induced toxic epidermal necrolysis. *Ann Pharmacother* 1993; **27**: 467–9.

33 Vidal C, Gonzalez Quintela A, Fuente R. Toxic epidermal necrolysis due to vancomycin. *Ann Allergy* 1992; **68**: 345–7.

34 Hsu SI. Biopsy-proved acute tubulointerstitial nephritis and toxic epidermal necrolysis associated with vancomycin. *Pharmacotherapy* 2001; **21**: 1233–9.

35 Melde SL. Ofloxacin: a probable cause of toxic epidermal necrolysis. *Ann Pharmacother* 2001; **35**: 1388–90.

36 Ipuge YA, Rieder HL, Enarson DA. Adverse cutaneous reactions to thiacetazone for tuberculosis treatment in Tanzania. *Lancet* 1995; **346**: 657–60.

37 Azon-Masoliver A, Vilaplana J. Fluconazole-induced toxic epidermal necrolysis in a patient with human immunodeficiency virus infection. *Dermatology* 1993; **187**: 268–9.

38 Taylor B, Duffill M. Toxic epidermal necrolysis from griseofulvin. *J Am Acad Dermatol* 1988; **19**: 565–7.

39 Mion G, Verdon G, Le Gulluche Y *et al.* Fatal toxic epidermal necrolysis after griseofulvin. *Lancet* 1989; **2**: 1331.

40 Sturchler D, Mittelholzer ML, Kerr L. How frequent are notified severe cutaneous adverse reactions to Fansidar? *Drug Saf* 1993; **8**: 60–8.

41 Wharton JR, Laughlin C, Cockerell CJ. Toxic epidermal necrolysis occurring as a consequence of treatment with foscarnet. *Cutis* 1999; **63**: 333–5.

42 Smith HR, Croft AM, Black MM. Dermatological adverse effects with the antimalarial drug mefloquine: a review of 74 published case reports. *Clin Exp Dermatol* 1999; **24**: 249–54.

43 Murphy M, Carmichael AJ. Fatal toxic epidermal necrolysis associated with hydroxychloroquine. *Clin Exp Dermatol* 2001; **26**: 457–8.

44 Bodokh I, Lacour JP, Rosenthal E *et al.* Syndrome de Lyell ou necrolyse epidermique toxique et syndrome de Stevens–Johnson après traitement par fluoxetine. *Thérapie* 1992; **47**: 441.

45 Richard MA, Fiszenson F, Jreissati M *et al.* Cutaneous adverse effects during selective serotonin reuptake inhibitors therapy: two cases. *Ann Dermatol Vénéréol* 2001; **128**: 759–61.

46 Lagnaoui R, Ramanampamonjy R, Julliac B *et al.* Fatal toxic epidermal necrolysis associated with tetrazepam. *Therapie* 2001; **56**: 187–8.

47 Knowles S, Gupta AK, Shear NH. The spectrum of cutaneous reactions associated with diltiazem: three cases and a review of the literature. *J Am Acad Dermatol* 1998; **38**: 201–6.

48 Hall VC, El-Azhary RA, Bouwhuis S, Rajkumar SV. Dermatologic side effects of thalidomide in patients with multiple myeloma. *J Am Acad Dermatol* 2003; **48**: 548–52.

49 Collins P, Rogers S. The efficacy of methotrexate in psoriasis: a review of 40 cases. *Clin Exp Dermatol* 1992; **17**: 257–60.

50 Primka EJ III, Camisa C. Methotrexate-induced toxic epidermal necrolysis in a patient with psoriasis. *J Am Acad Dermatol* 1997; **36**: 815–8.

51 Ozkan A, Apak H, Celkan T *et al.* Toxic epidermal necrolysis after the use of high-dose cytosine arabinoside. *Pediatr Dermatol* 2001; **18**: 38–40.

52 Wiener JS, Tucker JA Jr, Walther PJ. Interleukin-2-induced dermatotoxicity resembling toxic epidermal necrolysis. *South Med J* 1992; **85**: 656–9.

53 McIvor A. Fatal toxic epidermal necrolysis associated with etretinate (Letter). *BMJ* 1992; **304**: 548.

54 Cox NH. Acute disseminated epidermal necrosis due to omeprazole. *Lancet* 1992; **340**: 857.

55 Miralles ES, Nunez M, del Olmo N, Ledo A. Ranitidine-related toxic epidermal necrolysis in a patient with idiopathic thrombocytopenic purpura. *J Am Acad Dermatol* 1995; **32**: 133–4.

56 Brunner M, Vardarman E, Goldermann R *et al.* Toxic epidermal necrolysis (Lyell syndrome) following famotidine administration. *Br J Dermatol* 1995; **133**: 814–5.

57 Tidwell BH, Paterson TM, Burford B. Cimetidine-induced toxic epidermal necrolysis. *Am J Health Syst Pharm* 1998; **55**: 163–4.

58 Pfeiffer CM, Kazenoff S, Rothberg HD. Toxic epidermal necrolysis from atorvastatin. *JAMA* 1998; **279**: 1613–4.

59 Glasser DL, Burroughs SH. Valdecoxib-induced toxic epidermal necrolysis in a patient allergic to sulfa drugs. *Pharmacotherapy* 2003; **23**: 551–3.

60 Giglio P. Toxic epidermal necrolysis due to administration of celecoxib (Celebrex). *South Med J* 2003; **96**: 320–1.

61 Halevi A, Ben-Amitai D, Garty BZ. Toxic epidermal necrolysis associated with acetaminophen ingestion. *Ann Pharmacother* 2000; **34**: 32–4.

62 Shoss RG, Rayhanzadeh S. Toxic epidermal necrolysis following measles vaccination. *Arch Dermatol* 1974; **110**: 766–70.

63 Ball R, Ball LK, Wise RP *et al.* Stevens–Johnson syndrome and toxic epidermal necrolysis after vaccination: reports to the vaccine adverse event reporting system. *Pediatr Infect Dis J* 2001; **20**: 219–23.

64 Kaftori JK, Abraham Z, Gilhar A. Toxic epidermal necrolysis after excretory pyelography: immunologic-mediated contrast medium reaction? *Int J Dermatol* 1988; **27**: 346–7.

65 Lee ML, Chiu IS. Toxic epidermal necrolysis incriminating iopamidol in a child after cardiac catheterization. *Intl J Cardiol* 2002; **82**: 95–7.

66 Searles GE, Tredget EE, Lin AN. Fatal toxic epidermal necrolysis associated with use of terconazole vaginal suppository. *J Cutan Med Surg* 1998; **3**: 85–7.

67 Radimer GF, Davis J II, Ackerman AB. Fumigant-induced toxic epidermal necrolysis. *Arch Dermatol* 1974; **110**: 103–4.

68 Peck GL, Herzig GP, Elias PM. Toxic epidermal necrolysis in a patient with graft-vs-host reaction. *Arch Dermatol* 1972; **105**: 561–9.

69 Villada G, Roujeau J-C, Cordonnier C *et al.* Toxic epidermal necrolysis after bone marrow transplantation: study of nine cases. *J Am Acad Dermatol* 1990; **23**: 870–5.

70 Mandelcorn R, Shear NH. Lupus-associated toxic epidermal necrolysis: a novel manifestation of lupus? *J Am Acad Dermatol* 2003; **48**: 525–9.

Pathology

The histology of early lesions is characterized by moderate perivascular mononuclear cell infiltration in the papillary dermis, with epidermal spongiosis and exocytosis. Satellite cell necrosis, with close apposition of mononuclear cells to necrotic keratinocytes, may be seen. In established TEN (Fig. 74.4), there is full-thickness necrosis of the whole epidermis with blister formation. The necrotic process involves the epithelial lining of sweat ducts, while hair follicles are much less affected. There is little in the way of any dermal abnormality. Macrophages and dendrocytes with a strong immunoreactivity for TNF-α predominate in a cell-poor infiltrate [1]. TEN may be rapidly differentiated from the staphylococcal scalded skin syndrome (SSSS), in which blister formation results from intraepidermal subcorneal splitting caused by a toxin produced by *Staphylococcus aureus* group II, phage type 71, by examination of frozen sections of blister roof material [2,3]. The level of splitting is subcorneal in SSSS, while in TEN it is much lower, because the full thickness of the necrotic epidermis forms the roof of the blister. Differentiation from graft-versus-host disease may be difficult [4]. Direct immunofluorescence is negative, with the exception of a possible 'lupus band test' in cases associated with SLE.

REFERENCES

1 Paquet P, Pierard GE. Erythema multiforme and toxic epidermal necrolysis: a comparative study. *Am J Dermatopathol* 1997; **19**: 127–32.

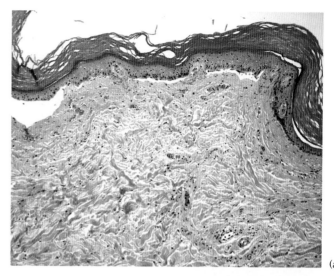

(a)

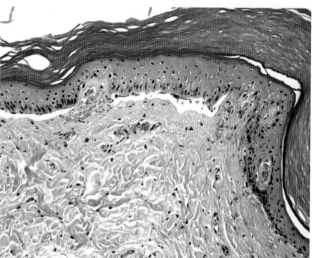

(b)

Fig. 74.4 (a,b) Histopathology of toxic epidermal necrolysis. Note full-thickness necrosis of epidermis, dermal–epidermal separation, and paucity of upper dermal cellular infiltration (H&E). (Courtesy of Dr E. Calonje, St John's Institute of Dermatology, London, UK.)

2 Amon RB, Dimond RL. Toxic epidermal necrolysis: rapid differentiation between staphylococcal- and drug-induced disease. *Arch Dermatol* 1975; **111**: 1433–7.

3 Ochsendorf FR, Schöfer H, Milbradt R. Diagnostik des 'Lyell-Syndroms': SSSS oder TEN? *Dtschr Med Wochenschr* 1988; **113**: 860–3.

4 Paquet P, Arrese JE, Beguin Y, Pierard GE. Clinicopathological differential diagnosis of drug-induced toxic epidermal necrolysis (Lyell's syndrome) and acute graft-versus-host reaction. *Curr Top Pathol* 2001; **94**: 49–63.

Clinical features

Stevens–Johnson syndrome [1–6]

SJS is a severe illness of usually sudden onset, associated with marked constitutional symptoms of high fever, malaise, myalgia, arthralgia and extensive erythema multiforme of the trunk, with occasional skin blisters and erosions covering less than 10% of the body's surface area.

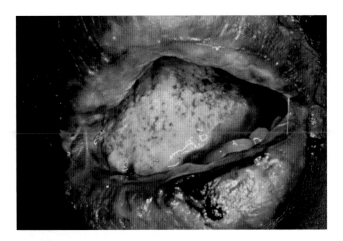

Fig. 74.5 Stevens–Johnson syndrome. Severe erosions at the lips.

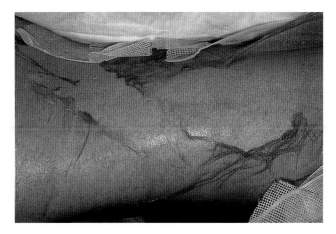

Fig. 74.6 Toxic epidermal necrolysis showing dusky erythema and stripping off of necrotic epidermis.

A prodromal systemic illness lasting 1–13 days before the eruption may occur. The skin lesions are variable in extent, and consist of typical maculopapular lesions of erythema multiforme, bullous or, rarely, pustular lesions. New crops of lesions develop over a period of 10 days, or sometimes 3–4 weeks. There is significant involvement of mucous membranes: the frequency in one review of 81 cases was oral mucosa 100%, eyes 91%, male genitalia 57% and anal mucous membrane 5%, while bronchitis and pneumonitis occurred in 6% and 23% of cases, respectively [6].

The oral mucous membrane shows extensive bulla formation followed by erosions and a greyish white membrane, so that the mouth and lips show characteristic haemorrhagic crusting (Fig. 74.5) [7]. The most common change in the eyes is a severe catarrhal or purulent conjunctivitis, but bulla formation may occur. Corneal ulceration is frequent, and anterior uveitis or panophthalmitis may occur. The eye changes often regress completely, but synechiae, corneal opacities and rarely blindness are possible sequelae. Genital lesions are frequent; retention of urine may occur, as may involvement of the bladder. Respiratory symptoms may occur, and often the radiological changes within the lungs are far greater than the symptoms. Abnormalities of liver function may be present. Renal involvement with haematuria or even renal tubular necrosis has been reported and may lead to progressive renal failure. Less common symptoms include diarrhoea, paronychia, shedding of nails, polyarthritis and otitis media. Untreated, this disease used to have a mortality of 5–15% from infection, toxaemia or renal damage, but the mortality rate is now lower. The eruption usually heals without sequelae, although the eyes may be permanently damaged.

Toxic epidermal necrolysis [8–17]

SJS should be differentiated from TEN, in which typically sheet-like erosions involve more than 30% of the body surface with widespread purpuric macules or flat atypical target lesions, and in which there is severe involvement of conjunctival, corneal, irideal, buccal, labial and genital mucous membranes [8–10]. SJS may, however, evolve into TEN.

Clinically, TEN presents with a prodromal period with flu-like symptoms (malaise, fever, rhinitis and conjunctivitis), sometimes accompanied by difficulty in urination, which usually lasts 2–3 days; however, it may last from 1 day to 3 weeks before signs of skin involvement develop. The acute phase of TEN is characterized by persistent fever, severe mucous membrane involvement and generalized epidermal sloughing to leave large raw painful areas, and lasts from 8 to 12 days. There may be an initial 'burning' maculopapular, urticarial or erythema multiforme-like eruption. This may start on the face and on the upper part of the body and rapidly extends. Most frequently, the initial individual skin lesions form poorly defined macules with darker purpuric or blistering centres, progressively merging on the chin, upper parts of chest and back. Less frequently, the initial manifestation may be a more confluent erythema. Sometimes the lesions are predominantly in photoexposed areas.

There is rapid progression to areas of confluent erythema, often starting in the axillae and groins, followed by blistering and sloughing of large areas of skin (Fig. 74.6). Nikolsky's sign, the ability to extend the area of superficial sloughing by gentle lateral pressure on the surface of the skin at an apparently unaffected site, may be positive. Detachment of the full thickness of the epidermis at sites of pressure or trauma, such as the back, shoulders or buttocks, leaves a dark red oozing dermis. In other areas, the pale necrotic epidermis remains *in situ*, with a wrinkled appearance. Blisters on the palms and soles may remain intact. However, the entire skin surface may be involved, with up to 100% of the epidermis sloughing off. Only the

Acute	Chronic
Similar to burns: depends on extent	*Ocular complications* (up to 35%)
Massive fluid and electrolyte loss (3–4 L/day)	Conjunctivitis, ectropion or entropion, corneal scarring
Prerenal renal failure	Symblepharon, Sjögren-like sicca syndrome
Bacterial infection and septicaemia	*Other mucous membrane involvement*
Hypercatabolism: insulin resistance	Oesophageal stricture
Diffuse interstitial pneumonitis	Phimosis
Mucous membrane involvement	Vaginal synechiae
	Oro-genital ulcers
	Miscellaneous
	Wound infection
	Pigmentary changes
	Nail dystrophy
	Hypohidrosis
	Scarring alopecia
	Contractures
	Development of melanocytic naevi

Table 74.4 Complications of toxic epidermal necrolysis.

hairy portion of the scalp is never affected. The process tends to occur in waves, over a 3–5-day period (sometimes a week), but involvement of the whole of the body surface occurs within 24 h in approximately 10% of cases.

Mucous membranes (particularly the buccal, and less commonly the conjunctival, genital, perianal, nasal, tracheal, bronchial, pharyngeal and oesophageal membranes) are involved in nearly all patients (85–95%). Widespread painful erosions cause crusted lips and increased salivation, and redness and soreness of the eyes is conspicuous, with photophobia. Mucous membrane lesions may precede the skin lesions by up to 3 days in one-third of cases [10]. Urethritis develops in up to two-thirds of patients, and may lead to urinary retention. Stomatitis and mucositis lead to impaired oral intake with consequent malnutrition and dehydration. Intestinal involvement has been documented [12]. Healing occurs by re-epithelialization; this may occur within a few days on the anterior thorax, but is slower on the back and at intertriginous areas. Most patients' skin lesions are completely healed in about 3–4 weeks, but mucosal lesions take longer and the glans penis may take up to 2 months to heal over.

Investigations. Approximately 50% of patients have a slight increase in aminotransferases, and approximately 10% have overt hepatitis. A rise in serum amylase is often present during the first few days, probably secondary to involvement of salivary glands. Anaemia is constant after a few days, and lymphopenia is usual, with a selective and transient depletion of CD4[+] T lymphocytes. Neutropenia is observed in approximately 30% of patients, and thrombocytopenia in 15%; eosinophilia is very unusual. Hypophosphataemia is nearly constant, and hyperglycaemia is frequent, as are increased urea and creatinine levels. Subclinical interstitial oedema is often noted on early chest X-rays.

Complications (Table 74.4). Acute complications are similar to those of extensive burns. The total daily fluid loss averages 3–4 L in adult patients with TEN affecting 50% of body surface area. It induces a reduction of intravascular volume and functional renal failure. If not corrected, hypovolaemia may lead to haemodynamic alterations and organic renal failure. Pneumonia or pneumonitis occurs in up to 30% of patients, contributed to by sloughing of the tracheobronchial tree [18]. Adult respiratory distress syndrome (ARDS) is one of the main complications. Anaemia or leukopenia, caused by selective depletion of CD4[+] helper T cells, is moderately common [16]. Oesophageal and intestinal erosions, with an endoscopic appearance reminiscent of ulcerative or pseudomembranous colitis, are recorded [19]; strictures may result. Disseminated intravascular coagulation is documented. Septicaemia, primarily the result of *Staphylococcus aureus* or *Pseudomonas* but on occasion caused by Gram-negative organisms or *Candida*, may result from infection of the skin, lungs, urinary tract catheters and intravenous (especially central) lines. Patients are usually febrile and shivering, even in the absence of infection. Hypothermia is infrequent and usually a marker of severe infection and irreversible septic shock. Protein loss, from skin lesions and increased catabolism, may reach 150–200 g/day. Inhibition of insulin secretion and/or insulin resistance in peripheral tissues is frequent, resulting in elevated plasma glucose levels and glycosuria.

Mucocutaneous complications of TEN [20,21] include wound infections, pigmentary changes (either hyper- or hypopigmentation) which may or may not resolve with time, nail shedding or dystrophy, hypohidrosis or hyperhidrosis, scarring alopecia and hypertrophic scarring which may lead to contractures. Development of melanocytic naevi has been reported [22]. Mucosal involvement may lead to chronic xerostomia, oesophageal strictures, phimosis, and chronic oro-genital erosions or vulvo-vaginal stenosis [23]. Appearances may resemble scarring from cicatricial pemphigoid or lichen planus.

Ocular complications occur in 40–50% of survivors [16], and include conjunctivitis, watery eyes because of tear duct obstruction, pseudomembrane formation, photophobia, ectropion, entropion with trichiasis, symblepharon and corneal vascularization, corneal opacities, and corneal ulceration and scarring [19]. Blindness may result. Lacrimal duct destruction may result in xerophthalmia. A Sjögren-like sicca syndrome may be seen [24]. A 'post-SJS/TEN' ocular syndrome with punctuate keratitis and formation of a corneal pannus may result in photophobia, burning eyes and visual impairment. Ankylosymblepharon (fusion of eyelids to each other and to the globe) may follow secondary infection.

REFERENCES

1 Kauppinen K. Cutaneous reactions to drugs: with special reference to severe mucocutaneous bullous eruptions and sulphonamides. *Acta Derm Venereol (Stockh)* 1972; **52** (Suppl. 68): 1–89.
2 Böttiger LE, Strandberg I, Westerholm B. Drug-induced febrile mucocutaneous syndrome: with a survey of the literature. *Acta Med Scand* 1975; **198**: 229–33.
3 Ruiz-Maldonado R. Acute disseminated epidermal necrosis types 1, 2, and 3: study of 60 cases. *J Am Acad Dermatol* 1985; **13**: 623–35.
4 Nethercott JR, Choi BC. Erythema multiforme (Stevens–Johnson syndrome): chart review of 123 hospitalized patients. *Dermatologica* 1985; **171**: 383–96.
5 Ting HC, Adam BA. Stevens–Johnson syndrome: a review of 34 cases. *Int J Dermatol* 1985; **24**: 587–91.
6 Ashby DW, Lazar T. Erythema multiforme exudativum major (Stevens–Johnson syndrome). *Lancet* 1951; **i**: 1091–5.
7 Rzany B, Hering O, Mockenhaupt M et al. Histopathological and epidemiological characteristics of patients with erythema exudativum multiforme major, Stevens–Johnson syndrome and toxic epidermal necrolysis. *Br J Dermatol* 1996; **135**: 6–11.
8 Bastuji-Garin S, Rzany B, Stern RS et al. A clinical classification of cases of toxic epidermal necrolysis, Stevens–Johnson syndrome, and erythema multiforme. *Arch Dermatol* 1993; **129**: 92–6.
9 Roujeau JC. The spectrum of Stevens–Johnson syndrome and toxic epidermal necrolysis: a clinical classification. *J Invest Dermatol* 1994; **102**: 28S–30S.
10 Roujeau JC. Stevens–Johnson syndrome and toxic epidermal necrolysis are severity variants of the same disease which differs from erythema multiforme. *J Dermatol* 1997; **24**: 726–9.
11 Lyell A. Toxic epidermal necrolysis (the scalded skin syndrome): a reappraisal. *Br J Dermatol* 1979; **100**: 69–86.
12 Rasmussen JE. Toxic epidermal necrolysis. *Med Clin North Am* 1980; **64**: 901–20.
13 Chan HL. Observations on drug-induced toxic epidermal necrolysis in Singapore. *J Am Acad Dermatol* 1984; **10**: 973–8.
14 Heng MCY. Drug-induced toxic epidermal necrolysis. *Br J Dermatol* 1985; **113**: 597–60.
15 Revuz J, Penso D, Roujeau J-C et al. Toxic epidermal necrolysis: clinical findings and prognosis factors in 87 patients. *Arch Dermatol* 1987; **123**: 1160–5.
16 Roujeau J-C, Chosidow O, Saiag P, Guillaume J-C. Toxic epidermal necrolysis (Lyell syndrome). *J Am Acad Dermatol* 1990; **23**: 1039–58.
17 Avakian R, Flowers FP, Araujo OE, Ramos-Caro FA. Toxic epidermal necrolysis: a review. *J Am Acad Dermatol* 1991; **25**: 69–79.
18 Lebargy F, Wolkenstein P, Gisselbrecht M et al. Pulmonary complications in toxic epidermal necrolysis: a prospective clinical study. *Intensive Care Med* 1997; **23**: 1237–44.
19 Chosidow O, Delchier J-C, Chaumette M-T et al. Intestinal involvement in drug-induced toxic epidermal necrolysis. *Lancet* 1991; **337**: 928.
20 De Felice GP, Caroli R, Auteliano A. Long-term complications of toxic epidermal necrolysis (Lyell's disease): clinical and histopathologic study. *Ophthalmologica* 1987; **195**: 1–6.
21 Sheridan RL, Schulz JT, Ryan CM et al. Long-term consequences of toxic epidermal necrolysis in children. *Pediatrics* 2002; **109**: 74–8.
22 Burns DA, Sarkany I. Junctional naevi following toxic epidermal necrolysis. *Clin Exp Dermatol* 1978; **3**: 323–6.
23 Meneux E, Wolkenstein P, Haddad B et al. Vulvovaginal involvement in toxic epidermal necrolysis: a retrospective study of 40 cases. *Obstet Gynecol* 1998; **91**: 283–7.
24 Roujeau J-C, Phlippoteau C, Koso M et al. Sjögren-like syndrome after drug-induced toxic epidermal necrolysis. *Lancet* 1985; **i**: 609–11.

Prognosis

There is an appreciable mortality as a result of TEN, increasing from 5% in SJS, to 10–15% in transitional SJS–TEN and 30–40% in TEN. ARDS and multiple organ failure are the usual causes of death [1]. They are often precipitated by sepsis with septicaemia, mainly resulting from *Staphylococcus aureus* and *Pseudomonas aeruginosa* [2]. Other causes of death are pulmonary embolism and gastrointestinal bleeding. Early withdrawal of the causative drug improves the prognosis, and drugs with a long half-life are associated with an increased risk of death [3,4]. Increased age in most [5] but not all [1] studies, extensive TEN, delay (more than 3–4 days) in referral to a regional centre [6], early thrombocytopenia and early empirical antibiotic treatment elsewhere are associated with a worse prognosis. It has been claimed that severe granulocytopenia is a poor prognostic indicator [7], although this has been disputed on the basis that lymphopenia is more usually found in severe TEN [8]. A specific severity-of-illness score to determine prognosis for cases of TEN (SCORTEN) based on seven independent risk factors for death as assessed on the first day of hospitalization, has been advocated (Table 74.5) [9].

Table 74.5 SCORTEN prognosis score.

Parameter*
Age > 40 years
Presence of a malignancy
Epidermal detachment > 30%
Heart rate > 120/min
Bicarbonate < 20 mmol/L
Urea > 10 mmol/L
Glycaemia > 14 mmol/L

1 point awarded for each parameter; SCORTEN derived by totalling scores

SCORTEN	Probability of death (%)
0–1	3
2	12
3	35
4	58
≥ 5	90

* Worst recorded value in the 24 h after admission.

REFERENCES

1 Schulz JT, Sheridan RL, Ryan CM *et al.* A 10-year experience with toxic epidermal necrolysis. *J Burn Care Rehabil* 2000; **21**: 199–204.
2 Roujeau J-C, Chosidow O, Saiag P, Guillaume J-C. Toxic epidermal necro-lysis (Lyell syndrome). *J Am Acad Dermatol* 1990; **23**: 1039–58.
3 Garcia-Doval I, LeCleach L, Bocquet H *et al.* Toxic epidermal necrolysis and Stevens–Johnson syndrome: does early withdrawal of causative drugs decrease the risk of death? *Arch Dermatol* 2000; **136**: 323–7.
4 Stern RS. Improving the outcome of patients with toxic epidermal necrolysis and Stevens–Johnson syndrome. *Arch Dermatol* 2000; **136**: 410–1.
5 Honari S, Gibran NS, Heimbach DM *et al.* Toxic epidermal necrolysis (TEN) in elderly patients. *J Burn Care Rehabil* 2001; **22**: 132–5.
6 McGee T, Munster A. Toxic epidermal necrolysis syndrome: mortality rate reduced with early referral to regional burn center. *Plast Reconstr Surg* 1998; **102**: 1018–22.
7 Westly ED, Wechsler HL. Toxic epidermal necrolysis: granulocytic leuko-penia as a prognostic indicator. *Arch Dermatol* 1984; **120**: 721–6.
8 Roujeau JC, Guillaume JC, Revuz J *et al.* Granulocytes, lymphocytes and toxic epidermal necrolysis. *Arch Dermatol* 1985; 121: 305.
9 Bastuji-Garin S, Fouchard N, Bertocchi M *et al.* SCORTEN: a severity-of-illness score for toxic epidermal necrolysis. *J Invest Dermatol* 2000; **115**: 149–53.

Diagnosis

Toxic shock syndrome, which usually occurs in menstru-ating women, may cause widespread erythema and desquamation, but skin tenderness and bullae are absent. Similarly, SSSS can generally be differentiated on clinical appearances and on the basis of histology. Linear IgA bullous dermatosis, whether idiopathic or drug-induced (e.g. vancomycin), may mimic TEN clinically [1], as may a widespread bullous fixed drug eruption [2,3]. The sub-corneal aseptic pustules of acute generalized exanthemat-ous pustulosis (AGEP) or acute pustular psoriasis (von Zumbusch) are usually distinctive but may coalesce to produce extensive superficial detachment mimicking TEN. Paraneoplastic pemphigus may closely resemble SJS, but direct immunofluorescence is positive.

Identification of the responsible drug is often difficult, because patients frequently take more than one medica-tion (an average of 4.4 in one series) [4,5]. A helpful guide-line is that most drugs that cause TEN have been first given between 1 and 3 weeks previously [6–8]; another very suggestive guide is that of recurrence within 48 h on administration of a drug previously recorded as having caused a similar reaction. A given drug is unlikely to be responsible for TEN if it was first given 24 h previously, or if the duration of treatment exceeds 3 weeks [4,7]. In case–control analyses, the risk with drugs used on a long-term basis was restricted to the first few weeks [8]. However, phenytoin-induced TEN may occur any time between 2 and 8 weeks after initiation of therapy, and may progress despite discontinuation of phenytoin days or weeks earlier [9]. Skin testing is unfortunately unreliable. Relevant positive patch tests were found in only 9% of 22 patients with SJS/TEN, compared with 50% of 14 patients with AGEP [10]. The *in vitro* lymphocyte transformation test is of no value [11]. In summary, there is no reliable test to confirm the aetiological role of a given drug in an individual case [6]. Re-exposure to drugs suspected of causing a reaction has resulted in fatality, and should not be carried out for diagnostic purposes [12].

REFERENCES

1 Dellavalle RP, Burch JM, Tayal S *et al.* Vancomycin-associated linear IgA bullous dermatosis mimicking toxic epidermal necrolysis. *J Am Acad Dermatol* 2003; **48**: S56–7.
2 Saiag P, Cordoliani F, Roujeau JC *et al.* Érythème pigmenté fixe bulleux disséminé simulant un syndrome de Lyell. *Ann Dermatol Vénéréol* 1987; **114**: 1440–2.
3 Baird BJ, De Villez RL. Widespread bullous fixed drug eruption mimicking toxic epidermal necrolysis. *Int J Dermatol* 1988; **27**: 170–4.
4 Guillaume J-C, Roujeau J-C, Penso D *et al.* The culprit drugs in 87 cases of toxic epidermal necrolysis (Lyell's syndrome). *Arch Dermatol* 1987; **123**: 1166–70.
5 Prendiville JS, Hebert AA, Greenwald MJ *et al.* Management of Stevens–Johnson syndrome and toxic epidermal necrolyis in children. *J Pediatr* 1989; **115**: 881–7.
6 Roujeau J-C, Chosidow O, Saiag P, Guillaume J-C. Toxic epidermal necro-lysis (Lyell syndrome). *J Am Acad Dermatol* 1990; **23**: 1039–58.
7 Avakian R, Flowers FP, Araujo OE, Ramos-Caro FA. Toxic epidermal necrolysis: a review. *J Am Acad Dermatol* 1991; **25**: 69–79.
8 Roujeau JC, Kelly JP, Naldi L *et al.* Medication use and the risk of Stevens–Johnson syndrome or toxic epidermal necrolysis. *N Engl J Med* 1995; **333**: 1600–7.
9 Kelly DF, Hope DG. Fatal phenytoin-related toxic epidermal necrolysis: case report. *Neurosurgery* 1989; **25**: 976–8.
10 Wolkenstein P, Chosidow O, Fléchet ML *et al.* Patch testing in severe cuta-neous adverse drug reactions including Stevens–Johnson syndrome and toxic epidermal necrolysis. *Contact Dermatitis* 1996; **35**: 234–6.
11 Roujeau J-C, Albengres E, Moritz SI. Lymphocyte transformation test in drug-induced toxic epidermal necrolysis. *Int Arch Allergy Appl Immunol* 1985; **78**: 22–4.
12 Bianchine JR, Macaraeg PVJ, Lasagna L *et al.* Drugs as aetiologic factors in the Stevens–Johnson syndrome. *Am J Med* 1968; **44**: 390–405.

Treatment [1–10]

The management of TEN is summarized in Table 74.6, and is perhaps best carried out on a dermatology intensive care or a burns unit. Clearly, presumptive causative drugs should be stopped as soon as possible. It should be remembered that HIV-1 infected patients with TEN are an occupational risk for health care workers [11]. The main principles of symptomatic therapy are the same as for major burns and include fluid replacement, anti-infectious therapy, aggressive nutritional support, warm-ing of environmental temperature and skin care with appropriate dressings. The extent of the detachment of the epidermis should be evaluated daily as a major pro-gnostic factor. It is expressed as a percentage of body sur-face area (BSA), using burn tables or the simple rule that one hand (palm and fingers) corresponds to 1% of the BSA. Hyperventilation and mild hypoxaemia on blood gas analysis indicate a high risk of progression to ARDS.

There is a significant incidence of disabling long-term complications in survivors, especially in relation to ocular and other mucous membranes. It is therefore particularly important to be aware of these and to take preventative

Table 74.6 Management of toxic epidermal necrolysis.

Intensive therapy or burns unit
Air-fluidized bed
Maintain fluid and electrolyte balance (replace up to 5 L/day)
Maintain body temperature
Maintain nutrition; oral hygiene
Frequent ophthalmological assessment
Antiseptic/antibiotic eye drops 2-hourly
Disrupt synechiae frequently
Limitation of infection
Neutropenia: reverse barrier nursing
Frequent cultures of erosions, and blood cultures
Culture tips of Foley catheters and intravenous lines
Prophylactic broad-spectrum systemic antibiotics (controversial)
Topical cleansing/antibacterial agents
0.5% silver nitrate solution on gauze *or* 10% chlorhexidine gluconate
    washes *or* saline washes *or* polymixin/bacitracin *or* 2% mupirocin
Avoid silver sulfadiazine
Wound care
Remove necrotic epidermis (controversial)
Paraffin gauze or hydrogel dressings
Biological dressings (xenografts, allografts, skin substitutes)

measures. Physical contact with patients during nursing procedures may produce loss of large sheets of skin, and the use of a turning frame or a ripple or air-fluidized bed will lessen discomfort and facilitate nursing care. Trauma, as with adhesive dressings or ECG electrode attachment pads, should be minimized. Eyelids and conjunctivae should be lubricated with soft paraffin, and gently separated to prevent the formation of adhesions. Opthalmological advice should be sought. Use of gas-permeable scleral contact lenses resulted in improved quality of life in 90% of patients by reducing photophobia and discomfort, and also improved visual acuity and healed corneal epithelial defects in 50% of patients [12]. Amniotic membrane has been used as a dressing for eye lesions in TEN [13]. Autologous germinal cells taken from the limbus and grafted on a support of amniotic membrane may be beneficial in the most severe cases [14]. Skin or other infection must be treated promptly. Good mouth care is important in preventing parotitis. Vaginal examination should be repeated in women and appropriate dressings used to avoid synechiae if erosions are seen. The issue of whether necrotic tissue should be removed is controversial; some authorities feel that this impairs healing. Eroded areas should be treated with biological [15] or synthetic dressings. Use of silver nitrate impregnated dressings [16] has been advocated.

There is no consensus on the merits of therapy with moderately high-dose corticosteroids for TEN. Some authorities maintain that high-dose steroid therapy promotes or masks the signs of infection, delays healing, precipitates gastrointestinal bleeding, prolongs hospitalization and increases mortality [1,2,17–19]. However, others favour steroid therapy on the basis that it may

reduce inflammation and keratinocyte necrosis [20]. It is generally agreed that if steroids, or any other immunosuppressive agent, are to be given, then they should be administered as early as possible in the evolution of the disease. There have been anecdotal reports on the beneficial use of plasmapheresis [21–23], but this has been questioned [24]. Both cyclophosphamide [25] and ciclosporin A [26–28] have produced improvement in anecdotal cases. Thalidomide therapy for TEN was associated with increased mortality [29]. *N*-acetyl cysteine has been documented to be useful in a few patients [30], perhaps because it enhances drug metabolism. On the basis that potential *Fas* (CD95) -mediated keratinocyte death in TEN might be blocked by naturally occurring *Fas*-blocking antibodies included in human immunoglobulin preparations, there have been several reports, mostly favourable, on human intravenous immunoglobulin (IVIG) therapy for TEN [31–39]. Early infusion of high-dose (1 g/kg/day for 3 days in adults) IVIG appears safe and well tolerated, but there may be variations in the efficacy of different batches of IVIG [36]. However, a recent report found no benefit from IVIG therapy [38], and there is currently no consensus on the best management for TEN [40]. There has been a single case report on the efficacy of treatment with monoclonal chimeric IgG anti-TNFα antibodies [41]. Because of the rarity of the condition, controlled trials assessing these different treatment approaches are very difficult to carry out.

Prevention and future use of drugs

Patients should be advised to avoid re-exposure to the suspect drug(s). Published cases of recurrences have all been attributed to the same generic drug or to compounds chemically closely related (e.g. aromatic anticonvulsants). Therefore, there is no rationale for restricting the use of all classes of 'high-risk drugs'. Because some familial cases have been reported, first-degree relatives should be alerted to their elevated risk of reaction to the same drug(s). Cases should be notified to regulatory agencies.

REFERENCES

1 Revuz J, Roujeau J-C, Guillaume J-C *et al.* Treatment of toxic epidermal necrolysis: Créteil's experience. *Arch Dermatol* 1987; **123**: 1156–8.
2 Roujeau J-C, Revuz J. Intensive care in dermatology. In: Champion RH, Pye RJ, eds. *Recent Advances in Dermatology*, Vol. 8. Edinburgh: Churchill Livingstone, 1990: 85–99.
3 Smoot EC III. Treatment issues in the care of patients with toxic epidermal necrolysis. *Burns* 1999; **25**: 439–42.
4 Eisen ER, Fish J, Shear NH. Management of drug-induced toxic epidermal necrolysis. *J Cutan Med Surg* 2000; **4**: 96–102.
5 Fritsch PO, Sidoroff A. Drug-induced Stevens–Johnson syndrome/toxic epidermal necrolysis. *Am J Clin Dermatol* 2000; **1**: 349–60.
6 Craven NM. Management of toxic epidermal necrolysis. *Hosp Med* 2000; **61**: 778–81.
7 Hansbrough JF, Muller P, Noordenbos J, Dore C. A 10-year experience with toxic epidermal necrolysis. *J Burn Care Rehabil* 2001; **22**: 97–8.

8 Spies M, Sanford AP, Aili Low JF *et al.* Treatment of extensive toxic epidermal necrolysis in children. *Pediatrics* 2001; **108**: 1162–8.

9 Palmieri TL, Greenhalgh DG, Saffle JR *et al.* A multicenter review of toxic epidermal necrolysis treated in US burn centers at the end of the twentieth century. *J Burn Care Rehabil* 2002; **23**: 87–96.

10 Ghislain PD, Roujeau JC. Treatment of severe drug reactions: Stevens–Johnson syndrome, toxic epidermal necrolysis and hypersensitivity syndrome. *Dermatol Online J* 2002; **8**: 5.

11 Descamps V, Tattevin P, Descamps DI. HIV-1 infected patients with toxic epidermal necrolysis: an occupational risk for healthcare workers. *Lancet* 1999; **353**: 1855–6.

12 Romero-Rangel T, Stavrou P, Cotter J *et al.* Gas-permeable scleral contact lens therapy in ocular surface disease. *Am J Ophthalmol* 2000; **130**: 25–32.

13 John T, Foulks GN, John ME, Cheng K, Hu D. Amniotic membrane in the surgical management of acute toxic epidermal necrolysis. *Ophthalmology* 2002; **109**: 351–60.

14 Tsai RJ, Li LM, Chen JK. Reconstruction of damaged corneas by transplantation of autologous limbal epithelial cells. *N Engl J Med* 2000; **343**: 86–93.

15 Pianigiani E, Ierardi F, Taddeucci P *et al.* Skin allograft in the treatment of toxic epidermal necrolysis (TEN). *Dermatol Surg* 2002; **28**: 1173–6.

16 Lehrer-Bell KA, Kirsner RS, Tallman PG, Kerdel FA. Treatment of the cutaneous involvement in Stevens–Johnson syndrome and toxic epidermal necrolysis with silver nitrate-impregnated dressings. *Arch Dermatol* 1998; **134**: 877–9.

17 Halebian PH, Corder VJ, Madden MR *et al.* Improved burn center survival of patients with toxic epidermal necrolysis managed without corticosteroids. *Ann Surg* 1986; **204**: 503–12.

18 Heimbach DM, Engrav LH, Marvin JA. Toxic epidermal necrolysis: a step forward in treatment. *JAMA* 1987; **257**: 2171–5.

19 Rzany B, Schmitt H, Schöpf E. Toxic epidermal necrolysis in patients receiving glucocorticosteroids. *Acta Derm Venereol (Stockh)* 1991; **71**: 171–2.

20 van der Meer JB, Schuttelaar ML, Toth GG *et al.* Successful dexamethasone pulse therapy in a toxic epidermal necrolysis (TEN) patient featuring recurrent TEN to oxazepam. *Clin Exp Dermatol* 2001; **26**: 654–6.

21 Kamanabroo D, Schmitz-Landgraf W, Czartnetski BM. Plasmapheresis in severe drug-induced toxic epidermal necrolysis. *Arch Dermatol* 1985; **121**: 1548–9.

22 Egan CA, Grant WJ, Morris SE, Saffle JR, Zone JJ. Plasmapheresis as an adjunct treatment in toxic epidermal necrolysis. *J Am Acad Dermatol* 1999; **40**: 458–61.

23 Bamichas G, Natse T, Christidou F *et al.* Plasma exchange in patients with toxic epidermal necrolysis. *Ther Apher* 2002; **6**: 225–8.

24 Furubacke A, Berlin G, Anderson C, Sjoberg F. Lack of significant treatment effect of plasma exchange in the treatment of drug-induced toxic epidermal necrolysis? *Intensive Care Med* 1999; **25**: 1307–10.

25 Heng MC, Allen SG. Efficacy of cyclophosphamide in toxic epidermal necrolysis: clinical and pathophysiologic aspects. *J Am Acad Dermatol* 1991; **25**: 778–86.

26 Renfro L, Grant-Kels JM, Daman LA. Drug-induced toxic epidermal necrolysis treated with cyclosporin. *Int J Dermatol* 1989; **28**: 441–4.

27 Arevalo JM, Lorente JA, Gonzalez-Herrada C, Jimenez-Reyes J. Treatment of toxic epidermal necrolysis with cyclosporin A. *J Trauma* 2000; **48**: 473–8.

28 Jarrett P, Rademaker M, Havill J, Pullon H. Toxic epidermal necrolysis treated with cyclosporin and granulocyte colony stimulating factor. *Clin Exp Dermatol* 1997; **22**: 146–7.

29 Wolkenstein P, Latarjet J, Roujeau JC *et al.* Randomised comparison of thalidomide versus placebo in toxic epidermal necrolysis. *Lancet* 1998; **352**: 1586–9.

30 Velez A, Moreno JC. Toxic epidermal necrolysis treated with *N*-acetylcysteine. *J Am Acad Dermatol* 2002; **46**: 469–70.

31 Viard I, Wehrli P, Bullani R *et al.* Inhibition of toxic epidermal necrolysis by blockade of CD95 with human intravenous immunoglobulin. *Science* 1998; **282**: 490–3.

32 French LE, Tschopp J. *Fas*-mediated cell death in toxic epidermal necrolysis and graft-versus-host disease: potential for therapeutic inhibition. *Schweiz Med Wochenschr* 2000; **130**: 1656–61.

33 Stella M, Cassano P, Bollero D *et al.* Toxic epidermal necrolysis treated with intravenous high-dose immunoglobulins: our experience. *Dermatology* 2001; **203**: 45–9.

34 Paquet P, Jacob E, Damas P, Pierard GE. Treatment of drug-induced toxic epidermal necrolysis (Lyell's syndrome) with intravenous human immunoglobulins. *Burns* 2001; **27**: 652–5.

35 Tristani-Firouzi P, Petersen MJ, Saffle JR *et al.* Treatment of toxic epidermal necrolysis with intravenous immunoglobulin in children. *J Am Acad Dermatol* 2002; **47**: 548–52.

36 Prins C, Kerdel FA, Padilla RS *et al.* Toxic epidermal necrolysis–intravenous immunoglobulin: treatment of toxic epidermal necrolysis with high-dose intravenous immunoglobulins—multicenter retrospective analysis of 48 consecutive cases. *Arch Dermatol* 2003; **139**: 26–32.

37 Trent JT, Kirsner RS, Romanelli P, Kerdel FA. Analysis of intravenous immunoglobulin for the treatment of toxic epidermal necrolysis using SCORTEN: the University of Miami Experience. *Arch Dermatol* 2003; **139**: 39–43.

38 Bachot N, Revuz J, Roujeau JC. Intravenous immunoglobulin treatment for Stevens–Johnson syndrome and toxic epidermal necrolysis: a prospective non-comparative study showing no benefit on mortality or progression. *Arch Dermatol* 2003; **139**: 33–6.

39 Wolff K, Tappeiner G. Treatment of toxic epidermal necrolysis: the uncertainty persists but the fog is dispersing. *Arch Dermatol* 2003; **139**: 85–6.

40 Majumdar S, Mockenhaupt M, Roujeau J, Townshend A. Interventions for toxic epidermal necrolysis. *Cochrane Database Syst Rev* 2002; **4**: CD001435.

41 Fischer M, Fiedler E, Marsch WC, Wohlrab J. Antitumour necrosis factor-α antibodies (infliximab) in the treatment of a patient with toxic epidermal necrolysis. *Br J Dermatol* 2002; **146**: 707–9.

Chapter 75

Topical Therapy

J. Berth-Jones

Dermatologists have the good fortune to work on the most accessible organ of the body. This gives us numerous advantages and greatly facilitates not only the diagnosis but also the treatment of skin disease. While systemic administration of drugs is often necessary in dermatology, many inflammatory and neoplastic conditions can be effectively managed using the wide range of externally applied physical or pharmacological modalities that are available, the latter being the subject of this chapter. Some of these are time-honoured treatments which have been used for a century or more, while others belong to the ever-expanding range of newer and increasingly potent agents constantly being developed and formulated for topical use.

Topical treatment offers the potential to achieve high concentrations of a drug in the skin with minimal exposure of other organs. This can greatly increase efficacy and also safety relative to systemic administration. When side effects do occur, they are most likely to take the form of localized reactions.

Prescribing topical treatment

Prescribing topical medication requires careful consideration of several factors if optimal results are to be achieved. When the treatment contains an active pharmaceutical agent it is necessary to specify the concentration of the drug, the vehicle and the frequency of application. The patient requires advice on the quantity to be used, precisely where it should be applied and often further explanation about precise timing of application in relation to bathing and other treatments. The prescriber needs to be aware of the hazards associated with a topical treatment, particularly the likelihood of the medication inducing irritant or allergic reactions. It is also important to understand the factors that influence systemic absorption.

Drug concentration

The conventions for defining the concentration of a drug in topical formulations are summarized in Table 75.1. The efficacy of a topically applied drug is usually not proportionate to the concentration. Doubling or halving the concentration of a drug often has a surprisingly modest effect on the response. In the case of topical corticosteroids, for example, different concentrations of active drug often have a similar biological effect [1]. However, the effect of changing the concentration in an individual case may be much greater than the apparent effect when two concentrations are compared in a clinical trial. There may also be differences between adults and children. The difference in efficacy between two concentrations of tacrolimus for example, appears to be larger in adults than in children.

Table 75.1 Prescribing conventions for specifying concentration.

1 The concentration of a drug contained in a topical medication is usually written as a percentage representing the proportion of the formulation, by weight, which is the active constituent. A concentration of 1% indicates that 1 g of drug will be contained in 100 g of the formulation. A wide range of concentrations can be specified in this way. Thus, salicylic acid may be used in concentration as high as 60% for treatment of plantar warts or corns, whereas calcitriol is used at a concentration of 0.003% in treatment of psoriasis. A very low concentration such as this is more often written as 3 µg/g

2 A frequently used alternative, especially for liquid preparations, is to express the percentage of the drug as a proportion of the volume of the formulation. Thus, a 1% solution contains 1 g of drug in 100 mL of the formulation. The abbreviations w/w (weight in weight) and w/v (weight in volume) are often employed to indicate which convention is being used

3 Another convention often used to describe the concentration of a solution is in 'parts'. Thus, a 1 part in 1000 solution of potassium permanganate contains 1 g in 1 L of solution, which could be expressed as 0.1% (w/v)

Choice of vehicle

Topical medication must be applied to the skin in a suitable vehicle. This term encompasses all the constituents of the formulation apart from the active pharmaceutical agent. The properties of some types of vehicle are summarized below. The choice of vehicle depends on the anatomical site to be treated and the condition of the skin. As a rule, acutely inflamed skin is best treated with fairly bland preparations, which are least likely to irritate. Moist or exudative eruptions are conventionally treated with 'wet' medications such as lotions or creams, while dry skin responds well to the occlusive action of ointments. Hair-bearing skin, especially the scalp, can be treated with medicaments formulated into shampoos, lotions, gels or mousses. The cosmetic properties of the vehicle assume particular importance when treating the face. Oily skin affected by acne is often best treated with lotions, while the more sensitive skin affected by rosacea may benefit from the emollient effect of a cream.

The characteristic features of various types of formulation are as follows (British Pharmacopoeia; BP).

Ointments. These are semi-solid vehicles composed of lipid; for example, white soft paraffin BP (petrolatum). They have useful occlusive and emollient properties. Some ointments contain emulsifying agents such as polyhydric alcohols (macrogols, polyethylene glycol) or cetostearyl alcohol (e.g. Emulsifying Ointment BP). The latter have the advantage of being less greasy, with good solvent properties, and are easily washed off. Ointments require fewer preservatives than other vehicles because they contain no water and do not sustain growth of microorganisms.

Creams. These are semi-solid emulsions containing both lipid and water. Emulsions are suspensions, either of lipid droplets in water or of water droplets in lipid (see emulsifiers, p. 75.7). In the former category are aqueous or vanishing creams (e.g. Aqueous Cream BP). These are water-miscible, cooling and soothing, and are well absorbed into the skin. In the latter category are water-in-oil creams (e.g. Oily Cream BP). These are immiscible with water and more difficult to wash off. They are emollient, lubricant and mildly occlusive (but less so than ointments).

Pastes. These are semi-solid preparations containing a high proportion of finely powdered material such as zinc oxide or starch. Protective (fatty) pastes are greasy and therefore messy and water insoluble. They are difficult to apply and remove, but their stiffness permits accurate localization of the paste and any constituent medication. They are occlusive, protective and hydrating. The consistency of these pastes can be 'softened' by adding oils or 'hardened' with hard paraffin. Drying pastes, also called cooling pastes, are mixtures of powder with liquid. These are non-greasy, water-miscible and easy to apply and remove. They are drying and soothing, and can be used in conjunction with dressings as paste bandages or as vehicles for active medicaments.

Lotions. These are liquid formulations that are usually simple suspensions or solutions of medication in water, alcohol or other liquids. Those containing alcohol often sting, especially when applied to broken skin. When left on the skin the liquid will evaporate, leaving a film of medication on the surface. Aqueous suspensions of powders such as calamine, which require shaking prior to each application, are known as *shake lotions*.

Gels. These are thickened aqueous lotions. They are semi-solid preparations containing high-molecular-weight polymers, such as carboxypolymethylene (Carbomer BP) or methylcellulose, and can be regarded as thickened aqueous lotions. Lotions and gels are especially suitable for treating the scalp and other hairy areas of skin. Like lotions, gels tend to dry when left on the skin. Gels can provide cosmetically acceptable formulations for use on the face.

Powders. These are applied directly to the skin and are also known as *dusting powders*. They can reduce friction (talc) or excessive moisture (starch). They are occasionally used to deliver drugs such as antifungal agents applied to the feet.

Paints. These are liquid preparations, either aqueous, hydro-alcoholic or alcoholic (*tinctures*), which are usually applied with a brush to the skin or mucous membranes and then evaporate. Collodion preparations are also sometimes referred to as paints.

Collodions. These (e.g. Flexible Collodion BP) are liquid preparations consisting of cellulose nitrate in organic solvent. They evaporate rapidly to leave a flexible film that can hold medicaments in contact with the skin. They are most frequently used to apply salicylic and lactic acids to warts. They may also be used as protectives to seal minor cuts and abrasions. They are easy to apply and are water repellent, but are inflammable.

Microsponges [2]. These are a novel approach to formulation, involving the use of porous beads, typically 10–25 μm in diameter, forming a reservoir loaded with the drug. This approach has been used for cosmetics and sunscreens as well as for medications such as benzoyl peroxide and retinoids. The aim is to provide sustained release of the drug while reducing irritation.

Liposomes. These are structures comprising an aqueous phase surrounded by a lipid capsule, ranging widely in diameter from several nanometers to several micrometers. They may contain several lipid layers so that the structure can be likened to that of an onion. Under certain conditions liposomes can release their contents close to a target cell, fuse with the cell membrane or be endocytosed by the cell [3]. They can be formulated into creams and gels. This technology is used in cosmetics but has so far had little impact on dermatological treatment. However, it may prove useful for reducing irritation from topical use of agents such as tretinoin, benzoyl peroxide and dithranol, and in reducing the staining of skin and clothes from the latter [3–5]. Liposomes do not appear to penetrate intact into the intracellular compartment of the epidermis, although an *in vitro* study using reconstructed human skin has suggested that liposomal lipids can be incorporated into the intercellular lipids of the stratum corneum and cell membranes in the uppermost viable layers of the epidermis [6].

Frequency of application

The frequency of application must be specified in order to maximize the response while avoiding side effects such as irritation. Excessive frequency of application may also result in unnecessary systemic exposure to the drug. Emollients should be applied frequently enough to maintain their physical effect. This may require several applications daily. Active preparations are usually applied just once or twice a day. As a general rule, twice daily application of drugs such as corticosteroids or deltanoids is only marginally more effective than once daily application, while requiring double the amount of medication and increasing systemic exposure to the drug. The pharmacological actions of a drug may persist long after it has left the surface of the skin. Thus, the ability of a potent topical corticosteroid to inhibit flares of atopic dermatitis

when applied just twice weekly [7] seems unlikely to be explained simply by persistence of a reservoir of the drug. Increasing the interval between applications can be a useful method of gradually reducing the intensity of a treatment, especially when it is difficult to do so by using a lower concentration or less potent agent.

Quantity to be applied

The total quantity to be dispensed should be specified, and it is helpful to inform the patient how long the prescribed quantity is expected to last. There is a tendency, especially in the case of topical steroids, for patients to be overcautious in their interpretation of the advice to 'apply sparingly' which will be found on the package insert. Minute quantities are rarely effective. Conversely, inappropriate use of active medicaments as emollients is not only wasteful but often hazardous. The potential for systemic absorption must be taken into account when prescribing, for example, topical corticosteroids, deltanoids or salicylic acid.

Estimates of the quantity of cream or ointment required for a single total body treatment of a male adult have varied considerably. In one study, a range of 12–27 g (average 18 g) was required for applications by 'trained operators' [8], while a range of 8–115 g (average 44 g) was required when the treatment was self-administered. In another study, in which treatment was applied by nurses, an average of 12 g of ointment was required [9]. In a more recent study, male patients treating themselves applied an average of 20 g of ointment, and females applied 17 g [10].

Based on these latter figures, the quantity required for 1 week of once daily application to the whole body would be approximately 140 g for males and 120 g for females, while for twice daily application, male and female patients require 280 and 240 g/week, respectively.

Table 75.2 provides approximate quantities required for single applications to specific anatomical regions in adults, while Table 75.3 provides a guide to total quantities required for a week of twice daily total body treatment for children of various ages. These guidelines can only be approximate and should be interpreted very flexibly. In addition to the obvious large differences between

Table 75.2 Approximate quantities (g) required for each application of medication to different anatomical regions. (Adapted from [10].)

Region	Males	Females
Trunk (including buttocks)	6.6	5.8
One leg	2.9	2.5
One foot	0.9	0.7
One arm and forearm	1.7	1.3
One hand	0.6	0.5
Face, neck and ears	1.3	0.9
Whole body	20	17

Table 75.3 Quantities (g) of medication required for twice daily application to the entire body at various ages. (Adapted from [13].)

Age	3 months	6 months	12 months	18 months	2 years	3 years	4 years	5 years	7 years	10 years	12 years
Daily requirement (g)	8	10	12	13	14	16	19	20	25	30	37
Weekly requirement (g)	56	67	84	93	95	112	135	140	172	210	256

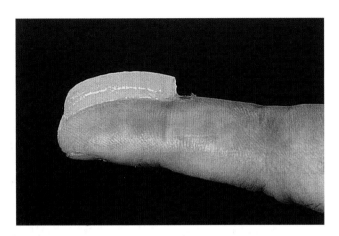

Fig. 75.1 The fingertip unit. From [13]. (Courtesy of Dr A.Y. Finlay and with permission from the Editor of *British Journal of Dermatology*.)

individuals of any age in body surface area, the condition of the skin may influence how far the medication will spread. Creams and ointments seem to cover a very similar area per unit of weight [8,9].

Simple practical guides to the quantity of a topical medication to apply are provided by the fingertip unit [10] and the rule of hand, as follows.

The *fingertip unit* is an approximate but practical measure of topical medication. It is the quantity of ointment extruded from a tube with a nozzle of 5 mm diameter (note that nozzles do vary somewhat) that extends from the distal crease of the forefinger to the ventral aspect of the fingertip (Fig. 75.1). This unit weighs approximately 0.49 g in males and 0.43 g in females [11] and covers, on average, an area of approxiamtely 300 cm². The number of units required for a single treatment of each anatomical region in adults and children of various ages is given in Table 75.4.

The '*rule of hand*' states that an area of the size that can be covered by four adult hands (including the digits) can be treated by 1 g of ointment or 2 fingertip units [12].

The figures discussed above are based on application of active medicaments. Emollients are applied for their physical properties rather than for delivery of a drug, and are generally used much more liberally. Emollient treatment of the whole body may require 100 g/day when the skin is very dry.

Advice to patients

Detailed instructions are often required as to the timing of applications. In many cases it is most convenient to apply the medication immediately after bathing. If other topical treatments are in use it is important to explain how the applications should be timed relative to each other. For example, application of an emollient immediately after application of an active agent will inevitably dilute the active medication and probably spread it over areas of skin where it is not required. When using a medication with a tendency to induce irritation it is helpful to warn patients about this in advance and to give advice on the best course of action when this occurs.

If it is planned to use any form of occlusion, bandaging or other dressing with topically applied medication, detailed instruction is required and this should ideally take the form of a demonstration by a specially trained nurse. Occlusion will invariably increase the level of penetration of a drug into the skin. The mechanism of this effect is not fully understood but seems to be partly the result of retaining a reservoir of the medication on the surface of the skin, and partly the effect of increased hydration of the stratum corneum. The simplest method of occlusion is the use of polythene gloves on the hands or 'clingfilm' on the feet or limbs. Self-adhesive hydrocolloid dressings can be very useful for limited areas on the limbs or trunk. 'Wet wrap' bandaging is described in the treatment of atopic dermatitis. Various additional types of bandaging (e.g. paste bandages) can be used to increase the penetration of topical medication and have the added benefit of preventing scratching.

Age	Face and neck	One upper limb	One lower limb	Trunk	Whole body
3–6 months	1	1	1.5	2.5	8.5
1–2 years	1.5	1.5	2	5	13.5
3–5 years	1.5	2	3	6.5	18
6–10 years	2	2.5	4.5	8.5	24.5
Adult	2.5	4.5	7.6	13.5	40

Table 75.4 Fingertip units required for a single treatment of various regions in children and adults. (Adapted from [10,13].) Note that the unit is measured using an adult finger.

When self-treatment fails, the efficacy of topical therapy can almost invariably be improved if the treatment can be applied by a specialist nurse in an outpatient department. Many dermatology departments are able to provide this service for patients with severe skin disease who are able to attend on a daily basis. The response to treatment is improved even further by admission to hospital for a period of rest and regular supervised treatment.

Hazards associated with topical treatment

The most frequent adverse effects associated with topical medication are localized irritant or allergic reactions. Irritant reactions can be minimized by applying treatment at the optimal concentration and treatment intervals and by selection of the correct vehicle. Sensitization is more difficult to anticipate and to prevent. Contact allergy can develop not only to the active medicament but also to constituents of the vehicle. Almost any component may sensitize: notable examples include ethylenediamine [14], propylene glycol [15], emulsifiers [16], sorbic acid [17,18], cetyl and stearyl alcohols [19] and fragrances [20]. Patients with chronic venous eczema or leg ulcers appear to be particularly susceptible [21,22]. Sensitivity to topical medication is often overlooked as the symptoms tend to be attributed to the disease being treated.

Systemic side effects from topically applied medication are relatively rare. Nonetheless, all topically applied drugs are absorbed to some degree and on occasions unexpected systemic toxicity occurs. Absorption varies very considerably depending on the region of skin being treated (Table 75.4) [23]. Occlusion greatly enhances absorption [24,25]. Systemic exposure can be greater than expected in children because of their relatively high ratio of skin surface to body mass. In the elderly, penetration of drugs may be increased as a result of changes in the structure of the skin. This effect is most pronounced on those drugs that are most hydrophilic [26]. Inflammation of the skin impairs barrier function and significantly increases drug absorption. This is especially significant in the erythrodermic patient [27–29].

REFERENCES

1 Stoughton RB, Wullich K. The same glucocorticoid in brand-name products: does increasing the concentration result in greater topical biologic activity? *Arch Dermatol* 1989; **125**: 1509–11.
2 Embil K, Nacht S. The Microsponge Delivery System (MDS): a topical delivery system with reduced irritancy incorporating multiple triggering mechanisms for the release of actives. *J Microencapsul* 1996; **13**: 575–88.
3 Schafer-Korting M, Korting HC, Braun-Falco O. Liposome preparations: a step forward in topical drug therapy for skin disease: a review. *J Am Acad Dermatol* 1989; **21**: 1271–5.
4 Patel VB, Misra AN, Marfatia YS. Preparation and comparative clinical evaluation of liposomal gel of benzoyl peroxide for acne. *Drug Dev Ind Pharm* 2001; **27**: 863–9.
5 Agarwal R, Saraswat A, Kaur I *et al*. A novel liposomal formulation of dithranol for psoriasis: preliminary results. *J Dermatol* 2002; **29**: 529–32.
6 Korting HC, Stolz W, Schmid MH *et al*. Interaction of liposomes with human epidermis reconstructed *in vitro*. *Br J Dermatol* 1995; **132**: 571–9.
7 Berth-Jones J, Damstra RJ, Golsch S *et al*. Twice weekly fluticasone propionate added to emollient maintenance treatment to reduce risk of relapse in atopic dermatitis: randomised, double blind, parallel group study. *BMJ* 2003; **326**: 1367–70.
8 Schlagel CA, Sanborn EC. The weights of topical preparations required for total and partial body inunction. *J Invest Dermatol* 1964; **42**: 253–6.
9 Maurice PDL, Saihan EG. Topical steroid requirement in inflammatory skin conditions. *Br J Clin Prac* 1991; **16**: 444–7.
10 Long CC, Finlay AY. The finger-tip unit: a new practical measure. *Clin Exp Dermatol* 1991; **16**: 444–7.
11 Finlay AY, Edwards PH, Harding KG. 'Fingertip unit' in dermatology. *Lancet* 1989; **11**: 155.
12 Long CC, Finlay AY, Averill RW. The rule of hand: 4 hand areas = 2 FTU = 1 g. *Arch Dermatol* 1992; **128**: 1129–30.
13 Long CC, Mills CM, Finlay AY. A practical guide to topical therapy in children. *Br J Dermatol* 1998; **138**: 293–6.
14 Fisher AA. Instructions for the ethylene diamine-sensitive patient. *Cutis* 1974; **13**: 27–8.
15 Hannuksela M, Pirilä V, Salo OP. Skin reactions to propylene glycol. *Contact Dermatitis* 1975; **1**: 112–6.
16 Hannuksela M, Kousa M, Pirilä V. Contact sensitivity to emulsifiers. *Contact Dermatitis* 1976; **2**: 201–4.
17 Brown R. Another case of sorbic acid sensitivity. *Contact Dermatitis* 1979; **5**: 268.
18 Saihan EM, Harman RRM. Contact sensitivity to sorbic acid in 'Unguentum Merck'. *Br J Dermatol* 1978; **99**: 583–4.
19 Blondeel A, Oleffe J, Achten G. Contact allergy in 330 dermatological patients. *Contact Dermatitis* 1978; **4**: 270–6.
20 Larsen WG. Perfume dermatitis: a study of 20 patients. *Arch Dermatol* 1977; **113**: 623–5.
21 Breit R, Bandmann HJ. Contact dermatitis. XXII. Dermatitis from lanolin. *Br J Dermatol* 1973; **88**: 414–5.
22 Wilkinson JD, Hambly EM, Wilkinson DS. Comparison of patch test results in two adjacent areas of England. II. Medicaments. *Acta Derm Venereol* 1980; **60**: 245–9.
23 Feldmann RJ, Maibach HI. Regional variation in percutaneous penetration of ^{14}C cortisol in man. *J Invest Dermatol* 1967; **48**: 181–3.
24 Sulzberger MB, Witten VH. Thin pliable plastic films in topical dermatologic therapy. *Arch Dermatol* 1961; **84**: 1027–8.
25 Bourke J, Berth-Jones J, Hutchinson PE. Occlusion enhances the efficacy of topical calcipotriol in psoriasis vulgaris. *Clin Exp Dermatol* 1993; **18**: 504–6.
26 Roskos KV, Maibach HI, Guy RH. The effect of aging on percutaneous absorption in man. *J Pharmacokinet Biopharm* 1989; **17**: 617–30.
27 Borzyskowski M, Grant DB, Wells RS. Cushing's syndrome induced by topical steroids used for the treatment of non-bullous ichthyosiform erythroderma. *Clin Exp Dermatol* 1976; **1**: 337–42.
28 Dwyer C, Chapman R. Calcipotriol and hypercalcaemia. *Lancet* 1991; **338**: 764–5.
29 Brubacher JR, Hoffman RS. Salicylism from topical salicylates: review of the literature. *J Toxicol Clin Toxicol* 1996; **34**: 431–6.

Formulation of topical treatment

The formulation of the vehicle in which a drug is delivered topically to the skin is critical in obtaining effective and consistent results. The vehicle has many roles. It must provide rapid delivery of the drug to the stratum corneum and into the viable layers of the skin. It must be soothing and comfortable to use and preferably also cosmetically acceptable. The vehicle must also provide a chemical environment in which the drug remains sufficiently stable prior to use to have a practical shelf life.

Most topical treatments are now commercially formulated in vehicles that have been carefully designed for optimal results. Some caution is therefore required when adding diluents or other medicaments to such a formulation. The role of the dermatologist in formulating topical treatment has been reduced over recent years by stricter financial, legislative and safety controls, which have resulted in the increasing reluctance of pharmacists to prepare extemporaneous or personalized formulations. Nonetheless, an understanding of the parts played by the various constituents of vehicles remains important. Only the most frequently used components are reviewed here. Further information regarding many of the materials and formulations discussed in this chapter is available in the British and US pharmacopoeias (BP, USP) and British Pharmaceutical Codex (BPC).

The simplest role of a vehicle is dilution of an active drug to the desired concentration. Agents such as beeswax, liquid paraffin, polyethylene glycol and powders are often added for their physical properties to adjust the thickness or texture of the medication. In addition to this, various constituents act as emollients, emulsifiers, fragrances, humectants, penetration enhancers, preservatives or solvents. Some of the constituents most often employed are listed in Table 75.5 and some are discussed further below. A single constituent often serves more than one function.

Lipids

Lipids incorporated into vehicles can act as diluents and solvents but are especially valuable as emollients: they have the ability to form a coating on the surface of the stratum corneum which inhibits evaporation of water, thus providing a softening and moisturizing effect. Generally speaking, the greater the proportion of lipid in the formulation, the greater will be the emollient action. Ointments are therefore more emollient than oily creams, which are more so than aqueous creams, while most lotions have no emollient effect. Lipids from a variety of sources are incorporated into topical treatments for skin disease.

Vegetable oils

Oils can be obtained from numerous vegetable sources by pressing or by solvent extraction. Vegetable oils are largely composed of triglycerides, which tend to contain large proportions of unsaturated fatty acids such as the 18-carbon fatty acids oleic acid (monoenoic) and linoleic acid (dienoic). The presence of these unsaturated fatty acids renders vegetable oils vulnerable to oxidation. This results in rancidity, which manifests as an unpleasant odour and is a major constraint on the use of vegetable oils in medicaments.

Arachis oil, derived from the groundnut or peanut, has been the subject of some concern recently over possible contamination with allergens that could cause hypersensitivity reactions in peanut-sensitive individuals. Cocoa butter, also known as theobroma oil, is a product of the cocoa bean and consists chiefly of the triglycerides of

Table 75.5 Frequently employed constituents of vehicles.

Lipids
Castor oil
Cetyl alcohol
Cocoa butter
Isopropyl myristate
Isopropyl palmitate
Lanolin
Liquid paraffin
Stearic acid
Stearyl alcohol
White soft paraffin (petrolatum)

Emulsifiers
Alkyl sulphates and sulphonates
Glyceryl monostearate
Lanolin and derivatives
Phosphoric acid esters
Polyethylene glycols
Polyvalent metallic soaps
Propylene glycol fatty acid esters
Quaternary ammonium cationic compounds
Sorbitan monolaurate, monopalmitate and mono-oleate
Triethanolamine oleate

Humectants
Glycerin
Propylene glycol
Urea
Pyrrolidone carboxylic acid
Gelatin
Sorbitol

Penetration enhancers
Azone
Dimethyl sulfoxide
Propylene glycol
Salicylic acid
Urea

Preservatives
Benzyl alcohol
Butylated hydroxyanisole
Butylated hydroxytoluene
Chlorocresol
Edetic acid/disodium edetate
Hydroxybenzoates (parabens)
Propylene glycol
Sodium metabisulphite
Sorbic acid/sorbates

Solvents
Acetone
Ethanol
Ether
Chloroform
Glycerin
Isopropyl alcohol
Methanol
Propylene glycol
Water

palmitic, stearic and oleic acids. It also contains antioxidants, which make it remarkably stable for a vegetable oil and which can even help to preserve other constituents with which it is compounded. It is brittle at room temperature but melts at between 30 and 35°C. Castor oil is obtained from the castor bean *Ricinus communis* and is composed almost entirely of triglycerides of the 18-carbon long-chain fatty acid ricinoleic acid. Olive oil contains a large proportion of oleic acid.

Mineral oils and greases

Extracts of crude oil (crude petroleum) resembling those we use today have been used for treatment of skin disease since a US patent was obtained, in 1872, by Robert Chesebrough for a product he called vaseline.

Emollient products extracted from crude oil can be produced as fluids, semi-solids or solids and include Liquid Paraffin BP, Mineral Oil USP, Yellow and White Soft Paraffin BP, Petrolatum USP. The extraction process involves treatments to remove elements other than hydrogen and carbon. Aromatic and unsaturated compounds are also eliminated, leaving a diverse range of hydrocarbon molecules, some straight chained, some branched and some polycyclic [1]. As a result of their fully saturated nature, these hydrocarbons are far more stable than the constituents of vegetable oils. They are remarkably inert and are not vulnerable to oxidation or rancidity. For this reason, mineral oils have substantially replaced vegetable oils as the lipids used in emollients and topical treatments.

Lanolin

The use of wool extracts for cosmetic and medicinal purposes dates back at least as far as ancient Greece. Lanolin (wool fat) is extracted from wool and is essentially the product of the sheep sebaceous gland [2]. It is available in abundance and, because its natural purpose is to protect the skin and wool of the sheep, it is perhaps an obvious choice of lipid material for use as an emollient.

Lanolin comprises a complex mixture of higher fatty acids esterified with mono- and dihydric alcohols, including aliphatic alcohols, and cholesterol and related sterols. Its precise composition varies qualitatively and quantitatively with humidity, temperature and method of collection. It is prone to auto-oxidation and is therefore often formulated with the antioxidant butylated hydroxytoluene. Lanolin is miscible with water and is a useful emulsifying agent when mixed with other lipids.

Lanolin has gained a reputation as a frequent contact sensitizer, although this remains questionable [3]. Small quantities of anionic detergent may be present in lanolin and may increase the apparent incidence of hypersensitivity [4]. It has also been suggested that misleadingly high proportions of positive patch tests to lanolin and wool alcohols have arisen partly because of selection of groups of patients who are particularly vulnerable to irritant reactions which are misinterpreted as allergy [3]. Sensitization to lanolin in the general population remains rare, of the order of 1 in a million, even though this material has so many applications that it is ubiquitous [3].

Partly because of its reputation as a sensitizer, numerous lanolin extracts and derivatives are often used instead of the natural material. These are produced by a range of processes including hydrolysis (to yield the constituent acids and alcohols), acetylation, ethoxylation and solvent fractionation. Eucerin (Wool Alcohols BP) is the wool alcohol fraction of wool fat, and contains cholesterol and isocholesterol. It is mixed with liquid, soft and hard paraffin to form Ointment of Wool Alcohols BP, which, on the addition of water, produces Hydrous Ointment BP, a vehicle for many water-in-oil (W/O) creams.

Fatty acids and alcohols

Long-chain fatty acids (e.g. palmitic and stearic acids and their alcohols, cetyl and stearyl) are very frequently used as emollients and, in creams, also serve as emulsifiers. Cetostearyl alcohol is a frequently used mixture of cetyl and stearyl alcohols. They can be obtained by hydrolysis of triglycerides from many different animal and vegetable fats and oils.

Waxes

Beeswax is secreted by worker bees to make the cell walls of the honeycomb. It has a melting point of approximately 60°C and is composed mainly of free cerotic acid and myricyl palmitate. It is used as a thickening agent for creams, ointments and lip salves. Emulsifying wax comprises cetostearyl alcohol, sodium lauryl sulphate and water. This is a constituent of emulsifying ointment BP.

Polyethylene glycols

Polyethylene glycols, also known as PEGs or macrogols, are dihydric alcohols. They are polymers of ethylene glycol linked by ether bonds with the general formula $H(O-CH_2-CH_2)_n-OH$ in which n may range from 2 to 90 000. PEGs can be designated by a number indicating the average molecular weight. At low molecular weights, up to 2000, they are hygroscopic. They variously serve as emollients, emulsifiers or thickeners and can also be used to impart a pleasant feel or texture to a formulation.

Cetomacrogols are cetylethers of polyethylene glycol (e.g. cetomacrogol 1000 is the monocetyl ether of polyethylene glycols with average molecular weight 1000). It is useful as a non-ionic emulsifying agent.

Emulsifiers

An emulsion is a two-phase system consisting of two immiscible components: one (the dispersed or inner phase) being suspended in the other (the continuous or outer phase) as small droplets. One phase is aqueous, the other oily. Stable emulsions remain in this form; unstable emulsions, with a large droplet size, tend to separate as cream does from milk. Production of a stable emulsion requires the presence of an emulsifier, which is a large molecule with both strongly polar (water-soluble) and non-polar (oil-soluble) groups allowing it to bridge the gap between polar and non-polar substances. A large and chemically diverse range of compounds can be used for this purpose; some examples are given in Table 75.5.

W/O systems result from the dispersion of an aqueous phase in an oily phase, as in Oily Cream BP. Oil-in-water (O/W) systems are formed when oil is the dispersed phase and water the continuous phase, as in Aqueous Cream BP. The former constitute, in general, oily creams or 'cold creams', the latter aqueous or 'vanishing creams'. It is sometimes possible to produce both types of emulsion in the same system [5]: these are called ambiphilic creams. Emulsions can be diluted with the outer (continuous) phase only. A simple method of determining the nature of an emulsion is to interpose on a filter paper a drop of the emulsion between one of oil and one of water. In 15 min the continuous phase will mix with, or be dispersed by, one or other of the neighbouring drops. Alternatively, it may be tested by adding a larger quantity of water. If the emulsion separates, it is of W/O type; if not, it is of O/W type, the continuous phase being (within limits) able to expand and still retain its contained disperse phase.

The relative affinity of an emulsifier for water and for oil is quantified by a value denoting its emulsification tendency known as the hydrophilic lipophilic balance (HLB) value [6]. Emulsifiers with an HLB value of 3–6 tend to give W/O systems and those with higher values O/W systems.

Humectants

These are compounds with a high affinity for water (hygroscopicity). They draw water into the stratum corneum and therefore have an emollient effect on dry skin. However, most of the water is drawn out from within the skin and in dry atmospheric conditions water loss from the skin surface may be increased by the presence of humectants.

Penetration enhancers

Agents that have been shown to enhance penetration of drugs through the skin include propylene glycol [7,8], azone [9], urea [10] and dimethyl sulfoxide (DMSO) and related compounds [11–14]. Mechanisms for this effect include hydration of the stratum corneum and keratolytic actions. The effect of salicylic acid as a penetration enhancing agent seems to be variable. *In vitro* studies have suggested that penetration of drugs is enhanced but this effect was not observed during *in vivo* studies of steroid penetration through normal skin [15,16]. However, in treatment of psoriasis, the addition of salicylic acid does seem to improve the response to topical corticosteroids [17,18].

DMSO is a highly polar, stable substance with exceptional solvent properties [19–23]. It releases histamine *in vivo* and may induce weals when applied topically. It reacts with water, liberating heat. The stratum corneum retains significant amounts of DMSO and, as most drugs are more soluble in DMSO than in water, this tends to promote percutaneous absorption [22]. This quality has been shown to be of particular value in increasing the effectiveness of idoxuridine in herpes simplex [24] and zoster [25]. Toxicological considerations have precluded its more widespread use.

Powders

Inorganic powders are an important component of many dermatological treatments and include zinc oxide, titanium dioxide, talc, bentonite and calamine. Organic powders include various starches and zinc stearate. *Zinc oxide* is widely used as a component of many dusting powders, shake lotions and pastes. It has covering and protective properties, gives consistency to creams and pastes, and is said to have cooling and slightly astringent properties. *Titanium dioxide* is chemically very inert and for this reason it can be used instead of zinc oxide in pastes containing salicylic acid. Like zinc oxide, it has useful UV-reflecting properties. *Talc* is inert magnesium polysilicate, with a very low specific gravity. It contributes 'slip' and has a cooling effect. *Calamine* may be either zinc carbonate or zinc oxide, coloured with a little ferric oxide, and has bland, soothing and antipruritic properties. *Starch* is more absorbent than inorganic powders, but tends to deteriorate and is prone to microbiological decomposition. Some powders, for example *bentonite* (colloidal hydrated aluminium silicate), *aluminium magnesium silicate*, *tragacanth*, *methylcellulose* and *carbomer* are used in gels or as stabilizers in shake lotions.

Preservatives

Ointments and some creams with oil as the continuous phase do not usually require preservatives. Lotions, O/W creams and gels, however, because they contain accessible water, are easily contaminated by moulds or bacteria. Animal and vegetable oils, unless protected from oxidation, tend to become rancid. The ideal preservative should be non-toxic, non-irritant, non-sensitizing, odourless, colourless and effective even at very low concentrations and under conditions of normal usage. In addition, it must be chemically compatible with both the vehicle and the active ingredients.

The parahydroxybenzoic acid esters (parabens) are effective and widely used preservatives. Because, individually, they are only sparingly water soluble, and as their effects are additive, mixtures are usually preferred. This also increases their spectrum of activity and lowers the risk of sensitization. Considering their widespread use, their sensitizing potential appears to be low [26].

Chlorocresol is a preservative used especially in the UK. It is more effective in acid than in alkaline solution. It has a low sensitizing potential. It is used in several corticosteroid creams.

Sorbic acid (2,4-hexadienoic acid) is also a good preservative, which maintains its activity in the presence of non-ionic detergents. It also has a low sensitization index. It can only be used, however, in preparations with a pH of less than 6.5.

Propylene glycol can inhibit the growth of moulds and fungi, and can therefore be used as a preservative.

Organic mercurials such as thiomersal are used as preservatives in many ophthalmic preparations and in some vaccines and prick-test solutions and are occasionally incorporated in some topical preparations [27]. Ethylenediaminetetra-acetate is a widely used preservative in ear, nose and eye drops. Gallates and other antioxidants such as butylhydroxyanisole and butylhydroxytoluene are used to prevent rancidity in oily and fatty preparations.

Other preservatives, including those mainly used in cosmetic products, are discussed in Chapters 19 and 20.

REFERENCES

1 Morrison DS. Petrolatum: conditioning through occlusion. In: Schueller R, Romanowski P, eds. *Conditioning Agents for Hair and Skin*. New York: Marcel Dekker, 1999.
2 Clark EW. The history and evolution of lanolin. In: Hoppe U, ed. *The Lanolin Book*. Hamburg: Beiersdorf, 1999: 9–50.
3 Kligman AM. The myth of lanolin allergy: lanolin is not a contact sensitizer. In: Hoppe U, ed. *The Lanolin Book*. Hamburg: Beiersdorf, 1999: 161–75.
4 Clarke EW, Cronin E, Wilkinson DS. Lanolin with reduced sensitizing potential: a preliminary note. *Contact Dermatitis* 1977; **3**: 69–76.
5 Clark R. In: Hibbot HW, ed. *Handbook of Cosmetic Science*. Oxford: Pergamon, 1963: 175–204.
6 Griffin WC. Calculation of HLB values of non-ionic surfactant. *J Soc Cosmet Chem* 1954; **5**: 249–56.
7 Ostrenga J, Haleblan J, Poulsen B *et al.* Vehicle for a new topical steroid, fluocinonide. *J Invest Dermatol* 1971; **56**: 392–9.
8 Polano MK, Ponec M. Dependence of corticosteroid penetration on the vehicle. *Arch Dermatol* 1976; **112**: 675–80.
9 Spruance SL, McKeough M, Sugibayashi K *et al.* Effect of azone and propylene glycol on penetration of trifluorothymidine through skin and efficacy of different topical formulations against cutaneous herpes simplex virus infections in guinea pigs. *Antimicrob Agents Chemother* 1984; **26**: 819–23.
10 Feldman RJ, Maibach HI. Percutaneous penetration of hydrocortisone with urea. *Arch Dermatol* 1974; **109**: 58–9.
11 Munro DD, Stoughton RB. Dimethylacetamide (DMAC) and dimethylform-amide (DMF) effect on cutaneous absorption. *Arch Dermatol* 1965; **92**: 585–6.
12 Feldman RJ, Maibach HI. Percutaneous penetration of C^{14} hydrocortisone in man. *Arch Dermatol* 1966; **94**: 649–51.
13 Stoughton RB. Dimethylsulfoxide (DMSO) induction of a steroid reservoir in human skin. *Arch Dermatol* 1965; **91**: 657–60.
14 Stoughton RB. Hexachlorophane deposition in human stratum corneum: enhancement by dimethylacetamide, dimethylsulfoxide and methylethylether. *Arch Dermatol* 1966; **94**: 646–8.
15 Tauber U, Weiss C, Matthes H. Does salicylic acid increase the percutaneous absorption of diflucortolone-21-valerate? *Skin Pharmacol* 1993; **6**: 276–81.
16 Wester RC, Noonan PK, Maibach HI. Effect of salicylic acid on the percutaneous absorption of hydrocortisone: *in vivo* studies in the rhesus monkey. *Arch Dermatol* 1978; **114**: 1162–4.
17 Koo J, Cuffie CA, Tanner DJ *et al.* Mometasone furoate 0.1%–salicylic acid 5% ointment versus mometasone furoate 0.1% ointment in the treatment of moderate-to-severe psoriasis: a multicenter study. *Clin Ther* 1998; **20**: 283–91.
18 Medansky RS, Cuffie CA, Tanner DJ. Mometasone furoate 0.1%–salicylic acid 5% ointment twice daily versus fluocinonide 0.05% ointment twice daily in the management of patients with psoriasis. *Clin Ther* 1997; **19**: 701–9.
19 Beger I, Lorenz D. Purification of analysis of dimethylsulphoxide. In: Martin D, Hauthal HG, eds. *Dimethyl Sulphoxide*. New York: Van Nostrand Reinhold, 1976: 41–8.
20 Jacob SW, Herschler R, eds. Biological actions of dimethyl sulphoxide. *Ann NY Acad Sci* 1975; **23**: 243.
21 Jacob SW, Bischel M, Herschler RJ. Dimethyl sulfoxide (DMSO): a new concept in pharmacotherapy. *Curr Ther Res* 1964; **6**: 134–5.
22 Katz M, Poulsen BJ. Absorption of drugs through the skin. In: Brodie BB, Gillette J, eds. *Handbook of Experimental Pharmacology*, Vol. 28. New York: Springer, 1971: 103–74.
23 Kligman AM. Dimethylsulfoxide. Part 2. *JAMA* 1965; **193**: 923–8.
24 MacCallum FO, Juel-Jensen BE. Herpes simplex virus skin infection in man treated with idoxuridine in dimethylsulphoxide: results of a double-blind controlled trial. *BMJ* 1966; **ii**: 805–7.
25 Juel-Jensen BE, MacCallum FO, MacKenzie AMR. Treatment of zoster with idoxuridine in dimethylsulphoxide: results of two double-blind controlled trials. *BMJ* 1970; **iv**: 776–80.
26 Schnuch A, Geier J, Uter W, Frosch PJ. Patch testing with preservatives, antimicrobials and industrial biocides: results from a multicentre study. *Br J Dermatol* 1998; **138**: 467–76.
27 Wilkinson DS. Thiomersal. *Contact Dermatitis* 1978; **5**: 58–9.

Topical treatments used in the management of skin disease

Antiperspirants

Most antiperspirants marketed for cosmetic purposes contain aluminium chloride hexahydrate. In contemporary products, refined formulations of aluminium chlorohydrates (or aluminium zirconium complexes) are often used to maximize precipitation of aluminium hydroxide within the sweat duct [1]. Cosmetic antiperspirants are often combined with antimicrobial agents that reduce axillary odour by inhibiting the action of bacterial metabolism on various components of apocrine sweat. Fragrances are often added to mask or adjust the odour in various ways [2].

In treatment of hyperhidrosis of the axillae, palms and soles, higher concentrations of aluminium chloride hexahydrate (e.g. 20–25% in ethanol) are generally used as first-line treatment. These are more effective, more irritant and more likely to damage clothing than cosmetic formulations. Blockage of the sweat duct is regarded as the principal mechanism of action [1,3], although secondary degeneration of the secretory cells may develop after long-term use as a result of the increased pressure in the duct [4]. For maximal efficacy, the treatment should be applied when the skin is dry and sweating is minimal. Application at night is often recommended; this also helps to minimize damage to clothing. Polythene occlusion may enhance efficacy and irritancy. Irritation often limits the use of this treatment but may settle with reduced frequency of application and with use of a mild or moderately potent topical steroid.

Traditional remedies that have fallen out of favour include the aldehydes. These are believed to work by a similar mechanism to aluminium salts. Aqueous glutaraldehyde solution (up to 10%) can be applied on a swab to the soles of the feet [5,6]. The keratin stains orange-brown when higher concentrations are used. Formaldehyde solution BP (1–3%), used as a twice daily soak, also helps mild cases. Both compounds are frequent sensitizers, and are therefore not ideal for prolonged use. Methenamine, an agent that releases formaldehyde and ammonia, seems to cause less sensitization and has been used as a 10% solution or at 5% concentration in a firm gel-stick formulation [7].

Anticholinergic agents inhibit the anomalous sympathetic (cholinergic) innervation of the sweat glands and can be applied topically to minimize the side effects associated with systemic administration. Poldine methylsulphate [8] and glycopyrronium bromide [9] can be very effective when administered by iontophoresis. Dry mouth is common and visual accommodation may be disturbed for 24–48 h following treatment. Iontophoresis with tap water is also effective, by an unknown mechanism [10,11], and avoids these side effects. Glycopyrrolate cream 2% or lotion has been used with success in patients suffering from severe gustatory sweating following parotidectomy [12].

Surgical treatments and injection of botulinum toxin are considered in Chapter 45.

REFERENCES

1 Fitzgerald JJ, Rosenberg AH. Chemistry of aluminium chlorohydrate and activated aluminium chlorohydrates. In: Laden K, ed. *Antiperspirants and Deodorants*, 2nd edn. New York: Marcel Dekker, 1999: 83–136.
2 Makin SA, Lowry MR. Deodorant ingredients. In: Laden K, ed. *Antiperspirants and Deodorants*, 2nd edn. New York: Marcel Dekker, 1999: 169–214.
3 Rosenberg AH, Fitzgerald JJ. Chemistry of aluminium-zirconium-glycine (AZG) complexes. In: Laden K, ed. *Antiperspirants and Deodorants*, 2nd edn. New York: Marcel Dekker, 1999: 137–68.
4 Holzle E, Braun-Falco O. Structural changes in axillary eccrine glands following long-term treatment with aluminium chloride hexahydrate solution. *Br J Dermatol* 1984; **110**: 399–403.
5 Juhlin L. Topical glutaraldehyde for plantar hyperhidrosis. *Arch Dermatol* 1968; **97**: 327–30.
6 Sato K, Dobson RL. Mechanism of the antiperspirant effect of topical glutaraldehyde. *Arch Dermatol* 1969; **100**: 564–9.
7 Cullen SI. Topical methenamine therapy for hyperhidrosis. *Arch Dermatol* 1975; **111**: 1158–60.
8 Hill BHR. Poldine iontophoresis in the treatment of palmar and plantar hyperhidrosis. *Aust J Dermatol* 1976; **17**: 92–3.
9 Abell E, Morgan K. The treatment of idiopathic hyperhidrosis by glycopyrrhonium bromide and tapwater iontophoresis. *Br J Dermatol* 1974; **911**: 87–91.
10 Grice K, Sattar H, Baker H. Treatment of idiopathic hyperhidrosis with iontophoresis of tap water and poldine methosulphate. *Br J Dermatol* 1972; **86**: 72–8.
11 Shrivastava SN, Singh G. Tap water iontophoresis in palmoplantar hyperhidrosis. *Br J Dermatol* 1977; **96**: 189–95.
12 May JS, McGuirt WF. Frey's syndrome: treatment with topical glycopyrrolate. *Head Neck* 1989; **11**: 85–9.

Antibiotics

Topical antibiotics are most frequently used in the treatment of superficial infections such as impetigo, superficially infected surgical wounds or infected leg ulcers, and also in acne vulgaris and rosacea.

When treating infected skin lesions it is important to establish the identity and antibiotic sensitivity of the organism whenever possible. Although staphylococcal infections are common, it should not be assumed that a cutaneous infection is brought about by this organism. Before using an antibiotic, consideration should always be given to the alternative of using an antiseptic, in order to reduce the risk of promoting antibiotic resistance. Antiseptics usually have the added advantage of covering a wider spectrum of organisms.

The value of many antibiotics is limited by their tendency to sensitize when used topically (e.g. chloramphenicol and neomycin). Once sensitization has developed this generally precludes future systemic use of the antibiotic. It is therefore preferable, when possible, to select an antibiotic for topical application that is not related to agents used systemically.

The topical antibiotics most used in treatment of acne and rosacea are tetracyclines, erythromycin and clindamycin. Topical metronidazole has proved useful in rosacea. In general, topical antibiotics work about as well as benzoyl peroxide or tretinoin in acne vulgaris. As in other indications, consideration should be given to alternatives to topical antibiotics, especially for long-term treatment, in order to reduce the emergence of resistant organisms. The detailed use of antibiotics in acne and rosacea is described in Chapters 43 and 44, respectively.

Bacitracin

This is an antibiotic that is too toxic for systemic use. Its antibacterial action is principally against Gram-positive organisms, so it is generally used topically in combination with other antibiotics, such as neomycin or polymyxin B. Allergic reactions of an anaphylactoid nature have been recorded [1]. In leg ulcer patients it was reported to be the most potent sensitizer of all the topical antibiotics tested [2].

Clindamycin

This is an effective topical treatment for acne vulgaris [3]. It is as effective as oral minocycline 50 mg twice a day [4], and oral tetracyline [5]. It was somewhat less effective than topical nicotinamide gel in a trial involving 76 patients [6]. It was found to be as effective as 5% benzoyl peroxide gel in patients with papular or pustular acne [7]; fewer side effects were seen with topical clindamycin. A small trial in rosacea has indicated that the response was comparable to that from oral tetracycline [8].

Erythromycin

Only the lipid-soluble forms (e.g. the base, propionate or stearate) are effective in acne vulgaris. Several authors have considered the problem of erythromycin-resistant propionibacteria [9,10]. It is equivalent in effect to topical clindamycin, is safe and well tolerated [11,12]. A topical 2% erythromycin gel has been shown to be as effective as 1% clindamycin phosphate in patients with mild to moderate acne [13], and 1.5% erythromycin and 1% clindamycin phosphate solutions were found to be equally effective [12].

Fusidic acid

Derived from *Fusidium coccineum*, this antibiotic is active against staphylococcal infections and effective in erythrasma [14]. It is used as a first-line treatment for pitted keratolysis [15] although there is surprisingly little published about this indication. It is also used in combination with topical steroids in the treatment of infected eczema.

Sensitization occurs only very rarely [16,17], but bacterial resistance is not uncommon.

Gentamicin sulphate

The particular dermatological value of gentamicin sulphate lies in its broad spectrum of activity, including against *Pseudomonas aeruginosa*. Contact allergy is fairly frequent in patients with chronic otitis externa [18] and, compared with other agents, it remains a common sensitizer [19]. Cross-sensitivity can develop with other aminoglycosides [20].

Metronidazole [19]

Metronidazole 0.75–1% has been shown to be a safe and effective treatment for rosacea [21,22]. Topical metronidazole has also been used with some success in patients with decubitus and other ulcers, eliminating malodour in 36 h [23]. In a double-blind placebo-controlled trial, topical metronidazole was ineffective in reducing the inflammatory lesions of acne [24].

Mupirocin

This topical antibiotic is derived from *Pseudomonas fluorescens* [25]. It is chemically unrelated to other antibiotics, and its mode of action in arresting bacterial protein synthesis is novel [26]. It is active against a wide range of Gram-positive organisms and some Gram-negative organisms [27]. Naturally, it is not active against *Pseudomonas* and may allow overgrowth of this organism. It can be highly effective in cutaneous bacterial infections [28,29]. It has also proved useful in the elimination of nasal carriage of staphylococci [30], including multiply-resistant organisms, but strains resistant to mupirocin are now an increasing problem.

Neomycin and framycetin
SYN. SOFRAMYCIN

These are aminoglycoside antibiotics with a broad spectrum of action against Gram-positive and Gram-negative organisms. Both are considered too toxic for systemic use. Many preparations containing one or other of these are marketed in the UK, and are widely used, although sensitization reactions are common, especially around leg ulcers, under occlusion and in patients with chronic otitis externa, pruritus ani or vulvae, or with recurrent eye problems. Neomycin was among the most common sensitizers reported by Wilkinson *et al.* [31]. Simultaneous contact allergy to neomycin, bacitracin and polymyxin has been reported [32].

Polymyxin B

This antibiotic is used in several proprietary topical formulations for application to skin, eyes and ears. It has useful activity only against Gram-negative organisms and is therefore usually combined with other antibiotics. The relatively low toxicity of polymyxin to keratinocytes may explain the good cosmetic results observed when it is used following dermabrasion [33].

Silver sulfadiazine

First introduced over 20 years ago [34,35], this compound has become established as a safe and convenient dressing for burns [35]. Even when applied over wide areas, systemic absorption is minimal and the risk of renal damage is thought to be slight [36]. It is applied as a 1% cream. It appears to have a low potential for sensitization and is useful in the management of leg ulcers where it provides good prophylaxis against *Staphylococcus aureus* and some Gram-negative organisms. Some patients may become sensitive to the cetyl alcohol contained in the base of one proprietary formulation. When sulphonamide-resistant Gram-negative bacilli were present, a silver nitrate/chlorhexidine cream was found to be of value [37].

Tetracyclines

These are used alone in the topical treatment of acne [38],

but are also present in several proprietary topical corticosteroid preparations. Bacterial resistance is common, especially in staphylococci. Tetracyclines tend to stain skin and clothing yellow.

REFERENCES

1 Vale MA, Connolly A, Epstein A. Metal/bacitracin induced anaphylaxis (Letter). *Arch Dermatol* 1978; **114**: 800.
2 Zaki I, Shall L, Dalziel KL. Bacitracin: a significant sensitizer in leg ulcer patients? *Contact Dermatitis* 1994; **31**: 92–4.
3 Kuhlman DS, Callen JP. A comparison of clindamycin phosphate 1% topical lotion and placebo in the treatment of acne vulgaris. *Cutis* 1986; **38**: 203–6.
4 Sheehan-Dare RA, Papworth-Smith J, Cunliffe WJ. A double-blind comparison of topical clindamycin and oral minocycline in the treatment of acne vulgaris. *Acta Derm Venereol (Stockh)* 1990; **70**: 543–7.
5 Katsambas A, Towaky AA, Stratigos J. Topical clindamycin phosphate compared with oral tetracycline in the treatment of acne vulgaris. *Br J Dermatol* 1987; **116**: 387–91.
6 Shalita AR, Smith JG, Parish LC et al. Topical nicotinamide compared with clindamycin gel in the treatment of inflammatory acne vulgaris. *Int J Dermatol* 1995; **34**: 434–7.
7 Schmidt JB, Neuman R, Fanta D et al. 1% Clindamycin phosphate solution versus 5% benzoyl peroxide gel in papular pustular acne. *Z Hautkr* 1988; **63**: 374–6.
8 Wilkin JK, De Witt S. Treatment of rosacea: topical clindamycin versus oral tetracycline. *Int J Dermatol* 1993; **32**: 65–7.
9 Bojar RA, Eady EA, Jones CE et al. Inhibition of erythromycin-resistant propionibacteria on the skin of acne patients by topical erythromycin with and without zinc. *Br J Dermatol* 1994; **130**: 329–36.
10 Harkaway KS, McGinley KJ, Foglia AN et al. Antibiotic resistance patterns in coagulase-negative staphylococci after treatment with topical erythromycin, benzoyl peroxide, and combination therapy. *Br J Dermatol* 1992; **126**: 586–90.
11 Schachner L, Pestana A, Kittles C. A clinical trial comparing the safety and efficacy of a topical erythromycin–zinc formulation with a topical clindamycin formulation. *J Am Acad Dermatol* 1990; **22**: 489–95.
12 Shalita AR, Smith EB, Bauer E. Topical erythromycin versus clindamycin therapy for acne: a multicenter, double-blind comparison. *Arch Dermatol* 1984; **120**: 351–5.
13 Leyden JJ, Shalita AR, Saajian CD et al. Erythromycin 2% gel in comparison with clindamycin phosphate 1% solution in acne vulgaris. *J Am Acad Dermatol* 1987; **16**: 822–7.
14 MacMillan AL, Sarkany I. Specific topical therapy for erythrasma. *Br J Dermatol* 1970; **82**: 507–9.
15 Tan E, Berth-Jones J. Pitted keratolysis. In: Lebwohl M, Heymann WR, Berth-Jones J, Coulson I, eds. *Treatment of Skin Disease: Comprehensive Therapeutic Strategies*. London: Mosby Harcourt, 2002: 469–71.
16 Baptista A, Barros MA. Contact dermatitis from sodium fusidate. *Contact Dermatitis* 1990; **23**: 186–7.
17 Romaguera C, Grimalt F. Contact dermatitis to sodium fusidate. *Contact Dermatitis* 1985; **12**: 176–7.
18 Holmes RC, Johns AN, Wilkinson JD et al. Medicament contact dermatitis in patients with chronic inflammatory ear disease. *J R Soc Med* 1982; **75**: 27–30.
19 Gollhausen R, Enders F, Przybilla B et al. Trends in allergic contact sensitization. *Contact Dermatitis* 1988; **18**: 147–54.
20 Forstrom L, Pirila V, Pirila L. Cross-sensitivity within the neomycin group of antibiotics. *Acta Derm Venereol Suppl (Stockh)* 1979; **59**: 67–9.
21 Aronson IK, Rumsfield JA, West EP et al. Evaluation of topical metronidazole gel in acne rosacea. *Drug Intell Clin Pharmacol* 1987; **21**: 346–51.
22 Erikson G, Nor CE. Impact of metronidazole on skin and colon microflora in patients with rosacea. *Infection* 1987; **15**: 8–10.
23 Witkowski JA, Parish LC. Topical metronidazole gel: the bacteriology of decubitus ulcers. *Int J Dermatol* 1991; **30**: 660–1.
24 Tong D, Peters W, Barnetson RS. Evaluation of 0.75% metronidazole gel in acne: a double-blind study. *Clin Exp Dermatol* 1994; **19**: 221–3.
25 Chain EB, Mellows C. Pseudomonic acid. I. The structure of pseudomonic CID A: a novel antibiotic produced by *Pseudomonas fluorescens*. *J Chem Soc Perkin Trans* 1977; **1**: 294–309.
26 Hughes J, Mellowes C. Interaction of pseudomonic acid A with *Escherichia coli* B isoleucyl t-RNA synthetase. *Biochem J* 1980; **191**: 209–10.
27 White AR, Beale AS, Boon RJ et al. Antibacterial activity of mupirocin, an antibiotic produced by *Pseudomonas fluorescens*. *R Soc Med Int Congr Symp Series* 1984; **80**: 43–55.
28 Lever R, Hadley K, Downey D, MacKie R. Staphylococcal colonisation in atopic dermatitis and the effect of topical mupirocin therapy. *Br J Dermatol* 1988; **119**: 189–98.
29 Mertz PM, Marshall DA, Eaglstein WH et al. Topical mupirocin treatment of impetigo is equal to oral erythromycin therapy. *Arch Dermatol* 1989; **125**: 1069–73.
30 Dacre JE, Emmerson AM, Jenner EA. Nasal carriage of gentamicin and methicillin resistant *Staphylococcus aureus* treated with topical pseudomonic acid. *Lancet* 1983; **ii**: 1036.
31 Wilkinson JD, Hambly EM, Wilkinson DS. Comparison of patch test results in two adjacent areas of England. II. Medicaments. *Acta Derm Venereol (Stockh)* 1980; **60**: 245–9.
32 Grandinetti PJ, Fowler JF Jr. Simultaneous contact allergy to neomycin, bacitracin, and polymyxin. *J Am Acad Dermatol* 1990; **23**: 646–7.
33 Berger RS, Pappert AS, Van Zile PS, Cetnarowski WE. A newly formulated topical triple-antibiotic ointment minimizes scarring. *Cutis* 2000; **65**: 401–4.
34 Fox CL. Pharmacodynamics of sulfadiazine and related topical antimicrobial agents. In: Frost P, Gomez EC, Zaias N, eds. *Recent Advances in Dermato Pharmacology*, New York: Spectrum, 1978: 441–56.
35 Fox CL. Silver sulfadiazide: a new topical therapy for *Pseudomonas* in burns. *Arch Surg* 1978; **96**: 184–8.
36 Delaveau P, Friedrich-Nove P. Absorption cutanée et l'elimination urinaire d'une combinaison sulfadiazine-argent utilisée dans le traitement de brûlures. *Therapie* 1977; **32**: 563–72.
37 Lowbury EJL, Babb JR, Bridges K. Topical chemoprophylaxis with silver sulfadiazine and silver nitrate chlorhexidine creams: emergence of sulphon-amide-resistant Gram-negative bacilli. *BMJ* 1976; **i**: 493–6.
38 Burton J. A placebo-controlled study to evaluate the efficacy of topical tetracycline and oral tetracycline in the treatment of mild to moderate acne. *J Int Med Res* 1990; **18**: 94–103.

Antifungal agents

Topical application of antifungal agents is used by dermatologists mainly for treatment of mild dermatophyte and yeast infections. As management of specific infections is described elsewhere, this chapter provides only a description of the antifungal agents available for topical application. Severe and extensive infections and infections of hair and nails are usually treated systemically (see Chapters 62 and 63). The most frequently prescribed topical antifungal agents are allylamines, imidazoles, morpholines and polyenes. Older compounds such as tolnaftate and undecylenate acid are mainly sold over-the-counter.

Allylamines

These inhibit fungal synthesis of ergosterol, an essential component of fungal cell membranes, by inhibiting squalene epoxidase. This also results in toxic accumulation of squalene within the organism, which is fungicidal. This class includes naftifine, butenafine (neither are marketed in the UK) and terbinafine. The fungicidal nature of these compounds results in rapid response of dermatophyte infection to topical application. Naftifine and butenafine also possess anti-inflammatory activity. Terbinafine is active topically against pityriasis versicolor as well as against dermatophytes.

It is of concern that a strain of *Trichophyton rubrum* apparently resistant to squalene epoxidase inhibitors has recently been reported [1].

Imidazoles

This is a large group of compounds which includes bifonazole, clotrimazole, econazole, fenticonazole, ketoconazole, isoconazole, miconazole, oxiconazole, sulconazole, terconazole, tioconazole and others. These have largely similar properties and act by inhibiting synthesis of ergosterol. They are fungistatic. They are active against a wide range of fungal organisms including *Candida* and *Pityrosporum* yeasts as well as dermatophytes. They also have potentially useful antibacterial properties and, at least *in vitro*, can suppress growth of *Staph. aureus* [2]. The range of formulations includes creams, powders, sprays, suspensions and nail lacquer.

There are also combined formulations available which contain imidazoles and corticosteroids. The precise role of these combined formulations is controversial. They can occasionally be useful to accelerate resolution of symptoms when infected skin is very inflamed and pruritic. However, it is also possible that they may impair the response to the antifungal agent [3] and the familiar hazards of topical corticosteroids include the potential to mask a persisting infection.

Morpholines

Amorolfine inhibits two separate stages in the synthesis of ergosterol and is fungicidal. It is marketed as a nail lacquer containing 5% amorolfine, for treatment of onychomycosis. An advantage of amorolfine in this application is that, in addition to efficacy against dermatophytes, it is also active against other filamentous fungi that cause onychomycosis, such as *Scytalidium* spp. and *Scopulariopsis* spp. The water-resistant properties of the lacquer allow the convenience of once or twice weekly application. Twice weekly application may be marginally more effective [4]. Cure rates are approximately 50% at 6 months. Amorolfine can act synergistically with other antifungal agents including azoles and allylamines, improving cure rates when topical amorolfine is combined with systemic itraconazole [5] or terbinafine for 3 months [6].

Polyenes

The important member of this group is nystatin—one of the earliest antifungal agents developed. It derives its name from the New York State health laboratory where it was discovered in the 1950s. Nystatin is a fungal metabolite with activity against *Candida albicans* and several other *Candida* species. It damages the fungal cell membrane by binding irreversibly to ergosterol, an action that is fungistatic at low concentrations and fungicidal at high concentrations. It is not effective against dermatophytes. It is a safe and well-tolerated compound which is not significantly absorbed when taken orally or when used topically on skin and mucous membranes. Nystatin is available in a range of formulations including cream, ointment, oral suspension, lozenges and pessaries. There are also a range of creams and ointments containing combinations of nystatin with antiseptics, antibiotics and various potencies of corticosteroids.

Ciclopirox olamine [7]

This hydroxypyridone compound has a different mode of action to most other antifungal agents and does not directly inhibit sterol synthesis. It binds with high affinity to trivalent cations such as Fe^{3+}, which are essential for the functioning of numerous enzymes including cytochromes. Several metabolic pathways are likely to be disrupted by this process, including mitochondrial electron transport. It demonstrates activity against a broad spectrum of dermatophytes, yeasts and moulds including *Scytalidium* spp. and *Scopulariopsis* spp. and is also effective against Gram-positive and Gram-negative bacteria including methicillin-resistant *Staph. aureus*. Ciclopirox is commercially formulated in a variety of creams, lotions, powder and as a nail lacquer but is not currently marketed in the UK.

Tolnaftate

This compound is available in a variety of formulations (creams, lotions, powder) that are generally sold over-the-counter for topical treatment of dermatophyte infections. It is a thiocarbamate derivative, chemically unrelated to other antifungal drugs, and is an inhibitor of squalene epoxidase. It is considered less effective than more recently developed agents but is superior to placebo [8].

Undecylenic acid

Undecylenic acid, a mono-unsaturated fatty acid, is largely used as an over-the-counter topical treatment for dermatophyte infection. In addition to its fungistatic activity, it has antiseptic and antiviral properties. Formulations include cream, ointment, paint, spray and powder. It is probably less effective than newer agents although it has proved superior to placebo and equivalent to tolnaftate in controlled trials [8,9]. Sensitization is occasionally reported.

Other topical antifungal agents

Whitfield's ointment, a combination of 6% benzoic acid and 3% salicylic acid, is effective in treatment of superficial dermatophyte infections. Studies in the tropics suggest that cure rates are quite acceptable when very low cost is a priority [10]. However, this formulation is not very cosmetically acceptable.

The antiseptic properties of benzoyl peroxide have been put to use in treatment of dermatophyte infection and pityriasis versicolor, although this compound is irritant and bleaches clothing so some caution is required [11].

Zinc pyrithione 1% and selenium disulphide 2.5% are used in shampoos to treat dandruff and seborrhoeic dermatitis. Both compounds have also been shown in placebo-controlled trials to be effective in treatment of pityriasis versicolor in the same concentrations. Zinc pyrithione shampoo can be lathered over the affected skin for 5 min then rinsed off every day for 2 weeks [12]. Selenium sulphide has been shown to be effective used in the same way but applied for 10 min/day for 7 days [13]. Some irritation may develop.

Resorcinol (1,3 dihydroxybenzene) is an antiseptic agent and preservative which is also added to some shampoos to suppress dandruff by inhibition of *Pityrosporum* yeasts.

Azelaic acid demonstrates antifungal properties and is discussed under the heading of depigmenting agents.

REFERENCES

1 Mukherjee PK, Leidich SD, Isham N *et al.* Clinical *Trichophyton rubrum* strain exhibiting primary resistance to terbinafine. *Antimicrob Agents Chemother* 2003; **47**: 82–6.
2 Jones BM, Geary I, Lee ME, Duerden BI. Comparison of the *in vitro* activities of fenticonazole, other imidazoles, metronidazole, and tetracycline against organisms associated with bacterial vaginosis and skin infections. *Antimicrob Agents Chemother* 1989; **33**: 970–2.
3 Alston SJ, Cohen BA, Braun M. Persistent and recurrent tinea corporis in children treated with combination antifungal/corticosteroid agents. *Pediatrics* 2003; **111**: 201–3.
4 Reinel D, Clarke C. Comparative efficacy and safety of amorolfine nail lacquer 5% in onychomycosis, once-weekly versus twice-weekly. *Clin Exp Dermatol* 1992; **17** (Suppl. 1): 44–9.
5 Lecha M. Amorolfine and itraconazole combination for severe toenail onychomycosis: results of an open randomized trial in Spain. *Br J Dermatol* 2001; **145** (Suppl. 60): 21–6.
6 Baran R. Topical amorolfine for 15 months combined with 12 weeks of oral terbinafine, a cost-effective treatment for onychomycosis. *Br J Dermatol* 2001; **145** (Suppl. 60): 15–9.
7 Gupta AK, Skinner AR. Ciclopirox for the treatment of superficial fungal infections: a review. *Int J Dermatol* 2003; **42** (Suppl. 1): 3–9.
8 Battistini F, Cordero C, Urcuyo FG *et al.* The treatment of dermatophytoses of the glabrous skin: a comparison of undecylenic acid and its salt versus tolnaftate. *Int J Dermatol* 1983; **22**: 388–9.
9 Fuerst JF, Cox GF, Weaver SM, Duncan WC. Comparison between undecylenic acid and tolnaftate in the treatment of tinea pedis. *Cutis* 1980; **25**: 544–6, 549.
10 Gooskens V, Ponnighaus JM, Clayton Y *et al.* Treatment of superficial mycoses in the tropics: Whitfield's ointment versus clotrimazole. *Int J Dermatol* 1994; **33**: 738–42.
11 Kligman AM, Leyden JJ, Stewart R. New uses for benzoyl peroxide: a broad-spectrum antimicrobial agent. *Int J Dermatol* 1977; **16**: 413–7.
12 Fredriksson T, Faergemann J. Double-blind comparison of zinc-pyrithione shampoo and its shampoo base, in the treatment of tinea versicolor. *Cutis* 1981; **31**: 436–7.
13 Sanchez JL, Torres VM. Double-blind efficacy study of selenium sulfide in tinea versicolor. *J Am Acad Dermatol* 1984; **11**: 235–8.

Antiparasitic agents

The principles of treatment of lice infestations and scabies are discussed in Chapter 33. Insecticide resistance has emerged as a significant problem in the treatment of head lice [1] and may necessitate treatment with a second agent or by using non-pharmacological approaches.

Pyrethroids

Pyrethroids are highly effective [2,3] and are now probably the most widely used agents. These are insecticides that are neurotoxic to parasites. Permethrin 5% cream is a first-line treatment for scabies. It should be applied from the neck down for 12 h. The 5% 'dermal cream' for treatment of scabies should not be confused with the 1% 'creme rinse' marketed for treatment of head lice. This has caused treatment failure in scabies [4]. The creme rinse is applied to the scalp for 10 min to treat head lice. For pubic lice, the 5% cream should be used as for scabies.

Phenothrin is another pyrethroid used for head and pubic lice. For head lice, the formulations available include in an aqueous 0.5% lotion (washed off after 12 h), an alcoholic 0.2% lotion (washed off after 2 h) and a 0.5% concentration in a mousse (washed off after 30 min). For pubic lice, the aqueous lotion should be applied to the whole body for 12 h.

Whether treating head lice, pubic lice or scabies, two treatments at an interval of 1 week are generally recommended for both these agents.

Malathion

Malathion is an organophosphorus cholinesterase inhibitor that paralyses parasites. In treatment of scabies, a 0.5% aqueous lotion is applied to the skin for 24 h and repeated after 1 week. For head lice, 0.5% aqueous or alcoholic lotions can be applied for 12 h on three occasions at 3-day intervals. For crab lice, the aqueous preparation should be applied all over the body for 12 h and repeated after 7 days.

Other antiparasitic agents

Benzyl benzoate is also believed to be neurotoxic to parasites. It can be used as a scabicide in a 25% emulsion applied daily for 3 days but is somewhat irritant. Carbaryl is another organophosphorus insecticide that can be used for head and pubic lice. It is available as 1% aqueous and 0.5% alcoholic lotions which are usually left on the skin for 12 h. A single application may be effective but is often repeated after 7 days. Gamma benzene hexachloride (lindane), used as a 1% lotion, is an effective scabicide although it has been withdrawn in the UK as a result of concern over systemic absorption and possible neurotoxicity [5]. It is applied for 12 h and this is sometimes repeated after 1 week. The risks seem small but are relatively greater in infants and young children, and when multiple applications are used. Both topical and oral ivermectin have been successfully used for both scabies and head lice [6–8]. A 1% solution in propylene glycol applied twice with a 1-week interval has proved highly effective in scabies [9]. Crotamiton has weak scabicidal activity and is an antipruritic. It is often used as a follow-up treatment to other therapies.

REFERENCES

1 Downs AM, Stafford KA, Hunt LP et al. Widespread insecticide resistance in head lice to the over-the-counter pediculocides in England, and the emergence of carbaryl resistance. Br J Dermatol 2002; **146**: 88–93.
2 Taplin D, Meinking TL. Permethrin: sexually transmitted diseases—advances in diagnosis and treatment. Curr Probl Dermatol 1996; **24**: 255–60.
3 Taplin D, Meinking TL, Porcelain SL et al. Permethrin 5% dermal cream: a new treatment for scabies. J Am Acad Dermatol 1986; **15**: 995–1001.
4 Cox NH. Permethrin for scabies: importance of the correct formulation. BMJ 2000; **320**: 37–8.
5 Franz TJ, Lehman PA, Franz SF et al. Comparative percutaneous absorption of lindane and permethrin. Arch Dermatol 1996; **132**: 901–5.
6 Youssef MY, Sadaka HA, Eissa MM et al. Topical application of ivermectin for human ectoparasites. Am J Trop Med Hyg 1995; **53**: 652–3.
7 Glaziou P, Cartel JL, Alzeiu P et al. Comparison of ivermectin and benzyl benzoate for treatment of scabies. Trop Med Parasitol 1993; **44**: 331–2.
8 Glaziou P, Nyguyen LN, Moulia-Pelat JP et al. Efficacy of ivermectin for the treatment of head lice (Pediculosis capitis). Trop Med Parasitol 1994; **45**: 253–4.
9 Victoria J, Trujillo R. Topical ivermectin: a new successful treatment for scabies. Pediatr Dermatol 2001; **18**: 63–5.

Antiviral agents

There are few topical agents available with specific antiviral activity although many antiseptics, especially povidone iodine [1,2], are known to inactivate viruses. The use of imiquimod, 5-fluorouracil and podophyllin in treatment of viral warts is discussed elsewhere in this chapter. Aciclovir, penciclovir and idoxuridine are used topically in management of herpes simplex and the latter is also used for herpes zoster.

Aciclovir and penciclovir

Topical aciclovir is used in the treatment of primary and recurrent herpes simplex types I and II [3]. The drug is a nucleoside analogue and is phosphorylated by a viral thymidine kinase to an active form that inhibits effective replication of viral DNA. A recommended regimen is application of 5% aciclovir cream at 4-hourly intervals for 5 days. Both labial and genital lesions can respond. Severe episodes are best treated systemically. Some protective effect may be obtained by regular prophylactic application of aciclovir cream [4]. Penciclovir has a similar mechanism of action. This is applied as a 1% cream 2-hourly for 4 days. Both of these agents should be applied as early as possible in the course of the episode.

Idoxuridine

Idoxuridine was the first agent to become available for topical treatment of herpes infections. It is a thymidine analogue that inhibits viral DNA replication. It is effective in reducing symptoms in treatment of herpes simplex [5] and zoster infections [6] applied topically at concentrations of 5–15%. A 5% solution in DMSO can be applied to affected areas of skin with a brush 4 times daily for 4 days. At lower concentrations, idoxuridine appears effective in treatment of genital warts [7]. Topical use of idoxuridine can occasionally sensitize [8].

REFERENCES

1 Kawana R, Kitamura T, Nakagomi O. Inactivation of human viruses by povidone–iodine in comparison with other antiseptics. Dermatol 1997; **195** (Suppl. 2): 29–35.
2 Simmons A. An open-label study conducted to evaluate the efficacy of Betadine cold sore paint. Dermatology 1997; **195** (Suppl. 2): 85–8.
3 Wagstaff AJ, Faulds D, Goa KL. Aciclovir: a reappraisal of its antiviral activity, pharmacokinetic properties and therapeutic efficacy. Drugs 1994; **47**: 153–205.
4 Gibson JR, Klaber MR, Harvey SG et al. Prophylaxis against herpes labialis with acyclovir cream: a placebo-controlled study. Dermatologica 1986; **172**: 104–7.
5 Spruance SL, Stewart JC, Freeman DJ et al. Early application of topical 15% idoxuridine in dimethyl sulfoxide shortens the course of herpes simplex labialis: a multicenter placebo-controlled trial. J Infect Dis 1990; **161**: 191–7.
6 Burton WJ, Gould PW, Hursthouse MW et al. A multicentre trial of Zostrum (5% idoxuridine in dimethyl sulphoxide) in herpes zoster. N Z Med J 1981; **94**: 384–6.
7 Happonen HP, Lassus A, Santalahti J et al. Topical idoxuridine for treatment of genital warts in males: a double-blind comparative study of 0.25% and 0.5% cream. Genitourin Med 1990; **66**: 254–6.
8 Thormann J, Wildenhoff KE. Contact allergy to idoxuridine: sensitization following treatment of herpes zoster. Contact Dermatitis 1980; **6**: 170–1.

Astringents

Astringents are compounds used to reduce exudation, acting by precipitation of protein. Those most frequently employed are aqueous solutions of potassium permanganate, aluminium acetate and silver nitrate.

Potassium permanganate

This is an oxidizing agent with antiseptic and fungicidal activity. It is used at concentrations of 1 : 4000–1 : 25 000. It can be applied as a rinse or soak or as a bath. A bath containing 1 : 25 000 $KMnO_4$ can be prepared by adding 2 g to each 50 L of water. The astringent and antiseptic properties of this solution are invaluable in treatment of very acute exudative eczematous dermatoses. However, it is messy and stains the skin and other materials.

Aluminium acetate

Also known as Burow's solution, this astringent is also mildly antiseptic and has the advantage of not causing the

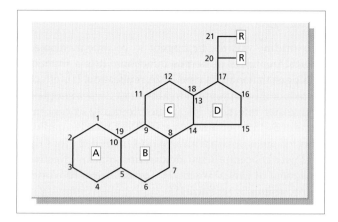

Fig. 75.2 The configuration of the basic corticosteroid structure.

staining associated with potassium permanganate. The solution is prepared using aluminium sulphate, acetic acid, tartaric acid and calcium carbonate. The solution contains 5% aluminium acetate and is diluted 1 : 10–1 : 40 with water for use in soaks, rinses or wet dressings.

Silver nitrate

In concentrations of 0.1–0.5% silver nitrate is an effective astringent and antiseptic, often used in management of leg ulcers and burns. Higher concentrations may cause pain. Silver nitrate causes staining of skin and most other materials.

Corticosteroids

Topical corticosteroids have now been in use for treating skin disease for over half a century, since the introduction of 'compound F' or hydrocortisone (cortisol) in 1952 [1]. Their impact has been immense. In addition to becoming the mainstay of treatment in eczematous dermatoses, they are used, either regularly or occasionally, in the management of most inflammatory skin diseases.

During the decades since hydrocortisone was introduced, numerous analogues have been developed from this molecule. The basic structure of the steroid moiety is shown in Fig. 75.2. Modifications to both the ring structure and the side-chains have increased specificity of action, increased penetration, dramatically increased potency and, to some degree, reduced side effects.

Hydrocortisone has considerable mineralocorticoid activity, which can be reduced by methylation or hydroxylation at position 16. Esterification at positions 16, 17 and 21 increases lipid solubility, promoting greater penetration of the stratum corneum barrier. This strategy lead to the development of highly lipophilic compounds such as betamethasone dipropionate and triamcinolone acetonide. Fluorination of the 9α position, the introduction of

an unsaturated bond between the first two carbon atoms and changes in the nature of the side-chains, particularly in the 21 position, brought about enhanced glucocortioid activity [2]. Fluticasone propionate has a fluoride thioester carbothiate at C21, a propionate ester at C17 and a methyl group at C16; this molecule is inactivated rapidly on first passage through the liver, confering greater systemic safety. Similar properties are demonstrated by methylprednisolone aceponate and mometasone furoate, while systemic exposure to prednicarbate is minimized by metabolism within the skin.

In view of the great differences in potency between different corticosteroids, it is essential for the dermatologist to be able to rank or classify them by potency in order to predict the response and possible adverse effects. This classification ideally needs to take account not only of the relative potency of the molecules, but also factors such as the concentration and the nature of the vehicle, which can significantly alter penetration.

Perhaps the ideal approach would be a large series of clinical trials to compare clinical efficacy of all the available corticosteroids. However, even if this were possible, it is by no means certain that the same ranking would be obtained in two different diseases. Many different approaches have therefore been developed to compare potencies of topical corticosteroids. Some of these employ various animal models of inflammation such as the implantation of a pellet of cotton into a subcutaneous pocket in rats. The potency of the antimitotic action of steroids can be assayed by applying the compound to the skin of hairless mice and measuring the level of suppression of the mitotic index after tape stripping [3]. However, the most widely used approach has been the vasoconstrictor assay, which depends upon the vasoconstricting property of glucocorticosteroids. This has the advantage of using human subjects and evaluates not only the intrinsic potency of the molecule but also its ability to penetrate the stratum corneum from a specific vehicle and even takes into account certain aspects of the removal and metabolism of the drug [4,5]. The degree of pallor produced following application of a compound to the skin seems to correlate fairly well with clinical potency and with the potential for side effects such as atrophogenicity. Typically, pallor reaches a peak at around 9–12 h after application and then falls, initially fairly rapidly over the next 10 h, then more slowly [6]. The total duration of action varies considerably between different compounds.

The various classifications adopted to provide a guide to the relative potencies of different compounds are substantially based on the vasoconstrictor assay but also take into account other evidence such as comparative clinical trials. The *British National Formulary* employs a four-point scale: mild, moderate, potent and very potent. In the USA, topical corticosteroids are ranked using a scale ranging from class 1 (super potent) to class 7 (mild).

Mechanism of action

Corticosteroids diffuse through the stratum corneum barrier and through cell membranes to reach the cytoplasm of keratinocytes and other cells present in the epidermis and dermis. Diffusion through the stratum corneum is generally considered to be the rate-limiting step in delivery of the drug. In the cytoplasm they bind to a specific receptor, the glucocorticoid receptor (GR). Clinical potency of corticosteroids seems to be strongly related to receptor binding affinity, which is very sensitive to certain structural changes in the steroid. Thus, the introduction of a double bond in the A ring, esterification in the 17α position, and fluorination at position 9α increase binding affinity, whereas esterification in the 21 position reduces binding affinity (Fig. 75.2).

The glucocorticoid receptor (glucocorticoid receptor α; $GR\alpha$) is a protein of molecular weight 330 kDa and is a member of the same receptor superfamily as receptors for other classes of steroid, thyroid hormone, calcitriol, etc. When not associated with a steroid ligand, this receptor is found in the cytoplasm as a component of a heterotetrameric structure containing two molecules of the 90 kDa heat shock protein hsp90, and a 59-kDa protein p59. Interestingly, p59 seems to belong to the family of immunophilins that interact with other immunosuppressant drugs. The binding of the receptor to its ligand results in activation of the receptor, which dissociates from the other components of the tetrameric complex [7]. The ligand-bound receptor then enters the nuclear compartment and interacts with specific response elements on the genome, glucocorticoid response elements (GREs). This modulates transcription of numerous genes. In addition, the ligand-bound receptor can inhibit, directly or indirectly, the activity of other transcription factors including NFκB, AP-1 and NFAT [8]. These interactions lead to changes in the expression of a wide range of genes, resulting in diverse cellular effects, which include suppression of the production of inflammatory cytokines, inhibition of T-cell activation, changes in the function of endothelial cells, granulocytes, mast cells and fibroblasts, and inhibition of proliferation. Part of the anti-inflammatory activity of corticosteroids may be explained by their ability to induce synthesis of lipocortin [9,10], a family of glycoproteins that regulate the activity of phospholipase A_2. This enzyme effects the production of arachidonic acid, the precursor for leukotrienes and prostaglandins.

The transcriptional activity of the steroid receptor seems likely to be regulated by an alternative isoform of the receptor known as glucocorticoid receptor β (GRβ), formed by alternative splicing. GRβ is an endogenous inhibitor of glucocorticoid action, which does not bind steroid ligands but competes with ligand-bound receptor for binding to GREs [11]. Staphylococcal superantigen can up-regulate expression of GRβ [12], providing a potential mechanism by which these bacteria might induce corticosteroid resistance.

Side effects of topical corticosteroids

The potential side effects of topical corticosteroids are significant but must be kept in proportion. When these compounds are prescribed appropriately, they can be of enormous benefit and clinically significant side effects are rare, especially in the short term (over a few days or weeks). Dermatologists have been very successful in making pharmacists, general practitioners and the public aware of the hazards. Patients are now frequently encountered whose dermatosis requires potent corticosteroids but who are denied effective treatment by the inappropriate prescription of hydrocortisone or simple emollients. Others apply the medication so 'sparingly' that it is completely ineffective. At times, the fear of using topical corticosteroids can be quite out of proportion to the likelihood of side effects developing. This situation is often termed 'steroid phobia'.

With the exception of structural changes introduced to minimize systemic exposure to topical corticosteroids, it has proved difficult to separate the various unwanted actions of these compounds from those that are so desirable. The side effects of topical steroids are directly related to their potencies. It is often appropriate to use more than one compound simultaneously so that mild or moderate steroids are used on areas where they are often effective, such as the face and flexures, while the more potent preparations are used only where they are required.

Local effects

The most common side effects are localized to application sites. The most worrying is cutaneous atrophy because this may become permanent. Other problems include the development of contact allergy and the risk of promoting infection. When treating the face, there are the additional risks of inducing acneiform eruptions. There are also potential risks from absorption and systemic exposure to the steroid.

Atrophic changes affect both the epidermis and the dermis. The epidermis becomes thinned. This results initially from a reduction in the size of epidermal cells, which reflects a reduction in metabolic activity [13]. After intense or prolonged steroid exposure, the number of cell layers is reduced, the stratum granulosum disappears and the stratum corneum is thinned [14–16]. There is suppression of many aspects of cell metabolism including the synthesis of stratum corneum lipids, synthesis of keratohyalin granules and the formation of corneodesmosomes required for structural integrity of the stratum corneum [17]. Inhibition of melanocyte function may develop, giving rise to localized hypopigmentation. This complication is

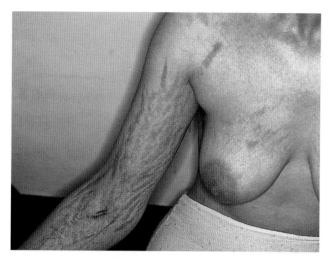

Fig. 75.3 Atrophy and striae induced by topical steroids. (Courtesy of St John's Institute of Dermatology, London, UK.)

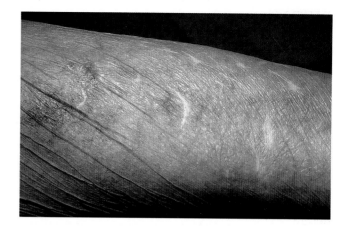

Fig. 75.4 Atrophy and scars induced by topical steroids. (Courtesy of St John's Institute of Dermatology, London, UK.)

Table 75.6 Relative levels of absorption of hydrocortisone applied at various sites. (Adapted from [23].)

Forearm	1
Sole	0.1
Ankle	0.4
Palm	0.8
Back	1.7
Scalp	3.5
Axilla	3.6
Forehead	6
Scrotum	42

most likely to occur with steroids applied under occlusion or with intracutaneous steroid injections [18,19].

In the dermis, topical corticosteroids induce resorption of mucopolysaccharide ground substance. This is likely to explain the rapid development of thinning, which reaches approximately 15% reduction in skin thickness after 3 weeks of treatment under occlusion with 0.1% betamethasone valerate [20]. Collagen synthesis is suppressed within 3 days of treatment with this compound [21]. Even mild corticosteroids such as hydrocortisone have been shown to inhibit collagen synthesis [22,23]. In a study in which betamethasone valerate was applied for 3 days there was still significant inhibition of collagen synthesis 2 weeks after treatment was discontinued [24]. When steroid exposure persists, thinning becomes clinically evident and fragility and striae may develop. The loss of connective tissue support for the dermal vasculature results in erythema, telangiectasia and purpura. With long-term use of potent preparations, these atrophic changes can become irreversible (Figs 75.3 & 75.4). The areas most vulnerable to developing atrophy are those where the skin is already relatively thin, including the flexures and especially the face (Table 75.6). In general, potent steroids should be used on the face only when treating severe dermatoses such as chronic discoid lupus erythematosus.

Contact allergy may develop to corticosteroids as well as to preservatives and other components of the vehicle. Contact sensitivity to hydrocortisone was first reported in 1959 but was initially considered a rare problem [25]. It is now clear that this is, in fact, a common event. In a large series of patients who were patch tested, 4.9% yielded positive results to one or more corticosteroids [26]. Tixocortol pivalate, considered the best patch test reagent for screening, was positive in just over 90% of those with a positive test to one or more corticosteroids. The most

frequent sensitizers in this series were hydrocortisone, budesonide and hydrocortisone butyrate. Sensitivity to more than one topical corticosteroid is common and four groups have been identified within which cross-reactivity is most likely to occur (Table 75.7) [27]. Reactivation of contact dermatitis after inhalation of a corticosteroid may also be under-recognized [28].

Caution is required when applying topical corticosteroids in the presence of infection as there is a risk of exacerbation. Clinically unequivocal bacterial superinfection of eczema is usually treated prior to use of topical corticosteroids. However, there is evidence that colonization with *Staph. aureus* can be reduced by improving the condition of the skin with potent or very potent topical corticosteroid treatment [29,30]. It is advisable to avoid the use of topical corticosteroids, whenever possible, in the presence of active viral infection including lesions of herpes simplex, viral warts or molluscum contagiosum. When dermatophyte infections are inadvertently treated with corticosteroid, the symptoms and signs may transiently improve, giving rise to the situation known as tinea incognito. Scabies presents a similar trap, as the pruritus can be improved by topical corticosteroids while the infestation persists unless a scabicidal treatment is also applied. However, topical corticosteroids are invaluable for treating the eczema associated with scabies. Infantile gluteal

Table 75.7 Groups of topical corticosteroids within which cross-sensitization is most likely to occur [27].

Group A
Cloprednol
Cortisone
Cortisone acetate
Fludrocortisone
Hydrocortisone
Hydrocortisone acetate
Methylprednisolone acetate
Prednisolone
Prednisolone acetate
Prednisone
Tixocortol pivalate

Group B
Amcinonide
Budesonide
Desonide
Fluocinolone acetonide
Fluocinonide
Halcinonide
Triamcinolone acetonide
Triamcinolone alcohol

Group C
Betamethasone
Betamethasone sodium phosphate
Dexamethasone
Dexamethasone sodium phosphate
Fluocortolone

Group D
Alclometasone dipropionate
Betamethasone valerate
Betamethasone dipropionate
Clobetasol-17-propionate
Clobetasone-17-butyrate
Flucortolone caproate
Flucortolone pivalate
Fluprednidene acetate
Hydrocortisone-17-butyrate
Hydrocortisone-17-valerate

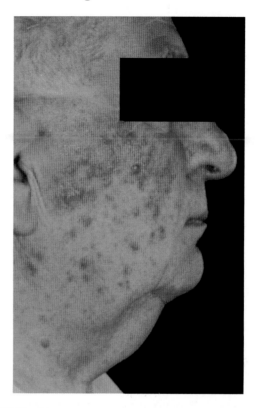

Fig. 75.5 Steroid rosacea.

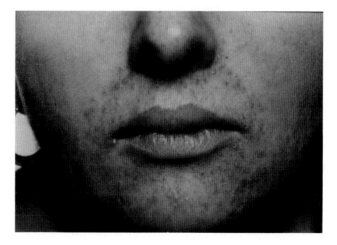

Fig. 75.6 Perioral dermatitis induced by a potent topical steroid. (Courtesy of St John's Institute of Dermatology, London, UK.)

granuloma (see Chapter 14) is found only in infants who wear napkins (diapers) and is often associated with the use of topical corticosteroids. Impairment of the immune response to *Candida* by steroids has been suggested as the cause [31].

The use of topical corticosteroids on the face can result in eruptions resembling rosacea (Fig. 75.5) and perioral dermatitis (Fig. 75.6) (see Chapter 44). Eruptions of inflammatory papules may also develop around the eyes and have been termed periocular dermatitis [32]. On other occasions, an eruption more closely resembling acne vulgaris, comprising inflammatory papules and pustules as well as comedones, may develop in treated areas of skin, usually on the face or upper trunk. Comedones have also been induced in perianal skin by the application of potent steroids [33]. The mechanisms involved in these eruptions are not well understood.

It is possible that the use of topical corticosteroids on the eyelids and periorbital skin can result in some exposure of the eye to the steroid. The use of corticosteroid eye drops is known to raise intraocular pressure, increase risk of cataract formation and to aggravate infections, especially herpes simplex. There have been only occasional reports of such ocular complications arising from the use of topical steroids applied around the eyes to treat skin disease [34–36]. Glaucoma has also been reported in a patient regularly treating hand eczema with betamethasone valerate at night, presumably resulting from inadvertent contamination of the eyes with the steroid [37]. These scant reports should be offset against the benefit of treating periocular skin disease, especially atopic dermatitis which is associated with keratoconus (probably as a result of frequent rubbing around the eyes) [38].

Locally applied corticosteroids have been demonstrated to impair wound healing and re-epithelialization in a variety of animal and humans models [39–41].

The question of whether tachyphylaxis develops during continued treatment with corticosteroids remains controversial. It is certainly common for patients to report that a topical corticosteroid which was highly effective during the first few days of application has subsequently lost efficacy. On occasions, withdrawal of corticosteroids is followed by a flare of disease. The hypothesis that these phenomena are caused by tachyphylaxis is supported by data from vasoconstrictor assays showing that successive applications of topical corticosteroids are associated with a decreasing response [42]. Furthermore, inhibitory effects on epidermal cell proliferation decreased during repeated administration of topical corticosteroids to hairless mice [43].

However, tachyphylaxis has not been shown to occur in clinical trials of corticosteroids in treatment of atopic dermatitis or psoriasis. It has therefore been proposed that patients report that the effect of the corticosteroid is diminishing when the underlying disease activity is increasing. Physicians observing patients intermittently may mistake stable disease activity for a failure to improve, even when there has been improvement from baseline, and may interpret this as tachyphylaxis. In a survey of dermatologists with 70 respondents, 57% believed that tachyphylaxis occurred within 8 weeks of initiating treatment of chronic plaque psoriasis with a potent corticosteroid. When this was put to the test in a clinical trial of 12 weeks' treatment duration, tachyphylaxis was not observed [44].

Rebound phenomena when topical corticosteroids are withdrawn have principally been of concern in the management of psoriasis. In several cases, withdrawal of treatment with potent or very potent corticosteroids has been followed by the eruption of severe generalized pustular psoriasis. This seems to have been especially likely to happen after potent or very potent corticosteroids have been used in large quantities or applied under occlusion [45]. In these cases it is likely that significant systemic exposure to the steroid was occurring and this was consequently withdrawn at the same time. The risk of this happening when unoccluded treatment with topical corticosteroids is used for chronic plaque psoriasis of moderate severity and disease extent are clearly very small, as this treatment has been so widely used, especially in the USA, yet generalized pustular psoriasis remains rare. Nonetheless, this phenomenon has resulted in a general reluctance of dermatologists in the UK to rely on topical steroids in the treatment of psoriasis vulgaris and this approach has the undoubted benefit of sparing patients other side effects such as cutaneous atrophy.

Vascular effects of corticosteroids include initial vasoconstriction of the superficial small vessels, followed by a phase of rebound vasodilatation. After prolonged treatment the vasodilation may become fixed and more conspicuous as a result of dermal and epidermal atrophy (Fig. 75.6) [46].

Systemic effects

Inhibition of the pituitary–adrenal axis by excessive application of moderately potent topical steroids or by relatively modest use of stronger steroids is well documented [47]. Temporary reversible suppression was seen after using 49 g/week of superpotent steroids for 2 weeks [48] in eight out of 40 patients, and similar results were seen in two further studies [49,50]. Significant suppression was reported in three patients using less than 50 g/week [51]. Recommended weekly dosage is less than 50 g of superpotent steroids and 100 g of potent steroids. In addition, prolonged usage at this level is best avoided. Children and babies have a high ratio of surface area to body volume and are more vulnerable to pituitary–adrenal suppression as a result of systemic absorption. Even hydrocortisone applied topically may suppress the adrenocortical response in some children [52]. Cushingoid features may be seen in infants inappropriately treated [53]. Severe medical problems are fortunately rare despite alarmingly abnormal biochemical parameters.

Vehicles and formulations

There is a large range of topical formulations of corticosteroids on the market. At first glance this may seem more than necessary but it is undoubtedly helpful to have a range of compounds available in a range of formulations. It is clearly important to be able to adjust the potency of the steroid being used so that the least potent compound that is effective can be employed at each site and at each stage in the progression of the dermatosis. It is necessary to be able to avoid corticosteroids to which patients are known or suspected to be sensitized. It is also helpful to have a range of formulations for each compound. Thus, ointments are helpful when eczema is dry, while creams are more effective if the eruption is moist or exudative. Lotions, gels or a mousse formulation are useful for the scalp. When the distribution is limited, as is often the case in lichen simplex chronicus or prurigo, the use of a steroid-impregnated tape will simultaneously prevent scratching and increase drug penetration by effective occlusion [54].

Several antimicrobial agents are commercially formulated in combination with topical steroids including clioquinol, clotrimazole, fusidic acid, miconazole, neomycin and nystatin. These compound formulations are the subject of some controversy. They can be helpful when there is a clear indication for each constituent but are probably used more often when the diagnosis is unclear in the hope of 'covering all the possibilities'. The latter approach is not recommended. Disadvantages include the risks of obscuring the diagnosis, promoting development of microbial resistance to antibiotics and sensitization of patients to antimicrobial agents that may then be impossible to use topically or systemically in future. The aminoglycosides, including neomycin, carry a particularly high risk of sensitization [55].

The case for use of these combinations is much stronger in the treatment of eczemas with evidence of secondary infection, although many dermatologists still prefer to give an antibiotic systemically. It seems very likely that some cases of atopic dermatitis are exacerbated by the presence of *Staph. aureus* on the skin. Superantigen production by these bacteria may have a role in this exacerbation of the disease [56] and may also have the effect of reducing sensitivity to corticosteroids [12].

There is also a special case for combining clioquinol with topical steroids in treatment of nickel dermatitis. This antiseptic is a potent chelating agent that can effectively inactivate nickel [57].

There are also commercially developed formulations combining corticosteroids with other active constituents. Mixtures containing tar, salicylic acid or calcipotriol can be useful in treatment of psoriasis. As in the case of antimicrobial agents, it is important that these compounds should only be used when there is a clear indication for each constituent and potent corticosteroids should only be used when they are really necessary.

Many dermatologists have found it useful to create their own formulations by dilution of proprietary products or addition of other medicaments such as tar and salicylic acid. There are some disadvantages to these practices. The stability of the steroid in a different formulation is unpredictable [58]. Changes in the vehicle may also alter levels of steroid penetration into the skin and systemic absorption [59].

Occlusion and topical steroids

The penetration of a topical corticosteroid can be greatly increased by occlusion using polythene film or gloves, or by using hydrocolloid dressings [60]. Polythene gloves are most easily used overnight, although they are uncomfortable, especially in warm weather. A similar occlusive effect is obtained when a steroid is covered by paste bandages and by the use of wet wrap bandaging in the treatment of atopic dermatitis. Using corticosteroids in this way will undoubtedly increase adverse as well as beneficial effects. However, judicious use of occlusion can be an invaluable strategy in the management of pompholyx, a refractory plaque of psoriasis on the leg, or a patch of lichen simplex. The incorporation of a corticosteroid such as fludroxycortide (flurandrenolone) into the adhesive of a plastic tape provides another effective method of using occlusion.

Whole-body occlusion of corticosteroids was formerly used, but adverse effects were common so this has fallen out of favour.

Intralesional steroids

Recalcitrant dermatoses (e.g. alopecia areata, keloid scars, lichen simplex, nodular prurigo) may respond to injection of steroid into the lesions. Triamcinolone is often used, but dermal atrophy and leukoderma may occur.

Indications for topical corticosteroids

The anti-inflammatory, immunosuppressant and anti-proliferative properties of corticosteroids find numerous applications in dermatology, which are considered in more detail in the relevant sections of this text. Table 75.8 lists some of these applications together with the potencies of compounds that are most often used and the level of evidence available to support their efficacy [61].

REFERENCES

1 Sulzberger MB, Witten VH. The effect of topically applied compound F in selected dermatoses. *J Invest Dermatol* 1952; **19**: 101–2.
2 Carson-Jurica MA, Schrader WT, O'Malley BW. Steroid receptor family: structure and functions. *Endocr Rev* 1990; **11**: 201–20.
3 Marks R, Pongsehirun D, Saylan T. A method for the assay of topical corticosteroids. *Br J Dermatol* 1973; **88**: 69–74.
4 McKenzie AW, Stoughton RB. Method for comparing percutaneous absorption of steroids. *Arch Dermatol* 1962; **86**: 608–10.
5 Barry BW, Woodford R. Activity and bioavailability of topical steroids: *in vivo/in vitro* correlations for the vasoconstrictor test. *J Clin Pharm* 1978; **3**: 43–65.
6 Barry BW, Woodford R. Comparative bio-availability and activity of proprietary topical corticosteroid preparations: vasoconstrictor assays on 31 ointments. *Br J Dermatol* 1975; **93**: 563–71.
7 Gehring U. The structure of glucocorticoid receptors. *J Steroid Biochem Mol Biol* 1993; **45**: 183–90.
8 Almawi WY, Melemedjian OK. Molecular mechanisms of glucocorticoid antiproliferative effects: antagonism of transcription factor activity by glucocorticoid receptor. *J Leukoc Biol* 2002; **71**: 9–15.
9 Blackwell GJ, Canuccio R, Di Rosa M *et al*. Macrocortin: a polypeptide causing the anti-phospholipase effect of glucocorticoids. *Nature* 1980; **287**: 147–9.
10 Hammarstrom S, Hamberg M, Duell EA *et al*. Glucocorticoid in inflammatory proliferative skin disease reduces arachidonic and hydroxyeicosatetraenoic acids. *Science* 1977; **197**: 994–5.
11 Bamberger CM, Bamberger AM, de Castro M, Chrousos GP. Glucocorticoid receptor β, a potential endogenous inhibitor of glucocorticoid action in humans. *J Clin Invest* 1995; **95**: 2435–41.
12 Hauk PJ, Hamid QA, Chrousos GP, Leung DY. Induction of corticosteroid insensitivity in human PBMCs by microbial superantigens. *J Allergy Clin Immunol* 2000; **105**: 782–7.

Table 75.8 Indications for topical corticosteroids, efficacy and potency of preparations generally employed.

Indication	Potency	Evidence grade	Occlusion and intralesional use
Actinic prurigo	P, VP	C	
Alopecia areata	P, VP	B	Ocl, I/L
Aphthous stomatitis	P	A	
Atopic eczema	M, Mod, P	A	
Bullous pemphigoid	P, VP	D	
Chronic actinic dermatitis	Mod, P	C	
Contact allergic dermatitis	Mod, P	B	
Contact irritant dermatitis	M, Mod, P, VP	C	
Cutaneous T-cell lymphoma	Mod, P	B	
Discoid eczema	P, VP	C	
Discoid lupus	P, VP	B	I/L
Geographic tongue	P	C	
Granuloma annulare	P, VP	E	Ocl, I/L
Granuloma faciale	Mod, P	E	Ocl, I/L
Grover's disease	P	D	
Hailey–Hailey disease	M, Mod, P	C	
Juvenile plantar dermatosis	Mod, P	C	
Langerhans' cell histiocytosis	Mod, P	C	
Lichen nitidus	P	E	
Lichen planopilaris	P, VP	D	I/L
Lichen planus	P, VP	C	Ocl, I/L
Lichen sclerosus	P, VP	A	
Lichen simplex	P, VP	A	Ocl, I/L
Lymphocytoma cutis	P	E	I/L
Lymphomatoid papulosis	P, VP	E	
Morphoea	P	E	I/L
Necrobiosis lipoidica	P	D	Ocl, I/L
Pemphigoid gestationis	P, VP	C	
Pityriasis rosea	Mod, P	E	
Pompholyx	P, VP	A	Ocl
Polymorphic eruption of pregnancy	P	B	
Pretibial myxoedema	P	C	Ocl
Prurigo nodularis	P, VP	E	Ocl, IL
Pruritus ani	M, Mod	A	I/L
Pruritus vulvae	Mod, P	B	
Psoriasis	M, Mod, P, VP	A	Ocl
Pyoderma gangrenosum	P, VP	D	
Sarcoidosis	P, VP	C	Ocl, I/L
Scleromyxoedema	P	E	Ocl, I/L
Seborrhoeic eczema	M, Mod	A	
Strawberry haemangioma	VP	D	
Subacute cutaneous lupus	Mod, P	E	
Subcorneal pustular dermatosis	Mod, P	D	
Sweet's syndrome	P	D	I/L
Urticaria pigmentosa	P, VP	C	Ocl
Vitiligo	P, VP	A	

Potency generally employed: M, mild; Mod, moderate; P, potent; VP, very potent.
Level of evidence available for efficacy [61]: A, double-blind trial; B, clinical trial; C, small trial or more than 20 cases reported; D, at least five cases reported to respond; E, less than five cases reported.
Modalities other than simple external application: Ocl (occlusion) and I/L (intralesional injection) indicate that these approaches have been reported to be useful in selected cases.

13 Delforno C, Holt PJ, Marks R. Corticosteroid effect on epidermal cell size. *Br J Dermatol* 1978; **98**: 619–23.
14 Lehmann P, Zheng P, Lavker RM, Kligman AM. Corticosteroid atrophy in human skin: a study by light, scanning, and transmission electron microscopy. *J Invest Dermatol* 1983; **81**: 69–76.
15 Sheu HM, Chang CH. Alterations in water content of the stratum corneum following long-term topical corticosteroids. *J Formos Med Assoc* 1991; **90**: 664–9.
16 Sheu HM, Lee JY, Chai CY, Kuo KW. Depletion of stratum corneum intercellular lipid lamellae and barrier function abnormalities after long-term topical corticosteroids. *Br J Dermatol* 1997; **136**: 884–90.
17 Kao JS, Fluhr JW, Man MQ *et al.* Short-term glucocorticoid treatment compromises both permeability barrier homeostasis and stratum corneum integrity: inhibition of epidermal lipid synthesis accounts for functional abnormalities. *J Invest Dermatol* 2003; **120**: 456–64.

18 Arnold J, Anthonioz P, Marchand JP. Depigmenting action of corticosteroids. *Dermatologica* 1975; **151**: 274–80.

19 McCormack PG, Ledesma CN, Vaillant JC. Linear hypopigmentation after intra-articular corticosteroid injection. *Arch Dermatol* 1984; **120**: 708–9.

20 Lubach D, Bensmann A, Bornemann U. Steroid-induced dermal atrophy: investigations on discontinuous application. *Dermatologica* 1989; **179**: 67–72.

21 Oikarinen A, Haapasaari KM, Sutinen M, Tasanen K. The molecular basis of glucocorticoid-induced skin atrophy: topical glucocorticoid apparently decreases both collagen synthesis and the corresponding collagen mRNA level in human skin *in vivo*. *Br J Dermatol* 1998; **139**: 1106–10.

22 Haapasaari KM, Risteli J, Karvonen J, Oikarinen A. Effect of hydrocortisone, methylprednisolone aceponate and momethasone furoate on collagen synthesis in human skin *in vivo*. *Skin Pharmacol* 1997; **10**: 261–4.

23 Nuutinen P, Riekki R, Parikka M, Salo T *et al*. Modulation of collagen synthesis and mRNA by continuous and intermittent use of topical hydrocortisone in human skin. *Br J Dermatol* 2003; **148**: 39–45.

24 Haapasaari KM, Risteli J, Oikarinen A. Recovery of human skin collagen synthesis after short-term topical corticosteroid treatment and comparison between young and old subjects. *Br J Dermatol* 1996; **135**: 65–9.

25 Burckhardt W. Kontaktekzem durch Hydrocortison. *Hautarzt* 1959; **10**: 42–3.

26 Burden AD, Beck MH. Contact hypersensitivity to topical corticosteroids. *Br J Dermatol* 1992; **127**: 497–500.

27 Coopman S, Degreef H, Dooms-Goossens A. Identification of cross-reaction patterns in allergic contact dermatitis from topical corticosteroids. *Br J Dermatol* 1989; **121**: 27–34.

28 Isaksson M, Bruze M. Allergic contact dermatitis in response to budesonide reactivated by inhalation of the allergen. *J Am Acad Dermatol* 2002; **46**: 880–5.

29 Nilsson E, Henning C, Hjorleifsson ML. Density of the microflora in hand eczema before and after topical treatment with a potent corticosteroid. *J Am Acad Dermatol* 1986; **15**: 192–7.

30 Nilsson EJ, Henning CG, Magnusson J. Topical corticosteroids and *Staphylococcus aureus* in atopic dermatitis. *J Am Acad Dermatol* 1992; **27**: 29–34.

31 Bonifazi E, Garofalo L, Lospalluti M. Granuloma gluteale infantum with atrophic scars: clinical and histological observations in 11 cases. *Clin Exp Dermatol* 1981; **6**: 23–9.

32 Velangi SS, Humphreys F, Beveridge GW. Periocular dermatitis associated with prolonged use of a steroid eye ointment. *Clin Exp Dermatol* 1998; **23**: 297–8.

33 Oliet EJ, Estes SA. Perianal comedones associated with chronic topical fluorinated steroid use. *J Am Acad Dermatol* 1982; **7**: 407.

34 Cubey RB. Glaucoma following the application of corticosteroid to the skin of the eyelids. *Br J Dermatol* 1976; **95**: 207–8.

35 Zugerman C, Saunders D, Levit F. Glaucoma from topically applied steroids. *Arch Dermatol* 1976; **112**: 1326.

36 Nielsen NW, Sorensen PN. Glaucoma induced by application of corticosteroids to the periorbital region. *Arch Dermatol* 1978; **114**: 953–4.

37 Schwartzenberg GW, Buys YM. Glaucoma secondary to topical use of steroid cream. *Can J Ophthalmol* 1999; **34**: 222–5.

38 Bawazeer AM, Hodge WG, Lorimer B. Atopy and keratoconus: a multivariate analysis. *Br J Ophthalmol* 2000; **84**: 834–6.

39 Marks JG Jr, Cano C, Leitzel K, Lipton A. Inhibition of wound healing by topical steroids. *J Dermatol Surg Oncol* 1983; **9**: 819–21.

40 Levy JJ, von Rosen J, Gassmuller J *et al*. Validation of an *in vivo* wound healing model for the quantification of pharmacological effects on epidermal regeneration. *Dermatology* 1995; **190**: 136–41.

41 Eaglstein WH, Mertz PM. New methods for assessing epidermal wound healing: the effects of triamcinolone acetonide and polyethelene film occlusion. *J Invest Dermatol* 1978; **71**: 382–4.

42 du Vivier A, Stoughton RB. Tachyphylaxis to the action of topically applied corticosteroids. *Arch Dermatol* 1975; **111**: 581–3.

43 du Vivier A. Tachyphylaxis to topically applied steroids. *Arch Dermatol* 1976; **112**: 1245–8.

44 Miller JJ, Roling D, Margolis D, Guzzo C. Failure to demonstrate therapeutic tachyphylaxis to topically applied steroids in patients with psoriasis. *J Am Acad Dermatol* 1999; **41**: 546–9.

45 Baker H. Corticosteroids and pustular psoriasis. *Br J Dermatol* 1976; **94** (Suppl. 12): 83–8.

46 Smith JG, Wehr RF, Chalker DK. Corticosteroid induced cutaneous atrophy and telangiectasia. *Arch Dermatol* 1976; **112**: 1115–7.

47 Cornell RC, Stoughton RB. Six month controlled study of effect of desoximetasone and betamethasone-17-valerate on the pituitary–adrenal axis. *Br J Dermatol* 1981; **105**: 91–5.

48 Katz HI, Hien NT, Prawer SE *et al*. Superpotent topical steroid treatment of psoriasis vulgaris: clinical efficacy and adrenal function. *J Am Acad Dermatol* 1987; **16**: 804–11.

49 Walsh P, Aeling JL, Huff L *et al*. Hypothalamus–pituitary–adrenal axis suppression by superpotent topical steroids. *J Am Acad Dermatol* 1993; **29**: 501–3.

50 Weston WL, Fennessey PV, Morelli J *et al*. Comparison of hypothalamus–pituitary–adrenal axis suppression from superpotent topical steroids by standard endocrine function testing and gas chromatographic mass spectrometry. *J Invest Dermatol* 1988; **90**: 532–5.

51 Ohman EM, Rogers S, Meenan FO *et al*. Adrenal suppression following low-dose topical clobetasol propionate. *J R Soc Med* 1987; **80**: 422–4.

52 Turpeinen M. Adrenocortical response to adrenocorticotrophic hormone in relation to duration of topical therapy and percutaneous absorption of hydrocortisone in children with dermatitis. *Eur J Paediatr* 1989; **148**: 729–31.

53 Borzvkowski M, Grant DB, Wells RS. Cushing's syndrome induced by topical steroids used for the treatment of non-bullous ichthyosiform erythroderma. *Clin Exp Dermatol* 1976; **1**: 337–42.

54 Cattaneo M, Betti R, Lodi A. Evaluation of efficacy and tolerability of K-SA fluocinolone acetonide tape. *Int J Clin Pharmacol Res* 1987; **7**: 279–82.

55 Morris SD, Rycroft RJ, White IR, Wakelin SH, McFadden JP. Occlusion and topical corticosteroid: comparative frequency of patch test reactions to topical antibiotics. *Br J Dermatol* 2002; **146**: 1047–51.

56 Skov L, Baadsgaard O. Bacterial superantigens and inflammatory skin diseases. *Clin Exp Dermatol* 2000; **25**: 57–61.

57 Memon AA, Molokhia MM, Friedmann PS. The inhibitory effects of topical chelating agents and antioxidants on nickel-induced hypersensitivity reactions. *J Am Acad Dermatol* 1994; **30**: 560–5.

58 Ryatt KS, Feather JW, Mehta A *et al*. The stability and blanching efficacy of betamethasone-17-valerate in emulsifying ointment. *Br J Dermatol* 1982; **107**: 71–6.

59 Harding SM, Sohail S, Busse MJ. Percutaneous absorption of clobetasol propionate from novel ointment and cream foundations. *Clin Exp Dermatol* 1985; **10**: 13–21.

60 David M, Lowe NJ. Psoriasis therapy: comparative studies with a hydrocolloid dressing, plastic film occlusion and triamcinolone cream. *J Am Acad Dermatol* 1989; **21**: 511–4.

61 Lebwohl M, Heymann WR, Berth-Jones J, Coulson I, eds. *Treatment of Skin Disease: Comprehensive Therapeutic Stratgies*. London: Mosby, 2002.

Cytotoxic and antineoplastic agents

Bleomycin

Bleomycin is a cytotoxic agent with antitumour, antibacterial and antiviral activity. It binds to DNA, causing strand scission and elimination of pyrimidine and purine bases.

A number of reports document successful treatment of recalcitrant viral warts with intralesional injections of 0.1% bleomycin [1–3]. Two large double-blind placebo-controlled trials gave similar results [2,3]. Seventy-five to 95 per cent of warts on the hands and 60% of plantar warts cleared following 1–3 injections. Local pain is significant, but tolerated by patients who had previously received many unsuccessful treatments. The mechanism of action in warts is not yet known. The small volumes used do not cause systemic toxicity. Treatment of a periungual wart resulted in a permanent nail dystrophy [4]; Raynaud's phenomenon may occur after treatment on digits. The compound must be handled with care.

Bleomycin has also been used in treatment of oral leukoplakia. A 1% solution in DMSO administered for 5 min over 14 consecutive days reduced the size of lesions and histological dysplasia in a trial with 22 patients [5].

5-Fluorouracil

This pyrimidine analogue is an antimetabolite that inhibits pyrimidine metabolism and DNA synthesis.

In the form of a 5% cream, 5-fluorouracil (5-FU) is a very effective treatment for multiple solar keratoses. Lesions on the scalp and face respond more readily than lesions on the limbs. A commonly used regimen comprises twice daily application for 2 weeks but there are many variations on this which are used to improve tolerability. A single daily application is sometimes adequate. Some dermatologists suggest a 1 week on, 1 week off regimen, or use the treatment for 1 week each month, or use it continuously but omit treatment at the weekend. Some patients require longer periods of treatment, and others are cleared only by occlusion of the agent with polyethylene film. A brisk inflammatory response should occur within the keratoses, otherwise clearing is incomplete. Severe ulcerative reactions occur in a few patients. Combination with a fluorinated steroid has been shown to limit the intensity of the inflammatory response without reducing the efficacy of 5-FU [6]. Combination of topical 5-FU applied twice daily with oral isotretinoin 20 mg/day for a median treatment duration of 21 days proved highly effective in a series of cases with disseminated actinic keratoses [7]. Actinic cheilitis and keratosis of the lip can be improved, although the treatment may cause some transient discomfort and dysplastic changes can persist histologically after apparently satisfactory clinical response [8].

5-FU can be effective in Bowen's disease, with 24 out of 26 lesions being cured in a series with 10-year follow-up [9]. However, a recent comparison with photodynamic therapy indicated that the latter was more effective [10]. Bowenoid papulosis can be treated with 5-FU and erythroplasia of Queyrat can also respond [11].

In treatment of basal cell carcinoma (BCC), topical 5-FU is considered most useful for low-risk lesions on the trunk and lower limbs [12]. It has proved successful in reducing the number of lesions appearing in the basal cell naevus syndrome [13]. Intralesional 5-FU has also been used with success in this indication [14].

5-FU, applied daily under adhesive plasters, proved effective in a placebo-controlled trial for the treatment of common viral warts [15]. Applied once or twice a week it has also been shown to be effective and well tolerated in curing resistant vaginal condylomas [16]. A proprietary combination of 5-FU and salicylic acid, applied on a daily basis, resulted in complete healing of genital warts in an average of 12 days [17].

5-FU can also be effective in extramammary Paget's disease [18]. It has been used with variable results in naevoid keratotic conditions including Darier's disease [19], and in superficial actinic porokeratosis [20].

T4 endonuclease V

This is a bacterial DNA repair enzyme that excises damaged sections of DNA. This is the initial step in repair of a DNA strand that has sustained photodamage. Remarkably, in a placebo-controlled study of 1 year duration, a liposomal formulation containing this enzyme has been demonstrated to reduce the occurrence of new neoplasms in patients with xeroderma pigmentosum [21]. This has implications not only for patients with this rare group of diseases; if one enzyme can be delivered into cells simply by application to the skin within liposomes, then it is possible that many other enzyme treatments might be delivered in similar vehicles.

Mechlorethamine

Mechlorethamine (mustine, nitrogen mustard) is a cytotoxic drug that is highly active when applied topically. It is an alkylating agent and acts by binding covalently to DNA and thus inhibiting replication. Its use is often constrained by its marked tendency to induce contact allergic dermatitis. Immediate hypersensitivity reactions can also occur but are less common. It is also potentially carcinogenic, although the precise level of risk is difficult to establish as many groups of treated patients have received additional carcinogenic treatments. Mechlorethamine has a number of dermatological applications.

The most frequent use is probably in the treatment of cutaneous T-cell lymphoma. Concentrations used most frequently are 0.01–0.02% and the treatment is applied once daily [22]. Aqueous solutions and also ointment formulations are highly effective. The latter seem to carry a lower risk of sensitization, although irritant reactions still occur. In a large, recently published series, 137 patients with stage T1 or T2 disease were treated with topical mechlorethamine alone for a median period of 5 years. Complete remission was achieved in the majority and only four progressed to a more advanced stage [22].

Topical mechlorethamine 0.02% can be highly effective and seems to be well tolerated in children with Langerhans' cell histiocytosis [23]. In this series, treatment was initially applied daily to affected areas of skin and the children were bathed to remove excess medication 10 min after the application was completed. The frequency of application was later reduced to every second or third day as the skin improved. Only two out of 20 children treated developed an irritant dermatitis [24].

Topical mechlorethamine has been recognized as effective in the treatment of psoriasis since a placebo-controlled trial was published in 1970 [25]. A solution containing 0.05% was effective after weekly application for 4–20 weeks but most patients eventually became sensitized and this has proved a major disadvantage. Some patients have successfully maintained long-term control of the disease using a concentration of 0.02% [26]. The risk of sensitization can be reduced by concurrent use of ultraviolet B (UVB) [27] or psoralen with UVA (PUVA) [28].

An encouraging report of alopecia areata and totalis responding to topical mechloethamine 0.02% has not yet been followed up by further reports of success [29]. In a subsequent report, no response was obtained in seven patients with alopecia totalis, although the treatment was well tolerated [30]. However, a recent study on a mouse model of alopecia areata did yield a positive response [31].

In single cases, pyoderma gangrenosum [32], and ulcerating lesions of chronic granulocytic leukaemia [33], have been reported to respond to topical mechlorethamine.

Imiquimod

This interesting compound belongs to a group known as imidazoquinolones. The actions of these compounds seem likely to be mediated by the Toll-like receptor 7 (TLR-7) [34]. This is a cell surface receptor found on cells of monocyte lineage. The naturally occurring ligands for TLRs are highly conserved microbial products, essential for microbial survival, which are responsible for stimulating the relatively primitive innate immune response. Interaction of TLR-7 with ligands activates a signalling pathway leading to release of large amounts of interferon-α, interleukin-12 (IL-12), tumour necrosis factor-α (TNF-α) and other potent cytokines. In addition to stimulating the innate response, these cytokines promote the development of antigen-specific cell-mediated immune responses. Imiquimod is therefore viewed as an immune response modulator.

The first clinical application in which imiquimod proved useful was for treatment of genital warts. In large placebo-controlled [35] and open-label [36] trials, imiquimod 5% cream applied three times weekly for 16 weeks produced complete clearance in 48–50% of patients. Relapse rates in those who had cleared (relapse being defined as recurrence of at least one visible wart) were 13% at 3 months [35] and 23% at 6 months post treatment [36]. Common warts may also respond. Thirty per cent of patients were cleared in a series of 50 treated with 5% imiquimod cream on 5 days each week for up to 16 weeks [37]. Sixteen of 18 children with warts of 2–7 years' duration were cleared of lesions after applying 5% imiquimod cream twice daily for 2–11 months [38]. Facial planar warts responded convincingly in a report of a single case [39]. In one case, stucco keratoses responded to imiquimod [40]; interestingly, human papillomavirus was detected in the lesions. Molluscum contagiosum has also been reported to respond in an uncontrolled study [37].

Imiquimod would seem to have potential in many additional applications including treatment of *in situ* malignancy. Actinic keratoses have been shown to respond in a placebo-controlled trial. Eighty-four per cent of patients were cleared after using imiquimod three times weekly for up to 12 weeks [41]. There was no response to the vehicle control. Fourteen of 15 patients with Bowen's disease had no residual lesion after daily application for up to 16 weeks [42]. Local skin reactions were common but these are thought to reflect the immune response to the tumour. In a series of similar size, actinic cheilitis responded well to imiquimod applied three times weekly for up to 6 weeks [43]. Partial and complete responses have been observed in treatment of cervical, vaginal and vulvar intraepithelial neoplasia and Bowenoid papulosis, although results have not been consistent [44–46]. Extramammary Paget's disease resolved in response to imiquimod in two cases treated daily or on alternate days, as tolerated, for 7.5 and 16 weeks [47]. Both of these patients experienced systemic symptoms (flu-like illness and nausea). Complete resolution was reported in a case of porokeratosis [48].

Trials on BCC have demonstrated unequivocal efficacy in dose ranging and placebo-controlled studies. In superficial BCC, resolution occurred in 81–88% of lesions treated daily, or on 5 days per week, for 6 or 12 weeks [49,50]. Treatment for 6 weeks appeared as effective as 12 weeks. Applying imiquimod on 3 days weekly for 6 weeks produced cure rates of 76%, or 87% when occluded [51]. In nodular BCC, daily treatment has yielded somewhat lower cure rates at 71% or 76% after 6 weeks or 12 weeks, respectively [52]. Treatment on 3 days weekly cured 50%, and 65% with the use of occlusion [51].

Imiquimod may find at least a palliative role in treatment of lentigo maligna and melanoma. In treatment of lentigo maligna, several cases and small series have reported apparently complete clinical resolution [53–55], in some cases confirmed histologically. However, one report describes lentigo maligna that apparently resolved following treatment with imiquimod but the course of the resolution was complicated by the development of a nodular melanoma and microsatellites; these were excised with the patient remaining disease-free after 17 months of follow-up [56]. Complete clinical and histological resolution has been reported in two cases of cutaneous metastatic melanoma [57], while marked improvement has been observed in additional cases [58,59]. In a further case, the cutaneous metastases resolved but lymph node metastasis developed [60].

Imiquimod may prove effective in suppressing the recurrence of keloids following excision. In an uncontrolled study with 12 subjects, the cream was applied nightly for 8 weeks, starting immediately after excision [61]. No recurrences were seen at 6 months.

Diclofenac

This compound is a non-steroidal anti-inflammatory drug that appears to be effective in topical treatment of actinic keratoses. A gel formulation containing 3% diclofenac and 2.5% hyaluronic acid has been developed specifically for this purpose. The mechanism of action remains uncertain. It has been proposed that excessive arachidonic acid metabolism resulting from overactivation of cyclo-oxygenase enzymes is carcinogenic [62]. If so, diclofenac may help suppress actinic keratoses by inhibition of cyclo-oxygenase.

In an open-label study, this formulation was applied twice daily until patients were clear, or for up to 180 days. Twenty-two (81%) of 27 patients who completed the study, and were assessed 30 days after treatment was discontinued, had a complete response and another four (15%) showed marked improvement [63]. These results have been supported by double-blind trials in which 3% diclofenac gel has been applied twice daily for 30–90 days and proved superior to vehicle in clearing solar keratoses [62,64,65]. Consistently, the largest and most statistically significant difference between diclofenac and vehicle has been observed at follow-up 30 days after treatment has been discontinued. This has occurred even when the difference has not been significant at the end of treatment [65]. As assessed at this follow-up visit, the proportions of patients completely cleared have been approximately 16% when treatment duration was 30 days [52], 31% when this was 60 days [52], 38% for 12 weeks [65] and 47% when the duration was 90 days [64]. It would therefore seem that the clearance rate continues to increase with increasing treatment duration.

The treatment seems to be well tolerated, although pruritus has not been uncommon and dermatitis, confined to the treated site, has developed occasionally.

Podophyllin and podophyllotoxin

Podophyllin (podophyllum) is a plant extract traditionally used to treat genital warts. Podophyllotoxin is the most active constituent. This is now available in standardized formulations free of the unwanted constituents of podophyllin. Podophyllotoxin is an antimitotic agent which arrests cells in metaphase by binding to tubulin. Podophyllin is known to be highly mutagenic and although podophyllotoxin may be less hazardous, both of these treatments should be avoided in pregnancy. Irritant reactions are common with these agents.

Podophyllin 0.5% in ethanol may be applied on 3 consecutive days each week to treat penile warts [66]. Podophyllin 10–25% in tincture of benzoin compound may be applied once or twice a week to genital or perianal warts (washed off after 6–12 h). Podophyllotoxin can be used at a 0.5% concentration in ethanol as a once daily application. It will clear 60–70% of genital warts within 3–5 days [67]. A cream formulation containing 0.15% podophyllotoxin is also available and can be applied twice daily for 3 days each week.

REFERENCES

1 Cordero AA, Guglielmi HA, Woscoff A. The common wart: intra-lesional treatment with bleomycin sulfate. *Cutis* 1980; **26**: 319–20.
2 Bunney HH, Nolan MW, Buxton PK *et al.* The treatment of resistant warts with intralesional bleomycin: a controlled clinical trial. *Br J Dermatol* 1984; **110**: 197–207.
3 Shumer SM, O'Keefe EJ. Bleomycin in the treatment of recalcitrant warts. *J Am Acad Dermatol* 1983; **9**: 91–6.
4 Miller RAW. Nail dystrophy following intralesional injections of bleomycin for periungual wart. *Arch Dermatol* 1984; **120**: 963–4.
5 Epstein JB, Wong FL, Millner A *et al.* Topical bleomycin treatment of oral leukoplakia: a randomized double-blind clinical trial. *Head Neck* 1994; **16**: 539–44.
6 Breza T, Taylor R, Eaglestein WH. Non-inflammatory destruction of actinic keratoses by fluorouracil. *Arch Dermatol* 1977; **112**: 1256–8.
7 Sander CA, Pfeiffer C, Kligman AM, Plewig G. Chemotherapy for disseminated actinic keratoses with 5-fluorouracil and isotretinoin. *J Am Acad Dermatol* 1997; **36**: 236–8.
8 Warnock GR, Fuller RP Jr, Pelleu GB Jr. Evaluation of 5-fluorouracil in the treatment of actinic keratosis of the lip. *Oral Surg Oral Med Oral Pathol* 1981; **52**: 501–5.
9 Bargman H, Hochman J. Topical treatment of Bowen's disease with 5-fluorouracil. *J Cutan Med Surg* 2003; **7**: 101–5.
10 Salim A, Leman JA, McColl JH *et al.* Randomized comparison of photodynamic therapy with topical 5-fluorouracil in Bowen's disease. *Br J Dermatol* 2003; **148**: 539–43.
11 Goette DK, Carson TE. Erythroplasia of Queyrat: treatment with topical 5-fluorouracil. *Cancer* 1976; **38**: 1498–502.
12 Telfer NR, Colver GB, Bowers PW. Guidelines for the management of basal cell carcinoma. *Br J Dermatol* 1999; **141**: 415–23.
13 Strange PR, Lang PG Jr. Long-term management of basal cell naevus syndrome with topical tretinoin and 5-fluorouracil. *J Am Acad Dermatol* 1992; **27**: 842–5.
14 Miller BH, Shavin JS, Cognetta A *et al.* Non-surgical treatment of basal cell carcinomas with intralesional 5-fluorouracil/epinephrine injectable gel. *J Am Acad Dermatol* 1997; **36**: 72–7.
15 Hursthouse MW. A controlled trial on the use of topical 5-fluorouracil on viral warts. *Br J Dermatol* 1975; **92**: 93–6.
16 Krebs HB. Treatment of vaginal condylomata acuminata by weekly topical application of 5-fluorouracil. *Obstet Gynecol* 1987; **70**: 68–71.
17 Djawari D. Fluorouracil treatment on condyloma acuminata. *Z Hautkr* 1986; **61**: 463–9.
18 Bewley AP, Bracka A, Staughton RC *et al.* Extramammary Paget's disease of the scrotum: treatment with topical 5-fluorouracil and plastic surgery. *Br J Dermatol* 1994; **131**: 445–6.
19 Knulst AC, De La Faille HB, Van Vloten WA. Topical 5-fluorouracil in the treatment of Darier's disease. *Br J Dermatol* 1995; **133**: 463–6.
20 Shelley WB, Shelley ED. Disseminated superficial porokeratosis: rapid therapeutic response to 5-fluorouracil. *Cutis* 1983; **32**: 139–40.
21 Yarosh D, Klein J, O'Connor A *et al.* Effect of topically applied T4 endonuclease V in liposomes on skin cancer in xeroderma pigmentosum: a randomised study. *Lancet* 2001; **357** (9260): 926–9.
22 Kim YH, Martinez G, Varghese A, Hoppe RT. Topical nitrogen mustard in the treatment of mycosis fungoides. *Arch Dermatol* 2003; **139**: 165–73.
23 Sheehan MP, Atherton DJ, Broadbent V, Pritchard J. Topical nitrogen mustard: an effective treatment for cutaneous Langerhans' cell histiocytosis. *J Pediatr* 1991; **119**: 317–21.
24 Hoeger PH, Nanduri VR, Harper JI *et al.* Long-term follow up of topical mustine treatment for cutaneous Langerhans' cell histiocytosis. *Arch Dis Child* 2000; **82**: 483–7.
25 Epstein E, Ugel AR. Effects of topical mechlorethamine on skin lesions of psoriasis. *Arch Dermatol* 1970; **102**: 504–6.
26 Taylor JR, Halprin K. Topical use of mechlorethamine in the treatment of psoriasis. *Arch Dermatol* 1972; **106**: 362–4.
27 Nusbaum BP, Edwards EK, Horwitz SN, Frost P. Psoriasis therapy: the

effect of UV radiation on sensitization to mechlorethamine. *Arch Dermatol* 1983; **119**: 117–21.

28 Maduit G, Silvestre O, Thivolet J. PUVA therapy prevents sensitization to mechlorethamine in patients with psoriasis. *Br J Dermatol* 1985; **113**: 515–21.

29 Arrazola JM, Sendagota E, Harto A, Ledo A. Treatment of alopecia areata with topical nitrogen mustard. *Int J Dermatol* 1985; **24**: 608–10.

30 Harrison PV, Latona J, Jovanovic M. Alopecia totalis and topical mustine. *Arch Dermatol* 1993; **129**: 514.

31 Tang L, Cao L, Bernardo O *et al.* Topical mechlorethamine restores auto-immune-arrested follicular activity in mice with an alopecia areata-like disease by targeting infiltrated lymphocytes. *J Invest Dermatol* 2003; **120**: 400–6.

32 Tsele E, Yu RCH, Chu AC. Pyoderma gangrenosum: response to topical nitrogen mustard. *Clin Exp Dermatol* 1992; **17**: 437–40.

33 Murphy WG, Fotheringham GH, Busuttil A *et al.* Skin lesions in chronic granulocytic leukemia: treatment of a patient with topical nitrogen mustard. *Cancer* 1985; **55**: 2630–3.

34 Stanley MA. Imiquimod and the imidazoquinolones: mechanism of action and therapeutic potential. *Clin Exp Dermatol* 2002; **27**: 571–7.

35 Edwards L, Ferenczy A, Eron L *et al.* Self-administered topical 5% imiquimod cream for external anogenital warts. *Arch Dermatol* 1998; **134**: 25–30.

36 Garland SM, Sellors JW, Wikstrom A *et al.* Imiquimod 5% cream is a safe and effective self-applied treatment for anogenital warts: results of an open-label, multicentre Phase IIIB trial. *Int J STD AIDS* 2001; **12**: 722–9.

37 Hengge U, Esser S, Schultewolter T *et al.* Self-administered topical 5% imiquimod for the treatment of common warts and molluscum contagiosum. *Br J Dermatol* 2000; **143**: 1026–31.

38 Grussendorf-Conen E-I, Jacobs S. Efficacy of imiquimod 5% cream in the treatment of recalcitrant warts in children. *Pediatr Dermatol* 2002; **19**: 263–6.

39 Khan Durani B, Jappe U. Successful treatment of facial plane warts with imiquimod. *Br J Dermatol* 2002; **147**: 1018.

40 Stockfleth E, Rowert J, Arndt R *et al.* Detection of human papillomavirus and response to topical imiquimod in a case of stucco keratosis. *Br J Dermatol* 2000; **143**: 846–50.

41 Stockfleth E, Meyer T, Benninghoff B *et al.* A randomized, double-blind, vehicle-controlled study to assess 5% imiquimod cream for the treatment of multiple actinic keratoses. *Arch Dermatol* 2002; **138**: 1498–502.

42 MacKenzie-Wood A, Kossard S, de Launey J. Imiquimod 5% cream in the treatment of Bowen's disease. *J Am Acad Dermatol* 2001; **44**: 462–70.

43 Smith KJ, Germain M, Yeager J, Skelton H. Topical 5% imiquimod for the therapy of actinic cheilitis. *J Am Acad Dermatol* 2002; **47**: 497–501.

44 Diaz-Arrastia C, Arany I, Robazetti SC *et al.* Clinical and molecular responses in high grade intraepithelial neoplasia treated with topical imiquimod 5%. *Clin Cancer Res* 2001; **7**: 3031–3.

45 Todd R, Etherington I, Luesley D. The effects of 5% imiquimod cream on high-grade vulval intraepithelial neoplasia. *Gynecologic Oncol* 2002; **85**: 67–70.

46 Porter WM, Francis N, Hawkins D *et al.* Penile intraepithelial neoplasia: clinical spectrum and treatment of 35 cases. *Br J Dermatol* 2002; **147**: 1159–65.

47 Zampogna JC, Flowers FP, Roth WI, Hassenein AM. Treatment of primary limited cutaneous extramammary Paget's disease with topical imiquimod monotherapy: two case reports. *J Am Acad Dermatol* 2002; **47**: S229–35.

48 Agarwal S, Berth-Jones J. Porokeratosis of Mibelli: successful treatment with 5% imiquimod cream. *Br J Dermatol* 2002; **146**: 338–9.

49 Marks R, Gebauer K, Shumack S *et al.* Imiquimod 5% cream in the treatment of superficial basal cell carcinoma: results of a multicentre 6 week dose–response trial. *J Am Acad Dermatol* 2001; **44**: 807–13.

50 Geisse J, Rich P, Pandya A *et al.* Imiquimod 5% cream for the treatment of superficial basal cell carcinoma: a double-blind randomized vehicle-controlled study. *J Am Acad Dermatol* 2002; **47**: 390–8.

51 Sterry W, Ruzicka T, Herrera E *et al.* Imiquimod 5% cream for the treatment of superficial and nodular basal cell carcinoma: randomized studies comparing low-frequency dosing with and without occlusion. *Br J Dermatol* 2002; **147**: 1227–36.

52 Shumack S, Robinson J, Kossard S *et al.* Efficacy of topical 5% imiquimod cream for the treatment of nodular basal cell carcinoma. *Arch Dermatol* 2002; **138**: 1165–71.

53 Ahmed I, Berth-Jones J. Imiquimod: a novel treatment for lentigo maligna. *Br J Dermatol* 2000; **143**: 843–5.

54 Bryden AM, Evans A, Dawe RS *et al.* A pilot investigative study of imiquimod in the treatment of lentigo maligna. *Br J Dermatol* 2003; **149** (Suppl. 64): 42.

55 Epstein E. Histologic resolution of melanoma *in situ* (lentigo maligna) with 5% imiquimod cream. *Arch Dermatol* 2003; **139**: 944–5.

56 Fisher GH, Lang PG. Treatment of melanoma *in situ* on sun-damaged skin with topical 5% imiquimod cream complicated by the development of invasive disease. *Arch Dermatol* 2003; **139**: 945–7.

57 Wolf IH, Smolle J, Binder B *et al.* Topical imiquimod in the treatment of metastatic melanoma to skin. *Arch Dermatol* 2003; **139**: 273–6.

58 Steinmann A, Funk JO, Schuler G, von den Driesch P. Topical imiquimod treatment of a cutaneous melanoma metastasis. *J Am Acad Dermatol* 2000; **43**: 555–6.

59 Bong AB, Bonnekoh B, Franke I *et al.* Imiquimod, a topical immune response modifier, in the treatment of cutaneous metastases of malignant melanoma. *Dermatology* 2002; **205**: 135–8.

60 Ugurel S, Wagner A, Pfohler C *et al.* Topical imiquimod eradicates skin metastases of malignant melanoma but fails to prevent rapid lymphogenous metastatic spread. *Br J Dermatol* 2002; **147**: 621–4.

61 Berman B. Pilot study of the effect of postoperative imiquimod 5% cream on the recurrence rate of excised keloids. *J Am Acad Dermatol* 2002; **47**: S209–11.

62 Rivers JK, Arlette J, Shear N *et al.* Topical treatment of actinic keratoses with 3.0% diclofenac in 2.5% hyaluronan gel. *Br J Dermatol* 2002; **146**: 94–100.

63 Rivers JK, McLean DI. An open study to assess the efficacy and safety of topical 3% diclofenac in a 2.5% hyaluronic acid gel for the treatment of actinic keratoses. *Arch Dermatol* 1997; **133**: 1239–42.

64 Wolf JE Jr, Taylor JR, Tschen E, Kang S. Topical 3.0% diclofenac in 2.5% hyaluronan gel in the treatment of actinic keratoses. *Int J Dermatol* 2001; **40**: 709–13.

65 Gebauer K, Brown P, Varigos G. Topical diclofenac in hyaluronan gel for the treatment of solar keratoses. *Australas J Dermatol* 2003; **44**: 40–3.

66 Maiti H, Hayl KR. Treatment of condyloma accuminata with podophyllin resin. *Practitioner* 1985; **229**: 37–9.

67 Von Krogh G. Topical self-treatment of penile warts with a 0.5% podophyllotoxin in ethanol for 4–5 days. *Sex Transm Dis* 1987; **14**: 135–40.

Depigmenting agents

Depigmenting agents are most frequently used by dermatologists in the treatment of melasma. Hydroquinone, used alone in concentrations usually ranging from 2 to 5%, or in combination with retinoic acid in 0.025–0.1%, is currently the most widely used treatment for this indication.

Post-inflammatory hyperpigmentation is another commonly encountered problem and this is particularly difficult to treat as much of the pigment is often contained in dermal melanophages. Nonetheless, depigmenting compounds such as tretinoin, hydroquinone or azelaic acid are sometimes prescribed.

In severe cases of vitiligo when depigmentation is already extensive, depigmenting agents can improve the appearance of the skin by removing residual patches of normal pigmentation.

Solar lentiginosis is another indication for which depigmenting agents can prove useful. Retinoic acid has the best evidence base in this indication.

There is also a demand among populations with pigmented skin for agents to reduce the intensity of pigmentation for purely cosmetic purposes. In parts of Africa, treatments abused for this purpose include very potent topical corticosteroids, mercury compounds and high concentrations of hydroquinone [1–3].

Hydroquinone

Hydroquinone (1,4 dihydroxybenzene) is widely used as a depigmenting agent both in clinical and cosmetic contexts.

The efficacy of 4% hydroquinone cream in treatment of melasma was demonstrated in a placebo-controlled trial in which treatment was applied nightly for 3 months [4]. Higher concentrations are sometimes used in extemporaneous formulations for severe or resistant cases of chloasma or for post-inflammatory hyperpigmentation. The efficacy of hydroquinone in post-inflammatory hyperpigmentation is likely to be highly variable as this is a very heterogeneous entity. Hydroquinone is used at 5% concentration as a constituent of Kligman cream (see below) [5]. It can cause both irritant and allergic reactions. The addition of a weak topical steroid reduces the irritant effect. It is unstable and tends to darken as a result of auto-oxidation. Hydroquinone probably reduces pigmentation, at least partly, as a result of inhibition of melanin synthesis, because it is known to inhibit tyrosinase. However, the mechanism is not fully understood. It has also been proposed that its action may be partly mediated by release of free radicals. In animal models, the effect of the drug is potentiated by the use of buthionine sulfoxime or cystamine to inhibit synthesis of the protective free radical scavenger glutathione [6].

Epidemiological studies indicate that a very large proportion of the African population (perhaps the majority of women) have used hydroquinone cosmetically as a skin lightening agent [1–3]. This practice has been strongly associated with the development, in these black-skinned individuals, of exogenous ochronosis [1–3,7,8]. This disease, like endogenous ochronosis (alkaptonuria), derives its name from the colour of the cutaneous pigment deposits that characterize these conditions (Greek *ochro*, yellow). When these are examined histologically they appear yellow or brown, although clinically the pigment appears dark brown or black. Endogenous ochronosis is an inborn error of metabolism in which deficiency of homogentisic acid oxidase results in accumulation of homogentisic acid, a metabolite of tyrosine and phenylalanine. Oxidation products of homogentisic acid are thought to constitute the pigment deposited in the skin, cartilage and elsewhere.

The pigment in exogenous ochronosis strongly resembles that in the endogenous form and may result from inhibition of homogentisic acid oxidase by hydroquinone. Milder cases show only macular sooty pigmentation while more advanced cases develop irregular stippling, papulation and pigmented colloid milia [8,9]. These features tend to be most prominent over the areas of skin most intensely exposed to the sun. Histologically, deposits of pigment are observed in the papillary and reticular dermis and probably represent accumulations of the pigment in association with degenerated collagen [9,10]. In many countries, the concentration of hydroquinone in cosmetic products has been legally restricted to 2% with the aim of reducing the risk of causing ochronosis. However, it is not established that this risk is dependent on the concentration [11].

In striking contrast to Africa, exogenous ochronosis seems to be rare in the USA, even though hydroquinone-containing compounds are widely used there [12,13]. Possible explanations put forward for this paradox include under-reporting, combined use with other compounds in Africa, the need for intense solar irradiation as a synergistic factor, the use of different formulations (especially hydroalcoholic solutions) in Africa, or that the use of these compounds in the USA may be relatively cautious.

Exogenous ochronosis occurs almost entirely in black skin. It does not seem to be a hazard in white skin, although occasional cases have occurred in Hispanics. The relatively high levels of enzyme activity associated with melanin synthesis in black skin and additional stimulation of these pathways by intense sun exposure seem to be required for ochronosis to develop.

Monobenzyl ether of hydroquinone

Skin bleaching with 20% monobenzyl ether of hydroquinone (monobenzone) is generally reserved for treatment of carefully selected cases of vitiligo. The resulting depigmentation may be permanent so this treatment is only suitable for those with extensive disease in whom the appearance of the skin would be improved by removing the residual pigment. Patients should be warned that results are unpredictable. Treatment may need to be prolonged and is not always successful [14]. Depigmentation may be permanent and may occur at sites other than those being treated. Conversely, spontaneous repigmentation may occur unexpectedly after cessation of the treatment, slowly or rapidly, at both treated and untreated sites [15]. Contact dermatitis can develop [14,16]. It has also been reported that this treatment may cause corneal and conjunctival pigmentation [17].

The addition of monobenzone to cosmetic skin lightening preparations caused an epidemic of leukomelanoderma in South Africa during the early 1970s [9].

Additional phenol derivatives

Mequinol (4-hydroxyanisole, 4-methoxyphenol) is another phenol derivative with depigmenting properties. It is a constituent of a commercially formulated solution containing 2% mequinol and 0.01% retinoic acid marketed for treatment of solar lentiginosis. In trials with treatment duration of 24 weeks, this combination appeared more effective than either of the constituents used alone, or than placebo [18]. Mequinol 20% cream has been successfully used to remove residual pigmentation in severe vitiligo with efficacy considered comparable to monobenzone [19].

N-acetyl-4-*S*-cysteaminylphenol (*N*-Ac-4-*S*-CAP) produces reversible depigmentation in the Yucatan pig model [20,21]. In one report of its use in melasma, 8% of patients showed complete depigmentation, 66% marked improvement and 25% moderate improvement [22].

Retinoic acid

Retinoic acid (tretinoin) has been successfully used to reduce pigmentation in a variety of disorders including melasma [23], solar lentiginosis [24,25] and post-inflammatory hyperpigmentation [26]. In most trials, tretinoin 0.1% cream has been used for 40 weeks. Retinoid dermatitis is a common side effect and may result in post-inflammatory hyperpigmentation. Some mild reduction of pigment may occur in normal skin surrounding the treated areas. The mechanism of action is not fully understood but may be at least partly explained by reduction in melanogenesis consequent upon reduction of tyrosinase activity [27].

Attempts have been made to use other retinoids for this purpose with variable results. All-*trans* retinol gel 10% proved effective, although irritant, in a Japanese study [28]. A study on the use of topical 0.05% isotretinoin in melasma showed no difference from placebo after 40 weeks [29].

Kligman cream

This formulation comprises 5% hydroquinone, 0.1% tretinoin and 0.1% dexamethasone in hydrophilic ointment [5]. It has been widely used as a depigmenting treatment, especially for melasma. The combined formulation is considered more effective than any of the individual constituents.

Azelaic acid

This dicarboxylic acid is a relatively safe, although mildly irritant agent, with several roles in dermatology.

As a depigmenting agent, azelaic acid is moderately effective in treatment of melasma. The proposed mechanism is direct or indirect inhibition of tyrosinase [30]. Azelaic acid 20% cream proved more effective than 2% hydroquinone cream after 24 weeks of treatment [31]. In two other studies with the same treatment duration, 20% azelaic acid proved equivalent in efficacy to 4% hydroquinone cream [32,33]. Another study on facial hyperpigmentation in darker skinned individuals compared a combination of azelaic acid 20% cream with glycolic acid 15% or 20% lotion, versus 4% hydroquinone cream; similar efficacy was observed from the two regimens [34]. The addition of tretinoin enhances the depigmenting effect [1,2]. Azelaic acid has also proved effective in treatment of Kitamura's reticulate acropigmentation [35].

Azelaic acid also has antineoplastic properties, inhibiting mitochondrial function and DNA synthesis [36], and has been used as a palliative treatment for lentigo maligna and malignant melanoma [37–39]. However, because some cases of lentigo maligna have progressed to invasive melanoma while using this treatment, it must be regarded as purely palliative in these indications [37].

Azelaic acid 20% cream is effective in treatment of acne vulgaris [40]. This is likely to be a result of a combination of antimicrobial and anti-inflammatory properties. It can inhibit growth of *Propionibacterium acnes* and *Staphylococcus epidermidis* and inhibits production of free radicals by polymorphs [41]. The latter property may also explain why it is effective in rosacea [42,43]. It may also prove to have a role as an antimycotic inhibiting growth of dermatophytes [44,45], and as a topical antimicrobial agent with activity against antibiotic-resistant *Staph. aureus* [46].

Kojic acid

This is a fungal metabolite known to inhibit tyrosinase [47]. It is a constituent of over-the-counter depigmenting creams sold mainly in Japan. In treatment of melasma, 1% kojic acid proved equally effective as 2% hydroquinone when each was used in combination with glycolic acid [48].

Liquiritin

This compound, which can be extracted from liquorice (*Glycyrrhiza glabra*) and other herbal sources, has been reported to effectively reduce the pigmentation of melasma in a double-blind trial [49].

REFERENCES

1 Adebajo SB. An epidemiological survey of the use of cosmetic skin lightening cosmetics among traders in Lagos, Nigeria. *West Afr J Med* 2002; **21**: 51–5.
2 Del Giudice P, Yves P. The widespread use of skin lightening creams in Senegal: a persistent public health problem in West Africa. *Int J Dermatol* 2002; **41**: 69–72.
3 Mahe A, Ly F, Aymard G, Dangou JM. Skin diseases associated with the cosmetic use of bleaching products in women from Dakar, Senegal. *Br J Dermatol* 2003; **148**: 493–500.
4 Haddad AL, Matos LF, Brunstein F *et al.* A clinical, prospective, randomized, double-blind trial comparing skin whitening complex with hydroquinone vs. placebo in the treatment of melasma. *Int J Dermatol* 2003; **42**: 153–6.
5 Kligman AM, Willis I. A new formula for depigmenting human skin. *Arch Dermatol* 1975; **111**: 40–8.
6 Bolognia JL, Sodi SA, Osber MP *et al.* Enhancement of the depigmenting effect of hydroquinone by cystamine and buthionine sulfoximine. *Br J Dermatol* 1995; **133**: 349–57.
7 Bentley-Phillips B, Bayles MA. Cutaneous reactions to topical application of hydroquinone: results of a 6-year investigation. *S Afr Med J* 1975; **49**: 1391–5.
8 Hardwick N, van Celder LW, van der Merwe CA *et al.* Exogenous ochronosis: an epidemiological study. *Br J Dermatol* 1989; **120**: 229–38.
9 Findlay CH, Morrison JCL, Simson IW. Exogenous ochronosis and pigmented colloid milium from hydroquinone bleaching creams. *Br J Dermatol* 1975; **93**: 613–22.
10 Snider RL, Thiers BH. Exogenous ochronosis. *J Am Acad Dermatol* 1993; **28**: 662–4. [A case occurring in a black American woman using hydroquinone 2–4% for 'many years'.]
11 Williams H. Skin lightening creams containing hydroquinone: the case for a temporary ban. *BMJ* 1992; **305**: 903–4.

12 Grimes P. Melasma: aetiologic and therapeutic considerations. *Arch Dermatol* 1995; **131**: 1453–7.

13 Burke PA, Maibach HI. Exogenous ochronosis: an overview. *J Dermatol Treat* 1997; **8**: 21–6.

14 Mosher DB, Parrish JA, Fitzpatrick TB. Monobenzylether of hydroquinone: a retrospective study of treatment of 18 vitiligo patients and a review of the literature. *Br J Dermatol* 1977; **97**: 669–79.

15 Oakley AM. Rapid repigmentation after depigmentation therapy: vitiligo treated with monobenzyl ether of hydroquinone. *Australas J Dermatol* 1996; **37**: 96–8.

16 Lyon CC, Beck MH. Contact hypersensitivity to monobenzyl ether of hydroquinone used to treat vitiligo. *Contact Dermatitis* 1998; **39**: 132–3.

17 Hedges TR III, Kenyon KR, Hanninen LA, Mosher DB. Corneal and conjunctival effects of monobenzone in patients with vitiligo. *Arch Ophthalmol* 1983; **101**: 64–8.

18 Fleischer AB Jr, Schwartzel EH, Colby SI, Altman DJ. The combination of 2% 4-hydroxyanisole (Mequinol) and 0.01% tretinoin is effective in improving the appearance of solar lentigines and related hyperpigmented lesions in two double-blind multicenter clinical studies. *J Am Acad Dermatol* 2000; **42**: 459–67.

19 Njoo MD, Vodegel RM, Westerhof W. Depigmentation therapy in vitiligo universalis with topical 4-methoxyphenol and the Q-switched ruby laser. *J Am Acad Dermatol* 2000; **42**: 760–9.

20 Jimbow M, Marusyk H, Jimbow K. The *in vivo* melanocytotoxicity and depigmenting potency of *N*-2,4-acetoxyphenyl thioethyl acetamide in the skin and hair. *Br J Dermatol* 1995; **133**: 526–36.

21 Alena F, Dixon W, Thomas P *et al.* Glutathione plays a key role in the depigmenting and melanocytotoxic action of *N*-acetyl-4-*S*-cysteaminylphenol in black and yellow hair follicles. *J Invest Dermatol* 1995; **104**: 792–7.

22 Jimbow K. *N*-acetyl-4-*S*-cysteaminylphenol as a new type of depigmenting agent for the melanoderma of patients with melasma. *Arch Dermatol* 1991; **127**: 1528–34.

23 Griffiths CEM, Finkel LJ, Ditre CM *et al.* Topical tretinoin (retinoic acid) improves melasma: a vehicle-controlled, clinical trial. *Br J Dermatol* 1993; **129**: 415–21.

24 Rafal ES, Griffiths CE, Ditre CM *et al.* Topical tretinoin (retinoic acid) treatment for liver spots associated with photodamage. *N Engl J Med* 1992; **326**: 368–74.

25 Griffiths CE, Goldfarb MT, Finkel LJ *et al.* Topical tretinoin (retinoic acid) treatment of hyperpigmented lesions associated with photo-aging in Chinese and Japanese patients: a vehicle-controlled trial. *J Am Acad Dermatol* 1994; **30**: 76–84.

26 Bulengo-Ransby SM, Griffiths CE, Kimbrough-Green CK *et al.* Topical tretinoin (retinoic acid) therapy for hyperpigmented lesions caused by inflammation of the skin in black patients. *N Engl J Med* 1993; **328**: 1438–43.

27 Romero C, Aberdam E, Larnier C, Ortonne JP. Retinoic acid as modulator of UVB-induced melanocyte differentiation: involvement of the melanogenic enzymes expression. *J Cell Sci* 1994; **107**: 1095–103.

28 Yoshimura K, Momosawa A, Aiba E *et al.* Clinical trial of bleaching treatment with 10% all-*trans* retinol gel. *Dermatol Surg* 2003; **29**: 155–60.

29 Leenutaphong V, Nettakul A, Rattanasuwon P. Topical isotretinoin for melasma in Thai patients: a vehicle-controlled clinical trial. *J Med Assoc Thai* 1999; **82**: 868–75.

30 Schallreuter KU, Wood JW. A possible mechanism of action for azelaic acid in the human epidermis. *Arch Dermatol Res* 1990; **282**: 168–71.

31 Verallo-Rowell VM, Verallo V, Graupe K *et al.* Double-blind comparison of azelaic acid and hydroquinone in the treatment of melasma. *Acta Derm Venereol* 1989; **143** (Suppl.): 58–61.

32 Piquero Martin J, Rothe de Arocha J, Beniamini Loker D. Double-blind clinical study of the treatment of melasma with azelaic acid versus hydroquinone. *Med Cutan Ibero Latin Am* 1988; **16**: 511–4.

33 Baliña LM, Graupe K. The treatment of melasma: 20% azelaic acid versus 4% hydroquinone cream. *Int J Dermatol* 1991; **30**: 893–5.

34 Kakita LS, Lowe NJ. Azelaic acid and glycolic acid combination therapy for facial hyperpigmentation in darker-skinned patients: a clinical comparison with hydroquinone. *Clin Ther* 1998; **20**: 960–70.

35 Kameyama K, Morita M, Sugaya K *et al.* Treatment of reticulate acropigmentation of Kitamura with azelaic acid: an immunohistochemical and electron microscopic study. *J Am Acad Dermatol* 1992; **26**: 817–20.

36 Breathnach AS. Azelaic acid: potential as a general antitumoural agent. *Med Hypotheses* 1999; **52**: 221–6.

37 McLean DI, Peter KK. Apparent progression of lentigo maligna to invasive melanoma during treatment with topical azelaic acid. *Br J Dermatol* 1986; **114**: 685–9. [Five cases improved, one of them cleared.]

38 Sowden J, Paramsothy Y, Smith AG. Malignant melanoma arising in the scar of lupus vulgaris and response to treatment with topical azelaic acid. *Clin Exp Dermatol* 1988; **13**: 353–6. [An *in situ* lesion partially responded histologically.]

39 Vereecken P, Heenen M. Recurrent lentigo maligna melanoma: regression associated with local azelaic acid 20%. *Int J Clin Pract* 2002; **56**: 68–9.

40 Graupe K, Cunliffe WJ, Gollnick HP *et al.* Efficacy and safety of topical azelaic acid (20% cream): an overview of results from European clinical trials and experimental reports. *Cutis* 1996; **57** (Suppl. 1): 20–35.

41 Fitton A, Goa KL. Azelaic acid: a review of its pharmacological properties and therapeutic efficacy in acne and hyperpigmentary skin disorders. *Drugs* 1991; **41**: 780–98.

42 Carmichael AJ, Marks R, Graupe KA, Zaumseil RP. Topical azelaic acid in the treatment of rosacea. *J Derm Treat* 1993; **4** (Suppl. 1): 19–22.

43 Maddin S. A comparison of topical azelaic acid 20% cream and topical metronidazole 0.75% cream in the treatment of patients with papulopustular rosacea. *J Am Acad Dermatol* 1999; **40**: 961–5.

44 Brasch J, Friege B. Dicarboxylic acids affect the growth of dermatophytes *in vitro*. *Acta Derm Venereol (Stockh)* 1994; **74**: 347–50.

45 Brasch J, Christophers E. Azelaic acid has antimycotic properties *in vitro*. *Dermatology* 1993; **186**: 55–8.

46 Maple PA, Hamilton-Miller JM, Brumfitt W. Comparison of the *in vitro* activities of the topical antimicrobials azelaic acid, nitrofurazone, silver sulphadiazine and mupirocin against methicillin-resistant *Staphylococcus aureus*. *J Antimicrob Chemother* 1992; **29**: 661–8.

47 Kahn V. Effect of kojic acid on the oxidation of DL-DOPA, norepinephrine, and dopamine by mushroom tyrosinase. *Pigment Cell Res* 1995; **8**: 234–40.

48 Garcia A, Fulton JE Jr. The combination of glycolic acid and hydroquinone or kojic acid for the treatment of melasma and related conditions. *Dermatol Surg* 1996; **22**: 443–7.

49 Amer M, Metwalli M. Topical liquiritin improves melasma. *Int J Dermatol* 2000; **39**: 299–301.

Depilatories

Depilation can be defined as temporary removal of hair, while epilation denotes permanent destruction of the follicle. Epilation therefore requires physical methods of destruction of the follicle such as electrolysis, lasers and intense pulsed light. Depilation can be achieved by shaving, waxing, plucking, threading and by use of topical depilatory creams. Systemic androgen antagonists have a part to play in some cases. All these techniques are described further in Chapter 63; only topical treatments are discussed here.

Traditional depilatory creams depend upon breaking the disulphide bonds in hair. Three main classes are currently used. The oldest are various sulphides, which have a powerful effect but may irritate, and which in the presence of water generate hydrogen sulphide which has an unpleasant odour. Strontium or barium sulphide 20% are widely used. They are effective on the terminal hair in the axillae. Thioglycollates are being used more frequently, but they are slower to work than sulphides. Concentrations of 2.5–4% produce an effect in 5–15 min. Substituted mercaptans (thioalcohols) are most widely used. They work slowly, but are suitable for use on the face.

Eflornithine hydrochloride is an irreversible inhibitor of ornithine decarboxylase, an enzyme required for hair growth. This is marketed as a 13.9% cream, which can slow the growth of facial hair. A response takes 4–8 weeks to develop and the effect wears off over a similar period when the treatment is discontinued. The benefit seems to be rather modest in many cases, with only 32% of patients reporting marked improvement [1,2]. Some irritation may occur.

REFERENCES

1 Shapiro J, Lui H. Vaniqa–eflornithine 13.9% cream. *Skin Therapy Lett* 2001; **6**: 1–3, 5.
2 Balfour JA, McClellan K. Topical eflornithine. *Am J Clin Dermatol* 2001; **2**: 197–201.

Dithranol

Dithranol (anthralin) [1] is a time-honoured topical treatment for psoriasis, similar in its irritating and staining properties to chrysarobin, which it supplanted in the early 20th century, but more effective. It is used in ointments, pastes, creams and as a pomade for use on the scalp.

The mechanism of action of dithranol is still uncertain. It inhibits glycolytic enzymes *in vitro* [2]. Reactive oxygen species are generated during auto-oxidation of dithranol [3] and these may inhibit mitochondrial function [4]. It has been suggested that enzyme inactivation may result from lipid peroxidation, leading to cross-linkage of enzyme proteins [5]. *In vitro* studies with human skin showed decreased oxygen consumption and inhibition of the pentose phosphate shunt [6]. The level of cyclic guanosine monophosphate is known to be increased in psoriasis. Dithranol has been shown to restore cyclic nucleosides in skin to normal levels [7]. It induces a marked antiproliferative effect [8,9].

The use of dithranol has proved remarkably safe. Staining of the skin and of other materials is certainly inconvenient although, as a result, the appearance of the skin provides a reliable guide to compliance (Fig. 75.7). Local reactions are common and irritation of normal skin accidentally contaminated with dithranol can be severe (Fig. 75.8). However, there is no evidence of systemic toxicity and it is not considered to be carcinogenic.

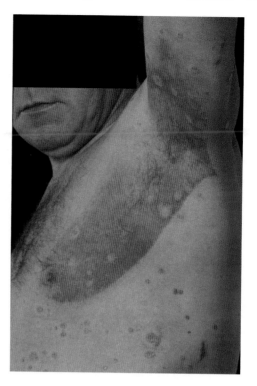

Fig. 75.8 An irritant reaction following accidental contamination of normal skin with dithranol.

Dithranol, especially when incorporated in zinc oxide, is slowly oxidized by alkaline impurities to an inactive pink anthrone [10]. The effect of salicylic acid in preventing this has been known for a long time [11–13]. Salicylic acid neutralizes hydroxyl ions in an alkaline medium, and perhaps reacts with free zinc ions to form an inactive zinc–dithranol complex. It has been found that zinc ions and salicylic acid, like dithranol itself, inhibit glucose-6-phosphate dehydrogenase, thus further justifying the time-honoured combination of these three agents [6]. The combination of tar with dithranol is said to reduce dithranol irritancy without inhibiting therapeutic effect [14]. The use of a water-soluble antioxidant, ascorbic acid, has allowed the production of stable dithranol cream preparations [10]. These are not as therapeutically potent as equivalent strengths of pastes or ointments but show much greater patient acceptability for home usage [15]. The development of lipid-encapsulated cream formulations also seems likely to increase acceptability by further reducing staining and irritation [16,17].

Short-contact applications of strong dithranol pastes or creams are known to be almost as effective as prolonged contact and facilitate treatment on an outpatient basis and self-treatment at home [18–20].

Dithranol has also been used to stimulate an inflammatory response and regrowth of hair in patients with alopecia areata [21], and for the treatment of warts [22].

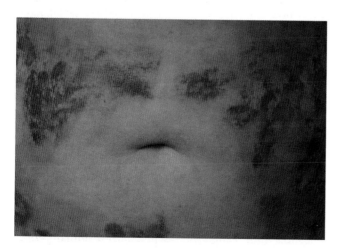

Fig. 75.7 Staining of the skin resulting from dithranol treatment.

REFERENCES

1 Shroot B, Schaefer J, Juhlin L. Editorial. Anthralin: the challenge. *Br J Dermatol* 1981; **105** (Suppl. 20): 3–5.

2 Rassner G. Enzymaktivitätshemmung *in vitro* durch Dithranol (Cignolin). *Arch Dermatol Res* 1972; **243**: 47–51.

3 Muller K. Antipsoriatic anthrones: aspects of oxygen radical formation, challenges and prospects. *Gen Pharmacol* 1996; **27**: 1325–35.

4 Fuchs J, Zimmer G, Wolbling RH, Milbradt R. On the interaction between anthralin and mitochondria: a revision. *Arch Dermatol Res* 1986; **279**: 59–65.

5 Diezel W, Mefferth H, Sonnichsen N. Untersuchungen zum Wirkungsmechanismus von Dithranol: Erhöhte Lipidperoxidation und Enzymhemmung. *Dermatologica* 1975; **150**: 154–62.

6 Raab WP. Dithranol (anthralin) versus triacetoxyanthracene. *Br J Dermatol* 1976; **95**: 193–6.

7 Saihan EM, Albano J, Burton JL. The effect of steroid and dithranol therapy on cyclic nucleotides in psoriasis epidermis. *Br J Dermatol* 1980; **102**: 565–9.

8 Swinkels OQ, Prins M, Gerritsen MJ *et al.* An immunohistochemical assessment of the response of the psoriatic lesion to single and repeated applications of high-dose dithranol cream. *Skin Pharmacol Appl Skin Physiol* 2002; **15**: 393–400.

9 Fisher LB, Maibach HI. The effect of anthralin and its derivatives on epidermal cell kinetics. *J Invest Dermatol* 1975; **64**: 338–41.

10 Whitefield M. Pharmaceutical formulations of anthralin. *Br J Dermatol* 1981; **105** (Suppl. 20): 28–32.

11 Luckacs S, Braun-Falco O. Uber das Verhalten von Dithranol (Cignolin) in Pasten und Lösungen und seine Beeingflussbarkeit durch Salicylsäure. *Hautarzt* 1973; **24**: 304–9.

12 Ponec-Waelsh M, Hulsebotsch HJ. Further studies on the interaction between anthralin, salicylic acid and zinc oxide in pastes. *Arch Dermatol Res* 1974; **249**: 141–52.

13 Raab WP, Gmeiner B. The inhibition of glucose-6-phosphate dehydrogenase activity by dithranol (anthralin), zinc ions/or salicylic acid. *Arch Dermatol Res* 1974; **251**: 87–94.

14 Schulz HJ, Schander S, Mahrle G *et al.* Combined tar-anthralin versus anthralin treatment lowers irritancy with unchanged antipsoriatic efficacy. *J Am Acad Dermatol* 1987; **17**: 19–24.

15 Wilson PD, Ive FA. Dithrocream in psoriasis. *Br J Dermatol* 1980; **103**: 105–6.

16 Thune P, Brolund L. Short- and long-contact therapy using a new dithranol formulation in individually adjusted dosages in the management of psoriasis. *Acta Derm Venereol Suppl* 1992; **172**: 28–9.

17 Agarwal R, Saraswat A, Kaur I *et al.* A novel liposomal formulation of dithranol for psoriasis: preliminary results. *J Dermatol* 2002; **29**: 529–32.

18 Runne V, Kunze J. Short duration ('minutes') therapy with dithranol for psoriasis: a new out-patient regimen. *Br J Dermatol* 1982; **106**: 135–9.

19 Runne V, Kunze J. Minute therapy of psoriasis with dithranol and its modifications: a critical evaluation based on 315 patients. *Hautarzt* 1985; **36**: 40–6.

20 Ryatt KS, Statham BN, Rowell NR. Short-contact modification of the Ingram regime. *Br J Dermatol* 1984; **111**: 455–9.

21 Fiedler-Weiss VC, Buys CM. Evaluation of anthralin in the treatment of alopecia areata. *Arch Dermatol* 1987; **123**: 1491–3.

22 Flindt-Hansen H, Tikjob G, Brandrup F. Wart treatment with anthralin. *Acta Derm Venereol (Stockh)* 1984; **64**: 177–9.

Emollients

The word emollient is derived from the Latin verb *mollire*, to soften. The term is used by dermatologists to denote materials that soften and moisturize the surface of the skin. Most of the formulations used as emollients are creams, ointments, bath oils or soap substitutes. Emollient creams and ointments are formulated using the various materials described earlier in this chapter as constituents of vehicles and are essentially vehicles without a drug to deliver. They are applied to the skin purely to take advantage of their physical properties (protecting, lubricating and moisturizing effects). The efficacy of an emollient is not related to the cost, although this may have some impact on cosmetic acceptability. The most effective emollient is probably white soft paraffin (petrolatum).

The value of bath oils is not well established, although these are widely used in the UK. Most contain lipids such as liquid paraffin, which probably help reduce the drying effect of bathing by protecting the stratum corneum with a layer of lipid. Some also contain antiseptics and antipruritic compounds which can be of additional value. The use of bath oils is best avoided for elderly patients as they tend to make the bath slippery.

The use of soaps on inflamed skin, especially in atopic dermatitis, is generally considered harmful and likely to exacerbate damage to the stratum corneum [1,2]. Compounds used as soap substitutes are lipid materials containing emulsifiers such as Aqueous Cream BP or Emulsifying Ointment BP. Most emollient creams can be used in this way. These can effectively remove lipid-soluble dirt and contamination from the skin surface while avoiding the damage done to the stratum corneum by irritant surfactants. Patients with dry skin conditions report that soap substitutes improve the condition of the skin [3]. Paradoxically, the introduction of washing with common toilet soap was accompanied by improvement in atopic dermatitis in one study [4], possibly reflecting increased compliance with other aspects of treatment.

REFERENCES

1 Van der Valk PGM, Nater JP, Bleumink E. Vulnerability of the skin to surfactants in different groups of eczema patients and controls as measured by water vapour loss. *Clin Exp Dermatol* 1985; **10**: 98–103.

2 White MI, McEwan Jenkinson D, Lloyd DH. The effect of washing on the thickness of the stratum corneum in normal and atopic individuals. *Br J Dermatol* 1987; **116**: 525–30.

3 Berth-Jones J, Graham-Brown RAC. How useful are soap substitutes? *J Dermatol Treat* 1992; **3**: 9–11.

4 Uehara M, Takada K. Use of soap in the management of atopic dermatitis. *Clin Exp Dermatol* 1985; **10**: 419–25.

Immunomodulators

SYN. CALCINEURIN INHIBITORS

Several topical medications alter immune responses, but are discussed elsewhere in this chapter—for example, corticosteroids or imiquimod, which is viewed as an immune response modulator. This section considers the calcineurin inhibitors.

These compounds have been developed for topical treatment of atopic dermatitis but seem likely to find numerous additional applications. There are currently two agents, tacrolimus and pimecrolimus, available in this class and others are likely to follow. The mechanism of action is similar to that of ciclosporin. Lymphocyte activation is suppressed by inhibition of calcineurin, a calcium- and calmodulin-dependent serine/threonine phosphatase. This cytoplasmic enzyme activates the

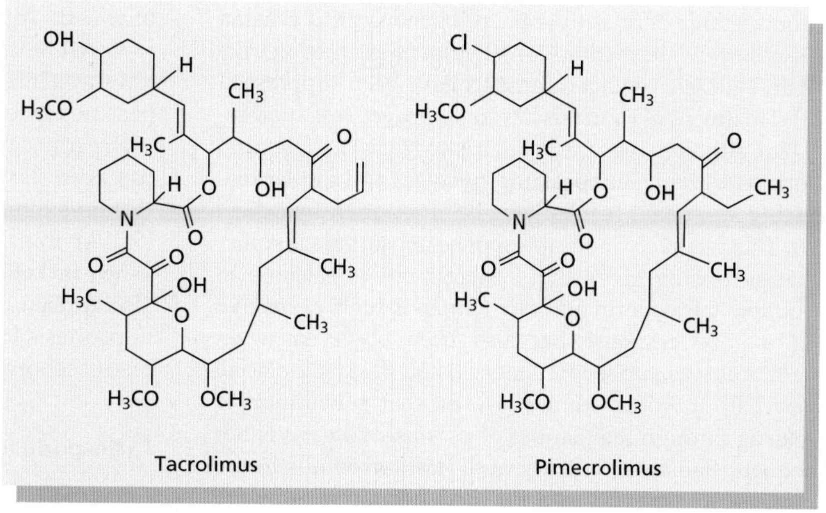

Fig. 75.9 The structures of tacrolimus and pimecrolimus.

nuclear factor of activated T cells (NFAT), a transcription factor regulating numerous lymphokines in both Th1 and Th2 lymphocyte subsets, and constitutes an important link in signal transduction from the T-cell receptor to the nucleus [1]. Similar mechanisms operating in other cell types, including mast cells [2,3], antigen-presenting cells [4] and keratinocytes [5], may provide additional targets for these drugs. In contrast to ciclosporin, these molecules have a sufficiently low molecular weight to penetrate the stratum corneum, at least when barrier function is impaired as is the case in atopic dermatitis. They are therefore active when applied topically. Both compounds have been under investigation in clinical trials for over 9 years now. A notable advantage of these agents is that they do not induce cutaneous atrophy [6,7], even with long-term regular application [8–10], and it is therefore possible to apply them to facial and flexural areas where prolonged use of topical corticosteroids causes concern. Theoretically, the local immunosuppression related to these compounds could increase the risks of infections and neoplasia. In the numerous trials on atopic dermatitis, infections have not been more frequent than expected. The risk of neoplasia also remains theoretical.

Tacrolimus

Tacrolimus (FK-506) is a macrolide lactam antibiotic (macrolactam) discovered in Japan where it was first isolated from a soil fungus, *Streptomyces tsukubaensis*. It has been used systemically in transplantation for over 15 years and is known to be effective, used systemically, in treatment of psoriasis [11]. It has a molecular weight of 822 Da and a complex structure (Fig. 75.9). The efficacy of tacrolimus in atopic dermatitis has been demonstrated in several placebo-controlled trials in both adults [12,13] and

children [14,15]. In comparative trials, tacrolimus ointment 0.1% applied twice daily is comparable in efficacy to potent topical corticosteroids such as hydrocortisone butyrate 0.1% [16] and betamethasone valerate 0.12% ointment [17]. It is been more effective than hydrocortisone acetate 1% ointment in children [15] and was more effective than the moderately potent alclometasone dipropionate 0.1% ointment in treatment of eczema on the face and neck in adults [18]. In children, a lower concentration of 0.03% tacrolimus has proved nearly as effective as 0.1% [14,15], while in adults there is a more marked difference between these concentrations and 0.1% is clearly more effective [16,19]. The most frequently encountered side effect is a burning sensation lasting for a few minutes after application. This tends to resolve after a few days and is rarely of sufficient severity to require withdrawal of the treatment. Systemic exposure is low and drug levels in blood are usually too low to measure [14,20,21]. Using data obtained from application of 0.3% tacrolimus ointment, systemic bioavailability has been estimated at 0.5% of that obtained by intravenous administration [21]. It is therefore unlikely that topical application of tacrolimus will exhibit systemic activity. Furthermore, systemic exposure tends to fall as the eczema improves, indicating that penetration of the drug is reduced as barrier function is restored [22].

Additional applications for topical tacrolimus have currently been less formally investigated and it should be noted, in particular, that extensive safety data relating to systemic exposure are available only for atopic dermatitis. The use of topical tacrolimus in Netherton's syndrome (ichthyosis linearis circumflexa) can result in clinically significant systemic exposure to the drug [23], indicating that some care is required.

Reports indicate that topical tacrolimus is effective in

treatment of several other varieties of eczema including chronic actinic dermatitis [24], endogenous hand eczema [25] and eyelid dermatitis [26]. In a guinea pig model, irritant and allergic contact dermatitis have been suppressed [27]. Treatment of psoriasis has so far proved less successful [28], although the author has treated facial and flexural psoriasis with unequivocal improvement and similar reasonably successful results have been reported by others [29]. This relatively modest response in psoriasis is somewhat surprising given that systemic use of calcineurin inhibitors (ciclosporin and tacrolimus) is highly effective and a good response has also been observed when tacrolimus was applied under occlusion in a microplaque assay [30]. It would seem, however, that penetration of the drug through the plaques of psoriasis vulgaris is not adequate. Sadly, the efficacy of topical tacrolimus in the Dundee experimental bald rat model of alopecia areata [31] has not so far been reproduced in the treatment of human cases of this disease. Development of a more appropriate formulation might improve results in psoriasis and alopecia areata.

There are more encouraging reports of efficacy of topical tacrolimus in a variety of other dermatoses including oral and genital erosive lichen planus [32–36], pyoderma gangrenosum [37–39], cutaneous graft-versus-host disease [40], rheumatoid leg ulceration [41], cutaneous sarcoidosis [42], steroid-induced rosacea [43], uraemic pruritus [44], vitiligo [45,46], discoid lupus erythematosus [47], eosinophilic folliculitis [48] and epidermolysis bullosa [49]. Oral and perineal lesions of Crohn's disease have responded [50] and topical tacrolimus has been effective in suppression of skin allograft rejection [51]. Improvement has been observed in Netherton's syndrome [23,52], although, as discussed above, significant systemic absorption may occur in this disease. Three cases of erosive pustular dermatosis of the legs responded to topical tacrolimus [53].

Pimecrolimus

Pimecrolimus (SDZ ASM 981) is another macrolactam with a structure similar although not identical to tacrolimus and molecular weight 810 Da (Fig. 75.9). The relatively small differences in structure compared to tacrolimus confer greater lipophilicity but reduce potency. Most of the clinical research on this compound has so far been in atopic dermatitis. Placebo-controlled trials have demonstrated efficacy and safety of pimecrolimus 1% cream in adults [54–56] and children from 3 months of age upward [57,58]. In a comparative study, this treatment was less effective than betamethasone valerate 0.1% cream [55]. Used in long-term studies, pimecrolimus has effectively inhibited flares of the disease and reduced the requirement for topical corticosteroids [56,58]. Systemic absorption of pimecrolimus has been low and usually undetectable

[59,60]. Topical pimecrolimus has been safe and well tolerated. Although a burning sensation is sometimes reported in the treated areas, this usually resolves after a few days. Infections have not been increased and there has been no evidence of increased neoplasia.

Experience with pimecrolimus in other skin diseases has been very limited so far. In animal models, pimecrolimus inhibits induction of contact allergic dermatitis [61]. An initial report suggests that it may suppress established nickel dermatitis [62]. Used systemically [63] and also applied topically under occlusion, it can be effective in psoriasis [64]. A response has also been reported in a case of seborrhoeic dermatitis [65].

Ciclosporin (cyclosporin)

Despite the best endeavours of many investigators over the years to develop topical uses for ciclosporin, this has failed to find any consistently useful role. Ciclosporin has a high molecular weight of 1202 Da and this is probably the reason why it does not penetrate through the skin in sufficient concentration to be effective. Early reports of efficacy in oral erosive lichen planus may have been the result of significant systemic absorption. A controlled study using triamcinolone as comparator found no difference between the treatments and the improvement observed was only modest [66].

REFERENCES

1 Ruzicka T, Assmann T, Homey B. Tacrolimus: the drug for the turn of the millenium? *Arch Dermatol* 1999; **135**: 574–80.
2 De Paulis A, Stellato C, Cirillo R et al. Anti-inflammatory effect of FK-506 on human skin mast cells. *J Invest Dermatol* 1992; **99**: 723–8.
3 Zuberbier T, Chong S-U, Grunow K et al. The ascomycin macrolactam pimecrolimus (Elidel, SDZ ASM 981) is a potent inhibitor of mediator release from human dermal mast cells and peripheral blood basophils. *J Allergy Clin Immunol* 2001; **108**: 275–80.
4 Wollenberg A, Sharma S, von Bubnoff D et al. Topical tacrolimus (FK506) leads to profound phenotypic and functional alterations of epidermal antigen-presenting dendritic cells in atopic dermatitis. *J Allergy Clin Immunol* 2001; **107**: 519–25.
5 Al-Daraji WI, Grant KR, Ryan K, Saxton A, Reynolds NJ. Localization of calcineurin/NFAT in human skin and psoriasis and inhibition of calcineurin/NFAT activation in human keratinocytes by cyclosporin A. *J Invest Dermatol* 2002; **118**: 779–88.
6 Reitamo S, Rissanen J, Remitz A et al. Tacrolimus ointment does not affect collagen synthesis: results of a single-centre randomized trial. *J Invest Dermatol* 1998; **111**: 396–8.
7 Queille-Roussel C, Paul C, Duteil L et al. The new topical ascomycin derivative SDZ ASM 981 does not induce skin atrophy when applied to normal skin for 4 weeks: a randomized, double-blind controlled study. *Br J Dermatol* 2001; **144**: 507–13.
8 Kapp A, Papp K, Bingham A et al. Long-term management of atopic dermatitis in infants with topical pimecrolimus, a non-steroid anti-inflammatory drug: flare reduction in eczema with Elidel (infants) multicenter investigator study group. *J Allergy Clin Immunol* 2002; **110**: 277–84.
9 Wahn U, Bos JD, Goodfield M et al. Efficacy and safety of pimecrolimus cream in the long-term management of atopic dermatitis in children. *Pediatrics* 2002: **110**: e2.
10 Kang S, Lucky AW, Pariser D et al. Long-term safety and efficacy of tacrolimus ointment for the treatment of atopic dermatitis in children. *J Am Acad Dermatol* 2001; **44**: S58–64.

11 Rappersberger K, Meingassner JG, Fialla R *et al*. Clearing of psoriasis by a novel immunosuppressive macrolide. *J Invest Dermatol* 1996; **106**: 701–10.

12 Nakagawa H, Etoh T, Ishibashi Y *et al*. Tacrolimus ointment for atopic dermatitis. *Lancet* 1994; **344**: 883.

13 Ruzicka T, Bieber T, Schopf E *et al*. A short-term trial of tacrolimus ointment for atopic dermatitis. *N Engl J Med* 1997; **337**: 816–21.

14 Paller A, Eichenfield LF, Leung DY *et al*. A 12-week study of tacrolimus ointment for the treatment of atopic dermatitis in pediatric patients. *J Am Acad Dermatol* 2001; **44** (Suppl. 1): S47–57.

15 Reitamo S, Van Leent EJ, Ho V *et al*. Efficacy and safety of tacrolimus ointment compared with that of hydrocortisone acetate ointment in children with atopic dermatitis. *J Allergy Clin Immunol* 2002; **109**: 539–46.

16 Reitamo S, Rustin M, Ruzicka T *et al*. Efficacy and safety of tacrolimus ointment compared with hydrocortisone butyrate ointment in adult patients with atopic dermatitis. *J Allergy Clin Immunol* 2002; **109**: 547–55.

17 FK-506 Ointment Study Group. Phase III comparative study of FK-506 ointment versus betamethasone valerate ointment in atopic dermatitis of the trunk and extremities. *Nishinihon J Dermatol* 1997; **59**: 870–9.

18 FK-506 Ointment Study Group. Phase III comparative study of FK-506 ointment versus alclometasone dipropionate ointment in atopic dermatitis of the face and neck. *Hifuka Kiyo* 1997; **92**: 277–88.

19 Hanifin JM, Ling MR, Langley R *et al*. Tacrolimus ointment for the treatment of atopic dermatitis in adult patients. I. Efficacy. *J Am Acad Dermatol* 2001; **44** (Suppl. 1): S28–38.

20 Bekersky I, Fitzsimmons W, Tanase A *et al*. Non-clinical and early clinical development of tacrolimus ointment for the treatment of atopic dermatitis. *J Am Acad Dermatol* 2001; **44**: S17–27.

21 Soter NA, Fleischer AB, Webster GF *et al*. Tacrolimus ointment for the treatment of atopic dermatitis in adult patients. II. Safety. *J Am Acad Dermatol* 2001; **44**: S39–46.

22 Alaiti S, Kang S, Fiedler VC *et al*. Tacrolimus (FK506) ointment for atopic dermatitis: a phase I study in adults and children. *J Am Acad Dermatol* 1998; **38**: 69–76.

23 Allen A, Siegfried E, Silverman R *et al*. Significant absorption of topical tacrolimus in three patients with Netherton syndrome. *Arch Dermatol* 2001; **137**: 747–50.

24 Suga Y, Hashimoto Y, Matsuba S *et al*. Topical tacrolimus for chronic actinic dermatitis. *J Am Acad Dermatol* 2002; **46**: 321–3.

25 Schnopp C, Remling R, Mohrenschlager M *et al*. Topical tacrolimus (FK506) and mometasone furoate in treatment of dyshidrotic palmar eczema: a randomized, observer-blinded trial. *J Am Acad Dermatol* 2002; **46**: 73–7.

26 Krupnick A, Clarke J, Fadness D, Singer G, Lebwohl M. Tacrolimus 0.1% ointment in the treatment of eyelid dermatitis. *J Invest Dermatol* 2001; **117**: 533.

27 Lauerma AI, Stein BD, Homey B *et al*. Topical FK506: suppression of allergic and irritant contact dermatitis in the guinea pig. *Arch Dermatol Res* 1994; **286**: 337–40.

28 Zonneveld IM, Rubins A, Jablonska S *et al*. Topical tacrolimus is not effective in chronic plaque psoriasis: a pilot study. *Arch Dermatol* 1998; **134**: 1101–2.

29 Yamamoto T, Nishioka K. Topical tacrolimus is effective for facial lesions of psoriasis. *Acta Derm Venereol* 2000; **80**: 451.

30 Remitz A, Reitamo S, Erkko P *et al*. Tacrolimus ointment improves psoriasis in a microplaque assay. *Br J Dermatol* 1999; **141**: 103–7.

31 McElwee KJ, Rushton DH, Trachy R, Oliver RF. Topical FK506: a potent immunotherapy for alopecia areata? Studies using the Dundee experimental bald rat model. *Br J Dermatol* 1997; **137**: 491–7.

32 Vente C, Reich K, Rupprecht R, Neumann C. Erosive mucosal lichen planus: response to topical treatment with tacrolimus. *Br J Dermatol* 1999; **140**: 338–42.

33 Lener EV, Brieva J, Schachter M *et al*. Successful treatment of erosive lichen planus with topical tacrolimus. *Arch Dermatol* 2001; **137**: 419–22.

34 Rozycki TW, Rogers RS III, Pittelkow MR *et al*. Topical tacrolimus in the treatment of symptomatic oral lichen planus: a series of 13 patients. *J Am Acad Dermatol* 2002; **46**: 27–34.

35 Kaliakatsou F, Hodgson TA, Lewsey JD. Management of recalcitrant ulcerative oral lichen planus with topical tacrolimus. *J Am Acad Dermatol* 2002; **46**: 35–41.

36 Kirtschig G, Van Der Meulen AJ, Ion Lipan JW, Stoof TJ. Successful treatment of erosive vulvovaginal lichen planus with topical tacrolimus. *Br J Dermatol* 2002; **147**: 625–6.

37 Reich K, Vente C, Neumann C. Topical tacrolimus for pyoderma gangrenosum. *Br J Dermatol* 1998; **139**: 755–7.

38 Jolles S, Niclasse S, Benson E. Combination oral and topical tacrolimus in therapy-resistant pyoderma gangrenosum. *Br J Dermatol* 1999; **140**: 564–5.

39 Lyon CC, Stapleton M, Smith AJ *et al*. Topical tacrolimus in the management of peristomal pyoderma gangrenosum. *J Dermatol Trea* 2001; **12**: 13–7.

40 Choi CJ, Nghiem P. Tacrolimus ointment in the treatment of chronic cutaneous graft-vs-host disease: a case series of 18 patients. *Arch Dermatol* 2001; **137**: 1202–6.

41 Schuppe H, Richter-Hintz D, Stierle HE *et al*. Topical tacrolimus for recalcitrant leg ulcer in rheumatoid arthritis. *Rheumatology (Oxford)* 2000; **39**: 105–6.

42 Katoh N, Mihara H, Yasuno H. Cutaneous sarcoidosis successfully treated with topical tacrolimus. *Br J Dermatol* 2002; **147**: 154–6.

43 Goldman D. Tacrolimus ointment for the treatment of steroid-induced rosacea: a preliminary report. *J Am Acad Dermatol* 2001; **44**: 995–8.

44 Pauli-Magnus C, Klumpp S, Alscher DM *et al*. Short-term efficacy of tacrolimus ointment in severe uremic pruritus. *Perit Dial Int* 2000; **20**: 802–3.

45 Grimes PE, Soriano T, Dytoc MT. Topical tacrolimus for repigmentation of vitiligo. *J Am Acad Dermatol* 2002; **47**: 789–91.

46 Smith DA, Tofte SJ, Hanifin JM. Repigmentation of vitiligo with topical tacrolimus. *Dermatology* 2002; **205**: 301–3.

47 Walker SL, Kirby B, Chalmers RJ. The effect of topical tacrolimus on severe recalcitrant chronic discoid lupus erythematosus. *Br J Dermatol* 2002; **147**: 405–6.

48 Dale S, Shaw J. Clinical picture: eosinophilic pustular folliculitis. *Lancet* 2000; **356**: 1235.

49 Carroll PB, Rilo HL, Abu Elmagd K *et al*. Effect of tacrolimus (FK506) in dystrophic epidermolysis bullosa: rationale and preliminary results. *Arch Dermatol* 1994; **130**: 1457–8.

50 Casson DH, Eltumi M, Tomlin S *et al*. Topical tacrolimus may be effective in the treatment of oral and perineal Crohn's disease. *Gut* 2000; **47**: 436–40.

51 Yuzawa K, Taniguchi H, Seino K *et al*. Topical immunosuppression in skin grafting with FK506 ointment. *Transplant Proc* 1996; **28**: 137–9.

52 Suga Y, Tsuboi R, Hashimoto Y *et al*. A case of ichthyosis linearis circumflexa successfully treated with topical tacrolimus. *Arch Dermatol* 2000; **42**: 520–2.

53 Brouard MC, Prins C, Chavaz P *et al*. Erosive pustular dermatosis of the leg: report of three cases. *Br J Dermatol* 2002; **147**: 765–9.

54 Van Leent EJM, Graber M, Thurston M *et al*. Effectiveness of the ascomycin macrolactam SDZ ASM 981 in the topical treatment of atopic dermatitis. *Arch Dermatol* 1998; **134**: 805–9.

55 Luger T, Van Leent EJ, Graeber M *et al*. SDZ ASM 981: an emerging safe and effective treatment for atopic dermatitis. *Br J Dermatol* 2001; **144**: 788–94.

56 Meurer M, Folster-Holst R, Wozel G *et al*. Pimecrolimus cream in the long-term management of atopic dermatitis in adults: a 6-month study. *Dermatology* 2002; **205**: 271–7.

57 Eichenfield LF, Lucky AW, Boguniewicz M *et al*. Safety and efficacy of pimecrolimus (ASM 981) cream 1% in the treatment of mild and moderate atopic dermatitis in children and adolescents. *J Am Acad Dermatol* 2002; **46**: 495–504.

58 Kapp A, Papp K, Bingham A *et al*. Long-term management of atopic dermatitis in infants with topical pimecrolimus, a non-steroid anti-inflammatory drug. *J Allergy Clin Immunol* 2002; **110**: 277–84.

59 Harper J, Green A, Scott G *et al*. First experience of topical SDZ ASM 981 in children with atopic dermatitis. *Br J Dermatol* 2001; **144**: 781–7.

60 Van Leent EJM, Ebelin M-E, Burtin P *et al*. Low systemic exposure after repeated topical application of pimecrolimus (Elidel®, SDZ ASM (981) in patients with atopic dermatitis. *Dermatology* 2002; **204**: 63–8.

61 Meingassner JG, Grassberger M, Fahrngruber H *et al*. A novel anti-inflammatory drug, SDZ ASM 981, for the topical and oral treatment of skin diseases: *in vivo* pharmacology. *Br J Dermatol* 1997; **137**: 568–76.

62 Queille-Roussel C, Graeber M, Thurston M *et al*. SDZ ASM 981 is the first non-steroid that suppresses established nickel contact dermatitis elicited by allergen challenge. *Contact Dermatitis* 2000; **42**: 349–50.

63 Rappersberger K, Komar M, Ebelin ME *et al*. Pimecrolimus identifies a common genomic anti-inflammatory profile, is clinically highly effective in psoriasis and is well tolerated. *J Invest Dermatol* 2002; **119**: 876–87.

64 Mrowietz U, Graeber M, Brautigam M *et al*. The novel ascomycin derivative SDZ ASM 981 is effective for psoriasis when used topically under occlusion. *Br J Dermatol* 1998; **139**: 992–6.

65 Crutchfield CE III. Pimecrolimus: a new treatment for seborrheic dermatitis. *Cutis* 2002; **70**: 207–8.

66 Sieg P, Von Domarus H, Von Zitzewitz V *et al*. Topical cyclosporin in oral lichen planus: a controlled, randomized, prospective trial. *Br J Dermatol* 1995; **132**: 790–4.

Retinoids

The retinoids can be defined either as compounds related structurally to retinol (vitamin A) or as compounds that are able to interact with retinoid receptors. The latter definition has become more useful as an increasing number of synthetic 'retinoids' are developed with diverse structures. Topical retinoic acid has been used in treatment of acne vulgaris for over three decades. During this period much has been learned about the fundamental part played by endogenous retinoids in the regulation of cell differentiation and proliferation and about the mechanisms involved. Retinoids are now used for many indications including psoriasis, photo-ageing and numerous disorders of keratinization as well as for suppression of dysplasia and malignancy.

The activity of endogenous retinoids within the cell is regulated by binding proteins known as cellular retinol binding proteins (CRBP I and II), and cellular retinoic acid binding proteins (CRABP I and II). These proteins are widely distributed throughout the body in many cell types. CRABP II predominates in skin, and is found in keratinocytes and fibroblasts [1]. This protein is up-regulated by retinoic acid [2] and by other compounds demonstrating retinoid activity, and is believed to have a role in regulating the availability of free retinoic acid within the cell.

Within the nucleus, retinoids bind to specific receptors, retinoic acid receptors (RAR α, β and γ) and retinoid X receptors (RXR α, β and γ). Alternative splicing of each of these receptors generates further diversity (the subtypes being known as RAR-α1, RAR-α2, etc.) [3]. All-*trans* retinoic acid is the endogenous ligand for the RARs while 9-*cis* retinoic acid is the endogenous ligand for the RXRs. The receptors most abundantly expressed in the epidermis are RAR-γ and RXR-α, while RAR-α and RXR-β are present at relatively low levels. These receptors bind to specific elements of DNA, known as response elements, within the regulatory regions of numerous genes and this interaction may increase or decrease transcription of the gene. There are usually several such response elements involved in regulating the transcription of any single gene. The retinoid receptors are mainly active as heterodimers of RXR and RAR. RXRs can also dimerize with several other similar receptors such as the vitamin D receptor, the thyroid receptor and orphan receptors (which have no established endogenous ligand). This range of different receptors and their dimers, the various possible states of binding with different ligands and the wide range of different response elements allows for the highly diverse and complex signalling required to regulate cellular metabolism. The end result of these processes acting on numerous different genes is that retinoids demonstrate a tendency to normalize keratinocyte differentiation in diverse circumstances where this is disturbed.

Metabolism of retinoids takes place within keratinocytes. The initial step is usually 4-hydroxylation by cytochrome P-450 enzyme systems, such as CYP 2S1 and CYP 26, which can be induced by their substrate and may show considerable interindividual variation [4]. This variation may explain some of the variability between individuals in responses to topical retinoids.

Systemic retinoids are known to be highly teratogenic when administered in doses sufficient to induce the mucocutaneous symptoms associated with hypervitaminosis A. This has led to some concern about the potential for the topical application of retinoids to exert teratogenic effects. Fortunately, this risk is entirely hypothetical. Systemic exposure to retinoids applied topically seems to be minimal [5,6], but it is generally recommended that even the topical use of retinoids should be avoided during pregnancy.

The naturally occurring 'endogenous' retinoids include retinol, which is metabolized within most cells, including keratinocytes, to retinoic acid. This process seems to be regulated by a variety of mechanisms so that the level of free retinoic acid is tightly controlled. Retinoic acid can isomerize to 13-*cis* and 9-*cis* retinoic acid, a process that occurs readily in the presence of visible light.

The synthetic retinoids currently used in the topical treatment of skin disease are adapalene, bexarotene and tazarotene. All these compounds are effectively absorbed into the epidermis when applied topically.

Retinol
SYN. VITAMIN A

Retinol is used widely in cosmetic products and tends to be regarded as a vitamin supplement rather than a medicament in this context. However, it is clear that retinol applied topically to the skin is absorbed into the epidermis and exhibits many of the pharmacological properties of retinoic acid. Topical application of retinol increases levels of retinyl esters within the epidermis [7]. These are esters of retinol with long-chain fatty acids which constitute an intracellular reservoir of inactive retinol. Esterification of retinol is induced by retinoic acid and this probably represents an autoregulatory mechanism that inhibits excess synthesis of retinoic acid [8]. In addition, topically applied retinol induces 4-hydroxylase activity, and thus increases metabolism and inactivation of retinoic acid [9]. Levels of CRABP II and CRBP are also induced by topical application of retinol [7].

Retinol increases epidermal thickness in a manner similar to retinoic acid but causes much less irritation [7,10]. Retinol 10% gel has been used as a component of a depigmenting regimen with results considered comparable to those obtained from retinoic acid. However, this high concentration was irritant [11].

Retinoic acid

SYN. TRETINOIN; ALL-*TRANS*-RETINOIC ACID; VITAMIN A ACID

Retinoic acid is well absorbed into the skin when applied topically and exerts potent local effects on cellular metabolism. This is the endogenous ligand for the RARs. Isomerization of retinoic acid results in formation of 13-*cis* and 9-*cis* retinoic acid [12], the latter being the naturally occurring ligand for the RXRs. These isomerizations are accelerated in visible light.

Retinoic acid is most frequently used in treatment of acne vulgaris. It is normally applied once or twice daily at a concentration of 0.01–0.025% in a lotion, cream or gel. Higher concentrations (e.g. 0.1%) have often been used in the past. It is particularly effective in reducing comedones [13,14] and is therefore often used in cases where these non-inflammatory lesions are prominent. It may cause some initial exacerbation of the symptoms for the first 6 weeks of treatment. During this period comedones are expelled and then prevented from reforming if its use is continued. Inflammatory lesions of acne are also reduced, possibly as a secondary event following the reduction in comedones. Irritant reactions are common and may even accelerate the response. However, neither erythema nor peeling is essential for response to be achieved [15]. The irritation can be managed by reducing the concentration or frequency of application. Topical retinoic acid is also effective for treatment of comedonal acne induced by systemic corticosteroids [16].

Topical retinoic acid improves several features of photo-ageing including fine and coarse wrinkling, and dyspigmentation [17]. The clinical improvement is accompanied by reversal of epidermal atrophy and dysplasia, and increasing collagen synthesis in the papillary dermis [18]. Similar effects can also be induced in intrinsically aged skin [19]. Treatment may need to be applied daily for 4 months or more to achieve these effects. A formulation containing 0.05% retinoic acid in an emollient cream base is marketed specifically for treatment of photo-ageing. Lower concentrations can also be effective [20].

Tretinoin has both a therapeutic and prophylactic effect on chemically induced skin tumours, and may be both a promoter and inhibitor of UVB carcinogenesis. Clinically, it exhibits an antineoplastic effect, and may be used to treat small solar keratoses either alone [21] or in combination with 5% 5-FU cream [22]. It also has a 'normalizing' effect on the histological appearance of dysplastic naevi [23].

Despite theoretical mechanisms and early claims that it could be effective, topical application of retinoic acid has not found a role in the treatment of psoriasis.

Retinoic acid can be effective in reducing various forms of hyperpigmentation (see depigmenting agents above).

Another interesting property of tretinoin is its ability to accelerate wound healing [24]. It needs to be applied before wounding, preferably for several weeks. Results of application after wounding have not been consistent, probably because of the irritant effect. The ability of retinoic acid to promote healing has been used to improve results from procedures such as chemical peeling [25] and dermabrasion [26].

A number of other conditions have been treated with topical retinoic acid with varying success. It is of value in the treatment of senile comedones [27]. Comedo and warty naevi may show some response, as may plane warts and reactive perforating collagenosis. Some cases of Darier's disease respond, especially if mild or localized [28]. Keratosis pilaris was reported to respond by eight of 49 respondents in a patient survey [29]. Of the ichthyoses, the lamellar variety appears to be helped most, although ichthyosis vulgaris was also responsive in a four-centre trial [30], as was erythrokeratoderma variabilis [31]. It can be useful in oral lichen planus [32], and in geographic tongue [33]. Fox–Fordyce disease (apocrine miliaria) has been effectively treated with a 0.1% solution [34]. Hydrocortisone cream (1%) has been recommended to control the associated axillary discomfort [35]. Hypertrophic scars and keloids have been reported to respond to a daily application of a 0.05% solution [36,37].

Although sensitization to retinoic acid has been reported this seems to be a rare event [38].

Isotretinoin

SYN. 13-*CIS* RETINOIC ACID

Isotretinoin is readily isomerized to tretinoin and vice versa. It therefore exhibits a similar receptor specificity to tretinoin, interacting with RARs. Isotretinoin is used both topically and systemically for treatment of acne vulgaris. When used topically it is considered somewhat less irritant than tretinoin but may be more so than adapalene [39]. The efficacy of isotretinoin 0.05% gel in acne vulgaris has been confirmed in comparison with placebo [40], and seems similar to that of retinoic acid [41]. In a trial comparing topical isotretinoin with benzoyl peroxide, the latter treatment improved inflammatory lesions more rapidly, although both comedones and inflammatory lesions eventually responded to a similar degree [42]. Topical isotretinoin is believed to work mainly by inhibiting comedogenesis, although it is also known to penetrate into sebaceous glands [43] and may reduce sebum secretion [44].

Isotretinoin cream does not appear effective in treatment of chronic plaque psoriasis [45]. However, it shares with tretinoin the ability to reduce features of photoageing [46,47]. It also demonstrates antineoplastic properties. A limited degree of response is seen in treatment of actinic keratoses when applied twice at a concentration of 0.1% for up to 24 weeks [48], and a degree of efficacy was shown in a trial on topical treatment of BCC although complete regression was only observed in four out of 50 cases treated [49].

In isolated reports, topical isotretinoin has proved helpful in treatment of perifolliculitis capitis abscedens et suffodiens [50], oral [51] and vulval [52] leukoplakia, oral lichen planus [53], hyperkeratosis of the nipple [54] and actinic granuloma [55]. It has not proved effective in melasma [56]. In treatment of Darier's disease, isotretinoin can prove helpful in treatment of small areas of hyperkeratosis but is also irritant [57,58].

Adapalene

Adapalene is a synthetic retinoid that has been developed for treatment of acne vulgaris. In randomized comparative trials, adapalene gel 0.1% has proved equally effective and better tolerated than retinoic acid gel 0.025% [39]. In comparison with topical isotretinoin, adapalene was slightly more effective and less irritant [59,60]. Adapalene appears to retain comedolytic activity while showing less potential for irritancy than retinoic acid. It exhibits specificity for RAR-β and -γ receptors with low affinity for RAR-α relative to retinoic acid [61]. It is highly lipophilic, a property likely to enhance efficacy by increasing penetration of the hair follicle. In addition, adapalene has anti-inflammatory properties that may improve both efficacy and tolerability [61]. Formulations available are cream, aqueous gel, lotion and single use pledgets, all containing 0.1% adapalene.

Bexarotene

Bexarotene is a novel synthetic retinoid with specificity for RXRs. Compounds with this pattern of receptor specificity are sometimes called rexinoids. It has proved helpful in the treatment of cutaneous T-cell lymphoma and can be used orally as well as topically in this indication. In a study on early (plaque stage) cutaneous T-cell lymphoma, topical treatment with bexarotene gel in concentrations ranging up to 1% applied up to four times daily achieved complete clinical clearance in 21% of cases and partial response in a further 42% [62]. The median time to response was 20 weeks. Topical bexarotene is produced as a 1% gel formulation. Treatment is usually commenced cautiously with applications on alternate days and gradually stepped up to four times daily [63].

Tazarotene

Tazarotene is a synthetic retinoid. It is a pro-drug that is rapidly hydrolysed to its active form, tazarotenic acid. The molecule has a rigid structure, in contrast to that of retinoic acid which can undergo conformational changes. Tazarotene exhibits a degree of receptor specificity, interacting with RAR-α, -β and -γ. The latter receptor is likely to be most important in the epidermis. Tazarotene does not bind to RXRs and, unlike retinoic acid, it is not susceptible to isomerization into a conformation that might do so [64].

It has been developed mainly for treatment of psoriasis and acne vulgaris. It is also known to be effective in treatment of psoriasis when administered orally.

The efficacy of topical tazarotene in psoriasis has been established in placebo-controlled trials, around 65% of patients showing 50% or greater improvement after 12 weeks of treatment with 0.1% tazarotene gel once daily [65]. In more recent studies investigating a cream formulation, 39–51% of patients were reported to experience clinical success after application of 0.1% tazarotene cream once daily for 12 weeks [66]. In a comparative study, the global improvement on 0.1% tazarotene gel applied once daily was slightly less than that obtained from 0.05% fluocinonide cream applied twice daily. In all these trials, and in contrast to fluocinonide, the response to tazarotene was notably well maintained during the 12 weeks after treatment was stopped [67]. Psoriatic onycholysis and nail pitting were improved by tazarotene in a small controlled trial [68]. Irritant reactions at the application site are common so tazarotene is sometimes used in conjunction with a topical corticosteroid. It has also been used with phototherapy. There are isolated reports of severe genital ulceration [69] and of pyogenic granuloma developing during topical treatment of psoriasis with tazarotene. The latter is a well-recognized side effect associated with systemic retinoids [70].

Tazarotene 0.1% gel has been shown to be effective in acne vulgaris in a placebo-controlled trial even when applied once daily for short contact periods of 30 s to 5 min [71]. In comparison with tretinoin in a 0.1% microsponge gel, tazarotene 0.1% gel proved more effective. The tolerability of the two treatments was considered comparable [72]. In a comparative study using once daily applications, tazarotene 0.1% gel proved more effective than adapalene 0.1% gel although it was also slightly more irritant [73].

Tazarotene seems to share with retinoic acid the ability to improve photo-ageing. In a trial of 1 year treatment duration, 0.1% tazarotene cream applied once daily significantly improved several features of photo-aged skin [74].

In small trials, tazarotene 0.1% gel was effective in management of oral lichen planus [75], and an O/W emulsion containing 0.01% tazarotene applied each night for up to 8 weeks proved helpful in keratosis pilaris [76]. In single cases or small series, useful responses to topical application of tazarotene have been reported in lamellar ichthyosis [77–79], X-linked ichthyosis and ichthyosis vulgaris [78], confluent and reticulate papillomatosis [80], elastosis perforans serpiginosa [81], Darier's disease [82,83] and warty dyskeratoma [84], pseudoacanthosis nigricans [85], spiny keratoderma [86], keratoderma blenorrhagica [87] and discoid lupus erythematosus [88].

Tazarotene is produced in gel and cream formulations at concentrations of 0.1 and 0.05%. The higher concentration appears more effective in psoriasis but also more irritant. In treatment of acne, the higher concentration is used most frequently.

REFERENCES

1 Astrom A, Tavakkol A, Pettersson U et al. Molecular cloning of two human cellular retinoic acid-binding proteins (CRABP). Retinoic acid-induced expression of CRABP-II but not CRABP-I in adult human skin *in vivo* and in skin fibroblasts *in vitro*. *J Biol Chem* 1991; **266**: 17662–6.

2 Elder JT, Cromie MA, Griffiths CE et al. Molecular cloning of two human cellular retinoic acid-binding proteins: stimulus-selective induction of CRABP-II mRNA—a marker for retinoic acid action in human skin. *J Invest Dermatol* 1993; **100**: 356–9.

3 Craven NM, Griffiths CEM. Topical retinoids and cutaneous biology. *Clin Exp Dermatol* 1996; **21**: 1–10.

4 Smith G, Wolf CR, Deeni YY et al. Cutaneous expression of cytochrome P-450 CYP 2S1: individuality in regulation by therapeutic agents for psoriasis and other skin diseases. *Lancet* 2003; **361**: 1336–43.

5 Chen C, Jensen BK, Mistry G et al. Negligible systemic absorption of topical isotretinoin cream: implications for teratogenicity. *J Clin Pharmacol* 1997; **37**: 279–84.

6 Johnson EM. A risk assessment of topical tretinoin as a potential human developmental toxin based on animal and comparative human data. *J Am Acad Dermatol* 1997; **36**: S86–90.

7 Kang S, Duell EA, Fisher GJ et al. Application of retinol to human skin *in vivo* induces epidermal hyperplasia and cellular retinoid binding proteins characteristic of retinoic acid but without measurable retinoic acid levels or irritation. *J Invest Dermatol* 1995; **105**: 549–56.

8 Kurlandsky SB, Duell EA, Kang S et al. Auto-regulation of retinoic acid biosynthesis through regulation of retinol esterification in human keratinocytes. *J Biol Chem* 1996; **271**: 15346–52.

9 Duell EA, Kang S, Voorhees JJ. Retinoic acid isomers applied to human skin *in vivo* each induce a 4-hydroxylase that inactivates only *trans* retinoic acid. *J Invest Dermatol* 1996; **106**: 316–20.

10 Duell EA, Kang S, Voorhees JJ. Unoccluded retinol penetrates human skin *in vivo* more effectively than unoccluded retinyl palmitate or retinoic acid. *J Invest Dermatol* 1997; **109**: 301–5.

11 Yoshimura K, Momosawa A, Aiba E et al. Clinical trial of bleaching treatment with 10% all-*trans* retinol gel. *Dermatol Surg* 2003; **29**: 155–60.

12 MacKenzie RM, Hellwege DM, McGregor ML et al. Separation and identification of geometric isomers of retinoic acid and methyl retinoate. *J Chromatogr* 1978; **155**: 379–87.

13 Kligman AM, Fulton JE Jr, Plewig G. Topical vitamin A acid in acne vulgaris. *Arch Dermatol* 1969; **99**: 469–76.

14 Pedace FJ, Stoughton R. Topical retinoic acid in acne vulgaris. *Br J Dermatol* 1971; **84**: 465–9.

15 Gunther S. Vitamin-A acid in acne vulgaris: association between peeling effect and improvement. *Dermatol Wochenschr* 1974; **160**: 215–8.

16 Mills OH, Leyden JJ, Kligman AM. Tretinoin treatment of steroid acne. *Arch Dermatol* 1973; **108**: 381–4.

17 Leyden JJ, Grove GL, Grove MJ et al. Treatment of photodamaged facial skin with topical tretinoin. *J Am Acad Dermatol* 1989; **21**: 638–44.

18 Kligman AM, Grove GL, Hirose RL et al. Topical tretinoin for photodamaged skin. *J Am Acad Dermatol* 1986; **15**: 836–59.

19 Kligman AM, Dogadkina D, Lavker RM. Effects of topical tretinoin on non-sun-exposed protected skin of the elderly. *J Am Acad Dermatol* 1993; **29**: 25–33.

20 Nyirady J, Bergfeld W, Ellis C et al. Tretinoin cream 0.02% for the treatment of photodamaged facial skin: a review of two double-blind clinical studies. *Cutis* 2001; **68**: 135–42.

21 Epstein JH. All-*trans*-retinoic acid and cutaneous cancers. *J Am Acad Dermatol* 1986; **15**: 772–8.

22 Robinson TA, Kligman AM. Treatment of solar keratoses of the extremities with retinoic acid and 5-fluorouracil. *Br J Dermatol* 1975; **92**: 703–6.

23 Meyskens FL Jr, Edwards L, Levine MS. Role of topical tretinoin in melanoma and dysplastic naevi. *J Am Acad Dermatol* 1986; **15**: 822–5.

24 Popp C, Kligman AM, Stoudemayer TJ. Pretreatment of photo-aged forearm skin with topical tretinoin accelerates healing of full-thickness wounds. *Br J Dermatol* 1995; **132**: 46–53.

25 Hevia O, Nemeth AJ, Taylor JR. Tretinoin accelerates healing after trichloroacetic acid chemical peel. *Arch Dermatol* 1991; **127**: 678–82.

26 Mandy SH. Tretinoin in the preoperative and postoperative management of dermabrasion. *J Am Acad Dermatol* 1986; **15**: 878–9, 888–9.

27 Kligman AM, Plewig G, Mills OH Jr. Topically applied tretinoin for senile (solar) comedones. *Arch Dermatol* 1971; **104**: 420–1.

28 O'Malley MP, Haake A, Goldsmith L, Berg D. Localized Darier disease: implications for genetic studies. *Arch Dermatol* 1997; **133**: 1134–8.

29 Poskitt L, Wilkinson JD. Natural history of keratosis pilaris. *Br J Dermatol* 1994; **130**: 711–3.

30 Muller SA, Belcher RW, Esterley NB. Keratinizing dermatoses. *Arch Dermatol* 1977; **113**: 1052–4.

31 Van der Wateren AR, Cormane RH. Oral retinoic acid as therapy for erythro-keratoderma variabilis. *Br J Dermatol* 1977; **97**: 83–5.

32 Gunther S. Vitamin A acid in treatment of oral lichen planus. *Arch Dermatol* 1973; **107**: 277.

33 Helfman RJ. The treatment of geographic tongue with topical Retin-A solution. *Cutis* 1979; **24**: 179–80.

34 Tkach JR. Tretinoin treatment for Fox–Fordyce disease. *Arch Dermatol* 1979; **115**: 1285.

35 Giacobetti R, Caro WA, Roenigk JR. Fox–Fordyce disease: control with tretinoin cream. *Arch Dermatol* 1979; **115**: 1365–6.

36 Janssen De Limpens AMP. The local treatment of hypertrophic scars and keloids with topical retinoic acid. *Br J Dermatol* 1980; **103**: 319–23.

37 Panagerie-Castaings H. Retinoic acid in the treatment of keloids. *J Dermatol Surg Oncol* 1988; **14**: 1275–6.

38 Lindgren S, Groth O, Molin L. Allergic contact response to vitamin A acid. *Contact Dermatitis* 1976; **2**: 212–7.

39 Cunliffe WJ, Poncet M, Loesche C, Verschoore M. A comparison of the efficacy and tolerability of adapalene 0.1% gel versus tretinoin 0.025% gel in patients with acne vulgaris: a meta-analysis of five randomized trials. *Br J Dermatol* 1998; **139** (Suppl. 52): 48–56.

40 Chalker DK, Lesher JL Jr, Smith JG Jr. et al. Efficacy of topical isotretinoin 0.05% gel in acne vulgaris: results of a multicenter, double-blind investigation. *J Am Acad Dermatol* 1987; **17**: 251–4.

41 Elbaum DJ. Comparison of the stability of topical isotretinoin and topical tretinoin and their efficacy in acne. *J Am Acad Dermatol* 1988; **19**: 486–91.

42 Hughes BR, Norris JF, Cunliffe WJ. A double-blind evaluation of topical isotretinoin 0.05%, benzoyl peroxide gel 5% and placebo in patients with acne. *Clin Exp Dermatol* 1992; **17**: 165–8.

43 Tschan T, Steffen H, Supersaxo A. Sebaceous-gland deposition of isotretinoin after topical application: an *in vitro* study using human facial skin. *Skin Pharmacol* 1997; **10**: 126–34.

44 Plewig G, Ruhfus A, Klovekorn W. Sebum suppression after topical application of retinoids (arotenoid and isotretinoin). *J Invest Dermatol* 1983; **80**: 357.

45 Bischoff R, De Jong EM, Rulo HF et al. Topical application of 13-*cis*-retinoic acid in the treatment of chronic plaque psoriasis. *Clin Exp Dermatol* 1992; **17**: 9–12.

46 Sendagorta E, Lesiewicz J, Armstrong RB. Topical isotretinoin for photodamaged skin. *J Am Acad Dermatol* 1992; **27**: S15–8.

47 Maddin S, Lauharanta J, Agache P et al. Isotretinoin improves the appearance of photodamaged skin: results of a 36-week, multicenter, double-blind, placebo-controlled trial. *J Am Acad Dermatol* 2000; **42**: 56–63.

48 Alirezai M, Dupuy P, Amblard P et al. Clinical evaluation of topical isotretinoin in the treatment of actinic keratoses. *J Am Acad Dermatol*, 1994; **30**: 447–51.

49 Sankowski A, Janik P, Jeziorska M et al. The results of topical application of 13-*cis*-retinoic acid on basal cell carcinoma: a correlation of the clinical effect with histopathological examination and serum retinol level. *Neoplasma* 1987; **34**: 485–9.

50 Karpouzis A, Giatromanolaki A, Sivridis E, Kouskoukis C. Perifolliculitis capitis abscedens et suffodiens successfully controlled with topical isotretinoin. *Eur J Dermatol* 2003; **13**: 192–5.

51 Piattelli A, Fioroni M, Santinelli A, Rubini C. *bcl-2* expression and apoptotic bodies in 13-*cis*-retinoic acid (isotretinoin) -topically treated oral leukoplakia: a pilot study. *Oral Oncol* 1999; **35**: 314–20.

52 Markowska J, Janik P, Wiese E, Ostrowski J. Leukoplakia of the vulva locally treated by 13-*cis*-retinoic acid. *Neoplasma* 1987; **34**: 33–6.

53 Giustina TA, Stewart JC, Ellis CN *et al*. Topical application of isotretinoin gel improves oral lichen planus: a double-blind study. *Arch Dermatol* 1986; **122**: 534–6.

54 Toros P, Onder M, Gurer MA. Bilateral nipple hyperkeratosis treated successfully with topical isotretinoin. *Australas J Dermatol* 1999; **40**: 220–2.

55 Ratnavel RC, Grant JW, Handfield-Jones SE, Norris PG. O'Brien's actinic granuloma: response to isotretinoin. *J R Soc Med* 1995; **88**: 528P–529P.

56 Leenutaphong V, Nettakul A, Rattanasuwon P. Topical isotretinoin for melasma in Thai patients: a vehicle-controlled clinical trial. *J Med Assoc Thai* 1999; **82**: 868–75.

57 Burge SM, Buxton PK. Topical isotretinoin in Darier's disease. *Br J Dermatol* 1995; **133**: 924–8.

58 McKenna KE, Walsh MY, Burrows D. Treatment of unilateral Darier's disease with topical isotretinoin. *Clin Exp Dermatol* 1999; **24**: 425–7.

59 Griffiths CEM, Elder JT, Bernard BA *et al*. Comparison of CD271 (adapalene) and all-*trans* retinoic acid in human skin: dissociation of epidermal effects and CRABP II m-RNA expression. *J Invest Dermatol* 1993; **101**: 325–8.

60 Ioannides D, Rigopoulos D, Katsambas A. Topical adapalene gel 0.1% vs. isotretinoin gel 0.05% in the treatment of acne vulgaris: a randomized open-label clinical trial. *Br J Dermatol* 2002; **147**: 523–7.

61 Michel S, Jomard A, Demarchez M. Pharmacology of adapalene. *Br J Dermatol* 1998; **139** (Suppl. 52): 3–7.

62 Breneman D, Duvic M, Kuzel T *et al*. Phase 1 and 2 trial of bexarotene gel for skin-directed treatment of patients with cutaneous T-cell lymphoma. *Arch Dermatol* 2002; **138**: 325–32.

63 Liu HL. Bexarotene gel: a Food and Drug Administration-approved skin-directed therapy for early stage cutaneous T-cell lymphoma. *Arch Dermatol* 2002; **138**: 398–9.

64 Chandraratna RA. Tazarotene: first of a new generation of receptor-selective retinoids. *Br J Dermatol* 1996; **135** (Suppl. 49): 18–25.

65 Weinstein GD, Krueger GG, Lowe NJ *et al*. Tazarotene gel, a new retinoid, for topical therapy of psoriasis: vehicle-controlled study of safety, efficacy, and duration of therapeutic effect. *J Am Acad Dermatol* 1997; **37**: 85–92.

66 Weinstein GD, Koo JY, Krueger GG *et al*. Tazarotene cream in the treatment of psoriasis: two multicenter, double-blind, randomized, vehicle-controlled studies of the safety and efficacy of tazarotene creams 0.05% and 0.1% applied once daily for 12 weeks. *J Am Acad Dermatol* 2003; **48**: 760–7.

67 Lebwohl M, Ast E, Callen JP *et al*. Once-daily tazarotene gel versus twice-daily fluocinonide cream in the treatment of plaque psoriasis. *J Am Acad Dermatol* 1998; **38** (5 Part 1): 705–11.

68 Scher RK, Stiller M, Zhu YI. Tazarotene 0.1% gel in the treatment of fingernail psoriasis: a double-blind, randomized, vehicle-controlled study. *Cutis* 2001; **68**: 355–8.

69 Wollina U. Genital ulcers in a psoriasis patient using topical tazarotene. *Br J Dermatol* 1998; **138**: 713–4.

70 Dawkins MA, Clark AR, Feldman SR. Pyogenic granuloma-like lesion associated with topical tazarotene therapy. *J Am Acad Dermatol* 2000; **43**: 154–5.

71 Bershad S, Kranjac Singer G, Parente JE *et al*. Successful treatment of acne vulgaris using a new method: results of a randomized vehicle-controlled trial of short-contact therapy with 0.1% tazarotene gel. *Arch Dermatol* 2002; **138**: 481–9.

72 Leyden JJ, Tanghetti EA, Miller B *et al*. Once-daily tazarotene 0.1% gel versus once-daily tretinoin 0.1% microsponge gel for the treatment of facial acne vulgaris: a double-blind randomized trial. *Cutis* 2002; **69** (Suppl.): 12–9.

73 Webster GF, Guenther L, Poulin YP *et al*. A multicenter, double-blind, randomized comparison study of the efficacy and tolerability of once-daily tazarotene 0.1% gel and adapalene 0.1% gel for the treatment of facial acne vulgaris. *Cutis* 2002; **69** (Suppl.): 4–11.

74 Phillips TJ, Gottlieb AB, Leyden JJ *et al*. Efficacy of 0.1% tazarotene cream for the treatment of photodamage: a 12-month multicenter, randomized trial. *Arch Dermatol* 2002; **138**: 1486–93.

75 Petruzzi M, De Benedittis M, Grassi R *et al*. Oral lichen planus: a preliminary clinical study on treatment with tazarotene. *Oral Dis* 2002; **8**: 291–5.

76 Gerbig AW. Treating keratosis pilaris. *J Am Acad Dermatol* 2002; **47**: 457.

77 Stege H, Hofmann B, Ruzicka T, Lehmann P. Topical application of tazarotene in the treatment of non-erythrodermic lamellar ichthyosis. *Arch Dermatol* 1998; **134**: 640.

78 Marulli GC, Campione E, Chimenti MS *et al*. Type I lamellar ichthyosis improved by tazarotene 0.1% gel. *Clin Exp Dermatol* 2003; **28**: 391–3.

79 Hofmann B, Stege H, Ruzicka T, Lehmann P. Effect of topical tazarotene in the treatment of congenital ichthyoses. *Br J Dermatol* 1999; **141**: 642–6.

80 Bowman PH, Davis LS. Confluent and reticulated papillomatosis: response to tazarotene. *J Am Acad Dermatol* 2003; **48** (Suppl.): S80–1.

81 Outland JD, Brown TS, Callen JP. Tazarotene is an effective therapy for elastosis perforans serpiginosa. *Arch Dermatol* 2002; **138**: 169–71.

82 Oster-Schmidt C, Stucker M, Altmeyer P. Follicular dyskeratosis: successful treatment with local retinoid. *Hautarzt* 2000; **51**: 196–9.

83 Burkhart CG, Burkhart CN. Tazarotene gel for Darier's disease. *J Am Acad Dermatol* 1998; **38**: 1001–2.

84 Abramovits W, Abdelmalek N. Treatment of warty dyskeratoma with tazarotenic acid. *J Am Acad Dermatol* 2002; **46** (Suppl. 2, Case reports): S4.

85 Weisshaar E, Bonnekoh B, Franke I, Gollnick H. Successful symptomatic tazarotene treatment of juvenile acanthosis nigricans of the familial obesity-associated type in insulin resistance. *Hautarzt* 2001; **52**: 499–503.

86 Helm TN, Lee J, Helm KF. Spiny keratoderma. *Cutis* 2000; **66**: 191–2.

87 Lewis A, Nigro M, Rosen T. Treatment of keratoderma blennorrhagicum with tazarotene gel 0.1%. *J Am Acad Dermatol* 2000; **43**: 400–2.

88 Edwards KR, Burke WA. Treatment of localized discoid lupus erythematosus with tazarotene. *J Am Acad Dermatol* 1999; **41**: 1049–50.

Sensitizing agents

These chemicals (dinitrochlorobenzene, squaric acid, diphencyprone, etc.) are known as universal sensitizers. Almost every individual will develop allergic dermatitis after repeated contact with these substances on the skin. Animals are also readily sensitized. For many years dermatologists have tried to use the induction of contact sensitization, using these and other allergens, to manipulate immune responses to advantage in a wide variety of benign and malignant skin diseases [1]. Numerous attempts have been made, with some reported success, to use sensitizers to stimulate an immune response to malignancies including melanoma [1,2]. Currently, topical sensitizers have found two main roles in dermatology: for the treatment of alopecia areata and viral warts [1]. The sensitizers that have been most intensively investigated are dinitrochlorobenzene (DNCB), squaric acid dibutylester and diphencyprone. The earliest of these to be used was dinitrochlorobenzene, which was found to be mutagenic. The use of squaric acid dibutylester or diphencyprone avoids this hazard and diphencyprone has the advantage of a practical shelf life. The latter has therefore become the most widely used sensitizer for treatment of alopecia areata and warts. Diphencyprone does not cross-sensitize patients to any other household or medicinal substances. An additional advantage of this compound is that it is photochemically unstable and degrades in the presence of visible light, so accidental spills will not indefinitely contaminate the environment; however, it also follows that diphencyprone must be stored in the dark.

The precise mechanisms by which induction of contact allergy can induce hair regrowth in alopecia areata have not been established. It seems likely that regulatory mechanisms activated to modulate the contact allergic reaction also down-regulate the autoimmune reaction responsible for the alopecia. Increased production of IL-10 may explain this effect [3]. There is no doubt that these agents can stimulate regrowth of hair. DNCB [4], squaric acid dibutyl ester [5] and diphenylcyclopropenone [6] have all been shown to stimulate hair regrowth on treated areas of the scalp in studies using untreated areas as a control. The same effect has been achieved, in sensitized individuals, by use of *Primula* leaves [7] or by nickel patch-test reagent [8]. The demonstration of hair regrowth on one side of the scalp that has been treated with allergen, while there is none on the other side, constitutes a well-controlled experiment which has been repeated regularly by the author. Sensitization can usually be achieved by application of 2% or higher concentration of diphencyprone to a small area of the scalp once weekly until a reaction is seen. Subsequent treatment can begin with a 0.01% solution and usually continues on a weekly basis, adjusting the concentration as required to maintain mild dermatitis. Attempts have been made to achieve the same effect by use of a simple inflammatory response induced by contact irritants. Phenolics, cantharides, camphor and other irritants have been used for many years, mostly without controlled trials [9]. Trials using croton oil and retinoic acid have not confirmed a response to these irritants [8,10]. With the possible exception of dithranol [11], it has proved difficult to establish the efficacy of irritants.

The efficacy of topical sensitizers in treatment of warts is still not so clearly established. Published controlled trials have been small and inconclusive [1,12]. Uncontrolled data are fairly convincing but inconsistent, perhaps because treatment regimens have also been variable [1]. The best results with diphencyprone have been obtained by first sensitizing patients at a site remote from the warts and then applying diphencyprone 0.01–6% to the lesions at intervals of 1–4 weeks. Complete clearance was reported in 70% of patients with this method [13]. Again, the mechanism of action has not been fully clarified but it is likely that the induction of an inflammatory reaction within the wart induces an influx of immunocompetent cells which can then promote an appropriate immune response to the infecting human papillomavirus.

The induction of contact allergic dermatitis is occasionally complicated by the development of pigmentary disturbances including vitiligo. This treatment modality is therefore probably best reserved for patients with white skin.

REFERENCES

1 Buckley DA, Du Vivier AWP. The therapeutic use of topical contact sensitizers in benign dermatoses. *Br J Dermatol* 2001; **145**: 385–405.
2 Wack C, Kirst A, Becker JC *et al*. Chemoimmunotherapy for melanoma with dacarbazine and 2,4-dinitrochlorobenzene elicits a specific T cell-dependent immune response. *Cancer Immunol Immunother* 2002; **51**: 431–9.
3 Hoffmann R, Wenzel E, Huth A *et al*. Cytokine mRNA levels in alopecia areata before and after treatment with the contact allergen diphenylcyclopropenone. *J Invest Dermatol* 1994; **103**: 530–3.
4 Daman LA, Rosenberg EW, Drake L. Treatment of alopecia areata with dinitrochlorobenzene. *Arch Dermatol* 1978; **114**: 1036–8.
5 Chua SH. Topical squaric acid dibutylester therapy for alopecia areata: a double-sided patient-controlled study. *Ann Acad Med Singapore* 1996; **25**: 842–7.
6 Happle R, Hausen BM, Wiesner-Menzel L. Diphencyprone in the treatment of alopecia areata. *Acta Derm Venereol* 1983; **63**: 49–52.
7 Rhodes EL, Dolman W, Kennedy C *et al*. Alopecia areata regrowth induced by *Primula obconica*. *Br J Dermatol* 1981; **104**: 339–40.
8 Suarez Martin E. Treatment of alopecia areata profiting from 'natural' allergy to nickel. *Arch Dermatol* 1984; **120**: 1138–9.
9 Swanson NA, Mitchell AJ, Leahy MS *et al*. Topical treatment of alopecia areata. *Arch Dermatol* 1981; **117**: 384–7.
10 Ashworth J, Tuyp E, MacKie RM. Allergic and irritant dermatitis compared in the treatment of alopecia totalis and universalis: a comparison of the value of topical diphencyprone and tretinoin gel. *Br J Dermatol* 1989; **120**: 397–401.
11 Schmoeckel C, Weissmann I, Plewig G, Braun-Falco O. Treatment of alopecia areata by anthralin-induce dermatitis. *Arch Dermatol* 1979; **115**: 1254–5.
12 Gibbs S. Topical immunotherapy with contact sensitizers for viral warts. *Br J Dermatol* 2002; **146**: 705.
13 Buckley DA, Keane FM, Munn SE *et al*. Recalcitrant viral warts treated by diphencyprone immunotherapy. *Br J Dermatol* 1999; **141**: 292–6.

Sunscreens

It is likely that in the early evolution of *Homo sapiens*, pigmentation of the skin developed primarily as protection from the risk of sunburn. Subsequent migration away from our equatorial origins reduced the risk of sunburn and skin pigmentation was lost in order to facilitate adequate penetration of UVB into the skin for photochemical synthesis of vitamin D. The adverse consequences of this loss of endogenous sunscreen may not have impaired reproductive potential of the species because the deleterious effects of sunlight tend to occur mainly in later life. However, individuals with white skin are clearly at greater risk from malignant melanoma, non-melanoma skin cancer, preneoplastic disorders and the premature ageing effects of UV irradiation. The sadly fashionable trend over recent decades to purposely expose the skin to solar irradiation in order to obtain a suntan has undoubtedly increased the frequency of these diseases.

It seems a logical approach to attempt to replace the pigment with an exogenous sunscreen applied to the skin surface and a large number of formulations are marketed for this purpose. Used properly, these compounds can reduce UV exposure and probably also the risks associated with photodamage, notably neoplasia. Regrettably, sunscreens are often used in such a way as to make it possible for individuals with pale skin, who could not normally withstand any significant sun exposure without burning, to lie in the sun for hours on end. Such 'abuse' of sunscreens seems likely to be harmful because it can result in significantly greater cumulative UV irradiation than would otherwise be possible. This is especially likely to happen if sunscreens with low sun protection factor ratings (see below) are used.

The ideal sunscreen should completely block the transmission of both UVB (280–315 nm) and UVA (315–400 nm) while at the same time being cosmetically acceptable and pleasant to use. Additional important properties are durability on the surface of the skin and water resistance. The latter is especially important if the sunscreen is

Table 75.9 Compounds used as active constituents of sunscreens.

Physical agents	Chemical agents
Zinc oxide	*Para*-aminobenzoic acid (PABA) and derivatives UVB
Titanium dioxide	Anthranilates UVA
Ferrous oxide	Cinnamates UVB
	Salicylates UVB
	Octocrylene UVB
	Benzotriazoles (Tinosorb) UVB, UVA
	Dibenzoylmethanes (Parsol 1789) UVA
	Benzophenones UVA
	Camphor derivatives (Mexoryl) UVA

to be used when swimming. Sunscreens are generally more effective in blocking UVB than UVA but effective filtration of UVA is important because these wavelengths contribute to photo-ageing [1], cutaneous immunosuppression [2,3] and carcinogenesis [4], and can have a central role in photodermatoses such as polymorphic light eruption [5]. No single compound can achieve all the desired aims so most commercial formulations contain a mixture of active constituents. These fall into two broad categories: physical sunscreens which act by reflecting and scattering UV light, and chemical agents which absorb UV light [6–8]. Frequently used compounds are listed in Table 75.9.

Physical agents such as titanium dioxide and zinc oxide can block a broad spectrum of UVB, UVA and visible light (ability to block the latter can be useful in some photodermatoses). However, their efficacy against UVA and visible light depends on particle size. Larger particle size results in superior efficacy but reduced cosmetic acceptability because of the increased whitening of the skin (which is, of course, reflection of visible light). There has been some concern over the potential for the interaction of both zinc and titanium oxides with UV light to release free radicals [9] but fortunately the harmful effects of these seem likely to be very limited as the oxide particles do not seem to penetrate below the surface layers of the stratum corneum into viable skin [10].

Chemical agents are each effective against a different range of wavelengths of UV light. Some absorb UVB and others UVA. Relatively few absorb long-wave UVA approaching the visible range, exceptions being butyl methoxydibenzoylmethane which has an absorption spectrum of 320–400 nm, and terephthalylidene dicamphor sulphonic acid, with absorption spectrum 290–400 nm. Chemical sunscreens can occasionally cause dermatitis. Irritant, allergic, phototoxic or photoallergic reactions may occur and may be caused not only by the active constituents but also by the base or by additives such as fragrances and stabilizers. Benzophenones are probably the most common sensitizers, while dibenzoylmethanes, *para*-aminobenzoic acid (PABA) and cinnamates may cause photoallergic dermatitis [11,12].

The concept of sun protection factors (SPF) was introduced to help consumers evaluate the level of protection from UVB and the risk of sunburn. Unfortunately, different systems of assay are used in different countries, making direct comparisons very misleading. However, all depend on deriving a ratio of the time or the amount of energy to reach a given end-point (such as minimal erythema) when using the screen, compared with that required without using the screen. Thus:

$$SPF = \frac{\text{Dose of UVB radiation producing minimal erythema with sunscreen}}{\text{Dose of UVB radiation producing minimal erythema without sunscreen}}$$

It should be noted that the SPF is based on application of an adequate quantity of the sunscreen, usually 2 mg/cm^2 of skin. This is probably more than is routinely applied by most users. As a guide, SPFs of up to 10 can be regarded as mild, 10–15 as medium and over 15 as strong protectors. International agreement is needed to standardize endpoints, light sources and conditions of testing. As a result, the classification of sunscreens into the broad categories listed above is helpful but comparisons between one product and another are not as accurate as they might appear. This is especially true of comparisons between products with high SPF values (above 15). There is currently even less standardization of the assessment of protection against UVA. Measurement of resistance to water has also not been standardized but can be assessed by several methods [13,14].

While it would seem likely that correct use of sunscreens will reduce the risk of malignancy, this has not been easy to confirm, especially in retrospective studies. Part of the difficulty is the likely association between use of a sunblock and sun exposure.

Suncreens have been shown to reduce UV-induced immunosuppression, which is considered to have a role in cutaneous carcinogenesis. Both the sensitization [15] and elicitation [2] phases of immune responses can be preserved by sunscreens.

In a placebo-controlled trial on a high-risk population, appropriate strength sunscreens have been shown to be effective in reducing the incidence of actinic keratoses [16]. In an Australian prospective controlled study, regular use of sunscreen reduced the total number of SCCs but not of BCCs [17]. A study of BCCs indicated that there were fewer p53 mutations in those BCCs that developed in patients who had used sunscreen. This might be indicative of effective protection against UV-induced DNA mutation by the sunscreen [18], while some BCCs develop as a result of other causes.

The prevention of melanoma by the use of sunscreens is a further controversial topic because two case–control studies have linked sunscreen usage to a higher incidence of melanoma [19,20]. This may be related in part to the likelihood that the subjects studied had previously used sunscreens that provided protection against UVB radiation alone, and exposed themselves to higher doses of solar radiation than those who did not use sunscreen. Other studies have examined the development of naevi as a marker for risk of melanoma. A retrospective epidemiological study from Israel found that use of sunscreen was associated with a higher number of naevi [21]. Conversely, a prospective controlled trial from Vancouver demonstrated a reduced rate of development of naevi over a 3-year period in children provided with sunblock and instructed on its use. The effect was especially evident in those children who were freckled [22].

In addition to the protection of healthy skin, sunscreens have an important role in the management of patients with photodermatoses. The most common of these, polymorphic light eruption, often seems to show rather limited benefit from sunscreens but may be effectively prevented by formulations that block a broad spectrum of UVA including longer wavelengths [5]. Sunscreens effective in blocking the offending wavelengths of UV light can also be helpful in management of less common photodermatoses including actinic prurigo, chronic actinic dermatitis, hydroa vacciniforme, lupus erythematosus, porphyrias and solar urticaria (see Chapter 24).

Whether sunscreens are applied to prevent solar damage to healthy skin or to alleviate a photodermatosis, it is important that these should not be regarded as the only means of limiting sun exposure. Staying indoors during the hours of peak sunlight intensity and, when outdoors, covering the skin with suitable clothing and headwear, constitute more effective strategies than using sunscreens.

REFERENCES

1 Seite S, Moyal D, Richard S *et al.* Effects of repeated suberythemal doses of UVA in human skin. *Eur J Dermatol* 1997; **7**: 204–9.
2 Moyal DD, Fourtanier AM. Efficacy of broad-spectrum sunscreens against the suppression of elicitation of delayed-type hypersensitivity responses in humans depends on the level of ultraviolet A protection. *Exp Dermatol* 2003; **12**: 153–9.
3 Seite S, Zucchi H, Moyal D *et al.* Alterations in human epidermal Langerhans' cells by ultraviolet radiation: quantitative and morphological study. *Br J Dermatol* 2003; **148**: 291–9.
4 Wang SQ, Setlow R, Berwick M *et al.* Ultraviolet A and melanoma: a review. *J Am Acad Dermatol* 2001; **44**: 837–46.
5 Allas S, Lui H, Moyal D, Bissonnette R. Comparison of the ability of two sunscreens to protect against polymorphous light eruption induced by a UV-A/UV-B metal halide lamp. *Arch Dermatol* 1999; **135**: 1421–2.
6 Shaath NA. The chemistry of sunscreens. In: Lowe NJ, Shaath NA, eds. *Sunscreens: Development, Evaluation and Regulatory Aspects*. New York: Marcel Dekker, 1990: 211–33.
7 Kaidbey KH, Kligman AM. An appraisal of the efficacy and substantivity of the new high-protection sunscreens. *J Am Acad Dermatol* 1981; **4**: 566–70.
8 Klein K. Formulating suncreen products. In: Lowe NJ, Shaath NA, eds. *Sunscreens: Development, Evaluation and Regulatory Aspects*. New York: Marcel Dekker, 1990: 235–66.
9 Yamamoto Y, Imai N, Mashima R *et al.* Singlet oxygen from irradiated titanium dioxide and zinc. *Methods Enzymol* 2000; **319**: 29–37.
10 Lademann J, Weigmann H, Rickmeyer C *et al.* Penetration of titanium dioxide microparticles in a sunscreen formulation into the horny layer and the follicular orifice. *Skin Pharmacol Appl Skin Physiol* 1999; **12**: 247–56.
11 English JS, White IR, Cronin E. Sensitivity to sunscreens. *Contact Dermatitis* 1987; **17**: 159–62.

12 Bilsland D, Ferguson J. Contact allergy to sunscreen chemicals in photosensitivity dermatitis/actinic reticuloid syndrome (PD/AR) and polymorphic light eruption (PLE). *Contact Dermatitis* 1993; **29**: 70–3.
13 Kraft ER, Hoch SG, Quisno RA *et al.* The importance of the vehicle. *J Soc Cosmet Chem* 1982; **23**: 383–91.
14 Thompson C, Maibach H, Epstein J. Allergic contact dermatitis from sunscreen preparations complicating photodermatitis. *Arch Dermatol* 1977; **113**: 1252–3.
15 Whitmore SE, Morison WL. Prevention of UVB-induced immunosuppression in humans by a high sun protection factor sunscreen. *Arch Dermatol* 1995; **131**: 1128–33.
16 Naylor MF, Boyd A, Smith DW *et al.* High sun protection factor sunscreens in the suppression of actinic neoplasia. *Arch Dermatol* 1995; **131**: 170–5.
17 Green A, Williams G, Neale R *et al.* Daily sunscreen application and betacarotene supplementation in prevention of basal-cell and squamous-cell carcinomas of the skin: a randomized controlled trial. *Lancet* 1999; **354**: 723–9.
18 Rosenstein BS, Phelps RG, Weinstock MA *et al.* P53 mutations in basal cell carcinomas arising in routine users of sunscreens. *Photochem Photobiol* 1999; **70**: 798–806.
19 Westerdahl J, Olsson H, Masback A *et al.* Is the use of sunscreens a risk factor for malignant melanoma? *Melanoma Res* 1995; **5**: 59–65.
20 Autier P, Dore JF, Schifflers E *et al.* Melanoma and use of sunscreens: an EORTC case–control study in Germany, Belgium and France. *Int J Cancer* 1995; **61**: 749–55.
21 Azizi E, Iscovich J, Pavlotsky F *et al.* Use of sunscreen is linked with elevated naevi counts in Israeli school children and adolescents. *Melanoma Res* 2000; **10**: 491–8.
22 Gallagher RP, Rivers JK, Lee TK *et al.* Broad-spectrum sunscreen use and the development of new naevi in white children: a randomized controlled trial. *JAMA* 2000; **14**: 2955–60.

Tars

Tars are distillation products of organic material. There are three main sources of therapeutic tars: wood, shale and coal.

Wood tars

Oils of cade (juniper), beech, birch and pine are widely used, particularly in Scandinavian countries. Wood tars lack certain basic chemical structures characteristic of coal tars, such as pyridine, quinoline and quinaline rings [1]. They may sensitize but do not photosensitize.

Wood tars are used for treating eczema and psoriasis in some countries. Oil of cade is particularly used in scalp preparations or when tar preparations are needed on the face. They are normally applied in 1–10% strength in ointments or pastes, or as a paint in 95% alcohol.

Shale tars

Oils were extracted from shale (sedimentary rock containing fossilized fish) for centuries before crude oil became available. Various extracts and distillates have long been used for medicinal purposes. Ichthammol (ichthyol) is a shale tar (bituminous tar). This contains a very high proportion of sulphur (about 10%), as compounds of thiopen. Shale tars have antiseptic and anti-inflammatory properties but are generally less effective than coal tars and may have a different mode of action. They are not photosensitizers. Ichthammol is often used in paste bandages for treating atopic eczema.

Coal tar

Coal tar [2–4] is a black, viscous fluid with a characteristic smell. Attempts to remove the colour, odour, photosensitizing property and carcinogenicity have not been entirely successful [5], and variations in this natural product have made the assessment of active ingredients particularly difficult [3,4]. Of some 10 000 different constituents believed to make up coal tar, only 400 have been identified. These constitute 55% of the whole.

All coal tars are products of different distillates of heated coal. The content of the tar depends on the type of coal used and the temperature of the distillation. 'Low-temperature' tar was found to contain a greater number of components but to be less effective in producing orthokeratosis in mouse-tail skin than 'high-temperature' tar [3,4]. It was also more irritating. However, a comparison of high- and low-temperature tars showed no eventual difference in effect in the treatment of psoriasis itself, although crude (high-temperature) coal tar gave quicker results [6]. This suggests that the reversal of parakeratosis is only one factor in the control of psoriasis. The authors of this study point out that dithranol was not very effective in the mouse-tail test [7].

The hydrocarbons, which constitute about half the composition of tar, include benzol, naphthalene and anthracene. The high-boiling-point tar acids (phenolics) include isomers of substituted polyhydroxyphenols, and it seems likely that it is such phenols which may be responsible for the therapeutic effect of tar [3,4,8]. However, the exact mechanism by which tar exerts its effect remains unknown. These high-temperature fractions may have a direct effect on the granular layer by release of lysosomes followed by mitotic stimulation. Low-temperature extracts appear to cause epidermal thickening without restitution of the granular layer [3,4], and may be the reason for the indifferent action of some synthetic and proprietary tar preparations [3,4,9]. Until a more suitable preparation is available, many dermatologists will continue to believe that crude tar remains therapeutically superior [9,10].

The combination of tar with UV light (the Goeckerman regimen) has long been known to be helpful in psoriasis. In recent years, attempts have been made to identify the critical wavelengths of radiation involved [11,12]. Generally, UVB radiation has been found to be more effective than UVA [13,14]. Refined tars are less phototoxic than the crude product, but phototoxicity is directly related to therapeutic efficacy. UVA [15] did not appear to be a useful adjunct to tar and UVB in the treatment of psoriasis in one study. Laboratory studies have shown that tar plus UV light reduces epidermal DNA synthesis [12,16]. This may be related to the formation of cross-links between opposite strands on the DNA double helix [17].

A cytostatic effect of crude coal tar has also been postulated [18] following the finding that prolonged application to normal skin produces epidermal thinning associated with retention hyperkeratosis. More studies are still required, particularly to identify the more active fractions of tar distillates.

The well-established carcinogenicity of pitch and heavy tar fractions has aroused renewed interest in the current climate of therapeutic conservatism. Concerns about the oncogenic potential of polycyclic hydrocarbons [19] and consumer protection [20,21] have been fuelled by reports that urine from patients with psoriasis using crude coal tar was mutagenic to certain bacterial strains [5]. Reports of malignant tumours in humans in relation to tar therapy are rare. Rook *et al.* [22] reported five cases and Greither *et al.* [23] reported 13. Most had genital or groin involvement, but these are nowadays unlikely sites for tar application. Reassuringly, several large long-term follow-up studies have shown no increased incidence of skin tumours [14,24–27].

Coal tar is now mainly used in treatment of psoriasis and is the basis of the Goeckerman regimen (see Chapter 35). Prior to the advent of topical corticosteroids, coal tar was widely used in treatment of eczematous dermatoses and it can still prove useful as a steroid-sparing agent and antipruritic. Coal tar can be added to paste bandages although ichthammol is often preferred.

REFERENCES

1 Obermeyer ME, Becker SA. A study of crude coal tar and allied substances. *Arch Dermatol Syphilol* 1935; **31**: 796–810.
2 Muller SA, Kierland RR. Crude coal tar in dermatologic therapy. *Mayo Clin Proc* 1964; **39**: 275–80.
3 Wrench R, Britten AZ. Evaluation of coal tar fractions for use in psoriasiform diseases using the mouse tail test. I. High and low temperature tars and their constituents. *Br J Dermatol* 1975; **92**: 569–74.
4 Wrench R, Britten AZ. Evaluation of coal tar fractions for use in psoriasiform diseases using the mouse tail test. II. Tar oil, acids. *Br J Dermatol* 1975; **92**: 575–9.
5 Wheeler LA, Soperstein MD, Lowe NJ *et al.* Mutagenicity of urine from psoriatic patients undergoing treatment with coal tar and ultraviolet light. *J Invest Dermatol* 1981; **77**: 181–5.
6 Chapman RS, Finn OR. An assessment of high and low temperature tars in psoriasis. *Br J Dermatol* 1976; **94**: 71–4.
7 Wrench R, Britten AZ. Evaluation of dithranol and a 'synthetic tar' as antipsoriatic treatments using the mouse tail test. *Br J Dermatol* 1975; **93**: 75–8.
8 Hellier FF, Whitefield M. The treatment of psoriasis with triacetoxyanthracene. *Br J Dermatol* 1967; **79**: 491–6.
9 Young E. An external treatment of psoriasis: a controlled investigation of the effects of coal tar. *Br J Dermatol* 1970; **82**: 510–5.
10 Champion RH. Treatment of psoriasis. *BMJ* 1966; **ii**: 993–5.
11 Fischer T. Comparative treatment of psoriasis with UV-light, trioxsalen plus UV-light and coal tar plus UV-light. *Acta Derm Venereol (Stockh)* 1971; **57**: 345–50.
12 Stoughton RB, Dequoy P, Walters JF. Crude coal tar plus near ultraviolet light suppresses DNA synthesis in epidermis. *Arch Dermatol* 1978; **114**: 43–5.
13 Parrish JA, Morison WL, Gonzalez E. Therapy of psoriasis by tar sensitization. *J Invest Dermatol* 1978; **70**: 111–2.
14 Petrozzi JK, Barton JO, Kaidbey KK. Updating of the Goeckerman regime for psoriasis. *Br J Dermatol* 1978; **98**: 437–44.
15 Diette KM, Momtaz K, Stern RS *et al.* Role of ultraviolet A in phototherapy for psoriasis. *J Am Acad Dermatol* 1984; **11**: 441–7.
16 Walter JF, Stoughton RB, Dequoy PR. Suppression of epidermal proliferation by ultraviolet light, coal tar and anthralin. *Br J Dermatol* 1978; **99**: 89–96.

17 Pathak MA, Biswas RK. Skin photosensitization and DNA cross-linking ability of photochemotherapeutic agents. *J Invest Dermatol* 1977; **68**: 236.
18 Lavker RM, Grove GL, Kligman AM. The atrophogenic effect of crude coal tar on human epidermis. *Br J Dermatol* 1981; **105**: 77–82.
19 Gilman AG, Rall TW, Nies AS *et al.* eds. *Goodman and Gilman's The Pharmacological Basis of Therapeutics*, 8th edn. New York: Pergamon, 1990.
20 Zackheim HS. Should therapeutic coal tar preparations be available over-the-counter? *Arch Dermatol* 1978; **14**: 125–6.
21 Stern RS, Laird N. Carcinogenic risk of treatments for severe psoriasis. *Cancer* 1994; **73**: 2760–3.
22 Rook AJ, Gresham GA, Davis RA. Epithelioma possibly induced by therapeutic application of tar. *Br J Cancer* 1967; **10**: 17–23.
23 Greither A, Gisbertz C, Ippen H. Teerbehandlung und Krebs. *Zeitschr Haut Geschlkr* 1967; **42**: 631–5.
24 Jones SK, Mackie RM, Holt DJ *et al.* Further evidence of the safety of tar in the management of psoriasis. *Br J Dermatol* 1985; **113**: 97–101.
25 Pittelkow MR, Perry HO, Muller SA *et al.* Psoriasis treated with coal tar: 25-year follow-up study. *Arch Dermatol* 1981; **117**: 465–8.
26 Maughan WZ, Muller SA, Perry HO *et al.* Incidence of skin cancers in patients with atopic dermatitis treated with coal tar. *J Am Acad Dermatol* 1980; **3**: 612–5.
27 Schmid MH, Korting HC. Coal tar, pine tar and sulphonated shale oil preparations: comparative activity, efficacy and safety. *Dermatology* 1996; **193**: 1–5.

Vitamin D analogues (deltanoids, secosteroids)

The therapeutic potential of vitamin D in psoriasis has been recognized for many years. Systemic use of these compounds can be highly effective but requires monitoring to avoid causing disturbance of calcium homoeostasis. Used topically, considerable efficacy can be maintained with a wide safety margin. The advent of calcipotriol in the early 1990s has greatly increased the use of this modality. Tacalcitol and calcitriol, which were known to be effective even earlier, have only more recently become widely available for treatment of psoriasis. The novel analogue maxacalcitol is also known to be effective.

Vitamin D is not strictly a vitamin because an exogenous source is not essential. Photochemical cleavage of 7-dehydrocholesterol to form vitamin D (cholecalciferol) takes place in the skin and requires fairly minimal exposure to UVB to generate physiological quantities of the product. It is this break in the steroid nucleus that characterizes vitamin D and its analogues and gives rise to the term secosteroids. Cholecalciferol requires two hydroxylations for activation. The first is 25-hydroxylation, which takes place mainly in the liver and is not a tightly controlled step [1]. 25-Hydroxycholecalciferol is the main storage form of vitamin D within the body. This is finally 'activated', mainly in the kidney, by a very tightly regulated hydroxylation to 1α,25-dihydroxycholecalciferol [2,3]. As the latter has three hydroxyl groups, it is also known as calcitriol (Fig. 75.10). Calcitriol is a potent hormone first characterized by its ability to increase calcium absorption from the gut. It has subsequently become recognized that the receptor for this potent hormone is expressed in virtually all types of cell. Calcitriol is of

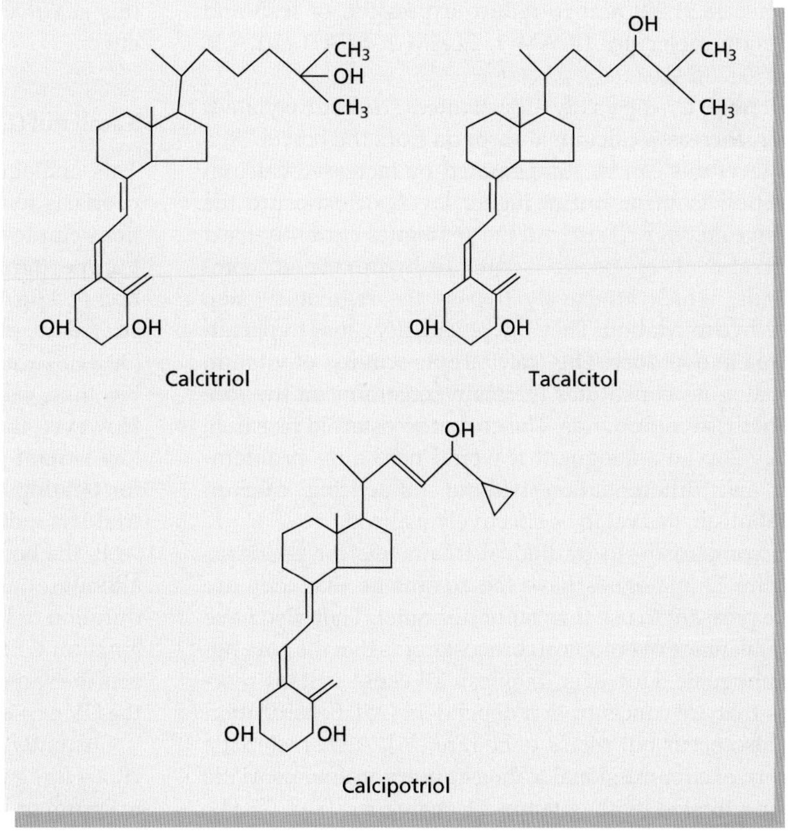

Fig. 75.10 Formulae of calcitriol, tacalcitol and calcipotriol.

fundamental importance in the regulation of differentiation and proliferation.

The vitamin D receptor is a phosphopeptide with molecular weight of approximately 60 kDa, able to move freely between the cytoplasm and the nucleus. It is a member of the steroid receptor superfamily, being similar in structure to the retinoid receptors, the thyroid hormone (T_3) receptor and receptors for other classes of steroid hormone. It is active mainly as a heterodimer in combination with the RXR [4]. The vitamin D receptor complex regulates transcription of numerous genes by binding to regulatory regions of DNA–vitamin D response elements. These are specific but heterogeneous regions of DNA generally situated upstream of regulated genes [4].

The therapeutic actions of vitamin D appear to result from a potent antiproliferative effect [5–8], the ability to promote differentiation [9–12] and perhaps also from immunosuppressive activity. *In vitro* secosteroids inhibit IL-2 release and lymphocyte activation [13,14], and release of IL-8 [15]. They also up-regulate expression of the receptor for the anti-inflammatory cytokine IL-10 [16]. They inhibit monocyte differentiation into dendritic cells, possibly by promoting expression of colony-stimulating factor 1 [17]. They inhibit keratinocyte synthesis of RANTES and IL-8 [18]. *In vivo*, they have been shown to inhibit expression of IL-8 [19], IL-6 [20] and other cytokines. During treatment of psoriasis they have been reported to reduce infiltration with lymphocytes and neutrophils [8,21,22] and to reduce expression of IL-8 and adhesion molecules (ICAM 1, ELAM 1, LFA 1, VLA 3, VLA 6) [23,24].

Vitamin D, especially in activated (1α-hydroxylated) forms, increases calcium absorption from the bowel. At a low level this can be compensated by increased calcium excretion in urine but at higher levels of exposure the serum calcium will rise. All the analogues currently used in treatment of psoriasis are 1α-hydroxylated compounds, which effectively bypass the regulatory step of 1α-hydroxylation. They can potentially cause hypercalcaemia in overdose. This 'calciotropic activity' of vitamin D analogues constitutes the main constraint on the safe use of these compounds. The goal of secosteroid research, to develop an analogue that would normalize proliferation and differentiation without influencing calcium metabolism, has yet to be effectively realized.

In comparison to traditional treatments for psoriasis, vitamin D analogues have the advantage that they are more pleasant to use than tar or dithranol. They also have the advantage over topical corticosteroids that they are not atrophogenic. However, they can all cause irritant reactions that are concentration dependent [25]. Sensitization can also occur but seems to be rare [26]. A characteristic pattern of circumlesional scaling appears around psoriatic lesions treated with vitamin D analogues (Fig. 75.11), which gives a guide to compliance almost as reliable as the

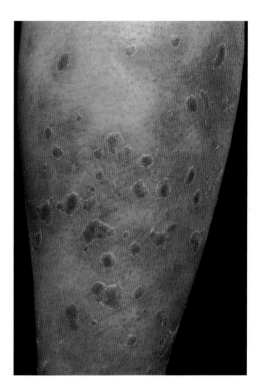

Fig. 75.11 Circumlesional scaling characteristic of psoriasis lesions treated with vitamin D analogues.

staining produced by dithranol [27]. It is not clear whether this is a manifestation of irritancy or a pharmacological effect.

Tacalcitol (1,24 dihydroxycholecalciferol)

This analogue has been used for topical treatment of psoriasis for many years in Japan, where the concentrations employed have ranged from 1 to 20 µg/g [28,29]. In Europe, tacalcitol is often used once daily at a concentration of 4 µg/g. Efficacy of this regimen has been demonstrated in placebo-controlled and dose-ranging studies [30,31]. Tacalcitol 4 µg/g applied once daily is less effective than calcipotriol 50 µg/g applied twice daily [32]. However, the lower concentration of tacalcitol results in a low irritant potential and it can therefore be safely used for treating facial or flexural psoriasis [33]. A long-term trial has indicated that, in patients who have responded well, the benefit can be maintained for up to 18 months, although only 64 out of 299 subjects completed the full duration of this trial [34]. Tacalcitol has been used in conjunction with both UVB [35] and PUVA [36] and accelerates the response to these treatments, potentially reducing the UV exposure required.

Currently, the recommended maximum dose of tacalcitol 4 µg/g is 10 g/day. However, no significant increase in serum or urine calcium was observed with daily doses of 15–20 g for up to 26 days [37]. It also appears safe to use tacalcitol at the higher concentration of 20 μg/g [29]. Hypercalcaemia has not yet been reported in association with topical application of this analogue. Sensitization may rarely occur [38].

Other indications in which topical tacalcitol has been employed with reported success include Nekam's disease [39], confluent and reticulate papillomatosis [40], Grover's disease [41], subcorneal pustular dermatosis [42], Hailey–Hailey disease [43], disseminated superficial actinic porokeratosis [44] and prurigo [45].

Calcitriol (1,25 dihydroxycholecalciferol)

Calcitriol is the naturally occurring form of activated vitamin D. This is known to be active both topically and systemically in treatment of psoriasis [46,47]. Like other analogues, it is rarely used systemically because of the need to monitor calcium homoeostasis although the hazards are probably not out of proportion to the potential benefit.

Calcitriol has been used topically at various concentrations ranging from 0.3 to 15 μg/g [48,49]. At the higher end of this range, changes are seen in urine and/or serum calcium levels, especially when large areas of skin are treated. At the lower end, efficacy is very limited. When applied twice daily at a concentration of 3 μg/g, controlled trials have demonstrated that a degree of efficacy can be maintained with minimal risk of effects on calcium homoeostasis [50]. The efficacy of this regimen was comparable to that of short-contact dithranol therapy in an 8-week trial with 114 subjects, although the overall improvement was not very impressive in either group, suggesting that the dithranol regimen may not have been optimal [50]. Calcitriol 3 μg/g is less effective than calcipotriol 50 μg/g [51]. In a long-term study, it was disappointing that only 75 out of 253 subjects continued to use the treatment for 1 year. Lack of efficacy was given as the main reason for withdrawal by 108 of the subjects. Twice daily treatment with calcitriol has shown a dose-sparing effect on UVB exposure when used in conjunction with broad-band phototherapy [52]. Calcitriol ointment 3 μg/g seems to have very little potential for irritancy or sensitization [53].

Calcipotriol (calcipotriene, MC 903)

Although developed relatively recently, calcipotriol has now been more intensively investigated than any other secosteroid for the treatment of psoriasis. The molecule has a cyclopropane group at the end of the side-chain, which facilitates rapid metabolism (Fig. 75.10). It is therefore ideal for topical administration and can be safely used in higher concentration than calcitriol or tacalcitol [54]. Placebo-controlled and dose-ranging trials demonstrated maximal response at the concentration of 50 μg/g

[55,56]. Virtually all subsequent research has investigated the use of calcipotriol at this concentration.

Efficacy and safety of calcipotriol in childhood psoriasis has been confirmed in trials on children from 2 years upwards [57,58]. It has also proved useful in an infant [59].

Reports indicate that topical calcipotriol can be useful in generalized pustular psoriasis [60,61] and in erythrodermic psoriasis [62,63]. However, absorption of the drug can be significantly higher in these circumstances and careful monitoring is required. In one case, generalized pustular psoriasis was thought to have been precipitated by calcipotriol [64]. Acrodermatitis continua [65] and nail psoriasis [66,67] may respond, although results are not consistent.

In comparative studies, calcipotriol 50 μg/g generally compares well to other topical treatments for psoriasis [68]. It has shown efficacy similar to potent topical corticosteroids such as betamethasone-17-valerate [69] and superior to tacalcitol 4 μg/g [31], calcitriol 3 μg/g [50] and to self-treatment with dithranol [70]. The response has been relatively well sustained over time in long-term trials [71,72]. It is notable, however, that only 26% of the patients on this treatment are able to discontinue the vitamin D analogue altogether (the rest requiring continuous treatment).

The use of calcipotriol has also been investigated in a wide range of combinations with other antipsoriatic medication. Combinations with topical corticosteroids can be particularly useful to increase efficacy and reduce irritation. When each medication is applied once daily, the combination with moderately potent or potent steroid reduces irritation and a potent steroid increases efficacy relative to twice daily application of calcipotriol alone [73]. A combined formulation (Dovobet®) containing betamethasone dipropionate 0.05% and calcipotriol 50 μg/g has proved more effective applied once daily than twice daily application of calcipotriol alone. The combined formulation was also less irritant [74]. A regimen combining short contact dithranol with twice daily application of calcipotriol proved more effective than dithranol alone [75].

Topical calcipotriol can also be used concomitantly with second-line therapies and exerts a useful dose-sparing effect when combined with UVB [76,77], PUVA [78–80], ciclosporin [81], retinoids [82] and fumaric acid esters [83].

Occlusion with polythene or hydrocolloid dressings can be used to augment the efficacy of calcipotriol [84]. This technique can be particularly useful for refractory plaques of psoriasis on the shins. Systemic absorption is also likely to be increased.

Calcipotriol not uncommonly induces irritant reactions, especially when applied to the face. Sensitization can also occur to calcipotriol although this seems to be rare [85–87]. In one case, propylene glycol in the base was responsible for the reaction [88].

The maximum recommended rate of usage is 100 g/ week of ointment. Exceeding this dose can induce hypercalcaemia although the safety margin seems reasonable and the use of higher doses can improve efficacy [89]. It is advisable to monitor urine and serum calcium in situations where there is a risk of inducing hypervitaminosis D (e.g. when the recommended dose is exceeded or when calcipotriol is used for indications other than psoriasis vulgaris, especially if large areas of skin are treated). Monitoring of serum calcium presents little difficulty but measurement of urine calcium excretion depends on obtaining accurate 24-h urine collections.

There are now a wide range of dermatoses in addition to psoriasis that have been reported to respond to calcipotriol, although the evidence is largely anecdotal in nature. These include confluent and reticulate papillomatosis [90], disseminated superficial actinic porokeratosis [91], erythema annulare centrifugum [92], extragenital lichen sclerosus [93], Flegel's disease [94], Grover's disease [95,96], inflammatory linear verrucous epidermal naevus [97], keratosis lichenoides chronica [98], lichen amyloidosus [99], lichen planus [100], nodular prurigo [101], naevoid hyperkeratosis of the nipple [102], morphoea [91], pityriasis rubra pilaris [91], Reiter's syndrome [91], ichthyoses [103,104], vitiligo [105] and Vorner's syndrome (epidermolytic palmoplantar keratoderma) [106].

Calcipotriol has not proved beneficial in trials on actinic keratosis [107], alopecia totalis [108], Darier's disease [103], hereditary palmoplantar keratoderma [103], keratosis pilaris [103] or seborrhoeic dermatitis [109].

Maxacalcitol (22-oxa-calcitriol)

This is an effective but currently unmarketed analogue with efficacy similar to calcipotriol [110].

REFERENCES

1 Ponchon G, Kennan AL, DeLuca HF. 'Activation' of vitamin D by the liver. *J Clin Invest* 1969; **48**: 2032–7.
2 Fraser DR, Kodicek E. Unique biosynthesis by kidney of a biological active vitamin D metabolite. *Nature* 1970; **228**: 764–6.
3 Boyle IT, Gray RW, DeLuca HF. Regulation by calcium of *in vivo* synthesis of 1,25-dihydroxycholecalciferol and 21,25-dihydroxycholecalciferol. *Proc Natl Acad Sci USA* 1971; **68**: 2131–4.
4 Carlberg C. Mechanisms of nuclear signaling by vitamin D$_3$: Interplay with retinoid and thyroid hormone signaling. *Eur J Biochem* 1995; **231**: 517–27.
5 Smith EL, Walworth NC, Holick MF. Effect of 1α,25-dihydroxyvitamin D$_3$ on the morphologic and biochemical differentiation of cultured human epidermal keratinocytes grown in serum-free conditions. *J Invest Dermatol* 1986; **86**: 709–14.
6 Ohta T, Mimura H, Kiyoki M. Effect of 1,24-dihydroxyvitamin D$_3$ on proliferation stimulated by epidermal growth factor in cultured mouse epidermal keratinocytes. *Arch Dermatol Res* 1996; **288**: 415–7.
7 De Mare S, De Jong EGJM, Van de Kerkhof PCM. DNA content and KS8.12 binding of the psoriatic lesion during treatment with the vitamin D$_3$ analogue MC 903 and betamethasone. *Br J Dermatol* 1990; **123**: 291–5.
8 Berth-Jones J, Fletcher A, Hutchinson PE. Epidermal cytokeratin and immunocyte responses during treatment of psoriasis with calcipotriol and betamethasone valerate. *Br J Dermatol* 1992; **126**: 356–61.

9 Hosomi J, Hosoi J, Suda T, Kuroki T. Regulation of terminal differentiation of cultured mouse epidermal cells by 1α,25-dihydroxyvitamin D$_3$. *Endocrinology* 1983; **113**: 1950–7.
10 Glade CP, Van Erp PEJ, Van Hooijdonk CAEM *et al.* Topical treatment of psoriatic plaques with 1α,24 dihydroxyvitamin D$_3$: a multiparameter flow cytometrical analysis of epidermal growth, differentiation and inflammation. *Acta Derm Venereol* 1995; **75**: 381–5.
11 Gerritsen MJP, Rulo HFC, Van Vlijmen-Willems I *et al.* Topical treatment of psoriatic plaques with 1,25-dihydroxyvitamin D$_3$: a cell biological study. *Br J Dermatol* 1993; **128**: 666–73.
12 Gerritsen MJP, Van Erp PEJ, Van de Kerkhof PCM. Transglutaminase-positive cells in psoriatic epidermis during treatment with calcitriol (1α,25 dihydroxy vitamin D$_3$) and tacalcitol (1α,24 dihydroxy vitamin D$_3$). *Br J Dermatol* 1995; **133**: 656–9.
13 Binderup L, Latini S, Binderup E *et al.* 20-Epi-vitamin D$_3$ analogues: a novel class of potent regulators of cell growth and immune responses. *Biochem Pharmacol* 1991; **42**: 1569–75.
14 Rigby WFC, Stacy T, Fanger MW. Inhibition of T lymphocyte mitogenesis by 1,25-dihydroxyvitamin D$_3$ (calcitriol). *J Clin Invest* 1984; **74**: 1451–5.
15 Zhang JZ, Maruyama K, Ono T, Iwatsuki K, Kaneko F. Regulatory effects of 1,25-dihydroxyvitamin D$_3$ and a novel vitamin D$_3$ analogue MC903 on secretion of interleukin-1α (IL-1α) and IL-8 by normal human keratinocytes and a human squamous cell carcinoma cell line (HSC-1). *J Dermatol Sci* 1994; **7**: 24–31.
16 Michel G, Gailis A, Jarzebska-Deussen B *et al.* 1,25-(OH)2-vitamin D$_3$ and calcipotriol induce IL-10 receptor gene expression in human epidermal cells. *Inflamm Res* 1997; **46**: 32–4.
17 Zhu K, Glaser R, Mrowietz U. Vitamin D$_3$ and analogues modulate the expression of CSF-1 and its receptor in human dendritic cells. *Biochem Biophys Res Commun* 2002; **297**: 1211.
18 Fukuoka M, Ogino Y, Sato H *et al.* RANTES expression in psoriatic skin, and regulation of RANTES and IL-8 production in cultured epidermal keratinocytes by active vitamin D$_3$ (tacalcitol). *Br J Dermatol* 1998; **138**: 63–70.
19 Reichrath J, Perez A, Muller SM *et al.* Topical calcitriol (1,25-dihydroxyvitamin D$_3$) treatment of psoriasis: an immunohistological evaluation. *Acta Derm Venereol* 1997; **77**: 268–72.
20 Oxholm A, Oxholm P, Staberg B, Bendtzen K. Expression of interleukin-6-like molecules and tumour necrosis factor after topical treatment of psoriasis with a new vitamin D analogue (MC 903). *Acta Derm Venereol* 1989; **69**: 385–90.
21 De Jong EMGJ, van de Kerkhof PCM. Simultaneous assessment of inflammation and epidermal proliferation in psoriatic plaques during long-term treatment with vitamin D$_3$ analogue MC 903: modulations and interrelations. *Br J Dermatol* 1991; **124**: 221–9.
22 Gerritsen MJP, Boezeman JBM, van Vlijmen-Willems IMJJ *et al.* The effect of tacalcitol (1,24 (OH2) D$_3$) on cutaneous inflammation, epidermal proliferation and keratinization in psoriasis: a placebo-controlled, double-blind study. *Br J Dermatol* 1994; **131**: 57–63.
23 Mozzanica N, Cattaneo A, Schmitt E *et al.* Topical calcipotriol for psoriasis: an immunohistochemical study. *Acta Derm Venereol Suppl* 1994; **186**: 171–2.
24 Cagnoni ML, Ghersetich I, Lotti T *et al.* Treatment of psoriasis vulgaris with topical calcipotriol: is the clinical improvement of lesional skin related to down-regulation of some adhesion molecules? *Acta Derm Venereol Suppl* 1994; **186**: 55–7.
25 Fullerton A, Serup J. Topical D vitamins: multiparametric comparison of the irritant potential of calcipotriol, tacalcitol and calcitriol in a hairless guinea pig model. *Contact Dermatitis* 1997; **36**: 184–90.
26 Kimura K, Katayama I, Nishioka K. Allergic contact dermatitis from tacalcitol. *Contact Dermatitis* 1995; **33**: 441–2.
27 Berth-Jones J. Circumlesional scaling induced by vitamin D: a guide to compliance. *Br J Dermatol* 2000; **143**: 206–7.
28 Kato T, Rokugo M, Terui T, Tagami H. Successful treatment of psoriasis with topical application of active vitamin D$_3$ analogue, 1α,24-dihydroxycholecalciferol. *Br J Dermatol* 1986; **115**: 431–3.
29 Miyachi Y, Ohkawara A, Ohkido M *et al.* Long-term safety and efficacy of high-concentration (20 µg/g) tacalcitol ointment in psoriasis vulgaris. *Eur J Dermatol* 2002; **12**: 463–8.
30 Van de Kerkhof PC, Werfel T, Haustein UF *et al.* Tacalcitol ointment in the treatment of psoriasis vulgaris: a multicentre, placebo-controlled, double-blind study on efficacy and safety. *Br J Dermatol* 1996; **135**: 758–65.
31 Baadsgaard O, Traulsen J, Roed-Petersen J, Jakobsen HB. Optimal concentration of tacalcitol in once-daily treatment of psoriasis. *J Dermatol Treat* 1995; **6**: 145–50.

32 Veien NK, Bjerke JR, Rossmann-Ringdahl I, Jakobsen HB. Once daily treatment of psoriasis with tacalcitol compared with twice daily treatment with calcipotriol: a double-blind trial. *Br J Dermatol* 1997; **137**: 581–6.

33 Schlotmann K, Ortland C, Neumann NJ *et al*. Placebo-controlled evaluation of the irritant potential of tacalcitol (1α,24-dihydroxyvitamin D$_3$) in healthy volunteers. *Contact Dermatitis* 2000; **42**: 260–3.

34 Van de Kerkhof PC, Berth-Jones J, Griffiths CE *et al*. Long-term efficacy and safety of tacalcitol ointment in patients with chronic plaque psoriasis. *Br J Dermatol* 2002; **146**: 414–22.

35 Messer G, Degitz K, Plewig G, Rocken M. Pretreatment of psoriasis with the vitamin D$_3$ derivative tacalcitol increases the responsiveness to 311-nm ultraviolet B: results of a controlled right/left study. *Br J Dermatol* 2001; **144**: 628–9.

36 Tzaneva S, Honigsmann H, Tanew A. A comparison of psoralen plus ultraviolet A (PUVA) monotherapy, tacalcitol plus PUVA and tazarotene plus PUVA in patients with chronic plaque-type psoriasis. *Br J Dermatol* 2002; **147**: 748–53.

37 Ahmed I, Berth-Jones J. High-dose tacalcitol in the treatment of extensive psoriasis. *J Eur Acad Dermatol Venereol* 2000; **14** (Suppl. 1): 258–9.

38 Kimura K, Katayama I, Nishioka K. Allergic contact dermatitis from tacalcitol. *Contact Dermatitis* 1995; **33**: 441–2.

39 Nijsten T, Mentens G, Lambert J. Vascular variant of keratosis lichenoides chronica associated with hypothyroidism andresponse to tacalcitol and acitretin. *Acta Derm Venereol* 2002; **82**: 128–30.

40 Ginarte M, Fabeiro JM, Toribio J. Confluent and reticulated papillomatosis (Gougerot–Carteaud) successfully treated with tacalcitol. *J Dermatolog Treat* 2002; **13**: 27–30.

41 Hayashi H. Treatment of Grover's disease with tacalcitol. *Clin Exp Dermatol* 2002; **27**: 160–1.

42 Kawaguchi M, Mitsuhashi Y, Kondo S. A case of subcorneal pustular dermatosis treated with tacalcitol (1α,24-dihydroxyvitamin D$_3$). *J Dermatol* 2000; **27**: 669–72.

43 Aoki T, Hashimoto H, Koseki S *et al*. 1α,24-dihydroxyvitamin D$_3$ (tacalcitol) is effective against Hailey–Hailey disease both *in vivo* and *in vitro*. *Br J Dermatol* 1998; **139**: 897–901.

44 Bohm M, Luger TA, Bonsmann G. Disseminated superficial actinic porokeratosis: treatment with topical tacalcitol. *J Am Acad Dermatol* 1999; **40**: 479–80.

45 Katayama I, Miyazaki Y, Nishioka K. Topical vitamin D$_3$ (tacalcitol) for steroid-resistant prurigo. *Br J Dermatol* 1996; **135**: 237–40.

46 Smith EL, Pincus SH, Donovan L, Holick MF. A novel approach for the evaluation and treatment of psoriasis. *J Am Acad Dermatol* 1988; **19**: 516–28.

47 Morimoto S, Yoshikawa K, Kozuka T *et al*. An open study of vitamin D$_3$ treatment in psoriasis vulgaris. *Br J Dermatol* 1986; **115**: 421–9.

48 Rizova E, Corroller M. Topical calcitriol: studies on local tolerance and systemic safety. *Br J Dermatol* 2001; **144** (Suppl. 58): 3–10.

49 Langner A, Stapor W, Ambroziak M. Efficacy and tolerance of topical calcitriol 3 µg/g^{-1} in psoriasis treatment: a review of our experience in Poland. *Br J Dermatol* 2001; **144** (Suppl. 58): 11–6.

50 Hutchinson PE, Marks R, White J. The efficacy safety and tolerance of calcitriol 3 µg/g ointment in the treatment of plaque psoriasis: a comparison with short-contact dithranol. *Dermatology* 2000; **201**: 139–45.

51 Bourke JF, Featherstone S, Iqbal SJ, Hutchinson PE. A double-blind comparison of topical calcitriol (3 µg/g) and calcipotriol (50 µg/g) in the treatment of chronic plaque psoriasis vulgaris. *Br J Dermatol* 1995; **133** (Suppl. 45): 17.

52 Ring J, Kowalzick L, Christophers E *et al*. Calcitriol 3 µg/g^{-1} ointment in combination with ultraviolet B phototherapy for the treatment of plaque psoriasis: results of a comparative study. *Br J Dermatol* 2001; **144**: 495–9.

53 Queille-Roussel C, Duteil L, Parneix-Spake A *et al*. The safety of calcitriol 3 µg/g ointment: evaluation of cutaneous contact sensitization, cumulative irritancy, photoallergic contact sensitization and phototoxicity. *Eur J Dermatol* 2001; **11**: 219–24.

54 Mortensen JT, Lichtenberg J, Binderup L. Toxicity of 1,25-dihydroxyvitamin D$_3$, tacalcitol, and calcipotriol after topical treatment in rats. *J Invest Dermatol Symp Proc* 1996; **1**: 60–3.

55 Kragballe K, Beck HI, Sogaard H. Improvement of psoriasis by a topical vitamin D$_3$ analogue (MC 903) in a double-blind study. *Br J Dermatol* 1988; **119**: 223–30.

56 Kragballe K. Treatment of psoriasis by the topical application of the novel cholecalciferol analogue calcipotriol (MC 903). *Arch Dermatol* 1989; **125**: 1647–52.

57 Darley CR, Cunliffe WJ, Green CM *et al*. Safety and efficacy of calcipotriol

ointment (Dovonex®) in treating children with psoriasis vulgaris. *Br J Dermatol* 1996; **135**: 390–3.

58 Oranje AP, Marcoux D, Svensson A *et al*. Topical calcipotriol in childhood psoriasis. *J Am Acad Dermatol* 1997; **36**: 203–8.

59 Travis LB, Silverberg NB. Psoriasis in infancy: therapy with calcipotriene ointment. *Cutis* 2001; **68**: 341–4.

60 Berth-Jones J, Bourke JF, Bailey K *et al*. Generalised pustular psoriasis responds to topical calcipotriol. *BMJ* 1992; **305**: 868–9.

61 Matsubara K, Kanauchi H, Imamura S. Successful treatment of generalized pustular psoriasis with calcipotriol [1α,24 (R)-(OH)-2D$_3$] ointment. *Acta Dermatol Kyoto* 1995; **90**: 447–52.

62 Dwyer C, Chapman RS. Calcipotriol and hypercalcaemia. *Lancet* 1991; **338**: 764–5.

63 Russell S, Young MJ. Hypercalcaemia during treatment of psoriasis with calcipotriol (Letter). *Br J Dermatol* 1994; **130**: 795–6.

64 Georgala S. Generalised pustular psoriasis precipitated by topical calcipotriol cream. *Int J Dermatol* 1994; **33**: 515–6.

65 Emtestam L, Weden U. Successful treatment for acrodermatitis continua of Hallopeau using topical calcipotriol. *Br J Dermatol* 1996; **135**: 644–6.

66 Kokelj F, Lavaroni G, Piraccini BM, Tosti A. Nail psoriasis treated with calcipotriol (MC 903): an open study. *J Dermatolog Treat* 1994; **5**: 149–50.

67 Petrow W. Treatment of a nail psoriasis with topical calcipotriol. *Aktuelle Dermatologie* 1995; **21**: 396–400.

68 Ashcroft DM, Po AL, Williams HC, Griffiths CE. Systematic review of comparative efficacy and tolerability of calcipotriol in treating chronic plaque psoriasis. *BMJ* 2000; **320**: 963–7.

69 Cunliffe WJ, Berth-Jones J, Claudy A *et al*. Comparative study of calcipotriol (MC 903) ointment and betamethasone 17-valerate ointment in patients with psoriasis vulgaris. *J Am Acad Dermatol* 1993; **26**: 736–43.

70 Berth-Jones J, Chu AC, Dodd WAH *et al*. A multicentre, parallel-group comparison of calcipotriol ointment and short-contact dithranol therapy in chronic plaque psoriasis. *Br J Dermatol* 1992; **127**: 266–71.

71 Ramsay CA, Berth-Jones J, Brundin G *et al*. Long-term use of topical calcipotriol in chronic plaque psoriasis. *Dermatology* 1994; **189**: 260–4.

72 Poyner T, Hughes IW, Dass BK *et al*. Long-term treatment of chronic plaque psoriasis with calcipotriol. *J Dermatolog Treat* 1993; **4**: 173–7.

73 Kragballe K, Barnes L, Hamberg KJ *et al*. Calcipotriol cream with or without concurrent topical corticosteroid in psoriasis: tolerability and efficacy. *Br J Dermatol* 1998; **139**: 649–54.

74 Guenther L, Van de Kerkhof PC, Snellman E *et al*. Efficacy and safety of a new combination of calcipotriol and betamethasone dipropionate (once or twice daily) compared to calcipotriol (twice daily) in the treatment of psoriasis vulgaris: a randomized, double-blind, vehicle-controlled clinical trial. *Br J Dermatol* 2002; **147**: 316–23.

75 Monastirli A, Georgiou S, Pasmatzi E *et al*. Calcipotriol plus short-contact dithranol: a novel topical combination therapy for chronic plaque psoriasis. *Skin Pharmacol Appl Skin Physiol* 2002; **15**: 246–51.

76 Kerscher M, Volkenandt M, Plewig G, Lehmann P. Combination of phototherapy of psoriasis with calcipotriol and narrow-band UVB. *Lancet* 1993; **342**: 923.

77 Kokelj F, Plozzer C, Guadagnini A. Topical tacalcitol reduces the total UVB dosage in the treatment of psoriasis vulgaris. *J Dermatolog Treat* 1996; **7**: 265–6.

78 Frappaz A, Thivolet J. Calcipotriol in combination with PUVA: a randomized double-blind placebo study in severe psoriasis. *Eur J Dermatol* 1993; **3**: 351–4.

79 Speight EL, Farr PM. Calcipotriol improves the response of psoriasis to PUVA. *Br J Dermatol* 1994; **130**: 79–82.

80 Kiriyama T, Danno K, Uehara M. Combination of topical tacalcitol and PUVA for psoriasis vulgaris. *J Dermatolog Treat* 1997; **8**: 62–4.

81 Grossman RM, Thivolet J, Claudy A *et al*. A novel therapeutic approach to psoriasis with combination calcipotriol ointment and very low-dose cyclosporine: results of a multicentre placebo-controlled study. *J Am Acad Dermatol* 1994; **31**: 68–74.

82 Van de Kerkhof PCM, Hutchinson PE. Topical use of calcipotriol improves outcome in acitretin treated patients with severe psoriasis vulgaris. *Br J Dermatol* 1996; **135** (Suppl. 47): 30.

83 Gollnick H, Altmeyer P, Kaufmann R *et al*. Topical calcipotriol plus oral fumaric acid is more effective and faster acting than oral fumaric acid monotherapy in the treatment of severe chronic plaque psoriasis vulgaris. *Dermatology* 2002; **205**: 46–53.

84 Bourke J, Berth-Jones J, Hutchinson PE. Occlusion enhances the efficacy of topical calcipotriol in psoriasis vulgaris. *Clin Exp Dermatol* 1993; **18**: 504–6.

85 Frosch PJ, Rustemeyer T. Contact allergy to calcipotriol does exist: report of an unequivocal case and review of the literature. *Contact Dermatitis* 1999; **40**: 66–71.

86 Yip J, Goodfield M. Contact dermatitis from MC 903: a topical vitamin D₃ analogue. *Contact Dermatitis* 1991; **25**: 139–40.

87 Bruynzeel DP, Hol CW, Nieboer C. Allergic contact dermatitis to calcipotriol. *Br J Dermatol* 1992; **127**: 66.

88 Fisher DA. Allergic contact dermatitis to propylene glycol in calcipotriene ointment. *Cutis* 1997; **60**: 43–4.

89 Bourke JF, Berth-Jones J, Hutchinson PE. High-dose topical calcipotriol in the treatment of extensive psoriasis vulgaris. *Br J Dermatol* 1993; **129**: 74–6.

90 Kurkcuoglu N, Celebi CR. Confluent and reticulated papilomatosis: response to topical calcipotriol. *Dermatology* 1995; **191**: 341–2.

91 Thiers BH. The use of topical calcipotriene/calcipotriol in conditions other than plaque-type psoriasis. *J Am Acad Dermatol* 1997; **37**: S69–71.

92 Gniadecki R. Calcipotriol for erythema annulare centrifugum. *Br J Dermatol* 2002; **146**: 317–9.

93 Kreuter A, Gambichler T, Sauermann K et al. Extragenital lichen sclerosus successfully treated with topical calcipotriol: evaluation by *in vivo* confocal laser scanning microscopy. *Br J Dermatol* 2002; **146**: 332–3.

94 Bayramgurler D, Apaydin R, Dokmeci S, Ustun M. Flegel's disease: treatment with topical calcipotriol. *Clin Exp Dermatol* 2002; **27**: 161–2.

95 Keohane SG, Cork MJ. Treatment of Grover's disease with calcipotriol (Dovonex®). *Br J Dermatol* 1995; **132**: 832–3.

96 Mota AV, Correia TM, Lopes JM, Guimaraes JM. Successful treatment of Grover's disease with calcipotriol. *Eur J Dermatol* 1998; **8**: 33–5.

97 Gatti S, Carrozzo AM, Orlandi A, Nini G. Treatment of inflammatory linear verrucous epidermal naevus with calcipotriol. *Br J Dermatol* 1995; **132**: 837–9.

98 Chang SE, Jung EC, Hong SM et al. Keratosis lichenoides chronica: marked response to calcipotriol ointment. *J Dermatol* 2000; **27**: 123–6.

99 Khoo BP, Tay YK, Goh CL. Calcipotriol ointment vs. betamethasone 17-valerate ointment in the treatment of lichen amyloidosis. *Int J Dermatol* 1999; **38**: 539–41.

100 Bayramgurler D, Apaydin R, Bilen N. Limited benefit of topical calcipotriol in lichen planus treatment: a preliminary study. *J Dermatolog Treat* 2002; **13**: 129–32.

101 Wong SS, Goh CL. Double-blind, right/left comparison calcipotriol ointment and betamethasone ointment in the treatment of prurigo nodularis. *Arch Dermatol* 2000; **136**: 807–8.

102 Bayramgürler D, Bilen N, Apaydin R, Erçin C. Naevoid hyperkeratosis of the nipple and areola: treatment of two patients with topical calcipotriol. *J Am Acad Dermatol* 2002; **46**: 131–3.

103 Delfino M, Fabbrocini G, Sammarco E et al. Efficacy of calcipotriol versus lactic acid cream in the treatment of lamellar ichthyosis and X-linked ichthyosis. *J Dermatolog Treat* 1994; **5**: 151–2.

104 Kragballe K, Steijlen PM, Ibsen HH et al. Efficacy, tolerability and safety of calcipotriol ointment in disorders of keratinization. *Arch Dermatol* 1995; **131**: 556–60.

105 Parsad D, Saini R, Verma N. Combination of PUVAsol and topical calcipotriol in vitiligo. *Dermatology* 1998; **197**: 167–70.

106 Lucker GPH, van de Kerkhof PCM, Steijlen PM. Topical calcipotriol in the treatment of epidermolytic palmoplantar keratoderma of Vorner. *Br J Dermatol* 1994; **130**: 543–5.

107 Smit JV, Cox S, Blokx WA et al. Actinic keratoses in renal transplant recipients do not improve with calcipotriol cream and all-*trans* retinoic acid cream as monotherapies or in combination during a 6-week treatment period. *Br J Dermatol* 2002; **147**: 816–8.

108 Berth-Jones J, Hutchinson PE. Alopecia totalis does not respond to the vitamin D analogue calcipotriol. *J Dermatolog Treat* 1991; **1**: 293–4.

109 Berth-Jones J, Adnitt PI. Topical calcipotriol is not effective in facial seborrhoeic dermatitis. *J Dermatolog Treat* 2001; **12**: 179.

110 Barker JNWN, Ashton REA, Marks R et al. Topical maxacalcitol for the treatment of psoriasis vulgaris: a placebo-controlled, double-blind, dose finding study with active comparator. *Br J Dermatol* 1999; **141**: 274–8.

Traditional remedies

Camphor

Camphor is an extract from the camphor laurel *Cinnamonum camphora*, best known as a moth repellant. It is sometimes added to lotions for its antipruritic and cooling effects. It is widely used in proprietary chilblain preparations.

Dyes

Gentian (crystal) violet. This is a triphenylmethane dye, which has antiseptic properties against bacteria and yeasts. Employed for many years as a topical treatment for bacterial and fungal skin infections, its use was drastically curtailed after experimental studies demonstrated that it interacted with DNA of living cells [1] and was linked to malignancies in mice [2]. No reports of human malignancy attributed to the use of gentian violet on the skin have been found in the recent literature. It is now licensed for topical application, as a 0.5% aqueous solution, to unbroken skin, and is not recommended for application to mucous membranes or open wounds. It has the advantages of being cheap, chemically stable and easy to prepare.

Brilliant green. This is also a triphenylmethane dye and has properties similar to gentian violet. It was often used in combination with the latter but does not seem to increase the spectrum of activity [3]. It has suffered similar restrictions in usage, as have other members of the group, such as malachite green.

Magenta. Magenta, or basic fuchsin, is a major component of Castellani's paint. It is known to have activity against Gram-positive bacteria and fungi, but is no longer used because of potential carcinogenicity. Colourless Castellani's paint, the same formula without the magenta (boric acid, resorcinol, phenol), has been used to reduce secondary bacterial contamination in onycholysis and in chronic paronychia.

Eosin. This is the disodium salt of tetrabromofluorescein. It is used as an astringent for areas of weeping eczema or superficial ulcers, and in dermatoses such as seborrhoeic dermatitis. Efficacy equivalent to flumethasone pivalate 0.02% has been demonstrated in infantile seborrhoeic dermatitis [4], and greater than clobetasone butyrate 0.05% in napkin dermatitis [5]. It has the advantage of being used in aqueous solution (usually 2%), which avoids problems with stinging, but allergy can occur, especially in patients with leg ulceration [6].

Menthol

Menthol is still mainly extracted from the Japanese mint (*Mentha arvensis*) although synthetic sources are now available. It is added to calamine and other lotions and creams to induce a cooling sensation and relieve pruritus.

REFERENCES

1 Rosenkranz HS, Carr HS. Possible hazard in use of gentian violet. *BMJ* 1971; **3**: 702–3.
2 Food Advisory Committee. Final report on the review of the Colouring Matter in Food Regulations 1973: Fd AC\REP\4. London: HMSO, 1987.
3 Bakker P, Van Doorne H, Booskens V *et al.* Activity of gentian violet and brilliant green against some microorganisms associated with skin infections. *Int J Dermatol* 1992; **31**: 210–3.
4 Shohat M, Mimouni M, Varsano I. Efficacy of topical application of glucocorticoids compared with eosin in infants with seborrhoeic dermatitis. *Cutis* 1987; **40**: 67–8.
5 Arad A, Mimouni D, Ben Amitai D *et al.* Efficacy of topical application of eosin compared with zinc oxide paste and corticosteroid cream for diaper dermatitis. *Dermatology* 1999; **199**: 319–22.
6 Le Coz CJ, Scrivener Y, Santinelli F, Heid E. Sensibilisation de contact au cours des ulcères de jambe. *Ann Dermatol Vénéréol* 1998; **125**: 694–9.

Miscellaneous agents

Capsaicin

Capsaicin is a remarkably potent compound extracted from hot peppers and responsible for the gustatory discomfort they induce. It is a very stable alkaloid probably produced by these plants to prevent the seeds being eaten by animals. Capsaicin stimulates release of substance P, which is subsequently depleted in sensory neurones [1]. It is also a potent ligand of the vanilloid receptor (VR1), which is expressed on sensory neurones [2]. Stimulation of this receptor by capsaicin can result in a refractory state in the neurone, probably explaining the hypoalgesia that can be induced by capsaicin.

The first application to be established for this drug was in treatment of post-herpetic neuralgia [3]. However, an increasing range of conditions are being reported to benefit including diabetic neuropathy [4], glossodynia [5], nodular prurigo [6], notalgia paraesthetica [7], pruritus ani [8], and pruritus caused by pityriasis rubra pilaris [9], psoriasis [10,11], PUVA [12] or uraemia [13].

REFERENCES

1 Buck SH, Burks TF. The neuropharmacology of capsaicin: review of some recent observations. *Pharmacol Rev* 1986; **38**: 179–226.
2 Szallasi A. Vanilloid (capsaicin) receptors in health and disease. *Am J Clin Pathol* 2002; **118**: 110–21.
3 Watson CP, Evans RJ, Watt VR. Post-herpetic neuralgia and topical capsaicin. *Pain* 1988; **33**: 333–40.
4 Forst T, Pohlmann T, Kunt T *et al.* The influence of local capsaicin treatment on small nerve fibre function and neurovascular control in symptomatic diabetic neuropathy. *Acta Diabetol* 2002; **39**: 1–6.
5 Epstein JB, Marcoe JH. Topical application of capsaicin for treatment of oral neuropathic pain and trigeminal neuralgia. *Oral Surg Oral Path* 1994; **77**: 135–40.
6 Stander S, Luger T, Metze D. Treatment of prurigo nodularis with topical capsaicin. *J Am Acad Dermatol* 2001; **44**: 471–8.
7 Wallengren J, Klinker M. Successful treatment of notalgia paresthetica with topical capsaicin: vehicle-controlled, double-blind, crossover study. *J Am Acad Dermatol* 1995; **32**: 287–9.
8 Lysy J, Sistiery-Ittah M, Israelit Y *et al.* Topical capsaicin: a novel and effective treatment for idiopathic intractable pruritus ani: a randomised, placebo controlled, crossover study. *Gut* 2003; **52**: 1323–6.
9 Neess CM, Hinrichs R, Dissemond J. Treatment of pruritus by capsaicin in a patient with pityriasis rubra pilaris receiving RE-PUVA therapy. *Clin Exp Dermatol* 2000; **25**: 209–11.
10 Bernstein JE, Parish LC, Rapaport M *et al.* Effects of topically applied capsaicin on moderate and severe psoriasis vulgaris. *J Am Acad Dermatol* 1986; **15**: 504–7.
11 Ellis CN, Berberian B, Sulica VI *et al.* A double-blind evaluation of topical capsaicin in pruritic psoriasis. *J Am Acad Dermatol* 1993; **29**: 438–42.
12 Kirby B, Rogers S. Treatment of PUVA itch with capsaicin. *Br J Dermatol* 1997; **137**: 152.
13 Cho YL, Liu HN, Huang TP, Tarng DC. Uraemic pruritus: roles of parathyroid hormone and substance P. *J Am Acad Dermatol* 1997; **36**: 538–43.

Minoxidil

This vasodilating agent was initially introduced as a systemic treatment for hypertension and was found to cause hypertrichosis. Subsequently, lotions containing minoxidil have been employed in various situations where hair is wanting. Formulations containing 2% and 5% solutions of minoxidil are currently available commercially. The most established indication is androgenetic alopecia although results are usually modest. Minoxidil can also accelerate hair regrowth after chemotherapy and there is possibly some modest benefit in patients with alopecia areata.

Topical application of minoxidil has proved remarkably safe. One potential hazard arising from long-term use is sensitization to the minoxidil or to components of the vehicle. A more common problem is hypertrichosis, usually on the face but sometimes more generalized [1]. This seems most likely to result from contamination of facial skin with minoxidil but systemic absorption has also been proposed to explain the most generalized cases. It is more problematic in female patients and is more likely to occur when the higher concentration is used.

The mechanism by which minoxidil stimulates hair growth remains to be established. It may exert direct effects on keratinocyte differentiation and proliferation within the hair follicle [2], it may alter the pattern of androgen metabolism in the dermal papilla [3] and it may improve vascularization of the papilla [4].

Androgenetic alopecia shows a positive although modest response to topical minoxidil in males and females. In a double-blind multicentre trial of 2% minoxidil in the USA, 256 females with androgenetic alopecia were treated for 32 weeks. Terminal (non-vellus) hairs increased from 140 to 163/cm^2 compared with a rise from 139 to 149/cm^2 in the placebo group. At the end of the study no dense regrowth was observed. Investigators reported moderate regrowth in 13% of the patients on active treatment and minimal regrowth in 50%, whereas the patients' assessments were more optimistic at 20% and 40%, respectively. The patients receiving placebo reported moderate and minimal regrowth in 7% and 33%, respectively [5]. In a similar European trial involving 294 female subjects, there was an increase in non-vellus hair of 33/cm^2 in the active group and $19/cm^2$ in the placebo group [6]. In an Australian trial on males with early pattern alopecia, only 12% had moderate regrowth after 48 weeks [7]. Response to the 5% lotion is somewhat better. In a recent study of 48 weeks' treatment duration completed by 351 male subjects, 5% solution was superior to 2% lotion and placebo from 8 weeks onward. At 48 weeks the mean terminal hair count had risen from 151 to $170/cm^2$ in the 5% group, from 144 to 156 in the 2% group and from 152 to 156 in the placebo group [8]. In male patients topical minoxidil is sometimes combined with oral finasteride [9].

Alopecia areata is sometimes treated with topical minoxidil, although cosmetically useful responses have not been frequent in most studies. The best results were reported by Fenton *et al.* [10] who conducted a double-blind crossover trial in which 30 subjects applied 1% minoxidil (lotion or ointment) or placebo twice daily, each for 3 months. By the end of the study 16 patients had grown cosmetically acceptable terminal hair, only one of them while on placebo. In a subsequent trial of very similar design on 23 patients, 13 demonstrated some degree of regrowth on the active medication while none did so on placebo—however, the result was cosmetically satisfactory in only one case [11]. In another study using 1% lotion on 48 subjects with severe disease, no difference was detected from placebo [12]. Similarly, no difference was observed between placebo and 3% minoxidil lotion after 3 months in a trial on 30 subjects with extensive disease [13]. In a study comparing 1% and 5% solutions, a total of 66 patients applied treatments twice daily [14]; patients with extensive (75% or greater) scalp hair loss showed a response, defined as terminal hair growth, in 38% of cases with 1% minoxidil versus 81% with 5% minoxidil. However, even in this high-dose group, only 6% showed a cosmetically acceptable response. A slightly higher rate of cosmetic response, 11%, was observed in an uncontrolled study in which 45 patients with severe disease applied 5% minoxidil twice daily and 0.5% dithranol (anthralin) cream once daily for 6 months [15]. Application of 2% minoxidil three times daily appeared to prolong the response to a 6-week tapering course of prednisolone in a double-blind study, although the numbers were too small to achieve statistical significance relative to placebo [16].

Other applications for topical minoxidil have included reduction in the duration of alopecia caused by chemotherapy. In a controlled trial on patients undergoing chemotherapy for breast carcinoma, the duration of baldness was 87 days in patients applying 2% minoxidil solution twice daily, versus 137 days in those applying placebo [17]. Additional applications have included stimulation of growth in hair transplants [18] and prevention of hair loss that may occur as a complication of cosmetic surgery [19].

REFERENCES

1 Peluso AM, Misciali C, Vincenzi C, Tosti A. Diffuse hypertrichosis during treatment with 5% topical minoxidil. *Br J Dermatol* 1997; **136**: 118–20.
2 Boyera N, Galey I, Bernard BA. Biphasic effects of minoxidil on the proliferation and differentiation of normal human keratinocytes. *Skin Pharmacol* 1997; **10**: 206–20.
3 Sato T, Tadokoro T, Sonoda T *et al.* Minoxidil increases 17β-hydroxysteroid dehydrogenase and 5α-reductase activity of cultured human dermal papilla cells from balding scalp. *J Dermatol Sci* 1999; **19**: 123–5.
4 Lachgar S, Charveron M, Gall Y, Bonafe JL. Minoxidil upregulates the expression of vascular endothelial growth factor in human hair dermal papilla cells. *Br J Dermatol* 1998; **138**: 407–11.
5 DeVillez RL, Jacobs JP, Szpunar CA, Warner ML. Androgenetic alopecia in the female: treatment with 2% minoxidil solution. *Arch Dermatol* 1994; **130**: 303–7.
6 Jacobs JP, Szpunar CA, Warner ML. Use of topical minoxidil therapy for androgenetic alopecia in women. *Int J Dermatol* 1993; **32**: 758–62.
7 Connors TJ, Cooke DE, De Launey WE *et al.* Australasian trial of topical minoxidil and placebo in early male pattern baldness. *Australas J Dermatol* 1990; **31**: 17–25.
8 Olsen EA, Dunlap FE, Funicella T *et al.* A randomized clinical trial of 5% topical minoxidil versus 2% topical minoxidil and placebo in the treatment of androgenetic alopecia in men. *J Am Acad Dermatol* 2002; **47**: 377–85.
9 Khandpur S, Suman M, Reddy BS. Comparative efficacy of various treatment regimens for androgenetic alopecia in men. *J Dermatol* 2002; **29**: 489–98.
10 Fenton DA, Wilkinson JD. Alopecia areata treated with topical minoxidil. *BMJ* 1983; **287**: 1015–7.
11 Frentz G. Topical minoxidil for extended areate alopecia. *Acta Derm Venereol* 1985; **65**: 172–5.
12 Vesty JP, Savin JA. A trial of 1% minoxidil used topically for severe alopecia areata. *Acta Derm Venereol* 1986; **66**: 179–80.
13 Price V. Topical minoxidil (3%) in extensive alopecia areata, including long-term efficacy. *J Am Acad Dermatol* 1987; **16**: 737–44.
14 Fiedler-Weiss VC. Topical minoxidil solution (1% and 5%) in the treatment of alopecia areata. *J Am Acad Dermatol* 1987; **16**: 745–8.
15 Fiedler VC, Wendrow A, Szpunar GJ *et al.* Treatment-resistant alopecia areata: response to combination therapy with minoxidil plus anthralin. *Arch Dermatol* 1990; **126**: 756–9.
16 Olsen EA, Carson SC, Turney EA. Systemic steroids with or without 2% topical minoxidil in the treatment of alopecia areata. *Arch Dermatol* 1992; **128**: 1467–73.
17 Duvic M, Lemak NA, Valero V *et al.* A randomized trial of minoxidil in chemotherapy-induced alopecia. *J Am Acad Dermatol* 1996; **35**: 74–8.
18 Avram MR. The potential role of minoxidil in the hair transplantation setting. *Dermatol Surg* 2002; **28**: 894–900.
19 Eremia S, Umar SH, Li CY. Prevention of temporal alopecia following rhytidectomy: the prophylactic use of minoxidil—a study of 60 patients. *Dermatol Surg* 2002; **28**: 66–74.

Nicotinamide [1]

The marked anti-inflammatory properties of topical nicotinamide, the amide derivative of vitamin B_3 (niacin), have been used to treat acne vulgaris. A 4% alcoholic gel is available. It is not yet certain by what mechanism the preparation exerts its anti-inflammatory effect. In a multicentre trial, it gave a global reduction in acne of 82% compared with 68% for 1% clindamycin gel over an 8-week period. An advantage of nicotinamide is that it avoids the problem of antibiotic resistance.

REFERENCE

1 Shalita AR, Smith JG, Parish LC *et al.* Topical nicotinamide compared with clindamycin gel in the treatment of inflammatory acne vulgaris. *Int J Dermatol* 1995; **34**: 434–7.

Chapter 76

Radiotherapy and Reactions to Ionizing Radiation

M.F. Spittle & C.G. Kelly

Introduction

The clinical effects of ionizing radiation on the skin have been known since the discovery of X-rays in 1895 [1]. At first, the physical aspects of dosimetry were little understood—a fact that did not hamper the enthusiasm with which both benign and malignant diseases were irradiated. Both the dosage and indications for irradiation were initially empirical, and the dermatologist may still see the late effects on the skin and subcutaneous tissues of overdosage due to inexperience. Indications for treating benign disease by irradiation have declined since the advent of topical steroids. If the effect of irradiation is understood, this treatment still has a specific place in the dermatologist's armamentarium for patients in whom disease is otherwise refractory to treatment [2,3].

Since the introduction of supervoltage irradiation, which gives a maximum dose below the surface of the skin, the acute skin reaction is rarely seen in the treatment of deep-seated malignant disease. However, if the skin is particularly at risk from recurrence as, for example, in the primary treatment of breast cancer, it can be fully treated.

It is in the best interest of patients suffering from skin tumours to be seen in a clinic where the expertise of specialists in radiotherapy and oncology, plastic surgery and micrographic surgery, as well as dermatology, are present.

REFERENCES

1 Goldschmidt H, Sherwin WK. Reactions to ionizing radiation. *J Am Acad Dermatol* 1980; **3**: 551–79.
2 Rowell NR. A follow-up study of superficial radiotherapy for benign dermatoses: recommendations for the use of X-rays in dermatology. *Br J Dermatol* 1973; **88**: 583–90.
3 Rowell NR. Ionizing radiation in benign dermatoses. In: Rook AJ, ed. *Recent Advances in Dermatology*, Vol. 4. Edinburgh: Churchill Livingstone, 1977: 329–50.

Types of ionizing radiation

X-rays are part of the electromagnetic spectrum. They have a shorter wavelength and are more energetic and penetrating than ultraviolet (UV) radiation.

Orthovoltage radiation includes beams softer than 1 million electron volts (MeV).

Grenz (German for border) rays are the most poorly penetrating ionizing rays. At 6–15 kV, these are at the borderline with non-ionizing radiation. As 90% of this radiation is absorbed in the upper 1 mm of the skin, it is important to treat only diseases of very superficial pathology with this beam. Dose-dependent pigmentation of the skin may occur, but alopecia will not, as the energy of the beam does not reach the depth of the hair follicle. Doses of 100–300 Gy have rarely been associated with malignancy [1], but there is a wide margin of safety with Grenz rays. However, the minimum voltage consistent with the depth of pathology should be chosen.

The most commonly used forms of radiotherapy in dermatological practice are superficial X-rays and electron beams.

Superficial X-rays, up to 100 kV, are used in the management of benign skin disease. The higher voltages are used for hypertrophic disease needing treatment to a greater depth, for example keloids. Fall-off of energy below the surface of the skin occurs in an exponential manner (Fig. 76.1) and there can still be substantial dose delivered at several centimetres depth.

Beta rays are electrons and can be derived from radioactive isotopes, such as ^{90}strontium or be produced by a linear accelerator. The energy of electrons is almost totally absorbed at a depth proportional to the given voltage. A useful treatment depth in centimetres is approximately one-third of the MeV energy, so a 4.5-MeV electron beam will be useful for treating to 1.5 cm and a 9-MeV beam to 3 cm (Fig. 76.2).

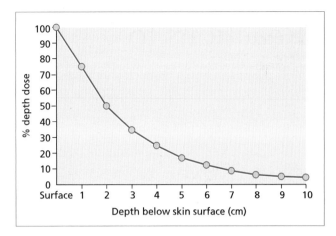

Fig. 76.1 Approximate per cent depth dose values for 90 kV superficial X-ray beam.

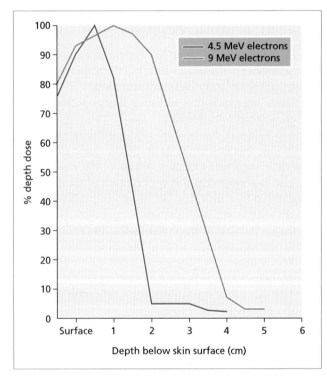

Fig. 76.2 Approximate per cent depth dose curves for 4.5 and 9 MeV electron beams.

As can also be seen in Fig. 76.2, the width of the peak of the beam also increases with electron energy. The peak can also be shifted to the left by the use of tissue equivalent material placed on the skin surface and acting as a degrader.

It is possible to irradiate the whole skin area with an electron beam. The minimal depth dose characteristics that may be achieved avoid the irradiation of subcutaneous structures which would occur if X-ray therapy that is absorbed exponentially was used. This technique is used in the treatment of mycosis fungoides [2]. Multiple radi-

ation fields are combined to give a homogeneous dose to the whole skin down to a depth of approximately 1 cm.

Electron-beam therapy is used to irradiate skin cancers in sites where the malignant lesion to be treated is large or overlying cartilage or bone. The mode of absorption of high-energy X-rays produced from a linear accelerator or of gamma rays is relatively independent of the atomic number of the tissue irradiated. Low-voltage X-rays are absorbed disproportionately in high-atomic-number materials. If this fact is not understood, necrosis may occur in cartilage or bone underlying large superficial lesions. Therefore, superficial X-ray therapy should be avoided when treating lesions overlying the nose, ear, hand and tibia to a radical dose. Modern high-voltage electron therapy is indicated in these sites [3].

Conventional photon beams or other less commonly used forms of radiotherapy such as fast neutron beams are rarely indicated in dermatological radiotherapy.

REFERENCES

1 Mortensen AC, Kjeldsen H. Carcinomas following Grenz ray treatment of benign dermatoses. *Acta Derm Venereol (Stockh)* 1987; **67**: 523–5.
2 Fuks A, Bagshaw MA. Total-skin electron treatment of mycosis fungoides. *Radiology* 1971; **100**: 145–50.
3 Spittle MF. Mycosis fungoides: electron beam therapy in England. *Cancer Treat Rep* 1979; **63**: 639–41.

Dose

The SI unit of absorbed dose is 1 J/kg and is called the gray. Note that 100 rad = 1 J/kg = 1 Gy; 1 rad = 1 cGy (centigray). The dose prescription is defined by the total dose given, the energy of the beam, the number of fractions given, the total number of days over which treatment is given and the volume or area treated. For example, a typical prescription for the treatment of a small basal cell carcinoma (BCC) might be '35 Gy using 90 kV SXT beam given in five fractions over 5 days to a 3-cm area'. This time–dose relationship is crucial to understanding the biological effect.

Radiosensitivity

All radiation is destructive. Abnormal cells repair radiation damage less well than normal cells. This inability to repair is reflected in death at mitosis. Anaplastic cells and those with a high mitotic index are more radioresponsive than differentiated cells. Radioresponsiveness and radiocurability are dissimilar and are functions of differences in cell population kinetics. Radiotherapy is usually given as a fractionated course, as the intervals between doses allow for the recovery of normal cells. The effect of a dose of radiation is reduced by increasing the number of fractions in which it is given or by lengthening the total overall treatment time. The effect of irradiation can be modified by anoxia, infection, oedema, trauma and any inborn genetic susceptibility. The face tolerates irradiation well, and radical dosages may be accompanied by good cosmetic results [1].

When benign conditions are being irradiated, the minimum dose and the lowest voltage appropriate to achieve the desired effect should be chosen. The threat of radiation carcinogenesis must clearly be seen in the context of the clinical indication for treatment. There is a threshold for somatic radiation changes which need not be breached in the treatment of benign conditions. The late radiation sequelae of treatment given many years ago are inexcusable with modern standards of dosimetry and equipment, and should not be seen in the treatment of benign diseases [2].

REFERENCES

1 Fitzpatrick PJ, Thompson GA, Easterbrook WM *et al*. Basal and squamous cell carcinoma of the eyelids and their treatment by radiotherapy. *Int J Rad Oncol Biol Phys* 1984; **10**: 449–54.
2 Traenkle HL. X-ray induced skin cancer in man. *Natl Cancer Inst Monogr* 1963; **10**: 423–32.

Indications for radiotherapy

Benign disease

Radiotherapy is used much less now in the management of benign skin conditions than formerly and then usually only after other treatment modalities have failed or are contraindicated. In some conditions such as psoriasis and eczema there is a response to radiotherapy but this is often only temporary [1]. Coupled with the risk of late radiation-induced malignancy, this has led to a decline in its use in all but the most refractory of cases. It is also still used occasionally in the management of keratoacanthoma where the differentiation from squamous cell carcinoma cannot be made with complete confidence [2–4]. Other rare uses are in Darier's disease [5], familial benign chronic pemphigus [5] and acrodermatitis continua of Hallopeau. Radiotherapy was used in the management of acne and rosacea in the past, and there may be patients still presenting with radiation sequelae or late radiation-induced tumours resulting from treatments given years ago for these benign conditions, and others such as ringworm [6].

REFERENCES

1 Fairris GM, Jones DH, Mack DP *et al*. Conventional superficial X-ray versus Grenz ray therapy in the treatment of constitutional eczema of the hands. *Br J Dermatol* 1985; **112**: 339–41.
2 Caccialanza M, Sopelana N. Radiation therapy of keratoacanthomas: results in 55 patients. *Int J Rad Oncol Biol Phys* 1988; **16**: 475–7.
3 Donahue B, Cooper JS, Rush S. Treatment of aggressive keratoacanthomas by radiotherapy. *J Am Acad Dermatol* 1990; **23**: 489–93.
4 Koster W, Nasemann T, Reimlinger S *et al*. Röntgendifferentialtherapie des Keratoakanthoms—ein kasuistischer Beitrag. *Z Hautkr* 1985; **60**: 215–8.
5 Mortensen AC, Kjeldsen H. Carcinomas following Grenz ray treatment of benign dermatoses. *Acta Derm Venereol (Stockh)* 1987; **67**: 523–5.
6 Shore RE, Albert RE, Reed M *et al*. Skin cancer incidence among children irradiated for ringworm of the scalp. *Radiat Res* 1984; **100**: 192–204.

Keloids

This is probably the most common benign condition now treated with radiotherapy. Keloids resistant to intralesional steroids or other conventional treatment may respond well to radiation. Excision of the keloid with early irradiation of the scar and stitch marks is more successful, but in some sites—for example, the tip of the shoulder and the upper middle chest, where surgery is inadvisable— good response of pain, itch and redness can be achieved, with some regression of the keloid itself. Relatively high doses are necessary; these will cause temporary hyperpigmentation, which will remain for many months in pigmented skin. Doornbos *et al*. [1] noted that 17 of 18 unexcised keloids that were less than a year old regressed with 1500 cGy given in three treatments over 6 days at 120 kV. Older keloids respond less well to irradiation. The most satisfactory management of keloids is postexcision irradiation, where a dose–response relationship can be seen. Total doses less than 900 cGy, irrespective of fractionation and postsurgical interval, did not prevent recurrence. Three doses of 400 cGy were given by Kovalic and Perez [2], with a 73% success rate. Using the commonly employed dose of 900 cGy, Lo *et al*. [3] described an 85% success rate and Borok *et al*. [4] a 96% response rate. No late sequelae or carcinogenesis was described by any of the previously quoted authors with follow-up in excess of 30 years.

As well as using superficial X-rays, treatment can be given using a radioactive iridium wire implant. At the time of excision a small plastic tube is inserted beneath the incision, with both ends of the tube exposed. The patient is then transferred to the radiotherapy department within 24 h, and the tube is loaded with iridium wire, and the scar irradiated to a dose of 20 Gy at 2 mm from the wire over 2 days. Escarmant *et al*. [5] describe the results of treating 783 keloid scars in 544 patients with interstitial iridium implants.

REFERENCES

1 Doornbos JF, Stoffel SJ, Hass AC *et al*. The role of kilovoltage irradiation in the treatment of keloids. *Int J Rad Oncol Biol Phys* 1990; **18**: 833–9.
2 Kovalic JJ, Perez C. Radiation therapy following keloidectomy: a 20-year experience. *Int J Rad Oncol Biol Phys* 1989; **17**: 77–80.
3 Lo TCM, Seckel BR, Salzman FA *et al*. Single-dose electron beam irradiation in treatment and prevention of keloids and hypertrophic scars. *J Radiother Oncol* 1990; **19**: 267–72.
4 Borok TL, Bray M, Sinclair I *et al*. Role of ionizing irradiation for 393 keloids. *Int J Rad Oncol Biol Phys* 1988; **15**: 865–70.
5 Escarmant P, Zimmermann S, Amar A *et al*. The treatment of 783 keloid scars by iridium-192 interstitial irradiation after surgical excision. *Int J Rad Oncol Biol Phys* 1993; **26**: 245–51.

Malignant disease

Radiotherapy for the common skin cancers

For most small BCC or squamous cell cancers without nodal involvement, surgical excision or radiotherapy will give excellent cure rates [1–4]. The decision as to which is the most appropriate modality will depend on several factors. These include the size and location of the tumour, any involvement of underlying tissues, and the likely functional and cosmetic outcome of either treatment. The patient's overall condition is important, as is the complexity of any surgery required; even the distance from the patient's home to the radiotherapy centre may play a role in determining the choice of treatment. The decision as to which modality of treatment to use should not be made solely on the basis of the patient's age.

Radiotherapy has a role to play in the treatment of almost all malignant skin conditions. Its use has been variable for several reasons. In some areas, traditional referral patterns have curtailed its use and the siting of radiotherapy departments in the larger conurbations has not given universal access to all patients. The past experience of radiation and lack of multidisciplinary meetings and clinics where the results of carefully considered fractionated radiotherapy could be seen by all attending have also reduced its use in appropriate cases [5]. Radiation damage, with skin atrophy, telangiectasia, necrosis and ulceration, occurred in the past, but this is now rare with better dosimetry, a wider range of radiotherapy modalities and more careful fractionation.

There is little difference in outcome between external beam radiotherapy with either superficial X-rays or an electron beam [6]. Locally placed moulds or applicators have also been used for malignant skin tumours, placing a radioactive source over the tumour and leaving this in position for a predetermined period [7,8].

Radiotherapy can be especially useful for tumour sites around the nose, ears and the eyelids, where surgical removal may result in a poor cosmetic result or loss of function [9]. The areas which have traditionally been considered as not suitable for radiotherapy, such as over the nose, pinna, dorsum of the hand or anterior lower leg can be treated if careful consideration is given to the volume treated, the total dose and the fractionation. It is also important to consider the general state of the patient and the condition of the skin in the site to be treated [10–13].

There are some patients who, for practical reasons, cannot have radiotherapy. If patients are unable to lie still because of confusion or neurological disease, then it can be impossible to deliver radiotherapy effectively and safely.

Radiotherapy doses for skin cancer

Radiotherapy doses have evolved empirically over a long

Table 76.1 Commonly used superficial radiotherapy dosage regimens for skin basal cell carcinoma and squamous cell carcinoma.

Total dose (Gy)	No. of fractions	Fractionation interval
18	1	–
28	2	7 weeks apart
35	5	Daily (for tumours less than 4 cm in diameter)
45	10	Daily (for tumours more than 4 cm in diameter)

These fractionation regimens are only examples. Many centres will have other similar but locally derived dose fraction regimens.

period of time and there is a wide range in use around the UK. As a rule, the greater the fractionation employed, that is the more the total dose is broken down into smaller fractions, the better the cosmetic effect (Table 76.1). This is obviously very important to some patients, but others are content to accept a poorer cosmetic effect if it allows fewer visits to hospital.

REFERENCES

1 Locke J, Karimpour S, Young G et al. Radiotherapy for epithelial skin cancer. Int J Radiat Oncol Biol Phys 2001; **51**: 748–55.
2 Morrison WH, Garden AS, Ang KK. Radiation therapy for nonmelanoma skin carcinomas. Clin Plast Surg 1997; **24**: 719–29.
3 Goldschmidt H, Breneman JC, Breneman DL. Ionizing radiation therapy in dermatology. J Am Acad Dermatol 1994; **30**: 157–82.
4 Ashby MA, McEwan L. Treatment of non-melanoma skin cancer: a review of recent trends with special reference to the Australian scene. Clin Oncol (R Coll Radiol) 1990; **2**: 284–94.
5 Motley RJ, Gould DJ, Douglas WS, Simpson NB. Treatment of basal cell carcinoma by dermatologists in the United Kingdom. British Association of Dermatologists Audit Subcommittee and the British Society for Dermatological Surgery. Br J Dermatol 1995; **132**: 437–40.
6 Griep C, Davelaar J, Scholten AN et al. Electron beam therapy is not inferior to superficial X-ray therapy in the treatment of skin carcinoma. Int J Radiat Oncol Biol Phys 1995; **32**:1347–50.
7 Guix B, Finestres F, Tello J et al. Treatment of skin carcinomas of the face by high-dose-rate brachytherapy and custom-made surface molds. Int J Radiat Oncol Biol Phys 2000; **47**: 95–102.
8 Berridge JK, Morgan DA. A comparison of late cosmetic results following two different radiotherapy techniques for treating basal cell carcinoma. Clin Oncol (R Coll Radiol) 1997; **9**: 400–2.
9 Petrovich Z, Kuisk H, Langholz B et al. Results and patterns of failure in 646 patients with carcinoma of the eyelids, pinna, and nose. Am J Surg 1987; **154**: 147–50.
10 Silva JJ, Tsang RW, Panzarella T et al. Results of radiotherapy for epithelial skin cancer of the pinna: the Princess Margaret Hospital experience, 1982–1993. Int J Radiat Oncol Biol Phys 2000; **47**: 451–9.
11 Avila J, Bosch A, Aristizabal S et al. Carcinoma of the pinna. Cancer 1977; **40**: 2891–5.
12 Lim JT. Irradiation of the pinna with superficial kilovoltage radiotherapy. Clin Oncol (R Coll Radiol) 1992; **4**: 236–9.
13 Bertelsen K, Gadeberg C. Carcinoma of the eyelid. Acta Radiol Oncol Radiat Phys Biol 1978; **17**: 58–64.

Radiotherapy for particular skin tumours

Basal cell carcinoma. Radiotherapy is useful for the primary treatment of small BCCs or larger lesions where surgery will leave a poor functional or cosmetic result. Radiotherapy also has a role to play after primary surgery if the margins are ambiguous and further surgery is thought not to be appropriate for the patient. It should not be used for re-treating BCCs which have recurred after previous radiotherapy. The morphoeic BCC subtype and the presence of underlying bone or cartilage involvement are relative contraindications to the use of radiation treatment; but even in the latter situation, radiotherapy can be given safely and effectively [1].

Squamous cell carcinoma. As with BCC, radiotherapy can be used as either the primary modality of treatment or as adjuvant treatment after surgery if there is a narrow surgical margin of clearance, the margin often being determined by the particular anatomical site of the tumour. The technique and dose are the same as those for treating BCC, but a wider margin is taken around the tumour and the patient is subjected to a more frequent and longer follow-up. If the squamous cell carcinoma has developed on the face, it is mandatory to check for cervical lymphadenopathy. Radiotherapy can be useful in palliation of advanced skin tumours and in some patients give long-term survival [2].

Bowen's disease. Radiotherapy can be a very effective treatment for Bowen's disease [3], but lesions on the leg have to be treated with more caution [3,4], as there is a danger of ulceration and very slow healing if large areas are treated. This condition can also be treated with a local mould, although this would be a relatively uncommon treatment modality.

Malignant melanoma. Malignant melanoma cells are not insensitive to radiotherapy, as is sometimes stated (Fig. 76.3a,b), but they do require higher dose-per-fraction regimens to overcome their ability to sustain more sublethal damage than other cell lines. Treatments may be hypofractionated, with patients receiving larger single doses in fewer fractions—for example, treatment being given three times rather than five times per week. Radiotherapy is also useful for palliation of both cutaneous and visceral metastases from melanoma [5].

There have not been any published prospective randomized controlled trials comparing surgery in melanoma with surgery and adjuvant radiotherapy, but there have been studies suggesting improved local control if postoperative radiotherapy is given [6,7].

Lentigo maligna and lentigo maligna melanoma. Radiotherapy has been used very successfully in both of these conditions. In one German study, there was no recurrence in any of 42 patients with lentigo maligna, with a mean follow-up of 15 months, and only two patients with lentigo maligna melanoma out of 22 showed local recurrence.

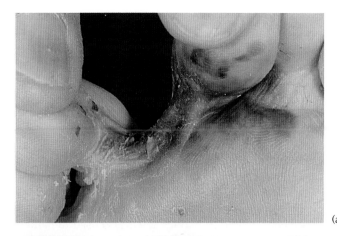

(a)

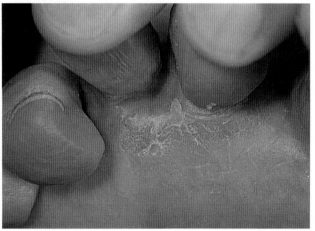

(b)

Fig. 76.3 A patient with malignant melanoma treated with primary radiotherapy. (a) Before treatment; (b) after treatment.

Cosmetic results were also reported as good or excellent in the majority of patients [8]. Similar complete responses for lentigo maligna were seen in studies from Australia [9] and Canada [10], again with good cosmetic results.

Merkel cell carcinoma. These tumours of neuroendocrine origin are most common on the head and neck, but can occur elsewhere on the skin. They have a tendency to recur locally after surgical removal and improved local control has been shown with a combination of wide excision and adjuvant post-operative radiotherapy [11–16].

Some authors even advocate irradiating the draining lymphatic nodes, especially if sentinal node biopsy is not performed. These are radiosensitive tumours and radiotherapy has been used as a primary treatment [16].

Cutaneous T-cell lymphoma. Radiotherapy can be used as both a localized treatment for isolated patches or plaques and for treating all of the skin by whole-body electron beam therapy [17–19]. With the latter, the patient takes up standard pre-determined poses for a number of fields allowing maximum cutaneous exposure to the beam. If treated early in the course of the disease, the patient can remain well and disease-free for a considerable period of time, but there is still doubt as to whether patients can be cured with this technique [20]. The eyes are shielded and the patient is made aware that he or she will lose their nails with this technique. Despite its drawbacks, radiotherapy is the most effective modality in achieving a complete response to treatment in cutaneous lymphomas.

Cutaneous Kaposi's sarcoma. It is well known that these tumours are sensitive to radiotherapy. Either superficial X-rays or electron beams can be used, depending on the thickness of the lesion(s) and consequently the depth of treatment required. Radiotherapy is also used to palliate systemic disease such as pulmonary masses [21,22].

Dermatofibrosarcoma protuberans. This low-grade sarcomatous tumour has a propensity to recur after surgery alone, and local control is improved by giving adjuvant radiotherapy [23,24].

Carcinoma metastatic to the skin from other primaries. Skin metastases tend to originate from the most common parenchymal tumours such as breast, colon and lung, but occasionally isolated skin metastasis occurs from tumours originating in the thyroid or urinary system. The latter two sites should be borne in mind if a patient presents with a single bizarre metastasis with no obvious evidence of previous primary tumour.

REFERENCES

1 Petrovich Z, Kuisk H, Langholz B *et al.* Treatment of carcinoma of the skin with bone and/or cartilage involvement. *Am J Clin Oncol* 1988; **11**: 110–13.
2 Lee WR, Mendenhall WM, Parsons JT, Million RR. Radical radiotherapy for T4 carcinoma of the skin of the head and neck: a multivariate analysis. *Head Neck* 1993; **15**: 320–4.
3 Dupree ML, Kiteley RA, Weismantle K *et al.* Radiation therapy for Bowen's disease: lessons for lesions of the lower extremity. *J Am Acad Dermatol* 2001; **45**: 401–4.
4 Cox NH, Dyson P. Wound healing on the lower leg after radiotherapy or cryotherapy of Bowen's disease and other malignant skin lesions. *Br J Dermatol* 1995; **133**: 60–5.
5 Seegenschmiedt MH, Keilholz L, Altendorf-Hofmann A *et al.* Palliative radiotherapy for recurrent and metastatic malignant melanoma: prognostic factors for tumor response and long-term outcome: a 20-year experience. *Int J Radiat Oncol Biol Phys* 1999; **44**: 607–18.
6 Burmeister BH, Smithers BM, Davis S. Radiation therapy following nodal surgery for melanoma: an analysis of late toxicity. *Aust NZ J Surg* 2002; **72**: 344–8.
7 O'Brien CJ, Petersen-Schafer K, Papadopoulos T, Malka V. Evaluation of 107 therapeutic and elective parotidectomies for cutaneous melanoma. *Am J Surg* 1994; **168**: 400–3.
8 Schmid-Wendtner MH, Brunner B, Konz B *et al.* Fractionated radiotherapy of lentigo maligna and lentigo maligna melanoma in 64 patients. *J Am Acad Dermatol* 2000; **43**: 477–82.
9 Harwood AR. Conventional radiotherapy in treatment of lentigo maligna and lentigo maligna melanoma. *J Am Acad Dermatol* 1982; **6**: 310–6.
10 Tsang RW, Liu FF, Wells W, Payne DG. Lentigo maligna of the head and neck: results of treatment by radiotherapy. *Arch Dermatol* 1994; **130**: 1008–12.
11 Eich HT, Eich D, Staar S *et al.* Role of postoperative radiotherapy in the management of Merkel cell carcinoma. *Am J Clin Oncol* 2002; **25**: 50–6.
12 Medina-Franco H, Urist MM, Fiveash J *et al.* Multimodality treatment of Merkel cell carcinoma: case series and literature review of 1024 cases. *Ann Surg Oncol* 2001; **8**: 204–8.
13 Fenig E, Brenner B, Katz A *et al.* The role of radiation therapy and chemotherapy in the treatment of Merkel cell carcinoma. *Cancer* 1997; **80**: 881–5.
14 Kokoska ER, Kokoska MS, Collins BT *et al.* Early aggressive treatment for Merkel cell carcinoma improves outcome. *Am J Surg* 1997; **174**: 688–93.
15 al-Ghazal SK, Hong A. Merkel cell carcinoma of the skin treated by primary radiotherapy. *Br J Dermatol* 1997; **136**: 640–1.
16 Suntharalingam M, Rudoltz MS, Mendenhall WM. Radiotherapy for Merkel cell carcinoma of the skin of the head and neck. *Head Neck* 1995; **17**: 96–101.
17 Kirova YM, Piedbois Y, Haddad E. Radiotherapy in the management of mycosis fungoides—indications, results, prognosis: twenty years' experience. *Radiother Oncol* 1999; **51**: 147–51.
18 Kirova YM, Piedbois Y, Le Bourgeois JP. Radiotherapy in the management of cutaneous B-cell lymphoma: our experience in 25 cases. *Radiother Oncol* 1999; **52**: 15–18.
19 Micaily B, Miyamoto C, Kantor G. Radiotherapy for unilesional mycosis fungoides. *Int J Radiat Oncol Biol Phys* 1998; **42**: 361–4.
20 Stallmeister T, Dieckmann K, Rehberger A, Jurecka W. Long-term remission of tumor-stage mycosis fungoides following total-skin electron-beam radiotherapy. *Eur J Dermatol* 1998; **8**: 240–2.
21 Kirova YM, Belembaogo E, Frikha H. Radiotherapy in the management of epidemic Kaposi's sarcoma: a retrospective study of 643 cases. *Radiother Oncol* 1998; **46**: 19–22.
22 Harrison M, Harrington KJ, Tomlinson DR, Stewart JS. Response and cosmetic outcome of two fractionation regimens for AIDS-related Kaposi's sarcoma. *Radiother Oncol* 1998; **46**: 23–8.
23 Ballo MT, Zagars GK, Pisters P, Pollack A. The role of radiation therapy in the management of dermatofibrosarcoma protuberans. *Int J Radiat Oncol Biol Phys* 1998; **40**: 823–7.
24 Haas RL, Keus RB, Loftus BM. The role of radiotherapy in the local management of dermatofibrosarcoma protuberans. Soft Tissue Tumours Working Group. *Eur J Cancer* 1997; **33**: 1055–60.

Acute radiodermatitis [1]

The minimal single dose that produces an observed erythema is called the 'erythema dose', and before the existence of other measurements much importance was placed on the dose needed to achieve this end. However, there is great individual variation, and field size, quality of radiation, area of skin irradiated, sex, race and age of the patient are some of the many factors affecting this parameter. The erythema dose was superseded by the roentgen and then the rad. The international unit of radiation dose is now the gray—the centigray is often used clinically.

The clinical course of the acute radiation reaction depends on the size of the dose and fractionation used. Large single fractions of irradiation are rarely given in clinical practice. An initial erythema and oedema may be seen within 24 h of irradiating the skin, and then a secondary and progressive erythema is manifest on the third to the sixth day. If the dose has been sufficiently high, vesicles and bullae may form, which subsequently dry and desquamate. The desquamated skin is usually dark. The perifollicular cells appear more resistant to radiation, and re-epithelialization is initiated in the perifollicular areas, which coalesce to cover the denuded surface. Postinflammatory pigmentation may occur at the periphery of the field and within the field in dark skins, and this pigmentation may last for many months. If the epithelium is irradiated to a high dose, it will appear atrophic and smooth, it is unable to form pigment, and is devoid of hair, sweat and sebaceous glands. This thin epithelium reacts poorly to trauma and has less tolerance of further radiation. Hyperkeratosis, telangiectasia and dyspigmentation may eventually occur, and malignant lesions supervene.

Treatment. There is little which influences the natural history of the acute radiation reaction. Trauma, heat, cold, friction and infection may cause ulceration, as such skin cannot readily repair damage. Mild steroid creams may give some symptomatic relief. Vigorous and repeated washing should be avoided in the acute stage.

Chronic radiodermatitis

The skin is atrophic and shows telangiectasia due to dilatation of a reduced or poorly supported skin vasculature. Dyspigmentation occurs; pigmentation usually is reduced or absent, but there may be small islands of increased pigment production and retention. Decreased sebaceous activity is invariable. The skin is usually atrophic, but increased fibrosis occasionally causes stiffening and tethering. Radionecrotic ulceration may occur, especially in areas of moisture and trauma, and is found in the most poorly vascularized central area of the irradiation scar. Areas of ulceration often show irregular new vessel growth, and histological examination may reveal pseudoepitheliomatous hyperplasia at the edge of an area of extreme atrophy or necrosis. Where there is underlying bone sequestration, radical surgery is necessary to obtain healing.

Chronic radiation change may be confused with a recurrence of a malignant lesion, but the severe pain associated with radiation necrosis is seldom seen with the malignant disease. The effects of normal ageing and sun exposure may combine with the effects of ionizing radiation, and produce accelerated changes of atrophy, necrosis or malignant change. This may also be seen when psoralens and UVA (PUVA) are used on irradiated skin.

Late radiation changes leading to necrosis should never be seen when modern techniques of fractionation to a radical dose for skin malignancies are used. Orthovoltage irradiation of skin overlying subcutaneous bone or cartilage, as on the lower leg, nose and ear, may occasionally result in radionecrosis, as there is a disproportionate absorption of radiation in these high-density tissues, and as cartilage has a particularly poor blood supply. Thus, supervoltage irradiation should be used in these sites. Radionecrosis typically occurs approximately 1 year following complete healing of the skin after radiotherapy, and is often precipitated by trauma or infection. Excision and grafting provide the only satisfactory treatment of extensive radionecrosis. Small areas may slowly heal with conservative management.

Histopathology

In acute radiodermatitis, there is oedema and sparseness of connective tissue beneath the epidermis. There may be flattening and loss of epidermal rete ridges with separation of the elastic tissue from the basal layer. Capillary endothelium may be hypertrophic and congested capillaries a feature. Haemorrhage and thrombosis are often observed.

Special stains may show subtle changes in the DNA–RNA structure of epithelial cells as early as the third day [1,2]. During the healing phase, the patchiness of the pathology is a striking feature. Atrophy may be bordered by epidermal hyperplasia, pigmentation is very irregular, and blood vessels are of variable size and shape; deeper vessels may be fibrosed. The fundamental pathology of chronic radiodermatitis is fibrosis of the vessels, with occlusion and varying degrees of homogenization of the connective tissue. Residual vessels may be enormously dilated. Bizarre, large, stellate fibroblasts may be seen in the dermal connective tissue in some cases. Fibrosis of the deep dermis and subcutaneous tissue may occasionally occur after supervoltage radiotherapy [3].

The changes in the epidermis vary from simple atrophy to acanthosis and extreme dyskeratosis. There is usually loss of adnexa such as hair follicles.

REFERENCES

1 Kurban AK, Farah FS. Effects of X-irradiation of the skin. *Acta Derm Venereol (Stockh)* 1969; **49**: 64–71.
2 Black MM, Wilson Jones E. Dermal cylindroma following X-ray epilation of the scalp. *Br J Dermatol* 1971; **85**: 70–2.
3 James WD, Odom RB. Late subcutaneous fibrosis following megavoltage radiotherapy. *J Am Acad Dermatol* 1980; **3**: 616–8.

Radiation-induced tumours

The type of tumour induced by radiation depends on both the cellular structure and the anatomical location of the damaged tissues. Basal cell epitheliomas occur following radiation to the face, scalp and trunk, whereas on the hands squamous cell tumours may occur. These are much more rarely seen since the development of more sophisticated radiotherapy machinery and a greater knowledge of radiobiology. It has not been possible to demonstrate any precise quantitative relationship between the development of cutaneous epitheliomas and the amount of radiation received on the skin surface, nor is it known what total dose or fractionation regimen would be most carcinogenic. It has long been known that carcinomas occur more profusely in areas subjected to many small doses administered at intervals over a long period. Multiple basal cell epitheliomas on the skin over the spine following radiotherapy to the lumbar spine for ankylosing spondylitis have been reported [1]. Some may show the histological appearances of the pre-malignant fibro-epithelioma of Pinkus. Radiation-induced basal cell epitheliomas of the scalp may be seen 20–50 years following X-ray epilation for ringworm infection. Late radiation changes are not always visible on the scalps of these patients, and hair growth may be relatively normal.

The doses of radiation used to treat benign dermatological conditions should never produce late radiation damage of even mild type [2]. In general, radiation-induced cancers have occurred after inappropriate doses, often of many thousands of centigray, given over a long period, frequently by lay therapists for conditions such as hirsutism or greasy skin and large pores [3], which are not indications for treatment by radiotherapy today. Shielding of structures especially sensitive to irradiation—for example, the adolescent thyroid [4]—was not routinely carried out. Although a greater knowledge of the limitations and effectiveness of radiation should prevent the occurrence of late radiation damage including carcinogenicity, the long latent period often demonstrated in those cases warns against early complacency [5,6].

Treatment. Most radiation-induced tumours should be excised. However, where there is no radiation damage evident on the skin, a subsequent radical dose of radiotherapy can be tolerated, but this would be indicated in very limited clinical circumstances.

Atypical fibroxanthoma
SYN. PSEUDOSARCOMA OF THE SKIN

This tumour, seen particularly in fair-skinned males who have suffered actinic damage, may also follow radiation damage [7–9]. It usually occurs on the face, but occasionally on the trunk or limbs. The clinical course is benign, despite the highly anaplastic histological appearance. Twenty-one tumours initially labelled as spindle cell squamous carcinomas were found by Hudson and Winkelmann [7] to be atypical fibroxanthoma.

Fibrosarcoma

Sarcoma appears to arise in irradiated skin much less frequently than carcinoma, and many of the tumours are low grade, showing no tendency to produce distant metastases [10]. At least some of the reported sarcomas are in reality spindle cell carcinomas [11]; this may be shown by the attachment of the tumour to the epidermis or by the presence of horny pearls. Radiation fibromatosis [12] is a diffuse proliferation in which bizarre and sometimes monstrous fibroblasts appear in the dermal connective tissue; the appearance can easily be mistaken for fibrosarcoma. Only exceptionally does fibromatosis undergo malignant change. It does appear that irradiation of an already chronically inflamed skin is more likely to be followed by a fibrosarcoma than irradiation of normal skin.

The fibrosarcomas, like the carcinomas following radiation, appear usually after repeated exposures to low-voltage rays and rarely from supervoltage radiation. The latent period in one series [13] averaged 26 years.

REFERENCES

1 Meara RH. Superficial basal-cell epitheliomata following radiotherapy. *Br J Dermatol* 1964; **76**: 294–6.
2 Lukacs S, Goldschmidt H. Radiotherapy of benign dermatoses: indications, practice and results. *J Dermatol Surg Oncol* 1978; **4**: 620–5.
3 Martin H, Strong E, Spiro RH. Radiation induced skin cancer of the head and neck. *Cancer* 1970; **25**: 61–71.
4 Goldschmidt H. Dermatologic radiotherapy and thyroid cancer. *Arch Dermatol* 1977; **113**: 362–4.
5 Fuks A, Bagshaw MA. Total-skin electron treatment of mycosis fungoides. *Radiology* 1971; **100**: 145–50.
6 Martin H, Strong E, Spiro RH. Radiation induced skin cancer of the head and neck. *Cancer* 1970; **25**: 61–71.
7 Hudson AW, Winkelmann RK. Atypical fibroxanthoma of the skin: a reappraisal of 19 cases in which the original diagnosis was spindle-cell squamous carcinoma. *Cancer* 1972; **29**: 413–22.
8 Kemmett D, Gawkrodger DJ, McLaren KM *et al.* Two atypical fibroxanthomas arising separately in X-irradiated skin. *Clin Exp Dermatol* 1988; **13**: 382–4.
9 Kempson RL, McGavran MH. Atypical fibroxanthomas of the skin. *Cancer* 1964; **17**: 1463–71.
10 Stout AP. Fibrosarcoma: the malignant tumor of fibroblasts. *Cancer* 1948; **1**: 30–63.
11 Traenkle HL. X-ray induced skin cancer in man. *Natl Cancer Inst Monogr* 1963; **10**: 423–32.
12 Stout AP. Juvenile fibromatosis. *Cancer* 1954; **7**: 953–78.
13 Russell B. Fibrosarcomata of the skin and subcutaneous tissues. *Trans Rep St John's Hosp Derm Soc Lond* 1959; **42**: 15–8.

Chapter 77

Physical and Laser Therapies

N.P.J. Walker, C.M. Lawrence & R.J. Barlow

Cryosurgery

Various methods of freezing skin have been described [1]. These achieve the following minimum temperatures: salt–ice mixture ($-20°C$); carbon dioxide snow ($-79°C$); dimethyl ether and propane (Histofreezer; $-50°C$); nitrous oxide ($-70°C$) and liquid nitrogen ($-196°C$). Because of its very low temperature, liquid nitrogen works faster than other methods. It is also easy to use, inexpensive and readily available. Liquid nitrogen is therefore the most widely used cryotherapy agent. All significant studies of cryotherapy technique have used liquid nitrogen, and it is the only agent discussed in this chapter. The effectiveness and freeze times of other cryogens has not been established.

Cryotherapy is believed to cause cell death in four ways.
1 Ice crystals formed in the cell damage cellular components [2]
2 Uneven intracellular ice formation during freezing leads to osmotic differences arising during thawing, which in turn cause cell disruption
3 Cold injury to small blood vessels results in ischaemic damage
4 Immunological stimulation produced by the release of antigenic components results in cell damage.

The extent of injury is determined by the rate of freezing, the coldest temperature reached, the freeze time and the rate of thawing. Maximum damage is produced by rapid freezing and slow thawing. Repeating the freeze–thaw cycle produces much greater tissue damage than a single freeze because the greater conductivity of the previously frozen skin and the already impaired circulation both allow a greater and faster depth of cold penetration.

It is suggested that a temperature of $-30°C$ is required to produce cell death. In practice, tissue temperatures achieved during cryotherapy do not need to be measured because clinical studies have determined the duration of liquid nitrogen spray freeze times for common skin conditions.

Clinical methods

In day-to-day use, liquid nitrogen *must* be kept in unsealed containers designed for the purpose. If containers are sealed, explosion will occur. One litre of liquid nitrogen held in an unsealed vacuum flask will last approximately 6 h. Liquid nitrogen can be applied using cotton wool swabs dipped into the liquid, but a liquid nitrogen spray is faster and more convenient.

Clinical uses

Liquid nitrogen cryotherapy has been used to treat a wide range of skin diseases (Table 77.1) [3]. The simplicity and speed of cryosurgery treatment are benefits, but cryotherapy can easily be performed incorrectly and ineffectively. The correct technique and freeze times are required to

Table 77.1 Skin conditions responsive to cryosurgery [3,13].

Naevi	Pigmented
	Epidermal
Lentigo	Benign
Vascular lesions	Telangiectasia
	Spider naevus
	Pyogenic granuloma
	Pseudopyogenic granuloma
	Kaposi's sarcoma
	Haemangioma
	Lymphangioma
Keratotic and preneoplastic	Viral warts
	Molluscum contagiosum
	Seborrhoeic keratosis
	Solar keratosis
	Cutaneous horn
	Keratoacanthoma
	Bowen's disease
Carcinoma [5–7]	Basal cell epithelioma
	Squamous cell epithelioma
	Lentigo maligna
Cysts	Epidermal
	Synovial
	Acne
	Mucous cyst
Leukoplakia	
Axillary hyperhidrosis	
Scarring	Keloid
	Acne (carbon dioxide snow, acetone 'slush')
Sebaceous hyperplasia	
Rhinophyma	

produce results similar to those described in published studies [4].

Cryosurgical treatment of basal cell epitheliomas gives cure rates that compare favourably with other modes of therapy [5–7], provided the correct technique is used and the treatment limited to small (less than 20 mm), well-defined, previously untreated tumours. Less favourable results are obtained with lesions on the inner canthus of the eye, nasolabial and retro-auricular folds and the hair-bearing scalp. The temperature reached and the number of freeze–thaw cycles are also critical. Debulking the tumour using curettage or electrosurgery prior to cryotherapy is advocated by some authors [8,9]. Lower leg Bowen's disease is best treated by curettage, which is superior to cryotherapy [10], which in turn is superior to radiotherapy [11].

Side effects [1]

Cryotherapy pain is significant but usually transient, and tissue swelling is common. Inflammation can be reduced with topical steroid applications [12]. Haemorrhagic blisters may occur but blister formation is not necessary for the cure of lesions such as viral warts. Sun-damaged and senile atrophic skin, and areas previously treated with topical steroids or X-irradiation, are more likely to blister or become necrotic after freezing. Skin necrosis is a desirable part of the treatment of neoplastic and many preneoplastic lesions, and several weeks may elapse before healing is complete. Hypopigmentation is common after liquid nitrogen cryosurgery, is particularly noticeable in dark-skinned patients and may be permanent [2,13]. Temporary post-inflammatory hyperpigmentation is to be expected following less severe freezing. Nerve damage resulting in paraesthesiae, distal anaesthesia and motor paralysis occasionally occurs [14]. Similarly, deep freezing over the lacrimal ducts may, very rarely, lead to permanent ductal obstruction [1].

REFERENCES

1 Dawber R, Colver G, Jackson A, Pringle F. *Cutaneous Cryosurgery: Principles and Clinical Practice.* London: Martin Dunitz, 1997.
2 Dawber RPR. Cold kills! *Clin Exp Dermatol* 1988; **13**: 137–50.
3 Kuflik EG. Cryosurgery updated. *J Am Acad Dermatol* 1994; **31**: 925–44.
4 McKenna DB, Cooper EJ, Kavanagh GM *et al.* Amelanotic malignant melanoma following cryosurgery for atypical lentigo maligna. *Clin Exp Dermatol* 2000; **25**: 600–4.
5 Kuflik EG, Gage AA. The 5 year cure rate achieved by cryosurgery for skin cancer. *J Am Acad Dermatol* 1991; **24**: 1002–4.
6 Torre D. Cryosurgery of basal cell carcinoma. *J Am Acad Dermatol* 1986; **5**: 917–29.
7 Holt PJA. Cryotherapy for skin cancer: results over a 5 year period using liquid nitrogen spray cryosurgery. *Br J Dermatol* 1988; **119**: 231–40.
8 Conclaves JC, Martins C. Debulking of skin cancers with radio frequency before cryosurgery. *Dermatol Surg* 1997; **23**: 253–6.
9 Nordic P. Curettage–cryosurgery for non-melanoma skin cancer of the external ear: excellent 5-year results. *Br J Dermatol* 1999; **140**: 291–3.
10 Ahmed I, Berth-Jones J, Charles-Holmes S *et al.* Comparison of cryotherapy with curettage in the treatment of Bowen's disease: a prospective study. *Br J Dermatol* 2000; **143**: 759–66.
11 Cox NH, Dyson P. Wound healing on the lower leg after radiotherapy or cryotherapy of Bowen's disease and other malignant skin lesions. *Br J Dermatol* 1995; **133**: 60–5.
12 Hinds TC, Spire J, Scott LV. Clobetasol propionate ointment reduces inflammation after cryotherapy. *Br J Dermatol* 1985; **112**: 599–602.
13 Graham GF, Deltas RL, Garrett AB *et al.* Guidelines of care for cryosurgery. *J Am Acad Dermatol* 1994; **31**: 648–53.
14 Faber WR, Naafs B, Sillevis Smitt JH. Sensory loss following cryosurgery of skin lesions. *Br J Dermatol* 1987; **117**: 343–7.

Curettage

Curettage is only possible when the curetted material is more fragile than normal skin (e.g. basal cell carcinoma; BCC), or there is a natural cleavage plane (e.g. seborrhoeic wart) between the lesion and the surrounding skin. On mobile or fragile skin areas, a starting point for curettage can be made by fulgurizing the rim. Stop bleeding using either a chemical haemostatic agent (e.g. aluminium chloride 30% in isopropyl alcohol), cautery or electrodesiccation. Do not use alcohol-based skin-cleansing solutions during cautery or electrodesiccation because of the fire

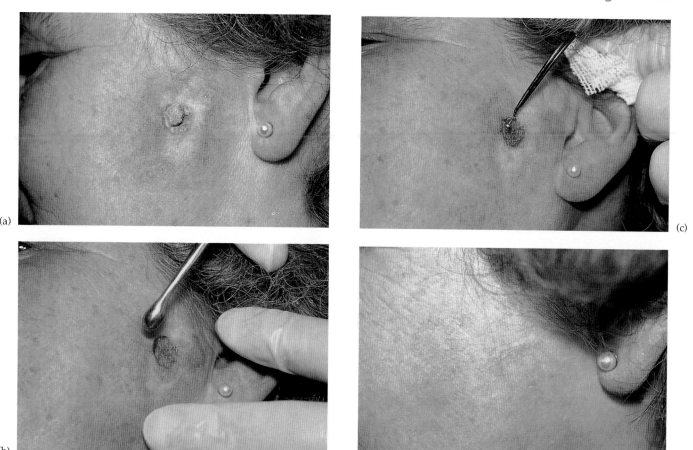

Fig. 77.1 Curettage and cautery of an actinic keratosis. (a) After local anaesthetic injection, this hyperkeratotic actinic keratosis was (b) curetted off and (c) the wound cauterized. (d) At 4 months the wound had healed leaving a barely visible scar.

risk. The resulting wound heals by re-epithelialization from the retained follicular and edge epithelium.

Benign lesions

Curettage of *viral warts* is sometimes effective. Treatment is painful and there is a risk of scarring and recurrence. Solitary warts on the face of adults can usually be removed by curettage, otherwise viral warts should only be curetted off when other methods have failed. Curettage is probably justifiable in painful plantar warts that have not responded to other therapies. Nerve block anaesthesia may be required [1]. There is a risk of painful scar formation. Peri- and subungual warts are difficult to curette off; the nail may have to be partially removed to allow adequate curettage. Genital or perianal warts that have not responded to cryotherapy, podophyllin or imiquimod can be curetted off. *Seborrhoeic warts* can be treated by cryotherapy or curetted off. In contrast, *pyogenic granulo-*

mas and *hypertrophic* or *solitary actinic keratoses* (Fig. 77.1) are best treated using curettage, as this provides material for histological confirmation of the diagnosis.

Non-melanoma skin cancers

The technique is the same for both BCC and squamous cell carcinoma (SCC) (Fig. 77.2). Tense the anaesthetized skin around the lesion and scrape off the bulk of the tumour using a small sharp curette [2]; the curette should not be so sharp that there is a risk of it slicing through the underlying dermis. The fragmented specimen should be mounted on a small piece of filter paper, where it is allowed to congeal slightly before being dropped into formalin. In this way the pathologist receives a single sample rather than multiple small floating fragments. Cauterize, using a hot wire with a beaded tip, or electrodesiccate the wound surface. Repeat the curettage using a smaller curette to search for residual pockets of tumour. At this stage, the curette will be scraping against the normal dermis and less material will be removed. If the curette penetrates the dermis and enters fat, curettage should be abandoned as it is impossible to distinguish between the softer tumour tissue and the underlying fat. The wound will need to be excised down to and including fat. Perforation of the

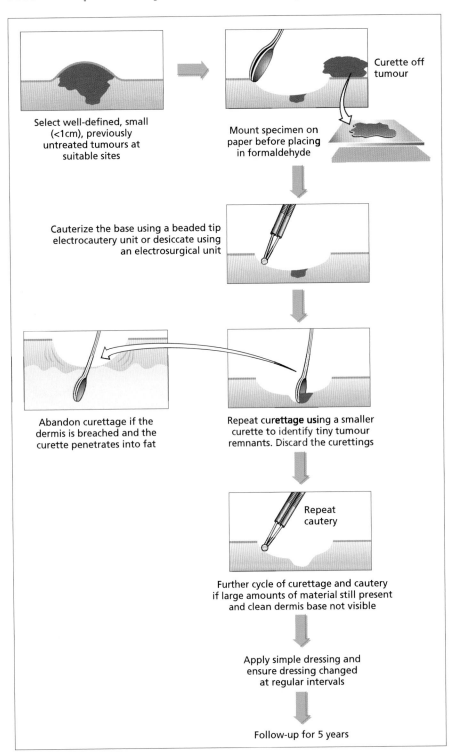

Select well-defined, small (<1cm), previously untreated tumours at suitable sites

Mount specimen on paper before placing in formaldehyde

Curette off tumour

Cauterize the base using a beaded tip electrocautery unit or desiccate using an electrosurgical unit

Abandon curettage if the dermis is breached and the curette penetrates into fat

Repeat curettage using a smaller curette to identify tiny tumour remnants. Discard the curettings

Repeat cautery

Further cycle of curettage and cautery if large amounts of material still present and clean dermis base not visible

Apply simple dressing and ensure dressing changed at regular intervals

Follow-up for 5 years

Fig. 77.2 Schematic diagram of the stages of curettage and cautery of a basal cell carcinoma. (From Lawrence [14].)

dermis is particularly likely to occur if an incisional biopsy has been taken prior to treatment. Repeat the cautery or electrodesiccation. A third cycle of curettage and cautery is required if a large amount of material is removed at the second stage. The histological specimen only confirms the diagnosis; it provides no indication about the adequacy of treatment. Do not curette recurrent tumours because of the high recurrence rates [3].

Basal cell carcinoma

Curettage of BCCs depends on the tumour being easier to scrape off than the surrounding normal tissue. Thus, if strands of fibrous tissue separate clumps of tumour (as occurs in morphoeic, recurrent or invasive BCCs) or the adjacent skin tears easily, cannot be tensed or hair roots impede curettage, the results will be poor and curettage

Table 77.2 Types of basal cell carcinoma (BCC) that should not be treated by curettage.

Large tumours (≥ 2 cm diameter)
Tumours at sites where curettage produces a poor cosmetic result, is technically difficult or is associated with a high risk of recurrence
Morphoeic, infiltrating or basisquamous BCCs
Recurrent tumours
Ill-defined tumours
Tumours penetrating muscle, fat, bone, etc.
Tumours where an incisional biopsy has been performed (risk of perforation of the dermal sling)

should be avoided. High recurrence rates occur after curettage of recurrent [3], morphoeic [4] or large tumours [4,5], or treatment by inexperienced operators (Table 77.2) [6]. When small (less than 20 mm diameter) [4–8] non-recurrent tumours [3,9,10] on suitable sites (Table 77.3) are curetted by experts [6,11], the 5-year cure rate is 95% or better (Table 77.4). Cautery and electrodesiccation can be used interchangeably and their use improves cure rates [12]. Paradoxically, despite these high cure rates, histological examination after curettage and electrodesiccation shows that some residual tumour is present in almost 30% of cases [13,14]. Thus, cure must also depend on other factors, such as residual tumour cell mass, inflammatory reaction and healing responses.

Squamous cell carcinoma

Experience shows [8,10,15] that well-differentiated, primary, slow-growing SCCs arising on sun-exposed sites can be cured by curettage and cautery (Table 77.5). However, SCCs with a higher risk of recurrence or metastasis should not be treated by curettage. These high-risk SCCs include lesions arising on scars, ears, lips, areas of radiation or thermal injury, chronic ulcers or sinuses, Bowen's disease and non-sun-exposed sites; and large (more than 20 mm), thick (more than 4 mm), poorly differentiated and recurrent SCCs, or those arising in an immunocompromised patient [16,17].

Intraepidermal carcinoma (Bowen's disease)

Intraepidermal carcinoma, especially on the lower leg, heals better after curettage than cryotherapy [18], as the extent of treatment is more predictably determined by the operator. Radiotherapy, 5-fluorouracil and excision are all alternatives.

REFERENCES

1 Eriksson E. *Illustrated Handbook in Local Anaesthesia*, 2nd edn. Philadelphia: Saunders, 1980: 112–4.
2 Bennett RG. *Fundamentals of Cutaneous Surgery*. St Louis: Mosby, 1988: 536–43.

Table 77.3 Sites to avoid curettage and cautery of basal cell carcinomas.

Sites with a high recurrence rate after all treatment modalities	Sites where curettage is technically difficult	Sites associated with poor cosmesis after curettage
Nose	Lips	Vermilion border
Nasolabial fold	Eyelid	Ala rim
Around the eye	Hair-bearing scalp	Nose tip
Around the ear		Chin
Scalp		

Table 77.4 Cure rates following curettage and cautery and/or electrodesiccation of primary basal cell carcinoma.

Author, year of publication	Number of tumours	Duration of follow-up (years)	Number of recurrences (%)	Tumour size
Simpson [9] 1966	495	2–5	35 (7)	ns
Williamson and Jackson [11] 1962	287	3	22 (7.6)	ns
Knox *et al.* [8] 1967	282	5	4 (1.4)	< 20 mm
Sweet [4] 1963	268	≥ 3	19 (7.1)	< 20 mm
Spiller and Spiller [7] 1984	208	5	3 (1.4)	< 20 mm
Tromovitch [10] 1965	75	≥ 5	(4)	ns

ns, not stated.

Table 77.5 Cure rates following curettage and cautery of primary squamous cell carcinoma (SCC).

Author, year of publication	Number of tumours	Duration of follow-up (years)	Percentage cure rate	Metastasis?	Tumour size (number greater and smaller than 2 cm)
Knox et al. [8] 1967	213	5	99	No record	185 < 2 cm 28 > 2 cm
Knox et al. [8] 1967	545	> 1	99	1	495 < 2 cm 50 > 2 cm
Tromovitch [10] 1965	29	5	96.6	Nil	No record
Freeman et al. [15] 1964	407	1–5	96–100	Nil	355 < 2 cm 52 > 2 cm

3 Menn H, Robins P, Knopf AW, Bart RS. The recurrent basal cell epithelioma: a study of 100 cases of recurrent retreated basal cell epithelioma. *Arch Dermatol* 1971; **103**: 628–31.

4 Sweet RD. The treatment of basal cell carcinoma by curettage. *Br J Dermatol* 1963; **75**: 137–48.

5 Dubin N, Kopf AW. Multivariate risk score for recurrence of cutaneous basal cell carcinomas. *Arch Dermatol* 1983; **119**: 373–7.

6 Kopf AW, Bart RS, Schrager D et al. Curettage–electrodesiccation treatment of basal cell carcinoma. *Arch Dermatol* 1977; **113**: 439–43.

7 Spiller WF, Spiller RF. Treatment of basal cell carcinoma by curettage and electrodesiccation. *J Am Acad Dermatol* 1984; **11**: 808–14.

8 Knox JM, Freeman RG, Duncan WC, Heaton CL. Treatment of skin cancer. *South Med J* 1967; **60**: 241–6.

9 Simpson JR. The management of rodent ulcers by curettage and cauterization. *Br J Dermatol* 1966; **78**: 147–8.

10 Tromovitch TA. Skin cancer: treatment by curettage and desiccation. *Calif Med* 1965; **103**: 107–8.

11 Williamson GS, Jackson R. Treatment of basal cell carcinoma by electrodesiccation and curettage. *Can Med Assoc J* 1962; **86**: 855–62.

12 Reymann F. Treatment of basal cell carcinoma of the skin with curettage. II. A follow-up study. *Arch Dermatol* 1973; **108**: 528–31.

13 Salasche SJ. Curettage and electrodesiccation in the treatment of mid-facial basal cell epithelioma. *J Am Acad Dermatol* 1983; **8**: 496–503.

14 Edens BL, Bartlow GA, Haghigi P et al. Effectiveness of curettage and electrodesiccation in the removal of basal cell carcinoma. *J Am Acad Dermatol* 1983; **9**: 383–8.

15 Freeman RG, Knox JM, Heaton CL. The treatment of skin cancer: a statistical study of 1341 skin tumours comparing results obtained with irradiation, surgery and curettage followed by electrodesiccation. *Cancer* 1964; **17**: 535–8.

16 Rowe DE, Carroll RJ, Day CL. Prognostic factors for local recurrence, metastasis, and survival rates in squamous cell carcinoma of the skin, ear and lip. *J Am Acad Dermatol* 1992; **26**: 976–90.

17 Motley R, Kersey P, Lawrence C. Multiprofessional guidelines for the management of the patient with primary cutaneous squamous cell carcinoma. *Br J Dermatol* 2002; **146**: 18–25.

18 Ahmed I, Berth-Jones J, Charles-Holmes S et al. Comparison of cryotherapy with curettage in the treatment of Bowen's disease: a prospective study. *Br J Dermatol* 2000; **143**: 759–66.

Electrosurgery

Electrosurgery includes electrodesiccation, electrofulguration, cutting diathermy (syn. electrosection, electroresection) and electrolysis [1,2]. Coagulation or tissue destruction is produced by the heat created as the electrical current passes through the tissue. Although not strictly an electrosurgical technique, electrocautery is usually also included because of its development from the established method of using heat in the form of hot oils, cautery irons, etc., to control bleeding.

Electrocautery

SYN. CAUTERY; HEAT CAUTERY; HOT-WIRE CAUTERY

The cautery machine power output should be controllable so that the tip temperature can be adjusted rather than being dependent on the battery power. A variety of tips are available. The *beaded tip* is best for haemostasis after curettage and shave biopsy; this should be just hot enough to char a cotton swab, but not red hot as the platinum tip may melt. If the beaded tip drags on the tissue as it is drawn across the wound, the tip temperature is too low. After use, any remaining debris should be burnt off the tip by briefly allowing it to become red hot. The needle-like end of the *cold point cautery tip* is heated, by conduction, via a wire coil, and is used to treat spider naevi. The *flat blade* can be used for pedunculated lesions or shave excisions, but has to be glowing red hot to cut through tissue, producing a heating artefact on the excised material. Furthermore, the red-hot blade has to be quickly passed through the skin to avoid excessive heat damage at the wound site, so the direction and depth of the cut cannot be adjusted easily and the blade may accidentally cut or burn deeper into the tissue than required.

Electrosurgery

SYN. SURGICAL DIATHERMY; COLD ELECTROCAUTERY

Waveform

Electrosurgical equipment converts domestic alternating current into high-frequency alternating current. When this passes through a high-resistance medium, such as the skin, heat is produced, resulting in tissue coagulation, desiccation or cutting, depending on the electrical waveform. A highly damped waveform (intermittent pulses of electrical discharge separated by intervals of zero voltage) results in electrodesiccation and/or fulguration. In contrast, a continuous waveform produces a cutting effect and a moderately damped or blended waveform (a mixture of continuous and highly damped waveforms) chiefly produces coagulation [3].

Unipolar/monoterminal/bipolar diathermy

Apart from the waveform produced, electrosurgery equipment also varies in the way the current is discharged and collected. Unipolar (monopolar) current is delivered via an active electrode, usually a needle or ball tip, resulting in a high concentration of current at the electrode tip. The current disperses through the patient's body and is collected via a dispersive (syn. indifferent, passive, return, earthing, ground) electrode with a large surface area. The current density falls with increasing distance from the active electrode and there is minimal risk of tissue damage as the current is collected over the large area of the dispersive electrode. If, because of faulty application or equipment, there is only a small area of skin–electrode contact, a burn may occur at the dispersive electrode. Also, if the current is channelled at narrow points along its path (e.g. the finger), an area of high-current density leading to tissue damage can occur. Bipolar electrodes avoid these hazards by producing and collecting the current using forceps so that current only travels in the tissue held between the tips. Monoterminal electrosurgical equipment (e.g. Birtcher Hyfrecator) produces a high-voltage low-amperage current, and is designed to be used without a dispersive electrode. However, there is a risk of a small but painful discharge occurring between the patient and the operator or other earthed point (e.g. the metal edge of an electrically insulated couch) [4]. This can be prevented by maintaining a large area of skin contact between the operator and patient during use, or using a dispersive electrode.

Electrodesiccation/electrofulguration

This is produced using a monoterminal or unipolar electrode. Electrodesiccation occurs when the needle remains in contact with the skin and no spark occurs. Because the current concentration is greater at the point of contact, the tissue damage is deeper compared with electrofulguration. During the latter, the needle tip is not in contact with the skin and a spark jumps between the skin and the needle, but its energy is spread over a greater area. The resulting heat causes superficial damage to the tissues and is an effective way of stopping bleeding. Various needle tips have been developed for specific circumstances [5]. Because of the risk of virus transmission, a different clean needle must be used for each patient [6].

Pacemakers and electrosurgery

There have been reports of electrosurgery interfering with pacemaker function temporarily and causing temporary asystole if there is no underlying cardiac rhythm, or caus-ing a demand pacemaker to switch to a fixed-rate mode [7]. The effect lasts only as long as the unit is being operated. When diathermy finishes, the pacemaker reverts to normal function. There are also anecdotal reports of the pacemaker failing shortly after electrosurgery [8]. Only older (pre-1990) pacemakers seem to be vulnerable. Modern pacemakers are considered to be resistant to these problems. All types of electrosurgical equipment, except cautery, can cause problems, although bipolar diathermy is the least hazardous. Short bursts (less than 5 s) should be used, the patient's heart rate can be monitored and resuscitation equipment should be available. Diathermy should not be performed within 15 cm of the heart, the pacemaker or its leads. If monopolar diathermy has to be used, the path from the active electrode (diathermy tip) to the dispersive electrode should be at least 15 cm from the heart, the pacemaker and its leads.

Spider naevi

Spider naevi are probably best treated using a pulsed dye laser. They can be also be destroyed using cold point cautery or electrodesiccation, but with greater risk of scarring.

Xanthelasma

Electrodesiccation and curettage of xanthelasma is relatively simple. The anaesthetized skin overlying the xanthelasma is fulgurized and disrupted. The underlying fatty deposits can be electrodesiccated, scraped off using a sharp curette and left to heal by second intention. Trichloracetic acid and ablative laser therapy can also be used.

Small seborrhoeic and plane warts

Eyelid seborrhoeic warts can be softened and removed by electrodesiccation, provided the anaesthetized eyelid margin is pulled away to prevent conjunctival damage.

Surgical paring and electrofulguration of rhinophyma

Cutting diathermy (syn. electrosection) using a unipolar diathermy and dispersive plate is particularly useful for treatment of rhinophyma, where bleeding can be a problem [9]. Re-epithelialization takes place, with surprisingly little scarring, from the abundant pilosebaceous follicles that remain in the dermis (Fig. 77.3). Carbon dioxide laser resection is also effective.

Electrolysis

Hair is not an electrical conductor and thus electronic tweezers do not produce permanent hair removal; this can only be achieved if the electrical current reaches the

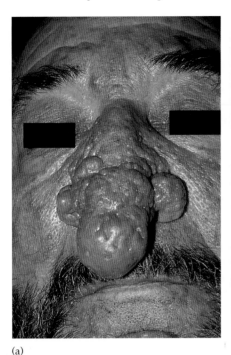
(a)

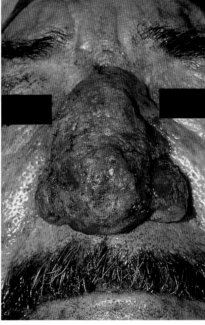
(b)

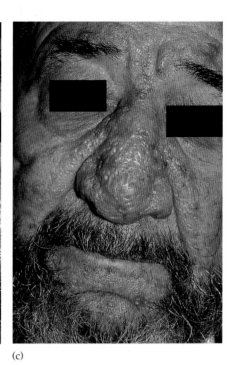
(c)

Fig. 77.3 Shave excision and electrosurgery of a rhinophyma.
(a) This disfiguring rhinophyma was reduced in size and (b) the
nose shape recreated by shave excision and electrodesiccation of
the bleeding surface under local anaesthetic, (c) resulting in an
acceptable cosmetic result at 4 months.

germinal bulb via a needle inserted to the correct depth
[10]. Galvanic electrolysis involves the use of low-voltage
low-amperage direct current passed down a needle
inserted into the follicle. The current causes dissolution of
the follicular epithelium and hence detachment of the hair
shaft. This technique is effective but time consuming.
High-frequency electrodesiccation is a faster alternative,
which destroys the follicle by heating. Insulated needles
deliver the electrical current to the base of the follicle. Side
effects of electrolysis include self-limiting redness and
wealing, post-inflammatory pigmentation, and scarring.
Compared with laser hair removal, electrolysis is better
for sparse hairs and fair hair.

REFERENCES

1 Jackson R. Basic principles of electrosurgery: a review. *Can J Surg* 1970; **13**:
354–61.
2 Elliott JA. Electrosurgery: its use in dermatology with a review of its development and technologic aspects. *Arch Dermatol* 1966; **94**: 340–9.
3 Boughton RS, Spencer SK. Electrosurgical fundamentals. *J Am Acad
Dermatol* 1987; **16**: 862–7.
4 Sebben JE. Patient 'grounding'. *J Dermatol Surg Oncol* 1988; **14**: 926–31.
5 Sebben JE. Modifications of electrosurgery electrodes. *J Dermatol Surg Oncol*
1992; **18**: 908–12.
6 Sheretz EF, Davis GL, Rice RW *et al*. Transfer of hepatitis B virus by contaminated reusable needle electrodes after electrodesiccation in simulated use.
J Am Acad Dermatol 1986; **15**: 1242–6.
7 Sebben JE. Electrosurgery and cardiac pacemakers. *J Am Acad Dermatol*
1983; **9**: 457–63.
8 Wajszczuk WJ, Mowry FM, Dugan NL. Deactivation of a dermal pacemaker by transurethral electrocautery. *N Engl J Med* 1969; **280**: 34–5.
9 Greenbaum SS, Krull EA, Watnick K. Comparison of CO₂ laser and electrosurgery in the treatment of rhinophyma. *J Am Acad Dermatol* 1988; **18**: 363–8.
10 Richards RN, Meharg GE. Electrolysis: observations from 13 years and 140
000 hours of experience. *J Am Acad Dermatol* 1995; **33**: 662–6.

Infrared coagulation [1–3]

The infrared coagulator produces ordinary light (non-
coherent) with a spectrum of 400–2700 nm. Power is
generated from a tungsten halogen bulb and is transmitted along a quartz glass light guide—at its end this has a
sapphire cap, which is placed in contact with the skin. The
heat imparted causes thermal injury to a depth dependent
on the duration of exposure, which can be set on an automatic timer and varied from 0 to 1.5 s; for example, a 1-s
exposure will remove tissue to a depth of approximately
0.75 mm.

The major characteristics are:
1 Non-laser radiation of maximum output 960 nm (near
infrared)
2 Tungsten halogen bulb power source—15 V, 150 W
3 Pulsed energy
4 Solid quartz glass light guide
5 Diameter of treated area 2–10 mm, the larger diameters
enabling more rapid treatment
6 Sapphire cap to light guide—sapphire is transparent to
near infrared but rapidly conducts away heat generated in
the upper dermis
7 Minimum optical hazard—the appearance of bright visible radiation causes aversion of the eyes if it is pointing in
their direction, thus preventing infrared damage
8 It is portable, and relatively cheap.

It has been used mainly for tattoos [1], a variety of superficial vascular lesions [2], warts and myxoid cysts of the digit. Tattoos [1] can be treated with remarkably little morbidity. The area to be treated is mapped into overlapping circles similar in diameter to the sapphire tip, and each circle is treated with a pulsed exposure of approximately 1.25 s. An ice cube applied to the skin for 5 s before and after treatment is used to minimize conducted heat damage to surrounding skin. The immediate appearance of the coagulated tissue is white and slightly contracted; the eschar, which develops over several days, drops off in 2–3 weeks. Serous exudate, pain and swelling during the healing phase are generally insignificant.

Telangiectases, port-wine stains and angioma serpiginosum have been treated using short exposure times (e.g. 0.75–0.875 s, also with ice). It is evidently less specific and probably less effective, with a greater risk of scarring, than an appropriate laser.

REFERENCES

1 Colver GB, Cherry GW, Dawber RPR, Ryan TJ. Tattoo removal using infrared coagulation. *Br J Dermatol* 1985; **112**: 481–5.
2 Colver GB, Cherry GW, Dawber RPR, Ryan TJ. Infrared coagulation for removing tattoos and vascular naevi. *Br J Dermatol* 1984; **111** (Suppl. 26): 27.
3 Burge S, Colver GB, Rayment R. *Simple Skin Surgery*, 2nd edn. Oxford: Blackwell Science, 1996: 69–70.

Caustics and chemical peeling

Caustics

In experienced hands, caustics provide a simple and readily available means of destroying many superficial skin lesions. The operator should be well acquainted with the action and degree of penetration of individual caustics, and the toxic effects that may result from absorption, especially if they are to be used on large areas, and particularly when applied to the face [1,2]. In treating individual lesions, caustics are usually applied by means of a cotton-bud applicator or a wool-tipped orange stick, pointed if necessary.

Aluminium chloride hexahydrate

A 20% solution (Driclor; Anhydrol Forte) usually applied on a cotton-bud is a very useful styptic for superficial wounds such as those following shave excision. Ferric subsulphate (Monsel's solution) is widely used, but may leave a pigmented scar.

Silver nitrate [3]

This is used in the form of a pencil or as a strong solution to suppress exuberant granulation. It is haemostatic and may be used to arrest bleeding after curettage. Repeated use tends to lead to unsightly staining of the skin.

Phenol (liquefied phenol)

This is a valuable superficial caustic, which should, however, be used cautiously. It should not be diluted as this increases its absorption and potency [4,5] and thus also its nephrotoxicity. Ochronosis may occur from prolonged absorption. It is not a haemostatic, and bleeding limits its effectiveness. When used as a treatment for ingrown toenails it is important that the phenol is applied to a 'dry' nail bed and that sufficient time is allowed for it to take effect [6].

Potential toxicity and cardiac arrhythmias remain a major concern, especially with more extensive use, and it should not be used during pregnancy. Phenol is used in a soap–croton oil–water mix for chemical face peels (see below). A glycol-spirit solution can be used for neutralization if required.

Trichloroacetic acid

This is an effective haemostatic caustic, which has many uses. The 30–50% concentration can be used as a styptic, and is frequently employed in conjunction with superficial curettage in the treatment of solar keratoses and seborrhoeic warts. The supersaturated solution can also be used on its own to treat many benign and dysplastic skin lesions. Trichloroacetic acid 50% is similar to phenol in its destructive effect on the epidermis.

Trichloroacetic acid may be a useful treatment for xanthelasmas and solar lentigos. It must be applied with great care, however, especially around the eyes. Its action is rapid, and a white 'frosting' occurs within a few seconds of application. The caustic action can be partially neutralized by applying alcohol, water or sodium bicarbonate-soaked gauze, but this is unlikely to have any effect once the acid has penetrated the skin.

Excess sebum should first be removed using detergent, ether or acetone. Trichloroacetic acid should then be applied with an 'almost dry' cotton applicator. The concentration to be used will vary according to site, the condition to be treated and whether the trichloroacetic acid is being used as a styptic or a superficial skin caustic.

Weaker solutions of trichloroacetic acid are sometimes used for treating wider areas of skin (see below). Because of deliquescence, trichloroacetic acid should be kept in a closed, coloured and corrosion-resistant bottle.

Dichloroacetic acid

This is also a powerful caustic and skin styptic.

Monochloroacetic acid

This should not be considered as a superficial caustic. It penetrates rapidly and may remove the whole epidermis by blister formation. It may be used for mosaic warts, and can also be used for resistant periungual warts.

Alpha-hydroxyacids [7]

These acids (e.g. glycolic acid) can be used to produce superficial or freshening peels and, at high concentration, medium-depth chemical peels.

Chemical peeling [1,2,7–10]

This procedure can be used to improve the appearance of ageing, wrinkled or sun-damaged skin. It is less effective in dealing with acne scars but is a valid dermatological manoeuvre for these and other superficial lesions on the face.

Chemical face peeling is used in conjunction with or as an alternative to dermabrasion. Patients with a dry skin and a fair complexion are the best subjects. A variety of preparations in differing concentration can be used alone or in combination, depending on the desired outcome [11]. Trichloroacetic acid is probably the most commonly used agent. Weak preparations (10–15%) may be used for light 'freshening' peels, and higher concentrations for medium-depth or deep peels. Alpha-hydroxy acids (mild), Jessner's solution (mild) and phenol (deep) may also be used. The neck should only be included with caution as the skin in this area is more prone to scarring and hyperpigmentation. Weaker preparations are generally used on eyelids, and care must be taken not to cause hypertrophic scars, which may occur around the mouth or mandible. Prolonged erythema and increased sensitivity to sunlight, and pigmentary changes (both hyperpigmentation and hypopigmentation) may follow the procedure.

REFERENCES

1 Brody HJ. *Chemical Peeling*. St Louis: Mosby Year Book, 1992.
2 Rubin MG. *Manual of Chemical Peels: Superficial and Medium Depth*. Philadelphia: Lippincott, 1995.
3 Jarson PO. Topical haemostatic agents for dermatologic surgery. *J Dermatol Surg Oncol* 1988; **14**: 623–32.
4 Conning DM, Hayes MJ. The dermal toxicity of phenol. *Br J Ind Med* 1970; **27**: 155–9.
5 Truppmann ES, Ellenberg JD. Major ECG changes during chemical facial peeling. *Plast Reconstr Surg* 1979; **63**: 44–8.
6 Frumkin A. Phenol cauterization of nail matrix remnants. *J Dermatol Surg Oncol* 1987; **13**: 1324–5.
7 Moy R, Luftman D, Kakita LS. *Glycolic Acid Peels*. New York: Marcel Dekker, 2002.
8 Lask GP, Parish LC, eds. *Aesthetic Dermatology*. New York: McGraw-Hill, 1991: 128–38.
9 McCollough G, Langsdon PR. *Dermabrasion and Chemical Peel*. New York: Thieme, 1988.
10 Stegman SJ, Tromovitch TA. *Cosmetic Dermatologic Surgery*, 2nd edn. Chicago: Year Book Medical, 1990.
11 Coleman WP, Futrell JM. The glycolic acid–trichloroacetic acid peel. *J Dermatol Surg Oncol* 1994; **20**: 76–80.

Intralesional therapy

Intralesional triamcinolone [1]

Aqueous suspensions of triamcinolone acetonide (10 mg/mL [Adcortyl] and 40 mg/mL [Kenalog]) [2] are available. Intralesional hydrocortisone acetate (25 mg/mL) can also be used. Triamcinolone acetonide 10 mg/mL is sufficient for all conditions except keloids. The amount injected ranges from 0.1 to 0.5 mL of 10 mg/mL solution, depending on the size and nature of the lesion. The injection should be given using a 27–30-gauge needle, deep in the dermis when possible, to minimize the risk of collagen atrophy. The manufacturers recommend that no more than 30 mg of triamcinolone acetonide should be given in one session, with a maximum of 5 mg at any one site. (Steroid equivalence: 5 mg prednisolone = 4 mg triamcinolone = 20 mg hydrocortisone.) Plasma cortisol levels are suppressed for a few days by 20 mg of intralesional triamcinolone acetonide given into various sites; higher doses suppress cortisol levels for longer [3]. Cushing's syndrome has occurred 2–3 weeks after a single treatment with 40 mg triamcinolone acetonide injected into keloids [4]. Local side effects include collagen atrophy [5], hypopigmentation [6], skin necrosis [6], perilymphatic linear depigmented and atrophic streaks [7,8], and telangiectasia [9].

Needleless injection of steroids

Intralesional triamcinolone is also given using a needleless injector (Dermojet or Portojet). The injection is slightly less painful but is principally employed because the injections can be given quickly [10]. There is a danger of intraocular injection if this technique is used around the eye [11]. Dose-for-dose, needleless injection of steroid appears to be less effective than needle injection, probably because some steroid solution spills onto the skin.

Uses

Intralesional triamcinolone therapy is used for inflammatory acne cysts, lichen planus, lichen simplex, lupus erythematosus [12], chondrodermatitis [13], orofacial granulomatosis [14], granuloma annulare, psoriasis and nail psoriasis [15], alopecia areata and many other steroid-responsive conditions [16].

REFERENCES

1 Callen JP. Intralesional corticosteroids. *J Am Acad Dermatol* 1981; **4**: 149–51.
2 Porter D, Burton JL. A comparison of intralesional triamcinolone hexacetonide and triamcinolone acetonide in alopecia areata. *Br J Dermatol* 1971; **85**: 272–3.

3 Potter RA. Intralesional triamcinolone and adrenal suppression in acne vulgaris. *J Invest Dermatol* 1971; **57**: 364–70.

4 Teelucksingh S, Balkaran B, Ganeshmoorthi A, Arthur P. Prolonged childhood Cushing's syndrome secondary to intralesional triamcinolone acetonide. *Ann Trop Paediatr* 2002; **22**: 89–91.

5 Krusche T, Worret WI. Mechanical properties of keloids *in vivo* during treatment with intralesional triamcinolone acetonide. *Arch Dermatol Res* 1995; **287**: 289–93.

6 Jarratt MT, Spark RF, Arndt KA. The effects of intradermal steroids on the pituitary–adrenal axis and the skin. *J Invest Dermatol* 1974; **62**: 463–6.

7 Kikuchi I, Horikawa S. Perilymphatic atrophy of the skin: a side-effect of topical corticosteroid injection therapy. *Arch Dermatol* 1974; **109**: 558–9.

8 Gupta AK, Rasmussen JE. Peri-lesional linear atrophic streaks associated with intralesional corticosteroid injections in a psoriatic plaque. *Pediatr Dermatol* 1987; **4**: 259–60.

9 Schetman D, Hambrick GW, Wilson CE. Cutaneous changes following local injection of triamcinolone. *Arch Dermatol* 1963; **88**: 820–8.

10 Abell E, Munro DD. Intralesional treatment of alopecia areata with triamcinolone acetonide by jet injector. *Br J Dermatol* 1973; **88**: 55–9.

11 Perry HT, Cohn BT, Nauheim JS. Accidental intraocular injection with Dermojet syringe. *Arch Dermatol* 1977; **113**: 1131.

12 Callen JP. Chronic cutaneous lupus erythematosus: clinical, laboratory, therapeutic and prognostic examination of 62 patients. *Arch Dermatol* 1982; **118**: 412–6.

13 Lawrence CM. The treatment of chondrodermatitis nodularis with cartilage removal alone. *Arch Dermatol* 1991; **127**: 530–5.

14 Sakuntabhai A, MacLeod RI, Lawrence CM. Intralesional steroid injection after nerve block anaesthesia in the treatment of orofacial granulomatosis. *Arch Dermatol* 1993; **129**: 477–80.

15 de Berker D, Lawrence CM. A simplified protocol of steroid injection for psoriatic nail dystrophy. *Br J Dermatol* 1995; **133** (Suppl. 45): 15.

16 Lebwohl M, Heymann WR, Berth-Jones J, Coulson I, eds. *Treatment of Skin Disease: Comprehensive Therapeutic Strategies*. London: Mosby, 2002.

Intralesional therapies for skin malignancies

Intralesional *methotrexate* is reported to be a painless and effective method of treating keratoacanthoma, with faster than spontaneous resolution [1,2]. Intralesional *5-fluorouracil* injections are very painful but when used for 4–6 weeks destroy small nodular BCCs [3] and some SCCs [4]. Intralesional *interferon-α2b* has been used to treat Bowenoid papulosis [5], melanoma [6], BCC [7,8] and SCC [9]. Up to 80% of small, solid or superficial BCCs injected, using high-dose therapy, appear to resolve, although adverse effects occur in 80% of patients at this dose. In contrast, only a minority of aggressive pattern, invasive BCCs respond [10]. Intralesional *interleukin* 2 in 1–4 weekly doses produced complete response in eight of 12 BCC patients treated [11]. Intralesional *bleomycin* followed by electrical stimulation (electrochemotherapy) has been used for a range of skin tumours, including SCC [12].

REFERENCES

1 Melton JL, Nelson BR, Stough DB *et al.* Treatment of keratoacanthomas with intralesional methotrexate. *J Am Acad Dermatol* 1991; **25**: 1017–23.

2 Hurst LN, Gan BS. Intralesional methotrexate in keratoacanthoma of the nose. *Br J Plast Surg* 1995; **48**: 243–6.

3 Miller BH, Shavin JS, Cognetta A *et al.* Non-surgical treatment of basal cell carcinoma with intralesional 5-fluorouracil/epinephrine injectable gel. *J Am Acad Dermatol* 1997; **36**: 72–7.

4 Kraus S, Miller BH, Swinehart JM *et al.* Intratumoural chemotherpy with fluorouracil/epinephrine injectable gel: a non-surgical treatment of cutaneous squamous cell carcinoma. *J Am Acad Dermatol* 1998; **38**: 438–42.

5 Gross G, Roussaki A, Schöpf E *et al.* Successful treatment of condylomata acuminata and Bowenoid papulosis with subcutaneous injections of low-dose recombinant interferon-α. *Arch Dermatol* 1986; **122**: 749–50.

6 Ishihara K, Hayasaka K, Yamazaki N. Current status of melanoma treatment with interferon, cytokines and other biologic response modifiers in Japan. *J Invest Dermatol* 1989; **92**: 326s–8s.

7 Edwards L, Tucker SB, Perednia D *et al.* The effect of an intralesional sustained-release formulation of interferon-α2b on basal cell carcinomas. *Arch Dermatol* 1990; **126**: 1029–32.

8 Cornell RC, Greenway HT, Tucker SB *et al.* Intralesional interferon therapy for basal cell carcinoma. *J Am Acad Dermatol* 1990; **23**: 694–700.

9 Edwards L, Berman B, Rapini RP *et al.* Treatment of cutaneous squamous cell carcinoma by intralesional interferon-α2b therapy. *Arch Dermatol* 1992; **128**: 1486–9.

10 Stenquist B, Wennberg AM, Gisslén H, Larkö O. Treatment of aggressive basal cell carcinoma with intralesional interferon: evaluation of efficacy by Mohs surgery. *J Am Acad Dermatol* 1992; **27**: 65–9.

11 Kaplan B, Moy RL. Effect of perilesional injections of PEG–interleukin 2 on basal cell carcinoma. *Dermatol Surg* 2000; **26**: 1037–40.

12 Mir LM, Glass LF, Sersa G *et al.* Effective treatment of cutaneous and subcutaneous malignant tumours by electrochemotherapy. *Br J Cancer* 1998; **77**: 2336–42.

Sclerotherapy (see also Chapter 50) [1]

The injection of sclerosant chemicals is a useful means of obliterating dilated superficial veins, particularly on the legs. The superficial vessels should only be treated after any proximal points of reflux have been dealt with. Patients who seek treatment therefore require a thorough assessment of their vascular system, and the history and physical examination may be supplemented with non-invasive venous assessment using ultrasonography.

There are a variety of sclerosants that can be used, and some are available in different concentrations. They may be divided into detergents (sodium morrhuate, sodium tetradecyl sulphate, polidocanol) [2], osmotic solutions (hypertonic saline) and chemical irritants (chromated glycerin). Each has advantages and disadvantages.

Side effects [3] include telangiectatic matting, post-inflammatory hyperpigmentation, ulceration, thrombophlebitis and, rarely, systemic reactions (urticaria, anaphylaxis).

REFERENCES

1 Goldman MP. Sclerotherapy. In: Roenigk RK, Roenigk HH, eds. *Dermatologic Surgery*, New York: Marcel Dekker, 1996: 1169–82.

2 Guex JJ. Indications for the sclerosing agent polidocanol (aetoxisclerol). *J Dermatol Surg Oncol* 1993; **19**: 959–61.

3 Goldman MP, Saddick NS, Weiss RA. Cutaneous necrosis, telangiectatic matting and hyperpigmentation following sclerotherapy: aetiology, prevention and treatment. *Dermatol Surg* 1995; **21**: 19–29.

Miscellaneous physical procedures

Keloid therapy

Keloids spread beyond the original wound and remain elevated, whereas hypertrophic scars are localized to the injured area and flatten spontaneously with time [1]. Both are more common in young individuals, Afro-Caribbeans and at particular sites, especially the central chest, back and posterior neck, followed by the ears, deltoid areas, anterior chest, beard area and the rest of the neck [2,3]. Patients with one keloid, except those on the earlobe [4], are believed to be at risk of further keloids. Many treatments have been suggested, including excision, superficial X-ray therapy (although this may provoke malignant tumours [5]), cryotherapy [6,7], pressure [8,9], ultrasound, laser excision [10], intralesional steroids, interferon-α2b [11] and verapamil [12]. Most reports have claimed partial benefit, few have admitted failure. Despite systemic or local side effects [13], intralesional steroid, in the form of triamcinolone 10–40 mg/mL, injected into the scar every 2–3 weeks, is probably the most effective therapy, particularly for presternal and small keloids. High pressure is required to inject steroids into hard keloids, and a Luer-lock glass or hubless disposable syringe is recommended [14].

Pedunculated or easily excised keloids (e.g. on the earlobe) are best treated by intramarginal excision and pre- and postoperative steroid injection [15]. On the earlobe, part of the skin covering the keloid can be salvaged to cover the defect created by removal of the latter [16]. Most authorities recommend a combination of surgery and triamcinolone injections. Some suggest that triamcinolone should be given before, during and after surgery [4], others use steroids during and after surgery [17], whereas others only use steroids postoperatively, to avoid the risk of wound dehiscence [18]. All agree that triamcinolone 40 mg/mL is usually required. On balance, it seems best to give steroids both intra- and postoperatively—approximately four times at 2–3-week intervals, starting 2–3 weeks after suture removal (which should be delayed for 10–14 days because of the risk of steroid-induced wound dehiscence). Freezing the keloid with liquid nitrogen before injection is said to make triamcinolone injection easier [19]. However, this may increase the risk of hypopigmentation. With repeated injections it becomes possible to inject more triamcinolone into the keloid, which can be felt to expand slightly as the steroid is injected. Remember that both cryotherapy and triamcinolone injections may produce skin depigmentation [4]. Alternative therapies include topical clobetasol propionate cream or flurandrenolone tape. The latter carries less risk of steroid atrophy of the adjacent skin because only the keloid is covered. Intralesional interferon-α2b appears to reduce keloid size and inhibit collagen production [11]. Intralesional verapamil is said to reduce keloid size [12] by inhibiting proline incorporation into collagen [20]. Silicone gel sheeting is advocated for larger keloids but the evidence that it is effective is not conclusive [21,22].

REFERENCES

1 Berman B, Bieley HC. Keloids. *J Am Acad Dermatol* 1995; **33**: 117–23.

2 Nemeth AJ. Keloids and hypertrophic scars. *J Dermatol Surg Oncol* 1993; **19**: 738–46.
3 Datubo-Brown DD. Keloids: a review of the literature. *Br J Plast Surg* 1990; **43**: 70–7.
4 Kelly AP. Keloid surgery. In: Robinson JK, Arndt KA, LeBoit PE, Wintroub BU, eds. *Atlas of Cutaneous Surgery*. Philadelphia: Saunders, 1996.
5 Hoffman S. Radiotherapy for keloids? *Ann Plast Surg* 1982; **9**: 265.
6 Rusciani L, Rossi G, Bono R. Use of cryotherapy in the treatment of keloids. *J Dermatol Surg Oncol* 1993; **19**: 529–34.
7 Shepherd JP, Dawber RP. The response of keloid scars to cryosurgery. *Plast Reconstr Surg* 1982; **70**: 677–82.
8 Nicolai JPA, Bos MY, Bronkhorst FB *et al*. A protocol for the treatment of hypertrophic scars and keloids. *Aesthetic Plast Surg* 1987; **11**: 29–32.
9 Mercer DM, Studd DM. 'Oyster splints': a new compression device for the treatment of keloid scars of the ear. *Br J Plast Surg* 1983; **36**: 75–6.
10 Kantor GR, Wheeland RG, Bailin PL *et al*. Treatment of earlobe keloid with carbon dioxide laser excision: a report of 16 cases. *J Dermatol Surg Oncol* 1985; **11**: 1063–5.
11 Granstein RD, Rook A, Flotte TJ *et al*. A controlled trial of intralesional recombinant interferon-γ in the treatment of keloidal scarring, clinical and histological findings. *Arch Dermatol* 1990; **126**: 1295–302.
12 Lawrence WT. Treatment of earlobe keloids with surgery plus adjuvant intralesional verapamil and pressure earring. *Ann Plast Surg* 1996; **37**: 167–9.
13 Krusche T, Worret WI. Mechanical properties of keloids *in vivo* during treatment with intralesional triamcinolone acetonide. *Arch Dermatol Res* 1995; **287**: 289–93.
14 Lawrence CM. *An Introduction to Dermatological Surgery*, 2nd edn. Edinburgh: Churchill-Livingstone, 2002.
15 Sharma BC. Keloids: a prospective study of 57 cases. *Med J Zambia* 1980; **14**: 66–9.
16 Salasche SJ, Grabski WJ. Keloids of the earlobes: a surgical technique. *J Dermatol Surg Oncol* 1983; **9**: 552–6.
17 Fewkes JL, Cheney L, Pollack SV. *Illustrated Atlas of Cutaneous Surgery*. Philadelphia: Lippincott, 1992: 22.5.
18 Bennett RG. *Fundamentals of Cutaneous Surgery*. St Louis: Mosby, 1988: 716–7.
19 Ceilley RI, Babin RW. The combined use of cryosurgery and intralesional injections of suspensions of fluorinated adrenocorticosteroids for reducing keloids and hypertrophic scars. *J Dermatol Surg Oncol* 1979; **5**: 54–6.
20 Lee RC, Ping J. Calcium antagonists retard extracellular matrix production in connective tissue equivalent. *J Surg Res* 1990; **49**: 463–6.
21 Phillips TJ, Gerstein AD, Lordan V. A randomized controlled trial of hydrocolloid dressing in the treatment of hypertrophic scars and keloids. *Dermatol Surg* 1996; **22**: 775–8.
22 Wittenberg GP, Fabian BG, Bogomilsky JL *et al*. Prospective, single-blind, randomized, controlled study to assess the efficacy of the 585-nm flash-lamp-pumped pulsed-dye laser and silicone gel sheeting in hypertrophic scar treatment. *Arch Dermatol* 1999; **135**: 1049–55.

Minor surgical procedures

Using an orange stick, small quantities of caustic agents can be precisely applied. When 90% liquid phenol is used to treat molluscum contagiosum or small cysts, the orange stick tip may need to be sharpened so that it just fits the cavity being treated. Remember that phenol melts some plastics.

Mollusca can be squeezed to express the cellular debris from the centre of the lesion before phenol application. The tip of the orange stick is dipped into the phenol, any excess wiped off, and the stick is then placed in the centre of the lesion and gently twisted. The solution does not need to be neutralized. After initial whitening, the molluscum becomes inflamed and then resolves 7–10 days later. Treatment is painful and not usually tolerated by small children.

Xanthelasma can be treated using the blunt end of an

orange stick, dampened with trichloroacetic acid, dabbed on to the affected area. *Multiple small facial epidermoid* or *acne cysts* can be treated in a similar way. The cyst is incised, the contents expressed and phenol carefully applied to the cyst lining using an orange stick. No dressing is required, but a local anaesthetic is necessary.

Milia are tiny keratin-filled epithelial-lined cysts with no connection to the overlying skin. They can be removed via a small skin incision made with a sterile no. 21 or 19 venesection needle. No anaesthetic is required. Prick the needle tip into the skin and, by pulling the cutting edge upwards, incise the skin overlying the milium. Hook or squeeze out the cyst through the skin incision.

Comedones may be emptied using a comedone expressor—a small metal instrument with a cup-shaped end, which has a central hole.

Haemostasis

Bleeding from open wounds can be stopped readily using an absorbable haemostatic dressing such as Surgicel (glucosic copolymer), Kaltostat (calcium alginate), Oxycel (oxidized cellulose) or Gelfoam (porous gelatin matrix), although the mechanism of action of these agents is poorly understood. These materials may behave like a foreign body while dissolving in the wound and increase the risk of infection, so large pieces should be removed before wound closure.

Chemical haemostatic agents [1] are effective on oozing skin wounds (e.g. after curettage and shave excision) but are ineffective in the presence of arterial bleeding, and should not be used in sutured wounds as they cause cell death, which predisposes to infection. Application should be followed by pressure on the wound for 2–3 min to allow haemostasis to occur without the chemical being washed away. Ferric subsulphate (Monsel's) solution carries the risk of iron tattooing [2]. Silver nitrate sticks are effective but caustic, and may leave scars. Aluminium chloride, either 35% in isopropyl alcohol or 20% in ethyl alcohol, is effective; occasionally, it causes histiocytic reactions in treated skin [3].

REFERENCES

1 Larson PO. Topical haemostatic agents for dermatologic surgery. *J Dermatol Surg Oncol* 1988; **14**: 623–32.
2 Olmstead PM, Lund HZ, Leonard DD. Monsel's solution: a histologic nuisance. *J Am Acad Dermatol* 1980; **3**: 492–8.
3 Barr RJ, Alpern KS, Jay S. Histiocytic reaction associated with topical aluminium chloride (Drysol reaction). *J Dermatol Surg Oncol* 1993; **19**: 1017–21.

Soft-tissue augmentation and facial line correction

The use of biocompatible materials to augment soft-tissue defects forms an integral part of a coordinated and planned approach to the management of the ageing face and rhytides. They can be used alone or in combination with botulinum toxin injections and peels. These materials may also be used to correct scars from conditions such as acne and chickenpox. A whole variety of materials is available [1], and patients for whom this type of treatment is being considered must be carefully evaluated and the techniques available discussed. Patients must be given realistic expectations. Some of the materials are biological or naturally occurring such as those based on collagen or hyaluronic acid—although they may be subject to complex manufacturing processes to produce the final material. Autologous fat can be used, although sometimes it does not persist, and there are currently over 60 autologous and synthetic products available. The choice of material will depend on the defect being treated, and requires a thorough knowledge of the aetiology of the defect and the materials available.

As fat is an autograft, *autologous fat implantation* (*microlipoinjection*) is potentially a useful method of soft-tissue augmentation, but it can only be placed subcutaneously. Fat injected into dermis does not survive [2]. The fat is harvested under tumescent anaesthesia using a syringe, via a wide-bore needle. Any contaminating blood is washed off and the fat reinjected using a 16–18-gauge needle. Intravascular injection, and infection, must be avoided. Microlipoinjection is used to increase lip size, obliterate age-related guttering on the hands, and in breast enlargement, melelabial sulci, idiopathic fat atrophy, after lupus profundus and for some acne scars, but cannot be used for small or superficial scars. Grafted fat persists for 1–2 years, although this varies with site and the cosmetic defect treated [3].

Bovine collagen (Zyderm I (35 mg/mL collagen) and Zyderm II (65 mg/mL)) has been used to correct superficial facial scars and wrinkles. The effect is temporary; after 6 months top-up treatment is required. Glutaraldehyde cross-linked collagen (Zyplast) was introduced with the aim of prolonging the effect, but appears to be little different [4]. Approximately 3% of patients react to the test injection [5]. Late allergic reactions are rare but may occur years after collagen injections [6,7]. Soft and distensible postoperative, chickenpox and acne scars respond well [8], unlike rigid fibrotic or ice-pick scars. Hyaluronic acid is also being developed for use in soft-tissue augmentation.

The use of permanent materials such as injectable medical grade *silicon* (polymerized dimethylsiloxane), *gelatin matrix implant* (*Fibrel*) and *polytetrafluoroethylene* (*Gore-Tex*) has lost favour because of permanent imperfect results and reports of inflammatory reactions [9,10].

REFERENCES

1 Klein AW. Skin filling, collagen and other injectables of the skin. *Dermatol Clin* 2001; **19**: 491–508.

2 Coleman WP, Lawrence N, Sherman RN *et al.* Autologous collagen? Lipocytic dermal augmentation: a histopathological study. *J Dermatol Surg Oncol* 1993; **19**: 1032–40.
3 Pinski KS, Roenigk HH. Autologous fat transplantation, long-term follow-up. *J Dermatol Surg Oncol* 1992; **18**: 179–84.
4 Matti BA, Nicolle FV. Clinical use of Zyplast in correction of age and disease related contour deficiencies of the face. *Aesthetic Plast Surg* 1990; **14**: 227–34.
5 Elson ML. Clinical assessment of Zyplast implant: a year of experience for soft tissue contour correction. *J Am Acad Dermatol* 1988; **18**: 707–13.
6 Hanke CW, Highley HR, Jolivette DM *et al.* Abscess formation and local necrosis after treatment with Zyderm or Zyplast collagen implant. *J Am Acad Dermatol* 1991; **25**: 319–26.
7 Moscona RR, Bergman R, Friedman-Birnbaum R. An unusual late reaction to Zyderm I injections: a challenge for treatment. *Plast Reconstr Surg* 1993; **92**: 331–4.
8 Varnavides CK, Forster RA, Cunliffe WJ. The role of bovine collagen in the treatment of acne scars. *Br J Dermatol* 1987; **116**: 199–206.
9 Clark DP, Hanke CW, Swanson NA. Dermal implants: safety of products injected for soft tissue augmentation. *J Dermatol Surg Oncol* 1989; **21**: 992–8.
10 Rapaport MJ, Vinnik C, Zarem H. Injectable silicone: cause of facial nodules, cellulitis, ulceration and migration. *Aesthetic Plast Surg* 1996; **20**: 267–76.

Lasers and flashlamps (intense pulsed light sources)

The term 'laser' is an acronym for *l*ight *a*mplification by *s*timulated *e*mission of *r*adiation. The first laser was developed by Maiman [1] in 1959, using a ruby crystal to produce red light of wavelength 694 nm. This was followed by the development of other laser systems, notably the neodymium:yttrium-aluminium-garnet laser (Nd:YAG) in 1961 [2], the argon laser in 1962 [3] and the carbon dioxide (CO_2) laser in 1964 [4]. Goldman *et al.* [5] established a role for lasers in dermatology by reporting the use of the ruby laser in the treatment of tattoos, the argon laser in the treatment of vascular lesions [6] and the Nd:YAG laser in the treatment of tattoos, port-wine stains and cutaneous malignancies [7]. In 1983, Anderson and Parrish [8] postulated the theory of selective photothermolysis, which has been applied in lasers and flashlamps to target chromophores such as haemoglobin and melanin, and treat superficial vascular malformations, tattoos and benign pigmented lesions. More recently, observations relating to light-assisted hair removal have been explained in terms of an 'extended theory of photothermolysis' [9,10]. Flashlamp technology is relatively recent, and produces high-intensity pulsed light in the 500–1200 nm range. Filters are used to remove shorter wavelengths where necessary.

Laser safety and laser–tissue interaction

Safety

Various safety measures are required to prevent accidents resulting from exposure to direct or reflected beams. These include the ignition of inflammable materials, including anaesthetic gases, and damage to the skin or eyes. Non-beam hazards include inhalation of the 'plume' arising from tissue destruction, contact with high-voltage electricity or fluid leakage from the laser cavity.

Physics

The generic name of a laser reflects the components of the solid, liquid or gas that constitutes its active medium and determines the wavelength(s) of the radiation produced. The beam may be continuous, pulsed or quality switched (Q-switched). Continuous wave light is a constant beam and has relatively low power. This can be interrupted to produce pulses with higher peak powers than in continuous mode and to allow cooling between pulses. Q-switching is a means of creating a very short pulse (nanosecond domain) with high peak power. The pulse width is varied so that it approximates the thermal relaxation time (see below) of the target chromophore.

The energy contained within light is expressed in joules and its fluence or energy density in J/cm^2. Power is the rate at which work is performed and is measured in Watts (W) or J/s.

The concept of selective photothermolysis has been applied to the removal of superficial vascular malformations, exogenous tattoos, certain benign pigmented lesions and hair. It postulates that light can be used to selectively damage or destroy a target chromophore if the following conditions are met.
1 Its wavelength is selected so that there is as big a difference as possible between the absorption coefficient of the target and the surrounding tissue.
2 The fluence is sufficiently high.
3 The pulse duration is less than or equal to the thermal relaxation time (TRT). The TRT is the time taken for the target to dissipate half of the incident thermal energy and is largely determined by the size of the chromophore. The TRT varies from a few nanoseconds (melanosomes) to several hundred milliseconds or more (leg venules).

It is likely that damage to large targets can be maximized by means of 'thermokinetic selectivity' [10]. Structures such as the hair follicle are relatively large but contain the same chromophore as smaller targets, in this example the melanosome, which one would want to protect during photoepilation. Because large structures cool slower than small structures, it is proposed that they reach higher and potentially damaging temperatures if the light source is manipulated appropriately. This is achieved by means of a pulse that is longer than the TRT of the epidermis and shorter than that of the follicle.

Some tissue targets, notably the hair follicle, are not uniform in their absorption of light, and it is possible that light-assisted hair removal is better explained by an 'extended theory of selective photothermolysis' [9]. This distinguishes between an 'absorber' chromophore (in which heat is generated) and a distant 'target', to which heat is transmitted and which is damaged as a result.

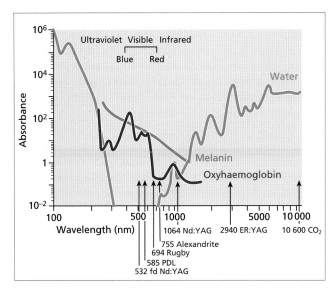

Fig. 77.4 Absorption spectra of principal tissue chromophores. (Reproduced with permission of Dr M. Waner.) Nd, neodymium; Er, erbium; YAG, yttrium-aluminium-garnet; PDL, pulsed dye laser; fd, frequency doubled.

The absorption spectra of important tissue chromophores are shown in Fig. 77.4 in relation to the wavelengths of the lasers widely used in dermatology [11]. As can be seen, haemoglobin has a number of different absorption peaks, whereas absorption by melanin diminishes in proportion to the wavelength of incident light. Consideration must also be given to the depth of the target structure and whether a long wavelength with deep penetration, albeit relatively poorly absorbed, may be preferable to a short wavelength with the opposite characteristics. In some situations, particularly in relation to melanin, a single wavelength may not be necessary and it may even be preferable to use flashlamps because of their broad emission spectrum (500–1200 nm). These are cheaper to manufacture than lasers and can be used with light filters (515–755 nm) to allow a potentially wide range of applications. It is possible to vary their pulse durations from 0.5 to 88.5 ms and to introduce intervals between pulses of 1–300 ms. At present they cannot substitute for lasers where focused high-energy beams are required.

Tissue cooling

Light wavelengths or spectra of 500–1200 nm are preferentially but not specifically absorbed by either haemoglobin or melanin, depending on the wavelengths employed. Epidermal melanin will therefore absorb both direct and back-scattered light from all such devices, whether or not it is the intended chromophore. Heat damage to the epidermis may result in blistering, dyspigmenta-

tion or scarring, and is particularly likely in pigmented skin. To reduce this risk, the wavelength should be optimized with respect to the absorption characteristics and depth of the target chromophore. Further enhancing safety in these patients is the use of long pulses [12] and cooling of the epidermis. The latter may be performed before, during or after the light pulse, or all three.

Cooling may take three forms:

1 *Cold air convection.* Air, chilled to temperatures as low as –30°C, is directed onto the area to be treated.

2 *Contact cooling.* This may involve simple application of ice-packs or more sophisticated systems that pass chilled water between colourless and transparent (usually sapphire) plates. Although a good method of cooling during light delivery, condensate on the plates can obscure the skin and require frequent wiping.

3 *Cryogen spray (dynamic) cooling.* A liquid cryogen is sprayed onto the skin immediately before the laser pulse. Evaporate cooling has a high heat transfer coefficient and this is therefore the most efficient way of precooling. With timed automated control this method is also relatively predictable and reproducible.

One important benefit of epidermal cooling has been to allow treatments at higher fluences than otherwise considered safe, and thereby to reduce the number of treatments required. It has also made possible or safer the treatment of patients with pigmented skin. Furthermore, cooling decreases the pain associated with treatment, thus reducing the need for topical or local anaesthetic. Cooling may, however, cause cryogen injury if used inappropriately.

REFERENCES

1 Maiman T. Stimulated optical radiation in ruby. *Nature* 1960; **187**: 493–4.
2 Johson LF. Optical laser characteristics of rare-earth ions in crystals. *J Appl Physiol* 1961; **34**: 897–909.
3 Bennett WR Jr, Faust WL, McFarlane RA *et al*. Dissociative excitation transfer and optical laser oscillation in NeO$_2$ and ArO$_2$ rf discharges. *Physiol Rev* 1962; **8**: 470–3.
4 Patel CKN, McFarlane RA, Faust WL. Selective excitation through vibrational energy transfer and optical laser action in N$_2$-CO$_2$. *Physiol Rev* 1964; **13**: 617–9.
5 Goldman L, Wilson R, Hornby P. Radiation from a Q-switched ruby laser: effect of repeated impacts of power output of 10 megawatts on a tattoo of man. *J Invest Dermatol* 1965; **44**: 69–71.
6 Goldman L, Dreffer R, Rockwell Jr, Perry E. Treatment of portwine marks by an argon laser. *J Dermatol Surg* 1976; **2**: 385–8.
7 Goldman L, Nath G, Schindler G *et al*. High power neodymium-YAG laser surgery. *Acta Derm Venereol (Stockh)* 1973; **53**: 45–9.
8 Anderson RR, Parrish JA. Selective photothermolysis: precise microsurgery by selective absorption of pulsed radiation. *Science* 1983; **220**: 524–7.
9 Altshuler GB, Anderson RR, Manstein D *et al*. Extended theory of selective photothermolysis. *Lasers Surg Med* 2001; **29**: 416–32.
10 Dierickx C, Alora MB, Dover JS. A clinical overview of hair removal using lasers and light sources. *Dermatol Clin* 1999; **17**: 357–66.
11 Waner M, Suen JY. Lasers in head and neck cancer. In: Suen JY, Myers E, eds. *Cancer of the Head and Neck.* New York: Saunders, 1996.
12 Battle EF, Suthamjariya K, Alora M *et al*. Very long-pulsed (20–2000 ms) diode laser for hair removal on all skin types. *Lasers Surg Med* 2000; **26** (Suppl. 12): 21 (Abstract).

Laser treatment of vascular and pigmented lesions and hair removal

Vascular lesions

Light–tissue interaction

A wavelength of 577 nm was used in early pulsed dye lasers for selective photothermolysis of superficial blood vessels because of its highly selective absorption by oxyhaemoglobin [1]. This has been replaced with 585–600 nm light, which has the advantage of deeper dermal penetration, although with reduced absorption at the longer wavelengths [2]. A pulse duration of approximately 0.45 ms was included in the design of early pulsed dye lasers (PDLs), on the basis of a calculated TRT of less than 1 ms for vessel diameters of 10–50 μm. The theoretical models may have slightly underestimated the TRT, which was measured in a subsequent *in vivo* study as 1–10 ms for vessel diameters of 30–150 μm [3]. As a consequence, newer PDLs allow pulse durations of up to 40 ms. Another laser useful for vascular anomalies is the potassium titanyl phosphate (KTP) laser (532 nm), light from which is well absorbed but is most useful for very superficial vessels. The alexandrite (755 nm) and Nd:YAG (1064 nm) lasers emit light with longer wavelengths and therefore relatively deep dermal penetration, the latter absorbed by a low absorption peak at 900–1000 nm.

Devices in common use

Pulsed dye lasers (585–600 nm) 4.5 and 1.5–40 ms

These contain a rhodamine dye, which is excited by a xenon flashlamp to produce light at 585–600 nm in pulses of 4.5 ms (short pulse PDL) or 1.5–40 ms (long pulse PDL). Light penetrates the dermis to a depth of 1.2 mm [4] and photocoagulates vessels of up to 100 μm in diameter. Purpura is associated with the short pulse width, which causes cavitation and rupture of the capillary wall.

Neodymium:yttrium-aluminium-garnet laser (1064 nm)

Used with long pulses (up to several hundred milliseconds) and epidermal cooling systems, the Nd:YAG laser may have a role in treating relatively deep and large vessels, including those on the legs.

Frequency doubled Nd:YAG or potassium titanyl phosphate crystal laser (532 nm)

Nd:YAG laser emissions can be passed through a KTP crystal to double the frequency to 532 nm. They may be flashlamp or diode pumped and are characterized by trains of short pulses that summate to give a wide pulse effect which is not associated with purpura. Light produced by KTP lasers is highly absorbed by haemoglobin (and melanin) but its wavelength penetrates only superficially. They are widely used, with or without cooling devices, to treat small facial vessels and superficial hypermelanosis.

Intense pulsed light source (500–1200 nm)

This device emits non-coherent light over a broad spectrum. Filters are used to eliminate wavelengths shorter than selected thresholds. There is contact cooling and its potential advantages are the large spot size and reduced likelihood of purpura.

Superficial vascular anomalies

Haemangiomas

These almost always appear after birth and may grow for months. They are often managed conservatively because most regress, sometimes leaving redundant atrophic skin. Intervention may be warranted when functional impairment results from the site and/or size of the haemangioma or where psychological development in childhood is a major consideration. Treatment with the short pulse PDL has been reported to reduce size and colour in up to 67% of superficial haemangiomas. Early proliferative haemangiomas associated with functional impairment or surface ulceration may respond to laser treatment with a reduction in size, together with improvement in the colour and integrity of overlying skin [5]. On the other hand, a randomized controlled study of 121 infants with early haemangiomas showed no advantage to PDL treatment over observation alone [6]. Where appropriate, treatment can be attempted with systemic corticosteroids, interferon or vincristine.

Port-wine stains, or capillary malformations

These may become thickened and darker because of progressive vascular ectasia. The 585 nm short pulse PDL is probably the treatment of choice for paediatric port-wine stains because vessel diameters are relatively small [7]. At 585 nm, the absorption coefficient of haemoglobin is a factor of five higher than at 595 nm and, used in conjunction with the long pulse, may be most suitable for resistant or adult port-wine stains (Fig. 77.5) [8]. Very exophytic lesions are probably best treated with the CO_2 laser [9]. Factors favouring a good response to PDL treatment are youth as well as flat and scarlet (as opposed to purple) port-wine stains on the head and neck (excluding the cheeks or midline) [10,11]. The use of spray cooling with higher fluences in both short [12] and long pulse (1.5–4.0 ms) [13] PDL has considerably expedited treatment of

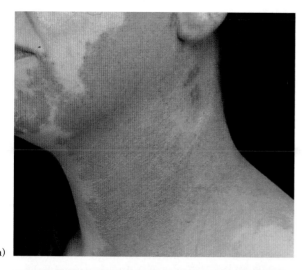

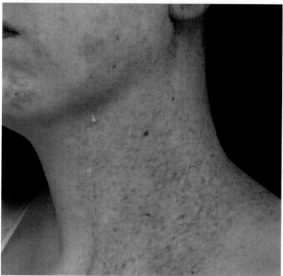

(a)

(b)

Fig. 77.5 Port-wine stain: (a) before, and (b) after treatment with a pulsed dye laser, showing considerable but incomplete lightening and polka dot patterning.

port-wine stains. Lesions immediately become purpuric if treated with adequate fluences and pulse durations of 10 ms or less. Although reduced by both cooling and long pulsing, a degree of post-treatment purpura formation is thought to be necessary for effective treatment of lesions [14]. Partial re-emergence may occur after successful treatment [15]. Flashlamps have also been used to treat port-wine stains with good effect [16].

Telangiectasiae

These are acquired capillary malformations and may occur in association with photoageing or as part of rosacea and erythrodysaesthesia. Although they respond to conventional PDL treatment [17,18], there is associated bruising and often subsequent 'polka dot' patterning. Treatments

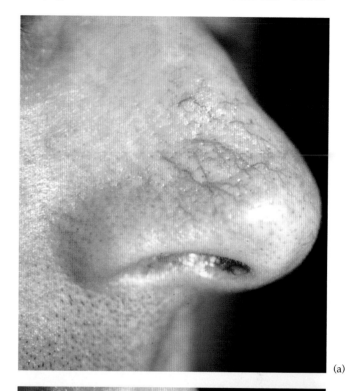

(a)

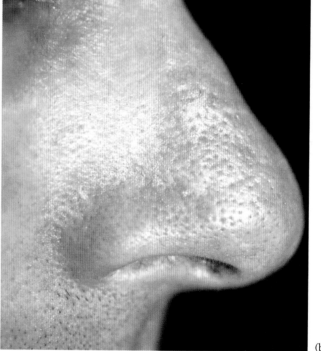

(b)

Fig. 77.6 Large nasal telangiectasiae: (a) before, and (b) immediately after KTP laser treatment, showing disappearance of vessels and absence of bruising.

with longer pulses and subpurpuric fluences are cosmetically preferable and may also be effective. Vessels can be treated individually (Fig. 77.6) or in groups, using small and large diameter KTP laser spot sizes, respectively

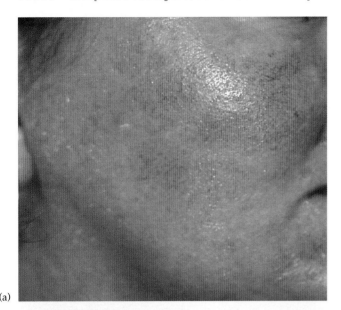

(a)

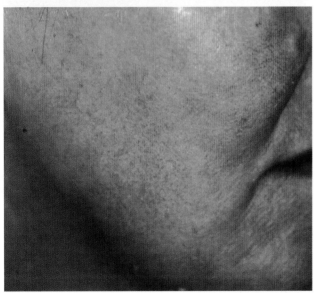

(b)

Fig. 77.7 Fine cheek telangiectasiae: (a) before, and (b) after one treatment with a flashlamp.

[19]. Flashlamps are an alternative non-bruising modality (Fig. 77.7), although several treatments may be required [20].

Leg venules

These are best treated by sclerotherapy because of their relatively high hydrostatic pressure and because of their depth and large size. If sclerotherapy is contraindicated, these vessels should respond best to large spot sizes (3–4 mm), high fluences (relative to wavelength) and long pulse durations, used in conjunction with effective cooling devices. Wavelength should be chosen according to the depth of the target vessel. Accordingly, long pulse

(1.5–4.0 ms) PDLs were developed with wavelengths in the 585–600 nm range and, used with fluences of 7–9 J/cm^2 [21,22], may sometimes be useful for superficial vessels less than approximately 0.5 mm in diameter. Longer wavelengths are used to target a different absorption peak of haemoglobin and achieve deeper penetration. The 3-ms alexandrite laser (755 nm), used with a fluence of 86 J/cm^2, has been reported to clear as many as 75% of leg vessels less than 3 mm in diameter [23]. Nd:YAG lasers with fluences higher than 100 J/cm^2 and with pulse durations of up to 1 s may be useful for larger vessels [24]. However, complications are common and include ulceration, dyspigmentation and scarring. The current consensus seems to be that laser therapy should be considered for patients in whom sclerotherapy is undesirable or contraindicated and who have small superficial single vessels. There are few data on the efficacy of the intense pulsed light source in this context but its emission spectrum and large applicator head would suggest a role in treating widespread fine telangiectasiae. Other cutaneous vascular lesions that have been reported to respond to laser treatment include venous lakes, angiofibromas, angiokeratomas and pyogenic granulomas [25,26].

Topical anaesthesia is usually satisfactory for treating facial lesions in adults but local or regional anaesthesia may be required. Treatment in other anatomical sites can usually be tolerated with topical or no anaesthesia. Depending on the size and site of the lesion, children under 12 years of age may need treatment under general anaesthetic. Emollients and analgesics relieve postoperative pain, swelling and erythema. Some patients develop crusting of the treated area. Complications resulting from PDL treatment include infection, dyspigmentation and both atrophic and hypertrophic scarring. Test treatments have been reported to be poor predictors of outcome.

REFERENCES

1 Anderson RR, Parrish JA. Microvasculature can be selectively damaged using dye lasers: a basic theory and experimental evidence in human skin. *Lasers Surg Med* 1981; **1**: 263–76.
2 Tan OT, Murray S, Kurban AK. Action spectrum of vascular specific injury using pulsed irradiation. *J Invest Dermatol* 1989; **92**: 868–71.
3 Dierickx CC, Casparian JM, Venugopalan V *et al.* Thermal relaxation of port-wine stain vessels probed *in vivo*: the need for 1–10 millisecond laser pulse treatment. *J Invest Dermatol* 1995; **105**: 709–14.
4 Spicer MS, Goldberg DJ. Lasers in dermatology. *J Am Acad Dermatol* 1996; **34**: 1–25.
5 Barlow RJ, Walker NPJ, Markey AC. Treatment of proliferative haemangiomas with the 585 nm pulsed dye laser. *Br J Dermatol* 1996; **134**: 700–4.
6 Batta K, Goodyear HM, Moss C *et al.* Randomized controlled study of early pulsed dye laser treatment of uncomplicated childhood haemangiomas: results of a 1-year analysis. *Lancet* 2002; **360**: 502–3.
7 Garden JM, Bakus AD. Laser treatment of port-wine stains and haemangiomas. *Dermatol Clin* 1997; **15**: 373–83.
8 Chang C-J, Kelly K, van Gemert MJC, Nelson JS. Comparing the effectiveness of 585 vs 595 nm wavelength pulsed dye laser treatment of port wine stains with cryogen spray cooling. *Lasers Surg Med* 2002; **31**: 352–8.
9 Ratz JL, Bailin PL, Levine HL. CO_2 laser treatment of portwine stains: a preliminary report. *J Dermatol Surg Oncol* 1982; **8**: 1039–44.

10 Renfro L, Geronemus RG. Anatomical differences of portwine stains in response to treatment with the pulsed dye laser. *Arch Dermatol* 1993; **129**: 182–8.

11 Fitzpatrick RE, Lowe NJ, Goldman MP *et al*. Flashlamp pulsed dye laser treatment of port wine stains. *J Dermatol Surg Oncol* 1994; **20**: 743–8.

12 Chang C-J, Nelson JS. Cryogen spray cooling and higher fluence pulsed dye laser treatment improve port-wine stain clearance while minimizing epidermal damage. *Dermatol Surg* 1999; **25**: 767–72.

13 Geronemus RG, Quintana AT, Lou WW, Kauvar AN. High-fluence modified pulsed dye laser photocoagulation with dynamic cooling of port-wine stains in infancy. *Arch Dermatol* 2000; **136**: 942–3.

14 Geronemus RG, Lou WW. Treatment of port-wine stains by variable pulse width pulsed dye laser: a preliminary study. *Dermatol Surg* 2001; **27**: 903–5.

15 Orten SS, Waner M, Flock S *et al*. Port wine stains: an assessment of 5 years of treatment. *Arch Laryngol Head Neck Surg* 1996; **122**: 1174–9.

16 Raulin C, Goldman MP, Weiss M, Weiss RA. Treatment of adult port-wine stains using intense pulsed light therapy (Photoderm VL): brief initial clinical report. *Dermatol Surg* 1997; **23**: 594–601.

17 Polla LL, Tan OT, Garden JM, Parrish JA. Tunable pulsed dye laser for the treatment of benign cutaneous vascular estasia. *Dermatologica* 1987; **174**: 11–7.

18 Decauchy F, Beauvais L, Meunier L, Meynadier J. Rosacea. *Rev Prat* 1993; **43**: 2344–8.

19 Goldberg DJ, Meine JG. Treatment of facial telangiectases with the diode pumped frequency doubled Q-switched Nd:YAG laser. *Dermatol Surg* 1998; **24**: 828–32.

20 Raulin D, Weiss RA, Schonermark MP. Treatment of essential telangiectasias with an intense pulsed light source (PhotoDerm VL). *Dermatol Surg* 1997; **23**: 941–6.

21 Kienle A, Hibst R. Optimal parameters for laser treatment of leg telangiectasia. *Lasers Surg Med* 1997; **20**: 346–53.

22 Hsia J, Lowery JA, Zelickson B. Treatment of leg telangiectasia using a long pulse dye laser at 595 nm. *Lasers Surg Med* 1997; **20**: 1–5.

23 Kauvar ANB, Lou WW. Pulsed alexandrite laser for the treatment of leg telangiectasia and reticular veins. *Arch Dermatol* 2000; **136**: 1371–5.

24 Weiss RA, Weiss MA. Early clinical results with a multiple synchronized pulse 1064 nm laser for leg telangiectasias and reticular veins. *Dermatol Surg* 1999; **25**: 399–402.

25 Tay YK, Weston WL, Morelli JG. Treatment of pyogenic granuloma in children with the flashlamp pumped pulsed dye laser. *Paediatrics* 1997; **99**: 368–70.

26 Ross BS, Levine VJ, Ashinoff R. Laser treatment of acquired vascular lesions. *Dermatol Clin* 1997; **15**: 385–96.

Other applications

Viral warts

PDLs are used to treat viral warts [1]. The rationale for this seems to be that photocoagulation of the underlying dermal vessels may compromise the viability of the abnormal epidermis [2]. Treatment of resistant warts, particularly if on plantar surfaces, is often only partly successful [3], in which case CO_2 laser ablation may be more effective, despite the greater likelihood of pain, infection and scarring [4].

Hypertrophic scars

PDLs have been reported to improve the colour and contour of erythematous and hypertrophic scars in studies that have sometimes been supported with objective measurements such as reflectance spectrometry and silicone profilometry [5]. The mechanism of action is unknown, although it is also possible that destruction of small vessels plays a part [6].

Psoriasis

Localized and resistant plaque psoriasis has been reported to respond in 21 patients who were treated at 2-week intervals with both the short and long pulse 585 nm PDL. No significant difference was found between the two lasers and 40% of treated areas were reported to be clear of psoriasis at 6 months postoperatively [7]. Although non-toxic, treatment is often painful and can cause dyspigmentation and scarring.

Narrow-band UVB treatment can also be administered to psoriatic patients by means of a 308-nm excimer laser, the advantages of which are sparing of uninvolved skin and fewer treatments than with conventional phototherapy [8].

REFERENCES

1 Jain A, Strorwick GS. Effectiveness of the 585 nm flashlamp pulsed tunable dye laser (PDTL) for treatment of plantar verrucae. *Lasers Surg Med* 1997; **21**: 500–5.

2 Tan OT, Hurwitz RM, Stafford TJ. Pulsed dye laser treatment of recalcitrant verrucae: a preliminary report. *Lasers Surg Med* 1993; **13**: 127–37.

3 Huilgol SC, Barlow RJ, Markey AC. Failure of pulsed dye laser therapy for resistant verrucae. *Clin Exp Dermatol* 1996; **21**: 93–5.

4 Logan RA, Zachary CB. Outcome of carbon dioxide laser therapy for persistent cutaneous viral warts. *Br J Dermatol* 1989; **121**: 99–105.

5 Alster TS, Williams CM. Treatment of keloid sternotomy scars with the 585 nm flashlamp pumped pulsed dye laser. *Lancet* 1995; **345**: 198–200.

6 Alster TS. Laser treatment of hypertrophic scars, keloids and striae. *Dermatol Clin* 1997; **15**: 419–29.

7 Zelickson BD, Mehregan DA, Wendelschfer-Crabb G *et al*. Clinical and histologic evaluation of psoriatic plaques treated with a flashlamp pulsed dye laser. *J Am Acad Dermatol* 1996; **35**: 64–8.

8 Feldman S, Mellen B, Housman TS *et al*. Efficacy of a 308-nm laser treatment of psoriasis: results of a multicenter study. *J Am Acad Dermatol* 2002; **46**: 900–6.

Tattoos and benign pigmented lesions

Laser–tissue interaction

Melanin absorbs light in the 500–1200 nm range (Fig. 77.4). At the shorter wavelengths absorption is higher and penetration less deep than the longer wavelengths. The Q-switch is an electro-optical device that is used to produce pulses of only a few nanoseconds. These are designed to be within the estimated TRT of melanosomes (0.5–1 µs) [1], although longer than that of tattoo particles, which is in the picosecond domain. Flashlamps can pulse within a millisecond range, which is relatively long in this context. Light may fragment and disperse melanin and tattoo ink, thereby altering its optical properties. It also seems likely that some is removed by transepidermal elimination and some by lymphatic drainage [2].

Devices in common use

Q-switched Nd:YAG laser (1064 nm) and frequency doubled Nd:YAG laser (532 nm)

The Q-switched Nd:YAG laser emits light that penetrates

2–3 mm into the dermis and is therefore suitable for the removal of deeper dermal pigmentation [3]. By passing the beam through a KTP crystal, the frequency is doubled and the wavelength halved (532 nm). The shorter wavelength penetrates less deeply and is therefore more useful for the removal of epidermal pigment.

Q-switched ruby laser (694 nm)

This laser emits red light (694 nm), which penetrates less than 1 mm into skin [4] but is better absorbed by melanin than longer wavelength light.

Q-switched alexandrite (755 nm) and diode lasers (810 nm)

These also emit red light at intermediate wavelengths, allowing somewhat deeper dermal penetration, although with some loss of absorption.

Intense pulsed light source (500–1200 nm)

These emit non-coherent light over a broad spectrum, with potential advantages in terms of penetration and absorption.

Tattoos

Q-switched treatment of tattoos is cosmetically superior to older destructive modalities [5]. Black or blue tattoo pigments absorb radiation across a broad range of wavelengths in the visible and near infrared spectrum. Green inks respond optimally to the Q-switched ruby (694 nm) [6] and Q-switched alexandrite (755 nm) lasers, but often persist [7]. Conversely, red pigments respond best to the green light emitted by the frequency doubled Nd:YAG laser (532 nm) [8]. The Nd:YAG laser is effective for blue or black tattoos but is relatively poorly absorbed by green pigments [9]. It has been successfully used to treat tattoos in pigmented skin [10]. Red, brown or flesh-toned inks may contain iron oxide or titanium oxide and can oxidize to a slate-grey or black colour during laser treatment. This may be exacerbated with subsequent treatments [11]. As these pigments may be used in cosmetic camouflage, tattoo test patches are important. Yellow and pastel colours are difficult to treat and complete resolution is unusual. Amateur tattoos usually require fewer treatments than professional tattoos [12].

Benign pigmented lesions

Epidermal pigmentation

Ephelides (freckles) and lentigines respond quickly and well to treatment with the Q-switched KTP (532 nm)

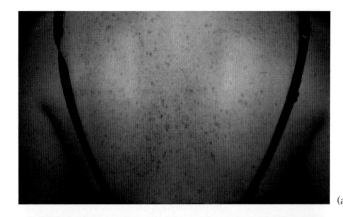

(a)

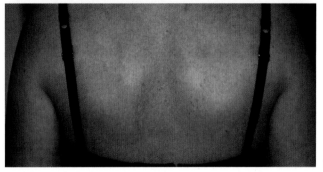

(b)

Fig. 77.8 Ephelides: (a) before, and (b) after treatment with a fd Q-switched Nd:YAG laser.

(Fig. 77.8) and Q-switched ruby laser (694 nm), although the former may bruise [13]. There are limited published data on the use of the intense pulsed light source in this context. Its emission spectrum and large beam diameter would suggest a useful role, even if the pulse width seems relatively long. Café-au-lait patches usually lighten in response to lasers, but pigmentation sometimes recurs.

Dermal pigmentation

In a study in which six patients with speckled and lentiginous naevi (naevus spilus) were treated with both a Q-switched ruby and Q-switched Nd:YAG laser, all showed 90% or greater clearance of the lesion after 1–5 treatments, the Q-switched ruby laser being the more effective. One patient is reported as showing transient hypopigmentation and another as developing hyperpigmentation peripheral to the treated lesion [14].

Naevus of Ota has been treated with the Q-switched ruby [15], alexandrite [16] and Nd:YAG lasers [17]. As might be expected, the relatively deep dermal pigmentation responds optimally and with fewer complications to treatment with the Q-switched Nd:YAG laser [18,19]. In some patients, pigmentation may re-emerge after treatment [20].

Both congenital and acquired melanocytic naevi have been treated with argon, ruby [21,22], alexandrite and

Nd:YAG lasers, although this remains controversial. The long-term effects of non-lethal laser irradiation on melanocytes are unknown, as is laser 'debulking' of congenital melanocytic naevi (CMN). Even after multiple treatments of CMN, many lesions repigment. In a study in which 31 CMN and clinically benign or atypical moles were treated with the Q-switched ruby laser, normal mode ruby laser or both, only 16 were visibly lighter 4 weeks after treatment. Subsequent excision for histological examination showed fibrosis and a decrease in melanocytes [23].

The Q-switched ruby laser appears to be ineffective in treating lentigo maligna and at least one such lesion has subsequently developed lentigo maligna melanoma [24]. It may also be relevant that *in vitro* studies of melanoma cells treated with Q-switched lasers have demonstrated an altered expression of cell surface receptors as well as altered cell migration [25]. Melasma does not in general respond to laser therapy and, as with post-inflammatory hyperpigmentation, laser therapy may darken lesions [26]. Haemosiderin seen in association with venous stasis will only occasionally respond to laser treatment [27]. Hyperpigmentation secondary to administration of minocycline [28,29] and amiodarone [30] responds readily to treatment with the Q-switched ruby, alexandrite and Nd:YAG lasers.

Light-assisted hair removal

The mechanism for light-assisted hair reduction remains incompletely understood. It is likely that the theory of selective thermolysis applies in this context. However, the targets are likely to be stem cells (mainly in the lower isthmus) and blood vessels in the papilla, whereas the absorbing chromophore is melanin in the hair shaft and matrix cells. For this reason, fair or white hair is largely resistant to treatment. Radiation in the 600–1200 nm spectrum is absorbed by melanin and penetrates the dermis further at longer wavelengths. The normal mode ruby (694 nm), alexandrite (755 nm) (Fig. 77.9) [31], diode (800 nm) [32] and Nd:YAG (1064 nm) [33] lasers have all been used with fluences of 20–60 J/cm^2, depending on spot size. The TRT of a 200–300 μm follicle is approximately 25–50 ms, but much shorter pulse durations seem to be effective. In an early study, follicular damage was demonstrated using a ruby laser (6 mm spot, 30–60 J/cm^2) with a pulse duration of only 270 μs. Six months later only four had less than 50% regrowth and five showed complete regrowth of hair [34]. These results were maintained at 2-year follow-up, suggesting that permanent loss of terminal hair is possible after one treatment with the normal mode ruby laser, albeit in a minority of patients [35]. Immediate follicular disruption has been shown to be followed by conversion of the anagen to the telogen phase with a subsequent increase in the number of miniaturized hair follicles.

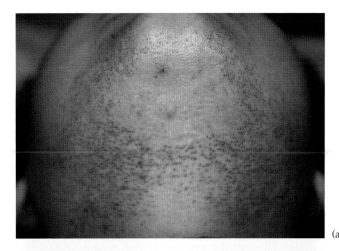

(a)

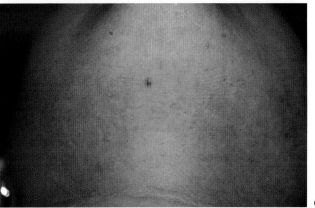

(b)

Fig. 77.9 Hirsutism on the neck of a female patient: (a) after a test treatment, and (b) after four treatments with a normal mode alexandrite laser, showing sparser and finer hairs.

It has recently been demonstrated that considerably longer pulses (30–400 ms) may be more effective in damaging the stem cells and papillary vessels, neither of which contains melanin nor is in direct contact with the melanin-rich components of the follicle. This observation has been explained in terms of an 'extended theory of selective photothermolysis' [36]. By using long pulses and by limiting the power of the light source, the heat generated by the 'absorber' (melanin in the hair shaft) can be kept below levels that would alter its structural and optical properties and thus interfere with further absorption of light. On the other hand, the heat generated may be high enough to diffuse into and denature the distant 'target' (the stem cells and papillary vessels). The delay between heating of the absorber chromophore and the distant target is referred to as the thermal damage time (TDT) and is significantly longer than the TRT.

In patients with pigmented skin, long wavelengths (1064 nm) and cooling devices are particularly important in reducing the risk of epidermal damage, with subsequent dyspigmentation or scarring. A small proportion of patients seem to experience a paradoxical increase in hair growth.

Flashlamps have been used to treat hypertrichosis [37] but it seems likely that subsequent blistering and dyspigmentation is more common than after laser treatment.

REFERENCES

1 Chang C-J, Nelson JS, Achauer BM. Q-switched ruby laser treatment of oculodermal melanosis (naevus of Ota). *Plast Reconstr Surg* 1996; **98**: 784–90.
2 Ara G, Anderson RR, Mandel KG et al. Irradiation of pigmented melanoma cells with high intensity pulsed radiation generates acoustic waves and kills cells. *Lasers Surg Med* 1990; **10**: 52–9.
3 Tse Y, Levine VJ, McClain SA, Ashinoff R. The removal of cutaneous pigmentary lesions with the Q-switched ruby laser and the Q-switched neodymium:yttrium-aluminium-garnet laser: a comparative study. *J Dermatol Surg Oncol* 1994; **20**: 795–800.
4 Grevelink JM, Leewan RL, Anderson RR, Byers R. Clinical and histological responses of congenital melanocytic naevi after single treatment with Q-switched lasers. *Arch Dermatol* 1997; **133**: 349–53.
5 Goldstein N, Penoff J, Price N et al. Techniques of removal of tattoos. *J Dermatol Surg Oncol* 1979; **5**: 901–10.
6 Kilmer SL, Anderson RR. Clinical use of the Q-switched ruby and the Q-switched Nd:YAG (1064 and 532 nm) lasers for treatment of tattoos. *J Dermatol Surg Oncol* 1993; **19**: 330–8.
7 Stafford TJ, Tan OT. 510 nm pulsed dye laser and alexandrite crystal laser for the treatment of pigmented lesions and tattoos. *Clin Dermatol* 1995; **13**: 69–73.
8 Goyal S, Arndt KA, Stern RS et al. Laser treatment of tattoos: a prospective, paired comparison study of the Q-switched Nd:YAG (1064 nm), frequency doubled Nd:YAG (532 nm) and Q-switched ruby lasers. *J Am Acad Dermatol* 1997; **36**: 122–5.
9 Kilmer SL, Lee MS, Grevelink JM et al. The Q-switched Nd:YAG laser effectively treats tattoos: a controlled dose–response study. *Arch Dermatol* 1993; **129**: 971–8.
10 Jones A, Roddey P, Orengo I, Rosen T. The Q-switched Nd:YAG laser effectively treats tattoos in darkly pigmented skin. *Dermatol Surg* 1996; **22**: 999–1001.
11 Anderson RR, Geronemus R, Kilmer SL et al. Cosmetic tattoo ink darkening: a complication of Q-switched and pulsed laser treatment. *Arch Dermatol* 1993; **129**: 1010–4.
12 Kilmer SL. Laser treatment of tattoos. *Dermatol Clin* 1997; **15**: 409–17.
13 Taylor CR, Anderson RR. Treatment of benign pigmented epidermal lesions by Q-switched ruby laser. *Int J Dermatol* 1993; **32**: 908–12.
14 Grevelink JM, Gonzalez S, Bonoan R et al. Treatment of naevus spilus with the Q-switched ruby laser. *J Dermatol Surg* 1997; **23**: 365–70.
15 Goldberg DJ, Nychay SG. Q-switched ruby laser therapy of naevus of Ota. *J Dermatol Surg Oncol* 1992; **18**: 817–21.
16 Alster TS, Williams CM. Treatment of naevus of Ota by the Q-switched alexandrite laser. *Dermatol Surg* 1995; **21**: 592–6.
17 Apfelberg DB. Argon and Q-switched neodymium:yttrium-aluminium-garnet laser treatment of naevus of Ota. *Ann Plast Surg* 1995; **35**: 150–3.
18 Chan HH, Ying SY, Ho WS et al. An *in vivo* trial comparing the clinical efficacy and complications of Q-switched alexandrite (QS alex) and Q-switched 1064 nm neodymium:yttrium-aluminium-garnet (QS 1064 Nd:YAG) lasers in the treatment of naevus of Ota. *Dermatol Surg* 2000; **26**: 919–22.
19 Chan HH, Leung RS, Ying SY et al. A retrospective study looking at the complications of Q-switched alexandrite (QS alex) and Q-switched neodymium:yttrium-aluminum-garnet (QS Nd:YAG) lasers in the treatment of naevus of Ota. *Dermatol Surg* 2000; **26**: 1000–6.
20 Chan HH, Leung RS, Ying SY et al. Recurrence of naevus of Ota after successful treatment with Q-switched lasers. *Arch Dermatol* 2000; **136**: 1175–6.
21 Waldorf HA, Kauvar AN, Geronemus RG. Treatment of small and medium congenital naevi with the Q-switched ruby laser. *Arch Dermatol* 1996; **132**: 301–4.
22 Ueda S, Imayama S. Normal-mode ruby laser for treating congenital naevi. *Arch Dermatol* 1997; **37**: 355–9.
23 Duke D, Byers R, Sober AJ et al. Treatment of benign and atypical naevi with the normal mode ruby laser and the Q-switched ruby laser. *Arch Dermatol* 1999; **135**: 290–6.
24 Lee PK, Rosenberg CN, Tsao H, Sober AJ. Failure of Q-switched ruby laser to eradicate atypical appearing solar lentigo: report of two cases. *J Am Acad Dermatol* 1998; **38**: 314–7.
25 van Leeuwen RL, Dekker SK, Byers HR et al. Modulation of $\alpha4\beta1$ and $\alpha5\beta1$ integrin expression: heterogeneous effects of Q-switched ruby, Nd:YAG, and alexandrite lasers on melanoma cells *in vitro*. *Lasers Surg Med* 1996; **18**: 63–71.
26 Grekin RC, Shelton RM, Geisse JK, Frieden I. 510 nm pigmented lesion dye laser: its characteristics and clinical uses. *J Dermatol Surg Oncol* 1993; **18**: 341–7.
27 Bekhor PS. The role of pulsed dye laser in the management of cosmetically significant pigmented lesions. *Australas J Dermatol* 1995; **36**: 221–3.
28 Tsao H, Busam K, Barnhill RL, Dover JS. Treatment of minocycline-induced hyperpigmentation with the Q-switched ruby laser. *Arch Dermatol* 1996; **132**: 1250–1.
29 Collins P, Cotterill JA. Minocycline induced pigmentation resolves after treatment with the Q-switched ruby laser. *Br J Dermatol* 1996; **135**: 317–9.
30 Karrer S, Hohenleutner U, Szeimies RM, Landthaler M. Amiodarone-induced pigmentation resolves after treatment with the Q-switched ruby laser. *Arch Dermatol* 1999; **135**: 251–3.
31 Finkel B, Eliezri YD, Waldman A, Statkine M. Pulsed alexandrite laser technology for non-invasive hair removal. *J Clin wLaser Med Surg* 1997; **15**: 225–9.
32 Campos VB, Dierickx CC, Farinelli WA et al. Hair removal with an 800 nm pulsed diode laser. *J Am Acad Dermatol* 2000; **43**: 442–7.
33 Bencini PL, Luci A, Galimberti M, Ferranti G. Long-term epilation with long-pulsed neodymium:YAG laser. *Dermatol Surg* 1999; **25**: 175–8.
34 Grossman MC, Dierickx CC, Farinelli WA et al. Damage to hair follicles by normal-mode ruby laser pulses. *J Am Acad Dermatol* 1996; **35**: 889–94.
35 Dierickx CC, Grossman MC, Farinelli WA, Anderson RR. Permanent hair removal by normal-mode ruby laser. *Arch Dermatol* 1998; **134**: 837–42.
36 Altshuler GB, Anderson RR, Manstein D et al. Extended theory of selective photothermolysis. *Lasers Surg Med* 2001; **29**: 416–32.
37 Gold MH, Bell MW, Foster TD, Street S. Long-term epilation using the EpiLight broad band, intense pulsed light hair removal system. *Dermatol Surg* 1997; **23**: 909–13.

Laser resurfacing and non-ablative resurfacing

Cutaneous ablation [1,2]

Light in the mid and far infrared region of the spectrum is rapidly absorbed by water and therefore by body tissue. There is no selectivity of effect. When the light strikes the body tissue, the cells are vaporized almost instantaneously. Although vaporization is limited to those cells immediately in the path of the beam, there is a narrow band of thermal damage around the treatment site whose width depends on the laser type, the power density and the exposure times. The CO_2 laser was the first laser to be used extensively in this way. Although initially the outcome could be compromised by unwanted thermal damage and scarring, this risk has been markedly reduced by the development of a variety of scanning devices. The CO_2 laser is the archetypal surgical laser. Using a high-power density, via a focusing handpiece, the depth of an incision is controlled by the speed with which the beam is moved over the surface, enabling excisions to be performed as easily as with a scalpel. Lower densities are now achieved by using a scanner, and this allows a variety of skin lesions to be treated (Table 77.6).

Resurfacing

The development of scanning systems has allowed the

Table 77.6 Some therapeutic applications of carbon dioxide laser radiation.

Keloids
Seborrhoeic keratoses
Epidermal naevi
Tumours
Warts, condylomas
Cheilitis
Tattoos

CO_2 laser to be used to treat extensive areas of skin damaged by photoageing or scarring, with good results [3,4]. This procedure is associated with prolonged morbidity, and lasers with even higher tissue absorption (erbium:YAG, 2940 nm), and therefore even less dermal damage, may offer advantages. Initial results were often disappointing when compared with the results following CO_2 laser treatment, but the introduction of newer modulated erbium:YAG lasers has led to an improvement in clinical results [5]. Furthermore, using the erbium:YAG laser to remove the thermally damaged layer following CO_2 laser treatment speeds healing and may improve the outcome [6].

REFERENCES

1 Alster TS, Lewis AB. Dermatologic laser surgery. *Dermatol Surg* 1996; **22**: 797–805.
2 Spicer MS, Goldberg DJ. Lasers in dermatology. *J Am Acad Dermatol* 1996; **34**: 1–25.
3 Lupton JR, Alster TS. Laser scar revision. *Dermatol Clin* 2002; **20**: 55–65.
4 Dover JS, Hruza GJ. Laser skin resurfacing. *Semin Cutan Med Surg* 1996; **15**: 177–88.
5 Sapijaszko MJA, Zachary CB. Er:YAG laser skin resurfacing. *Dermatol Clin* 2002; **20**: 87–96.
6 Fitzpatrick RE. Maximizing benefits and minimizing risk with CO_2 laser resurfacing. *Dermatol Clin* 2002; **20**: 77–86.

Non-ablative skin remodelling [1,2]

Although cutaneous 'resurfacing' can produce significant improvement in sun-damaged skin and scarring, this is not without a cost in terms of discomfort, a long period of recovery and significant risks. A number of lasers, intense pulsed light sources and radiofrequency devices are being investigated for their potential to improve sun-damaged, aged and scarred skin [3]. Studies using serial treatments at intensities that induce no more than a mild erythema lasting a few hours, have shown measurable improvement in vascular and pigmentary irregularities. There are some reports of improvements in fine wrinkles, although objectively the improvement is mild. There is a vast literature on the use of lasers for biomodulation and it is interesting that some of the studies of non-ablative skin remodelling show improvement at low intensities which is absent at higher ones [4]. As these technologies develop, they may find a place in the routine management of ageing skin in communities where this is considered a worthwhile use of resources.

REFERENCES

1 Hardaway CA, Ross EV. Non-ablative laser skin remodelling. *Dermatol Clin* 2002; **20**: 97–111.
2 Sadick NS. Update on non-ablative light therapy for rejuvenation: a review. *Lasers Surg Med* 2003; **32**: 120–8.
3 Ruiz-Esparza J, Gomez JB. The medical face lift: a non-invasive, non-surgical approach to tissue tightening in facial skin using non-ablative radiofrequency. *Dermatol Surg* 2003; **29**: 325–32.
4 Bjerring P, Clement M, Heickendorff L *et al.* Selective non-ablative wrinkle reduction by laser. *J Cutan Laser Ther* 2000; **2**: 9–15.

Photodynamic therapy

Photodynamic therapy (PDT) is based on a mechanism whereby topical porphyrin precursors are converted by skin cells into porphyrin, and light exposure activates the porphyrin, producing oxygen radicals which cause cell death. It has been used in the treatment of non-melanoma skin cancer.

5-Aminolevulinic acid (ALA) is a porphyrin precursor. When applied to the skin, ALA is absorbed and converted by intracellular enzymes, maximally 3–5 h later, to photoactive protoporphyrin IX. Protoporphyrin generates cytotoxic singlet oxygen when irradiated with non-coherent and coherent (i.e. laser) light sources in the 400–640 nm range. Some reports suggest that protoporphyrins are concentrated in tumour cells [1], others show no difference between tumour and normal perilesional skin porphyrin fluorescence [2]. Overall it seems likely that at most the porphyrin concentration in BCC is approximately twice as great as that found in adjacent uninvolved skin. These differences could be due to enhanced absorption through a defective overlying stratum corneum, hence the use of surface débridement before porphyrin precursor application.

Currently, although ALA, a naturally occurring haem precursor, is the most promising topical sensitizer [3], it is hydrophilic and this property may limit its penetration into thick BCCs. Lipophilic esters of ALA, e.g. methyl 5-aminolaevulinate, may be better [4]. Photosensitizers can be injected, e.g. meta-tetrahydroxyphenylchlorin [5], but this renders the patient temporarily photosensitive.

The tumour surface is scraped to remove crust or scale. A thick layer of porphyrin precursor cream is applied to the affected area plus a 5-mm margin of perilesional skin and covered with an adhesive occlusive dressing for 3–6 h. The area is then irradiated using a light source that contains 630-nm red light to coincide with the maximal absorption peak of protoporphyrin IX. Red light also has the advantage of penetrating more deeply into the skin than lower wavelengths. Treatment time is around 15 min for a non-laser source. The process is painful but most patients do not require injected local anaesthetic. The inflammatory reaction begins to appear almost immediately and discomfort may persist for 1–2 weeks. Complete healing takes 2–6 weeks. A second treatment is commonly given 2–3 months later if the first appears to have failed.

Bowen's disease and actinic keratoses

Thin *in situ* epidermal malignancies respond well with fewer side effects than are experienced after cryotherapy [6] or 5-fluorouracil (5-FU) therapy [7]. In comparison with these techniques, however, PDT is less easy to use over large areas.

BCC

In general, PDT is an unproven treatment for BCC. Most studies are small, give only 1–2-year follow-up and prefer to report cure rather than recurrence rates. PDT, using ALA, appears to work best on thin superficial BCCs, producing recurrence rates of around 10% [8–11]. Longer follow-up reveals a higher recurrence rate [12]. ALA penetrates BCCs > 2 mm thick poorly [13], resulting in high recurrence rates [14]. A recent randomized small study treating nodular BCCs showed a 10% 2-year recurrence rate after PDT compared with 2% for surgery. The poor results have led others to try two treatments 7 days apart [15], or use the lipophilic methyl 5-aminolaevulinate for PDT after first debulking the tumour by curettage [16]. These manoeuvres have not significantly improved the recurrence rates.

PDT is potentially a treatment option for large superficial BCCs or patches of Bowen's disease. However, as yet there is no convincing evidence that PDT is more cost effective than simple surgery, topical 5-FU, cryotherapy or superficial X-ray therapy for these lesions. PDT has the potential for fewer long-term side effects and better cosmesis. There is insufficient long-term cure rate evidence to justify its routine use in thick or nodular BCC.

REFERENCES

1 Svanberg K, Andersson T, Killander D *et al.* Photodynamic therapy of non-melanoma malignant tumours of the skin using topical delta-amino levulinic acid sensitization and laser irradiation. *Br J Dermatol* 1994; **130**: 743–51.
2 Martin A, Tope WD, Grevelink JM *et al.* Lack of selectivity of protoporphyrin IX fluorescence for basal cell carcinoma after topical application of 5-aminolevulinic acid: implications for photodynamic treatment. *Arch Dermatol Res* 1995; **287**: 665–74.
3 Szeimies RM, Landthaler M. Photodynamic therapy and fluorescence diagnosis of skin cancers. *Recent Results Cancer Res* 2002; **160**: 240–5.
4 Peng Q, Soler AM, Warloe T, Nesland JM, Giercksky KE. Selective distribution of porphyrins in skin thick basal cell carcinoma after topical application of methyl 5-aminolevulinate. *J Photochem Photobiol B* 2001; **62**: 140–5.
5 Baas P, Saarnak AE, Oppelaar H, Neering H, Stewart FA. Photodynamic therapy with meta-tetrahydroxyphenylchlorin for basal cell carcinoma: a phase I/II study. *Br J Dermatol* 2001; **145**: 75–8.
6 Morton CA, Whitehurst C, Moseley H *et al.* Comparison of photodynamic therapy with cryotherapy in the treatment of Bowen's disease. *Br J Dermatol* 1996; **135**: 766–71.
7 Salim A, Leman JA, McColl JH, Chapman R, Morton CA. Randomized comparison of photodynamic therapy with topical 5-fluorouracil in Bowen's disease. *Br J Dermatol* 2003; **148**: 539–43.
8 Rhodes LE, de Rie M, Enstrom Y *et al.* Photodynamic therapy using topical methyl aminolevulinate vs surgery for nodular basal cell carcinoma. *Arch Dermatol* 2004; **140**: 17–23.
9 Collins S, Ahmadi S, Murphy GM. Topical photodynamic therapy in dermatology—3 years experience at Beaumont Hospital. *Photodermatol Photoimmunol Photomed* 2002; **18**: 104.
10 Varma S, Wilson H, Kurwa HA *et al.* Bowen's disease, solar keratoses and superficial basal cell carcinomas treated by photodynamic therapy using a large-field incoherent light source. *Br J Dermatol* 2001; **144**: 567–74.
11 Morton CA, Whitehurst C, McColl JH, Moore JV, MacKie RM. Photodynamic therapy for large or multiple patches of Bowen disease and basal cell carcinoma. *Arch Dermatol* 2001; **137**: 319–24.
12 Fink-Puches R, Soyer HP, Hofer A, Kerl H, Wolf P. Long-term follow-up and histological changes of superficial non-melanoma skin cancers treated with topical delta-aminolevulinic acid photodynamic therapy. *Arch Dermatol* 1998; **134**: 821–6.
13 Orenstein A, Kostenich G, Malik Z. The kinetics of protoporphyrin fluorescence during ALA-PDT in human malignant skin tumours. *Cancer Lett* 1997; **120**: 229–34.
14 Morton CA, Brown SB, Collins S *et al.* Guidelines for topical photodynamic therapy: report of a workshop of the British Photodermatology Group. *Br J Dermatol* 2002; **146**: 552–67.
15 Haller JC, Cairnduff F, Slack G *et al.* Routine double treatments of superficial basal cell carcinomas using aminolaevulinic acid-based photodynamic therapy. *Br J Dermatol* 2000; **143**: 1270–5.
16 Soler AM, Warloe T, Berner A, Giercksky KE. A follow-up study of recurrence and cosmesis in completely responding superficial and nodular basal cell carcinomas treated with methyl 5-aminolaevulinate-based photodynamic therapy alone and with prior curettage. *Br J Dermatol* 2001; **145**: 467–71.

Chapter 78

Dermatological Surgery

C.M. Lawrence, N.P.J. Walker & N.R. Telfer

Introduction

The acquisition of basic dermatological surgery skills is an important component of dermatological training. This chapter covers simple excisional surgery and provides an introduction to more advanced techniques that dermatologists should be aware of and may practice. The reader is also referred to the specialist journal *Dermatologic Surgery*, and introductory [1–3] and intermediate textbooks [4–6]. Other books deal more specifically with cosmetic dermatological surgery [7,8] or general aspects of plastic surgery [9–11].

REFERENCES

1 Bennett RG. *Fundamentals of Cutaneous Surgery*. St Louis: Mosby, 1988.
2 Burge S, Colver GB, Rayment R. *Simple Skin Surgery*, 2nd edn. Oxford: Blackwell Science, 1996.
3 Lawrence CM. *An Introduction to Dermatological Surgery*, 2nd edn. St Louis: Mosby, 2002.
4 Roenigk RK, Roenigk HH, eds. *Dermatologic Surgery*, 2nd edn. New York: Marcel Dekker, 1996.
5 Eedy DJ, Breathnach SM, Walker NPJ. *Surgical Dermatology*. Oxford: Blackwell Science, 1996.
6 Zachary CB. *Basic Cutaneous Surgery: a Primer in Technique*. New York: Churchill Livingstone, 1991.
7 Parish LC, Lask GP. *Aesthetic Dermatology*. New York: McGraw-Hill, 1991.
8 Stegman SJ, Tromovitch TA. *Cosmetic Dermatologic Surgery*, 2nd edn. Chicago: Year Book Medical, 1990.
9 Grabbe WC, Smith JW. *Plastic Surgery*, 3rd edn. Boston: Little, Brown, 1979.
10 McGregor IA. *Fundamental Techniques of Plastic Surgery and Their Surgical Applications*. New York: Churchill Livingstone, 1975.
11 Sisson GA, Tardy MJ. *Plastic and Reconstructive Surgery of the Face and Neck*. New York: Grune & Stratton, 1977.

Critical anatomical areas

It is essential to have a working knowledge of the important clinical anatomy of each operation site. The following is only a brief introduction to some of the critical anatomical details with which the operator must be familiar. Excisions down to superficial fat will rarely result in exposure of or potential damage to functionally important structures, except in a very thin subject. Incisions to deep fat or fascia and the removal of large cysts or lipomas may result in exposure of important structures. On the head and neck, division of larger arteries and veins will not cause vascular complications because of the extensive collateral circulation. However, it is important to be aware of the position of large arteries and veins in order to be prepared to deal with bleeding from these vessels. Division of sensory nerves may produce annoying sensory loss, but this will have little functional impact on the head and neck. Knowledge of the anatomy of the supraorbital, infraorbital and mental sensory nerves is important, as these are commonly used in peripheral nerve blocks.

Division of motor nerves is potentially disabling and thus it is essential to know the anatomy of the vulnerable superficial cranial and peripheral motor nerves.

Skin tension lines and the orientation of scars

Incisions should be designed to follow the wrinkles or relaxed skin tension lines (syn. stress lines; favourable skin tension lines; maximal skin tension lines) as the resulting scars will be stronger and less likely to stretch [1]. Relaxed skin tension lines run perpendicular to the direction of contraction of the underlying muscles and parallel to the dermal collagen bundles [2]; cutting transversely across these weakens the skin much more than a cut running parallel to the collagen bundles [3]. In the absence of wrinkles, relaxed skin tension lines can be identified by asking the patient to grimace or by skin manipulation. Langer's lines [4] (syn. resting stress lines) were mapped on cadaver skin, and differ from relaxed skin tension lines on the limbs and trunk [3]; they should not be used for identifying the elective direction of excision.

Head and neck

Cosmetic units

Cosmetic results of surgery are better if all the incisions remain within a cosmetic unit [5]. These are areas of skin that share similar characteristics (e.g. the nose, cheek and periorbital skin). The junction lines separating these areas are also important because scars placed in junction lines are usually unobtrusive whereas scars that cross a junction line (bridge two cosmetic units) are very obvious. It is thus important to try to design a repair so that the scars follow relaxed skin tension lines and remain within the same cosmetic unit, or run in the junction lines between two adjacent cosmetic units.

Blood vessels and lymphatic supply of face

Larger vessels, particularly the temporal artery, can be avoided by hydrodissection (see p. 78.32). The facial artery (Fig. 78.1) at the nasolabial fold, and its continuation into the angular artery at the medial canthus, are frequently divided when excising tumours at these sites. The external jugular vein runs under the platysma muscle but on top of the sternocleidomastoid muscle, and may be easily damaged during superficial incisions on the neck at this site (Fig. 78.2a). Emissary veins, connecting the intracranial and extracranial venous circulation, run across the subgaleal space towards the back of the scalp (parietal emissary vein) and just above the forehead (frontal emissary vein) [6]. These veins may be damaged when undermining the subgaleal space at these sites. Lymphatic drainage sites should be examined for metastases during follow-up of patients treated for squamous cell carcinoma or melanoma [7]. Division of skin lymphatics during incisions under the eye may result in temporary but unavoidable lower eyelid lymphoedema. Postoperative lymphatic leakage sometimes occurs after lower limb or axillary excision. This resolves spontaneously with conservative management.

Sensory nerves of face

Nerve blocks. Sensation to the face is supplied by the trigeminal (Vth) cranial nerve. The three branches readily blocked in skin surgical procedures on the head and neck

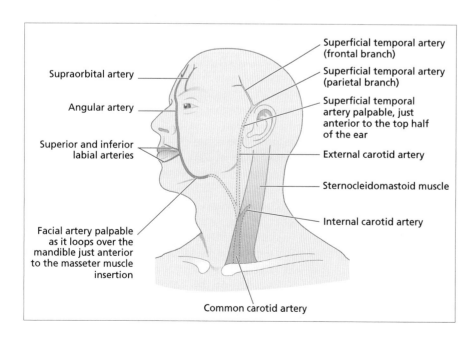

Fig. 78.1 Arteries of the head and neck encountered in skin surgery. The labial artery lies on the inside (mucosal) surface of the lip approximately 5 mm from the visible vermilion border. (---) Arteries rarely encountered; (—) arteries frequently identified during superficial skin surgery on the face.

Supraorbital artery

Angular artery

Superior and inferior labial arteries

Facial artery palpable as it loops over the mandible just anterior to the masseter muscle insertion

Superficial temporal artery (frontal branch)

Superficial temporal artery (parietal branch)

Superficial temporal artery palpable, just anterior to the top half of the ear

External carotid artery

Sternocleidomastoid muscle

Internal carotid artery

Common carotid artery

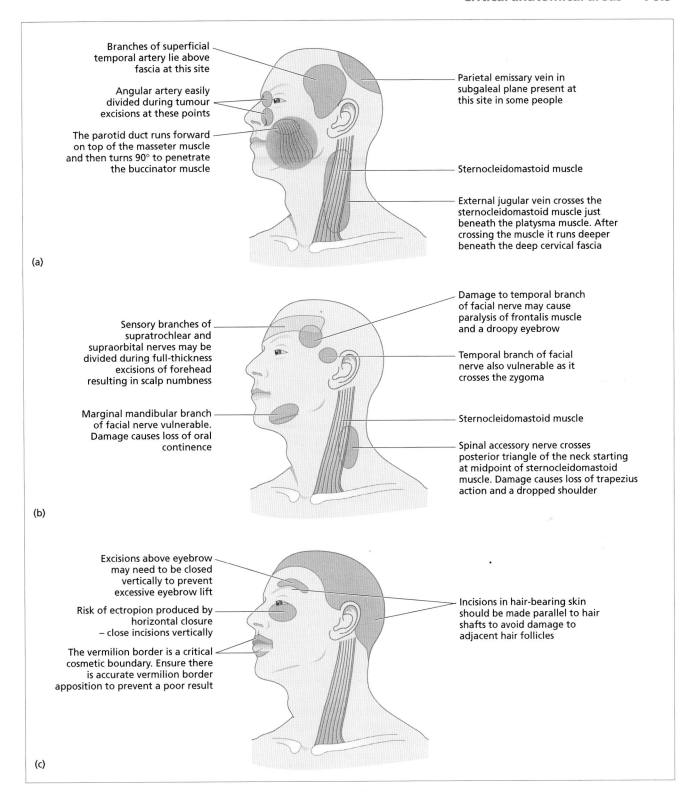

Fig. 78.2 Potential surgical hazard sites during skin surgery on the head. (a) Potential blood vessel and duct, (b) nerve and (c) cosmetic hazards on the head and neck. (From Lawrence [9].)

include the supraorbital, infraorbital and mental nerves (Fig. 78.3). These emerge from the skull via palpable foramina, which all lie in the same plane, just medial to a vertical line running through the pupil [8]. Blocking the great auricular, transverse cervical and lesser occipital

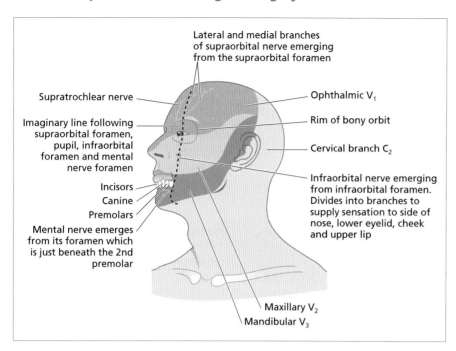

Fig. 78.3 Sensory nerves on the face used in nerve-block anaesthesia. Sensation on the face is served by the three main divisions of the trigeminal nerve: the ophthalmic, maxillary and mandibular divisions. Three important branches of these nerves—the supraorbital, infraorbital and mental nerves—emerge in the same plane along a vertical line running through the pupil.

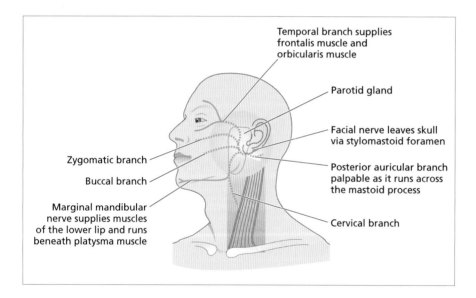

Fig. 78.4 Motor branches of the facial nerve vulnerable in skin surgery. (---) Nerves rarely encountered; (—) nerves at risk during superficial skin surgery on the face.

nerves as they emerge, approximately 10–20 mm above and below Erb's point, from the posterior border of the middle third of the sternocleidomastoid muscle [10] produces anaesthesia of a large portion of the scalp, neck and ear. Erb's point is identified by dropping a plumb line from the mid point of a line drawn between the mastoid process and the angle of the jaw. Where this line meets the posterior border of the sternocleidomastoid muscle is Erb's point. At this site, the spinal accessory (XIth) cranial nerve also emerges from behind the sternocleidomastoid muscle. This motor nerve is rarely affected by the local anaesthesia, as it lies deeper, on the floor of the posterior triangle, whereas the three named sensory branches of the cervical plexus curl round to lie on top of the sternocleidomastoid muscle [11].

Division of small sensory nerves. This is of little consequence, with the possible exception of scalp numbness following incisions on the forehead. Improvement in sensory loss can be expected for up to 1 year.

Motor nerves

Two branches of the facial (VIIth) cranial nerve, the marginal mandibular branch and the temporal branch, are vulnerable during skin surgery (Fig. 78.4). The temporal branch of the facial nerve supplies the frontalis and orbicularis muscles. Damage to the nerve supplying frontalis muscle results in difficulty raising the eyebrow, and the forehead furrows disappear. This can easily occur during excision of large tumours on the temple, lateral to the

Table 78.1 Undermining levels.

Site	Undermining level
Face	Mid-fat
Nose	Just above the periosteum and perichondrium
Forehead	Beneath the deep frontalis fascia (equivalent to the subgaleal plane)
Scalp	Subgaleal plane
Trunk and limb	
Small excisions	Deep fat
Large excisions	Just above the deep fascia

frontalis muscle, and as the nerve crosses the zygomatic arch. At both sites there is little tissue between the skin and periosteum (Fig. 78.2b). The marginal mandibular branch innervates muscles that move the lower lip. Damage can be devastating because it results in weakness of the lips, with dribbling when eating and drinking. The nerve is superficial and vulnerable as it emerges from under the parotid gland at the angle of the jaw, behind the point where the facial artery can be palpated as it crosses the mandible. More anteriorly, the nerve runs beneath the platysma muscle [12]. Variations in nerve position with age and neck position must also be considered. The remaining branches of the facial nerve are less vulnerable because they share several cross-connections and lie deeper. The other important motor cranial nerve is the accessory (XIth) nerve, which supplies the trapezius and sternocleidomastoid muscles. This may be damaged during dissection in the posterior triangle of the neck, causing weakness of the trapezius muscle and producing a dropped shoulder.

Undermining levels

When undermining to increase skin mobility, different levels are appropriate at different sites (Table 78.1).

Specific facial sites

If an incision runs across the vermilion of the *lip*, the vermilion border must be carefully marked before anaesthetic injection to avoid a poor cosmetic result (Fig. 78.2c). In older patients with poor lid elasticity, operations around the *lower eyelid* may result in ectropion if any downwards tension is applied to the lower eyelid. In a patient with poor lid elasticity, the procedure should be designed to increase rather than reduce eyelid tension; this usually means closing the wound vertically rather than horizontally. If an incision goes across the *hair line*, ensure that the scalp margin is reconstructed so that a smooth contour remains. Because hairs grow obliquely through the skin, any incision through *hair-bearing skin* should be made parallel to the hair shafts rather than vertically through the scalp so that fewer follicles are damaged.

Limbs

The only superficial motor nerve on the limbs is on the lateral aspect of the knee, where the common peroneal nerve (lateral popliteal) can be palpated against the bone as it winds round the neck of the fibula. Injury to the nerve at this site will produce a foot drop resulting from paralysis of foot dorsiflexors and elevators.

REFERENCES

1 Salasche SJ, Bernstein G, Senkarik M. *Surgical Anatomy of the Skin*. Norwalk: Appleton & Lange, 1988.
2 Borges AF, Alexander JE. Relaxed skin tension lines, Z-plasty on scars and fusiform excision of lesions. *Br J Plast Surg* 1962; **15**: 242–54.
3 Kraissl CJ. The selection of appropriate lines for elective surgical incision. *Plast Reconstr Surg* 1951; **8**: 1–28.
4 Langer K. On the anatomy and physiology of the skin. I. The cleavability of the cutis. Translated and republished in *Br J Plast Surg* 1978; **31**: 3–8, with covering editorial 1–2.
5 Summers BK, Siegle RJ. Facial cutaneous reconstructive surgery: general aesthetic principles. *J Am Acad Dermatol* 1993; **29**: 669–81.
6 Sobotta J. Head, neck upper limbs and skin. In: Staubesand J, ed. *Atlas of Human Anatomy*. Munich: Urban & Schwarzenberg, 1989.
7 Romanes GJ. *Cunningham's Manual of Practical Anatomy*, 15th edn, Vol. 3. Head and Neck and Brain. Oxford: Oxford University Press, 1986.
8 Scott DB. *Techniques of Regional Anaesthesia*. Norwalk: Appleton & Lange/ Mediglobe, 1989.
9 Lawrence CM. *An Introduction to Dermatological Surgery*. Oxford: Blackwell Science, 1996.
10 Lumley JSP. *Surface Anatomy, the Anatomical Basis of Clinical Examination*. Edinburgh: Churchill Livingstone, 1990.
11 Williams PL, Bannister LH, Berry M et al. eds. *Gray's Anatomy*, 38th edn. New York: Churchill Livingstone, 1995.
12 Summers BK, Siegle RJ. Facial cutaneous reconstructive surgery: facial flaps. *J Am Acad Dermatol* 1993; **29**: 917–41.

Equipment and sterilization [1–5]

Most dermatological surgical procedures can be safely performed in well-lit dedicated outpatient units using relatively simple equipment and surgical instruments [1–3]. However, the absence of a need for either expensive equipment or a completely sterile environment does not justify cutaneous surgery being performed in inadequate facilities or using inappropriate surgical equipment.

Dermatological surgery procedures range from superficial tissue destruction and removal through to surgical excision and complex wound repair. Consequently, a range of basic surgical instruments should be available to the skin surgeon, with selection depending upon the particular procedure being performed. The basic equipment, with optional items that should be available for more specialized procedures, is shown in Table 78.2. Advanced skin surgery (e.g. the removal and complex repair of difficult tumours and Mohs' micrographic surgery) requires both dedicated facilities and specialized surgical instruments to achieve the best results.

Most wound complications are associated with closure under excessive tension, haematoma formation and the presence of either necrotic tissue or foreign material. Wound infection, an uncommon complication of dermatological

Table 78.2 Essential and optional equipment. (From Burge *et al.* [1].)

Essential	Optional
The room	
An examination couch with adjustable backrest	Theatre table
A stool for the surgeon	
Good lighting: anglepoise lights	Overhead theatre lights
Equipment—preoperative preparation	
Autoclave for steam sterilization or electric oven for dry heat sterilization	
Skin preparation	
Chlorhexidine solution	
Chlorhexidine detergent (Hibiscrub®)	
Surgical gloves	
Sterile paper towels	Re-usable drapes
A window can be cut in the centre and the towel placed over the lesion	
Skin markers	Sterile pen and Indian ink
Gentian violet and pointed orange stick	
Skin marker pen	
Indelible felt-tip pen	
Anaesthetic	
Disposable syringes 2 mL, 5 mL fine needles	Dental syringe and fine needles
	Dental syringe vials
Lidocaine (lignocaine)	
1% and 2% plain and with epinephrine (adrenaline) 1 : 100 000 or 1 : 200 000	
Instruments	
Scalpel blades	
No. 15 for excision	
No. 22 for shave biopsy	
Scalpel handle	
Forceps	
Fine-toothed (e.g. Adson–Brown)	
Non-toothed	
Skin hook	
Can easily be constructed by pushing a sterile needle onto a sterile moistened cotton wool bud on an orange stick. Bend the needle into a curve	
Scissors	
Curved pointed iris scissors	
Blunt straight scissors	
Needle holders	
Small artery clamps	
Various sizes of absorbable and non-absorbable sutures attached to needles	Skin punch for biopsies, 3 mm and 4 mm
	Sharp ring curettes in various sizes
Haemostasis	
Gauze swabs	Hyfrecator
30–50% aluminium chloride in alcohol or Monsel's solution (67.5% basic ferric sulphate)	Electrocautery
	Diathermy
	Bipolar electrocoagulation
	Cryosurgery gun
	Supply of liquid nitrogen
	Silver nitrate sticks
Dressings	
Steri-strips	Opsite
Compound Benzoin tincture BP (Friar's balsam) for sticking plaster to skin	
Elastoplast	
Micropore	
Gauze	
Jelonet®	
Histopathology	
Specimen pots	EM fixative 4% glutaraldehyde
Fixative	
10% buffered formalin	Fixative or liquid nitrogen to store specimens for immunohistology

surgery, is more commonly related to surgical technique than poor operator cleanliness or instrument sterilization. However, correct hand washing techniques are vital to the prevention of cross-infection [4]. The tradition of protracted 'scrubbing up' is not essential prior to most dermatological surgical procedures—two washes in running water using 4% chlorhexidine or 10% povidine–iodine solution are sufficient. Between cases, alcohol-based [5] skin cleaning solutions are an alternative on clinically clean hands. The use of surgical gloves is mandatory for all procedures, and wearing eye protection is strongly recommended.

Dried tissue, pus or blood on instruments may harbour potentially dangerous organisms, and all instruments should be manually or ultrasonically cleaned and placed into sealed packs prior to autoclave sterilization [6,7]. Older methods of sterilization, for example boiling in water at atmospheric pressure and the use of various chemical agents (e.g. glutaraldehyde, phenolic agents) are no longer recommended [3]. The new variant Creutzfeldt–Jakob disease (vCJD) prion cannot be destroyed by sterilization, and equipment suspected of being contaminated must be quarantined. If contact is confirmed the equipment must be destroyed.

REFERENCES

1 Burge S, Colver GB, Rayment R. *Simple Skin Surgery*, 2nd edn. Oxford: Blackwell Science, 1996: 5–9.
2 Grande DJ, Neuberg M. Instrumentation for the dermatologic surgeon. *J Dermatol Surg Oncol* 1989; **15**: 288–97.
3 Diwan R. Instruments for dermatologic surgery. In: Lask GP, Moy RL, eds. *Principles and Techniques of Cutaneous Surgery*. New York: McGraw-Hill, 1996: 85–100.
4 Horton R. Hand washing: the fundamental infection control principle. *Br J Nursing* 1995; **16**: 928–33.
5 Parienti JJ, Thibon P, Heller R et al. Hand-rubbing with an aqueous alcoholic solution vs traditional surgical hand-scrubbing and 30-day surgical site infection rates: a randomized equivalence study. *JAMA* 2002; **288**: 722–7.
6 Sebben JE. Survey of sterile technique in dermatological surgeons. *J Am Acad Dermatol* 1988; **18**: 1107–14.
7 Sebben JE, Fazio MJ. Sterilization of equipment for dermatologic surgery. In: Lask GP, Moy RL, eds. *Principles and Techniques of Cutaneous Surgery*. New York: McGraw-Hill, 1996: 47–56.

Safety aspects

Certain basic safety measures and protocols are essential within a dermatological surgery unit in order to minimize the risks of infection and accidental injury to both patients and staff [1].

The routine use of aseptic technique minimizes the risk of bacterial colonization at the operation site, and prevents contamination from adjacent sites. Antisepsis and sterilization are discussed elsewhere (see p. 78.5). Control of blood-borne infections, especially human immunodeficiency virus (HIV) and hepatitis, has two main components: prevention of transmission from patient to patient, and protection of the surgical team [2]. It is now mandatory for all British medical and nursing staff to be adequately vaccinated against hepatitis B, and for hospitals to have both dedicated infection control staff and protocols to ensure instrument sterility. One approach suggested by the US Centers for Disease Control and Prevention (CDC) is to treat *all* patients as if they were infected with HIV, hepatitis B or other blood-borne pathogens and to adopt 'universal precautions' [3].

Needle-stick injuries and other sharp instrument cuts are particularly important, and all members of the surgical team should take extreme care with the use and disposal of 'sharps'. It is extremely dangerous to either leave uncapped needles on the instrument tray or to attempt needle recapping by the two-handed method. Ideally, the surgeon should make a habit of both disposing of used needles and syringes *immediately* after use and removing all sharp disposable instruments (e.g. needles, scalpel blades) from the tray after the operation, placing these directly into 'sharps disposal' boxes. All relatives and those theatre personnel not directly concerned with the procedure should be excluded from the operating room. Clothing should be specific for surgery—apart from potentially introducing a variety of organisms to the procedure room, clothes may become contaminated.

At the preoperative consultation, a careful history may identify certain potential problems (e.g. diabetes, epilepsy) and the presence of cardiac pacemakers [4]. A full drug history is important—aspirin and anticoagulants promote bleeding and non-selective β-blockers (e.g. propranolol) may rarely interact with epinephrine (adrenaline) in local anaesthetics, resulting in malignant hypertension. On direct questioning, some people may admit to a tendency to faint very easily, and some patients with epilepsy may have a history of fits triggered by surgery or dental procedures. As there is always a risk of patient collapse in operating rooms, there must be adequate space available for an emergency resuscitation to be performed. Resuscitation drugs and equipment, together with both suction and an oxygen supply should be readily available [5]. All theatre personnel should be trained in advanced resuscitation techniques, including emergency electrocardiography and cardiac defibrillation [6].

REFERENCES

1 Jackson M, Lynch P. An attempt to make an issue less murky: a comparison of four systems for infection prevention. *Infect Control Hosp Epidemiol* 1991; **12**: 48–9.
2 Maloney ME. Infection control. In: Lask GP, Moy RL, eds. *Principles and Techniques of Cutaneous Surgery*. New York: McGraw-Hill, 1996: 57–62.
3 CDC Update. Universal precautions for prevention of human immunodeficiency virus, hepatitis B virus, and other blood-borne pathogens in health-care settings. *Morb Mortal Wkly Rep* 1988; **37**: 377–82, 387–8.
4 Sebben JE. The hazards of electrosurgery. *J Am Acad Dermatol* 1987; **16**: 869–71.
5 Nagi C, Greenway HT. Emergency airway assessment and management: guide for office practice. *J Assoc Milit Dermatol* 1985; **9**: 66–8.
6 Cummins RO, Thesis W. Encouraging early defibrillation: the AHA and automatic defibrillators. *Ann Emerg Med* 1990; **19**: 1245–7.

Complications [1]

All dermatological surgical procedures may result in complications [1,2], most commonly bleeding, infection and poor wound healing (Table 78.3). Although complications will always occur, most can be prevented by a combination of thorough preoperative preparation and good surgical technique.

Patients on long-term anticoagulant therapy require careful assessment regarding the potential medical risks if therapy is temporarily discontinued to facilitate surgery and the risk of significant bleeding complications if therapy is unchanged [3]. In difficult cases, discussion with other specialists involved in the patient's care will often help resolve this issue. Drugs that block platelet function (e.g. aspirin, clopidogrel, ticlopidine) potentially

Table 78.3 Complications in wound healing.

Complications	Predisposing factors	Prevention
Infection	Infected lesions Poor sterility Steroids Adjacent infectious source Occlusive dressings Poor blood supply Fat, haematoma and foreign material Sutures Poor technique Excessive devitalized tissue from careless handling or electrocoagulation	Careful preoperative and operative techniques Sutureless closure Antibiotic sprays Prophylactic antibiotics for infected or potentially infected wounds
Delay in closure	Poor blood supply Excess movement Infection Tension Steroids Debilitated patient Poor nutritional status	Layered closure Gentle tissue handling Minimize devitalization of tissues Care in decision to operate Warmth Careful postoperative dressings
'Gaping scar'	Inadequate apposition Dermal instability Excess movement Infection Tension	Careful apposition Subcutaneous or subcuticular sutures Adequate postoperative support (e.g. antitension dressings)
Painful scars	Feet and fingers especially	Avoid pressure sites if possible Dressings to reduce subsequent pressure and/or movement Careful apposition
Hypertrophic scars	Site Tension Reaction to embedded material Trauma Individual susceptibility	Avoid 'cape' area if possible Good surgical technique including undermining of edges where necessary
Keloids	Previous history Black skin Upper half of body Tension	Avoid surgery where possible Antitension measures for 3 weeks Watch and prepare to treat
'Railroad tracks'	Skin sutures under too much tension	Good suture technique Use of 'non-reactive' suture material
Stitch marks 'abscess'	Sutures left in too long	Early suture removal
Wound edge inversion	Poor technique	Good surgical technique Occlusive or semi-occlusive dressings
Bleeding and/or haematoma formation	Bleeding tendency Aspirin Clopidogrel Ticlopidine Eptifibatid Tirofiban	Preoperative screening Good haemostasis Use of epinephrine (adrenaline) in local anaesthetic

increase the risks of bleeding complications. In most instances, aspirin can be continued without resulting in a worse surgical outcome, although intraoperative bleeding may take longer to control. However, at some sites (e.g. around the eye) or in procedures involving extensive undermining or complex wound reconstruction, it may be appropriate to withhold these drugs prior to procedures. If aspirin is stopped this must be done at least 10 days before surgery to allow a sufficient number of new platelets with normal clotting responses to be produced. Non-steroidal anti-inflammatory drugs (NSAIDs) present no significant problem and can be continued in all circumstances [4].

The use of epinephrine-containing local anaesthetics results in vasoconstriction and prolongs the duration of anaesthesia. Intra-operatively, bleeding can be controlled by a combination of electrosurgery, pressure and ligation. Postoperatively, the use of appropriate wound dressings is important—ranging from simple Band Aid dressings for superficial wounds to layered dressings with pressure pads for larger wounds where there is a significant risk of haematoma formation (e.g. following cyst or lipoma excision, widely undermined wounds). All patients should be given verbal and written information regarding wound care and how to contact the dermatology unit if problems arise. Haematoma formation may occur at various times after surgery and usually results in acute pain and swelling. The clinical appearances, together with the age and size of the haematoma, will dictate whether to open the wound, evacuate the haematoma and obtain haemostasis, or to manage the complication conservatively [5].

Wound infection is a major concern, but is fortunately relatively uncommon following skin surgery. If the risk of infection is higher than normal (e.g. following excision of an ulcerated tumour from a flexural site), prophylactic antibiotic therapy may be appropriate. Postoperative infection usually presents as erythema, pain and swelling in and around the wound, 4–8 days after the procedure. Depending upon the clinical appearances, management will range from wound care, topical and systemic antibiotics, through to incision and drainage of a frank wound abscess.

Other significant problems relate to both the cosmetic and functional results of surgery. The risks of scarring must be carefully explained prior to surgery, with special attention to the possibility of distortion of facial 'free margins' (e.g. vermilion, lower eyelid) and unsightly hypertrophic scars in high-risk body sites (e.g. upper arm, shoulders, chest). Altered pigmentation in and around the wound is an additional cosmetic risk in Asian and black patients. Nerve damage is a significant concern, as both sensory and motor nerves may be damaged during cutaneous surgery, particularly at certain 'high-risk' anatomical sites (see pp. 78.2–78.5).

REFERENCES

1 Stasko T. Complications of cutaneous procedures. In: Roenigk RK, Roenigk HH, eds. *Dermatologic Surgery*, 2nd edn. New York: Marcel Dekker, 1996: 149–75.
2 Harahap M, ed. *Complications of Dermatologic Surgery*. Berlin: Springer-Verlag, 1993.
3 Billingsley EM, Maloney ME. Considerations in achieving hemostasis. In: Robinson JK, Arndt KA, LeBoit PE, eds. *Atlas of Cutaneous Surgery*. Philadelphia: Saunders, 1996: 67–77.
4 Stables G, Lawrence CM. Management of patients taking anti-coagulant, aspirin, non-steroidal anti-inflammatory and other antiplatelet drugs undergoing dermatological surgery. *Clin Exp Dermatol* 2002; **27**: 432–5.
5 Telfer NR, Tong A, Moy RL. Skin flaps. In: Harahap M, ed. *Complications of Dermatologic Surgery*. Berlin: Springer-Verlag, 1993: 195–203.

Local anaesthetics [1]

Principles and types

An ideal local anaesthetic agent would be non-toxic, painless on injection, rapid in onset, highly effective and carry a low risk of sensitization. The best compromise is found in 0.5–2% lignocaine hydrochloride (lidocaine), an amide-type local anaesthetic, which is the agent of choice for most dermatological surgery. Other amide-type local anaesthetic agents include mepivacaine, bupivacaine and ropivacaine, which have a slower onset but more sustained duration than lidocaine (lignocaine) [1]. Local anaesthetics in 'multiuse' bottles generally contain parabens preservative, but those supplied in glass ampoules are often preservative-free.

Ester-type local anaesthetics, for example procaine (ester of *p*-aminobenzoic acid) are seldom used by dermatologists.

Epinephrine 1 : 80 000–1 : 200 000, when added to local anaesthetic solutions, prolongs the duration of anaesthesia and produces local vasoconstriction. By reducing absorption, it may reduce the risk of systemic lidocaine toxicity.

Toxic reactions [1,2]

Toxic reactions to lidocaine are rare, and more likely to occur with the use of high volumes of high-concentration solutions or if accidental intravascular injection occurs. Lidocaine toxicity usually presents as a sensation of numbness or tingling. Systemic reactions include vasodilatation, cardiac or respiratory depression, or central nervous system manifestations such as dizziness, drowsiness, tinnitus, slurring of speech, muscle twitching and seizures. These side effects are, to some extent, reversible with diazepam (Valium) but full resuscitation measures may be required.

Ester-type local anaesthetics should be used with caution in patients with renal impairment. They also cross-react with a number of drugs of the *p*-aminobenzoic acid ester type (e.g. sulphonamides, paraphenylenediamine)

[3,4]. Amide-type anaesthetics should be used with care in patients with hepatic impairment.

The maximum recommended dosage for lidocaine with epinephrine is 7 mg/kg or approximately 50 mL of a 1% lidocaine solution for an average adult. In practice, most dermatological procedures require substantially lower anaesthetic doses. In order to minimize the risk of accidental intravascular injection, it is a wise precaution to either aspirate prior to infiltration or, if using very fine (e.g. 30 gauge) needles, which will not aspirate blood, to keep moving the needle about in the skin while slowly infiltrating small volumes.

Systemic absorption of epinephrine may be associated with mild tachycardia and an excited state. More serious reactions are rare but, as with lidocaine toxicity, are more likely to occur with the use of high volume, high-concentration solutions or following accidental intravascular injection. The use of epinephrine in local anaesthetics should be avoided or used with caution during pregnancy, in combination with inhalation anaesthesia, or in patients suffering from severe glaucoma [5]. Interaction with non-selective β-blockers (e.g. propranolol) may rarely cause malignant hypertension [2], but this is not a risk with 'cardioselective' β-blockers (e.g. atenolol).

Patients should always be asked if they have had any untoward reactions to local anaesthetics (e.g. in dental procedures). These may have been nothing more than fainting, as vasovagal attacks are commonly associated with local anaesthesia, and should not be confused with serious toxic reactions. In cases of serious doubt, alternative methods of anaesthesia are necessary.

Methods

Local anaesthesia may be achieved *topically* using either tetracaine (amethocaine) cream (Ametop®) or a eutectic lidocaine–prilocaine cream (EMLA®) [4], or by *local infiltration*. Both EMLA® and Ametop® are applied under occlusion, 1–2 h before the procedure. Conjunctival anaesthesia is best achieved using proxymetacaine eye drops, which sting much less than tetracaine.

Other methods of anaesthesia include *field block* and *nerve block anaesthesia* [3,5], which produce temporary blockade of sensory nerve function in a given area. Field block involves infiltration of local anaesthetic at several points around surgical sites such as the nose and ear [2], and nerve block anaesthesia involves blockade of one or more major sensory nerves. The most useful facial nerve blocks in dermatological surgery involve branches of the trigeminal (Vth) cranial nerve (Fig. 78.3)—the supraorbital (forehead), supratrochlear (glabella), infraorbital (lower eyelid, nasal sidewall, upper lip) and mental (lower lip) nerves [4,5]. The choice of local anaesthetic method depends upon a number of factors, including the

procedure itself, anatomical site and expected duration of the operation.

Controversy surrounds the use of epinephrine in digital nerve block ('ring block') anaesthesia because of a real or theoretical risk of digital ischaemia. Some believe it is absolutely contraindicated [6], whereas others describe routine use without incident [7,8].

In order to minimize discomfort when administering a local anaesthetic injection, consideration should be given to using a relatively fine needle, injecting slowly, and using both verbal and tactile distraction techniques. Injecting into the subcutaneous fat is less painful than intradermal infiltration, although it does take longer for the skin surface to become anaesthetic. Whenever possible, anaesthetic solutions should be at room temperature, and epinephrine avoided if not considered useful for the particular procedure. Pain on injection is less when lidocaine solutions are buffered with sodium bicarbonate immediately prior to use [9].

Other anaesthetic agents include the following:

1 *Ethyl chloride* and *liquid nitrogen* spray give short-lived periods of anaesthesia by skin refrigeration. This may be sufficient for quick superficial procedures such as the incision of small cysts and milia, abscesses or the curettage of multiple small warts.

2 The anaesthetic effect of *antihistamines* (e.g. 1% diphenhydramine hydrochloride solution) can be used when hypersensitivity to other agents is present or strongly suspected.

3 The intradermal injection of *normal saline* produces a brief anaesthetic effect [2].

4 *Hypnosis* and *acupuncture* may be useful when performed by an experienced practitioner and in a suitable subject.

5 *General anaesthesia* is rarely used in dermatological surgery. Patients requiring a general anaesthetic (e.g. children requiring treatment of large facial birthmarks) are best admitted to hospital either as a day case or overnight.

REFERENCES

1 Auletta MJ, Grekin RC. *Local Anesthesia for Dermatologic Surgery*. New York: Churchill-Livingstone, 1991.
2 Skidmore RA, Patterson JD, Tomsick RS. Local anesthetics. *Dermatol Surg* 1996; **22**: 511–22.
3 Auletta MJ. Local anaesthesia for dermatologic surgery. *Semin Dermatol* 1994; **13**: 35–42.
4 Buckley MM, Benfield P. Eutectic lidocaine/prilocaine cream: a review of the topical anaesthetic/analgesic efficacy of EMLA. *Drugs* 1993; **46**: 126–51.
5 Adriani J. *Regional Anaesthesia: Techniques in Clinical Practice*. Springfield: Thomas, 1970.
6 Bennett RG. Anesthesia. In: Bennett RG, ed. *Fundamentals of Cutaneous Surgery*. St Louis: Mosby, 1988: 194–239.
7 Sylaidis P, Logan A. Digital block with adrenaline: an old dogma refuted. *J Hand Surg* 1998; **23**: 17–9.
8 Millard TP, James MP. Avoidance of adrenaline in peripheral local anaesthesia: a perpetuated medical myth? *Clin Exp Dermatol* 2001; **26**: 731–2.
9 Matarasso SL, Glogau RS. Local anaesthesia. In: Lask GP, Moy RL, eds. *Principles and Techniques of Cutaneous Surgery*. New York: McGraw-Hill, 1996: 63–75.

Biopsy techniques

Incisional and excisional elliptical biopsy

Elliptical excision biopsy is used for tumour or suspect mole removal. Incisional biopsy is used to take diagnostic biopsies of rashes and tumours before treatment is started. The technique has the advantage that the entire thickness of skin down to fat is excised. An appropriate margin can be selected if required and the incision line placed in the optimum direction [1].

For lesions on the face, orientate the ellipse so that the scar runs parallel to or within an existing skin crease (wrinkle line), or follows a boundary line between two adjacent cosmetic units. Excision direction is best assessed with the patient seated rather than lying flat, to allow for the effect of gravity on the skin crease lines. Wrinkle or smile lines can be exaggerated by asking the patient to grimace or smile, or by manipulating the skin [2]. In an excisional biopsy, measure the margin to be excised and mark the optimal line of closure before injecting the anaesthetic. When drawing on the skin, use a skin marker or Bonney's blue ink (a mixture of crystal violet and brilliant green), as other inks may tattoo the skin.

The ellipse length should be approximately three times the width, to produce an ellipse angle of approximately 30°, so that buckling does not occur when the wound is sutured (Fig. 78.5) [3]. A larger angle may suffice at some sites or in older people [4]. Make the incision as a single continuous sweep rather than a series of small nicks, and hold the blade at 90° to the skin, not angled inwards, so that the ellipse sides are vertical [5]. Ensure that the incision lines meet neatly without crossing over at the tip by starting and finishing each sweep with the blade held vertically. Incise down to fat. When the ellipse sides and tips are completely separate from the surrounding skin the ellipse should be sitting on a bed of fat. The fat under the ellipse should be cut through using scissors, while the ellipse is gently pulled away from the skin using a skin hook [6]. Undermine the edge at the appropriate level if there is any tension. Close the wound using both subcutaneous and surface sutures if necessary, using the correct suture technique.

Punch biopsy

Punch biopsy produces a core of skin down to fat. It is quick and easy to perform, and leaves only a small wound. The disadvantages include the potential for sampling error and the difficulty in stopping bleeding if a small arteriole is punctured at the base of the wound. Punch biopsies can also be used to excise naevi on the back. At this site, wounds can be allowed to heal by second intention, with better cosmetic results than primary closure produces [7]. Subcutaneous tissue lesions can be

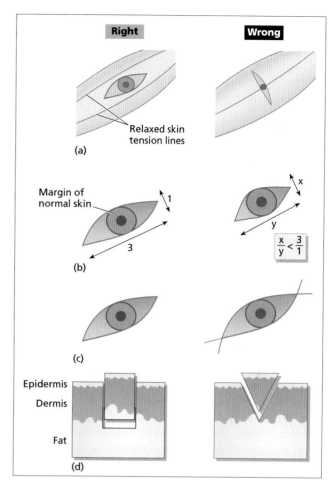

Fig. 78.5 Principles of elliptical excision. The ellipse is designed to follow skin-crease lines (a), and should be approximately three times as long as it is wide (b). Ensure that an appropriate margin of normal skin is also excised (b). At the ends of the ellipse, hold the blade vertically so that the incision lines do not cross over (c). The blade should be held at 90° to the skin when cutting the ellipse so that the wound has vertical sides down to fat. Do not bevel the blade towards the specimen as this makes the wound more difficult to close and may cut into the dermal component of the lesion (d). (From Lawrence [3].)

sampled using a punch biopsy by pinching up a fold of skin to include the subcutaneous tissue before the biopsy is taken [8].

Disposable and reusable 2–8 mm diameter punches are available. When the skin is numb, drill the blade down to fat with gentle downward pressure [5]. To minimize the scar size, stretch the skin at right angles to the wrinkle lines while taking the biopsy so that, when the tension is relaxed, an oval rather than a round wound is produced, with its long axis parallel to the wrinkle lines [6]. The skin core may pop up when the surrounding skin is pressed down, or it can be hooked out using a needle. Cut through the fat at the base with scissors and remove carefully to avoid crushing the specimen. The wound can be sutured or allowed to granulate; the latter produces an acceptable small round or oval scar. If the wound is to be allowed to heal by second intention, stopping bleeding using a collagen matrix dressing results in a better cosmetic result than using Monsel's solution [9].

Shave

Shave excision is a simple, rapid and effective method of removing benign papular naevi. It can also be used to obtain a tissue diagnosis in protuberant nodular skin tumours. Shave biopsy of dermatoses affecting the epidermis or high dermis results in adequate tissue for diagnosis, and the subsequent re-epithelialization from follicular epithelium produces a good cosmetic result.

Naevi

Inject the local anaesthetic directly into the naevus, as this stiffens the tissue and makes it easier to slice off. Holding a No. 15 blade horizontally, shave off the naevus flush with the skin. Stop bleeding using cautery, electrodesiccation or a chemical haemostatic agent. Any remaining wound edge tissue fragments can be destroyed using cautery or electrodesiccation. The wound will take 2–3 weeks to heal. In approximately 45% of head and neck and 30% of trunk naevi, no visible scar remains (Fig. 78.6). In the remainder, the scar is smaller than the original naevus on head, neck and limb sites and a little larger than the naevus on trunk sites. Pigmentation at the scar edge or centre remains in approximately 25% of initially pigmented naevi after shave excision; non-pigmented naevi rarely, if ever, leave a pigmented scar [10]. Persistent pigmentation is even more common when aluminium chloride haemostasis is used rather than cautery [11]. Recurrent or retained pigment does not need to be excised. If a further specimen is sent, the pathologist must be given the full history in order to interpret the changes correctly. Hairs remain in 25% of initially hairy naevi; these can be destroyed by electrolysis if necessary.

Skin tumours

Shave biopsy of a solid tumour is faster and easier than an incisional biopsy, which needs to be sutured. A fragment can be shaved off to confirm the diagnosis prior to definitive treatment. This type of biopsy will not help to distinguish a keratoacanthoma from a squamous cell carcinoma, and is unsuitable if histological examination of the deep margin or edge of a tumour is required to confirm the diagnosis. Bleeding can be stopped using silver nitrate stick coagulation, as the cosmetic outcome will be determined by the subsequent treatment. The fragile specimen should be mounted on paper before being placed in formalin.

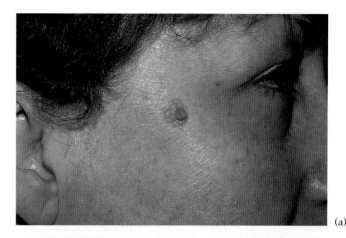

(a)

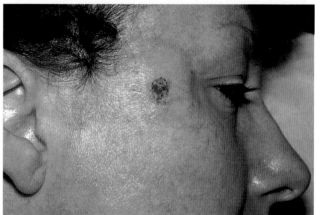

(b)

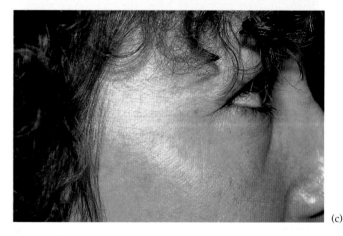

(c)

Fig. 78.6 Shave biopsy of benign papular naevi. (a) This patient had a benign tan-coloured naevus on the face (b) removed by shave excision followed by cautery, (c) resulting in a good cosmetic result 6 months later.

REFERENCES

1 Borges AF, Alexander JE. Relaxed skin tension lines, Z-plasty in scars and fusiform excisions of lesions. *Br J Plast Surg* 1962; **15**: 242–54.
2 Summers BK, Siegle RJ. Facial cutaneous reconstructive surgery: general aesthetic principles. *J Am Acad Dermatol* 1993; **29**: 669–81.
3 Lawrence CM. *An Introduction to Dermatological Surgery*, 2nd edn. St Louis: Mosby, 2002.
4 Hudson-Peacock MJ, Lawrence CM. Comparison of wound closure by

means of dog ear repair and elliptical excision. *J Am Acad Dermatol* 1995; **32**: 627–30.

5 Zachary CB. *Basic Cutaneous Surgery: a Primer in Technique.* New York: Churchill Livingstone, 1991.

6 Fewkes JL, Cheney ML, Pollack SV. *Illustrated Atlas of Cutaneous Surgery.* Philadelphia: Lippincott, 1992.

7 Barnett R, Stranc M. A method of producing improved scars following excision of small lesions of the back. *Ann Plast Surg* 1979; **5**: 391–4, 435.

8 Crollick JS, Klein LE. Punch biopsy diagnostic technique. *J Dermatol Surg Oncol* 1987; **13**: 839.

9 Armstrong RB, Nichols J, Pachance J. Punch biopsy wounds treated with Monsel's solution or a collagen matrix. *Arch Dermatol* 1986; **122**: 546–9.

10 Hudson-Peacock MJ, Bishop J, Lawrence CM. Shave excision of benign papular naevocytic naevi. *Br J Plast Surg* 1995; **48**: 318–22.

11 Hudson-Peacock MJ, Lawrence CM. Cosmetic outcome following shave excision of benign papular naevi using either electrocautery or aluminium chloride for haemostasis. *Br J Dermatol* 1995; **133** (Suppl. 45): 47.

Simple excision, suture technique and wound closure

Excision [1–3]

Skin biopsy specimens and cutaneous lesions can be removed using techniques other than elliptical excision, many of which (e.g. curettage, shave biopsy) do not result in a linear scar. Consequently, the decision to use formal surgical excision should balance the possible cosmetic advantages of other techniques (e.g. epidermal lesions and benign facial naevi) against the need to provide a full-thickness tissue specimen for histological examination (e.g. possible malignant melanoma).

Surgeon preparation

Dermatologists should be confident that they are competent to perform the proposed procedure and to manage any possible complications. If not, they should ask for a second opinion. The surgeon must be fully immunized against hepatitis B, and should observe safe practices with regard to handling sharps and tissue specimens. Surgical gloves should always be worn [4] and eye protection is strongly recommended.

Patient preparation

Patients should be fully aware of the significant risks, benefits and possible complications associated with the planned procedure. Informed consent [5] should be obtained, both verbally and in writing, for all invasive procedures. Usually, consent should be obtained from the parent or guardian in the case of minors, although some adolescents may be fully capable of both giving and withholding consent. Most patients about to undergo surgery are anxious and usually respond positively to appropriate reassurance as well as a calm and professional manner displayed by all members of the surgical team.

Examination and palpation of skin lesions will help to estimate their extent, depth and proximity to large blood vessels, nerves or other important structures. Langer's lines of skin tension [6] were previously used as a guide to incision, but the best cosmetic results are usually obtained by following the relaxed skin tension lines (RSTLs) [1,7], which tend to lie perpendicular to the major underlying muscles. Langer's lines and RSTLs often coincide, as on the neck. When they do not, as on the limbs, the choice depends on other factors. Excisions on the lower leg, for instance, close more easily along the long axis of the limb, rather than transversely. Testing for skin laxity by manipulating the skin usually clarifies the best direction in which to plan an excision. The size and type of excision made will also depend upon many factors, including the site and nature of the lesion to be excised and the nature of the planned skin closure.

The skin surface should be cleaned prior to operation with a detergent–antibacterial combination, most commonly containing either chlorhexidine [8] or povidone-iodine. This helps to reduce the risk of wound infection by removing pathogens and reducing the resident cutaneous bacterial flora [9].

Elliptical excision—general technique [2,3]

It can often be helpful to mark the planned lines of excision prior to cleaning the skin surface and infiltrating local anaesthetic. A reasonable period of time should be allowed for the anaesthetic to take full effect.

The small round-ended Gillette No. 15 blade is most commonly used to make two hemi-elliptical incisions perpendicular through the skin into the subcutaneous tissues. The length of the wound should be at least three times its breadth (the angles at the ends of the ellipse should not exceed 30°) taking care not to allow the incisions to cross each other ('fishtailing') at either end (Fig. 78.5). The skin ellipse is held firmly but gently with either fine-toothed forceps or a skin hook, and separated from its base. For both histological purposes and to facilitate wound closure the excised specimen should contain subcutaneous fat.

For standard histological processing the specimen should be placed in a formaldehyde–saline specimen bottle, clearly labelled with the patient's details. To prevent curling of small biopsy or excision samples, these may be placed on small squares of filter paper and floated into the formalin solution. When histological confirmation of tumour clearance is required, it can sometimes be helpful to 'colour code' or place a suture at the '12 o'clock' position of the surgical specimen to facilitate orientation and examination in the pathology department. For immunofluorescence or frozen section studies, specimens are placed on aluminium foil and immersed in liquid nitrogen.

Intraoperative bleeding is controlled by a combination of pressure, electrosurgery, clamping and ligation of vessels.

Depending upon the size of the defect and the body site, a variable degree of undermining of the wound edges will be necessary to facilitate the placing of subcutaneous absorbable sutures and to reduce wound tension. Finally, non-absorbable sutures are used to neatly appose and evert the wound edges [2,3].

The timing of suture removal depends upon the site and the amount of tension across the wound. With additional supporting surface tapes and buried sutures where appropriate, 4–5 days is usually sufficient for skin sutures on the face, 5–7 days for the scalp and neck and 10–14 days elsewhere.

REFERENCES

1 Baer RL, Kopf AW. Dermatologic office surgery. In: *Year Book of Dermatology 1963–64*. Chicago: Year Book Medical, 1964: 7–47.
2 Epstein E, Epstein E Jr, eds. *Skin Surgery*, 5th edn. Springfield: Thomas, 1982.
3 Stegman SJ. *Basics of Dermatologic Surgery*. Chicago: Year Book Medical, 1982.
4 Smith JG, Chalker DK. A glove upon that hand. *South Med J* 1982; **75**: 129–31.
5 Redden EM, Baker DC. Coping with the complexities of informed consent in dermatologic surgery. *J Dermatol Surg Oncol* 1984; **10**: 111–6.
6 Ridge MD, Wright V. The directional effects of skin: a bioengineering study of skin with particular reference to Langer's lines. *J Invest Dermatol* 1966; **46**: 341–6.
7 Kraissl CJ. The selection of appropriate lines for elective surgical excision. *Plast Reconstr Surg* 1951; **8**: 1–28.
8 Kaul AF, Jewitt JF. Agents and techniques for disinfection of the skin. *Surg Gynecol Obstet* 1981; **152**: 677–85.
9 Selwyn S, Ellis H. Skin bacteria and skin disinfection reconsidered. *BMJ* 1972; i: 136–40.

Sutures [1–4]

An ideal suture would have high tensile strength, handle easily, provide good knot security and cause no tissue reaction. Skin sutures are of two main types: *absorbable* and *non-absorbable*.

Now that catgut is rarely used, popular synthetic *absorbable sutures* include Vicryl™ (polyglactin-910), Dexon™ (polyglycolic acid), PDS (polydioxane sulphate), Maxon™ (polyglyconate) and Monocryl™ (poliglecaprone), all of which cause very little tissue reaction and dissolve completely in 90–120 days. Absorbable sutures are usually placed either subcutaneously in the subcutaneous fat to close off potential dead space or as subcuticular intradermal sutures to close and evert wound edges.

Non-absorbable sutures include braided silk and synthetic monofilament sutures such as nylon (Ethilon™) and polypropylene (Prolene™). Most dermatological surgeons prefer the better tensile strength and low tissue reactivity of the synthetic monofilament sutures. Braided sutures such as silk and Dacron™ have better knot-tying properties but tend to drag through tissue, and their braided nature may increase the risk of wound infection. For wounds that are likely to remain under constant tension, such as those on the back or shoulders, a non-absorbable suture such as nylon can be used to close the deep subcutaneous layer. Alternatively, a running subcu-

ticular Prolene suture can be left in place for long periods without leaving suture marks.

In general, skin suture needles are of the reverse cutting type (the sharp edge of the needle lies on the trailing rather than the leading edge). Suture sizes usually vary from 3/0 to 6/0, with suture selection depending on the wound size, anatomical site and surgeon preference.

Suture technique [2,3,5]

The ability to perform several different suture techniques is one of the skills needed in order to become proficient in dermatological surgery. The *simple interrupted suture* is the mainstay of final skin closure, although alternatives include a *running suture*, placed either as loops through the skin (*simple running suture*) or placed entirely within the dermis (*running subcuticular suture*). They are normally 4/0–6/0 gauge, and are placed close to the skin edge for fine approximation. If the wound tends to invert, then the deeper component of the suture can be placed more laterally to help evert the edges.

If there is tension across the wound, or a significant tendency to inversion, one or two *vertical mattress* sutures can be placed initially. A modification of this suture, the *half-buried mattress*, is also useful as a corner stitch when insetting the tips of skin flaps. The *horizontal mattress* suture (with or without bolsters) [6] can also be used to approximate long wounds or wounds under tension. Any wound tension must be managed by undermining and the use of buried sutures before the insertion of skin sutures. Failure to do this will increase the risks of infection and wound dehiscence, and often leave permanent unsightly, papular or linear suture marks.

There are various forms of *buried suture*, which are used to close off 'dead space' in a deep wound. Normally, this is obliterated by the use of interrupted *deep subcutaneous* or buried absorbable dermal sutures [7], or by using a '*purse-string*' variant of the horizontal mattress suture. Running sutures, both cutaneous and subcutaneous, can be used to save time, but may be less secure than interrupted sutures and can be tricky to remove. The running subcuticular suture, although difficult to learn, is an elegant suture technique, and it can be left in place for long periods without risk of leaving permanent suture marks.

Tape closures (e.g. Steri-Strips™) may be used in conjunction with interrupted sutures or on their own if there is good approximation and adequate subcutaneous or subcuticular support. They provide additional wound support both while skin sutures are in place and for the immediate period following suture removal. Cyanoacrylate tissue glues may also be useful, especially in children [8], and for securing skin grafts [9].

Stainless steel staples are a rapid and effective way to close longer skin incisions. They are strong, incite very little tissue reaction, and can be useful for closing scalp wounds and skin graft donor sites [10].

REFERENCES

1 Aston SJ. The choice of suture material for skin closure. *J Dermatol Surg Oncol* 1976; **2**: 57–61.
2 Dingman RO, Watanabe MJ, Izenberg PH. General principles of skin surgery. In: Epstein E, Epstein E Jr, eds. *Skin Surgery*, 5th edn. Springfield: Thomas, 1982: 74–107.
3 Stegman SJ. Suturing techniques for dermatologic surgery. *J Dermatol Surg Oncol* 1978; **4**: 63–8.
4 Swanson NA, Tromovitch TA. Suture materials, 1980s: properties, uses, and abuses. *Int J Dermatol* 1982; **21**: 373–8.
5 Stegman SJ, Tromovitch TA, Glogau RG. *Basics of Dermatologic Surgery.* Chicago: Year Book Medical, 1982.
6 Simmonds WL. Surgical gems: uses of bolsters in dermatologic surgery. *J Dermatol Surg Oncol* 1977; **3**: 281–2.
7 Albom MJ. Surgical gems: dermo-subdermal sutures for long, deep surgical wounds. *J Dermatol Surg Oncol* 1977; **3**: 504–5.
8 Ellis DAF, Shaikh A. The ideal tissue adhesive in facial plastic and reconstructive surgery. *J Otolaryngol* 1990; **19**: 68–72.
9 Craven NM, Telfer NR. An open study of tissue adhesive in full-thickness skin grafting. *J Am Acad Dermatol* 1999; **40**: 607–11.
10 Stegmaier OC. Use of skin stapler in dermatologic surgery. *J Am Acad Dermatol* 1982; **6**: 305–9.

Particular forms of excision

Variations in detail and technique apply to particular lesions and areas of the body.

Pilar or epidermal cysts [1]

Small cysts are often deeper than they appear and may be difficult to locate after infiltration with local anaesthetic. Careful preoperative skin marking will often help in their intraoperative location. Larger, tense cysts of the scalp often extend deeply and their removal may be accompanied by significant bleeding. Many cysts can be removed by making an elliptical incision into the overlying skin (surrounding the punctum, if present) and using blunt dissection to separate the cyst from the tissues while pulling gently on the ellipse and the attached cyst. If the cyst ruptures, the remaining contents should be expressed and the whole of the cyst wall removed. Irrigation of the wound prior to closure will remove residual cyst contents which might otherwise cause a granulomatous tissue reaction. Excision of large skin cysts leaves subcutaneous dead space, which must be obliterated with deep sutures to minimize the risks of haematoma formation, infection and wound dehiscence.

Lesions on the shoulder and upper back

Surgical excision on the shoulders, upper back and deltoid areas frequently results in poor cosmetic results, with the formation of stretched and frequently hypertrophic scars. Although meticulous surgical technique, appropriate undermining and careful suture technique may minimize these problems, patients should be carefully counselled and only offered surgical excision in these areas when it is absolutely necessary. One suggested alternative to excision and repair in these areas is to excise the lesion with a narrow margin of normal skin and allow healing by secondary intention [2].

Benign naevi

Surgical excision, even by experts, leaves scars and consequently benign naevi are best either left alone or removed by shave excision when possible.

Non-melanoma skin cancer: basal cell and squamous cell carcinomas

Many different surgical and non-surgical techniques may be used to treat non-melanoma skin cancer [3,4]. The choice of treatment is based upon various factors relating to both the tumour [5] and the patient [6].

Small primary well-defined lesions in areas of skin laxity are often best excised. An adequate margin should always be obtained, and prior skin marking following careful examination in good lighting is advisable [5]. Cure rates following surgical excision of such lesions can be excellent [7–9]. Some sites, such as the lips, ear, scalp and periocular and nasolabial areas, have a higher rate of recurrence, and (for squamous cell carcinoma) metastasis. Management of lesions in these sites, particularly if recurrent, poorly defined or showing infiltrative growth patterns, is best performed by a specialist dermatological surgeon [5,10].

Mucous membranes

Excision of lesions in the mouth and on the tongue, lips and genitalia can be difficult, with restricted access and often profuse bleeding. Consequently, only simple procedures should be attempted by non-specialists, and more complex cases referred to colleagues in oral surgery, urology and gynaecology as appropriate.

Keratoacanthoma

This is often difficult to differentiate, both clinically and histologically, from squamous cell carcinoma. Small lesions are often suitable for surgical excision, and larger lesions should be subjected to a transverse incisional biopsy passing from normal adjacent skin through the centre of the lesion and extending through the subcutaneous fat [11].

Pigmented lesions (see Chapter 38)

The diagnosis and management of pigmented lesions is a key component of clinical dermatology and forms an important part of the multidisciplinary treatment of malignant melanoma, also involving pathology, plastic surgery and clinical oncology.

Blue naevi, pigmented basal cell carcinomas, seborrhoeic

keratoses and dermatofibromas are usually easily recognizable to the trained eye, although diagnostic difficulties occasionally occur. When diagnostic doubt exists, and especially when malignancy is suspected, the lesion should be excised and submitted for histopathological examination. When the lesion is too large to excise and repair directly, an incisional biopsy may be indicated (e.g. possible malignant change in a large congenital naevus or facial lentigo). In these cases, if malignant melanoma is proven on biopsy, a second procedure, possibly involving complex wound reconstruction, will often be necessary. In such cases, an initial incisional biopsy does not appear to influence the overall prognosis [12], although determination of key prognostic features (e.g. growth phase, depth of invasion, presence of vascular invasion) can only be made accurately from examination of the full excision specimen.

Hypertrophic scars

Although these may occur at any site, they are especially common in certain anatomical sites such as the upper back, shoulders and deltoid areas. Most will slowly resolve with time and regular gentle wound massage. Intralesional steroid injections can be helpful, but may cause skin and fat atrophy and should be used with caution. Hypertrophic scars may also be treated (and possibly prevented) by the use of Z-plasty techniques [13], with pressure dressings or devices [14], and silicone gel sheet dressings [15].

REFERENCES

1 Roxburgh RA. Excision of sebaceous cysts and lipomas. *Br J Hosp Med* 1969; **2**: 866–7.
2 Barnett R, Stranc M. A method of producing improved scars following excision of small lesions of the back. *Ann Plast Surg* 1979; **3**: 391–4.
3 Dzubow L, Grossman D. Squamous cell carcinoma and verrucous carcinoma. In: Friedman RJ, Rigel DS, Kopf AW, Harris MN, Baker D, eds. *Cancer of the Skin*. Philadelphia: Saunders, 1991: 74–84.
4 Telfer NR, Colver GB, Bowers PW. Guidelines for the management of basal cell carcinoma. *Br J Dermatol* 1999; **141**: 415–23.
5 Breuninger H, Dietz K. Prediction of subclinical tumour infiltration in basal cell carcinoma. *J Dermatol Surg Oncol* 1991; **17**: 574–8.
6 Randle HW. Basal cell carcinoma: identification and treatment of the high-risk patient. *Dermatol Surg* 1996; **22**: 255–61.
7 Chernosky ME. Squamous cell and basal cell carcinomas: preliminary study of 3817 primary skin cancers. *South Med J* 1978; **71**: 802–3.
8 Marchac D, Papadopoulos O, Duport G. Curative and aesthetic results of surgical treatment of 138 basal-cell carcinomas. *J Dermatol Surg Oncol* 1982; **8**: 379–87.
9 Porte A, Molle B, Zumer L *et al.* Résultat du traitement de 250 épithéliomas cutanés. *Ann Chirurg Plast* 1979; **24**: 253–6 (Abstract).
10 Bart RS, Schrager D, Kopf AW *et al.* Scalpel excision of basal cell carcinomas. *Arch Dermatol* 1978; **114**: 739–42.
11 Owen C, Telfer N. Keratoacanthoma. In: Lebwohl M, Heymann WR, Berth-Jones J, Coulson I, eds. *Treatment of Skin Disease: Comprehensive Therapeutic Strategies*. London: Mosby, 2002: 315–8.
12 Epstein E, Bragg K, Linden G. Biopsy and prognosis of malignant melanoma. *JAMA* 1969; **208**: 1369–71.
13 Longacre JJ. *Scar Tissue: Its Use and Abuse*. Springfield: Thomas, 1972.
14 Carr JA. Pressure technique. In: Harahap M, ed. *Surgical Techniques for Cutaneous Scar Revision*. New York: Marcel Dekker, 2000: 447–60.
15 Sproat JE, Dalcin A, Weitauer N *et al.* Hypertrophic sternal scars: silicone gel sheet versus Kenalog injection treatment. *Plast Reconstr Surg* 1992; **90**: 988–92.

Wound closure [1–3]

A significant part of dermatological surgical practice involves the repair of surgical defects. Wounds can be allowed to heal by secondary intention healing, closed primarily, or repaired using skin grafts or skin flaps. Experience and careful consideration of the various wound closure options are necessary in order to offer patients the best possible cosmetic and functional results.

The M-plasty [4]

This is occasionally useful if one end of an elliptical excision will cross an important anatomical or cosmetic line. In this situation, an M-plasty will help to reduce the overall length of excision required by bringing the apex of the excision back within the original area to be excised.

'Dog-ear' repairs [5]

'Dog-ears' (folds or humps of skin) tend to occur when the length to width ratio of an excision is insufficient to prevent the skin at the poles from bulging outwards when the opposing skin edges are brought together. They tend to occur more commonly when there is limited laxity or movement in the surrounding tissues. Excisions where the angle at the apex exceeds 30° are also liable to produce 'dog-ears'. 'Pseudo-dog-ears' occur if too much fat is left at the poles of an excision.

There are several ways in which this problem can be surmounted [3].
1 The excision can be extended and the redundant overlapping skin excised.
2 One side of the pucker can be cut back flush with the skin and the excess skin from the other side identified by drawing it across the wound; this can then be cut off.
3 The excess skin of the 'dog-ear' can be removed by converting it into a T-plasty or an M-plasty. This is a useful technique when the length of the wound cannot be extended [6].

Wound edges of unequal lengths

This problem can often be resolved by using a halving technique: a suture is placed across the centre of the wound and subsequent sutures used to divide the two resultant defects into ever smaller compartments. Because of local skin elasticity, the shorter side tends to stretch to match the longer. For more disproportionate edges, a wedge may have to be removed from the longer side in order to make the sides of the resultant ellipse more equal,

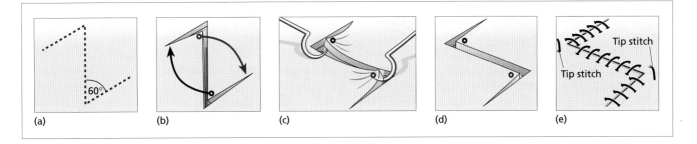

Fig. 78.7 Technique of Z-plasty. (From Eedy *et al.* [7].)

or the wound can be sutured in the normal way and a 'dog-ear' repair performed to remove the excess skin from one side.

Z-plasty

This is a technique that is used to treat scar contractures, skin 'webbing' and to break up or alter the direction of linear scars to try to improve the cosmetic or functional result. The size of the angle used determines the increase in the length of the scar that will result (Figs 78.7 & 78.8).

REFERENCES

1 Chernosky ME. Scalpel and scissor surgery as seen by the dermatologist. In: Epstein E, Epstein E Jr, eds. *Skin Surgery*, 5th edn. Springfield: Thomas, 1982: 189–229.
2 Stegman SJ. Planning closure of a surgical wound. *J Dermatol Surg Oncol* 1978; **4**: 390–3.
3 Stegman SJ. *Basics of Dermatologic Surgery*. Chicago: Year Book Medical, 1982.
4 Webster RC, Davidson TM, Smith RC *et al.* M-plasty techniques. *J Dermatol Surg Oncol* 1976; **2**: 393–6.
5 Gormley DE. The dog-ear: causes, prevention and correction. *J Dermatol Surg Oncol* 1977; **3**: 194–8.
6 Salasche SJ, Roberts LC. Dog-ear correction by M-plasty. *J Dermatol Surg Oncol* 1984; **10**: 478–82.
7 Eedy DJ, Breathnach SM, Walker NPJ. *Surgical Dermatology*. Oxford: Blackwell Science, 1996.

Dressings

Wound dressings are not essential [1], although optimizing wound care by using an appropriate dressing probably produces a predictably better result. An ideal dressing should meet the following criteria.
1 Soaks up excess exudate from the wound surface, thereby reducing the risk of bacterial penetration.
2 Maintains a moist wound–dressing interface to encourage migration of epidermal cells over the granulating tissue. Covered split-thickness wounds heal faster than dry wounds [2]. A scab is a poor barrier against loss of moisture from the dermal surface because it allows the surface to dry out, thus forcing the epidermis to grow under the dry wound surface. As the epidermal cells migrate, they secrete a proteolytic enzyme which dis-

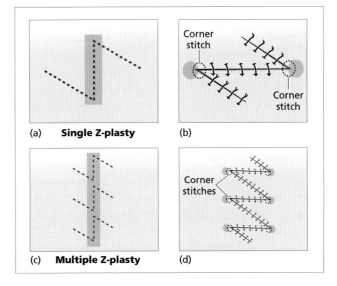

Fig. 78.8 Single and multiple Z-plasty. (a,b) Single Z-plasty. (c,d) Multiple Z-plasty. Note breaking up of zone of lateral tension (shaded areas) with multiple Z-plasty. (From Eedy *et al.* [7].)

solves the base of the scab; migration ceases when cell–cell contact occurs [3].
3 Does not contain organisms or fibres that may contaminate the wound. Cellulose-derived dressings may shed fibre fragments into the wound [4], causing a foreign body reaction and leading to increased risk of infection.
4 Is impermeable to bacteria.
5 Causes minimal injury to healing tissue when removed.
    It is often claimed that a dressing that permits increased oxygen permeability aids wound healing. Such dressings do aid healing in split-thickness wounds [5]. However, in full-thickness wounds the same synthetic wound dressings create hypoxic conditions at the healing surface [6]. Paradoxically, tissue hypoxia in full-thickness wounds appears to stimulate rather than retard granulation tissue formation [7].

Basic dressing [8]

This includes contact, absorbent and outer layers [9]. The layer in contact with the wound is non-adherent, either because it contains a greasy ointment (e.g. tulle dressing) or because it is made from a specially designed low-adherence material (e.g. polyethylene) [10]. The absorbent layer (e.g. cotton-wool, gauze) soaks up the excess wound exudate and cushions the wound. The outer layer (e.g. tubular bandage, elasticated tape) holds the other two layers in place and applies slight pressure. The basic dressing is left in place until suture removal, but needs to be changed if it gets wet or becomes saturated with exudate [11], as this greatly increases bacterial penetration. Many proprietary dressings combine two or all three components (e.g. Melolin® contains a polyethylene non-adherent layer attached to an absorbent cellulose component). The hydrogel (e.g. Vigilon®), hydrocolloid (e.g. Granuflex®), xerogel (e.g. dextranomer starch polymer), alginate (e.g. Kaltostat®) and synthetic foam dressings are designed to provide all three components, and these can also be used on pressure sores [12,13], leg ulcers [14] and full-thickness surgical wounds [15].

Pressure dressings

These are placed over the basic dressing. Most commonly, and on suitable sites, a piece of compressible padded dressing (e.g. cotton wool, sponge, eye pad) is pressed down onto the wound with an elasticated or *crepe bandage* for 48 h. Where bandage application is difficult, a *multi-tape dressing* can be used. Dental rolls are placed over and pressed down onto the dressing by using adhesive tape strips, and additional adhesive (e.g. collodion or tinct benz co.) is used to increase the tape adhesion. A *tie-over pressure dressing* is commonly applied over skin grafts, but can be used on any wound. Paired sutures are placed around the wound and tied together to hold down a three-layered contact, absorbent and compression dressing, so that the graft is held down onto the recipient site to prevent a haematoma forming beneath it.

Suggested dressing for wound types

Small full- or *partial thickness wounds* (shave and curettage sites) require a simple low-adherent dressing or paraffin tulle held in place with a conforming adhesive tape. Unsutured punch biopsy sites do not appear to benefit from occlusive dressings [16], but heal better with a collagen matrix dressing than they do after simply applying Monsel's solution to stop bleeding [17]. *Sutured wounds* (side-to-side closures and flaps) require a greasy antiseptic ointment application and an absorbent-backed, low-adherent dressing held in place with a conforming adhesive tape. A pressure dressing may also be required. After suture removal, apply adhesive tape strips for 5 days. On a *full-thickness graft*, apply a simple contact dressing (e.g. greasy antiseptic ointment and paraffin tulle) and then a tie-over pressure dressing which includes a sponge or cotton wool compressible pad. On *full-thickness wounds*,

a variety of wound management methods are used. If acceptable to the patient, the wound can be left without a dressing and simply cleaned two or three times daily, and a sterile white soft paraffin or vaseline-based antiseptic ointment applied. Alternatively, the wound can be cleaned less frequently if a combination contact/absorbent dressing is applied. During the initial exudative stage (the first 4 days) the dressing will need to be changed at least once a day. Thereafter, the dressing should be changed if the wound surface starts to dry out or the dressing becomes saturated, wet or otherwise dirty. The wound should be cleaned with a simple antiseptic (e.g. aqueous chlorhexidine, 10 vol. hydrogen peroxide) before being re-dressed using a vaseline-based antiseptic ointment (Polyfax®), and simple contact dressing (e.g. polyethylene/cellulose dressing; Melolin®) held in place with adhesive tape. Alternatively, a semi-permeable adhesive polyurethane [18] or gel, or colloid dressing can be used and changed as necessary. *Split-skin graft donor sites* heal faster with a dressing that maintains a moist wound–dressing interface; for example, a calcium alginate [19] or semi-permeable adhesive polyurethane film [20]. A pressure bandage applied over the wound is also required, but bleeding will still occur. The exudate can either be allowed to drain through puncture wounds made in the lower portion of the polyurethane film, or can be removed by changing the dressing more frequently, although this may introduce infection and is painful.

Wound healing is delayed by topical steroid application [21], tobacco smoking [22] and possibly age [23] via a decrease in skin blood flow with increasing arteriosclerosis [24].

REFERENCES

1 Mengert WF, Hermes RL. Simplified gynecologic care. *Am J Obstet Gynecol* 1949; **58**: 1109–16.
2 Hinman CD, Maibach H. Effect of air exposure and occlusion on experimental human skin wounds. *Nature* 1963; **200**: 377–8.
3 Harris DR. Healing of the surgical wound. I. Basic considerations. *J Am Acad Dermatol* 1979; **1**: 197–207.
4 Wood RAB. Disintegration of cellulose dressings in open granulating wounds. *BMJ* 1976; **1**: 1444–5.
5 Silver IA. Oxygen tension and epithelialization. In: Maibach HI, Rovee DT, eds. *Epidermal Wound Healing*. Chicago: Year Book, 1972.
6 Varghese MC, Balin AK, Carer M, Caldwell D. Local environment of chronic wounds under synthetic dressings. *Arch Dermatol* 1986; **122**: 52–7.
7 Knighton DR, Silver IA, Hunt TK. Regulation of wound healing angiogenesis: effect of oxygen gradients and inspired oxygen concentration. *Surgery* 1981; **90**: 262–70.
8 Bennett RG. *Fundamentals of Cutaneous Surgery*. St Louis: Mosby, 1988: 310–51.
9 Telfer NR, Moy RL. Wound care after office procedures. *J Dermatol Surg Oncol* 1993; **19**: 722–31.
10 Anonymous. Local applications to wounds. II. Dressings for wounds and ulcers. *Drug Ther Bull* 1991; **29**: 97–100.
11 Colebrook L, Hood AM. Infection through soaked dressings. *Lancet* 1948; **ii**: 682–3.
12 Engdahl E. Clinical evaluation of Debrisan on pressure sores. *Curr Ther Res* 1980; **28**: 377–80.
13 Gorse GJ, Messner RL. Improved pressure sore healing with hydrocolloid dressings. *Arch Dermatol* 1987; **123**: 766–71.

14 Handfield-Jones SE, Grattan CEH, Simpson RA, Kennedy CTC. Comparison of a hydrocolloid dressing and paraffin gauze in the treatment of venous ulcers. *Br J Dermatol* 1988; **118**: 425–7.

15 Eaglstein WH. Occlusive dressings. *J Dermatol Surg Oncol* 1993; **19**: 716–20.

16 Knudsen EA, Snitker G. Wound healing under plastic coated pads. *Acta Derm Venereol (Stockh)* 1969; **49**: 438–41.

17 Armstrong RB, Nichols J, Pachance J. Punch biopsy wounds treated with Monsel's solution or a collagen matrix. *Arch Dermatol* 1986; **122**: 546–9.

18 Hien NT, Prawer SE, Katz HI. Facilitated wound healing using transparent film dressing following Mohs micrographic surgery. *Arch Dermatol* 1988; **124**: 903–6.

19 Attwood AI. Calcium alginate dressing accelerates split skin graft donor site healing. *Br J Plast Surg* 1989; **42**: 373–9.

20 James JH, Watson ACH. The use of Op-site, a vapour permeable dressing on skin graft donor sites. *Br J Plast Surg* 1975; **28**: 107–10.

21 Eaglstein WH, Mertz PM. New method for assessing epidermal wound healing: the effects of triamcinolone acetonide and polyethylene film occlusion. *J Invest Dermatol* 1978; **71**: 382–4.

22 Silverstein P. Smoking and wound healing. *Am J Med* 1992; **93** (1A): 22S–4S.

23 Ashcroft GS, Horan MA, Ferguson MW. The effect of ageing on cutaneous wound healing in mammals. *J Anat* 1995; **187**: 1–26.

24 Tsuchida Y. The effect of ageing and arteriosclerosis on human skin blood flow. *J Dermatol Sci* 1995; **5**: 175–81.

Secondary intention healing

Full-thickness wounds remaining after malignant [1,2] or benign [3] tumour excision can be left to heal by second intention. The cosmetic result depends on wound site and patient age. The nasolabial fold, medial canthus, scalp and pre- and postauricular skin produce particularly good results, although the technique can be used in many sites, including the fingers [4]. Almost half of the reduction in wound size occurs because of scar contraction [5] and subsequent stretching of surrounding tissues [6]. Therefore, if the wound is next to a mucocutaneous junction, such as the lip, ala nasa or eyelid, scar contraction may distort this free margin, producing poor cosmesis and function. Most other head and neck sites heal well, although in general the cosmetic results are best on concave rather than convex skin surfaces [7]. The older the patient the better the result, probably because wound contraction is aided by the availability of loose adjacent skin and because hypertrophic scarring is less common in older patients. The method can be used if there is doubt about the adequacy of excision, or closure of the defect requires a larger or more complex procedure, which the patient will not tolerate. In some situations, such as excision of naevi on the back [3] or the treatment of acne keloidalis nuchae [8] and hidradenitis [9], secondary intention healing is the preferred method as it results in a superior cosmetic result.

When a tumour is being excised, the specimen is orientated with a marking suture before complete removal, so that if further excision is required the affected margin can be identified. When bleeding is controlled, a contact dressing is applied, and this is covered by a pressure dressing for 24–48 h. Thereafter, the dressing can be changed at 2–4-day intervals, depending on the amount of exudate. At each dressing change, the wound is cleaned to remove crust or debris and a greasy antiseptic ointment (e.g.

Polyfax®, Flamazine® or Betadine® ointment) and non-adherent dressing are applied. On average, a 25-mm diameter head and neck wound takes approximately 35 days to heal [10]. If histology shows that the tumour has been incompletely excised, the involved margin can be re-excised 1–2 weeks after the first excision. Because vertical sections are taken and the entire excision margin is not examined, the technique does not provide the same complete excision margin control as the horizontal sections of Mohs' surgery [1]. These wounds are surprisingly pain-free. Bacterial contamination may occur, but tissue infection is rare; when present the wound edge is tender, red and swollen. A yellow exudate is common in the first few days. Before granulation tissue appears, a yellowish fibrin clot covers the wound. Exposed periosteum and perichondrium must be kept moist and viable by using a saline-dampened alginate dressing. This encourages granulation tissue to migrate over the exposed area and also reduces the risk of bone desiccation and necrosis [11]. If the periosteum has been stripped off, the exposed bone can be fenestrated or abraded to encourage the formation of granulation tissue and hence enhance re-epithelialization [12]. When the wound first heals, the scar often contains large looped vessels, which slowly disappear as the scar thickens. A slightly elevated, red, hypertrophic scar is then present, and the cosmetic result is not optimum until approximately 1 year (Figs 78.9 & 78.10).

REFERENCES

1 Mohs FE. *Chemosurgery: Microscopically Controlled Surgery for Skin Cancer.* Springfield: Thomas, 1978.

2 Goldwyn RM, Rueckert F. The value of healing by secondary intention for sizeable defects of the face. *Arch Surg* 1977; **112**: 285–92.

3 Barnett R, Stranc M. A method of producing improved scars following excision of small lesions of the back. *Ann Plast Surg* 1979; **3**: 391–4, 435.

4 de Berker DAR, Dahl MGC, Malcolm AJ, Lawrence CM. Micrographic surgery for subungual squamous cell carcinoma. *Br J Plast Surg* 1996; **49**: 414–9.

5 Catty RHC. Healing and contraction of experimental full thickness wounds in the human. *Br J Surg* 1965; **52**: 542–8.

6 Lawrence CM, Comaish JS, Dahl MGC. Excision of skin malignancies without wound closure. *Br J Dermatol* 1986; **115**: 563–71.

7 Zitelli JA. Wound healing by secondary intention. *J Am Acad Dermatol* 1983; **9**: 407–15.

8 Glenn MJ, Bennett RG, Kelly AP. Acne keloidalis nuchae: treatment with excision and secondary intention healing. *J Am Acad Dermatol* 1995; **33**: 243–6.

9 Silverberg B, Smoot CE, Landa SJF, Parsons RW. Hidradenitis suppurativa: patients' satisfaction with wound healing by second intention. *Plast Reconstr Surg* 1987; **79**: 555–9.

10 Lawrence CM, Matthews JNS, Cox NH. The effect of ketanserin on healing of fresh surgical wounds. *Br J Dermatol* 1995; **132**: 580–6.

11 Snow SN, Stiff MA, Bullen R et al. Second intention healing of exposed facial-scalp bone after Mohs surgery for skin cancer: a review of 91 cases. *J Am Acad Dermatol* 1994; **31**: 450–4.

12 Latenser J, Snow SNP, Mohs FE et al. Power drills to fenestrate exposed bone to stimulate wound healing. *J Dermatol Surg Oncol* 1991; **17**: 265–70.

Skin grafts

Skin of varying thickness can be used for skin grafting. A

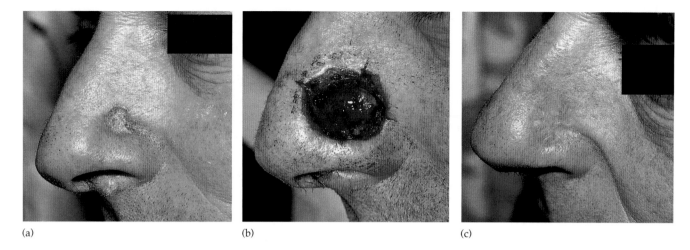

(a) (b) (c)

Fig. 78.9 (a) This man had a basal cell carcinoma on the side of the nose; (b) this was excised and the wound was allowed to heal by second intention. (c) The cosmetic result 4 months later was good.

Fig. 78.10 (a) This man had a basal cell carcinoma on the temple (b) excised. (c) Three months later the wound had healed but the scar was thick and red. (d) 15 months later this scar had become considerably less conspicuous.

split-skin graft is not limited in size, because the donor site regenerates. Full-thickness and composite skin grafts potentially produce better cosmetic results than split-skin grafts, but are limited in size by the amount of skin that can be removed from the donor site without creating problems. Compared with flaps, grafts are technically easier to perform, but generally produce inferior cosmetic results.

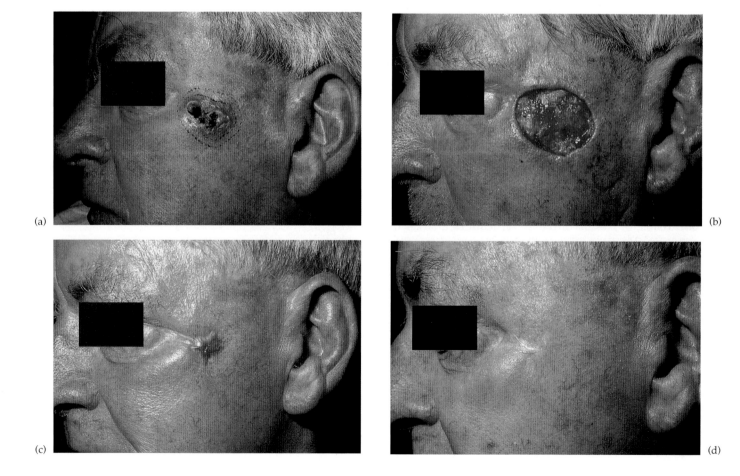

(a)

(b)

(c)

(d)

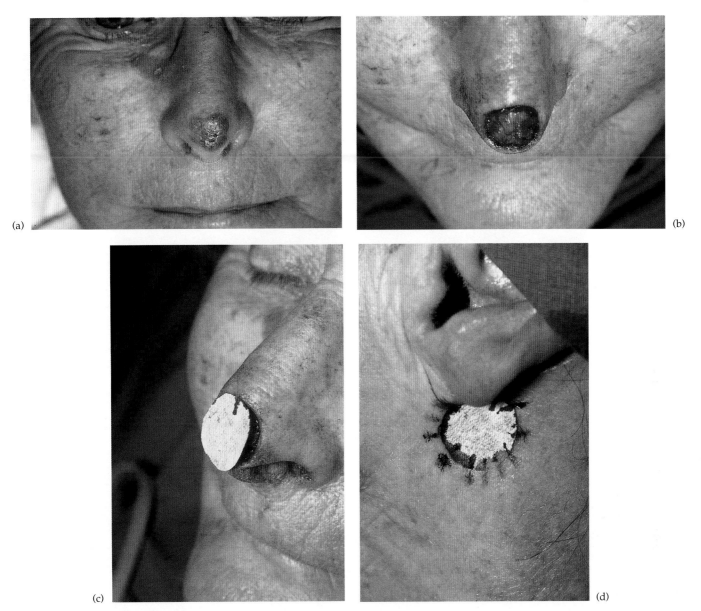

Fig. 78.11 Full-thickness graft on the nose. This basal cell carcinoma on the tip of the nose (a) was excised (b). The defect size and shape was recorded using a sterile paper template (c), the template was placed on the donor skin site (d) and the appropriate-sized piece of skin excised. The fat was trimmed off the undersurface of the donor skin, and this was sutured into place on the wound (e). A tie-over dressing was applied (f). Seven days later the dressing was removed and the graft was pink and had clearly taken (g). The subsequent cosmetic result at 3 months was excellent (h).

Full-thickness grafts

A full-thickness graft is used, in preference to a split-skin graft, when the cosmetic result and strength of the repair are important. Any site with matching and spare skin is a potential donor site [1]. Common donor sites include the skin behind and in front of the ear, nasolabial fold [2], upper eyelid, inner aspect of the upper arm, lower abdomen and supraclavicular fossa. The donor and graft sites should match for skin thickness, adnexal structures, surface markings, weathering and texture. After carefully assessing the amount and shape of skin required, the donor skin is excised down to fat [3]. The fat is then trimmed off the under surface of the graft to aid new blood-vessel penetration. Edge sutures are used to prevent shearing forces dislodging the graft, and a pressure dressing, usually held in place using tie-over sutures, is employed to prevent a haematoma lifting the graft off the recipient site (Fig. 78.11). In most instances, the donor site is chosen because there are redundant folds of skin present and the skin edges can be sutured easily after donor skin excision. At some sites (e.g. behind the ear), the donor

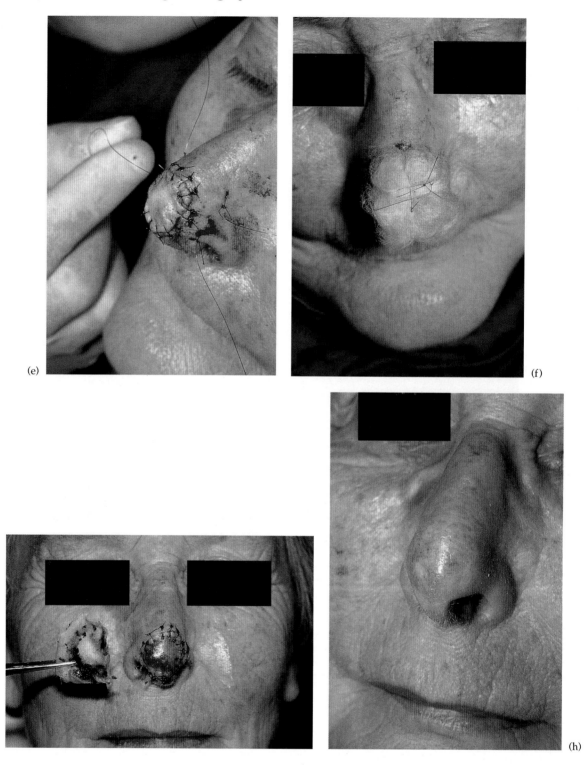

Fig. 78.11 (*cont'd*)

defect can be allowed to heal by second intention. Grafts take best on dermis and granulation tissue, will survive on fat, perichondrium and periosteum, but will perish on exposed bone or cartilage. Grafts fail because of infection or poor blood supply. The latter occurs because of faulty technique (e.g. incorrect haemostasis, suturing or wound care) or because the recipient site has an inadequate blood supply (e.g. previous radiotherapy or lower leg sites in people with compromised venous and/or arterial supply). All grafts contract, and near the lower eyelid this may lead to ectropion. Hence, at this and other critical sites, grafts should be 10–25% larger than the defect to compensate for this. Depressed graft scars may be elevated by injection of autograft fat under the graft [4].

Composite grafts

Composite grafts are defined as those comprising two or more germ layers. In dermatology, these are grafts containing skin and cartilage components. When used to repair full-thickness ala rim defects using skin taken from the helix rim, graft survival is unpredictable [5]. In contrast, composite grafts containing skin and perichondrium, or perichondrial cutaneous grafts, are claimed to be better than full-thickness grafts for nose, ear and periocular defects, as they contract less, induce new cartilage formation, and maintain their thickness and epidermal appendages [6].

Split-skin graft

Except in extreme circumstances (e.g. extensive burns) split-skin graft size is not limited by the amount of donor skin that can be harvested, because the donor skin site will re-epithelialize by regeneration from retained follicular remnants. Split-skin grafts can therefore be used to cover very large wounds. Because the skin is thin and relatively transparent, split grafts are also sometimes used to cover tumour excision sites where the adequacy of excision is dubious, because recurrence is more easily identified through the thinner graft than it would be after full-thickness or flap closure. The disadvantages of split-skin grafts compared with full-thickness grafts are the relatively poor cosmetic result and greater graft shrinkage [1]. When a split graft is taken, skin is sliced off through the dermis, leaving behind parts of the adnexal and follicular structures from which epidermis migrates to cover the donor site. Split-skin grafts can be taken using a hand-held knife or a mechanical dermatome (Fig. 78.12a). The latter is easier to use and produces a predictably good graft. *Meshing*, or cutting multiple parallel slits in the graft, allows it to expand rather like a fishnet stocking when stretched (Fig. 78.12b). The gaps are covered by epithelium migrating from the adjacent strips of the graft (Fig. 78.12c). A meshed graft will therefore cover a wider area, allow exudate to drain through the gaps (e.g. on the leg), and will conform to an uneven contour (e.g. ear). The common donor sites include the upper arm, upper thigh and abdominal wall. The donor site is best anaesthetized using EMLA® cream [7], and heals faster and painlessly with a dressing that maintains a moist wound–dressing interface (e.g. calcium alginate [8] and semi-permeable adhesive polyurethane film; Opsite®) [9].

Pinch grafts

Pinch grafts are occasionally useful for wounds of the

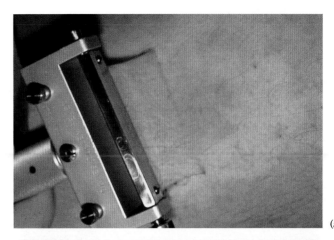
(a)

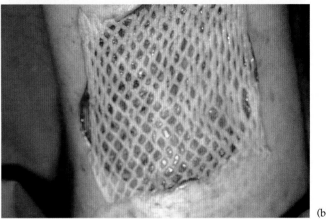
(b)

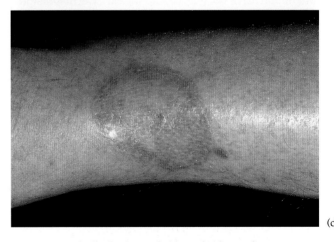
(c)

Fig. 78.12 Meshed split-skin graft. (a) A split-skin graft was harvested from the thigh skin using a power dermatome. (b) The skin was meshed on a mesher, and the meshed graft applied to the defect. (c) This was the appearance of the graft 11 months later.

lower leg, although the donor site heals leaving unsightly scars. The technique is simple [10], but without careful aseptic technique success rates are low [11]. The skin is elevated on a needle tip, the apex sliced off, and when multiple skin shaves have been harvested the grafts are placed at regular intervals on the clean granulating ulcer.

As with all leg-ulcer skin grafting, if the causative factors are not eradicated before grafting, the ulcer will recur even if the graft is initially successful.

Grafting techniques used for repigmentation of inactive vitiligo

Epidermal grafts containing viable melanocytes can be harvested using suction blisters [12], or very thin split-skin grafts [13]. Before grafting, the epidermis is removed from the hypopigmented skin by freezing to create a blister [12], or by dermabrasion [13]. Alternatively, *mini-grafts*, or tiny (1.2-mm diameter) full-thickness punch grafts of normally pigmented skin are grafted, at 2-mm intervals, into similar-sized punch wounds sited in the depigmented skin [14]. Because melanocytes migrate approximately 2 mm away from the graft site, there is no need to graft the whole area, and because the punch grafts are so small there is minimal cobblestone effect at the recipient site. In both techniques, a hidden donor site, such as the upper inner thigh or lower back, is used. Grafts of cultured autologous melanocytes have also been tried [15].

Acne scar punch grafts

Ice-pick acne scars can be excised using a punch biopsy blade, and the wound filled with a slightly bigger punch biopsy-shaped piece of donor skin taken from a matching but unobtrusive site (e.g. behind the ear). Dermabrasion is usually subsequently required to reduce the cobblestone effect [16].

REFERENCES

1 Skouge JW. *Skin Grafting: Practical Manuals in Dermatologic Surgery*. New York: Churchill Livingstone, 1991.
2 Booth SA, Zalla MJ, Roenigk RK, Phillips PK. The naso-labial fold donor site for full thickness skin grafts of nasal tip defects. *J Dermatol Surg Oncol* 1993; **19**: 553–9.
3 Roenigk RK, Zalla MJ. Full-thickness grafts. In: Robinson JK, Arndt KA, LeBoit PE, Wintroub BU, eds. *Atlas of Cutaneous Surgery*. Philadelphia: Saunders, 1996.
4 Hambley RM, Carruthers JA. Microlipoinjection for the elevation of depressed full-thickness grafts on the nose. *J Dermatol Surg Oncol* 1992; **18**: 963–8.
5 Lipman SH, Roth RJ. Composite grafts from earlobes for reconstruction of defects in noses. *J Dermatol Surg Oncol* 1982; **8**: 135–7.
6 Rohrer TE, Dzubow LM. Conchal bowl skin grafting in nasal tip reconstruction: clinical and histologic evaluation. *J Am Acad Dermatol* 1995; **33**: 476–81.
7 Goodacre TEE, Sanders R, Watts DA, Stoker M. Split skin grafting using topical local anaesthesia (EMLA): a comparison with infiltrative anaesthesia. *Br J Plast Surg* 1988; **41**: 533–8.
8 Attwood AI. Calcium alginate dressing accelerates split skin graft donor site healing. *Br J Plast Surg* 1989; **42**: 373–9.
9 James JH, Watson ACH. The use of Opsite, a vapour permeable dressing on skin graft donor sites. *Br J Plast Surg* 1975; **28**: 107–10.
10 Ceilley RI, Rinek MA, Zuehlke RL. Pinch grafting for chronic ulcers on the lower extremities. *J Dermatol Surg Oncol* 1977; **3**: 303–9.
11 Kirsner RS, Falanga V. Techniques of split skin grafting for lower extremity ulcerations. *J Dermatol Surg Oncol* 1993; **19**: 779–83.
12 Falabella R. Surgical techniques for repigmentation. In: Robinson JK, Arndt KA, LeBoit PE, Wintroub BU, eds. *Atlas of Cutaneous Surgery*. Philadelphia: Saunders, 1996.
13 Kahn AM, Cohen MJ. Vitiligo: treatment by dermabrasion and epithelial sheet grafting. *J Am Acad Dermatol* 1995; **33**: 646–8.
14 Boersma BR, Westerhof W, Bos JD. Repigmentation in vitiligo vulgaris by autologous minigrafting: results in 19 patients. *J Am Acad Dermatol* 1995; **33**: 990–5.
15 Olsson MJ, Juhlin L. Transplantation of melanocytes in vitiligo. *Br J Dermatol* 1995; **132**: 587–91.
16 Johnson WC. Treatment of pitted scars: punch transplant technique. *J Dermatol Surg Oncol* 1986; **12**: 260–5.

Flaps (Figs 78.13–78.16)

A flap is a section of full-thickness skin in which one portion, the pedicle, remains attached to the skin while the distal portion is undermined and moved to cover the defect [1]. The blood supply of any flap is therefore, at least initially, provided principally via its pedicle, and the broader the pedicle the better the blood supply. The length to width ratio of a flap should rarely exceed 3 : 1. The more closely a flap resembles a graft (thin, defatted skin) the greater is the contribution to its blood supply from the recipient site rather than the flap pedicle. The thinner the flap, however, the greater the contraction, and this is particularly important when using thin skin around the eye. Different techniques can be used for many repairs [2], although some techniques [3] are inherently suited to the nose [4,5], chin [6], eyelid [7,8], ear [9,10], forehead [11], scalp [12], cheeks [13] and lip [14,15].

Flaps can be confusingly categorized by the direction of movement, the name of the surgeon who first described the flap, the blood supply or the type of tissue moved. The most useful method relates to how the skin was moved to cover the defect—hence the description of advancement, rotation or transposition flaps (Table 78.4). Classification according to blood supply shows that dermatologists almost exclusively use random pattern flaps (the blood supply is inherent in the skin being moved). This may come from the dermal blood supply (reticular—the type most widely used by dermatologists), or the perforating vessels from the subdermal plexus (segmental, e.g. island pedicle flaps). In contrast, axial pattern flaps are designed to obtain their blood supply from one named artery. With the exception of the midline forehead flap [4], which is based on the supratrochlear artery, axial flaps are rarely used in dermatological surgery. Island pedicle flaps do not have a skin pedicle but get their blood supply from the tissue on the underside of the flap. This may be subcutaneous tissue, muscle or a named vessel.

As skin is moved to close the primary or original defect, a secondary defect is created which in turn also has to be covered. The essence of flap repair is to design the flap so that this secondary defect is created at a site where there is sufficient spare or loose skin to permit closure. On the face, loose skin is usually present in the middle of the forehead, the glabella region and bridge of the nose, the nasolabial fold, the front of the ear and the cheek. Hence, these areas of laxity will be exploited for most flaps.

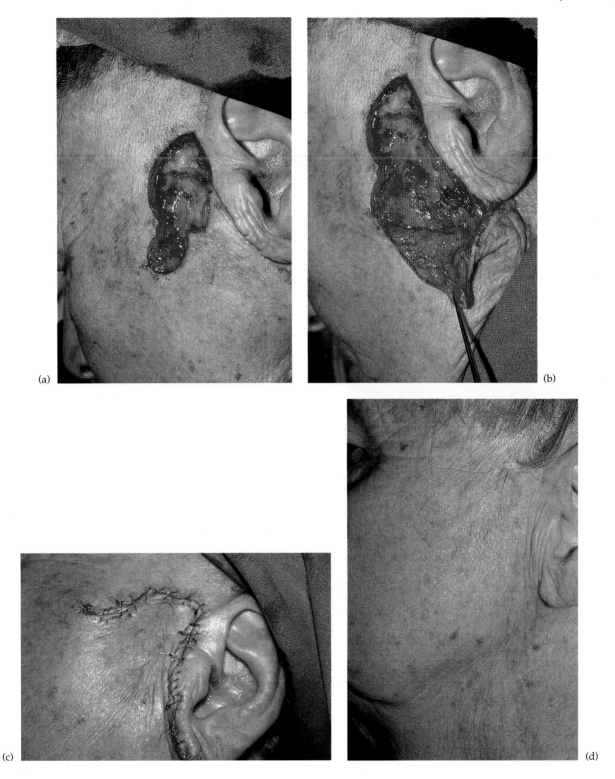

(a)

(b)

(c)

(d)

Fig. 78.13 Rotation flap on the pre-auricular skin. (a) This oddly shaped defect was closed (b) by rotating and advancing the loose skin under the chin up to cover the defect. (c) The incision line was placed in the skin crease at the anatomical boundary between the ear and the cheek, (d) and hence is inconspicuous 4 months later. The back cut was enhanced by Z-plasty under the ear (not shown).

Advancement flaps are used where skin must move in one direction from an area of laxity to cover the defect. Although simple to conceptualize they have limited use. The secondary defect is closed last, and the flaps have limited mobility. In many instances, defect coverage is only achieved by stretching the flap rather than transferring

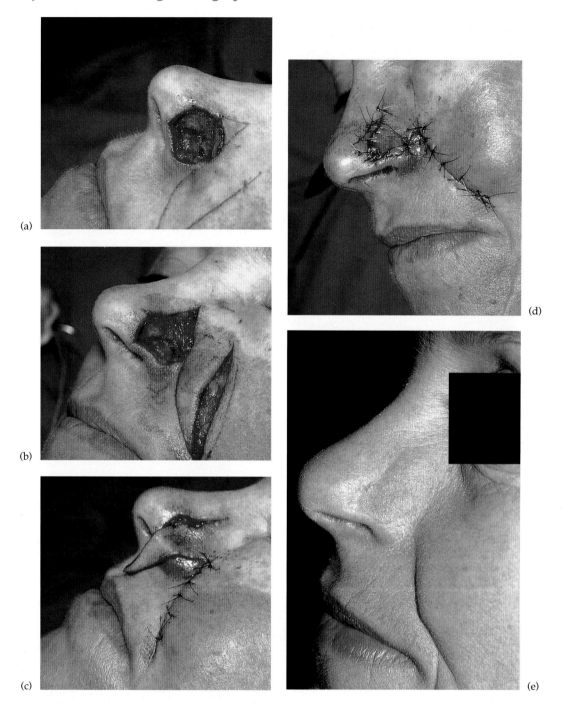

(a)

(b)

(c)

(d)

(e)

Fig. 78.14 Nasolabial fold flap. (a) This defect on the ala wall was covered by transposing a flap taken from the cheek skin (b). (c) The defect on the cheek was closed directly along the nasolabial fold, thus disguising the scar, and the flap of skin was then laid over the defect. (d) The flap was trimmed to shape and sutured into place. (e) The result 12 months later was good.

the tension to an area of lax skin. *Rotation flaps* usually require both advancement and rotation about a pivotal point on a broad pedicle (Fig. 78.13). Mobility is frequently limited, and long incisions and extensive undermining may be required to mobilize sufficient tissue; the second-ary defect is closed last. *Transposition flaps* provide the greatest mobility, and the secondary defect is closed first (Fig. 78.14). As a result, the flap is pushed rather than dragged into the defect, so that if a transposition flap is designed properly virtually all the tension can be placed on the secondary defect rather than the flap, thus reducing the risk of ischaemic necrosis. These advantages make transposition flaps the most widely used (Fig. 78.15). A wide variety of flaps based on these three simple designs have been described, each with careful refinements for different sites (Table 78.4).

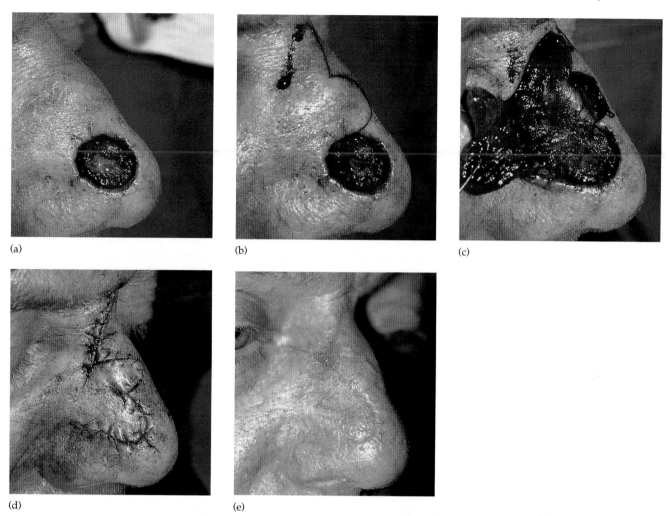

(a) (b) (c)

(d) (e)

Fig. 78.15 Bilobed flap on the nose. (a) This defect near the tip of the nose was covered using a bilobed flap designed to cover the defect by exploiting the looser skin higher up on the side of the nose (b). (c) Both parts of the flap were raised together, and were transposed into the defect and the secondary defect; (d) the tertiary defect was closed directly. (e) The cosmetic result at 6 months was good.

Complications

Ischaemic necrosis of the flap usually occurs because of excessive tension resulting from poor design or mobility. Secondary infection is also more common if the flap has a poor blood supply [29]. On the head and neck, blood supply is excellent at all sites, but on the trunk, and especially on the lower limb, attempts at flap repair frequently result in failure because of relatively poor blood supply. Cigarette smokers are more likely to suffer from flap or graft necrosis than non-smokers (Fig. 78.16), although this can be reversed if smokers significantly reduce cigarette consumption 2 days before and 7 days after surgery [30]. If the flap scar is obtrusive, particularly on the nose, it can

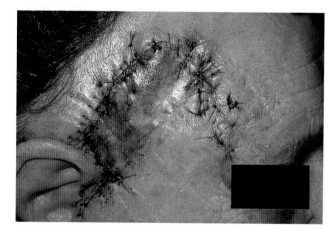

Fig. 78.16 Complications—flap necrosis in a cigarette smoker. Despite warnings, this patient continued to smoke before and after surgery. Possibly because of this, the rotation flap on her temple necrosed at 7 days.

be revised by dermabrasion, which is best performed 6 weeks after surgery [31]. Manual dermabrasion [32] or scalpel sculpturing [33] may be less hazardous to the operator and equally effective.

Table 78.4 Flap types and uses.

Flap type	Random pattern flaps (synonym/s)	Uses	Comments
Advancement	Crescentic advancement flap [16]	Cheek/nose, cheek/upper lip closures	In effect side-to-side closure with special attention to cosmetic boundaries. A useful technique
	Single advancement (U-plasty)	Cheek, temple, forehead [6], upper lip [15]	If designed with a broad base can be very effective on the cheek
	Double advancement (H-plasty)	Forehead defects, eyebrow repairs	Little mobility, multiple scars, numb scalp. Conceptually easy but difficult to get right
	Bipedical advancement [17]	Forehead, nasal side wall, chin	In effect side-to-side closure with parallel or V–Y relaxing incisions
	O–T-plasty (A–T-plasty, V–T-plasty, Dieffenbach's winged V-plasty [18])	Lower eyelid, upper lip [15], forehead [6]	A bilateral advancement flap useful around the eye, lip, nose [3] and hair margin
	Midline forehead island flap [19]	Medial canthus	A variety of island pedicle flap with a random pattern blood supply. Flap is tunnelled under the skin into the defect
	Island pedicle flap [20] (kite flap of Dufourmentel)	Upper lip [14], trunk and limb	Two pedicles can be used on the trunk and limb; one is used on repairs of the upper lip. The blood supply comes from the subcutaneous tissue attached to the underside of the skin. A similar design is used in an axial flap employed for defects on the nose tip and ala. The pedicle is based on the branch of the angular artery that supplies the nasalis muscle [21]
	Single advancement (unilateral Burow's wedge flap) [3]	Upper lip, temple, cheek, forehead	A useful flap which is both advanced and rotated into position and the redundant skin removed using a Burow's triangle
Rotation	Single rotation with back-cut (hatchet flap)	Cheek, temple, medial canthus	A useful technique [1] (Fig. 78.13)
	Sliding glabella rotation flap (V–Y advancement)	Medial canthus, dorsal nose [22]	Exploits the redundant skin in the glabella area. Skin movement includes both advancement and rotation as do many rotation or advancement flaps
	Double rotation (O–Z-plasty)	Forehead, scalp, chin [6]	Large area of undermining required. Only works on lax scalp
	Multiple rotation flaps (pinwheel design)	Scalp	Variant of O–Z-plasty
Transposition	Nasolabial flap [23]	Ala rim or side wall of the nose	Good results with careful attention to detail. Pincushioning can be a problem (Fig. 78.14)
	Basic transposition/rhombic flap	Cheek, nose, chin, medial canthus, upper lip	Rarely if ever used as the true geometric rhomboid. Basic transposition flaps are very useful and generally exploit the natural elasticity of the skin so that the flap shape adapts to fit the defect [24]. A Z-plasty adaptation [25] may enhance flap mobility [26]. The glabella transposition flap (banner flap) [27] is a named variant
	Median forehead pedicle flap	Nose tip or lower third of nose	Axial flap. Two-stage procedure; the flap knuckle or pedicle has to be separated later
	30° angle transposition flap [4] (Webster flap)	Dorsum of the nose	Not difficult. Bilateral and single flaps can be used
	Bilobed [28]	Nose side wall	A double transposition flap. Not as difficult to do as might appear (Fig. 78.15)

REFERENCES

1 Tromovitch TA, Stegman SJ, Glogau RG. *Flaps and Grafts in Dermatologic Surgery.* Chicago: Year Book, 1989.
2 Field LM. Combining flaps: medial canthal/lateral nasal root reconstruction utilising glabella 'fan' and cheek rotation flaps—an O–Z variation. *J Dermatol Surg Oncol* 1994; **20**: 205–8.
3 Summers BK, Siegle RJ. Facial cutaneous reconstructive surgery: facial flaps. *J Am Acad Dermatol* 1993; **29**: 917–41.
4 Salasche SJ, Grabski WJ. *Flaps for the Central Face.* New York: Churchill Livingstone, 1990.
5 Zitelli JA, Fazio MJ. Reconstruction of the nose with local flaps. *J Dermatol Surg Oncol* 1991; **17**: 184–9.
6 Wheeland RG. Reconstruction of the lower lip and chin using local and random pattern flaps. *J Dermatol Surg Oncol* 1991; **17**: 605–15.

7 Moy RL, Ashjian AA. Periorbital reconstruction. *J Dermatol Surg Oncol* 1991; **17**: 153–9.

8 Ross JJ, Pham R. Closure of eyelid defects. *J Dermatol Surg Oncol* 1992; **18**: 1061–4.

9 Cavanaugh EB. Management of lesions of the helical rim using a chondro-cutaneous advancement flap. *J Dermatol Surg Oncol* 1982; **8**: 691–6.

10 Mellette JR. Ear reconstruction with local flaps. *J Dermatol Surg Oncol* 1991; **17**: 176–82.

11 Siegel RJ. Forehead reconstruction. *J Dermatol Surg Oncol* 1991; **17**: 200–4.

12 Field LM. Scalp flaps. *J Dermatol Surg Oncol* 1991; **17**: 190–9.

13 Bennett RG. Local skin flaps on the cheeks. *J Dermatol Surg Oncol* 1991; **17**: 161–5.

14 Zitelli JA, Brodland DG. A regional approach to reconstruction of the upper lip. *J Dermatol Surg Oncol* 1991; **17**: 143–8.

15 Spinowitz AL, Stegman SJ. Partial-thickness wedge and advancement flap for upper lip repair. *J Dermatol Surg Oncol* 1991; **17**: 581–6.

16 Mellette JR, Harrington AC. Applications of the crescentic advancement flap. *J Dermatol Surg Oncol* 1991; **17**: 447–54.

17 Flint ID, Siegle RJ. The bipedical flap revisited. *J Dermatol Surg Oncol* 1994; **20**: 394–400.

18 Field LM. The forehead V to T plasty (Dieffenbach's winged V-plasty). *J Dermatol Surg Oncol* 1986; **12**: 560–2.

19 Field LM. Midline forehead island flap. *J Dermatol Surg Oncol* 1987; **13**: 243–6.

20 Skouge JW. Upper lip repair: the subcutaneous island pedicle flap. *J Dermatol Surg Oncol* 1980; **16**: 63–8.

21 Papadopoulos DJ, Pharis DB, Munavalli GS, Trinei F, Hantzakos AG. Nasalis myocutaneous island pedicle flap with bilevel undermining for repair of lateral nasal defects. *Dermatol Surg* 2002; **28**: 190–4.

22 Marchac D, Toth B. The axial frontonasal flap revisited. *Plast Reconstr Surg* 1985; **76**: 686–94.

23 Zitelli JA. The nasolabial flap as a single stage procedure. *Arch Dermatol* 1990; **126**: 1445–8.

24 Holt PJA, Motley RJ. A modified rhombic transposition flap and its application in dermatology. *J Dermatol Surg Oncol* 1991; **17**: 287–92.

25 Zachary CB. *Basic Cutaneous Surgery: a Primer in Technique.* New York: Churchill Livingstone, 1991: 87.

26 Johnson SC, Bennett RG. Double Z-plasty to enhance rhombic flap mobility. *J Dermatol Surg Oncol* 1994; **20**: 128–32.

27 Field LM. The glabella transposition 'banner' flap. *J Dermatol Surg Oncol* 1988; **14**: 376–8.

28 Zitelli JA. The bilobed flap for nasal reconstruction. *Arch Dermatol* 1989; **125**: 957–9.

29 Salasche SJ, Grabski WJ. Complications of flaps. *J Dermatol Surg Oncol* 1991; **17**: 132–40.

30 Goldminz D, Bennett RG. Cigarette smoking and flap and full-thickness graft necrosis. *Arch Dermatol* 1991; **127**: 1012–5.

31 Yarborough JM. Ablation of facial scars by programmed dermabrasion. *J Dermatol Surg Oncol* 1988; **14**: 292–4.

32 Zisser M, Kaplan B, Moy RL. Surgical pearl: manual dermabrasion. *J Am Acad Dermatol* 1995; **33**: 105–6.

33 Snow SNP, Stiff MA, Lambert DR. Scalpel sculpturing techniques for graft revision and dermatologic surgery. *J Dermatol Surg Oncol* 1994; **20**: 120–6.

Micrographic (Mohs') surgery [1–4]

The concept of controlling the excision margins of infiltrative skin tumours by microscopic examination of horizontal sections cut from the periphery of an excision specimen that had previously been fixed *in vivo* was developed by Mohs in the 1940s [5]. This fixed-tissue technique, which produced excellent cure rates even in some of the most difficult of tumours, has now largely been replaced by the fresh-tissue technique [6]. There are other techniques and adaptations, which aim to achieve 100% histological margin control, that may be more appropriate for tumours with difficult morphology or because of local circumstances [7,8].

The principle of the technique is that the maximum confidence as regards tumour clearance is combined with the minimum loss of surrounding normal tissue. This is particularly important for tumours with an infiltrative growth pattern, especially in critical anatomical sites, and for recurrent lesions. Essentially, the technique involves excision of the lesion and microscopic examination of sections cut from marked, anatomically orientated, segments of tissue, so that the entire periphery of the excision specimen is examined (Fig. 78.17) [9]. Immunofluorescence or immunoperoxidase staining with cytokeratin antibodies may help in the histological interpretation of infiltrative lesions [10].

One of the major disadvantages of Mohs' original technique, other than the prolonged nature of the procedure (possibly continuing over several days) and the pain and discomfort of the *in vivo* fixative, was the presence of a postoperative eschar, which precluded immediate reconstruction and necessitated healing by secondary intention. With the fresh-tissue technique all but the most extensive lesions can be excised in one session, usually under local anaesthesia, and the area can be repaired immediately. If paraffin sections are used, repair is best delayed until the microscopic sections have been examined. This is not to deny the value of secondary-intention healing in appropriate situations [11].

The results of micrographic surgery are impressive, with a 98–99% 5-year cure rate for basal cell carcinomas and a 94.4% 5-year cure rate for squamous cell carcinomas [12]. It should be considered the treatment of choice for the management of certain lesions. Tumours with infiltrative growth patterns or morphoeic histology may extend 7–10 mm beyond the clinically defined margins [13], and if such a tumour overlies a putative anatomical fusion plane (e.g. ala base), the use of horizontal frozen sections may be crucial in ensuring complete resection. Although the main indication is for basal cell carcinoma, the technique has been used for a wide variety of cutaneous malignancies [14].

REFERENCES

1 Bennett RG. Mohs' surgery. In: Bailin PL, Ratz JL, Wheeland RG, eds. *Advanced Dermatologic Surgery.* Philadelphia: Saunders, 1987: 409–28.

2 Drake LA, Dinehart SM, Goltz RW *et al.* Guidelines of care for Mohs' micrographic surgery. *J Am Acad Dermatol* 1995; **33**: 271–8.

3 Lawrence CM. Mohs' surgery of basal cell carcinoma: a critical review. *Br J Plast Surg* 1993; **46**: 599–606.

4 Swanson NA. Mohs' surgery. *Arch Dermatol* 1983; **119**: 761–73.

5 Mohs FE. Chemosurgery: a microscopically controlled method of cancer excision. *Arch Surg* 1941; **42**: 279–95.

6 Tromovitch TA, Stegman SJ. Microscopic-controlled excision of cutaneous tumours: chemosurgery, fresh tissue technique. *Cancer* 1978; **41**: 653–8.

7 Breuninger H, Schaumburg-Lever G. Control of excisional margins by conventional histopathological techniques in the treatment of skin tumours: an alternative to Mohs' technique. *J Pathol* 1988; **154**: 167–71.

8 Picoto A, Camacho F, Walker NPJ *et al.* Mohs' micrographic surgery: European experience. In: Roenigk RK, Roenigk HH, eds. *Surgical Dermatology,* London: Dunitz, 1993: 125–9.

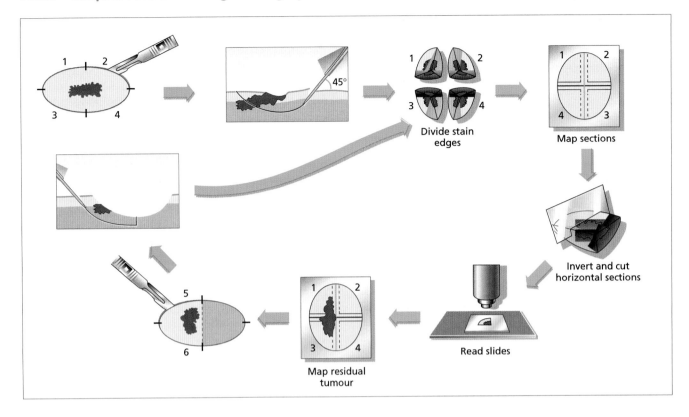

Fig. 78.17 The stages of Mohs' micrographic surgery.

9 Walker NPJ, Bailin PL. Dermatological surgery. In: Champion RH, ed. *Recent Advances in Dermatology*, Vol. 7. Edinburgh: Churchill Livingstone, 1986: 211–31.

10 Ramnarain N, Walker NPJ, Markey AC. Basal cell carcinoma: rapid techniques using cytokeratin markers to assist treatment by micrographic (Mohs') surgery. *Br J Biomed Sci* 1995; **52**: 184–7.

11 Zitelli JA. Wound healing by secondary intention. *J Am Acad Dermatol* 1983; **9**: 407–15.

12 Mohs FE. Chemosurgery: microscopically controlled surgery for skin cancer—past, present and future. *J Dermatol Surg Oncol* 1978; **4**: 41–54.

13 Lang PG, Maize JC. Histologic evolution of recurrent basal cell carcinoma and treatment implications. *J Am Acad Dermatol* 1986; **14**: 186–96.

14 Randle HW, Roenigk RK. Indications for Mohs' micrographic surgery. In: Roenigk RK, Roenigk HH, eds. *Dermatologic Surgery*, 2nd edn. New York: Marcel Dekker, 1996: 703–29.

Hair transplantation [1,2]

The punch autograft, originally described in 1939, was for many years the major procedure in this field. Other surgical techniques were developed, sometimes to be used alone or as adjuncts to punch grafting. These included strip and fusiform grafting, scalp reduction of balding areas with or without tissue expansion, and a variety of scalp flaps. Although these techniques could at times produce acceptable results, often patients were uneasy with the unnatural appearance which was achieved. The development in the 1980s of mini- and micrografts has extended to its logical conclusion with the use of follicular unit transplantation. Now, with repeated sessions of 1000–1500 grafts implanted into small slit or needle tunnel recipient sites, graft counts of 60–100 hairs/cm² can be achieved with excellent cosmetic results. The major condition for which these techniques are used remains androgenic alopecia in its various forms. Areas of focal scarring can also be treated.

Careful preoperative assessment of the mental and physical status of the patient is crucial. It is imperative to exclude those subjects with known functional psychoses, those who are dysmorphophobic or cannot comprehend the nature of the treatment and its effects, and those with physical illness that might compromise healing or satisfactory hair regrowth (e.g. bleeding disorders, steroid therapy and previous hypertrophic or keloid scars). Every patient accepted for transplantation or other surgical corrective treatment must have received clear instructions on the details of the operation and its potential side effects, and have a realistic expectation of outcome.

The details of the techniques will not be considered here. In treating androgenic alopecia, the exact techniques used will depend on the pattern of loss. The final outcome will depend as much on the design of the hairline and appropriate patient selection as on technique. Some patients are happy with frontal density correction and less dense grafting on other more posterior vertex areas. Several sessions are usually required to achieve a satisfactory result.

In general, most patients detect early hair growth in the eighth to 12th week after treatment, good growth usually being established at about the sixth month after graft insertion.

Complications are rare, and include arterial bleeding, arteriovenous and venous aneurysms, foreign body reactions, infection, poor graft survival and hypertrophic scarring.

REFERENCES

1 Norwood OT, Limmer BL. Advances in hair transplantation. *Adv Dermatol* 1999; **14**: 89–114.
2 Stough D, Whitworth JM. Methodology of follicular unit transplantation. *Dermatol Clin* 1999; **17**: 297–306.

Dermabrasion (surgical skin planing)
[1–4]

The abrasive (planing) technique for the removal of superficial lesions, rhinophyma, pitted or depressed scars, tattoos and foreign bodies was first clearly described by Kromayer [1]. Its main value lies in treating lesions on the face where regeneration of the epidermis proceeds rapidly, generally without scarring, because of the abundance of pilosebaceous structures from which repair occurs as long as destruction does not extend to the subcutis.

Considerable advances in the technique have taken place in the last 25 years, caused especially by the high-speed rotary drill and the use of more efficient refrigeration [2]. Care must be taken to follow details of the technique rigidly to avoid damage to the patient or operator. Briefly, the technique (allowing for many individual modifications) is as follows [2,4].

1 The patient is sedated, with, for example, 10–20 mg i.v. diazepam.
2 The area is prechilled with cold packs.
3 The skin is cleansed with spirit or some suitable substitute after washing with soap and water.
4 The ears and nostrils are plugged with ointment-impregnated gauze, and the hair and ears are carefully protected by clipped towels.
5 The eyes are carefully protected, for example by ointment and lead shields, by thick gauze held by an assistant, or by the plastic cups used by sunbathers to protect the eyes.
6 The area to be treated is frozen by a continuous stream of Freon (dichlorotetrafluoroethane), and the skin is abraded to the required depth. The degree of freezing and of abrasion necessary must be learnt by experience. The abrading wheels ('brushes') may be of stainless steel wires or diamond fraizes.

Bleeding occurs for 15–30 min after treatment. Paraffin gauze, dry dressings or non-adherent dressings are applied and removed in 1–24 h. The crusts separate in 7–10 days. Healing is usually completed within 3 weeks, particularly if the wound is left open and dry. The pain and crusting can be minimized and the rate of healing improved by the application of a biosynthetic dressing such as Opsite®, Biobrane® or Vigilon®. Preoperative topical retinoic acid may reduce the risk of postoperative milia formation and promote healing.

Infection following dermabrasion is rare, although herpes simplex can be devastating and aciclovir prophylaxis should be given to those at risk. Mild irritation or discomfort from sunlight or cosmetics may occur for a few weeks. Persistent erythema, hyperpigmentation, hypertrophic scars and dermatitis are occasional complications.

Dermabrasion can be considered as a very useful part of cosmetic dermatological practice. Its value in the minimizing of pitted acne scars of the face is undoubted (although the small 'ice-pick' scars respond less satisfactorily than coarse irregular scars). Other conditions for which it has been recommended include traumatic and surgical scars, tattoos, telangiectasia, melasma, epidermal naevi, angiofibromas in epiloia, actinic keratoses, syringomas, wrinkles, cysts and multiple milia [2]. It has been combined with topical steroids in hypertrophic lichen planus, lichen simplex and localized lichenified psoriasis.

REFERENCES

1 Kromayer E. *The Cosmetic Treatment of Skin Complaints*. Oxford: Oxford University Press, 1930.
2 Mandy SH. Dermabrasion. In: Lask GP, Moy RL, eds. *Principles and Techniques of Cutaneous Surgery*. New York: McGraw-Hill, 1996: 495–504.
3 Yarborough JM. Dermabrasion by wire brush. *J Dermatol Surg Oncol* 1987; **13**: 610–2.
4 Roenigk HH. Dermabrasion for rejuvenation and scar revision. In: Baran R, Maibach HI, eds. *Cosmetic Dermatology*. London: Dunitz, 1994: 451–66.

Botulinum toxins [1–3]

These potent neurotoxins have been used since 1979 for the treatment of strabismus and blepharospasm. They have been shown to be useful in the treatment of frown lines, disorders of the muscles of facial expression and hyperhidrosis [4]. The preparation of the toxin and its administration require great care, and although some authors advocate electromyographic guidance, most clinicians rely on clinical experience [5,6]. The effect of a single treatment may last up to 6 months, and with repeated injections the effect may become permanent. Botulinum toxin treatment is often a part of a structured approach to the management of the ageing face, which may include peels and dermal fillers.

REFERENCES

1 Carruthers JDA, Carruthers JA. Treatment of glabellar frown lines with *C. botulinum*-A exotoxin. *J Dermatol Surg Oncol* 1992; **18**: 17–21.
2 Garcia A, Fulton E. Cosmetic denervation of the muscles of facial expression with botulinum toxin. *Dermatol Surg* 1996; **22**: 39–43.
3 Sommer BG. *Botulinum Toxin in Aesthetic Medicine*. Oxford: Blackwell Science, 2001.
4 Naumann M, Flachenecker P, Bröcker E *et al*. Botulinum toxin for palmar hyperhidrosis. *Lancet* 1997; **349**: 252.

5 Lowe NJ, Maxwell A, Harper H. Botulinum-A exotoxin for glabellar folds: a double-blind, placebo controlled study with an electromyographic injection technique. *J Am Acad Dermatol* 1996; **35**: 569–72.
6 Klein AW. Complications, adverse reactions, and insights with the use of botulinum toxin. *Dermatol Surg* 2003; **29**: 549–56.

Miscellaneous surgical procedures

Techniques

Hydrodissection

The skin can be lifted away from underlying critical arteries and veins by hydrodissection. Approximately 20 mL of saline is injected into loose tissue below the lesion, thereby lifting the area to be excised off any underlying vital structures. The injection must be given after local anaesthesia, just before excision. The technique works best where there is a boundary that will delay the spread of the saline, for example on the temple and the ear [1].

Snip excision

Small tags can be snipped off with a pair of sharp scissors without the need for local anaesthetic [2]. The tag should be pulled away from the skin and snipped off at its base; bleeding usually stops spontaneously. Haemostasis may be a problem with larger polyps with a well-developed blood supply; hence, an anaesthetic will be required. The wounds can be left to heal by second intention, with excellent cosmetic results [3].

Relaxing incisions

Relaxing incisions are one of several techniques used to increase skin mobility. Multiple, small, full-thickness incisions are made parallel to the skin edge at the site of greatest wound tension [4]. These allow the skin to stretch like a meshed graft, resulting in small elliptical defects, which heal by second intention. The technique is particularly useful for excisions on the lower leg, where it produces surprisingly good cosmetic results with less morbidity than split- or full-thickness grafts. The technique can be used with other ways of improving skin mobility [5]. Other types of relaxing incision include the V–Y-plasty [6], which should not be confused with the V–Y island pedicle advancement flap (Table 78.4).

Wedge excision—lip, lid and ear

On the eyelid, lip and ear, a tumour can be excised and the defect readily closed by removing a full-thickness wedge with an appropriate margin of uninvolved skin. The different layers at the defect edges are then sutured, and thus the technique varies with the site. The inherent tissue elasticity of the eyelid and lip allows considerable defects

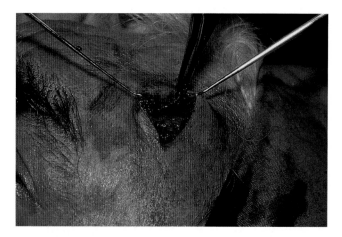

Fig. 78.18 Subfrontalis lipoma. This lipoma lies beneath the frontalis muscle. The muscle has been split vertically and is held back with forceps to reveal the lipoma.

to be repaired by direct closure without distorting the free margins of these structures. On the lip, defects smaller than one-third of the lip length can be closed directly following a wedge excision [7], if necessary using a W-plasty correction on the lower lip to avoid excessive distortion [8]. On the eyelid, defects of up to 50% can be closed directly, provided the correct technique is used [9]. However, a wedge excision on the ear reduces its size considerably, and buckling of the ear may occur unless the technique is modified to avoid this [10]. In most instances this type of defect is not a problem, as spectacles can still be supported by the ear and differences in ear size are rarely noticed.

Lipoma removal

Simple skin incision and lipoma excision ensures complete removal but produces a large scar. Scar size can be minimized by breaking up the lipoma into smaller fragments using blunt-ended forceps or a needle-holder inserted via a 4–6-mm punch biopsy wound made over the centre of the lipoma. The fragmented contents can then be squeezed out through the small wound. The fat can also be removed using liposuction [11]. A further development of this technique involves emulsification of the lipoma using an ultrasonic suction scalpel and removal of the fragments under endoscopic control [12]. A subfrontalis lipoma (Fig. 78.18) must be distinguished from a forehead epidermoid cyst. This can be particularly difficult to remove because of its site beneath the frontalis muscle of the forehead [13].

Tissue expansion

Tissue expansion may be helpful if there is insufficient local skin laxity to allow immediate closure and a graft would produce a relatively poor cosmetic result. The skin needed to fill the defect can be stretched to the required size by steadily expanding saline-filled plastic bags placed under the skin adjacent to the proposed defect. For 8–12 weeks after insertion the bags are filled at intervals to produce a mound that stretches the overlying skin. When the defect is excised, the adjacent distended skin is then available to cover the resulting defect [14]. Because the skin used is almost identical to the piece excised, the cosmetic result is potentially excellent. Expansion does not simply stretch existing skin but actually appears to induce basal layer mitotic activity, an increase in dermal collagen, and development of an enhanced blood supply from the fibrous capsule around the implant. Atrophy of adjacent fat and muscle also occurs. By contrast, immediate tissue expansion or stretching the skin at the time of operation using skin hooks, Foley catheters [15] or sutures [16] increases available skin in the short term but appears to result in greater shrinkage and hence scar stretching.

Circumcision

This simple surgical procedure [17] may be indicated in the management of lichen sclerosus et atrophicus.

REFERENCES

1 Salasche SJ, Giancola JM, Trookman NS. Surgical pearl: hydroexpansion with local anaesthetic. *J Am Acad Dermatol* 1995; **33**: 510–2.
2 Lawrence CM. *An Introduction to Dermatological Surgery.* Oxford: Blackwell Science, 1996: 66–8.
3 Fewkes JL, Cheney ML, Pollack SV. *Illustrated Atlas of Cutaneous Surgery.* Philadelphia: Lippincott, 1992.
4 Motley RJ, Holt PJA. The use of meshed advancement flaps in the treatment of lesions of the lower leg. *J Dermatol Surg Oncol* 1990; **16**: 346–8.
5 Kolbusz RV, Bielinski KB. The combined use of immediate intraoperative tissue expansion and meshing technique. *Arch Dermatol* 1993; **129**: 152–3.
6 Comaish JS. Dermatological surgery. In: Verbov JL, ed. *Dermatological Surgery.* Lancaster: MTP Press, 1986: 18.
7 Wheeland RG. Reconstruction of the lower lip and chin using local and random pattern flaps. *J Dermatol Surg Oncol* 1991; **17**: 605–15.
8 Jemec BIE. A short review of some methods of excisions from and reconstructions of lower lips. *J Dermatol Surg Oncol* 1981; **7**: 576–9.
9 Ross JJ, Pham R. Closure of eyelid defects. *J Dermatol Surg Oncol* 1992; **18**: 1061–4.
10 Tebbetts JB. Auricular reconstruction: selected single stage techniques. *J Dermatol Surg Oncol* 1982; **8**: 557–66.
11 Kaneko T, Tokushige H, Kimura N *et al.* The treatment of multiple angiolipomas by liposuction surgery. *J Dermatol Surg Oncol* 1994; **20**: 690–2.
12 Sawaizumi M, Maruyama Y, Onishi K *et al.* Endoscopic extraction of lipomas using an ultrasonic suction scalpel. *Ann Plast Surg* 1996; **36**: 124–8.
13 Salasche SJ, McCollough ML, Angeloni VL, Grabski WJ. Frontalis associated lipoma of the forehead. *J Am Acad Dermatol* 1989; **20**: 462–8.
14 Baker SR, Swanson NA. Reconstruction of midfacial defects following surgical management of skin cancer. *J Dermatol Surg Oncol* 1994; **20**: 133–40.
15 Auletta MJ, Matarasso SL, Glogau RG, Tromovitch TA. Comparison of skin hooks and Foley catheters for immediate tissue expansion. *J Dermatol Surg Oncol* 1993; **19**: 1084–8.
16 Liang MD, Briggs P, Heckler FR, Futrell JW. Pre-suturing a new technique for closing large skin defects—clinical and experimental studies. *Plast Reconstr Surg* 1988; **81**: 694–702.
17 Harahap ML, Siregar AS. Circumcision: a review and a new technique. *J Dermatol Surg Oncol* 1986; **14**: 383–6.

Specific diseases

Epidermoid cysts

Epidermoid cysts (sometimes incorrectly called sebaceous cysts) are lined by a keratinizing epithelium, which produces the cheesy, keratinous contents. Epidermoid cysts require excision if they are disfiguring or repeatedly infected. The inflamed tissue around an infected epidermoid cyst is friable, making it difficult to excise without fragmenting the cyst wall. An infected cyst should therefore be drained, and the patient treated with an appropriate antibiotic. When the inflammation settles the cyst can be excised. Cysts inflamed as a result of a foreign body giant cell reaction to released keratin are best treated by triamcinolone injection followed by subsequent removal. Freely mobile cysts can be easily shelled out through the smooth tissue plane that separates the very thin cyst wall from the surrounding tissue, although at this plane the cyst wall is easily punctured and must be handled gently. In all cases the entire cyst wall and punctum should be removed, the latter at the centre of a small skin ellipse, which can also be used to manipulate the cyst during removal. If the cyst ruptures during extraction, every effort should be made to remove residual wall fragments to prevent recurrence. To avoid long scars, very large cysts can be decompressed via a 4-mm punch biopsy before excision [1]. The wound is either left to heal for 4–6 weeks before definitive removal of the shrunken cyst or an attempt can be made to pull the cyst inside out through the circular wound using artery forceps [2]. Immobile cysts are surrounded by extensive scar tissue and usually have to be excised with the surrounding fibrotic tissue and overlying skin.

Hidradenitis

If medical treatment of hidradenitis suppurativa has failed, involved areas can be excised and the defects covered with skin grafts or flaps. However, cure rates of less than 20% are reported [3] and secondary infection is a frequent problem [4]. Alternatives such as excision followed by healing by second intention are well tolerated by the patient and produce good results [5]. An even simpler procedure involves deroofing the fistula leaving the floor of the track to re-epithelialize the wounded area. Excised tissue or suspect areas should be sent for histology because of the recognized complication of malignant change [6].

Vermilionectomy

This is sometimes called a mucosal advancement [7,8]. The vermilion, usually of the lower lip, is excised, principally because of actinic damage, and replaced by lip

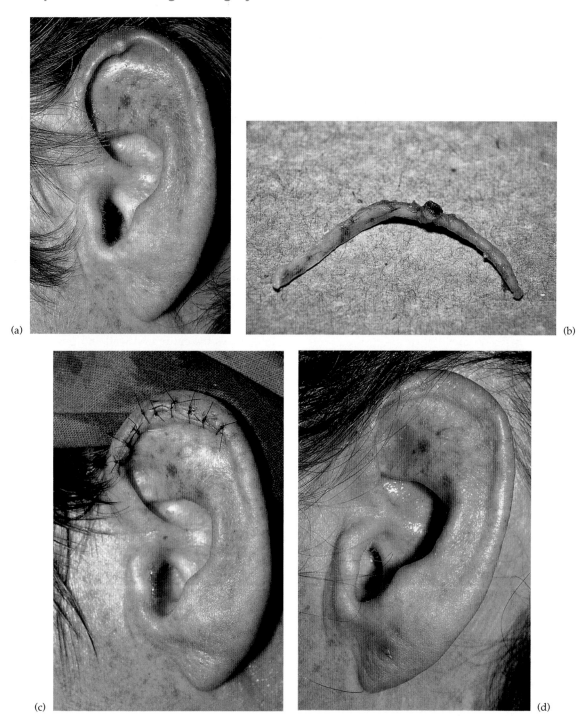

Fig. 78.19 Excision of chondrodermatitis nodularis helicis. (a) This helix nodule was treated by cartilage excision. An incision was made along the helix rim and the skin reflected to expose the cartilage. (b) A sliver of cartilage was taken to include the 3-mm punch biopsy of the skin nodule. Care was taken to ensure that the cartilage edges were smooth and gently shelving up to the uninvolved cartilage. (c) The skin edges were then sutured. (d) The result at 6 months was good.

mucosa pulled forward and sutured at the vermilion/skin border.

Split ear lobe

Split ear lobes may be congenital, or occur as a result of trauma or wearing heavy earrings. Simply de-epithelializing the sides of the cleft and suturing the exposed edges usually results in a notch appearing at the lobe edge. A full thickness or single-sided Z-plasty correction of the cut edges, depending on lobe thickness [9], is advocated as the best way to ensure good cosmesis, although many other methods are described [10].

Partial or incomplete clefts can be repaired by excising and suturing the enlarged hole. However, if there is only a narrow band of skin separating the hole from the lower pole of the lobe, it is probably best to create a complete defect by cutting the small bridge of skin and closing the defect accordingly. Earrings can be worn again only in patients with thick lobes. Some repairs incorporate reconstruction of a new earring hole at the same time as repair of the defect [11].

Chondrodermatitis nodularis

Intralesional and topical steroids help in approximately 25% of cases. Surgical excision of the affected cartilage without removal of skin (Fig. 78.19) will result in cure in over 90% of helix lesions and 70% of those on the antihelix [12]. Recurrences will occur if rough or protuberant edges of cartilage are left at operation, but can be treated using the same technique [13]. Other methods, including cryotherapy, curettage and laser ablation, have been used, but with mixed and unpredictable results.

Myxoid cysts

Myxoid cysts are ganglia arising as a result of joint fluid leakage from the distal interphalangeal joint into the surrounding tissues. The principle of treatment is that the connection between the cyst and the adjacent joint must be disrupted to prevent the cyst refilling. This is presumably what happens after successful cryotherapy [14], intralesional steroid therapy or curettage, although the cure rate of these procedures is relatively poor. The connection between the joint and the cyst can be identified by injection of dye into the joint [15]. Dye injection, however, is difficult and not essential. The joint fluid leakage site can be assumed to lie between the proximal portion of the cyst and the joint. A proximally based flap can be raised, to include the cyst and skin between the cyst and joint. The cyst is incised and drained. The flap is then resited (Fig. 78.20). The resulting scar presumably seals off the leak from the joint capsule [16].

Axillary vault excision and other remedies for hyperhidrosis

Axilla. If medical treatments fail (see Chapter 45), botulinum toxin (see p. 78.31) can be used, and this blocks sweating for 4–6 months [17]. Axillary hyperhidrosis can also be treated by excision of the sweat-gland bearing axillary skin [18]. The operation is not difficult, but wide

excision scars invariably stretch, and infections are common. Shelley described the use of a transverse excision in the centre of the hair-bearing dome of the axilla approximately 4.5 × 1.5 cm wide [19,20]. The sweat glands can be visualized on the undersurface of the adjacent skin and many of these can be snipped off or destroyed by electrodesiccation when the skin edges are undermined and everted. A light pressure dressing is applied for 24–48 h, and the wound is then left undressed and cleansed daily with a bactericidal antiseptic. Methods that attempt removal of the sweat glands using subcutaneous curettage [21] or liposuction [22], leaving the skin intact, are also described.

Palmar hyperhidrosis is difficult to treat. Endoscopic transthoracic sympathectomy [23] involves division of the sympathetic trunk running over the posterior wall of the chest cavity. However, side effects are significant, and over 80% of individuals develop compensatory sweating [24]. There is also a risk of Horner's syndrome and pneumothorax. In approximately 10% of cases [25], some recurrence of sweating occurs 1–2 years after surgery. The technique can also be useful in Raynaud's disease [26]. A similar approach can be used to reduce axillary sweating, when the second to sixth thoracic ganglia have to be destroyed. Access below the third thoracic ganglion is difficult, and this is believed to account for the poorer cure rate for axillary sweating [27]. Patients can also be successfully managed by repeated botulinum. Injections into the palm. The effects last about 6 months. Injections are painful. Transient weakness of the small hand muscles occurs in 40% [28].

REFERENCES

1 O'Keeffe PJ. Trephining sebaceous cysts. *Br J Plast Surg* 1972; **25**: 411–5.
2 Patton HS. An alternative method for removing sebaceous cysts. *Surg Gynecol Obstet* 1963; **117**: 645–6.
3 Jemec GBE. Effect of localised surgical excisions in hidradenitis suppurativa. *J Am Acad Dermatol* 1988; **18**: 1103–7.
4 Banerjee AK. Surgical treatment of hidradenitis suppurativa. *Br J Surg* 1992; **79**: 863–6.
5 Silverberg B, Smoot CE, Landa SJF, Parsons RW. Hidradenitis suppurativa: patients' satisfaction with wound healing by second intention. *Plast Reconstr Surg* 1987; **79**: 555–9.
6 Brown SCW, Kazzazi N, Lord PH. Surgical treatment of perineal hidradenitis suppurativa with special reference to recognition of the perianal form. *Br J Surg* 1986; **73**: 978–80.
7 Wheeland RG. Reconstruction of the lower lip and chin using local and random pattern flaps. *J Dermatol Surg Oncol* 1991; **17**: 605–15.
8 Field LM. An improved design for vermilionectomy with a mucous membrane advancement flap. *J Dermatol Surg Oncol* 1991; **17**: 833–4.
9 Reiter D, Alford EL. Torn earlobe: a new approach to management with a review of 68 cases. *Ann Otol Rhinol Laryngol* 1994; **103**: 879–84.
10 Blanco-Dávila F, Vásconez HC. The cleft earlobe: a review of methods of treatment. *Ann Plast Surg* 1994; **33**: 677–80.
11 Fayman MS. Split earlobe repair. *Br J Plast Surg* 1994; **47**: 293.
12 Lawrence CM. The treatment of chondrodermatitis nodularis with cartilage removal alone. *Arch Dermatol* 1991; **127**: 530–5.
13 Lawrence CM. Surgical treatment of chondrodermatitis nodularis. In: Robinson JK, Arndt KA, LeBoit PE, Wintroub BU, eds. *Atlas of Cutaneous Surgery*. Philadelphia: Saunders 1996: 201–6.

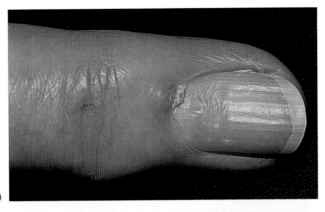
(a)

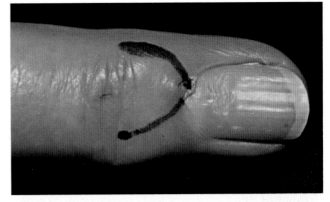
(b)

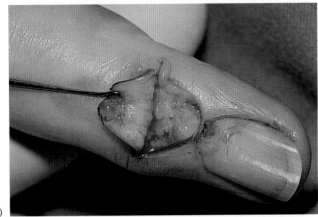
(c)

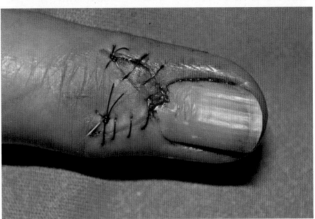
(d)

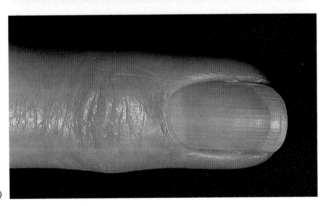
(e)

Fig. 78.20 Myxoid cyst surgical therapy. (a) The cyst is just under the proximal nail fold and producing a nail dystrophy. (b) A proximally based flap is designed to include the cyst and extend back to the distal interphalangeal joint. The flap is raised and the skin mobilized back to the DIP joint. (c) The cyst is incised and drained. No skin is excised. (d) The flap is resited and sutured. (e) The result 15 months later shows complete resolution and a normal nail plate.

14 Dawber RPR, Sonnex T, Leonard J, Ralfs I. Myxoid cysts of the finger: treatment by liquid nitrogen spray cryosurgery. *Clin Exp Dermatol* 1983; **8**: 153–7.

15 de Berker D, Lawrence C. Ganglion of the distal interphalangeal joint (myxoid cyst): therapy by identification and repair of the leak of joint fluid. *Arch Dermatol* 2001; **137**: 607–10.

16 Lawrence CM. Skin excision is not required in the surgical treatment of digital myxoid cysts. *Br J Dermatol* 2002; **147** (Suppl. 62): 30.

17 Wollina U, Karamfilov T, Konrad H. High-dose botulinum toxin type A therapy for axillary hyperhidrosis markedly prolongs the relapse-free interval. *J Am Acad Dermatol* 2002; **46**: 536–40.

18 Wen-Horng Wu, Sheih Ma, Jin-Teh Lin *et al.* Surgical treatment of axillary osmidrosis: analysis of 343 cases. *Plast Reconstr Surg* 1994; **94**: 288–94.

19 Hurley HJ, Shelley WB. A simple surgical approach to the management of axillary hyperhidrosis. *JAMA* 1963; **186**: 109–12.

20 Hurley HJ, Shelley WB. Axillary hyperhidrosis: clinical features and local surgical management. *Br J Dermatol* 1966; **78**: 127–40.

21 Jemec B. Abrasio axillae in hyperhidrosis. *Scand J Plast Reconstr Surg* 1975; **9**: 44–6.

22 Shenaq SM, Spira MS. Treatment of bilateral axillary hyperhidrosis by suction assisted lipolysis technique. *Ann Plast Surg* 1987; **19**: 548–51.

23 Drott C, Göthberg G, Claes G. Endoscopic transthoracic sympathectomy: an efficient and safe method for the treatment of hyperhidrosis. *J Am Acad Dermatol* 1995; **33**: 78–81.

24 Lin TS, Fang HY. Transthoracic endoscopic sympathectomy in the treatment of palmar hyperhidrosis: with emphasis on perioperative management (1360 case analyses). *Surg Neurol* 1999; **52**: 453–7.

25 Byrne J, Walsh TN, Hederman WP. Endoscopic transthoracic electrocautery of the sympathetic chain for palmar and axillary hyperhidrosis. *Br J Surg* 1990; **77**: 1046–9.

26 Nicholson ML, Hopkinson BR, Dennis MJS. Endoscopic transthoracic sympathectomy: successful in hyperhidrosis but can the indications be extended? *Ann R Coll Surg Engl* 1994; **76**: 311–4.

27 Gordon A, Colin J. Treating hyperhidrosis. *BMJ* 1993; **306**: 1752.

28 Schnider P, Moraru E, Kittler H *et al.* Treatment of focal hyperhidrosis with botulinum toxin type A: long-term follow-up in 61 patients. *Br J Dermatol* 2001; **145**: 289–93.

Cosmetic procedures

Scar revision including acne scar correction

Pitted or 'ice-pick' acne scars can be treated by dermabrasion [1], very deep pitted scars do well with punch grafting [2] and the wide depressed scars respond to soft-tissue augmentation techniques including collagen [3] and Fibrel injections [4]. The flat purple–pink scars are best left to improve with time. Scar revision after surgery includes dermabrasion, which is best done 6 weeks postoperatively [5], and the treatment of keloids or hypertrophic scars [6].

Liposuction (lipectomy)

This involves selective removal of subcutaneous fat using a small cannula and suction equipment to produce a slimmer body shape [7]. The technique can be used at almost any body site, and can produce impressive results when performed by an experienced physician. Tumescent anaesthesia [8] evolved from the need to do liposuction under local anaesthesia; as a consequence it has become apparent that higher maximal lidocaine doses are possible using dilute anaesthetic solutions [9]. Liposuction has also been used to treat lipomas [10] and insulin-induced fat hypertrophy [11], in flap undermining, lymphoedema [12], breast reduction, lipodystrophy [13] and axillary hyperhidrosis [14], and to remove haematomas or extravasated corrosive drugs [15].

Blepharoplasty

This involves the removal of redundant skin and orbital fat from the upper [16] and lower [17] eyelids in order to correct unsightly bags or skin folds. Selection of the correct procedure to take account of individual variations in eyelid anatomy, identification of pre-existing eye disease, meticulous technique and the ability to adapt or include other procedures depending on the coexisting abnormalities present make this an operation for the expert [18]. Complications include blindness [19], excessive sclera show or ectropion, and failure to correct the original defect.

REFERENCES

1 Alt TA. Technical aids for dermabrasion. *J Dermatol Surg Oncol* 1987; **13**: 638–48.
2 Solotoff SA. Treatment of pitted acne scarring: post-auricular punch grafts followed by dermabrasion. *J Dermatol Surg Oncol* 1986; **12**: 1079–84.
3 Varnavides CK, Forster RA, Cunliffe WJ. The role of bovine collagen in the treatment of acne scars. *Br J Dermatol* 1987; **116**: 199–206.
4 Millikan H, Banks K, Purkait B, Chungi V. A 5-year safety and efficacy evaluation with Fibrel in the correction of cutaneous scars following one or two treatments. *J Dermatol Surg Oncol* 1991; **17**: 223–9.
5 Yarborough JM. Ablation of facial scars by programmed dermabrasion. *J Dermatol Surg Oncol* 1988; **14**: 292–4.
6 Harahap M. Revision of a depressed scar. *J Dermatol Surg Oncol* 1984; **10**: 206–9.
7 Fournier PF. Why the syringe and not the suction machine. *J Dermatol Surg Oncol* 1988; **14**: 1062–71.
8 Coleman WP, Klein JA. Use of the tumescent technique for scalp surgery, dermabrasion and soft tissue reconstruction. *J Dermatol Surg Oncol* 1992; **18**: 130–5.
9 Samdal F, Amland PF, Bugge JF. Plasma lidocaine levels during suction-assisted lipectomy using large doses of dilute lidocaine with epinephrine. *Plast Reconstr Surg* 1994; **93**: 1217–23.
10 Kaneko T, Tokushige H, Kimura N *et al*. The treatment of multiple angiolipomas by liposuction surgery. *J Dermatol Surg Oncol* 1994; **20**: 690–2.
11 Hardy KJ, Gill GV, Bryson JR. Severe insulin-induced lipohypertrophy successfully treated by liposuction. *Diabetes Care* 1993; **16**: 929–30.
12 McO'Brien B, Khazanchi RK, Kumar PAV *et al*. Liposuction in the treatment of lymphoedema: a preliminary report. *Br J Plast Surg* 1989; **42**: 530–3.
13 Ketterings C. Lipodystrophy and its treatment. *Ann Plast Surg* 1988; **21**: 536–43.
14 Coleman WP. Non-cosmetic applications of liposuction. *J Dermatol Surg Oncol* 1988; **14**: 1085–90.
15 Martin PH, Carver N, Petros AJ. Use of liposuction and saline washout for the treatment of extensive subcutaneous extravasation of corrosive drugs. *Br J Anaesth* 1994; **72**: 702–4.
16 Perman KI. Upper eyelid blepharoplasty. *J Dermatol Surg Oncol* 1992; **18**: 1096–9.
17 Neuhaus RW. Lower eyelid blepharoplasty. *J Dermatol Surg Oncol* 1992; **18**: 1100–9.
18 Flowers RS. Blepharoplasty and periorbital aesthetic surgery. *Clin Plast Surg* 1993; **20**: 209–30.
19 Mahaffey PJ, Wallace AF. Blindness following cosmetic blepharoplasty: a review. *Br J Plast Surg* 1986; **39**: 213–21.

Index